Brain Injury Medicine

*Principles
and Practice*

Edited by

Nathan D. Zasler, MD
Douglas I. Katz, MD
Ross D. Zafonte, DO

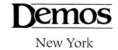

Demos

New York

Demos Medical Publishing, LLC, 386 Park Avenue South, New York, New York 10016

Visit our website at www.demosmedpub.com

Chapter 21, "The Older Adult" by Jeffrey Englander, David X. Cifu, and Trinh Tran, is an updated version of the chapter that originally appeared in the book, *Rehabilitation of the Adult and Child with Traumatic Brain Injury, Third Edition*, edited by M. Rosenthal, E.R. Griffith, J.S. Kreutzer, and B. Pentland, published by F.A. Davis in 1999.

Medicine is an ever-changing science undergoing continual development. Research and clinical experience are continually expanding our knowledge, in particular our knowledge of proper treatment and drug therapy. The authors, editors, and publisher have made every effort to ensure that all information in this book is in accordance with the state of knowledge at the time of production of the book.

Nevertheless, this does not imply or express any guarantee or responsibility on the part of the authors, editors, or publisher with respect to any dosage instructions and forms of application stated in the book. Every reader should examine carefully the package inserts accompanying each drug and check—if necessary, in consultation with a physician or specialist—whether the dosage schedules mentioned therein or the contraindications stated by the manufacturer differ from the statements made in this book. Such examination is particularly important with drugs that are either rarely used or have been newly released on the market. Every dosage schedule or every form of application used is entirely at the reader's own risk and responsibility. The editors and publisher welcome any reader to report to the publisher any discrepancies or inaccuracies noticed.

About the Cover: In vivo, noninvasive, three-dimensional reconstruction of the motor tract pathways using white matter tractography and diffusion tensor imaging techniques. Image courtesy of Dr. Mariana Lazar.

Cover design by Steven Pisano.

Library of Congress Cataloging-in-Publication Data

Brain injury medicine : principles and practice / edited by Nathan D. Zasler, Douglas I. Katz, Ross D. Zafonte.
    p. ; cm.
Includes bibliographical references and index.
    ISBN-13: 978-1-888799-93-4 (alk. paper)
    ISBN-10: 1-888799-93-5 (alk. paper)
  1. Brain—Wounds and injuries—Patients—Rehabilitation. 2. Brain—Wounds and injuries—Patients—Care. 3. Continuum of care.
  [DNLM: 1. Brain Injuries. 2. Continuity of Patient Care. WL 354 B81386 2006]
I. Zasler, Nathan D., 1958– II. Katz, Douglas. III. Zafonte, Ross D.
    RD594.B727 2006
    617.4'810443—dc22

                      2006006039

06 07 08 09 10   5 4 3 2 1

Manufactured in the United States of America

Acknowledgments

The three of us wish to thank all the contributors who agreed to take time to author chapters and share their expertise with the readers of this textbook. We hope that readers will be pleased with the quality and diversity of the various medical, rehabilitative, and other specialists who enabled this book to come to fruition. We believe the scope and multidisciplinary nature of this textbook add important dimensions to its overall value as a primary resource to you, the practitioner.

We would also like to thank the individuals at Demos Medical Publishing for their patience with this project. A special thanks to Dr. Diana Schneider for her leadership as well as her willingness to compromise. Additionally, we thank Craig Percy and Edith Barry who were essential along with other Demos staff in seeing this text come to completion.

Lastly, we would like to dedicate this book to all individuals with brain injuries, their families, and the professionals who are committed to serve and assist them in such a way as to optimize their potential to work, play, and love once again.

NZ, DK, RZ

As chief editor of this textbook, I would like to thank my co-editors, Dr. Douglas Katz of HealthSouth Braintree Rehabilitation Hospital and Boston University, Department of Neurology, and Dr. Ross Zafonte of University of Pittsburgh, Department of Physical Medicine and Rehabilitation, for their knowledge, patience, and expertise in assisting with the editing (and writing)

of this rather enormous undertaking. I know that each gentleman entered into the project never anticipating the tremendous amount of work and time that would ultimately be required. That said, I would like to thank each of you for your commitment to the project and your willingness to see it through.

I would like to personally thank a number of individuals who have served as professional role models in my career. One such individual is Dr. Henry S. Stonnington under whom I initially trained. He needs to be mentioned as a major guiding force for my decision to enter into the field of brain injury medicine and rehabilitation. I am deeply grateful to Dr. Stonnington for sharing his vision regarding brain injury care. I am also grateful for Dr. Stonnington's major contributions to the field, including founding the International Association for the Study of Traumatic Brain Injury which eventually merged with the International Brain Injury Association of which I currently serve as Chairperson. He was also the founder of the first major journal in the field of brain injury rehabilitation, *Brain Injury* (Taylor & Francis, London). I would also be remiss to not include Dr. Sheldon Berrol and Dr. Catherine Bontke, both now deceased, and Dr. Lawrence Horn as significant professional role models in molding my career goals and practice philosophy.

On a more personal note I would like to thank my beautiful and understanding wife, Lisa Nava Marcelle Zasler, for her love, vitality, and family values, and in particular her patience with regard to my level of professional commitment to my work. Without her as a stabilizing and energizing force in my life, I would certainly not have the ability to sustain such a level of professional motivation. I must also recognize my three beautiful children— Maia, Anya, and Aaron, who light up every single day of my life and make the world a much brighter place to live in. It is with great hope that by the time these children are adults, we will be much further along in assuring that individuals with brain injury and their families do not incur the type of sorrow, grief, lack of knowledge and/or resources, as well as long-term adverse consequences that so many of our patients today must often and unfortunately experience. I also hope that my brother Jonathan would be proud of my accomplishments, both personally and professionally. Most importantly, I want to thank my parents, Moshe and Joyce Zasler, who have always encouraged me to pursue my dreams and stood by me through "thick and thin." Thanks for being the best.

NZ

I also thank my co-editors, especially Dr. Nathan Zasler for setting high standards and keeping us moving forward and on target during this ambitious project. I would also like to acknowledge all those who have taught, influenced, supported, inspired, and collaborated with me throughout my career, especially my teachers, neurorehabilitation fellows, colleagues and fellow staff at Braintree Rehabilitation Hospital and Boston University. In particular, I would like to mention: Michael P. Alexander, MD, my mentor and colleague, who continues to serve as a teacher and role model for me; Virginia Mills, MS, PT, who, as a colleague, friend, and leader, has inspired me and taught me much about brain injury rehabilitation and how to do it right; T. Joy DePiero, MD, my neurorehabilitation partner at Braintree Rehabilitation Hospital, who has been an exceptional colleague, source of knowledge, and support over the last 20 years; my patients and their families who have taught me and inspired me so much over the years; and most importantly, my wonderful family: my wife Kim, my children Rachel and Daniel, and my parents Carol (1924–2004) and Warner, who have been a never-ending source of love and support during my time-consuming professional career.

DK

I would like to express my gratitude to my late parents, Albert and Grace. They instilled in me a desire to continually improve and to always maintain a sense of curiosity. My sincere appreciation goes toward my mentors, too numerous to mention, because they have helped shape my views and focus my enthusiasm throughout the years. To my wife, Cheryl, and son, Alexander, who have given their time to this and many other projects. I am struck by their patience and caring. Most of all, for this project I would like to acknowledge the people with brain injury whom I have had the opportunity to serve. We have grown and learned together, and we will continue to do so.

RDZ

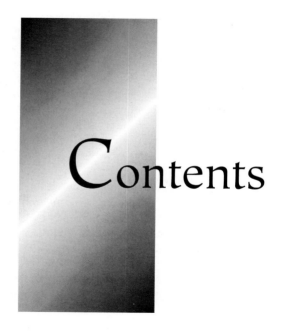

Contents

VI REHABILITATIVE CARE AND TREATMENT OF SPECIFIC POPULATIONS

VII NEUROLOGIC PROBLEMS

VIII   NEUROMUSCULOSKELETAL PROBLEMS

IX   MEDICAL MANAGEMENT ISSUES

X   COGNITIVE AND BEHAVIORAL PROBLEMS

XIV PSYCHOSOCIAL AND VOCATIONAL ISSUES

XV MEDICOLEGAL AND ETHICAL ISSUES

Preface

*B*rain Injury Medicine: Principles and Practice is designed as a comprehensive text for all clinicians dealing with the assessment, management, and rehabilitation of patients with traumatic brain injury (TBI) from "coma to community." This book examines numerous aspects of brain injury with perspectives from an internationally respected group of authors, who include both "in the trenches" practitioners as well as researchers. We hope that this text will serve as a "go-to reference" for clinical practitioners to use in day-to-day practice, students and trainees learning about TBI, and other professionals who need to learn more about TBI and its management.

The text opens with a description of the clinical continuum of care and the natural history of TBI, followed by perspectives on rehabilitative care in the United States and other countries, with discussions on training and research. Public health issues are discussed with chapters on epidemiology and prevention. The effects of trauma and recovery on the brain are described in chapters on pathophysiology, brain plasticity, and treatments that may influence neural recovery. Readers will learn up-to-date information on technologies to assess TBI, including structural and functional neuroimaging and electrophysiologic techniques. A series of chapters covers prognosis and outcome, including life-expectancy.

The bulk of the text deals with clinical care of patients with TBI—across the continuum of care, at different levels of severity, and among different age groups. There are discussions of the full gamut of medical assessment and management of neurologic, medical, physical, cognitive, and behavioral problems resulting from TBI. Given the biopsychosocial nature of TBI and its consequences, there are also chapters on the psychological, neuropsychological, psychosocial, ethical, and medicolegal aspects of this condition.

Ultimately, the 66 chapters in this comprehensive text will provide readers with a full complement of medical and interdisciplinary rehabilitation perspectives on the assessment and management of persons with mild to severe TBI. It is hoped that this text brings together knowledge, experience, and evidence-based medicine in a manner that will promote further cross-disciplinary practice and research in the field of TBI. Most of all, we hope that this book will result in individuals with TBI receiving timely and accurate assessments and appropriate management to optimize their outcomes as well as the quality of their lives and those who care for them.

Nathan D. Zasler, MD
Douglas I. Katz, MD
Ross D. Zafonte, DO

Foreword

We are what our brains allow us to be. A traumatic brain injury (TBI) changes a person as an individual and has an impact on the ability to interact with his or her environment. The neurorehabilitation of persons who have had a traumatic brain injury requires an extraordinarily diverse knowledge base and expertise in order to optimize both neurological and functional outcome and minimize medical, as well as psychosocial, morbidity. In an ideal scenario, the neurorehabilitationist facilitates maximal community independence, patient self-reliance, and community re-integration relative to work, leisure, and social interactions while maintaining psychoemotional health.

TBI may cause changes that affect cognition, behavior, language, somatic function, and neuromedical status. Such an injury can have a negative impact on the complex biopsychosocial relationships that we all have in our environment. Brain injury, in and of itself, can create additional and unexpected problems depending upon the age of the individual at the time of injury. Sometimes, these problems may not be readily apparent early after an injury, but may instead develop later, as the child "grows into" brain injury problems. The neurorehabilitation process should ideally start in the intensive care unit and continue through optimal community reintegration and medical stabilization. For some patients, this stage never comes, and chronic care is therefore necessary.

The neuromedical and rehabilitative management of TBI demands a vast knowledge of a multiplicity of fields including neurophysiology, neuroanatomy, neuropathology, neurology, neuropharmacology, neuropsychiatry, physiatry, psychology, neuropsychology, orthopedics, nursing, therapy specialties including occupational therapy, physical therapy, speech language pathology, and therapeutic recreation, among others. Based on extensive experience over the years, an interdisciplinary team approach clearly facilitates optimal neurorehabilitation. In order to optimize this process, all clinicians on the team must have a good understanding of how to optimize the efficacy of this treatment model and coordinate care in a manner that is most cost-efficient relative to achieving optimal functional outcomes.

Persons with TBI need to have a continuum of programs available in order to facilitate continuity of care and optimize their outcomes. The specific approaches may differ across the continuum of care, as might the medically indicated clinicians. Each of these stages potentially requires a different and evolving knowledge. Adequate appreciation of clinical nuances is paramount in being able to judge, document, and predict recovery and future neurorehabilitative needs. Functional gains can continue for years, even well after neurologic plateaus are reached. Even in scenarios where one finds that patients have functionally plateaued, there may still be opportunities to manipulate the environment and/or provide new treatment methodologies to further optimize quality-of-life and functional status.

Given the complexities in the medical management of this patient population and the need for a functional, holistic approach that utilizes a biopsychosocial model of care, clinicians need a source of information that brings together the myriad medical and allied health specialties involved in understanding TBI care and rehabilitation. This is the importance of *Brain Injury Medicine: Principles and Practice*. This book will provide readers with the most recent information and methodologies to facilitate clinical practice and optimize patient functional outcomes. The text provides the knowledge necessary to understand what is happening at various stages of recovery following TBI and, more importantly, what needs to be done during each stage. It is an excellent resource for both clinicians and non-clinicians alike. Medical physicians involved in neurorehabilitation, such as physiatrists or neurologists, as well as other rehabilitation team members, will find this book an invaluable resource. Physicians who deal with TBI in a non-neurorehabilitation context will certainly benefit from understanding brain injury from the perspective provided by this text, which will further facilitate use of rehabilitation resources in their own community. It is an outstanding and comprehensive book that can serve as the "bible" for each member of a team working with a TBI patient, allowing each of them to understand the reasons behind the decisions of their fellow team members.

We are what our brains allow us to be. The neurorehabilitation professional needs to have a standard by which to understand and advise patients, family members, fellow professionals, and payors regarding TBI-related issues. This book will significantly enable each professional to have access to this vast fund of knowledge.

Henry H. Stonnington, MBBS, MSc,
FRCPE, FAFRM (RACP), FAAPM&R
Medical Director, Rehabilitation Services,
Memorial Hospital
Clinical Professor, Section of PM&R,
Department of Internal Medicine
Louisiana State University Medical School

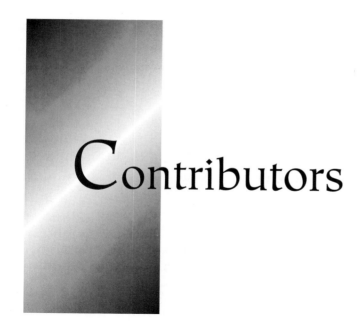

Contributors

Souheil G. Abou-Assi, MD
Gastrointestinal Specialists, Inc.
Richmond, Virginia
Chapter 36: Gastrointestinal and Nutritional Issues

Arthur Ameis, MD, FRCPC
Medical Director
Multi-Disciplinary Assessment Centre
Toronto, Ontario
Canada
Chapter 63: Ethical Issues in Clinicolegal Practice

Terri Antoinette, MHSA, CRRN
Chief Executive Officer
Legal Nurse and Clinical Services Consultants
Canonsburg, Pennsylvania
*Chapter 40: Neurorehabilitation Nursing of Persons
    with TBI: From Injury to Recovery*

David B. Arciniegas, MD
Director
Neurobehavioral Disorders Program
Associate Professor of Psychiatry and Neurology
University of Colorado School of Medicine
Medical Director
Brain Injury Rehabilitation Unit
HealthONE Spalding Rehabilitation Hospital
Aurora, Colorado
*Chapter 52: Pharmacotherapy of Neuropsychiatric
    Disturbances*
Chapter 53: Pharmacotherapy of Cognitive Impairment

Patricia M. Arenth, PhD
Assistant Professor
Department of Physical Medicine and Rehabilitation
University of Pittsburgh School of Medicine
Pittsburgh, Pennsylvania
Chapter 12: Functional Neuroimaging of TBI

John M. Barkley, MD
Staff Radiologist
Diagnostic and Interventional Radiology
The Methodist Hospital
Houston, Texas
*Chapter 11: Static Neuroimaging in the Evaluation of
    Traumatic Brain Injury*

Eli M. Baron, MD
Fellow
Cedars–Sinai Institute for Spinal Disorders
Los Angeles, California
*Chapter 18: TBI: Pathology, Pathophysiology, Acute
    Care and Surgical Management, Critical Care
    Principles and Outcomes*

Anna M. Barrett, MD
Associate Professor
Departments of Physical Medicine and Rehabilitation,
    Neurology, and Neurosciences
University of Medicine and Dentistry of New Jersey
New Jersey Medical School
Newark, New Jersey
Director of Stroke Rehabilitation
Kessler Medical Rehabilitation Research and Education
    Corporation
West Orange, New Jersey
Chapter 42: Cognitive Impairments After TBI

Kathleen R. Bell, MD
Professor
Department of Rehabilitation Medicine
University of Washington
Seattle, Washington
*Chapter 34: Complications Associated with Immobility
    After TBI*

Raquel Munitz Benabib, MS COVT
Psychologist, Vision Therapist
Centro de Aprendizaje de Cuernavaca
Cuernavaca Morelos, Mexico
Chapter 29: Evaluating and Treating Visual Dysfunction

Mark C. Bender, PhD
Rehabilitation Neuropsychologist
Medical Psychology Department
Sheltering Arms Rehabilitation
Richmond, Virginia
*Chapter 64: Assessment of Response Bias in Clinical
    and Forensic Evaluations of Impairment
    Following TBI*

Debra E. Berens, MS, CLCP
Private Practice
Rehabilitation Consultant/Life Care Planner
Atlanta, Georgia
*Chapter 66: Life Care Planning After TBI: Clinical and
    Forensic Issues*

Erin D. Bigler, PhD
Professor
Departments of Psychology and Neuroscience
Brigham Young University
Provo, Utah
Adjunct Professor of Psychiatry
University of Utah School of Medicine
Salt Lake City, Utah
*Chapter 15: Neuroimaging Correlates of Functional
    Outcome*

Shane S. Bush, PhD
Independent Practice
Smithtown, New York
Chapter 63: Ethical Issues in Clinicolegal Practice

Irvin V. Cantor, JD
Managing Director
Complex Litigation Group
Cantor Arkema, PC
Attorneys At Law
Richmond, Virginia
Chapter 62: Medicolegal Aspects of TBI

Freeman M. Chakara, PsyD
Clinical Neuropsychologist
Providence Behavioral Health
Leola, Pennsylvania
and
Lancaster Regional Medical Center
Lancaster, Pennsylvania
Chapter 42: Cognitive Impairments After TBI

Jerry Y.P. Chiang, MD
Research Fellow
Stanford University School of Medicine
Physical Medicine and Rehabilitation Service
VA Palo Alto Health Care System
Palo Alto, California
*Chapter 13: Electrophysiologic Assessment Techniques:
    Evoked Potentials and Electroencephalography*

Keith D. Cicerone, PhD
Director of Neuropsychology and Rehabilitation
    Psychology
Department of Physical Medicine and Rehabilitation
JFK Johnson Rehabilitation Institute
Edison, New Jersey
Chapter 41: Cognitive Rehabilitation

David X. Cifu, MD
The Herman J. Flax, MD Professor and Chairman
Department of Physical Medicine and Rehabilitation
Medical College of Virginia
Virginia Commonwealth University School of Medicine
Richmond, Virginia
Chapter 21: The Older Adult

Robert S.B. Clark, MD
Associate Professor
Departments of Critical Care Medicine and Pediatrics
University of Pittsburgh School of Medicine
Pittsburgh, Pennsylvania
Chapter 8: TBI: Pathobiology

Richard A. Clendaniel, PT, PhD
Assistant Professor
Doctor of Physical Therapy Division
Department of Community and Family Medicine
Duke University Medical Center
Durham, North Carolina
Chapter 28: Balance and Dizziness

Daniel M. Clinchot, MD
Associate Dean for Medical Education and Outreach
Medical Director of the Clinical Skills Education and
    Assessment Center
Associate Professor and Program Director
Department of Physical Medicine and Rehabilitation
The Ohio State University College of Medicine
Columbus, Ohio
*Chapter 19: Assessment, Early Rehabilitation
    Intervention, and Tertiary Prevention*

Carl A. Coelho, PhD
Professor and Chair
Communication Sciences Department
University of Connecticut
Storrs, Connecticut
*Chapter 48 : Cognitive-Communication Deficits
    Following TBI*

Michael W. Collins, PhD
Assistant Director
UPMC Sports Concussion Program
Assistant Professor
Department of Orthopedics
Division of Sports Medicine
University of Pittsburgh School of Medicine
Pittsburgh, Pennsylvania
Chapter 24 : Sport-Related Concussion

Victor G. Coronado, MD, MPH
Medical Officer
National Center for Injury Prevention and Control
Division of Injury Response
Centers for Disease Control and Prevention
Atlanta, Georgia
*Chapter 6: The Epidemiology of TBI: Implications for
    Public Health*

John D. Corrigan, PhD
Professor
Department of Physical Medicine and Rehabilitation
The Ohio State University College of Medicine
Columbus, Ohio
*Chapter 59: The Treatment of Substance Abuse in
    Persons with TBI*

Linda Creasey, RD, CNSD
Clinical Nutrition Supervisor
Food and Nutrition Services
Medical College of Virginia
Virginia Commonwealth University
Richmond, Virginia
Chapter 36: Gastrointestinal and Nutritional Issues

Numa Dancause, PT, PhD
Post-Doctorate Fellow
Department of Neurology
University of Rochester
Rochester, New York
*Chapter 49: Neuroscientific Basis for Occupational
    and Physical Therapy Interventions*

Alan M. Davis, MD, PhD
Assistant Professor
Department of Physical Medicine and Rehabilitation
University of Utah School of Medicine
Salt Lake City, Utah
Chapter 57: Complementary and Alternative Medicine

Steven M. Day, PhD
Senior Researcher
Life Expectancy Project
San Francisco, California
Chapter 17: Life Expectancy

Richard L. Delmonico, PhD
Chief, Neuropsychology
Kaiser Foundation Rehabilitation Center
Vallejo, California
Associate Clinical Professor
University of California, Davis
School of Medicine
Davis, California
*Chapter 37: Sexuality, Reproduction, and
    Neuroendocrine Disorders Following TBI*

Pedro Diaz-Marchan, MD
Associate Professor of Radiology
Associate Chair for Education
Program Director, Diagnostic Radiology Residency
Program Director, Neuroradiology Fellowship
Baylor College of Medicine
Chief of Neuroradiology
Ben Taub General Hospital
Houston, Texas
*Chapter 11: Static Neuroimaging in the Evaluation
    of TBI*

Marcel P.J.M. Dijkers, PhD
Associate Professor
Department of Rehabilitation Medicine
Mount Sinai School of Medicine
New York, New York
*Chapter 16: Functional Assessment in TBI
    Rehabilitation*

C. Edward Dixon, PhD
Director, Brain Trauma Research Center
Professor, Departments of Neurological Surgery,
Critical Care Medicine, Neurobiology,
and Physical Medicine and Rehabilitation
University of Pittsburgh School of Medicine
Pittsburgh, Pennsylvania
*Chapter 10: Advances in Innovative Therapies to
Enhance Neural Recovery*

Victor G. Dostrow, MD
Service Chief
Department of Neurology
Mississippi State Hospital
Whitfield, Mississippi
Clinical Associate Professor
Department of Neurology
University of Mississippi Medical Center
Clinical Assistant Professor
Department of Psychiatry
University of Mississippi Medical Center
Adjunct Associate Professor
Department of Pharmacy Practice
University of Mississippi School of Pharmacy
Jackson, Mississippi
Chapter 26: Post-Traumatic Seizures and Epilepsy

Elie P. Elovic, MD
Director, Traumatic Brain Injury Lab
Kessler Medical Rehabilitation Research and Education
    Corporation
Associate Professor
Department of Physical Medicine and Rehabilitation
University of Medicine and Dentistry of New Jersey
New Jersey Medical School
West Orange, New Jersey
Chapter 7: Primary Prevention
Chapter 31: Fatigue: Assessment and Treatment

Jeffrey Englander, MD
Vice Chair and Director of Brain Injury Rehabilitation
Co-Director, NIDRR TBI Model System of Care,
    Northern California
Santa Clara Valley Medical Center
San Jose, California
Chapter 21: The Older Adult

Paul J. Eslinger, PhD
Professor
Departments of Neurology, Neural and Behavioral
    Sciences,
Pediatrics and Radiology
Pennsylvania State University, College of Medicine and
    Milton S. Hershey Medical Center
University Hospital Rehabilitation Center
Hershey, Pennsylvania
Chapter 42: Cognitive Impairments After TBI

Alberto Esquenazi, MD
Director, Gait and Motion Analysis Laboratory
Co-Director, Neuroorthopedic Program MossRehab
Elkins Park, Pennsylvania
*Chapter 35: Assessing and Treating Muscle Overactivity
    in the Upper Motoneuron Syndrome*

Jonathan L. Fellus, MD
Assistant Clinical Professor
Department of Neurosciences
University of Medicine and Dentistry of New Jersey
New Jersey Medical School
Newark, New Jersey
Director of Brain Injury Services
Kessler Institute for Rehabilitation
West Orange, New Jersey
Chapter 31: Fatigue: Assessment and Treatment

Lisa P. Fugate, MD, MSPH
Assistant Professor
Department of Physical Medicine and Rehabilitation
The Ohio State University College of Medicine
Columbus, Ohio
*Chapter 19: Assessment, Early Rehabilitation
    Intervention, and Tertiary Prevention*

Michael Gaetz, PhD
Professor
UCFV Concussion Management Program
Kinesiology and Physical Education
University College of the Fraser Valley
Abbotsford, British Columbia
Canada
Chapter 22: Mild TBI
Chapter 24: Sport-Related Concussion

Joseph T. Giacino, PhD
Associate Director of Neuropsychology
JFK Johnson Rehabilitation Institute
New Jersey Neuroscience Institute
Edison, New Jersey
*Chapter 25: Assessment and Rehabilitative
    Management of Individuals with Disorders of
    Consciousness*

Daniel D. Gottlieb, OD
Director
Gottlieb Vision Group
Stone Mountain, Georgia
Chapter 29: Evaluating and Treating Visual Dysfunction

Brian Greenwald, MD
Assistant Professor
Department of Rehabilitation Medicine
Mount Sinai School of Medicine
New York, New York
*Chapter 16: Functional Assessment in TBI
    Rehabilitation*

Zeev Groswasser, MD, MPH
Head
Department of Brain Injury Rehabilitation
Loewenstein Rehabilitation Hospital
Ra'anana, Israel
Professor
Sackler Faculty of Medicine
Tel Aviv University
Tel Aviv, Israel
Chapter 3: International Perspectives on TBI
*   Rehabilitation*

Flora M. Hammond, MD
Brain Injury Program Director
Research Director
Department of Physical Medicine and Rehabilitation
Carolinas Rehabilitation
Charlotte, North Carolina
Chapter 30: Cranial Nerve Disorders

L. Anne Hayman, MD
Private Practice
Department of Radiology
Medical Clinic of Houston LLP
Houston, Texas
Chapter 11: Static Neuroimaging in the Evaluation of
*   Traumatic Brain Injury*

Jeffrey S. Hecht, MD
Associate Professor and Chief
Division of Surgical Rehabilitation
Department of Surgery
University of Tennessee Graduate School of Medicine
Medical Director
The Rehabilitation Center at Baptist Hospital
Medical Director
St. Mary's RehabCare Center
Knoxville, Tennessee
Chapter 55: Nutraceuticals
Chapter 57: Complementary and Alternative Medicine

Lawrence J. Horn, MD
Professor
Department of Physical Medicine and Rehabilitation
Wayne State University School of Medicine
Medical Director
Traumatic Brain Injury Program
Rehabilitation Institute of Michigan
Detroit, Michigan
Chapter 38: Post-Traumatic Pain Disorders: Medical
*   Assessment and Management*

Grant L. Iverson, PhD, RPsych
Professor
Department of Psychiatry
University of British Columbia
Coordinator of Psychology and Neuropsychology
    Services
Neuropsychiatry Program
Riverview Hospital
Vancouver, British Columbia
Canada
Chapter 22: Mild TBI
Chapter 23: Post-Concussive Disorder
Chapter 24: Sport-Related Concussion

Jack I. Jallo, MD, PhD
Associate Professor
Department of Neurosurgery
Temple University School of Medicine
Philadelphia, Pennsylvania
Chapter 18: TBI: Pathology, Pathophysiology, Acute
*   Care and Surgical Management, Critical Care*
*   Principles and Outcomes*

Joseph Jankovic, MD
Professor of Neurology
Director, Parkinson's Disease Center and Movement
    Disorders Clinic
Department of Neurology
Baylor College of Medicine
Houston, Texas
Chapter 27: Movement Disorders After TBI

Larry W. Jenkins, PhD
Associate Professor
Department of Neurosurgery
University of Pittsburgh School of Medicine
Pittsburgh, Pennsylvania
Chapter 8: Traumatic Brain Injury: Pathobiology

Robert L. Karol, PhD
Director
Department of Psychology and Neuropsychology
Program Director
Brain Injury Services
Bethesda Hospital
St. Paul, Minnesota
Chapter 44: Principles of Behavioral Analysis and
*   Modification*

Douglas I. Katz, MD
Associate Professor
Department of Neurology
Boston University School of Medicine
Boston, Massachusetts
Medical Director
Brain Injury Programs
Healthsouth Braintree Rehabilitation Hospital
Braintree, Massachusetts
Chapter 1: Clinical Continuum of Care and Natural History
Chapter 25: Assessment and Rehabilitative Management of Individuals with Disorders of Consciousness

Mary Ann E. Keenan, MD
Professor and Vice Chair of Graduate Medical Education
Chief, Neuro-Orthopedics Program
University of Pennsylvania Health System
Department of Orthopedic Surgery
Philadelphia, Pennsylvania
Chapter 35: Assessing and Treating Muscle Overactivity in the Upper Motoneuron Syndrome

Ofer Keren, MD
Director of Rehabilitation Department
Alyn Hospital
Pediatric and Adolescent Rehabilitation Center
Jerusalem, Israel
Professor
Sackler Faculty of Medicine
Tel Aviv University
Tel Aviv, Israel
Chapter 3: International Perspectives on TBI Rehabilitation

Donald F. Kirby, MD
Professor of Medicine, Psychiatry, Biochemistry and Molecular Physics
Chief, Section of Nutrition
Medical College of Virginia
Virginia Commonwealth University
Richmond, Virginia
Chapter 36: Gastrointestinal and Nutritional Issues

Kristi L. Kirschner, MD
Coleman Foundation Chair in Rehabilitation Medicine
Director, Donnelley Family Disability Ethics Program
Rehabilitation Institute of Chicago
Associate Professor
Departments of Physical Medicine and Rehabilitation and Medical Humanities and Bioethics
Northwestern University Feinberg School of Medicine
Chicago, Illinois
Chapter 65: Decision-Making Capacity After TBI: Clinical Assessment and Ethical Implications

Anthony E. Kline, PhD
Assistant Professor
Departments of Physical Medicine and Rehabilitation and Psychology
Associate Director of Rehabilitation Research
Safar Center for Resuscitation Research
University of Pittsburgh School of Medicine
Pittsburgh, Pennsylvania
Chapter 10: Advances in Innovative Therapies to Enhance Neural Recovery

Sally Kneipp, PhD
Director, Community Skills Program
Counseling and Rehabilitation, Inc.
Wyomissing, Pennsylvania
Counseling and Rehabilitation of New Jersey, Inc.
Marlton, New Jersey
Chapter 58: Community Re-entry Issues and Long-Term Care

Patrick M. Kochanek, MD
Professor and Vice Chairman
Department of Critical Care Medicine
Director, Safar Center for Resuscitation Research
University of Pittsburgh School of Medicine
Pittsburgh, Pennsylvania
Chapter 8: TBI: Pathobiology

Mary Jean Kotch MSN, CRRN-A
Clinical Nurse Specialist
Kaiser Foundation Rehabilitation Center and Hospital
Vallejo, California
Chapter 37: Sexuality, Reproduction, and Neuroendocrine Disorders Following TBI

Sunil Kothari, MD
Associate Director
Brain Injury and Stroke Program
The Institute for Rehabilitation and Research
Assistant Professor
Department of Rehabilitation Medicine
Baylor College of Medicine
Houston, Texas
Chapter 14: Prognosis After Severe Traumatic Brain Injury: A Practical, Evidence-Based Approach
Chapter 57: Complementary and Alternative Medicine
Chapter 65: Decision-Making Capacity After TBI: Clinical Assessment and Ethical Implications

Joachim K. Krauss, MD
Professor of Neurosurgery
Director and Chairman
Department of Neurosurgery
Medical University, MHH
Hannover, Germany
Chapter 27: Movement Disorders After TBI

Jeffrey S. Kreutzer, PhD, ABPP
Professor
Departments of Physical Medicine and Rehabilitation,
Neurosurgery, and Psychiatry
Virginia Commonwealth University School of Medicine
Richmond, Virginia
Chapter 43: Neuropsychological Assessment and
Treatment of TBI

Rael T. Lange, PhD
Research Scientist (Neuropsychology)
Department of Research
Riverview Hospital
Coquitlam, British Columbia
Canada
Chapter 22: Mild TBI
Chapter 23: Post-Concussive Disorder

Eun Ha Lee, MD, PhD
Research Fellow and Clinical Coordinator
Stanford University School of Medicine
Physical Medicine and Rehabilitation Service
VA Palo Alto Health Care System
Palo Alto, California
Chapter 13: Electrophysiologic Assessment Techniques:
Evoked Potentials and Electroencephalography

Henry L. Lew, MD, PhD
Clinical Associate Professor
Stanford University School of Medicine
Physical Medicine and Rehabilitation Service
VA Palo Alto Health Care System
Palo Alto, California
Chapter 13: Electrophysiologic Assessment Techniques:
Evoked Potentials and Electroencephalography

Lee A. Livingston, PsyD
Clinical Psychologist and Instructor
Department of Physical Medicine and Rehabilitation
Virginia Commonwealth University School of Medicine
Richmond, Virginia
Chapter 43: Neuropsychological Assessment and
Treatment of TBI

Lisa A. Lombard, MD
Assistant Professor
Medical Director, Traumatic Brain Injury Rehabilitation
Department of Physical Medicine and Rehabilitation
University of Pittsburgh School of Medicine
Pittsburgh, Pennsylvania
Chapter 54: Neuropharmacology: A Rehabilitation
Perspective

Jerilyn A. Logemann, PhD
Ralph and Jean Sundin Professor
Communication Sciences and Disorders
Northwestern University
Evanston, Illinois
Chapter 47: Evaluation and Treatment of Swallowing
Problems After TBI

David F. Long, MD
Brain Injury Program Director
Bryn Mawr Rehabilitation Hospital
Malvern, Pennsylvania
Chapter 33: Diagnosis and Management of Late
Intracranial Complications of TBI

Mark R. Lovell, PhD
Director
UPMC Sports Medicine Concussion Program
Associate Professor of Orthopedics
Division of Sports Medicine
University of Pittsburgh Medical Center
Pittsburgh, Pennsylvania
Chapter 24: Sport-Related Concussion

Michael F. Martelli, PhD
Director, Rehabilitation Neuropsychology
Concussion Care Centre of Virginia, Ltd.
and Tree of Life Services, Inc.
Glen Allen, Virginia
Medical College of Virginia
Virginia Commonwealth University School of Medicine
Richmond, Virginia
Chapter 38: Post-Traumatic Pain Disorders: Medical
Assessment and Management
Chapter 39: Psychological Approaches to
Comprehensive Pain Assessment and Management
Following TBI
Chapter 63: Ethical Issues in Clinicolegal Practice
Chapter 64: Assessment of Response Bias in Clinical
and Forensic Evaluations of Impairment
Following TBI

Brent E. Masel, MD
President and Medical Director
Transitional Learning Center at Galveston
Galveston, Texas
Chaper 30: Cranial Nerve Disorders

Nathaniel H. Mayer, MD
Emeritus Professor of Physical Medicine and
Rehabilitation
Temple University School of Medicine
Philadelphia, Pennsylvania
Director, Drucker Brain Injury Center and Motor
Control Analysis Laboratory
MossRehab Einstein at Elkins Park
Elkins Park, Pennsylvania
Chapter 35: Assessing and Treating Muscle Overactivity
in the Upper Motoneuron Syndrome

Thomas W. McAllister, MD
Professor of Psychiatry
Director of Neuropsychiatry
Department of Psychiatry
Dartmouth Medical School
Lebanon, New Hampshire
Chapter 45: Neuropsychiatric Aspects of TBI

James T. McDeavitt, MD
Senior Vice President
Division of Education and Research
Carolinas HealthCare System
Charlotte, North Carolina
Chapter 20: TBI: A Pediatric Perspective

Jacinta M. McElligott, MD
Director of Rehabilitation
National Rehabilitation Hospital
Dun Laoghaire
Co. Dublin, Ireland
Chapter 57: Complementary and Alternative Medicine

Robin McNeny, BS, OTR/L
Manager
Inpatient Occupational Therapy and Therapeutic
    Recreation
Occupational and Physical Therapy Department
Virginia Commonwealth University
Medical College of Virginia Hospitals Medical Center
Richmond, Virginia
*Chapter 51: Therapy for Activities of Daily Living:
    Theoretical and Practical Perspectives*

Jay M. Meythaler, MD, JD
Chairman and Professor
Department of Physical Medicine and Rehabilitation
Wayne State University
Specialist and Chief
Department of Physical Medicine and Rehabilitation
Detroit Medical Center
Detroit, Michigan
*Chapter 54: Neuropharmacology: A Rehabilitation
    Perspective*

Denise Morales, MD
Attending Physician
Department of Physical Medicine and Rehabilitation
Kaiser Foundation Rehabilitation Center
Vallejo, California
*Chapter 11: Static Neuroimaging in the Evaluation
    of TBI*

John A. Muenz, Jr., MD
Private Practice
Physical Medicine and Rehabilitation, Family Medicine
Associate Professor
Departments of Family Medicine, Orthopaedics, and
    Neurology
University of Florida—Jacksonville
Jacksonville, Florida
*Chapter 57: Complementary and Alternative
    Medicine*

Bruce E. Murdoch, PhD, DSc
Professor
Head School of Health and Rehabilitation Sciences
The University of Queensland
St. Lucia, Brisbane
Australia
*Chapter 46: Assessment and Treatment of Speech and
    Language Disorders in TBI*

W. Jerry Mysiw, MD
Associate Professor
Bert C. Wiley Chair and Vice Chair
Department of Physical Medicine and Rehabilitation
The Ohio State University College of Medicine
Columbus, Ohio
*Chapter 19: Assessment, Early Rehabilitation
    Intervention, and Tertiary Prevention*

Elena Napolitano, MD
Attending Physiatrist
Department of Physical Medicine and Rehabilitation
Shore Rehabilitation Institute
Brick, New Jersey
Chapter 7: Primary Prevention

Christine A. Nelson, PhD, OTR
Clinical Coordinator
Centro de Desarrollo
Cuernavaca, Mexico
*Chapter 29: Evaluating and Treating Visual
    Dysfunction*

Maureen R. Nelson, MD
Director, Pediatric Rehabilitation Services
Carolinas Rehabilitation
Physical Medicine and Rehabilitation
Charlotte, North Carolina
Clinical Associate Professor
Department of Physical Medicine and Rehabilitation
University of North Carolina
Chapel Hill, North Carolina
Chapter 20: TBI: A Pediatric Perspective

Keith Nicholson, PhD
Psychologist
Comprehensive Pain Program
The Toronto Western Hospital
University of Toronto
Toronto, Ontario
Canada
*Chapter 38: Post-Traumatic Pain Disorders: Medical
    Assessment and Management*
*Chapter 39: Psychological Approaches to
    Comprehensive Pain Assessment and Management
    following TBI*
*Chapter 64: Assessment of Response Bias in Clinical
    and Forensic Evaluations of Impairment
    Following TBI*

Randolph J. Nudo, PhD
Professor
Department of Molecular and Integrative Physiology
Director, Landon Center on Aging
The University of Kansas Medical Center
Kansas City, Kansas
*Chapter 49: Neuroscientific Basis for Occupational
    and Physical Therapy Interventions*

Kelly A. Ojdana, MS
Researcher
Life Expectancy Project
San Francisco, California
Chapter 17: Life Expectancy

William V. Padula, OD
Director
Padula Institute of Vision Rehabilitation
Guilford, Connecticut
Adjunct Faculty
Pennsylvania College of Optometry
Elkins Park, Pennsylvania
Chairperson, National Academy of Practice in
    Optometry (NAPO)
Founding President (Emeritus), Neuro-Optometric
    Rehabilitation Association (NORA)
Chapter 29: Evaluating and Treating Visual Dysfunction

Steven S. L. Pan, MD
Research Fellow
Stanford University School of Medicine
Physical Medicine and Rehabilitation Service
VA Palo Alto Health Care System
Palo Alto, California
*Chapter 13: Electrophysiologic Assessment Techniques:
    Evoked Potentials and Electroencephalography*

Amish R. Patel, DO
Resident
Department of Physical Medicine and Rehabilitation
Medical College of Ohio
Toledo, Ohio
*Chapter 32: Sleep Disturbances: Epidemiology,
    Assessment, and Treatment*

Thomas Politzer, OD
Private Practice
Golden, Colorado
Chapter 29: Evaluating and Treating Visual Dysfunction

Jeffrey Radecki, MD
Department of Physical Medicine and Rehabilitation
New York-Presbyterian
The University Hospital of Columbia and Cornell
New York, New York
Chapter 7: Primary Prevention

Cara Camiolo Reddy, MD
Traumatic Brain Injury Fellow and Clinical Instructor
Department of Physical Medicine and Rehabilitation
University of Pittsburgh School of Medicine
Pittsburgh, Pennsylvania
*Chapter 54: Neuropharmacology: A Rehabilitation
    Perspective*

Joseph H. Ricker, PhD
Associate Professor
Department of Physical Medicine and Rehabilitation
University of Pittsburgh School of Medicine
Pittsburgh, Pennsylvania
Chapter 12: Functional Neuroimaging of TBI

Allen J. Rubin, MD
The Center for Neuropsychiatry, LLC
Marlton, New Jersey
Adjunct Associate Professor of Clinical Psychiatry
Drexel University School of Medicine
Philadelphia, Pennsylvania
*Chapter 58: Community Re-entry Issues and
    Long-Term Care*

Michael Ruckenstein, MD
Associate Professor
Residency Program Director
Department of Otorhinolaryngology, Head and Neck
    Surgery
Hospital of the University of Pennsylvania
Philadelphia, Pennsylvania
Chapter 28: Balance and Dizziness

M. Elizabeth Sandel, MD
Chief, Physical Medicine and Rehabilitation
Napa Solano Service Area
Director, Research and Training
Kaiser Foundation Rehabilitation Center
Vallejo, California
Clinical Professor
Department of Physical Medicine and Rehabilitation
University of California, Davis, School of Medicine
Davis, California
*Chapter 37: Sexuality, Reproduction, and
    Neuroendocrine Disorders Following TBI*

Angelle M. Sander, PhD
Assistant Professor and Neuropsychologist
Department of Physical Medicine and Rehabilitation
Baylor College of Medicine/Harris County Hospital
  District
Associate Director
Brain Injury Research Center at The Institute for
  Rehabilitation and Research
Houston, Texas
*Chapter 60: A Cognitive-Behavioral Intervention for
  Family Members of Persons with TBI*

Joanne Scandale, PhD, CRC, CCM, LMHC
Program Director of Vocational Services
Department of Rehabilitation
Hutchings Psychiatric Center
Syracuse, New York
*Chapter 4: Training and Certification of Care
  Providers for Persons Sustaining TBI*

Nicholas D. Schiff, MD
Associate Professor
Department of Neurology and Neuroscience
Weill Medical College of Cornell University
New York, New York
*Chapter 25: Assessment and Rehabilitative Management
  of Individuals with Disorders of Consciousness*

Anbesaw Selassie, DrPH
Associate Professor of Epidemiology
Department of Biostatistics, Bioinformatics, and
  Epidemiology
Medical University of South Carolina
Charleston, Carolina
*Chapter 6: The Epidemiology of TBI: Implications for
  Public Health*

Robert M. Shavelle, PhD, MBA
Technical Director
Life Expectancy Project
San Francisco, California
Chapter 17: Life Expectancy

Neil T. Shepard, PhD
Professor
Department of Special Education and Communication
  Disorders
University of Nebraska, Lincoln
Lincoln, Nebraska
Chapter 28: Balance and Dizziness

Jonathan M. Silver, MD
Clinical Professor of Psychiatry
New York University School of Medicine
New York, New York
*Chapter 52: Pharmacotherapy of Neuropsychiatric
  Disturbances*
Chapter 53: Pharmacotherapy of Cognitive Impairment

Donald G. Stein, PhD
Asa G. Candler Professor
Department of Emergency Medicine
Emory University School of Medicine
Atlanta, Georgia
*Chapter 9: Concepts of CNS Plasticity and Their
  Implications for Understanding Recovery After Brain
  Damage*

David J. Strauss, PhD
Director
Life Expectancy Project
Emeritus Professor
University of California
San Francisco, California
Chaper 17: Life Expectancy

Katherine J. Sullivan, PhD, PT
Assistant Professor of Clinical Physical Therapy
Director, Entry-level Doctor of Physical Therapy
Department of Biokinesiology and Physical Therapy
University of Southern California
Los Angeles, California
*Chapter 50: Therapy Interventions for Mobility
  Impairments and Motor Skill Acquisition After TBI*

Andrew Sumich, MD
Private Practice
Physical Medicine and Rehabilitation
Carolina Neurosurgery and Spine Associates
Charlotte, North Carolina
Chapter 20: TBI: A Pediatric Perspective

Penelope S. Suter, OD
Optometrist in Private Practice
Research Associate
California State University
Bakersfield, California
*Chapter 29: Evaluating and Treating Visual
  Dysfunction*

Pam Targett, MEd
Rehabilitation Research and Training Center
Medical College of Virginia
Virginia Commonwealth University School of Medicine
Richmond, Virginia
Chapter 61: Returning to Work Following TBI

Laura A. Taylor, PhD
Licensed Clinical Psychologist
Village Family Psychiatry
Richmond, Virginia
*Chapter 43: Neuropsychological Assessment and
  Treatment of TBI*

Lora L. Thaxton, MD
Optimal Life Integrative Medicine Pain Center
Toledo, Ohio
*Chapter 32: Sleep Disturbances: Epidemiology,
Assessment, and Treatment*

John A. Thomas, OD
Adjunct Professor
Pacific University College of Optometry
Director
Head Trauma, Vision, Cognitive and Learning
   Disabilities Center
Denver, Colorado
Chapter 29: Evaluating and Treating Visual Dysfunction

David J. Thurman, MD, MPH
Neuroepidemiologist
National Center for Chronic Disease Prevention and
   Health Promotion
Centers for Disease Control and Prevention
Atlanta, Georgia
*Chapter 6: The Epidemiology of TBI: Implications for
Public Health*

Trinh Tran, MD
Clinical Instructor
University of California San Francisco School of
   Medicine
Laguna Hospital and Rehabilitation Center
San Francisco, California
Chapter 21: The Older Adult

Margaret A. Turk, MD
Professor
Department of Physical Medicine and Rehabilitation
Department of Pediatrics
SUNY Upstate Medical Center
Syracuse, New York
*Chapter 4: Training and Certification of Care
Providers for Persons Sustaining TBI*

Vincent Richard Vicci, Jr., OD
Staff Vision Care Consultant
Kessler Institute for Rehabilitation
West Orange, New Jersey
Staff Vision Care Consultant
Extended Recovery Unit
Robert Wood Johnson Rehabilitation Unit
JFK Memorial Hospital
Edison, New Jersey
Chapter 29: Evaluating and Treating Visual Dysfunction

Amy K. Wagner, MD
Assistant Professor
Department of Physical Medicine and Rehabilitation
Associate Director Rehabilitation Research
Safar Center for Resuscitation Research
University of Pittsburgh School of Medicine
Pittsburgh, Pennsylvania
*Chapter 5: Conducting Research in TBI: Current
Concepts and Issues*

Gary G. Wang, MD
Director
Traumatic Brain Injury Program
Erie County Medical Center
Buffalo, New York
*Chapter 56: Traditional Chinese Medicine Theory in
the Mechanism and Treatment of TBI*
Chapter 57: Complementary and Alternative Medicine

Roger O. Weed, PhD, CLCP
Professor and Coordinator
Graduate Rehabilitation Counseling Program
Department of Counseling and Psychological Services
Georgia State University
Atlanta, Georgia
*Chapter 66: Life Care Planning After TBI: Clinical and
Forensic Issues*

Michael West, PhD
Rehabilitation Research and Training Center
Medical College of Virginia
Virginia Commonwealth University School of Medicine
Richmond, Virginia
Chapter 61: Returning to Work Following TBI

Paul Wehman, PhD
Rehabilitation Research and Training Center
Medical College of Virginia
Virginia Commonwealth University School of Medicine
Richmond, Virginia
Chapter 61: Returning to Work Following TBI

Brooke-Mai Whelan, PhD
Research Fellow
Division of Speech Pathology
School of Health and Rehabilitation Sciences
The University of Queensland
St. Lucia, Brisbane
Australia
*Chapter 46: Assessment and Treatment of Speech and
Language Disorders in TBI*

Lezheng Wu, MD
Professor of Ophthalmology
Zhangshan Ophthalmic Center
Sun Yat-Sen University
Guangzhou, Canton
China
*Chapter 29: Evaluating and Treating Visual
Dysfunction*

Stuart A. Yablon, MD
Director, The Brain Injury Program
Methodist Rehabilitation Center
Jackson, Mississippi
Chapter 26: Post-Traumatic Seizures and Epilepsy

Satoko Yasuda, PhD
Rehabilitation Research and Training Center
Medical College of Virginia
Virginia Commonwealth University School of Medicine
Richmond, Virginia
Chapter 61: Returning to Work Following TBI

Ross D. Zafonte, DO
Professor and Chair
Department of Physical Medicine and Rehabilitation
University of Pittsburgh Medical Center
Pittsburgh, Pennsylvania
*Chapter 1: Clinical Continuum of Care and Natural
History*
*Chapter 54: Neuropharmacology: A Rehabilitation
Perspective*

Giuseppe Zappalà, MD
Behavioral Neurology and Cognitive Rehabilitation
Division of Neurology
Garibaldi Hospital
Catania, Italy
Chapter 42: Cognitive Impairments After TBI

Nathan D. Zasler, MD
CEO and Medical Director
Concussion Care Centre of Virginia, Ltd.
and Tree of Life Services, Inc.
Glen Allen, Virginia
Clinical Professor
Department of Physical Medicine and Rehabilitation
Medical College of Virginia
Virginia Commonwealth University School of Medicine
Richmond, Virginia
Clinical Associate Professor
Department of Physical Medicine and Rehabilitation
University of Virginia
Charlottesville, Virginia
Chairperson, International Brain Injury Association
*Chapter 1: Clinical Continuum of Care and Natural
History*
Chapter 22: Mild TBI
Chapter 23: Post-Concussive Disorder
*Chapter 38: Post-Traumatic Pain Disorders: Medical
Assessment and Management*
*Chapter 39: Psychological Approaches to
Comprehensive Pain Assessment and Management
Following TBI*
Chapter 63: Ethical Issues in Clinicolegal Practice
*Chapter 64: Assessment of Response Bias in Clinical
and Forensic Evaluations of Impairment
Following TBI*

George A. Zitnay, PhD, ABDA CBIS-CE
Director
National Brain Injury Research
Treatment and Training Foundation
Laurel Highlands Neurorehabilitation Center
Johnstown, Pennsylvania
*Chapter 2: Brain Injury Rehabilitation: Past, Present,
and Future?*

I

PERSPECTIVES ON REHABILITATIVE CARE AND RESEARCH

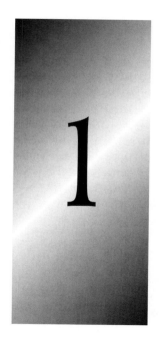

1 Clinical Continuum of Care and Natural History

Douglas I. Katz
Nathan D. Zasler
Ross D. Zafonte

SCOPE OF THE PROBLEM AND THE CHARACTERISTICS OF TRAUMATIC BRAIN INJURY

Systems of care for patients with traumatic brain injury (TBI) must account for the particular characteristics of this disorder. First, TBI is among the most common of serious, disabling neurological disorders. It is a significant problem in all societies. In the United States at least 1.4 million TBIs occur every year, and there are 5.3 million people living with disability from TBI (1–3). (See Thurman et al., Chapter 6, for a full discussion of the epidemiology of TBI). Systems of care must allocate resources for the large number of people who are affected by the disorder.

Second, TBI is largely a younger and older person's disorder (2). Individuals younger than 30, mostly males, make up the largest proportion of those affected. TBI usually impacts people who are in the later stages of adolescent development or in early adulthood. Therefore, TBI typically disrupts important periods of life involving educational and social development, emerging vocational productivity and adult independence, and beginning spousal relationships and family development. Older persons present particular problems related to aging including co-morbidities, slower and less complete recovery, and vulnerability to complications of injury and treatment (4) (see Englander et al., Chapter 21 on "The Older Adult").

Systems of care must address needs that include special educational requirements, independent living, vocational training and supports, and supports for family members.

Third, TBI commonly affects people with preexisting problems such as substance abuse, learning disabilities, behavioral disorders, psychiatric disorders and other risk factors that may make people more prone to injuries. In addition, persons with brain injury are more prone to psychiatric co-morbidities and psychosocial difficulties following injury. Systems of care must consider these pre-injury and post-injury issues with respect to injury prevention, their interactions with the clinical effects of injury and potential detrimental influence on recovery from TBI.

Fourth, the most important and consistent effects of TBI involve cognitive, emotional, and behavioral functioning. Motor and sensory perceptual problems also occur in varying amounts, more likely in those with more severe injuries. Cognitive and behavioral problems present more challenges to the health care system because they are often more difficult to recognize, characterize, and treat than traditional medical and physical problems. Persons with TBI, particularly less severe injuries, may not have any obvious physical markers of the injury, though there may be profound effects on the individual's ability to function, largely resulting from cognitive or behavioral dysfunction. Criteria for medical rehabilitation reimbursement, length of stay, and utilization decisions are often more focused on motor issues affecting function and less focused on cognitive and behavioral treatment issues. Some insurance payers even exclude coverage for cognitive rehabilitation, although there is evidence to support its efficacy (5, 6) (see Cicerone, Chapter 41 on cognitive rehabilitation). Systems of care must focus on proper assessment and treatment of cognitive and behavioral problems, even though they may not fit the characteristics of medical rehabilitative systems that were originally developed for medical and physical disabilities (see Chapters 41–45).

Fifth, TBI, especially more severe injuries, can have a relatively extended natural history and lifelong effects. Recovery from TBI may be more protracted, over a relative longer portion of the lifespan, than most other acquired injuries or neurological disorders that evolve more quickly or typically affect persons at later stages of life. Thus, systems of care for TBI need to recognize the potentially prolonged recovery timetable. Further, recovery after TBI has a somewhat predictable and characteristic course, with a variety of recognizable cognitive, behavioral, and sensorimotor syndromes at different stages. An appreciation of the natural history of TBI is essential to assessing the individual and to effectively applying treatment and services at different stages of recovery, as well to avoiding treatment that may be unnecessary or ineffective (see discussion on natural history below).

Finally, TBI is a disorder with a wide variety of pathophysiological effects, a range of severities, and a multitude of problems that may occur as the result of injury. Persons with apparently similar injuries may have significant variation in their presentation, course of recovery, response to interventions and ability to return to functioning. Systems of care should have a breadth of treatments and services to address the variety of problems that can occur after TBI, and the flexibility to move persons through the system in different ways depending on their individual needs at different times post-injury.

THE DEVELOPMENT OF SYSTEMS OF CARE

The provision of a comprehensive continuum of care for persons with TBI is an enormous challenge given the characteristics of TBI outlined above and the wide range of services that should be provided to large numbers of people, over relatively longer periods than most other disorders. The challenge confronts many groups: persons with TBI and their families; clinicians managing the care of the patient with TBI; service providers attempting to provide efficient and effective care; health insurance providers; public and other payers balancing coverage needs with financial pressures; and society at large, making choices about resource allocation and costs. Resources for patients with TBI include: acute and post-acute medical care; rehabilitative services in the hospital, at home, in the community, and in residential settings; psychosocial services; educational and vocational services; and a variety of other support services.

The development of systems of care for persons with TBI evolved in the 1970s and 1980s. In part, the systems that developed for care of patients with TBI were influenced by systems of care that were developed for those with spinal cord injury (SCI). Prior to development of specific programs for persons with TBI, patients were frequently treated in psychiatric facilities, nursing homes, or more general rehabilitation facilities. The Rehabilitation Services Administration and NIDHR (which was to become NIDRR), which had funded SCI model systems in the early 1970s, also funded two model system projects for TBI in 1978 at Stanford University and New York University (7). The recommendations from these projects helped to promote the development of interdisciplinary, dedicated TBI programs with services across the continuum of recovery. As programs began to develop, the lack of organized planning led to an initiative by the NIDRR under the Department of Education in 1987 to fund five TBI model systems demonstration projects (8). This has expanded to sixteen TBI Model Systems Projects throughout the country in part aimed at gathering information to improve comprehensive systems of care for patients with TBI. The components of these model systems of care includes emergency medical services, acute neurosurgical care, comprehensive rehabilitation services, long-term interdisciplinary follow-up and rehabilitation services, as well as what were termed optional services, including behavior modification programs, home rehabilitation services, case management and community living options (8). A key portion of this program has been longitudinal and project specific based research.

Beginning in the mid-1980s, the Commission on Accreditation of Rehabilitation Facilities (CARF) developed standards for TBI rehabilitative care by establishing specialized accreditation for TBI programs. It now accredits TBI programs in six categories: inpatient, outpatient, home- and community-based, residential, long-term residential, and vocational.

An important development in TBI care was the TBI Act of 1996 passed by Congress to "provide for the conduct of expanded studies and the establishment of innovative programs with respect to traumatic brain injury." Four provisions of the Act included surveillance and prevention under the CDC; basic and applied research to improve diagnosis, therapeutics and the continuum of clinical care conducted by the NIH; a planning and implementation grant program to the states under the Health Resources and Services Administration (HRSA); and a Consensus Conference conducted by the Center for Medical Rehabilitation and Research at NIH (9). The NIH consensus conference panel addressed the continuum of care for TBI in their conclusions. The recommendations included that "persons with TBI should have access to rehabilitation services through the entire course of recovery, which may last for many years after the injury" and that "community-based, non-medical services should be components of the extended care and rehabilitation available to persons with TBI" (10).

REALITIES OF THE MARKETPLACE

Although demonstration projects such as the TBI Model Systems have presented apparently effective systems of care for persons with TBI, the realities of the marketplace in the United States have presented challenges to providing such care and services to all those in need. Corrigan outlined 20 important challenges to meeting the needs of persons with TBI, within the categories of access, availability, appropriateness, and acceptability (9). With regard to access, the problems involve identifying and utilizing services, even if they are available. There may be difficulties accessing information about available resources. Sometimes it is difficult to determine what resources are covered by health insurance, and sometimes coverage is denied even after services are delivered. Families and care providers usually lack roadmaps to guide access to appropriate resources, and points of entry into publicly funded systems may be unclear. Service systems may have artificial barriers created by narrow eligibility criteria. Services are often fragmented and not well coordinated.

Corrigan pointed out a number of availability issues for which the main limiting factor is funding. Health insurance may not cover needed services that are available, or may direct individuals to centers that are less familiar with the care of persons with TBI. Further, lack of payer support may preclude the availability of some services to begin with. Many persons with TBI have no health care funding at all at the time of injury, and present state budget constraints are further threatening the Medicaid program. When available, health insurance typically fully covers acute care, but coverage for rehabilitative care becomes incrementally more difficult across the continuum of care, from inpatient to outpatient to residential and community services. Health insurance coverage also tends to be more restrictive for cognitive and behavioral services as opposed to more traditional physical rehabilitative and medical treatment. In many cases, coverage for services has to shift from private to public sources such as Medicaid and Medicare over the course of recovery because of limits in coverage for longer term care in many policies. Public funding has further restraints on long-term coverage. Several states have developed a system of Medicaid waivers to provide long-term home and community-based services that would otherwise be covered only for institutional settings, such as nursing

homes. The fragmentation and limitations in financing of care and services can create a nightmare of coordination for persons with brain injury, their families, and service providers. Clinicians who coordinate care for persons with brain injury must become aware of the complexities of reimbursement and the array of alternative sources of funding for TBI care and support in their community.

Other issues affecting the availability of services include geographic limitations; lack of transportation; a paucity of appropriate, affordable housing; limitations in resources for behavioral problems in children with special needs; and the long-term needs of persons with TBI (9). Patients with TBI in rural communities have special challenges in finding services within a reasonable distance. Even when available in a nearby area, transport to and from these services can be a major problem, and home services may not be available or sufficiently expert for this population. The ability to provide a full array of services to all age groups within a reasonable proximity, with full funding support, is an enormous challenge that may never be fully satisfied.

The appropriateness of available resources is also a common problem. Sometimes the reason for inappropriate services is dictated by payer constraints. For instance, because the main payer for long-term care services is Medicaid, if waivers to support home and community services are not available, patients with TBI who cannot return home may be placed in nursing homes, even though community-based services may be more appropriate. Even if services are available, programs and professional providers may lack the knowledge and expertise to serve this population. Generalists in a particular discipline or specialty may not have the skills for proper assessment or treatment of the patient with TBI. Accreditation programs such as CARF and the American Academy of Certified Brain Injury Specialists (AACBIS) have attempted to set standards and credentialing to assure appropriateness of programming and expertise. (See also Chapter 4 on training and certification.) Nevertheless, such expertise may simply not be available in some geographic areas or at certain levels of care. Sometimes erroneous services are applied because of this lack of expertise, but at times services may be improperly or needlessly applied even by those with expertise. Inaccurate diagnosis, inappropriate application of treatment at a particular stage of recovery, use of unproven or ineffective treatments, or application of effective treatment to those for whom it would not be of benefit are examples. Use of accurate diagnosis and prognosis is necessary to avoid some of these problems of inappropriate treatment (see below on natural history). Sometimes services are not fully relevant to a person's and family's needs at a particular time or in a particular environment. The acceptability of these services to the goals of the person with TBI and how services promote the persons self-actualization is another challenge to the TBI service marketplace (9).

ESSENTIAL COMPONENTS OF THE CLINICAL CONTINUUM

The continuum of care for patients with TBI occurs in a variety of settings. Figure 1-1 illustrates the different types of care and how patients may move through these components. The flow through these services may not be linear. Patients may enter or leave the system of care at different points, or reverse directions, based on individual needs or the dictates of the marketplace.

Prevention

The earliest aspect of the care continuum involves public health issues prior to injury occurrence. Injury prevention is an essential part of trauma care systems. The TBI Act of 1996 charged the CDC with the responsibility for prevention, in addition to surveillance, to assess factors that increase the risk of TBI and those that are protective. Injury prevention programs generally include three components: programs designed to alter behavior and improve decision-making to increase self-protection; product improvement to minimize the chance of injury or protect the individual

in an accident; and legislation and public policies that require individuals to follow safety guidelines. Prevention of TBI includes a number of efforts such as reducing alcohol-related injuries, preventing falls, preventing violence, promoting safe practices in sports, promoting helmet and seatbelt use, enhancing safe driving practices, and improving vehicle safety. (See Napolitano et al., Chapter 7, for a discussion of primary prevention.)

Emergency Medical Services

Since the 1980s, emergency trauma systems have developed throughout the United States and have led to improved survival and recovery (11–13). Mortality for those that reach the hospital has been reduced from nearly 50% to about 25% (13). Regional trauma systems have developed to promote quick evacuation using ground or air transport to level I and level II trauma centers from the field, or from level III and IV trauma centers when necessary for more serious injuries. The level I and II trauma centers have full-time intensive care, imaging, neurosurgical, and other trauma subspecialists. The Brain Trauma Foundation's (BTF) Guidelines for Prehospital

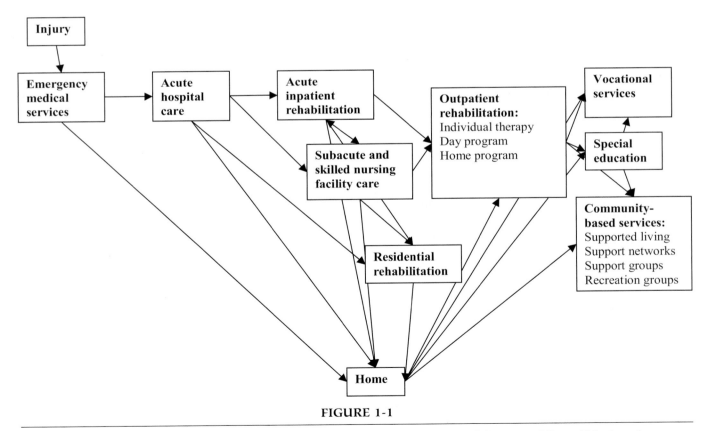

FIGURE 1-1

Usual flow of patients through the clinical continuum of care. Choices of services and direction of flow will be based on severity, stage of recovery, patient's needs, availability of resources, availability of home and community supports, and constraints of the marketplace

Management of Traumatic Brain Injury have played a role in improving emergency prehospital care (12). Although improved, proper diagnosis, patient education, and referral for appropriate follow-up is still lacking for many patients (14).

Acute Hospital Care

Patients with TBI who are admitted for acute hospital care range from those who need a period of observation to recognize secondary neurological deterioration and neurosurgical complications that may ensue after a delay, to those with co-morbidities that require hospital care, to those with more severe brain injury that requires intensive care management. Acute neurosurgical and intensive care for patients with TBI have improved over the last two decades with better survival and outcomes (15). Evidence-based guidelines for acute TBI care, including the use of intracranial pressure monitoring, have contributed to better outcomes (16–18). (See also Chapters 18 and 19 on acute care.)

Rehabilitation assessment and early rehabilitative interventions should take place a short time after admission, in the acute hospital setting. Subsequent decisions for rehabilitative care are made as the patient progresses toward medical and surgical stability, when the severity of the injury and the clinical rehabilitation needs become more apparent. The pathway toward acute inpatient rehabilitation versus outpatient or subacute care is largely based on injury severity and pace of recovery. Generally, patients with severe injuries (e.g., unconsciousness for a day or more, or post-traumatic amnesia and confusional states of at least days to weeks, or patients with large focal lesions) move to acute inpatient rehabilitation facilities. Constraints related to marketplace issues may affect this decision. For instance, some health care plans will not support admission to inpatient rehabilitation facilities if a patient has few traditional physical rehabilitation needs (e.g., needs little or no help ambulating) even if the patient has profound cognitive and behavioral disturbances related to the injury. Patients with mild injuries generally return home and may need outpatient rehabilitation services. A proportion of patients with moderate injury may benefit from at least a brief inpatient rehabilitation stay, depending on their circumstances. Patients who are slower to recover may require extended care in the acute hospital, or be transferred to subacute or skilled nursing facility (SNF) care instead of inpatient rehabilitation. In many systems such persons may be lost to the follow-up of those with a primary interest in caring for patients with TBI. Strong consideration should be given to transferring such patients to facilities with special expertise in the assessment and care of patients who are unconscious or minimally conscious (usually in acute inpatient rehabilitation or specialized subacute facilities), because these patients are vulnerable to secondary complications and may have significant potential for further recovery, albeit at a slower pace.

Acute Inpatient Rehabilitation

Acute inpatient rehabilitation may occur on general rehabilitation units or in dedicated brain injury units that are within acute care facilities or part of freestanding rehabilitation hospitals (inpatient rehabilitation facilities or long-term care hospitals). Admission criteria to hospital-based acute inpatient rehabilitation involve the following:

1. an intensity of medical and nursing care needs that requires full-time physician monitoring and specialized rehabilitative nursing expertise;
2. functional deficits that would benefit from a higher level of rehabilitation treatment intensity (usually designated at a minimum duration of 3 hours a day).

Patients are best served in programs dedicated to brain injury care or those with a significant proportion of staff with expertise in managing brain injury. Rehabilitation teams usually include: case managers; physical, occupational, and speech therapy staff; rehabilitation nurses; nursing assistants; psychologists; neuropsychologists; rehabilitation physicians (usually a physiatrist, rehabilitation neurologist, or neuropsychiatrist); primary care physicians; and a variety of other consultant medical specialists. Other disciplines such as social workers, rehabilitation technicians, therapy assistants, behavior specialists, recreation therapists, other subspecialty therapists, chaplains, and attorneys may also contribute to care.

Expertise in managing behavioral problems and assuring patient, family and staff safety is important because patients in agitated confusional states are usually managed at this level of care (see below). Family education to familiarize them with the problems and needs of persons with brain injury is essential at this level of care, especially for those that will transition home from acute inpatient rehabilitation. The decision regarding the next level of care depends on the patient's medical stability, level of dependency, safety, and whether the person's needs can be adequately met at home or requires further institutional care. Patients with severe TBI typically still require some supervision and, perhaps, physical assistance for self-care and mobility when they are ready to be discharged from acute inpatient rehabilitation.

Subacute and Skilled Nursing Facility Rehabilitation

Patients with TBI are usually admitted to this level of care from acute hospital care or acute inpatient rehabilitation. Therapies are provided at a lower level of intensity than in acute inpatient rehabilitation and the level of medical monitoring is less frequent than acute inpatient rehabilitation. There are many programs at this level that specialize in neurorehabilitation and it is certainly preferable if this level of care occurs in programs with special expertise in brain injury management. Specialized neurobehavioral treatment units in SNFs are available in some areas for patients with more persistent behavioral regulation problems.

As noted above, some SNFs may offer specialized care for patients with TBI with prolonged impairments of consciousness. The availability of specialized subacute and SNF facilities may be limited in some areas because of market constraints. Care for the needs of TBI patients in these settings may be costly, exceeding the usual reimbursement standards for this level of care. Alternative funding sources or variance in reimbursement standards may be necessary to maintain more specialized subacute or SNF care.

Often, SNF level rehabilitation care takes place in more general facilities, and frequently younger patients with TBI are in the minority among an older group of patients with other disorders, such as dementia. Lengths of stay at this level of care varies but usually lasts one or more months; a minority of patients transition to unskilled residential levels of care at the same facilities. A large proportion of patients transition home and may go on to outpatient rehabilitation or other outpatient services.

Outpatient Rehabilitation

Outpatient rehabilitation can take on a number of different forms. Sometimes it consists of individual therapies involving physical, occupational and speech therapists. There may be other available services including psychology, neuropsychology and therapeutic recreation. The team may be led by a case manager, and they may provide other coordinated activities such as group treatments. Usually rehabilitation at this level is less coordinated than inpatient treatment and therapists provide care more autonomously. This type of care may occur in the setting of the home through visiting nurse or other agencies, or on the premises of an acute hospital, a rehabilitation hospital, or an outpatient rehabilitation facility.

A more coordinated form of outpatient rehabilitation may take place in a day program, with a full array of therapies, group treatments and group activities, case management, and regular team meetings to set goals and review progress. More holistic programs may include a psychotherapeutic milieu associated with the therapy programming. These programs are often in naturalistic, community settings and take advantage of this location to set up activities to foster community reentry treatment goals.

The length and intensity of treatment is determined by the patient's needs but is largely constrained by health insurance payer contracts and public funding policies limiting duration of care and range of covered services.

Following outpatient rehabilitation, additional community-based services may be provided.

Residential Rehabilitation

Group residence programs may provide services at various stages after injury. These programs may offer individual therapies and group therapies, as well as resources to foster independent living skills. Residential programs may be aimed at patients recently discharged from acute hospital settings or acute inpatient rehabilitation, or those later in the process of recovery who cannot be in their own home setting, and who require a structured, supervised setting and specialized programming cannot be in their own home setting. There are usually only part-time nursing services and programs may or may not provide physician services. Those states with more generous auto insurance benefits tend to have more extensive residential programs. Staffing includes a mix of professional therapists, other professional disciplines, and lay staff. Patients may progress in levels of independence in these setting and go back home or to other long-term living arrangements, such as supported living (see "Other Community-Based Services" below), after this level of care.

Vocational Services

For most persons with TBI, the return to work is the most important long-term rehabilitation goal and measure of treatment success. Returning to some sort of productive activity is an essential part of societal reintegration and life satisfaction after brain injury and an important part of the continuum of care. In the United States, the states receive federal money to operate vocational rehabilitation programs to provide vocational rehabilitation services to individuals with disabilities. Services support reeducation, training and worksite support services. Even those with severe injuries, who may not qualify for regular marketplace jobs, are eligible for services under this mandate. Supported employment has become one of the important vocational rehabilitation strategies for getting persons with disabilities back to employment in regular work sites. These services are most successful when coordinated with outpatient rehabilitative care and assessments. Many of these programs have been underfunded and it has been a problem to provide the intensive ongoing supports that are necessary to keep some persons with TBI employed. Many states have adopted innovative programs to extend funding using resources such as Medicaid waivers to improve services and employment retention (19).

Special Education

Education services are a necessary component of the continuum of care for children and adolescents with TBI.

TBI became a part of the federal Individuals with Disability Education Act in 1990. This federal law mandates that the education needs of school age children with TBI, among other disabilities, will be provided in the public schools and must include any necessary rehabilitation services. Services should be planned and monitored using an individualized educational program (IEP). Students often transition from inpatient or outpatient rehabilitation to school-based services, sometimes beginning with home tutoring. Ylvisaker and colleagues have made a number of recommendations for assessment, intervention, student support, educator training, family support and system flexibility to better serve the particular educational and rehabilitative needs of students after TBI (20).

Other Community-Based Services

Persons with TBI may require other ongoing care and support after formal rehabilitative care has ended. These home and community-based services are more fragmented and less readily available. Patients who are unable to live independently, and who are not relying on home supervision by family or friends, require supported living environments. Previously, because Medicaid has been the primary funder of long-term care, this meant placement in nursing homes, usually a poor alternative for younger persons with TBI. A growing number of states with Medicaid waiver programs have been able to provide supported living services in the community using such models as supervised group homes, foster homes, and personal care attendants. A number of other models have been developed.

Community support networks and support groups for persons with TBI and their families are important resources. One such support network, the Clubhouse Model, adapted for persons with TBI in the 1980s from the psychiatric community, provides a setting for members and volunteers to participate in social, recreational, and work-related activities. It has been a cost-effective method to promote practical, functional living skills. Support groups for persons with TBI and their families are often sponsored by state chapters of the Brain Injury Association of America (BIAA).

Other necessary community services include provisions for transportation for those who are unable to drive or ride public transportation. Respite care to provide time-off for full-time caretakers of persons with severe disability after TBI is another important need. Legal services, financial and estate planning, mental health services, and treatment of substance abuse must also be considered part of community-based system of care for people with TBI.

Case Management

Fragmentation and lack of coordination of care is one of the major problems in finding and applying proper services for the individual with TBI. Case managers within institutions and in the community play an essential role in coordinating services. Case managers collaborate with others, including patients, families, providers, and payers to assess, plan, implement, coordinate and monitor services to meet an individual's needs and promote favorable outcomes in a cost-effective manner. In addition to coordinating care within the TBI system, case managers must coordinate treatment in other areas such as chronic pain, mental health and other medical specialty areas. Case managers and life care planners may develop proposals outlining the anticipated lifelong care needs of persons with TBI (see Weed and Berens, Chapter 66, on life care planning).

SERVICE DELIVERY IN RELATION TO NATURAL HISTORY OF TBI

Accurate diagnosis and an appreciation of the natural history of TBI are useful in formulating treatment plans and assuring appropriateness of services along the continuum of care. This effort involves assessing a person's brain injury in the context of pathophysiologic damage, associated clinical neurobehavioral syndromes, stage of recovery and anticipated course of recovery, based on knowledge of brain-behavior relationships and natural history (21). The formulation must also consider interaction with noninjury factors such as age and psychosocial issues, associated injuries, premorbid problems, co-morbidities, and later complications.

This understanding helps in determining where the patient is along the path of recovery and in projecting expectations for subsequent recovery to inform treatment planning with respect to treatment setting, treatment strategies, treatment goals, and length of stay. It may also help avoid unnecessary treatment of problems that may be expected to resolve as part of the natural course of recovery (e.g., post-traumatic amnesia or confusional agitation) or impairments with a poor prognosis that may not recover with direct treatment (e.g., amnesia after extensive, bilateral hippocampal injury or behavior dysregulation after massive bilateral orbital prefrontal and temporal polar damage).

Such an understanding of natural history also helps determine when clinical syndromes do not fit the expected path of recovery, suggesting possible secondary neurological complications (e.g. hydrocephalus, chronic subdural hematomas), the influence of noninjury factors (medical, iatrogenic or psychogenic), or misdiagnosis of injury type and severity. The clinical natural history of TBI can be defined in the context of focal or diffuse neuropathologic events. (See Kochenak et al., Chapter 8, for an extended discussion of TBI neuropathology.) The critical pathophysiologic factors are the type, distribution, severity, and location of these combined neuropatholog-ical events after brain injury.

Although focal and diffuse pathological processes are often intermingled and have common secondary and metabolic consequences, it is useful to consider them sep-arately for the purposes of clinical diagnosis. The preci-sion of diagnosis varies and may be challenging, especially with respect to diffuse and secondary injuries, for which there are as yet no readily available, direct clinical, diag-nostic probes.

Diffuse Injury

Diffuse axonal injury represents the main diffuse patho-logical process, but it is associated with a host of associ-ated pathophysiological phenomena (see Chapter 8). The natural history of diffuse injury is characterized by a rec-ognizable pattern of stages that occur across the wide spectrum of severity. Injury severity determines the dura-tion of recovery stages and levels of impairment at each stage of recovery. These stages can be combined into three principal phases of recovery from the acute to chronic stages:

1. loss of consciousness (LOC);
2. post-traumatic confusion and amnesia (PTA);
3. post-confusional restoration of cognitive function.

These form the basis for the main indices of clinical severity for TBI. These indices can help project a rough approximations for the time course of recovery and the probabilities for a particular outcome (22–26). The three phases of recovery appear to be proportionally related in patients with diffuse injury; each subsequent phase is typically several-fold longer than the previous one (22). Their proportionality in patients with diffuse injury, although variable, can contribute to predicting the time course of recovery. For instance, there was a predictable relationship between the duration of unconsciousness (LOC) and duration of confusion/PTA in a series of patients with diffuse injury defined by a linear regres-sion model that predicted nearly 60% of the variance — PTA (wks) = 0.4 × LOC (days) + 3.6 (22). This model was confirmed in a separate cohort of 228 patients (27). Longer PTA was observed in older patients, especially over age 40, or if a focal frontal lesion was present. Pre-dicting PTA may aid rehabilitative treatment planning with respect to length of stay decisions, treatment choices for confusional agitation, and other treatment issues at this stage of recovery.

Patients with the least severe diffuse injuries (mild concussion) evolve through LOC (if complete loss of con-sciousness occurs at all) in seconds to minutes and through PTA usually in minutes to hours, followed by a post-confusional phase typically lasting days to weeks. In mild TBI the transition through the earliest stages may be brief, unwitnessed, and difficult to document. Patients with severe TBI may require days to weeks to evolve through LOC, weeks to months to resolve confusion and PTA, and months to years to evolve through the post-confusional residual recovery phase. The course of recov-ery after severe TBI is among the longest observed after neurological damage. Dynamic changes in neuropsycho-logical functioning have been observed as long as 5 years post-injury (28–31). Some patients with very severe injuries may stall in recovery at some stage in this process (e.g., permanent vegetative state (32) or minimally con-scious state (33).

This pattern of recovery has been delineated in stages according to various schemas. The most widely used is the Rancho Los Amigos levels of cognitive functioning (34). (See Table 1-1.) Another schema, first proposed by Alexander (35) and further modified (referred to as the Braintree scale) (21, 36), follows more traditional neuro-logical nomenclature. (See Table 1-2.) As patients progress through these stages the principal defining cognitive lim-itations evolve from deficits in arousal and consciousness, to basic attention and anterograde amnesia, to higher-level attention, memory, executive functioning, processing speed, insight, and social awareness (37).

The first stage of recovery is *coma*, a state of uncon-sciousness without spontaneous eye opening. This corre-sponds to Rancho level I. Patients with diffuse axonal injury are unconscious at the outset, without lucid interval. The depth of coma in the time period shortly after injury, as measured by the Glasgow Coma Scale (GCS), is one of the common markers of injury severity and prognosis.

Almost all persons with severe TBI who survive resume spontaneous eye opening and sleep/wake cycles while still unconscious, a condition termed a *vegetative state* or Rancho level II. Except for the small percentage of very severely injured patients who remain permanently vegetative, evidence of awareness and purposeful behavior resume, often heralded by visual fixation and tracking. The ability to follow commands is the usual convincing

TABLE 1-1
Rancho Los Amigo Levels of Cognitive Functioning After TBI (34)

I.	No response
II.	Generalized responses
III.	Localized responses
IV.	Confused – agitated
V.	Confused – inappropriate
VI.	Confused – appropriate
VII.	Automatic – appropriate
VIII.	Purposeful and appropriate

TABLE 1-2

Braintree Neurologic Stages of Recovery from Diffuse TBI (and corresponding Rancho Los Amigos Scale Levels) [settings of care]

---

1. *Coma*: unresponsive, eyes closed, no sign of wakefulness (Rancho 1) [emergency medical services; acute inpatient hospital]
2. *Vegetative state/wakeful unconsciousness*: no cog-nitive awareness; gross wakefulness, sleep-wake cycles begin (Rancho 2) [acute hospital; acute inpatient rehabilitation; subacute rehabilitation]
3. *Minimally conscious state*: inconsistent, sim-ple purposeful behavior, inconsistent response to commands begin; often mute (Rancho 3) [acute hospital; acute inpatient rehabilitation; subacute rehabilitation]
4. *Confusional state*: interactive communication and appropriate object use begin; amnesic (PTA), severe basic attentional deficits, hypokinetic or agitated, labile behavior; later, more appropriate goal-directed behavior with continuing antero-grade amnesia (Rancho 4, 5, partly 6) [acute hospital; acute inpatient rehabilitation]
5. *Post-confusional/emerging independence*: marked by resolution of PTA; cognitive impairments in higher-level attention, memory retrieval and executive functioning; deficits in self-awareness, social awareness, behavioral and emotional regulation; achieving functional independence in daily self care, improving social interaction; developing independence at home (Rancho 6 & partly 7) [acute inpatient rehabilitation; subacute inpatient rehabilitation; outpatient rehabilitation; residential treatment; outpatient day hospital and community reentry]
6. *Social competence/community reentry*: marked by resumption of basic household independence; developing indepen-dence in community, household management skills and later returning to academic or vocational pursuits; recovering higher level cognitive abilities (divided attention, cognitive speed, executive functioning), self-awareness, social skills; developing effective adaptation and compensation for residual problems (Rancho 7& 8) [outpatient community reentry programs; community-based services – vocational; special education; supported living services; mental health services]

---

marker of restored consciousness. Almost all patients with some loss of consciousness will be evaluated and treated by emergency medical services. Those with brief alterations of consciousness (e.g., seconds or minutes) may be discharged home. Patients with more prolonged LOC or more complicated injuries (e.g., focal lesions, other injuries) will likely be admitted for acute inpatient care, often beginning in surgical intensive care units, usually supervised by neurosurgical or surgical trauma specialists.

For patients recovering slowly, cognitive respon-siveness may begin erratically and inconsistently, without any reliable interactive communication. This stage may be called a *minimally conscious state* and corresponds to Rancho level III (33). Many patients at this stage will con-tinue in acute medical care settings and some who are slower to recover will transition to rehabilitation facili-ties, including acute inpatient rehabilitation, subacute rehabilitation, long-term care hospitals or skilled nurs-ing facilities. (See also Chapter 25 on disorders of con-sciousness.)

When purposeful cognition is unequivocally estab-lished, basic attention and new learning remain severely impaired. This clinical condition may be labeled a *con-fusional state* and corresponds to Rancho levels IV, V, and part of VI. At this stage, patients are often highly dis-tractible, with poorly regulated behavior. They may rapidly escalate to agitated behavior (Rancho IV). Less often, patients may remain in a state of underactivated, hypokinetic, withdrawn behavior. Dense anterograde

amnesia also defines this stage; patients are disoriented, have little or no moment-to-moment episodic recall and display little or no ability to learn new information after even a brief delay (posttraumatic amnesia). As this stage evolves, patients are better able to focus attention and regulate behavior (Rancho V). The end of this stage is characterized by a significant improvement in focused and sustained attention, reliable orientation, and resumption of continuous, day-to-day memory, albeit still somewhat defective (Rancho VI). Patients at this period of recovery are appropriate for care in dedicated TBI units in acute inpatient rehabilitation. Towards the end of this period of recovery, transition to home and outpatient rehabili-tation programs should be contemplated. Patients who are transitioning slowly, or who still require significant amounts of supervision and assistance that may not be feasible at home, may require continued institutional treatment, perhaps at a skilled nursing facility or a resi-dential treatment facility. Some may transition to an outpatient day program.

The *post-confusional* stages of recovery are charac-terized by a gradual improvement in cognitive and behav-ioral functioning in those with more severe injuries. This phase of recovery may be further broken into stages of *emerging independence*, as patients' cognitive abilities, self-awareness, and insight allow independence in self-care and safe unsupervised activity at home (Rancho level VII), and a stage of *social competence and community reentry*, with restoration of the capacity for independent func-tion in the community or at the higher-level demands of school or the workplace (Rancho level VIII). Services at these stages of care include outpatient therapies, day programs, community-reentry programs, residential treatment, and a variety of community-based services.

Focal Injury

Focal cortical contusions, deep cerebral hemorrhages, and extraaxial (subdural and epidural) hemorrhages make up the majority of focal lesions after TBI. The time course of natural history of focal injury resembles that of vascular lesions of other causes, particularly hemorrhagic stroke, but the clinical consequences of focal injury after TBI are characteristic, owing to the predilection of lesions in the anterior and inferior portions of the frontal and temporal lobes. The acute phase involves edema and other early secondary pathophysiological phenomena which are maximal over the first few days post-injury. The resulting effects may include confusion and, perhaps, decreased arousal, especially if a mass effect compromises diencephalic and mesencephalic structures. Otherwise primary focal pathology is not directly associated with loss of consciousness.

As edema and other secondary effects wane over the first three weeks, more specific localizing effects of focal damage become more apparent. Recovery during this subacute phase is maximal over the first 3 months, but improvement may continue at a slower rate over many months. The size and depth of focal lesions, their laterality and the potential for reorganization within the neural networks affected by the damage, all in large part determine the time course and outcome.

Damage to limbic neocortical and heteromodal areas of the frontal and temporal lobes determines the usual effects of focal TBI on cognitive and behavioral functioning. The residual syndromes of prefrontal lesions include alterations in affect and behavior (e.g., disinhibition or apathy) impairment in attention, working memory and memory retrieval, and dysfunctional higher-level cognition (e.g., executive functions, insight, social awareness). Lesions in anterior and inferior temporal areas may also contribute to affective and behavioral disturbances. Larger lesions extending to medial temporal areas may produce specific impairments in memory encoding and retrieval (amnesia). Other localizing temporal syndromes involve extension of lesions into auditory association areas (e.g., aphasia, with left hemisphere lesions) and visual association areas (e.g., visual agnosias, especially with bilateral lesions).

The clinical syndromes associated with focal lesions are often embedded in the evolving effects of diffuse injury, if both types of injury are combined. Particularly with more severe and diffuse injuries, the overall outcome is driven largely by the effects of diffuse rather than focal injury (38). In patients with mild to moderate diffuse injury, large focal lesions may have more influence on recovery (39–41). Characterization of the localizing syndromes associated with focal lesions may be difficult until unmasked after resolution of post-traumatic confusion. Another difficulty in isolating the effects of focal lesions is that neurobehavioral syndromes may be identical to those related to diffuse injury (e.g., dysexecutive syndrome, behavioral dysregulation) because these same areas, especially their axonal projections, are affected by diffuse pathology (42).

Although the problems may be similar, recovery and prognosis may be different. For instance, features of the frontal lobe syndrome, may be more persistent in patients with frontal contusion (43, 44). Levin et al. (45) observed that although other aspects of recovery were similar, unilateral frontal lesions adversely affect psychosocial outcome in children with TBI compared to those without focal frontal lesions. These aspects of diagnosis and prognosis related to focal lesions should also help inform rehabilitation planning. For example, behavioral regulation problems related to bilateral frontal and temporal focal lesions may be more persistent and thus demand more active early intervention and treatment planning over a longer horizon than similar problems that might occur after diffuse injury, which may be expected to resolve more successfully as the stages of recovery evolve.

SUMMARY AND CONCLUSIONS

The provision of a continuum of care for persons with TBI is an enormous challenge given the numbers of people affected by the disorder (patients, family members, and others), the potential long-term course of recovery, the possible life-long effects (often beginning at an earlier stage of life), and the wide variety of types of brain damage, clinical effects, and associated problems. Systems of care for TBI involve coordination of numerous services utilizing many disciplines across the range of severities and course of recovery. These services include prevention; emergency, acute, early, and later rehabilitation; vocational, educational, and community support; and long-term care. A number of marketplace factors constrain the full development and availability of components of these systems for persons in need, most notably cost, payer support, and availability of resources. These constraints become progressively restrictive for services and supports beyond the acute treatment period.

An understanding of brain injury, its clinical consequences, associated problems and complications, and natural history of recovery helps in applying proper services for patients along the continuum of care, and helps assure more effective use of resources. Ongoing efforts at fruitful research to determine which interventions are most effective, for whom, and at what periods of time, will be essential to refine the best clinical practices possible along the continuum of care.

References

1. Langlois JA, Kegler SR, Butler JA, et al. Traumatic brain injury-related hospital discharges. Results from a 14-state surveillance system, 1997. *MMWR Surveill Summ* 2003;52:1–20.
2. Langlois JA, Marr A, Mitchko J, Johnson RL. Tracking the silent epidemic and educating the public: CDC's traumatic brain injury-associated activities under the TBI Act of 1996 and the Children's Health Act of 2000. *J Head Trauma Rehabil* 2005;20:196–204.
3. Thurman DJ, Alverson C, Dunn KA, Guerrero J, Sniezek JE. Traumatic brain injury in the United States: A public health perspective. *J Head Trauma Rehabil* 1999;14:602–615.
4. Coronado VG, Thomas KE, Sattin RW, Johnson RL. The CDC traumatic brain injury surveillance system: characteristics of persons aged 65 years and older hospitalized with a TBI. *J Head Trauma Rehabil* 2005;20:215–228.
5. Cicerone KD, Dahlberg C, Kalmar K, et al. Evidence-based cognitive rehabilitation: recommendations for clinical practice. *Arch Phys Med Rehabil* 2000;81:1596–1615.
6. Cicerone KD, Dahlberg C, Malec JF, et al. Evidence-based cognitive rehabilitation: updated review of the literature from 1998 through 2002. *Arch Phys Med Rehabil* 2005;86:1681–1692.
7. Cope DN, Mayer NH, Cervelli L. Development of systems of care for persons with traumatic brain injury. *J Head Trauma Rehabil* 2005;20:128–142.
8. Ragnarsson KT, Thomas JP, Zasler ND. Model systems of care for individuals with traumatic brain injury. *J Head Trauma Rehabil* 1993;8:1–11.
9. Corrigan JD. Conducting statewide needs assessments for persons with traumatic brain injury. *J Head Trauma Rehabil* 2001;16:1–19.
10. Rehabilitation of persons with traumatic brain injury. *NIH Consens Statement* 1998;16:1–41.
11. Rudehill A, Bellander BM, Weitzberg E, Bredbacka S, Backheden M, Gordon E. Outcome of traumatic brain injuries in 1,508 patients: impact of prehospital care. *J Neurotrauma* 2002;19: 855–868.
12. Watts DD, Hanfling D, Waller MA, Gilmore C, Fakhry SM, Trask AL. An evaluation of the use of guidelines in prehospital management of brain injury. *Prehosp Emerg Care* 2004;8:254–261.
13. Zink BJ. Traumatic brain injury outcome: concepts for emergency care. *Ann Emerg Med* 2001;37:318–332.
14. von Wild K, Terwey S. Diagnostic confusion in mild traumatic brain injury (MTBI). Lessons from clinical practice and EFNS—inquiry. European Federation of Neurological Societies. *Brain Inj* 2001;15:273–277.
15. Sumann G, Kampfl A, Wenzel V, Schobersberger W. Early intensive care unit intervention for trauma care: what alters the outcome? *Curr Opin Crit Care* 2002;8:587–592.
16. The Brain Trauma Foundation. The American Association of Neurological Surgeons. The Joint Section on Neurotrauma and Critical Care. Indications for intracranial pressure monitoring. *J Neurotrauma* 2000;17:479–491.
17. Bulger EM, Nathens AB, Rivara FP, Moore M, MacKenzie EJ, Jurkovich GJ. Management of severe head injury: institutional variations in care and effect on outcome. *Crit Care Med* 2002;30: 1870–1876.
18. Guidelines for the management of severe head injury. Brain Trauma Foundation, American Association of Neurological Surgeons, Joint Section on Neurotrauma and Critical Care. *J Neurotrauma* 1996;13:641–734.
19. Goodall P, Ghiloni CT. The changing face of publicly funded employment services. *J Head Trauma Rehabil* 2001;16:94–106.
20. Ylvisaker M, Todis B, Glang A, et al. Educating students with TBI: themes and recommendations. *J Head Trauma Rehabil* 2001;16: 76–93.
21. Povlishock JT, Katz DI. Update of neuropathology and neurological recovery after traumatic brain injury. *J Head Trauma Rehabil* 2005;20:76–94.
22. Katz DI, Alexander MP. Traumatic brain injury. Predicting course of recovery and outcome for patients admitted to rehabilitation. *Arch Neurol* 1994;51:661–670.
23. Haslam C, Batchelor J, Fearnside MR, Haslam SA, Hawkins S, Kenway E. Post-coma disturbance and post-traumatic amnesia

as nonlinear predictors of cognitive outcome following severe closed head injury: findings from the Westmead Head Injury Project. *Brain Inj* 1994;8:519–528.
24. Tate RL, Perdices M, Pfaff A, Jurjevic L. Predicting duration of posttraumatic amnesia (PTA) from early PTA measurements. *J Head Trauma Rehabil* 2001;16:525–542.
25. Zafonte RD, Mann NR, Millis SR, Black KL, Wood DL, Hammond F. Posttraumatic amnesia: its relation to functional outcome. *Arch Phys Med Rehabil* 1997;78:1103–1106.
26. Whyte J, Cifu D, Dikmen S, Temkin N. Prediction of functional outcomes after traumatic brain injury: a comparison of 2 measures of duration of unconsciousness. *Arch Phys Med Rehabil* 2001;82:1355–1359.
27. Katz DI, Otto RM, Agosti RM, MacKinnon DJ, Alexander MP. Factors affecting duration of posttraumatic amnesia after traumatic brain injury. *J Int Neuropsych Soc* 1999;5:139.
28. Hammond FM, Hart T, Bushnik T, Corrigan JD, Sasser H. Change and predictors of change in communication, cognition, and social function between 1 and 5 years after traumatic brain injury. *J Head Trauma Rehabil* 2004;19:314–328.
29. Millis SR, Rosenthal M, Novack TA, et al. Long-term neuropsychological outcome after traumatic brain injury. *J Head Trauma Rehabil* 2001;16:343–355.
30. Olver JH, Ponsford JL, Curran CA. Outcome following traumatic brain injury: a comparison between 2 and 5 years after injury. *Brain Inj* 1996;10:841–848.
31. Corrigan JD, Smith-Knapp K, Granger CV. Outcomes in the first 5 years after traumatic brain injury. *Arch Phys Med Rehabil* 1998;79:298–305.
32. Medical aspects of the persistent vegetative state (1). The Multi-Society Task Force on PVS. *N Engl J Med* 1994;330:1499–1508.
33. Giacino JT, Ashwal S, Childs N, et al. The minimally conscious state: definition and diagnostic criteria. *Neurology* 2002;58: 349–353.
34. Hagen C, Malkmus D, Durham P. Levels of cognitive functioning. Downey, CA: Ranchos Los Amigos Hospital, 1972.
35. Alexander MP. Traumatic brain injury. In: D.F. B, Blumer D, eds. *Psychiatric Aspects of Neurologic Disease.* New York: McGraw-Hill, 1982:251–278.
36. Katz DI. Neuropathology and neurobehavioral recovery from closed head injury. *J Head Trauma Rehabil* 1992;7:1–15.
37. Stuss DT, Buckle BA. Traumatic brain injury: neruopsychological deficits and evaluation at different stages of recovery and in different pathological subtypes. *J Head Trauma Rehabil* 1992; 7:40–49.
38. Ross BL, Temkin NR, Newell D, Dikmen SS. Neuropsychological outcome in relation to head injury severity. Contributions of coma length and focal abnormalities. *Am J Phys Med Rehabil* 1994;73:341–347.
39. van der Naalt J, Hew JM, van Zomeren AH, Sluiter WJ, Minderhoud JM. Computed tomography and magnetic resonance imaging in mild to moderate head injury: early and late imaging related to outcome. *Ann Neurol* 1999;46:70–78.
40. Levin HS, Williams DH, Eisenberg HM, High WM, Jr., Guinto FC, Jr. Serial MRI and neurobehavioural findings after mild to moderate closed head injury. *J Neurol Neurosurg Psychiatry* 1992;55:255–262.
41. Wilson JT, Hadley DM, Wiedmann KD, Teasdale GM. Neuropsychological consequences of two patterns of brain damage shown by MRI in survivors of severe head injury. *J Neurol Neurosurg Psychiatry* 1995;59:328–331.
42. Wallesch CW, Curio N, Galazky I, Jost S, Synowitz H. The neuropsychology of blunt head injury in the early postacute stage: effects of focal lesions and diffuse axonal injury. *J Neurotrauma* 2001;18:11–20.
43. Bigler ED. Quantitative magnetic resonance imaging in traumatic brain injury. *J Head Trauma Rehabil* 2001;16:117–134.
44. Wallesch CW, Curio N, Kutz S, Jost S, Bartels C, Synowitz H. Outcome after mild-to-moderate blunt head injury: effects of focal lesions and diffuse axonal injury. *Brain Inj* 2001;15:401–412.
45. Levin HS, Zhang L, Dennis M, et al. Psychosocial outcome of TBI in children with unilateral frontal lesions. *J Int Neuropsychol Soc* 2004;10:305–316.

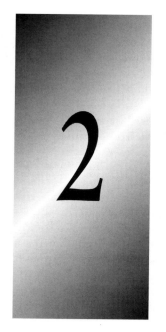

2

Brain Injury Rehabilitation: Past, Present, and Future?

George A. Zitnay

The ways that persons with disabilities have been viewed by society have changed significantly over the years, due mainly to economic, cultural, religious, and scientific influences. In most cultures, both in ancient and in earlier modern times, persons with a disability were negatively valued. Wolf Wolfensburger (1972) noted that historically persons with disability have been viewed as deviant. In ancient Greece and Rome, among Eskimos, and in Nazi Germany infanticide, abandonment, and extermination have been practiced on those perceived as deviant. Even in the United States, the U.S. Supreme Court upheld the states' right to sterilize persons with mental disability. Chief Justice Holmes declared "It is better for all the world, if instead of waiting to execute degenerate offspring for crime, or to let them starve for their imbecility, society can prevent those who are manifestly unfit from continuing their kind. [Three] generations of imbeciles are enough." *Buck v. Bell*, 274 U.S. 200 (1927).

Since earliest colonial times in America, persons with disabilities have been treated as offensive and frightening. Removal from society has been the way these individuals have been dealt with. During the Industrial Revolution, however, a degree of humanitarianism began to creep into the mainstream views of society as the incidence of occupational injuries increased. This was fueled by increasing public awareness about the issues of child labor, poor working conditions, and the large and growing number

of persons sustaining occupational injuries that left them with permanent disability. During World War I, the public concern over the large number of injured soldiers without means of support spurred on the creation of federal rehabilitation policies for military personnel.

Early pioneers in the emerging field of rehabilitation included Thomas Hopkins Galludet, who brought manual communication to Americans with speech and hearing impairments; Louis Braille, who developed a touch system for reading; Dorothea Dix, who championed the creation of asylums (mental hospitals) so that mentally ill persons would not be held in prisons; Edgar James Elms, who founded Goodwill Industries; Fred Albee, who provided rehabilitation services at his Reconstruction Hospital to return veterans with disabilities to useful civilian life; and many others such as Harvey Wilbur, Samuel Gridley Howe, and Jeremiah Milbank (1).

At the close of the nineteenth century, government responsibility to those with disabilities began to emerge. In 1910, the first workers compensation laws were passed because of industrial injuries; the National Defense Act of 1916 created the authority to assist soldiers in reentering civilian life by providing training in agriculture or mechanical arts (2). The Smith–Hughes Act of 1917 provided states with federal funds, to create vocational education programs, and the Soldiers Rehabilitation Act of 1918 authorized the development of vocational rehabilitation to veterans with disabilities. Two years later, the Act was extended to civilians (2). It was during these times that John Coulter, MD, established the first program in physical medicine at Northwestern University Medical School (1).

The next most significant public policy change occurred as a result of the Depression. With millions of Americans out of work, the Roosevelt Administration enacted the Social Security Act in 1935. The Act addressed the problems of unemployment, old age, poverty, and blindness. It also made vocational rehabilitation a permanent federal program (3).

World War II made a huge difference in the ways in which Americans perceived persons with disability, but also led to the formalization of physical medicine and rehabilitation as a medical specialty. Dr. Howard Kessler was a strong advocate of rehabilitation of veterans. He introduced the concept of a comprehensive medical-social-psychological-vocational approach to disability. It was during this time that Howard Rush, MD, a colonel in the U.S. Air Force, demonstrated the effectiveness of physical medicine with injured pilots. After World War II, when rehabilitation began to falter, Howard Kessler and Howard Rush persisted. The result was that the American Medical Association created a specialty board on physical medicine in 1944 (1).

The post-war expansion saw the growth of the federal government's role in rehabilitation. The Vocational Rehabilitation Amendments of 1954 forged a partnership between public and private organizations, including a federally assisted research program, and the training of professionals to staff public and private rehabilitation programs. The amendments authorized the construction of rehabilitation facilities. During this time, Mary Switzer served as the Federal Director of the Vocational Rehabilitation Department. She led the department until her retirement in 1970 (4).

During the 1960s and 1970s, there was a shift in focus from rehabilitation and disability program expansion to disability rights. Independent living, the concept of normalization, community-based rehabilitation, class action suits, and personal advocacy grew into a movement (5).

Looking back on the history of rehabilitation, we see the emergence of neurorehabilitation of persons with head injury. Howard Rush began providing neurorehabilitation to pilots injured in World War II, and he and Howard Kessler included psychosocial and psychological services as part of a comprehensive rehabilitation program. The early treatment of head injuries was also influenced by the discovery of new drugs. These psychopharmacological discoveries included lithium in 1949, chlorpromazine in 1952, the discovery of the antidepressant properties of iproniazid and imipramine in 1957 and the introduction of chlordiazepoxide in 1960. Neuropsychiatry began to show interest in patients with neurobehavioral problems following head injury. It wasn't until the 1970s, however, that what

is looked upon as the era of "head injury rehabilitation" began.

Many efforts emerged to address the needs of persons with disability. The Rehabilitation Act of 1973 (29 U.S.C. 780, et. seq.), which focused primarily on vocational rehabilitation, also established the National Council on Disability (NCD), an independent federal agency with 15 members appointed by the president and confirmed by the Senate. The NCD later to recommend to Congress that a civil rights law be enacted that was specific to persons with disability.

The Vietnam War made its mark on the history of disability rehabilitation as better medicine and the use of medevac helicopters resulted in soldiers surviving injuries they had not in earlier times.

One of the markers of the new era in brain injury rehabilitation was the development of the Glasgow Coma Scale and the Glasgow Outcome Scale by Graham Teasdale and Bryan Jennett (Lancet, 1974, 1975). This standardized method for assessing the severity of injury and predicting long-term outcomes following traumatic brain injury helped to make improvements in acute care and pushed brain injury rehabilitation to the forefront. Sheldon Berrol, Leonard Diller, and Yehuda Ben Yishay were pioneers in innovative rehabilitation, treatment, and organized research programs. This marked the beginning of patients being referred to specialized brain injury rehabilitation centers rather than being sent to nursing homes (6). According to Mitchell Rosenthal, this paradigm shift in care of persons with TBI occurred between 1975 and 1997. Soon, for-profit rehabilitation programs sprang up, and within five years (1980–1984) the number of TBI rehabilitation programs grew from approximately 10 to 500 (6). During this same time period the continuum of care expanded substantially to include day treatment, home programs, transitional living, residential care, behavior management, life care planning, vocational rehabilitation, independent living, coma stimulation programs, and support groups. Neuropsychological assessment, cognitive rehabilitation, computers, and other electronic devices for memory, attention, and organization were used in the treatment of many of the sequelae of TBI.

In April 1980, Marilyn and Martin Spivak hosted the first meeting of what was to become the National Head Injury Foundation (NHIF) at their home in Massachusetts. The purpose of the meeting was to discuss forming an organization to serve people who had survived TBI. During that year, a Board of Directors was selected and NHIF was incorporated as a not-for-profit organization. The founding goals have relevance even to this day. The goals of the NHIF were as follows:

- To stimulate public and professional awareness of the problem of head injury—the silent epidemic.

- To make the public aware of the nature and causes of head injury and the necessary steps that need to be taken to prevent them.
- To provide a central clearinghouse for information and resources for individuals with head injury and their families.
- To provide these individuals and their families with necessary information and support during and after crisis.
- To develop a support group network for both individuals with head injury and their families.
- To establish and promote specialized head injury rehabilitation programs.
- To help educate healthcare professionals about the unique needs of individuals with head injury.
- To advocate for increased research funding and more appropriate care for individuals with brain injury.

Later, in 1983 the goal of prevention was added.

It was during this time that the consumer movement in TBI really took hold. The establishment of NHIF chapters across the country helped to fuel this movement. The NHIF moved from Massachusetts to Washington, DC, to begin a new era of expansion. Soon the name was changed to the Brain Injury Association (BIA). While BIA was expanding into research and public policy, George A. Zitnay and Martin B. Foil, Jr., founded a new international organization in 1991. The International Brain Injury Association (IBIA) rapidly grew with the support of the World Health Organization (WHO). IBIA became a leader in multidisciplinary and interdisciplinary training and treatment with the establishment of the World Congress on Brain Injury, which has since been held in Denmark, Spain, Canada, Italy, and Sweden.

During the 1980s, with the increasing interest by professionals in brain injury rehabilitation, the American Congress of Rehabilitation Medicine created the Head Injury Interdisciplinary Special Interest Group (HI-ISIG). In the late 1980s two journals, *Brain Injury* and the *Journal of Head Trauma Rehabilitation,* began publishing, greatly expanding the scientific literature in TBI (6).

The 1980s were a tumultuous time for brain injury rehabilitation. In the early part of the decade, there was a huge increase in the development of for-profit rehabilitation programs aimed at attracting the families of persons with brain injury that had insurance, court settlements, or the ability to pay. Glossy brochures were published. Recruitment techniques included flying in whole families by private jet to visit programs. Facilities looked terrific. And executives were well paid. Some call this the "golden age." But others, particularly persons with brain injury, called it a time of shame.

In 1985, standards of care for brain injury rehabilitation were adopted by the Commission on Accreditation of Rehabilitation Facilities (CARF). These standards resulted from the work of the HI-ISIG. A milestone in brain injury rehabilitation was reached in 1987 when the U.S. Department of Education's National Institute on Disability and Rehabilitation Research funded five traumatic brain injury model systems of care (Thomas, 1988).

The 1980s can now be classified as a period of ups and downs, growth, investigation of fraud, decline, and then re-emergence as the decade closed with a period of downsizing, buyouts, closures, and finally settling into a period during which insurance companies questioned the value of rehabilitation and limited the amount and time for rehabilitation services. Emphasis was placed on home treatment, community-based rehabilitation, day services, independent living, and advocacy. By 2003, additional federal funding had expanded the program to include 16 participating sites throughout the United States.

In 1990, the Americans with Disabilities Act (ADA) was passed and signed into law by President George H. Bush. The Act proclaims that participation in the mainstream of daily life is the right of all Americans and calls for accommodation in housing and public spaces. The ADA was intended to foster independence and integration, affording persons with disability protection from antidiscrimination.

As important as the ADA was for antidiscrimination protection, however, it did not address many of the most pressing needs of persons with brain injury, such as assistance with access to appropriate care and rehabilitation. The ADA acknowledges that it is not so much the disability per se that makes life difficult for a person with a disability, but rather the way society responds to that disability. According to Justin Dart, the ADA seeks to change the status of people with disabilities by expecting a more enlightened attitude toward them. It rejects the long-standing and outmoded view of people with disabilities as being helpless and pitiful, and the primary role of the government as a charitable one—to take care of them through the provision of special programs and services. The ADA asserts that people with disabilities are full citizens who rightfully claim equal access and full participation, and that the role of government is to facilitate and support such claims (9).

The primary requirement of the ADA is the prohibition of discrimination. Antidiscrimination requirements for people with disabilities may be considered to have two central aspects: The first is that of not being treated in a prejudicial manner because of an individual, and often immutable, characteristic that has no bearing on the individual's skills or capabilities. The second requires paying particular attention to the individual's characteristics (e.g., race, sex, age or religion) to use the interaction between the individual and society to ameliorate or end the limitation or exclusion to equal access (10).

To focus greater attention on the wide spectrum of needs specific to persons with brain injury, BIA, under the direction of George A. Zitnay and with the help and support of Senator Edward Kennedy (D-MA), Senator Orrin Hatch (R-UT) and Congressman Jim Greenwood (R-PA), began work on writing the Traumatic Brain Injury (TBI) Act. Persons with brain injury provided leadership and input in the creation and passage of the TBI Act, including Sherrie Watson, Jean Ann McLaughlin, Maureen Campbell-Korves, Patsy Cannon, Gary Busey, and Marvel Vena. The TBI Act was signed into law by President Bill Clinton in 1996 (P.L. 104-166).

The TBI Act was the first federal law specifically for persons with brain injury. The law specifically established a federal grant program for states to create TBI Advisory Boards, conduct planning and assess the needs assessments of persons with TBI in order to improve access to services. The law directed the Centers of Disease Control and Prevention (CDC) to perform incidence and prevalence studies and establish educational and public awareness programs. The Act also required the National Institute of Child Health and Human Development of the federal National Institutes of Health to hold a consensus conference on the rehabilitation of persons with TBI. In 1998, an international panel of experts convened a conference, reaching a consensus that more research was needed on TBI rehabilitation.

The reauthorization of the TBI Act in 2000 (P.L. 106-310), included an expansion of the CDC's work with state registries to collect information that would help improve service delivery, expand incidence and prevalence studies to include persons of all ages as well as those in institutional settings and efforts to capture data on mild TBI. The new law also directed states to enhance "community-based service delivery systems that include timely access to comprehensive appropriate services and supports" as well as additional funding for the national Protection and Advocacy Systems to provide legal resources specifically for persons with TBI,

In 1999, the U.S. Supreme Court decision in *Olmstead* v. *L.C.* (527 U.S. 581), made a significant contribution to the movement toward community-based services. The court found that states are obligated under the ADA to provide appropriate settings for persons with disabilities in the "least restrictive environment." The court also found it to be discriminatory on the basis of disability for the state of Georgia to disallow the plaintiffs (persons with disabilities) to live in state-funded assisted living rather than the mental institution.

By the early part of the twenty-first century, various federal agencies were involved in brain injury research. The breadth of the federal government's commitment to furthering the science of TBI incidence and to improving rehabilitation increased. Federal efforts spanned from prevention through education under the CDC, to biomechanics research funded by the U.S. Department of Transportation, to battlefield studies and helmet studies by the U.S. Department of Defense, to 6 bench science research centers funded by the National Institute on Neurological Disorders and Stroke at NIH, to a Cooperative Multi Clinical Trials network of 8 sites funded by the National Center on Medical Rehabilitation Research at NIH, and 16 TBI Model Systems of Care funded by the U.S. Department of Education's National Institute on Disability Rehabilitation Research.

Finally, the late 1990s and early 2000s have come to be seen as a period of cost reduction, accountability, managed care, and the closing or merging of many programs in TBI rehabilitation. Length of stay, payment, and reimbursement have become real problems. While states have sought reimbursement solutions through waivers in the federal–state Medicaid program, the Medicare program—as the largest health insurer in the nation—has not kept up with medical advances and civil rights and expectations for recovery in its reimbursements to hospitals, nursing homes, and particularly specialized brain injury facilities.

The move toward empowering persons with disabilities has led to greater expectations for quality of life and consequently, greater efforts at finding innovative rehabilitation techniques and programs. This, combined with a better understanding of how the brain can heal, has helped shape the evolution of TBI rehabilitation.

Outcomes, evidence-based practice guidelines for management of acute care, penetrating head injury, and neurobehavioral sequelae of TBI have been developed by the Neurotrauma Foundation (NTF) and the National Brain Injury Research, Treatment, and Training Foundation (NBIRTT). This is in response to the need for accountability and improvement in quality of life. Currently an international group of rehabilitation specialists under the leadership of NBIRTT is working to create a new assessment tool to measure quality of life for persons with TBI. The QOLIBRI is currently being field-tested and will soon be available for widespread distribution.

To close this historical chapter, it is important to mention that research into new pharmacological agents, stem cells, and proteomics offer new hope for improving outcomes in rehabilitation.

What is the future of rehabilitation? Traditionally, rehabilitation has been a reactive rather than proactive profession. Rehabilitation education and similar activities have been based on past experience, often with little thought given to future needs. There is agreement in rehabilitation that several issues will profoundly affect the future. Those issues include changes in the nature of work in the United States; growing diversity in the workforce;

changes in the nature of disability; advances in rehabilitation and medical technology; and alterations in the nature of strategies of service delivery.

Constant changes in rehabilitation can be predicted with certainty. History suggests that rehabilitation practitioners, especially those working in brain injury, will continue to face budget cutbacks, resulting in staffing shortages, growing caseloads and changes in the structure and function of the rehabilitation system. To respond, the field must become proactive. This will involve networking with other rehabilitation professionals, facilities, agencies and consumers. There is and will continue to be a need to deliver efficient and effective rehabilitation services that can be measured and evaluated. Finally, we must continue to provide for continuous learning and education of professionals, consumers and policy makers." (14)

References

1. Dean, Russell. *New Life for Millions*, New York, 1972.
2. Obermann, C. Esco. *A History of Vocational Rehabilitation in America*, Minneapolis, 1967.
3. Hughes, Jonathan. *The Vital Few*, New York, 1986.
4. Rusalem, H. and Malikin, D. *Contemporary Vocational Rehabilitation*, New York, 1976.
5. Owens, Mary Jane. Consumer perspectives on the preparation of rehabilitation professionals. *J Vocational Rehabil*, 2 (1992): 4–11
6. Rosenthal, Mitchell, 1995 Sheldon Berrol, MD, Senior Lectureship in *Journal of Head Trauma Rehabilitation*, 1996; 11 (4): 88–95.
7. Spivak, M. A perspective of National Head Injury Foundation (NHIF) from 1980–1990. *TBI Challenge*, vol. 4, number 1, 2000.
8. Zitnay, G.A. *Encyclopedia of Disability and Rehabilitation*, New York, 1995.
9. Dart, Justin. ADA landmark declaration of equality." *Worklife: A Special Issue*, ed. Dick Dietl, Washington, DC, 1990.
10. Burgdorf, Robert L. History, in *The Americans with Disabilities Act: A Practical and Legal Guide to Impact Enforcement and Compliance*, Washington, DC, 1990.
11. Bérubé, Jean. A good first step towards assistance for persons with traumatic brain injury: The Traumatic Brain Injury Act of 1996, *J Head Trauma Rehabil*, 1997.
12. Bérubé, Jean. The TBI Act Amendments of 2000, *J Head Trauma Rehabil*, 2001.
13. *Olmstead* v. *L.C.* 527 U.S. 581 (1999).
14. Ward, Michael J., and Halloran, William D. Transition issues for the 1900s, *OSERS News in Print*, 1993.

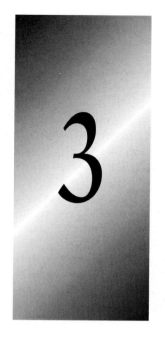

3 International Perspectives on TBI Rehabilitation

Zeev Groswasser
Ofer Keren

INTRODUCTION

Craniocerebral trauma has been linked historically with assault and war. Treatment of craniocerebral injuries by trephination was first described in the Edwin Smith surgical papyrus and by Hippocratic physicians. Some patients actually survived the trauma of the trephination, but most died. Over the years, the concept of cerebral compression by hemorrhage, originally described by Arabian physicians, gained recognition and eventually led to recognition of the need for decompression. Cushing (1) used meticulous debridement of penetrating brain injuries, which reduced mortality by 50 percent and resulted in a normal life expectancy for survivors. The introduction of antimicrobial and antibiotic agents, and the recognition that rapid intervention by trained neurosurgeons immensely decreased mortality from penetrating craniocerebral trauma, have both resulted in higher survival rates for patients.

Changes in lifestyle during the last century, especially the introduction of automobiles, became a major source for craniocerebral trauma. In motor vehicle accidents (MVA), brain injury is the cause of death in over 70 percent of fatal cases (2).

THE MODERN ERA OF TBI REHABILITATION

Interest in traumatic brain injury (TBI) has risen greatly since World War II. The number of publications devoted to what was then called "craniocerebral trauma" saw a threefold increase in the years 1956–1966 (3) and the topic has attracted increasing attention in national and international neurology and neurological surgery conferences. In the United States, the National Institute of Neurological Diseases and Blindness first designated craniocerebral trauma as a major topic of interest in October 1964. This paved the way for one of the first comprehensive conferences for the study of craniocerebral trauma that took place at the University of Chicago in 1966. The planning committee of that conference, chaired by Dr. Caveness, included neurosurgeons, neurologists, physiologists, and engineers, but no psychologists or physicians working in rehabilitation.

The translation from Russian into English of the works of A.K. Luria, *Human Brain and Psychological Processes* published in 1966 (4) and *The Working Brain*, first published in 1973, (5) led to rapid development of the field of neuropsychology, which plays a key role in the assessment and treatment of TBI patients today. In the last 20 years, TBI has become the accepted term for traumatic brain damage, and terms such as "craniocerebral trauma," used above, have disappeared altogether from the recent literature.

In the last 150 years, the structure/function relationship has provided one of the most intriguing research topics in the neurosciences. The localistic theories that emerged from the early studies of Broca and Wernicke in the nineteenth century were replaced in the 1930s by the holistic theory. Brain function and organization remained at center of interest, and in recent years current theories stress the dynamic aspects of brain function at the expense of the localistic or holistic approaches. The crucial role of the prefrontal cortex in human behavior has since gained increased recognition in modern neuropsychology. Historical illustrative case reports such as the case of Phineas Gage (first described in 1842) have became common knowledge (6).

Digital diagnostic brain imaging techniques introduced in the early 1970s in the form of computed tomography (CT), followed by magnetic resonance imaging (MRI), and in recent years by fMRI, PET, and SPECT have further promoted interest and research in the structure/function relationship following brain damage.

Tools developed in the field of neuropsychology have enabled a better assessment of cognitive deficits following TBI, which in turn has promoted various intervention processes designed to remedy the patients' cognitive deficits. It has become clear that the recovery processes may take longer than initially thought.

The drive to rehabilitate war veterans, probably driven by the feelings of guilt held by societies, exerted a profound effect on the rehabilitation of TBI patients. The basics of TBI rehabilitation were laid down in post–World War I Germany by K. Goldstein, who designed a center that included—in addition to the hospital—a psychology laboratory, a school, and later a vocational rehabilitation center, all for the purpose of providing comprehensive treatment (7). Goldstein evidently regarded the assessment of residual work potential and the prediction of vocational outcome as parts of the rehabilitation process (7). This type of rehabilitation approach was abolished altogether in 1933 after the Nazi takeover, especially because most of the leading physicians in these centers were Jewish. Goldstein himself left for the United States but did not pursue this line of work, described in his book *After-Effects of Brain Injuries in War*, which was published in 1942 (7). On the one hand, the state of rehabilitation in the United States at that time, and on the other hand the fact that Goldstein's main interest was aphasia and related disorders, created an atmosphere that hindered further progress along the original lines traced by Goldstein. It is noteworthy that the role of memory and attentional deficits as key sequelae influencing outcome following TBI became evident in the years after World War II.

It took almost 40 years for similar ideas regarding TBI rehabilitation to emerge, again because of war. The "Six-Day War" in 1967 and more so the "Yom Kippur War" in 1973 created the need and played the decisive role in the establishment, in December 1973, of the special medical unit devoted to TBI rehabilitation at the Loewenstein Rehabilitation Hospital (LRH) in Israel (8). TBI patients had been treated at LRH since the early

1960s. But it is worth noting that many of these patients were at that time still referred to mental hospitals because of severe behavioral deficits that may have dominated their condition.

The comprehensive model of treatment developed at LRH can be described as "Coma to Community" (Figure 3-1). It is a model of treatment that can be adopted easily by other countries. As a small country, Israel enjoys certain advantages in this respect because one center, located at the geographical center of the country, can serve the entire population. Patients with TBI had been admitted to LRH since the early 1960s, so it was a natural choice as the national center for TBI rehabilitation after the Yom Kippur War. After the war, patients with severe TBI from the civilian population, as well as victims of motor vehicle accidents (MVA) and work accidents, were referred almost exclusively to LRH. TBI patients in Israel have almost universal access to in-patient rehabilitation services. Victims of road accidents are almost always insured, while work accidents and other minor causes of TBI are covered by

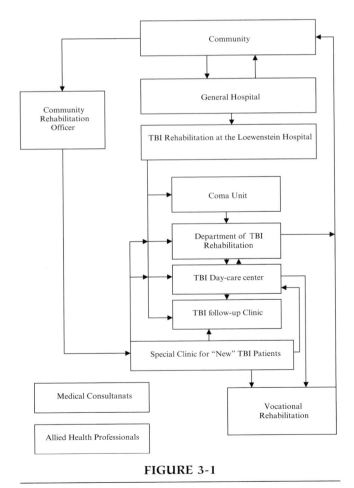

FIGURE 3-1

The LRH comprehensive "Coma to Community" TBI rehabilitation service the "sick funds." The establishment of a large rehabilitation center that serves almost all severe TBI patients in Israel has enabled the creation of a critical mass of knowledge regarding treatment and outcome, which was of utmost importance in the early years of modern TBI rehabilitation, before the existence of specialty conferences and journals devoted to this subject.

The LRH "Coma to Community" system provides inpatient rehabilitation facilities for about 220 severe TBI patients a year. The fact that patients are treated in a rehabilitation setting from an early stage has a beneficial effect on outcome (9–11). The out-patient program at LRH ensures continuity of care and prevents misunderstandings that often happen when patients change their place of treatment. The LRH experience suggests that large regional rehabilitation centers for TBI rehabilitation can provide a continuum of care that meets the changing needs of patients and is effective for both patients and healthcare providers. This model helps contain cost while building and maintaining trust with patients and healthcare providers alike.

Conferences

In the early 1970s, increasing interest in TBI rehabilitation encouraged an international exchange of ideas on this topic, especially because few books or journals were devoted to the subject at that time. The Glasgow Coma Scale (GCS), first published in 1974 by Teasdale and Jennett, exerted a strong influence on research of the effects following TBI by providing a reliable score that could be used to judge the initial severity of injury (12). This made it possible to recruit large numbers of patients for outcome studies, sometimes from several centers, and to compare various methods of treatment (13–15).

Several meetings on TBI research had been organized in the 1960s in the United States, but the first meeting in Europe regarding TBI rehabilitation was organized by Prof. Ö. Höök in Oslo in 1974. Some conferences became annual meetings such as the Williamsburg Annual Meeting and the Braintree Annual Traumatic Head injury Conference. The IX World Congress of Rehabilitation International took place in Israel in 1976. As a result of the involvement of the Loewenstein Rehabilitation Hospital staff, the local scientific committee included in the program a workshop on patients with brain injury. Since then, TBI rehabilitation has become a regular part of most, if not all, international conferences in rehabilitation medicine.

The foundation by Henry H. Stonnington of the International Association for the Study of Traumatic Brain Injury (IASTBI) spearheaded both research and collegial interchange among the international brain injury community. Subsequently, George Zitnay founded the International Brain Injury Association (IBIA). Due to the efforts of Nathan Zasler, Henry Stonnington, and

George Zitnay, these two organizations eventually merged, initially with IBIA becoming the scientific arm of IBIA. Over time, the IASTBI was simply folded into the IBIA organization, and its members were fully integrated within the latter organization. The IBIA continues to sponsor and plan a biannual international conference devoted to TBI. At these international meetings, experts as well as newcomers to the field meet each other, exchange formal and informal information, and help in the dissemination of information for the benefit of patients with TBI. In countries like the United States, it is not uncommon to have state TBI conferences performing similar functions, but on a smaller, local scale.

Journals

Research regarding TBI developed along two main lines. The first and more established line dealt with the acute phase. This was pursued primarily by neurosurgeons caring for patients in the early phase. These researchers already had established journals where they could publish their findings. Long-term care, which developed rapidly after the 1970s, posed different questions and research problems. Some peer reviewers described these problems as being of "limited interest," as described in editorial letters rejecting research findings and manuscripts regarding late sequelae of TBI. This situation led to the creation of special-interest groups such as IASTBI and IBIA, and also to the foundation of journals devoted entirely to TBI studies, such as *Brain Injury* and *The Journal of Head Trauma Rehabilitation*.

Recognition that the number of TBI patients in the community was growing and that rehabilitation techniques could improve a patient's condition beyond the course of natural recovery, helped to get data regarding TBI published in more general journals in medicine and neurology. In the Editorial of the first issue of *Brain Injury*, in 1987, McKinlay and Pentland wrote: "It is a commonplace that 15 or 20 years ago there was little interest in head injury, and only a small literature addressing the acute and long-term problems it presents. Nowadays there is an extensive literature ranging through epidemiology, pathophysiology, acute management, and rehabilitation, and *Brain Injury* is an expression of that greatly increased interest" (16). Other journals that take an interest in TBI, to mention but a few, are the *Journal of Neurotrauma*, *NeuroRehabilitation*, *Neurorehabilitation & Neural Repair*, and *Neuropsychological Rehabilitation*. The number of citations relevant to traumatic brain injury between the years 1988 and 1998 was 2563 (17).

Organizations

The increased interest in TBI, the growing number of people working in the field, and the belief that patients with

TBI present problems that are not well understood or treated by the general medical community, have created a genuine need for a "meeting place" for those involved in clinical care of these individuals. Professionals from various countries were involved in the foundation of IASTBI in the mid-1980s. As previously noted, an important role was played by the staff of the Department of Physical Medicine and Rehabilitation, Medical College of Virginia Hospital, Virginia Commonwealth University, from Richmond VA, headed by Henry H. Stonnington, who acted as the first chairperson of IASTBI and was also the first Editor-in-Chief of *Brain Injury* from 1987 to 2000. Subsequently, Jeffrey Kreutzer and Nathan Zasler were named co-editors of this journal.

TBI Support Groups

The Rationale for Support Groups for Post-TBI Patients
The growing interest in TBI in the medical community, the increased number of patients surviving the acute phase, and the understanding that severe TBI patients need treatment and support far beyond the first few months post-injury, have created a need for information resources. McMordie et al. found that many patients and their families indicated that inadequate information was provided regarding important consequences of TBI such as aftercare, referral resources, and prognosis (18). Areas of greatest informational deficit included post-hospitalization resources and expectations for outcome. Clergy proved to be by far more helpful in these respects to both patients and families than physiatrists (18).

Starting in the late 1970s and continuing into the early 1980s, the lack of resources for useful information such as books and journals, and the inadequate answers provided by the medical community, led to the foundation of support groups (SG) of patients for persons with TBI, as well as their families. These support groups were started initially by professionals treating such patients and by families of persons with TBI. The goals of such groups were to increase public awareness of the long-term impact of TBI on patients and their families, to stimulate the development of supportive services in the community, and to supply information regarding TBI (19). Peer support has been shown to be a promising approach to enhancing the coping skills of individual TBI patients and their families (20). Moreover, the impact of the cultural gap and feelings of stigma and social isolation have been shown to be universally experienced by TBI patients (21). Attentiveness, friendliness, and guidance on the part of the rehabilitation staff have been shown to have a significant positive impact on the well-being of TBI patients. Family conflicts have commonly deprived patients of familial support (21). A study of Hispanic TBI survivors demonstrated the importance of linguistic and ethnic factors in the implementation of support groups (22).

In many instances, regardless of the severity of TBI, the lives of the injured and their families are changed forever. These changes can produce a "catastrophic reaction." (11) The impact is often devastating both emotionally and financially. Support groups can be helpful by providing useful information that in many instances may otherwise be gained only by personal experience. This is one reason that individuals trust SGs. Information about the long-term effects of the injury, about available facilities, services, and programs specializing in patients with TBI are shared by these groups. This in turn has led to the establishment of national societies. The SGs are a social reference group, exerting a positive impact on the self-esteem of both TBI patients and their caregivers. The national groups, first in the United States and then in other countries (especially in Western countries), have been able to promote changes that acknowledge the long-term medical and social needs of this special patient population.

The sociopolitical atmosphere following the Vietnam War and the growing awareness regarding both individual and patient rights laid the groundwork for the necessary changes, especially because wounded war veterans and patients with TBI were generally young and had almost normal life expectancies. Understanding that these victims needed care for life helped to promote public awareness of their needs. The fact that most patients with severe TBI had some financial support from insurance companies attracted various organizations (both for and not for profit) to start TBI rehabilitation programs, which resulted in greater availability of such programs in the United States. Almost 700 such programs existed at one time in this country. But in light of the comprehensive "Coma to Community" treatment model set at LRH in Israel, it soon became clear that many of these programs were not able to bring together the critical mass of knowledge and experience needed to provide the long-term (at times life-long) integrative therapeutic milieu needed by TBI patients, and many of these programs survived for only relatively short periods of time.

With the development of electronic means of communication, opportunities for sharing and disseminating information have increased dramatically. Numerous websites can be found today that are operated by TBI SGs, and others contain a variety of sources of information regarding various aspects of TBI. Today, the Internet plays a key role in distributing information. Entering "TBI" in any search engine returns a large number of these sites. SGs are highly developed in the United States, Canada, and the United Kingdom

Support groups quickly understood the lack of public awareness regarding the long-term impact of acquired TBI on individuals, their families, and the community as a whole. This led to consolidation of local SGs into national organizations that are able to exert greater political influence on legislation, healthcare providers such as HMOs, and the insurance industry.

Structure of Brain Injury Support Groups Support groups can be nonprofit or for-profit organizations. Large state or national SGs often consist of local SGs. A TBI SG can be organized in different ways, depending on the objectives and composition of its board of directors. Directors may be appointed by the families, by healthcare providers (such as rehabilitation centers and organizations), or by interested parties such as attorneys' offices. In many cases, SGs are composed of all these various sources.

A successful model seems to be one in which all three elements combine into a well-coordinated group in which professionals in TBI rehabilitation (occupational, physical, therapeutic recreational, and speech therapists; vocational counselors; physicians; nurses; and family therapists) take an active role. The activities of individual SGs differ, but they all provide information about post-hospitalization community resources for further individual and family treatment and about vocational and recreational opportunities. Some of these groups have extended their goals and are involved in programs aimed at the prevention of TBI, reducing its overall incidence. TBI survivors are involved in many educational activities of the SGs, in many instances as part of their own rehabilitation program.

Long-term care for caregivers Long-term cognitive and especially behavioral changes affect not only the lives of TBI patients but also the lives of those living close to them, most notably that of the caregivers (23). Studies have shown that in many cases anxiety and dissatisfaction at five years post-injury are far more severe than at about three months or one year (24–26). With time, caregivers may need more support than in the early phase, which is often disregarded or neglected by the health providers who focus mainly on treating the patient. TBI programs, however, need to assign a professional staff to provide empathetic and functional help to the patient's caregivers (27). Because this type of intervention can be done for relatively short periods of time, voluntary organizations such as TBI SGs play a key role in providing this service in the later stages of treatment.

Some SGs provide newsletters treating such important subjects as social cognition, learning, and role-modeling processes. Others provide hotlines such as the Head Injury Hotline, which is a nonprofit clearinghouse that was founded by and has been operated by head injury activists since 1985, (28) with a team of consultants that includes individuals with TBI, family members, learning specialists, nurses, paraprofessionals, lawyers, neuropsychologists, and physicians specializing in emergency medicine and neurology. They offer consultations, research assistance, case management services, legal services, and in-service training. Their clientele consists of individuals with brain injuries and their families, U.S. government officials, agency heads, educators, medical and legal professionals,

and social workers. The activities of these groups include multiple and various aspects of TBI and are open to anyone interested.

Some SGs were organized by academic institutions such as Radford University's Waldron College in southwest Virginia, enabling students to take an active role in some of the programs (29). Some SGs have established Clubhouses for survivors of TBI to serve as a bridge between the past and a healing future. For example, the nonprofit program operated by the Long Island Head Injury Association, Inc. (30) provides a place for survivors to participate in meaningful work, and an opportunity to meet and build friendships and ultimately seek gainful employment within the community. Another example is the Jodi House, aimed at providing opportunities for each person to discover new paths to regain autonomy and purposefulness within their community (31).

Virtual support has also been developing in the last years. Examples of such activity can be found at the website of the TBI chat room (www.tbichat.org) which had an impressive increase of its use from 135,552 visits in 1998 to 554,244 in 2002. Such SGs help those who would enjoy attending SG meetings but are unable to do so because of problems of transportation or distance. A TBI survivor can contact the chat page 24 hours a day, participate in the general chat room, or enter one of several specialized chat rooms such as TBI in children. A chat room has been designed for children with TBI who are under age 17 years, as well as, their care providers and family members (32).

Today the Internet plays a key role in distributing information about resources regarding TBI rehabilitation. SGs have developed as a result of the understanding that patients and their caregivers require prolonged care, beyond what the health care systems and insurance can provide because of financial and knowledge barriers. Unfortunately, these groups are well developed and active only in countries in which rehabilitation medicine has become part and parcel of the routine medical service. It is hoped that other countries will soon recognize the special needs of TBI patients and provide for them. SGs can be instructive in bringing about this much needed change.

CONCLUDING REMARKS

The understanding and treatment of patients with traumatic brain injury has changed greatly in the last 35 years. As more patients survive the very acute phase and are referred to rehabilitation, the demand for rehabilitation services has been on the rise. Furthermore, recognition that these patients may need treatment and support for the rest of their lives increases the demand for rehabilitation services all over the world. Rational use of resources is a must, and the rapid dissemination of "how-to-do" information can promote the creation and improvement of TBI rehabilitation services for these individuals and their families, as well as society at large.

The established SGs and the national and international societies devoted to research and treatment of TBI, mostly active in Western countries, should become a source of inspiration for expanding services to these patients elsewhere in the world. Rehabilitation medicine is still one of the branches of medicine to which only a fraction of the people who need it have access. TBI rehabilitation, being more complex and expensive due to the large team needed for comprehensive treatment explains why in many countries these services are in their infancy. Today "how-to" data is becoming increasingly available, but communities and countries have to consider a different allocation of resources to properly implement TBI rehabilitation programs including prevention. Established TBI rehabilitation services are also under considerable financial pressure, which can promote research into more cost-effective prevention as well as treatment solutions. International cooperation in research will be essential in the coming years to achieve an evidence-based foundation for the practice of TBI rehabilitation. Ultimately our goal should be to provide cost-effective treatment that improves outcome, as well as, quality of life.

References

1. Cushing H. A study of a series of wounds involving the brain and its enveloping structures. *Br J Surgery* 5:558–684, 1918.
2. Walker AE. Introduction. In: *Head Injury*, Conference proceedings. Caveness WF, & Walker AE, (Eds.) Lippincott, Philadelphia, 1966, pp.13–26.
3. Caveness WF. Preface. In: *Head Injury*, Conference proceedings. Caveness WF, & Walker AE, (Eds.) Lippincott, Philadelphia, 1966.
4. Luria, AR. *Human Brain and Psychological Processes.* Harper & Row, New York, 1966.
5. Luria, AR. *The Working Brain.* Penguin, Harmondsworth, 1973.
6. Damasio H, Grabowski T, Frank R, Galaburda AM, Damamsio AR. The return of Phineas Gage: clues about the brain from the skull of a famous patient. *Science* 264:1102-1105, 1994.
7. Goldstein K. *After-effects of Brain Injuries in War.* Grune & Stratton, New York, 1942.
8. Boake C. History of cognitive rehabilitation following head injury. In: *Cognitive Rehabilitation for Persons with Traumatic Brain Injury,* Kreutzer JS & Wehman PH (eds.) Paul H. Brookes, Baltimore, MD, 1991 pp. 3–12.
9. Cope N, Hall KM. Head injury rehabilitation: benefits of early intervention. Archives of Physical Medicine and Rehabilitation, 63:433–437, 1982.
10. Mackay LE, Bernstein BA, Chapman PE, Morgan AS, Milazzo LS. Early intervention in severe head injury: long-term benefits of a formalized program. *Arch Phys Med Rehabil*, 73:635–641, 1992.
11. Groswasser, Z., Stern, J.M. A psychodynamic model of behavior after acute central nervous system damage. *J Head Trauma Rehabil* 13:69–79, 1998.
12. Teasdale G, Jennett B. Assessment of coma and impaired consciousness. Lancet, II:526–539, 1974.
13. Braakman R. Data bank of head injuries in three countries. Scottish Medical Journal, 23:107–108.
14. Jennett B, Teasdale G, Frey J, Braakman R, Heiden J. The efficacy of different therapies for severe head injuries. *Acta Neurochirurgica Suppl (Wien)* 28:210–212, 1979.
15. Jennett B, Teasdale G, Fry J Braakman R, Minderhoud J, Heiden J, Kurze T. Treatment for severe head injury. *J Neurol Neurosurg Psych,* 43:289–295, 1980.
16. McKinlay WW, Pentland B. Editorial: Developing rehabilitation services for the head injured: A UK perspective. *Brain Injury* 1:3–4, 1987.
17. Gordner, Ronald L., Tuel, Stephen M., compilers. Rehabilitation of persons with traumatic brain injury [bibliography online]. Bethesda (MD): National Library of Medicine; 1998 Sep. (Current bibliographies in medicine; no. 98-1). 2563 citations from January 1988 through August 1998, plus selected earlier citations. Available from: URL http://www.nlm.nih.gov/pubs/resources.html
18. McMordie WR, Rogers KF, Barker SL. Consumer satisfaction with services provided to head-injured patients and their families. *Brain Injury* 5:43–51, 1991.
19. http://abigroup.homestead.com.
20. Hibbard MR, Cantor J, Charatz H, Rosenthal R, Ashman T, Gundersen N, Ireland-Knight L, Gordon W, Avner J, Gartner A. Peer support in the community: initial findings of a mentoring program for individuals with traumatic brain injury and their families. *J Head Trauma Rehabil* 17:112–31, 2002.
21. Simpson G, Mohr R, Redman A. Cultural variations in the understanding of traumatic brain injury and brain injury rehabilitation. *Brain Injury* 14:125–140, 2000.
22. Armengol CG. A multimodal support group with Hispanic traumatic brain injury survivors. *J Head Trauma Rehabil* 14: 233–246, 1999.
23. Brooks DN, McKinlay W. Personality and behavioral change after severe blunt head injury—a relative's view. *J Neurol Neurosurg Psych* 46:336–44, 1983.
24. Brooks N, Campsie L, Symington C, Beattie A, McKinlay W. The five-year outcome of severe blunt head injury: A relative's view. *J Neurol Neurosurg Psych* 49:764–70, 1985.
25. Livingstone MG, Brooks DN, Bond M. Three months after severe head injury: psychiatric and social impact on relatives. *J Neurol Neurosurg Psych* 48:870–5, 1985.
26. Livingstone MG, Brooks DN, Bond M. Patient outcome in the year following severe head injury and relative's psychiatric and social functioning. *J Neurology, Neurosurg Psych* 48:876–81, 1985.).
27. Brodaty H, Green A. Who cares for the carer? The often forgotten patient. *Australian Family Physician* 3:833–836, 2002.
28. http://www.headinjury.com/aboutus.htm
29. http://www.radford.edu/NewsPub/February2002/0219support.html
30. http://lihia.org/CLUB.HTM
31. http://www.jodihouse.org/mission.htm
32. http://tbichat.org/index.html

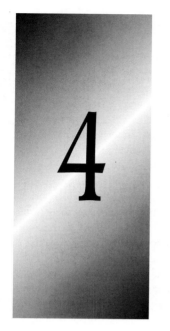

4 Training and Certification of Care Providers for Persons Sustaining TBI

Margaret A. Turk
Joanne Scandale

BACKGROUND

An increasing number of individuals have survived traumatic brain injury (TBI) as a result of advances in medical technology, emergency medical procedures, and neurosurgical techniques (1–3). An estimated 5.3 million Americans currently live with disabilities resulting from brain injury. This means that over 2 percent of the American population is living with disabilities caused by TBI (4). Estimates indicate that one million people are treated for head injuries and released from hospitals across the country each year, resulting in 80,000 people experiencing long-term disabilities. TBI is one of the most common childhood injuries (5).

TBI can significantly affect many physical, cognitive, and psychological processes, significantly disrupting the lives of individuals who experience such injuries. Survivors and their families require varying degrees of support along a continuum of disability. Early needs are usually met within the emergency department and/or acute care hospitalization, followed by acute rehabilitation. Medical and health professionals are the primary providers of service, interacting daily with patient and their families. Rehabilitation services are multidisciplinary, and the goals of care and service are restorative. Specialized programs and providers are sought to deliver quality care. Subacute and longer-term post-acute care needs may be very high, and may not always require health professionals. The services often are provided by different agencies and multiple health professionals, making coordination and continuity of services difficult. Post-acute care often focuses on behavioral plans, daily structure, and developing creative typical tasks. Support aides require communication skills and at least a knowledge base of behavior modification. With an increasing numbers of survivors, there is a greater need for trained and experienced providers for the acute through post-acute continuum.

Families are usually unprepared for their family member's injury, hospital course, and long-term rehabilitation. Changes in the family member are difficult to understand and difficult to deal with, despite educational efforts through rehabilitation programs. Often, these changes have a negative impact on families who then often become the primary caregivers after discharge from the hospital or acute rehabilitation programs (6, 7). Family caregivers of persons with brain injuries report high levels of depression and difficulties coping with the sequelae of brain injury (8–10). Family members are particularly challenged by the altered personalities and behavior changes exhibited by their loved ones (11).

Families may have to adjust their employment and social schedules in order to provide the level of care necessary for their family member with TBI. This may lead to feelings of social isolation, financial burden, and increased levels of stress. Employers, friends, and even family members may not believe that the individual has sustained a disability, thereby undermining the support necessary to assist him or her in adapting to life with a disability (2). Return to work and other previously held social roles might not be possible following injury, contributing to further disruption and stress within the family. Osberg and colleagues (12) suggest that with the necessary systems of support, family members can avoid some of the psychosocial problems that arise from caring for a family member with TBI.

Clinical practice, programs, and research in traumatic brain injury medicine have grown significantly over the past 35 years. Persons with TBI and their families, however, have reported the service system is "unorganized, uneducated, unresponsive, and uncaring." (13) A parent of a child with brain injury writes, "Another area of concern is the insufficient numbers of caregivers with training in ways brain injury differs from other neurologically impairing conditions. . . . Until caregivers better understand the cognitive and behavioral changes and learn more effective methods of dealing with deficits resulting form injury to the brain, we'll still be where we are today" (14). On a national and more general level, the Institute of Medicine (IOM) report, "To Err Is Human: Building a Safer Health System," notes the importance of communication among multiple providers and the need for standards for training and certification especially regarding safety and prevention of medical errors. At present, however, there exists no formal training or certification for medical health care providers within the field of brain injury medicine. Only recently has there been certification of brain injury care providers, those providing post-acute care within the community.

This chapter will review the state of the field regarding accreditation for programs, as well as training and certification of health care professionals and paraprofessionals providing front-line care and support in the community.

PROGRAM REVIEW AND ACCREDITATION

An initial attempt at standardizing rehabilitation care and assuring quality care was program evaluation and accreditation through the Commission on Accreditation of Rehabilitation Facilities (CARF). CARF was established in 1966 to ensure quality services for persons with disabilities and others receiving rehabilitation services. Improved safety, value, and quality of care of persons receiving services are a part of their mission. It is an international nonprofit accrediting body that accredits providers for specific services (e.g. behavioral health, employment and community services, medical rehabilitation). CARF standards are developed through leadership panels, advisory committees, focus groups, and field reviews. Persons served are also involved in the development of CARF standards.

The standards for brain injury programs were first offered in 1985, focusing on inpatient rehabilitation programs. Outpatient programs standards for accreditation were obtainable in 1988. Presently, there are standards for a variety of brain injury program services, beginning with inpatient rehabilitation at multiple levels and transitioning to residential and /or vocational services. CARF accredited programs serving persons who have sustained brain injury include over 100 inpatient rehabilitation programs, about 140 outpatient programs, more than 300 residential programs, almost 50 community services programs, and more than 70 vocational programs. Standards cover adult programs and programs for children and youth.

CARF has been responsive to the changing service needs over the last 25 years. As new services developed in the field, the Board of Directors has supported development of new standards. Standards are reviewed and updated on a routine basis. Program standards specifically for brain injury programs have provided some semblance of consistency for certain program elements, and are an initial step in assuring high quality care for persons who have sustained brain injuries.

MEDICAL AND HEALTH PROFESSIONAL CARE PROVIDERS

Brain injury rehabilitation has been provided for over 35 years in the United States, initially as a part of a larger rehabilitation program, and, increasingly since about the 1980's, as dedicated programs. Service provision has moved beyond hospitals and clinics, and into residences and communities. Advancements of medical science and vast improvements in medical and surgical care have presaged the growth of knowledge and practice. Patients often require the services of an interdisciplinary treatment team consisting of physicians, physical therapists, occupational therapists, speech language pathologists, rehabilitation counselors, psychologists, and social workers among other professional and paraprofessional staff. Interdisciplinary rehabilitation team members are typically guided by a set of standards of ethical practice for their particular professions (15). Physicians and health care professionals have risen to the challenge to provide high quality care, although subspecialization within disciplines has been acknowledged by acclamation and not certification.

Health professionals require standard training and licensure. Requirements of education and training regarding traumatic brain injury within each discipline now exist, although implementation may be uneven. Health professionals often gain experience by sharing information through team interactions, mentorship, or courses. Training and licensure for professionals does not require specialization in the care of persons who have sustained brain injury. There are no certification programs for specialization in the care of persons with brain injuries. Most disciplines do not have certification, but rather special interest groups in professional organizations (e.g. speech and language pathology). And where there may be special certification or plans for certification (e.g. physical therapy, psychology, occupational therapy), it is not specific to brain injury medicine or rehabilitation, but to a more general rehabilitation or components of a TBI service need.

The need for training and certification has been recognized increasingly nationally and internationally (16–19). The need to protect the public has been highlighted through the IOM report. The American Board of Medical Specialties (ABMS) has acknowledged this responsibility, and subsequently enacted implementation requirements of each member Board. These require programs of Maintenance of Certification within all represented specialties, and that subspecialty certification be reviewed through a vetted process.

There is a trend to formalize physician training in the management of persons who sustain brain injury. Physical Medicine & Rehabilitation (PM&R) residency programs developed formal training in Brain Injury Medicine during the 1980s and 1990s. A questionnaire survey report of PM&R residents and program directors conducted in 1991 concluded that two-thirds of programs either offer a formal rotation or require residents to participate in a clinical rotation in brain injury medicine (20). The findings of this and other surveys supported a need for more training in brain injury medicine for residents, including additional training sites across the continuum of care (19, 20). Bell and Massagli (19) reported that PM&R residents endorsed the position that a rotation in a skilled nursing unit providing services for individuals with brain injury offered unique clinical experiences. Currently, all PM&R residents must have formal training and competency in brain injury medicine, which is mandated through the Accreditation Council on Graduate Medical Education (ACGME) program requirements. Basic requirements for certification in PM&R include successful completion of an ACGME approved residency in addition to passing written and oral American Board of Physical Medicine & Rehabilitation (ABPMR) examinations. Because PM&R training and examinations require substantive coverage of brain injury medicine, certification in PM&R conveys a basic competence in brain injury medicine (BIM).

Beyond basic competency, there also exist formal (but not ACGME approved) Brain Injury Medicine Fellowships in PM&R. These fellowships and advanced clinical experience at academic and brain injury treatment centers provide the underpinnings for further expertise in BIM. The Brain Injury Special Interest Group (BISIG) of the American Academy of Physical Medicine & Rehabilitation (AAPM&R) supports these efforts. The BISIG

organized the development and writing of curricular materials for brain injury medicine fellowship programs. This material has been utilized by fellowship training program directors and mentors to provide structure and didactic content to fellowship training programs in existence or under development. The document has been updated, most recently in 2003.

Beyond PM&R, a number of other specialties engage in elements of brain injury medicine. Foremost among these are neurology and neurosurgery. These programs are most frequently focused on the immediate acute issues or subsequent co-morbidities (e.g. seizures, increased intracranial pressure). The clinical experience in post acute brain injury medicine is not required. Although some programs support this experience, the focus and intensity is widely variable. In general, the route to significant clinical participation in post acute Brain Injury Medicine is through fellowships, a limited number of which exist. These fellowships are not ACGME approved, nor is training sanctioned by their specialty Boards. Post residency training for neurologists is available in a number of fellowships providing clinical management and diagnostic experience across a variety of neurological diagnoses along with the associated therapy interventions.

None of the aforementioned fellowship programs are accredited through ACGME and there is no formal subspecialty certification in Brain Injury Medicine through ABMS. Therefore physicians who have completed the additional year of study are not formally certified by any ABMS Board.

The American Board of Physical Medicine and Rehabilitation is developing a Brain Injury Medicine subspecialty proposal for ABMS approval. The rationale for establishing this subspecialization is:

- To provide core competency standards of training for the evaluation and treatment of patients with brain injuries;
- To provide a high level of care for patients with acquired brain injury and their families in hospital and outpatient settings, and over the continuum of the process of recovery;
- To provide physicians with brain injury medicine administrative skills for activities such as program development, quality assurance, facilities planning, standards-setting;
- To promote and strengthen research for the advancement of the clinical science of brain injury medicine, including prevention, treatment, and restoration of function and outcomes research;
- To increase the number of expert clinicians, teachers, and investigators dedicated to the care of survivors of brain injury.
- To recognize physicians who have successfully completed additional training in brain injury medicine

programs beyond the primary residency training education in physiatry or neurology.

- To improve education in brain injury medicine for residents in physiatry and neurology, residents in other training programs, medical students, practicing physicians, and other medical personnel.
- To generate academic interest in the physiatric and neurological professional societies.

The formal process requires discussion and vetting through ABMS. The intention of ABPMR is to have an inclusive process with an opportunity for all physicians practicing Brain Injury Medicine to have access to the certification process.

There are many disciplines involved in the ongoing care, medical management, and rehabilitation of persons who have sustained brain injury. Although there are expert clinicians in the field, there is no formal certification for any of the professionals involved. Consumers and their families have made a strong case for the requirement of well trained and certified health care providers in the field of brain injury medicine.

COMMUNITY CARERS AND PARAPROFESSIONALS

Following discharge from the acute or sub-acute setting into the community, many persons with brain injury require ongoing care. Brain injury is a lifelong injury that impacts function across the lifespan. Support needs are typically very high, although social networks generally consist of only family members and service providers (13). Oftentimes, persons with brain injury continue to require the services of a multidisciplinary treatment team. Unfortunately, these services are often spread among several different provider agencies, making coordination and continuity of service a management nightmare.

Unlike the pre-existing community services for persons with mental illness or developmental disabilities, developed in the 1970s as part of deinstitutionalization, community services for persons with brain injury are relatively new. Further, attempts to "fit" persons with brain injury into pre-existing community service models (i.e. those for persons with developmental disabilities or mental illness) have attained limited success toward meeting the needs of persons with TBI. These factors contribute to the serious need for specialized training to meet the various needs of persons with brain injuries, caregivers, and their families.

Post-acute community based brain injury rehabilitation is not only a relatively new field, but is also impacted upon by misconceptions, cultural diversity, and inaccurate knowledge about TBI among community service providers. Many of the individuals who live in the community today would have likely not survived their injuries 25 years ago (16). The developments in emergency medical procedures, medical technology, and neurosurgical techniques, have sustained the lives of persons with brain injury, as the community services available for them are being established.

There is limited literature discussing the need for formalized training of providers of TBI services. However, the literature that is available speaks to the need for specialized provider training. The individuals who provide care to persons with TBI residing in the community are most often family members and direct care staff. Paid helpers can often lessen the stress placed upon family members, assuming the paid helper understands the nature of the injury and its sequelae.

Research on paid care work as it applies to persons with brain injury is virtually absent from the literature. McCluskey (21) found that agencies needed to increase efforts to train and orient new staff to the types of challenges they would face working with persons with brain injury. She also suggested that persons with brain injuries would benefit from closer contact between professionals and paid caregivers. Given the restrictions funding sources impose on treatment programs for persons with brain injuries there may be limited opportunities for professional intervention, placing greater emphasis on the importance of training care givers to implement activities to improve the functional performance of persons with brain injury (22).

The specific educational need areas that have been identified include several areas integral to the provision of rehabilitation services to persons with brain injury including; treatment of cognitive deficits, family and social issues, behavior modification techniques, and adjustment to brain injury (16, 18). The literature has also differentiated between the types of training and knowledge required by professionals and paraprofessionals and those with direct versus less direct care of the person with brain injury.

A demonstration project through the New York State Department of Health responded to the need for education of care providers and support for this difficult to serve population. Experts in the field of brain injury rehabilitation developed support for persons with brain injury, family members, friends, and community support staff. Additionally, the program offers an "apprentice" aspect that allows caregivers to receive intensive, contextualized training and coaching, enabling them to better serve persons with brain injury. The results of a preliminary cost-effectiveness study of the program (23) suggest that community supports for persons with behavioral issues resulting from TBI can be provided in a cost-effective manner, although recommendations are made for a systematic analysis of quality of life indicators before broader policies and programs are established.

The lifelong sequelae of TBI often exhaust private insurance funding streams early in the rehabilitation process. Therefore, public programs such as Medicaid and Medicare often become the primary sources of payment. Several states have established waiver programs for persons with TBI. These programs offer opportunities for designing integrated service plans for individuals with brain injury who would otherwise require some type of inpatient care. Care needs usually include support for specialists in case coordination and behavior management, not otherwise funded through typical private insurance. New York State's TBI Waiver Program offers long-term support focusing on post-rehabilitative care. The services offered by the waiver program are fashioned to offset several of TBI's sequelae. The services include: Service coordination, home and community support services, non-medical transportation, specialized medical equipment and supplies, home modifications, intensive behavioral supports, community integration counseling, substance abuse counseling, day programs, and independent living skills training. The services are based in a philosophy of individual choice, while accounting for the accompanying realities of needs, health and welfare issues, and budgets. One of the major challenges faced by provider agencies across the state has been the difficulty to attract and retain qualified staff. This may be a result of the lack of understanding of the behavioral and psychosocial sequelae associated with brain injury.

American Academy of Certified Brain Injury Specialists

A 1990 survey of 565 acute, subacute, and post-acute programs regarding the training needs of licensed and non-licensed staff brain injury services noted that seventy-five percent of the respondents (45 percent response rate) indicated that specialized training is needed for licensed staff, and 84 percent indicated that training is needed for non-licensed staff. This was further supported by Becker (18) who reported that respondents to their survey about education and training needs for staff endorsed specialized training for paraprofessionals, even more than for professionals.

As a result, the Brain Injury Association of America established the American Academy of Certified Brain Injury Specialists (AACBIS) as a standing committee of the association to address training needs. AACBIS operates under its own by-laws as approved by the Board of Directors of the Brain Injury Association of America. AACBIS Committee members are experienced professionals in the field of brain injury rehabilitation who volunteer their time and expertise to developing a certification program that meets the needs of the brain injury community. AACBIS currently offers certification for Brain Injury Specialists. The program is governed by

AACBIS and is administered by the Brain Injury Association of America in McLean, Virginia.

In 1996, AACBIS was established to assure the highest possible standards of rehabilitation and care for persons with brain injuries. The AACBIS is the only organization offering specialized training and certification programs for care givers of persons with brain injuries. AACBIS offers national certification programs improving the quality of care through the establishment of best practices for the education and training of individuals working in the field of brain injury services. The AACBIS offers a voluntary national certification program for both entry-level staff and experienced professionals working in brain injury services. AACBIS provides staff and professionals the opportunity to learn important information about brain injury, to demonstrate their learning in a written examination, and to earn a nationally recognized credential. Since its inception the program has certified more than 520 professionals. The AACBIS certification program is specially designed to address specific training issues in brain injury services and complement other credentials.

The AACBIS program is divided into three levels: Certified Brain Injury Specialist (CBIS)—Basic, CBIS—Instructor, and CBIS—Examiner. The curriculum includes units in the following areas:

- Brain Behavior Relationships
- Functional Impact of Brain Injury
- Health and Medical Issues
- Philosophy of Treatment
- Children and Adolescents with Brain Injury
- Brain Injury: A Family Perspective
- Legal and Ethical Issues

Critics of the examination focus on it being knowledge based when many of the skills integral for effective work with this population rely upon technique. Carnevale (24) developed a model that was both knowledge and practice based. The model utilized a mobile team approach, educating caregivers and persons with brain injury on how to implement and sustain home-based behavior management programs. The natural environment (e.g. home, community) brought to light the importance of flexible interventions that addressed both client and care giver needs. Training programs should focus on the "real life" or functional impact that brain injury has on an individual. Ideally, trainers could incorporate a model that includes visiting the settings in which the care giving is taking place or at least viewing videotapes of every day interactions between the person with the TBI and his/her environment. In short, at least a portion of training must be contextualized to increase the likelihood of positive impact given the cognitive and behavioral sequelae of TBI. Training programs specifically fashioned to provide knowledge and skills training regarding brain injury are needed to facilitate both the caregiver's and the person with brain injury's adjustment to providing/receiving services.

SUMMARY

With advancements in research and science, there have been improvements in acute and emergency medical care, with a significant increase in the numbers of persons who survive brain injury. Residual impairments from the brain injury include a variety of conditions, however cognitive impairments are often the most difficult to manage. Health professionals with expertise in brain injury medicine are required to provide ongoing services and support. Consumers and professionals recognize the importance of subspecialty training and certification.

Program accreditation has provided a base for delivery of quality services at a systems level. Individuals providing those services should also receive appropriate training, and ultimately certification, to further assure high quality care and avoidance of medical errors. The establishment of the American Academy for the Certification of Brain Injury Specialists (AACBIS) is a dynamic step toward addressing the needs and concerns of the brain injury community. Subspecialty training and certification in brain injury medicine and rehabilitation should be considered across all disciplines serving the needs of persons with brain injury. Programs offering such training narrow the information gap between healthcare professionals in the tertiary care hospitals and those in the long-term care facilities, contributing to the integration of brain injury services across the continuum of care. Partnerships among professional organizations, credentialing bodies, service agencies, and accrediting bodies must be forged in order to further integration of knowledge and skill sets into community based brain injury services.

References

1. Colantonio A, Dawson, DR, McLellan, BA. Head injury in young adults: long-term outcome. *Arch Phys Med Rehabil* 1999; 79:550–558.
2. Dixon TM, Layton BS. Traumatic brain injury. In MG Eisenberg, RLGlueckauf, HH Zaretsky (Eds.). *Medical Aspects of Disability: A Handbook for the Rehabilitation Professional*, Springer Publishing, 1999.
3. Thurman DJ, Alverson C, Dunn, KA, Guerrero, J, Sneizek, JE. Traumatic brain injury in the United States: a public health perspective. *J Head Trauma Rehabil* 1999; 14: 602–615.
4. Centers for Disease Control and Prevention (CDC). National Center for Injury Prevention and Control. Report to Congress on Mild Traumatic Brain Injury in the United States: Steps to Prevent a Serious Public Health Problem, Centers for Disease Control and Prevention : CDC 2003.
5. Gruskin KD, Schutzman SA. Head trauma in children younger than 2 years: are there predictors for complications? *Arch Pediatr Adolesc Med* 1999; 153:15–20.
6. Hawley CA, Ward AB, Magnay A R, Long J. Parental stress and burden following traumatic brain injury amongst children and adolescents. *Brain Inj* 2003; 17:1–23.
7. Kreutzer JS, Kolakowsky-Hayner SA, Demm SR, Meade MA. A structured approach to family intervention after brain injury. *J Head Trauma Rehabil* 2002; 17: 349–367.
8. Brooks DN. The head-injured family. *J Clin Exp Neuropsychol* 1991; 13:155–188.
9. Marsh NV, Kersel DA, Havill J H, Sleigh J W. Caregiver burden at 1 year following severe traumatic brain injury. *Brain Inj* 1998; 12:1045–1059.
10. Mitchley N, Gray JM, Pentland B. Burden and coping among the relatives and carers of brain-injured survivors. *Clin Rehabil* 1996; 10: 3–8.
11. Godfrey H, Harnett M, Knight R, Marsh M, Kesel D, Partridge F, Robertson R. Addressing distress in caregivers of people with traumatic brain injury (TBI): a psychometric study of the Head Injury Behavior Scale. *Brain Inj* 2003; 17: 427–435.
12. Osberg JS, Brooke MM, Baryza MJ, Rowe K, Lash M, Kahn P. Impact of childhood brain injury on work and family finances. *Brain Inj* 1997; 11:11–24.
13. Leith K, Phillips L, Sample P. Exploring the service needs and experiences of persons with TBI and their families: the South Carolina experience. *Brain Inj* 2004; 18:1191–1208.
14. Rocchio A. Where do we go from here? *Family News and Views*, A monthly Publication of the Brain Injury Association, 1997; 4(6).
15. Niemeier J, Burnett D, Whitaker D. Cultural competence in the multidisciplinary rehabilitation setting: Are we falling short of meeting needs? *Arch Phys Med Rehabil* 2003; 84:1240–1245.
16. Jackson H, Manchester D. Towards the development of brain injury specialists. *NeuroRehabilitation.* 2001; 16:27–40.
17. Swan IJ, Walker A. Who cares for the patient with head injury now? *Emerg Med J* 2001; 18:352–357.
18. Becker H, Harrell W, Keller L. A survey of professional and paraprofessional training needs for traumatic brain injury rehabilitation. *J Head Trauma Rehabil* 1993; 8:88–101.
19. Bell K, Massagli T. Subacute brain injury rehabilitation: an opportunity for medical education and training. *Brain Inj* 1996; 10:875–881.
20. Sandel M E, Finch M. The case for comprehensive residency training in traumatic brain injury. *Am J Phys Med Rehabil* 1993; 72:325–326.
21. McCluskey A. Paid attendant carers hold important and unexpected roles which contribute to the lives of people with brain injury. *Brain Inj* 2000; 14:943–957.
22. Sohlberg M, Glang A, Todia B. Improvement during baseline: three case studies encouraging collaborative research when evaluating caregiver training. *Brain Inj* 1998; 12:333–346.
23. Feeney TJ, Ylvisaker M, Rosen BH, Greene P. Community supports for individuals with challenging behavior after brain injury: An analysis of the New York State Behavioral Resource Project. *J Head Trauma Rehabil* 2000; 16:61–75.
24. Carnevale GJ, Natural-setting behavior management for individuals with traumatic brain injury: Results of a three-year caregiver training program. *J Head Trauma Rehabil* 1996; 11: 27–38.

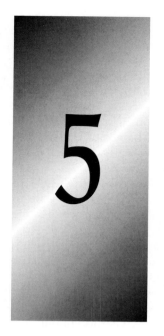

5 Conducting Research in TBI: Current Concepts and Issues

Amy K. Wagner

INTRODUCTION

The National Center for Injury Prevention and Control suggests that injuries have a substantial impact on the lives of individual Americans, their families, and society. The consequences of injuries can be extensive and wide ranging. They are physical, emotional, and financial; in the case of disabling injuries, the consequences are enduring (1). TBI is no exception to these consequences. TBI is an epidemic in the United States with an overall incidence of 200 per 100,000 per year (2). It has been well established that TBI causes chronic debilitation and functional loss over a lifetime. Unlike other disease processes with later onset, survivors of TBI often have many decades of productive life loss, costing themselves, their families, and society much with loss of the capability for competitive employment and other meaningful community roles. An estimated 5.3 million Americans, or 2 percent of the population, currently live with disabilities resulting from brain injury, and the national cost to society is estimated to be $48.3 billion per year (3). Injury is the leading cause of years of potential life lost before age 65, and TBI is responsible for a greater proportion of this mortality rate than most other types of injury (1). For survivors, TBI often results in disturbances of cognitive, behavioral, emotional, & physical functioning. Impairments within these domains can be a persistent & debilitating problem. Mild TBI is often undiagnosed, making the public health burden even larger than reported estimates indicate.

The magnitude of TBI related public health burden mandates that TBI researchers delineate the contributing mechanisms of injury and recovery, evaluate and implement effective treatments, and accurately prognosticate outcome with effective assessment tools. In the population with TBI, patients can have markedly different outcomes, despite similarities in the extent of the initial insult and in type of clinical management. Additionally, the population sustaining TBI is diverse, and a broad and complex range of internal and external factors can influence injury and recovery. These factors make accurate prognostication, sensitive outcome assessment, and effective conduct of clinical trials challenging issues in TBI research. To date, there is a paucity of proven interventions shown to significantly reduce morbidity and mortality or improve recovery and quality of life. Mechanisms of injury, neuroplasticity, and recovery are not fully understood, and outcome prognostication unrefined. In this chapter we discuss unique issues with conducting research in the population with TBI and appropriate outcome assessment in this population. We also highlight the importance of translational research and preclinical trials, evaluate challenges and pitfalls with condͮucting clinical trial research in this population, and outline issues with statistical approach and research design. Finally, we will discuss future considerations and pioneering directions for the field of TBI research.

Unique Aspects Associated with TBI Research

TBI is a complex disease involving both primary (focal and diffuse injuries) and secondary injury, with secondary injury involving complex biochemical cascades that lead to excitotoxicity (4–6), brain swelling (7), loss of cerebral blood flow autoregulation (8), oxidative injury (9, 10), inflammation (11, 12), and cellular necrosis and apoptosis (13, 14). Overlaid on this complex myriad of pathophysiological cascades are the influences of genetic make-up, and other premorbid and demographic characteristics that can influence the extent of injury or recovery. For instance, genetic polymorphisms associated with APOE have linked ApoE-4 expression to outcome after TBI (15–17). Other factors such as age, gender, minority status, and previous education may also impact outcome (18–21). Further, there is variability in the type and intensity of both acute and rehabilitation care that patients may receive. These factors are often influenced by treatment location, social supports, and source of payment (22–24). The multidisciplinary approach to therapies also provides unique challenges in understanding what portions of the rehabilitation process are crucial in improving a particular individual's recovery course. All of the differences in injury variables, personal characteristics, and treatments outlined above can create variability in recovery from TBI. This variability creates unique challenges for researcher in TBI to tease out the important mechanisms associate with injury and recovery, identify appropriate and effective therapeutic targets, and accurately prognosticate outcome.

Researching the Population with TBI

Researching the population with TBI poses other unique methodological challenges to researchers regarding recruitment, population characteristics and follow-up. Biases with recruitment may introduce systematic bias into the study population. One study evaluated this issue in mild TBI by comparing demographic, premorbid, and injury related characteristics of their population. Those who had more severe injuries, who were hospitalized, and who had a significant additional major injury were more likely to consent to participate in the study (25). In studies requiring the evaluation of patients who are unable to consent themselves for enrollment in a research study and/or the immediate implementation of a treatment intervention, obtaining consent can be a challenging issue that impacts recruitment and study design. Recently, one multicenter trial investigated the efficacy of early hypothermia treatment implemented within the first six hours from injury for patients with severe TBI. At the beginning of the study, informed consent was required for each study patient. During the course of the study, federal regulations changed to allow waived informed consent. Post-hoc analysis of this study population showed that with waived inform consent, time to randomization and treatment implementation decreased, patient accrual increased, and minority representation in the study population increased (26). This analysis illustrates the potential importance of waived informed consent on the integrity of early treatment interventions and in minimizing recruitment bias.

Alternatively, systematic bias may be introduced into a clinical data set through loss to follow-up. Loss to follow-up is an inherent problem when conducting research in the population with TBI. One study evaluating loss to follow-up using a variety of data sets, including a single center, multicenter, and statewide surveillance data set, found a loss to follow-up rate of approximately 37 percent and 58 percent one year and two years after injury respectively. Additionally, there appeared to be a selective bias to lose those who were socioeconomically disadvantaged, with violent etiologies of injury, and with a history of substance abuse (27). Systematic bias with loss to follow-up can significantly decrease the generalizeability of study findings and potentially confound apparent treatment efficacy with clinical trials.

A myriad of variables, including patient comorbidities and complications (28, 29), gender (18, 30, 31), cognitive reserve (32), injury severity (18, 32, 33), injury type (34–37) minority status (38), social supports (39) and acute discharge location (24) may all influence outcome. Additionally, patient recovery can occur over a prolonged period (40–42), and outcome assessment may vary with the type of individual (patient, caregiver, clinician) interviewed (43). Each of these issues must be considered carefully when designing studies. The appropriate use of covariate analysis, including time variables for longitudinal studies, and stratification is often necessary to avoid confounders obscuring research results. Time post injury is also an important consideration when designing clinical trials to minimize the effects of natural recovery on the apparent treatment effect.

Outcome Assessment Tools in TBI Research

The World Health Organization (WHO) has provided widely accepted definitions of impairment, disability, and handicap that have resulted in a conceptual framework by which world wide research has been conducted investigating the impact of injury and illness on individual function (44). This system more recently has been replaced by the International Classification of Functioning, Disability and Health (ICF) (45), providing an updated framework for rehabilitation research (46). Several existing TBI assessments measure outcome within more than one of these domains. Commonly utilized TBI outcome assessments vary in scope and mode of measurement. Some outcome assessments are general and designed to provide a global index of outcome, [e.g. Glasgow Outcome Scale-extended (GOS-E) (47), Disability Rating Scale (DRS) (48)]. Others are meant to measure functional abilities for daily activities [Functional Independence Measure (FIM) (49)] or community integration [Community Integration Questionnaire (CIQ) (50, 51)]. Assessments may also focus on quality of life (42, 52, 53), caregiver needs (54, 55), while others focus specifically on neuropsychological performance (41) or psychiatric dysfunction (56, 57). Finally, measurement tools may target specific populations, such as those with mild TBI (58). In particular, outcomes assessment is an important aspect of TBI rehabilitation research. However, studies often published in rehabilitation journals do not report the validity and reliability of the outcome measures used (59). Variable definitions and operationalization as well as associated social values and target population can be difficult to address when developing new or utilizing existing TBI outcomes assessments (60).

Multimodal assessments are often necessary to effectively reflect the complex range of factors affecting TBI outcome. However, no single measurement tool can encompass all relevant areas of TBI outcome. Additionally, there are limitations with the collection and analysis of many existing measurements. There are ceiling effects associated with some measures as individuals with TBI improve over time (61), and some outcome measures have a limited ability to measure group differences in function over long evaluation intervals (62). Attention to cultural, minority, age and gender related differences in response range for outcome assessments should also be considered when selecting assessments and interpreting results (19, 63–66). Choosing an appropriate primary outcome measure is of critical importance when designing clinical trials, selecting a proposed treatment effect size, and for developing effective models for prognostication. Appropriate and well validated outcome measures are often most effective when they target a population with a varied demographic profile and broad range of injury severity, are able to accurately place subjects in appropriate outcome categories at given time intervals, and are sensitive to change over time. Additionally good outcome assessments often link impairments to disability to handicap. For clinical trials, the GOS-E has gained popularity as a primary outcome assessment tool and is thought to be more sensitive than the standard GOS (47). However, The Functional Status Examination (FSE) is a well-validated new instrument that has been utilized in long-term studies for the population with moderate and severe TBI (42, 67). Its measurement properties are linked with other constructs such as family burden, depression, and satisfaction with functioning that make it an effective multi-modal assessment (42) that should also be considered when designing clinical studies.

Researchers should also examine prospective outcome assessments they plan to use to determine if appropriate steps have taken previously to validate that measure in their population of interest. Mode of assessment administration presents some unique concern regarding the validity of the assessment tool chosen. Some measures, including FIM (68) and CIQ (51) have been validated for administration over the telephone, however, many other measures have not been formally validated for multiple modes of administration, despite their widespread use in this manner. Telephone and mailings result in the study population becoming an unseen entity, which can introduce variability and bias into the responses generated.

Cognitive impairments of persons with TBI often make the use of proxies for outcome assessment and evaluation attractive. However, self-awareness of deficits for people with TBI (69) and participant-proxy differences in disability perceptions and quality of life (70) may preclude participant-proxy responses from being interchangeable. Some measures have been specifically evaluated for their reliability and accuracy when administered to both individuals with TBI and their proxies (68, 71), while others have not been evaluated for participant-proxy agreement. Recently, the intraclass correlations between participants with TBI and participant selected proxies on the Craig Handicap Assessment and Reporting Technique (CHART), the CIQ, and the FIM were evaluated. Results showed a high intraclass correlation for participants and proxies, with the highest values occurring on items assessing concrete or observable information (72). Other studies in a variety of patient populations also indicate that patient proxy agreement is generally better for questions regarding physical dimensions of functional status, and agreement is less consistent for questions regarding subjective or affective aspects of outcome assessment (70). Investigators should take time to carefully consider their primary outcome measure and choose their criteria for considering persons with TBI to be a capable respondent. The agreement between patient and proxy responses should be evaluated prior to an outcome assessment's inclusion in a study in order to avoid over or under estimation of treatment effects or invalid conclusions. Further, consistent criteria for the selection of a knowledgeable caregiver or significant other should be considered in the research design.

Clinical Trials in TBI

Randomized clinical trials are the gold standard by which researchers in any field of medicine test the efficacy and safety of treatment interventions. Clinical trials, particularly randomized clinical trials, provide a strong foundation for evidence based clinical practice and justification of payors to reimburse for treatments and therapies (73). However, in the area of TBI, there have been few clinical trials that have definitively identified any effective treatments for reducing morbidity or improving recovery. Numerous TBI clinical trials of acute pharmacological interventions, intended to improve functional & neuropsychological outcomes, have been conducted over the last 25 years, with often disappointing results (2, 74–80). The justification for virtually all of these trials were positive findings in animal studies, using rodent models, testing the trial drug or intervention that could not capture variables that may influence treatment outcome, such as, gender, age, and genetic variability (81, 82). As mentioned above, TBI is a heterogeneous disease, with a multitude of secondary injury cascades, affecting a diverse population. The complexity of the disease and diversity of the population it affects makes designing clinical trials in TBI particularly challenging.

For TBI rehabilitation research, double blind randomized control trials are particularly difficult to carry out. Sample sizes tend to be small, and the number of confounding variables are often quite high. There is a lack of consensus on appropriate outcome measures or how to objectively quantify rehabilitation based interventions, and (unlike acute care trials) post-intervention improvements may not be seen for months or years. Rehabilitation research also focuses on the improvement of functional abilities, participation in the community, and quality of life (46). For instance, social interventions such as caregiver education may improve community integration and quality of life for the population with TBI. Rehabilitation outcome often can be considered context specific and affected by a patient's physical environment, social environment, and personal attitudes and expectations (83). Contextual factors may influence rehabilitation outcome and decrease the generalizeability of clinical study results. Despite these challenges, some high quality rehabilitation based randomized clinical trials have occurred in the areas of seizure prophylaxis (84, 85), community based rehabilitation for long term survivors of TBI (86), Methylphenidate treatment (87), and cognitive rehabilitation (88). However, replication studies, studies with large population numbers, and the generalizability of findings to a large population are difficult to find in any area of TBI rehabilitation research.

A recent analysis regarding clinical trials in rehabilitation (89) suggests that characterizing participants in rehabilitation research studies is of critical importance to eliminate confounding, to ensure comparability across treatment conditions, and to adjust for differences in prognosis among participants. Additionally, the treatment or intervention must be adequately and objectively characterized in terms of mechanism of action, dose, route, intensity, and subject participation. Outcome measures utilized for characterizing treatment efficacy need to be sensitive and appropriate. Investigators should identify the appropriate target of their outcome assessment (e.g. disease, impairment, activity, participation, quality of life) and

ensure the measureability of their outcome target with the treatment intervention. Often, broadly defined outcomes such as quality of life have several factors that impact it. As such, a single intervention may impact specific impairments after TBI, but those changes may not be large enough to translate into a meaningful change in quality of life (89). Additional challenges in rehabilitation research occurs with blinding of physical treatments and with limitations of crossover designs when significant contamination of the study population from cross-training might dilute the effectiveness of the treatment intervention (90).

Multicenter clinical trials in TBI are considered necessary since the ability of a single center to recruit enough subjects to provide adequate statistical power is often limited. However, several statistical and design issues have been identified by investigators directing multi-center clinical trials that begin during emergency and intensive care. Intercenter variance in patient care and adherence to the research protocol has been a fatally flaw in some recent multicenter clinical trials. For example, it has been reported that intercenter variation, not explicable by injury severity or type, was responsible for approximately 40 percent of the variation in a multicenter clinical trial evaluating the effectiveness of tirilizad mesylate (77, 91). Intercenter variation was noted with a variety of intensive care treatments, including narcotic use for sedation, and with a number of physiological variables, including mean arterial pressure and cerebral perfusion pressure for a multicenter clinical trial evaluating the efficacy of hypothermia (92). Interestingly, recent studies with an experimental TBI model suggests that choice of anesthesia or sedation, including Fentanyl and Isoflurane, can have marked effects on outcome and in the context of hypothermia treatment (93, 94). This example demonstrates the potential impact that variation in standard care may play in recovery and outcome. Centers who can enroll small numbers of patients may contribute the most variability to standard care treatment regimens because they are often less likely to follow consensus recommendations for standard treatment (91). Misclassification of outcomes can also influence study results. Interestingly, one study reports, that as the numbers of outcome categories increase, the greater the likelihood of outcome misclassification and erroneous results (95). While dichotomous outcomes are not reasonable for each and every clinical trial, care must be taken to create effective algorithms for accurate data collection, and the use of pilot data may be helpful in determining an effective outcome measure with a minimum necessary requirement of categories. Subset analysis of data, even in negative multicenter trials, is recommended to identify potential subpopulations who might benefit from a particular treatment (96).

Recently, the NINDS May 2000 Clinical Trials in Head Injury Study Group identified and discussed many of the issues associated with failure to produce positive results with several recent trials (91). The Study Group concluded that in order for clinical trials to be effective, it is essential to: (i) establish that a drug or proposed intervention is having the desired effect on a specific mechanism of injury in vivo, (ii) to obtain adequate pre-clinical data, (iii) target subpopulations of patients most likely to benefit from the treatment, (iv) standardize clinical care, (v) choose appropriate outcome measures or endpoints, and (vi) have reasonable expectations for treatment effect (91). Priority should be placed on conducting experimental and clinical studies aimed at understanding mechanisms of injury and recovery, since they are critical when designing future clinical trials and identifying possible therapeutic targets. Evaluating the most effective window of treatment, dose response curves, drug pharmacokinetics and drug delivery to the brain, and multiple models of experimental TBI are needed for adequate pre-clinical trial data (91). Utilizing injury related prognostic variables in the selection criteria for studies may allow investigators to effectively target subpopulations for particular interventions. Functional status at the time of entry into rehabilitation trials may be more prognostic of outcome and a relevant way to group patients than injury variables (91). Other intrinsic variables such as age, gender, and genetic make-up are emerging as important variables to consider in trial design (15, 97). Strict adherance to clinical care guidelines, centralization of some study variables (e.g. CT scan interpretation), collection of concurrent medications, and collection of only essential study variables may improve the management of clinical trials. Finally, smaller effect sizes (5–7.5 percent), the careful design and use of sensitive outcomes as well as the judicious use of relevant proxy variables may allow investigators to appreciate subtle treatment effects for specific interventions (91).

Alternatives to Clinical Trials and Research Design

While randomized clinical trials are considered the gold standard for clinical research, they are not always feasible or practical for each research question. Ethical issues and the inability to obtain the resources necessary to conduct a full scale randomized clinical trials may preclude this study design (98). However, randomized clinical trials may have their own limitations in that they may not provide a representative measure of the effectiveness of the treatment in common clinical practice settings (99). Observational studies may be one alternative technique by which to study necessary research questions, particularly when treatment variables of interest are not assigned based on prognostic factors influencing outcome (98). Some reports suggest that effect sizes generated from well

done observational studies can be comparable to those obtained from randomized clinical trials (100) However, observational studies are vulnerable to confounding variables impacting the outcome variable of interest and require the use of covariate analysis. Common issues associated with exploratory analyses or observational studies, such as appropriate correction for multiple comparisons, avoiding type II experimental error, and appropriate sample size also need to be considered in the study design (101, 102), in order to provide accurate conclusions and a solid foundation for the design of a future clinical trial. Single subject research designs can be valuable, particularly in clinical practice, to determine effectiveness of treatments and lay the ground-work for larger studies (103).

Translational Research in TBI

Translational research is an important area of focus for TBI in that it identifies mechanisms of injury and recovery and lays the groundwork for the conduct of clinical trials. Advances in genomics and proteomics may provide a novel approach to identifying and exploring therapeutic targets (104, 105). Utilizing functional imaging technology (106–109) or quantitative EEG (110) may be some contemporary avenues by which to explore injury and recovery mechanisms directly in the clinical population with TBI. However, the majority of translational research requires the effective use of experimental models that reproduce the physiological and behavioral sequelae associated with injury. Several models, including fluid percussion (111) and controlled cortical impact (CCI) (112) are commonly used in rodents. Characteristics of the CCI model include not only a representative contusion, but also reproducible brain edema and marked changes in cerebral blood flow in surrounding cortex (113). Rodent models are cost effective, can provide a relevant and reproducible injury, and are effective in studying a variety of behavioral paradigms (114–117). Rodents, however, are not gyrocephalic animals, and the use of larger animal models, including primate models, may be necessary to fully characterize pathology associated with diffuse axonal injury. Experimental models of TBI have largely been utilized to study acute pathology and neuroprotection, however, they can be a useful approach for examining long term outcome, mechanisms of recovery, and relevant rehabilitation interventions. For example, the CCI model recently was utilized to study the differential effects of gender and environmental enrichment, an experimental correlate to therapy, on behavioral recovery (118). In order for TBI rehabilitation research to move forward, collaborative efforts with other basic science disciplines, such as neuroscience and psychology, to tackle complex issues such as cortical reorganization, neural plasticity, and the effects of rehabilitation strategies like forced use will be required (119). Future work will also require that researchers find ways to actively link studies involving acute mechanisms of injury and treatment inventions with central nervous system repair and recovery.

Priority Areas for TBI Rehabilitation Research

In 1999, an NIH consensus group identified and published some research priorities in the area of TBI (120). Highlighted among these priorities include a need for epidemiological studies targeting different demographic groups and to study mild TBI. The therapeutic window for treatment interventions needs to be studied, and the neurobiology of clinical TBI, using state-of the-art technology needs to be addressed. Specific prognostic equations should be developed, and the relationship between impairments and global outcome evaluated. Finally, the long term consequences of TBI and the developmental impact of TBI on children should also be a focus of study (120).

Several priority areas for TBI, injury prevention, and rehabilitation research have been set by primary federal organizations that fund TBI research. The National Institute for Disability and Rehabilitation Research's Long Range Plan has research priorities in the areas of employment outcomes, individual health and function, technology for access and function, and independent living and community integration (121). The development of sensitive and effective outcome measures is a priority. Research in rehabilitation science, disability studies, and disability policy are also current NIDRR research priorities. Investigators, particularly in the field of TBI rehabilitation research, have had a long history of utilizing NIDRR funding to evaluate important questions in the area of TBI outcome. The TBI model system centers (122, 123) have been an important part of this endeavor. NIDRR based collaborative networks for TBI research also foster increased interactions between a varied group of investigators and allow for the recruitment of large samples to answer important TBI rehabilitation research questions.

The Centers for Disease Control's (CDC) injury center interact with researchers in acute care and rehabilitation in order to "advance a broad based, multidisciplinary approach to injury" (1). Highlighted among their many priorities relevant to TBI are to (i) identify risk factors and develop and evaluate interventions for secondary conditions following TBI, particularly for patients not treated at state-of-the-art facilities; (ii) identify methods to ensure that people with TBI receive services; (iii) develop and apply methods for calculating population-based estimates of the incidence costs and consequences of those non-hospitalized after TBI; (iv) determine the impact of TBI on special populations; (v) develop and implement interventions for reducing disability after mild TBI; (vi) determine how the environment impacts disability after TBI;

and (vii) investigate the long-term effects of TBI on the health and longevity of persons with TBI. These priorities indicate that the CDC has a wide range of research opportunities for investigators to utilize that integrate aspects of secondary and tertiary injury control.

"Healthy People 2010" is a collection of national health objectives highlighted by the NIH as research priorities. The goals of Healthy People 2010 are designed to identify significant threats to national health and to establish goals aimed at reducing these threats. One priority of Healthy People 2010 is to eliminate health disparities among different segments of the population, including those with disabilities. In particular, Healthy People 2010 aims to "promote the health of people with disabilities, prevent secondary conditions, and eliminate disparities between people with and without disabilities in the U.S. population" (124). These particular aims suggest that National Institutes of Health (NIH) views disability related research, including research on assessing and preventing secondary conditions associated with TBI, as an important priority area of research.

In 2002, the NIH began developing its roadmap for medical research in the twenty-first century and identifying new pathways to discovery, research teams of the future, and re-engineering the clinical research enterprise (125). Future NIH funded TBI research will likely incorporate many of the new research paradigms outlined within this roadmap. TBI research teams of the future will likely be multidisciplinary in nature, integrating several distinct areas of science to evaluate broad research questions. NIH hopes to increase interactions between clinicians and basic scientist with the thought that this interaction will generate studies that are effectively able to translate basic research findings into meaningful changes in individual health. NIH is committed to training clinician researchers to take part in multidisciplinary and translational research endeavors. Contemporary and integrated networks of researchers able to conduct large-scale clinical trials to efficiently study relevant research questions and rapidly disseminate their findings in the context of best practices are a priority. Standardized data collection, sample sharing and the development of effective outcome measurements are also a priority. The NIH hopes to leverage significant advances in molecular biology, bioinformatics, computer science and engineering to encourage innovative ideas and perspectives that lead to seminal breakthroughs in scientific research that lead to improvements with human health. Finally, the NIH hopes to develop private-public partnerships to extend and accelerate research. As investigators incorporate this new vision into their scientific approach and programs of research, we will move forward in understanding key mechanisms of injury and recovery, and effectively identifying and implementing therapeutic strategies for the population with TBI.

References

1. CDC Injury Research Agenda. http://www.cdc.gov/ncipc/pub-res/research-agenda/agenda.htm. 2004.

2. Wolf AL, Levi L, Marmarou A, Ward JD, Muizelaar PJ, Choi S et al. Effect of THAM upon outcome in severe head injury: a randomized prospective clinical trial. *Journal of Neurosurgery* 1993; 78(1):54–59.

3. Thurman DJ, Alverson C, Dunn KA, Guerrero J, Sniezek JE. Traumatic brain injury in the United States: A public health perspective. *Journal of Head Trauma Rehabilitation* 1999; 14(6): 602–615.

4. Globus MY, Alonso O, Dietrich WD, et al. Glutamate release and free radical production following brain injury: effects of posttraumatic hypothermia. *Journal of Neurochemistry* 65, 1704–1711. 1995.

5. Danbolt NC. Glutamate uptake. [Review] [1082 refs]. *Progress in Neurobiology* 2001; 65(1):1–105.

6. Zipfel GJ, Babcock DJ, Lee JM, Choi DW. Neuronal apoptosis after CNS injury: the roles of glutamate and calcium. [Review] [158 refs]. *Journal of Neurotrauma* 2000; 17(10):857–869.

7. Roof RL, Duvdevani R, Heyburn JW, Stein DG. Progesterone rapidly decreases brain edema: treatment delayed up to 24 hours is still effective. *Experimental Neurology* 1996; 138(2):246–251.

8. Roof RL, Hall ED. Estrogen-related gender difference in survival rate and cortical blood flow after impact acceleration head injury in rats. *Journal of Neurotrauma* 17(12), 1155–1169. 2000.

9. Bayir H, Kagan VE, Tyurina YY, Tyurin V, Ruppel RA, Adelson PD, et al. Assessment of antioxidant reserves and oxidative stress in cerebrospinal fluid after severe traumatic brain injury in infants and children. *Pediatric Research* 2002; 51(5):571–578.

10. Kontos HA, Povlishock JT. Oxygen radicals in brain injury. *Central Nervous System Trauma* 3, 257–263. 1986.

11. Kushi H, Saito T, Makino K, Hayashi N. IL-8 is a key mediator of neuroinflammation in severe traumatic brain injuries. *Acta Neurochirurgica*, Supplement 2003; 86:347–350.

12. Frati A, Salvati M, Mainiero F, Ippoliti F, Rocchi G, Raco A, et al. Inflammation markers and risk factors for recurrence in 35 patients with a posttraumatic chronic subdural hematoma: a prospective study. *Journal of Neurosurgery* 2004; 100(1): 24–32.

13. Raghupathi R, Conti AC, Graham DI, Krajewski S, Reed JC, Grady MS, et al. Mild traumatic brain injury induces apoptotic cell death in the cortex that is preceded by decreases in cellular Bcl-2 immunoreactivity. *Neuroscience* 2002; 110(4):605–616.

14. Yakovlev AG, Faden AI. Caspase-dependent apoptotic pathways in CNS injury. [Review] [130 refs]. *Molecular Neurobiology* 2001; 24(1–3):131–144.

15. Friedman G, Froom P, Sazbon L, Grinblatt I, Shochina M, Tsenter J, et al. Apolipoprotein E-epsilon4 genotype predicts a poor outcome in survivors of traumatic brain injury. *Neurology* 1999; 52(2):244–248.

16. Chiang MF, Chang JG, Hu CJ. Association between apolipoprotein E genotype and outcome of traumatic brain injury. *Acta Neurochirurgica* 2003; 145(8):649–653.

17. Crawford FC, Vanderploeg RD, Freeman MJ, Singh S, Waisman M, Michaels L, et al. APOE genotype influences acquisition and recall following traumatic brain injury. *Neurology* 2002; 58(7):1115–1118.

18. Wagner AK, Hammond FM, Sasser HC, Wiercisiewski D, Norton HJ. Use of injury severity variables in determining disability and community integration after traumatic brain injury. *Journal of Trauma, Injury Infection & Critical Care* 2000; 49(3):411–419.

19. Rosenthal M, Dijkers M, Harrison–Felix C, et al. Impact of minority status on functional outcome and community integration following traumatic brain injury. *Journal of Head Trauma Rehabilitation* 11, 40–57. 1996.

20. Pennings JL, Bachulis BL, Simons CT, Slazinski T. Survival after severe head injury in the aged. *Archives of Surgery* 1993; 128(7):787–793.

21. Cifu DX, Kreutzer JS, Marwitz JH, Rosenthal M, Englander J, High W. Functional outcomes of older adults with traumatic brain injury: a prospective, multicenter analysis. *Archives of Physical Medicine & Rehabilitation* 1996; 77(9):883–888.

22. Mullins RJ, Veum–Stone J, Helfand M, Zimmer-Gembeck M, Hedges JR, Southard PA, et al. Outcome of hospitalized injured patients after institution of a trauma system in an urban area. *JAMA* 1994; 271(24):1919–1924.

23. Mullins RJ, Hedges JR, Rowland DJ, Arthur M, Mann NC, Price DD, et al. Survival of seriously injured patients first treated in rural hospitals. *Journal of Trauma, Injury Infection & Critical Care* 2002; 52(6):1019–1029.

24. Wagner AK, Hammond FM, Grigsby JH, Norton HJ. The value of trauma scores: predicting discharge after traumatic brain injury. *American Journal of Physical Medicine & Rehabilitation* 2000; 79(3):235–242.

25. McCullagh S, Feinstein A. Outcome after mild traumatic brain injury: an examination of recruitment bias. *J Neurol Neurosurg Psychiatry* 74, 39–43. 2003.

26. Clifton GL, Knudson P, McDonald M. Waiver of consent in studies of acute brain injury. *Journal of Neurotrauma* 2002; 19(10):1121–1126.

27. Corrigan JD, Harrison-Felix C, Bogner J, Dijkers M, Terrill MS, Whiteneck G. Systematic bias in traumatic brain injury outcome studies because of loss to follow-up. *Archives of Physical Medicine & Rehabilitation* 2003; 84(2):153–160.

28. Lew HL, Lee E, Date ES, Zeiner H. Influence of medical comorbidities and complications on FIM change and length of stay during inpatient rehabilitation. *American Journal of Physical Medicine & Rehabilitation* 2002; 81(11):830–837.

29. Wagner AK, Fabio A, Lombard LA, Zafonte RD, Peitzman AB. Patient premorbidity and acute care complications: associations with acute outcome and length of stay for persons with traumatic brain injury. *American Journal of Physical Medicine & Rehabilitation.* 83(3), 247. 2004.

30. Farace E, Alves WM. Do women fare worse: a metaanalysis of gender differences in traumatic brain injury outcome. [see comment]. *Journal of Neurosurgery* 2000; 93(4):539–545.

31. Wagner AK, Sasser H. Gender associations with disability and community integration after traumatic brain injury. *Archives of Physical Medicine and Rehabilitation* 81(9), 1267–1268. 2000.

32. Kesler SR, Adams HF, Blasey CM, Bigler ED. Premorbid intellectual functioning, education, and brain size in traumatic brain injury: an investigation of the cognitive reserve hypothesis. *Applied Neuropsychology* 2003; 10(3):153–162.

33. Zafonte RD, Mann NR, Millis SR, Black KL, Wood DL, Hammond F. Posttraumatic amnesia: its relation to functional outcome. *Archives of Physical Medicine & Rehabilitation* 1997; 78(10): 1103–1106.

34. Hanks RA, Wood DL, Millis S, Harrison-Felix C, Pierce CA, Rosenthal M, et al. Violent traumatic brain injury: occurrence, patient characteristics, and risk factors from the Traumatic Brain Injury Model Systems project. *Archives of Physical Medicine & Rehabilitation* 2003; 84(2):249–254.

35. Bushnik T, Hanks RA, Kreutzer J, Rosenthal M. Etiology of traumatic brain injury: characterization of differential outcomes up to 1 year postinjury. *Archives of Physical Medicine & Rehabilitation* 2003; 84(2):255–262.

36. Zafonte RD, Wood DL, Harrison-Felix CL, Valena NV, Black K. Penetrating head injury: a prospective study of outcomes. *Neurological Research* 2001; 23(2–3):219–226.

37. Wagner AK, Sasser HC, Hammond FM, Wiercisiewski D, Alexander J. Intentional traumatic brain injury: epidemiology, risk factors, and associations with injury severity and mortality. [erratum appears in *J Trauma* 2000 Nov;49(5):982]. *Journal of Trauma, Injury Infection & Critical Care* 2000; 49(3):404–410.

38. Sherer M, Nick TG, Sander AM, Hart T, Hanks R, Rosenthal M, et al. Race and productivity outcome after traumatic brain injury: influence of confounding factors. *Journal of Head Trauma Rehabilitation* 2003; 18(5):408–424.

39. Hibbard MR, Cantor J, Charatz H, Rosenthal R, Ashman T, Gundersen N, et al. Peer support in the community: initial findings of a mentoring program for individuals with traumatic brain injury and their families. [Review] [44 refs]. *Journal of Head Trauma Rehabilitation* 2002; 17(2):112–131.

40. Novack TA, Alderson AL, Bush BA, Meythaler JM, Canupp K. Cognitive and functional recovery at 6 and 12 months post-TBI. *Brain Injury* 2000; 14(11):987–996.

41. Millis SR, Rosenthal M, Novack TA, Sherer M, Nick TG, Kreutzer JS, et al. Long–term neuropsychological outcome after traumatic brain injury. *Journal of Head Trauma Rehabilitation* 2001; 16(4):343–355.

42. Dikmen SS, Machamer JE, Powell JM, Temkin NR. Outcome 3 to 5 years after moderate to severe traumatic brain injury. *Archives of Physical Medicine & Rehabilitation* 2003; 84(10):1449–1457.

43. Powell JM, Machamer JE, Temkin NR, Dikmen SS. Self-report of extent of recovery and barriers to recovery after traumatic brain injury: a longitudinal study. *Archives of Physical Medicine & Rehabilitation* 2001; 82(8):1025–1030.

44. Schuntermann MF. The International Classification of Impairments, Disabilities and Handicaps (ICIDH)—results and problems. [Review] [12 refs]. *International Journal of Rehabilitation Research* 1996; 19(1):1–11.

45. Bornman J. The World Health Organisation's terminology and classification application to severe disability. *Disability & Rehabilitation*. 26(3), 182–188. 2–4–2004.

46. Dahl TH. International classification of functioning, disability and health: an introduction and discussion of its potential impact on rehabilitation services and research. *Journal of Rehabilitation Medicine* 2002; 34(5):201–204.

47. Wilson JT, Pettigrew LE, Teasdale GM. Structured interviews for the Glasgow Outcome Scale and the extended Glasgow Outcome Scale: guidelines for their use. *Journal of Neurotrauma* 1998; 15(8):573–585.

48. Hall K, Cope DN, Rappaport M. Glasgow outcome scale and disability rating scale: comparative usefulness in following recovery in traumatic head injury. *Archives of Physical Medicine and Rehabilitation* 66(1), 35–37. 1985.

49. Cook L, Smith DS, Truman G. Using Functional Independence Measure profiles as an index of outcome in the rehabilitation of brain-injured patients. *Archives of Physical Medicine & Rehabilitation* 1994; 75(4):390–393.

50. Willer B, Rosenthal M, Kreutzer J, et al. Assessment of community integration following rehabilitation for traumatic brain injury. *Journal of Head Trauma Rehabilitation* 8, 75–87. 1993.

51. Willer B, Ottenbacher KJ, Coad ML. The community integration questionnaire. A comparative examination. *American Journal of Physical Medicine & Rehabilitation* 1994; 73(2):103–111.

52. Corrigan JD, Bogner JA, Mysiw WJ, Clinchot D, Fugate L. Life satisfaction after traumatic brain injury. *Journal of Head Trauma Rehabilitation* 2001; 16(6):543–555.

53. Dikmen S, Machamer J, Miller B, Doctor J, Temkin N. Functional status examination: a new instrument for assessing outcome in traumatic brain injury. *Journal of Neurotrauma* 2001; 18(2):127–140.

54. Sander AM, High WM, Jr., Hannay HJ, Sherer M. Predictors of psychological health in caregivers of patients with closed head injury. *Brain Injury* 1997; 11(4):235–249.

55. Struchen MA, Atchison TB, Roebuck TM, Caroselli JS, Sander AM. A multidimensional measure of caregiving appraisal: validation of the Caregiver Appraisal Scale in traumatic brain injury. *Journal of Head Trauma Rehabilitation* 2002; 17(2):132–154.

56. Levin H, Goldstein FC, MacKenzie EJ. Depression as a secondary condition following mild and moderate traumatic brain injury. *Semin Clin Neuropsychiatry* 2(3), 207–215. 1997.

57. Glenn MB, O'Neil-Pirozzi T, Goldstein R, Burke D, Jacob L. Depression amongst outpatients with traumatic brain injury. *Brain Injury* 2001; 15(9):811–818.

58. Collins MW, Iverson GL, Lovell MR, McKeag DB, Norwig J, Maroon J. On-field predictors of neuropsychological and symptom deficit following sports-related concussion. *Clinical Journal of Sport Medicine* 2003; 13(4):222–229.

59. Dijkers MP, Kropp GC, Esper RM, Yavuzer G, Cullen N, Bakdalieh Y. Reporting on reliability and validity of outcome measures in medical rehabilitation research. *Disability & Rehabilitation* 2002; 24(16):819–827.

60. Dijkers M. Measuring quality of life: methodological issues. [Review] [98 refs]. *American Journal of Physical Medicine & Rehabilitation* 1999; 78(3):286–300.

61. Hall K, Mann N, High W, Wright J, Kreutzer JS, Wood D. Functional measures after traumatic brain injury: ceiling effects of FIM, FIM+FAM, DRS, and CIQ. *Journal of Head Trauma Rehabilitation* 11(5), 27–39. 1996.

62. Hammond FM, Grattan KD, Sasser H, Corrigan JD, Bushnik T, Zafonte RD. Long-term recovery course after traumatic brain injury: a comparison of the functional independence measure and disability rating scale. *Journal of Head Trauma Rehabilitation* 2001; 16(4):318–329.

63. Schopp L, Shigaki C, Johnstone B, Kirkpatrick H. gender differences in cognitive and emotional adjustment to traumatic brain injury. *Journal of Clinical Psychology in Medical Settings* 8(3), 181–188. 2001.

64. Fenten G. The postconcussions syndrome: Social antecedents and psychological sequelae. *British Journal of Psychiatry* 162, 493–497. 1993.

65. O'Bryant SE, Hilsabeck RC, McCaffrey RJ, Drew GW. The Recognition Memory Test Examination of ethnic differences and norm validity. *Archives of Clinical Neuropsychology* 2003; 18(2):135–143.

66. Rosselli M, Ardila A. The impact of culture and education on nonverbal neuropsychological measurements: a critical review. *Brain & Cognition* 2003; 52(3):326–333.

67. Temkin NR, Machamer JE, Dikmen SS. Correlates of functional status 3–5 years after traumatic brain injury with CT abnormalities. *Journal of Neurotrauma* 2003; 20(3):229–241.

68. Segal ME, Gillard M, Schall R. Telephone and in-person proxy agreement between stroke patients and caregivers for the functional independence measure. *American Journal of Physical Medicine & Rehabilitation* 1996; 75(3):208–212.

69. Flashman LA, McAllister TW. Lack of awareness and its impact in traumatic brain injury. [Review] [85 refs]. *Neurorehabilitation* 2002; 17(4):285–296.

70. Weinfurt KP, Trucco SM, Willke RJ, Schulman KA. Measuring agreement between patient and proxy responses to multidimensional health-related quality-of-life measures in clinical trials. An application of psychometric profile analysis. *Journal of Clinical Epidemiology* 2002; 55(6):608–618.

71. Tepper S, Beatty P, DeJong G. Outcomes in traumatic brain injury: self-report versus report of significant others. *Brain Injury* 1996; 10(8):575–581.

72. Cusick CP, Gerhart KA, Mellick DC. Participant-proxy reliability in traumatic brain injury outcome research. *Journal of Head Trauma Rehabilitation* 2000; 15(1):739–749.

73. Fuhrer MJ. Overview of clinical trials in medical rehabilitation: impetuses, challenges, and needed future directions. [Review] [28 refs]. *American Journal of Physical Medicine & Rehabilitation* 2003; 82(10 Suppl):S8–15.

74. Muizelaar JP, Marmarou A, Ward JD, Kontos HA, Choi SC, Becker DP, et al. Adverse effects of prolonged hyperventilation in patients with severe head injury: a randomized clinical trial. *Journal of Neurosurgery* 1991; 75(5):731–739.

75. Muizelaar JP, Marmarou A, Young HF, et al. Improving the outcome of severe head injury with oxygen radical scavenger polyethylene glycol-conjugated superoxide dismutase: a Phase II trial. *Journal of Neurosurgery* 78, 375–382. 1993.

76. Clifton GL, Miller ER, Choi SC, Levin HS, McCauley S, Smith KR, Jr., et al. Lack of effect of induction of hypothermia after acute brain injury.[see comment]. *New England Journal of Medicine* 2001; 344(8):556–563.

77. Marshall LF, Maas AI, Marshall SB, Bricolo A, Fearnside M, Iannotti F, et al. A multicenter trial on the efficacy of using tirilazad mesylate in cases of head injury. *Journal of Neurosurgery* 1998; 89(4):519–525.

78. Ikonomidou C, Turski L. Why did NMDA receptor antagonists fail clinical trials for stroke and traumatic brain injury? [see comment]. [Review] [44 refs]. *Lancet Neurology* 2002; 1(6):383–386.

79. McIntyre LA, Fergusson DA, Hebert PC, Moher D, Hutchison JS. Prolonged therapeutic hypothermia after traumatic brain injury in adults: a systematic review. [see comment]. [Review] [58 refs]. *JAMA* 2003; 289(22):2992–2999.

80. Bullock MR, Lyeth BG, Muizelaar JP. Current status of neuroprotection trials for traumatic brain injury: lessons from animal

models and clinical studies. [Review] [82 refs]. *Neurosurgery* 1999; 45(2):207–217.

81. Clifton GL, Jiang JY, Lyeth BG, Jenkins LW, Hamm RJ, Hayes RL. Marked protection by moderate hypothermia after experimental traumatic brain injury. *Journal of Cerebral Blood Flow & Metabolism* 1991; 11(1):114–121.

82. Marion DW, White MJ. Treatment of experimental brain injury with moderate hypothermia and 21-aminosteroids. *Journal of Neurotrauma* 1996; 13(3):139–147.

83. Wade DT. Outcome measures for clinical rehabilitation trials: impairment, function, quality of life, or value? [Review] [11 refs]. *American Journal of Physical Medicine & Rehabilitation* 2003; 82 (10 Suppl):S26–S31.

84. Temkin NR, Dikmen SS, Wilensky AJ, Keihm J, Chabal S, Winn HR. A randomized, double-blind study of phenytoin for the prevention of post–traumatic seizures.[see comment]. New England Journal of Medicine 1990; 323(8):497–502.

85. Temkin NR, Dikmen SS, Anderson GD, Wilensky AJ, Holmes MD, Cohen W et al. Valproate therapy for prevention of post-traumatic seizures: a randomized trial. *Journal of Neurosurgery* 1999; 91(4):593–600.

86. Powell J, Heslin J, Greenwood R. Community based rehabilitation after severe traumatic brain injury: a randomised controlled trial. [see comment]. *Journal of Neurology, Neurosurgery & Psychiatry* 2002; 72(2):193–202.

87. Whyte J, Hart T, Schuster K, Fleming M, Polansky M, Coslett HB. Effects of methylphenidate on attentional function after traumatic brain injury. A randomized, placebo-controlled trial. *American Journal of Physical Medicine & Rehabilitation* 1997; 76(6):440–450.

88. Carney N, Chesnut RM, Maynard H, Mann NC, Patterson P, Helfand M. Effect of cognitive rehabilitation on outcomes for persons with traumatic brain injury: A systematic review. [see comment]. [Review] [45 refs]. *Journal of Head Trauma Rehabilitation* 1999; 14(3):277–307.

89. Whyte J. Clinical trials in rehabilitation: what are the obstacles? [Review] [12 refs]. *American Journal of Physical Medicine & Rehabilitation* 2003; 82(10 Suppl):S16–S21.

90. Terrin M. Fundamentals of clinical trials for medical rehabilitation. [Review] [9 refs]. *American Journal of Physical Medicine & Rehabilitation* 2003; 82(10 Suppl):S22–S25.

91. Narayan RK, Michel ME, Ansell B, Baethmann A, Biegon A, Bracken MB, et al. Clinical trials in head injury. [Review] [50 refs]. *Journal of Neurotrauma* 2002; 19(5):503–557.

92. Clifton GL, Choi SC, Miller ER, Levin HS, Smith KR, Jr., Muizelaar JP, et al. Intercenter variance in clinical trials of head trauma— experience of the National Acute Brain Injury Study: Hypothermia. [see comment]. *Journal of Neurosurgery* 2001; 95(5):751–755.

93. Statler KD, Kochanek PM, Dixon CE, Alexander HL, Warner DS, Clark RS, et al. Isoflurane improves long-term neurologic outcome versus fentanyl after traumatic brain injury in rats. *Journal of Neurotrauma* 2000; 17(12):1179–1189.

94. Statler KD, Alexander HL, Vagni VA, Nemoto EM, Tofovic SP, Dixon CE, et al. Moderate hypothermia may be detrimental after traumatic brain injury in fentanyl-anesthetized rats. *Critical Care Medicine* 2003; 31(4):1134–1139.

95. Choi SC, Clifton GL, Marmarou A, Miller ER. Misclassification and treatment effect on primary outcome measures in clinical trials of severe neurotrauma. *Journal of Neurotrauma* 2002; 19(1):17–22.

96. Choi SC, Bullock R. Design and statistical issues in multicenter trials of severe head injury. [Review] [8 refs]. *Neurological Research* 2001; 23(2–3):190–192.

97. Wagner AK, Bayir H, Ren D, Puccio A, Zafonte RD, Kochanek PM. Relationships between cerebrospinal fluid markers of excitotoxicity, ischemia, oxidative damage after severe TBI: the impact of gender, age, and hypothermia. *Journal of Neurotrauma* 21[2], 125–136. 2004.

98. Whyte J. Traumatic brain injury rehabilitation: are there alternatives to randomized clinical trials? *Archives of Physical Medicine & Rehabilitation* 2002; 83(9):1320–1322.

99. D'Agostino RB, Kwan H. Measuring effectiveness. What to expect without a randomized control group. [Review] [39 refs]. *Medical Care* 1995; 33(4 Suppl):AS95–105.

100. Benson K, Hartz AJ. A comparison of observational studies and randomized, controlled trials. [see comment]. *New England Journal of Medicine* 2000; 342(25):1878–1886.

101. Ottenbacher KJ. Statistical conclusion validity. Multiple inferences in rehabilitation research. *American Journal of Physical Medicine & Rehabilitation* 1991; 70(6):317–322.

102. Ottenbacher KJ, Barrett KA. Statistical conclusion validity of rehabilitation research. A quantitative analysis. *American Journal of Physical Medicine & Rehabilitation* 1990; 69(2):102–107.

103. Zhan S, Ottenbacher KJ. Single subject research designs for disability research. [Review] [32 refs]. *Disability & Rehabilitation* 2001; 23(1):1–8.

104. Jenkins LW, Peters GW, Dixon CE, Zhang X, Clark RS, Skinner JC, et al. Conventional and functional proteomics using large format two-dimensional gel electrophoresis 24 hours after controlled cortical impact in postnatal day 17 rats. *Journal of Neurotrauma* 2002; 19(6):715–740.

105. Marciano P, Eberwine JH, Raghupathi R, McIntosh TK. The assessment of genomic alterations using DNA arrays following traumatic brain injury: a review. [Review] [69 refs]. *Restorative Neurology & Neuroscience* 2001; 18(2–3):105–113.

106. Ricker JH, Hillary FG, DeLuca J. Functionally activated brain imaging (O–15 PET and fMRI) in the study of learning and memory after traumatic brain injury. [Review] [54 refs]. *Journal of Head Trauma Rehabilitation* 2001; 16(2):191–205.

107. Bigler ED. Quantitative magnetic resonance imaging in traumatic brain injury. [Review] [47 refs]. *Journal of Head Trauma Rehabilitation* 2001; 16(2):117–134.

108. Brooks WM, Friedman SD, Gasparovic C. Magnetic resonance spectroscopy in traumatic brain injury. [Review] [105 refs]. *Journal of Head Trauma Rehabilitation* 2001; 16(2):149–164.

109. Bergsneider M, Hovda DA, McArthur DL, Etchepare M, Huang SC, Sehati N, et al. Metabolic recovery following human traumatic brain injury based on FDG–PET: time course and relationship to neurological disability. *Journal of Head Trauma Rehabilitation* 2001; 16(2):135–148.

110. Wallace BE, Wagner AK, Wagner EP, McDeavitt JT. A history and review of quantitative electroencephalography in traumatic brain injury. [Review] [95 refs]. *Journal of Head Trauma Rehabilitation* 2001; 16(2):165–190.

111. Dixon CE, Lighthall JW, Anderson TE. Physiologic, histopathologic, and cineradiographic characterization of a new fluid-percussion model of experimental brain injury in the rat. *Journal of Neurotrauma* 1988; 5(2):91–104.

112. Dixon CE, Clifton GL, Lighthall JW, Yaghmai AA, Hayes RL. A controlled cortical impact model of traumatic brain injury in the rat. *Journal of Neuroscience Methods* 1991; 39(3):253–262.

113. Kochanek PM, Marion DW, Zhang W, Schiding JK, White M, Palmer AM, et al. Severe controlled cortical impact in rats: assessment of cerebral edema, blood flow, and contusion volume. *Journal of Neurotrauma* 12, 1015–1025. 1995.

114. Hamm RJ, Dixon CE, Gbadebo DM, Singha AK, Jenkins LW, Lyeth BG, et al. Cognitive deficits following traumatic brain injury produced by controlled cortical impact. *Journal of Neurotrauma* 1992; 9(1):11–20.

115. Whalen MJ, Clark RS, Dixon CE, Robichaud P, Marion DW, Vagni V, et al. Reduction of cognitive and motor deficits after traumatic brain injury in mice deficient in poly(ADP-ribose) polymerase. *Journal of Cerebral Blood Flow & Metabolism* 1999; 19(8):835–842.

116. Kline AE, Massucci JL, Marion DW, Dixon CE. Attenuation of working memory and spatial acquisition deficits after a delayed and chronic bromocriptine treatment regimen in rats subjected to traumatic brain injury by controlled cortical impact. *Journal of Neurotrauma* 2002; 19(4):415–425.

117. Wagner AK, Willard LA, Kline AE, Wenger MK, Bolinger BD, Ren D, et al. Evaluation of estrous cycle state and gender on behavioral outcome after experimental traumatic brain injury. *Brain Research* 998(1), 113–121. 2004.

118. Wagner AK, Kline AE, Sokoloski J, Ma X, Zafonte RD, Dixon CE. Environmental enrichment after experimental brain trauma enhances cognitive recovery in males but not females. *Neuroscience Letters*. 334, 165–168. 2002.

119. Taub E, Uswatte G, Elbert T. New treatments in neurorehabilitation founded on basic research. [Review] [92 refs]. *Nature Reviews Neuroscience* 2002; 3(3):228–236.

120. NIH Consensus Development Panel on Rehabilitation of Persons with Traumatic Brain Injury. Rehabilitation of Persons with Traumatic Brain Injury. *JAMA*. 282(10), 974–983. 9–8–1999.

121. NIDRR Long Range Plan. http://www.ncddr.org/new/announcements/nidrr_lrp/index.html. 2004.

122. TBI model system. http://www.tbindc.org/. 2004.

123. Bushnik T. Introduction: the Traumatic Brain Injury Model Systems of Care. *Archives of Physical Medicine & Rehabilitation* 2003; 84(2):151–152.

124. Heatlhy People 2010. http://www.healthypeople.gov. 2004.

125. National Institutes of Health. NIH Roadmap. http://nihroadmap.nih.gov/. 2003.

II

EPIDEMIOLOGY, PREVENTION, NEUROPATHOLOGY, AND NEURAL RECOVERY

6 The Epidemiology of TBI: Implications for Public Health

David J. Thurman
Victor Coronado
Anbesaw Selassie

INTRODUCTION

In the United States, traumatic brain injury (TBI) has been associated with more than 50,000 deaths annually, which is a third of all injury-related deaths. In addition, annually there are some 230,000 hospitalizations for nonfatal TBI, with an estimated 80,000 resulting in long-term disability (1). The incidence of TBI in the world population is unknown, but its magnitude is suggested by the *Global Burden of Disease Study* (2), which estimated the incidence of several categories of TBI severe enough to warrant medical care or result in death. For 1990, the estimates totaled over 9,500,000, but this may be conservative, as some categories (e.g., fall-related TBIs with short-term consequences) were not included. The uncertainty of these estimates notwithstanding, TBI clearly imposes a great burden on public health throughout the world. The purpose of this chapter is to characterize this burden by summarizing studies of the epidemiology of TBI, emphasizing findings about its frequency, risk factors, severity, and outcomes in populations. An understanding of the epidemiology of TBI is essential for developing effective prevention programs and for planning appropriate health care services for those injured.

DEFINITIONS

Traumatic Brain Injury

Case definitions for TBI have varied among epidemiologic studies, creating some difficulties in comparing their findings (3). For example, not all of the studies have included cases with skull fracture that lacked other documentation of neurologic symptoms or brain injury per se. In addition, the term "head injury" has often been used in place of TBI. An effort to standardize the epidemiologic case definition of TBI (as well as methods of data collection) led to the publication of *Guidelines for Surveillance of Central Nervous System Injury* by the Centers for Disease Control and Prevention (CDC) in 1995 (4). The CDC defined TBI as craniocerebral trauma, specifically, an occurrence of injury to the head (arising from blunt or penetrating trauma or from acceleration/deceleration forces) that is associated with any of these symptoms attributable to the injury: decreased level of consciousness, amnesia, other neurologic or neuropsychologic abnormalities, skull fracture, diagnosed intracranial lesions, or death.*

The guidelines also provided a standard case definition for data systems, which includes International Classification of Diseases, Ninth Revision (ICD-9) (5), or International Classification of Diseases, Ninth Revision, Clinical Modification (ICD-9-CM) (6), diagnostic codes in the ranges 800.0–801.9, 803.0–804.9, and 850.0–854.1 for cases regardless of survival status, with the addition of codes 873.0–873.9, 905.0, and 907.0 for cases resulting in death. Since the publication of the guidelines, most surveillance of TBI in the United States has relied on these definitions (7,8).

Severity

In epidemiologic reports, TBI severity refers to the amount of acute disruption of brain physiology or structure. Assessments of severity derive from clinical evaluations conducted early in the course of acute medical care; sometimes they also take into account the results of neuroimaging tests. Epidemiologic studies have used various classifications of TBI severity, such as the Glasgow Coma Scale (GCS) (9), the Abbreviated Injury Severity Scale (AIS) (10), and ICDMAP (11,12), an approximation of the AIS based on ICD-9-CM diagnostic codes. Severity is of interest to the extent that it helps to predict the course and eventual outcome of the injury, but should not be confused with outcome.

The ordinal categories of these severity scales are sometimes combined into the broader categories of mild (or minor), moderate, and severe TBI (13,14). Defining the boundaries of these categories has been difficult, especially defining the minimum criteria of a mild TBI. To address the latter issue, CDC recently convened an expert panel; the consensus-based definition they developed may be summarized as follows:

Mild TBI is an injury to the head (arising from blunt trauma or acceleration or deceleration forces) that results in one or more of the following: any period of confusion, disorientation, or impaired consciousness; any dysfunction of memory around the time of injury; loss of consciousness lasting less than 30 minutes; or the onset of observed signs or symptoms of neurological or neuropsychological dysfunction (15).

The term "mild" can be misleading if interpreted to mean inconsequential injury or injury with only minimal and transient effects. Clinical data indicate that some mild injuries have significant sequelae; the frequency with which these occur among people experiencing mild TBI remains to be determined by epidemiologic studies.

Outcome

TBI outcome refers to survival status after injury and to the extent of impairment and disability after there has been an opportunity for recovery. Because of methodologic difficulties, relatively few epidemiologic studies have addressed TBI outcomes. Some of these have used the Glasgow Outcome Scale (GOS), a five-point ordinal measure of global outcome (16).

Incidence and Prevalence

The measurement of TBI incidence (rate of occurrence of new cases) and prevalence (proportion of a population with TBI-related disability) requires population-based studies focused either on the entire population of interest or a representative sample of that population. Such epidemiological studies differ from descriptive studies of hospital case series, which constitute most of the clinical literature on TBI. Clearly, the latter cannot be assumed to reflect the entire population of persons with brain injury. Thus, such case series cannot accurately describe incidence rates or distribution of risk factors, causes, or severity in the entire population.

Public Health Surveillance

Surveillance is the ongoing, systematic collection and analysis of information to monitor health problems (17,18). Recent TBI surveillance has often focused on temporal trends in the incidence of these injuries (8,19).

METHODOLOGICAL ISSUES

Availability of Data

Several data sources in the United States provide quantitative data for population-based assessment of TBI (20). The most easily obtainable of these sources are designed for other administrative purposes, e.g., hospital billing, and thus they contain only limited information regarding the clinical manifestations and causes of TBI. The information they include can sometimes be enhanced by linkage with other data sources, e.g., data abstracted separately from medical records. The following data sources

---

*The CDC case definition of TBI was developed as a tool for public health surveillance, not clinical practice. As such, it attempts to identify not only cases of craniocerebral trauma where transient or persistent sequelae are noted but also cases where sequelae are possible. For this reason, the definition includes skull fractures in which medical records lack indications of neurologic injury per se, and also includes mild injuries in which records document only minimal and transient neurologic symptoms. The definition does not assume that the outcomes in such cases are necessarily adverse or of significant neurologic effect.

are widely available and useful for epidemiologic studies or surveillance.

Mortality The National Center for Health Statistics (NCHS) collects death certificate data from vital statistics records from all U.S. states and territories. These Multiple Causes of Death Data (MCDD) include information on demographics as well as the nature and external causes of injury, coded according to the International Classification of Diseases. The recent tenth revision of this classification (ICD-10) (21), incorporated major changes by forming new cause-of-death titles and codes and a restructuring of the leading causes of death (22). The effect of these changes on the comparability of mortality data collected before and after the implementation of ICD-10 has not yet been evaluated.

Most countries that belong to the World Health Organization (WHO) maintain some form of national death records using the ICD coding system. In general, developed countries have more reliable reporting systems than less-developed countries. Thus, comparisons of TBI mortality between countries must be made with caution, taking into account variability in the completeness of reporting systems and coding criteria.

Morbidity Developed countries often have national or regional data sets that allow descriptions of TBI-related hospital admissions, accurate to the extent that coding practices and reporting are reliable in individual hospitals. International comparisons of TBI using hospital discharge data systems are possible when uniform case definitions are used. The WHO *Standards for Surveillance of Neurotrauma* (23) contains such case definitions; these are consistent with CDC case definitions. The WHO Department of Injuries and Violence Prevention Program has many collaborating nations that provide aggregate data for international comparisons.

In the United States, the availability of such morbidity data is limited because the health care system is not centralized. Even so, several U.S. data sources are available:

The National Health Interview Survey (NHIS), conducted by NCHS, is an annual interview of a sample of households that in some years includes supplemental questions on injury. These allow estimates of TBI incidence, stratified by the level of care received (e.g., physician visit, hospital emergency department visit, or hospital admission). Survey data are limited by the accuracy of the information recalled by respondents.

The National Hospital Discharge Survey (NHDS), also conducted by NCHS, is an annual survey of patient discharges from a sample of

nonfederal hospitals. NHDS provides information on primary diagnosis and up to six secondary diagnoses, length of stay, payer information, and demographics. This enables estimates of the incidence of TBIs that result in hospital admission.

Many states aggregate claims data for hospital care to create hospital discharge data (HDD) sets. These data are standardized and coded according to the Uniform Billing form (UB-92), promulgated in 1992 by the U.S. Health Care Financing Administration (now the Center for Medicare and Medicaid Services). As long as states require all hospitals within their jurisdiction to report these data, HDD sets can enable reliable estimates of the incidence of TBI-related hospital discharges, and thus, they have become increasingly popular as primary sources of information for surveillance. These administrative claims data provide only limited information, however. In some state surveillance programs, additional information on severity, circumstances of injury, and short-term outcome is obtained by abstracting medical records in a representative sample of TBI cases identified from HDD sets.

Some emergency department data are also available with which to estimate the incidence of TBI among persons not admitted to hospitals. Since 1992, the NCHS's National Hospital Ambulatory Medical Care Survey (NHAMCS) has included a national sample of visits to emergency and outpatient departments of noninstitutional general and short-stay hospitals (24). In addition, some states maintain aggregate statewide emergency department visit data sets that can also be used for estimates of TBI incidence.

The NCHS National Ambulatory Medical Care Survey (NAMCS), another annual survey, provides information on ambulatory medical care provided by offices of physicians who are not federally employed. Although this data source affords some opportunity to estimate the incidence of injuries treated in an outpatient setting, the accuracy of physician office coding for specific diagnoses such as TBI has not been evaluated.

In many states, data on outpatient visits are available from state employee and workers' compensation insurance programs. These data sources provide detailed information on outpatient encounters for subscribers and their families. These sources may have limited use for the surveillance of minor injuries.

Quality of Data Sources

The quality of the data that come from vital and health care data systems is limited for several reasons. First, because such data sets are often collected for nonresearch purposes, such as reimbursement, they may omit some important clinical information, such as indicators of outcome. Second, these data are often collected on a large scale and recorded, coded, and transcribed by many persons with varying degrees of skill. Third, diagnostic coding may reflect a need to maximize reimbursement. Finally, many hospitals and health care systems may lack the means to validate the coding derived from the medical record and ensure high quality data.

The availability of medical care and medical technologies, the integration of health care systems, the quality of the public health infrastructure (including vital records and medical examiner or coroner systems), and the availability of information technologies can all affect the completeness of TBI diagnosis and reporting. Not surprisingly, these vary greatly among nations and regions, and thus, international comparisons of TBI have to be carefully interpreted with consideration given to bias in case-ascertainment and information.

Although mortality data systems are less prone to error from duplicate reports, morbidity data aggregated from HDD sets may be subject to overreporting due to hospital readmissions and inter-hospital transfers, unless data can be linked to identify these occurrences.

The incompleteness of data elements that are critical for understanding TBI occurrence is a major problem in hospital discharge and emergency department data systems. ICD-9-CM external-cause-of-injury coding (E-coding) is usually incomplete in hospital discharge data sets (25,26), rarely exceeding 90 percent unless augmented by medical record review. In addition, the 5th-digits of ICD-9-CM codes, which provide additional clinical detail, are often incomplete. These are particularly useful, if coded correctly, to assess severity. Other crucial data that are often missing include source of admission, secondary payers, secondary E-codes that describe place of occurrence, and information regarding impairments and disability noted at the time of hospital discharge.

Finally, there are substantial limitations in the quality of clinical information that health care providers record, upon which accurate ICD-9-CM coding (including 5th digit information) depends. Notably, Glasgow Coma Scale scores are not recorded in about 40 percent of hospital medical records of people with TBI (8). Sometimes this is due to inherent difficulties in applying the GCS; for example, it may be difficult to assign an accurate score in the presence of injury complications or medical interventions such as periorbital swelling, intubation, or the use of drugs (e.g., sedatives or paralytic agents). Also, the GCS does not account for the amount of stimulation needed to obtain a response, which may affect its reproducibility (27). In addition, the GCS is often not scored at consistent intervals following injury. Furthermore, numeric scales that are ordinal in nature, such as the GCS, are not linear. Thus, a 1-point change in a lower range of these scales may not represent the same degree of functional change as a 1-point change in a higher range (28). As well, the apparent simplicity of the GCS is misleading because it can be interpreted variously, even among neurosurgeons (29). Finally, its predictive value, especially when applied early, is limited (30).

PUBLISHED POPULATION-BASED STUDIES

Trends in TBI Incidence—United States

The incidence rates reported in selected epidemiological studies of TBI-related hospitalizations or TBI-related hospitalizations and death in U.S. localities are summarized in Table 6-1 (7, 8, 31–45). The rates should be compared with caution, because criteria for including cases and the use of rate adjustments vary (3). Still, these studies suggest that rates of TBI related hospitalization have decreased substantially in the last two decades.

From 1979 through 1992, the TBI-associated death rate in the United States decreased 22 percent, from 24.6 per 100,000 population to 19.3 per 100,000 (46). Most of the decrease resulted from a 42 percent decline in motor vehicle-related deaths, from 11.4 per 100,000 in 1979 to 6.6 per 100,000 in 1992. During the same period, firearm-related TBI deaths increased 9 percent, from 7.7 to 8.5 per 100,000, thus surpassing transportation crashes as the leading cause of TBI mortality. Rates of TBI-associated death due to falls and other causes decreased slightly during this period.

In contrast, an analysis of data from the NHDS for 1980 through 1995 documented a steep decline of 51 percent in TBI-related hospital discharge rates; they decreased from 199 to 98 per 100,000 per year over this period (47). The decline in rates of discharge occurred mainly among injuries classified as non-life-threatening. A comparison of findings in the 1979–1992 and the 1980–1995 analyses indicates a disproportionately large reduction in rates of nonfatal TBI resulting in hospitalization. This decrease may reflect some success in injury prevention, but it appears also to be the result of recent changes in admission policies that discourage inpatient care for less severe injuries (47). The apparent shift away from inpatient care underscores the need for surveillance of TBI patients treated in emergency departments and other outpatient settings.

TBI-Related Hospitalizations and Deaths—Other Countries

The incidence rates reported in selected epidemiological studies of TBI-related hospitalizations or TBI-related hospitalizations and death are shown for other developed

TABLE 6-1
Selected U.S. Studies of TBI Incidence

| Year Completed | Location | Rate / 100,000 | Cases Included* | | | Investigators |
			A	B	C	
1974	Olmsted Co., Minnesota	193	X	X	X	Annegers et al. (31)
1974	United States	200	X	X		Kalsbeek et al. (32)
1978	San Diego Co., California	294	X	X	X	Klauber et al. (33)
1978	North Central Virginia	175	X	X		Jagger et al. (34)
1980	Inner-city Chicago, Illinois	403	X	X	X	Whitman et al. (35)
1980	Rhode Island	152	X	X		Fife et al. (36)
1981	United States	136	X	X		Fife (37)
1981	Bronx, New York	249	X	X	X	Cooper et al. (38)
1981	San Diego Co., California	180	X	X	X	Kraus et al. (39)
1986	Maryland	132	X	X	X	MacKenzie et al. (40)
1992	Utah	108	X	X	X	Thurman et al. (41)
1992	Colorado	101	X	X	X	Gabella et al. (42)
1993	Colorado, Missouri, Oklahoma, and Utah	102	X	X	X	Centers for Disease Control and Prevention (43)
1993	Alaska	130	X	X		Warren et al. (44)
1993	Iowa	93	X	X	X	Schootman et al. (45)
1994	Seven states†	92	X	X	X	Thurman et al. (7)
1997	Fourteen states‡	70	X			Langlois et al. (8)

* TBI cases reported include: A, live hospital discharges; B, hospital inpatient fatalities; C, non-hospitalized fatalities (determined from vital records).

† Arizona, Colorado, Minnesota, Missouri, New York (excluding New York City), Oklahoma, and South Carolina.

‡ Alaska, Arizona, California, Colorado, Louisiana, Maryland, Minnesota, Missouri, Nebraska, New York, Oklahoma, Rhode Island, South Carolina, and Utah.

TABLE 6-2
Selected International Studies of TBI Incidence in Developed Countries

Year Finished	Location	Incidence Rate*	Investigators
1974	Scotland	313	Jennet and MacMillan (48)
1974	Akershus County, Norway	236	Nestvold et al. (49)
1980	Trøndelag, Norway	200	Edna and Cappelen (50)
1986	Aquitaine, France	281	Tiret et al. (51)
1987	South Australia, Australia	322	Hillier et al. (52)
1988	New South Wales, Australia	100	Tate et al. (53)
1988	Cantabria, Spain	91	Vazquez-Barquero et al. (54)
1993	Finland	97	Alaranta et al. (55)
1993	Denmark	157	Engberg and Teasdale (56)

* TBI-related hospitalizations or both hospitalizations and deaths per 100,000 population per year.

countries (48–56) in Table 6-2 and developing countries (57–61) in Table 6-3. Variations in case definitions, criteria for hospital admission, access to hospital care, and quality of national or regional health data sources, as well as different methods of identifying cases and collecting data hinder comparisons between these studies. These problems are especially difficult in developing countries (62). At present, there are too few published studies to form confident conclusions about TBI incidence worldwide or to describe international trends. Population-based studies from South Africa, India, and Taiwan suggest higher rates in developing countries, however, with a predominance of road traffic injuries, but clearly more data are needed. The dissemination and adoption of international standards for TBI surveillance such as those published by WHO (23) should improve the amount and quality of international data.

TABLE 6-3
Selected International Studies of TBI Incidence in Developing Countries

Year Finished	Location	Incidence Rate	Investigators
1983	Six cities, China	55*	
1985	Rural areas, China	64*	Zhao and Wang (57)
1986–1987	Johannesburg, South Africa	316†	Brown and Nell (58)
			Nell and Brown 59)
1991–1992	Bangalore, India	122†	Gururaj (60)
1988–1994	Taipei, Taiwan	220†	Chiu et al. (61)

* TBIs reported by household survey, number per 100,000 population per year.
† TBI-related hospitalizations or both hospitalizations and deaths per 100,000 population per year.

Recent Epidemiological Findings from the United States

Mortality   A recent report from the CDC summarizes information on TBI deaths, using data from NCHS MCDD collected from 1989 through 1998 (19). During that decade, an annual average of 53,288 deaths were associated with TBI, a rate of 20.6 per 100,000 population. During this interval, TBI-related death rates declined 11.4 percent, from 21.9 to 19.4 per 100,000. Most of these deaths were related to firearms, transportation (involving motor vehicle occupants, pedestrians, bicyclists, motorcyclists, and others), or falls.

According to this CDC study, death rates among males were 3.4 times as high as among females (33.0 per 100,000 males and 9.8 per 100,000 females). Rates were highest among persons aged 75 years and older, with a smaller peak among those aged 15–24 years. The leading causes of TBI-associated death varied with age, with firearm-related injuries ranking first among persons aged 20–74 years, transportation-related injuries first among those under 20, and falls the leading cause among persons 75 and older. Rates for males were consistently higher than those for females: for firearm-related rates they were 6 times as high (14.5 versus 2.4 per 100,000); motor vehicle-related rates, over 2.3 times as high (9.9 versus 4.3 per 100,000); and fall-related rates, 2.5 times as high (3.2 versus 1.2 per 100,000). TBI-associated death rates for the 1989–1998 period differed by race as well: per 100,000 they were 27.2 for American Indians and Alaska Natives, 25.0 for African Americans; 20.1 for whites; and 11.9 for all other racial groups combined.

Morbidity and Mortality   In the last decade, CDC has supported statewide surveillance of TBI-related hospitalizations and deaths in several states, using standard case definitions and methods noted above. An epidemiologic analysis of TBIs occurring in 1994 in Arizona, Colorado, Minnesota, Missouri, Oklahoma, New York (excluding New York City), and South Carolina (7) revealed an annual incidence rate of TBI for the combined population of 91.8 per 100,000 (age adjusted to the 1990 U.S. population). This rate included TBI-related deaths (20.7 per 100,000), leaving an age-adjusted rate of 71.1 per 100,000 TBI-related live hospital discharges. For hospitalizations and fatalities combined, the median age at the time of injury was 32 years. The incidence rate was highest among persons 75 years and older (191.1 per 100,000) and among persons aged 15–24 years (145.1 per 100,000) (Figure 6-1). Two-thirds of TBIs (66.7 percent) occurred among males, with the crude rate among males about twice that among females (124.1 versus 59.1 per 100,000).

Transportation-related crashes (involving motor vehicles, bicycles, pedestrians, and recreational vehicles) accounted for 49 percent of all TBIs in the seven states; falls accounted for an additional 26 percent (Figure 6-2). Firearm use accounted for another 10 percent, and assaults not involving firearms accounted for 8 percent. Nearly two-thirds of firearm-related TBIs (66.5 percent) were classified as suicidal in intent. The leading causes of TBI varied by age in the seven states (Figure 6-3); falls were by far the leading cause among persons aged 75 years and older (126.6 per 100,000), while transportation-related crashes led the list for persons aged 15–24 (97.9 per 100,000).

A more recent report describes similar findings for nonfatal brain injuries admitted to hospitals in 14 states during 1997 (8).* The age-adjusted TBI-related live hospital discharge rate for this 14-state population was 69.7 per 100,000, with age and sex distributions similar to those described in the earlier report from seven states. The more recent report describes differences in age-adjusted rates of TBI by race, with somewhat higher rates among American Indians/Alaska Natives (76.7 per 100,000) and African Americans (74.2 per 100,000) than among whites (63.0 per 100,000).

---

*Alaska, Arizona, California, Colorado, Louisiana, Maryland, Minnesota, Missouri, Nebraska, New York, Oklahoma, Rhode Island, South Carolina, and Utah.

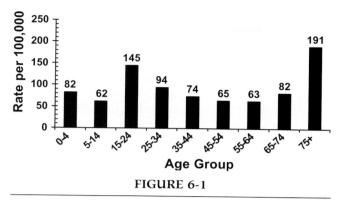

FIGURE 6-1

Rates of TBI-related hospitalization and death by age group*—seven states,† 1994

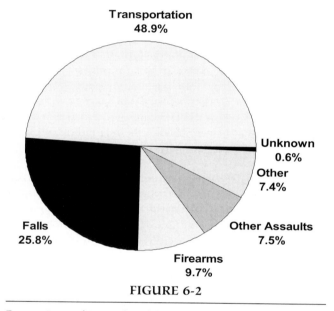

FIGURE 6-2

Proportions of TBI-related hospitalizations and deaths by external cause—seven states,† 1994

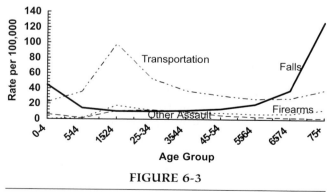

FIGURE 6-3

Rates of TBI-related hospitalization and death by age group and external cause of injury*—seven states,† 1994

---

* Rates not adjusted by sex.
† AZ, CO, MN, MO, NY (excluding NYC), OK, and SC.

Nonfatal TBIs Not Admitted to Hospitals   In the United States, the NCHS's NHIS has provided some information on TBI treated on an outpatient basis (63). In 1991, an estimated 1.54 million noninstitutionalized U.S. civilians sustained a brain injury that resulted in loss of consciousness but was not severe enough to cause death or long-term institutionalization, according to self-reported NHIS data collected with the 1991 Injury Supplement. Of these 1.54 million persons, 25 percent received no medical care for their TBI; 49 percent, care in an emergency department or other outpatient site, and 9 percent, overnight hospital care; 16 percent were admitted to a hospital for 2 or more days. The limitations of the survey methods and respondent recall may limit the accuracy of these estimates. Data from the NHAMCS of 1995–1996 may provide a more accurate estimate of the incidence of nonfatal TBIs in which the patient was treated and released from hospital emergency departments (64). This analysis indicates an average annual incidence rate of 392 such emergency department visits per 100,000 population, or about 1 million visits annually.

Severity and Outcome   Several measures of TBI severity have been used in epidemiological studies. The case fatality rate, which is the proportion of cases resulting in death, is the simplest epidemiological measure of severity as well as outcome. In the study of TBI-related hospitalizations and deaths in seven states during 1994, (7) 22.6 percent of all reported TBIs were fatal within the acute period of injury. Of all persons with reported TBIs, 16.9 percent died without being admitted to a hospital, while 5.6 percent died while receiving acute inpatient care. The case fatality rate varies greatly by cause; in this study, 90.4 percent of firearm-related TBIs resulted in death, but only 10.2 percent of fall-related TBIs proved fatal.

In the analysis of NHDS data for 1980–1995 described earlier, the authors used ICDMAP-generated ICD/AIS scores to estimate the severity distributions of hospitalized cases (47). In the NHDS data for the last 2 years of the study period (1994–1995), 52 percent were *mild* (ICD/AIS score 2), 21 percent were *moderate* (ICD/AIS score 3), 19 percent were *severe* (ICD/AIS score 4–6), and 7 percent were unknown. The proportion of TBIs classified as mild among the 1994–95 cases was considerably smaller than the corresponding proportion of 1980–1981 cases and was also smaller than proportions reported in earlier studies (3). These findings support a conclusion that persons in the United States with less severe TBI are now less likely to be admitted to the hospital.

Incidence of TBI-Related Disability   Few studies have addressed the incidence of TBI-related disability. From limited available epidemiological data, Kraus estimated that in 1990 about 83,000 or more U.S. residents were disabled by TBI. (3) The CDC published a similar estimate based on 1994 data from the NHDS and 1996–1997 data from the Colorado TBI Registry and Follow-up System (1, 65). The latter system surveyed TBI survivors one year after injury and measured long-term disability with the Functional Independence Measure (66). NHDS data indicate that during 1994, 230,000 persons hospitalized with TBI survived, and data from the Colorado TBI Registry and Follow-up System indicate that approximately 35 percent of hospitalized survivors of TBI are disabled 1 year after injury (7). Combining these figures suggests that more than 80,000 persons in the United States experience the onset of long-term disability each year following hospitalization for TBI. This estimate may be conservative, however, because it excludes the unknown number persons who are not hospitalized after TBI but still experience long-term disability as a consequence of their injury.

Prevalence of TBI-Related Disability   Despite the recent publication of reports on the incidence of TBI-related hospitalization in several countries, few reports are available on the population-based prevalence of TBI-related disability and relatively little of the published data was collected with sufficient rigor to enable confident estimates. Most studies of disability occurrence after TBI have examined series of patients admitted to research hospitals. Such studies, by not including persons hospitalized in nonresearch and community hospitals, may not be representative of the underlying population. In addition, they do not address the outcomes of TBIs that are treated only in hospital emergency departments. These limitations notwithstanding, several of such studies—reviewed in other chapters of this book—have a sufficiently broad inclusion of participants to permit important generalizations regarding outcomes following TBI-related admission. Such studies document high proportions of patients who experience long-term sequelae, including substantial psychosocial and physical disabilities that are often associated with cognitive impairments (67).

The information obtained from population-based follow-up studies in Colorado and South Carolina is expected to enable more accurate estimates of disability associated with those TBIs severe enough to warrant hospitalization. In addition, the CDC has provided a provisional estimate of the prevalence of disability from TBI in the United States, based on preliminary follow-up data from the Colorado TBI Registry and Follow-up System and historical and current estimates of national TBI incidence. Together these sources suggest that approximately 2 percent of the U.S. population (5.3 million in 1996) are living with disability as a result of a TBI. (7) This estimate does not, however, account for disability among people with TBI who visited emergency departments or outpatient clinics but were not admitted. Improvements

on this estimate can be expected as more data are obtained and analyzed from these studies.

Using Severity Indicators in TBI Surveillance to Predict Outcome   The Glasgow Coma Scale score is a widely used predictor of outcome, both mortality and disability (68–71), and yet its ability to predict the latter is limited in the population of TBI survivors who receive rehabilitation (72). Some research indicates that the prediction of the distribution of TBI disability outcomes in population-based studies may be improved by supplementing GCS data with information about computed tomography (CT) findings (73). Currently, state surveillance programs in the United States collect both GCS and CT scan data, but population distributions of severity based on the combination of these data elements have not yet been published. Other research has found predictive value in the duration of post-traumatic amnesia (74–78), and Nell and Yates proposed an enhancement of the GCS that incorporates a measure of duration of post-traumatic amnesia in persons with little or no depression of consciousness (79). Population-based studies that describe TBI severity with these measures have not yet been published; when available, such studies will help to predict the magnitude of ongoing health care needs among people with TBI.

Economic Costs   Max and colleagues, who analyzed 1985 U.S. incidence and cost data for TBIs that resulted in hospital admission or death (80), estimated that total lifetime costs for those injured were approximately $37.8 billion, with 12 percent for direct costs of medical care (hospital, extended, and other medical care and services); 55 percent, injury-related work loss and disability; and 34 percent, lost income resulting from premature death. A reexamination of this study that adjusted its estimates for inflation and more recent TBI incidence data, yielded total lifetime costs of $56.3 billion for injuries sustained in 1995 (81). New studies are needed that use recent healthcare cost data to update this estimate.

Studies of trends in the economic cost of TBI are of particular interest in pubic health. The Model Systems Traumatic Brain Injury program, funded by the U.S. Department of Education's National Institute on Disability and Rehabilitation Research, collects data from multiple centers, enabling trend analyses of the cost of medical care for enrolled TBI patients. A recent study indicates that from 1990 to 1996, average daily inpatient charges in this group of patients increased by 98 percent for acute care and 41 percent for rehabilitation (82). During this interval, however, these increases were offset by reductions in average lengths of stay of 42 percent in acute care and 38 percent in rehabilitation. The authors note that the steady downward trends in length of stay for both acute care and rehabilitation raise concerns about diminishing availability of health care services to persons with

TBI. The generalizability of their findings is uncertain, however, because they came from a study population that was likely skewed toward more serious injuries. Still, these findings support the need for current population-based assessments of trends in costs and care for TBI.

APPLYING FINDINGS TO PUBLIC HEALTH: PREVENTING TBI

The evidence reviewed in this chapter makes clear the great importance of TBI to public health. Despite progress in reducing the incidence of these injuries—especially those associated with motor vehicle crashes (19,46)—the need for more effective primary prevention programs remains. To be most effective, such programs must be guided by current findings regarding the principal causes of TBI—transportation injuries, falls, and violence—as well as an understanding of populations at increased risk and individual risk factors.

Because the primary prevention of TBI occurrence is incomplete, an effective public health response to TBI also requires concerted programs to minimize adverse outcomes and disability. Such secondary and tertiary prevention comprises acute care and rehabilitation of persons with TBI, the subjects of other chapters in this book. To this end we need comprehensive strategies to ensure that people with TBI have access to appropriate care and services and we need effective policies to promote their independence and integration into the community.

To help persons living with deficits from TBI, we need better information on the nature and scope of these disabilities, including who experiences disability, which rehabilitation treatment methods are most effective, and what services are useful and readily available. Population-based follow-up surveillance is needed to provide more precise information on the longer-term impacts of these injuries. Standard measures for TBI outcomes need to be refined so they will readily identify the types of impairment and disability most amenable to prevention through rehabilitation and social support. Better understanding of the relationship between the initial severity of an injury and its long-term outcome will help identify those persons who need ongoing medical care, rehabilitation, and other services. Such information will also help health practitioners and policy makers ensure that these services are available in the community.

SUMMARY

This chapter has reviewed epidemiological measures and estimates of TBI incidence, severity, long-term outcomes, and cost. All of these findings indicate that these injuries have a major impact on public health. Effective primary prevention programs are needed that are informed by accurate epidemiologic data regarding causes and the populations at highest risk. Doing this requires improved public health data systems that record those TBIs that do not result in hospital admission as well as those that do. More basic and clinical research is needed to improve the acute care and rehabilitation of TBI. Finally, more epidemiological research regarding TBI outcomes and disability is needed to develop policies that will ensure the availability of effective acute care, rehabilitation, and other services that will minimize disability among injured persons and promote their reintegration into the community.

References

1. Centers for Disease Control and Prevention. *Traumatic Brain Injury in the United States: A Report to Congress.* Atlanta, GA: Centers for Disease Control and Prevention, 1999.
2. Murray C JL, Lopez AD. *Global Health Statistics: A Compendium of Incidence, Prevalence and Mortality Estimates for Over 200 Conditions.* Cambridge, MA: Harvard University Press, 1996.
3. Kraus JF, McArthur DL. Epidemiologic aspects of brain injury. *Neurol Clin* 1996;14:435–450.
4. Thurman DJ, Sniezek JE, Johnson D, et al. *Guidelines for Surveillance of Central Nervous System Injury.* Atlanta, GA: National Center for Injury Prevention and Control, Centers for Disease Control and Prevention, U.S. Department of Health and Human Services, 1995.
5. World Health Organization. *International Classification of Diseases,* 9th Revision. Geneva: World Health Organization, 1977.
6. U.S. Department of Health and Human Services. *International Classification of Diseases, 9th Revision, Clinical Modification,* 3rd Edition. Washington, D.C.: U.S. Department of Health and Human Services, 1989.
7. Thurman DJ, Alverson C, Dunn KA, Guerrero J, Sniezek JE. Traumatic brain injury in the United States: a public health perspective. *J Head Trauma Rehabil* 1999;14:602–615.
8. Langlois JA, Kegler SR, Butler JA, et al. Traumatic brain injury-related hospital discharges: results from a 14-state surveillance system, 1997. *MMWR* 2003;52(SS-4):1–20.
9. Teasdale G, Jennett B. Assessment of coma and impaired consciousness a practical scale. *Lancet* 1974;2:81–84.
10. Association for the Advancement of Automotive Medicine (AAAM), *The Abbreviated Injury Scale,* 1990 Revision. Des Plains, IL: Association for the Advancement of Automotive Medicine, 1990.
11. MacKenzie EJ, Steinwachs DM, Shankar B. Classifying trauma severity based on hospital discharge diagnoses. Validation of an ICD-9-CM to AIS-85 conversion table. *Med Care* 1989; 27:412–422.
12. Center for Injury Research and Policy of the Johns Hopkins University School of Public Health, *ICDMAP-90 Software.* Baltimore, MD: The Johns Hopkins University and Tri-Analytics, Inc., 1997.
13. Rimel RW, Giordani B, Barth JT, Boll TJ, Jane JA. Disability caused by minor head injury. *Neurosurgery* 1981;9:221–228.
14. Rimel RW, Giordani B, Barth JT, Jane JA. Moderate head injury: completing the clinical spectrum of brain trauma. *Neurosurgery* 1982;11:344–351.
15. CDC National Center for Injury Prevention and Control. *Report to Congress on Mild Traumatic Brain Injury in the United States: Steps to Prevent a Serious Public Health Problem.* Atlanta, GA: Centers for Disease Control and Prevention, 2003.
16. Jennett B, Bond M. Assessment of outcome after severe brain damage. *Lancet* 1975;1:480–484.
17. Buehler JW. Surveillance. In: Rothman K and Greenland S (eds.). *Modern Epidemiology,* 2nd Edition. Philadelphia: Lippincott-Raven, 1998, pp. 435–457.

18. Centers for Disease Control and Prevention. Updated guidelines for evaluating public health surveillance systems. *MMWR* 2001;50(RR-13):1–35.

19. Adekoya N, Thurman DJ, White DD, Webb KW. Surveillance for traumatic brain injury deaths—United States, 1989–1998. MMWR *Surveill Summ* 2002;51(10):1–14.

20. Gable CB. A compendium of public health data sources. *Am J Epidemiol* 1990;131:381–394.

21. World Health Organization. *International Statistical Classification of Diseases and Related Health Problems*, Tenth Revision. Geneva: World Health Organization, 1992.

22. Hoyert DL, Arias E, Smith BL, Murphy SL, Kochanek KD. Deaths: final data for 1999. *Nat Vital Stat Rep* 2001;49(8):1–113.

23. WHO Advisory Committee on Neurotrauma Prevention. *Standards for Surveillance of Neurotrauma*. Geneva, Switzerland: World Health Organization, 1996.

24. Ly N, McCaig LF. National Hospital Ambulatory Medical Care Survey: 2000 outpatient department summary. *Adv Data* 2002 (327):1–27.

25. Sniezek JE, Finklea JF, Graitcer PL. Injury coding and hospital discharge data. *JAMA* 1989;262:2270–2272.

26. Hall MJ, Owings MF. Hospitalizations for injury: United States, 1996. *Adv Data* 2000 (318):1–9.

27. Muizelaar JP, Marmarou A, De Salles AAF, et al. Cerebral blood flow and metabolism in severely head-injured children. Part 1: relationship with GCS score, outcome, ICP, and PVI. *J Neurosurg* 1989;71:63–71.

28. Stein SC. Classification of head injury. In Narayan RK, Wilberger JE, Povlishock JT (eds.): *Neurotrauma*. New York: McGraw-Hill, 1996, pp. 31–41.

29. Marion DW, Carlier PM. Problems with initial Glasgow Coma Scale assessment caused by prehospital treatment of patients with head injuries: results of a national survey. *J Trauma* 1994; 36:89–95.

30. Waxman K, Sundine MJ, Young RF. Is early prediction of outcome in severe head injury possible? *Arch Surg* 1991;126:1237–1241.

31. Annegers JF, Grabow HD, Kurland LT, Laws ER Jr. The incidence, causes and secular trends of head trauma in Olmsted County, Minnesota, 1935–1974. *Neurology* 1980;30:912–919.

32. Kalsbeek WD, McLaurin RL, Harris BS 3rd, Miller JD. The National Head and Spinal Cord Injury Survey: major findings. *J Neurosurg* 1980;53 (Suppl):19–31.

33. Klauber MR, Barrett-Connor E, Marshall LF, Bowers SA. The epidemiology of head injury: a prospective study of an entire community San Diego County, California, 1978. *Am J Epidemiol* 1981;113:500–509.

34. Jagger J, Levine Jl, Jane JA, Rimel RW. Epidemiologic features of head injury in a predominantly rural population. *J Trauma* 1984;24:40–44.

35. Whitman S, Coonley-Hoganson R, Desai BT. Comparative head trauma experience in two socioeconomically different Chicago-area communities: a population study. *Am J Epidemiol* 1984; 4:570–580.

36. Fife D, Faich G, Hollinshead W, Boynton W. Incidence and outcome of hospital-treated head injury in Rhode Island. *Am J Public Health* 1986;76:773–778.

37. Fife D. Head injury with and without hospital admission: comparisons of incidence and short-term disability. *Am J Public Health* 1987;77:810–812.

38. Cooper KD, Tabaddor K, Hauser WA, et al. The epidemiology of head injury in the Bronx. *Neuroepidemiol* 1983;2:70–88.

39. Kraus JF, Black MA, Hessol N, et al. The incidence of acute brain injury and serious impairment in a defined population. *Am J Epidemiol* 1984;119:186–201.

40. MacKenzie EJ, Edelstein SL, Flynn JP. Hospitalized head-injured patients in Maryland: incidence and severity of injuries. *Md Med J* 1989;38:725–32.

41. Thurman DJ, Jeppson L, Burnett CL, Beaudoin DE, Rheinberger MM, Sniezek JE. Surveillance of traumatic brain injuries in Utah. *West J Med* 1996;164:192–196.

42. Gabella B, Hoffman RE, Marine WW, Stallones L. Urban and rural brain injuries in Colorado. *Ann Epidemiol* 1997: 7:207–12.

43. Centers for Disease Control and Prevention. Traumatic brain injury: Colorado, Missouri, Oklahoma, and Utah, 1990–1993. *MMWR* 1997:46:8–11.

44. Warren S, Moore M, Johnson MS. Traumatic head and spinal cord injuries in Alaska (1991–1993). *Alaska Med* 1995;37:11–19.

45. Schootman M, Harlan M, Fuortes L. Use of the capture–recapture method to estimate severe traumatic brain injury rates. *J Trauma* 2000;48:70–75.

46. Sosin DM, Sniezek JE, Waxweiler RJ. Trends in death associated with traumatic brain injury, 1979 through 1992. Success and failure. *JAMA* 1995;273:1778–1780.

47. Thurman DJ, Guerrero JL. Trends in hospitalization associated with traumatic brain injury. *JAMA* 1999;282:954–957.

48. Jennett B, MacMillan R. Epidemiology of head injury. *Br Med J* 1981;282: 101–104.

49. Nestvold K, Lundar T, Blikra G, Lonnum A. Head injuries during one year in a central hospital in Norway: a prospective study. Epidemiologic features. *Neuroepidemiol* 1988;7:134–144.

50. Edna TH. Cappelen J. Hospital admitted head injury. A prospective study in Trøndelag, Norway, 1979-80. *Scand J Soc Med* 1984. 12:7–14.

51. Tiret L, Hausherr E, Thicoipe M, et al. The epidemiology of head trauma in Aquitaine (France), 1986: a community-based study of hospital admissions and deaths. *Int J Epidemiol* 1990: 19:133–140.

52. Hillier SL, Hiller JE, Metzer J. Epidemiology of traumatic brain injury in South Australia. *Brain Inj* 1997;11:649–659.

53. Tate RL, McDonald S, Lulham JM. Incidence of hospital-treated traumatic brain injury in an Australian community. *Aust N Z J Public Health* 1998;22:419–423.

54. Vazquez-Barquero A, Vazquez-Barquero JL, Austin O, Pascual J, Gaite L, Herrera S. The epidemiology of head injury in Cantabria. *Eur J Epidemiol* 1992;8:832–837.

55. Alaranta H, Koskinen S, Leppanen L, Palomaki H. Nationwide epidemiology of hospitalized patients with first-time traumatic brain injury with special reference to prevention. *Wien Med Wochenschr* 2002;150:444–448.

56. Engberg Aa W, Teasdale TW. Traumatic brain injury in Denmark 1979–1996. A national study of incidence and mortality. *Eur J Epidemiol* 2001;17:437–442.

57. Zhao YD, Wang W. Neurosurgical trauma in People's Republic of China. *World J Surg* 2001;25:1202–1204.

58. Brown DS, Nell V. Epidemiology of traumatic brain injury in Johannesburg—I. Methodological issues in a developing country context. *Soc Sci Med* 1991;33:283–287.

59. Nell V, Brown DS. Epidemiology of traumatic brain injury in Johannesburg. II. Morbidity, mortality and etiology. *Soc Sci Med* 1991;33:289–296.

60. Gururaj G. An epidemiological approach to prevention-prehospital care and rehabilitation in neurotrauma. *Neurol India* 1995;43 (Suppl.): 95–106.

61. Chiu WT, Yeh KH, Li YC, Gan YH, Chen HY, Hung CC. Traumatic brain injury registry in Taiwan. *Neurol Res* 1997;19: 261–264.

62. Chiu WT, Laporte RE, Gururaj G, et al. Head Injury in developing countries. In Narayan RK, Wilberger JE Jr, Povlishock JT (eds.). *Neurotrauma*. New York: McGraw-Hill, 1996, pp. 36–42.

63. Sosin DM, Sniezek JE, Thurman DJ. Incidence of mild and moderate brain injury in the United States, 1991. *Brain Inj* 1996; 10:47–54.

64. Guerrero JL, Thurman DJ, Sniezek JE. Emergency department visits associated with traumatic brain injury: United States, 1995–1996. *Brain Inj* 2000;14:181–186.

65. Brooks CA, Gabella B, Hoffman R, Sosin D, Whiteneck G. Traumatic brain injury: designing and implementing a population-based follow-up system. *Arch Phys Med Rehabil* 1997;78 (8 Suppl):S26–S30.

66. Research Foundation, State University of New York. Guide for use of the uniform data set for medical rehabilitation including the functional independence measure (FIM) and functional assessment measure (FAM), version 4.0. Buffalo, New York: State University of New York, 1995.

67. NIH National Institute of Child Health and Human Development. *Report of the NIH Consensus Development Conference on the Rehabilitation of Persons with Traumatic Brain Injury.* Bethesda, MD: U.S. Department of Health and Human Services, 1999.

68. Levin HS, Gary HE Jr, Eisenberg HM, et al. Neurobehavioral outcome 1 year after severe head injury. Experience of the Traumatic Coma Data Bank. *J Neurosurg* 1990;73:699–709.

69. Zink BJ. Traumatic brain injury outcome: concepts for emergency care. *Ann Emerg Med* 2001;37:318–332.

70. Tilford JM, Simpson PM, Yeh TS , et al. Variation in therapy for pediatric head trauma patients. *Crit Care Med* 2001; 29:1056–1061.

71. White JR, Farukhi Z, Bull C, et al. Predictors of outcome in severely head-injured children. Crit Care Med 2001;29: 534–540.

72. Zafonte RD, Hammond FM, Mann NR, Wood DL, Black KL, Millis SR. Relationship between Glasgow coma scale and functional outcome. *Am J Phys Med Rehabil* 1996;75:364–369.

73. Williams DH, Levin HS, Eisenberg HM. Mild head injury classification. *Neurosurgery* 1990;27:422–428.

74. Levin HS, O'Donnell VM, Grossman RG. The Galveston Orientation and Amnesia Test. A practical scale to assess cognition after head injury. *J Nerv Ment Dis* 1979;167:675–684.

75. Katz DI, Alexander MP. Traumatic brain injury: Predicting course of recovery and outcome for patients admitted to rehabilitation. *Arch Neurol* 1994;51:661–670.

76. Wilson JT, Teasdale GM, Hadley DM, Wiedmann KD, Lang D. Post-traumatic amnesia: still a valuable yardstick. *J Neurol Neurosurg Psychiatry* 1994;57: 198–201.

77. McFarland K, Jackson L, Geffe G. Post-Traumatic amnesia: consistency-of-recovery and duration-to-recovery following traumatic brain impairment. *Clin Neuropsychol* 2001;15:59–68.

78. van der Naalt J, van Zomeren AH, Sluiter WJ, Minderhoud JM. One year outcome in mild to moderate head injury: the predictive value of acute injury characteristics related to complaints and return to work. *J Neurol Neurosurg Psychiat* 1999;66: 207–213.

79. Nell V, Yates DW, Kruger J. An extended Glasgow Coma Scale (GCS-E) with enhanced sensitivity to mild brain injury. *Arch Phys Med Rehabil* 2000;81:614–617.

80. Max W, MacKenzie EJ, Rice DP. Head injuries: costs and consequences. *J Head Trauma Rehabil* 1991;6:76–91.

81. Thurman DJ. The epidemiology and economics of head trauma. In Miller LP and Hayes RL (eds.). *Head Trauma: Basic, Preclinical, and Clinical Directions.* New York: John Wiley & Sons, 2001.

82. Kreutzer JS, Kolakowsky-Hayner SA, Ripley D, et al. Charges and lengths of stay for acute and inpatient rehabilitation treatment of traumatic brain injury 1990–1996. *Brain Inj* 2001;15:763–774.

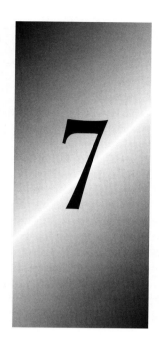

7 Primary Prevention

Elena Napolitano
Jeffrey Radecki
Elie P. Elovic

INTRODUCTION

The intent of this chapter is to review common prevention strategies and their overall effectiveness in this patient population, with an emphasis on the need for further preventative measures. The importance of these efforts will be obvious to readers after the following discussion that addresses the data on the incidence, severity, and consequences of traumatic brain injury (TBI).

Injury is the leading source of death for Americans under age 44 (1) and one-third of all injury-related deaths from 1979 to 1992 were associated with a TBI (2). Approximately 1.5 million Americans sustain a TBI every year (3). From 1979 to 1992, 50,000 American deaths and 230,000 hospitalizations occurred annually as a result of TBIs (2). In addition, each year over 80,000–90,000 people develop long-term disability secondary to TBI with approximately 14 million days of restricted activity secondary to TBI (4–6). The number of Americans who have some form of disability as a result of TBI is estimated to be around 5.3 million (7,8). The annual overall cost to the United States was estimated to be $37.8 billion in 1985 and $44 billion in 1988 (9).

In 1996, approximately 150,000 children and adolescents were left permanently disabled and in need of long-term follow-up as a result of unintentional injuries including brain and spinal cord injury (10). Injury mainly affects the younger population and encompasses more years of potential life lost than any other cause with estimates yearly totaling 3.5 million years (1). Most individuals who have sustained a TBI are unable to return to work and if they do return, their work capacity is limited. The estimated morbidity cost (injury related work loss and disability) was approximately $20.6 billion in 1985 (9).

There was a decrease in the incidence of TBI related death and hospitalization from 1979 to 1992. From 1974 to 1986, TBI incidence, morbidity, and death rate was approximately 50 percent higher than current estimates. Currently the TBI hospitalization incidence is about 100/100,000 (5). This differs from previous reports rates of 200/100,000 that were reported between 1974 and 1986 (7,11–13). The decrease may in part be a result of a decrease in severity of injury, overall change in admission policies, and a push to treat these injuries in the outpatient environment as well as possible benefit from prevention efforts. In 1980, the rate of TBI related mortality in the United States was 24.7/100,000; this had fallen 20 percent by 1994 to a rate of 19.8, with motor vehicle related mortality showing the greatest decline. With various prevention efforts such as use of air bags, seat belts, and child safety seats, mortality dropped 38 percent from 11.1 to 6.9/100,000 between 1980 and 1994.

TRAUMATIC BRAIN INJURY VS. OTHER DISABLING CONDITIONS

TBI has often been called the silent, or invisible, epidemic (7), a stepchild that has only received minimal public awareness and dedication of financial resources to its treatment and prevention. This is a grave mistake, as the annual incidence of TBI is greater than that of the more widely known conditions of spinal cord injury, breast cancer, multiple sclerosis, and HIV (See Figure 7-1.). For example, there are 50,000 deaths per year as a result of a traumatic brain injury versus 16,273 deaths reported in 1999 as a result of HIV (14). The mortality rate for HIV has dropped over the past few years, which can be mainly attributed to public awareness, dedication to preventative measures, research, and treatment. The same trend is potentially possible in TBI if efforts are directed to awareness and prevention. It may take multiple strategies, targeting various communities, to enhance public awareness (15). Meeting communities' individual needs can possibly lead to implementation of more effective preventative measures.

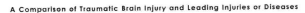

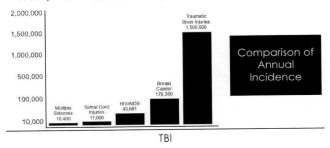

FIGURE 7-1

ECONOMICS OF TBI: COSTS, BURDEN, AND ITS PREVENTION

There are monumental economic costs associated with TBI, when one includes both direct medical care and indirect costs such as loss of productivity. It was estimated that in 1985 the lifetime cost of injury amounted to $38 billion for those injured enough to result in death or hospitalization (9). Ten years later, approximately $260 billion dollars was spent on injury in the United States (16).

With the growing medical costs in today's world, the cost/benefit ratio of a prevention program is an issue of importance. Some of the more accepted preventative measures such as Hepatitis B vaccinations in newborns, child safety belts, bicycle helmets, and smoke detectors have proven to be very cost effective. Injury prevention programs vary in their cost effectiveness; however, many of them have shown their worth. In regards to TBI, programs such as zero alcohol tolerance for drivers under 21 years of age and graduated licensing have also proven to be of benefit (1).

A study that examined the time and money spent counseling families of young children regarding injury prevention efforts, reported that $13 was saved for every dollar spent on counseling (17). Emphasis must be placed on community education for better public awareness. There appears to be a correlation between public awareness and the listener's educational level and income. This is an important point in patient education that should not be overlooked and should be factored into injury prevention programs.

There is a significant need to increase funding for prevention efforts. This may be problematic as funding may actually decrease as a result of an increased pressure to reduce spending by the federal government. As a result, it is probable that funding from the Preventative Health Services Block Grant will be reduced, which is a major funding source for injury prevention programs and chronic disease prevention (10).

WHAT IS PREVENTION?

Prevention can be subdivided into primary, secondary, and tertiary prevention. Primary prevention efforts are designed to prevent the actual injury. Examples of primary prevention include screening tests, fall-proofing homes, traffic laws and their enforcement, salting of ice-covered roads, and education on topics such as drinking and driving. Primary preventative measures has been shown to work with other conditions. Adjusting workstations for individual workers have had an impact on decreasing musculoskeletal disorders and injury from their use (18). Secondary prevention is described as lessening the impact of the damage resulting from injury. Examples include engineering methods, such as automobile seatbelts and airbags, which have had a significant effect at controlling injury (18). Developments of advanced trauma care and emergency management services are examples of tertiary prevention, with their purpose being to lessen the secondary sequalae of injury (1).

The USPS Task Force was a large four-year multidisciplinary effort to assess various preventative health measures. The summarized assessment contained 169 interventions in three different areas: screening, counseling and immunization/chemoprophylaxis. The predominant finding was that personal health behavior, such as smoking, diet and exercise, is the main contributor to mortality and disability. The task force emphasized the importance of physicians educating their patients while simultaneously giving them more responsibility for their own health. It was recommended that various strategies should be used to counsel the patients including support groups, written material and audiovisual aids (19).

INJURY CONTROL THEORY

Originally, the general belief was that TBI was a result of accidents, which implied that all persons had equal probability of sustaining injury (20,21). After a review of TBI epidemiology literature it appears that this may not be the case. Careful consideration must be made to a person's age, sex, and other individual risk factors that increase the likelihood of sustaining an injury (19). For example, falls among the elderly may be secondary to sedatives, antidepressants, lower extremity disability or balance impairments (5). There has been substantial work devoted to the identification of people at risk and developing effective preventive countermeasures (21,22) and as a result there has been a substantial increase in the science of injury control theory over the last 50 years

THE HADDON MATRIX

The Haddon Matrix is a model that divides injury into various components including a host, vector and the environment, both physical and social, that the host and vector interact within. An elderly person falling on the ice and breaking their hip can serve as an example. In this case, the host is the injured human, the vector the age of the person and the environment is the weather conditions during the time of injury.

Haddon also identifies three different phases of injury, the pre-injury, injury and post-injury phases. This is comparable to the primary, secondary and tertiary prevention efforts mentioned above (1). Using these sets of variables a table can be created where each cell represents an area and a temporal component. All the different variables that contribute to an injury can be placed into one of the table's cells.

To best illustrate this concept, consider the factors related to a motor vehicle accident in the preinjury phase. Age and alcohol use would be placed in the host pre-crash or pre-injury cell, the vector would include the condition of the vehicle and the environmental cell would contain the roadway design. The cell, which includes the socio-economic environment, takes into account the affordability to the consumer and their safety risks. It would account for risks associated with purchasing an older cheaper vehicle without safety features or poorer road handling capabilities.

By studying the epidemiology of injury, efforts can be made at breaking various injury patterns in the different phases. Potentially the most efficacious way to prevent an injury is to target the vector or injuring agent and thereby alter the mechanism of energy transmission. Creating better designed cars, better engineered roads and improving conditions of the vehicle would greatly impact injury prevention.

APPROACH TO HEALTH MAINTENANCE

To address the important issue of health maintenance there must be a comprehensive approach at controlling injury and promoting health. It must include passive and active strategies, education and legislation. Passive strategies include those in which the host does not have an active role in its use (23). By nature, they offer protection to a larger percentage of the population and have the advantage of demonstrating effect without requiring any effort by the host that requires protection (24). Some examples of these include airbags, road barriers, fingerprint based gunlocks and car safety engineering. Active strategies are ones that require the host's participation, with the donning of a seat belt, avoiding driving when under the influence, motorcycle helmet usage and car seats as examples. Active prevention is dependent upon the public's awareness of such measures and their overall compliance with them. It may take a tremendous amount of societal effort to encourage the host to adopt these active measures of prevention. While this is a disadvantage as compared to passive measures, their potential for increased efficacy makes them potentially both important and possibly extremely effective when used in combination with passive measures.

In regards to education, professional health organizations are groups comprised of individuals who have met a standard of training and whose purpose is to serve the public. It is only natural that these groups use their position and expertise to further educational efforts to educate the lay community. This can be implemented through journals, publications and testimonies to legislative groups. The American Cancer Society, founded in 1913, is an example of a nonprofit voluntary health agency, organized to spread knowledge about cancer and is supported by voluntary donation (25). The Center for Disease Control is a federal agency responsible for surveillance of communicable diseases in the United States, investigation of epidemic diseases and promotes immunization and health education programs (18). On a smaller scale, education at the community and individual level by both physicians and other health care professionals must be emphasized as it can have a tremendous impact on injury prevention (15).

In general, changing human behavior can be a very challenging endeavor and there is still some controversy on the appropriate approach. Haddon stated that targeting the vector with passive interventions and the environment may be the most effective in decreasing death and injury. This does not negate the potential benefit of using a combined approach, of active and passive measures of intervention. An example of this is the use of seatbelts in combination with airbags. Each prevention method has shown its benefit, however using both together has been shown to be more effective than either one by themselves.

If one factors in legislation, to increase compliance with active prevention efforts further benefits can be attained. The states that strengthened existing seatbelt laws and adopted primary enforcement seatbelt legislation had an estimated 79 percent compliance with belt use in 1998. This was an increase from 62 percent seat belt compliance in 1992 prior to the addition of primary enforcement legislation (1,26).

DEVELOPMENT OF A COMPREHENSIVE INJURY PREVENTION PROGRAM

The components critical to development of a comprehensive injury prevention program are active and passive strategies, education and legislation. Engineering solutions are an important component of the passive interventions and include items such as energy absorbing car bodies, road barriers and air bags. Active strategies, such as education, are also critical, both at the individual and community level (1). Some of the most effective interventions include hands on demonstrations and reinforcement at subsequent visits (27). However, the listener is more inclined to change their behavior if there is some incentive to do so.

It has been shown that if only education is used then the general public may not change their overall behavior (28). Community based intervention programs combining education with legislative options has been shown to be effective in increasing bicycle helmet usage (15). Work performed in three separate Maryland counties explored bike helmet usage by children under three separate conditions. In one county, helmet use improved significantly when education and legislation were combined (43 percent increase). Another county, which used education alone, showed only an 11 percent increase, which was not statistically significant (29). The third county, which did nothing, actually demonstrated a decreased rate of helmet use from 19 to 4 percent.

Enforcement of legislation is critical to maximize its potential benefit, with seatbelts being an example. By 1984 passenger cars were required to have seatbelts, but only 15 percent of people used them while driving. By 1987 education combined with seatbelt legislation increased this rate to 42 percent. This was further increased to 62 percent when secondary enforcement laws were enacted for nonuse. A secondary enforcement law is one that allows the giving of a citation when the driver has been pulled over for another traffic offense. This rate stayed the same through 1998 in the states that used secondary enforcement laws. When some states increased legislation and enforcement efforts with the enactment of primary enforcement legislation, which allowed ticketing when the only infraction was seatbelt nonuse, compliance increased to 79 percent (26).

In summary, a comprehensive approach to injury control including active and passive measures, education at both the community and individual level and appropriate legislation is the most efficacious way to facilitate injury prevention. It is necessary to take a multifaceted approach, targeting as many components of the Haddon Matrix as possible to promote injury prevention.

MOTOR VEHICLE

To begin the exploration of TBI prevention efforts, it is most fitting to approach this issue by examining the leading cause of TBI in the United States: motor vehicle accidents (7). Motor vehicle accidents are the most common cause of brain trauma in the United States and are responsible for approximately half of all brain injuries each year (30). The prevention strategies that have targeted motor vehicles have resulted in a decreased occurrence of transportation related brain trauma. There has been a 38 percent decrease in motor vehicle related deaths from 1980 to 1994 (7). In 1970, there were 4.6 highway fatalities per 100 million passenger miles traveled. This number dropped 50 percent to 2.3 fatalities per 100 million passenger miles by 1989 (31). The reason for this reduction in fatalities is multifaceted and includes airbags, seatbelts, safety features and a higher legal drinking age, all of which will be further addressed in this discussion. Transportation related TBI prevention efforts could be approached, using both passive and active methods and, as with other preventative measures, the more comprehensive the approach, the better the overall effectiveness.

AIRBAGS AND SEATBELTS

Airbags are designed to rapidly and automatically deploy during a frontal vehicle collision with the intent of creating an absorptive impact barrier between the vehicle's occupants and the automobile's front interior paneling. This barrier allows for the safer transfer of energy that occurs with impact. An airbag is deployed after the vehicle either comes into contact with a fixed obstacle, such as a brick wall, at 15 miles per hour or when it collides with an equally sized vehicle at 20 to 30 miles per hour. The entire cycle of deployment and subsequent deflation of airbags occurs within one second. It takes merely 1/20th of a second to inflate after impact with the deflation portion beginning within 4/20th of a second. The advantages of this rapid cycle lie in the ability of the driver to maintain control of the vehicle and also prevent trapping of passengers (32).

Advocacy for airbags has resulted in their installation as standard equipment in all passenger cars. Jagger has stated early in the 1990's that making airbags standard equipment would be of greater benefit in the prevention of TBI than any other prevention method (30). She surmised that of the number of patients admitted to a hospital who had acquired TBI, 25 percent could have been prevented by the use of airbags. While they have been of some benefit, Jagger's prediction has been somewhat off the mark as will be discussed later in this section.

Airbags are designed to protect against frontal impact collisions and are not designed to prevent ejection from the vehicle, a major cause of vehicle collision mortality, which requires seatbelt usage to prevent. Another issue, is that they were designed to be effective with frontal injuries and are less beneficial with impact that do not occur between 11 and 1 O'clock with 12 O'clock as direct head on collision (32). Newly developed side impact bags are being introduced into the market that provide much needed protection against side and rear impact collisions and vehicle rollovers. The issue of side air bags is important because it is thought of as an important way of protecting the torso in a side impact collision. It is an alternative to padding as it occupies less space in the car. There are still challenges with perfecting this method of prevention such as the timing of deployment of the bag and length of time for inflation. The best location of deployment also needs to be determined to minimize the risk of injury, particularly those of the upper extremities (33). It is important to ensure that the bag does not deflate too rapidly and become stiff because as the volume of the bag decreases, it automatically gets stiffer (34). Women are particularly vulnerable as they tend to sit closer to the steering wheel. One must be careful in the design of an airbag system as excessive stiffness may result in head injury (35). It is also difficult to make a side bag that would be appropriate for all torso sizes. It was suggested by Parkin et al. that the ideal "smart" restraint system would be programmed for the sex and age of the patient. The literature is yet to determine if side airbags will prevent brain injury. They continue to hold promise as frontal airbags are not foolproof and have limitations in the area of the body that they protect and the type of collision it protects against. Further research in this area is both exciting and still warranted.

The combined utilization of seatbelts and airbags has been proven to be the most protective. In the National Highway Safety Administration's Third Report to Congress in 1996, airbags were reported to reduce fatalities in pure frontal crashes, excluding rollovers, by 34 percent and 18 percent in near frontal collisions. In this analysis, the fatality rate using airbags alone was reduced by 13 percent taking all crashes into consideration. This is in comparison to a 45 percent reduction rate using lap-shoulder belts alone and 50 percent reduction using both modalities (32).

The National Highway Traffic Safety Administration's Crashworthiness Data System reported interesting information regarding the efficacy of airbag and seatbelt use in moderate and severe injuries. Tests studying the effects of airbags alone did not demonstrate a statistically significant result as moderate and severe injuries were reduced by merely 18 percent and 7 percent, respectively, when looking at all organ systems. This was in sharp contrast to the reported reduction of 49 percent and 59 percent with the use of a lap-shoulder belt system. Interestingly, the combination of both systems reduced risk by 60 percent. From this information one might conclude that airbags provide very little added benefit to the use of lap-shoulder belt system restraints. However, while injury severity to different body systems must be taken into consideration, TBI has been shown to be the major source of mortality in the multiple trauma occupant (36). With this in mind, a restraint system that protects against head and brain injury is of great importance. The use of manual lap-shoulder belt and airbags in combination resulted in an 83 percent and 75 percent reduction in moderate and severe head injuries, respectively. This data is significant when compared to the risk reduction of 59 percent and 38 percent with the use of a lap-shoulder belt alone. Although much of the risk reduction results from the use of the lap-shoulder belt alone, it is important to realize that lap-shoulder belts must be "used," which differs from the automatic deployment of an airbag restraint system.

The preventative benefits of seatbelts and airbags are clearly demonstrable. However, there have been a number of injuries associated with their use. Some of these injuries include spinal, brachial plexopathy, liver lacerations, small bowel tears, traumatic hernias, aortic tears, ocular and facial trauma, neck sprains, kidney trauma, sternal fractures, lung perforation, and placental/fetal injury (37–55). Airbags have also been reported to cause a number of injuries including skull fracture and facial injury (56–58), ocular trauma (59–63), burn injuries (64–66), reflex sympathetic dystrophy (67,68), extremity fracture (69, 70), chest injuries, spinal injury (71,72), ear and hearing loss (73,74). There is substantial evidence that children are most susceptible to injury due to airbag deployment (59,71,75–81). These injuries have been severe and even fatal in situations where children have been both properly and improperly positioned (59,71, 75, 80,82,83). Efforts are currently underway to ensure that the protective benefits of airbags are extended to include children.

MOTORCYCLES

TBI due to motorcycle accidents is a serious problem in the United States. Although motorcycle accidents account for only 6 percent of all related transportation accidents, it may very well be the most dangerous form of transportation (84). There have been nearly 10,000 deaths related to motorcycle accidents from 1989 to 1991(85) with an additional 15,000 motorcycle deaths associated with head injury from 1979 to 1986 (21). A fatality rate of 1.2/100,000 and a hospitalization rate of 24.7/100,000 were reported in a study from Connecticut with 22 percent of injuries occurring to the head, brain, or spinal areas (86). Comparatively, a study reported from New Zealand found a higher mortality rate of 3.6/100,000 and hospitalization rate if 80.4/100,000 related to motorcycle accidents (87).

Factors related to motorcycle fatalities include driver error (76 percent), most commonly excessive speed (21), failing to wear a helmet, and elevated blood alcohol levels. Amongst all methods of transportation, alcohol seems to be the greatest problem for motorcycle drivers with a study finding that they have the highest rates of both alcohol use and legal intoxication (88).

Probably the most critical mitigating factor relating to TBI and fatalities due to motorcycle accidents is the utilization of helmets. A study in 1982 reported that a helmetless rider has a 2.3 times greater likelihood of having head, neck, or facial injury and are 3.19 times as likely to suffer a fatality than those who wear helmets (89). Bachulis et al. (90). found the rate of brain injury to be double and severe brain injury six times more likely in helmetless riders. Similar findings were reported by Gabella et al. (91). with brain injury occurring 2.5 times as often in riders without helmets. The benefits of helmet use laws have also been demonstrated. After the implementation of a mandatory helmet law in Spain a 25 percent reduction in fatalities due to motorcycles related accidents was observed (92), as well as a decrease in injury severity, shorter hospital lengths of stay and better outcomes. Similar legislation passed in Taiwan resulted in a 33 percent reduction in head injuries (93). Similar findings have been reported from other areas of the world after mandatory helmet laws were enacted. The overwhelming result of this legislation has led to a reduced rate of overall fatalities, TBI related fatalities, overall TBI incidence, injury severity (92–99), length of hospitalization (96,97). and overall cost to society (96,97,100).

Despite this strong evidence from countries around the world, there are still a number of states across the United States that have not enacted mandatory helmet laws. In 2001, there were three states with no helmet legislation, 27 states with helmets required solely for teenage riders and only 20 states with mandatory helmet use for all motorcycle riders (100). Many states have had mandatory helmet laws in the 1970s that have since been repealed or revised.

In 1967, the Federal Government required states to pass a motorcycle helmet law in order to continue to receive federal safety funds. As a result, by 1975, 47 states had passed legislation requiring the use of helmets. However, as opposition mounted against the use of helmets, Congress overturned the helmet requirement. Following this action, more than half of all states with mandatory helmet laws revised their laws (101), with a resultant

decrease use of helmets in those states. Within 9 months of the repeal, the states of Texas and Arkansas saw a decline in helmet usage from 97 percent to 66 percent and 52 percent, respectively. There was a concomitant increase in overall motorcycle injuries, head injuries, and an increased proportion of those injured having suffered head injuries according to data obtained from the Arkansas Trauma Registry (101). This trend was also seen in Miami Dade County with an increased incidence of TBI and fatalities in the post repeal era that saw helmet usage dropping from 83 percent to 56 percent (102). Bledsoe et al. (103). reported on the Arkansas experience of helmet law repeal. A 6-year retrospective review of the trauma registry compared the results of the three years prior to repeal as compared to the three years afterwards. There was no statistical change in total and fatal collisions; however there was a major increase in nonhelmeted deaths at the scene of the accident. The nonhelmeted had significantly higher Abbreviated Injury Scores involving the head and neck, more expensive, longer ICU stays and substantially higher nonreimbursed hospital charges. This of course was a cost borne by the remainder of the community.

As mentioned above, the financial costs to society following the repeals of mandatory helmet laws have been substantial. A study in Texas concluded the median cost of motorcycle related injury increased 300 percent to $22,531 per event, with TBI costs increasing 75 percent to over $32,000. Most of these costs exceed limits set by insurance coverage and, so, the financial burden often falls on society (104).

Another issue that also arises is the relationship between alcohol and motorcycle driving. Since handling a motorcycle requires more coordination and judgment than driving a car, there may be a need to lower the blood alcohol level that classifies a motorcyclist as being under the influence. This is supported by a study that examined the blood alcohol levels of drivers of motorcycles and cars brought to trauma centers, with the motorcyclists having lower levels (105). This may indicate that a lower level of acceptable blood alcohol levels may be needed to determine when a motorcyclist is considered to be under the influence.

ROADWAY DESIGN

Accident prevention can also be achieved by identifying hazardous road locations with specific collision patterns. Various approaches can be used to correct these accident-prone areas through road engineering and technology. The first step in this area was in the 1930's when skidding resistance was added to wet roads (106). It was not until 20 years ago that a major movement in developing safer roads was initiated. *The Road Safety Code of Good*

Practice was a publication from the Local Authority Associations that included engineering in addition to education and enforcement, the three E's, for better road safety (107). One study attempted to identify crash problems on various urban arterial streets in Washington, DC (108). Data was retrieved from police reports of a total of 2013 crashes. The locations that had a large number of crashes were analyzed to identify pre-crash movements and travel directions of the crash – involved vehicles. It was found that, at some intersections, drivers had difficulty turning left from a private driveway whereas some intersections had extremely high traffic speeds with crashes likely to occur at the end of a ramp. Left turn signals were not provided at some of the intersections. Based on the analysis of the accident data recommendations were then provided. Changes made included the addition of left turn signals, prohibition of left turns from a driveway, improvement of storm drainage, increased pavement skid resistance as well as the initiation of pavement milling. It was also noted that stopped buses obstructed drivers' visual fields. Relocating bus stops, as well as removing large fixed objects, was a simple intervention that was effective in reducing accidents.

Sabey suggested that the use of four investigative techniques could be the foundation for intervention and treatment of the problem. These four areas included *single sites* where accidents cluster or "blackspots", *mass action* or locations that have common accident factors, *route action* or lengths of road with above average accident rates and *area action* including areas requiring a more global approach aimed at dealing with scattered accidents. He also provided examples of proposed treatments for each of the four variables. For instance, route action could be addressed with road marking to deter overtaking, increasing skidding resistance or installing roundabouts at key junctions to provide access to adjacent neighborhoods. In one trial of a 3km road with a large number of accidents per year, a roundabout was added as well as a new light to control crossings in addition to right turn bans. This resulted in a 12 percent reduction in accidents that resulted in injury (106).

Rear end collisions can also be reduced by engineering methods. In British Columbia, road factors account for about a third of collisions (109). The Insurance Corporation of British Columbia (ICBC) has provided funding for road improvement programs and countermeasures for rear end collisions since 1993, with the amount of funding from the ICBC having been increased substantially from 1993 to 1996. Some interventions that resulted from this movement included creating left or right turn lanes in areas where there are a large number of turning vehicles, acceleration/deceleration lanes, medians with turn protections, prohibiting turns and/or providing a special phase for left turning vehicles. These interventions resulted in a decrease of rear end collisions by 20–40 percent (109).

Simple techniques such as enhancing signal visibility also resulted in a decrease frequency of rear end collisions.

Speed bumps may be of value but this is controversial. Some argue that alone they may not reduce a driver's speed but may be effective if used in combination with other traffic control techniques (110). Further studies are still warranted. Other intervention methods such as matured in-service red light cameras (RLC) at T-intersections have also shown to result in an increased stopping frequency at these junctions. One study looked at three T-intersections in Singapore and found that the odds ratio to stop when approaching a camera was slightly higher than 17 times that if there were no camera surveillance (111).

The "three E's" education, engineering and enforcement are all important parts of injury prevention. Although there have been improvements noted in the roads over the past few years, there is still a need for further efforts, including assessment and treatment of accident-prone locations. There still is a strong need for further funding and legislation in this critical area of injury prevention in the United States.

FALLS

Falls have consistently been identified as the second most common cause of TBI (11–13,112–115). They occur in the greatest number among young children under the age of 5 and in the elderly (21). Younger children have a much larger head-to-body ratio and thus the head strikes the ground more frequently during play (116). Also as a result, a fall of only a few feet can have serious consequences in young children (117). Over two decades ago, falls from extreme heights accounted for 12 percent of all unintentional traumatic deaths in New York City children. Overall, in the United States, it has been estimated that falls comprise almost 9 percent of pediatric trauma deaths (118). Benoit et al. demonstrated that falls accounted for 41 percent of admissions to a suburban hospital for children age 0 to 14 years of age (119). Turning our attention to the elderly, fatalities as a result of TBI are most common over age 75 and falls are the number one cause of TBI in the elderly (7). Jagger et al. found that there was a stable pattern of occurrence of fall related TBI up to about 59 years old. Between the ages of 60–69, there was a dramatic rise in the occurrence, which continued to rise in those 70 years old and older (13). The financial burden from falls is enormous. In 1994 the estimated cost in the United States from falls approached $20.2 billion (120).

Efforts at fall prevention have been effective with legislation and education. In 1972, the New York City Department of Health developed a health education program termed "Children Can't Fly." This initiated installment of window guards in all New York City apartments that had children less that 11 years old residing in them. This resulted in a 96 percent decrease in falls from windows after implementation (118). The use of safety devices for windows in suburban areas has also shown to be helpful (119). There have been positive results in fall prevention both abroad such as in Sweden (121), as well as in American urban neighborhoods (122,123).

The issue of playground related falls can be addressed by the use of protective surfaces including adding a safe 12 inch border of a soft material such as wood chips, and sand or rubber around the play area (123–125). Adult supervision and education of the parents is still critical. Educational efforts directed at both children and the communities have also been shown to have benefits (126,127).

Fall prevention in the elderly requires several strategies that often require a doctor's input. Physicians must identify various factors that may contribute to falls in the elderly population. Miller et al. (128), mentioned four common issues that have been implicated in increasing the risk of falls in the elderly. They are postural hypotension, gait and balance instability, polypharmacy and the use of sedating medications. Other host related factors that have been associated with falls include musculoskeletal or neurological abnormalities, visual disturbances, dementia (129) and frailty (130).

Balance deficits in the elderly appear to be related to the deterioration of various input systems necessary for postural control. It has been demonstrated that in subjects over 70 years of age, there is a 40 percent reduction in sensory cells of the vestibular system (131). These elderly adults are more likely to fall if other systems required for postural control, such as vision and proprioception, are impaired (132). Impaired balance in the elderly can also be attributed to multiple deficits in the neuromuscular system. It has been consistently shown that disuse atrophy; motor weakness, deconditioning, abnormal tone and posturing contribute to impaired balance in the elderly (133,134). There may be generalized slowing of central-processing areas in the elderly that involve integration and coordination of multiple inputs and outputs in the brain including the motor cortex, basal ganglia, and cerebellum (133). Lesions within these pathways, such as that sustained by an ischemic stroke or intracerebral hemorrhage, may compound the problem. It is also important to realize that approximately one third of patients with severe closed head injury experience subsequent postural imbalance due to disruption of these various pathways (135).

Assessing patients for balance dysfunction is an important component in prevention. Various measures at measuring body sway have been looked at for reliability and repeatability in assessing our elderly population. One method, such as the posturographic quiet standing test, has been referred to in the literature. Helbostad et al.

evaluated subjects after asking them to stand as still as possible for thirty seconds. Task conditions were performed in random order amongst the subjects and included both eyes open or closed, wide or narrow stance and firm or compliant surface. Some patients were also asked to perform a cognitive task. It appears across all domains one can consistently and appropriately assess the frail elderly with repeated testing. Clinicians need to develop simple assessment measures, such as those described, that can be taken into the office setting. In this manner clinicians can initiate preventative measures once frail elderly patients at risk for balance instability and falls are identified (136).

Prevention must then be aimed at the various contributing factors. Balance training in physical therapy can be directed at lower extremity strengthening as well as proprioceptive and visual system training with repetitive feedback and continual cueing. Various approaches have been tried to enhance balance in therapy. The utilization of force-plate biofeedback system to improve standing ability has been reported to have positive effects (137). There is no standard physical therapy program or protocol for balance training and more research in this area is warranted. In addition to targeting the physical aspects, one must address a common, iatrogenic and possibly avoidable cause of balance impairment in the aged population and that is identification of polypharmacy. It appears the prevalence of inappropriate medication use in the elderly appears to be 20 percent in both the US and various countries in Europe. The result may lead to balance instability, sedation and confusion in our elderly population. Physician awareness of those at increased risk, such as elders treated with psychotropic medications and those with depression is important as it allows us to target modifiable variables as well as to avoid inappropriate prescription writing. Physicians must constantly readdress prescription medication to avoid both inappropriate use and polypharmacy (138). It is important to review all medications and try to decrease or eliminate the medications that may not be absolutely necessary (139).

The environment plays an important part in falls of the elderly. Speechley, M & Tinetti, M (130). found in a sample community of elderly persons that 15 percent of fallers did not have a chronic intrinsic risk factor and would not be considered frail. It appeared that environmental risk factors played a major role in the robust elderly population of fallers. Thus the elderly population must be counseled on safe performance of certain physical activities, such as climbing stairs and ladders and avoiding hazardous obstacles around the house such as throw rugs. The national bureau of standards has identified various household factors contributing to falls in the elderly. It was estimated that highly waxed floors, loose rugs, sharp furniture, poor lighting or problems with tubs and showers have contributed to 18–50 percent of falls (21). One study demonstrated that 10 hours of non-skilled time and $93 of supplies per person was all that was needed to make an elderly person's environment substantially safer (140).

Physicians can play an important role in fall prevention, especially after a first fall. More aggressive efforts at assessing the cause of falls are needed by physicians. Risk factors for osteoporosis should be identified as low bone mineral density (BMD) has been shown to contribute to falls. BMD screening must be considered in high risk patients such as chronic steroid users, those with a sedentary lifestyle and patients on antiepileptic medications. In one study, approximately 75 percent of women have never been screened for bone loss and less than 1/3 ever received recommendations for BMD screening. Osteoporosis prevention strategies including calcium supplementation can then be initiated when appropriate. It has been shown that most people in the US have inadequate calcium intake, making education with each visit necessary in our clinics. Education on the reduction of alcohol and caffeine intake in addition to the encouragement of weight bearing exercises should also part of our management plan. It is also important to address hormone status in addition to frequency and dose duration of steroids in chronic steroid users (141).

SPORTS AND RECREATIONAL INJURY

Recreational and sporting activities can be a significant cause of TBI with the majority of injuries being concussions (11,12,21,113). Unlike musculoskeletal training the brain cannot be conditioned to withstand the energy assault that is the cause of concussion (142). Therefore preventative efforts must instead be directed at improving equipment safety, behavior of the athlete, development of rules to mitigate risks and rigorous enforcement of rules and regulations to promote safety and prevent injury. This includes proper equipment design such as helmets for contact sports, sport rules that discourage dangerous activities and training and educational efforts for coaches and participants.

CYCLING

Bicycle related TBI is a significant concern given their large numbers each year. Every year 1,300 people die from bicycle related accidents, almost half of them under 21 years of age (120,143). Financially, the cost of non-fatal bicycle injuries in children under 14 years of age approaches $113 million every year (120). Fife et al. in a study conducted in Dade County Florida found that serious injuries related to bicycle riding were sustained in 676 out of 1,252 total injuries. Almost half of the serious injuries were located in the head and neck region (144). In patients admitted to a hospital secondary to a head injury the risk of death was 20 times higher for those who were not wearing a helmet (145). Spence et al. (146). evaluated fatal bicycle accidents in children aged 0–15 years old in Ontario from 1985–1989. They found that 70 percent of the accidents were a result of the cyclists themselves. In a similar study, the cyclist was responsible for 78 percent of all bicycle accidents with the major errors reported as riding through a stop sign (22 percent) and emerging from a minor road without caution (27 percent) (147). It was pointed out by Spence et al. that children this young might not have the psychomotor skills to ride safely in traffic. Instead the goal should be to prevent these children from riding on busy streets.

The most effective way to immediately protect the cyclist is to have him wear a helmet. In five case controlled studies that were reviewed, the data demonstrated that wearing a bicycle helmet had a large impact on reducing the risk of head or brain injury during a crash or collision. Estimates regarding the effectiveness of helmet use is that they decrease the risk of brain injury by 88 percent, severe brain injury by at least 75 percent and facial injury, particularly in the upper and mid facial regions, by 65 percent (148).

Thompson et al. (149). performed an extensive review of the literature to evaluate risk reduction for cyclists and helmet use during riding. The authors found that helmets were beneficial in the reduction of head, brain and severe brain injury in all age groups and included not only bicycle injuries but also motor vehicle and other types of crashes. The reduction in risk was estimated to be approximately 70 percent. This is a conservative value when compared to the numbers suggested by Koplan et al. in their CDC sponsored work, which reported a risk difference of 85 percent for head injury and 88 percent for TBI (120).

Helmet usage is only one component of the Haddon Matrix in regards to cycling injuries. As stated previously, a comprehensive approach is the most effective intervention for injury control and this must be incorporated for bicycle injuries. Passive measures such as helmets, road engineering, bicycle lanes and speed bumps must be employed (120). Active strategies such as modifying cyclists behavior and counseling children on safety skills while riding must be aggressively pursued. Helmet use should be mandatory for all child cyclists and legislation is still warranted in all states given its overall effectiveness.

BOXING

As expected the sport of boxing where the participants attempt to give each other concussions has the highest rate of TBI. Atha et al. (150). compared the blow thrown by a top quality heavyweight to a 13-pound mallet swung at 20 miles an hour. In this sport record keeping in regards to brain injury has not been as precise as in football but between the period of 1945 and 1979 there was documentation of 335 deaths from boxing related head injury (151). In one report, the incidence of TBI in professional boxers was estimated to be approximately 20 percent (152). In 1983 it was reported that minor head injury rate for amateurs was 5 percent which increased to 6.3 percent at the professional level (153). Fatalities at both levels are substantial (154). Various risk factors that have been identified that increase the chances that a boxer will sustain brain injury include career length, number of bouts, poor showings in the ring and apolipoprotein (APOE) genotype.

There has been an increase in the public's awareness of boxing related brain injury with Muhammed Ali's illness over the years. Various preventative measures have been attempted such as guidelines for determining when a player should return to play after a head injury. For instance, The National Amateur Athletic Union (AAU) Junior Olympic Boxing Program specifies the length of time a participant must remain out of competition after a knockout. Wilberger and Maroon. noted that the New York State Boxing Commission enforced a mandatory suspension of 45 days for mild concussions and 60 and 90 days for moderate and severe concussions (151). A problem identified with professional boxing is that there is not enough consistency between the various states. A boxer who has been suspended in one state may be able to participate in another state without any restrictions. Other preventative measures such as changes to increase ring safety and improved monitoring by the referee and an on site physician have resulted in decreased mortality (154). There is a strong need for physicians to take a more active role in education of both the amateur and professional athletes as well as all others such as all referee's and ring side physicians. LeClerc and Herrera (155) have suggested that physicians must take an active role in educating the public regarding the risks of boxing. Their statement," a watchful agnostic position among sport physicians is no longer justifiable" is a call to arms for health care providers to work diligently to educate the public concerning the dangers of boxing. While abolishing boxing may be an ultimate, but unrealistic goal, one must at a minimum strongly advocate for even greater safety measures (21).

FOOTBALL

The game of football has been associated with an increased risk of sustaining a TBI. The National Football Head and Neck Injury Registry reported 59 intracranial football injuries that resulted in death between the years of 1971 and 1975. In 1974, Blyth and Mueller (156) reported that while TBI accounted for only 5 percent of overall football injuries it accounted for 70 percent of the fatalities, with 75 percent of them occurring during tackling. The estimates for football related TBI are up to 250,000 concussions and 8 fatalities every year nationally. From 1985 to 1994, high school players sustained 81 percent of head injuries and 100 percent of cervical spine injuries (157). Furthermore, up to 20 percent of high school football players sustain a concussion per season played (1,158,159).

Given the popularity of the sport and interest to play among high school athletes, it is a sport that will likely continue to have many fans and participants. The focus must therefore be on injury prevention in addition to good clinical judgment in removing players from play at the greatest risk. The highest percentage of head and cervical spine fatalities associated with football was between 1965 and 1974. There was a significant decrease in head fatalities from 1985 through 1994 representing 5.4 percent of the fatalities from 1985 to 1994 (157). This is attributed to the multidisciplinary team involved in the football family including coaches, administrators, athletic trainers, physicians, national organizations; all of whom have provided education and public awareness.

Prevention efforts utilized for football have been effective. The issue of legislation and enforcement as well as passive and active strategies should again be revisited. With immediate punishment and consequences from illegal plays called by the officials, illegal dangerous plays can be discouraged and their incidence greatly reduced. There was a key rule change in 1976 that played a role in reducing head and spine fatalities. The rule prohibited initial contact with the helmet, also known as "head butting", or face mask, also known as "face tackling", when tackling or blocking. Tackling was responsible for 40.6 percent of all head fatalities from 1985–1994 and it is therefore imperative to adhere to this rule as a violation of it may result in a serious injury (157). There have been other important preventative efforts associated with football which include preseason conditioning, safe use of equipment and training for proper technique (160). In addition, proper fitting of helmets and physician evaluation post injury are also key components to any prevention program (21).

Second impact system is a potentially fatal complication that can result from repeated injuries prior to recovery from previous injury. It is important to mention this syndrome in the discussion of football related injuries. It may be missed clinically and appear as a minor injury but can be associated with massive cerebral edema, resultant brainstem compression and possible death (161). There are very few warning signs that would clue a physician to make the diagnosis of second impact syndrome. It is therefore important to abide by guidelines published by the Colorado Medical Society regarding assessing concussive symptoms during play. These are considered the best guidelines for return the play post concussion (158).

SOCCER

Another major sport that can account for a significant number of TBI is soccer or football to the rest of the non North American world. It has been estimated that head injuries account for between 4 and 22 percent of soccer injuries (162). Soccer is increasing in popularity and is considered to be the most popular sport worldwide. There were more than 40 million amateur participants noted in 1989 (163). Due to the large number of participants worldwide, the number of potential injuries can be significant, even if the rate of injury, may be lower than that of other higher contact sport (164). There is one Australian study the estimated injury rate occurred 96 per 1000 player hours (165). In Sweden, soccer is the number one source of recreational related injury with a rate of 39 percent reported (166). Data collected in Norway over an eight-year period, noted that 45 percent of all sports related head injuries were accounted for by soccer (167). Tysvaer and Storli looked at 69 active soccer players and 37 former players of a Norwegian national team and found that one third of the players had central cerebral atrophy and 81 percent had some form of neuropsychological impairment (162,168,169). Dvorak et al. have worked out both a risk analysis for prediction of injuries and the development of a prevention program focusing on the trainers, medical professionals and players. Recommendations included structured training, better medical supervision, player reaction time, rule design and enforcement that could result in an overall decrease in injury (170).

The use of controlled head contact with the ball is an important part of soccer. Some would argue that it plays a major role in TBI but this remains a controversial issue (1). It has been shown that older leather balls absorb water and increase the weight of the ball by 20 percent or more making them more dangerous (171). Soccer balls are now made of waterproof synthetic leather covered with urethane which repels water, which has decreased the injury potential (172). Head gear that has been designed to protect players playing soccer has been of limited value (173). A review of the literature has suggested that heading the ball plays a very small part of in soccer related TBI. Instead, accidental unplanned contact against goalposts, head to head contact, elbow contact and a ball kicked directly at the head are more likely to be the source of problems (1, 174). Tysvaer and Storli also noted that the younger players with less experience heading the ball had greater EEG, radiographic and neuropsychologic changes than their older more experienced counterparts (162).

Prevention efforts therefore should be directed to better training techniques, proper coaching, adhering to return to play guidelines, medical supervision post injury, rule changes and enforcement. These strategies would minimize unintentional head contact. The use of protective headgear by goalies and development of better head protection would also add to better injury control (172,174).

HOCKEY

Another sport that can be extremely rough and place the player at a high risk of TBI is hockey (175). Studies have estimated that the range for the incidence of head and neck injuries, excluding facial lacerations, was 6.3 percent to 45.12 percent (176,177). As in football the vast majority of these injuries are concussive in nature. However, in contrast to football, where most injuries occur at the high school level, hockey injuries occur throughout the spectrum of competition; including small children, high school, college and the elite professional teams (178).

The majority of injuries occur during checking, both legal and illegal (179,180). In one study it was found that 57 percent of children with ice hockey related injuries resulted from checking and that more than half of these injuries were considered significant (180). It was also found that the children were not educated on safety and injury prevention as 45 percent of the children reported that they could not sustain a TBI with a helmet on.

Attempts have been made at decreasing injury associated with the game of hockey. There was some thought previously that the use of face masks in hockey players may increase head and neck injuries because the players were more aggressive during play once the mask was on. This has proven to be a fallacy. In one study it was found that there was no significant increase in head and neck injuries with the use of face masks and there was an overall decreased incidence of facial lacerations (181) There have been other reports that mandatory facemasks reduced both facial injuries and TBI (178,182). It has been demonstrated that more hockey injuries occur early in the season, late in the periods and in the final period of games suggesting that conditioning may assist in injury prevention (183).

Education at the younger level is imperative and the emphasis should not be entirely on winning. In one study it was alarming that almost a third of the children would check illegally to win and 6 percent would intentionally injure another player to win (180). Parental attitudes should encourage nonviolence so these behaviors can be learned by their children and taken into adolescence and adulthood.

On the professional level, statistics show that in the Stanley Cup Finals the team with the least penalties secondary to violent behavior win the majority of the series (184).

In summary, sport related injuries account for a significant number of head injuries, which can be severe, fatal, result in long-term debility and/or be the cause of the termination of a player's career. It is important to stress a multifaceted approach to prevention of injury including education, rule enforcement, improvement in safety equipment and better-conditioned athletes with encouragement of nonviolent behaviors.

VIOLENCE AND SUICIDE

Violence in the United States is a major cause of morbidity and mortality and the statistics raise a significant amount of concern. The fatalities in children and adolescents from firearms have increased from an estimated 3000 fatalities per year in the mid-1980's to 4500 fatalities per year in 1992 (118). Approximately 73 percent of people who sustained a gunshot injury die at the scene, 12 percent die within three hours and 7 percent die after three hours (185). It has been estimated that 90 percent of all persons who sustain a gunshot wound to the head die (186). Upon review of the literature, self-inflicted injuries range from 11–50 percent, with an unclear percentage being accidental (187,188). There are strong demographic factors that contribute to firearm mortality (189). There is a reported tenfold higher rate of homicide in black males related to firearms between the ages of 15 to 19 years old when compared to white males in the same age group (118).

GUN CONTROL

Handguns continue to be purchased and remain in many American homes. They contribute to a significant amount of morbidity and mortality in the United States annually. Depending on the specific region, it has been estimated that between 15.7 percent and 30.1 percent of all homes contain a handgun (190,191).

Dresang evaluated gun deaths in urban and rural areas and it was found that in rural areas there was a higher amount of shotgun and rifle injuries with handguns accounting for more than 50 percent of gun deaths (192). Those who own handguns are twice as likely to have their gun loaded than an owner of any other type of firearm (193). Homicide risk is increased by threefold and suicide by fivefold among those with a gun in the home (194,195).

It still remains controversial how to enforce handgun control. There have been attempts at legislation, education and safety devices. However more strict regulation is warranted. For example, sales of firearms at gun shows still occur outside of the realm of regulation (196). It is important to realize that more legislation may not meet that much resistance from the general public. In one report, a large percentage of the public (68 percent) would support government regulation of handgun safety (197). Some believe that only the power of litigation will result in better prevention (196). Past legislation has proven to have a positive effect on injury control. One report noted that a 2-week ban on handguns in parts of Columbia was associated with a reduction in homicide rates in those cities (198). There was also a reported decrease in the number of accidental and home deaths in Maryland after handgun legislation was enacted in Maryland in 1987 (118).

GUN SAFETY

There continues to be a significant portion of the public that wants to keep a handgun in their homes. In one survey, 29 percent of respondents felt that owning a gun made their homes safer (199). Education of the public should be one of the major components of our preventative measures regarding handgun related injuries. Community based education programs have had some success in encouraging proper storage of firearms (200).

Different technological approaches have been tried to improve handgun safety. Safety locks (trigger lock being the most common), manual thumb safeties, loaded chamber indicators and magazine disconnectors are all attempts to prevent unintentional injuries (201). However, these devices do not protect from intentional injuries such as suicide or homicide. A grip safety feature is a passive preventative method designed to protect children from using the gun. Young children do not have the strength, coordination or hand size to press the safety lever and pull the trigger at the same time. Personalized handguns, a new developing technology, allow only the authorized owner to use the gun. Its features include a built-in locking system and the ability to recognize the authorized user. There are still some concerns regarding its use such as reliability, maintenance and cost. However there is a strong public desire for legislation requiring handguns to be personalized (197). There is no real possibility of an immediate answer to the issue of gun related violence. Zakcos has noted that only legislative lobbying has been linked to organizational resources (202). While Rodriguez stated that only the power of litigation will bring some response to these issues (196).

OTHER SOURCES OF VIOLENT INJURY

Violence continues to be a major contributing factor to TBI. This continues to be a major concern in urban areas. However it must be noted that there is a reasonable amount of violence in rural areas as well. Jagger et al.

evaluated the epidemiology of head injury in the rural area of north central Virginia. It was found that interpersonal violence accounted for 23/100,000 of head injuries in this area. This number was more than half of that seen for falls alone and overall was a fairly large number (13). The highest number of these types of injuries was in the 30–39 age group. Interpersonal violence included injuries with firearms, blunt weapons, knives or battery without a weapon. These other types of injuries are a worldwide problem. Stab wound injuries, for instance, are extremely high in parts of South Africa (203). Blunt trauma specifically can be mostly attributed to fists, baseball bats, bricks and bottles (204). There have been very little in the way of preventative measures and public education to minimize these other sources of injury.

DEPRESSION, SUICIDE, AND TBI

There have been reports that intentional TBI has been associated with gender, minority status, age, substance abuse and low socioeconomic status, with the most predictive of these variables being minority status and substance abuse (205). Additionally, a major concern is the risk of suicide among those with TBI. It has been estimated that suicide rates in the TBI population are 2.7 and 4 times higher than the general population when matched for age and sex (206). It has been shown that suicide risk is greater among patients with physical illness than among the general population (207). Simpson and Tate identified various factors of suicide risk in TBI outpatients including hopelessness (35 percent), suicide ideation (23 percent) and suicide attempts (18 percent) (208). A study of several disability groups noted 25 percent of patients had major depression and 7.3 percent reported clinically significant suicidal ideation (209).

There is considerable variability in TBI prevention worldwide. Although there is agreement about goals including general knowledge about suicide and development of skills in suicide risk assessment and management, prevention programs have a wide range of variability (210). The length of training programs for those with professionals and nonprofessional backgrounds range from 1 hour to 16 hours (211,212). Instructional materials used include anything from written materials, self-instructional videos to other methods such as didactic sessions. Some suicide preventative programs are broader and include a more general disabled population. If the TBI population is targeted and appropriate intervention occurs early then some suicides may be prevented. Physicians need to identify risk factors such as suicidal ideation, perform further research on other prognostic factors and be able to manage these patients once their risk has been identified. Simpson et al. created a training workshop for suicide assessment and management for staff in a rehabilitation center in New South Wales. The length of the workshop totaled approximately 5.25 hours of training in one day. There was improved staff knowledge and skills in suicide assessment and management (210). A larger more multifaceted approach is warranted. In addition to staff training including appropriate agency policies and procedures, collection of appropriate funding and involving more community support (213).

DRUGS AND ALCOHOL

Recreational pharmaceutical agents greatly complicate the problem of TBI. There have been several reports that head injuries and fractures are the two most common alcohol related types of trauma (214). In its white paper released in 1988 the National Head Injury Foundation Substance Abuse Task Force stated," neither age, nor occupation, nor any other factors place an individual at a greater risk of a TBI than does alcohol" (215). Many factors contribute to alcohol's exacerbation of TBI. First is the fact that a large minority of the consumers of alcohol are heavy consumers. With Kreutzer et al. estimating that 12 percent of American drinkers can be classified as "problem drinkers" (216). In addition to the large numbers of problem consumers, there is the additional problem of greater injury risk (217). The presence of intoxication at the time of trauma admission increased the odds ratio of a repeat trauma admission within the next 2 years, 2.5 times. In 1999 (218), there were 15,786 deaths and 300,000 injuries as a result of alcohol related MVA. Legal intoxication has been reported in up to 51 percent of people involved in TBI while up to 2/3rd have some history of drug or alcohol abuse (219–221). Positive testing for drugs or alcohol as high as 70 percent has been reported (222). While Anderson reported that 51 percent of non-belted passengers had alcohol on board. High School students demonstrated very significant risk tasking behavior in regards to alcohol It is alarming that over third of high school students would ride with a driver who had been drinking and over 17 percent would drive after they themselves had been drinking (223).

The importance of preventing teenage drinking has been further clarified by the work of Hingson's group (224). They conducted a survey of college students and demonstrated that there was a relationship between getting drunk for the first time before the age of 19 and drinking and driving, driving after five or more drinks, riding with a driver who was high or drunk and, after drinking, sustaining injuries that required medical attention. In another publication (225) the authors estimated that among college students there were over half a million full-time college students who were unintentionally injured while under the influence of alcohol and over 600,000 assaulted by another student who had been drinking.

Alcohol and drugs can also be involved in other etiologies of TBI. The commencement of drinking prior to age 17 tripled the likelihood that an individual would be involved in a physical fight in the last year (226). A survey performed by Gerhart et. al. demonstrated that alcohol abusers were more likely to sustain a violent TBI as compared to other TBI populations as well as having a worse outcome (227). The incidence of alcohol use in both TBI and SCI patients preinjury is very high. In one report it has been estimated the rate for heavy drinking was 42 and 57 percent respectively (228,229).

There is still some controversy regarding the effect of alcohol on outcomes in the acute setting. Some authors have reported an increased risk of pulmonary complications (230) while other studies have not supported the idea. Cornwell et al. (221). reported that sepsis, complications and mortality were correlated with injury severity and not to the presence or absence of alcohol or drugs. In regards to rehabilitation, Sparedo and Gill (231) reported an association between acute intoxication and lower functional levels at discharge as well as a longer period of post-traumatic agitation. Acute intoxication has also been correlated with longer acute hospitalization and a longer period of posttraumatic amnesia (232). There have also been reports that reported a positive correlation of impaired verbal memory and visiospatial function in those with positive alcohol and drug screens on trauma admission (233,234).

The performance of alcohol screens is not universally performed on all trauma patients (220), with some studies reporting less than 1/2 the trauma patients being tested. This may in part be secondary to a fear of a patient being subject to legal prosecution or denial of insurance coverage if tests are positive. However, this practice is problematic as this hinders both clinical care as well as further research efforts.

While a clear relationship has been established between alcohol and brain injury in the literature, questions still arise as to the most effective means of preventing alcohol related TBI. Prevention efforts must be directed at both passive and active measures as passive efforts alone have had a limited effect. Passive efforts such as breathalyzer testing, mental status or coordination testing prior to starting a car has been discussed for years but have not become a reality. Another intervention, that is passive to the alcohol consumer is the modification of the server's behavior. This is part based on the concept that many people who drink and drive are consuming alcohol at bars, clubs and restaurants (218).It has been reported that about half of the people who received a DUI left a place that served alcohol (235, 236). Efforts that focus on educating servers to carefully screen underage drinkers, refuse service to rapid drinkers, calling taxi services for consumers that seem unfit to drive and the offering of food to those drinking are all ways to delay potential intoxication and driving under the influence. Currently there is no uniformity between the educational programs across the country with some states having mandatory programs, while others voluntary educational programs for servers. The programs are not standardized across the country and address different issues such as legislation regarding intoxication, DUI, recognizing the signs of intoxication as well as liability issues. The fear of litigation may assist the management structure of these establishments to be supportive of their employees' efforts to mitigate this national problem and run a safer establishment (218).

These programs have been proven to be effective in both improving servers' decision making abilities (237) and in decreasing patrons' level of intoxication (238–240). Holder et al. (241). demonstrated that using these measures in three experimental communities resulted in a 10 percent reduction in alcohol related traffic accidents and significantly reduced the sale of alcohol to minors. These interventions have been shown to only be effective for about a year with some drop off after 15 months (242), It is therefore important to recognize the need for continuing education, which may be needed on a yearly basis. Mandatory legislation is still warranted for continuing education targeting servers.

Significant progress has been achieved due to alcohol related prevention programs. Since 1982, the rate of alcohol related MVA fatality has steadily dropped from a rate of 57 percent to 38 percent (218). Zobeck et al. also reported similar findings with a 10 percent decrease in alcohol related MVA fatalities from 1979–1990 (243). Not only that, but fatality rates per 100 million vehicles miles traveled, and per 100,000 population, registered vehicles and licensed drivers have decreased even more sharply. This may be due the multifaceted approach of various interventions such as public education, community programs, legislation and enforcement.

Recently, The Internal Medicine News has reported about the decrease in the use of alcohol and illicit drugs in the young. Kirn reported results of a national survey that questioned 50,000 students that were attending either public or private schools regarding their usage of illicit drug within the previous month. It demonstrated a 7 percent decrease in illicit drug use from 2003 to 2004. In addition he reported an overall decline in drug use over the past three years among high school seniors and the last eight years for younger teens (244). Jancin reported on the potential value of early recognition of young children who are at risk for developing problems with substance abuse later in life; in particular, evaluating preschoolers for the presence of temperament traits such as aggressiveness, impulsivity, poor attentiveness. Once these "red flags" are identified, some suggest that early comprehensive psychological evaluation with early intervention may help reduce the risk of problems later on in the teen and adolescent years (245)

Community programs such as Mothers Against Drunk Driving (MADD) have been instrumental in having the legal drinking age raised to 21 throughout the United States (21). However, raising the legal drinking age to 21 has not totally eliminated alcohol as a problem for teenage drivers. Alcohol has clearly been found in adolescents involved in trauma (246). In 1997, 21 percent of those killed driving while driving intoxicated were 15–20 years of age (120). In addition, 41 percent of college students report episodes of binge drinking during the previous 2 weeks (247). Control of access clearly is not enough to address the problem of alcohol related MVA.

Active preventative measures have been suggested to prevent TBI. Previously suggested strategies include involving survivors in policy making, working with journalists to improve media coverage of head injury and speaking to high-risk groups to encourage use of protective gear (248). Although all survivors cannot participate in every domain suggested, simple tasks associated with office maintenance, for example, could still contribute to head injury prevention. It is therefore important to channel the brain injury community to programs that facilitate education, legislation, public policy, lobbying, advertising and media, all aspects of prevention that need to be addressed by both survivors and health care professionals (214).

Preinjury family dynamics must be addressed after a TBI. A brain injury may magnify a dysfunctional family structure. There must be strategies for the family to learn how to cope with substance abuse and brain injury. This may help prevent a second injury or repetitive abuse behavior (219). The family must be involved in collaborative approaches between the health care provider and abuser. There must be consistent use of support groups with family participation. The family must be educated on the risk factors for abuse as well as be provided with coping mechanisms on how to handle and separate TBI related issues from abuse issues.

It is estimated that there are over 1.4 million DUI arrests every year in the Unites States. While this seems like a large number it is relatively small when it is compared to the number of actual occurrences. There are estimates of up to 126 million episodes of DUI that actually occurs every year in the United States (120). The original threshold for determining that one was driving while intoxicated or under the influence laws was 0.10 grams per deciliter. Evidence arose that even lower levels of blood alcohol could impair ones driving ability and in 1983 Utah and Oregon were the first two states that lowered the level to 0.08 grams per deciliter. By May 2001 24 states had lowered the acceptable blood alcohol level to less than 0.08 gm/deciliter for drivers 21 years of age (218). For those 20 and under a zero tolerance policy was adopted and any evidence of blood alcohol is considered illegal and subject to legal sanction (218,249).

Several studies have addressed the impact of this lowering of acceptable blood alcohol levels (250–258). which have been reviewed by Shults et al. (218). As a result of these changes, the overall rate of alcohol related MVA fatality dropped by 7 percent . In California and some of the other states, immediate confiscation of licensure, called administrative license revocation (ALR) was also implemented. In an effort to isolate the effects Hingson et al. looked at the effect of the BAC change in states which already had ALR rules on the books and noted a 5 percent decrease in alcohol related fatalities when the lower BAC rule was instituted (253). Voas et al. used a statistical approach to separate the different factors. Using multivariate analysis he demonstrated that there was a reduction of 8 percent in alcohol related fatalities as a result of lowering of the acceptable BAC level by itself (258). There are great cultural, demographic and geographical differences between the states studies so it is assumed that the results of these studies are likely to be representative of the United States (218). The U.S. Congress has been impressed enough by the evidence to require all states to lower the BAC to 0.08 gm /dl by October 2003 or they will lose federal highway funds (259).

Younger drivers, partake in other risk taking behaviors and are at greater risk of MVA than their more experienced counterparts. This may be a result of decreased experience or partaking in other risk taking behaviors that are associated with alcohol ingestion. The work of Anderson et al. that demonstrated that over half of non seat belt wearing drivers involved in a MVA were positive for alcohol as compared to 22 percent of those wearing shoulder belts serves as an example (260). Similarly, there is a much lower use of restraints among those who ingest alcohol. This is especially true with adolescents where only 7 percent with positive alcohol screens were using a restraint system as compared to 22 percent that had no alcohol (246). While, Peek-Asa and Kraus (88) demonstrated that motorcyclists involved in accidents who tested positive for alcohol were more likely to be speeding and not be wearing a helmet. Finally, Zador et al. (261). demonstrated that a 16 to 20 year old male who had a BAC level between 0.08 and 0.1 had a 24 times greater chance of dying from a MVA as compared to a BAC of zero. The benefit of Congressional mandates was again noted when its threat to withhold highway funding, prompted all states to pass legislation that requiring a BAC level of less than 0.02 for all drivers under 21 years of age (220). The minimum drinking age was first raised to 21 in several states by the 1970s. By 1987, all 50 states had raised the minimum drinking age to 21 (218). As a result of this change a double-digit decrease in both fatal and non-fatal MVA's was noted.

Legislation requires enforcement to be effective. There is a need to improve these efforts to facilitate prevention efforts. Sobriety checkpoints are an effective means of addressing this issue. There are two types of sobriety checkpoints, random breath testing (RBT) and selective breath testing (SBT). RBT has been used with Australia and Europe with great benefit. It is not currently available in the Unites States because of a lack of "probable cause." Instead in the United States only SBT sobriety checkpoints are utilized. With SBT checkpoints, the officer must have reasonable suspicion of intoxication in order for breath testing to be performed. Because of the nature of these checkpoints, they better serve the purpose of deterrence rather than actual identification of offenders (218).

SBT checkpoints have proven their efficacy and have been shown to reduce fatal car crashes 20–26 percent (262), as well as reducing overall crashes anywhere from 5 to 23 percent (218). RBT has been tested and has shown similar results (263–271). The studies of RBT showed a reduction in fatal crashes between 13–36 percent (264, 268,269,271) and 11–20 percent for all crashes (263, 265–271). RBT has also be shown to modify drivers' behavior in regards to drinking and driving. Work from Australia reported a 13 percent drop in drivers with any detectable alcohol on board and a 24 percent decrease in BAC level over 0.08 with RBT (223). The literature has shown that both the selective and random method of testing has been useful in reducing crashes of all types. While RBT is more sensitive that SBT relative to detecting elevated BAC, the literature has not demonstrated any difference in efficacy between the two methods relative to crash prevention (218). Technologic breakthroughs such as the addition of passive sensors that can sample for the presence of alcohol are being developed which may further increase the sensitivity of SBT by 50 percent which will further increase the sensitivity of SBT (272).

Even with proven efficacy, these programs face resistance as a possible violation of an individuals civil rights. The United States Supreme Court has weighed in and ruled on the appropriateness of a properly performed brief sobriety check The sense of the court was that this minor intrusion on human rights was more than balanced out by the public benefit of reducing DUI (273). Cost benefit issues is another issue raised regarding the use of SBT and the cost benefit ratio of having police officers man these checkpoints. Miller et al. (274). have addressed this issue. In their model of a community of 100,000 licensed drivers and assumed that the intervention would reduce accidents by 15 percent, a number chosen after reviewing the literature on SBT. Incorporating all of the costs of alcohol related MVA including medical, property etc, and their estimates were that $9.2 millions would be saved with an expenditure of $1.6 million with a ratio of nearly 6 to 1. An actual study performed in California was even more promising. Four communities introduced SBT for over ninth months at a relatively small cost of $165,000 The savings that resulted from this intervention resulted in a 23 times as large a benefit of $3.86 million. RBT testing may be more effective than SBT financially. Work from Australia and New South Wales has suggested that at an annual cost of $4 million per year a savings of $228 million was realized as a result of accident prevention (264). The efficacy of these programs both from a financial as well as from crash prevention requires society to take a look at these papers.

PEDIATRIC HEAD TRAUMA

Pediatric injuries are a significant cause of morbidity and mortality throughout the world. Approximately 600,000 children are hospitalized every year and more than 15 million children are seen in the emergency room each year because of their injuries (116). Head trauma accounts for over 500,00 emergency department visits annually (275). The annual costs exceed over 1 billion annually and 29,000 children sustain permanent disabilities.

CHILD ABUSE

Homicide from child abuse is the leading cause of death in infants in the United States (118). In 1999, approximately 4.1 percent of children less than 18 years old were victims of physical, emotional or sexual abuse (276). In a survey of pediatric head trauma, abuse accounted for 19 percent of cases and was associated with a higher rate of subdural hematoma (SDH), subarachnoid hemorrhage, as well as retinal hemorrhages (277). Child abuse is not only a form of violence but contributes to adverse consequences in maltreated children. Abuse in childhood has been associated with early pregnancy, drug abuse, school failure, mental illness, suicidal and aggressive behavior and violence later in life. Center (276).

Shaken baby syndrome results from severe movements of a child's head, can result in retinal hemorrhages, cerebral axonal injury, occult cervical injury, and coagulopathy (278,279). Young infants have weak neck muscles leaving them vulnerable to sustain SDH and shearing injuries. For a retinal hemorrhage to occur, it takes an extraordinary force and is usually not associated with an accidental injury (280). There are many educational programs in place to educate the community of the severe danger of shaking infants.

Child abuse has been associated with single-parent homes, low-income families and parents with alcohol and drug abuse and many home visitation programs in the United States are therefore directed toward the these high risk populations. The Center of Disease Control and Prevention noted that preventative programs delivered by nurses demonstrated a median reduction in child abuse of 48.7 percent and programs delivered by mental health workers demonstrated a median reduction in child abuse of 44.5 percent (276). In one study sample evaluating the cost-benefit ratio of home visits to low-income mothers, there was a net benefit of $350 dollars per family in 1997. Clinicians should also continue to target high-risk populations such as teenage parents, single mothers, families of low socioeconomic status and parents with alcohol, drug or mental health problems. Further programs are warranted to reach the goal of reduction of homicides from 6.5 to 3.0 per 100,000 populations by 2010 (281).

CAR SEATS AND AIR BAGS

Motor vehicle accidents are the major cause of death in children and adolescents. It has been estimated that motor vehicle accidents and traffic-related injuries account for 56 percent of injury fatalities (118), with front seat passengers appearing to be at the highest risk. There was legislation early on in the 1990's that focused its attention on placing young children in the back seat in addition to standardized three point restraints in all vehicles. The 1990s saw a decline in front seating of children in vehicles involved in fatal crashes likely attributed to public awareness and education and legislation (282). However children ages 6 to 12 remained at high risk for being front seated (282). Pediatric air bags systems pose a threat to the front-seated child passenger, with resultant cranial and cervical spine trauma (79). Patterns of injury in the child or adolescent will be different than that for an adult given the seat location, height and weight of the individual type of restraint and the biomechanics at impact placing the child closer to the deploying air bag all have an effect (283). Both age and weight of the child determine the appropriate restraint system. There has been legislation regarding child restraint system utilization, however, the poor compliance with these devices is concerning (284).

It has been estimated that 500 deaths and 53,000 injuries could be prevented each year if there were 100 percent compliance with existing state law and there was proper use of child safety belts (118). It is encouraging that education and legislation, including passive and active strategies, can result in a decrease in childhood injury.

PLAYGROUND AND RECREATIONAL INJURIES

In 1986, the United States Consumer Product Safety Commission estimated that approximately 7,000 children under the age of 15 had sustained a playground related injury that required hospitalization (116). Between 1990–1994, more than 200,000 playground injuries were reported (285). It has been estimated that 8 percent of

sport and recreation related head injuries are playground related (286).

A large proportion of injuries are related to climbing activities including monkey bars, jungle gyms, swings and slides, with approximately 25 percent of such injuries requiring hospitalization (287). In one study of Boston's playgrounds, 34 percent of playground hazards were related to climbers, 30 percent with slides and 22 percent with swings (288). Lillis & Jaffee evaluated all children injured on playground equipment in a metropolitan center in Canada. It was found that 39 percent of the children were under age 5 and 58 percent of those younger than 5 years old had head and cervical injuries (116).

Lessening the incidence and consequences of falls from playground equipment is a promising potential target for prevention efforts (289). Multifaceted efforts are important. Parents need to be educated and provide appropriate supervision in the playground environment. One study suggests one of the main contributing factors to playground injury is "lack of active competent adult supervision." (290) Educating children not to jump off a moving swing or walk behind a moving swing must be reinforced to the parents. The use of equipment by older children designed for younger children such as certain slides and climbing equipment that are very narrow can be dangerous. As a result the older child may slip or fall. Some slides are elevated 10–15 feet off the ground and the danger of the slide increases with increasing height. Unfortunately, the drive for safer design of playground sites has been pushed more by litigation than public policy.

The riding bicycles by children is another important area for prevention efforts and the use of helmets during bicycle riding is critical. It has been estimated that wearing helmets resulted in a 88 percent less risk of brain injury compared to those people who did not wear helmets (149). The problem is that use of helmets by North American children is less than 1 percent (146). This may be because children may feel like they do not fit in with their peers. If so, this is a strong reason to make helmet use mandatory and legislation is warranted to mandate helmet use in children. Legislation in addition to education of parents and children may improve compliance with helmet use. Skateboards are a common source of head injuries in the pediatric population. It appears that the rate of injury secondary to skateboards has surpassed that of bicyclists for those under 25 (291). The role of helmets in preventing serious injury related to skateboarding is also critical.

CONCLUSION

Traumatic brain injury is a major health problem for society. It is an area where prevention efforts can make a substantial difference in the overall public health. Prevention efforts must be directed at many different components that include legislation, education and motivation of the public to control this area of injury. There has been a tremendous progress made in TBI prevention over the last few decades. However, there is still a large amount of work needed to target all the different aspects, or "cells" in the Haddon Matrix, that contribute to TBI. Health care providers must continue to educate the lay public and assist politicians in recognizing the benefits of injury control. Hopefully as public awareness, technology and legislation improve so will prevention efforts.

References

1. Nguyen VQC, Cruz TH, McDeavitt JT. Traumatic brain injury and the science of injury control. State-of-the-art reviews: *PM&R* 2001 Jun; 213–27.

2. Sosin DM, Sniezek JE, Waxweiler RJ. Trends in death associated with traumatic brain injury, 1979 through 1992. Success and failure. *JAMA* 1995 Jun 14;273(22):1778–80.

3. Sosin DM, Sniezek JE, Thurman DJ. Incidence of mild and moderate brain injury in the United States, 1991. *Brain Inj* 1996 Jan;10(1):47–54.

4. Fife D. Head injury with and without hospital admission: comparisons of incidence and short-term disability. *Am J Public Health* 1987 Jul;77(7):810–2.

5. Thurman DJ, Alverson C, Dunn KA, Guerrero J, Sniezek JE. Traumatic brain injury in the United States: A public health perspective. *J Head Trauma Rehabil* 1999 Dec;14(6):602–15.

6. McDeavitt JT. Preface traumatic brain injury. Physical medicine and rehabilitation: State-of-the-art reviews 2001 Jun;15(2):ix-x.

7. Center for Disease Control and Prevention. Traumatic Brain Injury in the United States: A report to Congress. www.cdc.gov/ncipc/pub-res/tbicongress.htm 2001 [cited 2001 Nov 30];

8. McGarry LJ, Thompson D, Millham FH, Cowell L, Snyder PJ, Lenderking WR, et al. Outcomes and costs of acute treatment of traumatic brain injury. *J Trauma* 2002 Dec;53(6):1152–59.

9. Max W, MacKenzie EJ, Rice DP. Head injuries: costs and consequences. J Head Trauma Rehabil 1991;6:76–91.

10. Miller TR, Romano EO, Spicer RS. The cost of childhood unintentional injuries and the value of prevention. *Future Child* 2000;10(1):137–63.

11. Annegers JF, Grabow JD, Kurland LT, Laws ER, Jr. The incidence, causes, and secular trends of head trauma in Olmsted County, Minnesota, 1935–1974. *Neurology* 1980 Sep;30(9):912–9.

12. Kraus JF, Black MA, Hessol N, Ley P, Rokaw W, Sullivan C, et al. The incidence of acute brain injury and serious impairment in a defined population. *Am J Epidemiol* 1984 Feb;119(2): 186–201.

13. Jagger J, Levine JI, Jane JA, Rimel RW. Epidemiologic features of head injury in a predominantly rural population. *J Trauma* 1984 Jan;24(1):40–4.

14. U.S. Department of Health and Human Services. *HIV Aids Surveillance Reports*. www cdc gov/hiv/stats/hasr1102 pdf 2001 [cited 1 A.D. Dec 1];

15. Klassen TP, MacKay JM, Moher D, Walker A, Jones AL. Community-based injury prevention interventions. *Future Child* 2000;10(1):83–110.

16. Committee on Injury Prevention and Control DoHPaDPIoM. *Reducing the Burden of Injury: Advancing Prevention and Treatment*. Washington, D.C.: National Academy Press; 1999.

17. Miller TR, Galbraith M. Injury prevention counseling by pediatricians: a benefit-cost comparison. *Pediatrics* 1995 Jul;96(1 Pt 1):1–4.

18. Last JM, Gunther R. *Maxcy-Rosenau-Last Public Health and Preventative Medicine*. 13th ed. Norwalk, CT.: Appelton and Lange; 1992.

19. U. S. Preventative Services (USPS) Task Force. *Guide to Clinical Preventative Services: Report of the US Preventative Services Task Force*. 2nd ed. Baltimore, MD: WIlliams & WIlliams; 1989.

20. Guyer B, Gallagher SS. An approach to the epidemiology of childhood injuries. *Pediatr Clin North Am* 1985 Feb;32(1):5–15.

21. Elovic E, Antoinette T. Epidemiology and primary prevention of traumatic brain injury. In: Horn LJ, Zasler ND, editors. *Medical Rehabilitation of Traumatic Brain Injury*.Philadelphia: Hanley & Belfus; 1996. p. 1–28.

22. Teutsch SM. A framework for assessing the effectiveness of disease and injury prevention. *MMWR Morb Mortal Wkly Rep* 1992 Mar 27;41(RR-3):1–12.

23. Gielen AC, Girasek DC. Integrating perspectives on the prevention of unintentional injuries. In: Schneiderman N, Speers MA, Silva JM, Tomes H, Gentry JH, editors. *Integrating Behavioral and Social Sciences with Public Health*. Washington D.C.: American Psychological Association; 2001. p. 203–27.

24. Karlson TA. Injury control and public policy. *Crit Rev Environ Contr* 1992;195–241.

25. American Cancer Society. Cancer facts and figures, selected cancers. www.cancer.org/statistics/cff99/selectedcancers.html (2001).

26. National Highway Traffic Safety Administration. Standard enforcement saves lives; The case for strong seatbelt laws. Washington, D.C.: U.S. Department of Transportation; 1999.

27. DiGuiseppi C, Roberts IG. Individual-level injury prevention strategies in the clinical setting. *Future Child* 2000;10(1):53–82.

28. Roberston LS, Kelley AB, O'Neill B, Wixom CW, Eiswirth RS, Haddon W. A controlled study of the effect of television messages on safety belt use. *Am J Publ Health* 1974;1071–80.

29. Cote TR, Sacks JJ, Lambert-Huber DA, Dannenberg AL, Kresnow MJ, Lipsitz CM, et al. Bicycle helmet use among Maryland children: effect of legislation and education. *Pediatrics* 1992 Jun;89(6 Pt 2):1216–20.

30. Jagger J. Prevention of brain trauma by legislation, regulation and improved technology: A focus on motor vehicles. *Neurotrauma* 1992;9S:313–6.

31. National Highway Traffic Safety Administration. U.S. Department of Transportation DOT HS 808 841 (1990).

32. National Highway Traffic Safety Administration. Third Report to Congress: Effectiveness of occupant protection systems and their use. National Highway Traffic Safety Administration 1996 [cited 1 A.D. Dec 17]; Available from: URL: www.nhtsa.dot.gov/people/injury/airbags/208con2e.html

33. Duma SM, Boggess BM, Crandall JR, Hurwitz SR, Seki K, Aoki T. Upper extremity interaction with a deploying side airbag: a characterization of elbow joint loading. *Accid Anal Prev* 2003 May;35(3):417–25.

34. King AI, Yang KH. Research in biomechanics of occupant protection. *J Trauma* 1995 Apr;38(4):570–6.

35. Parkin S, Mackay GM, Cooper A. How drivers sit in cars. *Accid Anal Prev* 1995 Dec;27(6):777–83.

36. Gennarelli TA, Champion HR, Sacco WJ, Copes WS, Alves WM. Mortality of patients with head injury and extracranial injury treated in trauma centers. *J Trauma* 1989 Sep;29(9): 1193–201.

37. Agran PF, Dunkle DE, Winn DG. Injuries to a sample of seatbelted children evaluated and treated in a hospital emergency room. *J Trauma* 1987 Jan;27(1):58–64.

38. Appleby JP, Nagy AG. Abdominal injuries associated with the use of seatbelts. *Am J Surg* 1989 May;157(5):457–8.

39. Arajarvi E, Santavirta S, Tolonen J. Abdominal injuries sustained in severe traffic accidents by seatbelt wearers. *J Trauma* 1987 Apr;27(4):393–7.

40. Blacksin MF. Patterns of fracture after air bag deployment. *J Trauma* 1993 Dec;35(6):840–3.

41. Bourbeau R, Desjardins D, Maag U, Laberge-Nadeau C. Neck injuries among belted and unbelted occupants of the front seat of cars. *J Trauma* 1993 Nov;35(5):794–9.

42. Chandler CF, Lane JS, Waxman KS. Seatbelt sign following blunt trauma is associated with increased incidence of abdominal injury. *Am Surg* 1997 Oct;63(10):885–8.

43. Hall CE, Norton SA, Dixon AR. Complete small bowel transection following lap-belt injury. *Injury* 2001 Oct;32(8):640–1.

44. Holbrook JL, Bennett JB. Brachial plexus injury associated with chest restraint seatbelt: case report. *J Trauma* 1990 Nov;30(11):1413–4.

45. Immega G. Whiplash injuries increase with seatbelt use. *Can Fam Physician* 1995 Feb;41:203–4.

46. Johnson DL, Falci S. The diagnosis and treatment of pediatric lumbar spine injuries caused by rear seat lap belts. *Neurosurgery* 1990 Mar;26(3):434–41.

47. Kaplan BH, Cowley RA. Seatbelt effectiveness and cost of noncompliance among drivers admitted to a trauma center. *Am J Emerg Med* 1991 Jan;9(1):4–10.

48. Lubbers EJ. Injury of the duodenum caused by a fixed three-point seatbelt. *J Trauma* 1977 Dec;17(12):960.

49. May AK, Chan B, Daniel TM, Young JS. Anterior lung herniation: another aspect of the seatbelt syndrome. *J Trauma* 1995 Apr;38(4):587–9.

50. Restifo KM, Kelen GD. Case report: sternal fracture from a seatbelt. *J Emerg Med* 1994 May;12(3):321–3.

51. Santavirta S, Arajarvi E. Ruptures of the heart in seatbelt wearers. *J Trauma* 1992 Mar;32(3):275–9.

52. Shoemaker BL, Ose M. Pediatric lap belt injuries: care and prevention. *Orthop Nurs* 1997 Sep;16(5):15–22.

53. Verdant A. Abdominal injuries sustained in severe traffic accidents by seatbelt wearers. *J Trauma* 1988 Jun;28(6):880–1.

54. Warrian RK, Shoenut JP, Iannicello CM, Sharma GP, Trenholm BG. Seatbelt injury to the abdominal aorta. *J Trauma* 1988 Oct;28(10):1505–7.

55. Yarbrough BE, Hendey GW. Hangman's fracture resulting from improper seat belt use. *South Med J* 1990 Jul;83(7):843–5.

56. Bandstra RA, Carbone LS. Unusual basal skull fracture in a vehicle equipped with an air bag. *Am J Forensic Med Pathol* 2001 Sep;22(3):253–5.

57. Murphy RX, Jr., Birmingham KL, Okunski WJ, Wasser T. The influence of airbag and restraining devices on the patterns of facial trauma in motor vehicle collisions. *Plast Reconstr Surg* 2000 Feb;105(2):516–20.

58. Rozner L. Air bag-bruised face. Plast Reconstr Surg 1996 Jun;97(7):1517–9.

59. Lueder GT. Air bag-associated ocular trauma in children. *Ophthalmology* 2000 Aug;107(8):1472–5.

60. Stein JD, Jaeger EA, Jeffers JB. Air bags and ocular injuries. *Trans Am Ophthalmol Soc* 1999;97:59–82.

61. Ruiz-Moreno JM. Air bag-associated retinal tear. *Eur J Ophthalmol* 1998 Jan;8(1):52–3.

62. Zabriskie NA, Hwang IP, Ramsey JF, Crandall AS. Anterior lens capsule rupture caused by air bag trauma. *Am J Ophthalmol* 1997 Jun;123(6):832–3.

63. Ghafouri A, Burgess SK, Hrdlicka ZK, Zagelbaum BM. Air bag-related ocular trauma. *Am J Emerg Med* 1997 Jul;15(4):389–92.

64. Ulrich D, Noah EM, Fuchs P, Pallua N. Burn injuries caused by air bag deployment. *Burns* 2001 Mar;27(2):196–9.

65. White JE, McClafferty K, Orton RB, Tokarewicz AC, Nowak ES. Ocular alkali burn associated with automobile air-bag activation. *CMAJ* 1995 Oct 1;153(7):933–4.

66. Conover K. Chemical burn from automotive air bag. *Ann Emerg Med* 1992 Jun;21(6):770.

67. Guarino AH. More on reflex sympathetic dystrophy syndrome following air-bag inflation. *N Engl J Med* 1998 Jan 29;338(5):335.

68. Shah N, Weinstein A. Reflex sympathetic dystrophy syndrome following air-bag inflation. *N Engl J Med* 1997 Aug 21;337(8):574.

69. Kirchhoff R, Rasmussen SW. Forearm fracture due to the release of an automobile air bag. *Acta Orthop Scand* 1995 Oct;66(5):483.

70. Ong CF, Kumar VP. Colles fracture from air bag deployment. *Injury* 1998 Oct;29(8):629–31.

71. Giguere JF, St Vil D, Turmel A, Di Lorenzo M, Pothel C, Manseau S, et al. Airbags and children: a spectrum of C-spine injuries. *J Pediatr Surg* 1998 Jun;33(6):811–6.

72. Traynelis VC, Gold M. Cervical spine injury in an air-bag-equipped vehicle. *J Spinal Disord* 1993 Feb;6(1):60–1.

73. Morris MS, Borja LP. Air bag deployment and hearing loss. *Am Fam Physician* 1998 Jun;57(11):2627–8.

74. Kramer MB, Shattuck TG, Charnock DR. Traumatic hearing loss following air-bag inflation. *N Engl J Med* 1997 Aug 21;337(8):574–5.

75. Air-bag-associated fatal injuries to infants and children riding in front passenger seats—United States. *MMWR* 1995 Nov 17;44(45):845–7.

76. From the Centers for Disease Control and Prevention. Air-bag-associated fatal injuries to infants and children riding in front passenger seats—United States. JAMA 1995 Dec 13;274(22):1752–3.

77. From the Centers for Disease Control and Prevention. Update: fatal air bag-related injuries to children—United States, 1993–1996. JAMA 1997 Jan 1;277(1):11–2.

78. Angel CA, Ehlers RA. Images in clinical medicine. Atloido-occipital dislocation in a small child after air-bag deployment. *N Engl J Med* 2001 Oct 25;345(17):1256.

79. Marshall KW, Koch BL, Egelhoff JC. Air bag-related deaths and serious injuries in children: injury patterns and imaging findings. *AJNR Am J Neuroradiol* 1998 Oct;19(9):1599–607.

80. McCaffrey M, German A, Lalonde F, Letts M. Air bags and children: a potentially lethal combination. *J Pediatr Orthop* 1999 Jan;19(1):60–4.

81. Totten VY, Fani-Salek MH, Chandramohan K. Hyphema associated with air bag deployment in a pediatric trauma patient. *Am J Emerg Med* 1998 Jan;16(1):102–3.

82. Morrison AL, Chute D, Radentz S, Golle M, Troncoso JC, Smialek JE. Air bag-associated injury to a child in the front passenger seat. *Am J Forensic Med Pathol* 1998 Sep;19(3):218–22.

83. Willis BK, Smith JL, Falkner LD, Vernon DD, Walker ML. Fatal air bag mediated craniocervical trauma in a child. *Pediatr Neurosurg* 1996 Jun;24(6):323–7.

84. Flint S. *Prevention Matters*. Brain Injury Association; 2001.

85. Head injuries associated with motorcycle use—Wisconsin, 1991. *MMWR Morb Mortal Wkly Rep* 1994 Jun 17;43(23):423, 429–3, 431.

86. Braddock M, Schwartz R, Lapidus G, Banco L, Jacobs L. A population-based study of motorcycle injury and costs. *Ann Emerg Med* 1992 Mar;21(3):273–8.

87. Begg DJ, Langley JD, Reeder AI. Motorcycle crashes in New Zealand resulting in death and hospitalisation. I: Introduction methods and overview. *Accid Anal Prev* 1994 Apr;26(2):157–64.

88. Peek-Asa C, Kraus JF. Alcohol use, driver, and crash characteristics among injured motorcycle drivers. *J Trauma* 1996 Dec;41(6):989–93.

89. Heilman DR, Weisbuch JB, Blair RW, Graf LL. Motorcycle-related trauma and helmet usage in North Dakota. *Ann Emerg Med* 1982 Dec;11(12):659–64.

90. Bachulis BL, Sangster W, Gorrell GW, Long WB. Patterns of injury in helmeted and nonhelmeted motorcyclists. *Am J Surg* 1988 May;155(5):708–11.

91. Gabella B, Reiner KL, Hoffman RE, Cook M, Stallones L. Relationship of helmet use and head injuries among motorcycle crash victims in El Paso County, Colorado, 1989–1990. *Accid Anal Prev* 1995 Jun;27(3):363–9.

92. Ferrando J, Plasencia A, Oros M, Borrell C, Kraus JF. Impact of a helmet law on two wheel motor vehicle crash mortality in a southern European urban area. *Inj Prev* 2000 Sep;6(3):184–8.

93. Chiu WT, Kuo CY, Hung CC, Chen M. The effect of the Taiwan motorcycle helmet use law on head injuries. *Am J Public Health* 2000 May;90(5):793–6.

94. Fleming NS, Becker ER. The impact of the Texas 1989 motorcycle helmet law on total and head-related fatalities, severe injuries, and overall injuries. *Med Care* 1992 Sep;30(9):832–45.

95. Kraus JF, Peek C, McArthur DL, Williams A. The effect of the 1992 California motorcycle helmet use law on motorcycle crash fatalities and injuries. *JAMA* 1994 Nov 16;272(19):1506–11.

96. Muelleman RL, Mlinek EJ, Collicott PE. Motorcycle crash injuries and costs: effect of a reenacted comprehensive helmet use law. *Ann Emerg Med* 1992 Mar;21(3):266–72.

97. Rowland J, Rivara F, Salzberg P, Soderberg R, Maier R, Koepsell T. Motorcycle helmet use and injury outcome and hospitalization costs from crashes in Washington State. *Am J Public Health* 1996 Jan;86(1):41–5.

98. Sosin DM, Sacks JJ, Holmgreen P. Head injury—associated deaths from motorcycle crashes. Relationship to helmet-use laws. *JAMA* 1990 Nov 14;264(18):2395–9.

99. Tsai MC, Hemenway D. Effect of the mandatory helmet law in Taiwan. *Inj Prev* 1999 Dec;5(4):290–1.

100. Vaca F, Berns SD. National Highway Traffic Safety Administration. Commentary: Motorcycle helmet law repeal—a tax assessment for the rest of the United States? *Ann Emerg Med* 2001 Feb;37(2):230–2.

101. Vaca F, Berns SD, Harris JS, Jolly BT, Runge JW, Todd KH. National Highway Traffic Safety Administration. Evaluation of the repeal of motorcycle helmet laws. *Ann Emerg Med* 2001 Feb;37(2):229–30.

102. Hotz GA, Cohn SM, Popkin C, Ekeh P, Duncan R, Johnson EW, et al. The impact of a repealed motorcycle helmet law in Miami-Dade County. *J Trauma* 2002 Mar;52(3):469–74.

103. Bledsoe GH, Schexnayder SM, Carey MJ, Dobbins WN, Gibson WD, Hindman JW, et al. The negative impact of the repeal of the Arkansas motorcycle helmet law. *J Trauma* 2002 Dec; 53(6):1078–86.

104. National Highway Traffic Safety Administration. *Evaluation of Motorcycle Helmet Law Repeal in Arkansas and Texas*. Washington, D.C.: US Department of Transportation; 2000.

105. Sun SW, Kahn DM, Swan KG. Lowering the legal blood alcohol level for motorcyclists. *Accid Anal Prev* 1998 Jan;30(1):133–6.

106. Sabey B. Engineering safety on the road. *Inj Prev* 1995 Sep; 1(3):182–6.

107. Local Authority Associations. *Road Safety Code of Good Practice*. London, England: Association of County Councils; 1989.

108. Retting RA, Weinstein HB, Williams AF, Preusser DF. A simple method for identifying and correcting crash problems on urban arterial streets. *Accid Anal Prev* 2001 Nov;33(6):723–34.

109. Navin F, Zein S, Felipe E. Road safety engineering: an effective tool in the fight against whiplash injuries. *Accid Anal Prev* 2000 Mar;32(2):271–5.

110. Pau M, Angius S. Do speed bumps really decrease traffic speed? An Italian experience. *Accid Anal Prev* 2001 Sep;33(5):585–97.

111. Lum KM, Wong YD. A study of stopping propensity at matured red light camera T-intersections. *J Safety Res* 2002;33(3): 355–69.

112. Cooper K, Tabaddor K, Hauser WA, et al. The epidemiology of head injury in the Bronx. *Neuroepidemiology* 1983;2:70–88.

113. Whitman S, Coonley-Hoganson R, Desai BT. Comparative head trauma experiences in two socioeconomically different Chicago-area communities: a population study. *Am J Epidemiol* 1984 Apr;119(4):570–80.

114. Sosin DM, Sacks JJ, Smith SM. Head injury-associated deaths in the United States from 1979 to 1986 [see comments]. *JAMA* 1989 Oct 27;262(16):2251–5.

115. Tiret L, Hausherr E, Thicoipe M, Garros B, Maurette P, Castel JP, et al. The epidemiology of head trauma in Aquitaine (France), 1986: a community-based study of hospital admissions and deaths. *Int J Epidemiol* 1990 Mar;19(1):133–40.

116. Lillis KA, Jaffe DM. Playground injuries in children. *Pediatr Emerg Care* 1997 Apr;13(2):149–53.

117. Kotch JB, Chalmers DJ, Langley JD, Marshall SW. Child day care and home injuries involving playground equipment. *J Paediatr Child Health* 1993 Jun;29(3):222–7.

118. Stylianos S, Eichelberger MR. Pediatric trauma. Prevention strategies. *Pediatr Clin North Am* 1993 Dec;40(6):1359–68.

119. Benoit R, Watts DD, Dwyer K, Kaufmann C, Fakhry S. Windows 99: a source of suburban pediatric trauma. *J Trauma* 2000 Sep;49(3):477–81.

120. Koplan JP, Thacker SB. Working to prevent and control injury in the United States. *Fact Book for the Year 2000*. Centers for Disease Control and Prevention National Center for Injury Prevention and Control; 2000.

121. Bjerre B, Schelp L. The community safety approach in Falun, Sweden—is it possible to characterise the most effective prevention endeavours and how long-lasting are the results? *Accid Anal Prev* 2000 May;32(3):461–70.

122. Davidson LL, Durkin MS, Kuhn L, O'Connor P, Barlow B, Hegarty MC. The impact of the Safe Kids/Healthy Neighborhoods Injury Prevention Program in Harlem, 1988 through 1991. *Am J Public Health* 1994 Apr;84(4):580–6.

123. Durkin MS, Olsen S, Barlow B, Virella A, Connolly ES, Jr. The epidemiology of urban pediatric neurological trauma: evaluation of, and implications for, injury prevention programs. *Neurosurgery* 1998 Feb;42(2):300–10.

124. Consumer Product Safety Commission. *Home Playground Safety Tips*. www cpsc gov/cpscpub/pubs/323 html 2001 [cited 1 A.D. Feb 1];

125. Consumer Product Safety Commission. Public playground safety checklist. www cpsc gov/cpscpub/pubs/327 html 2001 [cited 1 A.D. Feb 1].

126. Gresham LS, Zirkle DL, Tolchin S, Jones C, Maroufi A, Miranda J. Partnering for injury prevention: evaluation of a curriculum-based intervention program among elementary school children. *J Pediatr Nurs* 2001 Apr;16(2):79–87.

127. Jeffs D, Booth D, Calvert D. Local injury information, community participation and injury reduction. *Aust J Public Health* 1993 Dec;17(4):365–72.

128. Miller KE, Zylstra RG, Standridge JB. The geriatric patient: a systematic approach to maintaining health. *Am Fam Physician* 2000 Feb 15;61(4):1089–104.

129. National Center for Injury Prevention and Control. Falls and Hip Fractures Among Older Adults. http://www.cdc.gov/ncipc/factsheets/falls.htm 2002 [cited 2 A.D. Feb 1].

130. Speechley M, Tinetti M. Falls and injuries in frail and vigorous community elderly persons. *J Am Geriatr Soc* 1991 Jan;39(1): 46–52.

131. Rosenthall U, Rubin W. Degenerative changes in the human vestibular sensory epithelia. *Acta Otolaryngol (Stockh)* 1975; 79:67–80.

132. Manchester D, Woollacott M, Zederbauer-Hylton N, Marin O. Visual, vestibular and somatosensory contributions to balance control in the older adult. *J Gerontol* 1989 Jul;44(4):M118– M127.

133. Hasselkus BR. Aging and the human nervous system. *Am J Occup Ther* 1974 Jan;28(1):16–21.

134. Sinclair AJ, Nayak US. Age-related changes in postural sway. *Compr Ther* 1990 Sep;16(9):44–8.

135. Wober C, Odler W, Kollegger H, Prayer L, Baumgatner C, Wober-Bingol C, et al. Posturographic measurement of body sway in survivors of severe closed head injury. *Arch Phys Med Rehabil* 1993;74(11):1151–6.

136. Helbostad JL, Askim T, Moe-Nilssen R. Short-term repeatability of body sway during quiet standing in people with hemiparesis and in frail older adults. *Arch Phys Med Rehabil* 2004 Jun;85(6):993–9.

137. Shumway-Cook A, Anson D, Haller S. Postural sway biofeedback: its effect on reestablishing stance stability in hemiplegic patients. *Arch Phys Med Rehabil* 1988 Jun;69(6):395–400.

138. Fialova D, Topinkova E, Gambassi G, Finne-Soveri H, Jonsson PV, Carpenter I, et al. Potentially inappropriate medication use among elderly home care patients in Europe. *JAMA* 2005 Mar 16;293(11):1348–58.

139. Brain Injury Association. Falls. www biausa org 2001 [cited 1 A.D. Dec 1].

140. Plautz B, Beck DE, Selmar C, Radetsky M. Modifying the environment: a community-based injury-reduction program for elderly residents. *Am J Prev Med* 1996 Jul;12(4 Suppl):33–8.

141. Smeltzer SC, Zimmerman V, Capriotti T. Osteoporosis risk and low bone mineral density in women with physical disabilities. *Arch Phys Med Rehabil* 2005 Mar;86(3):582–6.

142. Johnston KM, McCrory P, Mohtadi NG, Meeuwisse WH. Evidence-based review of sport-related concussion: Clinical science. *Clin J Sport Med* 2001;11:150–9.

143. Friede AM, Azzara CV, Gallagher SS, Guyer B. The epidemiology of injuries to bicycle riders. *Pediatr Clin North Am* 1985 Feb;32(1):141–51.

144. Fife D, Davis J, Tate L, Wells JK, Mohan D, Williams A. Fatal injuries to bicyclists: the experience of Dade County, Florida. *J Trauma* 1983 Aug;23(8):745–55.

145. Think First Foundation. Think first fact sheet bicycle safety. 2000.

146. Spence LJ, Dykes EH, Bohn DJ, Wesson DE. Fatal bicycle accidents in children: a plea for prevention. *J Pediatr Surg* 1993 Feb;28(2):214–6.

147. Williams AF. Factors in the initiation of bicycle-motor vehicle collisions. *Am J Dis Child* 1976 Apr;130(4):370–7.

148. Thompson DC, Rivara FP, Thompson R. Helmets for preventing head and facial injuries in bicyclists. *Cochrane Database Syst Rev* 2004;2.

149. Thompson DC, Rivara FP, Thompson R. Helmets for preventing head and facial injuries in bicyclists. *Cochrane Database Syst Rev* 2000;(2):CD001855.

150. Atha J, Yeardon MR, Sandover J, Parsons KC. The damaging punch. *BMJ* 1985;291:21–8.

151. Wilberger JE, Maroon JC. Head Injuries in Athletes. *Clin Sports Med* 1989;8:1–9.

152. Jordan BD. Chronic traumatic brain injury associated with boxing. *Semin Neurol* 2000;20(2):179–85.

153. Brain injury in boxing. Council on Scientific Affairs. *JAMA* 1983 Jan 14;249(2):254–7.

154. Ryan AJ. Intracranial injuries resulting from boxing: a review (1918–1985). *Clin Sports Med* 1987 Jan;6(1):31–40.

155. Leclerc S, Herrera CD. Sport medicine and the ethics of boxing. *Br J Sports Med* 1999 Dec;33(6):426–9.

156. Blyth CS, Mueller F. Football injury survey: Part 1 when and where players get hurt. *Physician Sportsmed* 1974;45–52.

157. Mueller FO. Fatalities from head and cervical spine injuries occuring in tackle football: 50 years experience. *Clin Sports Med* 1998;17:169–82.

158. Kelly JP, Nichols JS, Filley CM, Lillehei KO, Rubinstein D, Kleinschmidt-DeMasters BK. Concussion in sports. Guidelines for the prevention of catastrophic outcome. *JAMA* 1991 Nov 27; 266(20):2867–9.

159. Wilberger JE. Minor head injuries in American football. Prevention of long-term sequelae. *Sports Med* 1993 May;15(5):338–43.

160. Porter CD. Football injuries. *Phys Med Rehabil Clin N Am* 1999 Feb;10(1):95–115.

161. McCrory PR, Berkovic SF. Second impact syndrome. *Neurology* 1998 Mar;50(3):677–83.

162. Tysvaer AT. Head and neck injuries in soccer. Impact of minor trauma. *Sports Med* 1992 Sep;14(3):200–13.

163. Fields KB. Head injuries in soccer. *Physician Sportsmed* 1989;17(1):69–73.

164. Dvorak J, Junge A. Football injuries and physical symptoms. A review of the literature. *Am J Sports Med* 2000;28(5 Suppl): S3–S9.

165. Shawdon A, Brukner P. Injury profile of amateur Australian rules footballers. *Aust J Sci Med Sport* 1994 Sep;26(3–4):59–61.

166. Lindqvist KS, Timpka T, Bjurulf P. Injuries during leisure physical activity in a Swedish municipality. *Scand J Soc Med* 1996 Dec;24(4):282–92.

167. Ytterstad B. The Harstad injury prevention study: the epidemiology of sports injuries. An 8 year study. *Br J Sports Med* 1996 Mar;30(1):64–8.

168. Powell JW, Barber-Foss KD. Traumatic brain injury in high school athletes. *JAMA* 1999 Sep 8;282(10):958–63.

169. Tysvaer A, Storli O. Association football injuries to the brain. A preliminary report. *Br J Sports Med* 1981 Sep;15(3): 163–6.

170. Dvorak J, Junge A, Chomiak J. Risk factor analysis for injuries in football players. *Am J Sports Med* 2000;28:S69–S74.

171. Smodlaka VN. Medical aspects of heading the ball in soccer. *Physician Sportsmed* 1984;12(2):127–31.

172. Dailey SW, Barsan WG. Head Injuries in Soccer. A case for protective headgear? *The Physician and Sports Med* 1992;20(8): 79–82.

173. McIntosh AS, McCrory P. Impact energy attenuation performance of football headgear. *Br J Sports Med* 2000 Oct;34(5): 337–41.

174. Kirkendall DT, Jordan SE, Garret WE. Heading and head injuries in soccer. *Sports Med* 2001;31(5):369–86.

175. Biasca N, Simmen HP, Bartolozzi AR, Trentz O. Review of typical ice hockey injuries. Survey of the North American NHL and Hockey Canada versus European leagues. *Unfallchirurg* 1995 May;98(5):283–8.

176. Downs JR. Incidence of facial trauma in intercollegiate and junior hockey. *Physician Sportsmed* 1979;7(2):88–92.

177. Hayes D. Hockey injuries: How, why, where and when? *Physician Sportsmed* 1975;3(1):61–5.

178. Honey CR. Brain injury in ice hockey. *Clin J Sport Med* 1998 Jan;8(1):43–6.

179. Dryden DM, Francescutti LH, Rowe BH, Spence JC, Voaklander DC. Epidemiology of women's recreational ice hockey injuries. *Med Sci Sports Exerc* 2000 Aug;32(8):1378–83.

180. Reid SR, Losek JD. Factors associated with significant injuries in youth ice hockey players. *Pediatr Emerg Care* 1999 Oct;15(5): 310–3.

181. LaPrade RF, Burnett QM, Zarzour R. The effect of the mandatory use of face masks on facial laceration and head and neck injuries in ice hockey. *Am J Sports Med* 1995;23:773–5.

182. Voaklander DC, Saunders LD, Quinney HA, Macnab RB. Epidemiology of recreational and old-timer ice hockey injuries. *Clin J Sport Med* 1996 Jan;6(1):15–21.

183. Pinto M, Kuhn JE, Greenfield ML, Hawkins RJ. Prospective analysis of ice hockey injuries at the Junior A level over the course of one season. *Clin J Sport Med* 1999 Apr;9(2):70–4.

184. McCaw ST, Walker JD. Winning the Stanley Cup Final Series is related to incurring fewer penalties for violent behavior. *Tex Med* 1999 Apr;95(4):66–9.

185. Siccardi D, Cavaliere R, Pau A, Lubinu F, Turtas S, Viale GL. Penetrating craniocerebral missile injuries in civilians: a retrospective analysis of 314 cases. *Surg Neurol* 1991 Jun;35(6):455–60.

186. Kaufman HH, Makela ME, Lee KF, Haid RW, Jr., Gildenberg PL. Gunshot wounds to the head: a perspective. *Neurosurgery* 1986 Jun;18(6):689–95.

187. Krieger MD, Levy ML, Apuzzo ML. Gunshot wounds to the head in an urban setting. *Neurosurg Clin N Am* 1995 Oct;6(4): 605–10.

188. Nagib M, Rockswold G, Sherman R. Civilian gunshot wounds to the brain; prognosis and management. *Neurosurgery* 1986; 18:533–7.

189. Harrison-Felix C, Zafonte R, Mann N, Dijkers M, Englander J, Kreutzer J. Brain injury as a result of violence: preliminary findings from the traumatic brain injury model systems. *Arch Phys Med Rehabil* 1998 Jul;79(7):730–7.

190. Cook PJ, Ludwig J. *Guns in America: Results of a Comprehensive National Survey on Firearms Ownership and Use.* Washington, D.C.: Police Foundation; 1996.

191. Nelson DE, Grant-Worley JA, Powell K, Mercy J, Holtzman D. Population estimates of household firearm storage practices and firearm carrying in Oregon. *JAMA* 1996 Jun 12;275(22):1744–8.

192. Dresang LT. Gun deaths in rural and urban settings: recommendations for prevention. *J Am Board Fam Pract* 2001 Mar;14(2): 107–15.

193. Weil DS, Hemenway D. Loaded guns in the home. Analysis of a national random survey of gun owners. JAMA 1992 Jun 10; 267(22):3033–7.

194. Kellermann AL, Rivara FP, Somes G, Reay DT, Francisco J, Banton JG, et al. Suicide in the home in relation to gun ownership. *N Engl J Med* 1992 Aug 13;327(7):467–72.

195. Kellermann AL, Rivara FP, Rushforth NB, Banton JG, Reay DT, Francisco JT, et al. Gun ownership as a risk factor for homicide in the home. *N Engl J Med* 1993 Oct 7;329(15):1084–91.

196. Rodriguez MA, Gorovitz E. The politics and prevention of gun violence. *West J Med* 1999 Nov;171(5–6):296–7.

197. Teret SP, Webster DW, Vernick JS, Smith TW, Leff D, Wintemute GJ, et al. Support for new policies to regulate firearms. Results of two national surveys. *N Engl J Med* 1998 Sep 17;339(12): 813–8.

198. Villaveces A, Cummings P, Espitia VE, Koepsell TD, McKnight B, Kellermann AL. Effect of a ban on carrying firearms on homicide rates in 2 Colombian cities. *JAMA* 2000 Mar 1;283(9): 1205–9.

199. Howard KA, Webster DW, Vernick JS. Beliefs about the risks of guns in the home: analysis of a national survey. *Inj Prev* 1999 Dec;5(4):284–9.

200. Coyne-Beasley T, Schoenbach VJ, Johnson RM. "Love our kids, lock your guns": a community-based firearm safety counseling and gun lock distribution program. *Arch Pediatr Adolesc Med* 2001 Jun;155(6):659–64.

201. Milne JS, Hargarten SW. Handgun safety features: a review for physicians. *J Trauma* 1999 Jul;47(1):145–50.

202. Zakocs RC, Earp JA, Runyan CW. State gun control advocacy tactics and resources. *Am J Prev Med* 2001 May;20(4): 251–7.

203. Campbell NC, Thomson SR, Muckart DJ, Meumann CM, Van M, I, Botha JB. Review of 1198 cases of penetrating cardiac trauma. *Br J Surg* 1997 Dec;84(12):1737–40.

204. Zafonte RD, Mann NR, Millis SR, Wood DL, Lee CY, Black KL. Functional outcome after violence related traumatic brain injury. *Brain Inj* 1997 Jun;11(6):403–7.

205. Wagner AK, Sasser HC, Hammond FM, Wiercisiewski D, Alexander J. Intentional traumatic brain injury: epidemiology, risk factors, and associations with injury severity and mortality. *J Trauma* 2000 Sep;49(3):404–10.

206. Teasdale TW, Engberg AW. Suicide after traumatic brain injury: a population study. *J Neurol Neurosurg Psychiatry* 2001 Oct;71(4):436–40.

207. Mackenzie TB, Popkin MK. Suicide in the medical patient. *Int J Psychiatry Med* 1987;17(1):3–22.

208. Simpson G, Tate R. Suicidality after traumatic brain injury: demographic, injury and clinical correlates. *Psychol Med* 2002 May;32(4):687–97.

209. Kishi Y, Robinson RG, Kosier JT. Suicidal ideation among patients during the rehabilitation period after life-threatening physical illness. *J Nerv Ment Dis* 2001 Sep;189(9):623–8.

210. Simpson G, Winstanley J, Bertapelle T. Suicide prevention training after traumatic brain injury: evaluation of a staff training workshop. *J Head Trauma Rehabil* 2003 Sep;18(5):445–56.

211. Tierney RJ. Suicide intervention training evaluation: a preliminary report. *Crisis* 1994;15(2):69–76.

212. McIntosh JL, Hubbard RW, Santos JF. Suicide facts and myths: a study of prevalence. *Death Stud* 1985;9:267–81.

213. Potter LB, Powell KE, Kachur SP. Suicide prevention from a public health perspective. *Suicide Life Threat Behav* 1995;25(1): 82–91.

214. Jernigan DH. Alcohol and head trauma: strategies for prevention. *J Head Trauma Rehabil* 1991;6(2):48–59.

215. NHIF Professional Council Substance Abuse Task Force. NHIF Professional Council Substance Abuse Task Force White Paper. Washington, D.C.: National Head Injury Foundation; 1988.

216. Kreutzer JS, Doherty KR, Harris JA, Zasler ND. Alcohol use among persons with a traumatic brain injury. *J Head Trauma Rehabil* 1990;5(3):9–20.

217. Rivara FP, Koepsell TD, Koepsell TD, Jurkovich GJ, Gurney JG, Soderberg R. The effects of alcohol abuse on readmission for trauma. *JAMA* 1993;270:1962–4.

218. Shults RA, Elder RW, Sleet DA, Nichols JL, Alao MA, Carande-Kulis VG, et al. Reviews of Evidence Regarding Interventions to Reduce Alcohol-Impaired Driving. *Am J Prev Med* 2001;21(4S): 66–88.

219. Seaton JD, David CO. Family role in substance abuse and traumatic brain injury rehabilitation. *J Head Trauma Rehabil* 1990;5(3):41–6.

220. Corrigan JD. Substance abuse as a mediating factor in outcome from traumatic brain injury. *Arch Phys Med Rehabil* 1995;76: 302–9.

221. Cornwell EE, III, Belzberg H, Velmahos G, Chan LS, Demetriades D, Stewart BM, et al. The prevalence and effect of alcohol and drug abuse on cohort-matched critically injured patients. *Am Surg* 1998 May;64(5):461–5.

222. Madan AK, Yu K, Beech DJ. Alcohol and drug use in victims of life-threatening trauma. *J Trauma* 1999 Sep;47(3):568–71.

223. Everett SA, Shults RA, Barrios LC, Sacks JJ, Lowry R, Oeltmann J. Trends and subgroup differences in transportation-related injury risk and safety behaviors among high school students, 1991–1997. *J Adolesc Health* 2001 Mar;28(3):228–34.

224. Hingson R, Heeren T, Zakocs R, Winter M, Wechsler H. Age of first intoxication, heavy drinking, driving after drinking and risk of unintentional injury among U.S. college students. *J Stud Alcohol* 2003 Jan;64(1):23–31.

225. Hingson RW, Heeren T, Zakocs RC, Kopstein A, Wechsler H. Magnitude of alcohol-related mortality and morbidity among U.S. college students ages 18–24. *J Stud Alcohol* 2002 Mar; 63(2):136–44.

226. Hingson R, Heeren T, Zakocs R. Age of drinking onset and involvement in physical fights after drinking. *Pediatrics* 2001 Oct;108(4):872–7.

227. Gerhart KA, Mellick DC, Weintraub AH. Violence-related traumatic brain injury: a population-based study. *J Trauma* 2003 Dec;55(6):1045–53.

228. Kolakowsky-Hayner SA, Gourley EV, III, Kreutzer JS, Marwitz JH, Cifu DX, Mckinley WO. Pre-injury substance abuse among persons with brain injury and persons with spinal cord injury. *Brain Inj* 1999 Aug;13(8):571–81.

229. Bombardier CH, Rimmele CT, Zintel H. The magnitude and correlates of alcohol and drug use before traumatic brain injury. *Arch Phys Med Rehabil* 2002 Dec;83(12):1765–73.

230. Gurney JG, Rivara FP, Mueller BA, Newell DW, Copass MK, Jurkovich GJ. The effects of alcohol intoxication on the initial treatment and hospital course of patients with acute brain injury. *J Trauma* 1992 Nov;33(5):709–13.

231. Sparedo FR, Gill D. Effects of Prior Alcohol Use on Head Injury Recovery. *J Head Trauma Rehabil* 1989;4(1):75–82.

232. Kaplan CP, Corrigan JD. Effect of blood alcohol level on recovery from severe closed head injury. *Brain Inj* 1992 Jul;6(4): 337–49.

233. Tate PS, Freed DM, Bombardier CH, Harter SL, Brinkman S. Traumatic brain injury: influence of blood alcohol level on post-acute cognitive function. *Brain Inj* 1999 Oct;13(10):767–84.

234. Kelly MP, Johnson CT, Knoller N, Drubach DA, Winslow MM. Substance abuse, traumatic brain injury and neuropsychological outcome. *Brain Inj* 1997 Jun;11(6):391–402.

235. O'Donnell MA. Research on drinking locations of alcohol-impaired drivers: implications for prevention policies. *J Public Health Policy* 1985;6:510–25.

236. Lang E, Stockwell TR. Drinking locations of drink-drivers: an analysis of accident and non-accident cases. *Accid Anal Prev* 1991;573–84.

237. Gliksman L, McKensie D, Single E, Douglas R, Brunet S, Moffatt K. The role of alcohol providers in prevention: an evaluation of a server intervention programme. *Addiction* 1993;88: 1195–203.

238. Saltz RF. The role of bars and restaurants in preventing alcohol-impaired driving: an evaluation of server intervention. *Eval Health Professions* 1987;10:5–27.

239. Russ NW, Geller ES. Training bar personnel to prevent drunken driving: a field evaluation. *Am J Public Health* 1987;77: 952–4.

240. Lang E, Stockwell TR, Rydon P, Beel A. Can training bar staff in responsible serving practices reduce alcohol-related harm? *Drug Alcohol Rev* 1998;17:39–50.

241. Holder HD, Saltz RF, Grube JW, Treno AJ, Reynolds RI, Voas RB, et al. Summing up: lessons from a comprehensive community prevention trial. *Addiction* 1997 Jun;92 Suppl 2:S293-S301.

242. Buka SL, Birdthistle IJ. Long-term effects of a community-wide alcohol server training intervention. *J Stud Alcohol* 1999 Jan; 60(1):27–36.

243. Zobeck TS, Grant BF, Stinson FS, Bertolucci D. Alcohol involvement in fatal traffic crashes in the United States: 1979–90. *Addiction* 1994 Feb;89(2):227–33.

244. Kirn T. Teens' Use of Drugs, Tobacco Continues Decline. *Internal Medicine News* 2005;38(4):23.

245. Jancin B. Trajectory for Teen Substance Abuse Can Begin in Preschool. *Internal Medicine News* 2005;38(4):23.

246. Spain DA, Boaz PW, Davidson DJ, Miller FB, Carrillo EH, Richardson JD. Risk-taking behaviors among adolescent trauma patients. *J Trauma* 1997 Sep;43(3):423–6.

247. National Center for Alcohol and Drug Information. *Traumatic Brain Injury and Alcohol, Tobacco, and Other Drugs and the College Experience.* Washington, D.C.: U.S. Department of Health & Human Service; 1999.

248. Hatten J, Lambert S, McLoufhlin E. Involving survivors of acquired brain injury in injury prevention work. *J Head Trauma Rehabil* 1991;6(2):71–5.

249. Brain Injury Association. Understanding and Preventing Adolescent Brain injury: the teenage years. www biausa org 2002 [cited 1 A.D. Dec 31].

250. Apsler R, Char AR, Harding WM, Klein TM. *The Effects of .08 BAC Laws.* DOT HS 808 892. Washington,D.C.: U.S. Department of Transportation, National Highway Traffic Safety Administration, National Center for Statistics and Analysis, Community Preventive Services. Methods for systematic reviews of economic; 1999. [AU: Please check: Is this correct? Seems cut off.]

251. Foss RD, Stewart JR, Reinfurt DW. Evaluation of the effects of North Carolina's 0.08 percent BAC law. www.nhtsa.dot.gov/people/ncsa/nc08.html 2001

252. Hingson R, Heeren T, Winter M. Lowering state legal blood alcohol limits to 0.08 percent: the effect on fatal motor vehicle crashes. *Am J Prev Med* 1996;86:1297–9.

253. Hingson R, Heeren T, Winter M. Effects of recent 0.08 percent legal blood alcohol limits on fatal crash involvement. *Inj Prev* 2000;6:109–14.

254. Johnson D, Fell J. The impact of lowering the illegal BAC limit to .08 in five states. 1995 Oct 16; Chicago, IL: 39th Annual Proceedings, Association for the Advancement of Automotive Medicine; 1995.

255. Research and Evaluation Associates. The effects following the implementation of an 0.08 BAC limit and administrative per se law in California. Washington, D.C.: U.S. Department of Transportation, National Highway Traffic Safety Administration, National Center for Statistics and Analysis,. 1991.

256. Rogers PN. The general deterrent impact of California's 0.08 percent blood alcohol concentration limit and administrative per se license suspension laws. Sacramento, CA: California Department of Motor Vehicles, Research and Development Section, 1995.

257. Scopatz RA. Methodological study of between-states comparisons, with particular application to .08 percent BAC law evaluation. Washington, D.C.: 1998.

258. Voas RB, Tippetts AS, Fell J. The relationship of alcohol safety laws to drinking drivers in fatal crashes. *Accid Anal Prev* 2000 Jul;32(4):483–92.

259. Congressional Record. Volume 146 Page H9018. 2000.

260. Andersen JA, McLellan BA, Pagliarello G, Nelson WR. The relative influence of alcohol and seatbelt usage on severity of injury from motor vehicle crashes. *J Trauma* 1990 Apr;30(4):415–7.

261. Zador PL, Krawchuk SA, Voas RB. Alcohol-related relative risk of driver fatalities and driver involvement in fatal crashes in relation to driver age and gender: an update using 1996 data. *J Stud Alcohol* 2000 May;61(3):387–95.

262. Castle SP, Thompson JD, Spataro JA. *Early Evaluation of a Statewide Sobriety Checkpoint Program.* 39th annual proceedings.Chicago, IL: Association for the Advancement of Automotive Medicine, 1995. p. 65–78.

263. Armour M, Monk K, South D, Chomiak G. *Evaluation of the 1983 Melbourne Random Breath Testing Campaign: Interim Report, Casualty Accident Analysis.* N8–85. Melbourne, Australia: Victoria Road Traffic Authority; 1985.

264. Arthurson RM. Evaluation of random breath testing. Sydney: Research Note RN 10/85. Traffic Authority of New South Wales, 1985.

265. Cameron.M., Diamantopolou K, Mullan N, Dyte D, Gantzer S. Evaluation of the country random breath testing and publicity program in Victoria, 1993–1994. Report 126. Melbourne, Australia: Monash University Accident Research Center; 1997.

266. Dunbar JA, Penttila A, Pikkarainen J. Drinking and driving: choosing the legal limits. *Br Med J (Clin Res Ed)* 1987 Dec 5;295(6611):1458–60.

267. Hardes G, Gibberd RW, Lam P, Callcott R, Dobson AJ, Leeder SR. Effects of random breath testing on hospital admissions of traffic-accident casualties in the Hunter Health Region. *Med J Aust* 1985 Jun 10;142(12):625–6.

268. Henstridege J, Homel R, Mackay P. *The Long-Term Effects of Random Breath Testing in Four Australian States: A Time Series Analysis.* No. CR 162. Canberra, Australia: Federal Office of Road Safety; 1997.

269. Hormel R, Carseldine D, Kearns I. Drink-driving countermeasures in Australia. *Alcohol Drugs Driving* 1988;4:113–44.

270. McLean AJ, Clark MS, Dorsch MM, Holubowycz OT, McCaul KA. Random breath testing in South Australia: effects on drink-driving: HS 038 357. Adelaide, South Australia: NHMRC Road Accident Research Unit, University of Adelaide.; 1984.

271. Ross HL, McCleary R, Epperlein T. Deterrence of drinking and driving in France: an evaluation of the law of July 12, 1978. *Law Soc Rev* 1981;16:345–74.

272. Voas RB, Holder HD, Gruenewald PJ. The effect of drinking and driving interventions on alcohol-involved traffic crashes within a comprehensive community trial. *Addiction* 1997 Jun;92 Suppl 2:S221-S236.

273. Supreme Court Ruling. Michigan Department of State Police v Sitz, 496 U.S. 444, 110 L. Ed. 2d 412, 1990 U.S. LEXIS 3144, 110 S. Ct. 2481, 58 U.S.L.W. 4781. 1990.

274. Miller TR, Galbraith MS, Lawrence BA. Costs and benefits of a community sobriety checkpoint program. *J Stud Alcohol* 1998 Jul;59(4):462–8.

275. Schutzman SA, Greenes DS. Pediatric minor head trauma. Ann Emerg Med 2001 Jan;37(1):65–74.

276. Centers for Disease Control and Prevention. *Morbidity and Mortality Weekly Report. First Reports Evaluating the Effectiveness of Strategies for Preventing Violence: Early Childhood Home Visitation and Firearm Laws.* Findings from the Task Force on Community Preventative Services. 2003.

277. Reece RM, Sege R. Childhood head injuries: accidental or inflicted? *Arch Pediatr Adolesc Med* 2000 Jan;154(1):11–5.

278. Shannon P, Smith CR, Deck J, Ang LC, Ho M, Becker L. Axonal injury and the neuropathology of shaken baby syndrome. *Acta Neuropathol (Berl)* 1998 Jun;95(6):625–31.

279. Hymel KP, Abshire TC, Luckey DW, Jenny C. Coagulopathy in pediatric abusive head trauma. *Pediatrics* 1997 Mar;99(3):371–5.

280. Johnson DL, Braun D, Friendly D. Accidental head trauma and retinal hemorrhage. *Neurosurgery* 1993 Aug;33(2):231–4.

281. U.S. Department of Health and Human Services. *Healthy People 2010: With Understanding and Improving Health and Objectives for Improving Health,* 2nd ed. Washington, DC: U.S. Department of Health and Human Services.; 2000.

282. Wittenberg E, Goldie SJ, Graham JD. Predictors of hazardous child seating behavior in fatal motor vehicle crashes: 1990 to 1998. *Pediatrics* 2001 Aug;108(2):438–42.

283. Tyroch AH, Kaups KL, Sue LP, O'Donnell-Nicol S. Pediatric restraint use in motor vehicle collisions: reduction of deaths without contribution to injury. *Arch Surg* 2000 Oct;135(10):1173–6.

284. Kunkel NC, Nelson DS, Schunk JE. Do parents choose appropriate automotive restraint devices for their children? *Clin Pediatr (Phila)* 2001 Jan;40(1):35–40.

285. Playground safety—United States, 1998–1999. *MMWR Morb Mortal Wkly Rep* 1999 Apr 30;48(16):329–32.

286. Kelly KD, Lissel HL, Rowe BH, Vincenten JA, Voaklander DC. Sport and recreation-related head injuries treated in the emergency department. *Clin J Sport Med* 2001 Apr;11(2):77–81.

287. Waltzman ML, Shannon M, Bowen AP, Bailey MC. Monkeybar injuries: complications of play. *Pediatrics* 1999 May;103(5):e58.

288. Bond MT, Peck MG. The risk of childhood injury on Boston's playground equipment and surfaces. *Am J Public Health* 1993 May;83(5):731–3.

289. Plunkett J. Fatal pediatric head injuries caused by short-distance falls. Am J Forensic Med Pathol 2001 Mar;22(1):1–12.

290. King K, Ball D. A Holistic *Approach to Accident and Injury Prevention in Children's Playgrounds.* London, England: London Scientific Services; 1989.

291. Illingworth CM, Jay A, Noble D, Collick M. 225 skateboard injuries in children. *Clin Pediatr (Phila)* 1978 Oct;17(10):781–9.

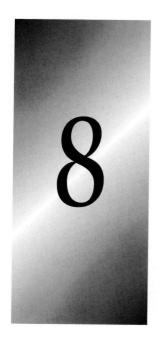

8 TBI: Pathobiology

Patrick M. Kochanek
Robert S.B. Clark
Larry W. Jenkins

INTRODUCTION

In the United States, over 50,000 people die and over 200,000 are hospitalized each year from traumatic brain injury (TBI) (1). Severe TBI is an important contributor to both this level of mortality and the associated morbidity. Treatment is usually supportive neurointensive care focused on the control of intracranial hypertension. Breakthroughs in the treatment of TBI have been hampered by a lack of understanding of the key mechanisms operating in the injured brain.

TBI involves a primary injury that includes direct disruption of brain parenchyma, and a secondary injury characterized by a cascade of biochemical, cellular, and molecular events involved in the evolution of secondary damage.

PRIMARY INJURY

Primary injury has traditionally been characterized as the damage that results directly from the shear forces at impact. Consequently, this topic has been of greater interest to investigators in the fields of injury prevention and biomechanics than those focused on the treatment of the evolution of secondary damage. A detailed discussion of the biomechanics of primary injury is beyond the scope of this chapter. Nevertheless, some insight into its

components is valuable. Key components of primary injury include cortical disruption, axonal injury, vascular injury, hemorrhage, and unusual, albeit important, miscellaneous forms of primary injury.

Primary injury has been modeled in vitro using approaches such as mechanical stretch of cultured neurons (2). Clinically, a number of aspects of primary injury can be appreciated when viewing the initial post-injury cranial computed tomographic (CT) scan or cranial magnetic resonance imaging (MRI) of patients. Direct cortical disruption seen in the initial minutes to hours after the insult represents primary injury that is not likely to be amenable to resuscitative therapy. In addition to direct cortical disruption, axonal injury and vascular disruption can result from primary injury. Indeed, because it is likely related to the anatomical association between axons and blood vessels, primary injury often results in coupled injury to these structures—and the commonly observed clinical picture of petechial hemorrhages in white matter signaling diffuse axonal injury (DAI) (3).

Classically, axonal disruption with retraction was believed to result only from direct shearing. However, work from the laboratory of Povlishock (4) over the past decade has identified a parallel secondary injury cascade in axons. Thus, as with gray matter injury, both primary and secondary axonal damage can occur after severe TBI. The concept of secondary axonal damage will be discussed in greater detail latter in this chapter. Finally, there are a number of miscellaneous forms of primary injury—and several of these can have critical consequences in the setting of acute injury. For example, pituitary stalk transection from shear forces has been reported (5) and leads to acute pituitary failure. Primary injury to the brain stem can also occur and often is associated with poor outcome (6). Similarly, primary injury from violent shaking in the setting of inflicted childhood neurotrauma (shaken baby syndrome) can include direct shearing of nerve roots in the upper cervical spine (7).

Another important aspect of primary injury is impact depolarization. At the time of severe injury, impact depolarization occurs, with massive increases in extracellular potassium ion and the indiscriminate release of the excitatory neurotransmitter glutamate (8). This immediate event initiates excitotoxicity—a key secondary mechanism that is discussed in detail latter in this chapter.

Although by definition, primary injury is not likely to be responsive to resuscitative approaches; it is interesting that our thinking on the lack of therapeutic approaches to primary injury may require reconsideration in the emerging era of tissue engineering and stem cell therapeutics (9). It is possible, that tissue replacement therapy in the future may allow successful therapeutic avenues even to lesions produced by primary injury and previously felt to lack therapeutic options. This could be particularly important as an adjunctive therapy in rehabilitation.

EVOLUTION OF SECONDARY INJURY

Secondary injury includes both the endogenous evolution of damage within the brain and the effects of secondary

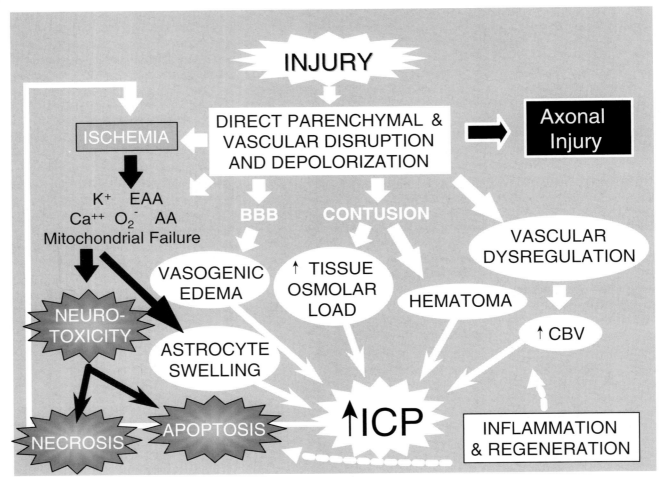

FIGURE 8-1

Categories of mechanisms proposed to be involved in the evolution of secondary damage after severe TBI in infants and children. Three major categories for these secondary mechanisms include (i) ischemia, excitotoxicity, energy failure, and cell death cascades; (ii) cerebral swelling; and (iii) axonal injury. A fourth category, inflammation and regeneration, contributes to each of these cascades. K^+ = potassium; EAA = excitatory amino acids; Ca^{++} = calcium; O_2^- = superoxide; AA = arachidonic acid; BBB = blood brain barrier; ICP = intracranial pressure; CBV = cerebral blood volume

extra-cerebral insults (i.e., hypotension, hypoxemia) from the injury scene through the intensive care unit (ICU).

Studies in models of TBI have begun to unravel the mechanisms producing secondary damage. Four categories of mechanisms can be defined (Figure 8-1), those associated with (i) ischemia, excitotoxicity, energy failure, and resultant cell death cascades; (ii) secondary cerebral swelling; (iii) axonal injury; and (iv) inflammation and regeneration. Within each category, a constellation of mediators of secondary damage, endogenous neuroprotection repair, and regeneration are involved. The quantitative contribution of each mediator to outcome and the interplay between these mediators remains poorly defined.

A variety of methods have been used to study the evolution of secondary damage in human head injury including (i) the analysis of brain biochemistry and molecular biology via of ventricular cerebrospinal fluid (CSF) drained in the treatment of intracranial hypertension, (ii) assessment of brain interstitial fluid by cerebral microdialysis, (iii) imaging techniques linked to assessment of cerebral blood flow (CBF) and cerebral metabolism, and (iv) the assessment of molecular markers in brain tissue obtained from patients treated with surgical decompression for refractory intracranial hypertension. We discuss these studies and cite the clinical evidence supporting proposed mechanisms of secondary damage. It is impossible to address all of the mediators that may be involved; however, key mechanisms will be considered.

POST-TRAUMATIC ISCHEMIA

Clinical studies in adults have indicated that soon after severe TBI, CBF is reduced and suggest that early post-traumatic ischemia might represent a therapeutic target (10,11). Clinical studies applying the stable xenon computed tomographic (CT) method of CBF assessment in the initial hours after severe TBI have been the most important in this regard. Early hypoperfusion or ischemia after severe TBI appears to represent a finding that is seen in most cases and is associated with poor outcome. The devastating consequences of secondary extra-cerebral insults early after injury (i.e., hypotension, hypoxemia) early post-trauma are also consistent with this possibility—because a hypoperfused brain is at high risk and may be incapable of mounting an appropriate vasodilatory response during these added insults (12). This is not to suggest that secondary insults are limited to the field or emergency department. Secondary ischemic insults can also occur in the ICU. This was best described in the classic report of Gopinath et al., (13) who used a jugular venous catheter to identify episodes of jugular venous desaturation (SjvO$_2$ < 50 percent for more than 10 minutes) in the ICU in 116 patients with severe TBI. In that study, 46 of the 116 patients had at least one episode of desaturation—suggesting ischemia. The causes of these episodes were either systemic such as hypotension or cerebral such as refractory intracranial hypertension. Episodes of desaturation were strongly associated with a poor neurological outcome. Just a single desaturation increased the incidence of poor outcome from 55 percent to 74 percent.

Numerous mechanisms may underlie the early post-traumatic hypoperfusion. Armstead reported reductions in the vasodilatory response to nitric oxide (NO), cGMP, cAMP, and prostanoids after experimental TBI in pigs, along with the release of superoxide anion (14,15). Also, greater injury-induced release of the potent vasoconstrictor peptide endothelin-1 in the newborn versus the juvenile pig was posed to mediate the hypoperfusion (16). Others have suggested a loss of either endothelial NO production, or reduced responsivity to NO as mediating hypoperfusion. Treatment with L-arginine (the substrate for NO production) improved CBF after TBI in rats (17). Similarly, treatment with L-arginine improved CBF and reduced contusion volume after TBI in rats (18). L-arginine is being tested in a clinical TBI trial in adults (personal communication, C. Robertson, MD). Loss of vasodilators and elaboration of vasoconstrictors, or other mechanisms, might be involved in producing early post-traumatic hypoperfusion (Figure 8-2).

Increases in metabolic demands, related to uptake of glutamate, as reflected by increases in brain tissue and CSF lactate, early after TBI have been reported in both models (19) and humans (20–22). Thus, reduced metabolic demands with a coupled CBF reduction in severely injured brain regions, early after injury, is an unlikely explanation for the hypoperfusion.

At more delayed times after injury (several hours to days), oxidative metabolism has been noted to be reduced to levels of ~50 percent of baseline for the

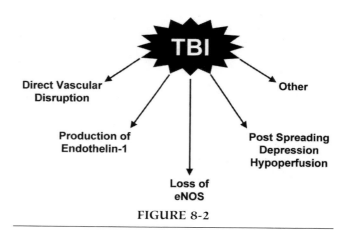

FIGURE 8-2

Schematic outlining putative mediators involved in the production of early post-traumatic hypoperfusion and/or ischemia after severe TBI. NOS = NO synthase. (See text for details.)

majority of the ICU course (20). The complex issue of issue alterations in metabolic demands after severe TBI is discussed in greater detail in the section on brain swelling later in this chapter.

EXCITOTOXICITY

Excitoxicity describes the process by which glutamate and other excitatory amino acids (EAAs) cause neuronal damage. Lucas and Newhouse (23) first described the toxicity of glutamate. Olney (24) subsequently reported that intraperitoneal administration of glutamate produces brain injury. Although glutamate is the most abundant neurotransmitter in the brain, exposure to toxic levels produces neuronal death (25).

Glutamate exposure produces neuronal injury in two phases. Minutes after exposure sodium-dependent neuronal swelling occurs (26). This is followed by delayed,

calcium-dependent degeneration. These effects are mediated through both ionophore-linked receptors, labeled according to specific agonists (N-methyl-D-aspartate [NMDA], kainate and α-amino-3-hydroxy-5-methyl-4-isoxazolepropionic acid [AMPA]), and receptors linked to second messenger systems, called metabotropic receptors. Activation of these receptors leads to calcium influx through receptor-gated or voltage-gated channels, or through the release of intracellular calcium stores. Increased intracellular calcium concentration is the trigger for a number of processes that can lead to cellular injury or death (Figure 8-3). One mechanism involves activation of constitutive NO synthase, leading to NO production, peroxynitrite formation and resultant DNA damage. Poly(ADP-ribose) polymerase (PARP) is an enzyme operative in DNA repair, and in the face of DNA damage, PARP activation leads to ATP depletion, metabolic failure and cell death (27). This may be important since PARP knockout mice exhibit improved outcome versus controls (28).

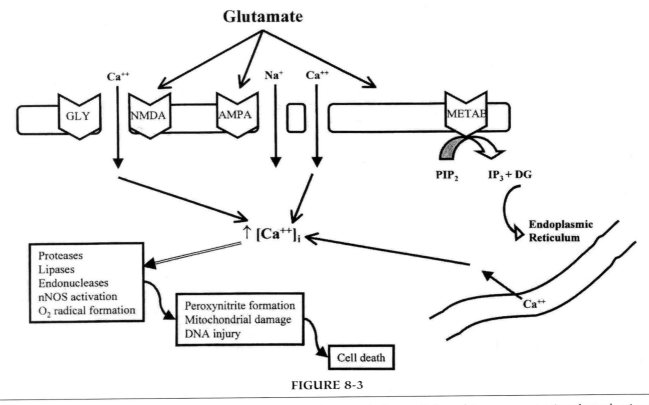

FIGURE 8-3

Mechanisms involved in excitotoxicity. Glutamate causes an increase in intracellular calcium concentration through stimulation of (i) the NMDA receptor with opening of the receptor-linked calcium ionophore, (ii) the AMPA receptor with opening of the voltage-gated calcium channels, and (iii) the metabotropic receptor, with the release of intracellular calcium stores via the second messengers inositol triphosphate and diacylglycerol. Increased intracellular calcium concentration leads to activation of proteases, lipases and endonucleases, along with neuronal NOS stimulation and production of oxygen radicals. This results in peroxynitrite formation, mitochondrial damage and DNA injury with subsequent cellular injury and death.

Abbreviations: GLY: glycine coagonist site; NMDA: N-methyl-D-aspartate receptor; AMPA: a-amino-3-hydroxy-5-methylisoazole-4-proprionic acid receptor; METAB: glutamate metabotropic receptor; PIP$_2$: phosphoinositide; IP$_3$: inositol triphosphate; DG: diacylglycerol

Recent evidence suggests that activation of PARP within mitochondria may contribute importantly to their failure (29).

Faden et al. (30) first reported an increase in interstitial EAAs to neurotoxic levels after experimental TBI. Antiexcitotoxic therapies improve outcome after experimental TBI. Pretreatment with NMDA antagonists (phencyclidine, MK-801) attenuate behavioral deficits after TBI in rats (31, 32). Other therapies that modify the glutamate-NMDA receptor interaction and improve outcome following experimental TBI are magnesium (33), glycine site antagonists (34), hypothermia (35), and pentobarbital (36).

Palmer et al. (37) first demonstrated increased concentrations of EAAs in ventricular CSF from adult patients with TBI. Glutamate concentrations were about 5-fold greater than in control patients (up to 7 μM)—levels sufficient to cause neuronal death in cell culture (38). However, CSF glutamate concentrations do not correlate to outcome after TBI in adults (39). Bullock et al. (40) characterized patterns of glutamate release by measuring EAAs by microdialysis after adult TBI. Patients with a normal head CT and no secondary ischemic events had interstitial concentrations of glutamate that were increased early in their course, then returned to normal, similar to the pattern seen in most experimental models. A second group of patients had an intermediate increase in glutamate concentration (5–20 μM) that declined over time, but remained higher than normal. Most of these patients had ischemic events or intracranial hypertension. A third group of patients had markedly increased concentrations of glutamate (over 20 μM). All patients with a progressively rising level of glutamate died.

Despite these findings, clinical trials with antiexcitotoxic therapies have been unsuccessful. This may be due to the fact that most therapies have been applied to all patients with TBI rather than those with excitotoxicity (41). Also, treatment may have been initiated too late. Inhibition of plasticity by anti-excitotoxic therapies may limit their efficacy—especially at the interface between the acute and subacute periods after injury (42).

ENDOGENOUS NEUROPROTECTANTS

Ischemia, excitotoxicity, or their combination is a key facet of secondary injury. These mechanisms are linked to calcium overload, oxidative stress, and mitochondrial failure. Studies have begun to define, in infants and children with severe TBI, the endogenous retaliatory response to these ischemic and excitotoxic insults. Space limitations have directed us to focus on two examples of this cascade—namely, adenosine and heat shock protein 70 (HSP 70). Endogenous neuroprotective responses related to the apoptosis, cell signaling, and inflammatory cascades are discussed later.

Adenosine is an endogenous neuroprotectant produced in response to both ischemia and excitotoxicity. Adenosine antagonizes a number of events thought to mediate neuronal death (43). Breakdown of adenosine triphosphate (ATP) leads to formation of adenosine, a purine nucleoside that decreases neuronal metabolism and increases CBF, among other mechanisms. Adenosine binding to A1 receptors decreases metabolism by increasing K^+ and Cl^- and decreasing Ca^{++} conductances in the neuronal membrane. A1 receptors are located on neurons in brain regions that are susceptible to injury (i.e., hippocampus) and are spatially associated with NMDA receptors (44). Thus, released adenosine minimizes excitotoxicity. Binding of adenosine to A2 receptors (on cerebrovascular smooth muscle) causes vasodilation, although binding to A2a receptors on neurons may be detrimental. Brain interstitial levels of adenosine are increased early after TBI in rats (45–47). In experimental TBI, brain interstitial adenosine increases immediately after injury to levels 50- to 100-fold greater than baseline (47). In clinical studies, marked increases in brain interstitial levels of adenosine in adults with TBI, were seen during episodes of jugular venous desaturation (secondary insults), supporting a role of adenosine as a "retaliatory" defense metabolite (48).

Another putative endogenous neuroprotectant that plays a role after severe TBI is HSP 70. This protein is induced as part of the classic preconditioning response in brain and has recently been shown to be increased in both CSF and brain tissue after severe TBI in humans (49–51). HSP 70 is believed to play an important role in optimizing protein folding as a molecular chaperone. It also inhibits pro-inflammatory signaling (52). Thus, the brain mounts an important endogenous defense response to TBI. Therapies designed to augment these pathways have not been examined adequately.

APOPTOSIS CASCADES

It is now increasingly clear from experimental models and human data that cells dying after TBI can be categorized on a morphological continuum ranging from necrosis to apoptosis (53,54). Apoptosis is a morphological description of cell death defined by cell shrinkage and nuclear condensation, internucleosomal DNA fragmentation, and the formation of apoptotic bodies (55). In contrast, cells dying of necrosis display cellular and nuclear swelling with dissolution of membranes. Apoptosis requires a cascade of intracellular events for completion of cell death; thus, "programmed-cell death" is the currently accepted term for the process of cell death that leads to apoptosis (56). In diseases with complex and multiple mechanisms, such as TBI, it is typically difficult to distinguish clinical apoptotic vs. necrotic cell death as classically defined (57).

Some cells may display DNA fragmentation and activation of proteases involved in programmed-cell death, despite having nuclear and cellular swelling. Dying cells with mixed phenotypes may represent particularly difficult therapeutic targets after TBI.

In mature tissues, programmed-cell death requires initiation via either intracellular or extracellular signals (see Figure 8-4). These signals have now been well characterized in vitro, and are becoming better characterized in vivo. Intracellular signaling appears to be initiated in mitochondria, triggered by disturbances in cellular homeostasis such as ATP depletion, oxidative stress, or calcium fluxes (58). Mitochondrial dysfunction leads to egress of cytochrome c from the inner mitochondrial membrane into the cytosol. Cytochrome c release can be blocked by anti-apoptotic members of the bcl-2 family (e.g., bcl-2, bcl-xL, bcl-w, and Mcl-1), and promoted by pro-apoptotic members of the bcl-2 family (e.g., bax, bcl-xS, bad, and bid) (59).

Cytochrome c in the presence of dATP and a specific apoptotic-protease activating factor (Apaf-1) in cytosol activates the initiator cysteine protease caspase-9 (60). Caspase-9 then activates the effector cysteine protease caspase-3, a key apoptosis effector that cleaves cytoskeletal proteins, DNA repair proteins, and activators of endonucleases (61).

An additional intracellular cascade of programmed cell death linked to mitochondrial injury is the apoptosis-inducing factor (AIF) pathway (62–66). This caspase-independent pathway is activated by mitochondrial permeability transition and results in the release of AIF from the mitochondrial membrane. AIF release leads to large-scale DNA fragmentation (50–700 kilo-base-pair in size). Recently, Zhang et al. (67) reported that the AIF pathway is activated in experimental TBI. To date, specific pharmacologic inhibitors of this pathway are lacking, however, this alternative form of delayed neuronal death may represent an important therapeutic target.

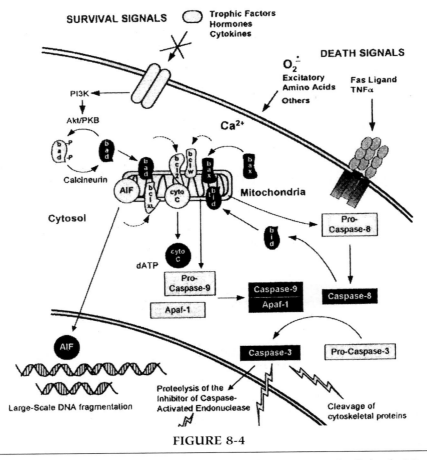

FIGURE 8-4

Simplified schematic depicting intracellular and extracellular pathways for programmed-cell death. Mitochondrial dysfunction caused by injurious stimuli such as oxidative stress or calcium fluxes can trigger release of cytochrome c or apoptosis inducing factor (AIF). Cytochrome c in the cytosol along with other enzymes and cofactors initiates activation of a cascade of caspases, culminating in apoptosis, with nucleosomal DNA cleavage. AIF triggers caspase-independent large-scale DNA fragmentation (see text for details). Programmed cell death can also be initiated by cell death receptors on the cell surface. Fas-ligand (Fas-L), either presented by an effector cell or in soluble form, binding to Fas-receptor (Fas-Rc), or TNF binding to TNF-receptor (TNF-Rc), can also initiate a cascade of caspases via intracellular death domains

Extracellular signaling of apoptosis occurs through the TNF superfamily of cell surface death receptors which include TNFR1 and Fas/Apo1/CD95 (68). Receptor-ligand binding of TNFR1-TNFα or Fas-FasL promotes formation of a trimeric complex of TNF- or Fas-associated death domains, respectively. These death domains contain caspase recruitment domains. The proximity of multiple caspases, in this case caspase-8, allows for activation of the effector cysteine protease followed by activation of caspase-3, where the mitochondrial- and cell death receptor-pathways converge. The cell death receptor pathway can also be regulated by soluble receptors and ligands that prevent and promote apoptosis, respectively, and by receptors lacking death domains. Finally, there is cross-talk between mitochondrial- and cell death receptor-pathways (69).

Bcl-2 is an important endogenous inhibitor of programmed-cell death in vitro (70). It is induced after experimental TBI (71) and reduces cortical tissue loss (72). Bcl-2 is increased in injured brain after severe TBI in humans (54). CSF levels of bcl-2 were increased ~4-fold in TBI compared with control patients. Moreover, CSF bcl-2 was associated with patient survival (73).

Clearly there is now substantial evidence, even in the clinical setting, for an important role for delayed neuronal death by apoptosis or mixed "apo-necrotic" phenotypes after severe TBI. This may represent a valuable opportunity for the development of new therapeutic approaches in the future.

CELL SIGNALING ABNORMALITIES IN NEURONAL DEATH

Neuronal death occurs after both experimental and clinical TBI. In addition to regions of brain directly contused, the hippocampus appears particularly vulnerable to TBI (74–78). As previously discussed, cell death execution pathways are activated by a sufficient severity of TBI involving mitochondrial injury, cytochrome C release with caspase activation, AIF release, and receptor-coupled pro-death pathways. Neurotransmitters, neurotrophins, cytokines, other growth factors, and oxidative stress activate multiple upstream signaling pathways linked to either pro-survival or pro-death activities (79). These receptors couple to signal transduction pathways involving interactions and cross-talk between multiple serine/threonine and tyrosine protein kinase cascades.

Many kinases involved in cell death process are serine/threonine protein kinases. Important participants in the cell death cascades include the mitogen activated protein kinases (MAPK). MAPKs cascades are complex and are mediated by successive protein kinases that sequentially activate each other by phosphorylation. They are importantly linked to two key components of the cell death cascade, jun kinase (JNK) and P38 MAPK (Figure 8-5). JNK and p38 MAPK pathways activate caspase-3 (80–82). Activation of JNK leads to induction of pro-death genes including FasL (81–83). JNK increases p53 and Bax levels which increase cell death. JNK and p38 function in different stress signaling pathways and both target similar nuclear transcription factors that can be activated by pro death stimuli such as oxidative stress (84). Studies in various TBI models have documented significant changes in both JNK, and p38 MAPKs that may be related to cell death and functional impairment after injury (85–87). MAPKs are also linked to survival signals through the ERK pathway, highlighting the complex cross-talk between these cascades (Figure 8-5).

Several protein kinase cascades play a major survival role. Phosphoinositide 3-kinase (PI3-K), protein kinase B (PKB), and protein kinase A (PKA) pathways are prototype examples (Figure 8-6). PKB is also called akt; the complex nomenclature of these kinases has evolved across many disease processes. PKB is activated upstream by PI3K in response to survival signals, and have numerous pro-survival, growth, differentiation and synaptic plasticity actions (88, 89). PKB affects survival by a number of mechanisms including the phosphorylation and inactivation of several pro-death mediators such as Bad. Bad, a member of the Bcl-2 family, is phosphorylated by PKB at ser136 resulting in Bad dissociation from Bcl-xL and binding to 14-3-3 proteins inhibiting cell death

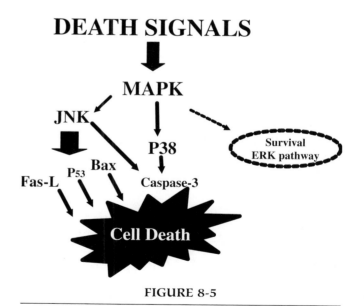

FIGURE 8-5

Cartoon showing the role of mitogen-activated protein kinases (MAPK) in transducing the signals involved in neuronal death. For example, oxidative stress triggers MAPK activation with resultant activation of jun kinase (JNK) which facilitates neuronal death mediated by a number of mechanisms including death receptors (Fas-Fas-L), P53 and Bax. MAPK also involves cross talk with some survival pathways such as ERK

SURVIVAL SIGNALS

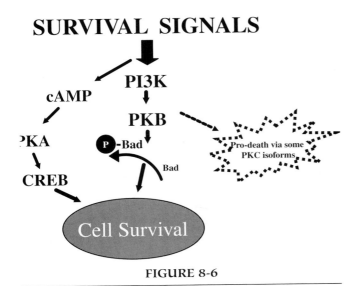

FIGURE 8-6

Cartoon showing the role of important survival signal-mediated kinase activation in promoting neuronal survival. Phospho-inositide 3-kinase (PI3-K), protein kinase B (PKB), and protein kinase A (PKA) pathways are involved. PKB affects survival by a number of mechanisms including the phosphorylation and inactivation of the pro-death mediator Bad. Phosphorylation of Bad results in its dissociation from Bcl-xL inhibiting cell death. CAMP-mediated activation of PKA can also lead to formation of the transcription factor "cAMP response element binding protein" (CREB), which also promotes cell survival

(Figure 8-6) (90). CAMP-mediated activation of PKA can also lead to formation of the transcription factor "cAMP response element binding protein" (CREB), which is similarly associated with cell survival. These pro-survival kinase pathways are outlined in Figure 6 (83). Survival signals are exemplified by growth factors, cytokines, hormones, cell–cell interactions as well as extracellular matrix adhesion molecules. Of course, inactivation of two pro-death members of the MAPK family, p38 and JNK/SAPK, have also been proposed as promoting survival by extracellular stimuli (91). Finally, activation of some PKC isoforms by PI3K can transduce pro-death signals, once again highlighting the complexity of these kinase cascades (Figure 8-6).

In summary, the complex but important kinase pathways are critically involved in the control of neuronal death and plasticity. Further insight into these cascades will likely lead to the development of powerful new tools to manipulate both neuronal death and rewiring after injury. Proteomics approaches may be essential to unraveling the cybernetic nature of these kinase pathways (92).

AXONAL INJURY

Traumatic axonal injury (TAI) encompasses the spectrum of mild to severe TBI, both clinically (93–96) and in

models (97–99). The extent and distribution of TAI depend on injury severity and category (focal versus diffuse) (100).

The classical view that TAI occurs due to immediate physical shearing is represented primarily in severe injury where frank axonal tears occur (93,94,101,102). However, recent experimental studies suggest that TAI predominantly occurs by a delayed process termed "secondary axotomy" (98,103,104). Two hypothetical sequences have attempted to explain secondary axotomy, one attributing axolemmal permeability and calcium influx as the initiating event (Figure 8-7), the other a direct cytoskeletal abnormality impairing axoplasmic flow (98,104,105). It has been posited that both forms of reactive axonal swelling take place but in different proportions depending on the severity of injury. Superimposed on these theories is the finding that hypoxic/ischemic insults can also produce axonal swelling that resembles retraction balls. As a result, differing as well as unifying theories for axonal injuries in brain injury have been proposed (98,104–107). Common mechanistic features include focal ion flux, calcium dysregulation, and mitochondrial and cytoskeletal dysfunction.

TAI contributes to the morbidity after TBI (98, 100–102). Until recently the contributions of TAI to morbidity, have remained speculative since TAI has remained refractory to treatment even in the laboratory. However, recent studies in experimental TBI models have shown that hypothermia or cyclosporin A can both reduce TAI (108,109). In contradistinction, hypothermia reduces growth factor signaling after experimental TBI (110,111) that could blunt regeneration. These therapeutic advances should help determine more definitively the contributions of TAI to secondary damage. Recent application of MRI to the study of TAI (112,113) and axonal connectivity (114,115) may improve our understanding of TAI and regeneration.

CEREBRAL SWELLING

In addition to cascades of neuronal death and axonal damage, brain swelling is a hallmark finding in severe TBI and results in the development of intracranial hypertension, which can have devastating consequences. Cerebral swelling and accompanying intracranial hypertension contributes to secondary damage in two ways. Intracranial hypertension can compromise cerebral perfusion leading to secondary ischemia. In addition, it can produce the devastating consequences of deformation through herniation syndromes. Intracranial hypertension results from increases in intracranial volume from a variety of sources, which are outlined in Figure 8-1. In some cases, such as with epidural, subdural or parenchymnal hematoma formation, an extra-axial or parenchymal blood collection is the key culprity—and is generally

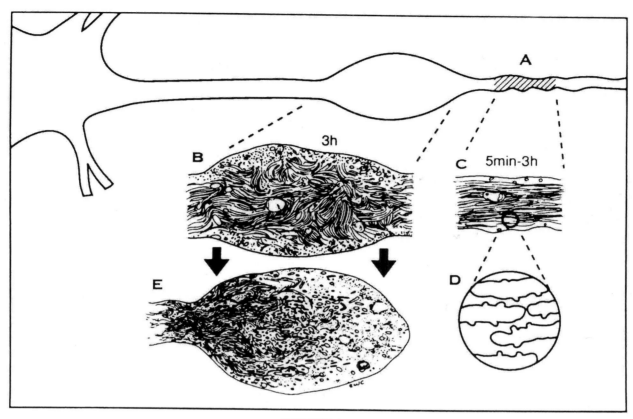

FIGURE 8-7

Reactive axonal swellings have been proposed to result from focal axolemmal disruption, ionic shifts and neurofilamentous compaction at site (A) results in a reactive swelling at site (B) in an upstream region of the axon. At the site of ionic influx, neurofilamentous compaction and mitochondrial swelling is seen (C). Neurofilament compaction is associated with neurofilament sidearm loss (D). Obstructed axonal transport results in upstream axonal enlargement, neurofilament misalignment, organelle accumulation, and formation of the typical reactive axonal swelling (E)

addressed by surgical evacuation (116). However, there are several important mechanisms that are more uniformly involved in the development of intracranial hypertension. These are related to either brain swelling from vasogenic edema, astrocyte swelling, and an increase in tissue osmolar load, or vascular dysregulation with swelling secondary to an increase in cerebral blood volume (CBV).

Recent data suggest that brain swelling after severe TBI results from edema rather than increased CBV. Marmarou et al. (117) measured both CBV and brain water in adults with TBI. Using a dye indicator technique (coupled to CT) to measure CBV and magnetic resonance imaging [MRI] to quantify brain water, increases in brain water were commonly observed, but were generally associated with reduced (not increased) CBV (Figure 8-8).

Thus, edema rather than increased CBV appears to be the predominant contributor to cerebral swelling after TBI. Both cytotoxic and vasogenic edema may play important roles in cerebral swelling. However, our traditional concept of cytotoxic and vasogenic edema is evolving.

There appear to be four putative mechanisms for edema formation in the injured brain. First, vasogenic edema may form in the extracellular space as a result of blood-brain barrier (BBB) disruption. Second, cellular swelling can be produced in two ways. Astrocyte swelling can occur as part of the homeostatic uptake of substances such as glutamate. Glutamate uptake is coupled to glucose utilization via a sodium/potassium ATPase, with sodium and water accumulation in astrocytes. Swelling of both neurons and other cells in the neuropil can also result from ischemia- or trauma-induced ionic pump failure. Finally, osmolar swelling may also contribute to edema formation in the extracellular space, particularly in contusions. Osmolar swelling, however, is actually dependent on an intact BBB or an alternative solute barrier.

Cellular swelling may be of greatest importance. Using a model of diffuse TBI in rats, Barzo et al. (118) applied diffusion-weighted MRI to localize the increase in brain water. A decrease in the apparent diffuse coefficient after injury suggested predominantly cellular swelling, rather than vasogenic edema, in the development

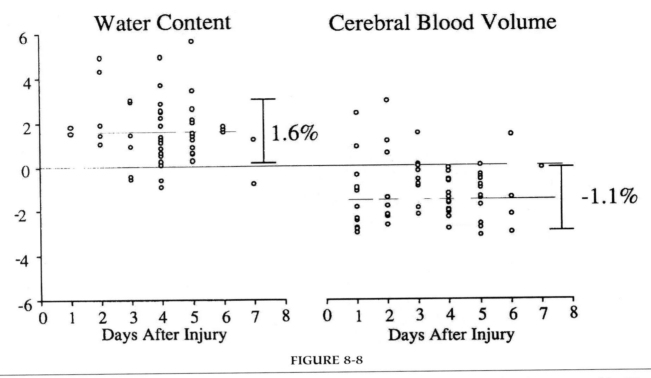

FIGURE 8-8

The percentage change in brain water content as assessed by MRI and cerebral blood volume (CBV) as measured by CT and indicatory dilution technique in 109 studies of adults with TBI. Brain water is increased and CBV is reduced in adults with severe TBI. Reprinted from the work of Marmarou et al. (121) with permission

of intracranial hypertension. Cellular swelling may be of even greater importance in the setting of TBI with a secondary hypoxemic-ischemic insult (119).

Katayama et al. (120) also suggested that the role of BBB in the development of post-traumatic edema may have been overstated—even in the setting of cerebral contusion. One intriguing possibility is that as macromolecules are degraded within injured brain regions, the osmolar load in the contused tissue increases. As the BBB reconstitutes (or as other osmolar barriers are formed), a considerable osmolar driving force for the local accumulation of water develops, resulting in the marked swelling so often seen in and around cerebral contusions (Figure 8-9).

In some cases, increases in CBV can be seen after TBI and contribute to intracranial hypertension. When an increase in CBV is seen, it may result from local increases in cerebral glycolysis "hyperglycolysis" as described by Bergsneider et al. (22). In regions with increases in glutamate levels, such as in contusions, increases in glycolysis are observed because astrocyte uptake of glutamate is coupled to glycolysis rather than oxidative metabolism. Recall that oxidative metabolism is generally depressed by ~50percent in comatose victims of severe TBI in the ICU (20). Hyperglycolysis results in a marked local increase in cerebral glucose utilization with a coupled increase in CBF and CBV and resultant local brain swelling. A detailed discussion of this topic is beyond the scope of this chapter.

As MRI and MR-spectroscopic methods continue to develop and become applied to critically ill patients (121) our "black box" knowledge of the mechanisms involved in cerebral swelling should greatly advance. It must be remembered that although neuronal and axonal injury are key downstream events in the evolution of damage after severe TBI, brain swelling and resultant intracranial hypertension is still the principal target for titration of therapy in the ICU.

INFLAMMATION AND REGENERATION

There appear to be both acute detrimental and subacute/chronic beneficial aspects of inflammation. There is robust acute inflammation after TBI. This has been shown in models of TBI (122–124), and in adult patients (125–128). NF-κB (129), TNFα (130, 131), IL-1β (132, 133), eicosanoids (134), neutrophils (123,135), and macrophages (136,137) contribute to both secondary damage and repair.

Markers of inflammation after TBI have been assessed in humans using two general strategies, (i) examination of inflammation in contused brain tissue resected from patients with refractory intracranial hypertension, and (ii) study of mediator levels in CSF. Consistent with a role for IL-1β in the evolution of tissue damage in

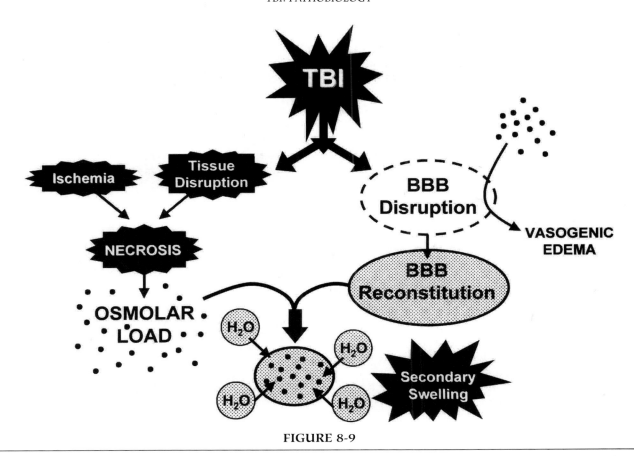

FIGURE 8-9

Schematic based on hypothesis of Katayama et al. (120) suggesting that as the osmolar load increases (breakdown of macromolecules in the region of contusion necrosis), a considerable driving force develops for the accumulation of water, resulting in the secondary swelling so often seen in and around cerebral contusions

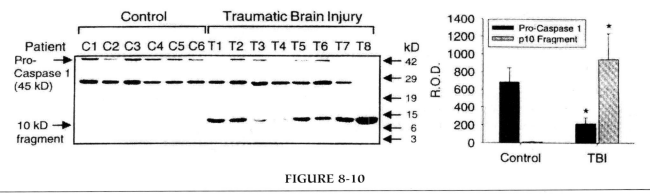

FIGURE 8-10

Evidence for activation of IL-1β converting enzyme (ICE) activation in cerebral contusions resected from adult patients with severe TBI and refractory intracranial hypertension. Western analysis demonstrating cleavage of the intact 45 kD pro-caspase-1 to the 10 kD fragment in each of eight victims of severe TBI but in none of 6 control brain samples from patients that died of non-CNS causes. Reprinted from Clark et al. (63) with permission

human TBI, Clark et al. (54) performed western analysis of brain samples resected from adults with refractory intracranial hypertension secondary to severe contusion. Interleukin-1-converting enzyme (ICE) was activated, as evidenced by specific cleavage in patients with TBI. ICE activation is critical to the production of IL-1β. ICE activation was not detected in patients that died of non-CNS etiologies (Figure 8-10). This supports the production of IL-1β, a pivotal pro-inflammatory mediator, in the traumatically injured brain in humans.

Studies of CSF further support a role for inflammation in TBI. Marion et al. (126) demonstrated increases in IL-1β in CSF after severe TBI in adults. These increases were attenuated by the use of moderate therapeutic hypothermia. Similarly, there are increases of a number of cytokines in CSF after severe TBI including IL-6, and IL-8 (128,138). Contusion and local tissue necrosis appear to be important to trigger neutrophil influx with resultant secondary tissue damage (123). Neutrophil influx is accompanied by increases in inducible nitric oxide synthase (iNOS) levels in brain (124) and is followed by macrophage infiltration, which peaks between 24–72 hours after injury (139). Macrophage infiltration and the differentiation of endogenous microglia into resident macrophages may signal the link between inflammation and regeneration, with elaboration of a number of trophic factors (i.e., nerve growth factor (NGF), nitrosothiols, vascular endothelial growth factor) (133, 138,140,141).

Kossmann et al (138) reported a link between IL-6 production and the production of neurotrophins, such as NGF. Cultured astrocytes treated with either IL-6, IL-8 or CSF from brain-injured adults, produced NGF. Cytokine production after TBI may be important to neuronal plasticity and repair, as discussed below.

Studies in models of TBI (131, 142) suggest beneficial aspects of inflammation on long-term outcome. Mice deficient in TNFα exhibit improved functional outcome (versus wild-type) early after TBI. However, the long-term consequences of TNFα deficiency on outcome are detrimental (131). Similarly, despite a detrimental role for iNOS in the initial 72 h posttrauma (143), iNOS deficient mice demonstrated impaired long-term outcome vs controls (142). iNOS is important in wound healing and iNOS-derived nitrosylation of proteins may play a role (141,144). Regeneration and plasticity play important roles in mediating beneficial long-term effects on recovery, and these responses are linked to inflammation.

The contribution of the inflammatory response to TBI remains to be determined. Although there are a few promising reports in models of the use of anti-inflammatory therapies in TBI and ischemia (targeting IL-1β, ICE, and TNFα) it is unclear whether anti-inflammatory therapies will improve outcome after clinical TBI. If inhibition of the inflammatory response is considered, exacerbation of infection risk must also be anticipated (145). Also, the link between inflammation and regeneration must be recognized.

CONCLUSIONS

Mechanisms involved in the evolution of secondary brain injury after TBI have been reviewed. Particular attention has been paid to studies at the bedside. Our understanding of the biochemical, cellular, and molecular responses has progressed—particularly with the application of molecular biology methods to human materials. Additional details on these mechanisms have also been reviewed in a companion article to this chapter which addresses the unique setting of pediatric TBI (146). Future investigation should integrate these findings with bedside physiology and an improved assessment of outcome. Finally, novel imaging and diagnostic methods, particularly MRI and MRS must be coupled with biochemical and molecular methods to clarify the mechanisms involved in secondary damage and the local effects of novel therapies.

ACKNOWLEDGEMENTS

The authors dedicate this chapter to the late Dr. Peter Safar for his vision and inspiration. We thank the National Institutes of Health/NINDS NS38087 (PMK), NS38620 (RSBC), NS 40049 (LJ) and NS30318 (PMK, RSBC), Center for Disease Control/University of Pittsburgh CIRCL (PMK), and the Laerdal Foundation for supporting this work. We thank Marci Provins and Fran Mistrick for preparation of the manuscript.

References

1. Waxweiler RJ, et al.: Monitoring the impact of traumatic brain damage: A review and update. In: *Traumatic Brain Injury: Bioscience and Mechanics*, Bandak FA, Eppinger RH, Ommaya AK (eds), Larchmont, NY, Mary Ann Liebert, Inc., pp. 1–8, 1996.
2. Engel DC, Slemmer JE, Vlug AS, Maas AI, Weber JT: Combined effects of mechanical and ischemic injury to cortical cells: Secondary ischemia increases damage and decreases effects of neuroprotective agents. *Neuropharmacology* 2005 Jul 23 [Epub ahead of print].
3. Pittella JE, Gusmao SN: Diffuse vascular injury in fatal road traffic accident victims: its relationship to diffuse axonal injury. *J Forensic Sci* 2003; 48:626–630.
4. Povlishock JT: Pathophysiology of neural injury: therapeutic opportunities and challenges. *Clin Neurosurg* 2000; 46:113–126.
5. Mark AS, Phister SH, Jackson DE Jr, Kolsky MP: Traumatic lesions of the suprasellar region: MR imaging. *Radiology* 1992; 182:49–52.
6. Hashimoto T, Nakamura N, Richard KE, Frowein RA: Primary brain stem lesions caused by closed head injuries. *Neurosurg Rev* 1993; 16:291–298.
7. Ghatan S, Ellenbogen RG: Pediatric spine and spinal cord injury after inflicted trauma. *Neurosurg Clin N Am* 2002; 13:227–233.
8. Katayama Y, Becker DP, Tamura T, Hovda DA: Massive increases in extracellular potassium and the indiscriminate release of glutamate following concussive brain injury. *J Neurosurg* 1990; 73:889–900.
9. Atala A: Tissue engineering for the replacement of organ function in the genitourinary system. *Am J Transplant* 2004; Suppl 6:58–73.
10. Marion DW, Darby J, Yonas H: Acute regional cerebral blood flow changes caused by severe head injuries. *J Neurosurgery* 1991; 74:407–414.
11. Bouma GJ, Muizelaar JP, Stringer WA, et al.,: Ultra-early evaluation of regional cerebral blood flow in severely head-injured patients using xenon-enhanced computerized tomography. *J Neurosurg* 1992; 77:360–368.
12. Chesnut RM, Marshall LF, Klauber MR, Blunt BA, Baldwin N, Eisenberg HM, Jane JA, Marmarou A, Foulkes MA: The role of secondary brain injury in determining outcome from severe head injury. *J Trauma* 1993; 34:216–222.

13. Gopinath SP, Robertson CS, Contant CF, Hayes C, Feldman Z, Narayan RK, Grossman RG: Jugular venous desaturation and outcome after head injury. *J Neurol Neurosurg Psychiatry* 1994; 57:717–723.

14. Armstead WM: Superoxide generation links protein kinase C activation to impaired ATP-sensitive K+ channel function after brain injury. *Stroke* 1999; 30:153–159.

15. Armstead WM: Brain injury impairs prostaglandin cerebrovasodilation. *J Neurotrauma* 1998; 15:721–729.

16. Armstead WM: Role of endothelin-1 in age-dependent cerebrovascular hypotensive responses after brain injury. *Am J Physiol* 1999; 277:H1884-H1894.

17. DeWitt DS, Smith TG, Deyo DJ, et al.: L-arginine and superoxide dismutase prevent or reverse cerebral hypoperfusion after fluid-percussion traumatic brain injury. *J Neurotrauma* 1997; 14:223–233.

18. Cherian L, Chacko G, Goodman JC, et al.: Cerebral hemodynamic effects of phenylephrine and L-arginine after cortical impact injury. *Crit Care Med* 1999; 27:2512–2517.

19. Hovda DA, Lee SM, Smith ML, et al.: The neurochemical and metabolic cascade following brain injury: Moving from animal models to man. *J Neurotrauma* 1995; 12:903–906.

20. Obrist WD, Langfitt TW, Jaggi JL, et al.: Cerebral blood flow and metabolism in comatose patients with acute head injury. Relationship to intracranial hypertension. *J Neurosurg* 1984; 61: 241–253.

21. DeSalles AAF, Kontos HA, Becker DP, et al.: Prognostic significance of ventricular CSF lactic acidosis in severe head injury. *J Neurosurg* 1986; 65:615–624.

22. Bergsneider M, Hovda DA, Shalmon E, et al.: Cerebral hyperglycolysis following severe traumatic brain injury in humans: a positron emission tomography study. *J Neurosurg* 1997; 86: 241–251.

23. Lucas DR, Newhouse JP: The toxic effect of sodium L-glutamate on the inner layers of the retina. *Arch Ophthalmol* 1957; 58: 193–201.

24. Olney JW: Brain lesions, obesity and other disturbances in mice treated with monosodium glutamate. *Science* 1969; 164:719–721.

25. Choi DW, Maulucci-Gedde M, Kriegstein AR: Glutamate neurotoxicity in cortical cell culture. *J Neurosci* 1987; 7:357–368.

26. Choi DW: Ionic dependence of glutamate neurotoxicity. *J Neurosci* 1987; 7:369–379.

27. Zhang J, Dawson VL, Dawson TM, et al.: Nitric oxide activation of poly(ADP-ribose) synthetase in neurotoxicity. *Science* 1994; 263:687–689.

28. Whalen MJ, Clark RSB, Dixon CE, et al: Reduction of cognitive and motor deficits after traumatic brain injury in mice deficient in poly(ADP-ribose) polymerase. *J Cereb Blood Flow Metab* 1999; 19:835–842.

29. Du L, Zhang X, Han YY, Burke NA, Kochanek PM, Watkins SC, Graham SH, Carcillo JA, Szabo C, Clark RS: Intra-mitochondrial poly (ADP-ribosylation) contributes to NAD+ depletion and cell death induced by oxidative stress. *J Biol Chem* 2003; 16;278: 18426–18433.

30. Faden AI, Demediuk P, Panter SS, et al.: The role of excitatory amino acids and NMDA receptors in traumatic brain injury. *Science* 1989; 244:798–800.

31. Hayes R, Jenkins L, Lyeth B, et al.: Pretreatment with phencyclidine, an *N*-methyl-*D*-aspartate receptor antagonist, attenuates long-term behavioral deficits in the rat produced by traumatic brain injury. *J Neurotrauma* 1988; 5:287–302.

32. McIntosh TK, Vink R, Soares H, et al.: Effects of noncompetitive blockade of N-methyl-D-aspartate receptors on the neurochemical sequelae of experimental brain injury. *J Neurotrauma* 1989; 6:247–259.

33. Smith DH, Okiyama K, Gennarelli TA, et al.: Magnesium and ketamine attenuate cognitive dysfunction following experimental brain injury. *Neurosci Lett* 1993; 157:211–214.

34. Huettner J: Indole-2-carboxylic acid: A competitive antagonist of potentiation by glycine at the NMDA receptor. *Science* 1989; 243:1611–1613.

35. Suehiro E, Fujisawa H, Ito H, et al.: Brain temperature modifies glutamate neurotoxicity *In Vivo* 1999; 16:285–297.

36. Goodman JC, Valadka AB, Gopinath P, et al.: Lactate and excitatory amino acids measured by microdialysis are decreased by pentobarbital coma in head-injured patients. *J Neurotrauma* 1996; 13:549–556.

37. Palmer AM, Marion DW, Botscheller ML, et al.: Increased transmitter amino acid concentration in human ventricular CSF after brain trauma. *NeuroReport* 1994; 6:153–156.

38. Meldrum BS, Garthwaite J: Excitatory amino acid neurotoxicity and neurodegenerative disease. *Trends Pharmacol Sci* 1990; 11: 379–387.

39. Brown JIM, Baker AJ, Konasiewicz SJ, et al.: Clinical significance of CSF glutamate concentrations following severe traumatic brain injury in humans. *J Neurotrauma* 1998; 15:253–263.

40. Bullock R, Zauner A, Woodward JJ, et al: Factors affecting excitatory amino acid release following severe human head injury. *J Neurosurg* 1998; 89:507–518.

41. Doppenberg EMR, Choi SC, Bullock R: Clinical trials in traumatic brain injury. What can we learn from previous studies? *Ann NY Acad Sci* 1997; 825:305–322.

42. Hendricson AW, Thomas MP, Lippmann MJ, Morrisett RA: Suppression of L-type voltage-gated calcium channel-dependent synaptic plasticity by ethanol: analysis of miniature synaptic currents and dendritic calcium transients. *J Pharmacol Exp Ther* 2003; 307:550–558.

43. Rudolphi KA, Schubert P, Parkinson FE, et al.: Neuroprotective role of adenosine in cerebral ischaemia. *Trends Pharmacol Sci* 1992; 13:439–445.

44. Deckert J, Jorgensen MB: Evidence for pre- and postsynpatic localization of adenosine A1 receptors in the CA1 region of rat hippocampus: a quantitative autoradiographic study. *Brain Res* 1988; 446:161–164.

45. Nilsson P, Hillered L, Ponten U, et al.: Changes in cortical extracellular levels of energy-related metabolites and amino acids following concussive brain injury in rats. *J Cereb Blood Flow Metab* 1990; 10:631–637.

46. Headrick JP, Bendall MR, Faden AI, et al.: Dissociation of adenosine levels from bioenergetic state in experimental brain trauma: Potential role in secondary injury. *J Cereb Blood Flow Metab* 1994; 14:853–861.

47. Bell MJ, Kochanek PM, Carcillo JA, et al.: Interstitial adenosine, inosine, and hypoxanthine, are increased after experimental traumatic brain injury in the rat. *J Neurotrauma* 1998; 15: 163–170.

48. Bell M, Robertson C, Kochanek P, et al.: Interstitial purine metabolites after traumatic brain injury in humans: evidence for energy failure during jugular venous desaturation. *J Neurotrauma* 1997; 14:791.

49. Dutcher SA, Underwood BD, Michael DB, Diaz FG, Walker PD: Heat-shock protein 72 expression in excitotoxic versus penetrating injuries of the rodent cerebral cortex. *J Neurotrauma* 1998; 15:421–432.

50. Seidberg NA, Clark RS, Zhang X, Lai Y, Chen M, Graham SH, Kochanek PM, Watkins SC, Marion DW: Alterations in inducible 72-kDa heat shock protein and the chaperone cofactor BAG-1 in human brain after head injury. *J Neurochem* 2003; 84:514–521.

51. Lai Y, Kochanek PM, Adelson PD, Janesko K, Ruppel RA, Clark RSB: Induction of the stress response after inflicted and non-inflicted traumatic brain injury in infants and children. *J Neurotrauma* 2004; 21:229–237.

52. Simon MM, Reikerstorfer A, Schwarz A, Krone C, Luger TA, Jaattela M, Schwarz T: Heat shock protein 70 overexpression affects the response to ultraviolet light in murine fibroblasts. Evidence for increased cell viability and suppression of cytokine release. *J Clin Invest* 1995; 95:926–933.

53. Rink A, Fung K-M, Trojanowski JQ, et al.: Evidence of apoptotic cell death after experimental traumatic brain injury in the rat. *Am J Pathol* 1995; 147:1575–1583.

54. Clark RS, Kochanek PM, Chen M, et al.: Increases in Bcl-2 and cleavage of Caspase-1 and Caspase-3 in human brain after head injury. *FASEB J* 1999; 13:813–821.

55. Kerr JF, Wyllie AH, Currie AR: Apoptosis: a basic biological phenomenon with wide-ranging implications in tissue kinetics. *Br J Cancer* 1972; 26:239–257.

56. Steller H: Mechanisms and genes of cellular suicide. *Science* 1995; 267:1445–1449.

57. Portera-Cailliau C, Price DL, Martin LJ: Excitotoxic neuronal death in the immature brain is an apoptosis-necrosis morphological continuum. *J Comp Neurol* 1997; 378:70–87.

58. Zamzami N, Susin SA, Marchetti P, et al.: Mitochondrial control of nuclear apoptosis. *J Exp Med* 1996; 183:1533–1544.

59. Adams JM, Cory S: The Bcl-2 protein family: arbiters of cell survival. *Science* 1998; 281:1322–1326.

60. Li P, Nijhawan D, Budihardjo I, et al.: Cytochrome c and dATP-dependent formation of Apaf-1/Caspase-9 complex initiates an apoptotic protease cascade. *Cell* 1997; 91:479–489.

61. Clark RSB, Kochanek PM, Watkins SC, et al.: Caspase-3 mediated neuronal death after traumatic brain injury in rats. *J Neurochem* 2000; 74:740–753.

62. Susin SA, Zamzami N, Castedo M, Hirsch T, Marchetti P, Macho A, Daugas E, Geuskens M, Kroemer G: Bcl-2 inhibits the mitochondrial release of an apoptogenic protease. *J Exp Med* 1996; 184:1331–1341.

63. Susin SA, Lorenzo HK, Zamzami N, Marzo I, Snow BE, Brothers GM, Mangion J, Jacotot E, Costantini P, Loeffler M, Larochette N, Goodlett DR, Aebersold R, Siderovski DP, Penninger JM, Kroemer G: Molecular characterization of mitochondrial apoptosis-inducing factor. *Nature* 1999; 397:441–446.

64. Susin SA, Daugas E, Ravagnan L, Samejima K, Zamzami N, Loeffler M, Costantini P, Ferri KF, Irinopoulou T, Prevost MC, Brothers G, Mark TW, Penninger J, Earnshaw WC, Kroemer G: Two distinct pathways leading to nuclear apoptosis. *J Exp Med 2000*; 192:571–580.

65. Hill IE, Murray C, Richard J, Rasquinha I, MacManus JP: Despite the intermucleosomal cleavage of DNA, reactive oxygen species do not produce other markers of apoptosis in cultured neurons. *Exp Neurol* 2000; 162:73–88.

66. Dumont C, Durrbach A, Bidere N, Rouleau M, Kroemer G, Bernard G, Hirsch F, Charpentier B, Susin SA, Senik A: Caspase-independent commitment phase to apoptosis in activated blood T lymphocytes: reversibility at low apoptotic insult. *Blood* 2000; 96:1030–1038.

67. Zhang X, Chen J, Graham SH, Du L, Kochanek PM, Draviam R, Guo F, Nathaniel PD, Szabo C, Watkins SC, Clark RSB: Intranuclear localization of apoptosis-inducing factor (AIF) and large-scale DNA fragmentation after traumatic brain injury in rats and in neuronal cultures exposed to peroxynitrite. *J Neurochem* 2002; 82:181–191.

68. Ashkenazi A, Dixit VM: Death receptors: signaling and modulation. *Science* 1998; 281:1305–1308.

69. Li H, Zhu H, Xu CJ, et al: Cleavage of BID by caspase 8 mediates the mitochondrial damage in the Fas pathway of apoptosis. *Cell* 1998; 94:491–501.

70. Hockenbery D, Nunez G, Milliman C, et al.: Bcl-2 is an inner mitochondrial membrane protein that blocks programmed cell death. *Nature* 1990; 348:334–336.

71. Clark RSB, Chen J, Watkins SC, et al.: Apoptosis-suppressor gene bcl-2 expression after traumatic brain injury in rats. *J Neurosci* 1997; 9:172–9182.

72. Raghupathi R, Fernandez SC, Murai H, et al.: BCL-2 overexpression attenuates cortical cell loss after traumatic brain injury in transgenic mice. *J Cereb Blood Flow Metab* 1998; 18:1259–1269.

73. Clark RSB, Kochanek PM, Adelson PD, et al.: Increases in bcl-2 protein in cerebrospinal fluid and evidence for programmed-cell death in infants and children following severe traumatic brain injury. J Pediatr 2000; 137:197–204.

74. Kotapka MJ, Graham DI, Adams JH, Gennarelli TA: Hippocampal pathology in fatal human head injury without high intracranial pressure. *J Neurotrauma* 1994; 11:317–324.

75. Jenkins LW, Lyeth BG, Lewelt W, Moszynski K, Dewitt DS, Balster RL, Miller LP, Clifton GL, Young HF, Hayes RL: Combined pre-trauma scopolamine and phencyclidine attenuate post-traumatic increased sensitivity to delayed secondary ischemia. *J Neurotrauma,* 1988; 5:275–287.

76. Forbes ML, Clark RS, Dixon CE, Graham SH, Marion DW, DeKosky ST, Schiding JK, Kochanek PM: Augmented neuronal death in CA3 hippocampus following hyperventilation early after controlled cortical impact. *J Neurosurg* 1998; 88:549–556.

77. Colicos MA, Dixon CE, Dash PK: Delayed, selective neuronal death following experimental cortical impact injury in rats: possible role in memory deficits. *Brain Res,* 1996; 739:111–119.

78. Graham DI, McIntosh TK, Maxwell WL, Nicoll JA, Recent advances in neurotrauma. *J Neuropathol Exp Neurol* 2000; 59:641–651.

79. Cross TG, Scheel-Toellner D, Henriquez NV, et al: Serine/threonine protein kinases and apoptosis. *Exp Cell Res* 2000; 256:34–41.

80. Orban PC, Chapman PF, Brambilla R: Is the Ras-MAPK signalling pathway necessary for long-term memory formation? *Trends Neurosci* 1999; 22:38–44.

81. Cross TG, Scheel-Toellner D, Henriquez NV, et al.: Serine/threonine protein kinases and apoptosis. *Exp Cell Res* 2000; 256:34–41.

82. Naor Z, Benard O, Seger R: Activation of MAPK cascades by G-protein-coupled receptors: the case of gonadotropin-releasing hormone receptor. *Trends Endocrinol Metab* 2000; 11:91–99.

83. Kaplan DR, Miller FD: Neurotrophin signal transduction in the nervous system. *Curr Opin Neurobiol* 2000; 10:381–391.

84. Ono K, Han J: The p38 signal transduction pathway: activation and function. *Cell Signal* 2000; 12: 1–13.

85. Dash PK, Mach SA, Moore AN: The role of extracellular signal-regulated kinase in cognitive and motor deficits following experimental traumatic brain injury, *Neuroscience* 2002; 114: 755–767.

86. Otani N, Nawashiro H, Fukui S, Nomura N, Shima K: Temporal and spatial profile of phosphorylated mitogen-activated protein kinase pathways after lateral fluid percussion injury in the cortex of the rat brain. *J Neurotrauma* 2002; 19:1587–1596.

87. Mori T, Wang X, Jung JC, Sumii T, Singhal AB, Fini ME, Dixon CE, Alessandrini A, Lo EH: Mitogen-activated protein kinase inhibition in traumatic brain injury: in vitro and in vivo effects. *J Cereb Blood Flow Metab* 2002; 22:444–452.

88. Nunez G, del Peso L: Linking extracellular survival signals and the apoptotic machinery, *Curr Opin Neurobiol* 1998; 8:613–618.

89. Konishi H, Matsuzaki H, Takaishi H, et al.: Opposing effects of protein kinase C delta and protein kinase B alpha on H(2)O(2)-induced apoptosis in CHO cells. *Biochem Biophys Res Commun* 1999; 264:840–846.

90. Coffer PJ, Jin J, Woodgett JR: Protein kinase B (c-Akt): a multi-functional mediator of phosphatidylinositol 3-kinase activation. *Biochem J* 1998; 335:1–13.

91. Xia Z, Dickens M, Raingeaud J, et al: Opposing effects of ERK and JNK-p38 MAP kinases on apoptosis. *Science* 1995; 270: 1326–1331.

92. Jenkins LW, Peters GW, Dixon CE, Zhang X, Clark RS, Skinner JC, Marion DW, Adelson PD, Kochanek PM: Conventional and functional proteomics using large format two-dimensional gel electrophoresis 24 hours after controlled cortical impact in postnatal day 17 rats. *J Neurotrauma* 2002; 19:715–740.

93. Adams JH, Graham DI, Murray LS, et al.: Diffuse axonal injury due to nonmissile head injury in humans: an analysis of 45 cases. *Ann Neurol* 1982; 12:557–563.

94. Adams JH, Doyle D, Ford I, et al.: Diffuse axonal injury in head injury: definition, diagnosis, and grading. *Histopathology* 1989; 15:49–59.

95. Christman CW, Grady MS, Walker SA, et al.: Ultrastructural studies of diffuse axonal injury in humans. *J Neurotrauma* 1994; 11:173–186.

96. Gennarelli TA, Thibault LF, Adams TH, et al.: Diffuse axonal injury and traumatic coma in the primate. *Ann Neurol* 1982; 12:564–574.

97. Povlishock JT: Traumatically induced axonal injury: pathogenesis and pathobiological implications. *Brain Pathol* 1992; 2:1–12.

98. Fitzpatrick MO, Maxwell WL, Graham DI: The role of the axolomma in the initiation of traumatically induced axonal injury. *J Neurol Neurosurg Psychiatry* 1998; 64:285–287.

99. Smith DH, Chen XH, Xu BN, et al.: Characterization of diffuse axonal pathology and selective hippocampal damage following inertial brain trauma in the pig. *J Neuropathol Exp Neurol* 1997; 56:822–834.

100. Gennarelli TA: Mechanisms of brain injury. *J Emerg Med* 1993; 11 Suppl 1:5–11.

101. Graham DI, Lawrence AE, Adams JH, et al.: Brain damage in fatal non-missile head injury without high intracranial pressure. *J Clin Pathol* 1988; 41:34–37.

102. Graham DI, Ford I, Adams JH, et al: Fatal head injury in children. *J Clin Pathol* 1989; 42:18–22.

103. Povlishock JT, Buki A, Koiziumi H, et al.: Initiating mechanisms involved in the pathobiology of traumatically induced axonal injury and interventions targeted at blunting their progression. *Acta Neurochir Suppl (Wien)* 1999; 73:15–20.

104. Povlishock JT, Jenkins LW: Are the pathobiological changes evoked by traumatic brain injury immediate and irreversible? *Brain Pathol* 1995; 5:415–426.

105. Maxwell WL, Povlishock JT, Graham DL: A mechanistic analysis of nondisruptive axonal injury: A review. J Neurotrauma 1997; 14:419–440.

106. Stys PK: Anoxic and ischemic injury of myelinated axons in CNS white matter: from mechanistic concepts to therapeutics. *J Cereb Blood Flow Metab* 1998; 18:2–25.

107. Kampfl A, Posmantur RM, Zhao X, et al.: Mechanisms of calpain proteolysis following traumatic brain injury: implications for pathology and therapy – implications for pathology and therapy: A review and update. *J Neurotrauma* 1997; 14:121–134.

108. Buki A, Koizumi H, Povlishock JT: Moderate post-traumatic hypothermia decreases early calpain-mediated proteolysis and concomitant cytoskeletal compromise in traumatic axonal injury. *Exp Neurol* 1999; 159:319–328.

109. Buki A, Okonkwo DO, Povlishock JT: Postinjury cyclosporin A administration limits axonal damage and disconnection in traumatic brain injury. *J Neurotrauma* 1999; 16:511–521.

110. Goss JR, Styren SD, Miller PD, et al.: Hypothermia attenuates the normal increase in interleukin 1b RNA and nerve growth factor following traumatic brain injury in the rat. *J Neurotrauma* 1995; 12:159–167.

111. DeKosky ST, Goss JR, Miller PD, et al.: Upregulation of nerve growth factor following cortical trauma. *Exp Neurol* 1994; 130:173–177.

112. Cecil KM, Hills EC, Sandel ME, et al.: Proton magnetic resonance spectroscopy for detection of axonal injury in the splenium of the corpus callosum of brain-injured patients. *J Neurosurg* 1998; 88:795–801.

113. McGowan JC, McCormack TM, Grossman RI, et al.: Diffuse axonal pathology detected with magnetization transfer imaging following brain injury in the pig. *Magn Reson Med* 1999; 41:727–733.

114. Xue R, van Zijl PC, Crain BJ, et al.: In vivo three-dimensional reconstruction of rat brain axonal projections by diffusion tensor imaging. *Magn Reson Med* 1999; 42:1123–1127.

115. Pajevic S, Pierpaoli C: Color schemes to represent the orientation of anisotropic tissues from diffusion tensor data: application to white matter fiber tract mapping in the human brain. *Magn Reson Med* 1999; 42:526–540.

116. Seelig JM, Becker DP, Miller JD, Greenberg RP, Ward JD, Choi SC: Traumatic acute subdural hematoma: major mortality reduction in comatose patients treated within four hours. *N Engl J Med* 1981; 304:1511–1518.

117. Marmarou A, Barzo P, Fatouros P, et al.: Traumatic brain swelling in head injured patients: brain edema or vascular engorgement? *Acta Neurochir Suppl (Wien)* 1997; 70:68–70.

118. Barzo P, Marmarou A, Fatouros P, et al.: Contribution of vasogenic and cellular edema to traumatic brain swelling measured by diffusion-weighted imaging. *J Neurosurg* 1997; 87:900–907.

119. Barzo P, Marmarou A, Fatouros P, et al.: MRI diffusion-weighted spectroscopy of reversible and irreversible ischemic injury following closed head injury. *Acta Neurochir Suppl (Wien)* 1997; 70:115–118.

120. Katayama Y, Mori T, Maeda T, et al.: Pathogenesis of the mass effect of cerebral contusions: Rapid increase in osmolality within the contusion necrosis. *Acta Neurochir Suppl (Wien)* 1998; 71:289–292.

121. Ashwal S, Holshouser BA, Shu SK, Simmons PL, Perkin RM, Tomasi LG, Knierim DS, Sheridan C, Craig K, Andrews GH, Hinshaw DB: Predictive value of proton magnetic resonance spectroscopy in pediatric closed head injury. *Pediatr Neurol* 2000; 23:114–125.

122. Rosomoff HL, Clasen RA, Hartstock R, et al.: Brain reaction to experimental injury after hypothermia. *Arch Neurol* 1965; 13:337–345.

123. Schoettle RJ, Kochanek PM, Magargee MJ, et al.: Early polymorphonuclear leukocyte accumulation correlates with the development of post-traumatic cerebral edema in rats. *J Neurotrauma* 1990; 7:207–217.

124. Clark RSB, Schiding JK, Kaczorowski SL, et al.: Neutrophil accumulation after traumatic brain injury in rats: Comparison of weight-drop and controlled cortical impact models. *J Neurotrauma* 1994; 11:499–506.

125. McClain C, Cohen D, Phillips R, et al.: Increased plasma and ventricular fluid interleukin-6 levels in patients with head injury. *J Lab Clin Med* 1991; 118:225–231.

126. Marion DW, Penrod LE, Kelsey SF, et al.: Treatment of traumatic brain injury with moderate hypothermia. *N Engl J Med* 1997; 336:540–546.

127. Kossmann T, Hans VHJ, Imhof H-G, et al.: Intrathecal and serum interleukin-6 and the acute-phase response in patients with severe traumatic brain injuries. *Shock* 1995; 4:311–317.

128. Kossmann T, Stahel PF, Lenzlinger PM, et al.: Interleukin-8 released into the cerebrospinal fluid after brain injury is associated with blood-brain barrier dysfunction and nerve growth factor production. *J Cereb Blood Flow Metab* 1997; 17:280–289.

129. Bethea JR, Castro M, Keane RW, et al.: Traumatic spinal cord injury induces nuclear factor-kB activation. *J Neurosci* 1998; 18:3251–3260.

130. Shohami E, Bass R, Wallach D, et al.: Inhibition of tumor necrosis factor alpha (TNFα) activity in rat brain is associated with cerebroprotection after closed head injury. J Cereb Blood Flow Metab 1996; 16:378–384.

131. Scherbel U, Raghupathi R, Nakamura M, et al.: Differential acute and chronic responses of tumor necrosis factor-deficient mice to experimental brain injury. *Proc Natl Acad Sci USA* 1999; 96:8721–8726.

132. Toulmond S, Rothwell NJ: Interleukin-1 receptor antagonist inhibits neuronal damage caused by fluid percussion injury in the rat. *Brain Res* 1995; 671:261–266.

133. DeKosky ST, Styren SD, O'Malley ME, et al.: Interleukin-1 receptor antagonist suppresses neurotrophin response in injured rat brain. *Ann Neurol* 1996; 39:123–127.

134. Shapira Y, Artru AA, Yadid G, et al.: Methylprednisolone does not decrease eicosanoid concentrations or edema in brain tissue or improve neurologic outcome after head trauma in rats. *Anesth Analg* 1992; 75:238–244.

135. Uhl MW, Biagas KV, Grundl PD, et al: Effects of neutropenia on edema, histology, and cerebral blood flow after traumatic brain injury in rats. *J Neurotrauma* 1994; 11:303–315.

136. Blight AR: Effects of silica on the outcome from experimental spinal cord injury: implication of macrophages in secondary tissue damage. *Neuroscience* 1994; 60:263–273.

137. Popovich PG, Guan Z, Wei P, et al.: Depletion of hematogenous macrophages promotes partial hindlimb recovery and neuroanatomical repair after experimental spinal cord injury. *Exp Neurol* 1999; 158:351–365.

138. Kossmann T, Hans V, Imhof H-G, et al.: Interleukin-6 released in human cerebrospinal fluid following traumatic brain injury may trigger nerve growth factor production in astrocytes. *Brain Res* 1996; 713:143–152.

139. Sinz EH, Kochanek PM, Heyes MP, et al.: Quinolinic acid is increased in CSF and associated with mortality after traumatic brain injury in humans. *J Cereb Blood Flow Metab (Rapid Communication)* 1998; 18:610–615.

140. Shore PM, Jackson EK, Wisniewski SR, Clark RS, Adelson PK, Kochanek PM: Vascular endothelial growth factor is increased in cerebrospinal fluid after traumatic brain injury in infants and children. *Neurosurgery* 2004; 54:605–611.

141. Bayir H, Kochanek PM, Siu SX, Arroyo A, Osipov A, Jiang J, Wisniewski S, Adelson PD, Graham SH, Kagan VE: Increased

S-nitrosothiols and S-nitrosoalbumin in cerebrospinal fluid after severe traumatic brain injury in infants and children: indirect association with intracranial pressure. *J Cereb Blood Flow Metab* 2003; 23:51–61.

142. Sinz EH, Kochanek PM, Dixon CE, et al.: Inducible nitric oxide synthase is an endogenous neuroprotectant after traumatic brain injury in rats and mice. *J Clin Invest* 1999; 104:647–656.

143. Wada K, Chatzipanteli K, Kraydieh S, et al.: Inducible nitric oxide synthase expression after traumatic brain injury and neuroprotection with aminoguanidine treatment in rats. *Neurosurgery* 1998; 43:1427–1436.

144. Yamasaki K, Edington HD, McClosky C, et al.: Reversal of impaired wound repair in iNOS-deficient mice by topical adenoviral-mediated iNOS gene transfer. *J Clin Invest* 1998; 101:967–971.

145. Heard SO, Fink MP, Gamelli RL, et al.: Effect of prophylactic administration of recombinant human granulocyte colony-stimulating factor (filgrastim) on the frequency of nosocomial infections in patients with acute traumatic brain injury or cerebral hemorrhage. *Crit Care Med* 1998; 26:748–754.

146. Kochanek PM, Clark RSB, Ruppel RA, Adelson PD, Bell MJ, Whalen MJ, Robertson CL, Satchell MA, Seidberg NA, Marion DW, Jenkins LW: Biochemical, cellular, and molecular mechanisms in the evolution of secondary damage after severe traumatic brain injury in infants and children: Lessons learned from the bedside. *Pediatr Crit Care Med* 2000; 1:4–19.

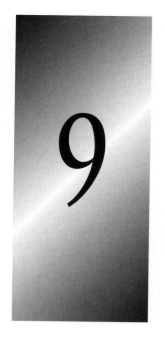

9 Concepts of CNS Plasticity and Their Implications for Understanding Recovery After Brain Damage*

Donald G. Stein

CONCEPTUAL AND THEORETICAL ISSUES IN RECOVERY OF FUNCTION: BACKGROUND

It is often taken for granted that after brain injury, "plasticity" and recovery may be possible, but their underlying mechanisms remain a matter of debate. The term "plasticity" is seldom explicitly defined in reports on neurorehabilitation. When any functional restitution or recovery after brain injury is observed, the assumption is that the inherent plasticity of the brain is responsible for the beneficial outcome. But what does this really explain about what is actually taking place in response to brain damage?

Until the 1960s, very few people in the field of neurorehabilitation supported the idea that the adult central nervous system (CNS) was capable of undergoing any substantial reorganization in response to brain damage, so any "recovery" was attributed to strategic behavioral tricks that brain-injured subjects were able to master in order to overcome their deficits (1). These were referred to as "compensatory strategies," but the argument was circular: you had behavioral recovery because of compensatory strategies which were inferred because you had behavioral recovery—hardly a meaningful explanation of mechanism!

One of the main dogmas that blocked substantive research and clinical understanding of the mechanisms of recovery in response to brain damage was promoted by the Nobel prize–winning neuroanatomist Ramon y Cajal (2), who forcefully argued that once development was over, any regeneration in the adult brain would be very limited, if it occurred at all. During that era, neuroanatomists who observed structural changes in the damaged adult brain—now considered characteristic of neuronal repair, such as axonal or dendritic sprouting, or even neurogenesis—often reported such changes as mere artifacts of histological techniques rather than as real evidence of CNS structural plasticity.

The paradigm shift that led to acceptance of the idea of CNS plasticity in response to injury began with the work of Raisman (3). Using then state-of-the-art electron microscopic techniques, Raisman first mapped the two primary afferent pathways into the subcortical structure he called the "septal nuclear complex" in adult rats. Once the pathways were identified, Raisman made separate and selective knife-cuts to disrupt one of the two paths to observe what changes would take place in the intact pathway in response to the injury. After waiting a suitable period of time he observed that (1) degenerating fibers

*This article is substantially revised from a previous version published as Stein DG, Hoffman SW: Concepts of CNS plasticity in the context of brain damage and repair, *J Head Trauma Rehabil* 18, 317–341, 2003.

caused by the cut left synapses in the septal nucleus vacated, and (2) fibers from the surviving pathway reoccupied the vacated synapses. Particularly interesting was that the new afferents were "heterotypic": they did not provide the same neurotransmitter to the septal cells as had the original fibers. Raisman concluded that:

> the finding that the distribution of one fibre pathway to the septum is altered by the destruction of another system of septal afferents suggests that synapses in the central nervous system of adult mammals may be far more labile than had been previously suspected. It is interesting to speculate why, in view of this anatomical plasticity, so little functional recovery accompanies lesions of the brain (p. 45).

Raisman and his colleagues did not follow up his remarkable observations with behavioral studies, but his work did lead others to change the view of the adult CNS from a static, phrenological collection of structures with fixed functions to a much more dynamic system capable of reorganization in response to injury (see, e.g., Cotman [4] and Steward [5]).

Although studies on promoting recovery of function appeared as early as the first few decades of the twentieth century (see Finger and Stein [6] for examples), until the early 1970s they were largely dismissed by the field as describing "anomalous" events not worthy of serious study. At the behavioral level, those adhering to the static view of the adult CNS could claim that when functional recovery was observed, it was simply because the tests being used were not sensitive enough to detect the underlying deficits.

The idea that recovery of function can be promoted by pharmacological agents, the transplantation of fetal or stem cell tissues, environmental stimulation, hormonal factors, and other means, is a very new concept in the history of the science and is still not completely accepted. For example, the indisputably best-selling textbook in neuroscience, used today in almost all comprehensive graduate neuroscience classes, is *Principles of Neural Science* (7). This work refers to plasticity only once (p. 34), and despite its comprehensive coverage and its heavy use by medical and biomedical professionals, it offers no discussion of recovery of function and its implications for thinking about the organization and adaptability of the brain in response to injury.

Grounds for cautious optimism may exist, however. In a new textbook closely modeled after Kandel et al., *Fundamental Neuroscience* (8), the authors do refer to "experience-driven plasticity" in the cortex and other neural systems, but they say nothing about any aspect of recovery of function and its potential underlying mechanisms. This blind spot in the basic education of young neuroscientists can have profound effects on the treatment of CNS injury and the allocation of resources for

research. Certainly no one is claiming that physiological repair of the damaged brain or spinal cord is going to occur under *all* conditions, but it is becoming impossible to ignore or deny the many hundreds of laboratory animal and human studies which have shown that some extent of repair, regeneration and functional recovery can be stimulated under some conditions. The focus should now be on determining what those conditions are, and applying them to achieve repair after degenerative or traumatic injuries to the brain or spinal cord.

The remainder of this chapter reviews several concepts of recovery that were proposed in the fields of neuropsychology and neurorehabilitation before there was much empirical and clinical data to support them. Given the large body of evidence we now have for dramatic reorganization and repair after injury, are these early concepts of functional recovery consistent with the well-accepted 'principle' of strict functional localization in the brain? Are plasticity concepts and localization dogma consistent with each other? Is localization dogma supported by the evidence, both modern high-tech data and the older intuitive clinical approach (9)?

First, is it clear what we mean when we use the term "neuroplasticity"? Is it a specific, well-defined phenomenon that can be applied as an explanatory construct? Over the last decade or so, there has been an explosion of interest in neuroplasticity and it is often taken for granted that what the term implies is well understood and accepted. PubMed, the National Institutes of Health's literature search engine, is a powerful tool for finding the most current articles in the biomedical sciences. Type in the word "neuroplasticity" and about *eleven thousand* articles appear. Neuroplasticity is applied to the symptoms of Alzheimer's disease, alterations in apolipoprotein E synthesis, chronic pain, mood disorders, recovery from stroke, long-term potentiation in the hippocampus, changes in memory in development and aging, allodynia, presynaptic neurotransmitter vesicle release, changes in synaptic terminal arborization, alterations during critical periods of development, alterations in glutamate receptors, changes in trans-cranial stimulation-induced excitability of the motor cortex, alterations in sensory-cortical maps, neurogenesis during development and aging, stem cell effects, axonal sprouting, epileptic seizure activity, and augmentation of immune-induced neural inflammatory response, all in the first twenty references that come up in PubMed! How can such ubiquitous use of the term be of any use in understanding what is actually occurring in the damaged nervous system in response to injury? One argument is that, clearly, 'plasticity' has manifold ways of expressing itself in both the intact and the damaged nervous system. But if every type of change in neural tissue is seen as plasticity, what then is NOT an example of the phenomenon?

Here is a case, taken from the field of neurogenesis, that illustrates the problem: recently, Parent and

Lowenstein (10) reviewed the literature on the effectiveness of stem cell proliferation in the adult nervous system of rodents. These authors reported that there is, indeed, a five- to tenfold increase in the number of dentate granule cells in the hippocampus following chemotoxic injury to the brain, and this could certainly be considered a dramatic example of injury-induced neuroplasticity. However, their review of the literature also showed that the neurogenesis was associated with increases in kindling and seizure activity in the hippocampus and with a later increase in apoptotic cell death. This is not to imply that, under all conditions, injury-induced neurogenesis would be detrimental. But this is a typical example of neuroplasticity that has a negative outcome. But if such a phenomenon (i.e., neurogenesis as a cause for post-traumatic epilepsy) is also an example of 'plasticity,' then just how useful is the concept for explaining recovery of function? Perhaps we need to distinguish between *negative* and *positive* plasticity and to think more critically about how we use the term to describe events in the central nervous system (CNS) associated with functional recovery and rehabilitation.

For the purposes of this review, "neuroplasticity" will be used only for verifiable examples of functional and adaptive recovery after brain injury. This is the behavioral concept that cognitive, sensory, or motor impairments gradually diminish or are eliminated over time rather than getting worse. Limiting the term in this way implies that there can be acute or chronic deficits which disappear spontaneously, or which can be reduced by pharmacological, physiological, surgical, or behavioral treatments over time (11–15).

"LOCALIZATION OF FUNCTION," RECOVERY OF FUNCTION, AND DEFINITIONS OF NEUROPLASTICITY

In the clinic, it may be difficult to accept a very limited definition of plasticity. This is because it is often necessary for brain-damaged patients to succeed in a variety of activities of daily living by substituting new behavioral strategies. This substitution is considered a form of 'compensation' or adaptation to a deficit. As noted earlier, some critics of the concept postulate that recovery of function does not really exist. They hold that all recovery is only a type of compensation (see [1] and [16] for a good discussion of this issue). This view is an offshoot of the idea that specific areas of the brain are genetically programmed to control or mediate behaviors, so the destruction or perturbation of a center in which such specific functions are localized leads to the permanent loss (or serious impairment) of that function.

The battle between those who argue for precise localization and those who think that functions are more widely distributed throughout the brain has been going on for more than a hundred years, and despite breakthroughs in brain imaging techniques, no resolution is in sight. Within this framework the limits or extent of localization seem to shift with the latest fashions in technology. For example, cortical maps grow or shrink according to how imaging methods are applied, and this determines how the loci of control are defined. As imaging studies proliferate, structures are added or subtracted at will to the number required to mediate a particular function, with the expansion taking place in the serial or parallel circuits so popular in computer-based metaphors of the brain. The more recovery observed, especially in the case of bilateral structural removal, the more structures have to be added to account for the observed plasticity. This issue is discussed further below.

Providing technical support for this conceptual approach to brain function is the rapid progress in molecular biological assays, which has led to a plethora of functional activities being assigned to the expression or inhibition of specific genes, a form of localization doctrine gone wild—a molecular biology of phrenology, so to speak, which is of growing concern to some investigators in this field. In an excellent brief review of the issue, Kosik cautions that:

> Genes, neurons and brain regions are annotated with functional descriptors that fail to capture the interactive nature of these units. The temptation is strong to jump beyond what a biological unit actually does, to a more encompassing functional label. For example, a mutant gene does not cause a disease; it merely encodes a mutant protein that leads to a cascade of events and, eventually, to a disease. The methodology to ascertain function can also be limiting. Just as the carpenter, whose only tool is a hammer, treats all objects like nails, so neurophysiologists and brain 'imagers' probe the brain with their own hammers and have cobbled a picture of brain function that is not explicitly integrated (17).

This discussion is not just an academic exercise, because one corollary of the 'strong' form of localization is that one can never expect to see any 'true' recovery of function, and perhaps it is because of this belief that recovery of function per se is rarely discussed in the major textbooks of basic neuroscience currently in use. These argue that subtle "tricks" must be used by the organism to perform effectively, and that the tricks may be too subtle to detect without sophisticated behavioral testing designed to reveal the underlying deficits and shifts in behavior (1). If no deficits are observed, it is because the tests are insensitive, or the wrong tests have been used, rather than because any true recovery of function has occurred. From this perspective, the job of the neuropsychological diagnostician is to tease out the deficits and prove the localization.

The only goal of rehabilitation, in this context, is to teach the patient new strategies to replace functions lost by the injury, and plasticity is defined by the extent to which such substitution is possible. For those who envision the nervous system as a kind of 'black box,' there is no need to speculate about underlying neural mechanisms or to worry about providing neuroprotection or enhancing neuroregeneration through a pharmacological or physiological substrate. The remaining brain tissue just does what it does to varying degrees of effectiveness, so why bother with trying to 'add' neurons or rebuild damaged circuits? Thus it is argued that while the brain-damaged patient may eventually accomplish the same goals as an intact individual, the means by which the task is accomplished may be very different.

EQUIPOTENTIALITY, VICARIATION, CNS REORGANIZATION AND RECOVERY OF FUNCTION

The assumption of substitution rather than restitution of function after brain damage fits well with the idea that intact parts of the brain can take over the functions of tissue lost or destroyed after injury or disease. In this paradigm, remaining healthy tissue is said to modulate its physiological activities to compensate for the damage to a specific area. But there is evidence to support a different model for response to injury. Thus, in laboratory rats and monkeys, if injury occurs during certain critical periods in early development, recovery of cognitive and motor functions can sometimes be greater than that seen in adults with similar kinds of CNS damage. Is this merely a form of compensatory strategy or is structural reorganization of the brain itself a major factor in the resulting plasticity?

In humans with early brain injury, the issues are more complex and controversial than for adult brain injury, especially with respect to intellectual skills, language and cognition. For example, there are many studies in both animals and children that provide strong substantiation that early brain damage is associated with long-term deficits and intellectual impairments in later life (18, 19). Other studies support what has been called the Kennard principle (20), that early brain lesions lead to much more sparing than the same injury in a more mature organism (21, 22).

How is it possible to reconcile these divergent findings? It now appears that there are a number of factors that can predispose to better recovery if injury occurs during early development, but there are also factors that can make matters worse. One of the most important of these factors appears to be a very specific, critical period for plasticity such that very early-occurring injury to the brain may be much worse than if the injury were to occur just

a few weeks or months later (23). Bryan Kolb and his colleagues have repeatedly demonstrated this phenomenon in laboratory rats. They also review evidence in human infants showing that if a cortical injury occurs within the first months of life, the results can be devastating, but if the same cortical area is damaged at around one to two years of age, there is much better recovery. Kolb and Cioe (24) found that even as little as one week of difference in age could have dramatic impact on morphogenesis and sparing of function after medial frontal cortical lesions in rats. Thus, if the lesions were done on post-natal day 2, animals tested as adults on spatial learning and reaching tasks were very impaired. If the same surgery was done on post-natal day 9, there was extensive recovery and apparently substantial generation of new neurons to replace those that were removed by the surgery. In development, then, the precise timing of the injury *may be critical* in determining whether or not recovery will be observed, and when or whether rebuilding of neuronal circuits may occur. Injuries occurring slightly or moderately later than immediately after birth, when one might assume the most plasticity, could lead to much better outcomes. This calls for a more modulated evaluation and interpretation of the Kennard Principle that the earlier the injury the better the outcome.

When such sparing of function is observed during development or at maturity, it is often attributed to the equipotentiality or vicarious function of cerebral (usually cortical) areas. Equipotentiality refers to the capacity of anatomically distinct areas of the brain to mediate a rather wide variety of functions. Despite the caveats discussed above, such plasticity is thought to be more likely when the brain is developing and not yet specialized for particular activities such as speech or patterned movement, but there is both historical and contemporary evidence to suggest that both equipotentiality and vicarious function can be induced in the adult organism as well.

The concept of neural vicariation implies that even the mature CNS has a certain number of redundant or backup subsystems that participate in this takeover of function (25). However, the mechanisms by which area *a* could "take over the function" of damaged area *b* and still perform function *a* are usually not described. If there is substitution or vicarious function, how can it be determined at the physiological and/or behavioral levels of analysis? In one study in adult squirrel and owl monkeys, Xerri, Merzenich, Peterson and Jenkins (26) trained the animals to retrieve small objects, used microelectrode techniques to map responsivity to afferent activity when the animals performed the tactile discrimination tasks, and then selectively damaged specific parts of the sensorimotor cortex by electrocoagulation of surface blood vessels. The brain tissue was then checked to make sure that it was completely unresponsive to any peripheral stimulation.

Immediately after the lesions the monkeys were retrained on the tasks and cortical remapping was performed. The resulting changes in post-injury behaviors were complex and highly individualistic, suggesting from the outset that early experience and perhaps genetic factors played a role in the extent of cortical reorganization and recovery of digit and hand use. Performance initially deteriorated, then started to get better with re-training, and appeared to be proportional to the difficulty of the task. In some cases, animals with large lesions actually recovered better than those with less damage. The two different strains of monkeys did not perform the same way, indicating that initial brain organization and reorganization may be different across strains.

Most dramatic was the fact that the post-lesion reorganization of the cortex was very variable across monkeys; completely new cortical fields representing the fingers emerged and were enlarged in cortical areas that are not normally responsive to cutaneous stimulation. The changes appeared to be due both to the lesion and to the training procedures. According to the authors, the representation of the hands in the SI region of the somatosensory cortex is topographically organized into discrete cytoarchitectonic and functional regions, so that when these regions are damaged, area-specific deficits can be observed. For example, damage to area 1 leads to deficits in the discrimination of textures, while damage to area 2 impairs recognition of size and shape. Damage to area 3 causes significant deficits in texture, size and shape discriminations. These observations suggest that areas not normally involved in mediating certain types of behaviors can 'take over' those functions under the right circumstances—an example of vicarious function as we have used it here. This means that when behavioral substitution occurs, there are specific physiological mechanisms to subserve the changes. More important, we also think it means that the brain is not just functioning as it did before but without a part. Rather, there is extensive permissive reorganization of neuronal activity (and structure) underlying vicarious function. These findings also highlight the importance of applying the appropriate rehabilitation strategies at the appropriate time to enhance adaptive cortical reorganization (27, 28).

Yet such reorganization may demand a high price: the emerging patterns could prevent true restitution of function by encumbering the brain with an experience-induced reorganization that would be difficult or impossible to undo. Until the recent development of sophisticated imaging and electrophysiological techniques, it was not possible to determine whether such equipotential, vicarious, or pluripotent systems did or did not exist. Recent studies using functional magnetic resonance imaging (fMRI) and other related techniques such as positron emission tomography (PET) scanning show that functional compensation may be due to extensive reorganization of activity in the damaged brain.

For instance, after an infarct in the striatum of human patients, a number of subcortical areas both ipsilateral and contralateral to the injury site become activated as behavioral recovery progresses. The activation, measured by increases in cerebral blood flow (CBF) and glucose metabolism, is not observed when normal, healthy volunteers are asked to perform the same motor tasks. Thus, if 'tricks' are being employed to compensate for lost functions, they could be mediated by shifts in the activity of cerebral structures that are not initially involved in the behaviors (or at least not in the same way) under normal circumstances. This type of reorganization can take weeks, months, or years to occur (29).

In an earlier report typical of studies on compensation, Castro-Alamancos, Garcia Segura and Borrell (30) showed that after bilateral injury of the sensory-motor cortex in rats there is a substantial deficit in bar-pressing response to prevent aversive stimulation. If the injury is followed by direct-brain stimulation of the ventral tegmental nucleus, substantial recovery of the bar-press behavior is observed. Under these conditions if the hindlimb sensory cortex in the recovered animals is ablated, the deficit returns. It is important to note that the ablation of this area in the first place does not cause the same deficit, and this is taken as evidence of compensatory shifts in cortical function; the hindlimb area "assumes the role of another area after induced recovery from brain damage".

In another example of shifts in function thought to be compensatory, Buckner et al. (31) used PET and fMRI scanning techniques to examine the preservation of speech using a variety of linguistic and cognitive tests in a 72-year-old patient one month after a stroke in the left-inferior frontal cortex. Although the patient was impaired in speech generation tasks, he was able to access words when given partial words as cues, a task that usually depends (according to the authors) on an intact left-inferior frontal cortex. The scanning during performance showed that the right-inferior prefrontal area was activated during the tasks. "This area is not typically activated by normal subjects performing word-stem completion and appears to be used (by the patient) to compensate for his damaged cortex" (p. 1253).

One of the most interesting forms of 'spontaneous' recovery in both animals and humans is seen in the 'serial lesion' effect (see [6] for a more detailed review). In this type of injury, lesions are inflicted in stages so that, for example, the left frontal cortex may be extirpated and then a second operation takes the homologous right frontal cortex thirty days later. Under these conditions, both animals and humans show remarkable and robust post-injury sparing of function compared to counterparts with the same damage inflicted in one stage [again, see [6]]. In humans, slow-growing injuries often do not lead to either the severity or sometimes even the appearance of the functional impairments noted when the same extent of injury occurs after a stroke or acute traumatic damage (32). Although there are numerous replications of the serial lesion effect in fully mature subjects, the research has not been the focus of much attention in contemporary neuroscience. This is probably because the instances of plasticity as demonstrated by considerable sparing of function *in the absence of special training or treatment* is problematic for current theories of highly organized modular function (see 6, 33–36 for examples). Thus, in the face of bilateral removal of a structure with no loss of function, it is difficult to sustain the notion that individual aggregates of cells or structures are critical for the expression of that function. Fortunately, current literature is beginning to take another look at what such plasticity implies for concepts about the organization of function in the adult CNS.

A few years ago, Seitz and Freund (37) reviewed human studies showing that slowly progressive lesions often remain asymptomatic for years because the space-occupying tumors cause a substantial reorganization of function as measured by regional CBF (rCBF) studies. These investigators studied a group of patients with brain tumors which invaded all of the hand/arm motor cortex, and who had developed seizures but were normal on neurologic examination. The rCBF showed that during finger movements the areas of activation were substantially displaced to more lateral positions, even to cortical areas outside the motor strip. The authors concluded that "the astonishing discrepancy between the functional consequences of acute versus chronic lesions of the nervous system raises the possibility that reorganization (of function) is not restricted to within-system recovery in the motor cortex" (p. 329). This type of slowly developing reorganization can be considered as evidence for equipotentiality or vicarious function in the broad sense. The authors also point out that over time, the patients learn to use and refine other behavioral strategies often seen in normal subjects. It is thought that such patients can be given substantial skill training to recruit other cortical areas into the functional reorganization produced by the demands on the damaged CNS.

Equipotentiality and vicarious function are perhaps most easily dramatized (and contested) in cases of brain injury during postnatal development. In the 1960's, the developmental psychologist Eric Lenneberg (38) proposed that, at birth, the two cerebral hemispheres are equipotential for cognitive and language functions, and only gradually become specialized as the child matures. This idea seemed to be supported by the now classic studies of Margaret Kennard in monkeys. She showed that animals with large cortical lesions inflicted early in life showed none of the extensive deficits seen when the same type of damage was inflicted at a later age (39). Subsequently, Patricia Goldman was able to show that early

brain lesions in monkeys led to substantially more sparing of cognitive functions than when the damage was inflicted in later life. Goldman and Galkin (40) reported that lesions of the frontal cortex in a fetal rhesus monkey operated on and returned to the womb until term not only showed complete sparing of cognitive function, but also demonstrated a radical reorganization of the entire cortical mantle evidenced by numerous ectopic gyri and sulci not seen in the intact animal.

It has become increasingly clear that the twin dogmas of specific localization and complete equipotentiality need to be re-evaluated in the face of better data and experimentation. In an excellent brief review of this literature, Vargha-Khadem et al. (41) reported that better testing of children has revealed residual deficits after early hemispheric removals. They note that some of these residual deficits could have been due to medications, seizures, and nutritional and other environmental factors. When such variables are controlled, the authors observe that, as equipotentiality theory would predict, the deficits are extremely mild considering the extent of tissue loss. According to Vargha-Khadem et al., either hemisphere does appear to be able to subserve linguistic and cognitive functions during the early stages of development; however, the cost of such 'compensation' may be a generally reduced level of such functions as visuospatial behaviors, caused by 'crowding' of the supposedly lateralized functions into the one remaining hemisphere (25).

DIASCHISIS, FUNCTIONAL INHIBITION, AND RECOVERY

More sophisticated imaging and electrophysiological techniques have been employed with increasing frequency to support the idea of diaschisis proposed by von Monakow at the beginning of the last century (42). In this early concept, brain injury triggers a form of long-lasting inhibition of neural activity that von Monakow called diaschisis. The inhibition is not limited to the site of injury but can spread to distal regions by means that were not clearly understood until fairly recently. Now we know that injury-induced biochemical and genomic alterations in protein synthesis can generate actions that are many synapses removed from the initial site of damage. The changes occur not only in the affected hemisphere, but also in the 'intact' contralateral homologues (see [51] below). Von Monakow postulated that recovery of function occurred as diaschisis dissipated over time, while permanent deficits were the result of permanent diaschisis.

Although the logic may appear circular, current research shows that injury to the brain does produce chronic suppression of activity associated with behavioral impairments (43–46). Agonist drugs which increase neurotransmitter activity or block inhibitory neurotransmitters have been used to promote functional recovery after stroke in both animal (47) and human (12) subjects. However, clinical trials with these agents have had apparently limited success (48). Can behavioral therapy (e.g., the forced-use paradigm) or treatment with stimulants (e.g., amphetamine) reduce or eliminate the diaschisis caused by the injury? Do other brain areas 'take over the function' of the area of stroke? Current evidence can be cautiously interpreted to suggest that this may be the case (14). It is often reported that a stroke (experimental or naturally induced) leads to functional reorganization in brain tissue immediately adjacent to the injured area, but there are also significant changes in the contralateral homologous regions. In one study, twelve patients with acute strokes had unilateral arm weakness and some ability to move the arm after one month. Six of the patients showed good recovery and six did not. The six with good recovery showed much more activation of the cerebellar hemisphere opposite the damaged corticospinal tract than did the poorly recovered patients (49). The authors suggested that the recovery could have been due to diaschisis, or unmasking, of the functions in the contralateral cerebellum.

In a recent review, Price and colleagues (50) introduce the concept of dynamic diaschisis. They suggest that the environmental context as well as the locus of damage can play a role in determining functional outcome (36). Price et al. propose that:

> the basic idea behind dynamic diaschisis is that an otherwise viable cortical region expresses aberrant neuronal responses when those responses depend on interactions with a damaged region. This effect might arise because normal responses in any given region depend upon driving and modulatory inputs from, and reciprocal interactions with, many other regions. The regions involved will depend on the cognitive and sensorimotor operation engaged in at any particular time (p. 419).

In other words, areas of the brain that are distant from the area of injury, even including the contralateral hemisphere, can show abnormal responses when the functional demand on the damaged tissue increases.

The authors conclude that dynamic diaschisis can be measured only with whole-brain functional imaging because one has to take into consideration the functional integration of many different brain regions. More important, "pathophysiological expression depends on the functional brain state *at the time the measurements are made*" ([50] p. 426, my italics). This can be taken to mean that brain structures may move 'in and out' of a state of disaschisis, depending on the functional demands made on them at a given time in the patient's experience. It is interesting to note that, well before there was sophisticated imaging, this same point was made by the neuropsychologist Alexander Luria in 1966 (51).

NEURONAL REORGANIZATION, UNMASKING, SPARING, LATENT SYNAPSES, AND FUNCTIONAL PLASTICITY

Thanks to refinements in microelectrode recording techniques, it has now been amply demonstrated in primates that certain brain areas such as the sensory motor cortex are capable of very rapid electrophysiological reorganization in response to brain injury. Thus, within very short periods of time after lesions of the afferent pathways or even after cortical damage, tissue adjacent to the affected areas reorganizes or expands its receptive fields to capture and mediate at least some of the original physiological activities that were destroyed by the injury. There is no doubt that such rapid reorganization occurs in a number of sensory and motor areas, but as noted earlier it must be emphasized that not all the reorganization is necessarily adaptive or beneficial to the organism.

Among the first to demonstrate injury-induced plasticity in the adult nervous system were Patrick D. Wall and his colleagues in the United Kingdom (52). Wall and his group first mapped the body surface of the ventral posterior lateral nucleus of the thalamus (VPL). This was done by tactile stimulation on the surface of the arms and legs of various laboratory animals. In a normal animal, the arm takes up two-thirds of the medial VPL and the leg occupies the lateral third. When inputs to the leg area were removed by unilateral excision of the gracile nucleus, the arm area expanded to "occupy two-thirds of the area previously responding to stimulation of the leg." This change was noted within three days of the lesion. While this is an example of reorganization and cellular plasticity in response to injury, it is hardly an adaptive response to have an area that previously subserved inputs from the leg area now responding primarily to stimulation of the arm. Using other forms of temporary "deafferentation" such as blockage of nerve conduction by ice, Wall's group was able to produce instantaneous remapping of cells in the lateral nucleus gracilis (LNG). Thus, the cells in the leg, normally activated by stimulation of the paws, now responded only to stimulation of the abdomen. In this case the unmasking of latent pathways was almost instantaneous, but, again, hardly adaptive with respect to behavioral utility.

Such changes in reorganization may be very long-lasting and dependent on post-injury experience. A number of years after the Wall experiments, Pons et al. were able to show that up to eleven years after a dorsal rhizotomy in adult rhesus monkeys, the brain region responding to stimulation of the hand (area 3b) responded instead to tactile stimulation of the face (53). In human patients, similar reorganization can be seen in phantom limb phenomena in response to amputation. This too has been taken as an example of neural plasticity in the adult nervous system (54, 55). These investigators found that tactile stimulation of the face often led to referred sensations somewhere out on the phantom limb. Thus "there was a topographically organized map of the hand on the lower face region and the referred sensations were modality specific," e.g., heat, cold, vibration, rubbing, etc. were felt as these same sensations at specific points on the phantom limb. The authors noted that this modality-specific referral from the face to the limb could occur only within a few hours after amputation, implying that the reorganized 'localization' of sensations must have been due to unmasking of previously silent pathways rather than any kind of structural or morphological changes per se.

Some patients report that, after a time, the phantom limb feels as if it is paralyzed or frozen into an excruciatingly painful clench with the fingers digging deeply into the palm. The patients cannot "will" the fingers to open and relieve the pain. Ramachandran and his group developed an ingeniously simple technique to provide relief, and in doing so again demonstrated the rapid reorganization of function that can occur in the appropriate context. Investigators asked patients to put their 'normal hand' into a box with a mirror in the saggital plane of the hand. This gave a mirror-image of the normal hand, so it looked to the patients as if they had two hands opposing one another in the mirror-box. Now the investigators asked the patients to slowly open and close the normal hand while looking at the image in the mirror so it would seem as if the phantom hand was now opening and closing. The patients were surprised to find that while doing this exercise they actually felt movements in the phantom hand, but, more important, a number of the patients reported that seeing the phantom hand paradoxically unclench (because it was the normal hand they were seeing) relieved the cramping pain. This observation indicates that the amputation-induced reorganization may be undone by training and experience, with a novel engram replacing the maladaptive one.

Phantom limb effects are dramatic examples of reorganizational plasticity in the adult brain, but similar mechanisms can be seen in the visual and auditory systems when injuries are inflicted during early development. Thus Rauschecker (56, 57) has shown that if the visual (occipital) cortex is deprived of its inputs from the optic nerves, that same cortex can then be stimulated by auditory input. In other words, the 'visual' cells are 'taken over' by the auditory and somatosensory nerve fibers and thus both the auditory and somatosensory cortex could be said to expand into the territory previously controlled and occupied by visual inputs. Likewise, if the auditory cortex is destroyed or the auditory nerve is cut, the auditory cortex will be captured by visual inputs that have expanded into the deafferented zone.

Rapid reorganization tends to be more robust during early development, and this may be one reason why young subjects with brain damage recover better than older counterparts with the same injury. Rauschecker asks what the post-recovery perception of animals brain-damaged during early development is like. Do they 'see' sounds and touches as in purported synesthesias, or does the visual cortex 'change' its functions to become auditory and/or somatosensory? What are the implications for the concepts of localization of function in the CNS during development and later in life?

Investigators also have shown that reorganization and expansion of functional cortical maps can be made to occur simply by providing intensive training experience in normal animals. Further, it appears that specific kinds of sensory training may be beneficial as rehabilitation therapy in brain-damaged subjects because it directly enhances the extent of rapid reorganization and functional plasticity. Nudo and his colleagues have recently reported that injury-induced reorganization and recovery of function can occur in the adult organism (58). Such recovery often requires experience-induced modifications in synaptic and cellular systems throughout the remaining healthy brain tissue that may not necessarily be contiguous to, or immediately involved in, the affected area and its functions. In other words, functions are widely distributed and in a constant state of dynamic interaction and change, not fixed and static as they are often represented in neuroscience texts.

It is clearly time to accept the idea that dynamic reorganization of functions is an ongoing event, not just a characteristic of the damaged brain, but a process that occurs in the course of normal activity and learning. Indeed, these changes may well serve as the basis for recovery mechanisms when there is an attack on the brain. For example, in accomplished musicians and athletes, somatosensory fields are markedly expanded compared to nontrained individuals. According to Nudo et al., highly repetitive practice on a tactile task in humans leads to marked expansion of the receptive field in the motor cortex which can persist for several months after the training is terminated. Maps also expand during the initial phases of training when the procedures are unfamiliar, and then shrink once explicit knowledge of the task has become habitual. (Nudo and his colleagues provide an excellent review of the various theories to account for this plasticity and the reader is urged to consult this paper.)

There are also apparently dramatic individual differences in the location and size of cortical receptive fields in normal individuals, which, in turn, vary in their degree of modifiability according to the subject's experiential history (59, 60). At the very least, the notion that neuronal pathways can be rewired by the use of drugs or stimulation needs to be approached carefully, because the wiring diagrams for each individual may be heavily influenced by early experience and training (60). In designing rehabilitation therapy, it should be noted that certain therapies or treatments used routinely in some rehabilitation settings could result in the formation of inappropriate connections and the prevention of functional recovery, even a form of learned helplessness (61). For instance, if the current paradigm of structure-function relationships is valid, it is hard to imagine how the capture of auditory input by visual fibers would automatically lead to an adaptive outcome.

In conjunction with electrophysiological experiments in primates, computer-assisted rapid fMRI studies in humans have shown that multiple systems throughout the brain become activated during selected cognitive tasks such as naming objects or performing simple mathematical calculations. Many neuroscientists now accept the view that widely distributed neural modules are involved in even simple cognitive or sensory processing. However, there is much less agreement as to the number of modules (brain areas) required to mediate even a simple behavior like reaching for a small piece of food. For example, over a period of about ten years, the number of CNS structures in the network said to be in control of 'vision' has increased from about 12 to well over 50. A corollary of this assumption is that highly focalized damage would cause very widespread changes both serially and in parallel throughout the brain. Therefore, recovery of behavioral functions may depend upon equally widespread changes in synaptic connectivity and their metabolic consequences.

WHAT HAVE WE LEARNED FROM CONSIDERING THE CONCEPTUAL ISSUES SURROUNDING NEURAL "PLASTICITY"?

"Those who forget history are condemned to repeat it" means as much in neuroscience as it does in political and social philosophy. Theories and hypotheses now in vogue rarely acknowledge early twentieth-century literature pleading for more acceptance of a dynamic and modular view of function to replace the idea that the adult nervous system is fixed and immutable in its structure-function relationships. In particular, in the 1960s, 1970s, and 1980s, many neurobiologists, dependent on molecular and reductionistic techniques, seemed to take pleasure in deriding the ideas of Karl Lashley, who wrote in 1937 that "the function of cells may be deduced from their position and connections, but their position is not therefore a necessary consequence of their function." Lashley goes on to say that "the mere existence of specialized regions in the brain is not conclusive evidence that the specialization is necessary or important for the integrative functions" (62). Given the subsequent observations of reorganizational changes in response to brain injury that we have discussed,

Lashley's position now has a contemporary ring. Writing just two years later, Goldstein (63), a German neurologist, stressed that

> the destruction of one part of the brain never leaves unchanged the activity of the rest of the organism, especially the rest of the brain. On the contrary, there usually occurs a widespread change of the distribution of excitation. Whether a certain symptom will appear on account of a local injury, especially whether it will become a permanent symptom, certainly depends on many other factors: the nature of the disease process, the condition of the rest of the brain, the difficulty of the performance requirements and the reaction of the entire organism to the defect. The localization of a performance (after an injury) no longer means an excitation in a certain place, but a dynamic process which occurs in the entire nervous system, even in the whole organism (pp. 258–259).

Thirty years after Goldstein, Alexander Luria argued that "the facts suggest that a disturbance of a particular form of activity may arise in far more extensive lesions than was hitherto supposed. Consequently, the performance of a given function necessitates the integrity of far more extensive and far more structurally varied zones of the cortex than was assumed by classical neurology" (51). Thus, almost four decades ago, Luria was arguing for a more dynamic view of nervous system function to account for how recovery from brain injury might occur. Luria felt it would eventually be recognized that "complex forms of psychological functions are never localized in isolated areas of the brain, but are always dependent on entire working constellations of cerebral zones, appearing in the course of postnatal development and changing dynamically as a particular functional system reaches a higher level of development." He predicted that the loss of any one link must inevitably lead to a disturbance of the normal working of the functional system as a whole (p. 70).

Luria's views were essentially ignored by the cerebral cartographers, who continued to add to the complexity of their diagrams without much concern for understanding how the parts worked together in the intact and the damaged brain. It was as if drawing the lines between anatomical components was a sufficient explanatory tool. Fortunately this view, so inimical to understanding the inherent plasticity of the CNS, is now being reconsidered in some quarters, although it is still far from extinction.

It must be said that contemporary research on localization of complex functions to specific areas of the cerebral cortex marshals some of neuroscience's most elegant techniques in support of its paradigm. This often entails careful testing of complex behaviors or components of behaviors while using microelectrodes to record from specific cells in anatomically defined loci. Testing for speech generation or cognitive responses in humans often uses highly sophisticated imaging techniques. Some of the most elegant work in this domain has been performed by Goldman-Rakic and her colleagues, who have focused on defining and elaborating the role of the prefrontal cortex in spatial performance, memory and cognition. Goldman-Rakic's work investigates the hypothesis that highly discrete areas of the frontal cortex are critical in the mediation of spatial and object cognition (64–67). Monkeys show significant increases in electrophysical activity in individual neurons in circumscribed areas of the prefrontal cortex. During object recognition, one set of neurons is activated, while in a spatial cognition task other cells in a different anatomical region become more active. Both electrophysiological and metabolic recording techniques are used to demonstrate changes in activity. In Goldman-Rakic's view, "a signal advance attributable to research in non-human primates over the past decades has been the fine-grained functional mapping of the cerebral cortex and the realization that cytoarchitectonically defined areas are not homogenous with respect to circuitry or to physiology . . . . It is to be confidently expected that functional specializations will surely follow the lines of these anatomical divisions when the appropriate tests are applied." She concludes, "In view of the parcellation of these fundamental information processing domains, it is far too early to reject cortical specialization so well grounded in cytoarchitectonic, hodological and neurochemical parcellation . . . ." (64). To be sure, the rigorous and refined techniques employed and the elegance of the results make for very compelling support for the doctrine of localization, but such findings and interpretations do not allow for the plasticity and reorganization seen after injury and are difficult to explain in the context of behavioral sparing or recovery of function in the adult organism. Studies not supporting parcellation theory are often dismissed as lacking technical sophistication or as having inappropriate behavioral tests.

Moreover, where plasticity of function is acknowledged it is often limited to the idea that immediately adjacent *cortical* tissue can be reorganized to mediate behaviors. Wall and Wang refer to these notions as "corticocentric theories," because plasticity is thought to be limited primarily to cortical structures, where the most dynamic changes in maps are registered (67). In a more radical approach, these authors argue that changes in response to injury are far more ubiquitous in both subcortical and cortical substrates and include molecular, morphological, neurochemical and anatomical changes that reorganize basically the entire functioning of the organism. The authors take a position similar to that of the neurologists of the mid-twentieth century, who believed that the deficits as well as the recovery seen were the result of such total organization, rather than the result of loss of a particular part in the brain.

> In response to injury initial multilevel changes emerge surprisingly rapidly. Functional changes can appear concurrently within minutes in spinal, brainstem, thalamic and cortical substrates. With the passage of time during the subsequent days, weeks, months and longer, acute changes in normal substrates apparently continue, spread and are further supplemented by subcortical and cortical abilities to regenerate and sprout new connections (pp. 204–205).

The perspective of Wall et al. is consistent with the earlier work of Jones (68) and Nudo (58). Jones presents evidence that even very small changes in subcortical organization caused by a peripheral or CNS injury can lead to highly amplified changes in the organizational maps of the cerebral cortex. Others such as Chen et al. (69) argue that the brain is constantly being modified by experience and that 'pre-determined' wiring diagrams do not represent the kinds of rapid and long-lasting injury-induced plasticity seen in developmental and adult brain damage. The authors also note that not all types of reorganization are beneficial and that one must distinguish between those changes that lead to recovery and those plastic changes that result in permanent impairments.

Although not always given the credit they deserve, the early investigators into plasticity of function—Lashley, Goldstein, Luria—had only their clinical and observational skills to evaluate patient behavior and draw conclusions that today are based on a wide variety of sophisticated molecular and physiological techniques. Nonetheless, their conclusions resonate well with those of contemporary neuroscientists.

For example, considering his own work on phantom limb plasticity, Ramachandran (54) concluded that new findings (on reorganization after amputation) "allow us to test some of the most widely accepted assumptions of sensory psychology and neurophysiology, such as Müller's law of specific nerve energies, 'pattern coding' versus 'place coding' (i.e., the notion that perception depends exclusively on which particular neuron fires rather than the overall pattern of activity)." Furthermore, the work showing that sensations associated with phantom limbs by training "suggests that the modular, hierarchical 'bucket brigade' model of the brain popularized by computer engineers needs to be replaced by a more dynamic view of the brain in which there is a tremendous amount of back-and-forth interaction between different levels in the hierarchy and across different modules" (p. 319). Finally, with respect to motor cortex damage, Nudo et al. (58) conclude their review of the literature by stating that "both human and animal studies have demonstrated both acute and chronic changes in functional topography and anatomy of intact cortical tissue adjacent to the injury, and of more remote cortical areas, including those of the contralateral (uninjured) hemisphere" (p. 1013).

Recent findings and the revised concepts of how adaptive and maladaptive plasticity occur in the adult human brain after injury clearly demonstrate that the adult CNS is capable of much more dynamic change in function and structure than had been thought over the last few decades of research in this area.

References

1. Goldberger ME: Recovery of movement after CNS lesions in monkeys. In Stein DG, Rosen JJ, Butters N (eds): *Plasticity and Recovery of Function in the Central Nervous System.* New York, Academic Press, 1974, pp. 265–338.
2. Cajal SR: *Degeneration and Regeneration of the Nervous System.* (May RM, tr. and ed.): London, Oxford University Press, 1928.
3. Raisman G: Neural plasticity in the septal nuclei of the adult rat. *Brain Res* 14:25–48, 1969.
4. Cotman CW (ed): *Neuronal Plasticity:* New York, Raven Press, 1978.
5. Steward O: Reorganization of neuronal connections following CNS trauma: Principles and experimental paradigms. *J Neurotrauma,* 6(2): 99–143, 1989.
6. Finger S, Stein DG: *Brain Damage and Recovery.* New York, Academic Press, 1982.
7. Kandel ER, Schwartz JH, Jessell TM: *Principles of Neural Science.* New York, McGraw-Hill, 2000.
8. Squire L, Bloom F, McConnell SK, Roberts, JL, Spitzer, NC, Zigmond MJ: *Fundamental Neuroscience.* San Diego, Academic Press, 2003.
9. Finger, S: *Origins of Neuroscience,* New York, Oxford University Press, 1994.
10. Parent JM, Lownstein DH: Seizure-induced neurogenesis: are more new neurons good for an adult brain? *Prog. Brain Res.* 135:121–131, 2002.
11. Fawcett JW, Rosser AE, Dunnett SB: *Brain Damage, Brain Repair.* Oxford, Oxford University Press, 2001.
12. Goldstein G, Beers SR: *Rehabilitation.* New York, Plenum Press, 1998.
13. Levin HS, Grafman J: *Cerebral Reorganization of Function after Brain Damage,* New York, Oxford University Press, 2000.
14. Stein DG, Brailowsky S, Will B: *Brain Repair.* New York, Oxford University Press, 1995.
15. Stuss DT, Winocur G, Robertson IH: *Cognitive Neurorehabilitation.* Cambridge, UK, New York, Cambridge University Press, 1999.
16. LeVere N, Gray-Silvia S, LeVere TE: Neural stystem imbalances and the consequence of large brain injuries. In Finger S, LeVere TE, Almli CR, Stein DG (eds): *Brain Injury and Recovery: Theoretical and Controversial Issues.* New York, Plenum, 1988, pp. 15–27.
17. Kosik KS: Beyond phrenology at last. *Nature Neuroscience Reviews* 4:234–239, 2003, p. 235.
18. Jordan FM, Murdoch BE: Linguistic status following closed head injury in children: a follow-up study. *Brain Inj* 4: 147–54, 1990.
19. Anderson VA, Catropps C, Rosenfeld J, Haritou F, Morse SA: Recovery of memory function following traumatic brain injury in pre-school children. *Brain Inj* 14:679–692, 2000.
20. Finger S, LeVere TE, Almli CR, Stein DG (eds): *Brain Injury and Recovery: Theoretical and Controversial Issues.* New York, Plenum, 1988.
21. Prinz M, Hovda DA: Mapping cerebral glucose metabolism during spatial learning: interactions of development and traumatic brain injury. *J Neurotrauma* 18:31–46, 2001.
22. Trudeau N, Poulin-Dubois D, Joanette Y: Language development following brain injury in early childhood: a longitudinal case study. *Int J Lang Commun Disord* 35:227–249, 2000.
23. Kolb B, Gibb R, Gorny G: Cortical plasticity and the development of behavior after early frontal cortical injury. *Devel Neuropsychol* 18:423–444, 2000.
24. Kolb B, Cioe J: Recovery from early cortical damage in rats, VIII. Earlier may be worse: behavioural dysfunction and abnormal cerebral morphogenesis following perinatal frontal cortical lesions in the rat. *Neuropharm* 39:756–764, 2000.
25. Slavin MD, Laurence S, Stein DG: Another look at vicariation. In Finger S, LeVere TE, Almli CR, Stein DG (eds): *Brain Injury and Recovery: Theoretical and Controversial Issues.* New York, Plenum, 1988, pp. 165–78.
26. Xerri C, Merzenich MM, Peterson BE, Jenkins W: Plasticity of primary somatosensory cortex paralleling sensorimotor skill recovery from stroke in adult monkeys. *J Neurophysiol* 79(4):2119–48, 1998.
27. Beaulieu CL: Rehabilitation and outcome following pediatric traumatic brain injury *Surg Clin North Am,* 82, 393–408, 2002.
28. Kolb B, Gibb, R, Gonzalez CL: Cortical injury and neuroplasticity during development. In Shaw C, McEachern JC (eds): *Toward a Theory of Neuroplasticity.* Philadelphia, Taylor & Francis, 2001, pp. 2223–2243.
29. York GK, Steinberg DA: Hughlings Jackson's theory of recovery. *Neurology* 45(4):834–8, 1995.
30. Castro-Alamancos MA, Garcia-Segura LM, Borrell J: Transfer of function to a specific area of the cortex after induced recovery from brain damage. *Eur J Neurosci* 4:853–863, 1992.
31. Buckner RL, Corbetta M, Schatz J, Raichle ME: Preserved speech abilities and compensation following prefrontal damage. *Proc Natl Acad Sci USA* 93:1249–1253, 1996.
32. Stein DG, Finger S, Hart T: Brain damage and recovery: problems and perspectives. *Behav Neural Biol* 37(2):185–222, 1983.
33. Stein DG: Some variables influencing recovery of function after central nervous system lesions in the rat. In Stein DG, Rosen JJ, Butters N (eds): *Plasticity and Recovery of Function in the Central Nervous System.* New York, Academic Press, 1974, pp. 265–338.
34. Star SL: *Regions of the Mind: Brain Research and the Quest for Scientific Certainty.* Stanford, California, Stanford UP, 1989.
35. Stein DG, Lewis ME, Functional recovery after brain damage. In Vital-Durand F and Jeannerod, M (eds): *Aspects of Neural Plasticity.* Paris, Institut national de la santé et de la recherche médicale, 1975, pp. 203–228.
36. Stein DG: In pursuit of new strategies for understanding recovery from brain damage: problems and perspectives. In Boll T and Bryant B (eds): *Clinical Neuropsychology and Brain Function: Research, Measurement, and Practice.* Washington DC, American Psychological Association, 1988, pp. 9–55.
37. Seitz RJ, Freund HJ: Plasticity of the human motor cortex: *Adv Neurol* 73:321–33, 1997.
38. Lenneberg EH: *Biological Foundations of Language.* New York, Wiley, 1967.
39. Kennard MA: Cortical reorganization of motor function. Studies on series of monkeys of various ages from infancy to maturity. *Archives of Neurology and Psychiatry* 148:227–40, 1942.
40. Goldman PS, Galkin TW: Prenatal removal of frontal association cortex in the fetal rhesus monkey: anatomical and functional consequences in postnatal life. *Brain Res* 152(3):451–85, 1978.
41. Vargha-Khadem F, Isaacs E, Muter V: A review of cognitive outcome after unilateral lesions sustained during childhood. *J Child Neurol* 9 Suppl 2:67–73, 1994.
42. Monakow Cv: *Die lokalisation im grosshirn und der abbau der funktion durch kortikale herde.* Wiesbaden, J.F. Bergmann, 1914.
43. Hausen HS, Lachmann EA, Nagler W: Cerebral diaschisis following cerebellar hemorrhage. *Arch Phys Med Rehabil* 78(5): 546–9, 1997.
44. Imahori Y, Fujii R, Kondo M, Ohmori Y, Nakajima K: Neural features of recovery from CNS injury revealed by PET in human brain. *Neuroreport* 10(1):117–21, 1999.
45. Laatsch L, Jobe T, Sychra J, Lin Q, Blend M: Impact of cognitive rehabilitation therapy on neuropsychological impairments as measured by brain perfusion SPECT: a longitudinal study. *Brain Inj* 11(12):851–63, 1997.
46. Rosen HJ, Petersen SE, Linenweber MR, Snyder AZ, White DA, Chapman L, et al.: Neural correlates of recovery from aphasia after damage to left inferior frontal cortex. *Neurology* 55(12):1883–94, 2000.

47. Feeney DM, Sutton RL: Pharmacotherapy for recovery of function after brain injury. *Crit Rev Neurobiol* 3(2):135–97, 1987.

48. Gladstone DJ, Black SE: Enhancing recovery after stroke with noradrenergic pharmacotherapy: a new frontier? *Can J Neurol Sci* 27(2):97–105, 2000.

49. Small SL, Hlustik P, Noll DC, Genovese C, Solodkin A: Cerebellar hemispheric activation ipsilateral to the paretic hand correlates with functional recovery after stroke. *Brain* 125(Pt 7):1544–57, 2002.

50. Price CJ, Warburton EA, Moore CJ, Frackowiak RS, Friston KJ: Dynamic diaschisis: anatomically remote and context-sensitive human brain lesions. *J Cogn Neurosci* 3(4):419–29, 2001.

51. Luria AR: *Higher Cortical Functions in Man.* New York, Basic Books, 1966, p. 13.

52. Merrill EG, Wall PD. Plasticity of connection in the adult nervous system. In Cotman CW (ed): *Neuronal Plasticity.* New York, Raven Press, 1978, pp. 97–111.

53. Pons TP, Garraghty PE, Ommaya AK, Kaas JH, Taub E, Mishkin M: Massive cortical reorganization after sensory deafferentation in adult macaques. *Science* 252(5014):1857–60, 1991.

54. Ramachandran VS, Blakeslee S: *Phantoms in the Brain: Probing the Mysteries of the Human Mind.* New York, William Morrow, 1998.

55. Ramachandran VS, Rogers-Ramachandran D: Phantom limbs and neural plasticity. *Arch Neurol* 57(3):317–20, 2000.

56. Rauschecker, JP: Compensatory plasticity and sensory substitution in the cerebral cortex. *Trends Neurosci* 18(1):317–20, 1995, 36–43.

57. Rauschecker, JP: Mechanisms of compensatory plasticity in the cerebral cortex. In Freund HJ, Sabel BA, Witte OW (eds): *Advances in Neurology.* Philadelphia, Lippincott-Raven, 1997, pp. 137–46.

58. Nudo RJ, Plautz EJ, Frost SB: Role of adaptive plasticity in recovery of function after damage to motor cortex. *Muscle Nerve* 24(8):1000–19, 2001.

59. Jenkins WM, Merzenich MM: Reorganization of neocortical representations after brain injury: a neurophysiological model of the bases of recovery from stroke. *Prog Brain* Res 71:249–66, 1987.

60. Merzenich M, Wright B, Jenkins W, Xerri C, Byl N, Miller S, et al.: Cortical plasticity underlying perceptual, motor, and cognitive skill development: implications for neurorehabilitation. *Cold Spring Harbor Symp Quant Biol* 61:1–8, 1996.

61. Wolf SL, Blanton S, Baer H, Breshears J, Butler AJ: Repetitive task practice: a critical review of constraint-induced movement therapy in stroke. *Neurolog* 8(6):325–38, 2002.

62. Lashley K: Functional determinants of cerebral localization. *Arch of Neurol and Psychia* 38:371–87, 1937.

63. Goldstein K: *The Organism, a Holistic Approach to Biology Derived from Pathological Data in Man.* New York, American Book Company, 1939.

64. Goldman-Rakic PS: Localization of function all over again. *Neuroimage* 11:451–457, 2000, p. 454.

65. Levy R, Goldman-Rakic PS: Segregation of working memory functions within the dorsolateral prefrontal cortex. *Exp. Brain Res* 133:23–32, 2000.

66. Adcock RA, Constable RT, Gore JC, Goldman-Rakic PS: Functional neuroanatomy of executive processes involved in dual-task performance. *Proc Natl Acad Sci (USA)* 97:3567–3572, 2000.

67. Wall JT, Xu J, Wang X: Human brain plasticity: an emerging view of the multiple substrates and mechanisms that cause cortical changes and related sensory dysfunctions of the sensory inputs from the body, *Brain Res. Rev.* 39:181–215, 2002, p. 182.

68. Jones EG: Cortical and subcortical contributions to activity-dependent plasticity in primate somatosensory cortex. *Ann Rev Neurosci* 23:1–37, 2000.

69. Chen R, Cohen LG, Hallett M: Nervous system reorganization following injury. *Neurosci* 111(4):761–73, 2002.

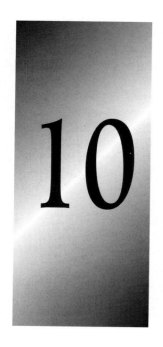

10 Advances in Innovative Therapies to Enhance Neural Recovery

C. Edward Dixon
Anthony E. Kline

This chapter reviews experimental neuroprotective agents, which are strictly defined as such if they have been reported to reduce morphological and/or functional deficits after traumatic brain injury (TBI). The categories below are not necessarily mutually exclusive. The pathways to cell dysfunction and death are not necessarily linear, but involve an intertwined network. The discussion also focuses on exogenous treatments rather then genetically induced manipulations (i.e., transgenic modification). Lastly, there will be no distinctions made between the various contemporary TBI models (1), although it is possible that the neuroprotective effects of some treatments may be model dependent.

EXCITOXICITY

Excitotoxicity is an important mechanism in secondary neuronal injury following TBI. Glutamate, aspartate, and glycine are amongst the most abundant excitatory neurotransmitters and the most commonly implicated in excitotoxic injury. Glutamate, the most prominent of these amino acids, activates receptors that are classified according to specific agonists. Receptors that modulate ionic channels are divided into those stimulated by N-methyl-D-aspartate (NMDA receptors) or those stimulated by α-amino-3-hydroxy-5-methylisoazole-4-proprionic acid (AMPA) or kainic acid (together referred to as non-NMDA receptors). Glutamate also acts at metabotropic receptors that act via second messenger systems (2). Excitotoxicity resulting from the TBI-induced release of excitatory amino acids and the damaging effects of increased intracellular calcium associated with glutamate receptor activation has been the target of intense investigation for over a decade.

Inhibiting Release of Excitoxins

Inhibiting glutamate release has been demonstrated to attenuate functional and morphological deficits after experimental TBI. Sun and Faden (3) reported that early treatment with 619C89, a sodium channel blocker that inhibits glutamate release, attenuates behavioral deficits and hippocampal neuronal loss. Riluzole (2-amino-6-trifluoromethoxy benzothiazole) has properties that include inhibition of glutamate release and has also been reported to attenuate functional (4) and morphological damage (5) after TBI. Treatment with galanin, a neuropeptide that inhibits neurotransmitter release by opening potassium channels and closing N-type calcium channels, attenuates motor, but not Morris water maze (MWM) deficits after TBI (6). However, blocking post-injury ion fluxes with tetrodotoxin was not found to be protective against behavioral deficits (7).

Blocking Receptor Activation

As summarized below, treatment with NMDA and non-NMDA receptor blockers has led to improved functional recovery and reduced hippocampal cell death and cortical damage after experimental TBI. NMDA-receptor blockade has been shown in several models of TBI to attenuate neurological deficits. Hayes et al. (8) reported behavioral protection by the noncompetitive NMDA antagonist phencyclidine after TBI. Studies by Faden et al. (9) found behavioral protection by dextromethorphan, a noncompetitive NMDA antagonist and 3-(2-carboxypiperazin-4-yl)propyl-l-phosphonic acid (CPP), a competitive NMDA antagonist. The NMDA-antagonist, MK-801, has been reported in numerous studies to be neuroprotective (10–13). Cortical and hippocampal damage is attenuated by both pretreatment with the NMDA antagonist CPP and the non-NMDA antagonist NBQX (14). Additionally, delayed treatment with NBQX, but not CPP, beginning 1 and 7 hr after TBI prevented hippocampal damage.

Remacemide hydrochloride, an NMDA receptor-associated ionophore blocker, has been reported to reduce post-traumatic cortical lesion volume, but not to improve MWM function (15). Gacyclidine, a noncompetitive NMDA receptor antagonist has been shown to attenuate neuronal death and deficits in MWM performance following frontal cortex contusion (16). Treatment with kynurenate, an NMDA and non-NMDA antagonist, has been reported to attenuate hippocampal CA_3 neuronal loss after TBI (17). Animals treated with HU-211, a synthetic, nonpsychotropic cannabinoid that acts as a noncompetitive NMDA receptor antagonist has been reported to enhance motor function recovery after TBI (18). The NMDA antagonist ketamine has been demonstrated to attenuate post-injury neurological (19) and cognitive deficits (20). Treatment with CP-98,113, an NMDA receptor blocker, has been shown to attenuate neurologic motor function and cognitive performance assessed in a MWM task (21). Increasing inhibitory function through stimulation of γ-aminobutyric acid (GABA(A)) receptors via bicuculline administration has been reported to attenuate MWM deficits after TBI (22).

In addition to playing an essential role in normal cell function, magnesium also has an antagonist effect on the NMDA receptor by blocking the NMDA receptor ion channel. The effects of magnesium after experimental TBI are presented in the "neutraceuticals" section of this chapter.

Many noncompetitive NMDA receptor antagonists have undesirable side effects. NPS 1506 is a noncompetitive NMDA receptor antagonist that appears less toxic than earlier agents (23). NPS 1506 has been reported to attenuate MWM performance and hippocampal CA_3 cell death, but not cortical lesion (23).

TBI-induced glutamate release can also damage tissue by activating metabotropic glutamate receptors (mGLuR), which are coupled to second messenger cascades through G-proteins. Modulation of mGLuRs has been shown to confer neuroprotection. Gong et al. (24) reported that intraventricular administration of α-methyl-4-carboxyphenylglycine (MCPG), a mGLuR antagonist, prior to TBI attenuated motor and MWM deficits. Administration of 2-methyl-6-(phenylethynyl)-pyridine (MTEP), a mGLuR5 antagonist, has been reported to reduce lesion volume and to attenuate motor and MWM deficits following TBI (25). Administration of a group II mGLuR agonist 30 min after TBI can improve behavioral recovery (26). Selective mGLuR1 antagonists have also been reported to attenuate motor deficits and MRI-assessed lesion volume (27). The compound ZJ-43, which inhibits Nacetylaspartylglutamate through selective activation of presynaptic Group II mGLuR3, has been recently shown to attenuate neuronal and glial degeneration after TBI (28).

Calcium Channel Blockers

Calcium channel blockers to reduce excessive accumulation of intracellular calcium have been examined as possible neuroprotective agents for TBI. Post-injury administration of the voltage-sensitive calcium channel blocker Ziconotide (also SNX-111 and CI-1009) has been reported to attenuate motor and cognitive deficits (29). Similarly, post-injury treatment of LOE 908, a broad-spectrum inhibitor of voltage-operated cation channels and store-operated cation channels has been demonstrated to reduce neuromotor and visuospatial memory deficits (30). Recently, treatment with the specific N-type voltage-gated calcium channel blocker SNX-185 has been shown to attenuate functional deficits and enhance neuronal survival after TBI (31). Pharmacologically blocking calcium entry has been another important strategy to reduce post-injury excitotoxicity. Treatment with (S)-emopamil, a calcium channel blocker, has been reported to attenuate post-injury motor deficits (32). Inhibiting polyamine-dependent calcium influx is another therapeutic target for attenuating post-injury excitotoxicity. Ifenprodil, a polyamine-site NMDA receptor antagonist, has been reported to reduce cortical morphology after TBI (33).

OXIDATIVE INJURY

Oxidative stress has been implicated in the pathology of TBI. Several agents with antioxidant properties have been evaluated in animal models of TBI. Hall and colleagues (34) reported that administration of a non-glucocorticoid 21-aminosteroid U74006F (tirilazad) enhanced neurological recovery in mice. Tirilazad has also been reported to attenuate axonal injury following TBI (35). Clifton et al. (36) reported that pretreatment and acute posttreatment with α-tocopherol succinate plus polyethylene glycol attenuated motor deficits following TBI. Analogues of α-tocopherol have also been reported to be neuroprotective in mice following TBI (37). Lidocaine, a local anesthetic, has been found to be a potent scavenger of hydroxyl radicals (38). Administration of lidocaine has been reported to attenuate postinjury neurological and motor function, but not cognitive function (39). Deferoxamine is an iron-chelating agent that can inhibit the iron-dependent hydroxyl radical production, and has been reported to improve spatial memory performance following TBI (40). Interestingly, deferoxamine was found not to improve functional outcome when combined with moderate hypothermia treatment (41). Superoxide dismutase (SOD) is a metalloenzyme, which catalyzes the dismutation of superoxide ion into oxygen and hydrogen peroxide. Administration of polyethylene glycol-conjugated SOD has been reported to reduce motor, but not MWM deficits following TBI (42). OPC-14117, is a superoxide scavenger that has been reported to attenuate tissue damage (43) and behavioral deficits (44,45) following TBI. Early treatment with LY341122, an inhibitor of lipid peroxidation and an antioxidant, has been reported to provide significant histopathological protection (46). Penicillamine is a scavenging compound that has been reported to improve motor performance in mice after TBI (47). The pineal hormone melatonin is a scavenger of free radicals has been found to reduce contusion volume following cortical impact in rats (48). Endothelin-1, a 21 amino acid peptide, has been closely linked to oxidative stress after TBI (49). The endothelin receptor subtype A antagonist, Ro 61-1790 has been show to attenuate Purkinje cell loss in the cerebellum after TBI. Kline and colleagues have recently shown that acute administration of the dopamine D2 receptor agonist bromocriptine, which exhibits significant antioxidant properties, reduced TBI-induced lipid peroxidation (i.e., oxidative stress) and enhanced spatial learning in a MWM task and increased hippocampal CA3 neuron survival after controlled cortical impact injury (50).

EXOGENOUS GROWTH FACTORS

Exogenous administration of several growth factors has been reported to produce beneficial effects on both cognitive performance and histological outcome measures after TBI. Sinson and colleagues have shown that nerve growth factor (NGF) attenuates cognitive dysfunction following fluid percussion brain injury (51). The same group has also reported an attenuation of cognitive deficits and cholinergic cell loss after fluid percussion injury and NGF infusion (52). Dixon et al. (53) have reported that intraventricular NGF infusion reverses the post-traumatic reduction in scopolamine-evoked ACh release, and significantly improves spatial memory retention following controlled cortical impact injury. Increasing NGF protein levels by intraventricular injections of liposome/NGF cDNA complexes similarly attenuates the loss of cholinergic neuronal immunostaining in the rat septum after TBI (54).

Utilizing the fluid percussion injury device, Frank and Ragel (55) demonstrated via histochemical quantification that at 48 hr after injury there is a significant difference in FGF-2-positive cells between the injured and contralateral cortex. Dietrich et al. (56) administered fibroblast growth factor-2 (FGF-2) intravenously for 3 hr beginning 30 min after fluid percussion injury and found a 50 percent decrease in the total number of necrotic neurons compared to controls. Furthermore, the overall contusion lesion volume was decreased by almost a third. Employing the same injury model, McDermott and colleagues (57) reported that post-injury FGF-2 treatment significantly attenuated post-traumatic memory dysfunction relative to vehicle-treated controls. However, no attenuation in histological damage was observed. In contrast to the beneficial effects reported by Dietrich et al. (56) and McDermott et al. (57) with FGF-2 treatment after fluid percussion injury, Guluma and colleagues failed to see a neurological improvement at 7 days after an injury of moderate severity in a similar same model (58). Using the controlled cortical impact injury model in rats, Yan and colleagues have shown that FGF-2 administration moderately improves MWM performance compared to controls, but has no effect on histological outcome (59). Recently, Yoshimura and colleagues reported that overexpression of FGF-2 increases neurogenesis in the adult mouse hippocampus after cortical impact injury and that neurogenesis is reduced in FGF-2 deficient mice (60). The authors conclude that supplementation of FGF-2 may be effective in treating TBI by simultaneously enhancing neurogenesis and reducing neurodegeneration.

Insulin-like growth factor 1 (IGF-1) is a mitogenic polypeptide structurally similar to insulin that is involved in repair and regeneration following injury to the brain. IGF-1 has been shown to be upregulated following cerebral cortical contusion via a weight drop injury model (61). A follow-up study found that the upregulation of IGF-1 mRNA levels can be blocked by NMDA receptor antagonists (62). Exogenous administration of IGF-1 has been demonstrated to improve neurological and cognitive outcome after fluid percussion brain injury in rats (63). IGF-1 has recently been evaluated in a unilateral penetration brain injury model. IGF-1 administration resulted in a significant decrease in Hsp70 and TUNEL positive cells in the peritrauma region. The neuroprotective effects of IGF-1 treatment were not limited to the cellular level, but also on behavioral outcome. Specifically, IGF-1 treated animals lost less postoperative weight and survived the trauma longer than controls (64).

HYPOTHERMIA

During the past decade, several experimental studies have provided evidence that mild to moderate hypothermia can provide behavioral protection following TBI. Studies employing multiple models have reported that moderate hypothermia can reduce neurological deficits (65–69) and improve cognitive function (59,65,67,69). Reports of histological protection by moderate hypothermia have been less consistent. Some investigators have reported reductions in contusion volume (70,71) decreased cortical necrotic neurons (70), reductions in axonal injury (72), and reduced ventricular enlargement (73). However, in a rat model of severe TBI with secondary insult, moderate hypothermia for 4 hr post-injury failed to improve motor function, cognitive function, lesion volume, or hippocampal neuronal survival (74). Furthermore, moderate hypothermia was found to be detrimental in fentanyl-anesthetized rats (75). Factors such as treatment window, injury severity, anesthesia, and rates of re-warming need to be further defined to optimize hypothermia treatment. (See Figure 10-1.)

PROTEASE INHIBITORS

Both intracellular proteases (e.g., calpains and caspases) and extracellular proteases (plasminogen activator and matrix metalloproteinase) are believed to contribute to the pathophysiology of neuronal cell death (76). Treatments that target these processes have been evaluated in experimental TBI. Post-injury uncontrolled activation of calpain, a calcium-dependent neutral protease, can destroy neurons. Calpain inhibitors have been the most researched target for TBI treatment. (Caspase inhibitors are reviewed below.) Saatman et al. (77) reported that treatment with the calpain inhibitorAK245 attenuated motor and cognitive deficits following TBI. A follow-up study found that AK245 did not attenuate cell death (78). Treatment with calpain inhibitor 2 has been demonstrated to reduce cortical loss following TBI (79). Administration of the calpain inhibitor SJA6017 has been found to inhibit functional deficits 24-hr postinjury (80). Treatment with the nonimmunosuppressive neuroimmunophilin (NIMM) ligand V-10,367 has been found to reduce calpain-mediated cytoskeletal damage (81). It has been recently

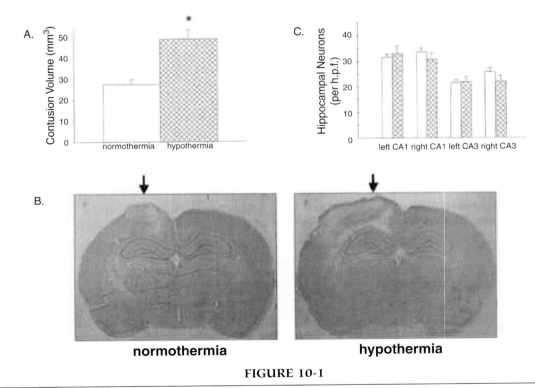

FIGURE 10-1

Histologic assessment performed 72 hr after traumatic brain injury in rats (*n* = 8 per group) treated with normothermia vs. hypothermia. *A,* surprisingly, contusion volume was markedly larger in hypothermic rats (*$p < 0.05$). *B,* representative coronal brain sections. The site of impact is marked by arrows. Contusion volume, demarcated by swollen, hypochromic cells, was nearly doubled in hypothermic rats. The hippocampus appeared largely unaffected in both experimental groups. *C,* hippocampal neuronal survival did not differ between experimental groups. Controlled cortical impact was delivered to the cortex overlying the left dorsal hippocampus. [From Statler et al., *Crit Care Med*, 2003; 31(4):1134–1139 (Ref. 75).]

demonstrated that preinjury administration of the calpain inhibitor MDL-28170 significantly reduced immunomarker of axonal injury after TBI (82).

INFLAMMATION

TBI can initiate a number of inflammatory processes that may contribute to secondary tissue damage. For instance, TBI can produce polymorphonuclear leukocyte migration into the brain that can result in neuronal damage. P-selectin blockade has been reported to reduce probe trial performance on a MWM task following TBI (83). Knoblach and Faden (84) demonstrated that anti-intracellular adhesion molecule-1 (ICAM-1) can attenuate motor deficits and neutrophil invasion after TBI. Systemic administration of a high, but not a low dose of interleukin-1 receptor antagonist has been reported to attenuate neurological recovery after TBI (85). The same study observed that motor function was impaired by the high dose of interleukin-1 receptor antagonist (85). Further work by Knoblach and Faden (86) failed to find a beneficial effect of selective IL-1 antagonists and suggested that the post-traumatic increases in IL-1-beta may not contribute to subsequent neurological impairment. Administration of anti-CD11B, a monoclonal antibody directed against the leukocyte adhesion molecules CD11B, reduced neurophil influx after TBI, but did not improve function (87). Nitric oxide (NO) derived from the inducible isoform of NO synthase (iNOS) is an inflammatory product implicated both in secondary damage and in recovery from brain injury. Sinz et al. (88) reported that rats treated with iNOS inhibitors aminoguanidine and L-N-iminothyl-lysine exacerbated functional outcome and histological damage thereby suggesting a beneficial role for iNOS in TBI. In contrast, Lu et al. (89) found that aminoguanidine treatment improved neurobehavioral outcome. Acute administration of a selective iNOS inhibitor, 1400W, has been shown to reduce lesion volume after lateral fluid percussion injury (90). Treatment with interleukin-10 has been reported to enhance neurological recovery following fluid percussion brain injury (91). However, the administration of interleukin-10 thirty min after experimental TBI via a controlled cortical impact was ineffective in attenuating functional and histopathological deficits with a dose that prevents neurotrophil accumulation in injured tissue (92). Cyclooxygenases (COX) play an important role in inflammatory cascades and increased expression of COX after experimental TBI has been well documented (93–96). Cernak et al. (95) found that chronic administration of the COX-2 inhibitor nimesulide improves cognitive function after TBI. Pre- and post-injury treatment with DFU has been shown to attenuate functional deficits and neuronal cell death after controlled cortical impact (97). At present, anti-inflammatory treatments remain a viable strategy.

ETHANOL

The neuroprotecive effects of ethanol have been disputed for years. Yamakami et al. (98) demonstrated that following severe brain injury, animals pretreated with high-dose ethanol showed significantly worsened neurological deficits at 24 hr postinjury. Shapira et al. (99) reported that acute, but not chronic, ethanol exposure increased neurological deficit and hemorrhagic necrosis volume in rats following TBI. Janis et al. (100) reported that low dose acute ethanol treatment could reduce MWM performance deficits. A low-dose of ethanol has been found to be associated with a marked attenuation of immediate post-injury hyperglycolysis and with more normal glucose metabolism in the injury penumbra over the ensuing 3 days post-injury (101). It was further observed that the reduction in CBF typically seen within the contusion core and penumbra after TBI is less severe when ethanol is present. In contrast, in a model of multiple episodes of mild TBI, acute ethanol intoxication acute ethanol treatment was not neuroprotective in rats (102). Acute pre-injury administration of ethanol has been shown to attenuate the cytokine response to injury (103). Recently, a treatment consisting of a low amount of ethanol combined with caffeine (caffeinol), has been found to be neuroprotective (104). If there is a beneficial effect of ethanol, the conditions by which it can be neuroprotective remain to be clarified.

HORMONAL AND GENDER INFLUENCES

It has been postulated in animal studies that the effects of female hormones may play a positive role in outcome from brain injury. Roof et al. (105) found that the presence of circulating endogenous or synthetic progesterone had a neuroprotective effect on the reduction of cerebral edema in female rats compared to males. However, in a temporal response study, Galani et al. (106) found that a 4 mg/kg dose of progesterone was more effective in reducing edema after medial frontal cortex contusions when given for 5 consecutive days versus 3 days. The authors speculate that the longer duration of progesterone treatment was more effective because there are two phases of edema—one that begins within hr after trauma and another that begins several days later (106). Apparently, the longer treatment was able to effectively attenuate the later phase of edema. In a similar study from the same group, 5 days of progesterone treatment was shown to protect against necrotic damage and behavioral abnormalities (107). Progesterone has also been reported to confer protection against lipid peroxidation and to facilitate cognitive recovery and reduce secondary neuronal loss after cortical contusion in male rats (105,108). It has recently been reported that allopregnanolone

(4,8, or 16 mg/kg), which is a metabolite of progesterone, and progesterone (16 mg/kg) administered at 1 and 6 hr after controlled cortical impact to the pre-frontal cortex and every day thereafter for 5 days resulted in less cell loss in the medio-dorsal nucleus of the thalamus and less learning and memory deficits compared with the vehicle-treated controls (109).

Animal studies also show that estrogen treatment immediately after TBI has a protective effect in males, but increases mortality and exacerbates outcome in females when assessing neurologic motor function one week after injury (110). Other studies (111,112) show a protective role of estrogen in maintaining cerebral blood flow, mortality, and cell death after experimental TBI. A recent study by Wagner et al. examined the effects of pre-injury hormonal status and gender on neurobehavioral and cognitive performance after controlled cortical impact injury. The results showed that females performed significantly better than males on motor performance measures, but were not significantly different on cognitive outcome as assessed in the MWM. Furthermore, there were no differences in performance between pro-estrous and non-proestrous females, suggesting that neither estrous cycle stage nor hormone level at the time of TBI have significant effects on behavioral recovery (113). These findings are supported by the results of a study in which nonovariectomized rats were subjected to a right parasagittal fluid percussion brain injury during either proestrous or nonproestrous and compared to ovariectomized female and male rats. Rats were sacrificed three days after TBI to assess neuropathology. The results showed that both the proestrous and nonproestrous rats had significantly smaller cortical lesions relative to males. In contrast, the ovarictomized females had contusion volumes that were significantly larger than both the proestrous and nonproestrous intact rats (114). Taken together, these data provide evidence that endogenous circulating hormones confer histopathological and behavioral protection after TBI.

MITOCHONDRIA

Sequestration of calcium loads within the mitochondrial matrix can open the mitochondrial permeability transition pore leading to cellular oxidative and metabolic stress. Acute treatment with cyclosporin A (CsA), an inhibitor of calcium-induced mitochondrial permeability transition pore, has been reported to reduce tissue damage following TBI in rats (115–117). CsA has also been found to enhance cognitive function after TBI (118). A single dose of CsA has also been reported to blunt axonal damage following TBI (119). Continuous infusion of CsA after TBI has be found to be reduce cortical damage (117). Improved mitochondrial function and

behavioral outcome has been achieved by treatment with ziconitide, a calcium channel blocker (120,121).

CATECHOLAMINE AGONISTS

The role that catecholamines play in promoting functional recovery after TBI is well documented (122–127). Feeney and colleagues have shown that a single dose of d-amphetamine administered 24 hr after a sensorimotor cortex injury produces an immediate and enduring acceleration in beam walking recovery in rats (122) and that multiple doses of amphetamine restore binocular depth perception in cats with bilateral visual cortex ablation (128). Beneficial effects of other catecholamine agonists on functional outcome in rat and/or cat following either weight drop cortical contusion or cortical aspirations have also been reported (129). Because the administration of norepinephrine antagonists block or reinstate deficits, the noradrenergic system has been implicated in the aforementioned studies. However, as suggested by the following reports, the dopaminergic system is also involved in the rehabilitative process.

The psychostimulant methylphenidate has been reported to have pharmacological properties similar to amphetamine, but without the undesirable sympathomimetic effect. A single administration followed by significant symptom relevant experience (i.e., beam walking experience) enhances recovery of motor function following sensorimotor cortex lesions (126). Moreover, daily methylphenidate treatments beginning as late as 24 hr after TBI in rats reveal significantly less spatial memory performance deficits versus saline treatment (127). Recently, the effect of daily administrations of amantadine beginning one day post-injury and continuing for 20 days was examined. Rats treated with amantadine had significantly less spatial memory performance deficits than their saline-treated counterparts (130). Biochemical studies have demonstrated that amantadine increases release of DA into extracellular pools by blocking reuptake and by facilitating the synthesis of DA (131–134). In addition to acting pre-synaptically, amantadine has been demonstrated to act post-synaptically to increase the density of post-synaptic DA receptors (134) or to alter their conformation (135). Evidence of a post-synaptic mechanism is clinically promising since the mechanisms of actions may not depend solely on the presence of surviving post-synaptic terminals. Because the mechanism of action of amantadine differs from other DA releasing drugs (see 136 for review), it is likely that the dopaminergic effects of amantadine are a combination of pre-synaptic and post-synaptic effects.

Rats receiving delayed and chronic pharmacological treatment with the dopamine D_2 receptor agonist bromocriptine exhibited both enhanced working memory

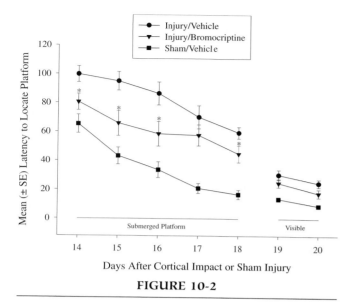

FIGURE 10-2

Mean (± SE) latency (sec) to locate a submerged platform in a spatial learning acquisition paradigm. *$P < 0.05$ vs. injury/vehicle. [From Kline et al., *J Neurotrauma* 2002; 19:415–425 (Ref. 50).]

and spatial acquisition in a MWM. Specifically, both injured groups exhibited significant impairments initially, but in marked contrast to the performance of the vehicle-treated group, the bromocriptine-treated animals required significantly less time to locate the platform (50). The dose of 5 mg/kg bromocriptine has been shown via microdialysis to increase extracellular DA levels in rats (137), suggesting that enhanced DA neurotransmission mediated the beneficial effects. However, as indicated in the "oxidative injury" section, the same dose of bromocriptine has also been reported to attenuate lipid peroxidation, suggesting that bromocriptine's antioxidant properties may also contribute to its therapeutic effects (50). (See Figure 10-2.)

The administration of selegiline (L-deprenyl) once daily for seven days beginning 24 hr after fluid percussion injury has been reported to improve cognitive function in the MWM and enhance neuroplasticity (138). L-deprenyl is used to enhance the action of DA by inhibiting its main catabolic enzyme in the brain, monoamine oxidase-B. Clinical studies also exist attesting to the benefits of DA augmentation following TBI (139,140).

These positive finding with delayed treatment suggests that strategies that enhance catecholamine neurotransmission during the chronic post-injury phase may be a useful adjunct in ameliorating some of the neurobehavioral sequelae following TBI in humans.

SEROTONIN AND TBI

Investigations regarding the role of serotonergic (5-HT) responses after TBI have not been as prolific as with other neurotransmitter systems. Utilizing a fluid percussion rat brain injury model, Busto et al. (141) reported that 5-HT levels increased from 18.85 ± 7.12 to 65.78 ± 11.36 pm/ml (mean ± SD) in the first 10 min after injury. The levels of 5-HT remained significantly higher than controls for the first 90-min sampling period. In parallel to the rise in 5-HT levels a significant 71 percent decrease in extracellular 5-HIAA levels was noted in the first 10 min after injury. These findings suggest that there is a rapid rise in extracellular 5-HT levels in cortical regions proximal to the injury site. Because 5-HT potentiation of excitatory amino acids has been reported in cat neocortex (142), the trauma-induced release of 5-HT might negatively impact recovery by promoting excitotoxic processes.

Serotonergic pathways originating in the raphe nuclei have extensive projections to brain areas involved in cognitive processing, and 5-HT receptor agonists and antagonists alter these processes (143,144). Of all the 5-HT receptors (5-HT R) characterized thus far ($5\text{-HT}_1 - 5\text{-HT}_7$), the 5-HT_{1A} is the most widely studied. 5-HT_{1A}Rs are abundantly expressed in brain regions, such as the cortex and hippocampus, that play key roles in learning and memory and that are susceptible to neuronal damage induced by brain injury (145,146). Numerous studies have reported on the effects of 5-HT_{1A}R agonists after focal or global cerebral ischemia in both rats and mice (145–150). These studies have focused on either pre or post-injury administration of various 5-HT_{1A}R agonists and their potential neuroprotective effects. What is generally found is that 5-HT_{1A}R agonism decreases histopathology after ischemic injury.

The investigation of 5-HT_{1A}R agonists on neurobehavioral and cognitive recovery after TBI produced by a well-established controlled cortical impact injury model, which produces deficits resembling those seen clinically, has only recently begun. Kline and colleagues have shown that a 4-hr continuous infusion of Repinotan HCL (BAY × 3702; 10 μg/kg/hr i.v.), a high-affinity, highly selective 5-HT_{1A}R agonist, commencing 5 min after cortical impact produced a marked attenuation of TBI-induced learning and memory deficits assessed in the MWM. Moreover, this treatment regimen attenuated hippocampal CA_1 and CA_3 cell loss, and decreased cortical lesion volume relative to vehicle-treated controls (151). Utilizing the same TBI model, Kline et al. (152) have also demonstrated that the classic 5-HT_{1A}R agonist 8-hydroxy-2-(di-*n*-propylamino)tetralin (8-OH-DPAT) produces similar effects on functional and histological outcome. Briefly, in a dose response study, a single dose of 0.5 mg/kg administered intraperitoneally 15 min following cortical impact significantly attenuated water maze performance relative to the vehicle controls. Additionally, 8-OH DPAT attenuated hippocampal CA_3 cell loss. The administration of the 5-HT_{1A} receptor antagonist WAY 100635 did not significantly impact functional or histological outcome following TBI. (See Figure 10-3.)

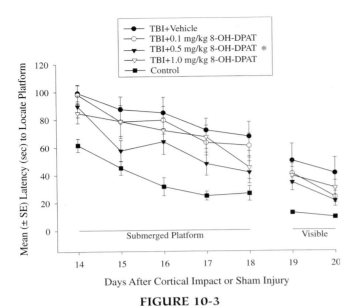

FIGURE 10-3

Mean (± SE) latency (sec) to locate either a submerged (hidden) or raised (visible) platform in a spatial learning acquisition paradigm in the Morris water maze. *$P < 0.05$ vs. TBI+Vehicle (Scheffé). [From Kline et al., *Neurosci Lett* 2002; 333:179–182 (Ref. 152).]

Although potential mechanisms contributing to the beneficial effects observed after a single treatment with 8-OH-DPAT in our TBI paradigm have not been reported, the results from other studies investigating 5-HT$_{1A}$R agonists suggest that it is via an attenuation of excitotoxicity. Electrophysiological studies have shown that 8-OH-DPAT, repinotan HCL, and other 5-HT$_{1A}$R agonists induce neuronal hyperpolarization by activating G-protein coupled inwardly rectifying K$^+$ channels (153,154) and decrease glutamate release after brain insult (145, 147,148). The latter effect is likely produced by activation of pre-synaptic 5-HT$_{1A}$ receptors on glutamatergic terminals (155,156). 5-HT$_{1A}$Rs activation may also contribute to neuroprotection by directly interacting with voltage-gated Na$^+$ channels to reduce Na$^+$ influx (157). 8-OH-DPAT and other 5-HT$_{1A}$R agonists also induce hypothermia (157–160), which may be another potential mechanism contributing to the neuroprotective effects observed in our studies. As indicated in a separate section of this chapter, hypothermia is a potent neuroprotective strategy after brain injury. However, we have recently reported that the beneficial effects observed with a single and early intraperitoneal injection of 8-OH-DPAT is not mediated by concomitant hypothermia. Briefly, following TBI and 8-OH-DPAT administration (same dose, route, and time frame as in the previous study, (152), we controlled temperature (normothermia) in one group of 8-OH-DPAT treated rats and allowed the other group to cool spontaneously. A comparison of both 8-OH-DPAT treatment groups did not reveal a difference in functional

or histological outcome, but both did perform significantly better than the vehicle control group (161).

ACUTE CHOLINERGIC TREATMENT

Acetylcholine (ACh) levels have been reported to change in brain and cerebral spinal fluid (CSF) following TBI. Gorman et al. (162) reported that hippocampal ACh levels (measured by microdialysis) increased signifcantly above control within 10 min after fluid percussion TBI. Saija et al. (163,164) found that ACh turnover rate (measured by a phosphoryl [^{2}H$_9$]choline method) increased significantly in the brainstem at 12 min and was still elevated at 4 hr after moderate fluid percussion TBI in the rat. Thus, moderate TBI appears to produce a transient release of ACh and increased cholinergic neuronal activity in some brain regions for several hr after injury.

Laboratory studies have demonstrated that excessive activation of acetylcholine (ACh) muscarinic receptors contribute significantly to functional deficits associated with experimental TBI in the rat. TBI induced muscarinic receptor activation mediates excitotoxic processes by modulating ionic fluxes via altered protein kinase C activity or inositol 1,4,5-triphosphate associated G-protein coupled PI turnover. The role of ACh in the induction of brain injury is further strengthened by evidence indicating that blockade of muscarinic cholinergic receptors during the acute phase can reduce injury and improve outcome. For example, pre-treatment (165,166) or immediate post-treatment (166) with the muscarinic receptor antagonist scopolamine has been demonstrated to significantly reduce functional motor deficits associated with TBI in the rat. Post-TBI administration of rivastigmine, an anticholinesterase drug that increases activity at both muscarinic and nicotinic receptors, has been shown to attenuate neurobehavioral and cognitive performance in mice.

In contrast, several lines of evidence indicate that experimental TBI in rats, in addition to transiently increasing ACh, also chronically decreases cholinergic neurotransmission, which may be related to disturbances in cognitive performance. Microdialysis studies at 2 weeks post-TBI have shown a reduction in the release of ACh evoked by the muscarinic autoreceptor antagonist, scopolamine (167,168). TBI can also produce increased sensitivity to disruption of spatial memory function by scopolamine that occurs concurrently with a reduction in scopolamine-evoked ACh release (169). A time-dependent loss of choline acetyltransferase (ChAT) enzymatic activity (162) and ChAT immunohistochemical staining (49,170,171) has also been reported after TBI. Dixon et al. (169) have reported a selective decrease in the V_{max} of choline uptake in the absence of any change in K_m after controlled cortical impact injury. However, alterations in synaptosomal choline uptake have not been reported at 1 week after closed head impact in rats (172). Ciallella and colleagues have reported chronic changes in vesicular ACh transporter (VAChT) and M_2 cholinergic muscarinic receptor, two proteins involved in cholinergic neurotransmission after TBI (173). Chronic mRNA changes in VAChT and M_2 have been evaluated at 4 weeks after moderate brain trauma in rats. VAChT and M_2 medial septal mRNA levels evaluated by RT-PCR revealed an increase in VAChT mRNA, but no significant change in M_2 mRNA levels compared to sham controls (174). Changes in VAChT and M_2 protein have been demonstrated to persist for up to one year following TBI (175). These changes may represent a compensatory response of cholinergic neurons to increase the efficiency of ACh neurotransmission chronically after TBI through differential transcriptional regulation.

Increasing levels of ACh pharmacologically can attenuate post-traumatic spatial memory performance deficits. For example, increasing ACh synthesis by increasing the availability of choline using CDP-choline treatment has been reported to enhance spatial memory performance (176). Additionally, chronic post-TBI administration of BIBM 99, a selective muscarinic M_2 receptor antagonist that increases ACh release by blocking pre-synaptic autoreceptors, has been reported to attenuate spatial memory deficits after TBI (177). Similarly, chronic post-TBI administration of MDL 26,479 (suritozole), a negative modulator at the γ-aminobutyric acid (GABA) receptor that enhances cholinergic function, attenuates spatial memory deficits after TBI (178). Several clinical reports have described beneficial effects on memory dysfunction with the acetylcholine-esterase inhibitor aricept (donepezil) after TBI in humans (179–182). Taken together, the studies described in this section suggest that therapies that attenuate the transient increase in ACh and/or alleviate the chronic decrease seen after TBI are capable of producing beneficial effects on functional outcome.

ENVIRONMENTAL ENRICHMENT

Exposing rats to complex, stimulatory and social housing (enriched environment (EE)) may be considered a rodent correlate of physiotherapeutic intervention and has been extensively studied in numerous experimental conditions. EE has been reported to increase brain weight, cortical volume, dendritic arborization, synaptogenesis, and neuronal survival (183,184). EE has also been shown to decrease apoptosis of neuronal precursor cells in the hippocampal dentate gyrus (185–187). Rats housed in EE for 30 days exhibit significantly higher levels of nerve growth factor mRNA in the rat visual cortex and hippocampus than those living in standard conditions (188). EE selectively increases 5-HT_{1A} receptor mRNA

expression and binding in the rat hippocampus (189). This finding demonstrates the importance of 5-HT-receptor subtypes in the effects of housing environment on hippocampal functions, such as synaptic plasticity. EE has also been shown to increase the expression of brain-derived neurotrophic factor mRNA in the rodent hippocampus, which correlates with improved spatial memory (190). Somatostatin levels (191), glucocorticoid receptor, and the nerve growth factor-induced immediate early gene NGFI-A (192) are also increased following exposure to an EE. In contrast to the studies observing increases in gene and neurotrophic expression (193,194), Hicks et al. (195) did not see alterations in BDNF, TrkB, or NT-3 gene expression in lateral fluid percussion injured rats exposed to an EE, but did see an attenuation of cognitive deficits. Hamm et al. (196) also reported improved MWM performance in rats exposed to an environment consisting of objects that provided motor, olfactory, tactile, and visual stimulation for 15 days following moderate fluid percussion injury. Furthermore, rats exposed to EE for 11 days after severe fluid percussion injury demonstrated improved MWM performance and reduced contusion lesion volume (197). EE has also been demonstrated to improve motor performance on a beam walk task or sensory neglect after cortical lesions (198–200). Wagner and colleagues have recently demonstrated that placing rats in an EE immediately after controlled cortical impact injury facilitates cognitive function in a spatial learning and memory task in the MWM (201). Briefly, as depicted in Figure 10.4, the rats in the EE (i.e., large cage with toys and objects designed to provide enhanced sensory stimulation) performed significantly better than the rats in standard conditions

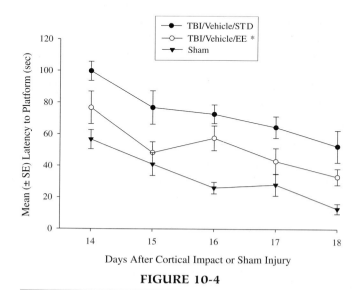

FIGURE 10-4

Mean (± SE) latency (sec) to locate a submerged platform in a spatial learning acquisition paradigm. *$P < 0.05$ vs. standard conditions. [From Wagner et al., *Neurosci Lett* 2002; 334:165–168 (Ref .201).]

(i.e., 2 rats per standard [STD] size cage with no enhanced sensory stimuli). Taken together, these reports attest to the beneficial effects conferred by EE after brain injury. Further studies investigating the combined effects of EE and pharmacotherapies known to also provide benefit after TBI, such as those outlined in this chapter, are warranted to examine this potentially efficacious, and perhaps synergistic, therapeutic approach. (See Figure 10-4.)

STEM CELL THERAPY

Multipotential stem cells are a contemporary choice for cell therapy TBI, as replacement of multiple cell types may be required for functional recovery. Several investigators have demonstrated that following TBI in adult rats, the number of proliferating cells labeled with bromodeoxyuridine is significantly increased in the bilateral subventricular zone and dentate gyrus (202–205). A better understanding of these endogenous neural stem cells may lead a less invasive model of stem cell therapy. There are several promising studies in which the transplantation of various progenitor cells have improved tissue survival and functional outcome. Bone marrow stromal cells, which normally give rise to bone, cartilage, adipose tissue, and hematopoiesis-supporting cells, have been shown to differentiate *in vitro* and *in vivo* into neural-like cells. Following TBI, treatment with bone marrow stromal cells has been shown to be functionally beneficial using intracerebral (206), intraarterial (207) and intravenous routes of administration (208). Transplantation of the neural stem cells (clone C17.2) has been reported to survive in the traumatically injured brain, differentiate into neurons and/or glia, and attenuate motor dysfunction after traumatic brain injury (209). Transplantation of embryonic stem cells has resulted in improved sensorimotor, but not cognitive function after TBI (210). Lu et al. (211) found that human umbilical cord blood cells injected i.v. into traumatic brain injured rats significantly reduced motor and neurological deficits compared with control groups by day 28 after the treatment. The cells were observed to preferentially enter the brain and migrate into the parenchyma and express the neuronal markers, NeuN and MAP-2, and the astrocytic marker, GFAP. These data suggest that the transplantation of progenitor cells into the brain may be a potential therapy for patients who have sustained traumatic brain injuries

NUTRACEUTICALS

Several empirical research studies have demonstrated that "natural" treatments can be effective in reducing some of the sequelae of TBI. An excellent example of a nutraceutical that has been extensively reported to reduce

secondary effects of TBI and improve behavioral outcome is magnesium (Mg^{2+}). Early work has shown that the administration of Mg^{2+} 30 min after a fluid percussion injury in rats provides significant improvement in neurological function when compared to saline-treated rats (212). Follow-up studies from the same group have shown that Mg^{2+} therapy is also effective in decreasing cognitive and motor deficits (58,213), histological damage (214,215), and expression of a gene (p53) associated with the induction of cell death (216). The beneficial effects of Mg^{2+} have been observed for up to 8-mo after TBI (217). Using an impact-acceleration model of severe traumatic diffuse axonal brain injury, Heath and Vink (218) have shown that intramuscular administration of $MgSO_4$ (750 μmol/kg) at 30 min or at 8, 12, or 24 hr after TBI significantly improves motor performance as assessed on a rotarod test vs. untreated-control animals. Although the rats treated at 24 hr displayed a slower rate of recovery during the early testing period, they eventually recovered significantly beyond the vehicle-treated group by the end of the testing session, suggesting that even delayed magnesium treatment is effective after TBI (218). A more recent finding by the same group reports that $MgSO_4$ (250 μmol/kg) at 30 min after diffuse TBI significantly improves sensorimotor function and learning performance (219). Mg^{2+} therapy has also been shown to facilitate functional recovery and prevent subcortical atrophy after lesions of the rat sensorimotor cortex (220).

Other nutraceuticals that have been reported to positively impact the neuroprotective and/or rehabilitative process after TBI include, but are not limited to, cytidinediphosphocholine (CDP-choline), creatine, and vitamins B3 and E. CDP-choline or citicholine is a naturally occurring endogenous nucleoside and an intermediate of phosphatidylcholine synthesis. When administered as a treatment after controlled cortical impact injury (100 mg/kg, 1–18 days post-TBI), CDP-choline-treated rats performed significantly better than vehicle-treated rats on both motor and cognitive tasks (176). Also utilizing the controlled cortical impact injury model, Baskaya et al. (221) demonstrated that intraperitoneal injections of CDP-choline (100 or 400 mg/kg twice after TBI) significantly decreased brain edema and BBB breakdown. In a more recent study, Dempsey and colleague reported that two treatments of CDP-choline (200 or 400 mg/kg, immediately post-TBI and 6 hr later) after cortical impact injury significantly prevented hippocampal neuron loss, decreased cortical contusion volume, and improved neurological recovery (222). Taken together, these studies indicate that CDP-choline is an effective neuroprotective agent on secondary injuries and neurobehavioral dysfunctions that are manifested after TBI. Creatine, a common food supplement used by individuals as a performance enhancer, has been demonstrated to attenuate the extent of cortical damage in mice and rats by as much as 36 percent and 50 percent, respectively (223). The authors suggested that protection might have been mediated by mechanisms involving creatine-induced maintenance of mitochondrial membrane potential, decreased intramitochondrial levels of reactive oxygen species and calcium, and preservation of adenosine triphosphate levels. In a study investigating the effects of vitamin B3, Hoane et al. (224) reported that a 500 mg/kg dose provided 15 min and 24 hr after TBI produced by a cortical contusion model significantly reduced the size of the lesion and glial fibrillary acidic protein positive astrocytes compared to saline-treated rats. Furthermore, vitamin B3 treatment also significantly improved behavioral outcome (224). The data suggest that vitamin B3 may have therapeutic potential for the treatment of TBI. In an investigation of vitamin E or α-tocopherol, Inci and colleagues have demonstrated that this neutraceutical also exhibits protective effects after TBI. Specifically, guinea pigs were subjected to a TBI utilizing a weight drop injury model and then administered 100 mg/kg of vitamin E. Lipid perixodation was measured using the thiobarbituric acid reactive substances method immediately, 1 hour, or 36 hr after trauma. The results indicated that α-tocopherol significantly suppressed the rise in lipid peroxide levels in traumatized brain tissue, suggesting that this treatment regimen has a protective effect against oxygen free radical-mediated lipid peroxidation after TBI (225).

CONCLUSIONS

The experimental control afforded with the utilization of animal models of TBI has allowed for the testing of several classes of neuroprotective therapies. Empirical studies have revealed several potential treatments that attenuate a range of neurobehavioral and morphological derangements. However, the translation of experimental neuroprotective treatments to humans has been limited. This situation may be improved be screening therapies under experimental conditions that better reproduce the clinical environment (e.g., ICU-like care, large animal models, etc.), and by conducting clinical trials that better mimic laboratory treatment administration protocols (e.g., earlier treatment windows).

*R*eferences

1. Kline AE, Dixon CE. Contemporary in vivo models of brain trauma and a comparison of injury responses. In: *Head Trauma: Basic, Preclinical and Clinical Directions*. Miller, L. P. and Hayes, R.L. (eds), John Wiley & Sons, New York, pp. 65–84, 2001.
2. Bittigau P, Ikonomidou C. Glutamate in neurologic diseases. *J Child Neurol* 1997; 12:471–485.
3. Sun FY, Faden AI. Neuroprotective effects of 619C89, a use-dependent sodium channel blocker, in rat traumatic brain injury. *Brain Res* 1995; 673:133–140.
4. McIntosh TK, Smith DH, Voddi J, Perri BR, Stutzmann JM. Riluzole, a novel neuroprotective agent, attenuates both neurologic

5. motor and cognitive dysfunction following experimental brain injury in the rat. *J Neurotrauma* 1996; 13(12):767–780.
5. Stover JF, Beyer TF, Unterberg AW. Riluzole reduces brain swelling and contusion volume in rats following controlled cortical impact injury. *J Neurotrauma* 2000; 17(12):1171–1178.
6. Liu S, Lyeth BG, Hamm RJ. Protective effect of galanin on behavioral deficits in experimental traumatic brain injury. *J Neurotrauma* 1994; 11(1):73–82.
7. Di X, Lyeth BG, Hamm RJ, Bullock MR. Voltage-dependent Na+/K+ ion channel blockade fails to ameliorate behavioral deficits after traumatic brain injury in the rat. *J Neurotrauma* 1996; 13(9):497–504.
8. Hayes RL, Jenkins LW, Lyeth BG, Balster RL, Robinson SE, Clifton GL, Stubbins JF, Young HF. Pretreatment with phencyclidine, an N-methyl-D-aspartate antagonist, attenuates long-term behavioral deficits in the rat produced by traumatic brain injury. *J Neurotrauma* 1988; 5(4):259–274.
9. Faden AI, Demediuk P, Panter SS, Vink R. The role of excitatory amino acids and NMDA receptors in traumatic brain injury. *Science* 1989; 244:798–800.
10. McIntosh TK, Faden AI, Yamakami I, Vink R. Magnesium deficiency exacerbates and pretreatment improves outcome following traumatic brain injury in rats: 31P magnetic resonance spectroscopy and behavioral studies. *J Neurotrauma* 1988; 5(1): 17–31.
11. McIntosh TK, Vink R, Yamakami I, Faden AI. Magnesium protects against neurological deficit after brain injury. *Brain Res* 1989; 482:252–260.
12. Hamm RJ, O'Dell DM, Pike BR, Lyeth BG. Cognitive impairment following traumatic brain injury: the effect of pre- and post-injury administration of scopolamine and MD-801. *Brain Res Cogn Brain Res* 1993; 1(4):223–226.
13. Lewen A, Fredriksson A, Li GL, Olsson Y, Hillered L. Behavioural and morphological outcome of mild cortical contusion trauma of the rat brain: influence of NMDA-receptor blockade. *Acta Neurochir (Wien)* 1999; 141(2):193–202.
14. Ikonomidou C, Turski L. Prevention of trauma-induced neurodegeneration in infant and adult rat brain: glutamate antagonists. *Metab Brain Dis* 1996; 11(2):125–141.
15. Smith DH, Perri BR, Raghupathi R, Saatman KE, McIntosh TK. Remacemide hydrochloride reduces cortical lesion volume following brain trauma in the rat. *Neurosci Lett* 1997; 231(3): 135–138.
16. Smith JS, Fulop ZL, Levinsohn SA, Darrell RS, Stein DG. Effects of the novel NMDA receptor antagonist gacyclidine on recovery from medial frontal cortex contusion injury in rats. *Neural Plast* 2000; 7:73–91.
17. Hicks RR, Smith DH, Gennarelli TA, McIntosh T. Kynurenate is neuroprotective following experimental brain injury in the rat. *Brain Res* 1994; 655:91–96.
18. Shohami E, Novikov M, Mechoulam R. A nonpsychotropic cannabinoid, HU-211, has cerebroprotective effects after closed head injury in the rat. *J Neurotrauma* 1993; 10(2):109–119.
19. Shapira Y, Lam AM, Eng CC, Laohaprasit V, Michel M. Therapeutic time window and dose response of the beneficial effects of ketamine in experimental head injury. *Stroke* 1994; 25(8):1637–1643.
20. Smith DH, Okiyama K, Gennarelli TA, McIntosh TK. Magnesium and ketamine attenuate cognitive dysfunction following experimental brain injury. *Neurosci Lett* 1993; 157:211–214.
21. Okiyama K, Smith DH, White WF, McIntosh TK. Effects of the NMDA antagonist CP-98, 113 on regional cerebral edema and cardiovascular, cognitive, and neurobehavioral function following experimental brain injury in the rat. *Brain Res* 1998; 792(2):291–298.
22. O'Dell DM, Gibson CJ, Wilson MS, DeFord SM, Hamm RJ. Positive and negative modulation of the GABA(A) receptor and outcome after traumatic brain injury in rats. *Brain Res* 2000; 861:325–332.
23. Leoni MJ, Chen XH, Mueller AL, Cheney J, McIntosh TK, Smith DH. NPS 1506 attenuates cognitive dysfunction and hippocampal neuron death following brain trauma in the rat. *Exp Neurol* 2000; 166(2):442–449.

24. Gong Q-Z, Delahunty TM, Hamm RJ, Lyeth BG. Metabotropic glutamate antagonist, MCPG, treatment of traumatic brain injury in rats. *Brain Res* 1995; 700:299–302.

25. Movsesyan VA, O'Leary DM, Fan L, Bao W, Mullins PGM, Knoblach SM, Faden AI. mGluR5 antagonists 2-methyl-6-(phenylethynyl)-pyridine and (E)-2-methyl-6(2-phenylethenyl)-pyridine reduce traumatic neuronal injury in vitro and in vivo by antagonizing N-methyl-D-aspartate receptors. *J Pharmacol Exp Ther* 2001; 296(1):41–47.

26. Allen JW, Ivanova SA, Fan L, Espey MG, Basile AS, Faden AI. Group II metabotropic glutamate receptor activation attenuates traumatic neuronal injury and improves neurological recovery after traumatic brain injury. *J Pharmacol Exp Ther* 1999; 290:112–120.

27. Faden AI, O'Leary DM, Fan L, Bao W, Mullins PG, Movsesyan VA. Selective blockade of the mGluR1 receptor reduces traumatic neuronal injury in vitro and improves outcome after brain trauma. *Exp Neurol* 2001; 167:435–444.

28. Zhong C, Zhao X, Sarva J, Kozikowski A, Neale JH, Lyeth BG. NAAG peptidase inhibitor reduces acute neuronal degeneration and Astrocyte damage following latral fluid percussion TBI in rats. *Neurotrauma* 2005; 22(2):266–276.

29. Berman RF, Verweu BH, Muizelaar JP. Neurobehavioral protection by the neuronal calcium channel blocker ziconotide in a model of traumatic diffuse brain injury in rats. *J Neurosurg* 2000; 93:821–828.

30. Cheney JA, Brown AL, Bareyre FM, Russ AB, Weisser JD, Ensinger HA, Leusch A, Raghupathi R, Saatman KE. The novel compound LOE 908 attenuates acute neuromotor dysfunction but not cognitive impairment or cortical tissue loss following traumatic brain injury in rats. *J Neurotrauma* 2000; 17(1):83–91.

31. Lee LL, Galo E, Lyeth BG, Muizelaar JP, Berman RF. Neuroprotection in the rat lateral fluid percussion model of traumatic brain injury by SNX-185, an N-type voltage-gated calcium channel blocker. *Exp Neurol* 2004; 190(1):70–78.

32. Okiyama K, Smith DH, Thomas MJ, McIntosh TK. Evaluation of a novel calcium channel blocker, (S)-emopamil, on regional cerebral edema and neurobehavioral function after experimental brain injury. *J Neurosurg* 1992; 77:607–615.

33. Dempsey RJ, Basaya MK, Dogan A. Attenuation of brain edema, blood-brain barrier breakdown, and injury volume by ifenprodiil, a polyamine-site N-methyl-D-aspartate receptor antagonist, after experimental traumatic brain injury in rats. *Neurosurgery* 2000; 47:399–404.

34. Hall ED, Yonkers PA, McCall JM, Braughler JM. Effects of the 21-aminosteroid U74006F on experimental head injury in mice. *J Neurosurg* 1988; 68:456–461.

35. Marion DW, White MJ. Treatment of experimental brain injury with moderate hypothermia and 21-aminosteroids. *J Neurotrauma* 1996; 13(3):139–147.

36. Clifton GL, Lyeth BG, Jenkins LW, Taft WC, DeLorenzo RJ, Hayes RL. Effect of D, α-tocopheryl succinate and polyethylene glycol on performance tests after fluid percussion brain injury. *J Neurotrauma* 1989; 6(2):71–81.

37. Grisar JM, Bolkenius FN, Petty MA, Verne J. 2,3-Dihydro-1-benzofuran-5-ols as analogues of α-tocopherol that inhibit in vitro and ex vivo lipid autoxidation and protect mice against central nervous system trauma. *J Med Chem* 1995; 38(3):453–458.

38. Das KC, Misra HP. (1992) Lidocaine: a hydroxyl radical scavenger and singlet oxygen quencher. *Mol Cell Biochem* 1992; 115(2):179–185.

39. Muir JK, Lyeth BG, Hamm RJ, Ellis EF. The effect of acute cocaine or lidocaine on behavioral function following fluid percussion brain injury in rats. *J Neurotrauma* 1995; 12(1):87–97.

40. Long DA, Ghosh K, Moore AN, Dixon CE, Dash PK. Deferoxamine improves spatial memory performance following experimental brain injury in rats. *Brain Res* 1996; 717:109–117.

41. Heegaard W, Biros M, Zink J. Effect of hypothermia, dichloroacetate, and deferoxamine in the treatment for cortical edema and functional recovery after experimental cortical impact in the rat. *Acad Emerg Med* 1997; 4(1):33–39.

42. Hamm RJ, Temple MD, Pike BR, Ellis EF. The effect of postinjury administration of polyethylene glycol-conjugated superoxide dismutase (pegorgotein, Dismutec) or lidocaine on behavioral function following fluid-percussion brain injury in rats. *J Neurotrauma* 1996; 13(6):325–332.

43. Mori T, Kawamata T, Katayama Y, Maeda T, Aoyama N, Kikuchi T, Uwahodo Y. Antioxidant, OPC-14117, attenuates edema formation, and subsequent tissue damage following cortical contusion in rats. *Acta Neurochir Suppl (Wien)* 1998; 71:120–122.

44. Kawamata T, Katayama Y, Maeda T, Mori T, Aoyama N, Kikuchi T, Uwahodo Y. Antioxidant, OPC-14117, attenuates edema formation and behavioral deficits following cortical contusion in rats. *Acta Neurochir Suppl (Wien)* 1997; 70:191–193.

45. Aoyama N, Katayama Y, Kawamata T, Maeda T, Mori T, Yamamoto T, Kikuchi T, Uwahodo Y. Effects of antioxidant, OPC-14117, on secondary cellular damage and behavioral deficits following cortical contusion in the rat. *Brain Res* 2002; 934(2):117–24.

46. Wada K, Alonso OF, Busto R, Panetta J, Clemens JA, Ginsberg MD, Dietrich WD. Early treatment with a novel inhibitor of lipid peroxidation (LY341122) improves histopathological outcome after moderate fluid percussion brain injury in rats. *Neurosurgery* 1999; 45(3):601–608.

47. Hall ED, Kupina NC, Althaus JS. Peroxynitrite scavengers for the acute treatment of traumatic brain injury. *Ann NY Acad Sci* 1999; 890:462–468.

48. Sarrafzadeh AS, Thomale UW, Kroppenstedt SN, Unterberg AW. Neuroprotective effect of melatonin on cortical impact injury in the rat. *Acta Neurochir (Wien)* 2000; 142:1293–1299.

49. Sato M, Noble LJ. Involvement of the endothelin receptor subtype A in neuronal pathogenesis after traumatic brain injury. *Brain Res* 1998; 809:39–49.

50. Kline AE, Massucci JL, Marion DW, Dixon CE. Attenuation of working memory and spatial acquisition deficits after a delayed and chronic bromocriptine treatment regimen in rats subjected to traumatic brain injury by controlled cortical impact. *J Neurotrauma* 2002; 19:415–425.

51. Sinson G, Voddi M, McIntosh TK. Nerve growth factor administration attenuates cognitive but not neurobehavioral motor dysfunction of hippocampal cell loss following fluid-percussion brain injury in rats. *J Neurochem* 1995; 65:2209–2216.

52. Sinson G, Perri BR, Trojanowski JQ, Flamm ES, McIntosh TK. Improvement of cognitive deficits and decreased cholinergic neuronal cell loss and apoptotic cell death following neurotrophin infusion after experimental traumatic brain injury. *J Neurosurg* 1997; 86:511–518.

53. Dixon CE, Flinn P, Bao J, Venya R, Hayes RL. Nerve growth factor attenuates cholinergic deficits following traumatic brain injury in rats. *Exp Neurol* 1997; 146:479–490.

54. Zou LL, Huang L, Hayes RL, Black C, Qiu YH, Perez-Polo JR, Le W, Clifton GL, Yang K. Liposome-mediated NGF gene transfection following neuronal injury: potential therapeutic applications. *Gene Ther* 1999; 6:994–1005.

55. Frank E, Ragel B. Cortical basic fibroblast factor expression after head injury: preliminary results. *Neurol Res* 1995; 17:129–131.

56. Dietrich WD, Alonso O, Busto R, Finklestein SP. Posttreatment with intravenous basic fibroblast growth factor reduces histopathological damage following fluid percussion brain injury in rat. *J Neurotrauma* 1996; 13:309–316.

57. McDermott KL, Raghupathi R, Fernandez SC, Saatman KE, Protter AA, Finklestein SP, Sinson G, Smith DH, McIntosh TK. Delayed administration of basic fibroblast growth factor (bFGF) attenuates cognitive dysfunction following parasagittal fluid percussion brain injury in the rat. *J Neurotrauma* 1997; 14:191–200.

58. Guluma KZ, Saatman KE, Brown A, Raghupathi R, McIntosh TK. Sequential pharmacotherapy with magnesium chloride and basic fibroblast growth factor after fluid percussion brain injury results in less neuromotor efficacy than that achieved with magnesium alone. *J Neurotrauma* 1999; 16:311–321.

59. Yan HQ, Yu J, Kline AE, Letart P, Jenkins LW, Marion DW, Dixon CE. Evaluation of combined fibroblast growth factor-2 and moderate hypothermia therapy in traumatically brain injured rats. *Brain Res* 2000; 887:134–143.

60. Yoshimura S, Teramoto T, Whalen MJ, Irizarry MC, Takagi Y, Qiu J, Haranda J, Waeber C, Breakefield XO, Moskowitz MA.

FGF-2 regulates neurogenesis and degeneration in the dentate gyrus after traumatic brain injury in mice. *J Clin Invest* 2003; 112:1202–1210.

61. Sandberg-Nordqvist AC, von Holst H, Holmin S, Sara VR, Bellander BM, Schalling M. Increase of insulin-like growth factor (IGF)-1, IGF binding protein-2 and -4 mRNAs following cerebral contusion. *Brain Res Mol Brain Res* 1996; 38:285–293.

62. Nordqvist AC, Holmin S, Nilsson M, Mathiesen T, Schalling M. MK-801 inhibits the cortical increase in IGF-1, IGFBP-2 and IGFBP-4 expression following trauma. *Neuroreport* 1997; 8: 455–460.

63. Saatman KE, Contreras PC, Smith DH, Raghupathi R, McDermott KL, Fernandez SC, Sanderson KL, Voddi M, McIntosh TK. Insulin-like growth factor-1 (IGF-1) improves both neurological motor and cognitive outcome following experimental brain injury. *Exp Neurol* 1997; 147:418–427.

64. Kazanis I, Bozas E, Philippidis H, Stylianopoulou F. Neuroprotective effects of insulin-like factor-1 (IGF-1) following a penetrating brain injury in rats. *Brain Res* 2003; 991:34–45.

65. Bramlett HM, Green EJ, Dietrich WD, Busto R, Globus MY, Ginsberg MD. Post-traumatic brain hypothermia provides protection from sensorimotor and cognitive behavioral deficits. *J Neurotrauma* 1995; 12(3):289–298.

66. Clifton GL, Jiang JY, Lyeth BG, Jenkins LW, Hamm RJ, Hayes RL. Marked protection by moderate hypothermia after experimental traumatic brain injury. *J Cereb Blood Flow Metab* 1991; 11:114–1121.

67. Dixon CE, Markgraf CG, Angileri F, Pike BR, Wolfson B, Newcomb JK, Bismar MM, Blanco AJ, Clifton GL, Hayes RL. Protective effects of moderate hypothermia on behavioral deficits but not necrotic cavitation following cortical impact injury in the rat. *J Neurotrauma* 1998; 15(2):95–103.

68. Lyeth BG, Jiang JY, Liu S. Behavioral protection by moderate hypothermia initiated after experimental traumatic brain injury. *J Neurotrauma* 1993; 10(1):57–64.

69. Markgraf CG, Clifton GL, Aguirre M, Chaney SF, Knox-Du Bois C, Kennon K, Verma N. Injury severity and sensitivity to treatment after controlled cortical impact in rats. *J Neurotrauma* 2001; 18(2): 175–186.

70. Dietrich WD, Alonso O, Busto R, Globus MY, Ginsberg MD. Post-traumatic brain hypothermia reduces histopathological damage following concussive brain injury in the rat. *Acta Neuropathol (Berl)* 1994; 87:250–258.

71. Palmer AM, Marion DW, Botscheller ML, Redd EE. Therapeutic hypothermia is cytoprotective without attenuating the traumatic brain injury-induced elevations in interstitial concentrations of aspartate and glutamate. *J Neurotrauma* 1993; 10(4):363–372.

72. Marion DW, White MJ. Treatment of experimental brain injury with moderate hypothermia and 21-aminosteroids. *J Neurotrauma* 1996; 13:139–147.

73. Bramlett HM, Dietrich WD, Green EJ, Busto R. Chronic histopathological consequences of fluid-percussion brain injury in rats: effects of post-traumatic hypothermia. *Acta Neuropathol (Berl)* 1997; 93:190–199.

74. Robertson CL, Clark RS, Dixon CE, Alexander HL, Graham SH, Wisniewski SR, Marion DW, Safar PJ, Kochanek PM. No long-term benefit from hypothermia after severe traumatic brain injury with secondary insult in rats. *Crit Care Med* 2000; 28:3218–3223.

75. Statler KD, Alexander HL, Vagni VA, Nemoto EM, Tofovic SP, Dixon CE, Jenkins LW, Marion DW, Kochanek PM. Moderate hypothermia may be detrimental after traumatic brain injury in fentanyl-anesthetized rats. *Crit Care Med* 2003; 31(4):1134–1139.

76. Lo EH, Wang X, Cuzner ML. Extracellular proteolysis in brain injury and inflammation: role for plasminogen activators and matrix metalloproteinases. *J Neurosci Res* 2002; 69(1):1–9.

77. Saatman KE, Murai H, Bartus RT, Smith DH, Hayward NJ, Perri BR, McIntosh TK. Calpain inhibitor AK295 attenuates motor and cognitive deficits following experimental brain injury in the rat. *Proc Natl Acad Sci USA* 1996; 93(8):3428–3433.

78. Saatman KE, Zhang C, Bartus RT, McIntosh TK. Behavioral efficacy of post-traumatic calpain inhibition is not accompanied by reduced spectrin proteolysis, cortical lesion, or apoptosis. *J Cereb Blood Flow Metab* 2000; 20(1):66–73.

79. Posmantur R, Kampfl A, Siman R, Liu J, Zhao X, Clifton GL, Hayes RL. A calpain inhibitor attenuates cortical cytoskeletal protein loss after experimental traumatic brain injury in the rat. *Neuroscience* 1997; 77:875–888.

80. Kupina NC, Nath R, Bernath EE, Inoue J, Mitsuyoshi A, Yuen PW, Wang KK, Hall ED. The novel calpain inhibitor SJA6017 improves functional outcome after delayed administration in a mouse model of diffuse brain injury. *J Neurotrauma* 2001; 18(11):1229–1240.

81. Kupina NC, Detloff MR, Dutta S, Hall ED. Neuroimmunophilin ligand V-10,367 is neuroprotective after 24-hour delayed administration in a mouse model of diffuse traumatic brain injury. *J Cereb Blood Flow Metab* 2002; 22(10):1212–1221.

82. Buki A, Farkas O, Doczi T, Povlishock JT. Preinjury administration of the calpain inhibitor MDL-28170 attenuates traumatically induced axonal injury. *J Neurotrauma* 2003; 20(3):261–268.

83. Grady MS, Cody RF Jr, Maris DO, McCall TD, Seckin H, Sharar SR, Winn HR. P-selectin blockade following fluid-percussion injury: behavioral and immunochemical sequelae. *J Neurotrauma* 1999; 16:13–25.

84. Knoblach SM, Faden AI. Administration of either anti-intercellular adhesion molecule-1 or a nonspecific control antibody improves recovery after traumatic brain injury in the rat. *J Neurotrauma* 2002; 19(9):1039–1050.

85. Sanderson KL, Raghupathi R, Saatman KE, Martin D, Miller G, McIntosh TK. Interleukin-1 receptor antagonist attenuates regional neuronal cell death and cognitive dysfunction after experimental brain injury. *J Cereb Blood Flow Metab* 1999; 19: 1118–1125.

86. Knoblach SM, Faden AI. Cortical interleukin-1 beta elevation after traumatic brain injury in the rat: no effect of two selective antagonists on motor recovery. *Neurosci Lett* 2000; 289(1):5–8.

87. Weaver KD, Branch CA, Hernandez L, Miller CH, Quattrocchi KB. Effect of leukocyte-endothelial adhesion antagonism on neutrophil migration and neurologic outcome after cortical trauma. *J Trauma* 2000; 48:1081–1090.

88. Sinz EH, Kochanek PM, Dixon CE, Clark RS, Carcillo JA, Schiding JK, Chen M, Wisniewski SR, Carlos TM, Williams D, DeKosky ST, Watkins SC, Marion DW, Billiar TR. Inducible nitric oxide synthase is an endogenous neuroprotectant after traumatic brain injury in rats and mice. *J Clin Invest* 1999; 104:647–656.

89. Lu J, Moochhala S, Shirhan M, Ng KC, Teo AL, Tan MH, Moore XL, Wong MC, Ling EA. Neuroprotection by aminoguanidine after lateral fluid-percussive brain injury in rats: a combined magnetic resonance imaging, histopathologic and functional study. *Neuropharmacology* 2003; 44(2):253–263.

90. Jafarian-Tehrani M, Louin G, Royo NC, Besson VC, Bohme GA, Plotkine M, Marchand-Verrecchia C. 1400W, a potent selective inducible NOS inhibitor, improves histopathological outcome following traumatic brain injury in rats. *Nitric Oxide* 2005;12(2): 61–69.

91. Knoblach SM, Faden AI. Interleukin-10 improves outcome and alters pro-inflammatory cytokine expression after experimental traumatic brain injury. *Exp Neurol* 1998; 153:143–151.

92. Kline AE, Bolinger BD, Kochanek PM, Carlos TM, Yan HQ, Jenkins LW, Marion DW, Dixon CE. Acute systemic administration of interleukin-10 suppresses the beneficial effects of moderate hypothermia following traumatic brain injury in rats. *Brain Res* 2002; 937(1–2):22–31.

93. Dash PK, Mach SA, Moore AN. Regional expression and role of cyclooxygenase-2 following experimental traumatic brain injury. *J Neurotrauma* 2000; 17(1):69–81.

94. Schwab JM, Seid K, Schluesener HJ. Traumatic brain injury induces prolonged accumulation of cyclooxygenase-1 expressing microglia/brain macrophages in rats. *J Neurotrauma* 2001; 18(9):881–890.

95. Cernak I, O'Connor C, Vink R. Inhibition of cyclooxygenase 2 by nimesulide improves cognitive outcome more than motor outcome following diffuse traumatic brain injury in rats. *Exp Brain Res* 2002; 147(2):193–199.

96. Kunz T, Marklund N, Hillered L, Oliw EH. Cyclooxygenase-2, prostaglandin synthases, and prostaglandin H2 metabolism in traumatic brain injury in the rat. *J Neurotrauma* 2002; 19(9):1051–1064.

97. Gopez JJ, Yue H, Vasudevan R, Malik AS, Fogelsanger LN, Lewis S, Panikashvili D, Shohami E, Jansen SA, Narayan RK, Strauss KI. Cyclooxygenase-2 specific inhibitor improves functional outcomes, provides neuroprotection, and reduces inflammation in a rat model of traumatic brain injury. *Neurosurgery* 2005; 56(3): 590–604.

98. Yamakami I, Vink R, Faden AI, Gennarelli TA, Lenkinski R, McIntosh TK. Effects of acute ethanol intoxication on experimental brain injury in the rat: neurobehavioral and phosphorus-31 nuclear magnetic resonance spectroscopy studies. *J Neurosurg* 1995; 82(5):813–821.

99. Shapira Y, Lam AM, Paez A, Artru AA, Laohaprasit V, Donato T. The influence of acute and chronic alcohol treatment on brain edema, cerebral infarct volume and neurological outcome following experimental head trauma in rats. *J Neurosurg Anesthesiol* 1997; 9(2):118–127.

100. Janis LS, Hoane MR, Conde D, Fulop Z, Stein DG. Acute ethanol administration reduces the cognitive deficits associated with traumatic brain injury in rats. *J Neurotrauma* 1998; 15(2):105–115.

101. Kelly DF, Kozlowski DA, Haddad E, Echiverri A, Hovda DA, Lee SM. Ethanol reduces metabolic uncoupling following experimental head injury. *J Neurotrauma* 2000; 17(4):261–272.

102. Biros MH, Kukielka D, Sutton RL, Rockswold GL, Bergman TA. The effects of acute and chronic alcohol ingestion on outcome following multiple episodes of mild traumatic brain injury in rats. *Acad Emerg Med* 1999; 6:1088–1097.

103. Gottesfeld Z, Moore AN, Dash PK. Acute ethanol intake attenuates inflammatory cytokines after brain injury in rats: a possible role for corticosterone. *J Neurotrauma* 2002; 19(3):317–326.

104. Dash PK, Moore AN, Moody MR, Treadwell R, Felix JL, Clifton GL. Post-trauma administration of caffeine plus ethanol reduces contusion volume and improves working memory in rats. *J Neurotrauma* 2004; 21(11):1573–1583.

105. Roof RL, Duvdevani R, Braswell L, Stein DG. Progesterone facilitates cognitive recovery and reduces secondary neuronal loss caused by cortical contusion injury in male rats. *Exp Neurol* 1994; 129:64–69.

106. Galani R, Hoffman SW, Stein DG. Effects of the duration of progesterone treatment on the resolution of cerebral edema induced by cortical contusions in rats. *Restor Neurol Neurosci* 2001; 18:161–166.

107. Shear DA, Galani R, Hoffman SW, Stein DG. Progesterone protects against necrotic damage and behavioral abnormalities caused by traumatic brain injury. *Exp Neurol* 2002; 178:59–67.

108. Roof RL, Hoffman SW, Stein DG. Progesterone protects against lipid peroxidation following traumatic brain injury in rats. *Mol Chem Neuropathol* 1997; 31:1–11.

109. Djebaili M, Hoffman SW, Stein DG. Allopregnanolone and progesterone decrease cell death and cognitive deficits after a contusion of the rat pre-frontal cortex. *Neuroscience* 2004; 123: 349–359.

110. Emerson SC, Headrick JP, Vink R. Estrogen improves biochemical and neurologic outcome following traumatic brain injury in male rats, but not females. *Brain Res* 1993; 608:95–100.

111. Roof RL, Hall ED. Estrogen-related gender differences in survival rate and cortical blood flow after impact-acceleration head injury in rats. *J Neurotrauma* 2000; 17:1155–1169.

112. Soustiel JF, Palzur E, Nevo O, Thaler I, Vlodavsky E. Neuroprotective anti-apoptosis effect of estrogens in traumatic brain injury. *J Neurotrauma* 2005; 22(3):345–352..

113. Wagner AK, Willard LA, Kline AE, Wenger MK, Bolinger BD, Ren D, Zafonte RD, Dixon CE. Evaluation of estrous cycle stage and gender on behavioral outcome after experimental traumatic brain injury. *Brain Res* 2004; 998:113–121.

114. Bramlett HM, Dietrich WD. Neuropathological protection after traumatic brain injury in intact female rats versus males or ovariectomized females. *J Neurotrauma* 2001; 18:891–900.

115. Okonkwo DO, Buki A, Siman R, Povlishock JT. Cyclosporin A limits calcium-induced axonal damage following traumatic brain injury. *Neuroreport* 1999; 10:353–358.

116. Scheff SW, Sullivan PG. Cyclosporin A significantly ameliorates cortical damage following experimental traumatic brain injury in rodents. *J Neurotrauma* 1999; 16(9):783–792.

117. Sullivan PG, Rabchevsky AG, Hicks RR, Gibson TR, Fletcher-Turner A, Scheff SW. Dose-response curve and optimal dosing regimen of cyclosporin A after traumatic brain injury in rats. *Neuroscience* 2000; 101:289–295.

118. Alessandri B, Rice AC, Levasseur J, DeFord M, Hamm RJ, Bullock MR. Cyclosporin A improves brain tissue oxygen consumption and learning/memory performance after lateral fluid percussion injury in rats. *J Neurotrauma* 2002; 19(7):829–841.

119. Buki A, Okonkwo DO, Povlishock JT. Postinjury cyclosporin A administration limits axonal damage and disconnection in traumatic brain injury. *J Neurotrauma* 1999; 16(6):511–521.

120. Verweij BH, Muizelaar JP, Vinas FC, Peterson PL, Xiong Y, Lee CP. Improvement in mitochondrial dysfunction as a new surrogate efficiency measure for preclinical trials: dose-response and time-window profiles for administration of the calcium channel blocker Ziconotide in experimental brain injury. *J Neurosurg* 2000; 93(5):829–834.

121. Berman RF, Verweu BH, Muizelaar JP. Neurobehavioral protection by the neuronal calcium channel blocker ziconotide in a model of traumatic diffuse brain injury in rats. *J Neurosurg* 2000; 93:821–828.

122. Feeney DM, Gonzalez A, Law WA. Amphetamine, haloperidol, and experience interact to affect rate of recovery after motor cortex injury. *Science* 1982; 217:855–857.

123. Goldstein LB, Davis JN. Clonidine impairs recovery of beam-walking after a sensorimotor cortex lesion in the rat. *Brain Res* 1990; 508:305–309.

124. Feeney DM. Pharmacologic modulation of recovery after brain injury: a reconsideration of diaschisis. *J Neuro Rehab* 1991; 5:113–128.

125. Feeney DM, Weisend MP, Kline AE. Noradrenergic pharmacotherapy, intracerebral infusion and adrenal transplantation promote functional recovery after cortical damage. *J Neural Transplant Plast* 1993; 4:199–213.

126. Kline AE, Chen MJ, Tso-Olivas DY, Feeney DM. Methylphenidate treatment following ablation-induced hemiplegia in rat: experience during drug action alters effects on recovery of function. *Pharmacol Biochem Behav* 1994; 48:773–779.

127. Kline AE, Yan HQ, Bao J, Marion DW, Dixon CE. Chronic methylphenidate treatment enhances water maze performance following traumatic brain injury in rats. *Neurosci Lett* 2000; 280: 163–166.

128. Hovda DA, Sutton RL, Feeney DM. Amphetamine-induced recovery of visual cliff performance after bilateral visual cortex ablation in cats: measurements of depth perception thresholds. *Behav Neurosci* 1989; 103:574–584.

129. Sutton RL, Feeney DM. A-noradrenergic agonists and antagonists affect recovery and maintenance of beam-walking ability after sensorimotor cortex ablation in the rat. *Restor Neurol Neurosci* 1992; 4:1–11.

130. Dixon CE, Kraus MF, Kline AE, Ma X, Yan HQ, Griffith RG, Wolfson BM, Marion DW. Amantadine improves water maze performance without affecting motor behavior following traumatic brain injury in rats. *Restor Neurol Neurosci* 1999; 14:285–294.

131. Gerlak RP, Clark R, Stump JM, and Vernier VG. Amantadine-dopamine interaction: possible mode of action in Parkinsonism. *Science* 1970; 169:203–204.

132. von Voigtlander PF, Moore KE. Dopamine: release from the brain in vivo by amantadine. *Science* 1971; 174:408–410.

133. Bak IJ, Hassler R, Kim JS, Kataoka K. Amantadine actions on acetylcholine and GABA in striatum and substantia nigra of rat in relation to behavioral changes. *J Neural Transm* 1972; 33: 45–61.

134. Gianutsos G, Chute S, Dunn JP. Pharmacological changes in dopaminergic systems induced by long-term administration of amantadine. *Eur J Pharmacol* 1985; 110:357–361.

135. Allen RM. Role of amantadine in the management of neuroleptic-induced extrapyramidal syndromes: overview and pharmacology. *Clin Neuropharmacol* 1983; 6:S64-S73.

136. Gualtieri T, Chandler M, Coons TB, Brown LT. Amantadine: a new clinical profile for traumatic brain injury. *Clin Neuropharmacol* 1989; 12:258–270.

137. Brannan T, Martinez-Tica J, DiRocco A, Yahr MD. Low and high dose bromocriptine have differential effects on striatal dopamine release: an in vivo study. *J Neural Transm Park Dis Dement Sect* 1993; 6:81–87.

138. Zhu J, Hamm RJ, Reeves TM, Povlishock JT, Phillips LL. Postinjury administration of L-deprenyl improves cognitive function and enhances neuroplasticity after traumatic brain injury. *Exp Neurol* 2000; 166:136–152.

139. Kraus MF, Maki PM. Effect of amantadine hydrochloride on symptoms of frontal lobe dysfunction in brain injury: case studies and review. *J Neuropsy Clin Neurosci* 1997; 9:222–230.

140. McDowell S, Whyte J, D'Esposito M. Differential effect of a dopaminergic agonist on prefrontal function in traumatic brain injury patients. *Brain* 1998; 121:1155–1164.

141. Busto R, Dietrich WD, Globus MY.-T, Alonso O, Ginsberg MD. Extracellular release of serotonin following fluid-percussion brain injury in rats. *J Neurotrauma* 1997; 14:35–42.

142. Nedergaard S, Engberg I, Flatman JA. The modulation of excitatory amino acid responses by serotonin in the cat neocortex in vitro. *Cell Mol Neurobiol* 1987; 7:367–379.

143. Barnes NM, Sharp T. A review of central 5-HT receptors and their function. *Neuropharmacology* 1999; 38:1083–1152.

144. Meneses A. 5-HT system and cognition. *Neurosci Biobehav Rev* 1999; 23:1111–1125.

145. De Vry J, Dietrich H, Glaser T, Heine H-G, Horv·th E, Jork R, Maertins T, Mauler F, Opitz W, Scherling D, Schohe-Loop R, Schwartz T. BAY x 3702. *Drugs of the Future* 1997; 22:341–349.

146. De Vry J, Jentzsch KR. Discriminative stimulus properties of the 5-HT$_{1A}$ receptor agonist BAY × 3702 in the rat. *Eur J Pharmacol* 1998; 357:1–8.

147. Mauler F, Fahrig T, Horv·th E, Jork R. Inhibition of evoked glutamate release by the neuroprotective 5-HT$_{1A}$ receptor agonist BAY × 3702 in vitro and in vivo. *Brain Res* 2001; 888:150–157.

148. Prehn JH, Welsch M, Backhauss C, Nuglisch J, Ausmeier F, Karkoutly C, Krieglstein J. Effects of serotonergic drugs in experimental brain ischemia: evidence for a protective role of serotonin in cerebral ischemia. *Brain Res* 1993; 630:10–20.

149. Semkova I, Wolz P, Krieglstein J. Neuroprotective effect of 5-HT$_{1A}$ receptor agonist, Bay × 3702, demonstrated in vitro and in vivo. *Eur J Pharmacol* 1998; 359:251–260.

150. Torup L, Møller A, Sager TN, Diemer NH. Neuroprotective effect of 8-OH-DPAT in global cerebral ischemia assessed by stereological cell counting. *Eur J Pharmacol* 2000; 395:137–141.

151. Kline AE, Yu J, Horvath E, Marion DW, Dixon CE. The selective 5-HT$_{1A}$ receptor agonist repinotan HCL attenuates histopathology and spatial learning deficits following traumatic brain injury in rats. *Neuroscience* 2001; 106:547–555.

152. Kline AE, Yu J, Massucci JL, Zafonte RD, Dixon CE. Protective effects of the 5-HT$_{1A}$ receptor agonist 8-hydroxy-2-(di-*n*-propylamino)tetralin (8-OH-DPAT) against traumatic brain injury-induced cognitive deficits and neuropathology in adult male rats. *Neurosci Lett* 2002; 333:179–182.

153. Prehn JH, Backhauss C, Karkoutly C, Nuglisch J, Peruche B, Rossberg C, Krieglstein J. Neuroprotective properties of 5-HT$_{1A}$ receptor agonists in rodent models of focal and global cerebral ischemia. *Eur J Pharmacol* 1991; 203:213–222.

154. Andrade R. Electrophysiology of 5-HT$_{1A}$ receptors in the rat hippocampus and cortex. *Drug Dev Res* 1992; 26:275–286.

155. Raiteri M, Maura G, Barzizza A. Activation of presynaptic 5-hydroxytryptamine1-like receptors on glutamatergic terminals inhibits N-methyl-D-aspartate-induced cyclic GMP production in rat cerebellar slices. *J Pharmacol Exp Ther* 1991; 257: 1184–1188.

156. Matsuyama S, Nei K, Tanaka C. Regulation of glutamate release via NMDA and 5-HT1A receptors in guinea pig dentate gyrus. *Brain Res* 1996; 728:175–180.

157. Melena J, Chidlow G, Osborne NN. Blockade of voltage-sensitive Na$^+$ channels by the 5-HT1A receptor agonist 8-OH-DPAT: possible significance for neuroprotection. *Eur J Pharmacol* 2000; 406:319–324.

158. Hjorth S. Hypothermia in the rat induced by the potent serotonergic agent 8-OH-DPAT. *J Neural Transm* 1985; 61: 131–135.

159. Millan MJ, Rivet JM, Canton H, Le Maouille-Girardon S, Gobert A. Induction of hypothermia as a model of 5-hydroxytryptamine 1A receptor-mediated activity in the rat: a pharmacological characterization of the actions of novel agonists and antagonists. *J Pharmacol Exp Ther* 1993; 264:1364–1376.

160. Cryan JF, Kelliher P, Kelly JP, Leonard BE. Comparative effects of serotonergic agonists with varying efficacy at the 5-HT$_{1A}$ receptor on core temperature: modification by the selective 5-HT$_{1A}$ receptor antagonist WAY 100635. *J Psychopharmacol* 1999; 13:278–283.

161. Kline AE, Massucci JL, Dixon CE, Zafonte RD, Bolinger BD. The therapeutic efficacy conferred by the 5-HT$_{1A}$ receptor agonist 8-hydroxy-2-(di-*n*-propylamino)tetralin (8-OH-DPAT) after experimental traumatic brain injury is not mediated by concomitant hypothermia. *J Neurotrauma* 2004; 21:175–185.

162. Gorman LK, Fu K, Hovda DA, Murray M, Traystman RJ. Effects of traumatic brain injury on the cholinergic system in the rat. *J Neurotrauma* 1996; 13:457–463.

163. Saija A, Hayes RL, Lyeth BG. Effect of concussive head injury on central cholinergic neurons. *Brain Res* 1988; 452:303–311.

164. Saija A, Robinson SE, Lyeth BG. Effect of scopolamine and traumatic brain injury on central cholinergic neurons. *J Neurotrauma* 1988; 5:161–169.

165. Robinson SE, Foxx SD, Posner MG, Martin RM, Davis TR, Guo HZ, Enters EK The effect of M1 muscarinic blockade on behavior and physiological responses following traumatic brain injury in the rat. *Brain Res* 1990; 511:141–148.

166. Lyeth BG, Dixon CE, Hamm RJ, Jenkins LW, Young HF, Stonnington HH, Hayes RL. Effects of anticholinergic treatment on transient behavioral suppression and physiological responses following concussive brain injury to the rat. *Brain Res* 1988; 488: 88–97.

167. Dixon CE, Liu SJ, Jenkins LW, Bhattacharjee M, Whitson J, Yang K, Hayes RL. Time course of increased vulnerability of cholinergic neurotransmission following traumatic brain injury in the rats. *Behav Brain Res* 1995; 70:125–131.

168. Dixon CE, Bao J, Long DA, and Hayes RL. Reduced evoked release of acetylcholine in the rodent hippocampus following traumatic brain injury. *Pharmacol Biochem Behav* 1996; 53:579–686.

169. Dixon CE, Hamm RJ, Taft WC, Hayes RL. Increased anticholinergic sensitivity following closed skull impact and controlled cortical impact traumatic brain injury in the rat. *J Neurotrauma* 1994; 11:275–287.

170. Leonard JR, Maris DO, Grady MS. Fluid percussion injury causes loss of forebrain choline acetyltransferase and nerve growth factor receptor immunoreactive cells in the rat. *J Neurotrauma* 1994; 11:379–392.

171. Schmidt RH, Grady MS. Loss of forebrain cholinergic neurons following fluid-percussion injury: implications for cognitive impairment in closed head injury. *J Neurosurg* 1995; 3:496–502.

172. Schmidt RH, Scholten KJ, Maughan PH. Cognitive impairment and synaptosomal choline uptake in rats following impact acceleration injury. *J Neurotrauma* 2000; 17:1129–1139.

173. Ciallella JR, Yan HQ, Ma X, Wolfson BM, Marion DW, DeKosky ST, Dixon CE. Chronic effects of traumatic brain injury on hippocampal vesicular acetylcholine transporter and M$_2$ muscarinic receptor protein in rats. *Exp Neurol* 1998; 142:11–19.

174. Shao L, Ciallella JR, Yan HQ, Ma X, Wolfson BM, Marion DW, Dekosky ST, Dixon CE. Differential effects of traumatic brain injury on vesicular acetylcholine transporter and M2 muscarinic receptor mRNA and protein in rat. *J Neurotrauma* 1999; 16:555–566.

175. Dixon CE, Kochanek PM, Yan HQ, Schiding JK, Griffith R, Baum E, Marion DW, DeKosky ST. One-year study of spatial memory performance, brain morphology and cholinergic markers after moderate controlled cortical impact in rats. *J Neurotrauma* 1999; 16:109–122.

176. Dixon CE, Ma X, Marion DW. Effects of CDP-choline treatment on neurobehavioral deficits after TBI and on hippocampal and neocortical acetylcholine release. *J Neurotrauma* 1997; 14: 161–169.

177. Pike BR, Hamm RJ. Post injury administration of BIBN 99, a selective muscarinic M$_2$ receptor antagonist, improves cognitive

performance following traumatic brain injury in rats. *Brain Res* 1995; 686:37–43.

178. O'Dell DM, Hamm RJ. Chronic post injury administration of MDL 26,479 (suritozol) a negative modulator at the GABAA receptor, and cognitive impairment in rats following traumatic brain injury. *J Neurosurg* 1995; 83:878–883.

179. Taverni JP, Seliger G, Lichtman SW. Donepezil medicated memory improvement in traumatic brain injury during post acute rehabilitation. *Brain Inj* 1998; 12:77–80.

180. Whelan FJ, Walker MS, Schultz SK. Donepezil in the treatment of cognitive dysfunction associated with traumatic brain injury. *Ann Clin Psychiatry* 2000; 12:131–135.

181. Masanic CA, Bayley MT, VanReekum R, Simard M. Open-label study of donepezil in traumatic brain injury. *Arch Phys Med Rehabil* 2001; 82:896–901.

182. Morey CE, Cilo M, Berry J, Cusick C. The effect of aricept in persons with persistent memory disorder following traumatic brain injury: a pilot study. *Brain Inj* 2003; 17:809–815.

183. Bennett EL, Rosenzweig MR, Diamond MC. Rat brain: effects of environmental enrichment on wet and dry weights. *Science* 1969; 163:825–826.

184. van Praag K, Kempermann G, Gage FH. Neural consequences of environmental enrichment. *Nat Rev* 2000; 1:191–198.

185. Kempermann G, Kuhn HG, Gage FH. More hippocampal neurons in adult mice living in an enriched environment. *Nature* 1997; 386:493–495.

186. Nilsson M, Perfilieva E, Johansson U, Orwar O, Eriksson PS. Enriched environment increases neurogenesis in the adult rat dentate gyrus and improves spatial memory. *J Neurobiol* 1999; 39:569–578.

187. Young D, Lawlor PA, Leone P, Dragunow M, During MJ. Environmental enrichment inhibits spontaneous apoptosis, prevents seizures and is neuroprotective. *Nat Med* 1999; 5:448–453.

188. Torasdotter M, Metsis M, Henriksson BG, Winblad B, Mohammed AH. Environmental enrichment results in higher levels of nerve growth factor mRNA in the rat visual cortex and hippocampus. *Beh Brain Res* 1998; 93:83–90.

189. Rasmuson S, Olsson T, Henriksson BG, Kelly PAT, Holmes MC, Seckl JR, Mohammed AH. Environmental enrichment selectively increases 5-HT1A receptor mRNA expression and binding in the rat hippocampus. *Mol Brain Res* 1998; 53:285–290.

190. Falkenberg T, Mohammed AK, Henriksson B, Persson H, Winblad B, Lindefors N. Increased expression of brain-derived neurotrophic factor mRNA in rat hippocampus is associated with improved spatial memory and enriched environment. *Neurosci Lett* 1992; 138:153–156.

191. Nilsson L, Mohammed AKH, Henriksson BG, Folkesson R, Winblad B, Bergstr^m L. Environmental influence on somatostatin levels and gene expression in the rat brain. *Brain Res* 1993; 628:93–98.

192. Olsson T, Mohammed AH, Donaldson LF, Henriksson BG, Seckl JR. Glucocorticoid receptor and NGFI-A gene expression are induced on the hippocampus after environmental enrichment in adult rats. *Mol Brain Res* 1994; 23:349–353.

193. Zhao LR, Mattsson B, Johansson B. Environmental influence on brain-derived neurotrophic factor messenger RNA expression after middle cerebral artery occlusion in spontaneously hypertensive rats. *Neuroscience* 2000; 97:177–184.

194. Zhao LR, Risedal A, Wojcik A, Hejzlar J, Johansson BB, Kokaia Z. Enriched environment influences brain-derived neurotrophic factor levels in rat forebrain after focal stroke. *Neurosci Lett* 2001; 305:169–172.

195. Hicks RR, Zhang L, Atkinson A, Stevenon M, Veneracion M, Seroogy KB. Environmental enrichment attenuates cognitive deficits, but does not alter neurotrophin gene expression in the hippocampus following lateral fluid percussion brain injury. *Neuroscience* 2002; 3:631–637.

196. Hamm RJ, Temple MD, O'Dell DM, Pike BR, Lyeth BG. Exposure to environmental complexity promotes recovery of cognitive function after traumatic brain injury *J Neurotrauma* 1996; 13:41–47.

197. Passineau MJ, Green EJ, Dietrich WD. Therapeutic effects of environmental enrichment on cognitive and tissue integrity following severe traumatic brain injury in rats. *Exp Neurol* 2001; 168:373–384.

198. Held JM, Gordon J, Gentile AM. Environmental influences on locomotor recovery following cortical lesions in rats. *Beh Neurosci* 1985; 99:678–690.

199. Gentile AM, Beheshti Z. Enrichment versus exercise effects on motor impairments following cortical removals in rats. *Beh Neural Biol* 1987; 47:321–332.

200. Rose FD, Davey MJ, Love S, Dell PA. Environmental enrichment and recovery from contralateral sensory neglect in rats with large unilateral neocortical lesions. *Beh Brain Res* 1987; 24:195–202.

201. Wagner AK, Kline AE, Sokoloski J, Zafonte RD, Capulong E, Dixon CE. Intervention with environmental enrichment after experimental brain trauma enhances cognitive recovery in male but not female rats. *Neurosci Lett* 2002; 334:165–168.

202. Dash PK, Mach SA, Moore AN. Enhanced neurogenesis in the rodent hippocampus following traumatic brain injury. *J Neurosci Res* 2001; 63(4):313–319.

203. Kernie SG, Erwin TM, Parada LF. Brain remodeling due to neuronal and astrocytic proliferation after controlled cortical injury in mice. *J Neurosci Res* 2001; 66(3):317–326.

204. Chirumamilla S, Sun D, Bullock MR, Colello RJ. Traumatic brain injury induced cell proliferation in the adult mammalian central nervous system. *J Neurotrauma* 2002; 19(6):693–703.

205. Rice AC, Khaldi A, Harvey HB, Salman NJ, White F, Fillmore H, Bullock MR. Proliferation and neuronal differentiation of mitotically active cells following traumatic brain injury. *Exp Neurol* 2003; 183(2):406–417.

206. Mahmood A, Lu D, Yi L, Chen JL, Chopp M. Intracranial bone marrow transplantation after traumatic brain injury improving functional outcome in adult rats. *J Neurosurg* 2001; 94(4):589–595.

207. Lu D, Li Y, Wang L, Chen J, Mahmood A, Chopp M. Intraarterial administration of marrow stromal cells in a rat model of traumatic brain injury. *J Neurotrauma* 2001; 18(8):813–819.

208. Lu D, Mahmood A, Wang L, Li Y, Lu M, Chopp M. Adult bone marrow stromal cells administered intravenously to rats after traumatic brain injury migrate into brain and improve neurological outcome. *Neuroreport* 2001; 12(3):559–563.

209. Riess P, Zhang C, Saatman KE, Laurer HL, Longhi LG, Raghupathi R, Lenzlinger PM, Lifshitz J, Boockvar J, Neugebauer E, Snyder EY, McIntosh TK. Transplanted neural stem cells survive, differentiate, and improve neurological motor function after experimental traumatic brain injury. *Neurosurgery* 2002; 51(4):1043–1052.

210. Hoane MR, Becerra GD, Shank JE, Tatko L, Pak ES, Smith m, Murashov AK. Transplantation of neuronal and glial precursors dramatically improves sensorimotor function but not cognitive function in the traumatically injured brain. *J Neurotrauma* 2004; 21(2):163–174.

211. Lu D, Sanberg PR, Mahmood A, Li Y, Wang L, Sanchez-Ramos J, Chopp M. Intravenous administration of human umbilical cord blood reduces neurological deficit in the rat after traumatic brain injury. *Cell Transplant* 2002; 11(3):275–281.

212. McIntosh TK, Vink R, Yamakami I, Faden AI. Magnesium protects against neurological deficit after brain injury. *Brain Res* 1989; 482:252–260.

213. Smith DH, Okiyama K, Gennarelli TA, McIntosh Magnesium and ketamine attenuate cognitive dysfunction following experimental brain injury. *Neurosci Lett* 1993; 157:211–214.

214. Bareyre FM, Saatman KE, Raghupathi R, McIntosh TK. Postinjury treatment with magnesium chloride attenuates cortical damage after traumatic brain injury in rats. *J Neurotrauma* 2000; 17:1029–1039.

215. Saatman KE, Bareyre FM, Grady MS, McIntosh TK. Acute cytoskeletal alterations and cell death induced by experimental brain injury are attenuated by magenesium treatment and exacerbated by magenesium deficiency. *J Neuropathol Exp Neurol* 2001; 60:183–194.

216. Muir JK, Raghupathi R, Emery DL, Bareyre FM, McIntosh TK. Postinjury magnesium treatment attenuates traumatic brain injury-induced cortical induction of p53 mRNA in rats. *Exp Neurol* 1999; 159:584–593.

217. Browne KD, Leoni MJ, Iwata A, Chen XH, Smith DH. Acute treatment with MgSO$_4$ attenuates long-term hippocampal tissue loss after brain trauma in the rat. *J Neurosci Res* 2004; 77(6):878–883.

218. Heath DL, Vink R. Improved motor outcome in response to magnesium therapy received up to 24 hr after traumatic diffuse axonal brain injury in rats. *J Neurosurg* 1999; 90:504–509.

219. Vink R, O'Connor CA, Nimmo AJ, Heath DL. Magnesium attenuates persistant functional deficits following diffuse traumatic brain injury in rats. *Neurosci Lett* 2003; 336:41–44.

220. Hoane MR, Irish SL, Marks BB, Barth TM. Preoperative regimens of magnesium facilitate recovery of function and prevent subcortical atrophy following lesions of the rat sensorimotor cortex. *Brain Res Bull* 1998; 45:45–51.

221. Baskaya MK, Dogan A, Rao AM, Dempsey RJ. Neuroprotective effects of citicholine on brain edema and blood-brain barrier breakdown after traumatic brain injury. *J Neurosurg* 2000; 92:448–452.

222. Dempsey RJ, Raghavendra Rao VL. Cytidinediphosphocholine treatment to decrease traumatic brain injury-induced hippocampal neuronal death, cortical contusion volume, and neurological dysfunction in rats. *J Neurosurg* 2003; 98:867–873.

223. Sullivan PG, Geiger JD, Mattson MP, Scheff SW. Dietary supplement creatine protects against traumatic brain injury. *Ann Neurol* 2000; 48:723–729.

224. Hoane MR, Akstulewicz SL, Toppen J. Treatment with vitamin B3 improves functional recovery and reduces GAP expression following traumatic brain injury in rats. *J Neurotrauma* 2003; 20:1189–1199.

225. Inci S, Ozcan OE, Kilinc K. Time-level relationship for lipid peroxidation and the protective effect of α-tocopherol in experimental mild and severe brain injury. *Neurosurgery* 1998; 43:330–335.

III

NEUROIMAGING AND NEURODIAGNOSTIC TESTING

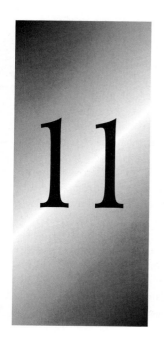

11 Static Neuroimaging in the Evaluation of TBI

John M. Barkley
Denise Morales
L. Anne Hayman
Pedro J. Diaz-Marchan

INTRODUCTION

Traumatic brain injury is a common problem in emergency facilities—especially in urban trauma centers. Surgical and medical management depend on the specific injuries a patient has sustained and a timely diagnosis at the time he or she enters the emergency center. Surgical and medical management also depends on both clinical data and imaging results. Both are essential for the appropriate selection of therapy.

Medical imaging has progressed substantially in the last several years, in part due to advances in neurological imaging. Imaging is a representation of the underlying vital structures that are deep below the skin. The human brain is a three-dimensional entity, but it is converted by hardware, software, and digital technology into a two-dimensional image that can be viewed on a sheet of film or at a computer workstation. One of the principal reasons that the field of radiology has advanced so much in the last several years has been the computer industry. The ability to digitally display and store high-resolution images has improved substantially.

Plain film radiography provides very little useful information for patients with traumatic brain injury (1). Plain films may be used to look for foreign bodies or visualize fractures, however computed tomography (CT) and magnetic resonance imaging (MRI) are essential for the accurate diagnosis and subsequent management of patients with traumatic brain injury. While MRI has made remarkable advances in the past 10 years, CT continues to be the initial imaging modality for the brain in the acute setting (2). Three-dimensional reconstructions of axial CT data may now be obtained, essentially eliminating plain film radiography from the imaging arsenal used in the workup of acute trauma.

One should understand the pathophysiology of different brain injuries and recognize these injuries in any form of imaging. While technology does change, the pathophysiology and appearance of these lesions remains the same. It is our hope that by the end of this chapter, the reader will have formed a sound understanding of the imaging appearance of the major pathologic entities of traumatic brain injury encountered in clinical practice. Both CT and MRI are described separately below, followed by the specific traumatic entities that are organized in a systematic fashion.

IMAGING TECHNIQUE

Modern digital imaging technology allows manipulation of data to reconstruct images in multiple planes. This manipulation of data allows the interpreting physician to gain three-dimensional information about the human brain from two-dimensional data. In addition, there are currently many three-dimensional techniques available for certain applications, although not practical in the acute setting. Imaging of the traumatically injured brain should be fast, reliable, diagnostic, and widely available. The workhorse of any facility continues to be CT scanning. Helical CT is extremely fast. It allows the technician to obtain whole-body images in a single breath hold. This is of paramount importance in patients who have sustained polytrauma of other organs in addition to brain injuries.

Many investigators have attempted to develop criteria for obtaining a CT scan in the acute setting for the evaluation of traumatic brain injury. The American College of Radiology (ACR) conducted a study in 1986 that ultimately divided neurologically traumatized patients into three groups of risk: low, moderate, and high. The low-risk group consisted of patients with minor symptoms without neurological deficits such as headache, dizziness, or scalp injuries. It was proposed that this group of patients could be observed without the need for imaging. The moderate- and high-risk groups included those patients with neurological deficits, altered consciousness, seizures, depressed skull fractures, or penetrating injuries. It was proposed that these patients should receive a non-contrast CT scan of the brain as part of the initial work-up (3). Although the ACR and others have attempted to define the indications for obtaining an imaging study in minor trauma, currently this is a multifactorial decision made in emergency centers across the country. Some researchers have also found that brain injuries detectable by CT imaging may occur in people with relatively minor complaints, normal neurological exam and/or a normal Glasgow Coma Scale (GCS) of 15 (4). Issues such as cost, risk-to-benefit ratio, and medical/legal concerns play roles in the decision to image patients with mild brain injuries or post-concussive disorders.

Computed Tomography

Sir Godfrey N. Hounsfield of Great Britain and Allan M. Cormack of the United States won the 1979 Nobel Prize in Medicine for their groundbreaking work that made CT a reality in the 1970s. A conventional CT scanner consists of a gantry, table, and computer workstation. Early CT scanners were slow and cumbersome. Only one slice could be acquired at a time. The incorporation of slip-ring technology in the 1990s allowed helical CT units with a continually rotating gantry to become available. With helical CT, the table and the patient are continually moving through the gantry. Many of these units also employ multiple detector arrays that increase the volume of tissue imaged and improve the speed with which the study is performed. Current multiple detector helical CT scanners produce remarkable images and allow versatile

reconstruction of volume data in multiple planes—axial, sagittal, coronal, and oblique projections. These units are four to six times faster than older helical units. An entire CT of the abdomen and pelvis may be performed in a trauma patient with a single breath hold in less than 30 sec. CT scans of the brain may be performed even faster.

The raw data obtained from CT detectors is mathematically manipulated using several algorithms and filters to obtain visual data that offers both spatial and contrast information. The visual contrast between different tissues when viewing a CT image is due to differences in the absorption of x-rays. The properties that govern x-ray absorption on plain films are identical for CT. As x-ray photons pass through air and tissue, the useful beam is subject to attenuation—or removal of photons (5). The x-rays may be attenuated (absorbed), scattered in a new direction, or pass through the tissue of interest.

The two extremes of air and metal have characteristic appearances on CT because no x-rays are absorbed by air while nearly all x-rays are absorbed by metal. Everything in between these two extremes has a spectrum of CT appearances. Visually, air is black, fat is dark, and soft tissue and fluid are shades of gray. Bone is white and metal is extremely bright—often causing streak artifact on the CT images. The Hounsfield Scale, named for the father of computed tomography, allows one to quantitate the actual tomographic densities of these different tissues. In fact, CT's ability to distinguish between subtle differences of similar tissues—or contrast resolution, is the true advantage of CT as an imaging modality. Hounsfield Units (HU) are numerical values that are assigned to each pixel (picture element) in a CT image. The scale is roughly −1000 to +3000. Water or simple fluid like cerebrospinal fluid (CSF) is set as the baseline of zero. Air is black, or −1000, while bright metal or iodinated contrast material is close to +3000. Soft tissue ranges from about −200 to +200. Gray matter of the brain is typically around 30–40 Hounsfield units. When interpreting a CT image of the brain, the density of surrounding structures or abnormalities is often compared to gray matter. A typical radiology report may read, "there is an intra-axial mass that is isodense (the same density) to gray matter."

Another advantage of CT is the ability to manipulate the raw data to augment certain visual characteristics for the person interpreting the image. Bone windows, brain windows, soft tissue windows, lung windows, and so on, are simply different ways of viewing the same raw data to take advantage of contrast differences. These different window settings are made by employing unique computer algorithms, or filters, to manipulate the raw data. These settings have both a window level and a window width. A window level is the center value of a certain setting, while the window width is the range around the center value. It is the window width that determines the visual contrast or "shades of gray" displayed for a certain setting (5). The window level accounts for the tissue brightness that is displayed (6).

The only absolute contraindication to obtaining a non-contrast CT is an unstable patient. Because CT imaging uses ionizing radiation, special care should be used with children and pregnant patients. Organs that are not included in the region of interest may be shielded with lead to protect them from unnecessary exposure to radiation. Although there is no danger with obtaining CT in patients with aneurysm clips or intracranial metal, these objects do create artifacts that render the interpretation of a CT difficult.

In order to perform a CT, the patient is placed in the supine position on the table and moved into the gantry. A CT scout image, or topogram, is obtained in order to determine the area that should be scanned. The scout image looks like a lateral plain film of the skull. The technologist can then orient the plane of the scan and set the slice thickness. Typically, the axial images are obtained parallel to the orbital roof. A trauma CT scan of the brain is performed without contrast in order to identify acute hemorrhage, which appears hyperdense (bright) on CT.

CT may also be obtained after the administration of intravenous, iodinated contrast material. Contrast is usually not needed in the evaluation of acute traumatic brain injury, unless screening of the vasculature is warranted. For suspected vascular injury, dedicated conventional angiography is often performed rather than CT angiography because of increased sensitivity and the ability for therapeutic intervention to be performed quickly if needed. Thus, routinely giving contrast for a CT in the acute setting for a patient with suspected brain injuries is a wasted step and may obscure underlying acute hemorrhage.

Contrast is administered in order to evaluate medical pathology for which the blood-brain barrier has been violated. These include inflammatory, infectious, vascular, and neoplastic abnormalities. Contrast is given to identify the enhancement patterns of intracranial mass, cerebral abscess, subdural empyema, encephalitis, and vasculitis. Contrast material is also required for performing CT angiography in order to visualize the enhancing arteries and veins.

With the advent of multidetector CT (MDCT), fast imaging of large volumes of tissue is possible, without sacrificing spatial resolution. MDCT with thin slices can be combined with software packages that optimize vascular enhancement. This allows one to control the intravenous bolus of contrast, specifying arterial phase and delayed venous phase scanning. This becomes important for CT angiography and evaluation of intracranial vasculature noninvasively. Post-processing techniques such as maximum intensity projection (MIP), volume rendering (VR), shaded surface display (SSD), and curved planar reformatted images allow one to manipulate the MDCT data to optimally display intracranial vascular

structures and detect pathology such as arterial occlusion, dissection, pseudoaneurysm formation, and vasospasm. Goldsher et al. evaluated 36 patients presenting with subarachnoid hemorrhage using MDCT angiography of the vertebrobasilar system. Their results suggest that cerebral MDCT angiography is a reliable, rapid, and minimally invasive diagnostic method, for assessing vasospasm of the posterior circulation in patients with subarachnoid hemorrhage (7). More studies are needed at large volume trauma centers to further define the role of MDCT angiography in the evaluation of traumatic intracranial vascular injury.

Sequential axial nonenhanced images of the brain are performed from the base of the skull through the vertex with slices that vary in thickness from 5 mm to 7 mm. Current helical scanners obtain overlapping voxels (volume elements) of tissue continuously from start to finish. The raw CT data is manipulated and sent to a workstation for processing. Images may then be viewed in different window settings on the workstation, film or Picture Archiving and Communication System (PACS). CT scans of the brain are often viewed in bone windows (window level: 700, window width: 3500), brain windows (window level: 40, window width: 100) and intermediate windows (window level: 80, window width 250)—for purposes of identifying subtle hemorrhages along the surface of the brain (1). Many hospitals are now converting to digital PACS systems in order to take advantage of the ability to manipulate data, eliminate film costs and allow clinicians to access a computer version of images and reports.

Magnetic Resonance Imaging

Magnetic Resonance Imaging (MRI) is an imaging technique that plays an adjunctive role in brain injury. The ability for tissue/fluid characterization and multiplanar imaging are advantages of MRI. While the imaging times of MRI have shortened with improved equipment and stronger magnets, performing an MRI is still much longer than performing a CT scan. Thus, the use of MRI in patients with acute traumatic brain injury is limited to certain patient populations. When compared to CT, MRI provides exquisite soft tissue detail, evaluation of the brainstem, skull base, and cranial nerves. It displays particularly well the posterior fossa, which is often obscured by a beam-hardening artifact that occurs with CT.

MRI is used primarily in the work-up of chronic conditions or for following the sequelae of traumatic brain injury. It is more accurate in assessing the general age of intracranial blood products. The appearance of evolving intracranial hemorrhage is described in detail later in the text. MR angiography is a technique that is useful to screen for concurrent vascular injuries in the head and neck. However, conventional angiography remains the gold standard in the evaluation of traumatic vascular injury, both for diagnosis and the opportunity for endovascular therapy such as embolization, angioplasty or stenting.

The human body is made up of water, natural elements, minerals and macromolecules such as proteins, fats, and carbohydrates. One of the main components is the hydrogen proton. Magnetic resonance imaging relies on the signal emitted by relaxing protons as they are disturbed by external magnetic fields and radiofrequency pulses. An MRI unit consists of a powerful external magnetic field, transmitting coils, receiving coils, patient table and a digital workstation (Figure 11-1). With the application of a strong external magnetic field, hydrogen protons in the body align themselves either parallel or anti-parallel with this field. Most of the protons align themselves with the lower energy parallel state, creating a net magnetic moment in the direction of the external magnetic field (8). This net magnetic moment in the direction of the external magnetic field is called the longitudinal vector.

Each proton has a spin and a motion called precession. The frequency with which the protons precess depend on the strength of the external magnetic field. The relationship between the precession frequency and the external magnetic field is described by the Larmor equation (5, 8):

$$\omega_0 = \gamma B_0$$
ω_0 is the precession frequency (Hz)
γ is the gyro magnetic ratio
B_0 is the strength of the external magnetic field (Tesla)

It can be derived from the equation that the precession of protons varies directly with the strength of the magnetic field. Stronger magnets produce faster precession.

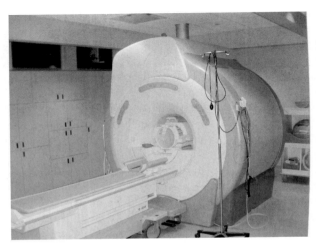

FIGURE 11-1

Standard 1.5 Tesla MRI gantry

This property allows for a higher signal and improved image quality. Most diagnostic quality magnets available in hospitals or outpatient facilities are in the 1.0–1.5 Tesla range. Magnets in the 3.0–7.0 Tesla range are now being used in academic centers for human and animal research. Stronger magnets will improve the quality, signal-to-noise ratio, and speed of acquisition of MR images in the future.

A radiofrequency pulse (RF) at the same frequency as the precessing protons is then turned on. This pulse disrupts the parallel/antiparallel equilibrium of the protons within the external magnetic field. Some protons are flipped into the higher-energy state, or antiparallel orientation. This eliminates the net magnetic longitudinal vector that had been in the direction of the external magnetic field. This disruption of the longitudinal vector, or transfer of energy from the RF pulse to the precessing protons is called *resonance* (8). The RF pulse results in a decrease or elimination of the longitudinal net magnetization and also allows the protons to precess in phase with one another. Because the protons are precessing in phase during the RF pulse, a net magnetization in the transverse direction is then created. Thus, after the RF pulse is turned on, the longitudinal magnetization in the direction of external magnetic field decreases, while a new transverse magnetization is created due to the protons now precessing in phase.

The RF pulse is then turned off. Protons gradually flip back to the lower-energy parallel orientation in the direction of the external magnetic field. The longitudinal magnetization vector gradually reappears. The reappearance of the longitudinal vector is called longitudinal relaxation and is described by the time constant T_1, or longitudinal relaxation time. The transverse magnetization that had been created by the protons precessing in phase disappears when the RF pulse is turned off. This is described by the transverse relaxation time, T_2. T_1 relaxation depends on the strength of the external magnetic field, tissue composition and structure. T_2 relaxation is affected by magnetic field inhomogeneities.

Each type of tissue has unique T_1 and T_2 properties that affect how they will appear on an MR image. When the RF pulse is turned off, special coils around the patient detect the signal of the increasing longitudinal vector and decreasing transverse vector (8). The decay and growth of these relaxation properties may be plotted on a graph. By changing different parameters and imaging times of the MRI sequence, one can take advantage of the different points along these relaxation curves, thereby affecting the signal of different tissues. These parameters can render an image T_1 weighted, T_2 weighted, or a combination of the two. In addition, each tissue has a certain proportion of protons per unit volume. Parameters can also be changed to take advantage of this proton density. For instance, water or fluid has a long T_1 and is typically dark on a T_1 weighted image and bright on a T_2 weighted image. Fat has a short T_1 and is typically bright on both T_1 and T_2 weighted images.

In order to localize the protons or the signal created within tissue, gradient magnetic fields are applied in a multiplanar fashion. The applied external magnetic field created by the MR gantry is fairly uniform or homogenous. Gradients are applied to the main magnetic field to create local differences across the area of interest. In other words, the magnetic field will change across the patient in several directions, determined by the gradients applied. These magnetic field gradients are imposed on the external field in order to change the precession frequency of each proton in the body slightly, allowing spatial localization to take place. Each proton can be identified in space and location because of its unique spin created by applying these known gradient fields across the regions of interest. The magnetic field gradients and radiofrequency excitations help to localize the signal from each voxel (volume element) within the patient being imaged (5, 8). It is beyond the scope of this chapter to describe the specific appearance of each tissue within a myriad of MR pulse sequences that seem to change daily.

CT is the dominant imaging modality for the detection of traumatic brain injury in the acute setting, while MRI is very helpful for the detection of occult lesions, follow-up and the long-term management of patients with traumatic brain injuries. Most initial decisions concerning management, such as surgery or no surgery in the emergency setting, are made based on the findings of a non-contrast CT of the brain. MRI may be obtained in the acute setting if there are clinical findings out of proportion to the CT findings, suggesting diffuse axonal injury or stroke. MRI also shows the chronic sequelae of the initial injury with excellent detail. Some common indications for obtaining an MRI in a post-traumatic work-up include chronic headaches, stroke, pseudoaneurysm, dementia, hydrocephalus, cranial nerve palsy, cavernous sinus injuries, persistent neurological deficits, or patients with diffuse axonal injury in light of a normal CT of the brain (1, 9, 10). The findings on MRI have implications on predicting patient outcome as well, and this topic will be discussed at the end of the chapter.

Gadolinium is a rare earth element with an atomic number of 64 that can be chelated to form MRI contrast material. Intravenous gadolinium chelate is non-iodinated and contrast reactions or renal failure are much less common than with iodinated contrast material. Gadolinium is paramagnetic, meaning that it affects the T_1 and T_2 characteristics in such a way that enhancement on post-contrast T_1 images can be seen. Gadolinium provides the same information that iodinated contrast provides on CT—it allows visualization of vasculature and areas of breakdown of the blood-brain barrier. MRI is often used in the subacute or chronic setting of relatively stable patients. Gadolinium is extremely safe and it is often used in many protocols after noncontrast MR images have been obtained.

BRAIN INJURY

Imaging technology changes quickly; thus it is advantageous to learn pathology in an organ-based fashion. No matter how the technology changes, the pathology remains the same. With the basic knowledge of pathophysiology, one can learn and adapt to how a particular condition appears within a myriad of changing imaging modalities. Imaging of patients with traumatic brain injury in the acute setting often begins with a noncontrast CT of the brain (6). All of the available data including history, physical exam, mechanism of injury, and vital signs are used in conjunction with the imaging evaluation to triage these patients into surgical or medical management. If surgery will be needed, decisions as to the timing of surgery are also made based on the clinical presentation and imaging results. These acute injuries may require early neurosurgical intervention and a timely interpretation of the imaging findings is advantageous in the emergency room setting (11).

When interpreting an emergent CT scan of the brain, particular attention should be paid to the midline structures, presence of shift, ventricles, basal cisterns, the presence of herniation, cerebral convexities, and mass effect (12). The skull of infants and young children has open sutures and fontanelles; thus there is more plasticity of the cranial vault, should pathology develop. The adult brain exists in a closed box, the densely ossified skull that does not yield to intracranial pathology. Skull fractures, particularly depressed fractures often herald underlying brain injuries. Another advantage of CT is the exsquisite bony detail it offers. Subtle, nondisplaced fractures in the plane of the scan may go undetected; however, these are felt by many researchers to be clinically insignificant (3,13). CT allows one to characterize fractures, the extent of bony injury and the sequelae of these fractures to the underlying brain parenchyma.

Air present within the skull or brain is termed pneumocephalus. The presence of pneumocephalus often heralds the presence of a fracture, usually communicating with air in the sinuses or outside of the skull. It is imperative to recognize fractures involving neurologically exquisite areas such as the orbit or the temporal bone. Temporal bone fractures, depending on type may lead to cerebrospinal fluid otorrhea, conductive hearing loss, sensorineural hearing loss or facial nerve paralysis. Other fractures such as nondisplaced calvareal fractures may be managed conservatively.

There is a finite amount of space within the adult skull. If something occurs within the skull to occupy the space, it occurs at the expense of the brain that is soft and very pliable. In response to a space-occupying intracranial lesion, the brain may become deformed, swollen or edematous. If the mass effect within the skull is severe enough, a herniation syndrome may result. The brain is made up of gray and white matter. The gray matter consists of the cerebral cortex, cerebellar cortex, and deep nuclei. The white matter consists of a network of axons—connections and tracts between these nuclei. Injuries involving the brain itself—the gray or white matter of the brain parenchyma, are called intra-axial injuries. The extra-axial space, on the other hand, is outside of the brain parenchyma. The brain is separated from the inner table of the calvarium by several layers of tissue called meninges.

The meninges are composed of different layers of connective tissue. The dura is the outer layer that is firmly attached to the inner table and periosteum of the skull. The arachnoid exists between the dura and the pia. The pia is a thin lining that covers the brain and spinal cord. It follows the cortex of the brain and lines each gyrus, while dipping into the intervening sulci. The subarachnoid space is the space bounded by the arachnoid layer and pia. It contains cerebrospinal fluid and blood vessels. There are several areas within the brain where the subarachnoid space expands to create cisterns. Abnormalities that affect the subarachnoid space may extend into these cisterns (14). The pia and arachnoid comprise the leptomeninges. Injuries outside of the brain parenchyma are called extra-axial injuries.

The brain and spinal cord are bathed in cerebrospinal fluid (CSF). This fluid is also present in the ventricles and cisterns of the brain. There are two lateral ventricles, with frontal, temporal, and occipital horns. The third and fourth ventricles are unpaired, midline structures. The lateral ventricles communicate with the third ventricle through the paired foramina of Monro. The third ventricle communicates with the fourth ventricle—which is in the posterior fossa of the brain through the cerebral aqueduct. In the normal state, the CSF volume remains relatively constant, although it is constantly in flux. A homeostasis is reached where the amount of CSF produced in the choroids plexus is the same as the amount of CSF being absorbed into the venous sinuses. Cerebral capillaries form an impermeable blood-brain barrier and the capillaries and ependymal cells form a blood-CSF barrier (14). These barriers may break down in pathological conditions such as trauma, infection or tumor. Injuries within the ventricles or CSF spaces, while inside the confines of the brain, are actually outside the brain parenchyma and thus are extra-axial injuries. Sometimes, it is difficult to determine whether a lesion is intra-axial or extra-axial, however there are signs on imaging that help to define the location of lesions.

In the sections that follow, several types of traumatic brain injury will be discussed. The injuries are organized according to location. Injuries involving the brain parenchyma, or intra-axial space will be discussed first, followed by a discussion of extra-axial manifestations of traumatic brain injury.

Intra-axial: Brain Contusions

Some authors have described brain injuries based on the mechanism of injury—such as impact injuries versus inertial injuries, or primary versus secondary injuries (15). The traumatic neuropathology described in this chapter will be divided into intra-axial injuries and extra-axial injuries. Injury of the brain may occur from blunt or penetrating forces. Lesions such as brain contusions or epidural hematomas occur due to direct force, while other injuries, described later, occur due to acceleration/deceleration or rotational forces.

Direct forces may impact on the skull and underlying brain to cause injury to the brain parenchyma. These manifest acutely as brain contusions (Figure 11-2). A contusion may be hemorrhagic (Figure 11-3) or nonhemorrhagic, and all involve the gray matter of the brain. The two main reasons for not giving contrast prior to imaging a patient with acute intracranial injuries are to perform the exam quickly and to look for intracranial blood products.

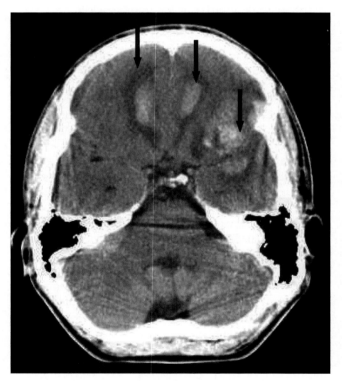

FIGURE 11-2

Intra-axial hematomas: Axial noncontrast CT demonstrates intra-axial contusions in the bilateral frontal lobes and left temporal lobe (arrows). There is associated vasogenic edema

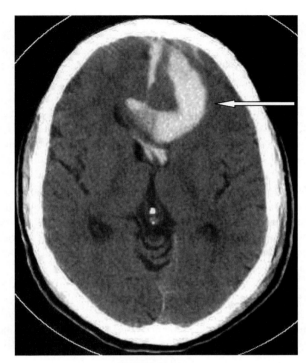

FIGURE 11-3

Hemorrhagic contusion: Axial noncontrast CT demonstrates a hemorrhagic contusion (arrow) in the left frontal lobe that extends across the midline and is associated with left to right shift and subfalcine herniation

Acute blood within the brain is bright on a non-contrast CT of the head, as is contrast material. Thus, contrast is withheld when evaluating the brain. The brightness of blood occurs due to the globin moiety of hemoglobin. Dehydration or an increase in hematocrit, may lead to a dense appearance of normal intracranial vasculature. In addition, hemorrhage may also appear denser than expected in these conditions (16).

Everything bright in the brain on CT may not always be due to acute hemorrhage. Calcification is also bright, and presents physiologically in the pineal gland and choroid plexus. In addition, the basal ganglia may exhibit calcification that is usually symmetrical from side to side. Dystrophic calcifications sometimes occur within the brain parenchyma due to prior infection or trauma. These dystrophic calcifications do not have mass effect or edema associated with them and will not enhance. Hemorrhagic contusions typically have a hypodense (dark) rim around them that represents edema (6). Arterial and venous malformations may also appear bright on CT, but are non-traumatic in nature. These conditions are associated with avid, tubular enhancement. In the case of an arterial-venous malformation, one may detect a nidus of tangled vessels that are associated with a prominent draining vein. These congenital or acquired vascular malformations are occasionally mistaken for traumatic injuries to the untrained eye. Follow-up imaging such as MRI or angiography are obtained to further characterize these lesions as vascular malformations.

Hypodense lesions on CT (dark lesions) usually indicate the presence of ischemia, infarction or contusions that are non-hemorrhagic (17). While bright contusions are hemorrhagic, non-hemorrhagic contusions are hypodense—or darker than the surrounding brain on noncontrast CT images. This is due to local edema and fluid. Small lesions are often nonhemorrhagic or the blood is beyond the resolution of CT and not visible on the image. These types of lesions may be missed on CT. Other dark, nontraumatic lesions such as lipomas, dermoids, or arachnoid cysts can be characterized as such due to the presence of fat or fluid density.

By definition, all brain contusions are intra-axial and involve the brain parenchyma. Specifically, they involve the gray matter of the brain cortex and typically occur in the anterior and basal aspects of the frontal, temporal, and occipital lobes. These regions are most susceptible to contusions because of the bony ridges immediately adjacent to the aforementioned locations. Temporal lobe injuries are adjacent to the petrous bone or greater wing of the sphenoid bone. Frontal lobe contusions are adjacent to the cribriform plate or lesser wing of the sphenoid bone (12). Contusions occur in 5–10 percent of patients with moderate or severe head trauma (18). They cause local mass effect of surrounding structures and efface adjacent sulci, ventricles and cisterns. When at the brain periphery, they form acute angles with the skull. If the contusion is located immediately adjacent to the site of external trauma, it is a coup injury. If the contusion is opposite to the site of external trauma, it is a contra-coup injury. If the contusions are large enough, they may cause severe mass effect, midline shift or herniation. These large contusions may require neurosurgical intervention to prevent secondary injuries to the remaining brain such as infarction due to vascular compression, hydrocephalus or cranial nerve palsy. Hemorrhages of the deep gray matter nuclei such as the basal ganglia sometimes occurs after severe mechanisms of injury due to rupture of perforating vessels.

In contrast to the CT appearance of hemorrhage—which depends upon the globin moiety of hemoglobin—the MRI appearance of hemorrhage is quite variable. MRI provides much more detailed information, regarding the chronicity of blood products. This is due to the ability of MRI to characterize, in a temporal fashion, the process of blood product degradation. The MRI imaging parameters, the timing of the hemorrhage and the oxidation of iron in hemoglobin all affect the appearance of blood products on MRI. Acute hemorrhage contains oxygenated hemoglobin, or oxyhemoglobin inside red blood cells. Acute blood within minutes after bleeding is composed of oxyhemoglobin appears similar to fluid (low T1, high T2).

Oxyhemoglobin is isointense (similar) to gray matter on T1-weighting, and hyperintense (bright) relative to gray matter on T2-weighting. Oxyhemoglobin is rarely detected with MRI unless the patient is actively bleeding or is sustaining intermittent bleeds prior to the MRI. Active bleeding is rarely appreciated on MRI because the exam is obtained in a delayed fashion, after the patient is stable. This is in contrast to CT, where patients are often imaged in the acute setting, and often require emergent therapy while in the gantry. Many of the treatment decisions prior to obtaining an MRI have already been made from the findings seen on noncontrast CT.

Within hours after acute intracranial hemorrhage, blood within the red blood cells becomes deoxygenated (8–72 hr), resulting in conversion from oxyhemoglobin to deoxyhemoglobin. This appears hypointense (dark) on both T1- and T2-weighting. During this phase, hemorrhage may be difficult to detect or qualify based on routine MRI parameters. Gradient echo sequences are often helpful in these instances, because of the magnetic susceptibility artifact caused by the iron moiety in hemoglobin (19). Magnetic susceptibility occurs due to drastic changes in tissue magnetization at tissue/air or tissue/metal interfaces (5). This entity causes a blooming appearance, or an enlarged hypointense (dark) halo around areas of metal, hemosiderin or air. The iron that becomes deposited within areas of hemorrhage is often detectable months after the injury on gradient echo MRI, when other MRI sequences have normalized (20).

After 3 to 7 days, intracellular deoxyghemoglobin becomes oxidized into intracellular methemoglobin, that appears hyperintense (bright) on T1-weighting and hypointense (dark) on T2-weighting. After 10 to 14 days, the red blood cells are broken down, releasing extracellular methemoglobin—that is, a paramagnetic substance and appears bright on both T1- and T2-weighting. Other substances that are bright on a T1 weighted image include gadolinium, fat, melanin and proteinaceous substances. Blood products are classically described as one of the causes of hyperintense (bright) foci on a precontrast T1-weighted MRI image. As stated earlier, because an MRI is usually obtained well after the acute insult, blood products are usually in the methemoglobin phase, which is bright on T1.

As white blood cells are mobilized to the site of chronic blood (months to years after hemorrhage), the extracellular methemoglobin is stored as ferritin and hemosiderin. Ferritin and hemosiderin appear hypointense (dark) to gray matter on both T1- and T2-weighting (1, 21–23). This appears as a dark ring—the hemosiderin ring around areas of old hemorrhage. Gradient echo and susceptibility sequences, as mentioned previously are exsquisitely sensitive to iron or metal. This allows the sequelae of prior hemorrhage to be detected months to years after the inciting injury. In addition, these sequences are good for detecting blood products or hemosiderin within the sulci and subarachnoid spaces—leptomeningeal hemosiderosis. Leptomeningeal hemosiderosis involves deposits of hemosiderin (iron) within the sulci, causing diffuse low signal intensity within sulci on T1 and T2 weighting.

In summary, the appearance of blood products on MRI is quite variable and depends on the timing of imaging in relation to when the injury occurred. The ability of MRI to image the physiologic degradation and evolution of hemorrhage allows one to more accurately describe the age of blood products. To review, hemorrhage evolves from hyperacute oxyhemoglobin (high T2) to acute deoxyhemoglobin (low T1, low T2) to early subacute intracellular methemoglobin (high T1, low T2) to late subacute extracellular methemoglobin (high T1, high T2), and finally to chronic hemosiderin (low T1/T2 ring; magnetic susceptibility).

Intra-axial: Shearing Injuries

Shearing injuries, like parenchymal contusions, may be either hemorrhagic or nonhemorrhagic. They typically occur at the gray/white matter junction, in a subcortical location. These injuries result from acceleration or deceleration of the brain during trauma. Shearing injuries may also occur in the brainstem, corpus callosum and septum pellucidum (24). Like any small abnormality in the brain, subtle lesions may not be appreciated with CT. Occasionally, shearing injuries are manifested as 1–5 mm petechial areas of hemorrhage. MRI has the advantage of gradient echo and magnetic susceptibility sequences that take advantage of the blooming phenomenon that occurs in areas of hemorrhage on MRI. Thus, MRI may detect a greater number of small hemorrhages that may not be seen with non-contrast CT (25). Shearing injuries may manifest clinically as neurological, cognitive or behavioral impairment. Shearing injuries may also occur in infants and young children due to non-accidental trauma. Shaken baby syndrome classically produces shearing injuries within the brain as well as retinal hemorrhages (26). Shearing injuries may also result from the rotational forces and impact injuries that occur during certain types of athletic pursuits, most notably contact sports (27).

A normal CT scan in light of a neurologically devastated patient is a classic finding in diffuse axonal injury (DAI). It is the most common cause of a post-traumatic vegetative state (1). DAI consists of innumerable shearing injuries that are often beyond the resolution of CT (28). The injuries typically occur at the gray-white matter junction in the frontal and temporal lobes. In very severe trauma, diffuse axonal injury may occur in the lobar white matter, corpus callosum and brainstem (Figure 11-4). In the brainstem, these shearing injuries are typically located in the dorsolateral aspects of the pons and midbrain. DAI occurs after acute acceleration/deceleration forces disrupt neuronal axons. The mechanism of injury is typically severe such as that seen in high-speed motor vehicle accidents. If the axonal injuries are nonhemorrhagic, they will likely not be seen on CT. Because CT often misses these injuries, follow-up MRI in patients with DAI may demonstrate bright T2 foci at the gray-white interfaces or even delayed petechial hemorrhages (23). MRI is much more sensitive in the detection of diffuse axonal injuries than is CT (Figure 11-5). Many of these injuries likely go undetected on any imaging modality. Gradient echo MR sequences are sensitive for subtle blood products by taking advantage of the blooming, or magnetic susceptibility artifact that iron containing compounds produce, as previously discussed. Gradient Recalled Echo (GRE) and fluid-attenuated inversion recovery (FLAIR) MRI sequences are very sensitive for the subtle findings seen in patients with petechial hemorrhage and diffuse axonal injury (29).

As mentioned earlier, CT markedly underestimates the extent of these injuries. The CT appearance may be normal or near normal. Patients who have sustained diffuse axonal injury have a worse long-term prognosis than those patients with gray matter contusions, thus it is helpful to employ MRI for diagnosis in these situations. Contusions often occur due to direct impact injuries that occur in focal locations. Shearing injuries and DAI, on the other hand, occur from global rotational forces imparted to the brain. These types of forces result in more extensive and generalized injuries to the brain. MRI is also useful for imaging the long-term sequelae of patients with

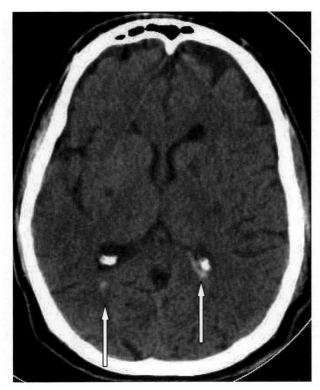

FIGURE 11-4

DAI: Axial noncontrast CT demonstrates shearing injuries involving the splenium of the corpus callosum and deep white matter (arrows)

(a)

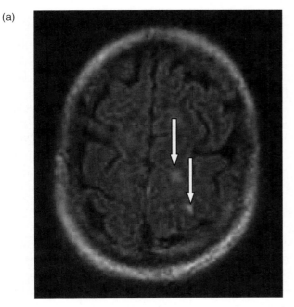

(b)

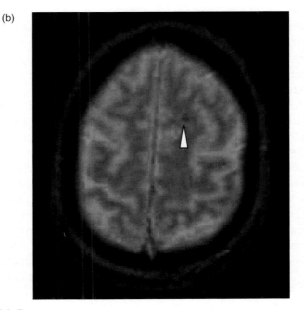

FIGURE 11-5

DAI: Axial FLAIR MRI (a) demonstrates foci of increased signal intensity within the deep bifrontal and left parietal white matter (arrows). Axial gradient echo (b) demonstrates a focus of magnetic susceptibility in the left frontal white matter (arrowhead). These foci are typical of petechial hemorrhages seen in DAI global brain injury. The long-term sequelae of DAI will be discussed in more detail at the end of the chapter.

Intra-axial: Herniation Syndromes

Severe intracranial injuries such as large hematomas or brain swelling, exert mass effect on the pliable brain within the closed-box of the adult cranium. The production of CSF and cerebral blood flow vary inversely with increasing intracranial pressure. Intracranial pressure will change if there are additions or subtractions to the fixed intracranial contents (brain, CSF, blood). This is called the Monro–Kellie Doctrine (14). Mechanical displacement of the brain, if severe enough, may lead to herniation syndromes. These include subfalcine, transtentorial, tonsillar, transsphenoidal, or external herniation.

Subfalcine herniation consists of midline shift of the cingulate gyrus under the midline dural reflection of the falx cerebri. This results in effacement of the ipsilateral lateral ventricle and noncommunicating hydrocephalus of the contralateral lateral ventricle (23). Dilation of the contralateral ventricle in subfalcine herniation occurs because of obstruction at the level of the foramen of Monro. If severe enough, cerebral infarction in the anterior cerebral artery distribution may occur because of compression of the vessels under the falx cerebri. Subfalcine herniation is the most common herniation syndrome (30).

If the uncal portion of the temporal lobe herniates across the tentorium (Figure 11-6), the midbrain is compressed, leading to injury of the contralateral cerebral peduncle (Kernohan's notch) or ischemia/infarction in the posterior cerebral artery distribution. Uncal herniation may also cause an ipsilateral cranial nerve III (occulomotor nerve) palsy. Uncal herniation may manifest clinically as ispsilateral dilated pupil and an ipsilateral hemiparesis, the latter due to compression of the contralateral cerebral peduncle.

Transtentorial herniation occurs in a cranial or caudal direction across the tentorium, that separates the posterior fossa contents from the supratentorial compartment. Descending herniation through the tentorium appears on CT as effacement of the suprasellar and perimesencephalic cisterns. Transtentorial herniation may lead to disruption of brainstem perforating vessels, causing petechial hemorrhages in the midline brainstem, Duret hemorrhages. If the cerebellum herniates upward through the tentorium, the basilar cisterns are effaced. This typically occurs due to a posterior fossa hemorrhage or mass.

Cerebellar tonsillar herniation occurs when the inferior portion of the cerebellum herniates downward through the foramen magnum. Tonsillar herniation may cause infarction in the posterior inferior cerebellar artery territory (PICA). Cerebellar tonsillar herniation occurs due to a posterior fossa mass, hemorrhage or swelling. This is important to distinguish from nontraumatic

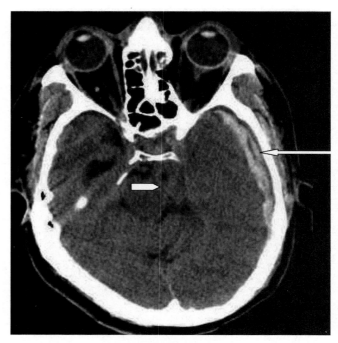

FIGURE 11-6

Uncal herniation: Axial noncontrast CT demonstrates a left-temporal subdural hematoma (arrow) associated with uncal herniation and compression of the midbrain (arrowhead). There is also contra-lateral dilatation of the temporal horn

cerebellar tonsillar herniation of greater than 5 mm through the foramen magnum—Chiari I malformation. Some of these patients with this congenital malformation are subject to trauma; however the herniation in these cases is not due to the trauma itself.

Transsphenoidal herniation occurs when the frontal or temporal lobes are displaced posteriorly or anteriorly across the greater wing of the sphenoid bone respectively. External herniation occurs when brain contents herniate through a bony defect—either fracture or surgical defect, outside of the calvarium. Any of the aforementioned herniation syndromes may occur due to mass effect from trauma, hemorrhage or neoplasm (12, 23). In some patients with severe mass effect, a combination of different herniation syndromes may result (Figure 11-7).

Intra-axial: Cerebral Edema

The term *cerebral edema* is often misused or misunderstood. Global cell injury or cell swelling has been called cerebral edema in the past. Multiple injuries to the brain or anoxic insult may present as diffuse abnormality, or brain swelling. Brain swelling occurs because of increased cerebral blood volume, loss of autoregulation of cerebral blood flow, or a generalized increase in tissue fluid. This manifests clinically as elevated intracranial pressure. Radiologically, brain swelling manifests as diffuse effacement of

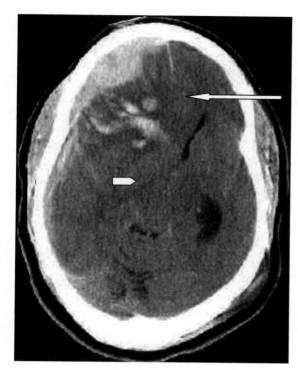

FIGURE 11-7

Herniation: Axial noncontrast CT demonstrates a right fronto-temporal subdural hematoma and right frontal hemorrhagic contusion associated with both subfalcine (arrow) and uncal herniation (arrowhead)

sulci, ventricles and cisterns. The normal appearing gray/white matter interface is also lost and the brain appears somewhat featureless throughout (Figure 11-8). As mentioned earlier, severe brain swelling may lead to herniation syndromes in the craniocaudal axis—transtentorial, or inferiorly through the foramen magnum.

The prior confusion of the term "cerebral edema" stems from the fact that there are many different types of edema that have specific pathophysiology. Cytotoxic edema occurs when there is cell injury, ischemia or death. Ion gradients that maintain cell homeostasis are lost, due to inactivation of the sodium/potassium ATP-ase. When ion gradients cannot be maintained, the cells eventually swell with fluid. An increase in water within the cell results in cytotoxic edema. This may be seen on CT as areas of subtle low density or loss of the normal gray/white interface—usually in a focal area or vascular territory. The visual density of gray and white matter on CT is abnormally uniform. Diffusion-weighted MRI (DWI) is very sensitive for areas of cytotoxic edema. Cytotoxic edema manifests as high signal on DWI sequences, or restricted diffusion (31). DWI has gained widespread use in the work-up of acute stroke, among other abnormalities that demonstrate restricted diffusion. An emerging role for DWI in predicting outcome of patients presenting with traumatic brain injury will be discussed later.

Vasogenic edema occurs when there is an increase in extracellular free water. This often occurs around masses, abscesses or hemorrhages. It manifests on CT and routine

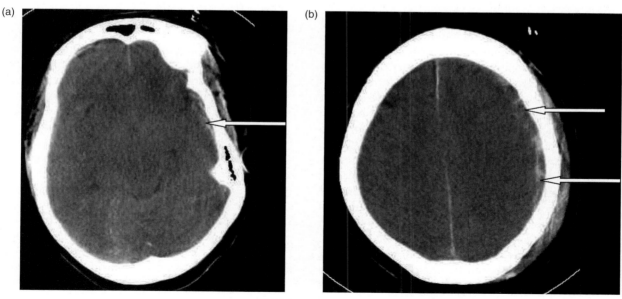

FIGURE 11-8

Brain Swelling: Axial noncontrast CT [(a) and (b)] demonstrate a left fronto-parietal subdural hematoma (arrow) and diffuse effacement of sulci and decreased gray/white matter differentiation. These findings are consistent with brain swelling

MRI sequences as fingerlike areas of hypodensity extending from the mass/hemorrhage into the adjacent white matter. Because vasogenic edema is free extracellular water, there is no restricted diffusion on diffusion-weighted MRI sequences. The diffusion MRI sequence and apparent diffusion coefficient (ADC) map, a calculated parameter, can distinguish between cytotoxic edema (irreversible) and vasogenic edema (reversible). Cytotoxic edema is high in signal intensity on DWI and low in signal intensity on the ADC map, while free water or vasogenic edema is low in signal intensity on DWI. DWI has properties that reflect relative T_2 weighting. Thus, anything that is bright on T_2 or FLAIR sequences, may be bright on DWI. This is termed T_2 shine-through. The ADC map image is devoid of T_2 weighting, and should always be checked in the setting of bright foci on DWI, to confirm that restricted diffusion of water is actually present.

Interstitial edema is seen in the setting of hydrocephalus and increased intracranial pressure. There is transependymal resorption of CSF from the dilated ventricles into the periventricular regions. There is also an increase in extracellular free water. On imaging, interstitial edema appears as hypodensity in the periventricular locations.

Extra-axial: Subdural Collections

Our discussion of the pathophysiology and imaging appearances of brain injury will now turn to the extra-axial space. As discussed earlier, the dura is a layer of tissue intimately applied to the inner table of the skull and periosteum. The arachnoid is a network of tissue between the outer dura and inner pia—which lines the cortex of the brain. A fundamental understanding of the dural vascular anatomy, including the middle meningeal artery and dural venous sinuses allows one to predict the etiology of an extra-axial hematoma (32). The subdural space is a potential space that becomes evident radiologically if there is fluid, hemorrhage or purulent material between the dura and arachnoid. Subdural collections are confined to the dural reflections and will not cross midline, although they may cross sutures. These boundaries are helpful if the collection is small and indeterminate. The midline dural reflection is the falx cerebri. Separating the cerebrum and cerebellum is the falx cerebelli. Subdural collections near the midline or cerebellum, may layer on these dural reflections. Sometimes it is difficult to characterize a collection as subdural or epidural in location. Furthermore, it may be difficult to characterize a hematoma as above or below the falx cerebri. In these instances, the indeterminate collections should be referred to as simply extra-axial.

A subdural hematoma is an extra-axial collection of blood that may occur if there is traumatic injury to the

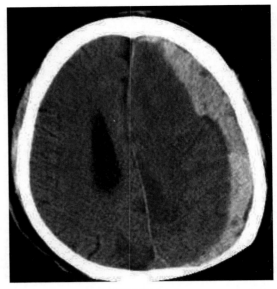

FIGURE 11-9

SDH: Axial noncontrast CT demonstrates an acute left fronto-parietal subdural hematoma with mass effect on the underlying cortex

bridging veins beneath the dura (Figure 11-9). These bridging veins travel within the subdural space, toward the main dural sinuses. Acceleration and deceleration forces may lead to tearing of the bridging veins and subsequently, a subdural hematoma. Arterial injury may rarely cause a subdural hematoma. Following vessel injury, blood collects between the dura and arachnoid. An acute subdural hematoma appears hyperdense (bright) on a noncontrast CT of the brain. It is often crescent-shaped and conforms to the inner table of the skull on axial images. Unlike the epidural space that is confined and may exert a tamponade effect to limit the size of the hematoma, subdural hematomas may become large because of the relatively unconfined nature of the subdural space, subarachnoid space and underlying brain. Because subdural hematomas may cross sutures, they are often seen layering along an entire hemisphere. If large enough, these hematomas will exert mass effect on the underlying brain, causing effacement of sulci, ventricles or even midline shift. Severe midline shift may progress to subfalcine herniation as described previously.

The natural evolution of a subdural hematoma may be followed with serial CT scans. The hematoma will become isodense (similar density) when compared to brain, making it difficult to detect between 5–20 days after injury (Figure 11-10). This decrease in density of a subdural hematoma is due to breakdown of hemoglobin and protein products within the collection. These subacute collections are subtle on imaging and secondary signs such as mass effect and sulcal effacement must be searched for in order to diagnose them. Eventually these

(a) 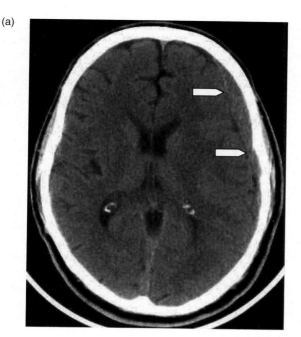 (b)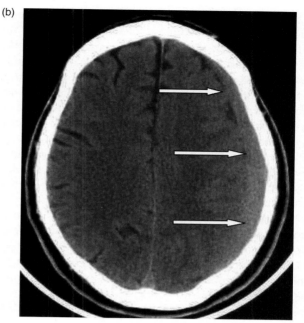

FIGURE 11-10

Subacute SDH: Axial noncontrast CT (10a) demonstrates subtle effacement of sulci on the left convexity (arrowhead). An image more superior (10b) shows the isodense left fronto-parietal SDH (arrows)

collections will become chronic and appear hypodense (dark) compared to underlying brain more than 3 weeks after injury (6, 18). Occasionally, a subacute or chronic subdural hematoma will rebleed, causing a heterogeneous appearance to the collection, with mixed areas of hyper and hypodensity. These collections composed of acute hemorrhage superimposed on chronic blood products appear as a blood-fluid levels in the supine patient. The blood-fluid level is due to differences in density of the blood, or the hematocrit effect. This leads to an appearance of acute, bright blood inferior to the more chronic, serous collection layering dependently.

The mortality rate from traumatic subdural hematomas may be lowered from 90 percent to 30 percent if diagnosis and treatment occur in a timely fashion, usually within the first 4 hr (33). The timing of surgical intervention depends on many factors such as co-existing injuries and the neurological status of the patient. Patients who receive early surgical evacuation of a symptomatic SDH have an improved neurological outcome with relief from increasing intracranial pressure (34).

Subdural hygromas are collections within the subdural space that are hypodense, much like chronic subdural hematomas. They are collections of cerebrospinal fluid (CSF) that result from traumatic leakage from the surface of the brain after injury to the arachnoid membrane (18). It may be difficult to distinguish a chronic subdural hematoma from a subdural hygroma or an expanded extra-axial space. This issue often arises when imaging elderly patients, who have some degree of atrophy and

expansion of the extra-axial spaces. MRI is helpful in these cases, for subdural hygromas and expanded extra-axial spaces will have identical signal characteristics with the CSF in the ventricles and cisterns on all MRI pulse sequences. Subdural hematomas, even if chronic will typically differ from CSF on one or more pulse sequences.

Extra-axial: Epidural Collections

The epidural space is another potential space that exists between the inner table of the skull and the closely adherent dura. Collections in the epidural space may dissect between these tissue layers to create an extra-axial epidural collection. Because of the firm attachment of the dura to the inner table of the skull, epidural hematomas tend to be smaller and more confined than the larger, subdural hematomas. Acute epidural hematomas result from injury to the middle meningeal artery or its branches due to fractures of the squamosal portion of the temporal bone (35). Occasionally, acute epidural hematomas contain air within them. These air containing epidural hematomas are associated with fractures that communicate with the sinuses or extra-cranially (36). Ninety-five percent of epidural hematomas are associated with skull fractures and are supratentorial, typically unilateral (1). Injuries of the dural venous sinuses may also lead to epidural hematomas (1). Injuries at the vertex of the skull may lead to disruption of the superior sagittal sinus, creating an epidural hematoma that crosses the midline. The collections typically appear biconvex, much like a lens, between the brain and skull on axial CT images. Unlike subdural hematomas, epidural hematomas can cross the midline. However, these collections are outside of the dura and cannot cross suture lines, for the dura is firmly attached to the skull at the sutures. If an acute epidural hematoma presents infratentorially, it is usually associated with trauma to the posterior fossa or fracture of the occipital bone (37, 38). An extra-axial hematoma in the posterior fossa is usually epidural in nature and typically unilateral (39). Rarely, acute epidural hematomas may be bilateral in approximately 5 percent of patients (Figure 11-11). When these collections are bilateral, they are often bifrontal in location (40).

Approximately one-third of patients with epidural hematomas are lucid clinically prior to neurological deterioration (35). Like all other forms of acute hemorrhage on CT, acute epidural hematomas are hyperdense (bright) compared to brain. These hematomas evolve to become isodense, then hypodense (dark) compared to brain over several days to weeks. Like any extra-axial collection, epidural hematomas will exert mass effect on the underlying brain and result in effacement of sulci and ventricles. When severe, these collections present with midline shift and herniation. In contrast to a peripherally located hemorrhagic contusion, epidural hematomas will typically form obtuse angles with the underlying brain, revealing their extra-axial location.

The mortality rate is lower for epidural hematomas (10 percent) when compared to subdural hematomas. The reported mortality rate is variable and ranges from 20 to 90 percent (1, 35, 41). Because of firm dural attachments, there is usually a tamponade effect for epidural hematomas, while subdural hematomas are less confined and may be larger or appear in a delayed fashion as discussed above. Most epidural hematomas are acute and are detected during the initial imaging work-up. Occasionally a patient may present subacutely with a delayed epidural hematoma. About 6–13 percent of epidural hematomas are delayed in presentation while some authors have reported this as high as 30 percent (42).

Extra-axial: Subarachnoid Hemorrhage

The subarachnoid space is the CSF containing space between the arachnoid membrane and the pia that covers the brain. CSF originates in the choroids plexus and flows from the ventricular system to the basilar cisterns, then finally to the surface of the brain. CSF is then absorbed by the small arachnoid granulations within the dural venous sinuses. CSF bathes the brain surface and extends into the sulci.

Subarachnoid hemorrhage (SAH) most commonly (90 percent) occurs secondary to a ruptured aneurysm involving the Circle of Willis. Usually subarachnoid hemorrhage secondary to a ruptured aneurysm is larger than bleeding caused by trauma. The locations are different as well. A ruptured aneurysm typically has most of the blood near the site of rupture. For example, if the aneurysm is located in the Circle of Willis, the basal cisterns usually fill with blood. Traumatic subarachnoid hemorrhage is

(a)

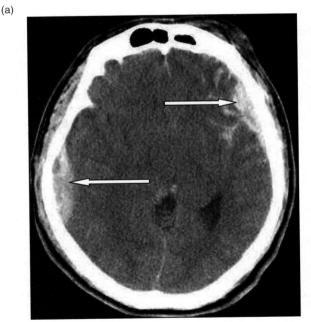

(b)

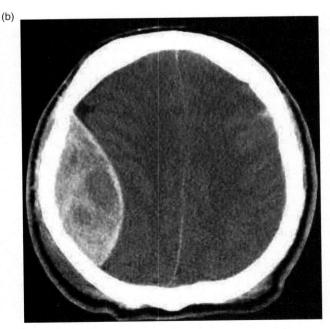

FIGURE 11-11

Acute EDH: Axial noncontrast CT (11a) demonstrates bilateral, biconvex epidural hematomas (arrows). An image more superior (11b) shows a large right-sided EDH with mixed, swirling density suggesting active bleeding

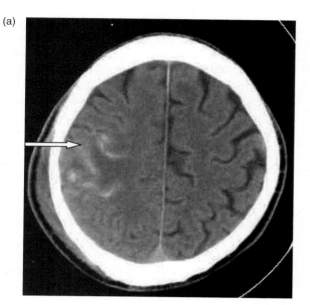 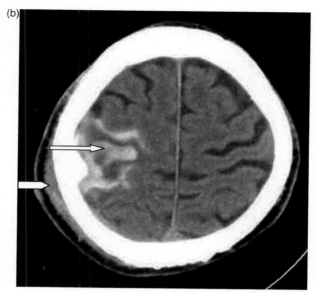

FIGURE 11-12

SAH: Axial noncontrast CT images [(a) & (b)] demonstrate traumatic subarachnoid hemorrhage filling right-sided sulci (arrows). Also note the right scalp soft tissue swelling (arrowhead)

much more variable in location. SAH presents on CT as hyperdense blood within the sulci (Figure 11-12) or basal cisterns. CT is very sensitive for the detection of acute SAH (18). MRI is less sensitive for the detection of acute SAH, however is very good for imaging chronic blood products or hemosiderin.

Besides a ruptured aneurysm or trauma, other causes of subarachnoid hemorrhage include arteriovenous malformations and coagulopathies (23). There are also many complications that may occur with SAH and follow-up imaging is recommended. These include vasospasm, stroke, communicating hydrocephalus, and arachnoiditis. MRI imaging in patients with SAH may show blood products in varying stages within the sulci or cisterns. Fluid attenuated inversion recovery (FLAIR) sequences employ a longer T1 and a 180-degree inversion pulse to reduce the signal level of CSF and detect abnormalities in the sulci such as SAH with a greater degree of certainty (5). As described earlier, chronic SAH may present on gradient echo or magnetic susceptibility sequences as leptomeningeal hemosiderosis—hypointense (dark) meninges on T_2-weighting (23).

Extra-axial: Intraventricular Hemorrhage

The intraventricular space is a CSF-containing space within the paired lateral, third and fourth ventricles. Intraventricular hemorrhage (IVH) may occur within any ventricle; however, often occurs in the lateral ventricles after trauma. It may be a primary event or secondary event such as extension from a parenchymal contusion or existing SAH. Primary IVH in the trauma patient is due to injury of the subependymal veins surrounding the ventricles. As described for mixed subdural hematomas with blood–blood levels, the acute intraventricular hematoma will layer in the dependent portions of the ventricle in a supine patient. If the hemorrhage is within the lateral ventricle, the blood is often seen in the occipital horns posteriorly. It has been reported to occur in 35 percent of patients with moderate to severe brain injury (1, 35). IVH may lead to a non-communicating hydrocephalus (described below) due to obstruction of CSF flow at the level of the foramina of Monro or the cerebral aqueduct (Figure 11-13).

Extra-axial: Hydrocephalus

Hydrocephalus is dilatation of the ventricles that contain cerebrospinal fluid (CSF). It involves an increase in the volume of CSF within the subarachnoid space, ventricles and cisterns (14). Ventriculomegaly is a generic radiological term meaning enlargement of the ventricles, while hydrocephalus implies a pathologic state that may lead to elevated intracranial pressure. Cerebral atrophy or old age may cause ventriculomegaly secondarily. The CSF-spaces dilate to compensate for the loss in brain parenchyma over time. Patients over the age of 65 usually have some degree of brain volume loss, or atrophy. The enlargement of the ventricles in this case is termed hydrocephalus ex vacuo. The ventricles, sulci and cisterns appear larger radiologically because of underlying brain parenchymal loss. Hydrocephalus ex vacuo occurs

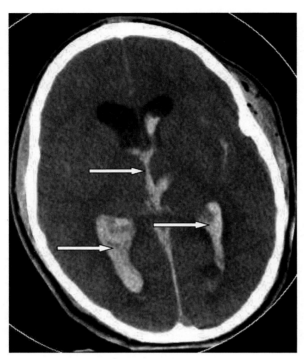

FIGURE 11-13

IVH: Axial noncontrast CT demonstrates intraventricular hemorrhage filling the third and lateral ventricles (arrows). There is also hydrocephalus present

physiologically and does not result in elevated intracranial pressure.

There are two types of pathological hydrocephalus: communicating hydrocephalus and noncommunicating hydrocephalus. In these conditions, there is an increase in CSF volume without brain atrophy. Communicating hydrocephalus is a global dilatation of all of the ventricles, while the connections between the ventricles remain patent. Typically, there is disruption of CSF reabsorption at the level of the arachnoid granulations of the dural venous sinuses. Conditions that cause communicating hydrocephalus include subarachnoid hemorrhage, meningitis and meningeal carcinomatosis (23). Communicating hydrocephalus can be differentiated from hydrocephalus ex vacuo by signs of elevated intracranial pressure and radiologically by dilated ventricles in the setting of cisternal and sulcal effacement.

Increased production of CSF may also cause communicating hydrocephalus, as in normal pressure hydrocephalus (NPH) and tumors of the choroid plexus. Prior to sampling CSF, clinicians often obtain an imaging study, usually a noncontrast CT of the brain to evaluate for hydrocephalus or mass effect. If too much CSF is removed in the acute setting, intracranial hypotension or herniation syndromes may develop (43–45).

Noncommunicating hydrocephalus is a condition in which there is obstruction of the ventricular system

somewhere between the lateral ventricles and the fourth ventricle. Congenital causes such as cerebral aqueductal stenosis may result in dilated lateral and third ventricles. Intraventricular hemorrhage, meningitis and infection may also result in obstruction of the ventricles. Obstruction may also occur at the level of the foramina of Monro leading from the paired lateral ventricles to the midline third ventricle. Thus, non-communicating hydrocephalus would be expected to cause asymmetric dilatation of the ventricles, while communicating hydrocephalus causes diffuse dilatation of the ventricular system on MRI and CT.

IMAGING: PREDICTING OUTCOME

As mentioned at the beginning of this chapter, it is important to understand the pathological conditions that occur within the skull and brain and the appearances of these injuries on CT and MRI. As the technology improves, the lexicon used for discussing imaging findings may change, however the pathology will not change. It is important to realize the limitations of CT and MRI and many injuries are currently beyond the resolution of any imaging modality. To review, CT is the initial imaging modality of choice in traumatic brain injury. The routine emergency non-contrast CT of the brain allows clinicians to rapidly decide if an injury requires emergent surgery, delayed surgery or only medical therapy.

CT also provides indirect signs of increased intracranial pressure through compression of brain stem cisterns, compression of the ventricles, midline shifts, and loss of gray-white matter differentiation (46). Because CT can be performed so quickly, there is less opportunity for motion artifacts that can ruin a study. In addition, there are essentially no contraindications other than an unstable patient, and CT can also be performed in patients with extensive life-support hardware.

After the initial work-up and management of neurologically traumatized patients occurs in the emergency room or intensive care unit settings, decisions must be made that concern the post-acute management of these patients. extra-axial collections, large contusions, midline shift and herniation syndromes are readily diagnosed with routine CT, and will allow the emergency room physician to appropriately triage these patients to surgery. As described previously, diffuse axonal injury (DAI) is often a neurologically devastating injury that may be missed in CT imaging. A normal CT scan in a patient that is comatose after sustaining traumatic brain injury is a classic finding. This is one of the reasons why clinical presentation and imaging are complementary and must be correlated with each another.

In a series of 448 patients with a GCS below 8, 70 patients had a normal CT scan on the day of admission and 47 of these remained normal with serial scanning.

This number represented 25 percent of those with DAI. Although 76 percent of those with normal scans made a good recovery, 19 percent had coma persisting longer than 2 weeks with subsequent severe disability. Brain atrophy at 6 months was a common result, despite the initial normal CT scan, implying diffuse injury. Delayed lesions (usually contusions) occurred in 24 patients, of which 9 had no clinical deterioration. Therefore, although a normal CT scan may be obtained initially in a patient with severe traumatic brain injury, abnormalities on serial imaging may evolve even in the absence of clinical deterioration. Likewise, abnormalities on CT imaging may appear in patients with very mild head injuries with few if any clinical findings (46).

To date, there is no agreed upon classification system for patients with head injury, the severity of clinical presentation, and the findings on imaging. Several different schemes, however, have been evaluated. One such classification is the National Traumatic Coma Data Bank (TCDB). This classification scheme is based on a multi-center study of patients with severe, blunt, traumatic head injuries. Clinically, all of these patients had a Glasgow Coma Scale of less than 8. The TCDB in these patients focused on the imaging findings of basal cistern effacement and midline shift, with the operative findings to predict mortality (47). Caroli et al identified several clinical and radiologic predictors of prognosis in patients with multiple post-traumatic intracranial lesions. The type of lesion—such as subdural hematoma or intracerebral hematoma, the Glasgow Coma Scale (GCS), the presence of prolonged increased intracranial pressure, and the absence of pupillary reflexes were found to all be statistically significant predictors of a poor outcome. Poor outcome in these patients was defined as death or a persistent vegetative state. The authors concluded that multiple lesions have the same prognosis as the corresponding single lesions and that management should be guided by the predominant pathology (48).

Toutant et al. noted that assessment of the basal cisterns can be used as an early noninvasive method to assist in determining prognosis. Compression of the basal cisterns in patients with traumatic brain injury was associated with a high mortality rate in both surgical and non-surgical patients. One-hundred percent of the deceased patients had cistern compression. The mortality rates were 77 percent, 39 percent, and 22 percent among patients with absent, compressed, and normal basal cisterns, respectively (49). Lannoo et al. studied patients with severe brain injury and the resulting mortality and morbidity in relation to age, and early (< 24 hr) clinical data and the imaging findings after CT. Patients with traumatic injuries to parts of the body other than the brain were used as controls. Of the group with traumatic brain injury, the mortality rate was 51 percent. Analyses combined 13 predictors into a model with an accuracy of 93 percent, a sensitivity of 90 percent, and a specificity of 95 percent. These 13 predictors included the following: 1, age; 2, GCS score; 3, pupillary reactivity; 4, blood pressure; 5, ICP; 6, blood glucose; 7, platelet count; 8, body temperature; 9, cerebral lactate; and 10, subdural; 11, intracranial; 12, subarachnoid; and 13, ventricular hemorrhage. Further analysis resulted in the GCS score being the best predictor of neuropsychological functioning, and pupillary reactivity being the most predictive for self-reported quality of life. Those factors important for predicting mortality such as elevated intracranial pressure and the CT observations failed to show any significant relationship with morbidity (50).

The anatomical location and mechanism of injury to the brain are crucial factors in determining future neurological functioning of patients. CT is the imaging study of choice in patients presenting acutely with penetrating injuries to the brain. Gonul et al. studied 35 patients presenting with penetrating orbitocranial gunshot injuries. This group found that anatomical location of injury, extent of injury and GCS score at presentation were the most important predictors of neurologic recovery following penetrating orbitocranial injuries (51). The anatomical location of an injury as determined by imaging also has implications on patient outcome. Blackman et al. evaluated the anatomical location of injuries involving 92 patients presenting with acute traumatic brain injury. They defined several levels of injury progressing from the cortex of the brain to the brainstem, a depth of injury level. Images were classified according to five depth of lesion levels (cortical to brainstem). Functional outcomes in mobility, self-care, and cognition were evaluated in conjunction with the depth of lesion encountered on imaging. Patients with deeper (brainstem) lesions tended to have longer lengths of stay in rehabilitation, however were able to eventually become equal with patients who had more superficial lesions. The authors suggested that one may not be able to predict outcome in the early acute phase in the intensive care unit on the basis of standard brain imaging alone. Patients with deeper lesions tended to enter rehabilitation at a more impaired level, although may eventually reach a level of functioning equal to peers with more superficial brain injuries. They also suggest that it may take a longer period of time to reach this level of functioning than for less severely injured individuals (52).

While many studies have evaluated the Glasgow Coma Scale or compared a different scale to the GCS, some authors have suggested that the 15-point GCS may not add any additional prognostic value over more simplified triage scales. Gill et al. evaluated the performance of GCS scores in a level 1 trauma center from 1990 to 2002, relative to four clinically relevant traumatic brain injury outcomes (emergency intubation, neurosurgical intervention, brain injury, and mortality). They evaluated a simplified 3-point scoring system (simplified verbal score: oriented = 2, confused conversation = 1, inappropriate words or less = 0; simplified motor score: obeys commands = 2, localizes pain = 1, withdrawal to pain or less = 0) with the total GCS and found that the simplified scoring system correlated well with the GCS for predicting outcome. This study suggests that the 15-point GCS may be needlessly complex for predicting neurological outcome (53).

While CT is most important in the acute triage of patients with traumatic brain injury, MRI is more helpful in evaluating the long-term sequelae of these patients. The value of MRI in predicting outcome of rehabilitation in patients with head injury appears promising in view of the relationship between MRI abnormalities and neuropsychological deficits (54). Post-traumatic seizures (PTS) and post-traumatic epilepsy (PTE) are well-documented sequelae of traumatic brain injury. Patients who have depressed skull fractures, acute intracranial hematomas, or seizures during the first week post-injury have an increased risk of developing PTE. Factors found to influence the likelihood of seizures include severe head injury (GCS 3 to 8), diffuse cerebral edema, acute SDH and depressed skull fractures (55). Information obtained through static neuroimaging techniques, and particularly MRI may help identify patients at increased risk for PTS or PTE (56, 57).

Mazzini et al. detected the risk factors for PTE in rehabilitation patients and found that the occurrence of PTE was significantly correlated with hypoperfusion in the temporal lobes, the degree of hydrocephalus, the evidence of intracerebral hematoma, and operative brain injury. Hypoperfusion in the temporal lobes was determined with single photon emission computed Tomography (SPECT), while hydrocephalus was diagnosed with MRI. This study sought to define the influence of PTE on late clinical and functional outcome. Findings revealed that the psychometric tests intended to explore memory, language, intelligence, attention, and spatial cognition did not show any significant difference between patients with and without epilepsy. PTE also was significantly correlated with a worse functional outcome 1 year after the trauma (58).

Pohlmann et al. identified clinical and neuroradiological variables in severe brain injury with predictive value for PTE and evaluated the influence of each risk factor for epilepsy. The authors found that of all patients with PTE in the study, 68.5 percent had their first seizure within two years after the trauma. Significant risk factors for PTE were focal signs in the first examination, missile injuries, frontal lesions, intracerebral hemorrhage, diffuse contusion, prolonged posttraumatic amnesia, depression fracture and cortical-subcortical lesions. The combination of the last three variables conferred a particularly high risk for PTE.

The authors concluded that the risk for PTE is clearly determined by variables that correlate with the severity, the extent of tissue loss and the penetrating nature of the brain injury. Combined seizure pattern, high seizure frequency, anti-epileptic drug noncompliance and alcohol abuse predicted poor seizure control (59).

While the use of MRI is well established in evaluating patients that present with PTE, some researchers have also studied the role of diffusion weighted MRI (DWI) in traumatic brain injury. As discussed earlier with cerebral edema, diffusion-weighted MRI (DWI) is very sensitive for areas of cytotoxic edema. Diffusion MRI is a sequence that has become very important in the imaging of acute and subacute stroke. It allows one to distinguish between cytotoxic edema that is present in cerebral infarction from vasogenic edema. In addition, the diffusion MRI helps to define at risk tissue and often is positive before the patient has CT findings to indicate a stroke. Schaefer et al. evaluated 26 patients presenting with diffuse axonal injury using diffusion weighted MRI. They found that the volume of lesions on diffusion-weighted MRI provides the strongest correlation with a score of subacute on modified Rankin scale at discharge (60). Goetz et al. evaluated 23 patients with traumatic brain injury using diffusion weighted MRI and specifically studied the role of the apparent diffusion coefficient (ADC). The ADC is a parameter used in diffusion MRI to distinguish between true diffusion restriction suggesting cytotoxic edema vs. "T2 shine-through," or anything that may be have increased signal on T2 weighted sequences. These researchers found reported a correlation between injury severity and increasing ADC ($p = 0.03$) but no correlation with either T1 or T2 weighted MRI, suggesting that the ADC used in diffusion MRI is a sensitive and independent marker of diffuse white matter tissue damage following traumatic insult (61).

Many of the studies discussing the use of MRI, and particularly diffusion MRI (DWI) have focused on subacute or chronic traumatic brain injuries. Some authors have also explored the use of MRI in the acute setting. Maeda et al. evaluated 10 patients with diffusion-weighted MRI, presenting in the acute setting with traumatic brain injury. Their study attempted to define the time frame for development of cerebral edema following acute brain injury. Within 3 hr post-trauma, diffusion MRI showed no remarkable pathology. Furthermore, the ADC values at 3 hr post injury were within the normal range (contused/normal brain = 1.00 ± 0.21). At 6 hr post-injury, diffusion-weighted MRI demonstrated a low signal intensity core in the contusion and a high signal intensity rim in the peripheral area of contusion. The ADC value at 6 hr increased in the contusion proper (contused/normal brain = 1.26 ± 0.13) and decreased in the peripheral area (contused/normal brain = 0.58 ± 0.19). These findings indicated that early cellular swelling in the peripheral area of contusion begins within 6 hr following injury. The authors also propose that the delayed occurrence of contusion-induced cellular swelling suggests that the cerebral blood flow does not decrease to ischemic levels immediately following injury (62).

Static imaging techniques may also be used to follow patients with brain injury for potential delayed complications. As discussed earlier, hemorrhagic or non-hemorrhagic contusions may occur in the brain due to blunt forces. The frontal and temporal lobes are particularly vulnerable to contusions secondary to the underlying bony ridges. Delayed bleeding may occur into these regions of perfused yet injured brain. These delayed complications may lead to neurological deterioration from edema, increasing mass effect, and herniation. Delayed hemorrhages into the orbital-frontal regions may also lead to neurological deterioration due to elevated intracranial pressure. Early diagnosis and aggressive therapy in these patients could potentially improve outcome (63). Several authors have examined the sequelae of delayed intra-cerebral hemorrhage and the role that static imaging plays (64, 65). Delayed intra-cerebral hemorrhage often occurs between 3 hr and 10 days after the inciting traumatic insult, particularly within the first 3 days. Thus, if these potential lesions are deemed clinically significant, static imaging performed within this time interval is likely to detect these delayed complications. There have been case reports of patients presenting with delayed hemorrhages as long as 168 days post-trauma (66). These occurrences are the exceptions rather than the rule. These delayed lesions may present with non-focal symptoms such as headache or vomiting. Thus, delayed intracerebral hemorrhage may be considered in the differential diagnosis in these patients if there has been a recent history of trauma.

CONCLUSION

This chapter has focused on the predominant static imaging modalities used in the evaluation of traumatic injury of the brain. In addition, the dominant injuries seen in clinical practice have been described, and their appearances on imaging have been reviewed. These injuries and their sequelae have been discussed in terms of clinical outcome.

In summary, imaging technology is rapidly progressing. There are advances being made daily in the fields of imaging physics, computers, computed tomography, and magnetic resonance imaging. These modalities become the tools that may be used by imagers and clinicians to evaluate, diagnose and treat traumatic injuries of the brain. What does not change, however, is the pathophysiology of brain injury. Thus, it is of paramount importance to learn the mechanisms, anatomy, physiology, and evolution of the different manifestations of traumatic brain injury.

References

1. Harris, JH & Harris, WH. *The Radiology of Emergency Medicine*, 4th Edition. Philadelphia: Lippincott, Williams & Wilkins, 2000; Pg 1–49.
2. Zee CS, Go JL. CT of head trauma. *Neuroimaging Clin N Am*. 1998; 8(3): 525–39.
3. *American College of Radiology Bulletin*. Reston, VA: American College of Radiology, 1986: 11: 8–9.
4. Vilke GM, Chan TC, Guss DA. Use of a complete neurological examination to screen for significant intracranial abnormalities in minor head injury. *Am J Emerg Med*. 2000; 18(2): 159–63.
5. Bushberg JT, Seibert JA, Leidholdt EM, Boone JM. *The Essential Physics of Medical Imaging*, 2nd edition. Philadelphia: Lippincott, Williams & Wilkins, 2002.
6. Cwinn AA, Grahovac SZ. *Emergency CT Scans of the Head: A Practical Atlas*. St. Louis: Mosby, 1998; pp. 3–52.
7. Goldsher D, Shreiber R, Shik V, Tavor Y, Soustiel JF. Role of multisection CT angiography in the evaluation of vertebrobasilar vasospasm in patients with subarachnoid hemorrhage. *AJNR Am J Neuroradiol* 2004; 25(9): 1493–1498.
8. Schild, HH. *MRI Made Easy*. Wayne, NJ: Berlex Laboratories, Inc., 1999.
9. Elster AD, Moody DM. Early cerebral infarction. gadopentetate dimeglumine enhancement. *Radiology* 1990; 177: 627–632.
10. Yuh WTC, Crain MR. Magnetic resonance imaging of acute cerebral ischemia. *Neuroimaging Clin N Am* 1992; 2: 421–439.
11. Stieg PE, Kase CS. Intracranial hemorrhage: diagnosis and emergency management. *Neurol Clin* 1998; 16(2): 373–90.
12. Brant WE, Helms CA. *Fundamentals of Diagnostic Radiology*, 2nd edition. Baltimore: Williams & Wilkins, 1999, pp. 25–65.
13. Thornbury JR, Campbell JA, Masters SJ, et al. Skull fractures and the low risk of intracranial sequelae in minor head trauma. *AJR* 1984; 143: 661–64.
14. Noback, CR, Strominger NL, Demarest RJ. *The Human Nervous System: Structure and Function*. 5th edition. Baltimore: Williams & Wilkins, 1996, pp. 67–82.
15. Pearl GS. Traumatic neuropathology. *Clin Lab Med*. 1998; 18(1): 39–64.
16. Rauch RA, Bazan C, Larsson EM, Jinkins JR. Hyperdense middle cerebral arteries identified on CT as a false sign of vascular occlusion. *AJNR Am J Neuroradiol* 1993; 14(3): 669–73.
17. Furuya Y, Hlatky R, Valadka AB, Diaz P, Robertson CS. Comparison of cerebral blood flow in computed tomographic hypodense areas of the brain in head-injured patients. *Neurosurgery*. 2003; 52(2): 340–45.
18. Gean AD. Concussion, contusion and hematoma. In: Gean AD. *Imaging of Head Trauma*. New York: Raven Press, 1994: 75–206.
19. Johnston KC, Marx WF Jr. Microhemorrhages on gradient echo MRI. *Neurology*. 2003; 60(3): 518.
20. Ripoll MA, Siosteen B, Hartman M, Raininko R. MR detectability and appearance of small experimental intracranial hematomas at 1.5 T and 0.5 T. A 6–7-month follow-up study. *Acta Radiol* 2003; 44(2): 199–205.
21. Gomori JM, Grossman RI, Goldberg HI, Zimmerman RA, Bilaniuk LT. Intracranial hematomas: imaging by high-field MRI. *Radiology* 1985; 157: 87–93.
22. Clark RA, Watanabe AT, Bradley WG, Roberts JD. Acute hematomas: effect of deoxygenation, hematocrit, and fibrin-clot formation and retraction on T2 shortening. *Radiology* 1990; 175: 201–206.
23. WeissLeder R, Rieumont MJ, Wittenberg J: *Primer of Diagnostic Imaging*, 2nd edition. St. Louis: Mosby, 1997, pp. 465–80.
24. Gentry LR, Godersky JC, Thompson BH. Traumatic brain stem injury: MR imaging. *Radiology* 1989; 171: 177–87.
25. Tong KA, Ashwal S, Holshouser BA, Shutter LA, et al. Hemorrhagic shearing lesions in children and adolescents with posttraumatic diffuse axonal injury: improved detection and initial results. Radiology 2003; 227(2): 332–39.
26. Guthrie E, Mast J, Richards P, McQuaid M, Pavlakis S. Traumatic brain injury in children and adolescents. *Child Adolesc Psychiatr Clin N Am*. 1999; 8(4): 807–26.

27. Cantu RC: Head injuries in sport. *Br J Sports Med* 1996; 30(4): 289–96.

28. Gean AD. White matter shearing injury and brainstem injury. In: Gean AD. *Imaging of Head Trauma*. New York: Raven Press, 1994: 207–48.

29. Hammoud DA, Wasserman BA. Diffuse axonal injuries: pathophysiology and imaging. *Neuroimaging Clin N Am* 2002; 12(2): 205–16.

30. Lane FJ, Sheden AI, Dunn MM, Ghatak NR. Acquired intracranial herniations: MR imaging findings. *AJR* 1995; 165: 967–73.

31. Mukherji SK, Chenevert TL, Castillo M. Diffusion-weighted magnetic resonance imaging. *J Neuroophthalmol.* 2002; 22(2): 118–22.

32. Shukla V, Hayman LA, Ly C, Fuller G, Taber KH. Adult cranial dura I: intrinsic vessels. *J Comput Assist Tomogr* 2002; 26(6): 1069–74.

33. Seely JM, Becker DP, Miller JD, et al. Traumatic acute subdural hematoma. *NEJM* 1982; 304: 123–32.

34. Sawauchi S, Beaumont A, Signoretti S, Tomita Y, Marmarou C, Marmarou A. Diffuse brain injury complicated by acute subdural hematoma in the rodents: the effect of early or delayed surgical evacuation. *Acta Neurochir Suppl.* 2002; 81: 243–44.

35. Gentry LR. Imaging of closed head injury. *Radiology* 1994; 191: 1–17.

36. Ersahin Y, Mutluer S. Air in acute extradural hematomas: report of six cases *Surg Neurol.* 1993; 40(1): 47–50.

37. Oliveira MA, Araujo JF, Balbo RJ Extradural hematoma of the posterior fossa. Report of 7 cases. *Arq Neuropsiquiatr.* 1993; 51(2): 243–46.

38. Holzschuh M, Schuknecht B. Traumatic epidural hematomas of the posterior fossa: 20 new cases and a review of the literature since 1961. *Br J Neurosurg* 1989; 3(2): 171–80.

39. Gelabert M, Prieto A, Allut AG. Acute bilateral extradural haematoma of the posterior cranial fossa. *Br J Neurosurg* 1997; 11(6): 573–5.

40. Gupta SK, Tandon SC, Mohanty S, Asthana S, Sharma S Bilateral traumatic extradural haematomas: report of 12 cases with a review of the literature. *Clin Neurol Neurosurg* 1992; 94(2): 127–31.

41. McCort JJ. Caring for the major trauma victim: the role for radiology. *Radiology* 1987; 163: 1–9.

42. Domenicucci M, Signorini P, Strzelecki J, Delfini R Delayed posttraumatic epidural hematoma. A review. *Neurosurg Rev.* 1995; 18(2): 109–22.

43. Samadani U, Huang JH, Baranov D, Zager E, Grady MS: Intracranial hypotension after intraoperative lumbar cerebrospinal fluid drainage. *Neurosurgery* 2003; 52(1): 148–51.

44. van Crevel H, Hijdra A, de Gans J. Lumbar puncture and the risk of herniation: when should we first perform CT? *J Neurol* 2002; 249 (2): 129–37.

45. Hasbun R, Abrahams J, Jekel J, Quagliarello VJ. Computed tomography of the head before lumbar puncture in adults with suspected meningitis. *N Engl J Med* 2001; 13 (24): 1727–33.

46. Katz DI, Black SE: Neurological and neuroradiological evaluation. In Rosenthal M, Griffith ER, Kreutzer JS, Pentland B: *Rehabilitation of the Adult and Child with Traumatic Brain Injury*. Philadelphia: F.A. Davis, 1999.

47. Zafonte RD. Neuroimaging in traumatic brain injury. In Horn LJ and Zasler ND. *Medical Rehabilitation of Traumatic Brain Injury*. Philadelphia: Hanley & Belfus, 1996.

48. Caroli M, Locatelli M, Campanella R, Balbi S, Martinelli F, Arienta C. Multiple intracranial lesions in head injury: Clinical considerations, prognostic factors, management and results in 95 patients. *Surg Neurol* 2001; 56(2): 82–88.

49. Toutant SM, Melville RK, Marshall LF, Toole BM, Bowers S, Seelig J, Varnell JB. Absent or compressed basal cisterns on first CT scan: ominous predictors of outcome in severe head injury. *J Neurosurg* 1984; 61: 691–694.

50. Lannoo E, Van Rietvelde F, Colardyn F, Lemmerling M, Vandekerckhove T, Jannes C, De Soete G. Early predictors of mortality and morbidity after severe closed head injury. *J Neurotrauma* 2000; 17(5): 403–414.

51. Gonul E, Erdogan E, Tasar M, Yetiser S, Akay KM, Duz B, Beduk A, Timurkaynak E. Penetrating orbitocranial gunshot injuries. *Surg Neurol* 2005; 63 (1): 24–30.

52. Blackman JA, Rice SA, Matsumoto JA, Conaway MR, Elgin KM, Patrick PD, Farrell WJ, Allaire JH, Willson DF. Brain imaging as a predictor of early functional outcome following traumatic brain injury in children, adolescents, and young adults. *J Head Trauma Rehabil* 2003; 18 (6): 493–503.

53. Gill M, Windemuth R, Steele R, Green SM. A comparison of the Glasgow Coma Scale score to simplified alternative scores for the prediction of traumatic brain injury outcomes. *Ann Emerg Medicine* 2005; 45 (1): 37–42.

54. Bontke CT, Boake CB. Principles of brain injury rehabilitation. In Braddom RL, et al,: *Physical Medicine and Rehabilitation*. Philadelphia: W.B. Saunders, 1996; pp. 1033–40.

55. Hahn YS, Fuchs S, Flannery AM, Barthel MJ, Mclone DG: Factors influencing post-traumatic seizures in children. *Neurosurgery* 1988; 22(5): 864–867.

56. Angeleri F, Majkowski J, Cacchio G, Sobieszek A, D'Acunto S, Gesuita R, Bachleda A, Polonara G, Krolicki L, Signorino M, Salvolini U: Posttraumatic epilepsy risk factors: one-year prospective study after head injury. *Epilepsia* 1999; 40 (9): 1222–30

57. Diaz-Arrastia R, Agostini MA, Frol AB, Mickey B, Fleckenstein J, Bigio E, Van Ness PC: Neurophysiologic and neuroradiologic features of intractable epilepsy after traumatic brain injury in adults. *Arch Neurol* 2000; 57 (11): 1611–6

58. Mazzini L, Cossa FM, Angelino E, Campini R, Patore I, Monaco F: Post-traumatic epilepsy: neuroradiologic and neuropsychological assessment of long-term outcome. *Epilepsia* 2003; 44 (4): 569–74.

59. Pohlmann-Eden B, Bruckmeir J: Predictors and dynamics of post-traumatic epilepsy. *Acta Neurol Scand* 1997; 95(5): 257–262.

60. Schaefer PW, Huisman TA, Sorensen AG, Gonzalez RG, Schwamm LH. Diffusion-weighted MR imaging in closed head injury: high correlation with initial Glasgow coma scale score and score on modified Rankin scale at discharge. *Radiology* 2004; 233 (1): 58–66.

61. Goetz P, Blamire A, Rajagopalan B, Cadoux-Hudson T, Young D, Styles P: Increase in apparent diffusion coefficient in normal appearing white matter following human traumatic brain injury correlates with injury severity. *J Neurotrauma* 2004; 21 (6): 645–54.

62. Maeda T, Katayama Y, Kawamata T, Koyama S, Sasaki J: Ultra-early study of edema formation in cerebral contusion using diffusion MRI and ADC mapping. *Acta Neurochir Suppl* 2003; 86: 329–31.

63. Lee TT, Villanueva PA. Orbital-frontal delayed hemorrhagic contusions: clinical course and neurosurgical treatment protocol. *Surg Neurol* 1997; 48 (4): 333–37.

64. Alvarez-Sabin J, Turon A, Lozano-Sanchez M, Vazquez J, Codina A. Delayed post-traumatic hemorrhage. "Spat-apoplexie." *Stroke* 1995; 26 (9): 1531–35.

65. Fukamachi A, Kohno K, Nagaseki Y, Misumi S, Kunimine H, Wakao T. The incidence of delayed traumatic intracerebral hematoma with extradural hemorrhages. *J Trauma* 1985; 25 (2): 145–49.

66. Kaplan M, Ozveren MF, Topsakal C, Erol FS, Akdemir I. Asymptomatic interval in delayed traumatic intracerebral hemorrhage: report of two cases. *Clin Neurol Neurosurg* 2003; 105 (3): 153–55.

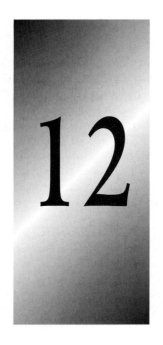

12 Functional Neuroimaging of TBI

Joseph H. Ricker
Patricia M. Arenth

INTRODUCTION

New technologies, as well as advances in existing technologies, have changed how both healthy and injured brains are evaluated in research and clinical settings. In combination with traditional neuromedical examination and psychometric testing, functional neuroimaging is providing a means through which additional information about brain structure, function, and recovery may be obtained. Enthusiasm for functional neuroimaging can be readily appreciated, yet it must be balanced by the need for empirical evidence and a healthy level of caution.

Increasingly, clinicians are using advanced imaging techniques (e.g., SPECT, PET, FMRI) with persons having traumatic brain injury (TBI), however, clinical application of most of these techniques still remains investigational, within the context of this population (1). The present chapter provides an overview of several functional neuroimaging procedures and their applications in the context of TBI. This chapter will also address many limitations of these procedures, with implications for exercising caution if they are utilized in clinical evaluation.

RESTING AND ACTIVATED FUNCTIONAL NEUROIMAGING

In functional neuroimaging, one can dichotomize the available techniques into two broad categories: "resting"

or "activated" (2). Resting paradigms are those that acquire functional images during nonactivated (i.e., "static" or baseline) conditions. Resting studies, by design, have no explicit or systematic requirements of the participant other than those required to successfully acquire a technically valid image, such as having the participant lie still, minimizing head movement, and eliminating extraneous stimuli (3). Although participants do not overtly engage in any specific task, there is no systematic way to "control" random or volitional covert mental activity during the image acquisition. There have been several studies that have applied resting functional neuroimaging across multiple populations, most of which have examined chronic glucose uptake (with positron emission tomography, PET), and resting cerebral blood flow (using PET or single photon emission computed tomography, SPECT). These studies will be discussed later in context.

In contrast to resting paradigms, activation studies require participants to systematically receive sensory input (e.g., a visual array) or engage in an activity (e.g., motor or cognitive) in order to elicit changes in brain physiology that are correlated with a specific stimulus or event in time (4). These tasks are usually administered in adherence to a strict protocol, typically with some form of overt response required in order to provide an objective correlate of the participant's active engagement in the task. Because of the physical properties of the dependent

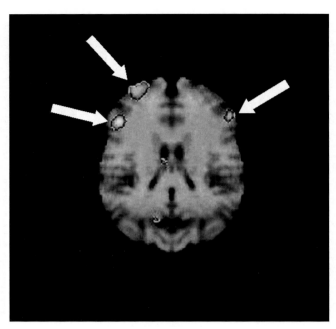

FIGURE 12-1

An Example of O-15 PET Combined with an Activation Paradigm. The participant is being asked to recall a previously learned list of words while being scanned. Regions of increased blood flow (indicated by the arrows) within the frontal lobes are associated with increased cerebral activity known to mediate retrieval of newly learned information

variables examined (e.g., briefer half-lives of radioisotopes, or transient changes in hemodynamic response), activation studies have much briefer time sampling windows than resting studies. Some technologies are even able to image changes across time in a relatively continuous manner (e.g., magnetoencephalography and event-related functional MRI). Given this improved level of control, activation studies permit examiners to make more accurate inferences about the cerebral activity correlated with the motor or cognitive process in question. Figure 12-1 presents an example.

SINGLE PHOTON EMISSION COMPUTED TOMOGRAPHY (SPECT)

SPECT is an approach to functional imaging that is based on the concept that regional changes in brain activity or chemistry can be measured indirectly via externally placed gamma radiation detectors (referred to as "cameras"), which detect the regional accumulations of tracer flow or receptor-binding isotopes. There is an emphasis on imaging changes in regional cerebral blood flow (rCBF), but relatively specific neuroreceptor imaging studies are also possible using SPECT (5).

The dependent variable in SPECT derives from the well-established principle of increased cerebral activity correlating with increased blood flow. That is, when neural activity in a region of the brain increases, related energy requirements also increase. Because the blood supply carries glucose and oxygen to the brain, the flow of blood to the active area increases (6). The radioisotopes themselves are absorbed into glial cells that are proximal to the active neurons, but these isotopes are not immediately excreted. Thus, the absorbed radioisotopes remain in greater concentration in the more active areas. Through normal radioactive decay, the isotope emits annihilated radioactive particles (i.e., photons), which are then detected by the external cameras. Computer-based reconstruction permits external representations to be derived that correlate with differences in blood flow.

SPECT is more widely available than PET or FMRI. In addition, many of the radioisotopes that are typically used with SPECT can be ordered and delivered in advance, thus precluding the necessity of an on-site cyclotron and chemist, as required for PET. SPECT has application in examining resting blood flow, but has more limited utility in imaging a change in blood flow from one point in time to another. SPECT can be used to image change in resting blood flow from one well-defined event to another (e.g., from pre-ictal to ictal state), but it is not appropriate for use in mapping blood flow changes that change rapidly over time (such as those encountered in most states of cognitive activity), or for making direct inferences about brain metabolism (4) due to the time require for radioactive decay of the isotopes: The most commonly used radioactive isotopes for SPECT are absorbed by the brain within 2 min, but may have half-lives of several hours. The effect of this is that after the tracer has been administered, the resulting images that may be acquired can remain the same for the next several hours.

SPECT is not as diverse as other imaging techniques, such as PET, but novel ligands are under continuous development. The compound 123-I–para iodoamphetamine (IAMP) provides a unique look at immediate and delayed perfusion. Other compounds such as 99m-Technetium–HMPAO are also being used for the same purpose. Recent technologic advances have provided for multiple-headed scanners, which offers improved spatial resolution.

As with all assessment tools SPECT has several sources of potential measurement error. Unlike PET, SPECT imaging requires that regional counts be normalized to an area that is ostensibly free from injury. Thus, *relative* flow values in SPECT are often based upon a region such as the thalamus or cerebellum. While such assumptions might be valid for some populations with focal lesions (e.g., stroke), they might not be valid for populations whose neuropathology is more diffuse, such as occurs in TBI. In addition, SPECT resolution currently does not yet approach that of PET imaging. Color SPECT imaging software can produce visually striking – but potentially misleading images, thus reliable and valid interpretation is best accomplished through quantitative pixel counts (7). It must also be noted that although SPECT *can* be used quantitatively, this is not the case in most clinical settings. Visual inspection of SPECT maps is a subjective, qualitative process, and interpretation may vary from clinician to clinician (8).

SPECT STUDIES OF BRAIN INJURY

Resting brain SPECT studies of individuals acquired months (or sometimes years) after moderate and severe brain trauma have demonstrated decreased cerebral blood flow, primarily within prefrontal cortex (9–10). In most of these studies, decreased blood flow and metabolism were generally beyond what might be expected based solely on findings from structural scans (i.e., CT and MRI). The presence of decreased resting blood flow or metabolism is not, however, in and of itself evidence of compromised or nonfunctional brain tissue (11).

Numerous investigations have demonstrated that SPECT is superior to CT and structural MRI in the detection of the presence and extent of trauma-related lesions. SPECT has been applied to mild brain injury and has demonstrated regionally decreased blood flow in the presence of normal acute CT scans, but there is much variability across individuals (i.e., no pathognomonic profile emerges). Positive SPECT findings have also sometimes been demonstrated in cases of below average neuropsychological test scores in cases of mild brain trauma, but it should be noted that SPECT findings are usually not very predictive of neuropsychological test performance (12–13).

In spite of advances in technology and data analysis, the utility of SPECT in characterizing specific injury states or predicting outcome remains controversial. SPECT has been shown particular utility when correlating neuropsychological parameters with the effects of brain injury (14–15), but caution must be exercised given that SPECT findings are routinely positive in a variety of medical and neurological disorders (16–19), learning disabilities (20), as well as in substance use and emotional disorders (e.g., 21–30). Some investigators have noted that when used in a *prospective* design, a negative SPECT scan is a good predictor of a favorable outcome after brain injury, and that SPECT overall correlates well with the severity of the initial trauma (31). Still, there are relatively few well-controlled prospective studies of SPECT (and for that matter, PET and FMRI) being used in differential diagnosis, prognosis, and intervention (2, 32). The use of normative data (8), rather than subjective impressions of SPECT images, will greatly facilitate such developments.

SPECT has been shown to be of use in research studies following brain injury, but there is no particular SPECT profile that is solely pathognomonic for any level of traumatic brain injury (2, 33). The Therapeutics and Technology Subcommittee of the American Academy of Neurology (34) rated SPECT as an *investigational* procedure for the study of brain trauma. More recently, the American College of Radiology (ACR) (1) has rated SPECT as inappropriate (a rating of 2 on a scale of 1 to 9, with 1 indicating "least appropriate") in clinically evaluating postconcussion symptoms. In spite of the absence of evidence supporting routine use of SPECT in brain injury, SPECT appears to be used frequently in clinical and forensic contexts as a means of supporting a diagnosis of brain injury. With increasing evidence and appropriately designed studies, however, and greater specificity of diagnostic criteria (particularly with mild head injury), SPECT is likely to be of improved clinical utility in the future (32, 35–36). For example, 99mTc SPECT has been used recently to examine the therapeutic effects of hyperbaric oxygen on recovery after TBI (37). SPECT has also recently been found to be predictive of post-traumatic amnesia acutely after TBI (38) and useful in assessing the efficacy of intraventricular shunt placement after TBI (39).

POSITRON EMISSION TOMOGRAPHY (PET)

Like SPECT, positron emission tomography (PET) is a radioisotope-based imaging technology. PET studies typically utilize intravenous tracers such as 18F-fluorodeoxyglucose (FDG) for the quantification of "resting" (i.e., nonactivated) regional brain metabolism (40). An exception is Xenon, which is an inhaled isotope. As they are catabolized, annihilation particles are emitted and are detected by an external scanner.

Resting blood flow changes (41) and dynamic changes associated with motor or cognitive activity (11) can be accomplished through the use of tracers such as oxygen-15 (O-15) labeled water. Radiolabeled ligands that bind selectively within dopaminergic, serotonergic, and other endogenous neurochemical systems have been developed and are seen as having great potential for future research (36). Genetically mediated transporter markers (e.g., for dopamine transport) are also available (42).

PET has been widely used as a research tool since the 1970s, but requires a cyclotron to be present on site for most radioisotopes and remains a very expensive procedure. Thus, its application to persons with traumatic brain injury has been minimally investigated. PET has the capability of demons\trating specific biochemical or physiologic processes associated with cerebral blood flow and metabolism. As with SPECT, clinical data from PET imaging are typically portrayed visually in the form of the spatial distribution of radioisotopes projected on to actual or standardized anatomic MRI templates.

PET STUDIES OF BRAIN INJURY

Acute O-15 PET studies of human brain trauma have shown that significant changes in regional (but not necessarily global) hemodynamics occur, such as lower contusional and pericontusional blood flow and flow-to-volume ratios (43). There is also heterogeneity in regional glucose metabolism (44). In addition, cerebral hyperglycolysis is a pathophysiological response that occurs in response to injury-induced neurochemical cascades and can be demonstrated via FDG-PET (45–46).

Several studies have demonstrated PET's ability to detect brain abnormalities that are not visualized on CT or standard MRI sequences in cases of moderate and severe brain injury (2). In addition, functional imaging data exist to suggest that there can be regions of physiological dysfunction beyond the boundaries of static lesions (e.g., contusions) seen with structural imaging. This has been demonstrated for many years using both FDG-PET (47) and Cobalt-55 PET (48). Such changes are seen acutely and occur more in grey matter relative to white matter (49). Acute metabolic changes often begin to resolve within the first month following injury, regardless of injury severity, but the correlation between the extent of change in disability and the changes in brain metabolism are minimal (46).

Although PET would appear intuitively to lend itself well to the many clinical issues that emerge after brain trauma, there are surprisingly few studies that have actually attempted to directly relate functional imaging findings with cognition after TBI. In most of these studies, the findings from neuropsychological and other assessments have been obtained at points in time that were quite disparate from the time at which imaging occurred. For example, one frequently cited paper (50) described FDG-PET and neuropsychological test scores among a selected group of 9 individuals that had experience mild head trauma. Their CT and MRI findings were negative, but PET imaging demonstrated a variety of regions of decreased FDG uptake, some (but not all) of which corresponded to decreased cognitive testing scores. Such findings have little generalizbility, however, given that subjects were specifically selected for inclusion based upon their outcome criteria rather than criteria selected a priori. In addition, scanning and the neuropsychological evaluation were separated in time by an average of 11 months, thus essentially negating the reliability of any correlation between PET and cognitive findings.

In more carefully designed studies, it has been noted that localized abnormal cerebral metabolic rates in frontal and temporal regions correlate with both subjective complaints and neuropsychological test results obtained during the chronic phase of recovery (51). In moderate and severe TBI, resting PET studies have demonstrated frontal hypometabolism, with related decreased performance on neuropsychological tests that are mediated by frontal lobe functioning (52). Recently, through the use of PET, an association between post-TBI anosmia and orbitofrontal hypometabolism has been demonstrated (53).

As described earlier in this chapter, activation studies are likely to be far more sensitive to the functional effects of brain injury or disease, as such paradigms introduce *in vivo* cognitive challenges (54). The first published PET study (55) to apply a cognitive activation paradigm with individuals that sustained brain injury demonstrated cerebral blood flow changes in the left prefrontal cortex among in individuals with TBI during a free recall task when compared to controls, but blood flow increases were noted in more posterior brain regions in TBI subjects during both free and cued recall. The change in allocation of neural resources during tasks with greater cognitive load may suggest increased cognitive effort among individuals with TBI (and thus greater blood flow within prefrontal cortex during task performance). In addition, it was demonstrated that during recognition tasks, both the controls and the individuals with TBI performed at comparable behavioral levels (and within normal limits), yet the individuals with TBI still demonstrated increased change in regional cerebral blood flow relative to the controls. This suggests that after brain injury, individuals must exert more cognitive effort than controls to attain the same level of overt behavior. Subsequently, a different group of investigators also demonstrated comparable findings in a larger sample of individuals with TBI, again using O-15 PET and a verbal memory task (56).

FUNCTIONAL MAGNETIC RESONANCE-BASED IMAGING (FMRI)

Techniques based on magnetic resonance imaging (MRI) capitalize on the presence of hydrogen in all of the body's tissues. When the nuclei of hydrogen atoms encounter a strong magnetic field, they align in parallel to that field's direction. In MRI, radiofrequency (RF) pulses are presented at an angle that is at 90° relative to the magnetic field. This causes roughly 1 percent of the hydrogen nuclei to realign and begin spinning in a different direction (a condition called "excitation"). When the RF pulse is then stopped, the nuclei return to their original alignment and spin (57). During the process of returning to previous resting status, an electrical signal is emitted from nuclei that is detectable by the scanner and allows reconstruction of static anatomic images.

Functional MRI (FMRI) is a variant of structural MRI. The primary difference, however, is that the dependent variable of interest in FMRI is the change in intensity of electrical signal emissions related to increases in blood flow (that are presumably caused by changes in neural activity). Thus, the focus of FMRI is on regional changes in brain activity rather than anatomic structure alone. As with O-15 PET, during FMRI specific stimuli or tasks are presented to the individual within the scanner in an attempt to elicit or increase brain activity. When neural activity increases in a brain region, there is a corresponding increase in blood flow to that region. In fact, this blood flow may increase by over 50 percent (58), beyond metabolic needs. This excess of flow to the region results in a localized surplus of oxyhemoglobin relative to deoxyhemoglobin in the cerebral venous and capillary beds. Oxyhemoglobin is naturally diamagnetic, while deoxyhemoglobin is paramagnetic (i.e., becomes readily magnetized within a magnetic field). With increased neural activity and concomitant increased blood flow, there is a net increase in diamagnetic material (oxyhemoglobin), and a net decrease in paramagnetic material (deoxyhemoglobin). This results in an increased signal intensity that can be detected externally, and is represented as higher signal intensity on $T2^*$ ("T2-star") weighted scans. This change in signal intensity is referred to as the blood oxygen level dependent—or "BOLD"—effect (59).

As compared with other neuroimaging techniques, FMRI utilizes the body's natural physical responses to high-strength magnetism, thus no exogenous radioisotopes or contrast agents are required. Anatomic resolution of fMRI is also superior to that of SPECT or PET. In addition, there are numerous activation paradigms that can be carried out in fMRI, and it allows for greater flexibility in paradigm with reference to repeatability and brevity of the overall scanning session in comparison to other techniques (2).

As with any imaging procedure, however, fMRI can be impacted by numerous variables, particularly in clinical populations such as TBI. Consideration must be made for head movement, normal high frequency noise within the scanner, morphologic brain abnormalities (e.g., frontal or temporal lobe resection secondary to trauma), claustrophobia, anxiety, boredom, or actual onset of sleep while in the scanner.

Although most contemporary MRI scanners can be adapted to perform FMRI, this technique is still investigational in most clinical populations, including brain injury (1). Thus, FMRI is primarily a research tool at this time and its availability is generally limited to academic medical centers. A single FMRI session generates a large volume of data, which necessitates considerations for computer hardware, data storage and data security. At present, FMRI protocols do not actually "automatically" or "objectively" yield brain maps, nor are there normative values for FMRI scans or activity levels. Resulting images

must therefore be carefully and skillfully reconstructed, and this reconstruction process should be considered as much of an art as science. The approach that one takes in reconstructing and displaying the data in the form of brain images data will impact the display, and potentially the interpretation, of the end product.

FMRI STUDIES OF BRAIN INJURY

At the time of this writing, there are very few FMRI studies of individuals with TBI, although there are several centers with active funding and ongoing protocols that will address this significant dearth in the scientific and clinical literature.

In the first FMRI studies of individuals with TBI (60–61), the investigators examined individuals with a very recent history of mild brain injury (i.e., within the previous 30 days). The individuals with mild TBI demonstrated intact behavioral performance on a verbal working memory task, but they did show right hemisphere lateralized FMRI activation in response to increased working memory load, as compared to healthy controls. In subsequent FMRI investigations of working memory following moderate and severe TBI (62–63), increased blood flow and more widespread dispersion of cortical activation was noted during working memory tasks. This again suggests that increased cognitive effort is reflected in increased brain activation on fMRI. In a study of working memory and response inhibition, FMRI was used to demonstrate increased recruitment of cerebral resources following severe diffuse TBI, particularly during response inhibition or when task difficulty was increased (64). This greater expenditure of effort to achieve overtly normal behavioral performance has also been demonstrated in an FMRI study of simple psychomotor execution (i.e., finger-tapping) among individuals with TBI examined several years after injury (65). One recent case study (66) has demonstrated correlations between changes in FMRI activations and improvement in cognitive status following rehabilitation of an individual with severe TBI, a compelling finding that warrants replication.

Although FMRI represents a very advanced approach to brain imaging vis-à-vis cognitive functioning when compared to SPECT or PET, it has not reached a sufficient threshold of evidence for routine use at any level of injury severity after head trauma. Given the paucity of FMRI research in TBI, the ACR has not fully evaluated FMRI and continues to classify this procedure as investigational in the examination of any level brain injury.

FUTURE RESEARCH

The past few years have seen tremendous advances in functional neuroimaging technologies and approaches to data analysis. In addition, there have been exploratory studies in several clinical populations, including TBI. In spite of these advances, these techniques remain investigational in most clinical applications (67). As with any technology, the transition from "investigational" to "routine" will not occur overnight, nor will it occur solely from the publication of a handful of case studies or small investigations drawn only from highly selected cases. It will occur after much additional, well-designed, systematic research (68). This should not be misinterpreted as a fatalistic statement, however. It is, in fact, the expectation of the authors that functional neuroimaging technologies will eventually demonstrate sufficient sensitivity and specificity to warrant routine clinical application, particularly among individuals with much potential to be helped by rehabilitation.

References

1. Davis PC, Drayer BP, Anderson RE, Braffman B, Deck MD, Hasso AN, Johnson BA, Masaryk T, Pomeranz SJ, Seidenwurm D, Tanenbaum L, Masdeu JC. American College of Radiology Appropriateness Criteria: Head Trauma. *Radiology* 2000; 215: 507–524.
2. Ricker JH. Functional neuroimaging in medical rehabilitation populations. In J. DeLisa & B. Gans (eds). *Rehabilitation medicine* (4th ed.), (Chapter 9: pp 229–242). Philadelphia: Lippincott, Williams & Wilkins, 2004.
3. Raichle ME. Functional neuroimaging: A historical and physiological perspective. In Cabeza R, Kingstone A (eds): *Handbook of functional neuroimaging of cognition* (pp. 3–26). Cambridge, MA: MIT Press, 2001
4. Huettell SA, Song AW, McCarthy G. *Functional magnetic resonance imaging.* Sinauer Associates, 2004
5. Kauppinen T, Ahonen A, Tuomivaara V, Hiltunen J, Bergstrom K, Kuikka J, Tornianinen P, Hillbom M. Could automated template based quantification of benzodiazepine receptors in brain single photon emission tomography with ^{123}I-NNC 13-8241 be used to demonstrate neuronal damage in traumatic brain injury? *Nuclear Medicine Communications*, 2002, 23, 1065–1072
6. Ingvar GH, Risberg J. Influence of mental activity upon regional blood flow in man. *Acta Neurol Scand* 1965; 14:183–186.
7. Audenaert K, Jansen HML, Otte A, Peremans K, Vervaet M, Crombez R, de Ridder L, van Heeringen C, Thiro J, Dierckx RA, Korf J. Imaging of mild traumatic brain injury using 57Co and 99mTc HMPAO SPECT as compared to other diagnostic procedures. *Med Sci Monit* 2003; 9(10): 112–117.
8. van Laere KJ, Warwick J, Versijpt J, Goethals I, Audenaert K, van Heerden B, Dierckx R. Analysis of clinical brain SPECT data based on anatomic standardization and reference to normal data: An ROC-based comparison of visual, semiquantitative, and voxel-based methods. *J Nucl Med* 2002; 43:458–469
9. Ricker JH, Zafonte RD. Functional neuroimaging in traumatic head injury: Clinical applications and interpretive cautions. *J Head Trauma Rehabil* 2000; 15(2):859–868
10. Ricker JH, Arenth PM. Traumatic brain injury. In M. D'Esposito (ed). *Functional Neuroimaging of the Nervous System* (Chapter 4). Taylor & Francis / CRC. In press.
11. Huettell SA, Song AW, McCarthy G. *Functional magnetic resonance imaging.* Sinauer Associates, 2004
12. Hofman PAM, Stapert SZ, van Kroonenburgh MJPG, Jolles J, de Kruijk J, Wilmink JT. MR imaging, single-photon emission CT, and neurocognitive performance after mild traumatic brain injury. AJNR *Am J Neuroradiol* 2001; 22:441–449
13. Umile EM, Plotkin RC, Sandel ME. Functional assessment of mild traumatic brain injury using SPECT and neuropsychological assessment. *Brain Inj* 1998; 12:577–594
14. Ichise M, Chung DG, Wang P, Wortzman G, Gray BG, & Franks W. Technetium-99m-HMPAO SPECT, CT, and MRI in the evaluation of patients with chronic traumatic brain injury: a correlation with neuropsychological performance. *J Nucl Med* 1994; 35:1217–1226
15. Audenaert K, Jansen HML, Otte A, Peremans K, Vervaet M, Crombez R, de Ridder L, van Heeringen C, Thiro J, Dierckx RA, Korf J. Imaging of mild traumatic brain injury using ^{57}Co and ^{99}mTc HMPAO SPECT as compared to other diagnostic procedures. *Med Sci Monit* 2003; 9(10):112–117
16. Dougherty DD, Rauch SL, Rosenbaum JF. *Essentials of neuroimaging for clinical practice.* Washington, DC: American Psychiatric Press, 2004
17. Garcia-Campayo J, Sanz-Carrillo C, Baringo T, Ceballos C. SPECT scan in somatization disorder patients: an exploratory study of eleven cases. *Aust NZ J Psychiatry* 2001; 35(3):359–363
18. Mountz JM, Liu HG, Deutsch G. Neuroimaging in cerebrovascular disorders: measurement of cerebral physiology after stroke and assessment of stroke recovery. *Semin Nucl Med* 2003; 33(1): 56–76
19. Pakrasi S, O'Brien JT. Emission tomography in dementia. *Nucl Med Commun* 2005; 26(3):189–196
20. Papanicolaou, A.C., Simos, P.G., Breier, J.I., Fletcher, J.M., Foorman, B.R., Francis, D., Castillo, E.M., & Davis, R.N. (2003). Brain mechanisms for reading in children with and without dyslexia. *Developmental Neuropsychology*, 24(2-3), 593–612.
21. Haldane M, Frangou S. New insights help define the pathophysiology of bipolar affective disorder: Neuroimaging and neuropathology findings. *Prog Neuropsychopharm Biol Psychi* 2004; 28(6):943–960
22. Kennedy SE, Zubieta JK. Neuroreceptor imaging of stress and mood disorders. *CNS Spectr* 2004; 9(4):292–301.
24. Ernst M, Kimes AS, Jazbec S. Neuroimaging and mechanisms of drug abuse: interface of molecular imaging and molecular genetics. *Neuroimaging Clin N Am* 2003; 13(4):833–849.
25. Pezawas L, Fischer G, Podreka I, Schindler S, Brucke T, Jagsch R, Thurnher M, Kasper S. Opioid addiction changes cerebral blood flow symmetry. *Neuropsychobiol* 2002; 45(2):67–73
26. Heinz A, Goldman D, Gallinat J, Schumann G, Puls I. Pharmacogenetic insights to monoaminergic dysfunction in alcohol dependence. *Psychopharmacology* 2004; 174(4):561–570
27. Browndyke JN, Tucker KA, Woods SP, Beauvais J, Cohen RA, Gottschalk PC, Kosten TR. Examining the effect of cerebral perfusion abnormality magnitude on cognitive performance in recently abstinent chronic cocaine abusers. *J Neuroimaging* 2004; 14(2):162–169.
28. Modell JG, Mountz JM. Focal cerebral blood flow change during craving for alcohol measured by SPECT. *J Neuropsychiat Clin Neurosci* 1995; 7(1):15–22
29. Malaspina D, Harkavy-Friedman J, Corcoran C, Mujica-Parodi L, Printz D, Gorman JM, Van Heertum R. Resting neural activity distinguishes subgroups of schizophrenia patients. *Biol Psychiatry* 2004; 56(12):931–937
30. Maron E, Kuikka JT, Ulst K, Tiihonen J, Vasar V, Shlik J. SPECT imaging of serotonin transporter binding in patients with generalized anxiety disorder. *Eur Arch Psychiatry Clin Neurosci* 2004; 254(6):392–396.
31. Jacobs A, Put E, Ingels M, Bossuyt A. Prospective evaluation of Technetium 99m HMPAO-SPECT in mild and moderate traumatic brain injury. *J Nucl Med* 1994; 35:942–947
32. Davalos DB, Bennett TL. A review of the use of single-photon emission computerized tomography as a diagnostic tool in mild traumatic brain injury. *Appl Neuropsychol* 2002; 9(2):92–105
33. Herscovitch P. Functional brain imaging: Basic principles and application to head trauma. In M Rizzo & D Tranel (eds), *Head injury and the postconcussive syndrome* (pp. 89–118). New York: Churchill Livingstone, 1996
34. Therapeutics and Technology Subcommittee of the American Academy of Neurology. Assessment of brain SPECT. *Neurology* 1996; 46:278–285
35. Bonne O, Gilboa A, Louzoun Y, Kempf-Sherf O, Katz M, Fishman Y, Ben-Nahum Z, Krausz Y, Bocher M, Lester H, Chisin R, Lerer B. Cerebral blood flow in chronic symptomatic

mild traumatic brain injury. *Psychiatr Res*: Neuroimaging 2003; 124:141–152

36. Cihangiroglu M, Ramsey RG, Dohrmann GJ. Brain injury: Analysis of imaging modalities. *Neurol Res* 2002; 24:7–18

37. Shi XY, Tang ZQ, Xiong B, Bao JX, Sun D, Zhang YQ, Yao Y. Cerebral perfusion SPECT imaging for assessment of the effect of hyperbaric oxygen therapy on patients with post-brain injury neural status. *Chin J Traumatol* 2003; 6(6):346–349.

38. Lorberboym M, Lampl Y, Gerzon I, Sadeh M. Brain SPECT evaluation of amnestic ED patients after mild head trauma. *Am J Emerg Med* 2002; 20:310–313.

39. Mazzini L, Campini R, Angelino E, Rognone F, Pastore I, Oliveri G. Posttraumatic hydrocephalus: a clinical, neuroradiologic, and neuropsychologic assessment of longterm outcome. *Arch Phys Med Rehabil* 2003; 84:1637–1641.

40. Buckner RL, Logan JM. Functional neuroimaging methods: PET and FMRI. In R Cabeza & A Kingstone (eds): *Handbook of functional neuroimaging of cognition*. Cambridge, MA: MIT Press, 2001

41. Coles JP, Fryer TD, Smielewski P, Rice K, Clark JC, Pickard JD, Menon DK. Defining ischemic burden after traumatic brain injury using 15-O PET imaging of cerebral physiology. *J Cereb Blood Flow Metabol* 2004; 24:191–201

42. Donnemiller E, Brenneis C Wissel J, Scherfler C, Poewe W, Riccabona G, Wenning GK. Impaired dopaminergic neurotransmission in patients with traumatic brain injury: a SPET study using 123I-fl-CIT and 123I-IBZM. *Eur J Nucl Med* 2000; 27: 1410–1414.

43. Hattori N, Huang SC, Wu HM, Yeh E, Glenn TC, Vespa PM, McArthur D, Phelps ME, Hovda DA, Bergsneider M. Correlation of regional metabolic rates of glucose with Glasgow Coma Scale after traumatic brain injury. *J Nucl Med* 2003; 44:1709–1716.

44. Hattori N, Huang SC, Wu HM, Weihsun L, Glenn TC, Vespa PM, Phelps ME, Hovda DA, Bergsneider M. Acute Changes in Regional Cerebral 18F-FDG Kinetics in Patients with Traumatic Brain Injury. *J Nucl Med* 2004; 45:775–783.

45. Bergsneider M, Hovda D, Shalmon E. Cerebral hyperglycolysis following severe traumatic brain injury in humans; a positron emission tomography. *J Neurosurg* 1997; 86:241–251.

46. Bergsneider M, Hovda DA, McArthur DL, Etchpare M, Huang SC, Sehati N, Satz P, Phelps ME, Becker DP. Metabolic recovery following human traumatic brain injury based on FDG-PET: Time course and relationship to neurological disability. *J Head Trauma Rehabil* 2001; 16(2):135–148.

47. Langfitt TW, Obrist WD, Alavia A, Grossman RI, Zimmerman R, Jaggi J, Uzzell B, Reivich M, Patton DR. Computerized tomography, magnetic resonance imaging, and positron emission tomography in the study of brain trauma. *J Neurosurg* 1986; 64: 760–767.

48. Jansen HML, van der Naalt J, van Zomeren AH. Cobalt-55 positron emission tomography in traumatic brain injury: A pilot study. *J Neurol Neurosurg Psychiatr* 1996; 60(2):221–224.

49. Wu HM, Huan, SC, Hattori N, Glenn TC. Vespa PM, Yu CL, Hovda DA, Phelps ME, Bergsneider M. Selective metabolic reduction in gray matter acutely following human traumatic brain injury. *J Neurotrauma* 2004; 21(2):149–161.

50. Ruff R, Crouch JA, Troester AI, Marshall LF, Buchsbaum MS, Lottenberg S, Somers LM. Selected cases of poor outcome following a minor brain trauma: comparing neuropsychological and PET assessment. *Brain Inj* 1994; 8(4):297–308.

51. Gross H, Kling A, Henry G, Herndon C, & Lavretsky H. Local cerebral glucose metabolism in patients with long-term behavioral and cognitive deficits following mild head injury. *J Neuropsychiatr Clin Neurosci* 1996; 8(3):324–334.

52. Fontaine A, Azouvi P, Remy P, Bussel B, Samson Y. Functional anatomy of neuropsychological deficits after severe traumatic brain injury. *Neurology* 1999; 53:1963–1968

53. Varney NR, Pinksont JB, Wu JC. Quantitative PET findings in patients with posttraumatic anosmia. *J Head Trauma Rehabil* 2001; 16(3):253–259.

54. Baron, J. C. Étude de la neuroanatomie functionelle de la perception par la tomographie à positons. *Revue Neurolog* 1995; 151:511–517.

55. Ricker JH, M,ller RA, Zafonte RD, Black K, Millis SR, Chugani H. Verbal recall and recognition following traumatic brain injury: A [15O]-water positron emission tomography study. *J Clinical Exp Neuropsychol* 2001; 23(2): 196–206.

56. Levine B, Cabeza R, McIntosh AR, Black SE, Grady CL, Stuss DT. Functional reorganisation of memory after traumatic brain injury: a study with H_2-^{15}O positron emission tomography. *J Neurol Neurosurg Psychiatr* 2002; 73(2):173–181.

57. Springer CS, Patlak CS, Playka I, Huang W. Principles of susceptibility contrast-based functional MRI: The sign of the functional response. In: Moonen CT, Bandettini PA (eds.), *Functional MRI*. Berlin: Springer-Verlag, 91–102, 2000.

58. Weisskoff RM. Basic theoretical models of BOLD signal change. In: Moonen CT, Bandettini PA (eds.), Functional MRI. Berlin / Heidelberg: Springer-Verlag, 115–123, 2000.

59. Chen, W. & Ogawa, S. (2000). Principles of BOLD functional MRI. In C.T. Moonen & P.A. Bandettini (Eds.), Functional MRI (pp. 103–112). Berlin: Springer-Verlag.

60. McAllister TW, Saykin AJ, Flashman LA, Sparling MB, Johnson SC, Guerin SJ, Mamourian AC, Weaver JB, Yanofsky N. Brain activation during working memory 1 month after mild traumatic brain injury: A functional MRI study. Neurology 1999; 53: 1300–1308.

61. McAllister TW, Sparling MB, Flashman LA, Guerin SJ, Mamourian AC, Saykin AJ. Differential working memory load effects after mild traumatic brain injury. *NeuroImage* 2001; 14:1004–1012.

62. Christodoulou C, DeLuca J, Ricker JH, Madigan N, Bly BM, Lange G, Kalnin AJ, Liu WC, Steffener J, Ni AC. Functional magnetic resonance imaging of working memory impairment following traumatic brain injury. *J Neurol Neurosurg Psychiatr* 2001; 71: 161–168.

63. Perlstein WM, Cole MA, Demery JA, Seighourel PJ, Dixit NK, Larson MJ, Briggs RW. Parametric manipulation of working memory load in traumatic brain injury: Behavioral and neural correlates. *J International Neuropsychol Soc* 2004; 10: 724–741.

64. Scheibel RS, Pearson DA, Faria LP, Kotrla KJ, Aylward E, Bachevalier J, Levin HS. An fMRI study of executive functioning after severe diffuse TBI. *Brain Inj* 2003; 17(11):919–930.

65. Prigatano GP, Johnson SC, Gale SD. Neuroimaging correlates of the Halstead Finger Tapping Test several years post-traumatic brain injury. *Brain Inj* 2004; 18(7):661–669.

66. Laatsch, L., Little, D., & Thulborn, K. (2004). Changes in fMRI following cognitive rehabilitation in severe traumatic brain injury: A case study. *Rehabil Psychol* 2004; 49: 262–267.

67. Bobholz J, Bilder R, Bookheimer S, Cole M, Mirsky A, Pliskin N, Rao S, Ricker JH, Saykin A, Mirsky A, Sweeney J, Westerveld M. Official position of the division of clinical neuropsychology (APA Division 40) on the role of neuropsychologists in clinical use of fMRI. *Clin Neuropsychol* 2004; 18:349–351.

68. Strangman G, O'Neil-Pirozzi TM, Burke D, Cristina D, Goldstein R, Rauch SL, Savage CR, Glenn MB. Functional neuroimaging and cognitive rehabilitation for people with traumatic brain injury. *Am J Phys Med Rehabil* 2005; 84:62–75.

13

Electrophysiologic Assessment Techniques: Evoked Potentials and Electroencephalography

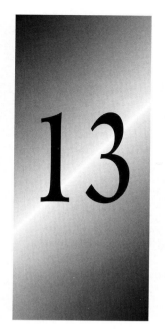

Henry L. Lew
Eun Ha Lee
Steven S. L. Pan
Jerry Y. P. Chiang

Various behavioral measures have been used to identify cognitive deficits as well as to predict functional outcome in traumatic brain injury (TBI). However, results among these studies have often conflicted (1, 2). Recently, advances in computer technology have facilitated electrophysiologic data acquisition and faster processing speed. As a result, electrophysiologic techniques have resurfaced as potentially powerful clinical measurements. As clinicians, we encounter persons with a variety of lesions in the nervous system. We are often expected to establish early diagnosis and treatment, as well as to provide continued monitoring of the recovery process. In this chapter, we summarize the potential applications of somatosensory evoked potentials (SEPs), brainstem auditory evoked potentials (BAEPs), conventional electroencephalography (EEG), P50, and P300 as objective measures in evaluating cognitive function, as well as their efficacy in predicting outcome in persons with TBI.

SOMATOSENSORY EVOKED POTENTIALS

The evoked potential (EP) is an electrophysiologic response of the nervous system that occurs as a result of repeated sensory stimulation (3). Different from conventional EEG, which shows continuously varying brain activity, EPs are averaged responses, which are temporally related to the incoming stimuli (4). Many EP measurements have been tested for their efficacy in clinical evaluation and in predicting functional outcome (5–7). Some tests provide reliable prediction of ominous outcomes (8, 9), while others prognosticate favorable outcomes (6, 7). SEPs seemed to belong to the former category (6, 9–13).

SEPs are responses of the nervous system to various sensory stimuli, including electrical, tactile, vibration, or painful stimulation. Among these stimuli, electrical stimulation has been most popular due to its ease of use. Short-latency SEP (SSEP) is a part of the SEP occurring within 50 msec after peripheral nerve stimulation in either upper or lower extremities (14). SSEPs are relatively independent from level of consciousness, while middle or long latency SEPs are influenced by cognitive status to a larger degree. Due to its reliability and stability, SSEP is commonly used for clinical evaluation and prognostication in TBI (4, 10). An example of normal SSEP from stimulation of median nerve is illustrated in Figure 13-1.

For traumatic coma in adults and adolescents, bilaterally absent cortical SEP responses predicted a 95 percent probability of non-awakening from coma (10, 15). Beca and colleagues studied SEPs within 4 days of coma onset in children with severe brain injury (16), and found that

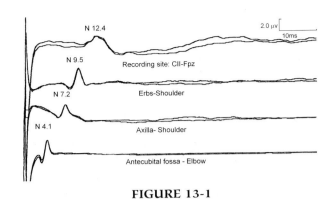

FIGURE 13-1

Normal SSEP waveforms from stimulation of left median nerve at the wrist

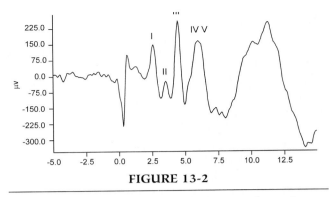

FIGURE 13-2

Normal brainstem auditory evoked potential waveform

absent SEPs had very high positive predictive values (92–100 percent) for unfavorable outcome. In children with TBI, the likelihood of awakening from coma despite bilaterally absent SEP response was approximately 7 percent (10, 15). In a recent study by Lew et al. (6), bilateral absence of cortically recorded median nerve SEP within 8 days of severe TBI (Glasgow Coma Scale ≤ 8) was strongly predictive ($p < 0.005$) of the worst functional outcome, namely, death or persistent vegetative state. In the above study, specificity and positive predictive values of absent SEP response for death or persistent vegetative state were as high as 100 percent at 6 months post-TBI.

In addition to SEP, there have been efforts to combine other evoked potential studies using so called "multimodality evoked potentials." Shin et al. performed BAEP and SEP in TBI patients, and compared the results with clinical outcome (11). Although neither of the electrophysiologic measurements showed significant correlation with the cognitive level at a one-year follow-up, SEP increased the predictive value of initial clinical parameters including Rancho Los Amigos Scale or age. As for visual evoked potential (VEP), it has been utilized independently to evaluate visual impairment such as post-traumatic vision syndrome after brain injury (17, 18).

Several factors must be taken into consideration during the interpretation and analysis of the SEP waveform. For example, peripheral neuropathy of the nerve being stimulated may prolong the latency of cortically recorded potentials. Evoked responses recorded from the brainstem and cervical spine should be reviewed to rule out concurrent spinal cord injury. To distinguish central pathology from peripheral pathology, central conduction time (from the brainstem or Erb's point to the cortical level) can be used (19). Increased level of sedation may reduce the amplitude of cortical SEP. Therefore, when the SEP amplitude is too small, it is prudent to repeat the test after removal of sedation (10). All things considered, decisions regarding continuation of life support should not depend totally upon SEP testing, but instead rely on overall clinical status, together with other laboratory findings and, most of all, family input.

BRAINSTEM AUDITORY EVOKED POTENTIALS

Brainstem Auditory Evoked Potentials (BAEPs, also known as BAER, brainstem auditory evoked response) represent the electrophysiologic response of the central nervous system to repeated click stimuli, and is characterized by a pattern of 5 neurogenic waves (20). The BAEP wave I originates from the cochlear nerve, and wave II arises from the cochlear nucleus. Waves III, IV, and V originate from the superior olivary complex, lateral lemniscus, and inferior colliculus, respectively. An example of normal BAEP waveform is illustrated in Figure 13-2.

Prolongations of interpeak intervals between I–III, III–V, or I–V have been reported in patients with TBI, (11, 21–24). The most ominous finding is complete absence of a repeatable waveform. In a study on comatose children and adolescents with traumatic brain injury, BAEP abnormality was found to be about 40 percent of the 62 patients tested (25). In a meta-analysis, it was concluded that normal BAEP obtained within the first week of TBI onset had a very good prognostic value for awakening from coma (26), while EEG did not have much clinical utility. However, another independent study showed that the presence of BAEP in post-coma unawareness patients did not have any significant prognostic value, because the presence of normal BAEP in these patients may merely suggest that the brainstem had been spared despite significant injury above the brainstem (27).

In mild TBI, prolongation of BAEP wave I and III latencies had been observed soon after concussion, and prolongation of BAEP interpeak intervals (between wave I and V) had been noted from the first day of TBI (28). In other studies of persistent post-concussion syndrome, no significant BAEP latency delays were found (29). In more severe cases of TBI, prolonged interpeak interval persisted for several weeks (28, 30, 31). It should also be noted that when more rigorous normative values were applied (abnormality defined as greater than 2.5 SD, rather than 2.0 SD, from the mean), no abnormalities in BAEP were noted after mild TBI (32). Also, in a group of amateur boxers (N = 47) who supposedly had repeated concussions, no differences in BAEP results were observed when compared to other athletes with low risk of TBI (33). There have been several studies on BAEP to determine its correlation with dizziness. In patients with post-concussion syndrome, the BAEP alterations were not associated with dizziness or abnormal vestibular function (34). In another study involving patients with mild head injury, significantly prolonged BAEP latency was observed. However it was not correlated with outcome after 3 months (35).

The value of BAEP for hearing screening has already been established in newborns because of its objective nature and ease of use (36, 37). Due to co-existing cognitive problems, it is sometimes difficult to detect hearing dysfunction in TBI patients, especially in the early stages of recovery (38). This may result in delays in audiological, surgical, and rehabilitative interventions. Review of literature from 1975 to 2001 showed that the incidence of hearing problems for various degrees of TBI varied from 7 to 50 percent (25, 39–43). A recent review of inpatient records from a TBI unit showed that 17 percent of moderate to severe TBI patients showed abnormal behavioral audiograms after the injury (44). If hearing screenings with BAEP were performed prospectively on all moderate-to-severe TBI patients, the incidence could be higher than 17 percent. In a study on 40 TBI patients (22), BAEP results were compared with behavioral audiometry, and the authors concluded that BAEP was more diagnostic than pure tone audiometry in the evaluation of brainstem dysfunction. In conclusion, the utility of BAEP in TBI may be limited to evaluation of brainstem dysfunction and hearing impairment (45).

ELECTROENCEPHALOGRAM

Conventional electroencephalogram (EEG) measures electrical activity generated by the brain via surface electrode recording. An example of ongoing EEG is illustrated in Figure 13-3. Traditional EEG studies typically involve subjective and qualitative analysis, although efforts are being made to objectively quantify the EEG data, such as Fourier Transform (FT) of the frequency bands. With advances in computer-based signal processing technology, quantitative EEG (QEEG) analyses may gain wider use in evaluating TBI patients (46).

Conventional EEG

There are four basic components in EEG waveforms. Alpha waves (8–12 Hz) are seen in the awake but relaxed

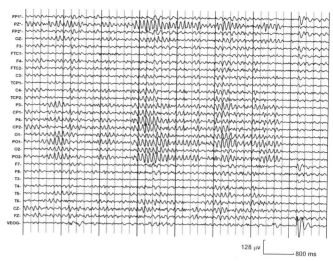

128 μv | 800 ms

FIGURE 13-3

Continuous electroencephalography recording by surface electrodes

state, while beta waves (12–30 Hz) are observed in the fully awake state. Delta waves are the slowest waves (less than 4 Hz), which are related to nondreaming deep sleep. Theta waves (4–8 Hz) also are associated with hypnotic or meditation states of consciousness. These waves are affected by age and recording sites. The pathologic brain wave patterns include focal or generalized spikes observed in patients with convulsive disorders. Other pathologic patterns vary from overall slowing to altered proportion of waves. Burst suppression pattern is characteristically seen during the induction stage of anesthesia. It is typically shown as a mixed pattern of high-voltage bursts and low-voltage suppression period, which are also related to anoxia, coma, and brain damage (47, 48).

EEG patterns have been empirically used to assess the severity of TBI and to predict their functional outcome (49). In 1973, Bricolo (49) reported that EEG is a useful evaluation tool for comatose TBI patients. They found that subjects with "spindle patterns" had relatively favorable prognosis, and patients with monophasic or slow disorganized electric activity patterns without response to environmental stimuli had much higher mortality rate. Synek (50) studied the EEG patterns of patients with cerebral anoxia or head injury, and concluded that those who responded to external stimuli were usually associated with good outcomes. Some other favorable EEG patterns included normal activity, rhythmic theta activity, frontal rhythmic delta activity, and spindle pattern. On the other hand, epileptiform activity, nonreactive, low-amplitude delta activity, and burst suppression patterns with interruptions of isoelectricity were associated with poor prognosis. Needless to say, patients with complete isoelectric EEG activity had the highest mortality.

Although EEG analyses may provide some prognostic information for patients with severe TBI, there are issues with their application in mild TBI. Jacome et al. (51) found no EEG abnormality in 24-hour ambulatory EEG monitoring of mild TBI patients. One and a half decades later, Voller et al. (52) did a combined EEG/MRI study. Again, no EEG abnormalities were observed in mild TBI patients. Even in patients with structural lesion per MRI, no focal change in EEG was noted. Based on the aforementioned studies, conventional EEG analysis is not highly regarded as either a diagnostic or prognostic tool in evaluating the patients with mild TBI.

Quantitative Electroencephalography

Quantitative electroencephalography (QEEG) is based on highly sophisticated computation of EEG signals. The fundamental element of QEEG is spectral analysis, which decomposes the complex EEG signal into various component frequencies. The amount of alpha (8–12 Hz), beta (12–30 Hz), delta (0–4 Hz), and theta (4–8 Hz) component activity contained in the EEG signals are quantitatively isolated and stored in digitized format for further analysis. Topographical mapping of different frequency bands (sometimes referred to as BEAM, brain electrical activity mapping) can be made based on the results of spectral analyses. QEEG has clinical value in certain neurologic abnormalities such as epilepsy, cerebrovascular disease, and dementia (53). However, experts in neurophysiology have not completely reached their consensus regarding the clinical utility of QEEG in mild head injury, moderate head injury, or post-concussion syndrome (53–56).

Due to the availability of digital recording and computer-based real-time quantitative analyses, many researchers have devoted their time and efforts to exploring QEEG as a tool for evaluating TBI patients. Bricolo et al. (57) first studied comatose TBI patients by spectral EEG analysis. They suggested that interhemispheric frequency band asymmetries were associated with poor outcome. In contrast, patients with spontaneous EEG power spectrum variability and persistence or return of EEG activity within the alpha or theta frequency were correlated with favorable prognosis. (58, 59).

Comparing the predictive values between QEEG and Glasgow Coma Scale (GCS) in severe TBI patients, Karnaze et al. (60) showed that altered spectral patterns were correlated with better survival, and its predictive value was equivalent to, but not significantly higher than that of GCS. Thatcher et al. (61) compared QEEG, GCS, brainstem auditory evoked potential (BAEP), and Computed Tomography (CT) in outcome prediction of 162 comatose TBI patients. EEG phase pattern was demonstrated to be the most prognostic, followed by EEG coherence, GCS, and brain CT, respectively. Alster et al. (62)

also demonstrated that spectral EEG analyses were more predictive of brain injury outcomes than GCS and BAEPs.

Thatcher et al. (63) compared QEEG patterns between patients with mild TBI and age-matched controls. An overall classification accuracy of 94.8 percent was reported. Mild TBI subjects showed increased coherence and reduced phase in frontal and temporal areas, decreased alpha band amplitudes in the parieto-occipital territories, and reduced spectral power difference across anterior/posterior cortical regions. Tebano (64) also performed spectral EEG analysis in persons with brain injury. Their results showed that mild TBI patients had a shift in peak alpha frequency band toward lower frequency values. Twelve years later, Cudmore (65) also demonstrated that EEG coherence pattern differentiated controls from patients with mild TBI. Increased alpha/theta ratio was observed in mild TBI patients (66), possibly due to reduced theta activity, with relatively stable alpha activities.

In summary, these studies imply that QEEG findings may be better than conventional EEG in studying mild TBI patients. However, inter-research comparison and meta-analysis are problematic due to lack of standardized techniques and inconsistent inclusion/exclusion criteria. In addition, QEEG analyses are derived from vast amount of data points over various recording electrodes, and researchers typically use multiple analyses to derive the results. Consequently, type I error is a major concern, and multiple inter-electrode comparisons may yield some "statistically significant" but not "clinically meaningful" results.

PAIN-RELATED POTENTIAL (P250)

Deep brain stimulation (DBS) of various brain regions (e.g., mesencephalic reticular formation or the thalamic center median-parafascicular (CM-Pf) complex) has been used to evaluate or even promote recovery from the persistent vegetative state (PVS). To monitor clinical utility of DBS, the late positive wave of cortical potentials elicited by painful stimuli (pain-related potential, P250) has been investigated (67–69). In chronic vegetative state, the depressed P250 was temporarily enhanced by DBS. A persistent enhancement of the P250 was also correlated with better clinical outcome (67). The P250 may provide objective and quantitative information regarding the level of cortical responsiveness to painful stimuli in persons in low level neurological states following brain injury.

P50

The P50-evoked response is the event-related potential (ERP) response around 50 msec to auditory stimuli (P50 ERP). This potential is recorded at the scalp, and reflects the cholinergically dependent, hippocampally mediated, and pre-attentive process of sensory gating to auditory stimuli (70, 71). Traditionally, paired auditory stimuli are used for P50 study. The procedure is as follows: First, hearing threshold (in dBSPL) is determined, and the auditory stimuli are presented at 25–45 dB SPL above the hearing threshold (72). Employing the International 10–20 System of Electrode Placement (73), the P50 potential is recorded at Cz-A1 with a ground electrode at A2. Pairs of auditory stimuli (1 msec duration, 20Hz–12kHz) are presented with certain intra-pair (around 0.5 sec) and inter-stimulus (around 10 sec) interval. An overall grand average is obtained for both the conditioning and test P50 responses. The P50 latency and amplitude can be identified by computer algorithm (72, 74).

The P50 ratio (in percentage) is the amplitude ratio of the test P50 to the conditioning P50. Examples of P50 suppression and nonsuppression are illustrated in Figure 13-4. It is used as an index for auditory sensory gating (72). P50 suppression is defined as a P50 ratio of ≤40 percent, and P50 nonsuppression is => 60 percent. P50 ratio between 40 and 60 is considered as an indeterminate P50 suppression (72). Arciniegas et al. reported that the P50 ratio was significantly increased in TBI (75). Interestingly, the P50 ratios of different TBI subgroups, categorized by duration of post-traumatic amnesia (PTA) did not show significant difference from one another. Those TBI subjects with similar level of cognitive impairment at the time of testing demonstrated similar amount of abnormal P50 suppression despite varying severity of initial brain injury. In another study (72), the frequency of P50 nonsuppression was investigated in patients with persistent posttraumatic attention and/or memory impairment. Preliminary analysis showed that the majority of TBI subjects have discernable P50 response, and that P50 nonsuppression is common among TBI patients with subjective symptoms of attention and memory

impairments, providing some evidence that clinically impaired auditory gating is variably correlated with P50 nonsuppression.

Regarding the source of P50 potential, it has been suggested that the generator is located at the hippocampus (74, 76, 77). Sensory gating process may facilitate stimulus selection and information processing, which are important for attention and memory function (72). It was suggested that impaired sensory gating cause attention and memory impairments after TBI (78), and that abnormal P50 findings may be a useful marker for cholinergic dysfunction (72, 75, 79, 80). In summary, these studies suggest that the P50 response may be useful not only for evaluating cognitive dysfunction, but also for monitoring pharmacological interventions in TBI.

EVENT-RELATED POTENTIALS/P300

Event-related potentials (ERPs) are cognitive potentials recorded over the scalp. They have been regarded by psychophysiologists as indicators of information processing, which may not be fully appreciated by measuring behavioral performance alone (6, 81, 82). In the active ERP paradigm, the subject is asked to discriminate a rare/target stimulus (typically with occurrence rate of 20 percent) from an interrupted series of frequent/nontarget stimuli (80 percent occurrence rate) (83). When averaged appropriately, the target stimuli generate a prominent positive peak (P300) approximately 300 msec after stimulus onset (83–85). The P300 response reflects active attention, working memory, and the ability to detect novel stimuli among a series of similar signals (81, 84, 86, 87). Amplitude of P300 reflects the amount of cerebral activity required to process information and maintain working memory as the controlled environment is updated with incoming sensory input (86). Studies have shown that the P300 latency is a reliable indicator of stimulus classification speed, which is independent from the response selection processes (88, 89). Traditionally, simple auditory and visual tasks such as tone and color recognition have been widely employed in ERP testing due to its ease of use (83, 86, 90, 91). Although these tasks are rather primitive when compared with other paradigms (e.g., word recognition, affect recognition), simpler tasks have the advantage of generating larger amplitudes and shorter latencies, which in turn simplify the data analysis process. An example of normal auditory P300 response is shown in Figure 13-5. The waveform was recorded at an Cz electrode, using an active oddball paradigm with pure tones as stimuli.

Not surprisingly, P300/ERP studies have been applied to patients with cognitive impairments (92) and psychiatric disorders (93, 94). For comatose patients who are unable to participate actively in the testing process, the passive ERP paradigm can be used (6, 95–98). Several brain

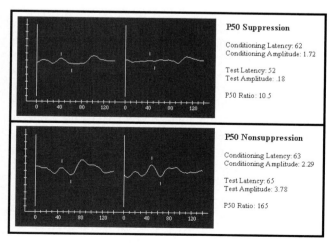

FIGURE 13-4

P50 suppression and nonsuppression (72)

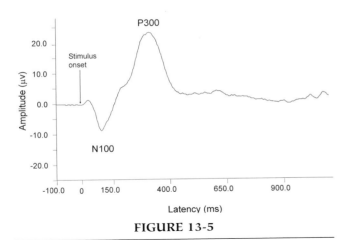

FIGURE 13-5

Normal auditory event-related potential (ERP) waveforms from pure tone (1000 Hz versus 500 Hz) discrimination task

injury studies utilized simple tones as stimuli (7, 95–99), which yielded P300 responses in about 30 percent of apparently comatose patients. Preserved P300 seemed to predict the emergence from coma (95, 99, 100) and higher chance of recovery (90 percent or higher) in long-term follow-up (95, 99, 101). However, the absence of P300 did not exclusively prognosticate ominous outcome (6).

Based on recent data published by various researchers (6, 101, 102), it was apparent that preserved P300 component was associated with good clinical outcomes, while it was coincidentally noted that the N100 component also correlated with favorable outcome. In one study (101), investigators recorded auditory P300 potentials using three different passive paradigms both in normal subjects and in patients with severe consciousness impairment after TBI. Results showed that the N100 latency was longer, with significantly depressed amplitude in TBI patients than in normal subjects. It suggested that cognitive processing of exogenous sensory stimuli may still take place, albeit with some delay, when the patients' level of consciousness appeared to be severely impaired. Although the N100 response was thought to be associated with passive perception of incoming sound (103), there is evidence to suggest its involvement with alertness and stimulus processing (81). Based on the above-mentioned studies, it is possible that both the N100 and P300 components are associated with active information processing (101, 102, 104).

To increase the ecologic validity of the ERP task, recent studies employed speech stimuli such as patients' names (6, 101, 105). From a theoretical standpoint, a person's own name would generate a more robust ERP response. By comparing three different speech targets (subject's own name, the word "mommy," and a meaningless speech sound), a recent study demonstrated that the subject's name was indeed a viable target for eliciting cognitive ERP (102).

ERP testing has also been used to monitor effects of caffeine, nicotine, alcohol intake, and various psychostimulants. Caffeine and nicotine increased the P300 amplitude and shortened the latency, while acute alcohol consumption decreased the amplitude and prolonged the latency (81). Anderer et al. compared the pharmacologic effects of various drugs in healthy subjects. While methylphenidate and citalopram enhanced P300 in various cortical regions, lorazepam and haloperidol depressed P300 component (106). From a theoretical perspective, ERP might be a useful tool in evaluating the pharmacologic effect of various so called "cognitive enhancers" after brain injury.

In summary, ERP may be valuable in investigating residual cognitive function of patients with TBI because of its noninvasive nature (107) and superior temporal resolution (108). Also, using multi-channel recording, ERP may contribute to localization of certain brain activities based on dipole theory. With advances in computer technology, ERP may complement behavioral testing in the comprehensive evaluation of cognitive function.

CONCLUSION

So far, we have discussed use of various electrophysiologic measurements for persons with TBI. SEP is a reliable prognosticator for ominous outcome after severe TBI. Combining ERP with SEP increases the power for predicting a favorable outcome. P300 and P50 are valuable in evaluating pharmacological effects of various drugs on cognitive function. The utility of BAEP in TBI is limited to evaluation of brainstem dysfunction and hearing impairment, rather than actual cognitive function. Although conventional EEG and QEEG have their inherent limitations, they may gain wider use as technology improves and more standardized studies are performed.

Neuro-imaging studies, such as MRI (magnetic resonance imaging) or fMRI (functional MRI) have been used to obtain structural information along with electrophysiologic information (109–112). While ERP measurement can provide high temporal resolution for evaluation of cognitive processing, fMRI detects regional changes of brain activity in response to specific task performance. However, most of these combination studies (using imaging and electrophysiologic measurements) have been performed on psychiatric patients, and have been rarely applied to persons with TBI. As for future research, the addition of electrophysiologic and neuro-imaging studies may provide comprehensive, objective, and valid assessments of cognitive status in persons with TBI, and may be useful in prognostication of long-term functional outcome.

References

1. Bezner JR, Hunter DL. Wellness perception in persons with traumatic brain injury and its relation to functional independence. *Arch Phys Med Rehabil* 2001, 82: 787–92.

2. Boake C, Millis SR, High WM, Jr., et al. Using early neuropsychologic testing to predict long-term productivity outcome from traumatic brain injury. *Arch Phys Med Rehabil* 2001, 82: 761–68.

3. Hallett M. Glossary of terms: EMG/EDX/clinical neurophysiology and the practice of medicine. *Muscle Nerve* 1992, 15: 1378–82.

4. Yamada T, Yeh M, Kimura J. Fundamental principles of somatosensory evoked potentials. In: Kraft GH, Lew HL, eds. *PM&R Clinics of North America*. Philadelphia: WB Saunders, 2004.

5. Houlden DA, Schwartz ML, Klettke KA. Neurophysiologic diagnosis in uncooperative trauma patients: confounding factors. *J.Trauma* 1992, 33: 244–51.

6. Lew HL, Dikmen S, Slimp J et al. Use of somatosensory-evoked potentials and cognitive event-related potentials in predicting outcomes of patients with severe traumatic brain injury. *Am J Phys Med Rehabil*. 2003, 82: 53–61.

7. Yingling CD, Hosobuchi Y, Harrington M. P300 as a predictor of recovery from coma. *Lancet* 1990, 336: 873.

8. Houlden DA, Li C, Schwartz ML, Katic M. Median nerve somatosensory evoked potentials and the Glasgow Coma Scale as predictors of outcome in comatose patients with head injuries. *Neurosurgery* 1990, 27: 701–7.

9. Sleigh JW, Havill JH, Frith R, Kersel D, Marsh N, Ulyatt D. Somatosensory evoked potentials in severe traumatic brain injury: a blinded study. *J Neurosurg* 1999, 91: 577–80.

10. Robinson LR, Micklesen PJ, Tirschwell DL, Lew HL. Predictive value of somatosensory evoked potentials for awakening from coma. *Crit Care Med* 2003, 31: 960–67.

11. Shin DY, Ehrenberg B, Whyte J, Bach J, DeLisa JA. Evoked potential assessment: utility in prognosis of chronic head injury. *Arch Phys Med Rehabil*. 1989, 70: 189–93.

12. Ozbudak-Demir S, Akyuz M, Guler-Uysal F, Orkun S. Postacute predictors of functional and cognitive progress in traumatic brain injury: somatosensory evoked potentials. *Arch Phys Med Rehabil*. 1999, 80: 252–57.

13. Haupt WF, Pawlik G. Contribution of initial median-nerve somatosensory evoked potentials and brainstem auditory evoked potentials to prediction of clinical outcome in cerebrovascular critical care patients: a statistical evaluation. *J Clin Neurophysiol* 1998, 15: 154–58.

14. Nuwer MR, Aminoff M, Desmedt J, et al. IFCN recommended standards for short latency somatosensory evoked potentials. Report of an IFCN committee. International Federation of Clinical Neurophysiology. *Electroencephalogr Clin Neurophysiol* 1994, 91: 6–11.

15. Robinson LR. Somatosensory evoked potentials in coma prognosis. In: Kraft GH, Lew HL, eds. *PM&R Clinics of North America*. Philadelphia: WB Saunders, 2004.

16. Beca J, Cox PN, Taylor MJ, et al. Somatosensory evoked potentials for prediction of outcome in acute severe brain injury. *J Pediatr* 1995, 126: 44–9.

17. Padula WV, Argyris S, Ray J. Visual evoked potentials (VEP) evaluating treatment for post-trauma vision syndrome (PTVS) in patients with traumatic brain injuries (TBI). *Brain Inj* 1994, 8: 125–33.

18. Sarno S, Erasmus LP, Lippert G, Frey M, Lipp B, Schlaegel W. Electrophysiological correlates of visual impairments after traumatic brain injury. *Vision Res* 2000, 40: 3029–38.

19. Keren O, Groswasser Z, Sazbon L, Ring C. Somatosensory evoked potentials in prolonged post-comatose unawareness state following traumatic brain injury. *Brain Inj* 1991, 5: 233–40.

20. Nuwer MR, Aminoff M, Goodin D, et al. IFCN recommended standards for brainstem auditory evoked potentials. Report of an IFCN committee. International Federation of Clinical Neurophysiology. *Electroencephalogr Clin Neurophysiol* 1994, 91: 12–17.

21. Aguilar EA, III, Hall JW, III, Mackey-Hargadine J. Neurootologic evaluation of the patient with acute, severe head injuries: correlations among physical findings, auditory evoked responses, and computerized tomography. *Otolaryngol Head Neck Surg* 1986, 94: 211–19.

22. Abd al-Hady MR, Shehata O, el Mously M, Sallam FS. Audiological findings following head trauma. *J Laryngol Otol* 1990, 104: 927–36.

23. Elwany S. Auditory brain stem responses (ABR) in patients with acute severe closed head injuries. The use of a grading system. *J Laryngol Otol*. 1988, 102: 755–59.

24. Hall JW, III, Huang-fu M, Gennarelli TA. Auditory function in acute severe head injury. *Laryngoscope* 1982, 92: 883–90.

25. Cockrell JL, Gregory SA. Audiological deficits in brain-injured children and adolescents. *Brain Inj* 1992, 6: 261–66.

26. Attia J, Cook DJ. Prognosis in anoxic and traumatic coma. *Crit Care Clin*. 1998, 14: 497–511.

27. Keren O, Sazbon L, Groswasser Z, Shmuel M. Follow-up studies of somatosensory evoked potentials and auditory brainstem evoked potentials in patients with post-coma unawareness (PCU) of traumatic brain injury. *Brain Inj* 1994, 8: 239–47.

28. Noseworthy JH, Miller J, Murray TJ, Regan D. Auditory brainstem responses in postconcussion syndrome. *Arch Neurol*. 1981, 38: 275–78.

29. Gaetz M, Weinberg H. Electrophysiological indices of persistent post-concussion symptoms. *Brain Inj* 2000, 14: 815–32.

30. McClelland RJ, Fenton GW, Rutherford W. The post-concussional syndrome revisited. *J Roy Soc Med* 1994, 87: 508–10.

31. Rizzo PA, Pierelli F, Pozzessere G, Floris R, Morocutti C. Subjective post-traumatic syndrome. A comparison of visual and brain stem auditory evoked responses. *Neuropsychobiology* 1983, 9: 78–82.

32. Werner RA, Vanderzant CW. Multimodality evoked potential testing in acute mild closed head injury. *Arch Phys Med Rehabil* 1991, 72: 31–4.

33. Haglund Y, Persson HE. Does Swedish amateur boxing lead to chronic brain damage? 3. A retrospective clinical neurophysiological study. *Acta Neurol.Scand* 1990, 82: 353–60.

34. Benna P, Bergamasco B, Bianco C, Gilli M, Ferrero P, Pinessi L. Brainstem auditory evoked potentials in post-concussion syndrome. *Ital J Neurol Sci*. 1982, 3: 281–87.

35. Soustiel JF, Hafner H, Chistyakov AV, Barzilai A, Feinsod M. Trigeminal and auditory evoked responses in minor head injuries and post-concussion syndrome. *Brain Inj* 1995, 9: 805–13.

36. Murray AD, Javel E, Watson CS. Prognostic validity of auditory brainstem evoked response screening in newborn infants. *Am J Otolaryngol* 1985, 6: 120–31.

37. Kramer SJ, Vertes DR, Condon M. Auditory brainstem responses and clinical follow-up of high-risk infants. *Pediatrics* 1989, 83: 385–92.

38. Fligor BJ, Cox LC, Nesathurai S. Subjective hearing loss and history of traumatic brain injury exhibits abnormal brainstem auditory evoked response: a case report. *Arch Phys Med Rehabil* 2002, 83: 141–43.

39. Lubinski R, Moscato BS, Willer BS. Prevalence of speaking and hearing disabilities among adults with traumatic brain injury from a national household survey. *Brain Inj* 1997, 11: 103–14.

40. Bergman M, Hirsch S, Solzi P. Interhemispheric suppression: a test of central auditory function. *Ear Hear* 1987, 8: 87–91.

41. Podoshin L, Fradis M. Hearing loss after head injury. *Arch Otolaryngol* 1975, 101: 15–8.

42. Griffiths MV. The incidence of auditory and vestibular concussion following minor head injury. *J Laryngol Otol* 1979, 93: 253–65.

43. Jury MA, Flynn MC. Auditory and vestibular sequelae to traumatic brain injury: a pilot study. *NZ Med J* 2001, 114: 286–88.

44. Lew HL, Lee EH, Miyoshi Y, Chang DG, Date ES, Jerger JF. Brainstem auditory-evoked pentials as an objective tool for evaluating hearing dysfunction in traumatic brain injury. *Am J Phys Med Rehabil* 2004, 83: 210–15.

45. Gaetz M, Bernstein DM. The current status of electrophysiologic procedures for the assessment of mild traumatic brain injury. *J Head Trauma Rehabil* 2001, 16: 386–405.

46. Wallace BE, Wagner AK, Wagner EP, McDeavitt JT. A history and review of quantitative electroencephalography in traumatic brain injury. *J Head Trauma Rehabil* 2001, 16: 165–90.

47. Young GB. The EEG in coma. *J Clin Neurophysiol* 2000, 17: 473–85.

48. Synek VM. Prognostically important EEG coma patterns in diffuse anoxic and traumatic encephalopathies in adults. *J Clin Neurophysiol* 1988, 5: 161–74.

49. Bricolo A, Turella G. Electroencephalographic patterns of acute traumatic coma: diagnostic and prognostic value. *J Neurosurg Sci.* 1973, 17: 278–85.

50. Synek VM. Value of a revised EEG coma scale for prognosis after cerebral anoxia and diffuse head injury. *Clin Electroencephalogr* 1990, 21: 25–30.

51. Jacome DE, Risko M. EEG features in post-traumatic syndrome. *Clin Electroencephalogr* 1984, 15: 214–21.

52. Voller B, Benke T, Benedetto K, Schnider P, Auff E, Aichner F. Neuropsychological, MRI, and EEG findings after very mild traumatic brain injury. *Brain Inj* 1999, 13: 821–27.

53. Nuwer M. Assessment of digital EEG, quantitative EEG, and EEG brain mapping: report of the American Academy of Neurology and the American Clinical Neurophysiology Society. *Neurology* 1997, 49: 277–92.

54. Nuwer MR. Assessing digital and quantitative EEG in clinical settings. *J Clin Neurophysiol* 1998, 15: 458–63.

55. Thatcher RW, Moore N, John ER, Duffy F, Hughes JR, Krieger M. QEEG and traumatic brain injury: rebuttal of the American Academy of Neurology 1997 report by the EEG and Clinical Neuroscience Society. *Clin Electroencephalogr* 1999, 30: 94–8.

56. Hoffman DA, Lubar JF, Thatcher RW, et al. Limitations of the American Academy of Neurology and American Clinical Neurophysiology Society paper on QEEG. *J Neuropsychiatry Clin Neurosci* 1999, 11: 401–7.

57. Bricolo A, Turazzi S, Faccioli F, Odorizzi F, Sciaretta G, Erculiani P. Clinical application of compressed spectral array in long-term EEG monitoring of comatose patients. *Electroencephal Clin Neurophys* 1978, 45: 211–25.

58. Cant BR, Shaw NA. Monitoring by compressed spectral array in prolonged coma. *Neurology* 1984, 34: 35–9.

59. Steudel WI, Kruger J. Using the spectral analysis of the EEG for prognosis of severe brain injuries in the first post-traumatic week. *Acta Neurochirurgica–Supplementum* 1979, 28: 40–2.

60. Karnaze DS, Marshall LF, Bickford RG. EEG monitoring of clinical coma: the compressed spectral array. *Neurology* 1982, 32: 289–92.

61. Thatcher RW, Cantor DS, McAlaster R, Geisler F, Krause P. Comprehensive predictions of outcome in closed head-injured patients: the development of prognostic equations. *Ann NY Acad Sci* 1991, 620: 82–101.

62. Alster J, Pratt H, Feinsod M. Density spectral array, evoked potentials, and temperature rhythms in the evaluation and prognosis of the comatose patient. *Brain Inj* 1993, 7: 191–208.

63. Thatcher RW, Walker RA, Gerson I, Geisler FH. EEG discriminant analyses of mild head trauma. *Electroencephal Clin Neurophys* 1989, 73: 94–106.

64. Tebano MT, Cameroni M, Gallozzi G, et al. EEG spectral analysis after minor head injury in man. *Electroencephal Clin Neurophys* 1988, 70: 185–9.

65. Cudmore LJ, Segalowitz SJ, Dywan J. EEG coherence shows altered frontal–parietal communication in mild TBI during a dual-task. *Brain Cogn* 2000, 44: 86–90.

66. Watson MR, Fenton GW, McClelland RJ, Lumsden J, Headley M, Rutherford WH. The post-concussional state: neurophysiological aspects. *B J Psychiatry* 1995, 167: 514–21.

67. Katayama Y, Tsubokata T, Yamamoto T, Hirayama T, Miyazaki S, Koyama S. Characterization and modification of brain activity with deep brain stimulation in patients in a persistent vegetative state: pain-related late positive component of cerebral evoked potential. *Pacing Clin Electrophysiol* 1991, 14: 116–21.

68. Yamamoto T, Katayama Y, Kobayashi K, Kasai M, Oshima H, Fukaya C. DBS therapy for a persistent vegetative state: ten years follow-up results. *Acta Neurochir Suppl* 2003, 87:15–8.

69. Yamamoto T, Katayama Y, Oshima H, Fukaya C, Kawamata T, Tsubokawa T. Deep brain stimulation therapy for a persistent vegetative state. *Acta Neurochir Suppl* 2002, 79:79–82.

70. Freedman R, Adler LE, Myles-Worsley M, et al. Inhibitory gating of an evoked response to repeated auditory stimuli in schizophrenic and normal subjects: human recordings, computer simulation, and an animal model. *Arch Gen Psychiatry* 1996, 53: 1114–121.

71. Adler LE, Hoffer LD, Wiser A, Freedman R. Normalization of auditory physiology by cigarette smoking in schizophrenic patients. *Am J Psychiatry* 1993, 150: 1856–61.

72. Arciniegas DB. Applications of the P50-evoked response to the evaluation of cognitive impairments following traumatic brain injury. In: Kraft GH, Lew HL, eds. *PM&R Clinics of North America.* Philadelphia: WB Saunders, 2004.

73. Laciga Z. [Proposal of an examination outline using electrodes with the system "10–20"]. *Cesk Neurol* 1968, 31: 236–38.

74. Nagamoto HT, Adler LE, Waldo MC, Freedman R. Sensory gating in schizophrenics and normal controls: effects of changing stimulation interval. *Biol Psychiatry* 1989, 25: 549–61.

75. Arciniegas D, Olincy A, Topkoff J, et al. Impaired auditory gating and P50 nonsuppression following traumatic brain injury. *J Neuropsychiatry Clin Neurosci* 2000, 12: 77–85.

76. Wilson CL, Babb TL, Halgren E, Wang ML, Crandall PH. Habituation of human limbic neuronal response to sensory stimulation. *Exp Neurol* 1984, 84: 74–97.

77. Reite M, Teale P, Zimmerman J, Davis K, Whalen J, Edrich J. Source origin of a 50-msec latency auditory evoked field component in young schizophrenic men. *Biol Psychiatry* 1988, 24: 495–506.

78. Arciniegas D, Adler L, Topkoff J, Cawthra E, Filley CM, Reite M. Attention and memory dysfunction after traumatic brain injury: cholinergic mechanisms, sensory gating, and a hypothesis for further investigation. *Brain Inj* 1999, 13: 1–13.

79. Arciniegas DB, Topkoff J, Silver JM. Neuropsychiatric aspects of traumatic brain injury. *Curr Treat Options Neurol* 2000, 2: 169–86.

80. Arciniegas DB. The cholinergic hypothesis of cognitive impairment caused by traumatic brain injury. *Curr Psychiatry Rep* 2003, 5: 391–99.

81. Lew H, Chmiel R, Jerger J, Pomerantz JR, Jerger S. Electrophysiologic indices of Stroop and Garner interference reveal linguistic influences on auditory and visual processing. *J Am Acad Audiol* 1997, 8: 104–18.

82. Segalowitz SJ, Dywan J, Unsal A. Attentional factors in response time variability after traumatic brain injury: an ERP study. *J Int Neuropsychol Soc.* 1997, 3: 95–107.

83. Polich J. P300 clinical utility and control of variability. *J Clin Neurophysiol* 1998, 15: 14–33.

84. Polich J, Kok A. Cognitive and biological determinants of P300: an integrative review. *Biol Psychol* 1995, 41: 103–46.

85. Bennington JY, Polich J. Comparison of P300 from passive and active tasks for auditory and visual stimuli. *Int J Psychophysiol* 1999, 34: 171–77.

86. Polich J, Herbst KL. P300 as a clinical assay: rationale, evaluation, and findings. *Int J Psychophysiol* 2000, 38: 3–19.

87. Viggiano MP. Event-related potentials in brain-injured patients with neuropsychological disorders: a review. *J Clin Exp Neuropsychol* 1996, 18: 631–47.

88. Ilan AB, Polich J. P300 and response time from a manual Stroop task. *Clin Neurophysiol* 1999, 110: 367–73.

89. McCarthy G, Donchin E. A metric for thought: a comparison of P300 latency and reaction time. *Science* 1981, 211: 77–80.

90. Polich J, Ellerson PC, Cohen J. P300, stimulus intensity, modality, and probability. *Int J Psychophysiol* 1996, 23: 55–62.

91. Polich J. Clinical application of the P300 event-related brain potential. In: Kraft GH, Lew HL, eds. *PM&R Clinics of North America.* Philadelphia: WB Saunders, 2004.

92. Olichney JM, Morris SK, Ochoa C, et al. Abnormal verbal event related potentials in mild cognitive impairment and incipient Alzheimer's disease. *J Neurol Neurosurg Psychiatry* 2002, 73: 377–84.

93. Ford JM, Mathalon DH, Kalba S, Marsh L, Pfefferbaum A. N1 and P300 abnormalities in patients with schizophrenia, epilepsy, and epilepsy with schizophrenialike features. *Biol Psychiatry* 2001, 49: 848–60.

94. Ford JM. Schizophrenia: the broken P300 and beyond. *Psychophysiology* 1999, 36: 667–82.

95. Kane NM, Curry SH, Rowlands CA, et al. Event-related potentials: neurophysiological tools for predicting emergence and early

outcome from traumatic coma. *Intensive Care Med* 1996, 22: 39–46.

96. Rappaport M, Clifford JO, Jr., Winterfield KM. P300 response under active and passive attentional states and uni- and bimodality stimulus presentation conditions. *J Neuropsychiatry Clin Neurosci* 1990, 2: 399–407.

97. Gott PS, Rabinowicz AL, DeGiorgio CM. P300 auditory event–related potentials in nontraumatic coma: association with Glasgow Coma Score and awakening. *Arch Neurol* 1991, 48: 1267–70.

98. Signorino M, D'Acunto S, Angeleri F, Pietropaoli P. Eliciting P300 in comatose patients. *Lancet* 1995, 345: 255–56.

99. Guerit JM, Verougstraete D, de Tourtchaninoff M, Debatisse D, Witdoeckt C. ERPs obtained with the auditory oddball paradigm in coma and altered states of consciousness: clinical relationships, prognostic value, and origin of components. *Clin Neurophysiol* 1999, 110: 1260–69.

100. Kane NM, Butler SR, Simpson T. Coma outcome prediction using event-related potentials: P(3) and mismatch negativity. *Audiol Neurootol* 2000, 5: 186–91.

101. Mazzini L, Zaccala M, Gareri F, Giordano A, Angelino E. Long-latency auditory-evoked potentials in severe traumatic brain injury. *Arch Phys Med Rehabil* 2001, 82: 57–65.

102. Lew HL, Slimp J, Price R, Massagli TL, Robinson LR. Comparison of speech-evoked vs. tone-evoked P300 response: implications for predicting outcomes in patients with traumatic brain injury. *Am J Phys Med Rehabil* 1999, 78: 367–71.

103. Pfefferbaum A, Wenegrat BG, Ford JM, Roth WT, Kopell BS. Clinical application of the P3 component of event-related potentials. II. Dementia, depression and schizophrenia. *Electroencephalogr Clin Neurophysiol* 1984, 59: 104–24.

104. Fioretto M, Gandolfo E, Orione C, Fatone M, Rela S, Sannita WG. Automatic perimetry and visual P300: differences between upper and lower visual fields stimulation in healthy subjects. *J Med Eng Technol* 1995, 19: 80–3.

105. Folmer RL, Yingling CD. Auditory P3 responses to name stimuli. *Brain Lang* 1997, 56: 306–11.

106. Anderer P, Saletu B, Semlitsch HV, Pascual-Marqui RD. Perceptual and cognitive event-related potentials in neuropsychopharmacology: methodological aspects and clinical applications (pharmaco-ERP topography and tomography). *Methods Find Exp Clin Pharmacol* 2002, 24 Suppl C:121–37.

107. Goodin D, Desmedt J, Maurer K, Nuwer MR. IFCN recommended standards for long-latency auditory event–related potentials. Report of an IFCN committee. International Federation of Clinical Neurophysiology. *Electroencephalogr Clin Neurophysio.* 1994, 91: 18–20.

108. Lew, H. L., Lee, E. H., Pan, S., and Date, E. S. Electrophysiologic abnormalities of auditory and visual information processing in patients with traumatic brain injury. *Am J Phys Med Rehabil* 2004, 83: 428433.

109. Ford JM, Gray M, Whitfield SL et al. Acquiring and inhibiting prepotent responses in schizophrenia: event–related brain potentials and functional magnetic resonance imaging. *Arch Gen Psychiatry* 2004, 61: 119–29.

110. Rangaswamy M, Porjesz B, Ardekani BA, et al. A functional MRI study of visual oddball: evidence for frontoparietal dysfunction in subjects at risk for alcoholism. *Neuroimage* 2004, 21: 329–39.

111. Pae JS, Kwon JS, Youn T, et al. LORETA imaging of P300 in schizophrenia with individual MRI and 128-channel EEG. *Neuroimage* 2003, 20: 1552–60.

112. Muller BW, Stude P, Nebel K, et al. Sparse imaging of the auditory oddball task with functional MRI. *Neuroreport* 2003, 14: 1597–601.

IV

PROGNOSIS AND OUTCOME

14 Prognosis After Severe TBI: A Practical, Evidence-Based Approach

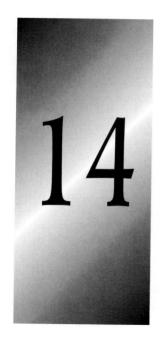

Sunil Kothari

It seems to be highly desirable that a physician should pay much attention to prognosis. If he is able to tell his patients when he visits them not only about their past and present symptoms, but also to tell them what is going to happen, as well as to fill in the details they have omitted, he will increase his reputation as a medical practitioner and people will have no qualms in putting themselves under his care.

Hippocrates

Like diagnosis and treatment, prognosis is a fundamental responsibility of all clinicians. This is especially true after a traumatic brain injury, when uncertainty about the future compounds the suffering already experienced by patients and families. Indeed, families have identified information about prognosis as one of their most important needs in the aftermath of a traumatic brain injury (1–3). Unfortunately, this need often goes unmet, as families report they were rarely provided adequate prognostic information (2,3).

Providing patients and families with this information can help in several ways. Knowing what the future might hold allows families to gain some cognitive control over a situation they otherwise feel powerless to affect. Moreover, there is a symbolic importance to prognosis: patients and families want to believe their condition is understood (4). Simply knowing that the clinician understands their condition can alleviate anxiety. Given the importance of prognosis for patients and families, some authors have even suggested that prognostication is an ethical *duty* for clinicians (4).

Despite its clear importance, clinicians often neglect prognosis. Some reasons for this neglect apply only to the delivery of *poor* prognoses: a lack of training in the delivery of "bad news", the emotionally demanding nature of providing a poor prognosis, a fear of extinguishing hope, and the fact that a poor prognosis highlights the limits of professional help (4). Other barriers can affect *any* act of prognosis: the belief that prognostication is arrogant or hubristic, a lack of facility in probabilistic reasoning, and the difficulty in extracting clinical guidelines from a large body of literature (4).

Because of this difficulty in developing guidelines based on the research literature, health care professionals often rely on their own clinical experiences in formulating prognoses. However, such an approach is of limited value: not only is a clinician's personal experience subject to selection bias, it is also prone to significant cognitive distortion (5,6). Many studies have shown that a clinician's "subjective" estimation of prognoses is often far less accurate than those derived from well designed studies (7–9).

Yet, providing prognostic information based on these studies can be difficult for TBI professionals. The literature is vast, with hundreds of studies reported, all varying in focus, design, and quality. Also, most of the studies were designed or reported in a way that makes it difficult to derive *clinically* useful guidelines. Often, they report only general associations (e.g., "outcome is related to the length of coma"). Even when these associations are quantified, it is done in a way that limits their applicability to individual cases (for instance, by using regression equations).

The purpose of this chapter is to address these obstacles and thereby derive accurate and useful guidelines from the relevant literature. It is hoped that this information will enable TBI professionals to make the most accurate prognoses possible, both to inform their own clinical decisions as well as to provide the desired information to patients and families. Of course, other reviews of this topic exist (10–24), including several excellent ones that have recently been published (25, 26). The review presented here differs from the others in three important ways. First, an attempt was made to review *all* available and relevant studies. Second, this is the first review to apply an evidence-based approach to this area. Finally, the primary aim was to develop guidelines that will be *clinically* useful.

The chapter is divided into five major sections:

- a summary of findings
- guidelines for communicating prognostic information
- a brief review of recent developments in the field
- an appendix on guidelines for evaluating studies on prognosis
- an appendix describing the methodology of the literature review

The core of the chapter is contained in the next two sections, which summarize the findings of the evidence-based review and provide guidelines on communicating this information to patients and families. The third section briefly describes developments in the area which will likely assume greater importance over the next several years. The first appendix provides a guide for evaluating future studies on prognosis. The second appendix provides a detailed description and justification for the methodology guiding this review. To maximize the usefulness of this chapter as a future reference, all the important information is summarized in the figures and tables. Therefore, after an initial reading of the entire chapter, readers can then simply refer to the tables and figures to review the essential information. This chapter does not address topics relevant to prognosis after TBI that are covered elsewhere in the textbook (see Figure 14-1).

SUMMARY OF FINDINGS

Medicine is a science of uncertainty and an art of probability.

William Osler

FIGURE 14-1

Topics Relevant to Prognosis Covered Elsewhere

Clinical Utility: The Concept of a "Threshold Value"

The primary purpose of this chapter is to provide clinicians with information that is not only evidence-based but also *practical*. The nature of the studies in this area makes this difficult, for several reasons. First, most of the relevant studies do not *directly* address issues of prognosis. Instead, they often have simpler aims, such as providing a description of the possible outcomes after TBI as well as the factors associated with these outcomes. As a result, the findings are reported in such a way that only the broadest generalizations are possible (e.g., that the initial Glasgow Coma Scale (GCS) score is correlated with outcome after a TBI). Although this knowledge does represent an advance in our understanding of TBI, it does little to help clinicians who are trying to prognosticate for individual patients. Even when these associations are quantified, it is in a form that is not clinically useful (e.g., as correlation coefficients).

This was a limitation even of those studies that directly addressed prognosis. For example, the relationship between a potential predictor variable and an outcome might be expressed as a path coefficient or the percentage of variance explained. Yet, both clinicians and laypeople are more used to thinking about, for instance, probabilities (e.g., "what are the chances that he will ever work again?"). Unfortunately, there is no straightforward way to translate results expressed as path coefficients, R^2, log-likelihood's, correlation matrices, etc., into prognoses that are meaningful to the clinician, let alone the family. For most clinicians, our knowledge begins and ends simply with the awareness that certain variables are associated with outcome (e.g., GCS, pupillary abnormalities, etc.), without knowing how to apply that information to individual cases. There were a handful of studies that actually did provide practical guidelines for clinicians (e.g., by using simple formulas, prediction trees, or scores from specially designed scales), but they did not meet the other inclusion criteria of this review.

To maximize the clinical utility of studies that did meet the inclusion criteria, the results were interpreted through the use of threshold values. These are values of a predictor variable above or below which a particular outcome was especially unlikely. For example, several studies reported that no one with a duration of PTA over three months achieved a good recovery as defined by the Glasgow Outcome Scale (GOS) (Figure 14-2). Thus, three months would be considered a threshold value for the duration of PTA, at least in terms of excluding the possibility of a good recovery on the GOS (Figure 14-3). Conversely, several studies found that no one who had a duration of PTA of *less than* two months ended up severely disabled (by GOS criteria); two months would then be the threshold value for excluding the possibility of severe disability.

As "milestones" in a patient's recovery, threshold values can be useful to clinicians. For instance, as the length of a patient's PTA extends beyond three months, rehabilitation clinicians can counsel family members about realistic expectations for the future. On the other hand, if two months have not yet elapsed since the injury, clinicians can give hope to families even if the patient is still in PTA.

Studies that reported their results in a way that allowed the determination of threshold values were especially important for this review. Unfortunately, less than a third of the included studies did so. In some cases this

---

- DEAD
- VEGETATIVE STATE ("alive but unconscious")
- SEVERE DISABILITY ("conscious but dependent")—unable to live alone for more than 24 hours: the daily assistance of another person at home is essential as a result of physical and/or cognitive impairments.
- MODERATE DISABILITY ("independent but disabled")—independent at home; able to utilize public transportation; able to work in a supported environment.
- GOOD RECOVERY ("mild to no residual deficits")—capacity to resume normal occupational and social activities, although there may be minor residual physical or mental deficits.

FIGURE 14-2

Glasgow Outcome Scale

A value of a predictor variable above or below which a certain outcome is especially likely or unlikely.

Example: *If post-traumatic amnesia (PTA) lasts more than three months, a person is very unlikely to achieve a "good recovery" on the Glasgow Outcome Scale (GOS).*

FIGURE 14-3

Definition of Threshold Value

---

was because the variable in question did not turn out to have a threshold value. This occurred when, regardless of the score or value, a prognostic factor was associated with all possible outcomes. For instance, for any initial GCS value between 3 through 8, all the outcomes on the GOS are possible, so there are no threshold values for this variable. With other factors, such as PTA, it does make sense to speak of threshold values. Even in these cases, however, only a minority of the studies were designed or reported so that one could determine what those threshold values actually were. The guidelines in this chapter relied heavily on these few studies, since they were the ones that provided the most useful information for clinicians.

Because of the limited number of studies involved, it was important to provide independent verification of the validity of their conclusions. This was done by determining if the results were consistent with the findings of the other, excluded, studies. For example, excluded studies were reviewed to determine if any of them reported a significant number of cases of good recovery on the GOS when the duration of PTA extended beyond three months (one of the threshold values derived from the included studies). If the excluded studies also converged on the same threshold values, one could be more sure of the validity of the original values. In fact, the results of the excluded studies were consistent with almost all the derived threshold values; the few exceptions were not clinically significant and are discussed in more detail below (in the sections on individual predictor variables).

The threshold values that were chosen were those that allowed one to exclude either a good recovery on the one hand or a severe disability on the other; no attempt was made to determine similar threshold values for moderate disability. This was motivated by the belief that, for most family members, it is the GOS categories of severe disability and good recovery that are of most interest in the subacute period. Families want to know how long they can still hope for a good recovery (and may not be as concerned, during that time, about whether the alternative is moderate disability or severe disability). Conversely, it is reassuring to families to hear it is unlikely the patient will be severely disabled (even if neither they nor the clinician knows whether the eventual outcome will be a good recovery or moderate disability).

Of course, interpreting threshold values is not unproblematic. There is a degree of statistical uncertainty for all calculated threshold values. For example, even if no one with a duration of PTA greater than three months had a good recovery in a particular study, such an outcome is still *statistically* possible. This statistical uncertainty can be quantified using confidence intervals. The lower end of the confidence interval would be zero (in a study where no one had the outcome of interest), while the upper end would represent the largest number of people who could have had the outcome of interest. The use of confidence intervals in this context is further explained in the second appendix.

There were also instances where two or more studies differed in the threshold values they identified (for instance, excluding the possibility of a good recovery after a PTA of two months in one study but not until a PTA of three months in another). As discussed below, a decision was made to err on the side of conservatism in these situations by choosing the value (larger or smaller, depending on the outcome), which minimized the possibility of an inaccurately pessimistic prognosis. So, in this example, one would choose three months of PTA as the threshold value in order to avoid discounting the possibility of a good recovery in those patients whose PTA lasted between two to three months.

Brief Comment on Methodology

The inclusion criteria are summarized in Figures 14-4 and 14-5. The second appendix provides a detailed review and justification for selecting these criteria. For present purposes, it is noted that the review focused on studies of adults who had sustained a moderate or severe TBI (either closed or penetrating). The predictor variables represented the information most likely to be available to rehabilitation clinicians: initial Glasgow Coma Scale score (GCS), length of coma, duration of post-traumatic amnesia (PTA), age, neuroimaging findings, and results of early neuropsychological testing. The outcomes of interest (assessed at 6 months or later) were vocational reentry, return to independent living, or the classification on the Glasgow Outcome Scale (GOS). The use of the GOS as the primary outcome of interest requires justification; this is provided in the second appendix.

Out of the hundreds of articles reviewed, there were only 35 studies that met all the inclusion criteria: 12 using neuroimaging predictors (27–38) (Table 14-1), 24 using clinical predictors (27, 29, 30, 33, 38–57) (Table 14-2), 2 focused on the elderly (58, 59) (Table 14-3), and 2 on

penetrating brain injury (60, 61) (Table 14-4) (the numbers add up to more than 35 because some studies investigated more than one prognostic factor). No studies that used early neuropsychological testing as a predictive variable met all the inclusion criteria. Neither did any studies that focused exclusively on moderate TBI. More importantly, of all the studies that were included, only a third allowed for the determination of threshold values. In particular, eight of the closed head injury studies reported threshold values with acceptable confidence intervals (0–12 percent): one for MRI, one for length of coma, two for length of PTA, and four for age. In what follows, the results of the studies are reviewed by predictor variable. The conclusions are summarized in Figure 14-6.

MRI

Summary   Two studies (32, 34) met the inclusion criteria, both using information from Magnetic Resonance Imaging (MRI) obtained within two weeks after injury. Both found the depth of the lesions correlated with outcome. Specifically, they discovered that lesions in the cortex or the white matter were not associated with worse outcome, whereas brain stem lesions were strongly associated with poor outcome. One study (34) also determined a

---

Outcomes studied should be relevant and meaningful to a layperson (e.g. family member) asking about prognosis.

Predictor variables should represent information easily accessible to rehabilitation clinicians.

The population studied should be similar to the population encountered by rehabilitation professionals.

The studies must meet minimal methodological criteria in terms of patient selection, follow-up, statistical analysis, etc.

FIGURE 14-4

General Guidelines for Inclusion of Studies

Population
1. Publication after 1983
2. Setting in North America, Western Europe, Australia, New Zealand, or Israel
3. Setting in either acute care or inpatient rehabilitation
4. Moderate and/or severe TBI (penetrating and/or closed)
5. Exclusively or primarily adult TBI

Predictors
6. Predictor variables: GCS (total), length of coma, PTA, age, neuroimaging (CT or MRI), and/or early neuropsychological testing.

Outcomes
7. Outcomes: GOS, vocational re-entry, and/or independent living
8. Outcomes assessed at 6 months or later

Methodology
9. Sample must represent consecutive admissions (whether done prospectively or retrospectively) or a random/neutral sampling of consecutive admissions
10. Sample size > 25
11. Follow-up greater than 80 percent
12. Statistical analysis performed (or, if not, enough information provided to analyze oneself)

FIGURE 14-5

Inclusion Criteria for Studies Population

TABLE 14-1
Neuroimaging

Study	Population	Number	Outcome	Predictor	Findings Associated with Worse Outcome	Statistics	Potential "Threshold" Values
Rao 1990	Inpatient rehab	79	Return to work (approx. 1.5 years)	CT (acute care)	Extent of CT damage (bilateral > unilateral > normal)	Univariate	None
Fearnside 1993	Severe; acute	315	GOS (6 months)	CT (admission)	Contusion, intracerebral hematoma & SAH	Multivariate	None
Kakarieka 1994	Severe; acute	414	GOS (6 months)	CT (admission)	Presence of SAH	Univariate & Multivariate	None
Walder 1995	Severe; acute	109	GOS (6 months)	CT (admission)	CT findings as characterized by Abbreviated Injury Scale and the Traumatic Coma Data Bank Classification	Univariate	None
Lobato 1997	Severe; acute	710	GOS (6 months)	CT (admission)	CT findings as characterized by Traumatic Coma Data Bank Classification	Univariate	None
Wedekind 1999	Severe; acute	57	GOS (> 6 months)	MRI (2 weeks)	Lesions in corpus callosum or basal ganglia or midbrain or total # of lesions	Univariate	None
Gomez 2000	Severe; acute	810	GOS (6 months)	CT (admission)	Status of cisterns, SAH, EDH, SDH, midline shift or contusion by univariate; status of cisterns, SAH, EDH & IVH by multivariate	Univariate & Multivariate	None
Firsching 2001	Severe; acute	102	GOS (2 years)	MRI (8 days)	Depth of lesion; (total # of lesions or corpus callosum lesions do not correlate w/outcome)	Univariate	No one with bilateral brainstem lesions achieved a good recovery (CI 0–8 percent)
Schaan 2001	All GCS (admitted to ICU); acute; isolated TBI	554	GOS (6 months)	CT (admission)	EDH, SDH, edema or contusion	Multivariate	None
Vos 2001	Severe; acute	63	GOS (6 months)	CT (admission)	CT findings as characterized by Traumatic Coma Data Bank Classification	Univariate	None
Mattioli 2003	All GCS (admitted to ICU); acute; included GSW	605	GOS (6 months)	CT (admission)	SAH	Multivariate	None
Rovlias 2004	Severe (isolated BI); acute	345	GOS (6 months)	CT (admission)	SAH; EDH; SDH	Multivariate	None

TABLE 14-2
Clinical Predictors

Study	Population/ Age [range (mean)]	Number	Outcome	Predictor	Findings Associated with Worse Outcome	Statistics	Potential "Threshold" Values
Born 1985	Severe; acute, 1–75 yo (23)	109	GOS (6 months)	Age	Older age	Univariate	None
Facco 1986	Severe; acute, 15–60 yo	56	GOS (6 months)	GCS; length of coma	Lower GCS	Univariate	None
Hans 1987	Severe; acute, 3–61 yo (23)	40	GOS (6 months)	Age; GCS	Older age; lower GCS	Univariate	None
Choi 1988	Severe; acute (30.8 yo)	523	GOS (6 months)	Age	Older age	Multivariate	None
Tate 1989	Severe; rehab, 15–45 yo (23.9)	100	GOS (6 years)	PTA; length of coma	Length of PTA; length of coma	Univariate	None
Narayan 1989	Severe; acute	133	GOS (>6 months)	Age; GCS	Older age; lower GCS	Multivariate	None
Rao 1990	Rehab, 17–66 yo (29)	79	Return to work (1 year)	Length of coma; age; PTA	Length of coma; older age; (length of PTA not correlated)	Univariate	None
Levin 1990	Severe; acute, 16–70 yo (27)	300	GOS (12 months)	GCS	Lower GCS	Univariate	None
Choi 1991	Severe; acute (30.9 yo)	617	GOS (12 months)	Age	Older age	Multivariate	None
Marshall 1991	Severe; acute (29.5 yo)	746	GOS (2 years)	GCS	Lower GCS	Univariate	None
Vollmer 1991	Severe; acute 15–80 yo	661	GOS (6 months)	Age	Older age	Univariate	No patient over 55 yo had a good recovery (CI 0–4 percent)
Bishara 1992	Severe; acute, 15–65 yo (25.7)	93	GOS (>6 months)	PTA; GCS; age	Length of PTA; lower GCS; (age not correlated)	Univariate and multivariate	No one had severe disability until PTA >2 months (CI 0–4 percent)
Godfrey 1993	Severe; acute (who survived acute care) 15–61 yo (25.38)	66	Return to work (>1 year)	PTA	Length of PTA	Univariate	None
Pennings 1993	Severe (GCS <5); acute, 20–92 yo	92	GOS (>6 months)	Age	Older age	Univariate	No patient over 60 yo had a good recovery (CI 0–7 percent)
Katz 1994	Rehab (with DAI), 8–89 yo	175	GOS (6 months)	GCS; PTA; Length of coma; age	Lower GCS, length of PTA, length of coma, older age (by univariate analysis); length of PTA, older age (by multivariate analysis)	Univariate and multivariate	No one with length of coma >2 weeks (CI 0–10 percent) or PTA >3 months (CI 0–11 percent) had a good recovery. Only 2 percent of patients with a PTA<2 months were severely disabled (CI .3–9 percent). Only 5 percent of length of coma <2 weeks were severely disabled (CI 2–12 percent)

TABLE 14-2
(continued)

Study	Population/ Age [Range (Mean)]	Number	Outcome	Predictor	Findings Associated with Worse Outcome	Statistics	Potential "Threshold" Values
Kakarieka 1994	Severe; acute 16–70 yo (36)	414	GOS (6 months)	Age	Older age	Multivariate	None
Walder 1995	Severe; acute 16–78 yo (26)	109	GOS (6 months)	Age	Older age	Univariate	None
Combes 1996	Severe; acute (38.5 yo)	198	GOS	Age	Older age	Multivariate	None
Ellenberg 1996	Severe; acute (that regained consciousness in acute care), 16- yo (29)	314	GOS (6 months)	PTA; length of coma; age	Length of PTA; length of coma; older age	Multivariate	None
Hawkins 1996	Rehab, 17–72 yo (27)	55	Return to work; independent living	GCS	None	Multivariate	None
Hellawell 1999	Moderate and severe; acute, 15–78 yo (39.2)	96	GOS (6 months)	GCS; PTA	Lower GCS; length of PTA	Univariate	None
Gomez 2000	Severe; acute, 15–>65 yo	810	GOS (6 months)	Age	Older age	Multivariate	None
Rovlias 2004	Severe; acute (isolated BI), 16- 70yo (40)	345	GOS (6 months)	GCS; age	GCS; age	Multivariate	None
Formisano 2004	Severe; rehab (coma >15 days), 11- 56 yo (26)	43	GOS (>1 year)	Length of coma; age	Length of coma; age	Univariate	None

TABLE 14-3
Elderly

Study	Population/ Age	Number	Outcome	Predictor	Findings Associated with Worse Outcome	Statistics	Potential "Threshold" Values
Ross 1992	Acute; all GCS; age >65 yo	195	GOS (6 months)	GCS	Lower GCS	Univariate	Only 3 percent of patients with an initial GCS <8 achieved a good recovery. (CI 1–9 percent)
Kilaru 1996	Acute; severe; >65 yo	40	GOS (38 months)	GCS	Lower GCS	Multivariate	No patient with admission GCS <8 achieved a good recovery. (CI 0–8 percent)

TABLE 14-4
Penetrating Missile Injury

Study	Population	Number	Outcome	Predictor	Findings Associated with Worse Outcome	Statistics	Potential "Threshold" Values
Grahm 1990	Acute; all GCS	100	GOS (>6 months)	GCS; CT	Lower GCS; bilateral or trans-ventricular injury on CT	Univariate	No patients with GCS < 8 or transventricular injury had good recovery (CI 0–4 percent)
Levy 1994	Acute ; GCS 3–5	190	GOS (6–12 months)	GCS; CT	Lower GCS; bilateral injury with IVH on CT	Multivariate	No patients with GCS 3–5 had a good recovery (CI 0–2 percent)

GCS:
- Lower scores associated with worse outcomes
- No threshold values

Length of Coma:
- Longer duration associated with worse outcomes
- Threshold values:
  - Severe disability unlikely when less than two weeks
  - Good recovery unlikely when greater than four weeks

PTA:
- Longer duration associated with worse outcomes
- Threshold values:
  - Severe disability unlikely when less than two months
  - Good recovery unlikely when greater than three months

AGE:
- Older age associated with worse outcomes
- Threshold values:
  - Good recovery unlikely when greater than 65 years

NEUROIMAGING:
- Certain features (e.g., depth of lesions) associated with worse outcomes
- Threshold values:
  - Good recovery unlikely when bilateral brainstem lesions present on early MRI

FIGURE 14-6

Summary of Studies of Nonpenetrating TBI

threshold for the possibility of a good recovery: no one in their study with bilateral brainstem lesions made a good recovery (95 percent CI: 0–8 percent) . Although the second study (32) reported a similar finding (i.e., no one with a lower brainstem lesion made a good recovery), the confidence interval was too large to be included. There were, however, some differences in the findings of the two studies. The study by Wedekind (32) found that lesions in the basal ganglia and corpus callosum, as well as the total lesion burden in the brain, were associated with a worse outcome; the later study (34) did not find these associations.

Discussion The advantage of conventional MRI (relative to CT scanning) is that it allows for better visualization of lesions, especially those in the brainstem. As a result, MRI is ideally suited to study the centripetal model of brain injury severity (62) which claims that the stronger the forces to which the brain is subjected, the more severe the injury and the deeper the lesions. The findings of these two studies (as well as others that did not meet the inclusion criteria) are consistent with this hypothesis: depth of lesion is associated with worse outcomes because it is a marker of brain injury severity.

Conclusions If an MRI from the first several weeks after a TBI is available, the depth of the lesions (and, possibly, the total lesion burden) are associated with worse outcome. In particular, the presence of bilateral brainstem lesions makes the possibility of a good recovery very unlikely.

CT

Summary Ten studies (27–31, 33, 35–38) met the inclusion criteria; all but one were conducted in the acute care setting. However, even the study from the rehabilitation setting made use of the acute care CT scan. Almost half of the studies used scales that included several different imaging variables, making it difficult to isolate how individual variables contributed to outcome (two of the studies used the Traumatic Coma Data Bank (TCDB) classification, one the intracranial severity score of the Abbreviated Injury Scale (AIS), and one a scale especially designed for the study). Nonetheless, certain patterns emerged.

Every study that looked at the presence of subarachnoid hemorrhage (SAH) as a variable found that it was associated with worse outcome. In addition, all but one of the studies that examined the presence of cisternal effacement or midline shift found they correlated with worse outcome. Finally, although the presence of epidural or subdural hematomas was correlated with worse outcome in the studies that included them as predictor variables, no more specific conclusions could be drawn, given the variation in how they were graded.

The two studies that used the TCDB classification reported threshold effects, although they differed in what they found. One study (31) found that no patient whose scan was classified as a "level VI" category (the worst rating) achieved a good recovery or moderate disability. The other study (36) found that no one with a "level I" scan (the best rating) did worse than moderate disability. However, the confidence intervals around both values were unacceptably large. In addition, neither study confirmed the finding of the other, rendering the reported thresholds unsupported across studies.

Discussion Since the acute care CT scan (or a report) is often available to rehabilitation professionals, it would have been helpful if the CT findings yielded more definitive prognoses. Unfortunately, although it is known that certain lesions are associated with worse outcomes, the nature of the relationship is such that more specific prognoses cannot be made. It may be that the use of more quantitative measures of CT lesions would yield better prognostic information, but this has not yet been demonstrated. Overall, all of these findings are consistent with those of the excluded studies.

Conclusions The presence of SAH, cisternal effacement, significant midline shift, EDH, or SDH on an acute care CT scan are all associated with worse outcomes. More specific conclusions about the implications of the lesions cannot be drawn, because each one individually can be associated with the full range of outcomes after TBI.

Initial GCS

Summary Of the studies that met the inclusion criteria, ten (38, 41, 42, 45, 46, 48, 50, 53, 56, 57) examined the relationship between GCS and outcome. As mentioned earlier, studies that used only a subset of the GCS (e.g., motor score) were excluded because, although rehabilitation professionals should have access to the initial GCS score, the individual subscores would be much less available. All but

one of the studies found an association between lower GCS scores and worse outcomes. Although the studies measured the GCS differently (e.g., admission, post-resuscitation, highest in the first 6–24 hr, etc.), none of them discovered threshold or cut-off values for outcomes. In other words, any particular initial GCS score could potentially be associated with any outcome (although the chances of having a good outcome diminish as the GCS score is lower).

Discussion Although providing a general idea of the severity of the injury, the GCS by itself does not yield definitive prognoses. This is true even when the accuracy of the GCS is increased by varying the timing and content of measurement. Even the most accurate of the methods did not improve accuracy enough to allow for more specific prognoses. Also, rehabilitation professionals are often limited in which GCS score they have access to (and often don't know exactly when it was obtained). For both these reasons, it did not seem worthwhile to look more closely at the accuracy of different ways of obtaining the GCS. All of these findings are consistent with the rest of the literature (that is, the studies that were excluded).

Conclusions Although the initial GCS score is associated with outcome and lower GCS scores are associated with worse outcomes, one cannot draw more specific conclusions solely from the GCS score.

Length of Coma

Summary Of the studies that met the inclusion criteria, there were six (27,39,41,44,53,55) that studied the relationship between the length of coma and outcome. Four of the six defined the length of coma as that period of time until the patient started following commands. The other two studies did not specify how coma duration was measured. All but one found a relationship between the duration of coma and outcome (the longer the duration of coma, the worse the outcome). In addition, one of the studies (53) reported its data in such a way that it was possible to determine a threshold value for excluding the possibility of a good recovery. Specifically, they found that no subject made a good recovery whose length of coma exceeded fourteen days (53).

Discussion Although the duration of coma has been defined several different ways (e.g., when GCS is 9 or above, when the eyes open, etc.), all the studies that reported their method of measurement used the time to follow commands. This was also the predominant method of measurement in the rest of the literature. Therefore, the rehabilitation clinician using the length of coma for prognostic purposes should follow the same guidelines. Only one study (53) reported a threshold value with an acceptable confidence interval. However, the value of 14 days they found seems too short. For instance, the Tate study (44) reported instances of a good recovery even after a month of coma. Other studies, excluded in the review, also converge on approximately one month as a cut-off point (beyond which the chances of a good recovery are small) (63–65). In these studies, it appears that, on average, only 7–8 percent of patients will make a good recovery who are not following commands beyond one month.

Conclusions   The longer the duration of coma (as measured by the time to follow commands), the more likely a worse outcome. In particular, a duration of coma greater than four weeks makes a good recovery unlikely.

PTA

Summary   Of the studies that met the methodological criteria, seven (27,44,50,51,53,55,57) investigated the relationship between the length of post-traumatic amnesia (PTA) and outcome. All but one found the two were associated (the longer the duration of PTA, the worse the outcome). Only two of the studies reported how they measured PTA (53,55); both of these studies relied on the Galveston Orientation and Amnesia Test (GOAT) to mark the end of PTA (i.e., a score of greater than 75 on two consecutive days). Two of the studies (50,53) reported their data in such a way that it was possible to determine threshold values for excluding the possibility of either a good recovery or a severe disability. Specifically, one of the studies found that no subject had an outcome of severe disability until their duration of PTA exceeded two months (CI 0–3.6 percent) (50). Similarly, the Katz study (53) found that only 2 percent of individuals with a duration of PTA less than two months was severely disabled (CI 0.3–8.8 percent). Although both studies converged on the period during which a severe disability was unlikely, they varied in when they were able to exclude the possibility of a good recovery. The longest reported duration of PTA before one could exclude a good recovery was three months (CI 0–11 percent) (53).

Discussion   The duration of PTA has long been considered one of the most powerful prognostic factors available to the rehabilitation clinician (66). Besides its power, the duration of PTA has other advantages that make it especially useful. For one, the duration of PTA lends itself to the identification of threshold values. Also, many of these thresholds are crossed while the patient is in inpatient rehabilitation, allowing the rehabilitation professional an opportunity to substantively address issues of prognosis during the rehabilitation stay. In addition, because these thresholds are often reached in rehabilitation, the rehabilitation professional has much more control over the measurement of this variable.

In general, the studies that reported thresholds converge on a duration of PTA of 2–3 months when the prognosis becomes much clearer. For instance, both the Bishara (50) and Katz (53) studies agreed that the possibility of severe disability was very unlikely when the duration of PTA was less than 2 months. Also, both the Bishara (50) study (whose confidence interval was too wide to include) and the Katz (53) studies converged on 2–3 months as the duration of PTA before the possibility of a good recovery becomes very unlikely. A review of the studies on PTA that did not meet the inclusion criteria revealed findings consistent with this value.

Conclusions   The longer the duration of PTA, the worse the outcome. In particular, it is unlikely that a person will have an outcome of severe disability if the duration of PTA is less than two months. Conversely, it is unlikely a person will have a good recovery when the duration of PTA extends beyond three months.

Age

Summary   Of the studies that met the inclusion criteria, seventeen (27,29,30,33,38,39,40,42,43,45,47,49,50,52–55) investigated the relationship between age and outcome. All but two (39,50) found the two were associated (the older the patient, the worse the outcome). There were differences in whether increasing age was seen as a continuous risk factor or whether the risk increased at certain ages ("inflection points"). Four of the studies (33,49,52,53) reported threshold values of an age above which a good recovery was extremely unlikely. However, there was variability in the exact age found to represent this cut-off point. Among patients with a severe TBI, two studies found that no patients had a good recovery after the ages of 55 (CI 0–4.1 percent) (49) and 60 (CI 0–6.9 percent) (52). Another study found that, although there were some patients with a good recovery after the age of 65, the probability was low (6 percent) (CI 2–14 percent) (33).

Discussion   Age is a powerful prognostic factor. Although the risk for adults appears continuous, the prognosis worsens significantly after the age of 65. This is discussed in more detail in the next section. A review of the excluded literature is consistent with these findings.

Conclusions   Older patients have a worse outcome after a severe TBI. In particular, in patients over 65, the chances of a good recovery after severe TBI are unlikely.

Special Populations: Elderly

Summary   There were two studies (58,59) meeting the inclusion criteria that examined prognostic factors in patients over the age of 65. Both studies found the initial

GCS was associated with outcome: the lower one's GCS score, the worse the outcome. One study (59) found that no subject with an admission GCS <8 had a good recovery at long-term follow-up (CI 0–8.2 percent). This is consistent with the studies mentioned previously (49,52) that also found no subjects over 65 who had a good recovery after a severe TBI.

The other study on the elderly (58), however, found that a subset of those with an admission GCS less than eight did have the potential to achieve a good recovery. Specifically, they reported that those patients who regained consciousness within 72 hours had the potential to achieve a good recovery (3 percent in their series) (CI 0.6–8.9 percent). This finding is consistent with the results of the other study mentioned previously (33) that found some patients over 65 who achieved a good recovery (6 percent in their series, with CI 2–14 percent).

Discussion The importance of TBI in the elderly is growing. This is not only because the incidence of TBI rises in the elderly but also because the percentage of the population over the age of 65 is growing. Although there may be confounding factors (e.g., co-morbidities), it is now clear that age is an independent risk factor in this population (67). There are many potential reasons for this, ranging from the nature of the injuries in the elderly (e.g., subdural hematomas) to changes in the brain as one ages (e.g., decreased functional reserve, less elasticity of blood vessels, etc.). These issues are discussed in more depth in the chapter on TBI in the elderly (Chapter 21).

For our purposes, the main point is that a good recovery after a severe TBI in a person over 65 is very unlikely. The increased likelihood of poor outcomes is also found in the other severity categories. In fact, several writers have noted that, in terms of outcome, a moderate TBI in the elderly resembles a severe TBI in a younger person (58, 68, 69). Even the outcomes of mild TBI in the elderly are much worse, with many never returning to their premorbid functional status (70).

Conclusions In patients over the age of 65, the lower the admission GCS, the worse the outcome. In particular, older patients who have sustained a severe TBI (GCS less than eight) are unlikely to achieve a good recovery.

Special Populations: Penetrating Injuries

Summary There were two studies (60, 61) that met the inclusion criteria which investigated prognostic factors in civilian patients with penetrating missile wounds. Both studies found the GCS was associated with outcome: the lower one's GCS score, the worse the outcome. Both studies also found that CT findings of bilateral injury or trans-ventricular injury were associated with worse outcomes. One study (60) found that no patients who had a

post-resuscitation GCS score <8 had a good recovery at long-term follow-up (CI 0–4.4 percent). The other study (61) only included patients with GCS scores of 3–5. No one in their series achieved a good recovery at long-term follow-up (CI 0–1.6 percent).

Discussion Penetrating injury differs from closed brain injuries in many ways, as discussed elsewhere in this textbook (Chapter 18). In terms of outcome, the early mortality rate after penetrating injury is much higher than that of closed head injury (71). Among the survivors, however, there are proportionally fewer people who are left vegetative or severely disabled (71). Although many prognostic factors have been studied in penetrating injuries (71), only the GCS is readily available to rehabilitation clinicians. Unlike closed head injury, where a range of outcomes is still possible with a GCS of 3–8, in penetrating injury it is very unlikely that patients with an initial GCS in this range will have a good recovery. These findings are consistent with those in the excluded studies; only one study reported any patients who achieved a good outcome with an initial GCS of 6–8 (8 percent) (72). However, they also found no one achieved a good recovery with an initial GCS of 3–5.

Conclusions In patients with a penetrating missile injury, lower GCS scores and CT findings of bilaterality or trans-ventricular injury are associated with worse outcomes. Moreover, those patients with a post-resuscitation GCS score of 8 or less are unlikely to achieve a good recovery.

Special Populations: Moderate TBI

The focus of this chapter is on severe TBI because it is with this group of patients that the most uncertainty exists about long-term prognosis. In contrast, outcomes after moderate TBI are much clearer (10,19): more than 90 percent of individuals with moderate TBI will achieve either a moderate disability or good recovery. This information is certainly useful for clinicians counseling family members, especially by reassuring them the odds are heavily in favor of at least independent living, if not a return to previous function.

There are certain risk factors associated with the poorer outcomes: lower GCS scores (e.g., 9 or 10), older age, and abnormalities on the CT scan (10,19). When these are present, patients are more likely to have a moderate disability (or, infrequently, even a severe disability) rather than a good recovery. This information can be used to adjust the content and tone of prognostic information provided to family members.

Although the prognosis after moderate TBI is good, it is here that the limits of the higher categories of the GOS are most obvious. Studies have shown that even individuals with a good recovery often have neurobehavioral problems that contribute significantly to the morbidity of moderate TBI (10,19). It is important to communicate this information to the family, although initially it may be in the most general of terms (e.g., "most people are able to at least live on their own after this type of brain injury, although they may have some other problems").

Neuropsychological Testing

Although early neuropsychological testing (performed within one month after injury or at the resolution of PTA) was originally included as a potential predictor variable, none of the studies reviewed met the methodological criteria, mainly because of limited follow-up. Still, because neuropsychological testing is so widely used in the rehabilitation setting, the findings of some of these studies (64,73–77) are reviewed here. Almost all the studies found an association between selected test results and long-term outcome, even when adjusted for demographic and injury severity variables (64). The specific tests found to be predictive varied between the studies, however, limiting the utility of the findings. Another feature of the studies that reduced their applicability was the use of statistical analyses that cannot easily be utilized in the clinical setting (e.g., correlation coefficients, principal components analysis, etc.).

Even when the findings were reported in a clinically useful way, the studies were still not helpful. This is because early neuropsychological testing, even when correlated with outcome, is not a particularly powerful predictor. In the language of the rest of the chapter, there were no threshold values that were found for neuropsychological test scores. For instance, one study (75) found that a normal score on one of ten tests identified as predictive still had less than a 50 percent chance of predicting productivity at one year or beyond. Even an impaired score, which was a more powerful prognosticator, predicted lack of productivity in only 70 percent of people. The utility of testing is further diminished by the fact that only a subset of patients are able to be tested subacutely; therefore, the results of these studies are not relevant to the significant number of patients who are not testable during inpatient rehabilitation.

In fact, this distinction between those who are testable or not (rather than the test scores themselves) turns out to be the most powerful predictor in these studies and one that could potentially serve as a threshold value for prognosis. In one of the two studies that examined this relationship (75), only 6 percent of patients who were unable to complete any test during inpatient rehabilitation were productive at one year. In the other study (64), only 6 percent of those who were not testable at one month were employed a year later. In contrast, being testable was not as predictive in either study, correctly classifying only about 40 percent-80 percent of those who

would be productive at one year. Although the inability to be tested in the subacute setting appears to be a potentially valuable prognostic variable, it does not provide significantly more information than the better supported use of length of coma or duration of PTA.

Indeed, it is likely that the findings in these studies were confounded by the length of coma or PTA. For instance, the first study was designed so that people were only tested when they emerged from post-traumatic amnesia. Thus, being testable was a marker for the length of PTA. The primary reason that patients who are not testable during inpatient rehabilitation do poorly is that they have a prolonged PTA. Assuming that most patients are discharged from inpatient rehabilitation about 2–3 months after their injury, those patients who are not testable during this period must have had lengths of PTA greater than 2–3 months, which was the threshold value identified in the previous studies. Similar considerations apply to the other studies (63,64). There was one study that did adjust for PTA duration; it found that neuropsychological test performance made a contribution to the prediction of productivity beyond that made by the duration of PTA (76). The exact improvement in predictive power made by the tests was not reported, however, and is unlikely to be clinically significant.

In conclusion, it is likely there is an association between early neuropsychological test performance and long-term outcome. More specific conclusions cannot be made because of the methodological limitations of the studies, the lack of consensus on which tests are most important, and because, even with the most robust results, there are no threshold values for test performance. The only statement that can be made with some confidence (within the constraints of the methodological limitations already discussed) is that not being testable early on is a poor prognostic sign for a productive long-term outcome. This subject is more extensively reviewed elsewhere (77).

Summary

The 35 studies were almost unanimous in finding that age, initial GCS score, length of coma, duration of PTA, and neuroimaging findings are correlated with outcome (Figure 14–6). However, this represents information that TBI clinicians already know. Of much greater interest is the existence of threshold values for several of the variables; these allow the clinician to formulate more fine-grained prognoses in individual cases. Specifically, age, length of coma, and duration of PTA all provide valuable information the clinician can use to mark milestones when either a severe disability or a good recovery are unlikely. These results are based on a small number of studies (less than a third of the total), however; this must be kept in mind when using this information in clinical situations. On the other hand, the fact that these results were consistent with those in the excluded studies increases one's confidence in the findings. In essence, the results are at least consistent with almost *all* the published literature.

There was only one minor exception to the general agreement between the included and excluded studies: the maximum length of coma after which a good recovery is extremely unlikely. The original review found a value of two weeks. However, as mentioned above, there were several excluded studies that found a significant number of individuals with a good recovery after two weeks of coma. These other studies seem to converge on the value of one month of coma as the time after which a good recovery is very unlikely. Because of the wish to err on the side of preserving hope, one month of coma was adopted as the final threshold value for length of coma (Figure 14-7).

Finally, the statistical uncertainty involved must be kept in mind. The upper limits of the confidence intervals for the threshold values averaged approximately 7 percent. This means that, on average, up to 7 percent of individuals could have outcomes that are considered unlikely (e.g., up to 7 percent of patients with a PTA greater than 3 months may have a good recovery on the GOS). This underscores the point that one should use terms such as "unlikely" or "very unlikely" rather than, for instance, "never" in talking with families. One may even want to convey the associated degree of uncertainty in quantitative terms.

Applying the Guidelines

The final guidelines are presented in Figure 14-7. They are based both on the results of the initial review as well as, for length of coma, the findings of the excluded studies. Also, only findings supported by more than one study were included; this meant the results of the MRI study were not part of the final guidelines. There are a few final points about applying these principles. The first is simply to recommend the use of the different sources of information at different times in the recovery process. For

example, if someone older than 65 years has a severe TBI, one knows fairly early that the chances of a good recovery are low, especially if they do not regain consciousness within a few days. For those under the age of 65, however, one will probably need to wait until the duration of coma is known (especially when it is less than two weeks or greater than 4 weeks). Later, because of its predictive power, the length of PTA should be used as the primary source of information.

This sequential use of different variables is important not only because the later variables are more powerful than the earlier ones. It is also necessary because there is not always a strong correlation between the variables (e.g., between the length of coma and duration of PTA). For instance, based on clinical experience, one can have a duration of coma of less than two weeks (which would imply a relatively good prognosis) with a protracted PTA of greater than 2–3 months (which implies a worse prognosis). In these cases, the prognosis based on the duration of PTA should be used as the primary source of information. It is also important to keep in mind some sense of the trajectory of recovery and adjust one's predictions accordingly. In someone who is still minimally conscious at two months, for instance, it is extremely unlikely they will become fully conscious and clear from PTA within the following month. Thus, one does not always have to wait until the passage of a full three months to infer that the likelihood of a good recovery is low.

Finally, it is also important to modify one's predictions based on the presence or absence of significant focal lesions. Although it is true that almost all the studies "correct" for the presence of focal lesions (by including both those with and without such lesions), knowledge of a significant focal lesion can help with prognostication in individual cases. Someone with a left anterior lesion and significant language deficits will likely have a worse outcome than patients who have similar lengths of coma, PTA, etc., but who don't have the same focal lesion. On the other hand, it has been shown that patients who primarily have diffuse axonal injury usually do worse than those whose primary lesions are focal (53). If the predominant underlying pathology is known, clinicians can use this information to modify what they tell patients and their families. In summary, application of the principles presented here involves the sequential use of the predictor variables, modified by knowledge of the larger trajectory of recovery as well as the presence or absence of significant focal lesions.

Severe disability (according to GOS) is unlikely when:
- Time to follow commands is less than two weeks
- Duration of PTA is less than two months

Good recovery (according to the GOS) is unlikely when:
- Time to follow commands is longer than one month
- Duration of PTA is greater than three months
- Age is greater than 65 years

---

* See text for important qualifications

FIGURE 14-7

---

*Summary of Evidence-Based Guidelines for Prognostication After Severe TBI**

COMMUNICATING PROGNOSES

Patients and their families will forgive you for wrong diagnoses, but will rarely forgive you for wrong prognoses.

David Seegal

Barriers to Communication

Formulating a prediction constitutes only part of the clinical act of prognosis; this information must then be communicated to patients and families. Clinicians' reluctance to communicate this information is just as responsible for the neglect of prognostication as is the difficulty in developing a prognosis in the first place. There are many reasons for this reluctance. Many health care professionals believe that patients and families don't want prognostic information (4). Yet, studies have shown that professionals significantly underestimate patients' and families' desire for this information (78–82). One study found that 88 percent of patients wanted prognostic information (83). Another study showed that, even when patients had not explicitly asked for prognostic information, they wished the clinician had discussed it with them (84).

Although none of these studies were specifically related to TBI (most were in oncology), there is no reason to believe the findings would be any different in brain injury. As mentioned earlier, families have identified information about the future as one of their greatest needs in the aftermath of a TBI (1–3). Of course, it is true some patients or their families sincerely do not want prognostic information (85). It may even be true that these preferences may vary by one's ethnic or cultural group (85). Therefore, one of the key steps in communicating prognoses is to find out how much information the patient or the family wants.

Another reason that rehabilitation professionals may be reluctant to discuss prognosis is the fear that families will interpret any discussion of uncertainty as evidence of the clinician's lack of competence (86). There is some support for this concern: one study found that the presentation of probabilities in discussing possible outcomes undermined patients' confidence in their physicians (87). In addition, there is evidence that clinicians themselves are unable to tolerate uncertainty (88); this is likely to contribute to their avoidance of prognosis.

Rehabilitation professionals may also believe that communicating a poor prognosis to patients or families causes too much pain, thereby extinguishing hope that might be needed to actively engage in rehabilitation. Yet studies in other contexts at least partially belie this concern. One study found that, although communicating a poor prognosis did result in short-term distress among cancer patients, they experienced less anxiety, more peace of mind, and better adjustment in the long-term (80). It might even be the case that not being told about a poor prognosis interferes with the grieving process by making it much more ambiguous (since one is not sure whether a loss has occurred). There is evidence this "ambiguous grief" results in more emotional distress than grief where the loss is both clear and acknowledged (89).

Finally, avoiding a discussion of prognosis can itself cause distress: the anxiety associated with uncertainty often compounds the suffering families experience. Of course, like everything else in medicine, the benefits of communication must be weighed against the risks; however, in most cases, it is probable that more is gained by open communication (4). This is not to say that minimizing distress and fostering hope are unimportant. Rather, it is to highlight the fact that the avoidance of prognosis is unlikely to achieve these goals. There are better means by which to foster hope; some of these ways will be discussed shortly.

Not only are clinicians concerned about the distress they might cause families, they themselves feel distress in communicating poor prognoses (4). Clinicians (especially physicians) might feel unprepared to deal with the emotions the patient or family might express. Also, it has been argued that conveying a poor prognosis reminds clinicians of the limits of their abilities (since they are powerless to change the outcome) and this also reduces their willingness to have these discussions. Finally, the fact remains that most clinicians (again, especially physicians) are simply not trained in "how to break bad news" (78). Their reluctance stems from not knowing *how* to proceed (compounded by their apprehension in publicly performing a skill they have not mastered).

It is hoped the guidelines presented here (summarized in Figures 14-8–14-10) will help allay some of this anxiety and improve the frequency and quality of communication of prognostic information. Several general guidelines for communicating prognostic information are presented in Figure 14-8; these guidelines will structure the discussion to follow.

Guidelines for Communicating Prognoses

Begin with the Patient and Family Although most patients and families want prognostic information, this is not universally true. Even those who want to discuss prognosis may differ in the amount of information desired as well as how its delivery is timed. Thus, if patients or families don't explicitly ask to discuss prognosis, it is important to ask if they are interested in the information. If so, one should explore in more detail what they are interested

---

- Begin with the family's desire for information as well as their current beliefs.
- Ensure that the meaning and content of the outcomes are understood.
- Present quantitative information in a manner that can be understood (see Figure 14-9).
- Foster hope.
- Pay attention to the process of communication (see Figure 14-10).

FIGURE 14-8

General Guidelines for Communicating Prognostic Information

- Try to use "natural frequencies" when communicating probabilistic information (e.g., "Eight out of ten people with this type of injury will make a good recovery")
- Present information both qualitatively as well as quantitatively (e.g., "This is a very good chance of a good recovery")
- Attempt to "frame" information in both a positive and negative manner (e.g., "That is the same as saying that two out of ten people with this type of injury will not make a good recovery")
- When possible, consider presenting the information visually.
- Ask person to restate, in their own words, their understanding of the information provided

FIGURE 14-9

Guidelines for the Communication of Quantitative Information

- Find a quiet, comfortable room without interruptions
- Sit close and speak face to face
- Have the family member's support network present, if wanted
- Present the information at a pace the family can follow
- Periodically summarize the discussion to that point
- Periodically ask family member to repeat or summarize what was said
- Keep the language simple but direct, without euphemism or jargon
- Allow time for questions

FIGURE 14-10

Guidelines for the Communication Process

in (for instance, in terms of possible outcomes). It is also helpful to begin by asking the family members what they already know and what their current perceptions are. This enables the clinician to build on the knowledge they already have or, if appropriate, correct any misinformation that might distort their understanding of the information to follow. Starting with the patient or family's desires and beliefs not only ensures that the discussion addresses their needs, but it also draws them into the conversation early (and thus hopefully makes it easier for them to articulate their concerns). It also gives them some sense of control in a situation where they often feel powerless.

Ensure Understanding of the Outcomes   It is important that families clearly understand the nature of the outcomes discussed. This is especially important when one is using studies that rely on the GOS. The names of the GOS

categories can be confusing. In particular, the terms moderate and severe disability may imply a far worse prognosis than might actually be the case. Most families would not necessarily consider someone who can live independently and use public transportation moderately disabled, even if they can't work. Or, a person who might be independent in mobility and self-care might not be considered severely disabled, even if they were unable to live independently for cognitive reasons. Given this ambiguity, it is best to avoid the GOS category names altogether, and simply describe concretely what the outcomes might be. It is also important to mention some of the limitations of the GOS. Families should be aware that patients who achieve a good recovery might still have significant emotional or behavioral issues. At the same time, they should also know that the category of severe disability does not automatically preclude a good quality of life. One study found that almost half of individuals classified as severely disabled by the GOS at one year were satisfied with their lives (and close to a third who had made a good recovery were dissatisfied with their lives) (90). Finally, it is important to stress to families that most of the studies on prognosis followed patients for only a year, on average, and that there is evidence for continued gains well beyond that time (15).

Present Statistical Information in an Understandable Manner   Prognostication is not only about the range of possible outcomes but also the likelihood of their occurring. Therefore, the ability to convey the numerical aspects of the information accurately is crucial. However, there are significant barriers to effective communication of quantitative information. The level of numerical literacy ("numeracy") in the general population is low (91). Even the understanding of the most elementary ideas of probability cannot be taken for granted. In one study, only half the respondents were able to predict the results of tossing a fair coin 1000 times. The same study found that only 16 percent of respondents correctly answered all three of a set of basic numerical questions (92). These findings have been reproduced in other studies (93).

People had the most difficulty with concepts such as relative risk (94), odds, rates (where the numerator is fixed at 1 and the denominator varies) (95), and proportions where the denominator was anything other than 10 or a 100. One common problem is that people often pay attention only to the numbers and not the form they are in. That is, they believe that the expression with the highest number must represent the highest probability, regardless of whether it is expressed as a rate, proportion, percentage, etc. In one study, subjects rated a health problem as riskier when told that it affects 1,286 out of 10,000 people compared to one that affects 24.14 out of 100 people (96). Other times it is not clear why people are having difficulty. For instance, in another study, half the respondents believed that 2.6/1000 was a larger number than 8.9/1000 (94). Converting between proportions and percentages was particularly difficult (92,97). In summary, there is a significant chance for confusion when the likelihood of outcomes is communicated by concepts such as rates, proportions, etc.

However, the most common way of communicating prognostic information, both in studies and in clinical practice, is through the uses of percentages (e.g., "there is a 70 percent chance he will be able to go back to work"). Yet the comprehension of even such a seemingly straightforward concept as percentages cannot be taken for granted. One study that assessed the understanding of the phrase "there is a 30 percent chance it will rain tomorrow" found that two thirds of the subjects misinterpreted the statement (for instance, believing it meant that it will rain just 30 percent of the day or in 30 percent of the area) (98). The problem here has less to do with numbers and more with an understanding of the referent class— what the percentage is about (e.g., believing that it refers to a portion of the day or the geographic area instead of the likelihood of any rainfall). Even when it seems clear to professionals what the referent class should be, patients can be confused. In one study where patients were told "your risk of developing breast cancer is 10 percent", one subject asked "10 percent of what?" (99). Besides confusion about the referent class, there are other logical or conceptual difficulties that people can have with percentages. For example, a study found that some people thought the risk of developing and dying of breast cancer was higher than the risk of simply developing breast cancer (100).

In addition to the conceptual issues, problems even arise with the numerical aspects of percentages. In looking at cumulative risks (which required addition), many subjects in one study ended up with totals greater than 100 percent (100). In another study of people who were "highly educated", 20 percent of the respondents were not able to state which represented the larger risk: 1 percent, 5 percent, or 10 percent (93). Thus, when communication about prognoses involves the use of percentages, it cannot be automatically assumed that patients or families understand this information.

The difficulty in understanding numerical information is further compounded by the quantified uncertainty associated with any prediction. That is, not only is the primary outcome itself expressed as a probability (e.g., "your son has a 70 percent chance of living independently . . ."), but this estimate itself is subject to uncertainty (". . . and we know this with 90 percent certainty"). Having to process two different levels of numerical uncertainty can overwhelm families and patients and, thus, ironically, end up disempowering decision-making rather than enabling it (87). These expressions of uncertainty can also undermine confidence in the clinician (87), as discussed earlier.

In the end, the numbers themselves may not even be used in decision making. Several studies have found that people immediately code numbers they hear into qualitative or ordinal categories such as high, medium, or low probability or even simply "likely" or "not likely" (86,94,96). Moreover, there is evidence the categories people use were better predictors of their decision making than the actual numbers they were given (94,96). Others have found the form of the information (numerical vs. qualitative) did not affect decision making (101). These findings raise the issue of whether professionals should be communicating numeric values to patients and their families in the first place, rather than using qualitative statements such as likely, unlikely, probable, etc.

In fact, studies have shown that about a third of people would prefer that information about the likelihood of future events be given in qualitative terms rather than numerically (102,103). The problem with qualitative information, however, is that there is a wide variation in the interpretation of the terms, both among patients as well as professionals. One study found that the range of values patients associated with the word "frequent" was 30 percent to 90 percent (102). A report on the understanding of these terms by professionals finds that, for example, the range of values associated with the term "unlikely" was .05 to 90 percent (104). A study that compared the understanding of clinicians and patients found that they differed by an order of magnitude in the numerical associations they made to the same qualitative terms (105). These findings suggest that any use of descriptive terms would need to be supplemented by numeric information, even for those patients who prefer that information be presented qualitatively.

In addition to numeric and qualitative *verbal* communication, there is evidence that graphic displays may also aid in communicating numeric information (106). However, very few studies have directly examined which format might be the most effective. One study that did investigate this question found that a row of ten human stick figures (shaded and unshaded to represent the percentages involved) was the most easily understood graphic and preferred by most of the subjects (99). This is an area needing further study.

So far the discussion has focused on how the quantitative content of information is presented, whether descriptively, numerically, graphically, etc. Yet, non-quantitative aspects of the message can also affect a person's perception of how likely an event is to occur. For example, one could state that a patient has a 10 percent chance of having a good outcome or a 90 percent chance of having a poor outcome. Almost universally, people perceived a good outcome as being more likely when presented with the "positive" statement ("10 percent chance of good outcome") than when presented with the "negative" statement, despite both being numerically equivalent. These findings are the result of "framing" effects, the most widely studied of which has been the "positive/negative" or "loss/gain" frame, as in the example above. A recent review found that, while framing effects did exist, their effect on patients' understanding was much less than that of the "innumeracy" described earlier (107). Still, the existence of framing effects has implications for how prognostic information might be communicated in TBI, as will be seen below.

Although the discussion so far has primarily been about patients and families, it should be pointed out that professionals, especially physicians, often have the same problems in handling quantitative information. Studies have found that physicians are subject to positive or negative framing effects in their treatment decisions: when the same numeric data were presented in a positive frame, physicians were more likely to undertake the treatment (108). Other studies have demonstrated that the way in which the results of clinical trials are reported will affect physician prescribing practices, even when the results themselves are identical (108). For instance, physicians are more likely to prescribe medications if efficacy is presented as a relative risk reduction instead of an absolute risk reduction (109,110). With regards to the qualitative use of probability terms, there is just as much variability in physicians' understanding of these terms as is found with laypeople (104). Finally, there is widespread acknowledgement of the difficulties most physicians have in understanding other statistical concepts, including concepts used routinely in journal articles and even clinical practice (111,112).

Practical Suggestions for Presenting Statistical Information Given the significant barriers to the communication and comprehension of numeric information, what is the best way for a professional to proceed? One solution would be to minimize the occasions in which this information would need to be presented. Clinicians could avoid these discussions during those periods of the recovery process when there are a wide range of possible outcomes. Because each of these outcomes will be associated with a different likelihood of occurring, a discussion would involve the presentation of many different probabilities, further compounding the difficulties patients and families have with quantitative information. One of the advantages of threshold values is that they minimize the cognitive demands on comprehension. To tell a family that it is extremely unlikely the patient will be severely disabled or, alternatively, that it is now extremely unlikely they will have a good recovery, is comprehensible and requires minimal numeric abilities to understand. During periods before these milestones are reached, clinicians could avoid discussing the probabilities of particular outcomes and rely on more general statements such as "All we can say at this point is that there is a chance that she

will be able to return to work; we will know more later, as further information becomes available".

Some families, however, will request detailed information even before milestones are reached. Or, even after a threshold has been crossed, they are interested in the likelihood of a moderate disability on the one hand and either a severe disability or good recovery, on the other. In these cases, there are some general principles that a TBI professional can follow to maximize the chances of comprehension (Figure 14-9). The first suggestion addresses the issue of what form the numeric information should be communicated in. As mentioned earlier, most people have significant difficulties with odds, rates, risks (especially relative risks), etc. Even percentages can be confusing for many people (100). The form of communicating numeric information that seems least susceptible to misunderstanding is the use of natural frequencies (98,99,112). In essence, a natural frequency describes the number of people out of an easily comprehensible set (e.g., 10 or 100) that have the outcome of interest. For instance, rather than state "There is an 80 percent chance your son will have a good recovery in a year", one would say "Out of 10 people like your son, eight of them will have a good recovery in a year" (98,99,112).

As professionals, we are so used to converting one expression into another that we may no longer perceive the differences between these two formulations. There are, however, two important differences between using natural frequencies and using percentages. First, from a numeric point of view, people have more difficulty with percentages than they do with proportions (as long as the denominator is either 10 or 100 and is kept constant). This is not the only issue, however. To see why, compare the two expressions: "Your son has an 8 out of 10 chance of having a good recovery" and "Out of 10 people like your son, eight of them will have a good recovery". Even though both formulations use proportions, people have much less difficulty with the second formulation.

This is because the second formulation specifies the referent class. By making it explicit that one is talking about people, the ambiguity that might result in questions such as "80 percent of what?" can be avoided. It also relevant that the referent class refers to persons instead of outcome categories. There is increasing evidence from cognitive psychology that people are better able to handle computations if they involve persons rather than abstract concepts (98,112). This was also seen when physicians were asked to solve questions of probability involving diagnostic testing (112).

Another suggestion to improve the communication of quantitative information would be to present the information through different routes; not just numerically, as just discussed, but also qualitatively and visually. Because most studies show that people are equally divided in how they wish to receive information, it would make sense to rely on more than one modality. And the fact that people might have difficulty even in their preferred modality justifies presenting the information in at least two different ways. So, in the example cited, after the information was presented numerically, one might say "This is a very good chance for a good recovery".

In addition, given the known effects of framing on the perception of information, one can consider framing the information both positively and negatively. One might say "This means that 2 out of 10 people in his situation will not have a good recovery". Although framing information both positively and negatively might ensure better understanding of the actual likelihood, it could be argued that clinicians should rely mainly on positive framing so as to maximize hope (see below). Finally, as with any other medical interaction, it is helpful to ask the patient or family members to state, in their own words, their understanding of the information.

Fostering Hope   The recommendation to foster hope may seem out of place in a discussion of *techniques* for communicating prognostic information. However, hope is an important part of this process. Of course, hope is most relevant when there is uncertainty. When the eventual outcome is fairly clear (e.g., PTA duration of several days), hope is less relevant precisely because of the certainty of the outcome. In contrast, when the outcome is uncertain (and an undesired outcome is possible), hope becomes correspondingly more important. Fostering hope has many advantages. For one, it may help patients and families to mobilize their energies and resources to engage fully in rehabilitation. In addition, when the prognosis is likely to be poor, even a little hope may "cushion the landing" and allow family members more time to process and come to terms with the probability of a poor outcome. Finally, based on clinical experience, most families seem far more upset with clinicians who offered them little or no hope when the outcome turned out well than those who offered some hope when the outcome was poor.

Of course, there are risks to offering hope, most notably the fear it might prevent family members from adequately preparing for a poorer outcome than they expect. However, the standard advice to families to "hope for the best but plan for the worst" (113) should allow most families to prepare for an undesired outcome without losing hope. When the concern about lack of adequate preparation persists, the clinician can always engage the family in another conversation, trying to shift their perspective. Overall, it appears that the benefits of offering hope in prognosis outweigh the risks (at least in most situations).

It was the commitment to fostering hope that was partly responsible for the emphasis on threshold values in this chapter. For instance, the interest in the longest period of PTA before one can reasonably exclude the possibility of a good recovery was motivated by the wish to preserve justified hope as long as possible. Likewise, being able to tell family members that the chances of severe disability were unlikely if a patient emerged from PTA within a particular time frame helps to allay fears about the possibility of an especially "bad" outcome. The disadvantage of threshold values is that one has to wait until the milestones are reached before one can provide families with more precise information. One way to minimize the frustration of families during the period before a threshold value is crossed is to describe concretely what the potential outcomes are. This is much more helpful and reassuring than saying "we'll just have to wait and see what happens". Knowing what the outcomes might be gives families some sense of control (if only cognitive), while preserving hope for a favorable outcome.

Another way in which to convey hope involves framing the information in a positive way by presenting the likelihood of the favorable outcome rather than the unfavorable outcome (e.g., by saying "he has an 80 percent chance of a good outcome" instead of "he has a 20 percent chance of a poor outcome"). One could also accentuate the positive aspects of less favorable outcomes. For instance, one could point out that someone with a severe disability may still be independent in mobility and self-care. Or that there is not a strong correlation between disability category and quality of life. Or that people with traumatic brain injury are usually fairly healthy. In addition, emphasizing that improvement continues beyond the first year (the end point for many of the studies discussed) is another way of providing encouragement. Even the uncertainty in the prognosis can help to foster hope; by carefully highlighting this uncertainty, one can salvage a little hope even when the prognosis is particularly poor. One could even provide a rough numerical estimation of this uncertainty, based on the confidence intervals discussed earlier (e.g., "Although it is possible that up to 5 percent of people in his condition could have a good recovery, it is extremely unlikely"). Finally, it is important to reassure the family they will not be abandoned and that the clinician will be available to them during the long period of recovery (if true).

Optimizing the Process   There have been several good reviews on improving the process by which this information is communicated, especially in the case of "bad news" (78–80). Some of these guidelines are summarized in Figure 14-10 and are self-explanatory.

RECENT DEVELOPMENTS

Predictions are difficult, especially about the future.
                                                                Yogi Berra

This chapter has focused on "classical" predictors of outcome after TBI. This was motivated by the wish to focus on variables that are easily accessible to rehabilitation professionals. In addition, there is a much larger body of literature available for these variables than for more recently discovered prognostic factors. Still, rehabilitationists should be aware of these recent developments as they are likely to affect clinical practice over the next several years. Several of the most promising of these prognostic variables are discussed below: magnetic resonance spectroscopy (MRS), serum 100b assays (s100b), and apolipoprotein E (APO E) status. The one other modality that might have been included here is the use of evoked potentials in prognostication; however, this topic is covered elsewhere in this book (see Chapter 13).]

MRS

Magnetic Resonance Spectroscopy (MRS) is a noninvasive modality that provides information about the neurochemical status of the brain. As such, it provides physiological information that appears to correlate more strongly with neuronal dysfunction than the structural information provided by conventional MRI. MRS allows one to measure the quantity of compounds thought to be markers of neuronal damage, whether from inflammation, impaired energy metabolism, neuronal death, myelin breakdown, etc. Examples include N-acetyl-aspartate (NAA), choline (Cho), and creatinine (Cr). Changes in the quantities of these compounds (or the ratio between them) correlate with the extent of cellular damage after neural insult.

Although this modality has been studied in many neurological disorders, its use in TBI is just beginning (114). Studies have already shown, however, that people with TBI and controls differ in the amount of these various compounds and that the relative concentrations correlate with *concurrent* neuropsychological performance (115) or GOS category (116). Other studies have demonstrated that certain variables (e.g., decreased NAA/Cr, decreased NAA/Cho, and increased Cho/Cr) correlate with other markers of injury severity (such as GCS and PTA) (117). Even more importantly, studies have shown that concentrations of these compounds seem to correlate with later outcomes, such as GOS at 6 months.

Several studies have found that MRS studies performed in the subacute period (approximately 6 weeks post-injury) correlated with outcome at 6 months or longer. For instance, either total gray matter NAA (118,119) or white matter NAA/Cr (120) correlated with both neuropsychological outcome (118,119) as well as outcome on the GOS (118,120), at 6 months. Other studies found that MRS scans done in the acute period also correlated with long-term outcome. One study found the NAA/Cr ratio acquired about two weeks after injury correlated with outcome on both the GOS and DRS at six months (121).

Besides the general finding that MRS variables correlate with later outcomes, several studies found threshold values that seem to discriminate between various possible outcomes. One study reported values of gray matter NAA above which no one had less than a good recovery and below which no one had a good recovery (118). Another study found minimal overlap in the white matter NAA/Cr values between those subjects with severe disability, moderate disability, and good recovery (121). Finally, several studies investigated the improvement in accuracy gained by using MRS data instead of traditional clinical variables. For instance, one study in children found the presence of early (one week) lactate correctly classified children into either a good recovery/moderate disability or a poor recovery 96 percent of the time (versus about 80 percent accuracy with traditional clinical variables) (122). Another investigation also found that early (one week) MRS variables improved accuracy over clinical variables from 72 percent to 84 percent (123).

Although the results of these studies are promising, several caveats must be kept in mind. First, all of these studies were exploratory and met few of the methodological criteria used in this chapter. In addition, although several of the studies demonstrated that acute MRS variables were more accurate than other acute variables (such as GCS, pupillary abnormalities, etc.), no study has compared the accuracy of MRS variables to the even more powerful clinical variables that are available later (e.g., duration of PTA). Despite these current limitations, MRS is potentially a powerful aid to clinical prognostication after TBI.

Serum 100b

Many serum markers have been proposed as prognostic factors after traumatic brain injury. These include serum 100b protein, neuron-specific enolase, interleukin 6, cleaved tau protein, and glial fibrillary acidic protein. Of these, the most promising work has involved serum 100b protein (S100b), which is found predominantly in astroglial cells. After a brain injury, increased levels of this compound are found in the blood as damaged glial cells release serum 100b across a disrupted blood-brain barrier. The protein is released immediately and peaks early; as a result, most investigators believe that only very early values (within hours after a TBI) are helpful in prognostication. As with MRS, serum 100b has also been studied in other neurological disorders such as anoxic brain injury.

Studies in traumatic brain injury have shown that early S100b levels correlate with the severity of injury (124,125) as well as the extent of abnormality seen on neuroimaging (125–129). More importantly, there are now many studies that suggest that early S100b values help predict long-term outcome as measured by the six month GOS category or neuropsychological test performance (127–133). Other studies have demonstrated that early S100b values are also correlated with outcome at one year, both on the GOS (134–136) as well as on quality of life measures (134).

Most of these studies reported cut-off values for S100b levels that help distinguish between favorable (usually moderate disability/good recovery) and unfavorable outcomes (usually severe disability or death). They also reported the sensitivity, specificity, vegetative state, and positive and negative predictive values of the different cut-off values chosen. In general, the values chosen had high specificities (over 90 percent) and moderate sensitivities (around 70 percent). In other words, when S100b values are higher than the threshold levels chosen, there is a 90 percent chance of an unfavorable outcome. On the other hand, serum values below the cut off values are not as helpful because as many as 30 percent of patients with values below the threshold can still have an unfavorable outcome. Of course, the values chosen can be adjusted to increase either the sensitivity or specificity (but always at the expense of the other). Most of the studies being discussed compared the accuracy of predictions based on S100b levels with those based on other variables such as GCS, imaging abnormalities, etc. In almost every case, the S100b value was the most powerful predictor of outcome (137). Finally, although the discussion so far has focused on severe injuries, there is interest in using S100b values to predict which patients are at the highest risk of developing persistent post-concussional symptoms after a mild TBI (138–141).

Although all of these results are encouraging, they are still preliminary. As with the studies on MRS, almost none of the studies met the methodological criteria used in this review. In addition, the studies that reported the relative superiority of S100b compared the accuracy of S100b levels to values of *isolated* acute care variables rather than to a *combination* of these factors (which are known to be more powerful). Another significant concern about the use of S100b assays is the accumulating evidence that there are significant extracranial sources of S100b. These include soft tissue and bone, which are often damaged by the same incidents that result in TBI (142). As a result, there is a concern that previous studies may not have adequately controlled for these extracranial sources of S100b; this issue is still being debated. Finally, since the serum 100b level must be drawn within a short period after the injury, it is only of use to the rehabilitationists if they have access to results from the acute care setting. Despite these concerns, S100b values are potentially a powerful aid to prognostication after TBI.

Apolipoprotein E

Apolipoprotein E plays a number of different roles in the human brain, many of which are not completely understood (143). Although its role in Alzheimer's disease has been known for a long time, there is now evidence this lipoprotein can affect outcome after TBI. Early studies suggested that possession of the E4 allele was associated with a worse outcome after TBI. One study found this allele over-represented in patients who were still vegetative after one year and that presence of the E4 allele was a better predictor of outcome than the duration of coma (144). In another early study, patients with the E4 allele were more than twice as likely to have an unfavorable outcome on the GOS as those without the allele, even when adjusted for age, CT findings, and initial GCS (145). A different study found that, although the risk of severe disability was not associated with the presence of the E4 allele, the chances of having a good outcome were lower in the E4 group, even when controlling for age or duration of unconsciousness (146).

Despite these early findings, more recent studies have demonstrated either a smaller effect of the E4 allele or no discernible effect. Although a recent study reported a lower FIM motor score in carriers of the E4 allele, the difference was clinically small and was not found in the cognitive FIM score (147). Other studies found no association between the presence of the E4 allele and GOS outcome at 6 months (148,143). However, in the latter study (143), this may have been a result of the population studied (South African blacks); all the previous studies were done in caucasian populations and it is known that the impact of the E4 allele varies by race, at least in Alzheimer's disease.

Thus, the results of the studies done so far have been inconsistent. It seems fairly clear that the E4 allele does modify some end-points such as hematoma size (149), performance on a few neuropsychological tests (150, 151), or the development of late post-traumatic seizures (148). Its effect on more global outcome measures, however, is less pronounced. More importantly, the effect is not large enough to significantly improve clinical prognostication. Rather, the value of these findings will more likely be in identifying targets for intervention in the pathophysiology of TBI.

Neural Networks

All the advances discussed above involved new types of information or data that were not previously available. But there is also some interest in different ways of analyzing already available information. All the studies discussed in this chapter used traditional statistical methodologies such as linear regression or decision trees. The use of newer statistical methodologies holds out the hope that more accurate predictions can be made than with conventional statistical methods. Probably the most promising of these new methods are neural networks. A neural network is a system of mathematical models that attempt to model the way the human brain processes information. One of its most distinctive features is that it "learns by experience".

That is, given a large data set and "training rules" about data relationships, the neural network can respond in novel ways to new inputs (such as data that were not used in the original "training"). The use of neural networks in clinical medicine is growing (152,153) and its use in TBI is being explored (154).

Two primary issues surround the use of neural networks in prognostication. The first is accuracy: does the use of the neural networks result in more accurate predictions than more traditional models? The evidence from other fields is mixed (152) and a study on TBI found no difference in accuracy between a neural network analysis and one based on logistic regression (154). The other issue surrounding the use of neural networks is ease of clinical use. The concern is that neural networks are "black boxes" because there is no way of making explicit how they generate their predictions. All one can know are the data inputs and the resultant outputs. In more traditional methods, the algorithm used is explicit and its conceptual bases understandable, even if its numeric aspects are not. It has been suggested that this lack of transparency would limit the use of neural networks by clinicians (153). Despite these concerns, the use of neural networks in outcome prediction after TBI holds promise and bears further investigation. Other statistical methods are also being evaluated; readers are directed elsewhere for more information (155,156).

CONCLUSIONS: SUGGESTIONS FOR FURTHER RESEARCH

There is still much work that needs to be done on prognosis after traumatic brain injury. For one, it would be helpful if a larger group, such as a task force, reviewed the literature in order to see if they could replicate the results of this chapter. Having a group of individuals involved, rather than a single author, might improve the quality of the criteria used, the scope of the literature search, as well as the classification of the studies. In addition, a larger group could expand the grading system that is used to include different levels of strength of evidence (as is common in most evidence based reviews). At the time of this writing, it appears that the American Congress of Rehabilitation Medicine has assembled a task force that may pursue these goals.

In addition to reviewing already existing studies, it is important that more studies be conducted in an attempt to confirm the findings of this review. However, these studies should be designed so as to build on the strengths of the current literature and to compensate for its weaknesses (in scope or design). This is crucial given how few studies formed the basis of the recommendations presented here. Most generally, it would be important for future studies to incorporate the concept of threshold

values to maximize their clinical utility. It would also be important to focus on those variables that have already shown promise as being clinically useful (such as the duration of coma or PTA, magnetic resonance spectroscopy, etc.) rather than those that are clearly not powerful enough to aid in clinical prognostication (such as initial GCS or CT imaging). It is noted that the utility of neuropsychological testing is still unclear, given the limitations of the studies done to date. It would be useful to have better studies in this area to determine the value of such testing.

In addition to selecting appropriate variables, it would be important for future studies to address shortcomings in the outcome measures used previously as well as to study more relevant populations. With regard to outcome measures, given the clear limitations of the Glasgow Outcome Scale, more studies should be conducted with newer, more promising measures such as the Community Integration Questionnaire. The duration of follow up should be longer as well, given what is now known about the possibility of clinically meaningful recovery that can occur a year or more after an injury. In terms of setting, more studies are needed that are based in inpatient rehabilitation (thus circumventing the problems that arise when attempting to extrapolate from the acute care setting to patients in rehabilitation).

Finally, it is important that studies be conducted that attempt to identify what types of prognostic information patients and families want. There have been very few studies that have explicitly addressed this issue (see the discussion in Appendix II). Yet, because prognostication is ultimately a *clinical* act (one directed at and meant to benefit patients and families), it is crucial that future studies on prognostication (as opposed to studies on outcomes more generally) be designed around the explicit needs of patients and their families.

APPENDIX I: EVALUATING AN ARTICLE ON PROGNOSIS

This section discusses some general guidelines that readers can use when evaluating individual studies on prognosis; these are summarized in Figure 14-11. Interested readers are referred to more detailed discussions of these issues (157–165). In general, three main principles guide the critical evaluation of an article on prognosis: the *quality* of the study, its *relevance* to one's own practice, and the *utility* of the findings. A study can be methodologically sound but inapplicable to one's practice, for instance if the study population is not similar to one's own. Or the reverse can happen: the study is relevant to one's practice but, because of problems in design, one cannot rely on the study's results. Finally, a relevant and methodologically sound study may still not be helpful because

Outcomes
- Is the outcome clinically important?
- Is the outcome measure validated?
- Is the outcome measure described well enough that it can be easily applied?
- Did an appropriate amount of time elapse before the outcome was measured?

Predictor Variables
- Are the predictor variables described well enough that they can be easily applied?
- Are the predictor variables easily accessible?
- Do the predictor variables have high reliability?

Sample
- Is the population described well enough to determine if they are similar in relevant aspects to your own (including the site)?
- Was their any bias in the selection of subjects (for instance, an inception cohort vs. a convenience sample)?
- Was the sample large enough?
- Was there minimal loss to follow up?
- Were the characteristics of those who were lost to follow up compared to those who completed the study?

Results
- Were the findings reported in a form that is useful for clinicians (e.g. absolute risk)?
- Was the precision of the estimates provided (e.g. confidence intervals)?
- Was there an evaluation of validity (replication of findings in same sample)?
- Have the findings been confirmed in other studies (reproducibility)?
- Are the findings believable on biological grounds?
- Do the findings represent an advance over already available prognostic tools?

FIGURE 14-11

Guidelines for Reading an Article on Prognosis

the results are reported in a way that makes it difficult to apply to clinical practice.

These principles of quality, relevance, and utility guide the questions that one should ask about the various components of the study: outcomes, predictors, sample, and results (Figure 14-11). It is also important to assess the statistical analysis performed, although this issue is only briefly addressed here. Many of the criteria listed in Figure 14-11 will be familiar: they are identical to the inclusion criteria for this review. The second appendix provides a detailed review of these criteria; therefore, they will not be discussed here. Rather, the focus will be on the new criteria listed. The following discussion is organized according to the topics mentioned earlier (outcomes, predictors, sample, results).

Outcomes

The outcomes must be of clinical relevance, one that would matter either to the clinician, the patient, or their family. Whatever outcome measure is used, it should be well described so clinicians can apply it to their own patients. The outcome should also be easy to measure in clinical practice. It should also be a measure that has either already been validated or, at least, has had some assessment of validity performed in the study itself. Finally, the outcome should be measured at an appropriate time (at least 6 months after a TBI).

Predictors

Many of the same criteria apply to the study's choice of predictor variables: they should be well described, have high reliability, and be easily accessible or easily performed by the clinician.

Sample

The sample should also be well described, so readers can decide if the subjects are similar to their own patients. In assessing this, it is also important to keep in mind the nature of the treatments received by the study population and whether one's own patients receive similar treatments. The study should be prospective, utilizing an inception cohort, rather than retrospective (e.g., a case-control design). The sample size should also be adequate. The size of the sample not only affects the precision of the estimates (e.g., the width of the confidence intervals) but also ensures the sample obtained is representative of the population. In addition, many of the statistical analyses performed require a sample of a certain size for the results to be valid (e.g., for multivariate analyses).

There should also be minimal loss to follow-up. Although most authors recommend the loss to follow-up should be no greater than 15–20 percent, the real issue is the number of people lost to follow-up relative to the number of people with the outcome of interest. One way of evaluating this would be to examine what would happen if everyone lost to follow-up ended up in each of the outcome categories. For instance, a 15 percent loss to follow-up in which the outcome categories were equally likely (e.g., 50 percent "good" and 50 percent "bad") would not affect the results significantly. Even if you assume that all of those lost to follow-up either had a good outcome or a bad outcome, the percentages would shift only slightly (e.g., to 57 percent and 43 percent in either direction), not enough to affect prognostication. On the other hand, in a study in which no one achieved a certain outcome (e.g., severe disability), a 15 percent loss to follow-up would be significant if all 15 percent were severely disabled. Finally, it would be ideal if the characteristics of those lost to follow-up were compared with those who remained in the study.

Results

The results have to be reported in a way that is clinically useful, so they can be used to formulate a prognosis for individual patients. In general, absolute risks or simple percentages are more useful than measures such as relative risk, likelihood ratios, odds, etc. There should also be some report of the precision of the estimate provided (e.g., the width of the confidence interval). Ideally, there should also be some assessment of the model's validity: both by replication of the findings in the original sample as well as, more importantly, replication at other sites. Although this assessment of validity represents the ideal, it is rarely met in studies of TBI. An exception that illustrates the importance of replication was a study done in the acute care setting (166). This study applied a previously published model (167) to their own patient population. Although the model was reported to be 100 percent accurate in the original study, the second study found it to be only about 65 percent accurate in their patient population.

Finally, the results of the study should be interpreted in the larger context of the available literature. Do the findings make sense based on what is known of the pathophysiology and natural history of TBI? Have other studies confirmed the findings? Do the findings provide for more accurate prognoses than is already possible?

APPENDIX II: METHODOLOGY

Methods

Extensive literature searches (based on the inclusion criteria described below) were performed on Medline, PsycInfo, and the personal database of a colleague of the author (which has over 20,000 TBI specific articles); the search covered the period from 1983 through 2004. Hundreds of articles were retrieved and their bibliographies then reviewed for further references. All the articles were then reviewed to determine whether they met the inclusion criteria. The inclusion criteria were developed after extensive discussions with various professionals (including, for instance, neurosurgeons and biostatisticians), as well as family members and survivors. The general principles that guided the selection of the inclusion criteria are presented in Figure 14-4. The inclusion criteria themselves are listed in Figure 14-5. The sections that follow explain the rationale for the criteria chosen.

Population

Severe TBI Patients with moderate and, especially, severe TBI make up most of those admitted to inpatient rehabilitation. Therefore, the original plan was to focus on both of these groups. However, there were no studies meeting the inclusion criteria that focused only on moderate TBI. Even among the studies that met the inclusion criteria, only a few included patients with moderate injuries and, even then, they only comprised a small percentage of the total number of patients. Moreover, these studies had other eligibility criteria that excluded many of the moderately injured patients (e.g., by only including patients who had been admitted to an ICU). For these reasons, this chapter focuses on patients with severe TBI. This seems appropriate given the limited evidence available for patients with moderate injuries, the generally good outcomes in this group (10), and because patients with severe injuries are the ones for whom prognostication is often the most difficult. Studies on civilian penetrating brain injury were evaluated separately from those on closed brain injury, given the substantial differences between these two populations.

Subacute Period After TBI (Acute Care and Rehabilitation) The focus of this chapter is on prognostication during the subacute period, which was defined as the period from the initial stabilization of the patient after the injury (usually in the first week) to approximately three months after the injury. It was felt that this period was of most concern to rehabilitation clinicians working with TBI. Certainly, there are other periods in which the question of prognosis is relevant. Most obviously, there is a great deal of concern about prognosis in the acute setting, early after a TBI. Similarly, survivors and family members often continue to have questions about "final" recovery many months or even years after a brain injury, during the chronic phase.

In this chapter, however, the focus is on prognostication during the time that lies between these two periods. There are various reasons for this focus. For one, the literature on prognostication is enormous, and it would be impossible to survey all of it in a single chapter. Besides, at least with regard to prognostication in the acute stage, there has already been a comprehensive evidence-based review (168). In addition, the focus in the immediate aftermath of a TBI is mostly on mortality rather than on broader outcomes. Rehabilitation professionals are less likely to be involved during the period immediately after the injury, although they often play a more important role after the patient is stabilized. Although rehabilitationists are the primary clinicians during the chronic phase (after approximately 6–12 months), the questions that arise during this period are often easier to answer because much more information is available by then.

In contrast, there is relatively little information during the subacute period, which is one reason why prognostication is so difficult then. At the same time, the need for prognostic information is greatest during this period.

Families have often been so focused on issues of survival during the acute care stage that they are just beginning to think about the long-term implications of the injury. This is especially true after patients are admitted to inpatient rehabilitation. In many ways, then, this period represents a pivotal point after a TBI and providing information about outcomes is one of the clinician's most important obligations during this time (2).

The question then arose as to whether to limit the review to only those studies done in the inpatient rehabilitation setting or to also include studies done in acute care. The populations are clearly different. The primary issue is that only a subset of all TBI patients admitted to acute care eventually goes to inpatient rehabilitation. Many patients die in the acute care setting. Of those patients that survive, some have improved to the point that they do not require inpatient rehabilitation and can be discharged with outpatient services. At the other end of the spectrum, many survivors of TBI have not made enough neurological progress to meet the criteria for admission to inpatient rehabilitation and are therefore often discharged to long-term care facilities or home. Thus, there is a concern that the acute care population would not necessarily be representative of patients seen in rehabilitation.

Despite these concerns, studies done in the acute care setting were included in this review. Since both acute care and inpatient rehabilitation usually occur during the subacute time period, it was felt that studies from both settings were needed to adequately represent this phase. Also, rehabilitation professionals often first encounter patients in the acute care setting and are often asked by other clinicians or family members about long-term prognosis early after a TBI. Additionally, despite differences between the two populations, the variables affecting prognosis seem to be similar; in fact, there were no appreciable differences in the findings of the studies done in the two settings.

The most important reason for including the acute care studies, however, is that there were only five studies conducted in the inpatient rehabilitation setting that met the inclusion criteria. Given the limited number of well designed rehabilitation studies, the choice was either to include acute care studies or to liberalize the inclusion criteria so more studies based in rehabilitation could be included. It was decided that well designed studies of prognosis from the acute care setting would be more useful than methodologically weaker studies based in the rehabilitation setting.

Studies Published After 1983 Beginning in the early eighties, changes in pre-hospital, neurosurgical, and ICU care have resulted in a steady decline in mortality from TBI (169–171). Whether functional outcome has also improved is less clear. There has been some concern that

although mortality has declined, the survivors are disproportionately severely disabled. Recent reports don't support these fears, however, and it now appears that functional outcomes have improved along with survival (172,173). Because of these changes in care, it was decided to exclude studies published before 1984, under the assumption that the care patients received before that time differed from current care in ways that directly impact outcome. Specifically, it is assumed that studies done before the early eighties would underestimate survival and function. Although acute medical and surgical care continued to improve after the early eighties, most of these changes have been relatively minor compared with those of twenty years ago. The primary changes over the past fifteen years have been the adoption of the new standards by an increasing number of non-academic centers (170,173).

Setting: North America/Western Europe/Australia/New Zealand/Israel Although there is some documented variation in TBI care *within* the United States (as well as between the U.S. and Europe) (174), care in the countries listed above was similar enough to justify grouping them together (175). Even though care in the excluded countries may be similar to that in the countries above, there is no evidence to support this. Because variations in care are likely to affect outcomes, studies originating in countries other than those listed were excluded.

Age: Adult Since pediatric TBI is discussed elsewhere the studies included in this review focused exclusively or predominately on *adult* TBI. Also, because age is such a powerful predictor of outcome, also included were studies on the elderly.

Subpopulations In general, studies that included a wide range of patients were preferred, since this would most closely resemble the typical patient population seen by most rehabilitation clinicians. In addition, beyond a certain point, it becomes difficult for clinicians to use a different set of guidelines for minor variations in pre-injury, injury, or post-injury factors. Some groups are so distinctive, however, that studies that focused exclusively on them were included. The most notable examples in this review were the studies on the elderly and those with civilian penetrating injuries. A few studies that focused on other subsets of the TBI population were included only if that subset made conceptual sense and was easily identifiable by a rehabilitation professional. For instance, included were studies that limited themselves to patients who regained consciousness in acute care as well as one that focused on TBI patients who did not sustain other injuries. However, studies that focused only on those patients with, for example, traumatic subarachnoid hemorrhage or a history of elevated intracranial pressure, were excluded under the assumption that this information was often not readily available and did not reflect conceptual categories that rehabilitation professionals routinely use.

Predictor Variables

The review is limited to the following predictor variables: age, initial Glasgow Coma Scale score (GCS), length of coma (LOC), duration of post-traumatic amnesia (PTA), and early neuroimaging (CT and MRI). There are several reasons for focusing exclusively on these predictors. First, these variables are among the most powerful predictors of outcome available. More importantly, they represent pieces of information that are either easily available to most rehabilitation clinicians (e.g., age, initial GCS, etc.) or can be prospectively determined in the rehabilitation setting (e.g., duration of PTA). Although there are other variables that can also have a significant impact on outcome (e.g., pupillary abnormalities, hypoxia, premorbid functioning, etc.), this information is often not readily available (for instance, because of the limited availability of medical records). Thus, studies that rely on utilizing this information may not be particularly useful for rehabilitation clinicians providing subacute prognostication.

Only those studies that used the *total* GCS score were included. Although there are compelling reasons for the use of just the motor score in prognostication (176), rehabilitation clinicians do not often have available to them a patient's GCS subscores. There were also many studies that combined the variables selected for this review with other variables to create a single predictive model (for instance: age, pupillary abnormalities, and GCS motor response). Although the clinical utility of these models is dependent on the *combination* of variables (some of which are not readily available to the rehabilitation clinician), the studies making use of these models were included because they provided evidence that the variable of interest (e.g., age in the example above) was, after a multivariate analysis, associated with outcome.

Although neuropsychological testing during inpatient rehabilitation was originally included as a predictor of interest, none of the studies on early neuropsychological testing met the methodological criteria. Although not discussed as part of the evidence based review, the studies that have been done are briefly reviewed in the body of the chapter.

Outcomes

Outcome Measures   One of the central issues in prognostication is to be clear about the outcome of interest. There are many outcome measures available: survival, physical impairment, ability to perform activities of daily living, cognitive and behavioral status, return to work,

independent living, quality of life, etc. (177,178). The outcome one chooses depends on the question(s) one is asking and whether these questions are being asked for research or clinical purposes. In particular, the interests of professionals (especially researchers) and families do not always coincide. For instance, there is evidence that the outcomes of most interest to family members, at least during the rehabilitation phase, have to do with broad conceptual categories such as independent living and return to work (179,180). Besides the intrinsic importance of these categories, there is a symbolic importance associated with them (181). That is, given the importance our culture places on employment and independent living, these roles come to symbolize our membership in the community at large. Even the concern with other outcomes (e.g., physical impairment, cognitive decline, etc.) is interpreted mainly by their impact on these more holistic functional categories (179,180).

Unfortunately, most studies do not use measures of these types of outcomes, for several different reasons. First, these outcomes are so broad that they can include a wide range of patients within a single category. For instance, the category of severe disability in the GOS would include both a minimally conscious patient as well as someone independent in basic activities of daily living who is unable to live alone because of cognitive deficits (182). These measures are also insensitive to changes that can occur beyond the first 6 months to a year, making them less useful in studying the longer term natural history of TBI (178,183). Third, the psychometric properties of these global outcome measures often are not as good as those of more fine-grained research measures. For example, there are concerns about inter-observer agreement in the clinical use of the GOS (15). Another concern with the GOS is the fact that what is documented is the rater's subjective impression of a person's abilities rather than actual outcome. For instance, the measure documents the rater's beliefs about a person's ability to work rather than actual employment (which may account for the finding that ratings on the GOS may not be as strongly correlated with measures of employment as one would expect) (177).

The broadness of categories such as return to work or independent living can obscure the underlying mechanisms that mediate the outcome. Although this is sometimes seen as an advantage of these measures (so that they "integrate" the effect of many deficits into a final outcome such as work) (184), this characteristic can also lead to the loss of valuable information. For instance, is the person unable to live independently because of executive dysfunction, impulsivity, or physical impairment? Or because of factors that have nothing to do with the brain injury (e.g., other disabling physical conditions, financial resources, family support, etc.) (25)? By collapsing these distinctions, the use of these outcome measures can obscure the underlying deficits that actually prevent people from living independently or returning to work.

There is also evidence that, at least early on, both patients and family members overestimate the contribution of certain outcomes to eventual quality of life (such as independent living) and underestimate the importance of others (such as social relationships). During the chronic phase of TBI, most studies show that emotional and behavioral issues are far more important to family members than, for instance, residence or occupational status (180,185–187). Even for patients, there is evidence the GOS categories do not correlate well with their own ratings of their quality of life (90). The broad categories of return to work, independent living, or the GOS are simply not designed to identify sequelae such as quality of life, social relationships, behavioral disturbances, etc.

However, although they will likely change their minds later, the fact remains that it is still these broad categories of functional outcome that families and patients are concerned with during the subacute period. To prognosticate about outcomes that are not yet relevant to them can lead to dissatisfaction and the perception that their needs for information are not being met. And since prognosis is ultimately a clinical act that tries to address the *current* needs of families and patients, their preferences have to be considered. For this reason, this review was limited to those studies that focused on return to work or independent living, either directly or through the GOS.

Despite its other limitations, the GOS actually seems to be one of the most useful measures of these sorts of outcomes. This is because the GOS utilizes outcome categories that correspond to those used by lay people, making results expressed in terms of its categories useful to clinicians. For instance, in discussing that their loved one will likely be "moderately disabled" in a year, the clinician can explain that the patient will likely be able to live independently but will have residual deficits precluding their being able to return to competitive employment. This outcome is understandable to family members since they, too, think in terms of independent living or employment.

In this respect, the GOS contrasts to measures such as the Disability Rating Scale (DRS) that either report a numerical score that has no real meaning to a layperson or is divided into categories (e.g., partial disability, moderately severe disability, etc.) that also have no clear conceptual correlates. Although it is true that information about living situation and employment can be extracted from the DRS, the data needed to do so is rarely reported in the literature (it is usually only the total score that is reported). The relatively clear meaning of the GOS categories is also an advantage relative to the results of neuropsychological testing. For most family members, a decline on a neuropsychological test is of little relevance except as it has an impact on "real-world" outcomes such as independent living.

Despite its advantages in addressing the needs of patients and families, there are still the many methodological limitations of the GOS mentioned earlier. There are newer measures that retain many of the advantages of the GOS while avoiding some of its limitations (e.g., the Community Integration Questionnaire). Unfortunately, there were no studies using these measures that also met all the other inclusion criteria. This fact reflects one of the primary reasons for the use of the GOS in this review. Because it is the most widely used measure in the TBI outcomes literature, including the GOS as an outcome measure significantly expanded the number of studies that could be included in this review. In fact, to exclude studies that used the GOS would have limited this review to less than a handful of studies (that met all the other criteria listed).

Outcome Measured at 6 Months or Later   For several reasons, this review is limited to studies that assess outcome no earlier than six months after injury. Waiting *at least* six months is uncontroversial given the well-known clinical observation that, for most individuals, significant improvement occurs during the first six months after an injury. It could be argued, however, that since recovery clearly continues after six months, it would be better to wait a longer period of time, for instance, at least a year. Indeed, there is growing evidence that some individuals can continue to have meaningful recovery even many years after their injury (188–190). Nonetheless, there are compelling reasons to include studies that assess outcome as early as six months. First, studies have shown that, despite continued improvement, it was rare for an individual's GOS category to improve after six months (191). More practically, if only studies that assessed outcome beyond six months were included, well over half of the studies would have been excluded, further limiting what is already a small evidence base.

Methodological Criteria

The methodological criteria adopted are, for the most part, self-explanatory. The review is limited to studies with consecutive admissions (or a random sample of consecutive admissions) to minimize the possibility of systemic bias (which might arise from sampling based on any other criteria). Likewise, the requirement of at least 80 percent follow-up minimizes the biases that might be encountered with high rates of drop-out. Historically, TBI outcome studies have been characterized by high rates of loss to follow-up (1/3 to 1/2 of the original sample); the implications of this for the validity of studies on outcome have been recently reviewed (192). Unfortunately, almost no studies analyzed the characteristics of those lost to follow-up to see if they differed substantially from those who were included. In the interest of having more than

1–2 studies to review, it was decided that an analysis of patients lost to follow-up would not be required of studies to be included.

The criterion specifying a minimum sample size was adopted from the AANS acute care prognostication review (168). Finally, the studies were reviewed to ensure that some form of statistical analysis was performed on the data of interest. If not, the study was still included if enough information was provided for the statistical analysis to be done by a knowledgeable reader. This was an issue for some of the older studies, where the distribution of outcomes was occasionally reported only in a descriptive manner. However, there was no attempt to screen studies based on the statistical models employed. The most commonly utilized models in this area are regression models and decision tress. The features and limitations of these approaches are detailed elsewhere (193–200).

There are some potential criteria not utilized in this review, either because they were not applicable or because they would have greatly limited the number of studies available. Most notably, a study was included even if it did not adjust for confounding factors (because so few did so). However, those studies that performed an univariate versus a multivariate analysis (or something else to adjust for confounding factors) are noted in the tables. More importantly, the fact that the studies that did not adjust for confounds came to the same conclusions as those that did increases the confidence in the findings of the review.

Threshold Values and Confidence Intervals

It cannot be automatically inferred that a particular outcome is impossible, just because no one over or under a particular threshold value had the outcome of interest in a particular study. This is because there is always a degree of statistical uncertainty, even when the outcome of interest does not occur. For example, even if no one with a duration of PTA greater than three months had a good recovery in a particular study, it might still be *statistically* possible that a certain percentage of them could have achieved that outcome. This possibility can be quantified by confidence intervals. In a study where no one had the outcome of interest, the lower end of the confidence interval would be zero, while the upper end would represent the largest number of people who could statistically be expected to develop the outcome of interest. The width of this confidence interval will depend on the sample size.

For instance, if no one out of a sample of 87 people achieved a good recovery on the GOS, the 95 percent confidence interval would be approximately 0 to 3 percent. That is, the findings are compatible (with 95 percent certainty) with up to 3 percent of that group achieving a good recovery. If, instead, no one out of a sample of only 17 people achieved a good recovery, the confidence interval would be much wider (approximately 0–16 percent). Therefore, the most that one can infer from the smaller study (with 95 percent certainty) is that anywhere from 0 to 16 percent of similar people could have had the outcome of interest. It is also important to keep in mind that a study in which no one had a particular outcome is not necessarily stronger evidence for a threshold value than a study in which some subjects had the outcome. It all depends on the width of the confidence interval. For instance, a study with a large sample (e.g., 150) that reported that 4 percent of subjects had a good recovery would actually have a smaller confidence interval (1–9 percent) than a study with a smaller sample (e.g., 27) in which no one achieved a good recovery (CI 0–11 percent).

Unfortunately, none of the studies that reported threshold values reported the associated confidence intervals. Therefore, the author calculated the confidence intervals for all the threshold values. However, only those threshold values with a 95 percent confidence interval of no greater than 0–12 percent are reported. This figure represented a balance between the limits of tolerability of error and the wish to include as many studies as possible.

References

1. NIH Consensus Development Panel on Rehabilitation of Persons with Traumatic Brain Injury. Rehabilitation of persons with traumatic brain injury. *JAMA* 1999; 282:974–983.
2. Holland D, Shigaki CL. Educating families and caretakers of traumatically brain injured patients in the new health care environment: a three-phase model and bibliography. *Brain Injury* 1998; 12(12)993–1009.
3. Junque C, Bruna O, Mataro M. Information needs of the traumatic brain injury patient's family members regarding the consequences of the injury and associated perception of physical, cognitive, emotional, and quality of life changes. *Brain Injury* 1997; 11(4):251–258.
4. Christakis NA. *Death Foretold*. Chicago: The University of Chicago Press 1999.
5. Dawes RM, Faust D, Meehl PE. Clinical versus actuarial judgment. *Science* 1989; 243:1668–1674.
6. Knaus WA, Wagner DP, Lynn J. Short-term mortality predictions for critically ill hospitalized adults: science and ethics. *Science* 1991; 254:389–393.
7. Perkins HS, Jonsen AR, Epstein WV. Providers as predictors: using outcome predictions in intensive care. *Crit Care Med* 1986; 14(2): 105–110
8. Poses RM, Bekes C, Copare FJ, et al. The answer to "what are my chances, doctor?" depends on who is asked: prognostic disagreement and inaccuracy for critically ill patients. *Crit Care Med* 1989; 17(8): 827–833
9. Chang RW, Lee B, Jacobs S, et al. Accuracy of decisions to withdraw therapy in critically ill patients: clinical judgment versus a computer model. *Crit Care Med* 1989; 17(11):1091–1097
10. van der Naalt J. Prediction of outcome in mild to moderate head injury: a review, *J Clin Exper Neuropsych*. 2001; 23(6):837–851.
11. Sherer M, Madison CF, Hannay HJ. A review of outcome after moderate head injury with an introduction to life care planning. *J Head Trauma Rehabil* 2000; 15(2):767–782.
12. Levin HS. Prediction of recovery from traumatic brain injury. *J Neurotrauma* 1995; 12(5):913–922.
13. Macniven E. Factors affecting head injury rehabilitation outcome: premorbid and clinical parameters. In Finlayson MA,

Garner SH (eds.). *Brain Injury Rehabilitation: Clinical Considerations*. Baltimore: Williams & Wilkins 1994:57–82.

14. Mack A, Lawrence JH. Functional prognosis in traumatic brain injury. *Phys Med & Rehab: State of the Art Reviews* 1989; 3(1): 13–26.

15. Sandel ME, Labi MLC. Outcome prediction: clinical and research perspectives. *Phys Med & Rehab: State of the Art Reviews* 1990; 4(3):409–420.

16. Jennett B. Assessment and Prediction of Outcome After Head Injury. In Macfarlane R, Hardy DG (eds.). *Outcome After Head, Neck and Spinal Trauma*. Oxford: Butterworth-Heinemann 1997.

17. Andrews BT. Prognosis in severe head injury. In Cooper PR, Golfinos JG (eds.). *Head Injury*. New York: McGraw-Hill 2000:555–563.

18. Marion DW. Outcome from severe head injury. In Narayan RK, Wilberger JE, Povlishock JT (eds.). *Neurotrauma*. New York: McGraw-Hill 1996:767–777.

19. Stein SC. Outcome from moderate head injury. In Narayan RK, Wilberger JE, Povlishock JT (eds.). *Neurotrauma*. New York: McGraw-Hill 1996:755–765.

20. Zafonte RD, Hammond FM, Peterson J. Predicting outcome in the slow to respond traumatically brain-injured patient: acute and subacute parameters. *NeuroRehab* 1996; 6:19–32.

21. Crepeau F, Scherzer P. Predictors and indicators of work status after traumatic brain injury: a meta-analysis. *Neuropsych Rehab* 1993; 3(1):5–35.

22. Yasuda S, Wehman P, Targett P, Cifu D, West M. Return to work for persons with traumatic brain injury. *Am J Phys Med Rehabil* 2001; 80(11):852–864.

23. Goldstein FC, Levin HS. Cognitive outcome after mild and moderate traumatic brain injury in older adults. *J Clin Exper Neuropsych* 2001; 23(6):739–753.

24. Rapoport MJ, Feinstein A. outcome following traumatic brain injury in the elderly: a critical review. *Brain Injury* 2000; 14(8): 749–761.

25. Wagner AK. Functional prognosis in traumatic brain injury. *Phys Med & Rehab: State of the Art Review* 2001; 15(2):245–267.

26. Shutter LA, Jallo JI, Narayan RK. Traumatic brain injury. In Evans R, Baskin D, Yatsu F (eds.). *Prognosis of Neurological Disorders*. 2nd ed. New York: Oxford University Press 2000; 335–365.

27. Rao N, Rosenthal M, Cronin-Stubbs D, et al. Return to work after rehabilitation following traumatic brain injury. *Brain Injury* 1990; 4(1):49–56.

28. Fearnside MR, Cook RJ, McDougall P, McNeil RJ. The Westmead Head Injury Project outcome in severe head injury. a comparative analysis of pre-hospital, clinical and CT variables. *Br J Neurosurgery* 1993; 7:267–279.

29. Kakarieka A, Braakman R, Schakel EH. Clinical significance f the finding of subarachnoid blood on CT scan after head injury. *Acta Neurochir* 1994; 129:1–5.

30. Walder AD, Yeoman PM, Turnbull A. The abbreviated injury scale as a predictor of outcome of severe head injury. *Intensive Care Med* 1995; 21:606–609.

31. Lobato RD, Gomez PA, Alday R, et al. Sequential computerized tomography changes and related final outcome in severe head injury patients. *Acta Neurochir* 1997; 139:385–391.

32. Wedekind C, Fischbach R, Pakos P, et al. Comparative use of magnetic resonance imaging and electrophysiologic investigation for the prognosis of head injury. *J Trauma* 1999; 47(1):44–49.

33. Gomez PA, Lobato RD, Boto GR, et al. Age and outcome after severe head injury. *Acta Neurochair (Wein)* 2000;142:373–381.

34. Firsching R, Woischneck D, Klein S et al. Classification of Severe Head Injury Based on Magnetic Resonance Imaging. *Acta Neurochir* 2001; 143:263–271.

35. Schaan M, Jaksche H, Boszczyk B. Predictors of outcome in head injury: proposal of a new scaling system. *J Trauma* 2002; 52(4): 667–674.

36. Vos PE, Van Voskuilen AC, Beems T, et al. Evaluation of the traumatic coma data bank computed tomography classification for severe head injury. *J Neurotrauma* 2001; 18(7):649–655.

37. Mattioli C, Beretta L, Gerevini S, et al. Traumatic subarachnoid hemorrhage on the computerized tomography scan obtained at admission: a multicenter assessment of the accuracy of diagnosis

and the potential impact on patient outcome. *J Neurosurg* 2003; 98:37–42.

38. Rovlias A, Kotsou S. Classification and regression tree for prediction of outcome after severe head injury using simple clinical and laboratory variables. *J Neurotrauma* 2004; 21(7):886–893.

39. Formisano R, Voogt RD, Buzzi MG et al. time interval of oral feeding recovery as a prognostic factor in severe traumatic brain injury. *Brain Injury* 2004; 18(1):103–109.

40. Born JD, Albert A, Hans P, et al. Relative prognostic value of best motor response and brain stem reflexes in patients with severe head injury. *Neurosurgery* 1985; 16(5):595–601.

41. Facco E, Zuccarello M, Pittoni G, et al. early outcome prediction in severe head injury: comparison between children and adults. *Child's Nerv Syst* 1986; 2:67–71.

42. Hans P, Albert A, Born JD. Predicting recovery from head injury. *Brit J Hospital Med* 1987 (June):535–540.

43. Choi SC, Narayan RK, Anderson RL, et al. Enhanced specificity of prognosis in severe head injury. *J Neurosurg* 1988; 69:381–385.

44. Tate RL, Lulham JM, Broe GA, et al. Psychosocial outcome for the survivors of severe blunt head injury: the results from a consecutive series of 100 patients. *J Neurol & Psych* 1989; 52: 1128–1134.

45. Narayan RK, Enas GG, Choi SC, et al. Practical techniques for predicting outcome in severe head injury. In Becker DP, Gudeman SK *Textbook of Head Injury*, Philadelphia: Saunders, 1989 pp. 420–425

46. Levin HS, Gary HE, Eisenberg HM, et al. Neurobehavioral outcome 1 year after severe head injury. *J Neurosurg* 1990; 73: 699–709.

47. Choi SC, Muizelaar JP, Barnes TY, et al. Prediction tree for severely head-injured patients. *J Neurosurg* 1991; 75:251–255.

48. Marshall LF, Gautille T, Klauber MR. The outcome of severe closed head injury. *J Neurosurg* 1991; 75:S28-S36.

49. Vollmer DG, Torner JC, Jane JA, et al. Age and outcome following traumatic coma: why do older patients fare worse? *J Neurosurg* 1991; 75:S37-S49.

50. Bishara SN, Partridge FM, Godfrey HPD, et al. Post-traumatic amnesia and Glasgow coma scale related to outcome in survivors in a consecutive series of patients with severe closed-head injury. *Brain Injury* 1992; 6(4):373–380.

51. Godfrey HPD, Bishara SN, Partridge FM, et al. Neuropsychological impairment and return to work following severe closed head injury: implications for clinical management. *NZ Med J* 1993; 106:301–303.

52. Pennings JL, Bachulis BL, Simons CT, et al. Survival after severe brain injury in the aged. *Arch Surg* 1993; 128:787–794.

53. Katz DI, Alexander MP. Traumatic brain injury: predicting course of recovery and outcome for patients admitted to rehabilitation. *Arch Neurol* 1994; 51:661–670.

54. Combes P, Fauvage B, Colonna M, et al. Severe Head Injuries: An Outcome Prediction and Survival Analysis. *Intensive Care Med* 1996; 22:1391–1395.

55. Ellenberg JH, Levin HS, Saydjari C. Posttraumatic Amnesia as a Predictor of Outcome After Severe Closed Head Injury. *Arch Neurol* 1996; 53:782–791.

56. Hawkins ML, Lewis FD, Medeiros RS. Serious Traumatic Brain Injury: An Evaluation of Functional Outcomes. *J Trauma* 1996; 41(2):257–264.

57. Hellawell DJ, Taylor R, Pentland B. Cognitive and Psychosocial Outcome Following Moderate or Severe Traumatic Brain Injury. *Brain Injury* 1999; 13(7):489–504.

58. Ross AM, Pitts LH, Kobayashi S. Prognosticators of Outcome After Major Head Injury in the Elderly. *J of Neuroscience Nursing* 1992; 24(2):88–93.

59. Kilaru S, Garb J, Emhoff T, et al. Long-Term Functional Status and Mortality of Elderly Patients with Severe Closed Head Injuries. *J Trauma* 2000; 142:373–381

60. Grahm TW, Williams, Jr FC, Harrington T, et al. Civilian Gunshot Wounds to the Head: A Prospective Study. *Neurosurgery* 1990; 27(5):696–700.

61. Levy ML, Masri LS, Lavine S et al. Outcome Prediction after Penetrating Craniocerebral Injury in a Civilian Population: Aggressive Surgical Management in Patients with Admission

Glasgow Coma Scale Scores of 3, 4, or 5. *Neurosurgery* 1994; 35(1):77–85.

62. Levin HS, Williams D, Crofford MJ et al. Relationship of Depth of Brain Lesions to Consciousness and Outcome After Closed Head Injury. *J Neurosurg* 1988; 69:861–866.

63. Dikmen, S.S., Ross, B.L., Machamer, J.E. One Year Psychosocial Outcome in Head Injury. *J of the Intl Neuropsych Society* 1995; 1:67–77.

64. Dikmen, S.S., Temkin N.R., Machamer, J.E., et al. Employment Following Traumatic Head Injuries. *Arch Neurol* 1994; 51: 177–179.

65. Groswasser Z., Sazbon L. Outcome in 134 Patients with Prolonged Posttraumatic Unawareness. *J Neurosurg* 1990; 72:81–84.

66. Greenwood R. Value of Recording Duration of Post-Traumatic Amnesia. *The Lancet* 1997; 349:1041–1042.

67. Jane, J.A., Francel, P.C. Age and Outcome of Head Injury. in Narayan R.K., Wilberger J.E., Povlishock J.T. (eds.). *Neurotrauma*. New York: McGraw-Hill 1996:723–741.

68. Pentland B, Jones PA, Roy CW et al. Head Injury in the Elderly. *Age and Aging* 1986; 15:193–202.

69. Rothweiler B, Temkin NR, Dikmen SS. Aging Effect on Psychosocial Outcome in Traumatic Brain Injury. *Arch Phys Med Rehabil* 1998; 79:881–887.

70. Maurice-Williams RS. Head Injuries in the Elderly. *British J of Neurosurg* 1999; 13(1):5–8.

71. Pruitt, Jr BA (ed.). Part 2: Prognosis in Penetrating Brain Injury. *J Trauma* 2001; 51:S44-S86.

72. Nagib, M.G., Rockswold, G.L., Sherman, R.S., et al. Civilian Gunshot Wounds to the Brain: Prognosis and Management. *Neurosurgery* 1986; 18(5):533–537.

73. Ip RY, Dornan J, Schentag C. Traumatic Brain Injury: Factors Predicting Return to Work or School. *Brain Injury* 1995; 9(5): 517–532.

74. Cattelani R, Tanzi F, Lombardi F et al. Competitive Re-employment After Severe Traumatic Brain Injury: Clinical, Cognitive and Behavioural Predictive Variables. *Brain Injury* 2002; 16(1):51–64.

75. Boake C, Millis SR, High WM et al. Using Early Neuropsychologic Testing to Predict Long-Term Productivity Outcome From Traumatic Brain Injury. *Arch Phys Med Rehabil* 2001; 82:761–768.

76. Sherer M, Sander AM, Nick TG et al. Early Cognitive Status and Productivity Outcome After Traumatic Brain Injury: Findings From the TBI Model Systems. *Arch Phys Med Rehabil* 2002; 83: 183–192.

77. Sherer M, Novack TA, Sander AM et al. Neuropsychological Assessment and Employment Outcome After Traumatic Brain Injury: A Review. *Clin Neuropsychologist* 2002; 16(2):157–178.

78. Buckman R. How to Break Bad News: A Guide for Healthcare Professionals. The Johns Hopkins University Press, Baltimore 1992.

79. Ptacek JT, Eberhardt TL. Breaking Bad News: A Review of the Literature. *JAMA* 1996; 276(6):496–502.

80. Girgis A, Sanson-Fisher RW. Breaking Bad News: Consensus Guidelines for Medical Practitioners. *J of Clinical Oncology* 1995; 13(9):2449–2456.

81. Lobb, E.A., Kenny D.T., Butow, P.N. Women's Preferences for Discussion of Prognosis in Early Breast Cancer. *Health Expectations* 2001; 4:48–57.

82. Blanchard C., Labrecque M., Ruckdeschel J. et al. Information and Decision-Making Preferences of Hospitalized Adult Cancer Patients. *Soc Sci Med* 1988; 27(11):1139–1145.

83. Butow P.N., Maclean M., Dunn S.M., et al. The Dynamics of Change: Cancer Patients' Preferences for Information, Involvement and Support. *Annals of Onc* 1997; 8:857–863.

84. Sanchez-Menegay, C., Stalder, H. Do Physicians Take into Account Patients' Expectations? *J Gen Intern Med* 1994; 9:404–406.

85. Blackhall, L.J., Murphy, S.T., Frank, G., et al. Ethnicity and Attitudes Toward Patient Autonomy. JAMA 1995; 274(10):820–825.

86. Bottorff, J.L., Ratner, P.A., Johnson, J.L., et al. Communicating Cancer Risk Information: *The Challenges of Uncertainty*. Pt. Ed. and Counseling. 1998; 33:67–81.

87. Fong, G.T., Rempel, L.A., Hall, P.A. Challenges to Improving Health Risk Communication in the 21st Century: *A Discussion Monogr Natl Cancer Inst* 1999; 25:173–176.

88. Gerrity, M.S., DeVellis, R.F., Earp, J.A. Physicians' Reactions to Uncertainty in Patient Care. *Medical Care* 1990; 28(8):724–736.

89. Boss P. *Ambiguous Loss*. Cambridge, Massachusetts. Harvard University Press 1999.

90. Kothari S, Sander AM, Contant C et al. The Relation Between Level of Disability and Satisfaction with Life in Individuals with Traumatic Brain Injury. *Arch Phys Med Rehabil* 2001; 82 (10): 1490

91. Paulos JA. *Innumeracy: Mathematical Illiteracy and its Consequences*. New York: Hill & Wang 1988.

92. Schwartz, L.M., Woloshin, S., Black, W.C., et al. The Role of Numeracy in Understanding the Benefit of Screening Mammography. *Ann Intern Med* 1997; 127(11):966–972.

93. Lipkus I.M., Samsa G., Rimer B.K. General Performance on a Numeracy Scale Among Highly Educated Samples. *Med Decis Making* 2001; 21:37–44.

94. Lloyd, A.J. The Extent of Patients' Understanding of the Risk of Treatments. *Quality in Health Care* 2001; 10(Suppl I): i14-i18.

95. Grimes DA, Snively GR. Patients' Understanding of Medical Risks: *Implications for Genetic Counseling*. Obstetrics & Gynecology 1999; 93(6):910–914.

96. Rothman, A.J., Kiviniemi, M.T. Treating People With Information: An Analysis and Review of Approaches to Communicating Health Risk Information. *Monogr Natl Cancer Inst* 1999; 25:44–51.

97. Sheridan, S.L., Pignone, M.P., Lewis, C.L. A Randomized Comparison of Patients' Understanding of Number Needed to Treat and Other Common Risk Reduction Formats. *J Gen Intern Med* 2003; 18:884–892.

98. Gigerenzer, G., Edwards, A. Simple Tools for Understanding Risks: From Innumeracy to Insight. *BMJ* 2003; 327:741–744.

99. Schapira, M.M., Nattinger, A.B., McHorney, C.A. Frequency or Probability? A Qualitative Study of Risk Communication Formats Used in Health Care. *Med Decis Making* 2001; 21:459–467.

100. Weinstein, N.D. What Does It Mean to Understand a Risk? Evaluating Risk Comprehension. *Monogr Natl Cancer Inst* 1999; 25:15–20.

101. Marteau, T.M. Communicating Genetic Risk Information. *British Med Bulletin* 1999; 55(2):414–428.

102. Edwards, A., Elwyn G. Understanding Risk and Lessons for Clinical Risk Communication About Treatment Preferences. *Quality in Health Care* 2001; 10(Suppl I):i9-i13.

103. Mazur, D.J., Hickam, D.H. Patients' Interpretations of Probability Terms. *J Gen Intern Med* 1991; 6:237–240.

104. Bryant, G.D., Norman, G.R. Expressions of Probability: Words and Numbers. *New England Journal of Medicine* 1980; 302(7):411

105. Paling, J. Strategies to Help Patients Understand Risks. *BMJ* 2003; 327:745–748.

106. Lipkus, I.M., Hollands, J.G. The Visual Communication of Risk. *Monogr Natl Cancer Inst* 1999; 25:149–63.

107. Moxey, A., O'Connell, D., McGettigan, P., et al. Describing Treatment Effects to Patients. *J Gen Intern Med* 2003; 18:948–959.

108. McGettigan P., Sly, K., O'Connell D., et al. The Effects of Information Framing on the Practices of Physicians. *J Gen Intern Med* 1999; 14:633–642.

109. Forrow, L., Taylor, W.C., Arnold, R.M. Absolutely Relative: How Research Results Are Summarized Can Affect Treatment Decisions. *Am J of Med* 1992; 92:121–124.

110. Naylor, C.D., Chen, E., Strauss, B. Measured Enthusiasm: Does the Method of Reporting Trial Results Alter Perceptions of Therapeutic Effectiveness? *Annals of Intern Med* 1992; 117:916–921.

111. Berwick, D.M., Fineberg, H.V., Weinstein, M.C. When Doctors Meet Numbers. *Amer J of Med* 1981; 71:991–998.

112. Gigerenzer, G. The Psychology of Good Judgment: Frequency Formats and Simple Algorithms. *Med Decis Making* 1996; 16: 273–280.

113. Back AL, Arnold RM, Quill TE. Hope for the Best, and Prepare for the Worst. *Ann Intern Med* 2003; 138:439–443.

114. Brooks W., Friedman S., Gasparovic C. Magnetic Resonance Spectroscopy in Traumatic Brain Injury. *J Head Trauma Rehabil* 2001; 16(2):149–164.

115. Friedman S., Brooks W., Jung R. et al. Proton MR Spectroscopic Findings Correspond to Neuropsychological Function in Traumatic Brain Injury. *Am J Neuroradiol* 1998; 19:1879–1885.

116. Choe B., Suh T., Choi K. et al. Neuronal Dysfunction in Patients with Closed Head Injury Evaluated by In Vivo 1H Magnetic Resonance Spectroscopy. *Investigative Radiology* 1995; 30(8): 502–506.

117. Garnett M., Blamire A., Rajagopalan B. et al. Evidence for Cellular Damage in Normal-Appearing White Matter Correlates with Injury Severity in Patients Following Traumatic Brain Injury: *A Magnetic Resonance Spectroscopy Study Brain* 2000; 123: 1403–1409.

118. Friedman S., Brooks W., Jung R. et al. Quantitative Proton MRS Predicts Outcome After Traumatic Brain Injury. *Neurology* 1999; 52(7):1384–1391.

119. Brooks W., Stidley C., Petropoulos H. et al. Metabolic and Cognitive Response to Human Traumatic Brain Injury: A Quantitative Proton Magnetic Resonance Study. *J Neurotrauma* 2000; 17(8):629–640.

120. Stinson G., Bagley L., Cecil K. et al. Magnetization Transfer Imaging and Proton MR Spectroscopy in the Evaluation of Axonal Injury: Correlation with Clinical Outcome after Traumatic Brain Injury. *Am J Neuroradiol* 2001; 22:143–151.

121. Garnett M., Blamire A., Corkill R. et al. Early Proton Magnetic Resonance Spectroscopy in Normal-Appearing Brain Correlates with Outcome in Patients Following Traumatic Brain Injury. *Brain* 2000; 123:2046–2054.

122. Ashwal S., Holshouser B., Shu S. et al. Predictive Value of Proton Magnetic Resonance Spectroscopy in Pediatric Closed Head Injury. *Pediatric Neurol* 2000; 23:114–125.

123. Shutter L., Colohan A. Magnetic Resonance Spectroscopy Increases the Accuracy of Predicting Functional Outcomes After Traumatic Brain Injury. *Abstract: American College of Surgeons* 2002 Clinical Congress.

124. Mussack T., Biberthaler P., Wiedemann E. et al. S-100b as a Screening Marker of the Severity of Minor Head Trauma (MHT)- a Pilot Study. *Acta Neurochir* 2000; [Suppl]76:393–396.

125. Herrmann M., Jost S., Kutz S. et al. Temporal Profile of Release of Neurobiochemical Markers of Brain Damage After Traumatic Brain Injury is Associated with Intracranial Pathology as Demonstrated in Cranial Computerized Tomography. *J of Neurotrauma* 2000; 17(2):113–122.

126. Romner B., Ingebrigtsen T., Kongstad P. et al. Traumatic Brain Damage: Serum S-100 Protein Measurements Related to Neuroradiological Findings. *J of Neurotrauma* 2000; 17(8):641–647.

127. Raabe A., Grolms C., Keller M. et al. Correlation of Computed Tomography Findings and Serum Brain Damage Markers Following Severe Head Injury. *Acta Neurochir* 1998; 140:787–792.

128. Raabe A., Grolms C., Seifert V. Serum Markers of Brain Damage and Outcome Prediction in Patients After Severe Head Injury. *British J Neurosurg* 1999; 13(1):56–59.

129. Raabe A, Volker S. Protein S-100B as a Serum Marker of Brain Damage in Severe Head Injury: Preliminary Results. *Neurosurg Rev* 2000; 23:136–138.

130. Chatfield D., Zemlan F., Day D. et al. Discordant Temporal Patterns of S100B and Cleaved Tau Protein Elevation After Head Injury: A Pilot Study. *British J Neurosurg* 2002; 16(5):471–476.

131. Elting J., de Jager A., Teelken A. et al. Comparison of Serum S-100 Protein Levels Following Stroke and Traumatic Brain Injury. *J Neurological Sciences* 2000; 181:104–110.

132. Pleines U., Morganti-Kossmann M., Rancan M. et al. S-100B Reflects the Extent of Injury and Outcome, Whereas Neuronal Specific Enolase is a Better Indicator of Neuroinflammation in Patients with Severe Traumatic Brain Injury. *J Neurotrauma* 2001; 18(5):491–498.

133. Herrmann M., Curio N., Jost S. et al. Release of Biochemical Markers of Damage to Neuronal and glial Brain Tissue is Associated with Short and Long Term Neuropsychological Outcome After Traumatic Brain Injury. *J Neurol Neurosurg Psychiatry* 2001; 70:95–100.

134. Woertgen C., Rothoerl R., Brawanski A. Early S-100B Serum Level Correlates to Quality of Life in Patients After Severe Head Injury. *Brain Injury* 2002; 16(9):807–816.

135. Mussack T., Biberthaler P., Kanz K. et al. Serum S-100B and Inter-leukin-8 as Predictive Markers for Comparative Neurologic Outcome Analysis of Patients After Cardiac Arrest and Severe Traumatic Brain Injury. *Crit Care Med* 2002; 30(12):2669–2674.

136. Rothoerl R., Woertgen C., Brawanski A. S-100 Serum Levels and Outcome After Severe Head Injury. *Acta Neurochir* 2000; [Suppl]76:97–100.

137. Woertgen C., Rothoerl R., Metz C. et al. Comparison of Clinical, Radiologic, and Serum Marker as Prognostic Factors after Severe Head Injury. *J Trauma* 1999; 47(6):1126.

138. Savola O., Hillborn M. Early Predictors of Post-Concussion Symptoms in Patients with Mild Head Injury. *European J Neurology* 2003; 10:175–181

139. Waterloo K., Ingebrigtsen T., Romner B. Neuropsychological Function in Patients with Increased Serum Levels of Protein S-100 After Minor Head Injury. *Acta Neurochir* 1997; 139:26–32.

140. Ingebrigtsen T., Waterloo K., Jacobsen E. et al. Traumatic Brain Damage in Minor Head Injury: Relation of Serum S-100 Protein Measurements to Magnetic Resonance Imaging and Neurobehavioral Outcome. *Neurosurgery* 1999; 45(3):468.

141. Ingebrigtsen T., Romner B., Marup-Jensen S. et al. The Clinical Value of Serum S-100 Protein Measurements in Minor Head Injury: A Scandinavian Multicentre Study. *Brain Injury* 2000; 14(12):1047–1055.

142. Anderson R., Hansson L., Nilsson O. et al. High Serum S100B Levels for Trauma Patients without Head Injuries. *Neurosurg* 2001; 48(6):1255–1260.

143. Nathoo N., Chetty R., van Dellen J. et al. Genetic Vulnerability Following Traumatic Brain Injury: The Role of Apolipoprotein E. *J Clin Pathol Mol Path* 2003; 56:132–136.

144. Sorbi S., Nacmias B., Piacentini S. et al. ApoE as a Prognostic Factor for Post-Traumatic Coma. *Nature Medicine* 1995; 1(9):852.

145. Teasdale GM, Nicoll JA, Murray G et al. Association of Apolipoprotein E Polymorphism with Outcome After Head Injury. *The Lancet* 1977; 350:1069–1071.

146. Friedman G., Froom P., Sazbon L. et al. Apolipoprotein E4 Genotype Predicts a Poor Outcome in Survivors of Traumatic Brain Injury. *Neurology* 1999; 52:244.

147. Lichtman S., Seliger G., Tycko B. et al. Apolipoprotein E and Functional Recovery from Brain Injury Following Postacute Rehabilitation. *Neurology* 2000; 55:1536–1539.

148. Diaz-Arrastia R., Gong Y., Fair S. et al. Increased Risk of Late Posttraumatic Seizures Associated with Inheritance of APOE E4 Allele. *Arch Neurol* 2003; 60:818–822.

149. Liaquat I., Dunn L., Nicoll J. et al. Effect of Apolipoprotein E Genotype on Hematoma Volume After Trauma. *J Neurosurg* 2002; 96:90–96.

150. Liberman J., Stewart W., Wesnes K. et al. Apolipoprotein E4 and Short-Term Recovery from Predominantly Mild Brain Injury. *Neurology* 2002; 58:1038–1044.

151. Crawford F., Vanderploeg R., Freeman M. et al. APOE Genotype Influences Acquisition and Recall Following Traumatic Brain Injury. *Neurology* 2002; 58:1115–1118.

152. Baxt, W.G. Application of Artificial Neural Networks to Clinical Medicine. *The Lancet* 1995; 346:1135–1177.

153. Hart A, Wyatt J. Evaluating black-boxes as medical decision aids: issues arising from a study of neural networks. *Med Inform* 1990; 15(3): 229–236

154. Lang EW, Pitts LH, Damron SL et al. Outcome After Severe Head Injury: An Analysis of Prediction Based Upon Comparison of Neural Network Versus Logistic Regression Analysis. *Neurol Research* 1997; 19:274–280.

155. Sakellaropoulos GC, Nikiforidis GC. Development of a Bayesian Network for the Prognosis of Head Injuries using Graphical Model Selection Techniques. *Meth Inform Med* 1999; 38:37–42.

156. Amin AP, Kulkarni HR. Improvement in the Information Content of the Glasgow Coma Scale for the Prediction of Full Cognitive Recovery After Head Injury Using Fuzzy Logic. *Surgery* 2000; 127(3):245–253.

157. Wasson JH, Sox HC, Neff RK, Goldman L. Clinical Prediction Rules: Applications and Methodological Standards. *New Eng J of Med* 1985; 313(13):793–799.

158. Laupacis A, Wells G, Richardson WS, Tugwell P. Users' Guides to the Medical Literature: V. How to Use an Article About Prognosis. *JAMA* 1994; 272(3):234–237.

159. Wyatt JC, Altman DG. Commentary: Prognostic Models: Clinically Useful or Quickly Forgotten? *BMJ* 1995; 311:1539–1541.

160. Braitman LE, Davidoff F. Predicting Clinical States in Individual Patients. *Ann Intern Med* 1996; 125(5):406–412.

161. Randolph AG, Guyatt GH, Richardson WS. Prognosis in the Intensive Care Unit: Finding Accurate and Useful Estimates for Counseling Patients. *Crit Care Med* 1998; 26(4):767–772.

162. Laupacis A, Sekar N, Stiell IG. Clinical Prediction Rules: A Review and Suggested Modifications of Methodological Standards. *JAMA* 1997; 277(6):488–494.

163. Justice AC, Covinsky KE, Berlin JA. Assessing the Generalizability of Prognostic Information. *Ann Intern Med* 1999; 130(6):515–524.

164. Simon R, Altman DG. Statistical Aspects of Prognostic Factor Studies in Oncology. *Br J Cancer* 1994; 69:979–985.

165. Altman DG, Royston P. What Do We Mean by Validating a Prognostic Model? *Statist Med* 2000; 19:453–473.

166. Feldman Z, Contant CF, Robertson CS et al. Evaluation of the Leeds Prognostic Score for Severe Head Injury. *The Lancet* 1991; 337:1451–1453.

167. Gibson RM, Stephenson GC. Aggressive Management of Severe Closed Head Trauma: Time for Reappraisal. *The Lancet* 1989:369–371.

168. Chestnut Rm, Ghajar J, Maas AIR, et al. Management and Prognosis of Severe Traumatic Brain Injury. Part 2: Early Indicators of Prognosis in Severe Traumatic Brain Injury. *J Neurotrauma* 2000; 17:557–627.

169. Wilberger JE. Emergency Care and Initial Evaluation. in Cooper PR, Golfinos JG (eds.). *Head Injury.* New York: McGraw-Hill 2000: 27–40 .

170. Ghajar J, Hariri RJ, Narayan RK et al. Survey of Critical Care Management of Comatose, Head-Injured Patients in the United States. *Critical Care Medicine* 1995; 23(3): 560–567.

171. Jennett B. Historical Perspective on Head Injury. in Narayan RK, Wilberger JE, Povlishock JT (eds.). *Neurotrauma.* New York: McGraw-Hill 1996:3–11.

172. Eker C, Schalen W, Asgeirsson B et al. Reduced Mortality After Severe Head Injury Will Increase the Demands for Rehabilitation Services. *Brain Injury* 2000; 14(7):605–619.

173. Bulger EM, Nathens AB, Rivara FP et al. Management of Severe Head Injury: Institutional Variations in Care and Effect on Outcome. *Crit Care Med* 2002; 30(8):1870–1876.

174. Hukkelhoven CWPM, Steyerberg EW, Farace E et al. Regional Differences in Patient Characteristics, Case Management, and Outcomes in Traumatic Brain Injury: Experience from the Tirilazad Trials. *J Neurosurg* 2002; 97:549–557.

175. Chui W. Head Injuries in Developing Countries. in Narayan RK, Wilberger JE, Povlishock JT (eds.). *Neurotrauma.* New York: McGraw-Hill 1996:

176. Stein SC. Classification of Head Injury. in Narayan RK, Wilberger JE, Povlishock JT (eds.). *Neurotrauma.* New York: McGraw-Hill 1996: 31–42

177. Boake C, High WM. Functional Outcome From Traumatic Brain Injury: Unidimensional or Multidimensional? *Phys Med & Rehabil* 1996; 75(2):105–113.

178. Hannay HJ, Sherer M. Outcome From Head Injury. in Narayan RK, Wilberger JE, Povlishock JT (eds.). *Neurotrauma.* New York: McGraw-Hill 1996:723–741.

179. Evans RW, Ruff RM. Outcome and Value: A Perspective on Rehabilitation Outcomes Achieved in Acquired Brain Injury. *J Head Trauma Rehabil* 1992; 7(4):24–36.

180. Condeluci A, Ferris LL, Bogdan A. Outcome and Value: The Survivor Perspective. *J Head Trauma Rehabil* 1992; 7(4):37–45.

181. Prigatano GP. Work, Love, and Play after Brain Injury. *Bull Menninger Clin* 1989; 53(5): 414–31.

182. Jennett B, Bond M. Assessment of Outcome After Severe Brain Damage: A Practical Scale. *Lancet* 1975; 1:480–484.

183. Baalen BV, Odding E, Maas AIR, Ribbers GM, Bergen MP, Stam HJ. Traumatic Brain Injury: Classification of Initial Severity and Determination of Functional Outcome. *Disability & Rehabil* 2003; 25(1):9–18.

184. Groswasser Z, Melamed S, Agranov E, Keren O. Return to Work as an Integrative Outcome Measure Following Traumatic Brain Injury. *Neuropsych Rehabil* 1999; 9(3/4):493–504.

185. Morton MV, Wehman P. Psychosocial and Emotional Sequelae of Individuals with Traumatic Brain Injury: A Literature Review and Recommendations. *Brain Injury* 1995;9(1):81–92.

186. Hoofien D, Gilboa A, Vakil E et al. Traumatic Brain Injury (TBI) 10–20 Years Later: A Comprehensive Outcome Study of Psychiatric Symptomatology, Cognitive Abilities and Psychosocial Functioning. *Brain Injury* 2001;15(3):189–209.

187. Campbell CH. Needs of Relatives and Helpfulness of Support Groups in Severe Head Injury. *Rehab Nursing* 88; 13(6):320–325.

188. Rappaport M, Herrero-Backe C, Rappaport ML et al. Head Injury Outcome Up to Ten Years Later. *Arch Phys Med Rehabil* 1989; 70:885–892.

189. Corrigan JD, Smith-Knapp K, Granger CV. Outcomes in the First 5 Years After Traumatic Brain Injury. *Arch Phys Med Rehabil* 1998; 79:299–305.

190. Olver JH, Ponsford JL, Curran CA. Outcome Following Traumatic Brain Injury: A Comparison Between 2 and 5 Years After Injury. *Brain Injury* 1996; 10(11):841–848.

191. Choi SC, Barnes TY, Bullock R, Germanson TA, Marmarou A, Young HF. Temporal Profile of Outcomes in Severe Head Injury. *J Neurosurg* 1994; 81:169–173.

192. Corrigan JD, Harrison-Felix C, Bogner J, Dijkers M, Sendroy-Terrill M, Whiteneck G. Systematic Bias in Traumatic Brain Injury Outcome Studies Because of Loss to Follow-Up. *Arch Phys Med Rehabil* 2003; 84:153–160.

193. Choi SC, Barnes TY. Predicting Outcome in the Head-Injured Patient. in Narayan RK, Wilberger JE, Povlishock JT (eds.). *Neurotrauma.* New York: McGraw-Hill 1996:779–790.

194. Concato J, Feinstein AR, Holford TR. The Risk of Determining Risk with Multivariable Models. *Ann Intern Med* 1993; 118(3):201–210.

195. Harrel, Jr HE, Lee KL, Matchar DB et al. Regression Models for Prognostic Prediction: Advantages, Problems, and Suggested Solutions. *Cancer Treatment Reports* 1985; 69(10):1071–1077.

196. Hosmer DW, Taber S, Lemeshow S. The Importance of Assessing the Fit of Logistic Regression Models: A Case Study. *Am J Pub Health* 1991; 81(12):1630–1635.

197. Diamond, G.A. What Price Perfection? Calibration and Discrimination of Clinical Prediction Models. *J Clin Epidemiol* 1992; 45(1):85–89.

198. Charlson, M.E., Ales, K.L., Simon, R., et al. Why Predictive Indexes Perform Less Well in Validation Studies. *Arch Intern Med* 1987; 147:2155–2161.

199. Andrews PJD, Sleeman DH, Statham PFX et al. Predicting Recovery in Patients Suffering from Traumatic Brain Injury by Using Admission Variables and Physiological Data: A Comparison Between Decision Tree Analysis and Logistic Regression. *J Neurosurg* 2002; 97:326–336.

200. McQuatt A, Sleeman D, Andrews PJD et al. Discussing Anomalous Situations Using Decision Trees: A Head Injury Case Study. *Methods Inf Med* 2001; 40:373–379.

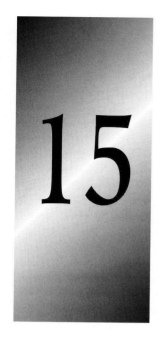

15 Neuroimaging Correlates of Functional Outcome

Erin D. Bigler

NEUROIMAGING CORRELATES OF FUNCTIONAL OUTCOME

How do neuroimaging findings best predict outcome once the brain has been injured? The answer is complicated. Even though many trauma-induced abnormalities can be identified by neuroimaging and such findings represent one of our best objective measures of brain injury, there are numerous variables (in addition to simply identifying neuroimaging abnormalities) that have to be considered. For example, imaging—even functional imaging—represents only a particular moment in time, yet predictions of outcome typically involve statistical statements of much broader timeframes involving the future, including the lifetime of the individual injured. Likewise, the recovery process is dynamic and ever changing, particularly in the first year of injury. A host of injury variables apply, including: the type of brain injury, the severity of injury, the brain regions most likely affected, the age at time of injury, as well as, the issues involving cognitive reserve and individual differences. Since the advent of contemporary neuroimaging the type, degree, location, and a host of other indicators of brain imaging abnormalities have been examined in an attempt to answer this question.

The chapter that follows will provide an update on this topic, by first offering an overview of the history of lesion-location research in predicting functional outcome from traumatic brain injury (TBI), followed by typical injury characteristics observed in neuroimaging of TBI that are predictive of functional outcome, along with current methods for establishing the best predictor of outcome and future implications of the clinical utility of neuroimaging in evaluating functional outcome from TBI. Because of rapid changes in technology and how brain scans can be analyzed (1), only a few studies have actually systematically addressed this issue with a mixture of qualitative and quantitative analyses in using neuroimaging to predict functional outcome (2–10). Basically, these studies demonstrate that presence of abnormalities in structural imaging are associated with more negative outcome, particularly when the abnormalities are shown to be chronic. This chapter will review these studies along with other clinical associations and methods for the use of structural imaging findings in the prediction of functional outcome in TBI.

HISTORICAL PERSPECTIVE AND AN INTRODUCTION TO THE PROBLEMS OF PREDICTING FUNCTIONAL OUTCOME BASED ON STRUCTURAL NEUROIMAGING

Clinical neurology, as did much of medicine, developed from a 'signs and symptoms' approach, where a particular neurological symptom (i.e., paralysis) had a clinical presentation (i.e., hemiplegia) that specified a particular pathophysiology (i.e., corticospinal tract damage potentially localized), depending on what other signs and symptoms were present. The motor system analogy is used here, because it was the first to be comprehensively examined resulting in established functional outcome using lesion-localization methods of neuropathologists and clinicians. Likewise, motor impairment has been the system most extensively examined from a traditional structural as well as functional neuroimaging perspective (see Figure 15-1) (11, 12) where clinical outcome has been related to underlying brain pathology. For example, using neuroimaging techniques, identification of damage within the corticospinal track (see Figure 15-2) typically leads to some type of motor impairment as shown in Figure 15-3; where this patient had left-side hemiplegia as a result of shear injury at the level of the internal capsule. Accordingly, knowing the location of the lesion within a dedicated neural pathway (i.e., corticospinal) for a specific function (in this case, motor) leads to a predictable functional outcome (impaired motor skills).

Extensive mapping of sensory-perceptual and some language based pathologies were the next to show lesion-location specificity and prediction of functional outcome depending on a signs and symptoms approach, particularly with primary sensory systems (13). Mapping of language function, however, turned out to be far more problematic than initially anticipated in light of what were thought to be well known "language" centers of the brain such as Broca's and Wernicke's areas. It became apparent that language was less dedicated to precise locations that could be consistently identified between individuals and was more loosely distributed than the more 'hard-wired' sensory and motor systems. So, instead of showing discrete lesions that consistently impaired language, studies generally found more extensive regions wherein damage anywhere within some boundary would result in language impairment. This is nicely demonstrated in Figure 15-4 taken from the work of Bates et al. (14), mapping out left-hemisphere lesions in right handed individuals that produce language impairment (deficits in word fluency and auditory comprehension). Figure 15-4 also shows that no uniform area that when damaged produced the same disturbance in language in all subjects, but rather damage across a broad range of the left hemisphere resulted in impaired language function. There were areas where the likelihood of language impairment was maximized, but this illustration also demonstrates individual differences in brain organization once outside of primary motor and sensory systems. The more distinct 1:1 correspondence between pathology and

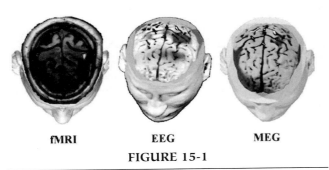

fMRI   **EEG**   **MEG**

FIGURE 15-1

Three images of the cortical activation related to a simple unilateral finger movement showing how functional imaging techniques can isolate motor cortex. *Left*: The cortical regions showing an increased hemodynamic response with respect to the rest period. Such hotspots are located over the primary motor cortex. *Center*: The spatial distribution of the estimated cortical current density distribution occurring over a reconstruction of the cortex 100 ms before the movement occurs. The cortical current density distribution is obtained by high-resolution EEG recordings with 128 electrodes. *Right*: The current density distribution is relative to the same time instant (100 ms before movement) but is estimated form the MEG recordings in the same subject. This demonstrates the focal nature of somatomotor function. Used with permission from Babiloni et al. (12). Accordingly, cortical damage outside this system does not impair direct motor functions of the hand

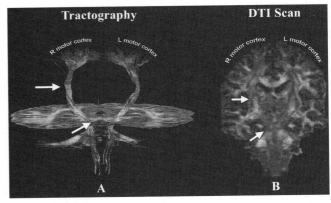

FIGURE 15-2

(Left, A) Diffusion tensor imaging (DTI) tractography is used to isolate the corticospinal tract (upper arrow), demonstrating its descent from motor cortex, down through the midbrain region (lower arrow). Arrows represent where injuries to this direct motor pathway resulted in the motor impairment and paralysis seen in the case presented in Figures 15-3 and 15-6. Although the fibers that comprise the corticospinal track involve only a very small region of the brain, damage anywhere along this pathway will result in some type of functional impairment in motor abilities. (Right, B) Colorized DTI scan image in coronal plane used to identify tract orientation used to perform the tractography to isolate the corticospinal tracks. Blue represents tissue aligned in vertical orientation which was the source to extract the fiber pathways depicted in A. Adapted from Lazar et al. (22) and Lainhart et al. (118) used with permission

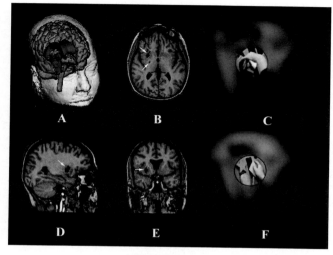

FIGURE 15-3

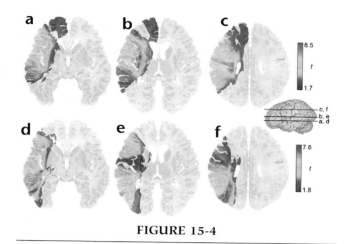

FIGURE 15-4

MR imaging showing residual small, focal shear lesions involving the basal ganglia (arrows in B, D, and E) and internal capsule (B, bottom arrow) in the right hemisphere (scans are in radiological perspective, with right on the viewer's left) that result in impaired motor function on the left side of the body (refer to C). In F, the patient has no difficulty placing blocks while blindfolded to successfully complete the Tactual Performance Test. In contrast, impaired motor performance is present in the left hand demonstrated by paralysis and posturing as shown in C. This figure demonstrates the impact of a strategically placed lesion (shown in red in A) to result in functional impairment. B, D and E represent the axial, sagittal and coronal views with arrows pointing to the focal lesions. The figure in A contains the 3-D reconstruction of the brain with the ventricle in blue, showing the location of the focal damage. Figure 15-6 (also from this patient) demonstrates atrophy of the cerebral peduncle, a consequence of damage to the corticospinal track and some focal hemorrhaging (petechial in nature) that occurred at the level of the midbrain

This illustration demonstrates the dispersion of left hemisphere regions that disrupt language function after a focal cerebrovascular accident. Representative slices from voxel-based lesion-symptom mapping (VLSM) computed for fluency and auditory comprehension performance of 101 aphasic stroke patients. These maps are colorized depictions of *t*-test results evaluating patient performance on a voxel-by-voxel basis. Patients with lesions in a given voxel were compared to those without lesions in that voxel on measures of fluency (a–c) or auditory comprehension (d–f). High *t*-scores (red) indicate that lesions to these voxels have a highly significant effect on behavior. Dark blue voxels indicate regions where the presence of a lesion had relatively little impact on the behavioral measure. Only voxels that were significant at $p = 0.05$ (controlling the expected proportion of false positive) are shown. Insert of brain depicts the level of each slice. Lesions within the insula (b) and deep parietal white matter (c) had the most impact on fluency, whereas injury to the middle temporal gyrus (d) produced the largest effect on measures of auditory comprehension. Used with permission from Bates et al. (14)

function as found in dedicated motor and sensory systems is less apparent once function is defined by some element of cognition or behavior. In general, widely dispersed neural regulatory systems underlie complex behaviors and therefore, structure-function relationships predictive of functional outcome outside of primary motor and sensory deficits are more difficult to establish (15). Nonetheless, general statements can be made about neuroimaging defined damage to certain brain regions or neuroregulatory centers and functional outcome.

Also, because of neural mechanisms that relate to recovery and adaptation, small lesions strategically placed within dedicated neural pathways may have pronounced effects upon functional outcome of motor or sensory abilities, such as complete paralysis, blindness or loss of smell or auditory processing. In contrast, extensive lesions that do not damage such dedicated primary systems may have no or minimal effect upon such functions, even though the

area of damage may encroach such regions. This is readily observed by comparing the case presented in Figure 15-3 to the one in Figure 15-5. In Figure 15-3 and in the additional imaging presented in Figure 15-6 the patient has distinct damage at the level of the internal capsule and basal ganglia on the right, as well as Wallerian degeneration at the level of the cerebral peduncle, reflective of generalized 'downstream' wasting of the corticospinal track. This is consistent with the left side motor involvement as shown in Figure 15-3. In contrast, the patient shown in Figure 15-5 received extensive focal damage to the left frontal region, which extends back towards motor cortex, but does not specifically involve motor systems, even though there is a small white matter (WM) lesion noted at the top of the internal capsule (see Figure 15-6). This patient had no motor deficits on a widespread neuropsychological battery of motor tasks, including the Tactual Performance Test on which the case in Figure 15-3 displayed distinct impairment. Additionally, even though there is extensive frontal

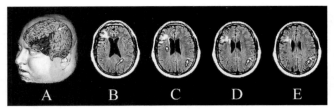

FIGURE 15-5

This case demonstrates extensive focal frontal pathology that resulted from a fall, that included frontal skull fracture and subdural hematoma that was surgically removed. Red represents the residuals from the coup injury or point of initial impact producing focal damage shown in the 3-D in A. Extensive frontal involvement is also depicted in the axial fluid attenuated inversion recovery images (FLAIR) images, but not only is the brain damaged in the region where focal impact occurred, but is damaged in a linear fashion directly opposite the point of focal impact, representing the contre coup injury as shown by the arrows. Unlike the case in Figures 15-3 and 15-6, this patient did not have paralysis, even though the focal frontal damage is very close to motor cortex (colored in green). Thus, extensive damage can occur to the cerebral cortex without causing functional impairment in motor function. Likewise, even though this patient had extensive left hemisphere damage, language function recovered to the point where he performed within normal limits, although probably below premorbid levels, even though some areas of damage overlap with the brain regions delimited in Figure 15-4 that would be expected to affect language

wasting in the patient presented in Figure 15-5, the patient had only minimal language deficits, despite considerable overlap of damage to frontal tissue that usually impairs language (see Figure 15-4). Other than subtly reduced word fluency and an occasional stuttering-like episode during conversational speech, the patient's performance on language tests was otherwise within normal limits.

Thus in attempting to predict functional outcome, a strategically placed lesion, albeit relatively small, may produce a distinct deficit if it involves a primary motor or sensory region of the brain. Oppositely, even large lesions such as that depicted in Figure 15-5 may not produce a consistent syndrome when damage is outside primary motor and sensory systems, due to individual differences in brain structure-function relationships. Neuroimaging methods have improved greatly over the last 20 years providing excellent macroscopic detection of brain pathology associated with TBI. As might be expected from the discussion in this section, while there are some generalities that can be established using lesion detection and localization methods to prognosticate about functional outcome (see Refs. 16, 17), there are also limitations when structural imaging is the only method used for predicting functional outcome.

Because contemporary magnetic resonance (MR) imaging so nicely depicts gross structural pathology, early neuroimaging studies were overly optimistic and assumed

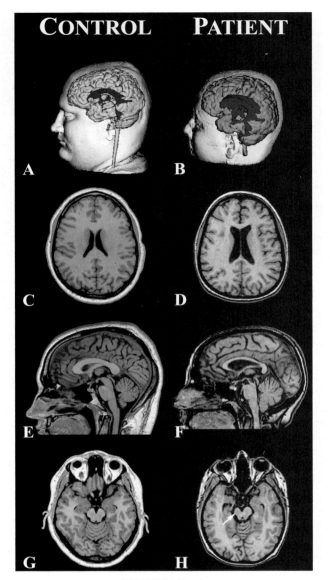

FIGURE 15-6

This is the same patient (shown on the right) as depicted in Figure 15-3, but with additional views compared to a non-brain injured control subject on the left. The axial view at the level of the body of the ventricle demonstrates ventricular dilation as a result of hydrocephalus ex vacuo. This is also a reflection of generalized cerebral atrophy, which is also demonstrated by the nonspecific loss in size of the corpus callosum (CC) as shown in F. Uniform CC reduction, as seen in this case, probably reflects uniform reduction of white matter pathways in the brain following severe TBI. In H, the cerebral peduncle on the right (viewer's left) shows atrophy, an indication of corticospinal involvement and consistent with the motor impairment shown in Figure 15-3. Also, at this level note the dilation of the temporal horns of the lateral ventricle, typically an indication of temporal lobe damage as well (see Bigler et al., Ref. 86). The 3-D image at the top show's the brain in flesh tone and the ventricle in blue. Clearly there is generalized ventricular dilation in the TBI patient as seen in B

that distinct lesion-behavior connections could be established, relating the presence of certain lesions with a typical functional outcome (see Ref. 18). However, initial studies were disappointing in their ability to predict outcome from TBI. As imaging technology improved, part of the reason for these disappointing findings became obvious, because what constitutes a 'lesion' depends on the imaging methods used and their resolution to detect abnormalities, as well as the underlying diffuse nature of TBI even when the only clinically identifiable abnormality is a focal lesion. This problem is shown in the case illustrated in Figures 15-3 and 15-6. Although distinctly focal lesions are clearly identified, generalized cerebral atrophy is also present and manifested by ventricular enlargement, wasting of the corpus callosum, and prominence of the cortical sulci. Thus, whatever effects occur from the focal injuries, do so within the backdrop of generalized damages.

From the perspective of actually detecting an abnormality with MR imaging, different MR weightings have different sensitivity in detecting pathology, which then influences how imaging findings relate to functional outcome. The problem of differences in sensitivity in detecting abnormalities and their relationship to functional outcome is presented in Figure 15-7. In this figure what shows up as an abnormality changes as to the type of MR image sequence used. For example, the T1 image provides excellent anatomical detail along with clearly defined areas of abnormal signal depicting multiple regions of damaged tissue, including prominent areas of encephalomalacia together with cystic formations in the frontal region. Although on initial review this may seem to capture the extent of the underlying damage, other imaging sequences

FIGURE 15-7

Multiple imaging sequences were performed on this subject with severe TBI, showing how each imaging sequences is sensitive to different types of pathology. In each case, the additional identification of abnormal signal from the separate imaging sequences has been superimposed upon a 3-D reconstruction of the brain. The ventricle is represented by blue. At the top of each figure is the image sequence (i.e., T1) and the colorization (i.e., red) depicting damage identified. Quantitative data demonstrating widespread atrophy is provided in Table 15-1

TABLE 15-1
Quantitative Analysis Comparing the Volumes of Different Brain Structures from a TBI* Patient to a Control

BRAIN MEASURE	TBI PATIENT	CONTROL
Whole brain (cc)		
Total cerebral spinal fluid	476.20	84.75
Total gray matter	635.04	886.70
Total white matter	224.22	386.60
Total temporal horn	7.54	0.71
Total lateral ventricles	75.54	17.20
Total third ventricle	4.29	0.77
Total fourth ventricle	3.41	3.13
Total ventricle	90.78	21.81
Total brain matter volume	859.26	1273.30
Ventricle to brain ratio	10.57	1.71
Total intracranial volume	1335.47	1358.05
Whole cerebellum (cc)		
Total gray matter	94.70	121.56
Total white matter	19.03	34.46
Total volume	113.72	156.02
Frontal lobe (cc)		
Dorso-lateral frontal grey and white matter total	16.13	55.66
Medio-lateral frontal grey and white matter total	34.26	81.02
Inferior orbital frontal grey and white matter total	1.85	7.51
Total csf	57.87	9.98
Total prefrontal grey matter	38.72	94.07
Total prefrontal white matter	13.53	50.13
Temporal lobe (cc)		
Total hippocampus	1.88	4.62
Total parahippocampal gyrus	4.57	7.07
Total fusiform gyrus	5.22	7.86
Total inferior temporal gyrus	6.19	13.36
Total middle temporal gyrus	9.77	14.49
Total superior temporal gyrus	14.03	24.79
Total temporal horn	5.59	0.72
Total gyri	41.66	72.19
Total sulci	11.33	3.48
Temporal poles (cc)		
Total gray matter	31.18	54.29
Total white matter	3.31	11.50
Total temporal pole	34.49	65.79
Basal ganglia (cc)		
Total caudate	3.58	7.76
Total putamen	4.04	10.05
Total globus pallidus	1.21	2.16
Total basal ganglia	8.83	19.97
Corpus callosum (mm²)		
Corpus callosum total	4.79	8.78
Brain stem (cc)		
Cerebral peduncle	0.19	0.37
Midbrain	1.05	1.31
Midbrain-tegmentum	2.79	4.20
Midbrain-tectum	0.51	0.74
Pons	7.95	11.26
Medulla	3.81	4.05

* TBI = traumatic brain injury.

demonstrate even greater pathology that simply cannot be ascertained from the T1 image. For example, the T2 images provide better delineation of abnormal CSF collections, conspicuously involving almost the entirety of the frontal region at the level viewed, better appreciated than the dark signal seen in the T1 images. However, neither the T1 nor T2 images fully depict the extent of disseminated white matter abnormalities, as shown in the fluid attenuated inversion recovery images (FLAIR) or the residual hemorrhagic lesions as shown by the gradient recalled echo (GRE) images. Not shown here are other methods that detect abnormalities such as MR spectroscopy, magnetization transfer and white-matter coherence determined by diffusion tensor imaging (DTI, 1, 19, 20) that would likely demonstrate even additional abnormalities if applied to a case like that shown in Figure 15-7. Finally, when a functional imaging tool is used, such as single photon emission computed tomography (SPECT; see Figure 15-7), further clarity of the extent of functional impairment is evident by the widespread perfusion defects, even in some tissue where more normal signal is observed on MR imaging. Thus, what is defined as abnormal is dependent on imaging sequences and technology used, where each imaging method has its own set of limitations. Without taking into consideration all of these abnormalities in the predication of functional outcome, functional outcome predicted strictly from neuroimaging becomes problematic.

Lastly, an even more potentially insurmountable limitation of contemporary neuroimaging in predicting functional outcome is that even with our best existing neuroimaging tools, microstructure cannot be imaged. Inferences can be made about neurochemical composition of tissue via MR spectroscopy (MRS, 4,21) and diffusion tensor imaging permits identification of aggregate white matter tracts (see Figure 15-2 and Ref. 22) and their 'coherence' where optimal white matter shows lower apparent diffusion and higher fractional anisotropic coefficients (see 23), but actual microstructure can not be imaged in vivo at this time. That is not to say that tremendous strides are not occurring in exploring methods of neuroimaging of microanatomy (see 24), but the application of such structural imaging techniques is just now being applied to the study of functional recovery from TBI and its predication. Because of these limitations with structural imaging, it is likely that many of the advances in predicting TBI outcome will come from the integration of structural and functional neuroimaging (25, 26).

At the microstructure level, post-mortem cases have clearly shown widespread histopathological abnormalities, particularly in moderate to severe TBI (27–29), especially involving axonal damage (27, 30, 31) and disrupted neurotransmitter systems, but also mild TBI where gross abnormalities based on visual inspection are either absent or minimal (32–36). Since in structural neuroimaging the threshold detection of abnormal signal using current MR technology is approximately a mm^3, whatever abnormality can be visualized in structural imaging represents the sum total of all underlying microstructure pathology. Returning to Figures 15-3 and 15-6, while the focal deficits are clearly evident, there is generalized damage. Presence of generalized damage suggests widespread microstructure pathology affecting the brain in a nonspecific fashion. This is not only readily depicted in the case shown in Figures 15-3 and 15-6 but can be shown by comparing the volumes of different brain structures from a TBI patient to a normative comparison as presented in Table 1, which was taken from the patient shown in Figure 15-7. Using quantitative methods, surface area measurements or actual volumes can be calculated from any brain region of interest (ROI) and compared to normative data, or an appropriately matched control (see Ref. 37). For the case presented in Figure 15-7 the patient's quantitative imaging findings are compared to an age and head size (i.e., intracranial volume) matched control subject. As can be seen, in all comparisons, including all of the subcortical structures, atrophy has occurred. As shown by the comparisons in Table 15-1, there is not a region that was spared 'injury', either directly or indirectly, in this case of severe TBI. This observation of widespread damage, both at the macroscopic (which neuroimaging can detect), as well as microscopic level in TBI, has led to the concept of diffuse brain injury (DBI), and will be described next. DBI may be the single most important factor that complicates predicting outcome from structural neuroimaging studies.

NEUROIMAGING OF TRAUMATIC BRAIN INJURY (TBI) AS A DIFFUSE BRAIN INJURY (DBI)

Graham et al. (29) discuss TBI in the context of underlying general neuropathology, often referred to as DBI (see also Refs. 31, 38, 39). This is a very important concept to understand in interpreting functional outcome from structural imaging and, as will be shown by the discussion that follows, ventricular dilation in combination with reduced brain volume are indicators of DBI (37).

As introduced above, hydrocephalus ex vacuo is a commonplace occurrence in moderate-to-severe (i.e., Glasgow Coma Score, GCS < 12) TBI. This occurs because ventricular CSF is under pressure, which in turn creates an outward pressure gradient within the ventricle, which under normal conditions is kept in balance by brain mass and CSF reabsorption, so that a constant equilibrium is maintained between brain and ventricle. However, following TBI induced neuronal cell loss, brain parenchymal volume is reduced but ventricular CSF pressure (provided that some type of occlusive hydrocephalus is not present) remains constant. With the loss of parenchymal volume there will be a natural, passive expansion of the ventricle. This is illustrated in all of the clinical cases presented so far (see Figures 15-3, 15-5, 15-6, and 15-7).

One of the most straightforward ways to quantify ventricular dilation or hydrocephalus ex vacuo in TBI patients is to compare the ratio of total ventricular volume to total brain volume, the so-called ventricle-to-brain ratio or VBR. Because the margins between the ventricular cavity and brain parenchyma are distinct on CT and/or MR imaging, VBR can be readily calculated using either imaging technology (Bigler, 1999). From mid-adolescence to late middle life, the VBR is relatively constant at about 1.5, with a standard deviation of approximately 0.5 (40, 41). This type of quantitative analysis can then be applied to scan findings at anytime post-injury in demonstrating trauma related DBI. For example, the case presented in Figure 15-8, demonstrates the use of VBR to show acute effects of cerebral edema (another potential generalized insult to the brain in TBI) and then ventricular expansion as an indicator of generalized parenchymal volume loss and DBI (42). This case is particularly helpful in demonstrating these points, as the patient had MR imaging done prior to injury, depicting normal ventricular size based on quantitative analyses. Increased levels of cerebral atrophy, as measured by VBR or other indices of parenchymal volume loss, relate negatively to overall outcome (43).

VBR is related to all severity of injury measures in a rather linear fashion, as shown in Figure 15-9, including GCS, loss of consciousness (LOC) and post trauma amnesia (PTA) (44) and any adverse systemic effects such as hypoxia (42). Unmistakably, ventricular dilation of the nature observed in TBI results from DBI and is likely the best single measure of DBI. Based on this assumption, larger VBR reflects generalized atrophy and therefore represents a severity marker of neuropathological changes. Larger VBR is associated with worse cognitive outcome and greater neurobehavioral sequela of acquired brain injury (37).

Unfortunately, quantitative analyses are often not available to the clinician, so how does one best evaluate ventricular dilation and cerebral atrophy, short of quantitative analyses? Actually, this can be readily performed with a straightforward visual inspection of either CT or MR findings, since small ventricular size is the norm in the noninjured brain until after the sixth decade of life (41). Since this is more completely addressed in a following section, only brief mention will be made here. Even when substantial acute pathological changes are present in the initial CT scan done on hospital admission following TBI, the DOI scan provides baseline information

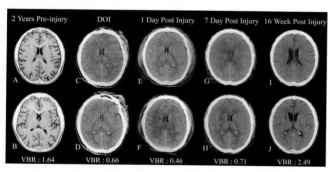

FIGURE 15-8

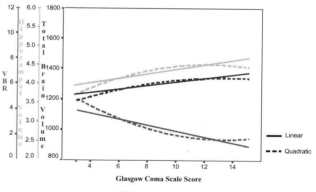

FIGURE 15-9

Axial MR (A, B) taken prior to injury, compared to follow-up computerized tomography (CT, images C-J)) imaging done on the day-of-injury (DOI, shown in C and D) and at different times post-injury. Note the compression of the ventricular system (smaller size) on the DOI scan, representative of generalized cerebral edema. The patient's pre-traumatic brain injury (TBI) ventricle-to-brain ratio (VBR), shown at the bottom, was well within normal limits (normal VBR ~1.5, standard deviation = 0.5), but on the DOI scan and the acute stage post-injury, VBR is significantly reduced, again another indicator of generalized cerebral edema. By four months post-injury (I, J) significant ventricular dilation has occurred and VBR has risen to approximately two standard deviations above the mean, reflective of generalized brain volume loss secondary to trauma induced generalized degermation. This patient had a Marshall et al., (65) level III (swelling) clinical rating of the DOI CT scan (see Table 15-2)

This illustration is from our ongoing traumatic brain injury (TBI) data base and represents 151 subjects with varying levels of severity of injury as defined by Glasgow Coma Scale (GCS). Plotting either brain volume, hippocampal volume, or the ventricle-to-brain ratio (VBR, a measure of global atrophy) results in linear and quadratic relationships that demonstrate brain or hippocampal atrophy is directly related to the severity of injury. Note that the relationship is best fit by a linear rather than quadratic function for whole brain volume (Blue color), the ventricle-to-brain ratio atrophy index (Red color) or hippocampal volume (Yellow color). The hippocampal data is based on a subset comprised of 46 subjects. In each case there is a linear loss of brain parenchymal volume directly related to severity of injury. Accordingly, loss of tissue is a function of severity of injury. Similar plots are achieved if PTA or LOC are substituted for GCS. Adapted from Bigler et al. (119)

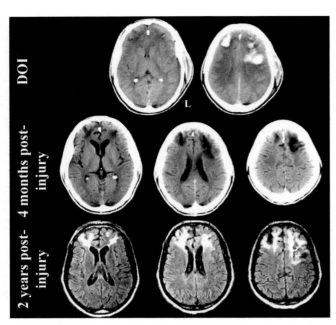

FIGURE 15-10

Day-of-injury (DOI) axial computerized tomography (CT) scans demonstrated multiple frontal hemorrhagic contusions and intraparenchymal areas of hemorrhage and edema, with compression of the anterior horns of the lateral ventricle. By four months post injury, follow-up CT demonstrates loss of density in frontal tissue, with corresponding dilation of the anterior horns of the lateral ventricle. However, the entire ventricular system is also showing expansion (hydrocephalus ex vacuo), reflective of generalized degeneration. By two years post-injury, fluid attenuated inversion recovery images (FLAIR) magnetic resonance (MR) imaging demonstrates generalized ventricular enlargement and extensive signal abnormality widely distributed across the frontal regions, bilaterally. This illustration demonstrates the utility of comparing DOI imaging to subsequent imaging studies and how this permits easy tracking of degenerative changes (i.e., ventricular dilation)

about preinjury ventricular size. As shown in Figure 15-10, this patient sustained a severe head injury as a consequence of an auto-pedestrian accident, and DOI CT findings demonstrated extensive frontal hemorrhagic lesions. Nonetheless, ventricular size can still be distinguished, even though generalized edema had developed by the time that the initial CT scan was obtained. On the DOI scan, small anterior horns of the lateral ventricular system can be readily identified, although somewhat effaced by the surrounding edema. In comparison, by the chronic stage, all follow up scans demonstrated ventricular dilation as well as changes in frontal parenchyma. Thus, clinicians should not only view the DOI imaging to identify acute pathology, but also as a benchmark for what the brain looked liked before injury. Another way to view trauma induced atrophy, or DBI, is by viewing the midsagittal plane, where not

only the body of the lateral ventricle can be observed, but the corpus callosum (CC) as exemplified in Figure 15-6. Figure 15-6 compares the midsagittal MR view and a 3-D comparison of the ventricular system in the case presented in Figure 15-3 to show the diffuse nature of moderate to severe TBI as expressed by ventricular dilation and CC atrophy. Regardless of how it is demonstrated (i.e., simple visual inspection and interpretation, quantitative measures such as increased VBR, increased clinical atrophy ratings [see below] or thinning of the CC, etc.), presence of generalized cerebral atrophy is a predictor of cognitive, neuropsychiatric and neurobehavioral sequelae (2, 5, 6, 37, 45, 46).

What has just been discussed brings up another issue that demonstrates the complexities and challenges of establishing brain-behavior relationships in predicting functional outcome in TBI. For those who survive significant brain injury and 'recover' whatever function or make whatever type of adaptation possible, structural imaging will mainly highlight the lesion or damage, which is probably not where functional reorganization is or has taken place (26, 47–49). For example, in the case presented in Figure 15-5 where extensive cortical wasting, particularly of the left frontal region, had occurred, frontal damage originally resulted in a generalized expressive aphasia that lasted several months. However, after an extended recovery and rehabilitation period, this patient eventually recovered verbal abilities to the point of obtaining a verbal IQ score of 100 and a normal score on confrontational naming, performances that reflect general intactness of language. He still had some diminished word fluency, but the more significant changes were in personality, drive and temperament, not language. Obviously, the abnormalities that reflect absence of and/or nonfunctional tissue do not necessarily represent the regions of the brain that have adapted. Research in this area has shown that functional reorganization occurs in regions that have been spared or less damaged, often distributed in a fashion that cannot be fully predicted due to individual differences, and often in regions not traditionally associated with such functions (50, 51).

This issue of functional adaptation has been nicely demonstrated by Mathias et al. (52) who has studied reaction time and speed of processing in mild to severe TBI. If white matter is particularly vulnerable to brain injury, structurally identified by reduced CC surface area, this would suggest disrupted interhemispheric white matter projection and interhemispheric transfer of information. However, Mathias et al. (52) as well as others (53–55) have shown that the degree of CC atrophy only modestly, and in many cases nonsignificantly, relates to deficits in interhemispheric transfer observed in patients with TBI. In other words, the CC is critical for transfer and integration of information between the two hemispheres and is clearly vulnerable in TBI (see Figure 15-6), but despite presence of CC lesions and atrophic changes, for the most part TBI patients recover the ability to carry on interhemispheric transfer of information and reaction time tasks, albeit slower than their non-TBI matched cohorts. Rarely do TBI patients have a lasting callosal syndrome (56). So, even though significant CC atrophy occurs in brain injury and is related to severity of injury, somehow the injured brain adapts and interhemispheric transfer of information occurs. When such adaptation occurs, using just structural neuroimaging as the basis for measuring the atrophy of the CC results in minimal power to predict impairment. The point here is that when some functional recovery has taken place, structural imaging of damaged tissue may not capture how the brain has adapted, it only measures the original region(s) of damage. Chapter 16 on functional imaging will have more to say about this problem, and the future of predicting functional outcome will probably come from the integration of structural and functional imaging.

In summary thus far, the mere presence of imaging abnormalities from trauma are not sufficient, by today's understanding of brain-behavior relationships to fully predict functional outcome. What may appear straight-forward (i.e., simply comparing 'lesions' to outcome) actually represents a very complex clinical question. Restrictions of current neuroimaging methods to fully integrate all levels and types of abnormalities from cerebral trauma into a prediction model, means that any one identified neuroimaging abnormality, by itself, often lacks robust relationship with functional outcome (57, 58). The exception here, as will be discussed later, is with brainstem abnormalities.

Vulnerability of Frontal and Temporal Regions

The earliest post-mortem TBI studies demonstrating the most likely regions of contusion confirmed the predilection for fontal and temporal locations (59). More contemporary neuroimaging studies have clearly demonstrated the greater likelihood of frontal-temporal damage over damage to any other brain region in cases of TBI (60) and can be shown when voxel-based morphometry (VBM) is used to compare those with brain injury versus control subjects as presented in Figure 15-11. A dorsal view of a skull, with the skull cap removed, is shown in Figure 15-12, clearly demonstrating the location of the

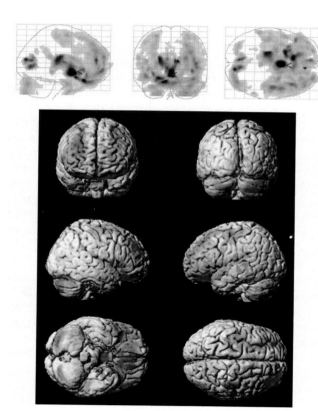

FIGURE 15-11

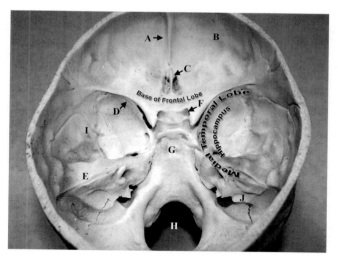

FIGURE 15-12

Statistical parametric mapping (SPM, top black and white plots) of a voxel-by-voxel quantification of damage (shown in red in the 3-D brain representations) from a group of TBI subjects who had sustained frontal or temporal lobe contrusions. VBM analyses where red represents decreased gray matter density in six TBI adolescents (mean age = 16 years old, standard deviation = 5.1) all with moderate-to-severe TBI (all had had GCS scores of 8 or below) compared to 18 control subjects of similar age (three control subjects per TBI patient within 2 years of age). Note the predominance of frontotemporal damage

Dorsal view of the open human skull (skull cap removed), where the skull cap has been removed. Top of the picture is just above the orbit. The general location of the base of the frontal lobe (jugum of the sphenoid bone) and location of the medial temporal lobe is outlined in bold letters. A: Frontal crest, B: Orbital part of frontal bone and anterior cranial fossa, C: Crista galli, D: Sphenoid, E: Petrous part of temporal bone, F: Anterior clinoid process, arrow points into the pituitary fossa or sella turcica, G: dorsum sellae above with clivus extending down, H: Foramen magnum, I: Middle cranial fossa, J: Posterior cranial fossa

anterior, middle and posterior cranial fossa. The ventral surface of the frontal lobe is situated in the anterior cranial fossa, the ventral surface of the temporal lobe in the middle cranial fossa and the cerebellum in the posterior cranial fossa. For slight movement and minimal impact, the three cranial fossa create protective factors to hold the brain in place. However, the soft, pliable brain is no match against the hard inner table of the skull once inertial forces exceed its tolerance limits. Mechanical deformation of the brain against bone, not only injures the parenchyma through mechanisms of compression and stretching (31), but increases the likelihood of contusion (61, 62). Using the integration of CT, that permits detailed identification of the bones of the skull, and MRI, that permits detailed identification of brain structures, the vulnerability of these regions is easy to appreciate because of how they are partially cradled and encapsulated by bone as shown in Figure 15-13. Thus, the undersurface of both the frontal and temporal regions become particularly vulnerable to mechanical deformation and/or contusion against boney structures as well as the anterior aspect of the temporal lobe against the sphenoid bone and the medial aspect of the temporal lobe against the sphenoid and petrous bones and clinoid process. Likewise, the basal forebrain sits just anterior to the clinoid process and the jugum of the sphenoid, both regions that have some potential for protrusion into the base of the frontal lobe. Likewise, more anteriorly, the frontal bone plate just above the nasal-orbital region, as shown in Figure 15-12, has several prominent ridges. Understanding this part of the

brain-skull interface becomes particularly important in understanding the behavioral significance of neuroimaging findings in TBI and the increased likelihood of inferior frontal and anteromedial temporal lobe damage (see 62), as clearly demonstrated by the VBM analysis shown in Figure 15-11.

Given that there is greater frontotemporal lobe damage associated with TBI, it is no surprise that the most common neuropsychological sequelae associated with TBI are those in the realm of memory and executive impairment (60). Since memory, particularly working memory, is central to all aspects of executive function, it may be that the single most important cognitive function typically disrupted by TBI is some aspect of memory (61, 63). Budson and Price (64) have recently reviewed the gross neuroanatomy associated with memory dysfunction as depicted in Figure 15-14. By comparing the illustration of the brain regions typically damaged in TBI, as shown by the VBM analysis presented in Figure 15-11, it should come as no surprise why some impairment in memory is such a common feature in TBI. Budson and Price (64) go on to provide more details as to key structures involved in various types of memory and that is presented in Figure 15-14. As can be seen major frontotemporolimbic regions and pathways are at the basis of the key structures that underlie memory function. What is of particular interest in linking TBI to neuroimaging findings and cognitive outcome, is that each structure depicted in Figure 15-14 has been shown to be affected by TBI and in the case presented in Table 15-1 and Figure 15-7, each of the areas key to memory function were damaged. Accordingly, Figure 15-14 can be used as a guide to the type of memory dysfunction that may result from a brain injury, depending of the location and extent of involvement of a particular brain region.

NEUROIMAGING OF ACUTE INJURY AND PREDICTION OF OUTCOME

Although from the above discussion, it is easy to see why the effects of TBI are more complicated than just location of a lesion(s) that predicts neurobehavioral outcome, it is still important to understand how lesions begin and evolve following trauma, and how the earliest lesions identified by neuroimaging relate to functional outcome. Using acute imaging compared to sub-acute and chronic imaging and tracking lesions and atrophic changes may yield far more important predictive statements about outcome, than just a single static image, usually during the chronic stage, to predict functional outcome. Since the first neuroimaging study of someone with a brain injury is typically a CT scan on the day-of-injury (DOI), this Chapter will next overview the relationship between the DOI CT scan and functional outcome. The DOI scan serves another purpose as well (as introduced above) that

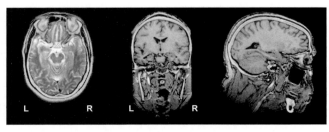

FIGURE 15-13

From left to right, fused spiral CT bone window imaging of the skull (shown in pink) interfaced with MRI in axial (T2), coronal (T1) and sagittal (T1). Bone is shown in pink to highlight how the brain is encapsulated by the cranium, particularly the anterior and middle cranial fossa. This patient sustained a moderate TBI with left temporal petrous bone fracture, that had healed by the time imaging was obtained. However, not the increased CSF in the anterior pole in the T2 Axial view shown on the left. Likewise, the coronal view in the middle demonstrates temporal lobe atrophy (temporal horn dilation, reduced size of hippocampus compared to the contralateral size of the hippocampus), reduced temporal stem. Quantitative analyses demonstrated overall reduced temporal lobe white matter volume, reduced since of entorhinal cortex, hippocampal and amygdala volumes

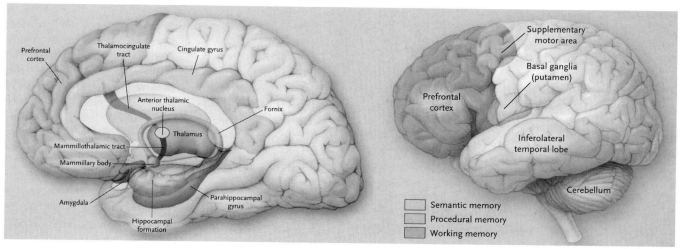

FIGURE 15-14

Left: The medial temporal lobes, including the hippocampus and parahippocampus, form the core of the episodic memory system. Other brain regions are also necessary for episodic memory to function correctly. *Right*: The inferolateral temporal lobes are important in the naming and categorization tasks by which semantic memory is typically assessed. However, in the broadest sense, semantic memory may reside in multiple and diverse cortical areas that are related to various types of knowledge. The basal ganglia, cerebellum, and supplementary motor area are critical for procedural memory. The prefrontal cortex is active in virtually all working memory tasks. Other cortical and subcortical brain regions will also be active, depending on the type and complexity of the working memory task. Used with permission of Budson and Price (64) and NEJM

of establishing a baseline to track changes overtime. Thus, comparing follow-up CT or MR imaging to the DOI scan (as in Figures 15-8 and 15-10) often provides more useful information relating to predication of outcome from brain injury; such comparisons will be the basis of the concluding topic.

Much of the interpretation of DOI CT scans has already been addressed in chapter 11 and therefore this section will concentrate not so much on lesion identification, but on the relationship between these lesions and functional outcome. Figure 15-15 summarizes the typical lesions seen on acute CT imaging in cases of cerebral trauma where CT imaging is positive. These types of abnormalities, as well as other common trauma related abnormalities, can be simply classified and rated, as shown in Table 15-2 based on the work of Marshall et al. (65). This guide can be used to establish severity of abnormalities as found in acute imaging, as will be discussed and elaborated upon in the next section, where acute imaging findings are used to predict functional outcome.

DAY-OF-INJURY (DOI) COMPUTERIZED TOMOGRAPHY (CT) AND PREDICTION OF OUTCOME

The scale established by Marshall et al. (65) attempted to characterize trauma induced acute abnormalities on a nominal rating scale grading computerized tomography (CT) abnormalities from not discernible (Grade I) to

diffuse (Grade IV), as well as whether a hematoma was present (Grade VI), or had to be evacuated (Grade V), along with presence of brainstem pathology (Grade VII). These classifications by Marshall et al. are more completely detailed in Table 15-2 and the different type of acute traumatic lesions seen on CT as presented in Figure 15-15, in turn result in distinct likelihood of frontotemporal atrophy as already shown in most of the previous examples given in this chapter, and specifically shown in Figure 15-16. The patient shown in Figure 15-16 sustained a moderate-to-severe TBI in an auto-pedestrian accident with bilateral temporal contusions and development of a subdural, which was evacuated. The neuroimaging done more than two years post injury demonstrates the frontotemporal locus of damage. This patient's initial DOI CT scan would have been rated a III by the standards outlined in Table 15-2.

In a comprehensive study that examined 240 consecutive admissions at a Trauma I hospital for head injury who survived sufficiently to progress to an inpatient rehabilitation unit, we were able to examine the predictability of CT findings based on the Marshall et al. (65) rating system to outcome at various stages during the recovery process (see Refs. 9, 66). For these 240 subjects the mean GCS was approximately 9, with an average of several days of unconsciousness and an average PTA of 2 to 3 weeks. Accordingly, as a group, these subjects generally sustained moderate-to-severe TBI and represented the typical course of outcome following inpatient rehabilitation. Using the Marshall et al. (65) classification method, the most common lesions present on the DOI CT scan were Level

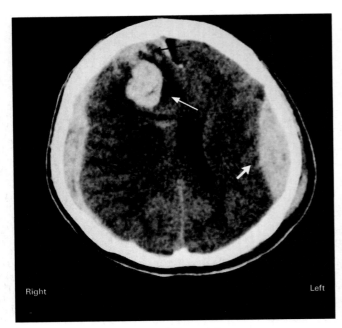

FIGURE 15-15

The axial section of a computerized tomography (CT) scan of the head at the level of the lateral ventricles, obtained without the addition of contrast medium, revealed four types of acute post-traumatic intracranial hemorrhage (Left is on the reader's right side); an epidural hematoma (thick white arrow) and a squamous temporal fracture (which is not shown) on the left side, a laminate subdural hematoma (thick black arrow) on the right side, right-sided periventricular and frontal-lobe contusions containing an intraparenchymal hematoma (thin white arrow), and a subarachnoid hemorrhage (thin black arrow) in the right frontal region. These injuries were sustained in a fall. (Reproduced with permission from Mattiello & Munz, (120) and the *New England Journal of Medicine*. Copyright © Massachusetts Medical Society.) Had this patient received a Marshall et al. (52) rating, it would be a level IV (see Table 15-2)

II (some diffuse swelling and presence of some petechial hemorrhages or small contusions). In fact amongst these 240 hospitalized subjects, almost 60 percent of all CT scans were so classified, whereas about 13 percent had Level I findings, 17 percent had Level III findings, approximately 4 percent with Level IV and 3 percent with Level VII. About 17 percent had some type of mass lesion. Since this study was based on the initial or DOI CT scan, no one had a mass lesion removed at that point, therefore no Level V subjects were part of this study. Despite clear-cut findings of pathology on the DOI CT scan (i.e., > Level II),

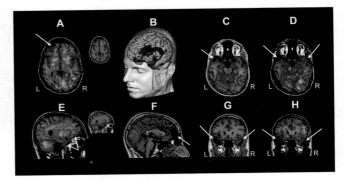

FIGURE 15-16

This illustration demonstrates the vulnerability of frontal and temporal regions for focal brain injury following traumatic brain injury (TBI). The 3-D reconstruction shown in B, highlights the frontotemporal damage in red as identified in multiple planes of magnetic resonance (MR) and fused MR-single photon emission computed tomography (SPECT) imaging, where arrows point to regions of focal encephalomalacia. D is the fused SPECT image with the axial MR shown in C and H represents the coronal fused MR-SPECT, where distinct focal temporal lobe encephalomalacia is evident in G. L designates left, R designates R. For A and E, the inset shows the level for the fused MR-SPECT image

---

TABLE 15-2≠

Descriptive Categories of Abnormalities Visualized on CT* Scanning

	LEVEL	DEFINITION
I	Diffuse Injury I (no visible pathology)	No visible intracranial pathology seen on CT scan
II	Diffuse Injury II	Cisterns are present with midline shift 0–5 mm and /or: lesion densities present; no high- or mixed-density lesion >25cc; may include bone fragments and foreign bodies
III	Diffuse Injury III (swelling)	Cisterns compressed or absent with midline shifts 0–5 mm; no high-or mixed-density lesion >25cc
IV	Diffuse Injury IV (shift)	Midline shift >5mm, no high- or mixed-density lesion >25cc
V	Evacuated mass lesion	Any lesion surgically evacuated
VI	Non-evacuated mass lesion	High- or mixed-density lesion >25cc, not surgically evacuated
VII	Brain stem injury	Focal brainstem lesion, no other lesion presenty

≠Based on Ref. 65.
*CT = computerized tomography.

such findings were not very predictive of outcome at the time of admission to rehabilitation, rehabilitation discharge, or one year followup using the Functional Independence Measure (67, 68) or the Disability Rating Scale (DRS, 69), except for those with abnormal brainstem findings on CT. Presence of a brainstem lesion was a negative predictor at all time periods post-injury and distinctly predictive of those with the worst outcome (see also Ref. 70). Thus, the mere presence or absence of CT abnormalities on the DOI scan was by itself not much of a predictor of neurobehavioral and or neuropsychiatric outcome, except for those with brainstem lesions. This is consistent with other studies that have attempted to use the DOI CT as a functional indicator of outcome (8, 71–73).

We next examined how DOI CT findings related to more long-term MR imaging findings, using quantitative measures, exploring the relationship of atrophy (i.e., increased VBR) determined at 25 days or later post-injury to outcome. One of the nice factors using the VBR metric is that it automatically corrects for head size differences (74), so no further adjustment in the ratio score is need in comparing subjects of different age, sex or physical characteristics. It may seem intuitive that with greater rating of acute CT abnormality that more prominent VBR would be the outcome. However, this was not the case. It appears that a threshold effect was present, where once injury equalled or surpassed a Marshall et al. (65) Level II rating (see Table 15-2), significant cerebral atrophy resulted that was indistinguishable from the other CT ratings. Another way of saying this is that once a Level II CT classification had been reached, DBI effects had occurred that ultimately resulted in generalized cerebral atrophy, but the degree of cerebral atrophy was rather independent of the CT rating. Interestingly, in the Katz and Alexander (8) study, presence of scan abnormalities, in association with the length of PTA, was the best predictor of outcome (see also 75). Again, it may simply mean that it is not so much the magnitude of DOI CT scan abnormalities, but rather the mere appearance of abnormalities in conjunction with certain markers of brain injury severity, such as PTA, that become predicative of functional outcome. Regardless of DOI CT ratings, by one-year follow-up, increased VBR was associated with greater deficits in FIM and DRS outcome. Presence of any DOI CT lesion has been shown to be associated with greater likelihood of developing MRI identified cerebral atrophy and greater atrophy is a risk factor for worse outcome (43).

When post-traumatic atrophy is substantial, especially in cases where acute injury is a Marshall et al. (65) CT rating of Level II or greater, tracking changes from the DOI CT scan can be most informative, simply by viewing the progression of change in the ventricular system and prominence of cortical sulci in imaging studies (either CT or MR; see Figures 15-8 and 15-10). Somewhere between 25 days post-injury and six months, the majority of atrophic changes that are likely to occur will have done so (see 40, 76), although degenerative changes may continue for up three years post-injury before the brain returns to its 'normal' age-related volume loss (see 77). Given these observations, if the clinician obtains the DOI CT and a follow-up CT or MR scans at least six weeks post-injury, presence of identified lesions or atrophic changes relate to poorer outcome. Suggested methods for easy clinical rating of these abnormalities will be offered in the next section.

In the study of TBI outcome, Dikmen et al. (78) have compiled a variety of measures they label as a "Functional Status Examination" (FSE, 78) that include the Glasgow Outcome Scale (GOS, 79), health and back-to-work questionnaires, psychosocial and emotional functioning, as well as two neuropsychological measures [i.e., Trail Making Test (80), California Verbal Learning Test (81)]. A single FSE composite score can be created from these different measures and then used to explore DOI CT relationships with outcome. Using the FSE, Temkin et al. (72) examined 209 adults with TBI all with CT abnormalities (i.e., 65, rating of Diffuse Injury II or greater) and only 20 percent of the cases reported no problems, which formed their 'good' functional status group, meaning that 80 percent had some residual impairment reflected in worse FSE composite scores. The majority of CT abnormalities in this 'good' outcome group where Marshall et al. (65) classification group II with regard to DOI CT abnormalities with the majority in the 'good' outcome group having GCS of 13–15, but minimal PTA. In contrast, the 80 percent in the Temkin et al. (72) study that had intermediate (i.e., some residual deficit) to poor FSE findings, also had Diffuse Injury II classification by Marshall et al. (65) standards as the most common rating with GCS also in the 13–15 range. They even had similar LOC duration but what distinguished this group with poorer outcome was longer PTA. Thus, long duration PTA and presence of at least a Marshall et al. rating of II, results in the worse functional outcome.

Katz and Alexander (8) examined 243 patients with TBI admitted to an inpatient rehabilitation unit and studied the global effects of abnormalities on either CT and/or MR imaging including petechial white matter hemorrhages, diffuse or localized edema, intraventricular or subarachnoid hemorrhaging, and cortical contusions. All imaging studies were based on clinical ratings of the scans and did not systematically employ the Marshall method for rating CT scans and included not only DOI scans but sub-acute scan information as well. Presence of scan abnormalities in association with duration of PTA was associated with greater deficit as measured by the GOS (79). Interestingly, focal lesions were not that predictive of outcome. Their study also addressed age where older individuals (i.e., >40 years of age) demonstrated worse outcome even though imaging and injury severity characteristics were not different. Integrating these findings with the Bigler et al. (9) and Temkin et al. (72) studies, discussed above, since of all the injury severity measures (i.e., LOC, PTA, GCS), PTA is the most predictive of VBR (see Figure 15-9) and, since Temkin et al. (72) and Katz and Alexander (8) both demonstrated the importance of PTA in defining outcome, PTA, in relationship to imaging findings, may provide the best indicators of functional outcome. Consequently, worse functional outcome is expected when structural neuroimaging on the DOI scan demonstrates presence of a Marshall et al. (65) level rating of II or greater in conjunction with extended duration PTA or when chronic findings of focal or generalized cerebral atrophy are found on follow-up imaging more than 25 days post-injury.

CLINICIAN BASED RATING METHODS FOR STRUCTURAL NEUROIMAGING IN PREDICITNG FUNCTIONAL OUTCOME

Lobular Atrophy and Functional Outcome

For a variety of reasons, including the configuration of the brain within the anterior and middle cranial fossa, frontal and temporal regions of the brain are particularly vulnerable to injury (82), as explained above and exemplified in Figure 15-16. Scheid et al. (83) found the frontal lobes to have at least three times the number of microbleeds than any other brain region, with the temporal lobe coming in second place for most frequent location for injury. This was graphically depicted in the group VBM analysis presented in Figure 15-11 and in an individual case as presented in Figure 15-16, where neuroimaging studies were performed several years after significant brain injury where the patient initially sustained frontal and temporal lobe contusions, leaving the patient with chronic lesions as areas of focal encephalomalacia that also exhibited perfusion defects on SPECT imaging. Because of the critical nature of frontal and temporal regions in regulating memory, executive and emotional functioning, damage to these areas typically affects such functions. A simple lobular rating method has been shown effective in establishing the degree of atrophy in frontal and temporal regions (84) that can be used by the clinician to forecast functional outcome relationships. The ratings are based on T1 weighted MR images, but other weightings could also be substituted, including CT imaging. Figures 15-17 and 15-18 demonstrate this clinical rating method and Figure 15-19 presents actual TBI cases and their functional outcome associated with the clinical rating methods for identifying frontal and temporal lobe atrophy using the guidelines shown in Figures 15-17 and 15-18. In studies that have employed this

method presence of frontal and/or temporal lobe atrophy was chiefly associated with neuropsychological deficits in memory as well as associated deficits in executive function and presence of neuropsychiatric symptoms, particularly depression and anxiety (84, 85). Because these rating methods only require visual inspection of the imaging studies, they can be performed in the clinicians office and provide a useful index for establishing brain-behavior relationships and functional outcome in TBI. One reason for the importance of identifying temporal lobe atrophy is because of the relationship of hippocampal atrophy (86) and the susceptibility of the hippocampus to injury (87).

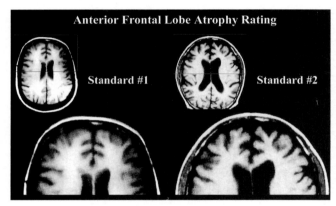

FIGURE 15-17

Anterior frontal lobe atrophy rating of T1-weighted axial images based on the method outlined by Victoroff et al. (117). In performing this rating, the frontal region has been isolated in red as shown in the axial view inset and the rating standards blown-up for the Standard #1 and #2 images. Presence of atrophy is visualized as a prominence in subarachnoid cerebral spinal fluid (CSF), which fills the widened sulci because of reduced gyral size. On the T1 image presented in this figure, CSF is represented by dark signal. Ratings focus on the cortex anterior to the frontal operculum (that is, anterior to the insula). Ratings assess the single image showing the lateral ventricles at the point of the longest visible anteroposterior connection or depending on the slice angle the image closest to the mid point of the genu of the corpus callosum where full view of the extent of the interhemispheric fissure can be viewed, example as shown. Atrophy is rated as follows: 0 = none or negligible (see Figure 15-19, control subject); 0.5 minimal, but less than seen in Standard #1; 1 = mild or moderate = equal to or greater than standard #1, or up to that equal to Standard #2; 2 = severe = definitely more than Standard #2. The key in making these ratings is to not focus on ventricular dilation, focal pathology of the frontal lobes or some other type of abnormality, other than the atrophy. The ratings can either be performed as a total frontal atrophy rating or by left and right. As shown in Figure 15-19, two clinical cases of severe traumatic brain injury (TBI) demonstrate the implementation of the rating in this figure and Figure 15-18

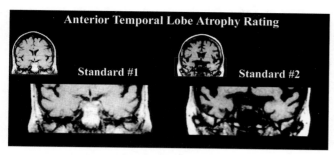

FIGURE 15-18

All of the clinical caveats given in the caption for Figure 15-17 also apply in rating the temporal lobe. Ratings are carried out on the T1 coronal image. Coronal images are used because they provide better visualization of medial temporal anatomy than axial images. Ratings assess the single image that is the first image, moving posteriorly, that definitely shows both temporal stems connecting the temporal and frontal lobes. This image usually shows the amygdalae and/or anterior aspect of the hippocampus (but neither the amygdala nor the hippocampus is rated). Ratings focus on gyral atrophy, attempting not to be influenced by the width of the Sylvian fissure (which might reflect parietal rather than temporal lobe atrophy). To get a total temporal lobe atrophy rating, both individual temporal lobe ratings can be summed. The rating following standards are used: 0 = none or negligible (see Figure 15-19); 0.5 = minimal, or up to that seen in Standard #1: 1 = mild or moderate = definitely more than standard #1, less than or equal to Standard #2: 2 = severe = definitely more than Standard #2. As an example, an actual rating of temporal lobe atrophy in a TBI patient is presented in Figure 15-19

White Matter Hyperintensities (WMHs) and Functional Outcome

Damage to white matter may show up as a hyperintensity on several types of MR imaging sequences (i.e., T2, intermediate, etc.) and relate to functional outcome (88–91). While such hyperintensities do occur in the normal population, are related to aging (92) and by themselves may not signify pathology (92, 93), they are more frequent in patients who have experienced a head injury (94). There are simple rating scales that can be used by the interested clinician to classify WMHs, typically in periventricular (PV) and centrum semi-ovale (CS) regions of the brain; these are described in Figure 15-20 and several TBI cases with WMHs are shown in Figure 15-21. In the study by Hopkins et al. (94), WMHs in frontal and/or temporal regions were associated with greater deficits in memory and executive function compared to TBI patients without WMHs. Additionally, TBI patients with WMHs endorsed more symptoms of depression and anxiety. The qualitative rating method of WMHs is straightforward to perform, and can be readily done in the clinicians office if the proper image sequences have been obtained. Simply stated, presence of WMHs in frontal and temporal brain regions is

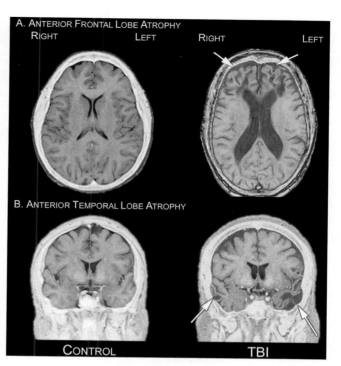

FIGURE 15-19

Using the rating method outlined in Figures 15-17 and 15-18, two different TBI patients, one with frontal atrophy (top right) and the other with temporal lobe atrophy (bottom right), were rated. For comparison, two non-brain injured age-matched controls are presented on the left, both received a 0.0 rating on their respective ratings. The frontal rating for atrophy (shown in A) was a 2, bilaterally. Note in comparison to the normal control, the prominence of the frontal sulci and interhemispheric fissure. For the temporal rating it was also a 2, but only on the left. It was 1 on the right. Both patients had poor outcome (impaired memory and executive function and at the time of imaging, both had received long-term antidepressant medication for mood management), particularly the one with such prominent frontal atrophy. These type of clinical ratings can be quickly performed on any patient and provide a meaningful qualitative rating for linking structural pathology to functional outcome. Adapted from Bergeson et al. (84)

associated with worse functional outcome in TBI. Since, the degree of WMH abnormality is related to severity of injury, and severity of injury is related to worse functional outcome, presence of WMHs becomes another rating index of severity of injury. The clinical cases using this method as shown in Figure 15-21, where all patients had significant residual neurobehavioral deficits in association with WMHs.

Clinical Rating of Ventricular Dilation as a Predictor of Outcome

Ventricular dilation, specifically hydrocephalus ex vacuo, as previously discussed, was the first trauma induced

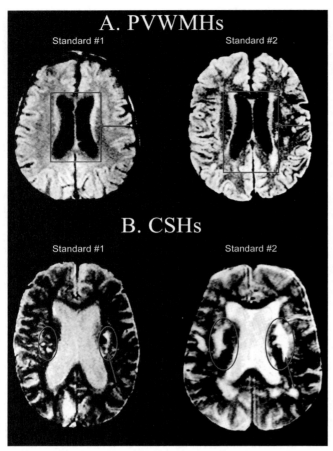

FIGURE 15-20

pathological change to be systematically investigated in TBI following the introduction of clinical CT imaging in the mid 1970s (see Refs. 95, 96). Ventricular dilation, as previously explained, is a sign of generalized cerebral atrophy where more dilation is associated with poorer outcome (2, 6). Unfortunately for the clinician, most of the work with ventricular dilation and outcome from TBI has been based on quantitative methods that require digital images along with hard and software for image analysis. However, a simple rating method can be performed, using data already presented in cases used in this Chapter. Since ventricular size is quite constant through the 6th decade of life (41, 97), this makes clinical rating relatively straightforward. Using a four-point scale, as discussed above with lobular atrophy and WMH ratings, where 0 represents 'within normal limits', .5 indicates slight dilation, 1.0 indicates mild to moderate and 2 represents moderate and beyond, ventricular dilation can be established by using the standards presented in Figure 15-22. Clinical ratings of 1 or higher are the ones most likely to be related to poorer outcome. Groswasser et al.'s (2) research suggests that this may be accomplished by just rating the III ventricle. Normal III ventricle size is rather slit-like (see Figure 15-23). Because of its midline position deep within the brain, III ventricle dilation may reflect atrophic changes of not only subcortical but cortical atrophy and may be very sensitive to parenchymal volume loss anywhere in TBI (98). Again taking from cases already presented in this chapter, Figure 15-23 shows the ease in viewing III ventricle

White matter hyperintensity rating methods are presented in this figure.(A.) *Method for rating periventricular white matter hyperintensities (PVWMHs)*: PVWMHs are defined as hyperintensities hugging the ventricle ("rims" and "caps") on the proton density (intermediate echo) axial image. The proton density images were used in the original Victoroff et al. (117) standardization because these images exhibit good contrast between the ventricles and PVWMHs, although T2-weighted images can also be used. Ratings assess the single image showing the lateral ventricles at the first level (going superiorly) that is definitely superior to the lateral bulges of hyperintensity created by the heads of the caudate nuclei. 0 = none or negligible; 0.5 = less than or equal to standard #1; 1 = mild or moderate = definitely more than standard #1, less than or equal to standard #2; 2 = severe = definitely more than standard #2. Note that in Standard #2, the signal is brighter and more extensive going beyond, in some cases, the length of the ventricle (see double arrow). For the standard, Victoroff et al. (117) used the highlighted image in the figure, rating only the left (views are in radiological perspective.)

(B.) *Method for rating centrum semi-ovale white matter hyperintensities (CSHs)*: CSHs are defined as deep white matter hyperintensities definitely separated from the ventricle on the T2-weights axial image. Hyperintense T2 lesions may be seen with or without corresponding hypointense T1 lesions. When corresponding lesions less than 0.5 cm are seen on both T1

and T2, particularly in the periventricular white matter and basal ganglia, they are regarded as probable Virchow-Robin spaces. Lesions greater than 0.5 cm seen on both T1 and T2 are regarded as probable completed infarctions. Both are excluded from the ratings of CSHs. Thus the CSH rating encompasses all hyperintense T2 lesions that do not have a matching hypointensity on the T1 image, regardless of size, degree of hyperintensity, or shape. Ratings assess the single image showing the lateral ventricles at the point of the longest visible anteroposterior connection. When in doubt, ratings are made by reference to one side (the left side, viewer's right) of the standard scans: 0 = none or negligible; 0.5 = less than or equal to the left side of standard #1; 1 = mild or moderate = definitely more than standard #1, less than or equal to the left side of standard #2; 2 = severe = definitely more than the left side of standard #2. Again, as in A., the standard image is highlighted.

Similar ratings can be made using this scheme when fluid attenuated inversion recovery images (FLAIR) and various susceptibility weighted MR images as they too have sensitivity to white matter abnormalities and presence of hemosiderin (as a marker of shear injury) in white matter. Figure 15-21 shows white matter injury with the above ratings in two TBI cases. These ratings can also be applied to white matter abnormalities that are outside the traditional region of the centrum semiovale. For ease in classification these are labeled CSH+. An example of this is presented in Figure 15-21

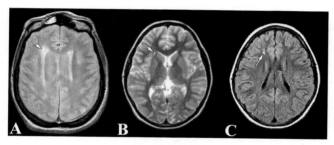

FIGURE 15-21

(A) Axial proton density magnetic resonance (MR) scan showing periventricular white matter hyperintensities (PVWMH; see arrow) in a traumatic brain injury (TBI) patient in the frontal region on the right (scans are in radiological perspective). (B) T2 weighted image showing white matter hyperintensities (CSH+) in right frontal region (arrow). (C) Fluid attenuated inversion recovery images (FLAIR) image showing CSH+ in another region of the frontal lobe in the same TBI patient as shown in B. Presence of these types of frontal lesions relate to impaired functional outcome in TBI and likely reflect focal disruption of white matter pathways and are a clinical manifestation of diminished white matter integrity

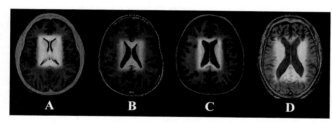

FIGURE 15-22

Using scans from different figures in this chapter, a simple, normal 'Ventricular Size' rating can be established by using the four figures and a four point rating scale. Ventricle Part A is from the control subject in Figure 15-19A. Part B is from the subject in Figure 15-13, although this body of the lateral ventricle view was not actually shown. Part C is from Figure 15-6D and part D is Figure 15-19A (traumatic brain injury, TBI, patient). Similar to the ratings for focal atrophy of the frontal (see Figure 15-13) or temporal lobe (see Figure 15-14) regions, the ventricular rating is based on a 0, 0.5, 1 and 2 rating, where A represents 0, B represents a 0.5 (greater than A but equal to or less than B), C represents a 1.0 (greater than B but equal to or less than C) and 2.0 is anything greater than C exemplified by D. The presence of increased ventricular size in TBI is associated with worse functional outcome

size and its relationship to brain injury severity and outcome.

Coup-Contre-Coup and Outcome

The coup-contre-coup phenomena in brain injury is a common form of injury (29) and actually represents another

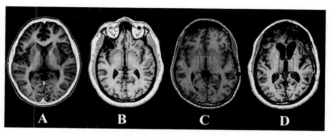

FIGURE 15-23

Using scans from different figures in this chapter, a simple 'Ventricular Size' rating of the III Ventricle can be established. (A) Using the axial MR view from Figure 15-8, with a reversed gray scale image, the III ventricle region is outlined in red. This represents a normal III ventricle size. (B) View (not previously shown) taken from the case presented in Figures 15-3 and 15-6 and shows a mild dilation (III ventricle outlined in red). (C) This view was taken from the case presented in Figure 15-16 and demonstrates a mild-to-moderate dilation (particularly the more posterior aspect of the III ventricle as outlined in red). (D) This was taken from the case in Figure 15-7 and demonstrates a moderate-to-severe dilation of the III ventricle (outlined in red). Applying the four point rating scale for III ventricle dilation A would be rated as 0; B at 0.5; C a 1; and D a 2. In each, classification incorporates the figure as equal to or less than the Standard. Increased III ventricle dilation in traumatic brain injury (TBI) is associated with worse outcome

factor that complicates the prediction of outcome using neuroimaging findings. As previously discussed this is excellently demonstrated in the neuroimaging depicted in Figure 15-5. This patient fell some 20 feet, striking the left frontal region, resulting in depressed skull fracture and development of a subdural hematoma that had to be neurosurgically removed. The residual focal effects of the left frontal injury are readily detected by the presence of focal atrophy, highlighted in red in the illustration. However, only on the FLAIR image, can the contre coup damage be detected in the right parietal area, in the form of abnormal signal intensity, not atrophy, particularly in white matter. The right parietal damage is in a linear path directly opposite the point of left frontal impact, where the skull fracture occurred. Although beyond the scope of full discussion in this chapter, an obvious implication of a contre coup injury such as that shown in Figure 15-5, some 10 cm completely opposite the point of impact, means that tremendous biomechanical forces of physical energy were transmitted through the brain on this plane (see Ref. 39). With such impact forces of injury transferred through the brain there typically are widespread microstructural changes within the sectors subjected to acceleration/deceleration injury that are not detected by neuroimaging, but only pathologically identified microscopically (see Ref. 29). With regards to functional outcome in the presence of coup/contre coup injuries, the very nature of these multi-focal injuries in association with DBI factors, makes prognostication difficult. This may be why in the Katz and Alexander (8) study presence of focal contusions was not strongly associated with outcome. When lobular atrophy is identified, as discussed above, additional imaging sequences should be obtained to explore whether contre coup injury is present and its relationship to functional outcome.

TBI, Anterior Commissure and Basal Forebrain Damage

Over the last decade, the clinical importance of the basal forebrain in neuropsychiatric disorders has been clearly established (99, 100) and discussed earlier in this chapter. As the name implies, the basal forebrain is a region at the posterior base of the frontal lobe, cradled in the anterior cranial fossa, situated just above and anterior to the clinoid process of the skull, making it vulnerable to impact injury at the skull-brain interface in this region (101). The location of the anterior commissure (AC) is typically considered part of one of the superior boundaries of the basal forebrain. The AC is comprised of a small band of white matter tracts that course between the two hemispheres that interconnects mesial temporal and orbitofrontal cortices (102). Although not specifically investigated, it probably shares a similar vulnerability as does the CC (103) and as recently shown by Wilde et al. (43) the ventral aspect of the frontal lobe is particularly vulnerable to injury. As shown in Figure 15-24 (this is the same patient as shown in Figure 15-16), in comparison to a normal control, a TBI patient with severe injury clearly demonstrates AC atrophy, as shown by the dilation of the suprachiasmatic recess compared to the control subject. What is also evident in this illustration is that all of the area under the AC exhibits atrophy as well. This region contains the critical origins of cholinergic innervation for all of cerebral cortex (104). The AC has traditionally been considered part of the upper boundary of the basal forebrain, so atrophic changes at the level of the AC and below, probably reflect basal forebrain damage. The basal forebrain regions at the AC level comprise critical structures of the limbic system and the ventral striatum including the extended amygdala, the basal nucleus of Meynert and the midline septal nuclei (99, 100). These brain regions have been shown to be critical for maintenance of emotional regulation and given its vulnerability to injury; it is likely that basal forebrain damage contributes to the common emotional changes associated with TBI (62, 105, 106). Lastly, as shown by the VBM analysis depicted in Figure 15-11, one of the areas of greatest change in gray matter density in this cohort of TBI subjects analyzed was in the basal forebrain region.

Medial Temporal Lobe Damage

As shown in Figure 15-13, the medial aspect of the temporal lobe butts up against the medial surface of the

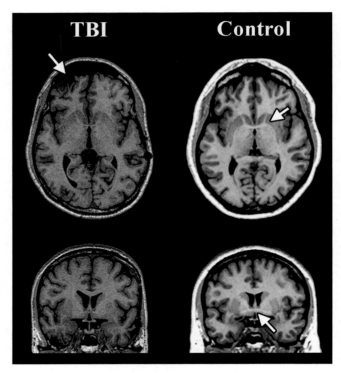

FIGURE 15-24

The TBI case on the left is the same as shown in Figure 15-16 and Figure 15-23C. The control subject on the right is the same as shown in Figure 15-6A. The arrows shown in the control subject point to the anterior commissure (AC) in axial (top right) and coronal (bottom right) planes, that is easily identified by the distinct and unmistakable band of white matter fiber projections. In the coronal view, the region beneath the AC, in part, defines the basal forebrain. In comparison to the TBI subject, it is clear that there is a diminution in the size of the AC. Also note in the TBI patient dilation of the III ventricle (see Figure 15-23) and enlargement of the suprachiasmatic recess, indicating volume loss of brain parenchyma in this area. The suprachiasmatic recess is just to the left margin of the arrow in the bottom coronal view of the control subject and is situated just above the optic chiasma. This is also the region of the substantia innominata, where in the nucleus basalis of Meynert exists and other critical structures of cholinergic innervation (121, 122). This TBI patient also had an area of focal encephalomalacia of the frontal region (arrow), as indicated by increased focal CSF in that region. Damage involving atrophy of the AC and inferior frontal region, including the basal forebrain likely results in significant changes in memory and mood regulation, as was the case with this patient

middle cranial fossa, formed in part by the clinoid and sphenoid bones. The medial surface of the parahippocampal gyrus houses both the entorhinal cortex and subiculum, which input the hippocampus. Hippocampal atrophy following TBI has been one of the most replicated findings in quantitative analysis of temporal lobe

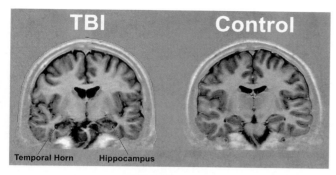

FIGURE 15-25

True inversion recovery sequence that highlights the distinction between white and gray matter and clearly shows the atrophy of the medial temporal lobe, expressed as reduced volume of the hippocampus (compare to control subjects at similar level) and temporal horn dilation. Loss of medial temporal lobe volume, and in particular volume loss of the hippocampus, gives rise to 'downstream' atrophy of the limbic projection system of the fornix, as shown in Figures 15-26 and 15-27

structures (63), but as shown in Figure 15-13, the atrophy of the medial temporal lobe and its underlying white matter pathways exhibits atrophy as well as the distinctly evident hippocampal atrophy. While memory outcome is one of the most replicated of the neurocognitive sequelae of TBI and relates to hippocampal atrophy (60), memory impairment following TBI could result from widespread medial temporal lobe damage as well (see Ref. 62). As shown in Figure 15-25, even though the hippocampus is clearly atrophic, so is entorhinal cortex and adjacent white matter. Since entorhinal cortex is the recipient of diverse inputs from all regions of cerebral cortex, the disruption of memory may have nonspecific factors associated with damage outside of the hippocampus, proper and this likely relates to only the modest relationship between hippocampal atrophy and memory outcome. Damage to the medial temporal lobe structures and the hippocampus, in turn disrupts input to the fornix, resulting in atrophy of the fornix, which may also be susceptible to mechanical deformation and shear/stretch effects as well (107), can be readily visualized in MR imaging as shown in Figures 15-26 to 15-27. Furthermore, fornix atrophy leads to reduced size of the mammillary body and the mammillothalamic tracks, as shown in Figure 15-26 and 15-27. Returning to Figure 15-14, all of these structures are critical to memory function and susceptible to injury in TBI.

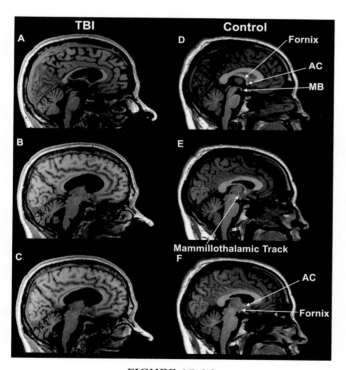

FIGURE 15-26

As labeled in the control subject, atrophy of the fornix, anterior commissure (AC), mammillary body (MB) and the mammillothalamic track can be readily identified in the TBI patient. The sagittal image is from a 3 Tesla scan and clearly shows ventricular dilation, thinning of the corpus callosum, marked shrinkage of the fornix, clear reduction in the size of the AC and MB with no ability to identify the mammillothalamic track. This patient sustained a severe TBI in a MVA, with his initial GCS rated at a 5

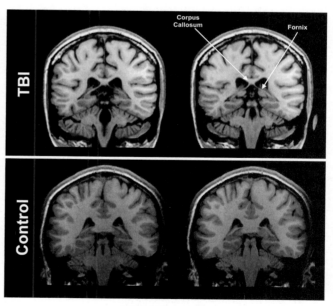

FIGURE 15-27

Fornix in coronal perspective as it comes off of the posterior aspect of the hippocampus at the level of the splenium of the corpus callosum. This patient sustained a severe TBI in a MVA where her initial GCS was reported to be a 4. This illustration demonstrates the ease with which fornix atrophy can be identified

THE INTEGRATION OF STRUCTURAL AND FUNCTIONAL IMAGING

The image of the brain generated by CT or MRI only represents gross brain structure. Although in the living individual structure is never devoid of function, neither CT nor MRI structural imaging provide a direct measure of function. However, as explained in Chapter 12 on functional imaging in this book, the principles of structural imaging can be applied to obtain functional measures of the brain. As already discussed, when structural changes are detected they merely depict where the macroscopic abnormalities are and not necessarily the totality of areas or systems that may be disrupted. However, structural imaging typically represents the very best method for projecting functional changes as nicely depicted in Figure 15-28 based on the studies by Lewine et al. (26, 49). As shown in this illustration, MR structural imaging is used as the format for demonstrating where SPECT and MEG abnormalities were found, both measures of functional impairment. As depicted in Figure 15-28, structural pathology in the inferior frontal region was obvious on MR imaging, likely from gliding-type contusions between the brain and the inner table of the skull, particularly the greater sphenoid and the boney protrusions of the interior surface of the frontal bone (i.e., crista galli). Despite the clarity of these distinct lesions, with relatively well demarcated boundaries as defined by the MR signal intensity returning to uniformity once outside the confines of the lesion, neural function was not normal in the 'normal' appearing tissue just outside of the well defined areas of damage. As such, these 'normal' areas, even though close to the lesion, do not exhibit abnormal MR signal and therefore, from strictly a structural imaging standpoint, would be interpreted as 'normal' brain parenchyma. However, when the perfusion defects of SPECT are superimposed, it is apparent that the area of dysfunction exceeds the distinct MR identified lesion boundaries. In other words, the actual area of 'damage' that disrupts function, as measured by SPECT imaging is greater than the lesion(s). More importantly, though, the SPECT abnormalities still do not encompass all the abnormalities as reflected in the MEG findings. Therefore, the true extent of the 'abnormality' will always be larger than the defined lesion. By integrating all three methods, MR, SPECT and MEG, a clearer picture of more generalized cerebral dysfunction involving a much larger area of cerebral cortex emerges. It may be that such integrated imaging methods will yield better prediction of functional outcome. Using the same type of techniques, essentially any imaging modality can be integrated with another, such as 3-D CT or MR images integrated with PET, MRS, quantitative EEG data and so forth. An example of this is presented in Figure 15-29 showing the presence of structural atrophy of the medial temporal area in

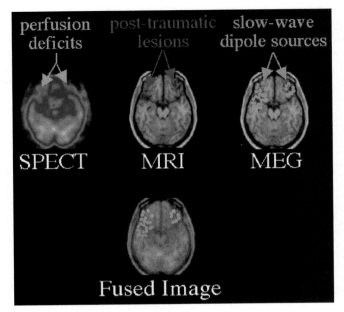

FIGURE 15-28

Data are shown for an 18-year-old male subject who suffered moderate head trauma in a motor vehicle accident at age 14. The subject had a Glasgow Coma Score (GCS) of 10 at the time of hospital admission. This patient sustained a moderate-to-severe traumatic brain injury (TBI) with post-injury neuroimaging being performed more than a year post-injury. The single photon emission computed tomography (SPECT) and magnetoencephalography (MEG) were co-registered with the coordinates of the magnetic resonance imaging (MRI), so that all three images could be reliably integrated where SPECT and MEG abnormalities are projected specifically on their corresponding regions on the MRI, as shown in the top row. This also permits the 'fusing' of all images, into a single integrated image showing all abnormalities in a single view. Normal SPECT perfusion is characterized by yellow-orange, more prominently observed toward the cortical surface, where gray matter is found. Blue represents less to absent perfusion, normal in regions of highly concentrated white matter (do to minimal metabolic activity in such regions) or in cerebral spinal fluid (CSF) filled spaces, because no perfusion occurs in such regions. Initial MR revealed by frontal and left temporal contusions and a left fronto-temporal sub-dural hematoma. At the time of SPECT/MRI/MEG imaging, the patient had a chronic post-concussive syndrome characterized by mild depression, frequent head aches, memory and attention problems, and general cognitive decline as characterized by low IQ and impaired processing speed and accuracy. MRI revealed focal bi-frontal and left temporal encephalomalacia, some generalized atrophy and ventricular dilation, and evidence of diffuse axonal injury. SPECT showed concordant hypoperfusion of right and left frontal regions and the left temporal lobe. SPECT also provided evidence of a mild generalized cortical atrophy and ventricular dilation. MEG revealed focal slow waves at concordant right and left frontal and left temporal regions. MEG also showed left parietal slow waves. MEG was the only imaging method to explicitly reveal parietal injury. (Reproduced with permission from Lewine et al., Ref. 26.)

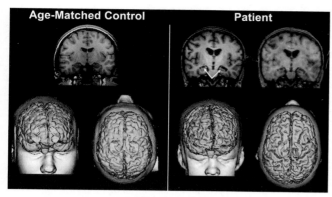

FIGURE 15-29

The T1 coronal image of the TBI patient presented on the right clearly demonstrates bilateral hippocampal atrophy (arrows) clearly defined by the shrunken appearance of the hippocampi and the dilated temporal horns of the lateral ventricle. The Fluorine-18 dioxyglucose (FDG) PET imaging fused with the structural MRI, as shown on the right demonstrates relatively normal cortical metabolic activity, except in the medial temporal lobe region and particularly in the bilateral hippocampal region. The hippocampus can be isolated in 3-D as shown below, where the control subject demonstrates the normal appearance of the hippocampus whereas in comparison to the patient's atrophic hippocampus. As would be expected, this patient exhibits significant deficits in short-term memory function, where some of his neuropsychological scores are below three standard deviations of where they were expected to be prior to injury

a child who sustained a severe TBI that resulted in bilateral hippocampal atrophy. Interfacing the PET imaging with the structural clearly shows significant defects in cerebral activation in the medial temporal region, that is actually asymmetric even though the appearance of the structural atrophy of the hippocampus and temporal lobes appear to by symmetric and bilateral.

NEW TECHNIQUES AND INTEGRATION ACROSS TECHNIQUES: THE FUTURE OF STRUCTURAL IMAGING IN PREDICTING FUNCTIONAL OUTCOME

Only a brief statement will be made on this topic, which should be obvious to the reader at this time. Detection of structural pathology will only improve with the introduction of new hard and software for structural image analysis (1, 108–114) More rapid and automated image analysis methods are being introduced on a regular basis (115). Accordingly, the predication of functional outcome in TBI will only improve in the future, particularly as functional imaging measures are integrated with structural (116).

SUMMARY AND CONCLUSIONS

Although predicting functional outcome from neuroimaging findings is a complex task fraught with many limitations, recent advancements in brain imaging have resulted in significant improvement and understanding of the relationship between structural neuroimaging findings and outcome. As a conclusion to this chapter, the following simplified outline is proffered as a clinician's guide in determining relationships between clinical neuroimaging findings and outcome. The rating begins with the DOI scan, typically a CT, compared to various CT and or MR follow-up scans, particularly more than 25 days post-injury.

1. If the DOI CT is a Level I according to the Marshall et al. (65) rating method (no discernible abnormality, as shown in Table 15-1) and there was minimal or no LOC or PTA and GCS was >13, structural neuroimaging will likely be interpreted as "clinically" normal and neither qualitative or quantitative analyses will be that predictive of functional outcome. In other words, a 'normal' scan does not necessarily mean normal or a good recovery but absence of abnormality, particularly with minimal PTA, tends to seen in those with the best chance for good functional outcome.

2. If the DOI CT is a Level I but there is positive LOC and PTA, the patient should have follow-up MR imaging (a minimum of 25 days post-injury) that includes protocols sensitive to blood byproducts, white matter integrity and CSF filled spaces. Normal scan findings at follow-up imaging will be predictive of better outcome than found in those with positive follow-up scans. Those with MR abnormalities in followup who show enlarged VBR as a sign of generalized atrophy, presence of focal frontal or temporal lobe atrophy or generalized white matter atrophy (i.e., callosal atrophy) or WMHs will have worse outcome. Functional neuroimaging may be particularly important in understanding outcome at this stage.

3. TBI patients with Level II CT findings or worse generally are more likely to have abnormalities identified on follow-up MR imaging and the degree of VBR identified atrophy will relate to outcome. More atrophy (i.e., larger VBR), generally the worse the outcome. Focal atrophy of the frontal and or temporal brain regions will relate to deficits in short-term memory and/or executive function and likewise, will be associated with a greater likelihood for neuropsychiatric disorder, particular in the domain of mood and anxiety based symptoms.

4. Independent of DOI CT rating, in TBI cases where frontal and or temporal lobe atrophy is identified and/or presence of white matter lesions and/or blood

byproducts (i.e., hemosiderin) in these region, using the method outlined in this chapter for rating of lobular atrophy and/or WMHs [i.e., based on the Victoroff et al. (117) method] will be associated with greater deficits in one or all of the following functions: executive, emotion and/or memory. Where focal atrophy is present, review of the scans for potential contre coup injury is recommended. Presence of contre coup injury complicates the prediction of functional outcome.

5. Presence of brainstem lesions on DOI CT carries the worst prognosis for functional outcome.

References

1. Kessler RM: Imaging methods for evaluating brain function in man. *Neurobiol Aging* 2003;24 Suppl 1:S21–35; discussion S37–39.
2. Groswasser Z, Reider G, II, Schwab K, Ommaya AK, Pridgen A, Brown HR, Cole R, Salazar AM: Quantitative imaging in late TBI. Part II: cognition and work after closed and penetrating head injury: a report of the Vietnam head injury study. *Brain Inj* 2002;16:681–90.
3. van der Naalt J: Prediction of outcome in mild to moderate head injury: A review. *J Clin Exp Neuropsychol* 2001;23:837–851.
4. MacKenzie JD, Siddiqi F, Babb JS, Bagley LJ, Mannon LJ, Sinson GP, Grossman RI: Brain atrophy in mild or moderate traumatic brain injury: a longitudinal quantitative analysis. *AJNR Am J Neuroradiol* 2002;23:1509–1515.
5. Reider-Groswasser I, Cohen M, Costeff H, Groswasser Z: Late CT findings in brain trauma: Relationship to cognitive and behavioral sequelae and to vocational outcome. *AJR* 1993;160: 147–152.
6. Reider-Groswasser II, Z G, Ommaya AK, K S, Pridgen A, Brown HR, Cole R, Salazar AM: Quantitive imaging in late traumatic brain injury. Part I: late imaging parameters in closed and penetrating head injuries. *Brain Inj* 2002;16:517–525.
7. Fontaine A, Azouvi P, Remy P, Bussel B, Samson Y: Functional anatomy of neuropsychological deficits after severe traumatic brain injury. *Neurology* 1999;53:1963–1968.
8. Katz DI, Alexander MP: Traumatic brain injury: Predicting course of recovery and outcome for patients admitted to rehabilitation. *Arch Neurol* 1994;51:661–670.
9. Bigler ED, Ryser DK, Gandhi P, Kimball J, Wilde E: Day of injury computerized tomography, rehabilitation status, and development of cerebral atrophy in persons with traumatic brain injury. *American Journal of Rehabilitation Medicine* 2006, in press.
10. van der Naalt J, Hew JM, van Zomeren AH, Sluiter WJ, Minderhoud JM: Computed tomography and magnetic resonance imaging in mild to moderate head injury: early and late imaging related to outcome. *Ann Neurol* 1999;46:70–8.
11. Toga AW, Mazziotta JC. *Brain Mapping: The Systems.* New York: Academic Press; 2000.
12. Babiloni F, Mattia D, Babiloni C, Astolfi L, Salinari S, Basilisco A, Rossini PM, Marciani MG, Cincotti F: Multimodal integration of EEG, MEG and fMRI data for the solution of the neuroimage puzzle. *Magn Reson Imaging* 2004;22:1471–6.
13. Kertesz A. *Localization and Neuroimaging in Neuropsychology.* San Diego, CA: Academic Press; 1994.
14. Bates E, Wilson SM, Saygin AP, Dick F, Sereno MI, Knight RT, Dronkers NF: Voxel-based lesion-symptom mapping. *Nat Neurosci* 2003;6:448–50.
15. Tomaiuolo F, Worsley KJ, Lerch J, Di Paola M, Carlesimo GA, Bonanni R, Caltagirone C, Paus T: Changes in white matter in long-term survivors of severe non-missile traumatic brain injury: a computational analysis of magnetic resonance images. *J Neurotrauma* 2005;22:76–82.
16. Ardaman MF, Hayman LA, Taber KH, Charletta DA: An imaging guide to neuropsychology. Part I: Visual object and face recognition,

17. spatial perception, voluntary actions and auditory word comprehension. *Int J Neuroradiol* 1996;2:296–308.
17. Ardaman MF, Hayman LA, Taber KH, Charletta DA: An imaging guide to neuropsychology. Part II: Word retrieval, sentence processing, speech production, reading, spelling, writing, calculation, memory, and problem solving. *Int J Neuroradiol* 1996; 2:374–388.
18. Bigler ED, Yeo RA, Turkheimer E, eds. Neuropsychological function and brain imaging: Introduction and overview. New York: Plenum Press; 1989.
19. Arfanakis K, Haughton VM, Carew JD, Rogers BP, Dempsey RJ, Meyerand ME: Diffusion tensor MR imaging in diffuse axonal injury. *AJNR Am J Neuroradiol* 2002;23:794–802.
20. Melhem ER, Itoh R, Jones L, Barker PB: Diffusion tensor MR imaging of the brain: effect of diffusion weighting on trace and anisotropy measurements. *AJNR Am J Neuroradiol* 2000;21:1813–19.
21. Sinson G, Bagley LJ, Cecil KM, Torchia M, McGowan JC, Lenkinski RE, McIntosh TK, Grossman RI: Magnetization transfer imaging and proton MR spectroscopy in the evaluation of axonal injury: correlation with clinical outcome after traumatic brain injury. *AJNR Am J Neuroradiol* 2001;22:143–51.
22. Lazar M, Weinstein DM, Tsuruda JS, Hasan KM, Arfanakis K, Meyerand ME, Badie B, Rowley HA, Haughton V, Field A, Alexander AL: White matter tractography using diffusion tensor deflection. *Hum Brain Mapp* 2003;18:306–21.
23. Goetz P, Blamire A, Rajagopalan B, Cadoux-Hudson T, Young D, Styles P: Increase in apparent diffusion coefficient in normal appearing white matter following human traumatic brain injury correlates with injury severity. *J Neurotrauma* 2004;21:645–54.
24. Fatterpekar GM, Naidich TP, Delman BN, Aguinaldo JG, Gultekin SH, Sherwood CC, Hof PR, Drayer BP, Fayad ZA: Cytoarchitecture of the Human Cerebral Cortex: MR Microscopy of Excised Specimens at 9.4 Tesla. *AJNR Am J Neuroradiol* 2002;23:1313–1321.
25. Strangman G, O'Neil-Pirozzi TM, Burke D, Cristina D, Goldstein R, Rauch SL, Savage CR, Glenn MB: Functional neuroimaging and cognitive rehabilitation for people with traumatic brain injury. *Am J Phys Med Rehabil* 2005;84:62–75.
26. Lewine JD, Davis JT, Bigler ED, Hartshorne M, Thoma R, Funke M, Sloan JH, Orrison WW: Multimodal brain imaging in mild and moderate head trauma: Integration of MEG, SPECT, and MRI. *J Head Trauma Rehabil.* (in press)
27. Medana IM, Esiri MM: Axonal damage: A key predictor of outcome in human CNS diseases. *Brain* 2003;126:515–530.
28. Gennarelli TA, Thibault LE, Graham DI: Diffuse axonal injury: An important form of traumatic brain damage. *Neuroscientist* 1998;4:202–215.
29. Graham DI, Gennarelli TA, McIntosh TK. Trauma. In: Graham DI, Lantos PI, eds. *Greenfield's Neuropathology.* Seventh ed. London: Arnold; Hodder Headline Group; 2002:823–882.
30. Murdoch I, Perry EK, Court JA, Graham DI, Dewar D: Cortical cholinergic dysfunction after human head injury. *J Neurotrauma* 1998;15:295–305.
31. Povlishock JT, Katz DI: Update of neuropathology and neurological recovery after traumatic brain injury. *J Head Trauma Rehabil* 2005;20:76–94.
32. Blumbergs P, Scott G, Manavis J, Wainright H, Simpson DA, McLean AJ: Staining of amyloid precursor protein to study axonal damage in mild head injury. *Lancet* 1994;344:1055–1056.
33. Geddes JF, Vowles GH, Nicoll JAR, Revesz T: Neuronal cytoskeletal changes are an early consequence of repetitive head injury. *Acta Neuropathol* 1999;98:171–178.
34. Geddes JF, Hackshaw AK, Vowles GH, Nickols CD, Whitwell HL: Neuropathology of inflicted head injury in children: I. Patterns of brain damage. *Brain* 2001;124:1290–1298.
35. Geddes JF, Vowles GH, Hackshaw AK, Nickols CD, Scott IS, Whitwell HL: Neuropathology of inflicted head injury in children: II. Microscopic brain injury in infants. *Brain* 2001;124:1299–1306.
36. Bigler ED: Neuropsychological findings in a case of autopsy confirmed neuropathology in mild traumatic brain injury. *JINS* 2003; 9:541–542.
37. Bigler ED: Quantitative magnetic resonance imaging in traumatic brain injury. *J Head Trauma Rehabil* 2001;16:1–21.

38. Runnerstam M, Bao F, Huang Y, Shi J, Gutierrez E, Hamberger A, Hansson HA, Viano D, Haglid K: A new model for diffuse brain injury by rotational acceleration: II. Effects on extracellular glutamate, intracranial pressure, and neuronal apoptosis. *J Neurotrauma* 2001;18:259–73.

39. Smith DH, Meaney DF, Shull WH: Diffuse axonal injury in head trauma. *J Head Trauma Rehabil* 2003;18:307–316.

40. Blatter DD, Bigler ED, Gale SD, Johnson SC, Anderson CV, Burnett BM, Ryser D, Macnamara SE, Bailey BJ: MR-based brain and cerebrospinal fluid measurement after traumatic brain injury: Correlation with neuropsychological outcome. *AJNR Am J Neuroradiol* 1997;18:1–10.

41. Blatter DD, Bigler ED, Gale SD, Anderson CV, Johnson SC, Burnett BM, Parker N, Kurth S, Horn SD: Quantitative volumetric analysis of brain MR: Normative database spanning 5 decades of life. *AJNR Am J Neuroradiol* 1995;16:241–251.

42. Hopkins RO, Tate DF, Bigler ED: Anoxic versus traumatic brain injury: amount of tissue loss, not etiology, alters cognitive and emotional function. *Neuropsychology* 2005;19:233–42.

43. Wilde EA, Hunter JV, Newsome MR, Scheibel RS, Bigler ED, Johnson JL, Fearing MA, Cleavinger HB, Li X, Swank PR, Pedroza C, Roberson GS, Bachevalier J, Levin HS: Frontal and temporal morphometric findings on MRI in children after moderate to severe traumatic brain injury. *J Neurotrauma* 2005;22: 333–44.

44. Bigler ED, Neeley ES, Ozonoff S, Coon H, McMahon W, Lainhart JE: Superior temporal gyrus and autism. *Brain Impairment* 2004;5:105–106.

45. Salazar AM. Traumatic brain injury: The continuing epidemic. In: Hachinski, ed. *Challenges in Neurology*. Philadelphia: Davis, F A; 1992:55–67.

46. Yount R, Raschke KA, Biru M, Tate DF, Miller MJ, Abildskov T, Gandhi PV, Ryser D, Hopkins RO, Bigler ED: Traumatic brain injury and atrophy of the cingulate gyrus. *J Neuropsychiatry Clin Neurosci* 2002;14:416–423.

47. Azouvi P: Neuroimaging correlates of cognitive and functional outcome after traumatic brain injury. *Curr Opin Neurol* 2000;13:665–9.

48. Levine B, Cabeza R, McIntosh AR, Black SE, Grady CL, Stuss DT: Functional reorganisation of memory after traumatic brain injury: a study with H(2)(15)0 positron emission tomography. *J Neurol Neurosurg Psychiatry* 2002;73:173–81.

49. Lewine JD, Davis JT, Thoma R, Bigler ED, Sloan JH, Funke M, Moore KR, Orrison WW: Long-term psychological consequences of mild and moderate head trauma: A magnetoencephalographic investigation. *Brain Inj*. (in press)

50. Dobkin BH: Functional rewiring of brain and spinal cord after injury: The three Rs of neural repair and neurological rehabilitation. *Curr Opin Neurol* 2000;13:655–659.

51. Stein DG, Hoffman SW: Concepts of CNS plasticity in the context of brain damage and repair. *J Head Trauma Rehabil* 2003; 18:317–341.

52. Mathias JL, Bigler ED: Information processing speed and its relationship to quantitative neuroimaging following moderate and severe traumatic brain injury. *Brain Inj* 2003;17:136.

53. Levin HS, Benavidez DA, Verger-Maestre K, Perachio N, Song J, Mendelsohn DB, Fletcher JM: Reduction of corpus callosum growth after severe traumatic brain injury in children. *Journal of Neurology, Neurosurgery, and Psychiatry* 2000;54:647–653.

54. Levin H: Corpus callosal atrophy following closed head injury: Detection with magnetic resonance imagery. *J Neurosurg* 1990;73: 77–81.

55. Johnson SC, Bigler ED, Burr RB, Blatter DD: White matter atrophy, ventricular dilation, and intellectual functioning following traumatic brain injury. *Neuropsychology* 1994;8:307–315.

56. Bigler ED, Orrison J, W. W. Neuroimaging in sports-related brain injury. In: Collins M, Lovell M, Barth JT, Echemendia RJ, eds. *Sports-Related Traumatic Brain Injury: An International Perspective*. Lisse, The Netherlands: Swets & Zeitlinger Publishers; 2003:in press.

57. Garnett MR, Blamire AM, Corkill RG, Cadoux-Hudson TAD, Rajagopalan B, Styles P: Early proton magnetic resonance spectroscopy in normal-appearing brain correlates with outcome in patients following traumatic brain injury. *Brain* 2000;123: 2046–2054.

58. Garnett MR, Blamire AM, Rajagopalan B, Styles P, Cadoux-Hudson TAD: Evidence for cellular damage in normal-appearing white matter correlates with injury severity in patients following traumatic brain injury: A magnetic resonance spectroscopy study. *Brain* 2000;123:1403–1409.

59. Gurdjian ES. *Impact Head Injury*. Springfield, Ill: Charles C. Thomas; 1975.

60. Bigler ED. Structural Imaging. In: Silver JM, McAllister TW, Yudofsky SC, eds. *Textbook of Traumatic Brain Injury*. Washington, DC: American Psychiatric Publishing; 2005:79–105.

61. Zafonte RD, Ricker J, Yonas H, Wagner A: Frontal contusions imaging and behavioral consequences. *Am J Phys Med Rehabil* 2005;84:197–8.

62. Van Hoesen GW, Augustinack JC, Redman SJ: Ventromedial temporal lobe pathology in dementia, brain trauma, and schizophrenia. *Ann N Y Acad Sci* 1999;877:575–94.

63. Serra-Grabulosa JM, Junque C, Verger K, Salgado-Pineda P, Maneru C, Mercader JM: Cerebral correlates of declarative memory dysfunctions in early traumatic brain injury. *J Neurol Neurosurg Psychiatry* 2005;76:129–31.

64. Budson AE, Price BH: Memory Dysfunction. *N Engl J Med* 2005;352:692–699.

65. Marshall LF, Marshall SB, Klauber MR, Clark M, Eisenberg HM, Jane JA, Luerssen TG, Marmarou A, Foulkes MA: A new classification of head injury on computerized tomography. *J Neurosurg* 1991;75:S14-S20.

66. Ryser DK, Bigler ED, Blatter D. Clinical and neuroimaging predictors of post TBI outcome. In: Ponsford J, Snow P, Anderson V, eds. *International Perspectives in Traumatic Brain Injury*. Bowen Hills: Australian Academic Press; 1998:79–83.

67. Linacre JM, Heinemann AW, Wright BD, Granger CV, Hamilton BB: The structure and stability of the Functional Independence Measure. *Arch Phys Med Rehabil* 1994;75:127–32.

68. Hall K, Hamilton B, Gordon W, Zasler N: Characteristics and comparisons of functional assessment indices: Disability Rating Scale, Functional Independence Measure, and Functional Assessment Measure. *J Head Trauma Rehabil* 1993;8:60–74.

69. Rappaport M, Hall KM, Hopkins K, et al: Disability rating scale for severe head trauma: Coma to community. *Arch Phys Med Rehabil* 1982;63:118–123.

70. Gentry LR, Godersky JC, Thompson BH: Traumatic brain stem injury: MR imaging. *Radiology* 1989;171:177–187.

71. Kido DK, Cox C, Hamill RW, Rothenberg BM, Woolf PD: Traumatic brain injuries: Predicitive usefulness of CT. *Radiology* 1992;182:777–781.

72. Temkin NR, Machamer JE, Dikmen SS: Correlates of functional status 3–5 years after traumatic brain injury with CT abnormalities. *J Neurotrauma* 2003;20:229–41.

73. Henry-Feugas M, Azouvi P, Fontaine A, Denys P, Bussel B, Maaz F, Samson Y, Schouman-Claeys E: MRI analysis of brain atrophy after severe closed-head injury: Relation to clinical status. *Brain Inj* 2000;14:597–604.

74. Bigler ED, Neeley ES, Miller MJ, Tate DF, Rice SA, Cleavinger H, Wolfson L, Tschanz J, Welsh-Bohmer K: Cerebral volume, cognitive deficit and neuropsychological performance: Comparative measures of brain atrophy: I. Dementia. *JINS* 2004;10:442–52.

75. Collins MW, Iverson GL, Lovell MR, McKeag DB, Norwig J, Maroon J: On-Field predictors of neuropsychological and symptom deficit following sports-related concussion. *Clin J Sports Med* 2003;13:222–229.

76. Bigler ED, Burr R, Gale S, Norman MA, Kurth SM, Blatter DD, Abildskov T: Day of injury CT scan as an index to pre-injury brain morphology. *Brain Inj* 1994;8:231–238.

77. Bigler ED, Tate DF: Brain volume, intracranial volume, and dementia. *Invest Radiol* 2001;36:539–546.

78. Dikmen S, Machamer J, Miller B, Doctor J, Temkin N: Functional status examination: a new instrument for assessing outcome in traumatic brain injury. *J Neurotrauma* 2001;18:127–40.

79. Jennett B, Bond M: Assessment of outcome after severe brain damage. *Lancet* 1975;1:480–4.

80. Reitan RM, Wolfson D. *The Halstead-Reitan Neuropsychological Test Battery: Theory and Clinical Interpretation*. Tuscon: Neuropsychology Press; 1993.

81. Delis DC, Kramer JH, Kaplan JH, Kaplan E. *California Verbal Learning Test.* San Antonio, TX: The Psychological Corporation; 1987.

82. Umile EM, Sandel ME, Alavi A, Terry CM, Plotkin RC: Dynamic imaging in mild traumatic brain injury: Support for the theory of medial temporal vulnerability. *Arch Phys Med Rehabil* 2002;83:1506–1513.

83. Scheid R, Preul C, Gruber O, Wiggins C, von Cramon DY: Diffuse axonal injury associated with chronic traumatic brain injury: Evidence from T2*-weighted gradient-echo imaging at 3 T. *AJNR Am J Neuroradiol* 2003;24:1049–1056.

84. Bergeson AG, Lundin R, Parkinson RB, Tate DF, Victoroff J, Hopkins RO, Bigler ED: Clinical rating of cortical atrophy and cognitive correlates following traumatic brain injury [Abstract]. *J Neuropsychiatry Clin Neurosci* 2003;15:276–277.

85. Cato M, Delis D, Abildskov TJ, Bigler ED: Assessing the elusive cognitive deficits associated with ventromedial prefrontal damage: A case of a modern-day Phineas Gage. *JINS* 2004;10: 453–465.

86. Bigler ED, Anderson CV, Blatter DD: Temporal lobe morphology in normal aging and traumatic brain injury. *AJNR Am J Neuroradiol* 2002;23:255–266.

87. Slemmer JE, Matser EJT, De Zeeuw CI, Weber JT: Repeated mild injury causes cumulative damage to hippocampal cells. *Brain* 2002;125:2699–2709.

88. Parkinson RB, Hopkins RO, Cleavinger HB, Weaver LK, Victoroff J, Foley JF, Bigler ED: White matter hyperintensities and neuropsychological outcome following carbon monoxide poisoning. *Neurology* 2002;58:1525–1532.

89. Spilt A, Geeraedts T, de Craen AJ, Westendorp RG, Blauw GJ, van Buchem MA: Age-related changes in normal-appearing brain tissue and white matter hyperintensities: more of the same or something else? *AJNR Am J Neuroradiol* 2005;26:725–9.

90. Inglese M, Bomsztyk E, Gonen O, Mannon LJ, Grossman RI, Rusinek H: Dilated perivascular spaces: hallmarks of mild traumatic brain injury. *AJNR Am J Neuroradiol* 2005;26:719–24.

91. Giugni E, Sabatini U, Hagberg GE, Formisano R, Castriota-Scanderbeg A: Fast detection of diffuse axonal damage in severe traumatic brain injury: comparison of gradient-recalled echo and turbo proton echo-planar spectroscopic imaging MRI sequences. *AJNR Am J Neuroradiol* 2005;26:1140–8.

92. Bigler ED, Kerr B, Victoroff J, Tate D, Breitner JCS: White matter lesions, quantitative MRI and dementia. *Alzheimer Dis Assoc Disord* 2002;16:161–170.

93. Atlas S. *Magnetic resonance imaging of the brain and spine.* 3rd ed. Hagerstown, MD: Lipponcott, Williams & Wilkins; 2001.

94. Hopkins RO, McCourt A, Cleavinger H, Parkinson RB, Victoroff J, Bigler ED: White matter hyperintensities and neuropsychological outcome following traumatic brain injury. *JINS* 2003;9:234.

95. Cullum CM, Bigler ED: Ventricle size, cortical atrophy and the relationship with neuropsychological status in closed head injury: A quantitative analysis. *J Clin Exp Neuropsychol* 1986;8: 437–452.

96. Levin HS, Neyers CA, Grossman RG, Sarwar M: Ventricular enlargement after closed head injury. *Arch Neurol* 1981;38: 623–629.

97. Scahill RI, Frost C, Jenkins R, Whitwell JL, Rossor MN, Fox NC: A longitudinal study of brain volume changes in normal aging using serial registered magnetic resonance imaging. *Arch Neurol* 2003;60:989–994.

98. Bigler ED. Neuroimaging in traumatic brain injury. In: Raymond MJ, Bennet LC, Hartlage LC, Cullum CM, eds. *Mild Traumatic Brain Injury. A Clinician's Guide.* Austin, TX: Pro-ED; 1999.

99. Heimer L: Basal forebrain in the context of schizophrenia. *Brain Res Brain Res Rev* 2000;31:205–235.

100. Heimer L: A new anatomical framework for neuropsychiatric disorders and drug abuse. *Am J Psychiatry* 2003;160:1726–1739.

101. Gean AD. *Imaging of Head Trauma.* New York: Raven Press; 1994.

102. Di Virgilio G, Clarke S, Pizzolato G, Schaffner T: Cortical regions contributing to the anterior commissure in man. *Exp Brain Res* 1999;124:1–7.

103. Takaoka M, Tabuse H, Kumura E, Nakajima S, Tsuzuki T, Nakamura K, Okada A, Sugimoto H: Semiquantitative analysis

of corpus callosum injury using magnetic resonance imaging indicates clinical severity in patients with diffuse axonal injury. *J Neurol Neurosurg Psychiatry* 2002;73:289–293.

104. Mesulam M: The cholinergic lesion of Alzheimer's disease: pivotal factor or side show? *Learn Mem* 2004;11:43–9.

105. Olver JH, Ponsford JL, Curran CA: Outcome following traumatic brain injury: a comparison between 2 and 5 years after injury. *Brain Inj* 1996;10:841–848.

106. Salmond CH, Chatfield DA, Menon DK, Pickard JD, Sahakian BJ: Cognitive sequelae of head injury: involvement of basal forebrain and associated structures. *Brain* 2005;128:189–200.

107. Tomaiuolo F, Carlesimo GA, Di Paola M, Petrides M, Fera F, Bonanni R, Formisano R, Pasqualetti P, Caltagirone C: Gross morphology and morphometric sequelae in the hippocampus, fornix, and corpus callosum of patients with severe non-missile traumatic brain injury without macroscopically detectable lesions: a T1 weighted MRI study. *J Neurol Neurosurg Psychiatry* 2004;75: 1314–22.

108. Zilles K, Palomero-Gallagher N, Grefkes C, Scheperjans F, Boy C, Amunts K, Schleicher A: Architectonics of the human cerebral cortex and transmitter receptor fingerprints: reconciling functional neuroanatomy and neurochemistry. *Eur Neuropsychopharmacol* 2002;12:587–99.

109. Hofman PAM, Stapert SZ, van Kroonenburgh MJPG, Jolles J, de Kruijk J, Wilmink JT: MR imaging, single-photon emission CT, and neurocognitive performance after mild traumatic brain injury. *AJNR Am J Neuroradiol* 2001;22:441–449.

110. Ashburner J, Csernansky JG, Davatzikos C, Fox NC, Frisoni GB, Thompson PM: Computer-assisted imaging to assess brain structure in healthy and diseased brains. *Lancet Neurol* 2003;2:79–88.

111. Zhang L, Ravdin LD, Relkin N, Zimmerman RD, Jordan B, Lathan WE, Ulug AM: Increased diffusion in the brain of professional boxers: A preclinical sign of traumatic brain injury? *AJNR Am J Neuroradiol* 2003;24:52–57.

112. Kumar R, Gupta RK, Rao SB, Chawla S, Husain M, Rathore RK: Magnetization transfer and T2 quantitation in normal appearing cortical gray matter and white matter adjacent to focal abnormality in patients with traumatic brain injury. *Magn Reson Imaging* 2003;21:893–899.

113. Grefkes C, Weiss PH, Zilles K, Fink GR: Crossmodal processing of object features in human anterior intraparietal cortex: an fMRI study implies equivalencies between humans and monkeys. *Neuron* 2002;35:173–84.

114. Bodegard A, Geyer S, Grefkes C, Zilles K, Roland PE: Hierarchical processing of tactile shape in the human brain. *Neuron* 2001; 31:317–28.

115. Makale M, Solomon J, Patronas NJ, Danek A, Butman JA, Grafman J: Quantification of brain lesions using interactive automated software. *Behav Res Methods Instrum Comput* 2002; 34:6–18.

116. Crafton KR, Mark AN, Cramer SC: Improved understanding of cortical injury by incorporating measures of functional anatomy. *Brain* 2003;126:1650–1659.

117. Victoroff J, Mack WJ, Grafton ST, Schreiber SS, Chui HC: A method to improve interrater reliability of visual inspection of brain MRI scans in dementia. *Neurology* 1994;44:2267–2276.

118. Lainhart JE, Lazar M, Bigler ED, Alexander AL. The brain during life in autism: Advances in neuroimaging research. In: Casanova M, ed. *Recent Developments in Autism Research.* New York: Nova Science Publishers; 2005.

119. Bigler ED: Neurobiology and neuropathology underlie the neuropsychological deficits associated with traumatic brain injury. *Arch Clin Neuropsychol* 2003;18:595–621.

120. Mattiello JA, Munz M: Four types of acute post-traumatic intracranial hemorrhage. *N Engl J Med* 2001;344:580.

121. Sasaki M, Ehara S, Tamakawa Y, Takahashi S, Tohgi H, Sakai A, Mita T: MR anatomy of the substantia innominata and findings in Alzheimer disease: a preliminary report. *AJNR Am J Neuroradiol* 1995;16:2001–7.

122. Hanyu H, Asano T, Sakurai H, Tanaka Y, Takasaki M, Abe K: MR analysis of the substantia innominata in normal aging, Alzheimer disease, and other types of dementia. *AJNR Am J Neuroradiol* 2002;23:27–32.

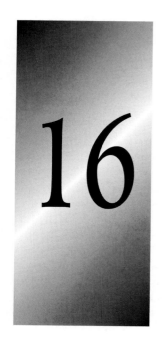

16 Functional Assessment in TBI Rehabilitation

Marcel Dijkers
Brian Greenwald

Chronic disease and injury often result in difficulties performing day-to-day activities, because of physical, cognitive or emotional impairments. The process of determining the type and degree of such problems, or the ability to perform normal acts, activities and roles, is typically designated "functional assessment". This is a misnomer, in that "assessment of function" or "functioning assessment" more clearly expresses the nature of this activity. Terms that overlap with "functional assessment" (FA) to a considerable degree are health status assessment, disability assessment or measurement, geriatric assessment, and others (1, 2). All of these activities aim to measure to what degree the person in his or her functioning deviates from "normal", where normal may refer to typical for persons without disorder (either all persons, or persons of the same age, gender, education, etc.), or the person's own pre-injury status.

Assessment in this context refers to quantification, where the exact position of the person on a continuum ranging from unable (complete lack of function) to very able (on a level with or even better than "average" or pre-injury) is determined and expressed in a number. This is the meaning of the term FA as commonly used in health care and rehabilitation practice and research. (From other perspectives, quantification is a more limited activity than assessment) (3). However, the term assessment has a second meaning, referring to evaluation or valuation: the

worth or meaning attached to the (amount of) function, by the person involved or by others. While the two types of "functional assessment" are strongly connected, the two are not synonymous. Whereas it is generally true that the value of a particular status increases with functional ability (being able to walk fast is more valuable than being able to walk only slowly), people may differ in how they valuate one ability compared to another (talking vs. reasoning), and in how they value one specific level of an ability compared to another level (4). These inter-individual differences come into play more, to the degree that the issue shifts from basic human functions (e.g. grasping) to more complex ones (holding down a job). Traditional methods of FA deal exclusively with the quantification issues (which are far from simple by themselves), and not with the valuation question. However, it is becoming increasingly clear that in order to assess with any level of adequacy what medical care and rehabilitation "produce", issues of valuation need to be dealt with (5). In this chapter, the reasons for and some methods of capturing the subjective valuing of functional states will be discussed, along with more traditional "functional assessment" methodologies and measures.

THE DISABLEMENT CONTINUUM

As suggested above, "functioning" may cover an extremely broad area, from simple functions involving a single body

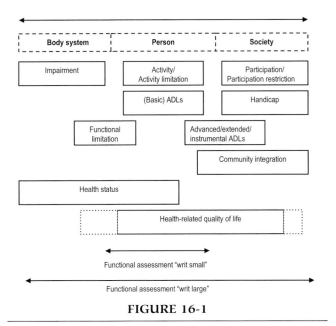

FIGURE 16-1

Aspects of functioning on a continuum

system to complex activities that are dependent on multiple physical and cognitive skills and are implemented in social interactions according to established social and cultural patterns. In Figure 16-1, the World Health Organization's International Classification of Functioning, Disability and Health (ICF) is used as a framework to delineate various concepts and terms encountered in the FA literature.

The WHO defines impairment as "problems in body function or structure as a significant deviation or loss"; in spite of the word "body", impairments include deficits in psychological functions (6) p.12. In a previous edition of the ICF, the International Classification of Impairments, Disabilities and Handicaps (ICIDH) (7) the same term was used; the taxonomy offered, however, did not make a clear distinction between deficits of structure and deficits of function at the impairment level. An FA instrument at the Impairment level often used in TBI care and research is the Glasgow Coma Scale (GCS) (8). At the level of the person, activity is characterized as "execution of a task or action by an individual"(6);p.14 its negative aspect, activity limitations, is defined as "difficulties an individual may have in executing activities"(6);p.14. The ICIDH used the term "disability" for this concept, which was defined very much similar to the current term "activity limitation". Within rehabilitation, the prototypical measure of activity limitations is the Functional Independence Measure (FIM) (9), but many other instruments have been used, within and outside traumatic brain injury rehabilitation. Finally, the person-in-interaction with others may have participation restrictions, which are defined as "problems an individual

may experience in involvement in life situations"(6)p.14; the positive counterpart is characterized as "involvement in a life situation";(6)p.14 In the ICIDH the term "handicap" was used for the negative aspect, which was defined in a manner quite different from the newer term. However, many of the measures developed to operationalize "handicap", such as the Craig Hospital Assessment and Reporting Technique (CHART) (10) are now used as measures of participation restrictions, including in the traumatic brain injury (TBI) literature.

Human activities range from simple acts such as stretching a leg to complicated pursuits such as running a household, and it is difficult to define the three concepts of impairment, activity (limitation) and participation (restriction) in a clear and non-overlapping way. The ICF offers separate concepts for the three domains of the disablement continuum, but only two taxonomies: one for Impairments, and one for Activities and Participation, with guidelines for users of the latter as to how the theoretical distinction might be implemented in practice, using the taxonomy. In some instances, it is even not simple to place any one act or activity in one of the three ICF baskets. Many measures of "functioning" such as the Disability Rating Scale (DRS) (11) overlap two or three of the concepts – intentionally or because the developers were not aware that the indicators they combined belonged to distinct conceptual classes.

FA "writ small" deals with Activities/Activity Limitations, and rehabilitation and other specialists have developed many measures to quantify self-care, mobility, everyday communication and other types of activities. We will focus on a limited number of measures commonly used in TBI services and research, but try to give the readers an overview of the concepts and techniques useful in understanding and evaluating instruments, and selecting them for clinical and research applications. FA "writ large" also includes measuring Impairments and Participation (12), and instruments that quantify those aspects of the latter two that are of relevance to TBI are included here.

Many terms developed prior to or outside the ICIDH/ICF can be placed on the same disablement continuum, as shown in Figure 16-1. The core interests of rehabilitation, Activities of Daily Living (ADLs) (sometimes designated basic ADLs) coincide with Activities. Extended (Instrumental, Advanced) ADLs (measured using e.g. the Frenchay Activities Index (FAI) (13) or the Adelaide Activities Profile (AAP) (14)) are generally defined to straddle the Activity-Participation distinction; on the other side of the continuum, Functional Limitations typically represent activities such as grasping and lifting that cross the divide between Impairments and Activities. Measures of Functional Limitations used in TBI care and research include the TEMPA(15) which assesses upper limb function. Developed and applied outside of TBI care are such UE measures as the CUE (16), and newer LE measures such as the WISCI (17). Community integration instruments, such as the CHART or, in TBI research more frequently, the Community Integration Questionnaire (CIQ) (18) quantify aspects of IADLs, and other facets of Participation, with emphasis on the social interactional components.

Health status, a term used by health outcomes researchers, typically is defined and operationalized as combining elements of Impairment and Activity Limitations, although some measures (such as the well-known Short-Form 36) (SF-36) (19) also includes indicators of Participation. The SF-36 now increasingly is used as a measure of quality of life (QOL). QOL has been defined in a number of ways;(20) most definitions and operationalizations of health-related QOL (HRQOL) overlap with Activities and Participation, and may even take in some aspects of Impairment. Many disease-specific HRQOL measures include symptoms, which typically are missing from Activity and Participation measures; however, many symptoms can be seen as Impairments, which suggests that HRQOL is somehow synonymous with "disablement", the term the ICIDH' authors used to represent the entire spectrum from Impairments through Handicaps.

THE STRUCTURE OF FUNCTIONAL ASSESSMENT INSTRUMENTS

At the simplest level, FA measures consist of a number of separate items, each one of which refers to a narrow or broad ability or skill – for instance, lifting overhead, transferring into a bathtub, or making telephone calls. On each item from two to as many as seven different levels or categories of "ability" are distinguished, which have quantitative values from 0 (or 1) to the highest. The lowest category corresponds to no ability/cannot do at all/need maximum help, and the highest to independence, "normal", or even above average. Additional metrics have been used, such as difficulty (21) and time needed (22). For measures of participation, metrics used include frequency of performing an activity (10), hours spent on an activity (23), share of activities performed (24), and others. The numbers a patient or subject receives on the constituent items typically are added together, and the total (with or without further arithmetical manipulation) reflects his or her functional status in the domain being measured. For some measures, the items all have the same number of steps and the same minimum and maximum value (e.g. FIM), but that is not necessarily the case – for instance, the Barthel Index(25) consists of some items with only two categories of ability, while the others items have three. Differential scoring of the categories from one item to the next can be used to express the relative

weight (importance) of the constituent skills for overall functioning, according to the instrument's creator. A separate weighting step prior to addition can be used to achieve the same purpose.

The numeric values of the categories (item scale steps) represent measurement on an ordinal scale – they only indicate relative order along the able-not able (or not participating-participating) continuum, but the differences between scale steps are not equivalent, and the values chosen for them are arbitrary. As a result, adding up the scores for the items to obtain the total score is not an operation that is allowed, based on the rules of mathematics. Therefore, total scores do not reflect position along a continuum that has a true zero point, and constant distances between scale points. (These constitute the definition of a ratio scale, which is what is required for calculating means for a group, or percentage improvement over time). However, research has shown that if the item category values are chosen "reasonably", the sum of ordinal items corresponds quite well to values on a true ratio scale, at least for intermediate levels of the continuum of total scores (26). Rasch analysis, a mathematical procedure based on Item Response Theory (IRT) has been used to transform a set of scores on ordinal FA items into a score on an interval scale (10, 21, 26). The theoretical assumptions and mathematical manipulations underlying Rasch Analysis-based FA instruments are beyond the scope of this chapter; good introductions to the technique and its application to FA may be found in Bond and Fox (27).

However, most FA measures used in TBI clinical services and research such as the GCS, DRS, and CIQ have never been subjected to Rasch analysis, let alone rescored on the basis of the findings of such an analysis. They may not be unidimensional, and increases from very low initial scores (e.g. a FIM total of 40) may be much easier to accomplish than apparently equally great increases (as expressed in score points) from medium or high starting points (e.g. a FIM of 90). As a result, one should be quite careful in interpreting FA instrument scores as applied to individuals, and to groups. Especially "percent improvement" and "change efficiency scores" should be considered as nothing but approximations of the mathematical precision they appear to offer. Calculation of means and all other operations that require interval scales (regression analysis, etc.) are somewhat less suspect, but the results also should be considered as approximations. Mathematical wizardry cannot make up for the basic problems created by ordinal measurement of skills and performances. In the years to come, more information on Rasch-analysis or IRT analysis of existing FA instruments will become available, and new instruments will be introduced that were developed using up-to-date IRT methods. We will be much more justified in treating the scores on those types of instruments as ratio scale numbers.

ISSUES IN FUNCTIONAL ASSESSMENT

Capacity and performance

Two aspects of functioning are commonly distinguished: capacity and performance (6). Capacity is what people can do under optimal circumstances – well rested, encouraged to their best, in a physical environment with minimal barriers. Performance is what they do do in everyday life. People who can do self-care not necessarily always do it, for a variety of reasons. One of the most common reason is that their environment is not accommodating, or that the energy and time a task requires preferentially are spent on other, more worthwhile endeavors – whether that is work or watching one's favorite soap opera. Studies with spinal cord injury patients have shown that many for whom self-care is a "marginal" skill prefer to have a personal care attendant or family member perform their care, so that they can get out of the house and get to their job (28). There are no clear parallels for cognitive-communicative skills after TBI, although it is likely that people with limited short-term memory and impaired ability to focus may leave it to others to read a bus schedule for them and tell them what time they need to catch the bus to make it to an appointment, even though with sufficient time and effort they could figure that out by themselves.

At the Impairment end of the disablement continuum, functional limitations tests tend to be performance focused. The ASIA motor scale(29) is based on the patient's ability to contract key muscles, and the physician and patient are hardly interested in the patient's actual frequency of contracting those muscles. At the other end of the continuum, measures of participation or community integration without exception quantify performance. It is either impossible to test capacity (how could one test "ability to function as a brain surgeon"), or not of interest: actual performance is of importance as the long-term outcome of rehabilitative efforts, not potential. It is in the middle ground, the domain of Activities, that a discrepancy between capacity and performance is most likely to be relevant, and performance is modifiable with environmental and other interventions.

Testing, observation and reporting on performance

Three methods are used to collect functional information. Testing involves requiring the patient or client (or research subject) to perform specific tasks or skills under the direct supervision of the test administrator, who times the test, assesses the amount of help from aids or aides that is needed, etc. This tends to occur in laboratory situations, but testing can also be done in the person's home or other setting where the activities involved are or should be performed (30). Depending on the degree to which the test situation approximates an optimal one, the resulting score quantifies optimal capacity, or capacity in the situation that is considered most relevant to the uses to which the functional information is to be put.

Observation of actual behavior is the basis for quantifying what the person does do, rather than what he or she can do. Most functional assessments of Activity reported as part of inpatient or outpatient rehabilitation programs is observation based – at least in theory. For instance, the Uniform Data System (UDS) FIM admission and discharge scores are based on what the patient does in the first three days after admission or the last three before discharge. In practice, there is continuous pressure on the patients to perform at their best, especially in treatment with PTs and OTs, and the measure of performance turns into a measure of capacity. Research using the LORS, for instance, has shown that scores reported by therapists are systematically lower than those reported by nurses (31). Nurses presumably report on what they observe the patients doing when going about their life on the nursing unit, while therapists only see them during scheduled hours, where they cannot waste time observing what the patients do naturally – the therapists need to optimize the patients' performance.

A third way of collecting FA information is through report by the patient, or a proxy such as a family member. These reports can involve capacity (for instance, in the CUE(16)), but more typically address performance. Questions are asked about how the person performs the various activities included in the FA measure in his or her daily routine. Using a standardized branching questionnaire, trained interviewers can reach a high-level of inter-rater (inter-interviewer) reliability. This is how data are typically collected for follow-up assessments in the UDS, and other program evaluation approaches.

All three methods have their advantages and disadvantages, in terms of cost, personnel needed, required ability of the patient to cooperate with the data collection, etc. If capacity data are of interest, testing is the preferred method; for true performance data, interviewing is the only feasible approach. Problems arise when the data obtained by two methods need to be linked. For instance, a typical question (clinically and in research) is whether the person manages to maintain or even improve on the skills he or she was discharged with from inpatient rehabilitation. The hospital data are typically collected using observation, in an environment that tends to be more accessible than the typical residence, and with overt or covert pressure to perform one's best. The home follow-up data are normally collected using interviews, concern performance in a different environment, in which there may be no incentive at all to use all the abilities taught in rehabilitation. If a change in functional performance is noted, is this due to the change in data collection method per se, or due to changes in the environment, or even because of changes in the true underlying capacity (continued neurological recovery)? This issue has hardly been studied, and we don't know enough about differences in scores for various data collection methods for various FA instruments to tease apart the various factors (32).

The nature of the items

In an IQ test, the person tested completes multiple arithmetic, similarities, and other items which in themselves are not of interest to the test administrator. The IQ score that results is of interest, because it gives an (imperfect) indication of the person's overall cognitive abilities. The focus is on the underlying trait – intelligence. In FA, however, the items most likely have intrinsic meaning, to the person performing the assessment and to the individual assessed: they reflect activities that are of importance in and of themselves – whether it is stair climbing or the ability to communicate a simple idea. FA "tends to occur within a realistic setting that approximates the one in which the actual criterion behavior will occur" (2) p101. That does not mean that there is no underlying construct "functional ability" that is of interest – but the underlying ability is of concern mostly because it informs on the functional items that were part of the assessment, and possibly on those that were not part of it. Because the primary interest is in the items (tasks, activities) themselves, there always is a tendency to include in FA measures the full panoply of acts that are part of normal human functioning. The Patient Evaluation and Conference System (PECS) in one of its versions included 97 items, of which as many as possible were to be completed as applicable to the patient (33, 34). Such an extensive menu is feasible when various staff report on patient status within their area of expertise (speech and language, neuropsychology, chaplaincy, etc.) but not in situations where subjects are tested, or are required to report on their performance. Maintaining a balance between feasibility and inclusion of those functional tasks that are key to living has always been a balancing act for FA instrument developers. Measures that cover "all areas of life" (or at least all aspects of Activities and Participation) tend to select fairly broadly defined tasks (e.g. "dressing"), and limit the number to 10 to 20. Instruments developed for use by specific disciplines are apt to include more narrowly defined tasks ("putting on a pull-over") and include a large number: The Klein-Bell ADL Scale contains 170 items to cover just six areas: dressing, mobility, elimination, bathing/hygiene, eating, and emergency telephone use (35).

When the focus of FA shifts from performance of individual tasks to the status of broad underlying abilities ("self care"; "motoric strength and coordination"), the need to include each and every possible item diminishes. Traditional psychometric methods can be used to show that the underlying construct can be measured with one set of items (indicators) as well as with another set,

and that the resulting total scores will have high correlations with one another. Some measures of functional limitations (the transition area between Impairments and Activities) do not attempt to "cover the waterfront"; they select activities that are representative of the entire universe of relevant items, and use those to score, for instance, upper extremity functioning. After all, once it is known how much difficulty a subject has picking up a can of soup, and how much picking up a ream of paper, it should be fairly clear how well she would do lifting a paperback book. To what degree this same reasoning applies at the other end of the disablement spectrum, Participation, is not yet known. The ICF distinguishes about 90 different aspects of "Participation", in 9 chapters covering communication, mobility, domestic life, etc. Is it necessary to obtain information on all of these to get a complete view of someone's level of Participation? Or is it possible to extrapolate from three household tasks to all others, and also to know quite adequately how well the person does in the civic responsibilities domain? That depends to a large degree on whether Participation is a single unidimensional construct, or a large collection of items that all reflect Participation in some way, but do not even represent multiple dimensions. There presumably are key Participation components that no FA instrument would want to omit (work, social relations with family), but the need to, and opportunity for, collecting information on all others is still not known. These and other problems involved in measuring Participation are discussed in greater detail in Dijkers et al. (36).

The presence of an unidimensional continuum underlying functional tasks makes it possible, for those whose interest is more in the patients'/clients'/subjects' status on the construct rather than their performance on each of the individual items, to use computer adaptive testing (CAT) and related techniques to administer very short, targeted sets of items, matched to the individuals' ability (performance) level, that produce the same quantity and quality of information as the more expansive sets of items from which these sets are drawn (37–39). To date, application of CAT to FA has been more demonstration of concept than use in daily clinical and research practice.

ISSUES IN MEASUREMENT: THE PSYCHOMETRIC CHARACTERISTICS OF FA INSTRUMENTS

Whenever we measure, error creeps into the resulting score, whether it is a small error in measuring simple concrete characteristics (for instance, the area of a room), or a large error in quantifying abstract concepts such as authoritarianism. FA is no exception, and the issue is not so much getting rid of the error (we never will be able to that completely), but being aware of the amount of error our data contain, and being aware what it means for any conclusions we draw and actions we undertake based on those data. Metrology (the science of measuring) is a major concern in all science disciplines, and the developers and users of FA instruments have mostly relied on the methodologies for instrument development originating in psychology. "Psychometrics" is a very technical and for most clinicians very boring subject, but knowledge of some of the basics is necessary for the fruitful use of FA instruments.

Traditionally, two aspects of the data reflecting the results of measurement have had most emphasis, validity and reliability, but in clinical applications such issues as sensitivity and practicality are increasingly getting attention. In theory, reliability is an aspect of validity, but most people tend to think of them as separate characteristics of instruments (or, more properly, of the data produced by instruments), and the techniques for quantifying validity and reliability are separate. "Validity" refers to the question: is this instrument measuring what it purports to measure? If it is targeting characteristic X, do the numbers reflect X, and not Y, or a little X with a lot of Z? "Reliability" refers to the question: how reproducible is this measurement – if we repeated the measurement operation, with the same or a similar "ruler", would we get the same result? As illustrated in Figure 16-2, an instrument can be very reliable without being valid. If it is not reliable at all, it by definition is not valid. The goal we are aiming for is instruments that are both valid (they measure what we want to measure) and reliable (they give results that are reproducible).

Over the years, a great many techniques have been developed to quantify validity and reliability, each applicable to different situations. Unfortunately, psychologists and social scientists have fallen into the habit of "inventing" new types of validity and reliability, by naming them after the techniques. However, there is no such thing as test-retest reliability or construct validity. There is only one validity and one reliability of each instrument, which are estimated using different techniques.

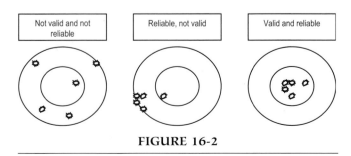

FIGURE 16-2

The relationship of reliability and validity

Reliability

Estimating the reliability of measures is the easiest to understand. The estimates all are based on some form of repeat measurement. If two clinicians at the same time rate the ability of patient X on the FIM Grooming item, they should come up with the same number – or else one or both are wrong. We can estimate the reliability of the FIM grooming item *as used by these two clinicians* by having the two rate a few hundred patients, and calculate how often they agree – completely, or almost so. A statistical formula such as coefficient kappa (or weighted kappa) can be used to express the result. All these formulas are constructed in such a way that the result, the reliability coefficient, varies between 0.00 (no reliability whatsoever) and 1.00 (perfect reliability). "Interrater reliability" can be estimated based on a few raters to represent all possible raters, so that we can have an idea as to how reliable this one-item instrument is in the hands of the average clinician.

If the same patients are rated by the same clinician twice, we similarly can calculate "intra-rater reliability", the degree to which she agrees with her earlier ratings. There are two scenarios for this – either the patients' performance is videotaped, or the rater observes the patients twice. In the latter case, it is of course important that we are sure these patients have not changed in the mean time. In both instances, the clinician should "forget" about her rating the first time around – which is not that difficult if large numbers of ratings are to be made.

Functional status is a fairly broad and abstract entity (a "construct", in psychometrical parlance), and it is unlikely that a single item such as Grooming can represent the entire construct. Typically, we select multiple indicators (items), and combine them to adequately operationalize the theoretical definition we may have. Use of multiple indicators has another advantage – any random measurement error involved with quantifying any one item is likely offset by the random error in another item. (For that reason, the more items there are in an instrument, the more reliable it will be, ceteris paribus, because the chance of random error being eliminated is increased. Any *systematic* error will just remain, however, and practical issues come into play if instruments are too long). Because each item in a FA instrument is a repeat measurement of the construct, like the two raters for Grooming are repeat measures, we can calculate the agreement between items, as yet another estimate of reliability. A number of formulas to estimate "internal consistency reliability" exist, the most frequently used of which is (Cronbach's) coefficient alpha. "Split-half" and "parallel forms" reliability are related formulas. All of them take values between 0.00 and 1.00.

The minimal level of reliability a measure needs to have depends on the purpose to which the data are to be put. A minimum of 0.90 for situations where decisions on an individual patient need to be made (discharge Mrs. Jones or extend her stay another week?) is often quoted, while 0.70 or 0.80 is a typical minimum required for group applications, such as in program evaluation and research. Longer instruments tend to be more reliable, but the trend is toward the use of short forms, such as the SF-12 and the CHART-SF rather than long ones, like their parents SF-36 and CHART. With better construction, new short instruments can offer reliability approximating that of older long ones. Another development is computer-adapted testing (CAT), in which only those questions that are targeted to the ability level of the person are being asked (39). For very simple instruments, paper-and-pencil adapted testing is possible (40, 41).

Validity

Validity cannot be estimated in such a simple way as reliability can, except in one unusual situation: there is an existing instrument that we are certain is perfectly valid. In that case, we can administer the old instrument and the new one to a sample, calculate the correlation between the two scores, and use that correlation as the estimate of the validity of the new measure. The issue of course is: if there is a perfectly good measure, why is there a need to develop a new one? (The importance of having a shorter scale may be the only acceptable reason). Less powerful methods are used in the more common situation: there is no existing measure, or the existing ones are problematic in themselves.

"Face validity" is (in the eyes of most authorities) not a form of validity determination, but an answer to the question: does the instrument "on the face of it" measure what those completing it expect to see – does a measure of X have questions about X that patients recognize as such? Some instruments have no or little face validity, but are perfectly valid – for instance, the Minnesota Multiphasic Personality Inventory (MMPI). In the arena of FA face validity is hardly an issue, because the constructs quantified, or at least the activities that are used as indicators, have a fairly low level of abstraction. The closely related term "content validity" refers to a measure covering the entire construct the developer is targeting, in the eyes of experts. It is generally determined by having the experts draw up lists of necessary content for a measure of X, or checking the content of the draft measure. Of course, this presumes there is a clear description (by the authors) of the concept they would like to operationalize – it makes no sense criticizing a painted portrait on realism if you don't know the person depicted. There are no standard formulas for calculating this validity aspect.

"Predictive validity" concerns the ability of a measure to predict a future state or event that is inherently linked to the characteristic being measured. A college entrance examination is said to have predictive validity if it can be used to accurately predict who in four (five, six) years will graduate. A parallel in FA would be the ability of a measure to predict who will be successfully discharged home versus to a nursing home. One problem with predictive validity assessment is the fact that there are no hard and fast rules as to what should be the minimum level of success in predicting. We know that many factors affect successful independent living – the accessibility of the home, family and other support available, the person's stubbornness and willingness to run risks of falling, etc. Does a FA instrument have adequate predictive validity if predictions based on it are correct 40% of the time? 50%?

"Known group validity" is based on differences in scale scores between two groups that are known to differ in the characteristic the instrument aims to measure. The average score of persons with TBI on a measure of physical functioning should be higher than the average of persons with SCI; in case of a measure of cognitive functioning, the situation should be reversed. If the data do not parallel these expectations, quite likely the instrument is not measuring what we think it is. Alternatively, a lot of systematic error (bias) is reflected in the data. A similar problem as mentioned above occurs with determining known group validity: how much of the variation in the functional status of the overall group should be explained by diagnostic category, TBI vs. SCI? If every person with TBI is known to have a higher physical functioning level than every person with an SCI, things would be easy: the variation explained should be 100%, and everything lower than that would mean less than perfect validity. However, the distributions for functioning ability of the SCI and TBI groups overlap, and the variation explained in a t-test reflects both the difference between group means, the standard deviations around those means, and the random and systematic error in the measure we use. Stating that a good functional measure should explain between 0% and 100% of variance is not very helpful in selecting or developing an instrument.

Lastly, "construct validity" concerns the relationships between the measurement data of a (highly abstract) construct and data for other constructs. Sometimes we have a basis in theory to predict that construct K should be strongly related to (yet not identical with) construct L, and be independent of construct M. (For instance, "ADL ability is related to community integration, but unrelated to political party preference"). If the data brings this out, the operationalization of K should be valid (and similarly the operationalizations of L and M). If the predicted association between K and L is minimal or absent, however, we don't know if the problem is with the theory, or the operationalization of K, or the measurement of L. And it is an unusual theory that specifies the exact strength of the relationship between K and L, predicated on perfect measurement of the constructs involved. "Strong" or "very strong" is the best we get, and those are not very good starting points for evaluating the level of validity of the instruments involved.

The above should make clear that the estimation of the validity of instruments always is less straightforward than the quantification of their reliability. Finding high values parallel to e.g. a 0.91 level of test-retest reliability just does not happen; validity coefficients are much lower, because all methods of validity estimation are roundabout. In practice, it is necessary to use all possible methods of estimating validity, and based on multiple findings "patch together" evidence supporting validity – which never will be iron-clad. Finding encouraging levels of the various types of validity distinguished here, in multiple studies, with patterns of correlations that make sense based on expert knowledge, is what typically occurs. Fortunately, in the case of FA, the construct being measured is fairly concrete, and the specialists involved have extensive knowledge of the determinants, correlates, intergroup differences etc. of various aspects of functional status, making the issue of assessing the quality of specific measures less problematic than the preceding list of issues might suggest.

"Ecological validity" does not concern validity proper, but the relevance of assessment data to real-life situations outside the testing situation. For instance, the Wisconsin card-sort test(42) is a measure of executive functioning (the ability to plan, initiate, execute, monitor and correct one's actions) often used by neuropsychologists to assess persons with TBI. Like all neuropsychological tests, it is administered in a quiet office after the person tested has had a good night's sleep and is still fresh, etc. How well do the results predict the patient's ability to make breakfast for her children while testing the middle schooler on history and finishing her own make-up before leaving for work, with the TV competing for attention?(43) Testing executive functioning in situations that resemble the real world would provide data that are more "ecologically valid", but the standardization of testing might suffer. Standardization of testing has always been a keystone of psychometric methods of assessing reliability and validity of neuropsychological instruments, and of quantifying the abilities of individual patients or clients – they are capacity measures. However, standardized environments tend to be dissimilar from the settings where people perform self-care, communicate, do work and all other things captured under the umbrella of functioning. Testing in a standardized environment almost always means in an optimal environment – and the results tend therefore to be more indicative of capacity than of performance.

Sensitivity.

It is easy to see that if a FA "measure" has just two categories: "able" and "unable", it lacks sensitivity: it cannot reflect fine distinctions in ability/performance, and it cannot be used to record minor but clinically significant changes. Sensitivity refers to the ability of an instrument to capture distinctions that are clinically relevant or small enough to be of importance in research, across the full extent of the range of ability of the cases to be measured. When sensitivity is discussed in relation to change, the term responsiveness is frequently used.

Floor effects and ceiling effects are one issue in sensitivity. The first terms refer to the lowest measurable level of performance on an FA instrument being higher than what is the status of the least able person to be measured. All individuals who have ability equal to the lowest measurable level or lower are clumped together and given the corresponding score. Vice versa, a ceiling effect means that the highest measurable level is lower than the level of at least some of the more able patients/clients. It should be noted that very often measures are developed for one population, in which they have no floor or ceiling effects, but then applied to another, in which they do. For instance, the FIM was designed to quantify functional status of rehabilitation inpatients, and any patient who achieves the maximum score on discharge was probably an inappropriate admission. However, a few years after onset of TBI many persons will score at the maximum of the Motor FIM subscale. The FIM was never designed to distinguish between people with minimal deficits that do not affect functioning, other mere mortals, and Superman. Thus, "lack of responsiveness" sometimes is a problem for which the instrument user is responsible, not the instrument developer.

Quantification of responsiveness is not done using formulas resulting in simple coefficients ranging from 0.0 (not responsive at all) to 1.0 (maximum responsiveness possible). All methods are mostly useful for comparing responsiveness of one measure with that of another, allowing one to select the most responsive one. A variety of indices are used, including effect sizes (the mean change between time 1 and time 2 divided by the standard deviation at time 1), the standardized response mean (the mean change between time 1 and time 2, divided by the standard deviation of change scores), receiver operating characteristic (ROC) analysis, and many others. Discussion of these indices is beyond the scope of this chapter; the reader is referred to the extensive literature (44–46). A particular subgroup of these indices involves a rating, typically by the patients themselves, that from time 1 to time 2 they have improved (or deteriorated) a little or a lot, or stayed the same; any FA score changes should correspond to these subjective "transition ratings" (47, 48), or else it lacks responsiveness.

Other psychometric characteristics

Beyond validity, reliability and sensitivity, there are a number of other characteristics of a FA measure that are relevant to its use in clinical, program and research applications, most of which have to do with practicality:

- Language: this is especially relevant to self-administered measures, such as the CIQ (18), but may also be an issue with observational and other measures. Both the reading level and a translation in a language the user is familiar with are of concern
- Training required: many observational FA instruments and test-type measures require the user to be trained, and sometimes certified (30), in order to produce reliable data
- Time and equipment required: measures that take inordinate time on the part of the subjects or the administrator, or that use special equipment (in some test-type measures such as the Tufts assessment of motor performance (TAMP) (49)) may not be suitable outside research applications

USES OF FUNCTIONAL ASSESSMENT

The origin of FA (writ small) in medical rehabilitation is in attempts by clinicians to express quantitatively the deficits patients had on admission to rehabilitation, and to monitor progress, or at least determine discharge status, so that there was some "proof" of the effectiveness of treatment, beyond the patient's simple report that he or she now could do things that were impossible or difficult before admission. The fore-runners of instruments such as the Barthel Index (BI) (25) were simple checklists for recording (lack of) problems with performing self-care and mobility activities (2). From these simple early efforts, measurement instruments of sometimes great sophistication have grown. In addition, the range of applications of these instruments has expanded tremendously, so that we now can describe uses in the care of individual patients, treatment programs as a whole, reimbursement, and research. The type of information needed in these various applications is somewhat different, and even when the basic instrument used is the same (the FIM is the "workhorse" of medical rehabilitation, and is used almost throughout all these types of applications), ideally there would be differences in scoring or other details.

Uses in care of individual patients

Decisions on admissions to inpatient and outpatient programs are often based on a formal FA, to see if the person has the types and degrees of deficits that the program is qualified and authorized to treat, either in general or for the specific person in question. The "baseline" assessment therefore often is communicated to the third party payor, who may use it to approve program admission and a certain duration or intensity of treatment. The pre-admission or admission assessment is frequently the basis for a prognosis, which is communicated to the patient and the payor, and ideally underlies goal setting. Many programs use an FA instrument such as the FIM to set goals, either for classes of patients or for individual patients. Software applications have been developed to assist case managers to make such predictions; they are based in large part on a data base that contains the data on many previous patients with the same rehabilitation diagnosis, age, gender and co-morbidities.

Goal setting ideally is more individualized than the limited number of constituent items and/or outcome levels of standard instruments allow. Several methodologies have been developed to allow more or less "customized" selection and quantification of goals, which then are the basis for treatment plan development. Results can be monitored to see if goals are reached (in the time span planned), or need to be modified based on new or initially unknown complicating factors. Goal Attainment Scaling (GAS) is a method originally developed in the mental health arena(50) that has been applied in medical rehabilitation, mostly for research purposes, it seems (51, 52).

In GAS, the client and therapist together set multiple goals, and for each determine the most likely outcome level, as well as two levels of lesser accomplishment, and two of better accomplishment. For instance, for the goal mobility, the target level could be "household walker – can ambulate 50 feet without walker, and without difficulty". Lower levels could reflect use of supports and/or lesser distance (scored as –1 and –2); higher levels greater distance and/or outdoors mobility (scored as +1 and +2). Each of the several goals (walking; bathing; doing dishes, etc.) is given an importance weight reflecting patient/client valuation. To calculate the overall outcome of treatment, the outcomes for the various goals are summed, after weighting by the importance factors. Thus, the GAS and derivative methods incorporate to some degree the individual valuation of functioning components, but do so only for those actions and activities that display major deficits, rather for all domains of functioning. The end result of the outcomes operationalization reflects success in terms of the goals set, not client functioning in terms of deviation from "normal". For that reason, these types of instruments may be more useful in clinical applications than in research on the determinants and consequences of functional deficits. Appropriate use of functional measures for goal setting must take into account premorbid function, patient resources (financial assets, family and community support), and known prognostic information. The Canadian Occupational Performance Measure (COPM) (53, 54) uses a methodology very similar to GAS. Ironically, much less is known about the reliability of individualized instruments such as the GAS and COPM than about the measurement qualities of standardized instruments such as the FIM.

Decisions on treatment termination should be based on a number of factors, that include not just functional status (achievement of treatment goal, plateauing) but also family factors, carry over and continuation or generalization of functional skills learned in therapy.

Treatment monitoring using a FA measure is applied in many rehabilitation programs, even if the goals have been set without patient input or without subjective a-priori weighting. Team rounds often exist of the reporting by "most responsible/ knowledgeable therapies" (nursing for bladder; speech for expression, etc.) of the current status of the patient on the numeric items offered by the FA instrument used in the facility. Even before powerful desk-top or hand-held computers existed, various facilities had developed computerized systems for collecting and displaying functional status information – e.g. the Rehabilitation Indicators project (55) and the PECS (33, 34, 56). Even if weekly or less frequent team meetings do not employ formal quantification, the status of the patient with respect to various skills and other aspects of Impairment, Activities and (in outpatient programs) Participation is typically discussed. Almost all rehabilitation programs quantify status on discharge, because that information is needed to document program results, and subsequently is used in program evaluation. While increasingly treatment termination decisions are based on "external" criteria (e.g. a maximal length of stay approved by a third party payor), ideally they are founded on either the accomplishment of goals, or plateauing of the patient in terms of overall functional ability. In both instances, measurement of patient status should be performed using an instrument that has minimal error so that (lack of) change can be reliably determined.

FA information may also be used to communicate about progress and outcomes of treatment with persons who are not part of the team. Patients themselves, their family members, referral sources, and payors have a keen interest in the functional aspects of the patient's status, especially where it concerns Activities and Participation. One additional use of FA for individual cases is long-term monitoring of a patient's status. Especially in the case of progressive diseases, this type of information is important to make decisions on new treatments, changes in patient environments, etc. In fact, this use of FA has led to a designation of functional status information as a sixth (after the standard four and pain) vital sign (57).

The foregoing issues suggest that the choice of an appropriate validated FA measure for the individual with TBI depends on a number of factors including: time after injury, rehabilitation setting, and goals of rehabilitation. When clinical improvement is seen, and goals and maybe even the rehabilitation setting (inpatient acute and subacute, etc.) are changed, the measurement tools should be reevaluated. The use of a scale that is insensitive to the improvement that is expected, or not measuring the progress toward an individual's goal, should be avoided.

Uses in program administration.

Most rehabilitation programs have as their overall goal something along the lines of: to improve quality of life by reducing impairments and increasing activities and participation level. Program evaluation aims to assess to what degree a program indeed accomplishes what it sets out to do – improve functional status of people with disablement. Basic questions are: do patients change for the better (program effectiveness), and if so, are resources used optimally in accomplishing this (program efficiency).

While change from admission to discharge from a program is common, it is unfortunately not easy to offer proof that the program deserves credit. For instance, a person with TBI may score higher on a post-test than on a pre-test for a number of reasons that have nothing to do with the selection, timing, quality and quantity of services received: natural recovery, improved test-taking ability, and many others (58). All rehabilitation programs face the same problem, and one solution that has been found is to compare outcomes between programs, under the assumption that not *all* change in *all* programs can be explained by causes other than treatment received, and the "excess" change in the best programs is truly the result of interventions. Longitudinal evaluation of a program's outcomes is facilitated by creation of a minimal data set for all programs that includes demographics, time since injury and measures of injury severity, in addition to specific scales of functioning, selection of which depends on program type and time of follow-up (59). The Uniform Data System (UDS) in which most inpatient rehabilitation facilities in the US participate, as well as some subacute facilities and nursing homes that offer rehabilitation, is one such data aggregator.

Comparisons between programs is fair only, of course, if their inputs (admission status) are the same; it may be much easier to bring an admit FIM score of 50 up to 100 for someone with SCI than for a patient with TBI. Thus, UDS and other aggregators produce reports that compare like with like, in terms of diagnostic group, co-morbidities, age, and other factors considered relevant to chances of program success. The focus tends to be on functional status change over time, as the key indicator of effectiveness. Because the better programs may achieve a certain level of change using much fewer resources than poorly organized ones, length of stay (LOS) is typically used as a gross indicator of resource use. Functional status change per day then is an indicator of program efficiency. (It may be worth repeating here that a number of assumptions, including interval-level measurement of functional status, are made that may not stand up to scrutiny). There are other methods of evaluating a program's effectiveness, e.g. by evaluating what percentage of the patients did achieve the goals that were set at admission. It is natural that a small percentage of patients do not progress as well as anticipated, e.g. due to inter-current illness. But if a large percentage fails to make the standardized or individualized functional goals set for them, the program is either selecting the wrong types of patients, or staff and programs are ineffective. Shifts in program admission policies, management or processes may be needed. Unfortunately, routine program evaluation data tend to be insufficient to indicate where exactly the problem is and how it can be fixed; additional studies are needed to obtain that information. However, routine outcome data can and should be communicated to stakeholders, including current and future patients, third party payors, and the local community. The Centers for Medicare and Medicaid Services (CMS) has started to post comparative functional outcomes for nursing homes on its website, and it is to be expected that similar "report cards" including functional FA information will be published in the future for many other facilities that offer rehabilitation of some type.

Choosing appropriate functional measures for the evaluation of a TBI program should be based on what point of the rehabilitation spectrum the program serves. Measures of impaired structure/function would be appropriate for acute inpatient care, with coma scales used for low level patients. Activity measures are most appropriate for acute or subacute inpatient care; Participation measures are needed to assess the effectiveness and efficiency of outpatient services in the community.

The Commission on Accreditation of Rehabilitation Facilities (CARF) (http://www.carf.org) is a widely recognized not-for profit accrediting organizations and programs, including TBI programs. It currently offers accreditation in seven categories of brain injury services, including inpatient hospital rehabilitation, residential services, and home and community-based services. Accreditation is based on documenting adherence to standards as well as a surveyors' evaluation. Depending on the level of care different criteria need to be met. Ensuring patient and family education as well as considering future rehabilitation needs are required components. Outcome measures include appropriate functional assessment during and after treatment. Patient and family satisfaction measures also play an important role.

In addition to program evaluation (which is a CARF-required activity) and accreditation, FA data are used in a variety of activities centering on improving program services quality. Whether they are called outcomes management, continuous quality improvement (CQI), or total quality management (TQM), they all involve considering the organization delivering services as a system, with parts and subsystems that all should be studied continuously to reduce inefficiencies, improve administrative and clinical procedures, and reduce risks and adverse events (3). FA information almost by definition plays a key role in making decisions in programs that deal with individuals with TBI or other disabilities. For instance, an

admission-to-discharge increase in functioning less than a specified minimum could be an indicator threshold violation that triggers an in-depth investigation whether a problem (opportunity to improve processes) exists. FA information could also function as a monitor that is collected routinely to indicate functioning of the program(s) – a vital sign for the organization.

Effective 2002, CMS has, under its Prospective Payment System (PPS), paid inpatient rehabilitation facilities (IRFs), fixed amounts for each patient discharged, rather than reimbursing (adjusted) charges, costs of operations or some other formula used in earlier years and still used by other payors. The fixed amounts are based in part on the functional status of the patient on admission, combined with diagnostic category (stroke, TBI, SCI, etc.) and age category. For functional status a minor variation on the FIM is used, which is embedded in the IRF-Patient Assessment Instrument (IRF-PAI). The combination of diagnosis, IRF-PAI functional status category and age defines a group whose rehabilitation requires unique resources, as acknowledged in the payment amount for each case (60). (This payment is further adjusted for comorbidities ("tiers"), salary levels in the region the facility is located, etc.). The PPS has given facilities financial incentive to hasten if not improve outcomes. Facilities need to ensure they are doing functional assessment accurately to document patient impairment.

The National Committee on Vital and Health Statistics (NCVHS) has recommended capturing and classifying functional status information as part of routine health care transactions, so that administrative databases could be mined and used for a variety of purposes, including monitoring overall population health, health care management, public health planning, predicting costs and financial management, and policy development (61). At the moment, only limited information on functioning is available, mostly through Medicare files, on special populations: those receiving inpatient rehabilitation (IRF-PAI), nursing home residents (Minimum Data Set – MDS), and people receiving home health (Outcome and Assessment Information Set – OASIS). The Subcommittee on Populations of the National Committee on Vital and Health Statistics which investigated these issues suggested that, with modifications, the ICF might be a useful taxonomic system (a "uniform code") to base such data collection across the continuum of care on. The uniform code would not prescribe *how* to measure functional status, but only specify *what* data elements need to be reported. (In this sense, it would be comparable with e.g. the ICD, which does not specify *how* to diagnose a particular disease, only *what* the disorders of interest are and how they are related to one another). A German group under the guidance of Stucki and associated with the WHO has begun the development of ICF "core sets" – listings of selected Impairments, Activity Limitations and Participation Restrictions that are of particular relevance to the care and management of a particular diagnostic group (62–64). The ICF allows coding the severity of Impairments, Activity Limitations and Participation Restrictions,(65) but these are very "primitive" methods that do not operationalize measurement. Presumably, productive use of the core sets, especially in applications beyond clinical care, requires a system or systems of functional assessment.

Uses in research

Program evaluation typically does not address what was done for individual patients (the "black box" aspect of rehabilitation) to explain changes in functional status and link those interventions to outcomes. It also does not systematically address alternative explanations for outcomes, and has no hard evidence for the effectiveness of traditional or innovative treatments. This is where research comes in. Per end June, 2005, Medline contained over 27,000 records classified under "Activities of Daily Living", which is used to classify papers on ADLs, (chronic) limitations of activity, independent living, and self care. Functional assessment papers are also indexed under other headings – for instance, "geriatric assessment" added another 2,000 plus unduplicated records. Of this total, only a small number addresses clinical application at the level of the individual (presumably less than 5%) and a slightly larger number (maybe 10%) concerns the program level uses of FA measures. Most published research concerns either the development of FA instruments, including assessing reliability, validity, sensitivity, and practicality characteristics, or the use of FA measures to evaluate the effects of rehabilitation, describe the natural course of disablement, assess the financial and social impact of disability, etc.

Because functioning is the central interest of rehabilitation providers and researchers, and their patients/clients, it is to be expected that much of their research uses FA information as either the "independent" (predictor) variable, or the "dependent" (outcome) one, or both. The same holds true with respect to TBI rehabilitation: FA measures, whether specific to individuals to this diagnostic group (CIQ,(18, 66) Disability Rating Scale (DRS),(11)) or generic (FIM) are used in a large percentage of the published research. In this literature one also finds application of very specialized measures (e.g. of functional communication) that will not be covered here. It is worthwhile to remember, though, that before any use is made of its results, this research needs to be assessed in terms of the applicability of the FA instruments selected, and their psychometric qualities.

SUBJECTIVE VALUATION OF FUNCTIONAL PERFORMANCE

A major criticism of most of the FA measures used in TBI clinical care, program evaluation and research is the fact that they do not reflect the subjective view of the person involved. "Normal functioning" may be a laudable goal, but not if that functioning detracts from the person's subjective QOL. For instance, O'Neill et al. found that persons with TBI may do better holding down part-time rather than (normative) full-time jobs. (67). Several studies have shown that measures of participation account for much more of the variance in life satisfaction or well-being measures than do measures of impairment or activity limitations (68–71). Thus, the nature of the fit between functional activities and the person's values, preferences and abilities needs to be considered and reflected in some way in FA instruments, especially in Participation measures. Corrigan noted that outcomes can be defined from three perspectives: that of the person with TBI, that of the healthcare professionals treating the injury, and that of society (72). The latter two perspective presumably are reflected, to some degree, in the FA measures commonly used. However, the point of view of the insider, the person with TBI, to date has not been investigated with any degree of the attention it deserves.

This case has been made most fervently by Brown and Gordon (5). They argue that in the measurement of social constructs, value judgments are involved, and the values of the insiders (here: persons with TBI) and the outsiders (persons without disability: clinicians, researchers) may be different. Power imbalances occur in measurement whenever the outsider's values and preferences are incorporated into the means-ends chain leading from interventions to immediate outcomes to ultimate outcomes, with few, if any, mechanisms for tapping into the values and preferences of the insider. Such power imbalances are of concern because the insider's perspective can vary significantly from that of the outsider.

While most instruments designed to measure aspects of "functioning" have concentrated on the "how independent" and "how much" of acts, actions and roles, a few have explored additional dimensions. GAS and the COPM, mentioned above, are semi-structured approaches by which rehabilitation service recipients formulate individualized goals for therapy and provide perceptions of the adequacy of their performance, their satisfaction with performance, and the importance of each goal to their lives. An importance-weighted sum of outcome serves as the key evaluation measure.

Given their open-ended nature, GAS and COPM goals specified can reflect performance in the domains of Participation and Activity, and even inclusion of Impairment aspects is possible. The choice of goals reflects individual valuation, as does the importance rating. A number of other instruments with standardized content have included importance ratings, such as the MACTAR (73) and many instruments traditionally classified as quality of life measures (74).

Three approaches to measuring participation with attention to both its objective and its subjective dimensions have been developed. Based on the (draft) CIQ-2, Johnston et al. derived a version in which subjects expressed their opinions and feelings about their participation (75). Each CIQ-2 question about objective aspects of everyday life was supplemented by three questions:

- "How satisfied or dissatisfied are you" with the activity? A 7-point rating scale was offered.
- "Would you like this to change?" Four response categories were offered: no; yes, want more; yes, want less; and yes, want a qualitative change.
- "How important would this change be to you?" Five response categories were offered.

A similar addendum was created by Cicerone et al. for the original CIQ (76). CIQ scores had no correlation with the Quality of Community Integration Questionnaire, and fairly weak correlations with the Satisfaction with Cognitive Functioning, suggesting that satisfaction with the underlying cognitive skills needed for participation not necessarily translates into satisfaction with participation per se, which may be restricted by non-cognitive impairments in the person, or societal barriers.

Similar conclusions were reached in a third study that evaluated a participation instrument we developed that incorporates both objective and subjective elements, the POPS (described below). Brown et al. found that persons with and without TBI rated the importance of the 26 items included in the POPS largely the same (23). At the individual item level, there was a fairly strong relationship between the level of involvement (PO), and desire for change (PS): those individuals (particularly those with TBI) who did little or nothing of an activity almost never wanted to do less, and more often wanted to do more. The PO total score was only weakly correlated with the PS total score (0.22 for the TBI group; 0.16 for the comparison group), again indicating that satisfaction with participation (as reflected in desire to change) is not predicted very well by overall level of participation in those activities that "society" typically declares part of the repertoire of its adult members – the normative view reflected in objective participation instruments.

Subjective measures of the type described have a number of shortcomings, according to critics. First, they typically involve the multiplication of two factors, one an importance rating, the other a satisfaction rating or a desire for change indicator. The critics claim that no measurement model applies to such a procedure, and that therefore the resulting item scores and total scores have no meaning, or at least cannot be considered reliable or valid. The measurement model of classical test theory and that of IRT only recognize simple items each measured on an ordinal scale as input to measurement instruments that operationalize constructs on a (pseudo) interval scale. Another criticism of individualized measures is that if

individuals can determine (by exclusion or even nomination) which particular activities should be included in a measure, and with what weight, the "content" of the construct varies from person to person, and performing averaging and other statistical manipulations makes no sense. However, if the *content* in all instances judged (by the researcher) to be relevant to the construct, there is no problem. Personal construct psychology adherents see this as a strength of the methodology, rather than a weakness.

SELECTION OF A FUNCTIONAL ASSESSMENT MEASURE

The selection of a FA measure to apply in a clinical, administrative or research situation is not straightforward. A first step always should be determining what one wants to measure: Activity (Limitation) only, or aspects of Impairment and Participation (Restriction) in addition? While there are a few instruments such as the Disability Rating Scale that cover all three domains, they do that often poorly, and using two or three separate instruments may be preferable. A second question is: what aspect of functioning is of interest, capacity or performance, and consequently what type of administration should be selected: testing in a laboratory or other setting, observation, or report by the patient or a proxy. This limits choices, and one's options might be even more restricted if the population one deals with has particular characteristics that make application of the most common instruments impossible – e.g. intubation. The resources available for administration – a special laboratory, administrator training, time of administrator and subject – typically play a major role. Lastly, metrology characteristics – reliability, validity, sensitivity - should inform the selection, although in some situations the choice of instruments is so limited that one needs to accept a measure with less than stellar characteristics.

The following sections offer thumbnail descriptions of some of the more common FA measures used in TBI rehabilitation and outcomes research, or in similar applications on broader groups. The information offered is necessarily limited. The TBI Model Systems of Care maintain a website, COMBI (Center on Outcome Measurement in Brain Injury) (http://www.tbims.org/combi/list.html) that in mid-2005 contained information on 27 instruments commonly used in TBI clinical services and research, including most of the ones listed below. (The ones covered are marked with an asterisk). For each instrument, the following are offered: the actual instrument (subject to copyright restrictions); a syllabus containing administration and scoring instructions; information on administrator training and testing required; a description of the psychometric qualities of the instrument, based on the published literature; and frequently asked questions. The various sections are kept up-to-date by experts, frequently the individual(s) who created the instrument involved. This resource is highly recommended to anyone needing more information on any of the measures listed below.

IMPAIRMENT/FUNCTIONAL LIMITATION MEASURES

Glasgow Coma Scale

The most commonly used and universally accepted TBI impairment instrument is the Glasgow Coma Scale (GCS) (8). The GCS was designed as a brief measure of the depth of coma that can be applied in the acute care setting. Three physical exam parameters are assessed: best visual, verbal, and motor responses. Eye opening is scored 1 to 4, verbal response is scored 1 to 5, and motor response is scored 1 to 6. Total scores, which can range from 3 to 15, typically are stratified into three levels: severe (GCS 3–8), moderate (GCS 9–12), and mild (GCS 13–15) (77). Of the three subscores, the GCS motor score has been found to be the most sensitive to long term outcome (78).

The GCS has been found to be a strong predictor of outcomes including as measured by acute care costs and mortality (79–86). In much research on outcomes of services provided in rehabilitation or the community, the GCS is used as a basic indicator of injury severity. Control for severity by using GCS as a covariate allows a better assessment of the impact of (experimental) treatment. However, it should be realized that the GCS score can be falsely low in the presence of drugs, alcohol, hypoxia or hypotension. Conversely it can be falsely high in the presence of an undetected expanding hematoma. Determining a GCS score may be difficult when a patient is intubated. Meredith published a study validating the accuracy of deriving a verbal score for intubated patients based on eye and motor subscores (87).

ACTIVITY/ACTIVITY LIMITATION MEASURES

Barthel Index

The Barthel Index (BI), developed in the fifties by Mahoney and Barthel(25) at one point in time was the major FA instrument in use in rehabilitation in the USA. It was improved upon and supplanted by the FIM, and now mostly has historic significance. However, clinicians and researchers in the United Kingdom, Australia and elsewhere still use the BI and modifications of it. The BI consist of 10 physical functioning items. Feeding, dressing, toilet transfer and stairs are scored on a 3-point scale: can do alone (10 points), can do with help (5), and cannot do at all (0). Grooming and washing/bathing are scored on a two-point scale: can do alone (10 points), can do with help or cannot do at all (0). Bladder control and bowel control are on a three-point scale: incontinent (0), accidents (5) and unimpaired (10). Chair/bed transfer is also on a three-point scale, but independence gets 15 points, help needed either 10 or 5 (if much help is needed). Lastly, walking 50 yards is on a two-point scale: 15 points if independent, 0 if needs help. If the person cannot walk, wheelchair propulsion is substituted, which has a maximum score of 5 for ability, with or without help. The highest BI score possible is 100, the minimum is 0, and intermediate points are interpreted as percent of maximum. Alternatives and extensions of the BI have been created that add items, make the scoring more sensitive, or otherwise improve on this rather crude but simple instrument (2).

*Functional Independence Measure

The Functional Independence Measure or FIM, the dominant FA (writ small) instrument in US and international medical rehabilitation for the last 20 years was created, as part of an effort to develop a uniform system to track rehabilitation data, to improve upon the BI (9). It maintained all the BI items, splitting some, and added tasks reflecting status in the socio-cognitive domain. Initially the FIM for all its components used four-point rating scales, but early on, at the request of clinicians who wanted greater sensitivity, these were replaced by seven-point scales, reflecting a range from total assistance (score 1) to complete independence (score 7). Some recent scholarship suggests that in practice, clinicians cannot reliably distinguish the seven categories, and that a four-category scale may be more useful (88). Extensive manuals have been published to guide raters in how to apply the rating scale in each domain, and how to handle unusual situations, such as: should the motor items be scored with or without the patient's orthosis in place (89).

There are 18 items in the FIM, 13 covering ADLs, bowel/bladder care, and mobility, and 5 reflecting everyday communication and cognition. Some applications calculate a single FIM total score by summing over the 18 items, resulting in a total between 18 (total lack of functional ability) to 126 (normal or almost normal), but a more common algorithm, that has considerable research support(26, 90) uses the 13 motor items to calculate a motor subscale score, and the 5 remaining items to calculate a (socio)cognitive subscale score. More fine-grained subscales have been distinguished in various studies,(91) but for "routine" applications the two-subscale method is satisfactory. Typical administration of the FIM is by observation for inpatient rehabilitation status, and standardized interview for follow-up. However, self-administered versions have been used, and one study even used testing on the entire instrument (92). Testing on individual items is commonly done in research.

Many studies have reported on the internal consistency, test-retest or interrater reliability, validity and other psychometrics of the FIM, which characteristics have generally been found to be satisfactory, for the motor component more so than for the socio-cognitive one. A quantitative summary of the research up to 1995 is provided by Ottenbacher et al (93). A criticisms of the FIM sometimes reported is that it has ceiling effects, either in all diagnostic groups, or in selected ones. However, it should be kept in mind that it was designed for quantifying functional status in acute rehabilitation inpatients; within that population, almost all persons are not at ceiling, although there are exceptions, e.g. for SCI patients on the socio-cognitive scale. Use of the FIM in routine rehabilitation practice follows the rule that if a patient is not observed performing a particular task, that task should be coded 1. For instance, many rehabilitation programs do not ask patients to do a tub transfer on admission, and stairs may never be attempted by some diagnostic groups on admission or discharge. This coding instruction causes "missing information" to coincide with "total assistance", causing serious distortions when these clinical data are used in research and other applications (60).

A separate version of the FIM has been developed for children, specifically those under 7 years of age, who for developmental reasons do not score maximal on the FIM items, even in the absence of disablement. The WeeFIM has the same 18 items, and the same 7 item categories for each, but the scoring instructions take developmental issues into account (94–96). Among TBI researchers, dissatisfaction with the limited coverage by the FIM of communicative, cognitive, and behavioral disturbances after brain injury lead to the creation of a "FIM-annex", the *Functional Assessment Measure (FAM), which offers an additional 12 items in these domains (97). The 30-item FIM+FAM has been subjected to limited testing of psychometric qualities, but appears a satisfactory measure (98).

PARTICIPATION/PARTICIPATION RESTRICTION MEASURES

"Social disability", "social adjustment", "social integration", "community integration" and "handicap" have been the organizing concepts for a number of measures that quantify participation in household and other productive activities, other social role performance, social relationships and similar activities now captured in the rubric "Participation" (36). Of the major "Participation" scales that are found in the (TBI) rehabilitation literature, the Craig Hospital Assessment and Recording Technique (CHART) (10), the Community Integration Questionnaire (CIQ) and the Mayo-Portland Adaptability Inventory (MPAI) (99) are based, to varying degrees, on the handicap concept of the ICIDH, the forerunner of the ICF. Three measures based on ICF concepts to date have not

or only on a limited basis been used in published studies with individuals with TBI: Life-H(100); POPS(23) and the Participation Measure for Post-Acute Care (PM-PAC) (101).

*Craig Handicap Assessment and Reporting Technique (CHART)

The Craig Handicap Assessment and Reporting Technique was designed to provide a simple, objective measure of the degree to which impairments and disabilities result in handicaps in the years after initial rehabilitation (10). The original CHART, developed in 1992, included domains to assess five of the WHO dimensions of handicap: physical independence, mobility, occupation, social integration, and economic self-sufficiency. Orientation (ability to orient self to one's surroundings) was added later (102). The revised CHART consists of 32 questions and employs up to seven questions in each of the six domains to quantify the extent to which individuals fulfill various social roles. The items focus on observable criteria and have been worded to minimize ambiguity and promote a consistent interpretation.

Each of the subscales of the CHART has a maximum score of 100 points, which indicates that roles within the domain are fulfilled at a level equivalent to that of the norm: an able-bodied person. High subscale scores indicate less handicap, or higher social and community participation. The CHART was designed to be administered by interview, either in person or by telephone, and takes approximately 15 minutes. Participant-proxy agreement across disability groups has provided evidence in support of the use of proxy data for persons with various types of disabilities. The CHART has been found to be an appropriate measure of handicap that can be used with individuals having a range of physical or cognitive impairments, including individuals with TBI. The instrument has been used for research by the developers,(103–108), and others,(109, 110).

A short form of the CHART (*CHART-SF) was developed using regression analysis and related statistical methods to select items, followed by rescoring so as to create the same 0–100 ranges as the original CHART displays. The Short Form has 19 items (instead of 32); its metric properties and equivalence to the CHART have not yet been evaluated.

*Community Integration Questionnaire (CIQ)

The Community Integration Questionnaire constitutes a measure of rehabilitation outcome after TBI which reflects the values and goals of individuals who have a disability. Willer and his associates developed the CIQ using the following design criteria: brevity; suitable for use in an in-person or telephone interview, conducted with the person with TBI him/herself (preferably), or with a proxy; focus on behaviors rather than feeling states; no biases resulting from age, gender or socioeconomic status; sensitive to a wide variety of living situations; and value neutral (18, 66, 111). Factor analysis was the basis for selecting from a larger pool of items 15 questions addressing home integration (H), social integration (S), and productive activities (P). These questions focus on involvement in roles and household chores, frequency of activities; one addresses the nature of leisure partners: family, friends with or without TBI. The CIQ has been used extensively in research on individuals with TBI, (67, 76, 108, 109, 112–117) as well as those with other types of acquired brain injury.

Dijkers reviewed the psychometric evidence available for the CIQ, and concluded that there were concerns with respect to reliability and validity; sensitivity and score distributions were problematic, and age and gender biases were prominent (24). He embarked on the development of an updated version (known as CIQ-2), which sought to rectify these problems, while maintaining as much of the old measure as possible. Items were added that broadened the scope of household and social activities, as well as travel and mobility; nature of companions and of the organization where the person works or goes to school were added. The final instrument, consisting of 37 questions, has not yet been published. A preliminary version was used in one published study that incorporated a modification that added a subjective participation component (75).

Participation Objective, Participation Subjective (POPS)

The Participation Objective, Participation Subjective (POPS) measure developed by Brown et al. (23) differs from typical participation instruments in several ways:

- It focuses solely on activities, not on non-activity indicators related to community functioning, e.g., income, whether one's companions are largely disabled or able-bodied. The 26 items range from sexual activity to work, and from paying bills to speaking to strangers.
- It generates two measures: the PO, comprising an "objective" measure of participation, and the PS, comprising a subjective measure.

Subjective assessment (the PS measure) incorporates the preferences of the person by gauging the individual's satisfaction with his/her level of engagement in each activity, weighted by his/her rating of the activity's importance. These product scores are averaged across the 26 items to calculate a total score. In addition, there are five subscores more-or-less paralleling the ICF Activity domains: Domestic life, Interpersonal interactions and relationships, Major

life areas (work, school, etc.), Transportation, and Community, recreational and civic life.

The PO gauges performance in terms of frequency or duration of engagement in activity in real environments, not in terms of degree of impaired functioning. Total score and domain subscores are calculated using an algorithm that takes into account the importance ratings that persons with TBI and non-disabled individuals gave to these items, reflecting "societal" values rather than individual ones. (23).

Participation Measure for Post-Acute Care (PM-PAC)

The Participation Measure for Post-Acute Care (PM-PAC) was designed to measure "participation outcomes of rehabilitation services provided in outpatient or home-care settings" From the literature and existing instruments the developers created or adopted a final set of 33 items in seven domains derived from the ICF: mobility; role functioning; community, social and civic life; domestic life; economic life; interpersonal relationships; and communication. (101). Items were written to "reflect a person's degree of perceived limitation in a particular life situation regardless of cause or means". Most items use a 5-point degree of limitation (not at all to extremely) response scale, but duration and degree of satisfaction are also used. Factor analysis and item response theory models were used to asses the dimensionality of the various subscales; some items needed to be reassigned, but in general the results indicated useful subscales ranging from three to nine items each, in which the "limitation", duration and satisfaction items combined well. Further research, including development of computer adapted testing (CAT) versions, is planned.

MEASURES THAT CROSS-CUT ICF DOMAINS

*Level of Cognitive Function Scale (LCFS)

The Rancho Los Amigos Level of Cognitive Function Scale (Rancho or LCFS) was designed to describe the typical stages of behavioral recovery following a severe TBI during inpatient rehabilitation (118). The Rancho consists of a single 8-level ordinal item in which each category corresponds to increasingly complex behaviors. (With just a single item, the LCFS differs from the other FA instruments discussed here, and technically is not a "scale"). The simplicity of the scale has brought it into wide use by healthcare providers and payers.

The Rancho has been shown to have a modest degree of validity and reliability (119). Scores on admission to rehabilitation correlate with 24-hour GCS score, length of coma, and duration of posttraumatic amnesia. In addition, the LCFS correlates with the DRS and the FIM and FAM cognitive items (120). Given the correlations between measures of severity and disability, it is not surprising that the Rancho score on admission to rehabilitation is associated with vocational outcomes (121, 122). When applying the Rancho scale, it should be recognized that it was devised only as a descriptor. Recovery from severe brain injury is not linear. In addition, patients may vary in their Rancho level depending on the time of day and other circumstances. The Rancho is not a particularly sensitive measure of recovery and it should not be used to measure recovery. Patients may skip levels or never go beyond a particular level, despite ongoing progress.

Thus, the Rancho scale is best used as it was initially designed, as a simple descriptive scale. It can offer some advantage in pre-admission screening and communication with healthcare providers/ payers. It can also alert rehabilitation teams to treatment issues they are likely to face.

*Disability Rating Scale (DRS)

Rappaport's Disability Rating Scale (DRS) has 8 items that address the three original World Health Organization categories of impairments, disability and handicap (7). The first three items of the DRS (eye opening, communication ability, and motor response) are slight modification of the Glasgow Coma Scale(8) and reflect impairment ratings. Cognitive ability for feeding, toileting, and grooming items reflect level of disability. Handicap is addressed with two items, ability to live independently and employability. Each of the areas of functioning is rated on a scale of 0 to either 3 or 5, with the highest scores representing the higher level of disability. The maximum score is 29 (extreme vegetative state); a person without disability would score zero. The DRS rating must be obtained while the individual is not under the influence of anesthesia, other mind-altering drugs, recent seizure, or recovering from surgical anesthesia.

The DRS is fairly easy to use and can generally be completed in under 5 minutes. It can be scored from direct observation, via clinical interview, or by telephone interview (123). No significant technical training is required to administer the scale. Subjective assessment by clinicians is required for cognitive capacity of self-care, rather than actual observation of self care items. This subjective rating is also used for rating employability and independent living potential. The DRS is more reliable than the Level of Cognitive Functioning Scale (119). It has been used to predict ability to return to employment based on admission and discharge DRS scores (122–124). The DRS has been shown to be an effective scale to track progress across the continuum of clinical services and the course of functional recovery (11, 123).

Many studies have reported good reliability and validity coefficients for the DRS (106, 119, 120, 122, 123, 125–127). Limitations of the DRS include its assessment of general functioning rather than specific functional changes, its lack of utility in patients with only physical disability, and its poor sensitivity to functional evaluation of mild or very severe impairment (DRS Score >22), where small functional changes may not be reflected in scores (120). Therefore, the DRS is more useful when used in conjunction with more detailed measures of function. For patients with Functional Independent Measure (FIM) scores >25, the FIM may have more sensitivity to changes in rehabilitation than the DRS (128). Subjectivity of rating cognitive capacity may also limit its use in mild or severe injuries. In addition, the DRS falls short in assessing patients with severe apraxia, aphasia, or aphonia as well as those who are "locked in" or have tracheostomies.

*Mayo-Portland Adaptability Inventory (MPAI)

The Mayo-Portland Adaptability Inventory (MPAI), developed from a modification of Lezak's Portland Adaptability Inventory, was designed to assist in the clinical evaluation of people during the post-hospital period following TBI, and to assist in the evaluation of rehabilitation programs designed to serve this population. The MPAI can be completed by professional staff, people with TBI and/or their significant others. In the most recent version, MPAI-4, items represent the range of physical, cognitive, emotional, behavioral, and social problems that people may encounter after TBI. MPAI-4 items also provide an assessment of major obstacles to community integration that may result directly from TBI, as well as features of the social and physical environment. The three subscales (Ability, Adjustment, and Participation) have good psychometric properties.

The MPAI-4 and its predecessors have been used in a number of studies initiated by the co-developer and his associates (99, 129–133). Unfortunately, the MPAI has found no use outside this group.

*Glasgow Outcome Scale (GOS)

The Glasgow Outcome Scale is a ordinal, single-item instrument used to describe outcome after TBI globally (134). It was commonly used before instruments such as the DRS and GCS were introduced. As a brief outcome scale it has been replaced by the DRS, which offers greater sensitivity to small changes or differences. However, the GOS it is still used occasionally, especially in neurosurgical studies of outcome after TBI. The five categories of the original scale are: dead, vegetative, severely disabled, moderately disabled, and good recovery. The *Extended Glasgow Outcome Scale (GOS-E), an expanded version of the scale, divides each of the latter three categories in two, creating eight categories and increasing sensitivity of the instrument. A structured interview was introduced to rectify a second problem of the GOS: fairly low inter-rater reliability (135). Adequate interrater reliability and content validity have been demonstrated for the GOS-E, and compared to the GOS, the GOS-E has been shown to be more sensitive to change in mild to moderate TBI (136). The validity of the GOS-E is also superior to that of the original measure (137).

References

1. Keith RA. Functional status and health status. *Arch Phys Med Rehabil* 1994;75:478–483.
2. Crewe NM, Dijkers M. Functional assessment. In: Scherer M, Cushman L, eds. *Psychological Assessment in Medical Rehabilitation Settings.* Washington DC: American Psychological Association; 1995:101–144.
3. Johnston MV, Eastwood E, Wilkerson DL, Anderson L, Alves A. Systematically asessing and improving the quality and outcomes of medical rehabilitation programs. In: Delisa JA, Gans BM, Walsh NE, eds. *Physical Medicine and Rehabilitation: Principles and Practice.* 4th ed. Philadelphia: Lippincott Williams Wilkins; 2005:1163–1192.
4. Stineman MG, Wechsler B, Ross R, Maislin G. A method for measuring quality of life through subjective weighting of functional status. *Arch Phys Med Rehabil* 2003;84:S15–22.
5. Brown M, Gordon WA. Empowerment in measurement: "muscle," "voice," and subjective quality of life as a gold standard. *Arch Phys Med Rehabil* 2004;85:S13–20.
6. World Health Organization. *International Classification of Functioning, Disability and Health: ICF.* Geneva: World Health Organization; 2001.
7. World Health Organization. *International Classification of Impairments, Disabilities and Handicaps. A Manual of Classification Relating to the Consequenses of Disease.* Geneva: World Health Organization; 1980.
8. Teasdale G, Jennett B. Assessment of coma and impaired consciousness. A practical scale. *Lancet* 1974;2:81–84.
9. Keith RA, Granger CV, Hamilton BB, Sherwin FS. The functional independence measure: A new tool for rehabilitation. *Adv Clin Rehabil* 1987;1:6–18.
10. Whiteneck GG, Charlifue SW, Gerhart KA, Overholser JD, Richardson GN. Quantifying handicap: A new measure of long-term rehabilitation outcomes. *Arch Phys Med Rehabil* 1992;73:519–526.
11. Rappaport M, Hall KM, Hopkins K, Belleza T, Cope DN. Disability rating scale for severe head trauma: Coma to community. *Arch Phys Med Rehabil* 1982;63:118–123.
12. Frey W. Functional assessment in the 80s: A conceptual enigma, a technical challenge. In: Halpern A, Fuhrer M, eds. *Functional Assessment in Rehabilitation.* Baltimore: Paul H. Brooks Publishing Co.; 1984:11–43.
13. Holbrook M, Skilbeck CE. An activities index for use with stroke patients. *Age Ageing.* 1983;12:166–170.
14. Clark MS, Bond MJ. The Adelaide Activities Profile: A measure of the life-style activities of elderly people. *Aging (Milano).* 1995;7:174–184.
15. Moseley AM, Yap MC. Interrater reliability of the TEMPA for the measurement of upper limb function in adults with traumatic brain injury. *J Head Trauma Rehabil* 2003;18:526–531.
16. Marino RJ, Shea JA, Stineman MG. The Capabilities of Upper Extremity instrument: Reliability and validity of a measure of functional limitation in tetraplegia. *Arch Phys Med Rehabil* 1998;79:1512–1521.
17. Ditunno JF,Jr, Ditunno PL, Graziani V, et al. Walking Index for Spinal Cord Injury (WISCI): An international multicenter validity and reliability study. *Spinal Cord* 2000;38:234–243.
18. Willer B, Ottenbacher KJ, Coad ML. The Community Integration Questionnaire. A comparative examination. *Am J Phys Med Rehabil* 1994;73:103–111.
19. Ware JE,Jr, Sherbourne CD. The MOS 36-item short-form health survey (SF-36). I. Conceptual framework and item selection. *Med Care.* 1992;30:473–483.
20. Dijkers MP. Quality of life after traumatic brain injury: A review of research approaches and findings. *Arch Phys Med Rehabil* 2004;85:S21–35.
21. Jette AM, Haley SM, Coster WJ, et al. Late life function and disability instrument: I. Development and evaluation of the disability component. *J Gerontol A Biol Sci Med Sci.* 2002;57:M209–16.
22. Gerrity MS, Gaylord S, Williams ME. Short versions of the timed manual performance test. Development, reliability, and validity. *Med Care.* 1993;31:617–628.
23. Brown M, Dijkers M, Gordon WA, Ashman T, Charatz H. Participation Objective, Participation Subjective: A measure of participation combining outsider and insider perspectives. *J Head Trauma Rehabil* 2004;19:459–481.
24. Dijkers M. Measuring the long-term outcomes of traumatic brain injury: A review of the Community Integration Questionnaire. *J Head Trauma Rehabil.* 1997;12:74–91.
25. Mahoney FI, Barthel DW. Functional evaluation: The Barthel Index. *Md State Med J* 1965;14:61–65.
26. Linacre JM, Heinemann AW, Wright BD, Granger CV, Hamilton BB. The structure and stability of the Functional Independence Measure. *Arch Phys Med Rehabil* 1994;75:127–132.
27. Bond TG, Fox CM. *Applying the Rasch Model. Fundamental Measurement in the Human Sciences.* Mahwah, NJ: Erlbaum;2001.
28. Martin C, Dijkers M, DeSantis N. Self-care skills: Learning and abandoning. Chicago: American Spinal Injury Association; 1994.
29. Marino RJ, Ditunno JF, Donovan WH, et al, eds. *International Standards for Neurological and Functional Classification of Spinal Cord Injury.* Chicago: 2000.
30. Park S, Fisher AG, Velozo CA. Using the Assessment of Motor and Process Skills to compare occupational performance between clinic and home settings. *Am J Occup Ther.* 1994;48:697–709.
31. Malzer RL. Patient performance level during inpatient physical rehabilitation: Therapist, nurse, and patient perspectives. *Arch Phys Med Rehabil* 1988;69:363–365.
32. Smith PM, Illig SB, Fiedler RC, Hamilton BB, Ottenbacher KJ. Intermodal agreement of follow-up telephone functional assessment using the Functional Independence Measure in patients with stroke. *Arch Phys Med Rehabil* 1996;77:431–435.
33. Jellinek HM, Torkelson RM, Harvey RF. Functional abilities and distress levels in brain injured patients at long-term follow-up. *Arch Phys Med Rehabil* 1982;63:160–162.
34. Harvey RF, Jellinek HM. Patient profiles: Utilization in functional performance assessment. *Arch Phys Med Rehabil* 1983;64:268–271.
35. Klein RM, Bell B. Self-care skills: Behavioral measurement with Klein-Bell ADL scale. *Arch Phys Med Rehabil* 1982;63:335–338.
36. Dijkers MP, Whiteneck G, El-Jaroudi R. Measures of social outcomes in disability research. *Arch Phys Med Rehabil* 2000;81: S63–80.
37. Webster K, Cella D, Yost K. The Functional Assessment of Chronic Illness Therapy (FACIT) measurement system: Properties, applications, and interpretation. *Health Qual Life Outcomes* 2003;1:79.
38. Andres PL, Black-Schaffer RM, Ni P, Haley SM. Computer adaptive testing: A strategy for monitoring stroke rehabilitation across settings. *Top Stroke Rehabil* 2004;11:33–39.
39. Dijkers MP. A computer adaptive testing simulation applied to the FIM instrument motor component. *Arch Phys Med Rehabil* 2003;84:384–393.
40. Bode RK, Heinemann AW, Semik P. Measurement properties of the Galveston Orientation and Amnesia Test (GOAT) and improvement patterns during inpatient rehabilitation. *J Head Trauma Rehabil.* 2000;15:637–655.
41. Cook KF, Roddey TS, Gartsman GM, Olson SL. Development and psychometric evaluation of the flexilevel scale of shoulder function. *Med Care* 2003;41:823–835.
42. Vayalakkara J, Backhaus SD, Bradley JD, Simco ER, Golden CJ. Abbreviated form of the Wisconsin Card Sort Test. *Int J Neurosci.* 2000;103:131–137.
43. Manchester D, Priestley N, Jackson H. The assessment of executive functions: Coming out of the office. *Brain Inj* 2004;18: 1067–1081.

44. Terwee CB, Dekker FW, Wiersinga WM, Prummel MF, Bossuyt PM. On assessing responsiveness of health-related quality of life instruments: Guidelines for instrument evaluation. *Qual Life Res.* 2003;12:349–362.

45. Ward MM, Marx AS, Barry NN. Identification of clinically important changes in health status using receiver operating characteristic curves. *J Clin Epidemiol.* 2000;53:279–284.

46. Diehr P, Chen L, Patrick D, Feng Z, Yasui Y. Reliability, effect size, and responsiveness of health status measures in the design of randomized and cluster-randomized trials. *Contemp Clin Trials.* 2005;26:45–58.

47. Fischer D, Stewart AL, Bloch DA, Lorig K, Laurent D, Holman H. Capturing the patient's view of change as a clinical outcome measure. *JAMA* 1999;282:1157–1162.

48. Guyatt GH, Norman GR, Juniper EF, Griffith LE. A critical look at transition ratings. *J Clin Epidemiol.* 2002;55:900–908.

49. Gans BM, Haley SM, Hallenborg SC, Mann N, Inacio CA, Faas RM. Description and interobserver reliability of the Tufts Assessment of Motor Performance. *Am J Phys Med Rehabil* 1988;67: 202–210.

50. Kiresuk TJ, Sherman RE. Goal Attainment Scaling: A general method for evaluating comprehensive community mental health programs. *Community Mental Health J.* 1968:4(6): 443–453.

51. Malec JF. Goal Attainment Scaling in rehabilitation. *Neuropsychological Rehabilitation.* 1999;9:253–275.

52. Rockwood K, Joyce B, Stolee P. Use of Goal Attainment Scaling in measuring clinically important change in cognitive rehabilitation patients. *J Clin Epidemiol.* 1997;50:581–588.

53. Law M, Baptiste S, McColl M, Opzoomer A, Polatajko H, Pollock N. The Canadian Occupational Performance Measure: An outcome measure for occupational therapy. *Can J Occup Ther.* 1990;57:82–87.

54. Pollock N, Baptiste S, Law M, McColl MA, Opzoomer A, Polatajko H. Occupational performance measures: A review based on the guidelines for the client-centred practice of occupational therapy. *Can J Occup Ther.* 1990;57:77–81.

55. Brown M, Diller L, Gordon WA, Fordyce W, Jacobs D. Rehabilitation indicators and program evaluation. *Rehabil Psychol.* 1984; 29:21–35.

56. Harvey RF, Jellinek HM. Functional performance assessment: A program approach. *Arch Phys Med Rehabil* 1981;62:456–460.

57. Bierman AS. Functional status: The sixth vital sign. *J Gen Intern Med* 2001;16:785–786.

58. Campbell DT, Stanley JC. *Experimental and Quasi-Experimental Designs for Research.* Chicago: Rand McNally and Company; 1963.

59. Hall KM, Johnston MV. Outcomes evaluation in TBI rehabilitation. part II: Measurement tools for a nationwide data system. *Arch Phys Med Rehabil* 1994;75:SC10–8.

60. Carter GM, Relles DA, Ridgeway GK, Rimes CM. Measuring function for medicare inpatient rehabilitation payment. *Health Care Financ Rev* 2003;24:25–44.

61. Iezzoni LI, Greenberg MS. Capturing and classifying functional status information in administrative databases. *Health Care Financ Rev* 2003;24:61–76.

62. Cieza A, Stucki G, Weigl M, et al. ICF core sets for low back pain. *J Rehabil Med* 2004;(Suppl 44):69–74.

63. Geyh S, Cieza A, Schouten J, et al. ICF core sets for stroke. *J Rehabil Med* 2004;(44 Suppl):135–141.

64. Stucki G, Cieza A, Geyh S, et al. ICF core sets for rheumatoid arthritis. *J Rehabil Med* 2004;(Suppl 44):87–93.

65. Ustun TB, Chatterji S, Kostansjek N, Bickenbach J. WHO's ICF and functional status information in health records. *Health Care Financ Rev* 2003;24:77–88.

66. Willer B, Rosenthal M, Kreutzer JS , Gordon WA, Rempel R. Assessment of community integration following rehabilitation for traumatic brain injury. *J Head Trauma Rehabil* 1993;8: 75–87.

67. O'Neill J, Hibbard MR, Brown M, et al. The effect of employment on quality of life and community integration after traumatic brain injury. *J Head Trauma Rehabil* 1998;13:68–79.

68. Heinemann AW, Whiteneck GG. Relationships among impairment, disability, handicap and life satisfaction in persons with

traumatic brain injury. *Journal of Head Trauma Rehabilitation.* 1995;10:54–63.

69. Pierce CA. Life satisfaction after traumatic brain injury and the WHO model of disablement. unpublished manuscript

70. Huebner RA, Johnson K, Bennett CM, Schneck C. Community participation and quality of life outcomes after adult traumatic brain injury. *Am J Occup Ther.* 2003;57:177–185.

71. Dijkers M. Quality of life after spinal cord injury: A meta analysis of the effects of disablement components. *Spinal Cord.* 1997; 35:829–840.

72. Corrigan JD. Community integration following traumatic brain injury. *NeuroRehabilitation.* 1994;4:109–121.

73. Tugwell P, Bombardier C, Buchanan WW, Goldsmith CH, Grace E, Hanna B. The MACTAR patient preference disability questionnaire—an individualized functional priority approach for assessing improvement in physical disability in clinical trials in rheumatoid arthritis. *J Rheumatol.* 1987;14:446–451.

74. Dijkers MP. Individualization in quality of life measurement: Instruments and approaches. *Arch Phys Med Rehabil* 2003;84: S3–14.

75. Johnston MV, Goverover Y, Dijkers MP. Community activities and individuals' satisfaction with them: Quality of life in the first year after traumatic brain injury. *Arch Phys Med Rehabil* 2005;86:735—745.

76. Cicerone KD, Mott T, Azulay J, Friel JC. Community integration and satisfaction with functioning after intensive cognitive rehabilitation for traumatic brain injury. *Arch Phys Med Rehabil* 2004;85:943–950.

77. Clifton GL, Hayes RL, Levin HS, Michel ME, Choi SC. Outcome measures for clinical trials involving traumatically brain-injured patients: Report of a conference. *Neurosurgery.* 1992;31:975–978.

78. Hall KM. Functional assessment in traumatic brain injury. In: Rosenthal M, Griffith ER, Kreutzer JS, Pentland B, eds. *Rehabilitation of the Adult and Child with Traumatic Brain Injury.* 3rd ed. Philadelphia: FA Davis; 1999:131–146.

79. Rocca B, Martin C, Viviand X, Bidet PF, Saint-Gilles HL, Chevalier A. Comparison of four severity scores in patients with head trauma. *J Trauma.* 1989;29:299–305.

80. Levati A, Farina ML, Vecchi G, Rossanda M, Marrubini MB. Prognosis of severe head injuries. *J Neurosurg.* 1982;57:779–783.

81. Pal J, Brown R, Fleiszer D. The value of the Glasgow Coma Scale and injury severity score: Predicting outcome in multiple trauma patients with head injury. *J Trauma.* 1989;29:746–748.

82. Katz DI, Alexander MP. Traumatic brain injury. Predicting course of recovery and outcome for patients admitted to rehabilitation. *Arch Neurol.* 1994;51:661–670.

83. Narayan RK, Greenberg RP, Miller JD, et al. Improved confidence of outcome prediction in severe head injury. A comparative analysis of the clinical examination, multimodality evoked potentials, CT scanning, and intracranial pressure. *J Neurosurg.* 1981;54: 751–762.

84. Choi SC, Narayan RK, Anderson RL, Ward JD. Enhanced specificity of prognosis in severe head injury. *J Neurosurg.* 1988;69: 381–385.

85. Changaris DG, McGraw CP, Richardson JD, Garretson HD, Arpin EJ, Shields CB. Correlation of cerebral perfusion pressure and Glasgow Coma Scale to outcome. *J Trauma.* 1987;27:1007–1013.

86. Lehmkuhl LD, Hall KM, Mann N, Gordon WA. Factors that influence costs and length of stay of persons with traumatic brain injury in acute care and inpatient rehabilitation. *J Head Trauma Rehabil* 1993;8:88–100.

87. Meredith W, Rutledge R, Fakhry SM, Emery S, Kromhout-Schiro S. The conundrum of the Glasgow Coma Scale in intubated patients: A linear regression prediction of the Glasgow verbal score from the Glasgow eye and motor scores. *J Trauma.* 1998;44:839–44;discussion 844–5.

88. Nilsson AL, Sunnerhagen KS, Grimby G. Scoring alternatives for FIM in neurological disorders applying Rasch analysis. *Acta Neurol Scand.* 2005;111:264–273.

89. Granger CV, Hamilton BB, Kayton R. Guide for the use of the Functional Independence Measure (WeeFIM) of the Uniform Data Set for medical rehabilitation. Buffalo: Research Foundation of the State University of New York; 1989.

90. Granger CV, Hamilton BB, Linacre JM, Heinemann AW, Wright BD. Performance profiles of the Functional Independence Measure. *Am J Phys Med Rehabil* 1993;72:84–89.

91. Stineman MG, Shea JA, Jette A, et al. The Functional Independence Measure: Tests of scaling assumptions, structure, and reliability across 20 diverse impairment categories. *Arch Phys Med Rehabil* 1996;77:1101–1108.

92. Karamehmetoglu SS, Karacan I, Elbasi N, Demirel G, Koyuncu H, Dosoglu M. The Functional Independence Measure in spinal cord injured patients: Comparison of questioning with observational rating. *Spinal Cord.* 1997;35:22–25.

93. Ottenbacher KJ, Hsu Y, Granger CV, Fiedler RC. The reliability of the Functional Independence Measure: A quantitative review. *Arch Phys Med Rehabil* 1996;77:1226–1232.

94. Ottenbacher KJ, Msall ME, Lyon NR, Duffy LC, Granger CV, Braun S. Interrater agreement and stability of the Functional Independence Measure for children (WeeFIM): Use in children with developmental disabilities. *Arch Phys Med Rehabil* 1997;78: 1309–1315.

95. Ottenbacher KJ, Taylor ET, Msall ME, et al. The stability and equivalence reliability of the Functional Independence Measure for children (WeeFIM). *Dev Med Child Neurol.* 1996;38: 907–916.

96. Msall ME, DiGaudio K, Rogers BT, et al. The Functional Independence Measure for children (WeeFIM). Conceptual basis and pilot use in children with developmental disabilities. *Clin Pediatr (Phila).* 1994;33:421–430.

97. Hall KM. The Functional Assessment Measure (FAM). *J Rehabil Outcomes Meas.* 1997;1:63–65.

98. Hawley CA, Taylor R, Hellawell DJ, Pentland B. Use of the Functional Assessment Measure (FIM+FAM) in head injury rehabilitation: A psychometric analysis. *J Neurol Neurosurg Psychiatry.* 1999;67:749–754.

99. Malec JF, Buffington AL, Moessner AM, Thompson JM. Maximizing vocational outcome after brain injury: Integration of medical and vocational hospital-based services. *Mayo Clin Proc.* 1995; 70:1165–1171.

100. Fougeyrollas P, Noreau L, Bergeron H, Cloutier R, Dion SA, St-Michel G. Social consequences of long term impairments and disabilities: Conceptual approach and assessment of handicap. *Int J Rehabil Res.* 1998;21:127–141.

101. Jette A, Haley SM, Andres PL, Coster WJ. Development and initial testing of the Participation Measure for Post-Acute Care (PM-PAC). unpublished manuscript.

102. Mellick D, Walker N, Brooks CA, Whiteneck G. Incorporating the cognitive independence domain into CHART. *J Rehabil Outcomes Meas.* 1999;3:12–21.

103. Cusick CP, Gerhart KA, Mellick D, Breese P, Towle V, Whiteneck GG. Evaluation of the home and community-based services brain injury medicaid waiver programme in colorado. *Brain Inj.* 2003;17:931–945.

104. Cusick CP, Brooks CA, Whiteneck GG. The use of proxies in community integration research. *Arch Phys Med Rehabil* 2001;82:1018–1024.

105. Cusick CP, Gerhart KA, Mellick DC. Participant-proxy reliability in traumatic brain injury outcome research. *J Head Trauma Rehabil* 2000;15:739–749.

106. Zhang L, Abreu BC, Gonzales V, Seale G, Masel B, Ottenbacher KJ. Comparison of the Community Integration Questionnaire, the Craig Handicap Assessment and Reporting Technique, and the Disability Rating Scale in traumatic brain injury. *J Head Trauma Rehabil* 2002;17:497–509.

107. Mellick D, Gerhart KA, Whiteneck GG. Understanding outcomes based on the post-acute hospitalization pathways followed by persons with traumatic brain injury. *Brain Inj.* 2003;17:55–71.

108. Hall KM, Bushnik T, Lakisic-Kazazic B, Wright J, Cantagallo A. Assessing traumatic brain injury outcome measures for long-term follow-up of community-based individuals. *Arch Phys Med Rehabil* 2001;82:367–374.

109. Corrigan JD, Smith-Knapp K, Granger CV. Outcomes in the first 5 years after traumatic brain injury. *Arch Phys Med Rehabil* 1998;79:298–305.

110. Hall KM, Dijkers M, Whiteneck G, Brooks CA, Krause JS. The Craig Handicap Assessment and Reporting Technique (CHART): Metric properties and scoring. *Top Spinal Cord Inj Rehabil* 1998;4:16–30.

111. Willer B, Linn R, Allen K. Community integration and barriers to integration for individuals with brain injury. In: Finlayson MAJ, Garner SH., eds. *Brain Injury Rehabilitation: Clinical Considerations.* Baltimore: Williams and Wilkins; 1994.

112. Bush BA, Novack TA, Malec JF, Stringer AY, Millis SR, Madan A. Validation of a model for evaluating outcome after traumatic brain injury. *Arch Phys Med Rehabil* 2003;84:1803–1807.

113. Seale GS, Caroselli JS, High WM,Jr, Becker CL, Neese LE, Scheibel R. Use of Community Integration Questionnaire (CIQ) to characterize changes in functioning for individuals with traumatic brain injury who participated in a post-acute rehabilitation programme. *Brain Inj.* 2002;16:955–967.

114. Bogner JA, Corrigan JD, Mysiw WJ, Clinchot D, Fugate L. A comparison of substance abuse and violence in the prediction of long-term rehabilitation outcomes after traumatic brain injury. *Arch Phys Med Rehabil* 2001;82:571–577.

115. Novack TA, Bush BA, Meythaler JM, Canupp K. Outcome after traumatic brain injury: Pathway analysis of contributions from premorbid, injury severity, and recovery variables. *Arch Phys Med Rehabil* 2001;82:300–305.

116. Willer B, Button J, Rempel R. Residential and home-based postacute rehabilitation of individuals with traumatic brain injury: A case control study. *Arch Phys Med Rehabil* 1999;80:399–406.

117. Harrison-Felix C, Zafonte R, Mann N, Dijkers M, Englander J, Kreutzer J. Brain injury as a result of violence: Preliminary findings from the traumatic brain injury model systems. *Arch Phys Med Rehabil* 1998;79:730–737.

118. Hagen C. Language and cognitive disorganization following closed head injury: A conceptualization. In: Trexler L, ed. *Cognitive Rehabilitation. Conceptualization and Intervention.* New York: Plenum Press; 1982:131–151.

119. Gouvier WD, Blanton PD, LaPorte KK, Nepomuceno C. Reliability and validity of the Disability Rating Scale and the Levels of Cognitive Functioning Scale in monitoring recovery from severe head injury. *Arch Phys Med Rehabil* 1987;68:94–97.

120. Hall KM, Hamilton BB, Gordon WA, Zasler ND. Characteristics and comparisons of functional assessment indices: Disability Rating Scale, Functional Independence Measure, and functional assessment measure. *J Head Trauma Rehabil* 1993;8:60–74.

121. Cifu DX, Keyser-Marcus L, Lopez E, et al. Acute predictors of successful return to work 1 year after traumatic brain injury: A multicenter analysis. *Arch Phys Med Rehabil* 1997;78:125–131.

122. Rao N, Kilgore KM. Predicting return to work in traumatic brain injury using assessment scales. *Arch Phys Med Rehabil* 1992;73: 911–916.

123. Rappaport M, Herrero-Backe C, Rappaport ML, Winterfield KM. Head injury outcome up to ten years later. *Arch Phys Med Rehabil* 1989;70:885–892.

124. Cope DN, Cole JR, Hall KM, Barkan H. Brain injury: Analysis of outcome in a post-acute rehabilitation system. part 1: General analysis. *Brain Inj.* 1991;5:111–125.

125. Eliason MR, Topp BW. Predictive validity of Rappaport's Disability Rating Scale in subjects with acute brain dysfunction. *Phys Ther.* 1984;64:1357–1360.

126. Fryer LJ, Haffey WJ. Cognitive rehabilitation and community readaptation: Outcomes from two program models. *J Head Trauma Rehabil* 1987;2:51–63.

127. Novack TA, Bergquist TF, Bennett G, Gouvier WD. Primary caregiver distress following severe head injury. *J Head Trauma Rehabil* 1991;6:69–77.

128. Bowers D, Kofroth L. Comparison: Disability rating scale and Functional Independence Measure during recovery from traumatic brain injury. *Arch Phys Med Rehabil* 1989;70:A58.

129. Malec JF. Impact of comprehensive day treatment on societal participation for persons with acquired brain injury. *Arch Phys Med Rehabil* 2001;82:885–895.

130. Malec JF. Comparability of Mayo-Portland Adaptability Inventory ratings by staff, significant others and people with acquired brain injury. *Brain Inj.* 2004;18:563–575.

131. Malec JF, Moessner AM, Kragness M, Lezak MD. Refining a measure of brain injury sequelae to predict postacute rehabilitation outcome: Rating scale analysis of the Mayo-Portland Adaptability Inventory. *J Head Trauma Rehabil* 2000;15:670–682.

132. Malec JF, Kragness M, Evans RW, Finlay KL, Kent A, Lezak MD. Further psychometric evaluation and revision of the Mayo-Portland Adaptability Inventory in a national sample. *J Head Trauma Rehabil* 2003;18:479–492.

133. Bohac DL, Malec JF, Moessner AM. Factor analysis of the Mayo-Portland Adaptability Inventory: Structure and validity. *Brain Inj.* 1997;11:469–482.

134. Jennett B, Snoek J, Bond MR, Brooks N. Disability after severe head injury: Observations on the use of the glasgow outcome scale. *J Neurol Neurosurg Psychiatry* 1981;44:285–293.

135. Wilson JT, Pettigrew LE, Teasdale GM. Structured interviews for the Glasgow Outcome Scale and the Extended Glasgow Outcome Scale: Guidelines for their use. *J Neurotrauma.* 1998;15:573–585.

136. Wilson JT, Pettigrew LE, Teasdale GM. Emotional and cognitive consequences of head injury in relation to the Glasgow Outcome Scale. *J Neurol Neurosurg Psychiatry* 2000;69:204–209.

137. Levin HS, Boake C, Song J, et al. Validity and sensitivity to change of the Extended Glasgow Outcome Scale in mild to moderate traumatic brain injury. *J Neurotrauma* 2001;18:575–584.

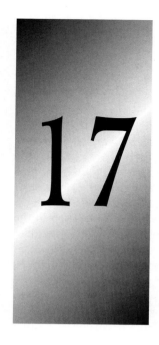

17 Life Expectancy

Robert M. Shavelle
David J. Strauss
Steven M. Day
Kelly A. Ojdana

1. INTRODUCTION

Rehabilitation needs and long-term planning for persons with severe traumatic brain injury (TBI) are covered in depth in other chapters of this volume. Here we consider one important aspect of long-term planning, namely longevity.

It is well known that mortality after severe TBI is exceptionally high in the acute post-injury period. It is perhaps less well known that long term mortality (2 years or more post-injury) is also increased, by comparison with the general population. It follows as a mathematical consequence that the life expectancy is reduced.

There are many studies of short-term survival after TBI. Detailed long-term data, however, and resulting research studies, are relatively sparse. The largest group studied on a long-term basis appears to be in the California Disabilities Database, which includes approximately 4,000 persons with disability secondary to TBI.

In this chapter we review what is known about life expectancy in TBI and present some new findings. Section 2 gives a brief review of key actuarial ideas needed for a discussion of life expectancy. Section 3 discusses the causes of death for which the risk is increased after a serious TBI, and reviews the literature. It is not always recognized that persons with TBI are subject to excess mortality risk from some of these causes. In section 4 we review the literature on life expectancy after TBI, focussing on recent research.

After this we discuss the factors that best predict life expectancy (section 5). It will be seen that, as in other types of chronic disability, the severity of motor dysfunction is the most important predictor of reduction in life expectancy. Later, in sections 6 and 7, we present some new findings on life expectancy and long-term decline in function after TBI. We discuss the effect of quality of care on life expectancy in section 8, the estimation of life expectancy in individual cases in section 9, and offer some conclusions in section 10.

2. TERMINOLOGY

It will prove helpful in the later sections to be familiar with the following terms:

- **Survival time:** the actual number of years lived by a given patient or member of a study population. A patient alive at the end of a study period is said to have a **censored** survival time as of that date.
- **Life expectancy:** the **average** survival time in a large group of similar persons. Note that this is not a prediction about any individual's actual survival time, as some survival times will be much longer and others much shorter than average.
- **Median survival time:** the time after which exactly half of a large group of persons are still alive. If all

the survival times are known (uncensored) and ordered from smallest to largest, the median is the middle value.

- **Exposure time:** the total number of person-years lived by all the members of a study population during the study period.
- **Mortality probability:** The chance of dying in a given period (e.g., a year). Like all probabilities, this number is between 0 and 1 inclusive.
- **Mortality rate:** The number of deaths in a study population divided by the number of person-years of exposure time. This is always larger than the mortality probability over the same period. Except in very high-risk populations, where the mortality rate could be greater than 1.0, however, the difference between the two is small.
- **Standardized mortality ratio (SMR):** the ratio of the observed number of deaths in a study population to the expected number, where the latter is what would arise from a suitably chosen reference group (often the age- and sex-matched general population in a given country). For example, an SMR of 2 means that the study population has twice the death rate of the reference group, after adjustment for age and sex differences. For further discussion, see Kahn & Sempos (1).
- **Relative risk (RR):** the ratio of the mortality rate in a study population to the mortality rate in the reference population. Unlike the SMR, the expected number is not standardized to the age and sex distribution in the reference population. The RR is often termed the **mortality ratio** (MR) in the actuarial literature.
- **Excess death rate (EDR):** the difference between the death rate in a study population and that in the reference population.
- **Life table:** a standard table summarizing mortality information about a group. Life tables are constructed for entire populations (2–6) or for suitably large subgroups (7–11). The table derives entirely from a set of age-specific mortality rates, and gives the life expectancy at every age. The median survival time can be easily computed from table entries (12, 13).

3. CAUSES OF DEATH AFTER TBI

It is clear from the published literature that there is an increase in long-term mortality in persons who have suffered a severe TBI. The published studies are, however, not entirely consistent on which causes of death account for the excess.

In the very short term, the primary cause of death is the brain damage itself. One of the largest studies was that of Sekulovic and Ceramilac (14), who summarized autopsies of 499 deaths occurring within 30 days of traumatic brain injury. They found that 78% of the deaths were due to injury to brain stem, brain edema, or brain compression. Of the remainder, the most frequent cause was pneumonia.

The definition of "longer term" varies among the studies. For example, Baguley et al. (15) considered patients who had been released from the hospital into rehabilitation facilities, while Shavelle et al. (16) considered one year or longer post injury.

The published studies make clear that, even in the long-term, death rates from many different causes are elevated for persons with TBI by comparison with the general population. These causes are considered below.

- **Epilepsy.** We refer here to post-traumatic epilepsy, rather than post-traumatic seizures. Post-traumatic epilepsy refers to recurrent long-term episodes often observed in persons with TBI, while the term post-traumatic seizures is generally applied to events in the first post-injury week.

  The classic studies of World War II veterans with TBI first documented the increased mortality risk from post-traumatic epilepsy (17). Later studies similarly addressed World War I veterans and reported the same finding (18, 19). This was confirmed in Roberts' long-term follow-up of patients in England during the 1960's and 70's (20, 21) and in Rish et al.'s study of veterans from the Vietnam war (22). More recently Shavelle et al., in their study of Californians with long-term mental disabilities from TBI, estimated a standardized mortality ratio (SMR) for seizures of 24 by comparison to the general population (16). Even patients with less severe disabilities were subject to an increased risk.

  The literature shows that epilepsy is more common in penetrating head injuries, such as gunshot wounds, than in non-penetrating injuries (23–27). One might expect that the severity of epilepsy would be greater, and therefore the mortality risk higher, for those with penetrating injuries. There does not appear to be any available evidence on this, however.
- **Suicide.** Roberts (20) found an increased suicide rate (SMR = 3) over the long term. A similar finding, and one documented in greater detail, was reported by Teasdale & Engberg (27). The latter authors, in their large study of Danish patients with TBI, found a suicide rate approximately four times that of the general population. They point out that persons with certain psychiatric conditions may be prone both to have accidents causing TBI and to commit suicide, though it seems unlikely that this could explain most of the association. A recent study by Pentland et al. (150) also found an increased proportion (1.3% of all deaths) due to suicide.

No increase in the suicide rate was observed by Walker and Blumer (28) or Shavelle et al. (16).

- **Respiratory infections and pneumonia.** Many studies document the increased risk of death due to these causes in patients with severe TBI. This is especially marked in persons who have become nonambulatory. Shavelle et al. (16) reported an approximately ten-fold increase in the mortality rate from respiratory causes, and Pentland et al. (150; Figure 2) found it to be the leading cause of death in this population after cardiac diseases. It appears that it is primarily the immobility, not the brain injury per se, that increases the risk; for example, a similar finding is reported in patients immobilized by spinal cord injury (29, 30).
- **Meningitis** was reported as an increased risk by Roberts (20), but not by other researchers (15, 16, 22).
- **Diseases of the circulatory system** are the leading cause of death in Western countries, and in the long-term the risk of death appears to be even higher in persons with severe TBI. Shavelle et al. (16) reported an approximately tripled mortality rate from these causes, by comparison with the general population, which by itself indicates a substantial reduction in life expectancy. Not surprisingly, the increase was largest among patients who had become nonambulatory. Weiss et al. (19) also found a long-term increase in the death rate from diseases of the circulatory system.

There are at least two mechanisms that could contribute to the increase in circulatory disease, and related deaths. First, persons confined to a wheelchair often take little exercise, and this alone increases the long-term risk of circulatory disease (31–35). Secondly, paraplegia appears to increase the risk of embolisms that travel from the lower body to the brain or lungs, and are often fatal. We are not aware of any studies that quantify these effects after TBI specifically, but a similar pattern of increased mortality has been observed in persons immobilized from spinal cord injury (29, 30) or cerebral palsy (59).

As with others who are immobile, persons suffering a TBI have an increased incidence of morbidity due to deep vein thrombosis, pressure sores, sepsis and urinary tract infections (36–48). However, there do not appear to be any studies documenting increased long-term mortality due to these causes. Of the 135 deaths described in Table 17-1 below, only one was due to any of the above (urinary sepsis).

Walker et al. (18) suggested that an injured brain makes the entire body more vulnerable to the stresses of aging. Lewin et al. (21, p. 1535) doubted Walker's hypothesis, pointing out that in their own study only a small number of causes of death appeared to be elevated

TABLE 17-1
Causes of Death for Persons Injured at Ages 10 or Older Who Died 5 or More Years Later

CAUSE OF DEATH (ICD-9 CODES)	NUMBER	%
Cancer (140–239)	9	7
Seizures (345, 436, 780.3)	14	10
Circulatory (390–459, except 436)	26	19
Respiratory (460–519)	15	11
Digestive (520–579)	6	4
Urinary/kidney (580–599)	4	3
Choking/suffocation (910–915)	3	2
Other external (800+, except 910–915)	13	10
All other causes, including missing	45	33
Total	135	100

in their TBI population. As noted earlier, however, the much larger study of Shavelle et al. (16) found increased mortality from most major causes other than cancer, which may support the view of Walker et al.

Table 17-1 shows causes of death for persons injured at ages 10 or older, who died 5 or more years after injury. The data are from the California Disabilities Database over the period 1988 to 1999 (49).

Excluding the "All other causes" category, the largest category was circulatory diseases. The comparatively small proportion of cancer deaths reflects the increased number of premature deaths to other causes; for example, there were more deaths due to respiratory diseases and seizures than to cancer.

4. RECENT LITERATURE ON LIFE EXPECTANCY

There is an abundant literature on short-term survival after TBI. The focus here is on the major recent studies on long-term survival. For a detailed history of studies prior to 1979 see Roberts (20, chapter 4).

- Walker and Erculei (17, 50) studied 364 World War II head-injured men from injury to 15 years later. The authors found a death rate 3 to 4 times greater than expected. They analyzed the frequency and severity of seizures, noting that men with post-traumatic seizures did not, on average, survive as long as those without seizures.
- Walker et al. (18) analyzed survival data through 1965 on 574 German World War I head-injured men. This ambitious study included a contemporary

control series of 581 unwounded veterans receiving meritorious medals. They constructed life tables and found a roughly 4-year reduction in life expectancy in the TBI group, with a larger reduction for those with epilepsy.

- Roberts (20) followed 469 patients who were amnesic or unconscious for a week or longer after a severe head injury. His analysis concentrated on the 366 who were discharged alive from hospital. He found that the chance of dying in the first 20 years after injury was elevated only in those injured at ages 5 to 25, and concluded that the effect of TBI on life expectancy was a 5-year reduction (20, p.146).

It appears from Roberts' Table 5.3 that some 80–90% of these persons could walk unassisted. If so, his conclusion would not apply to the most severely injured patients who were wheelchair-dependent or even bedridden. It has sometimes been inferred, incorrectly, that the Roberts' estimated 5-year reduction applied regardless of the severity of disabilities. Roberts himself evidently did not hold this view, as he reported that persons with the most extreme disabilities rarely survived ten years (20, p.142).

- Rish, Dillon and Weiss (22) studied 1127 Vietnam veterans who survived one week or longer after a penetrating head injury. The all-cause SMR over the 15-year study period exceeded 4 during years 1–3, ranged from 2 to 4 during years 4–11 and 13 post-injury, and was (probably because of the small sample size) less than 1 for years 12, 14 and 15. The authors concluded that the study population may have "approached the norm."

- Corkin, Sullivan and Carr (51) studied 190 World War II veterans with penetrating head injuries and a matched set of 106 with peripheral nerve injuries. They reported that head injury coupled with epilepsy reduced life expectancy compared to the control group, but that head injury alone did not.

- Walker and Blumer (28) studied 244 World War II head-injured men with post-traumatic epilepsy and found a death rate several times higher than in the general population.

- Strauss, Shavelle and Anderson (52) studied 946 children and adolescents aged 5 to 21 who suffered a TBI, following the subjects for up to 9 years. They constructed life tables stratified by a crude mobility scale (none, poor, fair/good). The resulting reductions in life expectancy, compared with the general population, ranged from very large (40 years) in persons with the most severe disabilities to quite small (2 years) in those who retained good mobility.

- Baguley et al. (15) studied 476 patients injured from 1986 to 1996. During the average follow up time of 5 years there were 27 deaths, compared to 6.7 expected, giving an SMR of 4.0. The difference was highly statistically significant, again demonstrating that life expectancy after TBI cannot be considered normal.

- Shavelle and Strauss (53) computed excess death rates for persons with TBI, beginning two years after injury. The population studied was the largest in the literature, with 2629 subjects and 268 deaths in the 1988 to 1997 study period. As in their previous studies, these authors found that excess death rates were relatively small for ambulatory persons, but much larger for those who had become nonambulatory.

- Brown et al. (151) followed up on 1,448 persons with TBI, of whom 164 (11%) were described as having moderate to severe injuries. They found that persons with mild TBI exhibited a small but statistically significant reduction in long-term survival. For those with moderate or severe TBI, long-term survival of those who survived the first six months was similar to those with mild TBI. A difficulty in interpreting this last finding is that the "moderate to severe" range presumably contained a mixture of persons with extremely severe disabilities (for whom the life expectancy is without question markedly decreased) and persons with much less severe disabilities. The overall effect therefore depends on the relative proportions.

- Harrison-Felix et al. (152) followed 2178 persons with TBI who completed inpatient rehabilitation in one of 15 National Institute on Disability and Rehabilitation Research-funded TBI Model Systems of Care. They estimated an average reduction in life expectancy of 7 years. In a follow up publication jointly written with the present authors (153), they indicated a general approach to estimating the life expectancy of an individual of a given age, sex, and score on the Disability Rating Scale. For example, according to the Model Systems data the life expectancy of a young adult with an "extremely severe" disability is 50% of normal. This again indicates how life expectancy after TBI varies greatly according to the severity of the injury.

While some of the studies — most notably, those of subjects without epilepsy — did not report a substantial reduction in life expectancy in some groups, this may be because persons in those groups were less severely disabled. There can be no question that mortality is markedly increased among the most severely disabled patients, a pattern well documented also in cerebral palsy (54–65) and spinal cord injury (19, 30, 66–70). In discussions of life expectancy of persons with TBI, therefore, it is important to consider the severity of disability.

Persons with more severe injuries are much more likely now than in the past to survive the early high-risk period (22). Other things being equal, it may therefore be that the more recent studies have a higher proportion of severely disabled persons. This would have obvious implications for the comparison of older and newer studies.

5. FACTORS RELATED TO SURVIVAL

The best predictors for survival in the *short* term are clinical measures such as the patient's Glasgow coma scale and duration of post-traumatic amnesia. The concern in this chapter, however, is with factors predictive of long-term survival.

For persons with TBI as well as in the general population, age is of course the most obvious determinant of life expectancy. Apart from age, the key factor is the severity of disability, especially motor dysfunction. This can be measured by simple functional items such as the patient's ability to walk, use hands, and self-feed. Other factors (such as preserved cognitive function or epilepsy) have a relatively small effect once motor function has been accounted for.

We now consider the factors that have been considered significant for life expectancy, citing the available evidence.

- **Age.** The increase in mortality of persons with TBI with age has been documented in many studies (52, 53, 71–74).
- **Sex.** In the general population, mortality of males at most ages is appreciably higher than that of females (2–6). For example, in the U.S. general population males age 30 to 60 have about twice the risk of death as females (2). Similar sex-differences have also been observed in persons with TBI (35). As would be expected, the difference is most marked in persons with milder disabilities and all but disappears at the most severe end of the spectrum. For example, no sex difference was been found in the survival of persons in the permanent vegetative state (75).
- **Time since injury** is certainly an important factor in the short-term. The mortality risk declines steadily during the first two years after injury as the patient's condition stabilizes. In the much longer term, however, there is no clear evidence of a trend, once severity of disability is taken into account. For example, mortality rates of persons 5 years post-injury do not seem markedly higher than otherwise comparable persons 10 years post-injury (49).

Because mortality after severe TBI is so high shortly after injury, it has sometimes been suggested that individuals vary greatly in their "toughness": only the tough survive the initial post-acute period, and these individuals are likely to survive much longer. No doubt individuals do vary to some extent in their abilities to survive major trauma. A more plausible explanation, however, is the well-known "healthy survivor" effect: persons with the most severe injuries die first, and the remainder have better survival because their injuries are, on average, less severe. This explanation is consistent with our finding that after the first few years, mortality rates are fairly constant over time once mobility and other factors are taken into account.

- **Mobility** is the most powerful predictor of long-term survival after TBI. Using the extensive California Disabilities Database, Strauss, Shavelle and Anderson (52) found a large difference in survival based on an overall mobility scale (none, poor, fair/good). The risk of death for persons with no mobility was approximately four times higher than those with fair or good mobility, even after adjustment for several other factors.

Shavelle and Strauss (53) subsequently computed age-specific mortality rates for three levels of ambulation (walks well alone; walks with support or unsteadily alone; does not walk). The age-specific mortality risks relative to the general population ranged from as low as 1.3 to as high as 17. Additional research indicates that, as would be expected, still more precise discrimination can be made based on more refined measures of motor function (49). Similarly, Baguley et al. (15) found that Functional Assessment Measure score was associated with survival.

- **Feeding ability.** Strauss, Shavelle and Anderson (52) found a sharp contrast in survival between four groups of persons: those requiring a feeding tube (RR = 6.6 compared to the best group), those fed orally by others (RR = 2.9), those who could finger feed (RR = 2.1), and those who could use utensils (the best group, with RR = 1 by convention). The inability to self-feed is an indirect measure of neurological compromise. It seems likely it is this compromise that causes the increased mortality, and the inability to self-feed is primarily a marker for it.
- **Need for ventilator support, oxygen, and/or frequent suctioning; history of respiratory problems.** We recently investigated the effect of these factors (49). Each was much more common in persons who could not walk and who required a feeding tube than in persons who were higher-functioning. In the former group, the univariate effect — that is, when no adjustment for mobility, etc. was made — was statistically significant and large: the relative risks for the factors ranged from 2 to 6. However, once age, sex, mobility and feeding were accounted for the (multivariate) relative risk was less than 1.2 for each factor.
- **Deficits in cognitive function and ability to communicate** are strongly correlated with severity of motor dysfunction. Although cognitive and communicative

functions are strong univariate predictors of mortality, their effects are modest when motor function is taken into account (49, 52). The same finding has been documented in persons with cerebral palsy (61, 62).

- **Epilepsy.** Many authors have found that epilepsy was strongly associated with reduced survival (17, 19, 50, 51). However, as others have suggested, this was likely because the presence of post-traumatic epilepsy is highly correlated with the extent of brain damage (17, 22). That is, epilepsy served as a marker for injury severity. Nevertheless, epilepsy is an independent risk factor for increased mortality. We recently confirmed this, and additionally found that in those who cannot walk, the relative risk of death for persons with generalized tonic-clonic seizures is 1.2 compared to others (49). In a separate study of people with minimal physical disabilities, Strauss et al. (76) similarly documented the increased mortality associated with recent seizures.

- **Calendar year.** The question is whether survival rates have improved over the years for a patient of given age and severity of disability. This would be termed a *secular trend*. The available data does not reveal any evidence of such a trend in recent (1980+) years (15, 49, 52). This may seem paradoxical because (i) as noted in other chapters of this volume, advances in rehabilitation have improved functional outcome after TBI, and (ii) as documented above, functional outcome, specifically mobility and feeding skills, are key factors associated with life expectancy. Thus it may well be that among patients with similar *initial* injuries, survival now is better than in previous decades because functional outcome is better. The cited research (15, 49, 52), however, looked at a different issue: comparison of survival now and in the past of patients who have the same *functional outcome*.

Several other factors should be mentioned as possible predictors of survival:

- **Poor education.** This factor was noted by Corkin, Sullivan and Carr (51). They suggest many reasons for the increased risk of death, including subsequent occupation and access to health care. To our knowledge other researchers have neither confirmed nor disproved this.

- **Depth of brain injury.** Weiss et al. (19) found that, as expected, the survival was poorer in persons with deeper (greater than 3 cm) brain injuries, although the difference was not statistically significant.

- **Penetrating versus closed head injuries.** Baguley et al. (15), in comparing the literature, concluded that there was no evidence of a difference. After controlling for functional abilities we too could find no difference, though the power of this comparison was low (49). Zafonte et al. (77) also found no difference in functional outcome at one year post-injury. On a related point, we found no difference in survival (49) between those who suffered skull fractures (ICD-9 codes 800–804) versus intracranial injuries (850–854). Finally, it may be that the effect of epilepsy is different in penetrating versus closed injuries, though evidence on this does not appear to be available.

- **Duration of unconsciousness.** Neither Shavelle and coworkers (49, 52) nor Weiss et al. (19) found this to be a significant factor. Lyle et al. (78) found that duration of coma was associated with both recovery and survival to 2 years, but it is not clear if this result would hold true if attention was restricted to those alive at 1 year post-injury, and if the functional outcome — e.g., mobility — was accounted for.

- **Glasgow coma scale (GCS) and the duration of post-traumatic amnesia (PTA).** Again, these factors are measures of the severity of the injury, are highly correlated with short-term survival, and therefore have a relationship to subsequent longevity. We are not aware of any evidence, however, that either of these factors is associated with subsequent long-term survival given the functional outcome one year post injury.

- **Maladaptive behaviors** – such as drug use, other substance abuse, suicide attempts, assault, aggression, self-injurious behavior, and lack of safety awareness – are much more common in those who have suffered a TBI or other central nervous system trauma than in the general population. For example, several studies report an association between CNS trauma and criminal behavior, especially violent crime (79–81). Such behaviour is also more frequent in persons with TBI than in others with comparable levels of functioning whose disabilities are due to cerebral palsy, autism, and other conditions (32).

These behaviors, with the exception of safety awareness, were *positive* factors for life expectancy when considered in isolation (49). That is, for example, persons who abused drugs had a *lower* mortality rate (and thus higher life expectancy) than those who did not. This is not surprising as those who could exhibit the behaviors were much less severely disabled, on average, than those who could not. In fact, these factors had a small *negative* effect on survival once functional abilities were taken into account (49).

Maladaptive behaviors in general have all been shown to be associated with increased mortality. For a review of the epidemiological data, see Harris & Barraclough (82). As these authors show, a major component of the increase is deaths due to unnatural causes, including accidents, suicide and homicide.

It may be that the reduced life expectancy of relatively high-functioning persons with TBI in part reflects an increased rate of unnatural deaths associated with behavioral problems.

- **APOE 4.** It is also possible that the APOE 4 allele plays a role. As noted by Baguley et al. (15) in citing Teasdale et al. (83) and Friedman et al. (84), patients with the APOE 4 allele are more likely to suffer unfavorable outcome after severe traumatic brain injury. Recent research (85, 86) on this issue has found that the presence of the APOE 4 allele is associated with poorer memory performance and rehabilitation outcome after TBI. Research by Liberman et al. (87), however, did not show a consistent influence of APOE genotype on outcome. We are not aware of any data on the independent effect of this allele on long-term survival.
- **Quality of care** is addressed separately in section 8.
- **Other factors relevant to life expectancy in the general population** are also relevant for persons with

TBI. These include pre-injury health status and history of smoking, alcohol and drug abuse, obesity, etc. Scientific literature on the effect of most of these factors is available.

- There are **factors uncommon in the general population** that can affect the mortality risk of persons with TBI. Examples are difficulties with chewing and swallowing, contractures, pressure sores (for persons with limited mobility), bowel and bladder dysfunction, frequency of infections, and psychological factors (attitude to the disability, depression, aggressive behavior, etc.). For many of these factors, published studies of the effect on mortality are not available.

6. NEW ESTIMATES OF LIFE EXPECTANCY IN TBI

Tables 17-2 and 17-3 show our most recent findings (49). These represent a refinement of the data presented in our

TABLE 17-2
Female Life Expectancy by Age and Severity of Disability

AGE	PVS[a]	CANNOT WALK FED BY OTHERS[b]	CANNOT WALK SELF FEEDS[c]	SOME WALKING ABILITY[d]	WALKS WELL ALONE[e]	GENERAL POPULATION
10	12	27	46	55	61	70.0
20	11	26	40	48	54	60.2
30	10	22	33	41	46	50.5
40	9	16	26	31	36	41.0
50	7	11	19	23	27	31.7

[a]Permanent vegetative state: No purposeful motor or cognitive function. Requires a feeding tube.
[b]Does not feed self, must be fed completely (either orally or by a feeding tube).
[c]Can feed self with fingers or utensils, with assistance and/or spillage.
[d]Walks with support, or unsteadily alone at least 10 feet but does not balance well.
[e]Walks well alone for at least 20 feet, and balances well.

TABLE 17-3
Male Life Expectancy by Age and Severity of Disability

AGE	PVS[a]	CANNOT WALK FED BY OTHERS[b]	CANNOT WALK SELF FEEDS[c]	SOME WALKING ABILITY[d]	WALKS WELL ALONE[e]	GENERAL POPULATION
10	12	27	46	50	56	64.3
20	11	26	40	44	49	54.7
30	10	22	33	37	41	45.4
40	9	16	26	28	32	36.2
50	7	11	19	20	23	27.4

[a]Permanent vegetative state: No purposeful motor or cognitive function. Requires a feeding tube.
[b]Does not feed self, must be fed completely (either orally or by a feeding tube).
[c]Can feed self with fingers or utensils, with assistance and/or spillage.
[d]Walks with support, or unsteadily alone at least 10 feet but does not balance well.
[e]Walks well alone for at least 20 feet, and balances well.

earlier publications, and take account of age, sex, and walking and feeding ability. For comparison, life expectancies in the permanent vegetative state (PVS) and the U.S. general population are also shown. As can be seen, the remaining life expectancy decreases both with age and with severity of injury.

At the most severe end of the disability spectrum, the permanent vegetative state (PVS), the life expectancy is at most 12 years, and no significant differences were found between the sexes. The PVS analyses are specific to persons with acquired injuries, including TBI and near-drowning, and who will require gastrostomy feeding for life. The corresponding figures (not shown) for persons with congenital conditions, degenerative diseases, or who require a ventilator are lower still.

Persons in the minimally conscious state (MCS) – a group that has received recent attention in the clinical literature (88–90) – have slightly higher cognitive function than those in the PVS. A study of infants who were immobile and in the MCS ("IMCS") found that their survival was only slightly better than those in the PVS (91). Thus, once again, mobility is seen to be a more important predictor of survival than cognitive function. A subsequent analysis of 2,534 children and adults who were in the IMCS gave the same finding (49).

The nonambulatory group covers a wide range of functional abilities. At the low end of the range are persons in the vegetative state, and those who are immobile and require gastrostomy feeding. At the high end are persons who feed themselves, and have reasonable self care skills, even though they cannot walk. Tables 17-2 and 17-3 include a simple stratification on the basis of self-feeding, an important predictor of life expectancy. Further distinctions can of course usefully be made.

It should be pointed out that there are persons whose residual TBI is so mild that they do not require services (e.g., occupational and physical therapy) on an ongoing basis. These persons would not be in the California data base, and their life expectancies may be higher than any group described above. In the best case, where the effects of the TBI are minimal, the life expectancy is of course essentially normal, or even better than normal (if, for example, the person was a nonsmoker, took regular exercise, maintained a good weight, etc.).

Persons in the highest functioning group of the table — those who can walk well alone and balance well — nevertheless have disabilities severe enough to require ongoing services. The aggregate life expectancy is reduced by 4 to 9 years compared to the general population. As expected, the difference is smallest for the oldest persons. Note that there is no sex difference in life expectancy in the most severely disabled category, but a substantial difference among the higher functioning groups.

The TBI figures in Tables 17-2 and 17-3 do not take account of whether the person needs a feeding tube. This need is uncommon in the higher-functioning groups, but about half of the persons over age 10 who cannot walk and cannot feed themselves do require a feeding tube, and their life expectancy is lower. Also not considered are specific fine and gross motor skills and cognitive ability, all of which affect life expectancy to some extent.

Technical Note   The scientific methods underlying the study of life expectancy are well-documented in the actuarial, epidemiological and statistical literature; see, for example, Singer (91), Kahn and Sempos (1), Collett (92), Schoen (93) and Anderson (12). Full details on the specific methods used to compute the results in Tables 17-2 and 17-3 are described elsewhere (75, 94, 95). A brief summary follows:

- The analyses were based on data from 1,723 persons at all ages (PVS) and 3,598 persons over age 10 (TBI).
- A data set of person-months was constructed — PVS: 56,229 person-months; TBI: 285,424 person-months. Each person-month was associated with the subject's age, severity of disability, etc., and an indicator variable for whether the person died in that month.
- Logistic regression was used to compute the annual mortality rates. The following factors were used:
  - **PVS analyses:** age, time since injury, etiology, and need for feeding tube.
  - **TBI analyses:** age, sex, time since injury, and the walking and feeding categories listed in the table.
- The PVS analyses provided mortality rates for all ages. The TBI analyses provided rates at the starting ages and a model was used to compute rates at subsequent ages. A life table or survival curve was then constructed, with the life expectancy obtained directly in the former case, and as the area beneath the curve in the latter.

7. LONG-TERM DECLINE IN FUNCTION

In the short term, patients with TBI often regain some functioning in the first year post-injury (96–98), but the rate of recovery slows thereafter (28, 99, 100). An exception is the elderly, who have a low rate of recovery even in the first year (101–104).

It appears that, over the long term, patients with TBI will lose functional abilities faster than those in the general population:

- Lewin et al. (21) reported progressive intellectual deterioration in their patients, more so than would occur in the general population.
- A relevant comparison may be with persons who have suffered repeated ("chronic") TBI, as contrasted to acute TBI. Chronic TBI can result from boxing

(105, 106) and possibly from "heading the ball" in soccer (107–110). It is an often-progressive neurological condition with many of the same pathological characteristics as Alzheimer's disease (110–112).

We investigated this issue of long-term decline in our TBI database, concentrating on one important functional measure: ambulation.

Figure 17-1 shows the long-term prognosis for a group of 100% who initially could walk with support (crutches, braces, etc.) two years post-injury. Of these, roughly 15% died within the next 8 years, 20% lost the ability to walk, 55% did not change, and 10% could walk well alone. That is, of those still alive twice as many declined in functioning as improved.

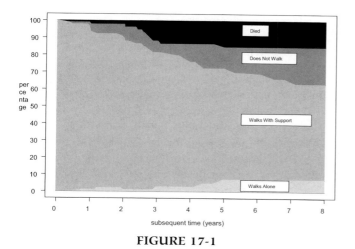

FIGURE 17-1

Long-term change in ambulation for adults aged 40 and over

Technical Note   The curves for the cohort, including the survival curve, were computed using the Aalen-Johansen estimator (113). This statistical method was developed as an extension of the usual Kaplan-Meier (114) estimator to address the case of multiple live states (115). Day (116) showed that, in statistical parlance, the estimator is consistent and more efficient than the extended Kaplan-Meier estimator proposed by Strauss and Shavelle (117). The latter has previously been used to produce similar diagrams involving improvement or decline in function of persons with developmental disabilities (62, 118).

8. QUALITY OF CARE AND LIFE EXPECTANCY

Quality of care is a rather vague term that is frequently raised in discussions of life expectancy. It seems to cover a variety of issues, including:

- The expertise of the caregivers, ranging from highly qualified professionals to relatively unskilled (and

low paid) staff. A complicating factor is that caregivers are often family members, who generally do not have formal qualifications but in some cases become highly skilled carers.
- The accessibility of physicians and emergency services.
- The quantity of care and equipment provided, which is often a reflection of the funds available.

The effect of quality of care on life expectancy surely depends on what is being compared. If, for example, it is good care versus negligent or even deliberately substandard care, the difference in life expectancy will doubtless be large. This comparison, however, is generally not of interest. The most relevant comparison is between:

a. The normal, standard care available in most Western societies, and
b. The care expected given that the patient has a carefully prepared and well-funded life care plan.

It might be argued that the care embodied in (b) represents the best case in practice, as one cannot forecast exactly what care the patient will receive, or will choose to receive, in the coming decades.

The issue is evidently a complex one and we do not attempt to draw any definitive conclusions. Nevertheless, these observations may be helpful:

- Some states or countries provide services to persons with disabilities as an entitlement. For example, California provides annual person-centered individual program plans plus provision of all indicated care. In such cases it may not be clear what is the difference, if any, between (a) and (b) above.
- Strauss et al. carried out a series of studies in California that compared mortality in large long-term state facilities, private group homes, and the patient's own family home (119–127). The authors found that mortality rates in the group homes and in family homes were comparable. Mortality rates in the state facilities, however, were generally lower, corresponding to modestly higher life expectancies. Reasons for the difference, which are related to quality of care, include round the clock supervision, continuity of care, centralized record keeping, and immediate access to medical attention (127).
- It is sometimes asserted that quality of care is the most important determinant of life expectancy. If the comparison is between (a) and (b) above, this assertion is incorrect: the most important determinant is undoubtedly the severity of the disability. For example, literature from many countries documents that young patients in the permanent vegetative state have mortality rates up to 500 times larger than in the general population (75, 128–136). If quality of

care is as important a determinant of mortality risk, then death rates under "standard" care would have to be 500 times higher than they would be under option (b). This is an extremely large ratio; to put it in perspective, heavy smokers are subject to mortality rates that are only 2–3 times that of the general population (137, 138).

- Researchers at The Dartmouth Atlas Project have found that more care (beyond what is reasonable and necessary) does not significantly prolong the life span of persons in the general population (139–142). Their website also provides an annotated list of 387 additional references supporting this conclusion (143).

- Finally, it may be noted that life insurance companies offer reduced premiums to persons with favorable risk characteristics, such as having ideal weight and being a nonsmoker. To our knowledge, (i) they do not give discounted rates to physicians or to the wealthy, both of whom have access to high quality health care, and (ii) life annuity underwriters do not routinely adjust for quality of care when pricing their structured settlements.

9. ESTIMATION OF LIFE EXPECTANCY IN INDIVIDUAL CASES

Life expectancy is an important factor in assessing the lifetime cost of future care for an individual with TBI. As we have seen, a sensible discussion requires, at a minimum, some familiarity with both the basic actuarial concepts and the relevant scientific literature. In practice, however, persons concerned with life expectancy assessment often lack this background, and as a result erroneous views are frequently advanced. We discuss some of the more significant issues below.

Much unnecessary confusion arises from the misuse of the term life expectancy when survival time is intended.

- For example, a terminally ill patient may ask the treating physician about life expectancy, but usually neither is interested in averages. Even in cases where the survival time will be limited to a few months or years, it is impossible to predict it with accuracy (144, 145). This forces the physician either to refuse to opine, and appear unhelpful, or to offer what is known about the average survival time in such cases. Even if the quoted average is appropriate, however, the patient's actual survival time will likely be very different and the doctor will appear to be "wrong" (146, 147).
- In the legal arena, on the other hand, predictions of actual survival time are generally not required. For example, it is impossible to predict the survival time

of a normal 70 year-old male: according to government statistics 10% of such males will die in the next 4 years while another 10% will live well into their 90's (2). But the *average* survival time — i.e., the life expectancy — is given by standard government life tables and is widely accepted by courts as the basis for compensation. It may be argued that the same reasoning should apply to persons with reduced life expectancy, including those with TBI.

- We note that if one insists upon making a prediction of survival time, then either the life expectancy or the median survival time is a possible choice. The latter has the useful interpretation of being the time at which the patient is as likely as not to be still alive. In the case of persons at high risk, such as those who are immobile and tube fed, the life expectancy is higher than the median (75).

A common misconception is that if a person's current mortality risk is low then the life expectancy is nearly normal.

- The argument runs, for example, that although a given patient has severe epilepsy he is unlikely to die of it, and therefore "on the balance of probabilities the epilepsy will not reduce his life expectancy." This argument again reflects confusion of life expectancy and survival time. In a very large group, *some* of the individuals will die of epilepsy, even though they are not the majority, and this reduces the *average* survival time – i.e., the life expectancy.
- An illustration of this point is the comparison of males and females. Males have life expectancies about 6 years shorter than females. It would thus be a mistake to argue that because a given 10 year-old boy is in perfect health and is currently subject to an extremely low mortality risk his life expectancy is the same as that of a 10 year-old girl.
- Further, the effect of even a moderate additional mortality risk on life expectancy is often underestimated. For example, if a 10 year-old girl has a medical condition that raises her mortality risk by only 5 deaths per 1000 persons per year for life, the result is a life expectancy reduction of 11 years.

It is often asserted that "Published studies are all based on large groups and it is impossible to predict the life expectancy of an individual."

- Confusion of life expectancy and survival time aside, the assertion is essentially that because a scientific analysis cannot take account of *every* factor relevant to life expectancy of a given individual, *nothing* scientific can be said about an individual's prognosis for survival.

- If this were true then standard government life tables would be irrelevant to an individual, and economists and others have been wrong to refer to them. It would also mean that life insurance actuaries and medical directors, who routinely decide whether to offer insurance to individuals and at what price, have no basis for making such decisions.

Frequently the view is expressed that high quality medical care will ensure a normal life expectancy. This is incorrect, as was discussed in the previous section.

The life expectancy literature on cerebral palsy, spinal cord injury and other conditions is extensive, and the comparison with these conditions to TBI may be helpful.

- The comparison with *cerebral palsy* (59–65) may provide a useful lower bound to the life expectancy in TBI, as persons with TBI appear to be subject to similar or slightly lower mortality risks than those with comparably severe cerebral palsy (52).

  For example, the life expectancy of a 15 year-old male with cerebral palsy who can lift his head when lying on his stomach but cannot roll over or sit independently, and who is fed orally by others, has been estimated to be 22.8 additional years (62). This may therefore be a reasonable approximation to, though perhaps a slight underestimate of, the life expectancy of a similar TBI patient.
- Similarly, comparison with the *spinally-injured* patient, though imperfect, may be useful. For example, the life expectancy of a young paraplegic has been well documented to be reduced by 10 years or more (66–69). Such persons are unable to walk, but generally have unimpaired cognitive function, no bulbar dysfunction, and have normal upper body function and self-care skills with their hands. They therefore compare favorably in most respects with persons with TBI who have lost the ability to walk. (Some caveat is necessary here because spinally-injured patients are more at risk of certain medical conditions, including spinal degeneration and bowel and bladder problems.)
- For a person with TBI who is cognitively near-normal and ambulatory but still has some permanent difficulties with motor function, there is still some modest reduction in life expectancy. This may be seen by comparison with *uninjured persons who live a sedentary life style*, whose life expectancy may be argued to represent an upper bound in many cases. A permanently sedentary lifestyle is known to lead to increased risk of heart disease and other conditions (148, 149), and can be shown to lead to a reduction of about 4 years.
- Finally, if the patient has only minimal physical disability but suffers *from mental disorder or severe*

behavioral problems, the literature on excess mortality in such conditions may be applicable (82).

Taking Account of Multiple Factors

Although ambulation and self-feeding are valuable predictors of expected longevity, there are other factors with some relevance. Some of these were discussed in section 5, and in addition there are refinements to mobility and self-care (can the subject roll over, sit or stand without support, carry on conversations, dress and bathe himself, etc.). Further, there are factors, such as bulbar dysfunction and hospital admissions for pneumonia, that must have some predictive value but for which there appears to be no relevant mortality data.

How can all these factors be incorporated into an estimate of a given individual's life expectancy? It is evidently not feasible to take them all into account in a scientific analysis. The rational approach is to work with the available data as far as possible – perhaps taking account of key factors such as mobility and self-care skills – and then to consider other factors for which data are not available. It may then be reasonable to argue for an adjustment, either upwards or downwards, to the evidence-based estimate. The input of a clinician can be very helpful in describing these factors and their effect on the individual's prognosis.

An alternative view is sometimes expressed: that the scientific approach should be abandoned because such an analysis cannot take account of *every* factor. Instead, a life expectancy is chosen on the basis of, for example, clinical introspection. It seems to us that this position is untenable: the existing mortality data should at least provide a *starting point* for any rational discussion.

10. CONCLUSIONS

An individual's *life expectancy* is the average number of additional years of life in a large group of similar persons. In many cases it can be estimated with some precision. Life expectancy should be distinguished from the individual's actual *survival time*, which is impossible to predict with accuracy, even in the uninjured general population.

We have seen that mortality is increased after TBI, many causes of death being more common than in the general population. These include pneumonia and other respiratory diseases, seizures, accidents (including choking), and – importantly – diseases of the circulatory system, related to immobility.

The key predictors of survival are mobility and self-care skills (notably, the abilities to walk and to self-feed). The life expectancy of persons who walk and self-feed is only modestly reduced by comparison with the general population, whereas nonambulatory persons with minimal self-care skills suffer a much greater reduction. An extreme case is a gastrostomy-dependent patient in the permanent vegetative state, where the life expectancy is 10 years or less.

To estimate a given individual's life expectancy one can use the literature and existing data to account for some key predictors. Subsequently, it is reasonable to consider additional factors, which have not been taken into account, and to argue for a further adjustment. The alternative approaches of simply assuming that general population figures apply, or of proposing an estimate solely on the basis of clinical intuition, lack scientific justification and are in our view untenable. The existing population data must surely provide at least a starting point.

Finally, we note two factors relevant to life expectancy that have been insufficiently studied. The first is the prospect for improvement in function after the first few post-injury years. Although it is sometimes stated that almost all the meaningful recovery in function occurs during the first two years, it is a matter of clinical observation that substantial improvement sometimes occurs considerably later. There have been cases of persons emerging from the vegetative state after three or more years, although remaining with severe motor and cognitive dysfunction. It appears that there are no studies documenting the frequency of these late recoveries, or the degree of improvement that may occur.

Second, little is known about the decline in function of persons with TBI in old age. For example, if a young adult suffers a TBI and after several years is able to walk unsteadily and to carry on conversations with somewhat slurred speech, what can be expected in the subsequent decades, and what is the expected pattern of decline in old age? Further research on these questions would be valuable.

References

1. Kahn HA, Sempos CT. *Statistical methods in epidemiology.* Oxford: Oxford University Press 1989.
2. Anderson RN. United States life tables, 1997. National Vital Statistics Reports; vol 47 no 28. Hyattsville, Maryland: National Center For Health Statistics 1999.
3. Statistics Canada. Gender-specific life tables, 1990–1992.
4. The Stationery Office. Interim life tables, 1996–1998. London: The Stationery Office 1999.
5. Australian Bureau of Statistics. Australian Life Table 1996–1998. Office of the Government Statistician 1998.
6. Hong Kong Life Tables 1996–2029. Demographic Statistics Section, Census and Statistics Department, Hong Kong Special Administrative Region, People's Republic of China.
7. Strauss DJ, Eyman RK. Mortality of people with mental retardation in California with and without Down syndrome, 1986–1991. *American Journal of Mental Retardation 1996;* 100:643–653.
8. Singer RB, Strauss DJ, Shavelle RM. Comparative mortality in cerebral palsy patients in California, 1980–1996. *Journal of Insurance Medicine* 1998;30:240–246.
9. Singer RB, Strauss DJ. Comparative mortality in mentally retarded patients in California, with and without Down's syndrome, 1986–1991. *Journal of Insurance Medicine* 1997;29:172–84.
10. Shavelle RM, Strauss DJ. Comparative mortality of persons with Autism in California, 1980–1996. *Journal of Insurance Medicine* 1998;30:220–225.
11. Eyman RK, Grossman HJ, Chaney RH, Call TL. The life expectancy of profoundly handicapped people with mental retardation. *New England Journal of Medicine* 1990;323:584–589.
12. Anderson, TW. *Life expectancy in court: A textbook for doctors and lawyers.* Vancouver, British Columbia: Teviot Press 2002.
13. Http://www.LifeExpectancy.com/LifeTable.shtml
14. Sekulovic N, Ceramilac A. Brain injuries-causes of death, and life expectancy. *Acta Neurochir Suppl (Wien)* 1979;28:203–204.
15. Baguley I, Slewa-Younan S, Lazarus R, et al. Long-term mortality trends in patients with traumatic brain injury. *Brain Injury* 2000;14:505–512.
16. Shavelle RM, Strauss D, Whyte J, Day SM, Yu YL. Long-term causes of death after traumatic brain injury. *American Journal of Physical Medicine and Rehabilitation* 2001;80:510–516;quiz 517–519.
17. Walker AE, Erculei F. Post-traumatic epilepsy 15 years later. *Epilepsia* 1970;11:17–26.
18. Walker AE, Leuchs HK, Lechtape-Gruter H, Caveness WF, Kretschman C. Life expectancy of head injured men with and without epilepsy. *Archives of Neurology* 1971;24:95–100.
19. Weiss GH, Caveness WF, Einsiedel-Lechtape H, McNeel ML. Life expectancy and causes of death in a group of head-injured veterans of World War I. *Archives of Neurology* 1982;39:741–743.
20. Roberts AH. *Severe accidental head injury: An assessment of long-term prognosis.* London: The Macmillan Press 1979.
21. Lewin W, Marshall TF, Roberts AH. Long-term outcome after severe head injury. *British Medical Journal* 1979;2:1533–1538.
22. Rish BL, Dillon JD, Weiss GH. Mortality following penetrating craniocerebral injuries. *Journal of Neurosurgery* 1983;59:775–780.
23. Temkin NR, Haglund MM, Winn HR. Causes, prevention, and treatment of post-traumatic epilepsy. *New Horiz* 1995;3:518–522.
24. Kuhl DA, Boucher BA, Muhlbauer MS. Prophylaxis of posttraumatic seizures. *DICP* 1990;24:277–285.
25. Weiss GH, Salazar AM, Vance SC, Grafman JH, Jabbari B. Predicting posttraumatic epilepsy in penetrating head injury. *Archives of Neurology* 1986;43:771–773.
26. Salazar AM, Jabbari B, Vance SC, Grafman J, Amin D, Dillon JD. Epilepsy after penetrating head injury. I. Clinical correlates: A report of the Vietnam Head Injury Study. *Neurology* 1985;35:1406–1414.
27. Teasdale TW, Engberg AW. Suicide after traumatic brain injury: A population study. *Journal of Neurology, Neurosurgery and Psychiatry* 2001;71:436–440.
28. Walker AE, Blumer D. The fate of World War II veterans with posttraumatic seizures. *Archives of Neurology* 1989;46:23–26.
29. Hartkopp A, Brønnum-Hansen H, Seidenschnur A-M, Biering-Sørensen. Survival and cause of death after traumatic spinal cord injury: A long-term epidemiological survey from Denmark. *Spinal Cord* 1997;35:76–85.
30. DeVivo DJ, Stover SL. Long-term survival and causes of death. In: SL Stover, JA DeLisa & GG Whiteneck (Eds), *Spinal cord injury: Clinical outcomes from the model systems.* Gaithersburg, MD: Aspen 1995.
31. Paffenbarger RS Jr, Hyde RT, Wing AL, Lee IM, Jung DL, Kampert JB. The association of changes in physical-activity level and other lifestyle characteristics with mortality among men. *New England Journal of Medicine* 1993;328:538–545.
32. Paffenbarger RS Jr, Hyde RT, Hsieh CC, Wing A. Physical activity, all-cause mortality, and longevity of college alumni. *New England Journal of Medicine* 1986;314:605–613.
33. Paffenbarger RS Jr, Hyde RT, Wing AL, Hsieh CC. Physical activity and longevity of college alumni. *New England Journal of Medicine* 1986;315:399–401.
34. Wei M, Kampert JB, Barlow CE, Nichaman MZ, Gibbons LW, Paffenbarger RS Jr, Blair SN. Relationship between low cardiorespiratory fitness and mortality in normal-weight, overweight, and obese men. *JAMA* 1999;282:1547–1553.
35. Paffenbarger RS, Hyde RT, Wing AL. Physical activity and physical fitness as determinants of health and longevity. In: Bouchard C, Shephard RJ, Stephens T, Sutton JR, McPherson BD (Eds).

Exercise, fitness, and health: A consensus of current knowledge. Champagne, Illinois: Human Kinetics Books, 1990, pp. 33–48.

36. Barnes MP. Rehabilitation after traumatic brain injury. *British Medical Bulletin* 1999, 55:927–943.

37. Perry J. Rehabilitation of the neurologically disabled patient: principles, practice, and scientific basis. *Journal of Neurosurgy* 1983; 58:799–816.

38. Cupitt JM. Prophylaxis against thromboembolism in patients with traumatic brain injury: A survey of UK practice. *Anaesthesia* 2001; 56:780–785.

39. Wagner RH, Cifu DX, Keyser-Marcus L. Functional outcome of individuals with traumatic brain injury and lower extremity deep venous thrombosis. *Journal of Head Trauma Rehabilitation* 1999; 14:558–566.

40. Burke DT. Venous thrombosis in traumatic brain injury. *Journal of Head Trauma Rehabilitation* 1999;14:515–519.

41. Velmahos GC, Nigro J, Tatevossian R, Murray JA, Cornwell EE 3rd, Belzberg H, Asensio JA, Berne TV, Demetriades D. Inability of an aggressive policy of thromboprophylaxis to prevent deep venous thrombosis (DVT) in critically injured patients: Are current methods of DVT prophylaxis insufficient? *Journal of the American College of Surgeons* 1998;187:529–533.

42. Hammond FM, Meighen MJ. Venous thromboembolism in the patient with acute traumatic brain injury: screening, diagnosis, prophylaxis, and treatment issues. *Journal of Head Trauma Rehabilitation* 1998;13:36–50.

43. Lai JM, Yablon SA, Ivanhoe CB. Incidence and sequelae of symptomatic venous thromboembolic disease among patients with traumatic brain injury. *Brain Injury* 1997;11:331–334.

44. Marin R. Physical medicine and rehabilitation in the military: the Bosnian mass casualty experience. *Military Medicine* 2001;166: 335–337.

45. Ferido T, Habel M. Spasticity in head trauma and CVA patients: etiology and management. *Journal of Neuroscience Nursing* 1988;20:17–22.

46. Pohl M, Ruckriem S, Strik H, Hortinger B, Meissner D, Mehrholz J, Pause M. Treatment of pressure ulcers by serial casting in patients with severe spasticity of cerebral origin. *Archives of Physical Medicine and Rehabilitation* 2002;83:35–39.

47. Alvi A, Doherty T, Lewen G. Facial fractures and concomitant injuries in trauma patients. *Laryngoscope* 2003, 113:102–106.

48. Shackford SR, Mackersie RC, Davis JW, Wolf PL, Hoyt DB. Epidemiology and pathology of traumatic deaths occurring at a Level I Trauma Center in a regionalized system: the importance of secondary brain injury. *Journal of Trauma* 1989;29:1392–1397.

49. Shavelle RM, Strauss DJ, Day SM, Ojdana KA. To avoid unnecessary repetition in the text, this citation refers to unpublished research by the Life Expectancy Project specifically for this chapter.

50. Walker AE, Erculei F. *Head injured men 15 years later.* Springfield, Ill: Charles C Thomas, 1968, page 106.

51. Corkin S, Sullivan EV, Carr FA. Prognostic factors for life expectancy after penetrating head injury. *Archives of Neurology* 1984;41:975–977.

52. Strauss DJ, Shavelle RM, Anderson TW. Long-term survival of children and adolescents after traumatic brain injury. *Archives of Physical Medicine and Rehabilitation* 1998;79:1095–1100.

53. Shavelle RM, Strauss DJ. Comparative mortality of adults with traumatic brain injury in California, 1988–97. *Journal of Insurance Medicine* 2000;32:163–166.

54. Hutton JL, Pharoah POD. Effects of cognitive, motor, and sensory disabilities on survival in cerebral palsy. *Archives of Disease in Childhood* 2002;86:84–89.

55. Hutton JL, Colver AF, Mackie PC. Effect of severity of disability on survival in north east England cerebral palsy cohort. *Archives of Disease in Childhood* 2000;83:468–474.

56. Hutton JL, Cooke T, Pharoah POD. Life expectancy in children with cerebral palsy. *British Medical Journal* 1994;309:431–435.

57. Eyman RK, Grossman HJ. Living with cerebral palsy and tube feeding [letter]. *Journal of Pediatrics* 2001;138:147.

58. Blair E, Watson L, Badawi N, Stanley FJ. Life expectancy among people with cerebral palsy in Western Australia. *Developmental Medicine & Child Neurology* 2001, 43:508–515.

59. Strauss DJ, Cable W, Shavelle RM. Causes of excess mortality in cerebral palsy. *Developmental Medicine and Child Neurology* 1999;41:580–585.

60. Shavelle RM, Strauss DJ, Day SM. Comparison of survival in cerebral palsy between countries [letter]. *Developmental Medicine & Child Neurology* 2001;43:574.

61. Strauss DJ, Shavelle RM, Anderson TW. Life expectancy of children with cerebral palsy. *Pediatric Neurology* 1998;18:143–149.

62. Strauss DJ and Shavelle RM. Life expectancy of adults with cerebral palsy. *Developmental Medicine and Child Neurology* 1998; 40:369–375.

63. Plioplys AV, Kasnicka I, Lewis S, Moller D. Survival rates among children with severe neurologic disabilities. *Southern Medical Journal* 1998;91:161–172.

64. Crichton JU, Mackinnon M, White CP. The life expectancy of persons with cerebral palsy. *Developmental Medicine and Child Neurology* 1995;37:567–576.

65. Evans PM, Evans SJW, Alberman E. Cerebral palsy: Why we must plan for survival. *Archives of Diseases in Childhood* 1990;65: 1329–1333.

66. Strauss DJ, DeVivo M, Shavelle RM. Long-term mortality risk after spinal cord injury. *Journal of Insurance Medicine* 2000; 32:11–16.

67. DeVivo MJ, Krause JS, Lammertse DP. Recent trends in mortality and causes of death among persons with spinal cord injury. *Archives of Physical Medicine and Rehabilitation* 1999;80:1411–1419.

68. Frankel HL, Coll JR, Charlifue SW, Whiteneck GG, Gardner BP, Jamous MA, Krishnan KR, Nuseibeh I, Savic G, Sett P. Long-term survival in spinal cord injury: A fifty year investigation. *Spinal Cord* 1998;36:266–274.

69. Yeo JD, Walsh J, Rutkowski S, Soden R, Craven M, Middleton J. Mortality following spinal cord injury. *Spinal Cord* 1998; 36:329–336.

70. DeVivo MJ, Ivie SC. Life expectancy of ventilator-dependent persons with spinal cord injuries. *Chest* 1995;108:226–232.

71. Johnstone B, Childers MK, Hoerner J. The effects of normal ageing on neuropsychological functioning following traumatic brain injury. *Brain Injury* 1998;12:569–576.

72. Teasdale TW, Skene A, Spiegelhalter D, et al. Age, severity and outcome of head injury. In RG Grossman and PL Gildenberg (Eds.) *Head Injury: Basic and clinicial aspects.* New York: Raven Press, 1982, pages 213–220.

73. Pentland B, Jones PA, Roy CW, Miller JD. Head injury in the elderly. *Age and Aging* 1986;15:193–202.

74. Coffey E. Traumatic brain injury in the elderly. Paper presented at the British Neuropsychiatric Association Annual Meeting, Oxford, England 1992.

75. Strauss DJ, Shavelle RM, Ashwal S. Life expectancy and median survival time in the permanent vegetative state. *Pediatric Neurology* 1999;21:626–631.

76. Strauss DJ, Day SM, Shavelle RM, Wu YW. Remote symptomatic epilepsy: Does seizure severity increase mortality? *Neurology* 2003;60:395–399.

77. Zafonte RD, Mann NR, Millis SR, Wood DL, Lee CY, Black KL. Functional outcome after violence related traumatic brain injury. *Brain Injury* 1997;11:403–407.

78. Lyle DM, Pierce JP, Freeman EA, et al. Clinical course and outcome of severe head injury in Australia. *Journal of Neurosurgery* 1986;65:15–18.

79. Rantakallio P, Koiranen M, Mottonen J. Association of perinatal events, epilepsy, and central nervous system trauma with juvenile delinquency. *Archives of Disease in Childhood* 1992;67(12): 1459–1461.

80. Sarapata M, Herrmann D, Johnson T, Aycock R. The role of head injury in cognitive functioning, emotional adjustment and criminal behaviour. *Brain Injury* 1998;12(10):821–842.

81. Turkstra L, Jones D, Toler HL. Brain injury and violent crime. *Brain Injury* 2003;17(1):39–47.

82. Harris EC, Barraclough B. Excess mortality of mental disorder. *British Journal of Psychiatry* 1998;173:11–53.

83. Teasdale GM, Nicoll JA, Murray G, Fiddes M. Association of apolipoprotein E polymorphism with outcome after head injury. *Lancet* 1997;350:1069–1071.

84. Friedman G, Froom P, Sazbon L, Grinblatt I, Shochina M, Tsenter J, Babaey S, Yehuda B, Groswasser Z. Apolipoprotein E-epsilon4 genotype predicts poor outcome in survivors of traumatic brain injury. *Neurology* 1999;52:244–248.

85. Crawford FC, Vanderploeg RD, Freeman MJ, Singh S, Waisman M, Michaels L, Abdullah L, Warden D, Lipsky R, Salazar A, Mullan MJ. APOE genotype influences acquisition and recall following traumatic brain injury. *Neurology* 2002;58: 1115–1118.

86. Lichtman SW, Seliger G, Tycko B, Marder K. Apolipoprotein E and functional recovery from brain injury following postacute rehabilitation. *Neurology* 2000;55:1536–1539.

87. Liberman JN, Stewart WF, Wesnes K, Troncoso J. Apolipoprotein E epsilon 4 and short-term recovery from predominantly mild brain injury. *Neurology* 2002;58:1038–1044.

88. Giacino JT, Ashwal S, Childs N, Cranford R, Jennett B, Katz DI, Kelly JP, Rosenberg JH, Whyte J, Zafonte RD, Zasler ND. The minimally conscious state: Definition and diagnostic criteria. *Neurology* 2002;58(3):349–353.

89. Ashwal S, Cranford R. The minimally conscious state in children. *Seminars in Pediatric Neurology* 2002;9:19–34.

90. Strauss DJ, Ashwal S, Day SM, Shavelle RM. Life expectancy of children in vegetative and minimally conscious states. *Pediatric Neurology* 2000;23:312–319.

91. Singer RB. The application of life table methodology to risk appraisal. In: RDC Brackenridge and WJ Elder (Eds), *Medical selection of life risks*, 3rd edition, pp. 51–78. New York: Stockton Press 1992.

92. Collett D. *Modelling survival data in medical research*. London: Chapman and Hall 1994.

93. Schoen R. *Modelling multigroup populations*, chapter 1. New York: Plenum 1988.

94. Strauss DJ, Shavelle RM, DeVivo MJ. Life tables for people with traumatic brain injury. *Journal of Insurance Medicine* 1999; 31:104–105.

95. Strauss DJ, Shavelle RM, DeVivo MJ, Day S. An analytic method for longitudinal mortality studies. *Journal of Insurance Medicine* 2000;32:217–225.

96. Hammond FM, Grattan KD, Sasser H, et al. Long-term recovery course after traumatic brain injury: a comparison of the functional independence measure and disability rating scale. *Journal of Head Trauma Rehabilitation* 2001;16:318–329.

97. Sander AM, Roebuck TM, Struchen MA, et al.. Long-term maintenance of gains obtained in postacute rehabilitation by persons with traumatic brain injury. *Journal of Head Trauma Rehabilitation* 2001;16:356–373.

98. Pierallini A, Pantano P, Fantozzi LM, et al. Correlation between MRI finding and long-term outcome in patients with severe brain trauma. *Neuroradiology* 2000;42:860–867.

99. Jaffe KM, Polissar NL, Fay GC, et al. Recovery trends over three years following pediatric traumatic brain injury. *Archives of Physical Medicine and Rehabilitation* 1995;76:17–26.

100. Chadwick O, Rutter M, Brown G, et al. A prospective study of children with head injuries: II. cognitive sequelae. *Psychological Medicine* 1981;11:49–61.

101. Susman M, Dirusso SM, Sullivan T, et al. Traumatic brain injury in the elderly: Increased mortality and worse functional outcome at discharge despite lower injury severity. *Journal of Trauma* 2002;53:219–223.

102. Berker E. Diagnosis, physiology, pathology and rehabilitation of traumatic brain injuries. *International Journal of Neuroscience*, 1996;85:195–220.

103. Asikainen I, Kaste M, Sarna S. Predicting late outcome for patients with traumatic brain injury referred to a rehabilitation programme: a study of 508 Finnish patients 5 years or more after injury. *Brain Injury* 1998;12:95–107.

104. Cifu DX, Kreutzer JS, Marwitz JH, Rosenthal M, Englander J, High W. Functional outcomes of older adults with traumatic brain injury: a prospective, multicenter analysis. *Archives of Physical Medicine and Rehabilitation* 1996;77:883–888.

105. Porter MD, Fricker PA. Controlled prospective neuropsychological assessment of active experienced amateur boxers. *Clinical Journal of Sport Medicine* 1996;6:90–96.

106. Haglund Y, Eriksson E. Does amateur boxing lead to chronic brain damage? A review of some recent investigations. *American Journal of Sports Medicine* 1993;21:97–109.

107. Jordan SE, Green GA, Galanty HL, et al. Acute and chronic brain injury in United States National Team soccer players. *American Journal of Sports Medicine* 1996;24:205–210.

108. Guskiewicz KM, Marshall SW, Broglio SP, et al. No evidence of impaired neurocognitive performance in collegiate soccer players. *American Journal of Sports Medicine* 2002;30:157–162.

109. Matser JT, Kessels AG, Jordan BD, et al. Chronic traumatic brain injury in professional soccer players. *Neurology* 1998;51: 791–796.

110. Jordan BD. Chronic traumatic brain injury associated with boxing. *Seminars in Neurology* 2000;20:179–185.

111. Jordan BD, Relkin NR, Ravdin LD, et al. Apolipoprotein E epsilon4 associated with chronic traumatic brain injury in boxing. *Journal of the American Medical Association* 1997;278: 136–140.

112. Roberts GW, Allsop D, Bruton C. The occult aftermath of boxing. *Journal of Neurology, Neurosurgery, and Psychiatry* 1990; 53:373–378.

113. Aalen OO, Johansen S. An empirical transition matrix for non-homogeneous Markov chains based on censored observations. *Scandinavian Journal of Statistics* 1978;5:141–150.

114. Kaplan EL, Meier P. Nonparametric estimation from incomplete observations. *Journal of the American Statistical Association* 1958, 58:457–481.

115. Anderson PK, Borgan O, Gill RD, Keiding N. *Statistical models based on counting processes*. New York: Springer-Verlag 1993.

116. Day SM. *Estimators of long-term transition probabilities of multistate stochastic processes*. Doctoral Dissertation, University of California at Riverside, December, 2001.

117. Strauss D, Shavelle R. An extended Kaplan-Meier estimator and its applications. *Statistics in Medicine* 1998;17:971–982.

118. Strauss D, Ashwal S, Shavelle R, Eyman RK. Prognosis for survival and improvement in function in children with severe developmental disabilities. *The Journal of Pediatrics* 1997;131: 712–717

119. Strauss DJ, Kastner TA. Comparative Mortality of People with Developmental Disability in Institutions and in the Community. *American Journal on Mental Retardation* 1996;101:26–40.

120. Strauss DJ, Eyman RK, Grossman HJ. The prediction of mortality in children with severe mental retardation: The effect of residential placement. *American Journal of Public Health* 1996; 86:1422–1429.

121. Strauss DJ, Shavelle RM. Mortality of persons with mental retardation in institutions in the community [Letter]. *American Journal of Public Health* 1997;87:1870–1871.

122. Strauss DJ, Shavelle RM, Baumeister AA, Anderson T. Mortality in persons with developmental disabilities after transfer into community care. *American Journal on Mental Retardation* 1998; 102:569–581.

123. Strauss DJ, Shavelle RM, Anderson T, Baumeister AA. External causes of death among persons with mental retardation: The effect of residential placement. *American Journal of Epidemiology* 1998;147:855–862.

124. Strauss DJ, Anderson T, Shavelle RM, Trenkle S, Sheridan F. Causes of death of persons with developmental disability placed from California institutions into community care. *Mental Retardation* 1998;36:386–391.

125. Strauss DJ, Kastner TA, Shavelle RM. Mortality of adults with developmental disabilities living in California institutions and community care, 1985–1994. *Mental Retardation* 1998;36: 360–371.

126. Shavelle RM, Strauss DJ. Mortality in persons with developmental disabilities after transfer into community care: A 1996 update. *American Journal on Mental Retardation* 1999;104: 143–146.

127. Strauss DJ, Shavelle RM. What can we learn from the California mortality studies? *Mental Retardation* 1998;36:406–407.

128. Multi-society task force on the persistent vegetative state. Medical Aspects of the Persistent Vegetative State, Part I. *New England Journal of Medicine* 1994;330:1499–1508.

129. Ashwal S, Eyman RK, Call TL. Life expectancy of children in a persistent vegetative state. *Pediatric Neurology* 1994;10: 27–33.

130. Higashi K, Sakata Y, Hatano M, Abiko S, Ihara K, Katayama S, Wakuta Y, Okamura T, Ueda H, Zenke M, Aoki H. Epidemiological studies on patients in persistent vegetative state. *Journal of Neurology, Neurosurgery and Psychiatry* 1977;40:876–885.

131. Higashi K, Hatano M, Abiko S, Ihara K, Katayama S, Wakuta Y, Okamura T, Yamashita T. Five year follow-up study of patients with persistent vegetative state. *Journal of Neurology, Neurosurgery and Psychiatry* 1981;44:552–554.

132. Sazbon L, Groswasser Z. Outcome in 134 patients with prolonged posttraumatic unawareness: I. parameters determining late recovery of consciousness. *Journal of Neurosurgery* 1990; 72:75–80.

133. Sazbon L, Groswasser Z. Medical complications and mortality of patients in the postcomatose unawareness (PC-U) state. *Acta Neurochirurgica* 1991;112:110–112.

134. Tresch DD, Sims FS, Duthie EH, Goldstein MD, Lane PS. Clinical characteristics of patients in the persistent vegetative state. *Archives of Internal Medicine* 1991;151:930–932.

135. Vollmer DG, Torner JC, Jane JA, Sadovnic B, Charlebois D, Eisenberg HM, Foulkes MA, Marmarou A, Marshall LF. Age and outcome following traumatic coma: Why do older patients fare worse? *Journal of Neurosurgery* 1991;75:S37–S49.

136. Zafonte RD, Hammond FM, Peterson J. Predicting outcome in the slow to respond brain-injured patient: Acute and subacute parameters. *NeuroRehabilitation* 1996;6:19–32.

137. Richards H, Abele JR. *Life and worklife expectancies.* Tucson: Lawyers & Judges 1999.

138. Hummer RA, Nam CR, Rogers RG. Adult mortality differentials associated with cigarette smoking. *Population Research and Policy Review* 1998;17:185–304.

139. Fisher ES, Welch HG. Avoiding the unintended consequences of growth in medical care: How might more be worse? *JAMA* 1999;281:446–453.

140. Fisher ES, Wennberg JE, Stukel TA, et al. Associations among hospital capacity, utilization, and mortality of US Medicare beneficiaries, controlling for sociodemographic factors. *Health Services Research* 2000;34(6):1351–62.

141. Skinner JS, Wennberg JE. How much is enough? Efficiency and Medicare spending in the last six months of life. In: DM Cutler (Ed.), *The Changing Hospital Industry: Comparing Not-for-Profit and For-Profit Institutions*, pp. 169–193, Chicago: The University of Chicago 2000.

142. Fisher ES, Wennberg DE, Stukel TA, Gottlieb DJ, Lucas FL, Pinder EL. The implications of regional variations in Medicare spending. Part 2: Health outcomes and satisfaction with care. *Annals of Internal Medicine* 2003;138:288–298.

143. Is more health care better? http://www.dartmouthatlas.org/ismorebetter/is_more_better_1.php. Accessed February 7, 2003. The bibliography includes citations and abstracts for articles relevant to the question of whether more care is better, and is also available from the authors.

144. Christakis NA, Lamont EB. Extent and determinants of error in doctors' prognoses in terminally ill patients: Prospective cohort study. *British Medical Journal* 2000;320:469–472.

145. Parkes CM. Accuracy of predictions of survival in later stages of cancer. *British Medical Journal* 1972;2:29–31.

146. Christakis NA. *Death foretold: Prophecy and prognosis in medical care.* Chicago: University of Chicago Press 1999, page 66.

147. Meadow W, Sunstein C. Statistics, not experts. *Duke Law Journal* 2001;51:629–646.

148. Wannamethee SG, Shaper AG, Walker M. Changes in physical activity, mortality, and incidence of coronary heart disease in older men. *The Lancet* 1998;351:1603–1608.

149. Schroll M. Physical activity in an ageing population. *Scandinavian Journal of Medicine & Science in Sports* 2003;13:63–69.

150. Pentland B, Hutton LS, Jones PA. Late mortality after head injury. *Journal of Neurology, Neurosurgery and Psychiatry* 2005;76: 395–400.

151. Brown AW, Leibson CL, Malec JF, Perkins PK, Diehl NN, Larson DR (2004). Long-term survival after traumatic brain injury: A population-based analysis, NeuroRehabilitation, 19:37–43.

152. Harrison-Felix C, Whiteneck G, DeVivo M, Hammond FM, Jha. A Mortality following rehabilitation in the traumatic brain injury model systems of care. *NeuroRehabilitation* 2004;19:45–54.

153. Strauss DJ, Shavelle RM, DeVivo MJ, Harrison-Felix C, Whiteneck GG Life expectancy after traumatic brain injury [letter]. *NeuroRehabilitation* 2004;19:257–258.

V

ACUTE CARE

18 TBI: Pathology, Pathophysiology, Acute Care and Surgical Management, Critical Care Principles, and Outcomes

Eli M. Baron
Jack I. Jallo

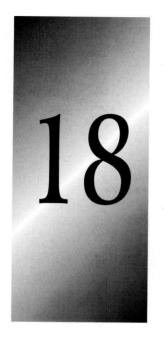

Traumatic brain injury (TBI) accounts for more than 50,000 deaths in the United States yearly and accounts for nearly 50 percent of all injury deaths (1, 2). TBI remains the leading cause of both injury death and disability among children and young adults (1). Recent observations suggest a decline in both TBI-related hospitalization and TBI-related deaths (2). This is largely due to a 40% decline in TBI related deaths in motor vehicle accidents, attributed to both the increased use of seat belts and an increase in use of safety equipment (3). Nevertheless, there remains a substantial social and economic burden related to TBI, with 1.5 million Americans sustaining a TBI yearly and 250,000 Americans being hospitalized yearly for TBI (4, 5). Of these, 80 to 90,000 people yearly experience long-term disability (6). Costs of acute hospitalization in 1997 to 1999 ranged from over $8000 on average for moderately injured patients to over $33,000 on average for patients with TBI requiring critical care (5). In 1995 the total direct and indirect costs of TBI in America was estimated at $56.3 billion (7). Further, at least 5.3 million Americans (~2% of the population) live with TBI related disabilities (6). Thus TBI presents an enormous medical and socioeconomic burden and is certainly one of the leading public health problems in the United States.

A recent study reviewing the hospital discharge data over the year 1997 revealed motor-vehicle crashes, falls, and assaults as the leading causes of injury for TBI-related discharges (27.9, 22.5, and 7.3/100,000 respectively). Rates were highest for American Indians and Alaska Natives (75.3/100,000) and Blacks (74.4/100,000), reflecting lower socioeconomic status. The age-adjusted rate for males was about twice as high as for females (91.9 versus 47.7/100,000 respectively). For both sexes, the rates were highest among those aged between 15 and 19 years and ≥ 65 years, reflecting increased risk taking in the younger population (e.g. drinking and driving, driving without seatbelts, etc.) and confirming that TBI is a very important health problem among the elderly (8). Another larger study confirmed an alarming increase in the rate of fall related TBI deaths in the elderly from 1989–1998 (9). A decline of nearly 50% in terms of hospitalization has been observed since 1980, that has been attributed in part to injury prevention and to changes in hospital admission practices where more patients with mild TBI are managed in outpatient settings (6, 10).

An emphasis has been made regarding the mortality rates in severe TBI falling from the 50% range in the 1970's to the 30% range in the 1990's, with a concomitant increase in the number of good to moderately disabled survivors (as opposed to those severely disabled or vegetative). This his been proposed to be due to multiple factors including improved rescue systems, enhanced emergency care in trauma facilities, rapid surgical treatment and improvement in critical care (11). One controversial area regarding improvement in mortality statistics is intracranial pressure (ICP) monitoring and its role in the management of severe brain injury. ICP monitoring has become a cornerstone in the modern day management of severe head injury. Much emphasis has been made in terms of classifying the resultant brain injury resulting from the initial traumatic insult as primary brain injury and subsequent insults as secondary injury. Secondary injury results from entities such as hypotension, hypoxia and ICP elevation. ICP monitoring may allow clinicians to intervene earlier in terms of treating ICP elevations, which are associated with an increased mortality. A basic understanding of injury mechanisms, morphology, pathophysiology, clinical presentation, therapeutic options and expected outcomes is necessary for the clinician involved in the rehabilitation of those sustaining TBI. The present discussion focuses on the diagnosis and management of the adult with traumatic brain injury with a review of head injury morphology, pathophysiology, surgical indications, ICP monitoring, ICU care, and outcomes.

HEAD INJURY MORPHOLOGY

Head injuries can be classified as blunt or penetrating injuries. Blunt TBI includes motor vehicle accidents and falls, and is responsible for the majority of TBI in this country. *Coup* and *contrecoup* injuries respectively refer to damage resulting from blunt trauma, where coup injuries occur adjacent to the area struck by an object and countercoup injuries occur on the opposite side, usually due to resultant acceleration of the brain after being subject to a force and striking the calvarium or skull base of the opposite side. Penetrating injuries include bladed weapons and both low velocity and high projectiles such as handguns and assault rifles. The majority of injuries are either homicides or suicides, although accidental firearms injuries contribute significantly to this number. Injury resulting from gunshot wounds occurs as a result of energy transfer from the projectile to impacted tissue. Initially, injury starts by the direct crushing and lacerating of tissues as the missile enters the skull and brain, taking with it bone and tissue fragments. A pulsating temporary cavity, with lower intracavitary pressures is formed, where the cavity may be many times larger than the diameter of the bullet. This may generate pressure waves radiating to locations away from the bullet path, causing stretching and tearing wounds (12). Penetrating injuries also carry with them a theoretically increased risk of infection, especially if bone and particulate matter enter the neural substance. Despite recent advances in neurosurgical and critical care, the prognosis for patients sustaining gunshot wounds to the head remains dismal, with an overall mortality rate of patients presenting to hospitals alive being near 60% (12).

Head injuries are further classified by their pathologic and morphologic descriptions. Skull fractures are frequently seen with head injury. The more severe the injury, the more likely the presence of skull fractures. In one series of patients sustaining TBI, 3% of emergency room attendees, 65% of neurosurgical ICU admission and 80% of fatalities sustained skull fractures (13). Skull fractures are an important entity since they carry a much higher association with intracranial hemorrhages than TBI without the presence of skull fractures (13, 14).

Skull fractures can be associated with a variety of trauma related complications. They can be a source of infection and pathologic communication with the exterior. Cerebrospinal fluid rhinorrhea results from a fracture in the cribriform plate. Otorrhea results from fractures within the mastoid air cells or temporal bone (14). These entities carry a 2–9% risk of associated meningitis (15, 16). Depressed skull fractures carry a long-term risk of late posttraumatic seizures of 31% (17). Temporal bone fractures can be associated with seventh nerve damage and/or hearing loss.

Basilar skull fractures are associated in general with greater forces than simple cranial vault fractures. Classic signs of these include raccoon eye's, representing cribriform plate fractures and Battle's sign, representing ecchymoses over the mastoid process associated with an ipsilateral skull fracture.

Cerebral contusions most commonly occur in the frontal and temporal poles adjacent to bony surfaces of the skull base, resulting from the brain striking these upon traumatic acceleration (Figure 18-1). Gliding contusions of the

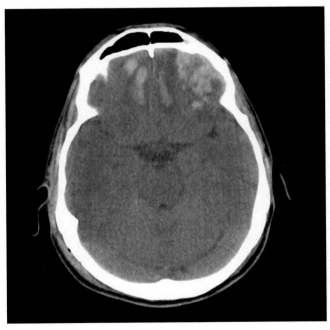

FIGURE 18-1

Axial noncontrast CT scan demonstrating bilateral frontal contusions grey white junction represent considerably greater forces acting on the brain with associated rotational/acceleratory vectors (14). Clinically, contusions can range from asymptomatic lesions to massive pulped areas of brain with resulting herniation. Cortical lacerations occur with penetrating injuries including depressed skull fractures.

Epidural hemorrhages usually occur in the middle fossa via laceration of the middle meningeal artery, although they can also occur in the anterior and posterior fossae. They are usually lenticular shaped and are bounded by suture lines where the pericranial layer of dura attaches to the skull (Figure 18-2). Epidural hemorrhages are most commonly associated with an overlying skull fracture (14). Though classically described with an associated lucid interval prior to clinical deterioration, only about half of patients undergoing surgical intervention present this way. These are important injuries to identify; if detected early they are usually associated with a good outcome and have a mortality of less than 10% (18).

Acute subdural hemorrhages are usually associated with a much poorer prognosis than epidural hemorrhages. This is because they often represent much more severe underlying brain damage (19). They usually result from torn bridging veins or from associated contusions hemorrhaging into the subdural space. Subdural hemorrhages tend to follow the shape of the convexities and tend to cover the entire hemisphere (Figure 18-3) (13). The present discussion pertains to acute subdural

hemorrhages in traumatic settings. Chronic subdural hemorrhages represent a different pathophysiologic condition where an initial small subdural hematoma enlarges secondary to transudative forces or repeated small hemorrhages because of associated chronic membranes. These tend to occur in older adults and are also most commonly related to an initially tearing of bridging veins.

Trauma is also the most common cause of subarachnoid hemorrhage. Often this occurs locally over convexities affected by coup type of injuries or the frontotemporal poles affected by contrecoup injuries (Figure 18-4). Subarachnoid hemorrhage from trauma can also occur in the interhemispheric fissure and in the basilar cisterns. At times it can be difficult to discern from aneurysmal subarachnoid hemorrhage, but usually the history is very suggestive of the etiology. Traumatic subarachnoid hemorrhage can result in hydrocephalus, defined as abnormal ventricular expansion with associated raised intracranial pressure (13). Hydrocephalus can also occur secondary to TBI in cases without frank intraventricular hemorrhage.

Diffuse axonal injury is a pathologic term referring to changes occurring in the brain post TBI as a result of rotational forces. The term shear injury is often used synonymously. These terms refer to classic pathologic changes including focal lesions in the corpus callosum, focal lesions of various sizes in the posterolateral quadrants of the

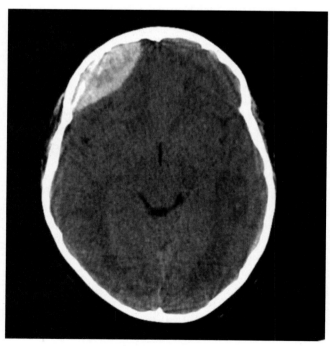

FIGURE 18-2

Axial noncontrast CT scan demonstrating a right frontal epidural hematoma. Note the lenticular shape

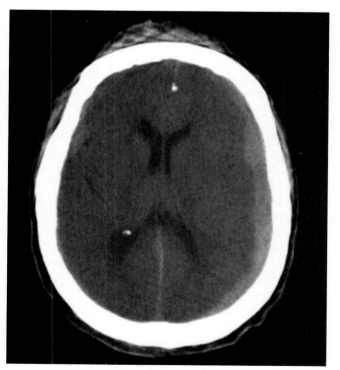

FIGURE 18-3

Axial noncontrast CT scan demonstrating a left sided acute subdural hematoma. Note that this spans the length of the convexity

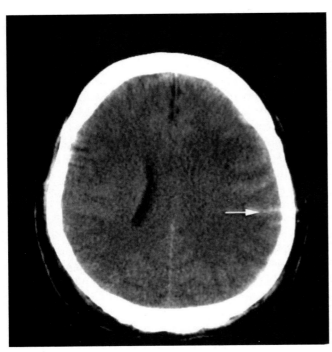

FIGURE 18-4

Axial noncontrast CT scan demonstrating a small amount of left convexity traumatic subarachnoid hemorrhage. Note its appearance as hyperdensity adjacent to the ipsilateral sulci (arrow)

brainstem next to the superior cerebellar peduncles and microscopic evidence of widespread damage to axons (13). Though MRI imaging may hint at it, the diagnosis is a tissue based one. Diffuse axonal injury is the most commonly cited cause, in the absence of hemorrhages or ICP elevations, of prolonged depressed consciousness and of severe disability in brain injured individuals. Three grades for diffuse axonal injury are widely used: Grade 1 abnormalities refer to scattered axonal bulbs through out the white matter of the brain; Grade 2 requires the presence of a corpus callosum lesion; in Grade 3 there is the additional lesion in the dorsolateral quadrant(s) of the rostral brain stem; Grade 3 lesions nearly always result in patients being in coma or a vegetative state until death (14).

CONCUSSION

The term concussion has been used to describe the brain injury phenomenon often resulting in very disabling symptoms following a mild to moderate TBI where no hematoma or other intracranial pathology is seen on imaging. Symptoms include headache, nausea, vomiting, difficulty concentrating, retrograde and/or anterograde amnesia and personality changes, among others. Numerous clinical definitions of this term have been used with some requiring a loss of consciousness and others not.

Even with a mild TBI, there can be widespread neuronal dysfunction and axonal injury, with the possibility of delayed axotomy occurring, all potentially contributing to the post concussive syndrome (see below)(20).

PATHOPHYSIOLOGY AND MOLECULAR BASIS FOR INJURY

Primary Injury

The events that occur at the moment of injury, although possibly preventable are not reversible. Brain contusions and hemorrhages, however, represent potentially avoidable causes of death and disability when evacuated promptly. These are often seen together.

Secondary Injury

Secondary neuronal injury after TBI has received much attention with new mechanisms being elucidated and previously described mechanisms being better understood. At a macroscopic level, secondary phenomena include edema, ischemia, necrosis, elevated intracranial pressure and inadequate cerebral perfusion. At a cellular level, energy failure occurs in association with a cascade of events that contribute to secondary injury such as elevated levels of intracellular calcium, release of excitatory amino acids, generation of free radicals, and breakdown of the cellular cytoskeleton and membrane with vascular dysfunction eventually leading to cell death (21).

Excitatory Amino Acids

The first event in this sequence is thought to be the release of excitatory amino acids; this mechanism of injury has been termed excitotoxic injury. Following brain injury, excitatory amino acids are released from injured cells. Of the excitatory amino acids, glutamate has been studied the most. Glutamate acts postsynaptically at five subtypes of receptors. These receptors are named based on the agent that specifically activates them. The NMDA (N-methyl-D-aspartate) receptor complex is an ion channel that allows passage of calcium and sodium ions. When activated by glutamate, the NMDA receptor allows calcium ions to enter the cell. Large influxes of calcium ions into neurons stimulate calcium dependent enzymes with activation of proteases, kinases, phospholipases, and nitric oxide synthase. If unchecked, these processes can eventually lead to cell death with breakdown of the cytoskeleton, free radical formation, alterations in gene expression and protein synthesis, and membrane dysfunction. Blocking the NMDA receptor improves neuronal survival in vitro and in animal models of neuronal injury (21). NMDA blockers failed to show efficacy in recent human trials for TBI. This has been thought to be due to glutamate exitotoxicity occurring immediately at injury time but afterwards glutatmate has important normal functions, such as promotion of neuronal survival. The administration of numerous NMDA antagonists in human trials may have been in the time period where glutamate had resumed its normal critical functions, rather than earlier when they would have possibly prevented excitotoxicty (22).

Free Radicals

Free radical formation is an important part of many mechanisms of secondary injury. The most common free radicals studied are superoxide (O_2^-), hydrogen peroxide (H_2O_2), hydroxyl (OH), and nitric oxide (NO). Free radicals are atoms or molecules possessing an unpaired electron in the outer orbit making them highly reactive. Free iron is a key catalyst of free radical mediated injury and is readily available in injured and contused brain tissue. Free radicals damage endothelial cells and injure the brain parenchyma. This results in disruption of the blood brain barrier and is partly responsible for both vasogenic and cytotoxic edema. Once initiated, free radical injury is a self-perpetuating process with increasing damage generating more free radicals. Cells attempt to minimize injury caused by free radicals by binding them with free radical scavengers such as vitamin E, ascorbic acid, superoxide dismutase, and others. Nevertheless, these coping mechanisms may be overwhelmed in areas of significant brain injury or ischemia. Pharmacological free radical scavenging agents have been effective in reducing neuronal damage in animal models of brain injury (21). Unfortunately, a human trial of a free radical scavenger (polyethylene glycol – superoxide dismutase) in severe head injury did not demonstrate an improved outcome (23). More recently, the cannabinoid dexanabinol has been proposed as a neuroprotective treatment for head injury. Mechanistically, dexanabinol most likely works as a noncompetitive NMDA antagonist in vitro and in vivo. It blocks NMDA stimulated calcium influx in primary neuronal culture, and head injury related calcium influx in rats. In addition, it is a potent free radical scavenger (24). Recently, however, a very large multicenter, Food and Drug Administration double-blind, randomized, placebo-controlled trial of dexanabinol vs. placebo failed to demonstrate efficacy of the drug in humans (25).

NITRIC OXIDE

Nitric oxide, a ubiquitous second messenger has been implicated in a variety of cellular processes including vascular relaxation, neurotransmitter effects, and cytotoxicity. Nitric oxide is formed by the conversion of L-arginine to L-citrulline and nitric oxide via nitric oxide synthase (NOS). The mechanism of nitric oxide cytoxicity is unclear, but is closely intermingled with NMDA, calcium, and free radical mediated injury. Inhibitors of nitric oxide synthase have been found to reduce neuronal injury in animal models of brain injury. A host of other mediators of secondary brain injury are under investigation including: catecholamines, adenosine, cytokines, opioid peptides, and thyrotropin releasing hormone (21).

PHYSIOLOGIC RESPONSE TO BRAIN INJURY

Brain Edema

The cellular mechanisms of secondary brain injury described above contribute to brain edema, and subsequently to elevations in intracranial pressure, decreased cerebral perfusion, and cerebral ischemia. Brain edema has been traditionally described as either vasogenic or cytotoxic. *Vasogenic edema* results from disruption of the blood brain barrier. The blood brain barrier is maintained by tight junctions between endothelial cells that line the vessels of the brain. Injury to these cells allows extravasation of fluid and proteins into the interstitial space of the brain parenchyma. Disruption of endothelial cells may be primary, resulting from the initial impact or subsequent hemorrhage, or secondary resulting from free radical generation, cytokines, and other secondary mechanisms of injury. *Cytotoxic* or *cellular edema* is edema of the cells themselves in contrast to vasogenic edema which is edema of the interstitial space. Cytotoxic edema results from failure of cellular ion homeostasis and membrane function. As previously mentioned, secondary injury at a cellular level results in loss of ion homeostasis and membrane dysfunction. The time course of brain edema is variable. It is thought, however, that vasogenic edema occurs early after injury and cytotoxic edema occurs in a more delayed fashion. Brain edema after traumatic brain injury is often maximal at 24 to 48 hours (26).

Edema of the brain is an important marker for injury and is also a cause of secondary injury. This is because the brain is confined by the skull, which acts as a closed container. Intracranial pressure is determined by the volume of three elements in the skull: the brain parenchyma volume, the blood volume, and the cerebrospinal fluid (CSF) volume. An increase in the volume of any of these elements will result in an increased intracranial pressure after compensatory mechanisms are exhausted. As intracranial pressure rises, there is an initial passive release of CSF into the spinal canal. There is also an innate compliance of the craniospinal axis that allows for an increase in intracranial contents without an initial increase in intracranial pressure. Once the compensatory reserve is exhausted, there is a precipitous rise in intracranial pressure (Figure 18-5) (21).

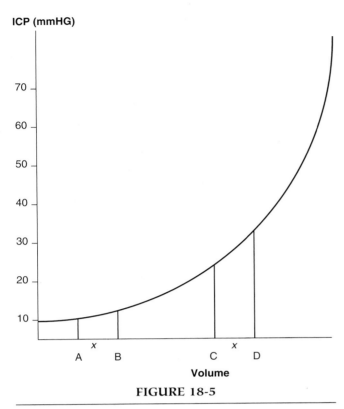

FIGURE 18-5

Pressure volume curve of the craniospinal axis demonstrating a precipitous rise in intracranial pressure associated with exhaustion of compensatory mechanisms. At a pressure of 10 mmHg a volume of *x* can be added with little change in ICP (represented by points A to B). Adding the same volume when the ICP is about 25 mmHg results in a much larger change in ICP (points C to D)

Intracranial Pressure and Cerebral Blood Flow

Intracranial pressure in an adult is ordinarily under 15 mmHg. Sustained elevations in intracranial pressure above 20 mmHg are poorly tolerated by the injured brain and have been associated with increased mortality (27, 28). Sustained elevation in intracranial pressure may result in cerebral ischemia if cerebral perfusion is hampered and, if severe, can result in brain herniation. Brain herniations may occur across the falx and involve the cingulate gyrus, across the tentorial hiatus and involve the uncus, or through the foramen magnum and involve the cerebellar tonsills. Cerebral ischemia results from inadequate cerebral perfusion. The ideal degree of cerebral perfusion in the injured brain is unknown. In the uninjured brain, cerebral blood flow is tightly regulated by myogenic, humoral, and neural mechanisms to maintain a constant flow despite changes in systemic arterial pressure and intracranial pressure. This autoregulation functions over a broad range of systemic arterial pressures ranging from a lower limit of 65mmHg and an upper limit of 140mmHg to maintain

cerebral blood flow at approximately 50ml/100gms/min. If blood flow falls beneath 25ml/100gms/min then electrical activity is lost and the EEG is flat, below 12ml/100gms/min brain stem evoked responses are lost and below 10ml/100gms/min brain failure results with loss of ion homeostasis and eventual cell death (21).

Cerebral Perfusion Pressure

It is of paramount importance that an adequate cerebral blood flow be maintained to the injured brain. Unfortunately, there is no simple technique that allows for reliable, continuous bedside measurement of cerebral blood flow. As a result, the concept of cerebral perfusion pressure is invoked when discussing cerebral blood flow to the injured brain. Cerebral perfusion pressure (CPP) is defined as the difference between mean arterial pressure (MAP) and intracranial pressure (ICP): CPP = MAP − ICP. The concept of autoregulation can be extended to discussions of cerebral perfusion pressure in the uninjured brain. Autoregulation in terms of perfusion pressure has a lower limit of 50mmHg and an upper limit of approximately 140mmHg. With a perfusion pressure below 50mmHg, cerebral arterioles are maximally dilated and perfusion cannot match the brains metabolic needs. If this state persists brain ischemia follows. As previously noted, the brain poorly tolerates ischemic conditions which aggravate secondary injury. With a perfusion pressure greater than 140mmHg, cerebral arterioles are maximally constricted and blood flow increases passively with perfusion pressure (Figure 18-6) (21).

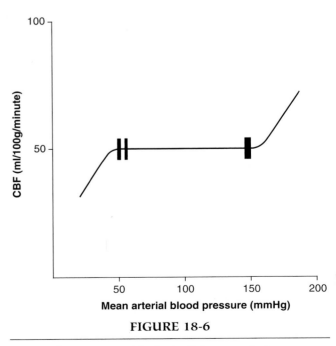

FIGURE 18-6

Autoregulation curve of the brain. Below a perfusion pressure of 50 mmHg and above a pressure of 140 mmHg blood flow passively correlates with perfusion pressure

Discussions of cerebral autoregulation are generally predicated on the brain's physiologic responses to changes in systemic arterial pressure. However, these discussions assume that the physiologic responses that are in effect in an uninjured brain are also in place after brain injury. This has been a topic of debate and study. Up to one-half of severely head injured patients will have some autoregulatory impairment. It appears as though the autoregulatory curve is shifted to the right with an increase in the lower limit at which autoregulation is effective (21). Patients with severe head injury probably require a CPP of 60mmHg to 70mmHg to maintain autoregulation of cerebral blood flow and prevent ischemic complications. In one study, outcome was shown to be significantly worse in patients with a CPP less than 60mmHg (29). Additionally, Rosner et al. (30) demonstrated more favorable outcomes when CPP was kept above 70mmHg. Current recommendations are to maintain cerebral perfusion pressure at 60mmHg to 70mmHg(31). Targeting CPP beyond 70 mmHg may increase the risk of adult respiratory distress syndrome, offsetting potential benefits from this therapy (32).

CLINICAL PRESENTATION AND MANAGEMENT

Head injury can present in a variety of manners and often requires a high index of suspicion to be diagnosed. While loss of consciousness or altered consciousness, headaches, anisocoria, nausea/vomiting/dizziness and/or witnessed obvious traumatic injury to the head usually prompt a clinical workup, often TBI presents more subtly. All patients with a loss of consciousness or posttraumatic disturbance in sensorium should undergo CT scanning of the brain. Particular attention should be paid to intoxicated individuals, even without obvious signs of external injury. Subdural hemorrhages can easily be missed in patients intoxicated with alcohol, who may have suffered unrecognized head injuries. Further, stimulant drugs may result in TBI related agitation being overlooked. The widespread availability of CT scanning should result in a very low threshold for imaging.

Head injury can be classified as mild, moderate and severe. This is conveniently done with the aid of the Glasgow Coma Scale (GCS)(Table 18-1). Initially intended as a tool for clinicians to communicate their assessment of a patient's level consciousness in an objective matter (33), the GCS has been widely adapted as a head injury scoring system and has also proven to be an effective prognosticator with regard to clinical outcomes. Mild TBI is classified as GCS 14–15, moderate as GCS 9–13 and severe as GCS 3–8 (19).

In the field patients should have their airway status, breathing and circulation addressed first. Hypotension and hypoxia in the field are proven secondary injury insults that are associated with poor outcomes, with hypotension being considerably more detrimental than hypoxia (34); both of these must be prevented if possible. Endotracheal intubation may be necessary in the field. Patients should have a GCS score assessed and pupillary exam prior to any sedation or paralytic being administered if possible. This can be done accurately by emergency medical personnel (35). Even if the patient has focal or lateralizing signs, such as a decreased sensorium and an enlarging pupil, current recommendations do not support ICP directed measures in the field, with the possible exception of hyperventilation in the intubated patient in neurologic extremis. Every effort to have TBI patients transported to the nearest facility possessing CT scanning, neurosurgical expertise and ICP monitoring capabilities, should be made(35). This can be most easily expedited in areas where neurotrauma systems are established. The spine should also be immobilized as there is a 4 to 8 percent association of cervical spine injury with TBI(36).

Upon arrival in the emergency room, the Advanced Trauma Life Support (ATLS) protocol, as per the American College of Surgeons, should be followed. This protocol stresses a systematic approach to trauma injury, where airway, breathing and circulation are assessed first. The assessment of the circulatory system should include attention to all sites of external bleeding including scalp lacerations which may be a source of exsanguination. Efforts should be made to control bleeding. In terms of fluid resuscitation crystalloid vs. colloid remains controversial. A recent large prospective randomized trial compared

TABLE 18-1	
Glasgow Coma Scale (from Teasdale and Jennet (129))	
Eye Opening:	
Spontaneous	E4
To voice	E3
To pain	E2
None	E1
Best Motor Response	
Obeys commands	M6
Localizes	M5
Withdrawal	M4
Abnormal flexion	M3
Extensor posture	M2
None	M1
Best Verbal Response	
Oriented	V5
Confused conversation	V4
Inappropriate words	V3
Incomprehensible sounds	V2
None	V3
Score is (E + M +V) = 3 to 15	

saline to albumin in the intravascular resuscitation of critically ill patients. Similar outcomes were seen in both groups in terms of mortality and length of stay. Seven of the study population constituted patients with TBI. Mortality was increased in the subgroup with TBI receiving albumin with a relative risk of 1.62 over the group receiving normal saline (95 percent confidence interval, 1.12 to 2.34; P = 0.009). The authors cautioned, however, that "such subgroup differences frequently occur by chance and the rate of death from any cause over a 28-day period is not considered the most appropriate outcome measurement with which to assess treatment effects in patients with brain injury (37)."

Once fluid resuscitation is addressed, a neurologic assessment is made in terms of GCS score, pupillary exam and lateralizing signs. This is preferably done prior to any sedation or paralytic being given. A lateral c-spine and chest x-ray should be performed. A CT scan is then performed as rapidly as possible in any patients with a suspected or confirmed loss of consciousness, skull fracture or abnormal neurologic/GCS exam. CT scanning has become the diagnostic procedure of choice for the initial assessment of intracranial injury. It accurately shows acute blood and identifies most skull fractures. Any coagulopathy requires correction in patients with acute blood on their CT scans.

Patients with mild traumatic brain injury who are neurologically normal with a negative head CT may be discharged home safely (38, 39). Other patients, especially those with altered mental status or collections on their CT scans should be admitted for observation and possible serial imaging. Patients with isolated skull fractures and normal neurologic exams can possibly be discharged to home, although this is controversial and must be assessed on a case to case basis (40–43).

SURGICAL TREATMENT OF HEAD INJURY

Operative therapy is indicated in patients where intracerebral collections are exerting significant mass effect. Traditionally this has been defined as greater than 5 mm of midline shift (19). Midline shift is measured on axial CT scan images in terms of displacement of the septum pellucidum from the midline at the level of the foramen of Monroe. A line is drawn at the midline of the skull in the sagittal plane and then a perpendicular line is extended to the septum pellucidum, which is measured and recorded as shift (Figure 18-7). Mass effect is also evaluated in terms of correlation of local effect of abnormal collections on more normal appearing adjacent brain. Similarly, the basilar cisterns are evaluated for compression.

Numerous surgical criteria for a variety of commonly seen TBI related pathologies have been proposed (18). Epidural hemorrhages greater than 30 cc in volume

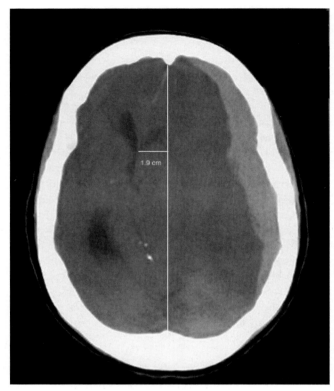

FIGURE 18-7

Midline shift measurement: the septum pelucidum is measured at the level of the foramen of Monroe. This scan demonstrates 1.9 cm of left to right shift

should be evacuated regardless of whether the patient is symptomatic. Those patients with a GCS score less than 9 with associated papillary dilation and an epidural hematoma should undergo decompression as soon as possible. Epidural hemorrhages less than 30 cc in volume and less than 1.5 cm in thickness, with less than 5 mm midline shift, may be managed by close observation and serial imaging in patients without focal deficits. Similarly, patients with acute subdural hemorrhages greater than 1 cm in thickness or subdural hemorrhages associated with greater than 5 mm of midline shift should undergo emergent evacuation. Smaller subdural hemorrhages may require evacuation in patients with neurologic deficits, in those deteriorating neurologically and in those with raised intracranial pressures. Both types of acute hemorrhages are best evacuated either through a craniotomy or craniectomy.

Intracerebral contusions may also be life threatening. Patients with intracerebral contusions with progressive neurologic deterioration referable to the contusion or resultant refractory intracranial hypertension should be treated operatively (Figure 18-8). Comatose patients with frontal or temporal contusions greater than 20 cc in volume with a midline shift of 5 mm and/or cisternal compression on CT scan, and those with a contusion

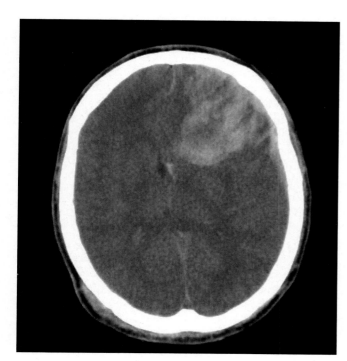

FIGURE 18-8

Axial noncontrast CT scan demonstrating life threatening left frontal intracerebral contusion which necessitated surgical evacuation.

greater than 50 cc in volume should be treated operatively. These numbers are general guidelines: patients with relatively good neurologic exams and contusions in eloquent cortex may be carefully watched, with medical treatment of ICP elevations if needed (18). Contusions are often associated with numerous other pathologic findings on CT scan such as significant cerebral edema with resultant cisternal compression and traumatic subarachnoid hemorrhage. In patients with severely contused frontal lobes with significant mass effect and resultant medically refractory intracranial hypertension, bifrontal decompressive craniectomy may be life saving; nevertheless, decompressive craniectomy for refractory ICP elevations remains a controversial area as discussed below.

Open depressed skull fractures greater than the thickness of the skull with evidence of dural laceration should be operated on acutely to lower the risk of infection. Nonoperative management may be an option for depressed skull fracture if there is no clinical or radiographic evidence of dural penetration, no evidence of significant intracranial hematoma, depression less than 1 cm thickness, no frontal sinus involvement, no gross cosmetic deformity, no evidence of wound infection, pneumocephalus or gross wound contamination. All open skull fractures, regardless of whether managed expectantly or surgically, should be treated with antibiotics. Closed skull fractures can be managed nonoperatively.

ICP MONITORING AND THE TREATMENT OF ELEVATED ICP

Per the Guidelines for the Management of Severe Traumatic Brain Injury (44), ICP monitoring is appropriate in patients with GCS scores post resuscitation < or = 8 with a head CT demonstrating hemorrhages, contusions, edema or compressed basilar cisterns. ICP monitoring may also be appropriate in patients with GCS scores post resuscitation < or = 8 with a normal head CT and 2 of the following: age > 40, motor posturing, or a systolic blood pressure of < 90 mmHg. These recommendations are largely based on the landmark paper by Narayan et al. (27) which defined which patients are likely to develop ICP elevations. There is a clear association between (abnormally) elevated ICP's and mortality (28, 45). While no significant prospective study to date has demonstrated that ICP monitoring leads to decreased mortality or improved clinical outcomes, there is considerable evidence favoring its use in the management of patients with severe TBI based on retrospective series and trauma data bank studies (46–49). Nevertheless, there remains some controversy regarding the efficacy of ICP monitoring based therapy vs. empiric therapies for head injury (e.g. empiric mannitol administration)(50–52). Despite this controversy, it has become a mainstay in the critical care management of patient's with severe TBI and may also be appropriate in some cases of moderate TBI.

Ventriculostomy (external ventricular drain) insertion is the ICP monitoring procedure of choice in adults with severe TBI. It permits both monitoring of pressure via transduction of a continuous fluid column from the ventricles and also permits CSF drainage (Figure 18-9). Other monitoring technologies such as fiberoptic monitors are also acceptable but do not permit cerebrospinal fluid drainage and are subject to measurement drift (53, 54).

A threshold of 20–25 mmHg can be used to define an elevated ICP. ICP elevation presenting as a change from lower more normal pressures must always prompt a search for a potential surgical mass lesion via a repeat head CT. Elevation of the head of the bed to 30 degrees promotes jugular venous drainage and lowers ICP (55). Preventing hyperthermia can also lower ICP. While a large recent trial found systemic hypothermia ineffective in improving outcomes in TBI (56), animal models have shown it to be neuroprotective and it may play a future role in TBI management. In patients where ICP management is of concern, a mechanical airway should be in place, allowing hyperventilation and sedation/paralysis to be used as needed. Steroids have not shown to be of benefit in reducing ICP elevations and are not recommended for use in TBI. Recently, the results of a very large randomized control trial where 10008 adults with head injury and a Glasgow coma score (GCS) of 14 or less within 8 h of injury were randomly allocated 48 h

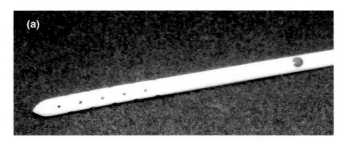

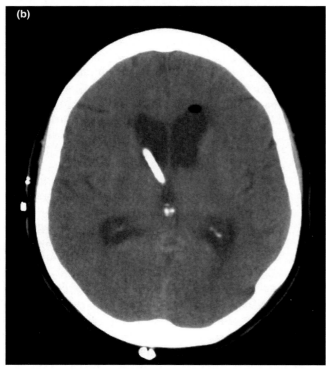

FIGURE 18-9

18-9(a): Ventriculostomy catheter: a silicon catheter used for measurement of ICP and ventricular drainage. 18-9(b) Axial noncontrast CT scan demonstrating ideal placement of a ventricular catheter at the foramen of monroe

infusion of corticosteroids (methylprednisolone) or placebo were published. Compared with placebo, the risk of death from all causes within 2 weeks was higher in the group allocated corticosteroids (1052 [21.1%] vs 893 [17.9%] deaths; relative risk 1.18 [95% CI 1.09–1.27]; p = 0.0001) (57). Based on the results of this trial a recent Cochrane review on the topic concluded that steroids should no longer be routinely used in people with traumatic head injury (58).

Mannitol is a very effective drug for lowering ICP and is a mainstay in this regard. It works by dehydrating the brain, especially areas of cerebral edema and by altering cerebral rheology. Unfortunately it loses some of its efficacy with time and has some potentially serious side effects including renal failure and pulmonary edema.

Mannitol is optimally given as a slow intravenous bolus. The dose is 1 mg/kg for immediate maximum effect and duration (19). High dose therapy is preferred in the presence of acute intracranial hematoma prior to surgery (59). Smaller doses are used as maintenance therapy for ICP elevation. Mannitol's effects may be augmented by other diuretics such as furosemide. A Foley catheter must be present to help monitor mannitol's diuretic effect. Serial serum osmolarties should also be measured, where osmolarities should be kept below 320 mOsm to reduce risk of renal failure (44).

While hyperventilation was advocated in the past to lower ICP, current recommendations are more modest in terms of its use. Hyperventilation works to lower ICP by causing cerebral vasoconstriction. This reduces ICP but can also exacerbate cerebral ischemia. Hyperventilation also loses efficacy with continued use. Current recommendations are for avoidance of the use of *prophylactic* hyperventilation in the first 24 hours after severe TBI. It is reserved for treatment of patients with established ICP elevations (e.g. PCO_2 30–35 mmHg) and more aggressive hyperventilation is for those patients with refractory ICP elevation and those in neurologic extremis (44, 60).

Sedation with short acting benzodiazepines such as midazolam and analgesic agents such as morphine maybe useful additional agents to manage elevated ICP. Similarly, paralytics maybe useful in the management of refractory ICP elevations. Barbiturates are considered the last line medical therapy for otherwise medically refractory intracranial hypertension. They require electroencephalogram monitoring in order to confirm burst suppression. Barbiturates have serious side effects including cardiac depression and increased infection risk. Because of barbiturates' cardiac effects, most centers use pulmonary artery catheters for hemodynamic monitoring.

In cases of medically refractory ICP elevation or in cases of significant intraoperative brain swelling decompressive unilateral or bilateral craniectomy with duraplasty has been advocated. In the operating room this decision maybe made for technical reasons (e.g. the brain is swelling so rapidly that traditional closure of the dura and bone is impossible). The use of this procedure to treat medically refractory ICP elevation is controversial. Various studies have found improved outcomes and decreased mortality in patients undergoing a craniectomy for refractory ICP vs. those medically managed (61–63). It remains to be proven, however, whether decompressive craniectomy is beneficial over maximal medical treatment.

In the presence of ICP elevation an attempt should be made to increase cerebral perfusion pressures to at least 60 mmHg in adults. CPP is defined as the difference between mean arterial pressure and ICP. In the presence of elevated ICP, cerebral autoregulation maybe deranged. Thus elevating CPP maybe critical for brain tissue at risk for ischemia. Nevertheless, it is important to remember that ICP elevation is itself detrimental; therefore ICP elevation should never be simply treated by elevation of CPP alone. Rather, its cause should be investigated and concomitantly treated.

CRITICAL CARE AND ADDITIONAL NEUROMONITORING TECHNOLOGIES

A brief discussion of some of the issues regarding TBI related neurocritical care is warranted. As stressed above, ICP monitoring has become a mainstay in the modern management of severe TBI. Efforts should be made to maintain CPP above 60 mmHg in patients with elevated ICP's. Knowledge of patients' hemodynamic and volume status can be very useful in the maintenance of appropriate blood pressures for CPP directed therapy. Thus a central venous catheter should be placed for central venous pressure monitoring. In patients' undergoing treatment with barbiturates, pulmonary artery catheterization is warranted. Current recommendations are for maintaining euvolemia. Intravenous fluids should be isotonic solutions such as normal saline. Dextrose containing solutions are avoided as hyperglycemia has been shown to be associated with worse outcomes in TBI (64).

Similarly, glucose abnormalities must be avoided as secondary insults. Electrolytes should be followed with at least daily laboratory studies. Particular attention should be paid to sodium values. Syndrome of inappropriate antidiuretic hormone, diabetes insipidus and cerebral salt wasting have all been described in association with TBI—all are potential sources of secondary brain injury (65).

Seizures are another potential source of secondary insult. *Early post traumatic seizures* are those that occur within the first 7 days after a TBI and *late posttraumatic seizures* are those that occur later. Early posttraumatic seizures are more common in younger people and their risk of occurrence is increased in the presence of hematomas, contusion, prolonged unconsciousness and focal neurologic signs. They are usually focal seizures with or without secondary generalization. Late posttraumatic seizures are associated with penetrating injuries, early seizures, intracranial hematomas/contusions, GCS score less than or equal to 10 and depressed skull fractures. They are usually generalized convulsive seizures(17). Current recommendations are for *prophylactic* treatment of seizures in the TBI patient undergoing craniotomy or at risk for seizures with phenytoin or carbamezapine for 1 week (17, 44, 66, 67). If late seizures do occur, they should be managed by a neurologist in accordance with standard approaches to new onset seizures(44).

Infection in the ICU setting represents a very common source of morbidity and mortality in the TBI patient population. Urinary tract infections are the most common ICU associated infection. Their most effective means of prevention is avoiding prolonged use of catheters. Secondary to the need for mechanical ventilation for a majority of these patients, and also their reduced airway protection mechanisms, pneumonia in the severe TBI patient population is the second most common nosocomial infection and the most common infectious cause of death (68). Several authorities have recommended early tracheostomy in these patients to promote pulmonary toilet, reduce infections and decrease length of stay in the ICU (69, 70). Aggressive attention to suctioning and maintaining the head of the bed elevated while administering tube feeds to minimize aspiration risk are mandatory as is strict hand washing (68). Immobile patients should be rolled every two hours to minimize the risk of skin breakdown. Early removal of patients' cervical collars may further avoid another source of decubitus ulcers (71). Perioperative antibiotics should be administered for trauma craniotomies (68). Additionally, antibiotic coated ventricular catheters may reduce infection rates in patients needing prolonged monitoring (72).

Nutrition should be initiated early in the critically ill TBI patient. This is preferably through a small intestine tube, with feedings starting within 2 to 3 days of injury (73, 74). Caution must be exerted when inserting nasal feeding tubes, as anterior skull base fractures may allow passage of the tube intracranially (75, 76). Nutritional needs in the TBI patient have been estimated to increase 40 percent over that calculated for uninjured people of similar age, sex and height. This is due to numerous factors including hormonal factors, cytokines and movement occurring post TBI. Despite high protein intake and appropriate caloric provision, during the early period post TBI, positive nitrogen balance cannot be achieved. A nutritional goal in the ICU should be the maintenance of adequate caloric and protein intake in an effort to improve nitrogen balance (77). Every severe TBI patient should have a formal nutrition assessment by an appropriately trained dietician. Markers such as prealbumin, nitrogen balance and liver function tests should be followed regularly. Gastrointestinal prophylaxis should also be routinely used in order to minimize the risk for stress ulcers.

Deep venous thrombosis is a common complication in the critically ill TBI population, with as many as 53.8% of patients experiencing this complication (78). Patients should have sequential compression boots and subcutaneous heparin used whenever possible. The safety of both subcutaneous heparin injections and low molecular weight heparins started early (within 24 to 72 hours) in severe TBI has been demonstrated (79, 80). Deep venous thrombosis should also be considered as source of fever. In cases of established thrombosis where anticoagulation is contraindicated, inferior vena cava filter placement should be considered.

Additional neuromonitoring technologies are used in selected centers. These include jugular bulb venous saturation monitoring, cerebral blood flow monitoring and regional tissue oxygen tension monitoring, among others. Jugular venous oxygen saturation monitoring is intended to detect increases in oxygen consumption (decreased jugular oxygen saturation) and as a result globally increased oxygen extraction by the brain. It is measured by placing a catheter tip (equipped with a fiberoptic monitor) in the dominant jugular bulb and is reserved for patients with severe TBI. Current recommendations are to maintain jugular venous saturation between 55% and 75%, with this range intended to allow for a margin of error. Desaturations below 50 percent are associated with significant increases in patient mortality (81). Any reported desaturation must be confirmed by a jugular venous bulb blood sample being sent for analysis to confirm the reading. If a desaturation is confirmed, a workup is pursued to find its cause in an effort to reverse any potential secondary insults contributing to the desaturation, including overly aggressive hyperventilation (82).

While jugular venous oxygen saturation monitoring may be reflective of global oxygenation, regional oxygenation is better measured by brain tissue oxygen tension monitors (83). These monitors can be inserted in normal brain or preferably in the penumbra of an intracerebral lesion. Therapy then can be directed towards improvement of cerebral oxygenation (84). Brain tissue oxygen tension monitors can be placed safely and they reliably measure oxygen tissue tension adjacent to insertion sites. Because brain tissue hypoxia has been related to poor outcomes, efforts should be made to prevent this. The effects of tissue oxygen tension directed therapy need to be studied further before this modality is globally recommended (85).

Various centers routinely use a host of methods to measure cerebral blood flow, which are considered experimental techniques in the management of severe TBI. These include intermittent measurement techniques such as xenon techniques (including inhalational, intravenous and xenon/CT scanning), nitrous oxide saturation techniques, single-photon emission tomography (SPECT) and positron emission tomography (PET) scanning, gradient-echo echo planar imaging (EPI) using magnetic resonance imaging (MRI) technology and transcranial doppler (TCD) monitoring. Other techniques measure continuous regional cerebral blood flow such as laser-doppler flowmetry and thermal diffusion flowmetry. Cerebral blood flow measurement represents a method of assessing brain function in an objective manner. In non-pathologic conditions, cerebral blood flow and brain metabolism tend to be coupled. Thus increased cerebral metabolism tends to increase cerebral blood flow and vice versa. In patients sustaining TBI, however, this coupling is retained only in 45 percent of cases (86). Reduced cerebral blood flow has been associated with worse neurologic outcomes (87, 88). Further, global cerebral blood flow may be different than regional blood flow (89),

misleading a clinician to think that perfusion is adequate when critical structures are being under perfused. These technologies may actually allow a clinician to make management decisions resulting in a different maneuver than routine ICP directed therapies alone (which could potentially worsen regional blood flow related secondary insults)(90). The routine use of global and regional cerebral blood flow measuring technologies has yet to be widely accepted.

Another potentially useful monitoring modality in the management of severe TBI patients in the ICU is continuous electroencephalography (EEG) monitoring. EEG can detect both convulsive and nonconvulsive status epilepticus, which often is an unsuspected cause for altered consciousness in patients with severe TBI. In one series nonconvulsive status epilepticus was demonstrated in 11% of patients (91). It may be associated with poor outcomes (92). Continuous EEG monitoring is also mandatory in the monitoring of barbiturate therapy.

OUTCOMES FROM TRAUMATIC BRAIN INJURY

Mild traumatic brain injury is noted for very often having an association with the troubling postconcussive syndrome. This can be described as having three categories of symptoms. These include cognitive complaints (e.g. decreased attention, poor concentration), somatic symptoms (e.g. headache, tinnitus, light sensitivity, etc.) and affective complaints, such as depression or irritability. These symptoms occur in 80 to 100% of individuals post mild TBI. These are paralleled by deficits in cognitive testing, with impaired speed and information processing and decreased performance on tests of memory and attention. At three months post injury, symptoms have resolved in two thirds of patients (20). Complicating the matter, many physicians are skeptical about the post concussive syndrome's existence, where often litigation is considered as a motive for continued symptoms. While secondary gain should always be considered in this group of patients, the majority of patients with post concussive symptoms have symptoms independent of litigation. Regardless of litigation, patient's with post concussive syndrome tend to have their symptoms improve with time (93). Despite the tendency for improvement with time, some people experience long term disability related to mild TBI including depression, sleep disturbances, post traumatic stress disorder and anxiety (20). A clinical evaluation by a neuropsychiatrist specializing in TBI can be very useful here where a combined educational and, if necessary, pharmacologic approach may prove beneficial.

Most patients with moderate TBI tend to improve neurologically. In one series following 79 patients, 67% of patients improved to GCS 15 by time of discharge.

At an average follow up of 27 months, Glasgow outcome scores (see below) were rated as good or moderate disability in the majority of survivors of moderate TBI, but only 74% of these patients who were employed prior to their TBI returned to work. The majority had significant cognitive and functional deficits, including memory problems, concentration difficulties and headaches, among others (94). Other reports have confirmed good recoveries in terms of general outcomes at 3 months but few patients are actually symptom free. When compared to patients who sustain mild TBI, those with moderate TBI recover less completely and more slowly. Patients tend to have difficulty with memory function and as many as 50 percent have some emotional or behavioral difficulty at 1-year post injury (95).

The mortality from severe TBI has fallen from the 50% range in the 1970's to the 30% range at present date. This is likely due to the implementation of prevention measures, safety legislation, public education initiatives, further improvements in and wider availability of emergency medical systems and regional trauma centers. Improvements in neurocritical care and the implementation of evidence-based treatment guidelines for severe head injury patients may also be responsible for improved survival rates(96). Advances in prehospital care may be contributing substantially to lower TBI mortalities. In San Diego county, California, from the years 1980 to 1982 there was a decline the head injury death rate by 24%. Similarly, the number of patients listed as dead on arrival at hospital emergency facilities decreased by 68%. This is believed to be due to a concurrent marked improvement in the county's ground and air emergency medical system(97). Becker et al. demonstrated a mortality in the 30% range in severe TBI patients managed with modern neurocritical care principals, including ICP monitoring, when compared with same era management at other institutions resulting in a mortality in the 50% range (47). Other series report similar mortalities from severe TBI in patients undergoing aggressive neurocritical care management(98, 99). Further, in patients with severe blunt TBI surviving beyond the emergency room, the mortality rate across the state of Pennsylvania for the years 1995–2000 was 34% for those undergoing ICP monitoring, while those managed without monitors had an overall mortality rate of 43% (100).

Numerous factors have been established as predictors of mortality in severe TBI. These include hypotension, hypoxia, decreasing GCS score, decreased GCS motor score, increased age, increased injury severity score, bilateral unreactive pupils, and abbreviated injury severity score of head among others. Head injury characteristics on CT have also been used as prognosticators regarding mortality in severe TBI. These include compression of the basilar cisterns, presence of traumatic subarachnoid hemorrhage, presence of midline shift and the presence of other intracranial lesions on CT (31).

Though numerous studies have focused on predicting mortality in patients' with severe TBI, as survival improves, the focus of outcome assessments must be directed towards quality of survival and any residual disability. In this direction the term 'functional outcome' is gaining acceptance.

The World Health Organization (WHO) model of disease impact provides guidance as to the direction of outcome measures (101). This model identifies four areas in which an injury can be assessed: pathology, impairment, disability and handicap. Pathology is the most well known area to the acute care physician. It is determined by the lesion characteristics. These include location, hemorrhage, diffuse axonal injury, and elevated intracranial pressure among others. Impairment in the TBI patient refers primarily to the neurological deficits, but associated problems may have an impact on the level of impairment. For example, a patient with significant orthopedic injuries may have weight bearing limitations that contribute to the level of impairment. Disability and handicap outcomes are more familiar to rehabilitation specialists. These domains make up some of the major long-term limitations for the TBI patient (102). Disability is usually described in terms of activities of daily living (ADL). A number of measurement tools have been developed to assess this area. These include the Glasgow Outcome Scale (GOS), the Disability Rating Scale (DRS) the Functional Independence Measure (FIM), the Functional Status Examination (FSE), socioeconomic measures, quality of life measures and caregiver burden measures.

The GOS is frequently used in the neurosurgical literature. It was created in an effort to provide a global assessment of disability post severe TBI. The GOS has 5 categories: good recovery, moderate disability, severe disability, vegetative state, and death (Table 18-2) (103). Good recovery and moderate disability are generally grouped together as favorable outcomes, with the other 3 categories making up the poor outcomes. It is a fairly reliable measure but lacks sensitivity due to its broad categories. Nevertheless, at 6 months post injury the GOS has been shown to correlate well with neuropsychological, psychosocial, and vocational functioning (104).

The DRS was developed as a quantitative instrument for assessing outcomes in severe head trauma. It was designed to be easily learned, be quickly completed, be valid and have high inter-rater reliability. It consists of 8 items divided into 4 categories: 1. Arousal and awareness; 2. Cognitive ability to handle self-care functions; 3. Physical dependence upon others; 4. Psychosocial adaptability for work, housework, or school. Scores range from 0, which signifies no disability to 30, which indicates death (105). The DRS is widely used as an outcome assessment. It has shown good reliability, better precision

---

TABLE 18-2

Glasgow Outcome Scale (from Jennet and Bond (103))

---

5 **Good Recovery**: resumption of normal life even
   though there may be some persistent neurologic and
   psychologic deficits

4 **Moderate Disability**: disabled but independent.
   Though these patients may have considerable neurologic deficit (e.g. hemiparesis) they can travel independently and work in sheltered environments

3 **Severe Disability**: conscious but disabled. These
   patients are dependent for daily support due to
   physical or psychological limitations

2 **Persistent Vegetative State**: Unresponsive and
   speechless individuals who have sleep wake cycles

1 **Death**

---

than the Glasgow Outcome Scale, and greater reliability than other measures (106).

The FIM is an 18 item, 7 level scale that rates the ability of person to perform independently in self care, sphincter control, transfers, locomotion, communication and social interaction. The scores range from 18 (minimally dependent) to 126 (maximally dependent). The score can further be divided by two subscales, motor (the sum of 15 components of the scale) and cognitive (the sum of 8 components of the scale)(10). While showing good reliability for spinal cord injury as an overall assessment of self-care and mobility, it is also useful for assessment of functional outcomes post TBI (106).

The FSE was developed to evaluate functional changes as a result of TBI. It covers physical, social, and psychological domains. The FSE consists of data gathered through a structured interview and is scored from 0–28, where 0 signifies no change from preinjury, 27 maximum dependence on others and 28 death. The FSE is significantly related to important constructs such as family burden, significant other depression, and sacrifices the family makes, as well as overall indices of recovery and satisfaction with level of functioning. The FSE correlates with overall recovery and patient level of satisfaction significantly better than the GOS (107).

Functional outcomes in patients sustaining severe TBI vary by report but overall ~ 30% are reported as having good outcome on the GOS at 1 year. In 1977, Becker et al. reported patients surviving severe TBI. At 3 months or more post injury, 36% made a good recovery, 24% were moderately disabled, 8% were severely disabled, 2% were vegetative and 30% were dead (47). Jiang et al. (108) studied 846 patients with severe TBI and at 1-year reported good recovery in 31.56%, moderate disability in 14.07%, severe disability in 24.35%, vegetative

status in 0.59%, and a 1-year mortality of 29.43%. Rudehill et al. (109) reported data from the Karolinska institute regarding severe TBI in terms of GOS "when no further improvement could be anticipated. This final condition usually occurred 3–12 months after injury." Forty one percent of patients with GCS scores 3–4 post resuscitation had GOS scores of 4–5, 21% had GOS scores of 2–3 and 38% had a score of 1 (death). Of patients with a GCS 5–8 post resuscitation, 70% had a GOS score of 4–5, 17% had a score of 2–3 and 13% had a score of 1. Data from the Trauma Coma Databank revealed GOS scores in patients sustaining severe TBI of 4–5 in 43%, 2–3 in 21%, and 1 in 36% (110).The European Brain Injury Consortium survey revealed GOS score in patients with severe TBI at 6 months post injury of 4–5 in 45% 2–3 in 19% and 1 in 36% (111). Thus, in modern series, the majority of severe TBI patients have favorable outcomes, with few patients surviving with severe disability or in vegetative states.

Nevertheless, few patients sustaining severe TBI return to their premorbid functioning and the majority have significant cognitive and emotional sequelae (112). Tate et al. (113) found that 75% of patients surviving severe TBI have major disability in terms of reintegration with regards to employment, interpersonal relationships, functional independence, social contacts and leisure interests. Even among those with GOS scores of good recovery and moderate disability, only 50% had good psychosocial reintegration. Another series found a 70% unemployment rate at 1 year and a 24% rate of depression following severe TBI. Of these patients, impatience was the most frequently described behavioral problem. Thirty percent of these patients had returned to live with their parents, and relationship breakdown occurred for 38% (114). In another series looking at patients at 3 years follow up, though only 5% of the patients had a GOS of 2 or 3, half of surviving patients were noted to have social handicaps and 78% were noted to have neuropsychological impairment. Half of these patients suffered from headaches (115). Severe TBI patients continue to experience significant cognitive difficulties at 1-year post injury. Kersel et al. (116) followed 65 patients with severe TBI and assessed their GOS and neuropsychological outcomes at 6 months and then at 1 year. They assessed pre-morbid intellectual level, current level of general intellectual functioning, simple and complex attention, verbal memory, executive functioning and perceptual functioning: despite 51% of patients having a good recovery and 20% having moderate disability on the GOS, at best 31% and up to 63 percent had difficulty in neurocognitive tests administered 1 year post injury. Impairment was most frequently seen in verbal memory tests , complex attention tests and executive functioning. General intelligence and perception were among the areas least affected 1year post-injury.

Depression, decreased social contact and loneliness remain persistent long-term problems for the majority of individuals with severe TBI (117). Hoofien et al. (118) assessed 67 patients at 10 to 20 years post TBI and noted serious psychiatric symptoms in this group. About half the patients had problems with hostility including temper outbursts and poor self control. Depression and anxiety were also very common. The psychological and emotional consequences of severe TBI present an enormous caregiver burden. Despite a high incidence of physical disability and cognitive impairment in severe TBI patients at 1 year, the presence of emotional difficulties may cause the most stress for care givers. Anger, dependency and apathy were all found in one series to be the most difficult emotional problems (in severe TBI patients) for caregivers to deal with; over one third of caregivers were found to have clinically significant anxiety and depression and over one quarter reported impairment in their own social adjustment such as problems in their marriages or continuing employment (119). Psychosocial problems and difficulties with re-entry into the community thus represent a major challenge in the rehabilitation of patients sustaining severe TBI (117).

THE ROLE OF THE REHABILITATION SPECIALIST IN PATIENTS SUSTAINING TBI

The rehabilitation specialist plays a pivotal role in the treatment of those sustaining TBI. While emergency medical service personnel/paramedics, emergency physicians, trauma surgeons, neurosurgeons and critical care specialists may be involved in the initial encounter and acute inpatient management of patients sustaining TBI, the rehabilitation specialist is essential in directing appropriate rehabilitative services to the patient sustaining brain injury. For mild TBI, a single early intervention may be appropriate or more intensive services involving neuropsychiatric intervention may be needed in some cases (20, 120).

For more severe TBI, extensive rehabilitation is often needed. This may be better started off early rather than later, with resultant improved mobility and decreased length of acute rehabilitation stay (121, 122). Intensive rehabilitation may also improve early functional outcome of TBI patients(123).

Acute rehabilitation for patients with severe TBI starts in the comatose and early arousal states, with the goals of preventing orthopedic and visceral complications. Subsequent inpatient rehabilitation is designed to help impairments recover and to teach patients to compensate for their disabilities. This includes both psychological and physical therapy. A third phase, and perhaps most difficult, is therapy "for achieving physical, domestic and social independence, reduction of handicaps and

re-entry into the community (124)." One controversial area is sensory stimulation which is intended to accelerate recovery or arousal in patients who are comatose or vegetative. There is little evidence to support or to challenge this practice (125).

Rehabilitation specialists need to be aware of the possible causes of readmission to acute care for patients sustaining TBI, including the possibility of patients requiring further neurologic workup. During the first year post TBI, the most common reasons for rehospitalization include orthopedic or reconstructive surgery, followed by infectious disorders and general health maintenance. After the first year, seizures and psychiatric problems represent a considerable portion of admissions (126). In the case of new onset post traumatic seizures, a detailed workup with neurologic consultation should be pursued. Posttraumatic hydrocephalus may be another problem seen late after TBI. Symptoms include arrest in clinical progress, dementia, gait disturbance and incontinence (127). The threshold to obtain a repeat CT scan should be low in the TBI patient with any neurologic deterioration. It should be kept in mind that even after one year post injury, patients sustaining severe TBI may significantly benefit from inpatient rehabilitation (128).

Conclusions

TBI remains an enormous problem despite advances in its management in the last 30 years. It represents a tremendous social and economic cost. The patient experiencing head injury should be evaluated in a systematic manner with attention being paid to the possibility of the presence of a mass lesion. This may mean the need for a mechanical airway, decompressive surgery and the possibility of ICP monitoring. Hypotension and hypoxia, in addition to elevated ICP, are critical secondary insults that must be avoided if possible. Outcomes from TBI continue to improve but are still hampered by significant psychological, cognitive and economic disability in survivors. The rehabilitation specialist plays a key role in the care of patients post severe TBI by being involved in acute care, inpatient rehabilitation, outpatient treatment, and, ultimately, societal reintegration.

References

1. MacKenzie EJ. Epidemiology of injuries: current trends and future challenges. *Epidemiol Rev* 2000; 22:112–119.
2. Thurman D, Guerrero J. Trends in hospitalization associated with traumatic brain injury. *Jama* 1999; 282:954–957.
3. Sosin DM, Sniezek JE, Waxweiler RJ. Trends in death associated with traumatic brain injury, 1979 through 1992. Success and failure. *Jama* 1995; 273:1778–1780.
4. Traumatic Brain Injury in the United States: A report to Congress, in. Atlanta, Center for Disease Control, 1999.
5. McGarry LJ, Thompson D, Millham FH, et al. Outcomes and costs of acute treatment of traumatic brain injury. *J Trauma* 2002; 53:1152–1159.

6. Thurman DJ, Alverson C, Dunn KA, et al. Traumatic brain injury in the United States: A public health perspective. *J Head Trauma Rehabil* 1999; 14:602–615.

7. Thurman D. The epidemiology and economics of head trauma, in Miller L, Hayes R (eds). *Head Trauma: Basic, Preclinical, and Clinical Directions.* New York: Wiley and Sons 2001.

8. Langlois JA, Kegler SR, Butler JA, et al. Traumatic brain injury-related hospital discharges. Results from a 14-state surveillance system, 1997. *MMWR Surveill Summ* 2003; 52:1–20.

9. Adekoya N, Thurman DJ, White DD, et al. Surveillance for traumatic brain injury deaths—United States, 1989–1998. *MMWR Surveill Summ* 2002; 51:1–14.

10. Bushnik T, Hanks RA, Kreutzer J, et al. Etiology of traumatic brain injury: characterization of differential outcomes up to 1 year postinjury. *Arch Phys Med Rehabil* 2003; 84:255–262.

11. Malik AS, Narayan RK. Critical Care Management of Severe Head Injury, in Kaye AH, Black PM (eds). *Operative Neurosurgery.* London: Churchill Livingstone 2002, pp. 207–216.

12. Trask T, Narayan RK. Civilan Penetrating Head Injury, in Narayan R, Wilberger J, Povlishock J (eds). *Neurotrauma.* New York: McGraw Hill 1996, pp. 869–889.

13. Graham DI. Neuropathology of Head Injury, in Narayan R, Wilberger J, Povlishock J (eds). *Neurotrauma.* New York: McGraw Hill 1996, pp. 43–59.

14. Adams J, Graham D. *An Introduction to Neuropathology.* Edinburgh, Churchill Livingstone, 1994.

15. Appelbaum E. Meningitis following trauma to the head and face. *Jama* 1960; 173:1818–1822.

16. Dagi TF, Meyer FB, Poletti CA. The incidence and prevention of meningitis after basilar skull fracture. *Am J Emerg Med* 1983; 1:295–298.

17. Temkin NR, Haglund M, Winn HR. Post-Traumatic Seizures, in Narayan R, Wilberger J, Povlishock J (eds). *Neurotrauma.* New York: McGraw Hill 1996, pp. 611–619.

18. Bullock MR, Chesnut RM, Ghajar J, et al. Surgical Management of Traumatic Brain Injury, in. New York, Brain Trauma Foundation.

19. Narayan RK. Head Trauma, in Krantz BE, Ali J, Aprahamian C, Bell RM, Boyle DE, Collicott PE, Felicianio DV, Jurkovich GI, Kellam JF, Maull KI, McManus WF, Morris JA, Parks SN, Narayan RK, Raemenofsky SA, Rinker C, Timberlarke GA (eds). *Advanced Trauma Life Support for Doctors.* Chicago: American College of Surgeons 1997, pp. 181–206.

20. McAllister TW, Arciniegas D. Evaluation and treatment of post-concussive symptoms. *NeuroRehabilitation* 2002; 17:265–283.

21. Jallo J, Narayan RK. Pathophysiology of Head Injury, in Webb AR, Shapiro MJ, Singer M, Suter P (eds). *Oxford Textbook of Critical Care.* Oxford: Oxford University Press 1999.

22. Ikonomidou C, Turski L. Why did NMDA receptor antagonists fail clinical trials for stroke and traumatic brain injury? *Lancet Neurol* 2002; 1:383–386.

23. Young B, Runge JW, Waxman KS, et al. Effects of pegorgotein on neurologic outcome of injury. A multicenter, randomized controlled. *Jama* 1996; 276:538–543.

24. Biegon A, Joseph AB. Development of HU-211 as a neuroprotectant for ischemic brain damage. *Neurol Res* 1995; 17: 275–280.

25. Dexanabinol Fails To Demonstrate Efficacy as Measured by Primary Clinical Outcome Endpoint, in PRNewswire-FirstCall. Iselin, Pharmos Corporation, 2004.

26. Marmarou A. Traumatic brain edema: an overview. *Acta Neurochir Suppl (Wien)* 1994; 60:421–424.

27. Narayan RK, Kishore PR, Becker DP, et al. Intracranial pressure: to monitor or not to monitor? A review of our experience with severe head injury. *J Neurosurg* 1982; 56:650–659.

28. Eisenberg HM, Frankowski RF, Contant CF, et al. High-dose barbiturate control of elevated intracranial pressure in patients with severe head injury. *J Neurosurg* 1988; 69:15–23.

29. Changaris DG, McGraw CP, Richardson JD, et al. Correlation of cerebral perfusion pressure and Glasgow Coma Scale to outcome. *J Trauma* 1987; 27:1007–1013.

30. Rosner MJ, Rosner SD, Johnson AH. Cerebral perfusion pressure: management protocol. *J Neurosurg* 1995; 83:949–962.

31. Bullock MR, Chesnut RM, Clifton GL, et al. Guidelines for the management of severe traumatic brain injury: Cerebral perfusion pressure, in. New York, Brain Trauma Foundation.

32. Robertson CS, Valadka AB, Hannay HJ, et al. Prevention of secondary ischemic insults after severe head injury. *Crit Care Med* 1999; 27:2086–2095.

33. Teasdale G, Jennett B. Assessment of coma and impaired consciousness. A. *Lancet* 1974; 2:81–84.

34. Chesnut RM, Marshall LF, Klauber MR, et al. The role of secondary brain injury in determining outcome from severe head injury. *J Trauma* 1993; 34:216–222.

35. Gabriel EJ, Ghajar JBG, Jagoda A, et al. Guidelines for Prehospital Management of Traumatic Brain Injury, in. New York, Brain Trauma Foundation, 1999.

36. Holly LT, Kelly DF, Counelis GJ, et al. Cervical spine trauma associated with moderate incidence, risk factors, and injury. *J Neurosurg* 2002; 96:285–291.

37. Finfer S, Bellomo R, Boyce N, et al. A comparison of albumin and saline for fluid resuscitation in the intensive care unit. *N Engl J Med* 2004; 350:2247–2256.

38. Ingebrigtsen T, Romner B. Routine early CT-scan is cost saving after minor. *Acta Neurol Scand* 1996; 93:207–210.

39. Shackford SR, Wald SL, Ross SE, et al. The clinical utility of computed tomographic examination in the management of patients with. *J Trauma* 1992; 33:385–394.

40. Hutchinson PJ, Kirkpatrick PJ, Addison J, et al. The management of minor traumatic brain injury. *J Accid Emerg Med* 1998; 15:84–88.

41. Greenes DS, Schutzman SA. Infants with isolated skull fracture: what are characteristics, and do they require. *Ann Emerg Med* 1997; 30:253–259.

42. Kadish HA, Schunk JE. Pediatric basilar skull fracture: do children findings and no intracranial injury require. *Ann Emerg Med* 1995; 26:37–41.

43. Vogelbaum MA, Kaufman BA, Park TS, et al. Management of uncomplicated skull fractures in admission necessary? *Pediatr Neurosurg* 1998; 29:96–101.

44. Bullock MR, Chesnut RM, Clifton GL, et al. Management and Prognosis of Severe Traumatic Brain Injury, in. New York, Brain Trauma Foundation.

45. Narayan RK, Greenberg RP, Miller JD, et al. Improved confidence of outcome prediction in severe head injury. A comparative analysis of the clinical examination, multimodality evoked potentials, CT scanning, and intracranial pressure. *J Neurosurg* 1981; 54:751–762.

46. Bowers SA, Marshall LF. Outcome in 200 consecutive cases of severe head injury treated in San Diego County: a prospective analysis. *Neurosurgery* 1980; 6:237–242.

47. Becker DP, Miller JD, Ward JD, et al. The outcome from severe head injury with early diagnosis and intensive management. *J Neurosurg* 1977; 47:491–502.

48. Ghajar JBG, Hariri RJ, Patterson RH. Improved Outcome from Traumatic Coma Using Only Ventricular Cerebrospinal Fluid Drainaing for Intracranial Pressure Control. *Advances in Neurosurgery* 1993; 21:173–177.

49. Lane PL, Skoretz TG, Doig G, et al. Intracranial pressure monitoring and outcomes after traumatic brain injury. *Can J Surg* 2000; 43:442–448.

50. Fleischer AS, Payne NS, Tindall GT. Continuous monitoring of intracranial pressure in severe closed head injury without mass lesions. *Surg Neurol* 1976; 6:31–34.

51. Stuart GG, Merry GS, Smith JA, et al. Severe head injury managed without intracranial pressure monitoring. *J Neurosurg* 1983; 59:601–605.

52. Smith HP, Kelly DL, Jr., McWhorter JM, et al. Comparison of mannitol regimens in patients with severe head injury undergoing intracranial monitoring. *J Neurosurg* 1986; 65:820–824.

53. Ostrup RC, Luerssen TG, Marshall LF, et al. Continuous monitoring of intracranial pressure with a miniaturized fiberoptic device. *J Neurosurg* 1987; 67:206–209.

54. Bavetta S, Norris JS, Wyatt M, et al. Prospective study of zero drift in fiberoptic pressure monitors used in clinical practice. *J Neurosurg* 1997; 86:927–930.

55. Feldman Z, Kanter MJ, Robertson CS, et al. Effect of head elevation on intracranial pressure, and cerebral blood flow in head. *J Neurosurg* 1992; 76:207–211.

56. Clifton GL, Miller ER, Choi SC, et al. Lack of effect of induction of hypothermia after acute brain injury. *N Engl J Med* 2001; 344:556–563.

57. Roberts I, Yates D, Sandercock P, et al. Effect of intravenous corticosteroids on death within 14 days in 10008 adults with clinically significant head injury (MRC CRASH trial): randomised placebo-controlled trial. *Lancet* 2004; 364:1321–1328.

58. Alderson P, Roberts I. Corticosteroids for acute traumatic brain injury. *Cochrane Database Syst Rev* 2005:CD000196.

59. Roberts I, Schierhout G, Wakai A. Mannitol for acute traumatic brain injury. *Cochrane Database Syst Rev* 2003:CD001049.

60. Marion DW, Firlik A, McLaughlin MR. Hyperventilation therapy for severe traumatic. *New Horiz* 1995; 3:439–447.

61. Polin RS, Shaffrey ME, Bogaev CA, et al. Decompressive bifrontal craniectomy in the treatment of severe refractory posttraumatic cerebral edema. *Neurosurgery* 1997; 41:84–92; discussion 92–84.

62. Kontopoulos V, Foroglou N, Patsalas J, et al. Decompressive craniectomy for the management of patients with refractory hypertension: should it be reconsidered? *Acta Neurochir (Wien)* 2002; 144:791–796.

63. Guerra WK, Piek J, Gaab MR. Decompressive craniectomy to treat intracranial hypertension in head injury patients. *Intensive Care Med* 1999; 25:1327–1329.

64. Rovlias A, Kotsou S. The influence of hyperglycemia on neurological outcome in patients with severe head injury. *Neurosurgery* 2000; 46:335–342; discussion 342–333.

65. Andrews BT. Fluid and electrolyte management in the head injured patient, in Narayan R, Wilberger J, Povlishock J (eds). *Neurotrauma*. New York: McGraw Hill 1996, pp. 331–344.

66. Temkin NR, Dikmen SS, Wilensky AJ, et al. A randomized, double-blind study of phenytoin for the prevention of post-traumatic seizures. *N Engl J Med* 1990; 323:497–502.

67. Temkin NR, Dikmen SS, Winn HR. Management of head injury. Posttraumatic seizures. *Neurosurg Clin N Am* 1991; 2:425–435.

68. Greenberg SB, Atmar RL. Infectious complications following head injury, in Narayan R, Wilberger J, Povlishock J (eds). *Neurotrauma*. New York: McGraw Hill 1996, pp. 703–722.

69. Gurkin SA, Parikshak M, Kralovich KA, et al. Indicators for tracheostomy in patients with. *Am Surg* 2002; 68:324–328; discussion 328–329.

70. Teoh WH, Goh KY, Chan C. The role of early tracheostomy in critically ill. *Ann Acad Med Singapore* 2001; 30:234–238.

71. Powers J. A multidisciplinary approach to occipital cervical collars. *J Nurs Care Qual* 1997; 12:46–52.

72. Zabramski JM, Whiting D, Darouiche RO, et al. Efficacy of antimicrobial-impregnated external ventricular drain catheters: a prospective, randomized, controlled trial. *J Neurosurg* 2003; 98:725–730.

73. Kirby DF, Clifton GL, Turner H, et al. Early enteral nutrition after brain injury by percutaneous endoscopic gastrojejunostomy. *JPEN J Parenter Enteral Nutr* 1991; 15:298–302.

74. Grahm TW, Zadrozny DB, Harrington T. The benefits of early jejunal hyperalimentation in the head-injured patient. *Neurosurgery* 1989; 25:729–735.

75. Fremstad JD, Martin SH. Lethal complication from insertion of basilar skull fracture. *J Trauma* 1978; 18:820–822.

76. Dees G. Difficult nasogastric tube insertions. *Emerg Med Clin North Am* 1989; 7:177–182.

77. Young B, Ott L. Nutritional and Metabolic Management of the Head Injured Patient, in Narayan R, Wilberger J, Povlishock J (eds). *Neurotrauma*. New York: McGraw Hill 1996, pp. 345–363.

78. Geerts WH, Code KI, Jay RM, et al. A prospective study of venous thromboembolism. *N Engl J Med* 1994; 331:1601–1606.

79. Kim J, Gearhart MM, Zurick A, et al. Preliminary report on the safety of heparin for prophylaxis after severe head injury. *J Trauma* 2002; 53:38–42; discussion 43.

80. Norwood SH, McAuley CE, Berne JD, et al. Prospective evaluation of the safety of thromboembolism in patients with intracranial. *Arch Surg* 2002; 137:696–701; discussion 701–692.

81. White H, Baker A. Continuous jugular venous oximetry in the brief review. *Can J Anaesth* 2002; 49:623–629.

82. Woodman T, Robertson CS. Jugular Venous Oxygen Saturation Monitoring, in Narayan R, Wilberger J, Povlishock J (eds). *Neurotrauma*. New York: McGraw Hill 1996, pp. 519–537.

83. Gopinath SP, Valadka AB, Uzura M, et al. Comparison of jugular venous oxygen saturation and brain tissue Po2 as monitors of cerebral ischemia after head injury. *Crit Care Med* 1999; 27:2337–2345.

84. Haitsma IK, Maas AI. Advanced monitoring in the intensive care unit: brain tissue oxygen tension. *Curr Opin Crit Care* 2002; 8:115–120.

85. van den Brink WA, van Santbrink H, Steyerberg EW, et al. Brain oxygen tension in severe head injury. *Neurosurgery* 2000; 46: 868–876; discussion 876–868.

86. Sioutos PJ, Orozco JA, Carter LP. Regional cerebral blood flow techniques, in Narayan R, Wilberger J, Povlishock J (eds). *Neurotrauma*. New York: McGraw Hill 1996, pp. 503–517.

87. Robertson CS, Contant CF, Gokaslan ZL, et al. Cerebral blood flow, arteriovenous oxygen difference, and outcome in head injured patients. *J Neurol Neurosurg Psychiatry* 1992; 55:594–603.

88. Kelly DF, Martin NA, Kordestani R, et al. Cerebral blood flow as a predictor of outcome injury. *J Neurosurg* 1997; 86:633–641.

89. Marion DW, Darby J, Yonas H. Acute regional cerebral blood flow changes. *J Neurosurg* 1991; 74:407–414.

90. Sioutos PJ, Orozco JA, Carter LP, et al. Continuous regional cerebral cortical blood flow head-injured patients. *Neurosurgery* 1995; 36:943–949; discussion 949–950.

91. Vespa PM, Nuwer MR, Nenov V, et al. Increased incidence and impact of nonconvulsive and convulsive seizures after traumatic brain injury as detected by continuous electroencephalographic monitoring. *J Neurosurg* 1999; 91:750–760.

92. Young GB, Jordan KG, Doig GS. An assessment of nonconvulsive seizures in the intensive care unit using continuous EEG monitoring: an investigation of variables associated with mortality. *Neurology* 1996; 47:83–89.

93. Evans RW. Postconcussion syndrome and whiplash injuries, in Narayan R, Wilberger J, Povlishock J (eds). *Neurotrauma*. New York: McGraw Hill 1996, pp. 593–609.

94. Vitaz TW, Jenks J, Raque GH, et al. Outcome following moderate traumatic brain injury. *Surg Neurol* 2003; 60:285–291; discussion 291.

95. Stein S. Outcome from moderate head injury, in Narayan R, Wilberger J, Povlishock J (eds). *Neurotrauma*. New York: McGraw Hill 1996, pp. 755–765.

96. Kelly DF, Becker DP. Advances in management of neurosurgical trauma. *World J Surg* 2001; 25:1179–1185.

97. Klauber MR, Marshall LF, Toole BM, et al. Cause of decline in head-injury mortality rate in San Diego County, California. *J Neurosurg* 1985; 62:528–531.

98. Miller JD, Butterworth JF, Gudeman SK, et al. Further experience in the management of severe head injury. *J Neurosurg* 1981; 54:289–299.

99. Marshall LF, Smith RW, Shapiro HM. The outcome with aggressive treatment in severe head injuries. Part I: the significance of intracranial pressure monitoring. *J Neurosurg* 1979; 50:20–25.

100. Baron EM, Gaughan JP, Gopez J, et al. Intracranial pressure monitoring in patients sustaining severe blunt head injury in pennsylvania: risk factors and outcomes in hospitalized patients over 5 years (1995–2000). Presented at Congress of Neurologic Surgeons, Denver, CO, 2003.

101. Organization WH. The international classification of imapairments, disabilities and handicaps, in. Geneva, World Health Organization.

102. Jallo J, Narayan RK. Assessment of Head Injury, in Webb AR, Shapiro MJ, Singer M, Suter P (eds). *Oxford Textbook of Critical Care*. Oxford: Oxford University Press 1999.

103. Jennett B, Bond M. Assessment of outcome after severe brain damage. *Lancet* 1975; 1:480–484.

104. Satz P, Zaucha K, Forney DL, et al. Neuropsychological, psychosocial and vocational correlates of the Glasgow Outcome Scale at 6 months post-injury: a study of moderate to severe traumatic brain injury patients. *Brain Inj* 1998; 12:555–567.

105. Rappaport M, Hall KM, Hopkins K, et al. Disability rating scale for severe head trauma: coma to community. *Arch Phys Med Rehabil* 1982; 63:118–123.

106. Ditunno JF, Jr. Functional assessment measures in CNS trauma. *J Neurotrauma* 1992; 9 Suppl 1:S301–305.

107. Dikmen S, Machamer J, Miller B, et al. Functional status examination: a new instrument for assessing outcome in traumatic brain injury. *J Neurotrauma* 2001; 18:127–140.

108. Jiang JY, Gao GY, Li WP, et al. Early indicators of prognosis in 846 cases of severe traumatic brain injury. *J Neurotrauma* 2002; 19:869–874.

109. Rudehill A, Bellander BM, Weitzberg E, et al. Outcome of traumatic brain injuries in 1,508 patients: impact of prehospital care. *J Neurotrauma* 2002; 19:855–868.

110. Marshall LF, Gautille T, Klauber MR, et al. The outcome of severe closed head injury. *J Neurosurg* 1991; 75:S28–S36.

111. Murray GD, Teasdale GM, Braakman R, et al. The European Brain Injury Consortium survey of head injuries. *Acta Neurochir (Wien)* 1999; 141:223–236.

112. Marion DW. Outcome from severe head injury, in Narayan R, Wilberger J, Povlishock J (eds). *Neurotrauma.* New York: McGraw Hill 1996, pp. 767–777.

113. Tate RL, Lulham JM, Broe GA, et al. Psychosocial outcome for the survivors of severe blunt head injury: the results from a consecutive series of 100 patients. *J Neurol Neurosurg Psychiatry* 1989; 52:1128–1134.

114. Kersel DA, Marsh NV, Havill JH, et al. Psychosocial functioning during the year following severe traumatic brain injury. *Brain Inj* 2001; 15:683–696.

115. Annoni JM, Beer S, Kesselring J. Severe traumatic brain injury—epidemiology and outcome after 3 years. *Disabil Rehabil* 1992; 14:23–26.

116. Kersel DA, Marsh NV, Havill JH, et al. Neuropsychological functioning during the year following severe traumatic brain injury. *Brain Inj* 2001; 15:283–296.

117. Morton MV, Wehman P. Psychosocial and emotional sequelae of individuals with traumatic brain injury: a literature review and recommendations. *Brain Inj* 1995; 9:81–92.

118. Hoofien D, Gilboa A, Vakil E, et al. Traumatic brain injury (TBI) 10–20 years later: a comprehensive outcome study of psychiatric symptomatology, cognitive abilities and psychosocial functioning. *Brain Inj* 2001; 15:189–209.

119. Marsh NV, Kersel DA, Havill JH, et al. Caregiver burden at 1 year following severe traumatic brain injury. *Brain Inj* 1998; 12:1045–1059.

120. Paniak C, Toller-Lobe G, Reynolds S, et al. A randomized trial of two treatments for mild traumatic brain injury: 1 year follow-up. *Brain Inj* 2000; 14:219–226.

121. Lipper-Gruner M, Wedekind C, Klug N. Functional and psychosocial outcome one year after severe traumatic brain injury and early-onset rehabilitation therapy. *J Rehabil Med* 2002; 34:211–214.

122. Wagner AK, Fabio T, Zafonte RD, et al. Physical medicine and rehabilitation consultation: relationships with acute functional outcome, length of stay, and discharge planning after traumatic brain injury. *Am J Phys Med Rehabil* 2003; 82:526–536.

123. Zhu XL, Poon WS, Chan CH, et al. Does intensive rehabilitation improve the functional outcome of patients with traumatic brain injury? Interim result of a randomized controlled trial. *Br J Neurosurg* 2001; 15:464–473.

124. Mazaux JM, Richer E. Rehabilitation after traumatic brain injury in adults. *Disabil Rehabil* 1998; 20:435–447.

125. Lombardi F, Taricco M, De Tanti A, et al. Sensory stimulation for brain injured individuals in coma or vegetative state. *Cochrane Database Syst Rev* 2002:CD001427.

126. Cifu DX, Kreutzer JS, Marwitz JH, et al. Etiology and incidence of rehospitalization after traumatic brain injury: a multicenter analysis. *Arch Phys Med Rehabil* 1999; 80:85–90.

127. Bontke CF, Zasler ND, Boake C. Rehabiliation of the head-injured patient, in Narayan R, Wilberger J, Povlishock J (eds). *Neurotrauma.* New York: McGraw Hill 1996, pp. 841–858.

128. Tuel SM, Presty SK, Meythaler JM, et al. Functional improvement in severe head injury after readmission for rehabilitation. *Brain Inj* 1992; 6:363–372.

129. Teasdale G, Jennett B. Assessment and prognosis of coma after head injury. *Acta Neurochir (Wien)* 1976; 34:45–55.

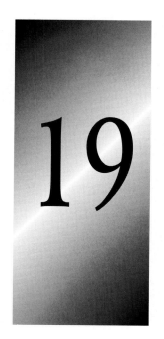

19 Assessment, Early Rehabilitation Intervention, and Tertiary Prevention

W. Jerry Mysiw
Lisa P. Fugate
Daniel M. Clinchot

An estimated 5.3 million Americans live with a combination of chronic physical, cognitive and neurobehavioral impairments secondary to traumatic brain injury (TBI) that adversely affects daily function, social participation and/or quality of life (1). The annual economic impact for the direct care of TBI survivors, excluding inpatient care, has been estimated at $25 billion.1 Also, the annual incidence of TBI is estimated at 180–220 per 100,000 population. As the subsequent fatality rate is estimated at 10%, that suggests that approximately 550,000 persons are hospitalized annually in the United States with brain injury. The vast majority of survivors with a mild TBI are expected to have a good recovery, but as many as two thirds of survivors with a moderate TBI and approaching 100% of severe TBI survivors are left with permanent impairments and disabilities (1–2). It is apparent that the societal impact of TBI will continue to grow when one considers these statistics together with the observation that TBI primarily occurs in young adults.

Some of the impairments and disabilities after TBI can be attenuated by tertiary preventative measures such as early and adequate treatment directed at arresting the ongoing injury process, preventing complications and by the early use of comprehensive rehabilitative interventions. The role of early and comprehensive rehabilitation in achieving these goals is increasingly supported in the neuroscience and neurorehabilitation literature that studies aspects of brain plasticity in both animal models and clinical paradigms. These areas of research have documented the importance of enriched environments and physical activity to neurogenesis and cell survival (3). Animal and clinical studies have also documented the negative impact on outcome secondary to chemical and physical restraints relative to participation in rehabilitation (3–5).

The initial physiatric evaluation of a traumatic brain injury survivor should, therefore, ideally occur within the first twenty-four hours of the event. That is, rehabilitation should no longer be considered the final stage of the recovery process but rather rehabilitative assessment and intervention should be implemented during the acute recovery period and continue through the subacute and chronic stages for a comprehensive rehabilitation program that maximizes functional outcome. Indeed, a small yet compelling body of evidence continues to evolve supporting the concept that early application of rehabilitation strategies shortens the length of hospitalization and enhances the quality of outcome (3,6,7).

The issues that a physiatrist needs to consider during the initial evaluation of a patient with a moderate to severe traumatic brain injury include: 1) an assessment of residual impairments, 2) an estimation of prognosis, 3) initiation of early rehabilitation intervention emphasizing preparation for ongoing rehabilitation needs and prevention of complications, and 4) formulation of a long-term treatment plan that will address the rehabilitation and reintegration needs of the survivor. This chapter will review those issues that are most germane to the physiatrist during the acute care phase of intervention after a traumatic brain injury.

ASSESSMENT

Residual Impairments

The impairments incurred secondary to a severe traumatic brain injury can be broadly categorized as physical, cognitive and neurobehavioral. Potential impairments are numerous and have been comprehensively reviewed elsewhere. (8) A thorough documentation of all impairments and deficits during the initial physiatric evaluation is often neither practical nor possible in a coma emerging patient where arousal, awareness or communication may be compromised. However, attention should certainly be directed to those impairments that have prognostic implications and those that have an impact upon the immediate rehabilitation strategies. Because the majority of traumatic brain injuries result from motor vehicle accidents, (9) associated injuries that can have a significant impact on survival and functional outcomes are found in 60% of patients (10–12). Hence, it is incumbent upon the rehabilitation team to be cognizant of medical issues such as fractures, that may have been undetected during the acute stabilization (10).

The physical consequences of neurotrauma most critical for assessment and early intervention are those that effect swallowing, communication, mobility and locomotion. Preliminary swallowing evaluation and treatment recommendations can be done at bedside while the patient is still in the intensive care unit and completed as the patient becomes more alert. The establishment of a consistent communication system is a prerequisite for determining the extent of cognitive deficits and thus appropriate rehabilitation interventions. Disorders affecting mobility and locomotion are often the primary focus of the family and render the survivor at risk for secondary complications.

Cognitive deficits have a greater impact on functional outcome than the residual physical deficits in longitudinal studies (13). However, the specific cognitive deficits that most profoundly effect long-term outcome remain to be determined through further research. Thus, the cognitive skills most appropriate for screening during the initial assessment are those that effect communication and the ability to learn basic functional skills.

Neurobehavioral sequellae of severe traumatic brain injury can have similar global effects in all functional spheres and may have the greatest impact in long-term outcome (8). Agitation, the most dramatic behavioral disor-der observed in the coma emerging brain trauma survivor, has significant impact on the initial type of rehabilitation services. Both the presence and presentation of agitation have long-term prognostic implications (14,15).

Prognosis

Predicting outcome after TBI serves several practical purposes. Estimating prognosis permits the development of a more meaningful individualized rehabilitation plan. The family and subsequently the patient benefit from the prognostic information as part of their adjustment to the catastrophic event. Finally, the ability to accurately predict outcome is important for program evaluation purposes and in designing studies targeted to influence functional outcome. To date, the studies designed to identify significant prognostic variables have resulted in two general observations. First, no single variable is adequate to predict an outcome from an injury as complex and heterogeneous as TBI. Second, the importance of prediction variables is predicated on the outcome of interest. For example, injury severity variables predict rehabilitation readiness and, to some extent, rehabilitation outcome, but these variables are less robust at predicting vocational outcome (2,6,16–19). Similarly, vocational outcome prediction involves knowledge of premorbid, social and disability variables that are not immediately critical to the early assessment of the TBI survivor (17–19).

At the initial physiatric evaluation, a number of prognostic variables are available that include premorbid, injury severity, impairments and functional characteristics (Table 19-1) (2, 20–22).

Age at the time of injury appears to be the most powerful premorbid prognostic indicator of both mortality and functional outcome. Studies stratifying severe TBI patients at 50, 60, 65 and 70 years of age have consistently shown that mortality dramatically increases with increasing age. This prognostic indicator remains significant even when the severity of the injury is controlled for by using the Glasgow Coma Scale (GCS), the Injury Severity Scale, or other measures of trauma severity (23). Mortality as high as

TABLE 19-1
Early Predictors of Outcome
Age
Primary brain injury
Secondary brain injury
Glagow Coma Scale
Pupillary response
CT scan
Sitting balance
Functional Independence Measure
Post-traumatic amnesia

79% has been described in patients greater than 60 years old, and 33% has been described in those under 40 years of age (6). This same study compared outcome at 6 months and found that a good outcome in the greater than 60 years old group was limited to 2%. In the under 40 years old group, 38% had a good outcome. Finally, age remained a significant prognostic indicator even after controlling for past medical history (24).

The type of central nervous system lesion incurred at the time of trauma has been correlated with both survival and functional outcome. For example, the presence of a mass lesion implies a higher mortality and a poorer functional outcome (2,25). Most studies agree that the injury with the highest mortality rate and the poorest functional outcome is the subdural hematoma (25,26). Other acute computed tomography (CT) scan changes that carry prognostic implications include the presence of third ventricle and/or basal cistern abnormalities, implying raised intracranial pressure in excess of 20 millimeters; the functional outcome of survivors with this acute CT scan finding remains poor at 6 months post-injury (27). Temporal lobe lesions, with a resulting midline shift of more than 4 millimeters, carry negative prognostic implications for both survival and functional outcome (28). Finally, basal ganglion hemorrhages are rare CT abnormalities after a severe traumatic brain injury. As a primary lesion, basal ganglion hemorrhages carry a fairly good prognosis with the majority of patients achieving a moderate or good functional outcome (29).

The most comprehensive assessment of the predictive value of early CT scan findings and functional outcome at one year looked at 849 patients who were admitted to inpatient rehabilitation and followed for 1 year (20). This observational study found that a midline shift of greater than 5 mm or a subcortical contusion resulted in greater assistance requirements for activities of daily living (ADL), ambulation and supervision, whereas, bilateral cortical contusions were associated with significant global supervision needs but not ADL or ambulation assistance needs (20).

Both coma duration and coma depth are important markers of injury severity with prognostic implications, but coma duration may be a better predictor of motor and cognitive recovery than coma depth (30–33). Coma duration and outcome, assessed by the Glasgow Outcome Scale, have been found to be correlated in that functional outcome is proportionately worse at 1-year post injury with increasing length of coma and patients who remain comatose for greater than 2 weeks rarely achieve a good recovery (34). At the other end of the spectrum, coma durations as little as 1 hour have also been found to effect outcomes such as subsequent employment (34). This relationship between coma duration and outcome is more prominent with diffuse axonal injury and appears somewhat linear in that there is no clear cut-off that predicts outcomes assessed by the Glasgow Outcome Scale (30).

Coma depth, as measured by the Glasgow Coma Scale (GCS), has been an important prognostic indicator of mortality and to a lesser extent, outcome. Glasgow Coma Scale scores during the first 24 hours post-injury appear to be better predictors of survival than scores after the first 24 hours, but GCS scores 2–3 days post-injury are better predictors of functional outcome. A review of the prognostic importance of the Glasgow Coma Scale by the Brain Trauma Foundation concluded that there is an increasing probability of poor outcome with decreasing GCS scores in a continuous stepwise manner (2). However, most of these studies collapse the Glasgow Outcome Scale into two or three outcome categories; the predictive value of the initial GCS score is poor when trying to be more precise in using all five Glasgow Outcome Scale variables (2). Early GCS scores have limited prognostic value for acute inpatient rehabilitation outcome. The initial and lowest 24-hour GCS score has limited value as a predictor of rehabilitation admission and discharge Rancho Los Amigos Levels of Cognitive Functioning Scale, Functional Independence Measure and Disability Rating Scale scores (35). Another study found that the GCS score did not predict the degree of improvement in the Functional Independence Measure score during inpatient rehabilitation (36). A more recent analysis of GCS scores found that the admission GCS score during a period between 1997 and 2001 was not as predictive of the Glasgow Outcome Scale score at six months post-injury as had been observed between 1992 and 1997 (37). These data appear to reflect a change in the early management of TBI patients with more aggressive resuscitation. For prognostic purposes, GCS scores should be obtained after the patient has been resuscitated and after pharmacologic sedating and paralytic agents are metabolized (2).

The duration of post-traumatic amnesia (PTA) is thought to have an even stronger relationship with outcome than depth or duration of coma. Periods of post-traumatic amnesia ranging from 1 hour to several days have resulted in impairment of divided attention as determined by the Paced Auditory Serial Addition Task (PASAT) that persist for 15 and 40 days post-injury, respectively (30). The duration of post-traumatic amnesia has also been found to be predictive of functional outcome as measured by the rehabilitation admission and discharge Functional Independence Measure and Disability Rating Scale scores (22). Data from the International Data Coma Bank have demonstrated that less than 2 weeks of PTA resulted in 80% of patients achieving a good recovery and 0% remaining in the severe disability functional outcome category; after 4 weeks of PTA, functional outcome diminished to 27% achieving a good recovery and 30% remaining severely disabled (34). Others have demonstrated that greater than 4 weeks of PTA results in virtually no patients achieving a good recovery. After 12 weeks of PTA, severe cognitive deficits and a very poor prognosis for functional independence at 1 year are observed (30). As a caveat, the importance of PTA duration on functional prognosis is most translatable to injuries involving primarily diffuse axonal injury. The relationship between PTA duration and outcome in patients with predominantly focal pathology is less clear (34).

Two forms of secondary brain injury have been correlated with outcome, raised intracranial pressure and hypotension. Raised intracranial pressure has been shown to be a strong predictor of outcome per the Glasgow Outcome Scale (2,34,38). The effect of raised intracranial pressure on neuropsychological function is less clear. Both initial and maximum intracranial pressure have prognostic significance, however, maximum intracranial pressure better predicts outcome (39). The impact of intracranial pressure on outcome is unrelated to the age of the survivor, the GCS scores or the type of CNS lesion. Hypotension is perhaps the secondary brain injury most detrimental to survival and functional outcome. Hypotension, along with age, intracranial lesion, pupillary reactively and post-resuscitation GCS score, is considered as one of the five most powerful predictors of outcome during the injury through resuscitation period (2). The presence of hypotension with systolic pressures of less than 90 mmHg or a cerebral perfusion pressure less than 70 mmHg at the time of resuscitation increases the mortality and significantly decreases functional outcome (40–43). In contrast hypoxia, although more prevalent than hypotension at resuscitation, results in only a slight increase in mortality and may have little impact on long term outcome (40).

Increasingly, studies have explored the relationship between impairments and extent of disability at the time of presentation to rehabilitation with functional outcome. One study looked at CT scan abnormalities present at the time of admission to acute rehabilitation; an association was noted with functional outcome and disposition at discharge from rehabilitation (44). Normal CT scans implied an 83% chance of achieving independent living skills, independent mobility and returning to home. On the other hand, large ventricles implied a very poor prognosis for independence in self-care skills and mobility. Only half of the latter patients were able to return to home (44). In addition, FIM scores at the time of initiating rehabilitation have been found to be useful predictors of discharge FIM score and rehabilitation length of stay (6). Similarly, FIM scores have been highly predictive of minutes of required assistance and the extent of supervision needs (45). The impairments that have a significant impact on FIM gain and efficiency are varied but include cognition, balance and medical comorbidities (15,16,21,46).

In summary, traumatic brain injury outcome is too complicated to be predicted accurately with one or several variables. Also, this literature is limited in that the overwhelming preponderance of studies exploring the impact of premorbid, acute injury and post-injury indicators on functional outcome have utilized the Glasgow Outcome Scale as the primary outcome measure; the Glasgow Outcome Scale, however, provides limited information concerning functional skills and limited insight into the comprehensive cognitive, behavioral, and physical deficits common after a traumatic brain injury. Increasingly, studies are examining the prognostic information available at the time of presentation to rehabilitation. At this time, the strength of these predictors remains inadequate to dictate the rehabilitation programming needs of an individual. Hence, the increasing availability of good prognostic information assist the physiatrist in developing an appropriate comprehensive rehabilitation plan, but the data to date remain inadequate to supercede clinical judgment.

Early Rehabilitation Intervention

The significance of early and more aggressive rehabilitation on improving functional outcome has been supported through the observations that prolonged acute care length of stay and a subsequent delay in the onset of multidisciplinary rehabilitation is associated with a longer rehabilitation hospitalization and lower functional outcome (7,47,48). However, functional outcome between the early admission and the late admission groups appears comparable at 2 years (47). These observations, however, cannot exclude the impact of other TBI comorbidities on observed outcomes. Another study examined early intervention on a neurotrauma service while the patient was still on a ventilator (49). Early intervention resulted in shorter rehabilitation stays, higher Rancho levels at discharge from rehabilitation, improvement in the percentage of subsequent patients requiring institutional placement after acute rehabilitation and perhaps most remarkably, shorter durations of coma. Similarly, studies have found that earlier physiatric involvement after TBI is associated with better functional outcome presumably due to the subsequent earlier initiation of multidisciplinary rehabilitation interventions (50). Studies such as these are of enormous significance because the role of rehabilitation in decreasing impairments, disability and handicap while also decreasing long-term health care expenditures has never been directly proven. These studies, however, are part of a growing body of evidence that support the important role of early rehabilitation intervention.

Management of the Minimally Responsive Patient

Definable stages of recovery have been reported for patients emerging from traumatic coma. These stages have been most lucidly outlined by Hagen, Malkmus and

---

TABLE 19-2
Rancho Los Amigos Levels of Cognitive Functioning

I. No response
II. Generalized response
III. Localized response
IV. Confused – agitated
V. Confused – inappropriate
VI. Confused – appropriate
VII. Automatic – appropriate
VIII. Purposeful – appropriate

Durham who developed the Rancho Los Amigos Scale of Cognitive Functioning (Table 19-2) (51).

This scale uses behavioral observation to categorize a patient's level of cognitive functioning; it works well as a simple means by which clinicians can communicate an individual's level of cognitive functioning and develop appropriate rehabilitation strategies.

The initial three Rancho stages represent the low level, or minimally responsive, brain injury survivor. A patient emerging into Level III begins to demonstrate localized responses such as tracking, pulling tubes, restlessness and the beginning of command following. Responses initially are inconsistent, and become more reliable as the patient progresses through stage IV. Recovery through Rancho Levels I, II and III may be protracted in one of eight severe TBI survivors (52). Therefore, objective means to document progress, monitor cognitive status and determine the therapeutic efficacy of intervention becomes an important adjunct in the clinical management of vegetative or low level, coma emerging populations. Examples of two scales utilized for the monitoring of vegetative or low functioning, coma emerging survivors are the Western Neurosensory Stimulation Profile and the Coma/Near Coma Scale.

The Coma/Near Coma Scale consists of eight parameters each with a specified number of stimuli and trials (53). Based on the numerical scoring system, patients are stratified into 1 of 5 categories: no coma, near coma, moderate coma, marked coma and extreme coma. The Coma/Near Coma Scale can be administered quickly. The Western Neuro Sensory Stimulation Profile is a more extensive instrument that consists of 32 items that assess arousal, attention, response to stimuli and expressive communication (54). This instrument, however, requires 20–40 minutes to complete. Both instruments have good interrater reliability and documented construct validity. However, the literature describing the utility of these or other instruments for monitoring the clinical course of vegetative or coma emerging patients remains limited.

Coma rehabilitation, or multisensory stimulation programs are rehabilitation programs designed for patients that are in coma, coma emerging or a vegetative state that have as a primary purpose the prevention of complications associated with prolonged immobilization and the creation of an environment in which the patient has the maximum chance to emerge. This is accomplished by means of a multidisciplinary program involving medical and nursing interventions, sensory stimulation, regular exercise and family education (55,56). It is believed that in this environment, central nervous system pathways will begin to be able to process information with increasing complexity. Advocates of these programs profess that their intervention potentiates the maximum chance of recovery, allows close monitoring of cortical function and facilitates the development of the best overall care plan for the patient. However, a recent review of sensory stimulation literature for brain injured patients could find no adequate clinical trials or evidence to support, or for that matter, rule out the effectiveness of multisensory programs for patients in coma or vegetative states (56).

Multisensory stimulation programs typically stimulate the five senses directly and the patient responses are assessed with the intent of advancing the stimulations as the complexity of response increases (55). However, the optimal nature and frequency of stimulation remains to be defined and varies considerably through the literature. Programs range in intensity between two sessions of 10 minutes each per day to 36 repetitions of the sensory stimulation procedure per day, 7 days per week (55–58). In addition to the lack of consensus as to the nature of the intervention program, interpretation of the available literature suffers from a lack of consistency in definitions of coma or the vegetative state (56). Frequently, the outcome measures were either not objective or lacked clinical significance. These methodologic issues lead one to conclude that there is no compelling evidence to support or refute the possibility that the multisensory stimulation interventions are more effective than standard multidisciplinary rehabilitation at arousing the patient from coma or reducing the time to recover from coma (56). However, in view of the medical, psychological, economic and social implications associated with the treatment of this population, well designed investigation of multisensory stimulation after brain injury is warranted to determine if this strategy should be incorporated as a standard of care.

Post-Traumatic Amnesia

Post-traumatic amnesia (PTA) represents a form of delirium that is both unique to traumatic brain injury survivors and universal in that all survivors of moderate and severe TBI experience post-traumatic amnesia. The period of post-traumatic amnesia has considerable clinical significance. Prognostic information can be discerned from this stage of recovery and both the cognitive and behavioral characteristics of post-traumatic amnesia have an immediate impact on rehabilitation intervention strategies.

The definition of post-traumatic amnesia has evolved over time. Initially it was described by Russell as indicating a period of impaired consciousness after head injury (59). Later post-traumatic amnesia was defined as "taken to end at the time from which the patient can give a clear and consecutive account of what was happening around him" (60). Others have described post-traumatic amnesia as an absence of continuous memory or an inability to retain new information. Today, post-traumatic amnesia suggests the broader syndrome of disorientation to time, place and person, confusion, diminished memory and reduced capabilities for attending and responding to environmental cues (61).

Symonds in 1928 was the first to identify length of coma as an estimate of prognosis after brain injury (62). In 1882, Ribot proposed a classification of amnesia that included both anterograde and retrograde amnesias (63). The concept and clinical significance of post-traumatic amnesia, however, was first suggested in 1932 by Russell (59). Retrograde amnesia implies an inability to retrieve information that was acquired prior to the onset of a specific pathologic event (64). Typically retrograde amnesia involves a gradient; events closer to the injury are less likely to be recalled than earlier memories occurring before the injury. As the patient improves and confusion clears, the duration of retrograde amnesia usually shrinks from perhaps years to approximately 30 minutes or so preceding the pathologic event. After the survivor clears post-traumatic amnesia, the retrieval of remote memory remains impaired but there is no longer a temporal gradient; that is, there is not selective sparing of the oldest memories (64,65). Retrograde amnesia is rarely an isolated event and typically, post-traumatic amnesia is significantly longer than the duration of retrograde amnesia (66).

Post-traumatic amnesia is rarely if ever complete (67). Levin, et al found that during post-traumatic amnesia, initial learning and accelerated forgetting are both problematic but forgetting is particularly accelerated whereas acquisition of new information is less impaired (68). Also, patients during post-traumatic amnesia can demonstrate long-term learning, especially involving tasks that require limited attention. For example, a patient may demonstrate learning during post-traumatic amnesia in situations where the probability of response is increased with repetition (69). A patient may also learn during post-traumatic amnesia through stimulus response training such as acquisition of motor skills (60). The concept of learning during post-traumatic amnesia is salient to the rehabilitation professional in that issues of self-care, mobility and locomotion can be successfully addressed during this amnestic stage. Similarly, problem behaviors can be addressed during this amnestic state with behavioral interventions that are consistent and repetitious.

The duration of post-traumatic amnesia is a marker of injury severity and carries significant prognostic implications. By 1961, the duration of post-traumatic amnesia was thought to represent "the best yardstick we have" of blunt head injury severity (70). Over the decades, it has been demonstrated that the length of post-traumatic amnesia is predictive of functional outcome, return to work, occurrence of post-traumatic epilepsy and cognitive recovery (19,22,71–79).

Predicting resolution of post-traumatic amnesia also carries significant therapeutic implications in that the resolution of post-traumatic amnesia is often associated with a marked improvement in behavior, a reduction in agitation, an improvement in attention, a readiness to tolerate the demands of a more comprehensive neuropsychological assessment, and an increase in capacity to more fully participate in a comprehensive rehabilitation program (80). Therefore, predicting whether and when a patient will clear post-traumatic amnesia is useful in establishing a survivor's programming needs. It has been speculated that the duration of post-traumatic amnesia is approximately four times the duration of coma, but other studies have failed to support the length of coma as a reliable a predictor of clearing post-traumatic amnesia (80,81). A younger age implies a greater likelihood of clearing post-traumatic amnesia but age does not accurately predict when the survivor will clear this stage. Finally, several attempts to predict post-traumatic amnesia duration early in the post-acute period utilizing validated instruments that prospectively measure post-traumatic amnesia duration have yielded mixed results. Specifically, time after trauma and the first weekly aggregate score assessed by the Orientation Group Monitoring System accounted for only 15.9% of the variance (80). However, a model utilizing the Modified Oxford PTA Scale found that a three variable regression model, consisting of day after trauma when testing was started, rate of change of post-traumatic amnesic scores over the first 5 days of testing and the score on the first day of testing accounts for 89% of the variance in observed length of post-traumatic amnesia (82).

Traditionally the duration of post-traumatic amnesia has been estimated retrospectively. This is potentially problematic in that islands of intact memory may develop when the patient otherwise is unable to sustain continuous memory (83,84). Therefore, retrospectively inquiring as to the time of the first intact memory post-injury could result in an underestimation of post-traumatic amnesia duration. Similarly, retrospectively inquiring as to the interval when orientation normalized can lead to a misleading estimate of post-traumatic duration; 10% to 20% of survivors may be oriented without having cleared post-traumatic amnesia (83,85).

The first instrument developed to prospectively assess the duration of post-traumatic was the Galveston Orientation and Amnesia Test (GOAT) (84). This instrument is

TABLE 19-3
Prospective Measures of Post-Traumatic Amnesia Duration

Galveston Orientation and Amnesia Test (68)
Oxford PTA Scale (25)
Orientation Group Monitoring System
Westmead PTA Scale (91)
Julia Farr Services PTA Scale (92)
Modified Oxford PTA Scale (24)

reliable (Kendell Correlation Co-efficient of 0.99). The core application for this instrument is the assessment of temporal orientation. This instrument can be administered daily at bedside during the course of a brief interview. Construct validity for the GOAT has been demonstrated through correlation with Glasgow Outcome Scale level, the severity of computed tomography findings, and functional outcome. Finally, the GOAT's brevity renders it more applicable to monitor recovery through PTA in the acute care setting than the other more extensive assessments of PTA such as the Orientation Group Monitoring System (86–89). Other instruments have subsequently been developed to prospectively measure the duration of post-traumatic amnesia (Table 19-3) (90–92).

Each instrument emphasizes different constructs of post-traumatic amnesia, and with the exception of the Orientation Group Monitoring System, are generally brief, lending themselves to bedside utilization. The Orientation Group Monitoring System is based on behavioral observations during a scheduled therapeutic orientation group and, therefore, is appropriate for an inpatient rehabilitation setting where its utility in the early detection of evolving medical complications that present as a decline in cognitive function can be utilized (89). The Galveston Orientation and Amnesia Test is the most widely utilized prospective assessment of post-traumatic amnesia with well established, sound psychometric properties (93).

Thus, the period of post-traumatic amnesia has important clinical significance. The duration of PTA carries prognostic implications concerning long-term outcome. During PTA, acquisition and storage of memory are impaired but under proper circumstances, new functional skills can be acquired. Finally, the behavioral and cognitive abnormalities characteristic of PTA carry significant therapeutic implications regarding supervision needs and formalized programming needs.

Agitation

Perhaps the most compelling behavioral change during post-traumatic amnesia is post-traumatic agitation. Denny-Brown (1945) first described restlessness as a natural sequela of traumatic brain injury (94). The classic example of agitation is the patient at Level IV of the Rancho Los Amigos Level of Functioning who is "confused-agitated" and functioning in a heightened state of activity and diminished capability for processing new information or responding to events in the environment. Various estimates of agitation incidence have ranged between 11%, 33% to over 50% (95,96). In part, this disparity was related to the absence of a consistent definition. In 1996, Sandel and Mysiw defined post-traumatic agitation as a subtype of delerium unique to TBI patients who are still in post-traumatic amnesia and who demonstrate excesses of behavior that include akathesia, aggression and emotional lability (97). This definition is consistent with the constructs defined in both the Agitated Behavior Scale, a reliable and valid instrument, designed to measure the severity and nature of post-traumatic agitation (98), and a survey of expert TBI rehabilitation physiatrists (99).

The initial approach to the agitated patient includes a comprehensive examination emphasizing other medical or neurologic etiologies for the observed behavior prior to initiating treatment strategies. Fractures, peripheral nerve injuries, skin lesions, J/G-tube sites and tracheotomy sites, for example, are potential sources of noxious stimuli that left untreated with appropriate analgesia may present as agitated behavior in the coma emerging, confused patient. In addition, all medical conditions that have the potential to result in a decline in mental status or cognitive function should be considered as studies have shown that cognition improves before agitation and a decline in cognition often results in an increase in agitation (15,100). Also, all pharmacologic interventions should be reviewed for evidence of toxicity or adverse reactions.

Management strategies utilized in treating agitated behavior include one-to-one monitoring, behavioral modification, physical restraints, environmental modification and pharmacologic intervention (101). As rehabilitation stays shorten, the prompt resolution of agitation becomes increasingly important so as to not interfere with other treatment goals (101). Therefore, pharmacologic intervention has also become increasingly important as an adjunct in the treatment of the agitated traumatic brain injury survivor.

There have been six randomized clinical trials published exploring pharmacologic treatment options for agitated aggressive behavior after brain injury (102–107). Four of these studies looked at the role of beta blockers, one studied methylphenidate and the sixth study utilized amantadine. The beta blockers did appear to be most effective, but the population studied was not limited to traumatic brain injury survivors. The methylphenidate study looked at an aspect of agitation, namely aggression, in a group of TBI survivors who cleared post-traumatic amnesia. The amantadine study utilized a behavioral outcome not ideally suited to the assessment of post-traumatic agitation.

The balance of the studies exploring the efficacy of pharmacologic interventions for post-traumatic agitation are primarily case reports or series that utilized an AB rather than ABA design and lacked a reliable outcome measure. Also, these studies fail to consider the impact of the pharmacologic intervention on outcome. As previously noted in the post-stroke population, evidence has begun to emerge that suggests that certain categories of pharmacologic agents utilized in the acute care setting, namely neuroleptics, do have a negative impact on cognitive recovery during the rehabilitation setting (108).

Several classes of medications are most commonly utilized in the management of post-traumatic agitation (Table 19-4).

A survey of the American Academy of Physical Medicine and Rehabilitation Brain Injury Special Interest Group in 1997 revealed that the five most frequently prescribed drugs to diminish the severity of post-traumatic agitation were carbamazepine, tricyclic antidepressants, trazodone, amantadine and beta-blockers (99). During episodes of extreme agitation, the literature appears to support abortive agents such as short-acting benzodiazepines or atypical antipsychotics (109).

Data suggest that as patients emerge from coma, improvement in cognition precedes resolution of agitation (15,87). This supports the clinical observation that agitation management strategies that diminish cognition may, in fact, prolong and exacerbate agitation. Therefore, the ideal pharmacologic management of post-traumatic agitation would include the simultaneous objective monitoring of both the agitation severity and cognitive function. The Agitated Behavior Scale has been validated to provide an assessment of agitation severity, duration and the relative contribution of aggression, disinhibition or lability to the observed behavior (98). Two instruments that lend themselves to monitoring cognitive recovery during pharmacologic intervention of agitation include the previously mentioned Galveston Orientation and Amnesia Test and the Orientation Group Monitoring System (84,86). In the rehabilitation setting, the Orientation Group Monitoring System does offer a distinct advantage over the GOAT through its increased sensitivity in detecting medical complications such as adverse drug effects, infections and hydrocephalus (88). The GOAT's brevity renders it the more useful instrument in the acute care setting.

In summary, multiple pharmacologic treatments have been proposed for the management of post-traumatic agitation; the efficacy and indications remain largely unproven. The optimal medication would: 1) control behavior without sedation; 2) augment or at least not delay or interfere with recovery of cognition; and 3) maintain a low side-effects profile. Given the heterogeneity of primary and secondary brain injury mechanisms, injury severity, presence of pre-existing conditions and the variable clinical presentation of post-traumatic agitation, it is unlikely that one pharmacologic agent will evolve as effective in the management of agitation in all or even a majority of survivors.

Cardiovascular Autonomic Disorders

Cardiovascular disorders associated with TBI may include rhythm disturbances, ischemic changes, cardiac contusion, hypotension and hypertension. Of these, hypertension is the most common and immediate cardiovascular disorder associated with severe head injury (110). In fact, autonomic dysfunction has been reported in 15–33% of acute brain injury survivors (111,112). The condition is most commonly found after brainstem or diffuse axonal injury. Although tachycardia, fever and hypertension represent the most frequent presenting signs, the physical findings could include any combination of autonomic disturbances. (Table 19-5).

This diagnosis of autonomic dysfunction is a diagnosis of exclusion (Table 19-6) (111,112).

In the event that the clinical picture primarily involves hypertension, then other etiologies can be considered such as increased intracranial pressure (113), hydrocephalus (114), or medications such as steroids or nonsteroidal anti-inflammatory drugs.

The presence of autonomic dysfunction is associated with morbidity, due to possible secondary myocardial infarction, intracerebral hemorrhage, rhabdomyolysis. The hypertension and associated medical instability may

---

TABLE 19-4

Classes of Medications Commonly Used to Treat Post-Traumatic Agitation

- Benzodiazepines
- Anticonvulsant
- Antidepressant
- Antipsychotics
- Buspirone
- Amantadine
- Beta-blockers
- Lithium

TABLE 19-5

Common Presentations of Autonomic Dysfunction After Brain Trauma

- Hypertension that is either constant or fluctuating
- Fever that may range from low grade to high
- Tachycardia
- Pupillary dialation
- Diaphoresis
- Dystonia or extensor posturing

TABLE 19-6
Differential Diagnosis of Autonomic Dysfunction After Brain Trauma

- Infection/sepsis
- Neuroleptic malignant syndrome
- Autonomic dysreflexia secondary to spinal cord injury
- Malignant hyperthermia
- Pheochromocytoma
- Thyroid storm
- Delirium tremens
- Lethal catatonia
- Serotonin syndrome

preclude initiation of most direct rehabilitative interventions. As such, patients who experience autonomic dysfunction are likely to require longer periods of inpatient rehabilitation and tend to have a longer period of post-traumatic amnesia, poorer Glasgow Outcome Scale score and lower Function Independence Measure score.

Again, although autonomic dysfunction is seen in 15–28% of TBI survivors acutely in the rehabilitation setting, the incidence is estimated to be between 10 and 15% and the prevalence diminishes rapidly to less than 3% after discharge (110,115). In Labi and Horn's retrospective study of 74 patients with no premorbid history of hypertension who were discharged from a rehabilitation hospital after their first TBI, only 11 (15%) developed hypertension during admission (115). Five (7%) were discharged on anti-hypertension medication, of whom 3 were able to discontinue or reduce medication at 1 month after discharge and 2 were lost to follow-up. In the interim, the treatment involves controlling the blood pressure with beta blockers or alpha blockers (116). In the more advanced forms of autonomic dysfunction, spasmolytics such as dantrolene, and analgesics such as opiates and either dopamine agonists or antagonists may prove effective at ameliorating some of these symptoms (117).

Hypotension in the rehabilitation setting is frequently associated with prolonged bed rest or medication adverse effects, volume depletion or neuroendocrine abnormalities. The most common medications causing orthostatic hypotension are anti-hypertensive, in particular diuretics, alpha blockers and vasodilators.

Electrocardiographic abnormalities commonly accompany early recovery from TBI. Incidence after severe head injury varies from greater that 80% during the acute medical admission (118) to approximately 20% during inpatient rehabilitation (110). ECG evidence suggesting myocardial ischemia, including prolonged QT interval, inverted T waves, and ST segment elevation has been well documented in the neurosurgical literature (113,118,119). Myocardial injury has been corroborated through laboratory medicine and at autopsy. CK-MB activity may remain elevated at least 3 days after injury (113). Histologic evidence of myocardial necrosis at autopsy has confirmed the presence of myocardial injury following head injury (120). In the absence of direct cardiac trauma, myocardial damage may be secondary to massive release of catecholamine from autonomic dysfunction (121).

Dysrhythmias appear to occur less commonly, although the incidence has not been studied after TBI. Case reports include life-threatening torsades de pointes, concomitant pulsus alternans and U-wave alternans, transient heart block ranging from prolonged PR intervals to high-grade AV block with ventricular escape rhythm (121–124). Most commonly seen in the rehabilitation setting are nonspecific ST and T wave changes (110). Given the potential for underlying myocardial damage, baseline EKG at the time of rehabilitation admission is a valuable screening exam and an important adjunct to a thoughtful cardiopulmonary evaluation.

Respiratory Disorders

Respiratory or pulmonary complications noted after traumatic brain injury include those directly related to trauma such as pneumothorax, hemothorax and flail chest. In addition, a number of pulmonary complications occur that are at least, in part, related to the subsequent neurologic dysfunction, including: respiratory failure, pneumonia, neurogenic pulmonary edema and tracheal/airway complications (125). Pulmonary complications are the most frequent complications occurring after the acute trauma through the rehabilitation hospital stay, with up to 60% of patients experiencing pneumonia, respiratory failure occurring in up to 43% and 39% requiring a tracheotomy (16,125–132).

In a British analysis of mortality after pediatric TBI, 93% of potentially preventable deaths prior to hospital admission were of respiratory etiology, predominantly aspiration (133). Following admission one quarter of all deaths were attributable to pulmonary abnormalities. Of those considered to be preventable deaths, nearly 60% were secondary to respiratory arrest or airway obstruction. More recent data has documented that the presence of respiratory failure, pneumonia and tracheotomies show a strong relationship to both acute and inpatient rehabilitation length of stay (16). In addition, those survivors without respiratory failure or who did not require a tracheotomy demonstrated a better one year outcome per the Disability Rating Scale and the Function Independence Measure (16).

Alcohol intoxication, frequently associated with TBI, is a significant risk factor for respiratory complications. In a study of 520 patients, nearly 40% were intoxicated at the time of admission (134). Although injury severity appeared similar to the non-intoxicated cohort, intoxicated patients were 30% more likely to require intubation prior to admission and 80% more likely to have respiratory distress requiring artificial ventilation during the acute care admission. Potential factors contributing to a 40% greater risk of pneumonia included ethanol related immune suppression, a higher likelihood of aspiration and/or a higher prevalence of pneumonia preceding the TBI. Of note, where alcohol intoxication was documented on admission, length of hospital stay was not extended unless pulmonary complications developed, specifically respiratory distress or pneumonia. Given the frequency of these complications, alcohol intoxication complicating TBI has obvious economic and public health ramifications.

The majority of patients who undergo tracheotomy will recover sufficient neurologic integrity to consider decannulation. Decannulation is pursued when the individual no longer requires ventilation, effectively manages their secretions and is thought to be at low risk for aspiration (125). There is no standardized protocol for decannulation. Usually this is accomplished in a stepwise fashion with incrementally decreasing the cannula diameter followed by a trial of plugging the tube; if the patient is asymptomatic, has an effective cough and manages their secretions, then the tube is finally removed and an occlusive dressing is applied (125). Prospective studies of patients with long term tracheotomy, using direct laryngeal visualization prior to decannulation have demonstrated an incidence of serious abnormalities which exceeds 30%, in both the acute and subacute setting (129–131). Tracheal stenosis, subglottic stenosis, glottic stenosis, tracheomalacia, tracheal granuloma are seen most frequently with varying degrees of clinical symptoms. In view of these complications, direct laryngoscopy prior to decannulation has been suggested.

Where studies have stratified by cognitive level, as expected, morbidity and mortality are much higher for decannulation at Rancho Levels II and III (129). Central respiratory lability and poor pulmonary toilet with resultant pneumonia leading to sepsis contribute significantly to the increased mortality in the vegetative and coma emerging patient. Hence, the appropriateness or merit of decannulating patients who remain severely neurologically compromised remains uncertain. On the other hand, predictors of successful decannulation include: 1) traumatic mechanism of brain injury; 2) younger age; and 3) alert cognitive status (130). Also, of those in whom adequate cough and swallowing reflexes have been documented, complications are not observed to correlate with age, diagnosis, Rancho scale or duration of tracheotomy (131).

Several factors may predispose to increasing laryngotracheal mucosal reaction following traumatic brain injury (129). Emergent intubation frequently occurs under less than optimal circumstances. The peri-injury and acute stabilization period are frequently complicated by hypotension and resultant tissue hypoxia (129). Cervical hyperextension associated with decerebrate or decorticate posturing can enable the posterior pharyngeal tissues to act a fulcrum for the rigid endotracheal tube (132). Head movement, potentially creating a see-sawing movement of the tube, may be marked with agitation (132).

Prolonged tracheal intubation is known to result in a number of complications. These complications can be diminished with proper choice of tube, meticulous attention to details of airway management to prevent excessive movement of the tube during turning, suctioning, and ventilator connection/disconnection, adequate sedation to prevent coughing, agitation and decerebrate or decorticate posturing, adequate humidification, use of soft nasogastric tubes, and prevention of tissue hypoxia, anemia and infection all of which further increase the risk of tissue injury.

Fever

A common acute complication after a severe traumatic brain injury is fever. Although frank fever of unknown origin (temperature elevation of greater than 38.2° C on several occasions over at least a 3 week period of time and an inability to diagnose the underlying etiology after at least 1 week of intensive investigation) (134) is unusual, a similar systematic approach to diagnose the underlying etiology is often warranted. The differential diagnosis for fever of unknown origin is extensive and includes infectious, neoplastic, autoimmune, granulomatosis, metabolic, inherited, psychogenic, periodic and thermoregulatory disorders (134). The list of likely sources of fever after a severe traumatic brain injury is less extensive but this framework is often useful for accurate diagnosis (135).

Urinary tract infections affect approximately 40% of traumatic brain injury survivors during the rehabilitation phase of recovery (110) Ureteral obstruction is seen in approximately 1% of patients after a traumatic brain injury. Other potential genitourinary sources of fever include pyelonephritis, perinephric abscess and prostatic abscess.

Approximately 34% of traumatic brain injury survivors develop respiratory complications that predispose them to pulmonary infections (110). Poor ventilation with secondary atelectasis is thought to be the most common pulmonary complication of trauma and a potential forerunner of pneumonia. Tissue necrosis secondary to lung trauma with subsequent formation of a pulmonary cavity may also predispose the patient to secondary lung infections (136). The presence of endotracheal or tracheotomy tubes predispose patients to bacterial colonization and a greater risk of secondary lung infection. Finally, tubes utilized for enteral feeding increase the probably of aspiration pneumonia by as much as 25%.

The head and neck area includes several other potential sources of fever after a traumatic brain injury.

For example, perinasal sinusitis after nasotracheal intubation has been estimated to occur in approximately 26% of patients (139,140). Also nasogastric intubation has been reported to cause a similar rate of sinusitis and fever in trauma survivors. Finally, within the head and neck area, dental abscess is a potential etiology secondary to teeth rendered non-viable by trauma (141).

Cardiovascular etiologies for fever include subacute and acute endocarditis (142), dissecting aortic aneurysm (143), intravenous line sepsis (144) and thromboembolic disease (145). The incidence of thromboembolic disease after traumatic brain injury has been reported to occur at a rate as low as 4% during the rehabilitation course. However, this incidence is possibly low due to the nonspecific clinical presentation of thromboembolic disorders and the concomitant issue of impaired arousal and cognition.

Other sources for fever include musculoskeletal etiologies such as heterotopic ossification, (146) which can mimic deep venous thrombosis in its presentation, and osteomyelitis from either hematogenous or contiguous spread (110). Perisplenic, pericardial and retroperitoneal cryptic hematomas have been associated with a prolonged fever after trauma (110,147). Adverse reactions to medications includes drug fever; an important and potentially life threatening example of this would be the neuroleptic malignant syndrome (148,149). Finally, neurologic etiologies for fever after trauma would include bacterial meningitis, infected intraventricular shunts, hyperthermia reactions to acute hydrocephalus, neurogenic hyperthermia and the post-ictal period (150–154).

Bladder and Bowel Function

Traumatic brain injury often results in injury to the frontal lobes resulting in loss of cortical control over urination and defecation (155). In addition, injury to the subcortial structures can result in the development of bladder dysnergia. In one large study of brain injury survivors, 38% of patients developed urinary tract infections. Although the majority of these patients had indwelling Foley catheters, 37% did not. Therefore, bladder dysfunction was seen in 8% of the cohort (110).

The incidence of urinary incontinence during the first 6 weeks after TBI has been found in approximately 62% of patients (156). Also, 9.5% of survivors are found to have evidence of urinary retention (156). Urodynamic studies primarily document an uninhibited over active bladder where the patient demonstrates loss of voluntary control over micturation, disturbed bladder perception and poor sphincter control to the extent that upon virtually the first sensation of filling, the patient develops almost immediate micturation (157).

The clinical significance of urinary incontinence and retention early in the coma emerging brain injured patient is that this increases the risk of urinary tract infection and

the development of skin ulcer (156,157). Also, the presence of urinary incontinence is associated with a poorer functional outcome at discharge from both acute care and inpatient rehabilitation and it increases the likelihood of requiring a long-term care disposition (156).

Treatment options for urinary incontinence after TBI includes behavioral strategies such as a timed voiding program (158). All predisposing factors to urinary tract infections such as Foley catheters, bladder retention, fecal incontinence, and inadequate hydration, are removed or addressed. A timed voiding program initially begins with toileting the patient frequently with gradual increases in interval length. For the patient who voids frequently in small amounts with low post-void residual volumes, anti-cholinergic agents can be considered as an adjunct (159). However, important possible adverse effects of anti-cholinergic agents include a slowing of cognitive recovery, worsening of delerium and the development of urinary retention.

Bowel dysfunction after traumatic brain injury often results from a loss of cortical control over the defecation reflex causing the patient to be incontinent. In addition, constipation is a frequent occurrence in the acute care setting due to lack of mobility, use of potentially constipating medication and alteration in normal diet. Stool softeners, osmotic laxatives, stimulant suppositories and adequate hydration are often helpful initially to maintain bowel regularity. As the patient recovers, the bowel program should be tailored to additionally utilize the gastrocolic reflex, approximately 30 minutes after eating, as well as gravity by having them sit in an upright position to defecate. As noted with urinary incontinence, the presence of bowel incontinence is associated with a more severe injury and poorer functional status at both acute care and other inpatient rehabilitation (160).

Diarrhea is a common occurrence in low level brain injury patients on enteral feedings. This can lead to loss of skin integrity, infect pressure sores and other wounds, and result in severe dehydration. Use of formulas high in fiber, and using isosmotic formulas are often helpful. Supplementing the enteral feeding with fiber compounds such as psyllium mucilloid can also be helpful in forming stool. The use of anti-diarrheal medications are not necessary and in the case of loperamide can be potentially sedating. Patients after severe traumatic brain injury often require antibiotic treatment for various infections, are debilitated, and in the hospital; thus they are at significant risk for the development of bowel infections. In the patient who has persistent diarrhea, infectious etiology should be considered (139).

Swallowing and Nutrition

Two primary nutritional issues confront the TBI survivor, the timing of initiating nutritional support and the optimal route of administration. After moderate or severe TBI, the patients demonstrate and increase in caloric requirements (161) due to hyper metabolism, increased energy expenditure and increased protein loss (162–164). This state can persist for up to 4 weeks (121). Studies have shown that early nutritional support prevents the loss of immune competence, decreases morbidity and mortality, shortens the length of hospital stay and may decrease subsequent disability (165–168).

The merits of enteral (gastrostomy versus jejunostomy) versus parenteral routes of nutritional support are not resolved. As arousal improves, swallowing evaluations involving a combination of bedside swallowing assessments or video fluoroscopy, are performed by a speech-language pathologist or occupational therapist, are warranted as swallowing disorders are estimated to occur in 25–30% of brain injury survivors (169,170). The video fluoroscopic evaluation is often an essential adjunct in the evaluation of these patients because physical findings alone are not sufficiently sensitive to predict the ability to safely swallow. In a study by Winstein, (170) 12% of patients with swallowing disorders had normal gag reflexes and 77% has a good voluntary cough reflex. Thus, the information provided by a comprehensive assessment helps the clinician to make important judgments about the patient's ability to begin oral feeding and which swallowing strategies would most facilitate safe swallowing.

At first, oral feeding is often restricted to therapeutic purposes and requires the direct supervision and intervention by a speech-language pathologist or occupational therapist. Safe therapeutic feeding is additionally predicated on the survivor's behavioral sequela; behaviors such as agitation, impulsivity, lack of initiation, and hyperphagia should be monitored for and, when present, treated using appropriate behavioral management interventions. After oral feeding has begun, it is sometimes difficult for the patient to maintain adequate caloric intake necessitating a combination of oral and enteral feeding and close monitoring of nutritional status. Attempts to advance oral feeding are intermittently slowed by the loss of appetite. In these instances, a specific etiology should be sought such as an evaluation of taste and smell due to cranial nerve or cortical dysfunction, as well as local trauma, leading to anosmia and/or gustatory dysfunction. Depression, neuroendocrine perturbations and pharmacologic interventions should also be considered as etiologies for decreased appetite.

Spasticity, Dystonia and Other Muscle Overactivity

After a traumatic brain injury, spasticity, dystonia and other forms of muscle overactivity are not limited to the limbs but can also present in the torsal, facial, and oral pharyngeal musculature. Interventions are clearly warranted when the muscle tone significantly interferes with achievement of rehabilitation goals. Otherwise, it is a commonly held tenet that spasticity should not be treated unless it interferes with function. However, the veracity of this approach in a coma emerging patient, where plasticity may be affected by the consequence of abnormal tone has not been adequately studied.

The first stage of treatment for spasticity involves physical modalities, range of motion, and exercise.

Cryotherapy has been found to be helpful in temporarily reducing spasticity for 1 to 3 hours after application (171). This is often sufficient time to allow for therapeutic interventions including serial casting, ambulation or range of motion exercises. Application of casts to preserve or increase range of motion has been shown to have a secondary beneficial affect on reducing spasticity (172). Thus, through the use of serial casting early in the care of brain injury patients, improvements in tone and maintenance of joint range of motion can be fostered.

If spasticity continues despite these interventions, pharmacologic therapy is indicated (173,174). Unfortunately, the use of anti-spasticity medications can have negative effects on cognition (88). In the traumatic brain injury population, dantrolene sodium becomes an attractive pharmacologic agent, primarily because of low potential for cognitive side-effects; however, routine blood monitoring is required because of potential toxic effects on the liver. Other anti-spasticity medications primarily include tizanidine, baclofen and the benzodiapines; a wide variety of other off-label agents exist with some value in tone reduction (173,174). Although these medications can all help with tone reduction, they require close monitoring because of the significant potential for impairing cognition.

If pharmacotherapeutic interventions are ineffective in reducing spasticity, motor point blocks, nerve blocks and botulinum toxin are effective in reducing tone in a specific group of muscles such as lower limb adductors or plantar flexors. Neurectomies and intrathecal infusion of baclofen have been shown to help with persistent hypertonicity (177,178). However, during the early rehabilitation assessment and intervention after TBI, these more invasive interventions are rarely indicated.

TERTIARY PREVENTION

Venous Thromboembolism

Deep venous thrombosis (DVT) represents a significant source of morbidity and potential mortality for patients with head trauma. Pulmonary embolism from DVT is apparently increasing in importance as a cause of death of inpatients with traumatic brain injury (179). The NIH Consensus Conference estimated the incidence of DVT after severe traumatic brain injury to be approximately

40% and the incidence of fatal pulmonary embolus is approximately 1% (180). The incidence of DVT in TBI patients upon admission to inpatient rehabilitation has been estimated as high as 20% (181,182). Despite these data, there is no standard of care for DVT prophylaxis, screening or treatment after TBI. In part, this is secondary to the safety concerns associated with the use of anticoagulation after trauma and a traumatic brain injury. However, there is increasing evidence to support the safety of initiating either heparin or low molecular weight heparin (LMWH) within 24–72 hours of severe head injury or intracranial bleed (183,184). Similarly, the value of screening for DVT at presentation to inpatient rehabilitation has been supported (185). The incidence of DVT can be significantly reduced using a specialized approach of prophylactic intervention in conjunction with routine monitoring in high risk patients. High risk categories include: 1) advanced age; 2) severe injury; 3) prolonged immobilization; 4) number of transfusions; 5) presence of clotting disorder (179,186–190).

In the event that prophylaxis against DVT is initiated, The Eastern Association for the Surgery of Trauma Practice Guidelines for the Prevention of Venous Thromboembolism in Trauma Patients in 2002 suggested that pneumatic compression devices may be of some benefit, LMWH is superior to heparin for prophylaxis in moderate to high risk trauma patients and duplex ultrasound is appropriate to diagnose symptomatic DVT and may be appropriate for screening of high risk asymptomatic patients (191). In those patients who are unable to receive these forms of prophylaxis, prophylactic Greenfield filter placement deserves strong consideration.

Contractures

Contractures of the limbs, as well as the axial skeleton can potentially have devastating implications on self-care, mobility and even vocalization. Persons who are at greatest risk for contractures are those with: 1) a long period of coma and immobilization; 2) severe brain injury; and 3) altered muscle tone. The best treatment of joint contractures is prevention of contractures by an ongoing program of range of motion exercises and maintenance of postural adaptation (i.e., sitting, lying prone or supine and standing). Serial casting has been shown to be useful in the prevention and treatment of contractures (172,192,193). The therapeutic benefit of continual casting versus casting/bi-valve splinting has been debated with the current literature suggesting that continuous casting has a slightly better therapeutic advantage (193). However, others question the therapeutic value of orthotics and actively discourage their utilization due to a concern that motor relearning may be affected (194).

Once contractures develop, treatment depends on the severity of the contractures. Treatment options include an aggressive stretching program in association with physical modalities, serial casting, and dynamic bracing. Pharmacologic interventions are initiated to address abnormal muscle tone. Other more focal interventions such as botulinum toxin, motor point blocks or neural blocks may be adequate and, thereby, minimize the potential adverse cognitive effects of antispasticity medications. In extreme cases, surgical release of the contracted tissue may be warranted to increase function. Surgical release of contracted tissue can improve skin care and hygiene, prevent the development and foster the healing of pressure sores, reduce pain and improve transfers and ambulation (186). However, such aggressive intervention for contractures is limited to the more chronic survivor who has failed conservative measures and are rarely if ever considered in the early course of the coma-emerging patient.

Fractures

The incidence of concurrent fractures in patients with traumatic brain injury is approximately 30% (195); approximately 11% of these fractures are initially undetected (196). In brain injury survivors with fractures, there is an associated high risk of developing heterotopic ossification (197). This occurs especially in patients with forearm (198) and hip fractures (195). In a cohort of patients with hip fractures after traumatic brain injury, 100% developed heterotopic ossification (187). Conventional treatment of fractures including splints and casting often results in less than desirable results. Uncontrolled limb motion is common in the brain injury survivor especially early in the recovery as the patient emerges from coma (195). Early definitive fixation of upper and lower limb fractures allows for a shorter period of immobilization, early range of motion activity and less overall nursing care (198). Early mobilization and range of motion activities reduces the likelihood of developing severe spasticity, contractures, and anklylosing heterotopic ossification. In addition, early definitive fixation diminishes the need for casting of limbs, which often interferes with rehabilitation intervention.

Peripheral Nerve Injuries

It has been estimated that 34% of patients admitted to a rehabilitation unit were diagnosed with previously undetected peripheral nerve injuries (199). Ulnar nerve entrapment in the cubital tunnel was found most frequently with brachial plexus injury and common peroneal compression neuropathies of slightly less frequency (199). Median nerve compression at the wrist has been reported in brain injury patients with wrist and finger flexor spasticity (200). Factors that are felt to contribute to compression neuropathies in the brain injury population include: 1) extrinsic pressure from a hematoma or heterotopic ossification; 2) prolonged coma; 3) severe spasticity; 4) improper positioning; 5) fractures; and 6) improperly applied casts (199–201).

It has been estimated that 50% of these neuropathies are preventable (199). Thus, in the acute care setting, preventive measures are incorporated to the rehabilitation intervention such as proper positioning, monitoring of cast application, and the early treatment of spasticity and heterotopic ossification.

Heterotopic Ossification

The risk of developing heterotopic ossification in the traumatic brain injury survivor is 20% and the risk increases as the severity of injury, length of immobilization and duration of coma increases (202). Also, the presence of spasticity and fractures increase the risk, especially if the fracture involves an open reduction, internal fixation or if there is a joint dislocation. Heterotopic ossification usually involves the large joints of the body (hips, elbows, shoulder and knees). Excess bone formation can result in significant disability by severely limiting the range of motion of a joint. Progressive loss of joint mobility and markers of increased osteoblastic activity such as an elevated fractionated alkaline phosphatase level warrants a comprehensive musculoskeletal examination, three phased bone scan and x-rays to confirm the presence, distribution and extent of heterotopic ossification (203). However, plain radiographs may not demonstrate the presence of heterotopic ossification for one to two months after the initial onset. Osteocalcin, another marker of osteoblastic activity, does not appear to be useful in the early detection of heterotopic ossification or in assessing its maturity (203). Heterotopic ossification often presents as a soft tissue swelling and loss of range of motion. The differential diagnosis the includes thrombophlebitis, cellulites, septic joint, fracture, hematoma or soft tissue trauma.

The treatment of heterotopic ossification initially involves preventive strategies; once heterotopic ossification formation has begun additional preventive and therapeutic interventions are initiated. Diphosphonates and indomethacin have been shown to prevent heterotopic bone formation (199,204). Diphosphonates may also minimize the extent of heterotopic ossification formation after its onset, but the role of diphosphonates in this setting remains controversial. The treatment of heterotopic ossification also includes physical modalities such as aggressive range of motion exercises in an attempt to reduce the likelihood of bony ankylosis (204,205). Other investigators discourage aggressive range of motion out of concern that the micro trauma or local hemorrhage may predispose the development of heterotopic ossification. In the relatively rare event that heterotopic ossification causes sufficient joint ankylosis to impede function, surgery is usually performed in combination with the radiation of

the involved area in the hope of regaining range of motion and arresting further bone development. However, surgery is often discouraged until one to two years after the onset of heterotopic ossification due to increased risk of recurrence during the active growth phase of the ectopic bone.

INDIVIDUALIZED REHABILITATION PLAN

After documenting the extent of impairments and estimating functional outcome, the physiatrist is charged with determining the most appropriate rehabilitation interventions for the survivor. Early rehabilitation is initiated while the survivor remains on the trauma or neurosurgical service. Rehabilitation options following this early stage are predicated on the nature of residual impairments (170). In the unlikely event that a survivor of a severe traumatic brain injury recovers sufficiently during acute care to permit rehabilitation management on an outpatient basis, individual outpatient services or a day-treatment program may be recommended. Typically day treatment rehabilitation offers survivors integrated programs of physical therapy, occupational therapy, speech pathology, cognitive remediation, vocational and psychological services up to 8 hours per day, 5 days per week.

If, at the time of discharge from acute care, the residual impairments are of such severity that the patient remains dependent, then options include either an acute or subacute rehabilitation program. The typical admission to a traumatic brain injury acute rehabilitation unit is an individual who is able to consistently follow a 1 step command, is commonly confused and disoriented, restless if not overtly agitated, and many have a combination of physical limitations or medical complications. Ideally, it is the goal of this phase of rehabilitation to assist the patient from the late stages of unconsciousness through clearing post-traumatic amnesia, resolution of agitation, and at least minimal independence in activities of daily living. For the individual and their family, the most salient goal of the acute rehabilitation phase is to regain optimal independence in activities of daily living. To remain in this rehabilitation environment, the patient must be able to tolerate and benefit from a minimum of 3 hours of therapy, 5 days per week.

Subacute rehabilitation programs are largely nursing home based. These programs do not require that a patient tolerate 3 hours of therapy per day. Consequently, subacute rehabilitation programs are most appropriate for survivors who remain in the "coma stages", responds to simple commands inconsistently or the rate of progress is slow. The typical length of stay is considerably longer than the present national average of approximately 21 days in acute rehabilitation. Largely because of staffing and overhead, subacute rehabilitation offers health care providers a less expensive form of specialized intervention. Although data exist supporting the importance of early rehabilitation interventions on outcome (43,44), virtually no data exist comparing acute versus subacute intervention outcome.

After inpatient rehabilitation, a number of post-acute management strategies are available. Again, if the patient can be managed at home, then rehabilitation options would include individual in home or outpatient therapy, or comprehensive day-treatment services. If a patient in an acute rehabilitation setting fails to achieve basic functional independence in a timely fashion, then a transfer to a subacute rehabilitation program may be warranted. In the event that behavioral problems such as agitation preclude discharge to the home, more specialized inpatient behavioral treatment programs are indicated.

Another level in the continuum of rehabilitation includes transitional living programs. These are typically residential, community based treatment alternatives for individuals with primarily cognitive and neurobehavioral deficits that preclude independent living. The length of stay in a transitional living program may last as long as 12 months with the ultimate goal being independent living.

The final stage in the rehabilitation continuum includes vocational rehabilitation. This stage in the recovery process is initiated a number of months post-acute injury. Hence, vocational rehabilitation, transitional living and even specialized behavioral programs are rarely relevant or pressing program options to consider during the initial physiatric evaluation.

References

1. Brain Injury Association of America. Fact Sheet, March 2001.
2. Bullock R, Chestnut R, Clyton G. Guidelines for the management of severe head injury. Brain Trauma Foundation, American Association of Neurologic Surgeons. Joint Section on Neurotrauma and Critical Care. *J Neurotrauma* 1996; 13:641–734.
3. Tukstra LS, Holland AL, Boys GA. The neuroscience of recovery and rehabilitation: What have we learned from animal research. *Arch Phys Med Rehabil* 2003; 84:604–12.
4. Feeny D, Gonzale ZA, Law W. Amphetamine, haloperidol and experience interact to affect rate of recovery after motor cortex injury. *Science* 1982; 217:855–7.
5. Feeny D, Sutton RL, Pharmacotherapy for recovery of function after brain injury. *CRC Crit Rev Neurobiol* 1987; 3:135–97.
6. Cowan TD, Meythaler JM, et al. Influence of early variables in traumatic brain injury on functional independence measure scores and rehabilitation length of stay and charges. *Arch Phys Med Rehabil* 1995; 76:797–800.
7. Sirois MJ, Lavoie A, Dionne CE. Impact of transfer delay to rehabilitation in patients with severe trauma. *Arch Phys Med Rehabil* 2004; 85:184–91.
8. Griffith ER. *Types of disability*. In: Rehabilitation of the Head Injured Adult. M Rosenthal, ER Griffith, MR Bond, JD Miller (Eds.). Philadelphia, PA: Davis, 1983, pp. 23–32.
9. Frankowski RF. *The demography of head injury in the United States*. In: Neurotrauma, Volume 1. M Miner, KA Wagner (Eds.). Boston: Butterworths, 1986, pp. 1–17.
10. Kushwaha VP, Garland DG. Extremity fractures in the patient with a traumatic brain injury. *J Am Acad Orthop Surg* 1998; 6:298–302.
11. Groswasser Z, Cohen M, Blankstein E. Polytrauma associated with traumatic brain injury: Incidence, nature and impact on rehabilitation outcome. *Brain Injury* 1990; 4:161–6.
12. Siegel JH. The effect of associated injuries, blood loss, and oxygen debt on death and disability in blunt traumatic brain injury: The need for early physiologic predictors of severity. *J Neurotrauma* 1995; 12:579–90.
13. Jennett B, Teasdale G. *Management of head injuries*. Philadelphia, PA: Davis, pp. 301–16.
14. Reyes RL, Bhattacharyya AK, Heler D. Traumatic head injury: Restlessness and agitation as prognosticators of physical and psychologic improvements in patients. *Arch Phys Med Rehabil* 1981; 62:20–23.
15. Bogner JA, Corrigan JD, Fugate LG, et al. Role of agitation in prediction of outcomes after traumatic brain injury. *Am J Phys Med Rehabil* 2001; 80:636–44.
16. Englander JS, Cifu DX, Wright J, et al. The impact of acute complications, fractures, and motor deficits on functional outcome and length of stay after traumatic brain injury: A multicenter analysis. *J Head Trauma Rehabil* 1996; 11:15–26.
17. Ponsford JL, Oliver JH, Curran C, Ng K. Prediction of employment status two years after traumatic brain injury. *Brain Injury* 1995; 9:11–20.
18. Felmingham KL, Baguley IJ, Crooks J. A comparison of acute and post discharge predictors of employment 2 years after traumatic brain injury. *Arch Phys Med Rehabil* 2001; 82:435–9.
19. Wagner AK, Hammond FM, Sasser HC, Wiercisiewski D. Return to production activity after traumatic brain injury: Relationship is the measure of disability, handicap and community integration. *Arch Phys Med Rehabil* 2002; 83:107–14.
20. Englander J, Cifu DX, Wright JM, Black K. The association of early computed tomography scan findings and ambulation, self-care, and supervision needs at rehabilitation discharge and at 1 year after traumatic brain injury.
21. Juneja G, Czyrny J, Linn RT. Admission balance and outcome of patients admitted for acute inpatient rehabilitation. *Am J Phys Med Rehabil* 1998; 77:388–93.
22. Zafonte RD, Mann NR, Millis SR, et al. Post-traumatic amnesia: Its relation to function outcome. *Arch Phys Med Rehabil* 1997; 78:1103–6.
23. Pennings JL, Bachulis BL, Simon CT, Slazinski T. Survival after severe brain injury in the aged. *Arch Surg* 1993; 128:787–94.
24. Broas PL, Stappaerts KH, Rommens PM, Louette LK, Gruwez JA. Polytrauma in patients of 65 and over: Injury patterns and outcome. *Int Surg* 1988; 73:119–22.
25. Gennarelli TA, Spielman GM, Langfitt TW, Gildenberg PL, et al. Influence of the type of intracranial lesion on outcome from severe head injury. *J Neurosurg* 1982; 56:26–32.
26. Takenaka N, Mine T, Sugu S, Tamura K, Sagou M, Hirose Y, Ogino M, Okuno T, Enomoto K. Interpeduncular high-density spot in severe shearing injury. *Surg Neurol* 1990; 34:30–38.
27. Colquhoun IR, Burrows EH. The prognostic significance of the third ventricle and basal cisterns in severe closed head injury. *Clin Radiology* 1989; 40:13–6.
28. Young B, Rapp RP, Norton JA, Haack D, Tibbs PA, Bean JR. Early prediction of outcome in head-injured patients. *J Neurosurg* 1981; 54:300–3.
29. Katz DI, Alexander MP, Seliger GM, Bellas DN. Traumatic basal ganglion hemorrhage: Clinicopathologic features and outcome. *Neurology* 1989; 39:897–904.
30. Mack H. Horn LJ. Functional prognosis in traumatic brain injury. In: Traumatic *Brain Injury: Physical Medicine and Rehabilitation State of the Art Reviews*, Volume 3. LJ Horn, DN Cope (Eds). Philadelphia: Hanley and Belphus, 1989, pp. 13–26.
31. MacPherson V, Sullivan SJ, Lambert J. Prediction of motor status 3 and 6 months post severe traumatic brain injury: A preliminary study. *Brain Injury* 1992; 6:489–98.
32. Wilson B, Vizor A, Bryant T. Predicting severity of cognitive impairment after severe had injury. *Brain Injury* 1991; 5: 189–97.
33. Vogenthaler DR, Smith KR Jr, Goldfader P. Head injury, a multivariate study: Predicting long-term productivity and independent living outcome. *Brain Injury* 1989; 3:369–85.

34. Katz DI. Neuropathy and neurobehavioral recovery from closed head injury. *J Head Trauma Rehabil* 1992; 7(2):1–15.

35. Zafonte RD, Hammond FM, Mann NR, et al. Relationship between Glasgow Coma Scale and functional outcome. *Am J Phys Med Rehabil* 1996; 75:364–9.

36. Toschlog EA, MacElligot J, Sagroves SG, et al. The relationship of Injury Severity Score and Glasgow Coma Score to rehabilitative potential in patients suffering traumatic brain injury. *Am Surg* 2003; 69:491–7.

37. Balestreri M, Czojnyka M, Chatfield D, et al. Predictive value of Glasgow Coma Scale after brain trauma: Change in trend over the past ten years. *J Neurol Neurosurg Psychiatry* 2004; 75:161–2.

38. Lane PL, Skoritz TG, Doig G, et al. Intracranial pressure monitoring and outcomes after traumatic brain injury. *Can J Surg* 2000; 43:442–8.

39. Nordby KH, Gunnerod N. Epidural monitoring of the intracranial pressure in severe head injury characterized by non-localizing motor response. *Acta Neurochir* 1985; 74:21–6.

40. Chesnut RM, Marshall LF, Klauber MR, Blunt BA, Baldwin N, Eisenberg HM, Jane JA, Marmarou A, Foulkes MA. The role of secondary brain injury in determining outcome from severe head injury. *J Trauma* 1993; 34:216–22.

41. Bouma GJ, Muizelaar JP, Choi SC, Newlon PG, Young HF. Cerebral circulation and metabolism after severe traumatic brain injury: The elusive role of ischemia. *J Neurosurg* 1991; 75:685–93.

42. Rosner MJ, Rosner SD, Johnson AH. Cerebral perfusion pressure: Management protocol and clinical results. *J Neurosurg* 1950; 83:949–62.

43. Struden MA, Hanney HJ, Contant CF, et al. The relation between acute physiological variable and outcome on the Glasgow Outcome Scale and Disability Rating Scale following severe traumatic brain injury. *J Neurotrauma* 2001;18:115–35.

44. Timming R, Orrison WW, Mikula JA. Computerized tomography and rehabilitation outcome after severe head trauma. *Arch Phys Med Rehabil* 1982; 63:154–9.

45. Corrigan JD, Smith-Knapp K, Granger CV. Validity of the functional independence measure for persons with traumatic brain injury. *Arch Phys Med Rehabil* 1997; 78:828–34.

46. Black K, Zafonte R, Millis S, et al. Sitting balance following brain injury: Does it predict outcome? *Brain Injury* 2000; 14:141–52.

47. Cope N, Hall K. Head injury rehabilitation: Benefit of early intervention. *Arch Phys Med Rehabil* 1982; 63:433–7.

48. High WM, Hall KM, Rosenthal M, et al. Factors affecting hospital length of stay and charges following traumatic brain injury. *J Head Trauma Rehabil* 1996; 11:85–96.

49. Mackay LE, Bernstein BA, Chapman PE, Morgan AS, Milazzo LS. Early intervention in severe head injury: Long-term benefits of a formalized program. *Arch Phys Med Rehabil* 1992; 73:635–41.

50. Wagner AK, Zafonte RD, Goldberg G, et al. Physical medicine and rehabilitation consultation: Relationships with acute functional outcome, length of stay, and discharge planning after traumatic brain injury. *Am J Phys Med Rehabil* 2003; 82:526–36.

51. Hagen C, Malkmus D, Durham P. Levels of cognitive functioning. In: *Rehabilitation of the Head Injured Adult: Comprehensive physical management.* Downey, CA: Professional Staff Association of Rancho Los Amigos Hospital, 1979.

52. Levin HS, Saydjari C, Eisenberg HM, et al. Vegetative state after head injury: A traumatic coma data bank report. *Arch Neurol* 1991; 48:580–5.

53. Rappaport M, Dougherty A, Kelting D. Evaluation of coma and vegetative states. *Arch Phys Med Rehabil* 1992; 73:628–34.

54. Ansell BJ, Keenan JE. The Western Neuro Sensory Stimulation Profile: A tool for assessing slow-to-recover head injured patients. *Arch Phys Med Rehabil* 1989; 70:104–8.

55. DeYoung S, Gross R. Coma recovery program. *J Rehab Nursing* 1991; 12:121–3.

56. Lombardi F, DeTanti M, Teloro E, Liberati A. Sensory stimulation for brain injured individuals in coma or vegetative state. *The Cochrane Database of Systematic Reviews.* The Cochrane Library, Volume (3), 2003.

57. LeWinn EB, Dimancescu MP. Environmental deprivation and enrichment in coma. *Lancet II* 1978; pp. 156–7.

58. Wilson SL, Powell GE, Elliott K, Thwaites H. Sensory stimulation in prolonged coma: Four single case studies. *Brain Injury* 1991; 5:393–400.

59. Russell WR. Cerebral involvement in head injury. *Brain* 1932; 55:549–603.

60. Symonds CP, Russell RW. Accidental head injuries. *Lancet* 1943; p. 187.

61. Jackson RD, Mysiw WJ, Corrigan JD. Orientation Group Monitoring System: An indicator for reversible impairments in cognition during posttraumatic amnesia. *Arch Phys Med Rehabil* 1989; 70:33–6.

62. Symonds CP. Observations on the differential diagnosis and treatment of cerebral states consequent upon head injuries. *British Medical Journal* 1928; 2:828–32.

63. Levin HS, Peters BH, Hulkonen DA. Early concepts of anterograde and retrograde amnesia. *Cortex* 1983; 19:427–40.

64. High WM, Levin HS, Gary HE. Recovery of orientation following closed head injury. *J Clin Exp Neuropsychology* 1990; 12:703–14.

65. Levin HS, High WM, Meyers CA, von Laufen A, Hayden ME, Eisenberg HM. Impairment of remote memory after closed head injury. *J Neurol Neurosurg Psychiatry* 1985; 48:556–63.

66. Kapur N, Ellison D, Smith MP, McLellan DL, Burrows EH. Focal retrograde amnesia following bilateral temporal lobe pathology: A neuropsychological and magnetic resonance study. *Brain* 1992; 115:73–85.

67. Hirst W, Volpe BT. Memory strategies with brain damage. *Brain Cognition* 1988; 8:379–408.

68. Levin HS, High WM Jr, Eisenberg HM. Learning and forgetting during post-traumatic amnesia in head injured patients. *J Neurol Neurosurg Psychiatry* 1988; 51:14–20.

69. Warrington EK, Weiskrantz L. Amnesia: A disconnection syndrome? *Neuropsychologia* 1982; 20:233–43.

70. Jennett B. Assessment of the severity of head injury. *J Neurol Neurosurg Psychiatry* 1976; 39:647–55.

71. Mysiw WJ, Corrigan JD, Carpenter D, Chock SKL. Prospective assessment of post-traumatic amnesia: A comparison of the GOAT and the OGMS. *J Head Trauma Rehabil* 1990; 5:65–72.

72. Brooks DN, Aughton ME, Bond MR, et al. Cognitive sequelae in relationship to early indices of severity of brain damage after severe blunt head injury. *J Neurol Neurosurg Psychiatry* 1980; 43:529–34.

73. Geffen GM, Encel JS, Forrester GM. Stages of recovery during post-traumatic amnesia and subsequent everyday memory deficits. *Neuro Report* 1991; 2:105–8.

74. Haslam C, Batchelor J, Fearnside MR, et al. Post-coma disturbance and post-traumatic amnesia as nonlinear predictors of cognitive outcome following severe closed head injury: Findings from Westmead Head Injury Project. *Brain Injury* 1994; 8:519–28.

75. Haslam C, Batchelor J, Fearnside MR, et al. Further examination of post-traumatic amnesia and post-coma disturbance as non-linear predictors of outcome after head injury. *Neuropsychology* 1995; 9:599–605.

76. Bishora SN, Partridge FM, Godfey HPD, Knight RG. Post-traumatic amnesia and Glasgow Coma Scale related to outcome in survivors in a consecutive series of patients with severe closed-head injury. *Brain Injury* 1992; 6:373–80.

77. McMillan TM, Jongen ELMM, Greenwood RJ. Assessment of post-traumatic amnesia after severe closed head injury: Retrospective or prospective? *J Neurol Neurosurg Psychiatry* 1996; 60:422–7.

78. Tate RL, Brae GA. Psychosocial adjustment after traumatic brain injury. What are important variables? *Psychological Med* 1999; 29:713–25.

79. Amed S, Bigsley R, Sheikh JI, Date ES. Post-traumatic amnesia after closed head injury: A review of the literature and some suggestions for future research. *Brain Injury* 2000; 14:765–80.

80. Saneda DL, Corrigan JD. Predicting clearing of post-traumatic amnesia following closed head injury. *Brain Injury* 1992; 6:167–74.

81. Jennett B, Teasdale G. Management of head injuries. Philadelphia: FA Davis, 1981, p. 90.

82. Tate RL, Perdias M, Pfaff A, Jurjevic L. Predicting duration of post-traumatic amnesia (PTA) from early PTA measurements. *J Head Trauma Rehabil* 2001; 16:525–42.

83. Crovitz HF. Techniques to investigate post-traumatic and retrograde amnesia after head injury. In: *Neurobehavioral Recovery from Head Injury.* HS Levin, J Grafman, HM Eisenburg (Eds.). New York: Oxford University Press, 1987, pp. 330–4.

84. Levin HS, O'Connell VM, Grossman RG. The Galveston Orientation and Amnesia Test. A practical scale to assess cognition after head injury. *J Nerv Ment Dis* 1979; 167:675–84.

85. Gronwell D, Wrightson P. Duration of post-traumatic amnesia after mild head injury. *J Clin Neuropsychology* 1980; 1:51–60.

86. Corrigan JD, Arnett JA, Houck LJ, Jackson RD. Reality orientation for brain injured patients: Group treatment and monitoring of recovery. *Arch Phys Med Rehabil* 1984; 66:675–84.

87. Corrigan JD, Mysiw WJ. Agitation following traumatic head injury: Equivocal evidence for a discrete stage of cognitive recovery. *Arch Phys Med Rehabil* 1988; 69:487–92.

88. Jackson RD, Mysiw WJ, Corrigan JD. Orientation Group Monitoring System: An indictor for reversible impairments in cognition during post-traumatic amnesia. *Arch Phys Med Rehabil* 1989; 70:33–6.

89. Mysiw WJ, Bogner JA, Arnett JA, et al. The Orientation Group Monitoring System for measuring duration of post-traumatic amnesia and assessing therapeutic interventions. *J Head Trauma Rehabil* 1996; 11:1–8.

90. Artiola, Fortuny L, Briggs M, Newcomb F, et al. Measuring duration of post-traumatic amnesia. *J Neurol Neurosurg Psychiatry* 1980; 43:377–90.

91. Shores EA, Marosszky JE, Sandonam J, Batchelor J. Preliminary validation of a clinical scale for measuring the duration of post-traumatic amnesia. *Med J Aust* 1986; 144:569–72.

92. Forrester G, Geffen G. Julia Farr Services. *Post-traumatic Amnesia Scales Manual.* Unley, South Australia: Julia Farr Foundation, Inc., 1995.

93. Bode RK, Heinemann AW, Semik P. Measurement properties of the Galveston Orientation Amnesia Test (GOAT) and improvement patterns during inpatient rehabilitation. *J Head Trauma Rehabil* 2000; 15:637–655.

94. Denny-Brown D. Disability arising from closed head injury. *JAMA* 1945; 127:429–36.

95. Mysiw WJ, Jackson RD, Corrigan JD. Amitriptyline for post-traumatic agitation. *Am J Phys Med Rehabil* 1988; 67:29–33.

96. Brooke MM, Questad KA, Patterson DR, Bashak KJ. Agitation and restlessness after closed head injury: A prospective study of 100 consecutive admissions. *Arch Phys Med Rehabil* 1992; 73:320–3.

97. Sandel ME, Mysiw WJ. The agitated brain injured patient. Part I: Definitions, differential diagnosis and assessment. *Arch Phys Med Rehabil* 1996; 77:617–23.

98. Corrigan JD. Development of a scale for assessment of agitation following traumatic brain injury. *J Clin Exp Neuropsychol* 1989; 11:261–77.

99. Fugate LP, Spacek LA, Kresty LA, et al. Measurement and treatment of agitation following traumatic brain injury: II. A survey of the brain injury special interest group of the American Academy of Physical Medicine and Rehabilitation. *Arch Phys Med Rehabil* 1997; 78:924–8.

100. Young GP. The agitated patient in the emergency department. *Emergency Med Clin North America* 1987; 5:765–81.

101. Whyte J, Rosenthal M. Rehabilitation of the patient with traumatic brain injury. In: *Rehabilitation Medicine: Principles and Practice.* JA DeLisa (Ed.). Philadelphia: JB Lippincott, 1993, pp. 825–60.

102. Brooke MM, Patterson DR, Questad KA, et al. The treatment of agitation during initial hospitalization after traumatic brain injury. *Arch Phys Med Rehabil* 1992; 73:917–21.

103. Greendyke RM, Kanter DR, Schuster DB et al. Propranolol treatment of assaultive patients with organic brain disease. A double-blind crossover, placebo-controlled study. *J Nerv Ment Dis* 1986; 174:290–4.

104. Greendyke RM, Kanter DR. Therapeutic effects of pindolol on behavioral disturbances associated with organic brain disease: A double-blind study. *J Clin Psychiatry* 1986; 47:423–6.

105. Greendyke RM, Berkner JQ, Webster JC, Gulya A. Treatment of behavioral problems with pindolol. *Psychosomatics* 1989; 30:161–5.

106. Mooney GF, Haas LJ. Effect of methylphenidate on brain-injury related anger. *Arch Phys Med Rehabil* 1993; 74:153–60.

107. Schneider WN, Drew-Cates J, Wong TM, Dombovy ML. Cognitive and behavioral efficacy of amantadine in acute traumatic brain injury: An initial double-blind placebo-controlled study. *Brain Injury* 1999; 13:863–72.

108. Mysiw WJ, Bogner JA, Corrigan JD, et al. The impact of acute care medications on rehabilitation outcome after traumatic brain injury. *Brain Injury,* in press.

109. Elovic EP, Lansang R, Li Y, Ricker JH. The use of atypical antipsychotics in traumatic brain injury. *J Head Trauma Rehabil* 2003; 18:177–95.

110. Kalisky Z, Morrison DP, Meyers CA, von Laufen AO. Medical problems encountered during rehabilitation of patients with head injury. *Arch Phys Med Rehabil* 1985; 66:25–9.

111. Baguley IJ, Nichols JL, Felmingham KL. Dysautonomia after traumatic brain injury: A forgotten syndrome? *J Neurol Neurosurg Psychiatry* 1999; 678:39–43.

112. Baguley IJ. Nomenclature of "paroxysmal sympathetic storms". *Mayo Clinic Proc* 1999; 74:105.

113. Hackenberry LE, Miner ME, Rea GL, Woo J, Graham SH. Biochemical evidence of myocardial injury after severe head trauma. *Crit Care Med* 1982; 10:641–4.

114. Mysiw WJ, Jackson RD. Relationship of new-onset systemic hypertension and normal pressure hydrocephalus. *Brain Injury* 1990; 4:233–8.

115. Labi ML, Horn LJ. Hypertension in traumatic brain injury. *Brain Injury* 1990; 4:365–70.

116. Robertson CS, Clifton GL, Taylor AA, Grossman RG. Treatment of hypertension associated with head injury. *J Neurosurg* 1983; 59:455–60.

117. Russo RN, O'Flaherty S. Bromocriptine for the management of autonomic dysfunction after severe brain injury. *J Paediatr Child Health* 2000; 36:283–5.

118. Miner ME. Systemic effects of brain injury. *Trauma* 1985; 2:75–83.

119. McLeod AA, Neil-Dwyer CH, Meyer CH, et al. Cardiac sequelae of acute head injury. *Br Heart J* 1982; 47:221–9.

120. Rose AG, Novitsky D, Cooper DK. Myocardial and pulmonary histopathologic changes. *Transplantation Proc* 20 1988; (Suppl):29–32.

121. Rotem M, Constantini S, Shir Y, Corteu S. Life threatening torsade de pointes arrhythmia associated with head injury. *Neurosurg* 1982; 23:89–92.

122. Lee YC, Sutton FJ. Concomitant pulses and U-wave alternans after head trauma. *Am J Cardiol* 1985; 55:851–2.

123. Wirth R, Fenster PE, Marcus FI. Transient heart block associated with head trauma. *J Trauma* 1988; 28:262–4.

124. Dire DJ, Patterson R. Transient first-degree AV block and sixth nerve palsy in a patient with closed head injury. *J Emer Med* 1987; 5:393–7.

125. Wiercisiewski DR, McDeavitt JT. Pulmonary complications in traumatic brain injury. *J Head Trauma Rehabil* 1998; 13:28–35.

126. Black KL, Hanks RA, Wood DL, et al. Blunt versus penetrating violent traumatic brain injury: Frequency and factors associated with secondary conditions and complications. *J Head Trauma Rehabil* 2002; 17:489–96.

127. Akers SM, Bartter TC, Pratter MR. Respiratory care. State of the Art Review. *Phys Med Rehabil* 1990; 4:527–42.

128. Becker E, Bar-Or O, Mendelson L, Najenson T. Pulmonary functions and responses to exercise of patients following craniocerebral injury. *Scand J Rehabil Med* 1978; 10:47–50.

129. Nowak P, Cohn AM, Guidice MA. Airway complications in patients with closed head injuries. *Am J Otolaryngol* 1987; 8:91–6.

130. Woo P, Kelly G, Kirshner P. Airway complications in the head injured. *Laryngoscope* 1989; 99:725–31.

131. Law JH, Barnhart K, Rowlett W, de la Rocha O, Lowenberg S. Increased frequency of obstructive airway abnormalities with long-term tracheotomy. *Chest* 1993; 104:136–8.

132. Klingbeil GE. Airway problems in patients with traumatic brain injury. *Arch Phys Med Rehabil* 1988; 69:493–5.

133. Sharples PM, Storey A, Aynsley-Green A, Eyre JA. Avoidable factors contributing to death of children with head injury. *British Med J* 1990; 300:87–91.

134. Gurney JG, Rivara FP, Mueller BA, Newell DW, Copass MK, Jurkovich GJ. The effects of alcohol intoxication on the initial treatment and hospital course of patients with acute brain injury. *J Trauma* 1992; 33:709–13.

135. Jackson RD, Mysiw WJ. Fever of unknown origin following traumatic brain injury. *Brain Injury* 1991; 5:93–100.

136. Carrol K, Cheeseman SH, Fink MP, Umali CB, Cohen LT. Secondary infection of post-traumatic pulmonary cavitary lesions in adolescents and young adults: Role of computed tomography and operative debridement and drainage. *J Trauma* 1984; 29:601–4.

137. Craven DE. Nosocomial pneumonia: New concepts on an old disease. *Infection Control Hospital Epidemiology* 1988; 9:57–8.

138. Watts C, Pulliam M. Problems associated with multiple trauma. In: *Neurologic Surgery*. JR Youcnau (Ed.). Philadelphia: WB Saunders, 1982; pp. 2475–2530.

139. O'Reilly MJ, Reddick EJ, et al. Sepsis from sinusitis in nasotracheally intubated patients. *Am J Med* 1979; 66:463–7.

140. Bell RM, Page GV, Bynoe RP, et al. Post-traumatic sinusitis. *J Trauma* 1988; 28:923–30.

141. Levinson SL, Barondess JA. Occult dental infection as a cause of fever of obscure origin. *Am J Med* 1979; 66:463–7.

142. Douglas A, Moore-Gillon J, Eykyn S. Fever during treatment or infective endocarditis. *Lancet* 1986; i:1341–3.

143. Murray HW, Mann JJ, Genecin A, McKusick VA. Fever with dissecting aneurysm of the aorta. *Am J Med* 1976; 61:140–4.

144. Cunha BA, Tu RP. Fever in the neurosurgical patient. *Heart Lung* 1988; 17:608–11.

145. Sasahara AA, Sharma GVRK, Barsamian EM, Schoolman M, Cella G. Pulmonary thromboembolism: Diagnosis and treatment. *Clin Cardiology* 1983; 249:2945–50.

146. Ragone DJ Jr, Kellerman WC, Bonner FJ Jr. Heterotopic ossification masquerading as deep venous thrombosis in head injured adult: Complication of anticoagulation. *Arch Phys Med Rehabil* 1986; 67:339–41.

147. Scott CM, Grasberger RC, Heeran TF, et al. Intra-abdominal sepsis after hepatic trauma. *Am J Surg* 1988; 155:284–8.

148. Mackowiak PA, Le Maistre CF. Drug fever: A critical appraisal of conventional concepts. *Annals Int Med* 1987; 106:728–33.

149. Cohen BM, Baldessarini RJ, Pope HG, et al. Neuroleptic malignant syndrome. *NEJM* 1985; 313:1293.

150. Buckwald FJ, Haud R, Hanselbout RR. Hospital acquired bacterial meningitis in neurosurgical patients. *J Neurosurg* 1977; 46:494–500.

151. Mancebo J, Domingo P, Blanch L, et al. Post-neurosurgical and spontaneous gram-negative bacillary meningitis in adults. *Scand J Inf Disease* 1986; 18:533–8.

152. Talman WT, Florek G, Bullard DE. A hyperthermic syndrome in two subjects with acute hydrocephalus. *Arch Neurol* 1988; 45:1037–40.

153. Benedek G, Toth-Daru P, Janaky J, et al. Indomethacin is effective against neurogenic hyperthermia following cranial trauma or brain surgery. *Canadian J Neurol Sci* 1987; 14:145–8.

154. Semel JD. Complex partial status epilepticus presenting as fever of unknown origin. *Arch Int Med* 1987; 147:1571–2.

155. Zasler ND, Horn LJ. Rehabilitative management of sexual dysfunction. *J Head Trauma Rehabil* 1990; 5(2):14–24.

156. Chuo K, Chuo A, Kong ICH. Urinary incontinence after traumatic brain injury: Incidence, outcomes and correlates. *Brain Injury* 2003; 17:469–78.

157. Oostra K, Ebraer K, Van Laere M. Urinary incontinence in brain injury. *Brain Injury* 1995; 10:459–64.

158. Garcia JG, Lam C. Treating urinary incontinence in a head-injured adult. *Brain Injury* 1990; 4:203–7.

159. Whyte J, Glenn MB. The care and rehabilitation of the patient in a persistent vegetative state. *J Head Trauma Rehabil* 1986; 1(1):39–53.

160. Foxx-Orenstein A, Kolakowsk-Haynor S, Morwitz JH, et al. Incidence, risk factors, and outcomes of fecal incontinence after acute brain injury: Findings from the Traumatic Brain Injury Model Systems national database. *Arch Phys Med Rehabil* 2003; 84:231–7.

161. Rapp RP, Young B, Twyman D, Bivins BA, et al. The favorable effect of early parenteral feeding on survival in head-injured patients. *J Neurosurg* 1983; 58:906–12.

162. Deutschman CS, Konstantinides FS. Physiological and metabolic response to isolated closed head injury. Part I: Basal metabolic state: Correlating of metabolic and physiological parameters with fasting and stressed controls. *J Neurosurg* 1986; 64:89–98.

163. Phillips R, Ott L, Young B, Walsh J. Nutritional support and measured energy expenditure of the child and adolescent with head injury. *J Neurosurg* 1987; 67:846–51.

164. Weekes E, Elia M. Observations on patterns of 24-hour energy expenditure changes in body composition and gastric emptying in head injured patients receiving nasogastric tube feeding. *J Paretr Enteral Nutr* 1996; 20:31–7.

165. Young B, Ott L, Twyman D, et al. The effect of nutritional support on outcome from severe head injury. *J Neurosurg* 1987; 67:668–76.

166. Hadley MN, Gram TW, Harrington T, et al. Nutritional support and neurotrauma: A critical review of early nutrition in forty-five acute head injured patients. *Neurosurg* 1986; 19:367–73.

167. Rapp RP, Young DB, Twyman D. The favorable effect of early parenteral feeding on survival in head-injured patients. *J Neurosurg* 1983; 58:906–12.

168. Taylor SJ, Fettes SB. Enhanced enteral nutrition in head injury: Effect on the efficacy of nutritional delivery, nitrogen balance, gastric residuals and risk of pneumonia. *J Human Nutr Dietetics* 1998; 11:391–401.

169. Winstein CJ. Neurogenic dysphagia: Frequency, progression, and outcome in adults following head injury. *Physical Therapy* 1983; 63:1992–7.

170. Price R, Lehmann JF, Boswell-Bessette S, Burleigh A, deLateur BJ. Influence of cryotherapy on spasticity at the human ankle. *Arch Phys Med Rehabil* 1993; 74:300–4.

171. Barnard P, Dill H, Eldredge P, et al. Reduction of hypertonicity by early casting in a comatose head-injured individual. *Physical Therapy* 1984; 64:1540–2.

172. Gracies JM, Elovic E, McGuire J, Sampson DM. Traditional pharmacological treatments for spasticity. Part I: Local treatments. *Muscle Nerve Suppl* 1997; 6:S61–91.

173. Gracies JM, Nauce P, Elovic E, et al. Traditional pharmacological treatments for spasticity. Part II: General and regional treatments. *Muscle Nerve Suppl* 1997; 6:S92–120.

174. Yablon SA, Agana BT, Ivanhoe CB, Boake C. Botulinum toxin in severe upper extremity spasticity among patients with traumatic brain injury: An open labeled trial. *Neurology* 1996; 47:939–44.

175. Easton JKM, Ozel T, Halpern D. Intramuscular neurolysis for spasticity in children. *Arch Phys Med Rehabil* 1979; 60:155–8.

176. Meythaler JM, Guin-Renfroe S, Grabb P, Hadley MN. Long-term continuously infused intrathecal baclofen for spastic-dystonic hypertonia in traumatic brain injury: 1 year experience. *Arch Phys Med Rehabil* 1999; 80:13–9.

177. Garland DE, Thompson R, Waters RL. Musculocutaneous neurectomy for spastic elbow flexion in non-functional upper extremities in adults. *J Bone Joint Surg* 1980; 62:108–12.

178. Dennis JW, Menawat S, Von Thron J, et al. Efficacy of deep venous thrombosis prophylaxis in trauma patients and identification of high-risk groups. *J Trauma* 1993; 35(1):132–9.

179. Consensus Conference: Prevention of venous thrombosis and pulmonary embolism. *JAMA* 1986; 256(6):744–9.

180. Cifu DX, Kaelin DL, Wall BE. Deep venous thrombosis: Incidence on admission to a brain injury rehabilitation program. *Arch Phys Med Rehabil* 1996; 77:1182–5.

181. Meythaler JM, DeVivo MJ, Hayner JB. Cost-effectiveness of routine screening for proximal deep venous thrombosis in acquired brain injury patients admitted to rehabilitation. *Arch Phys Med Rehabil* 1996; 77:1–5.

182. Kim J, Gearhart M, et al. Preliminary report on the safety of heparin for deep venous thrombosis prophylaxis after severe head injury. *J Trauma* 2002; 53:38–43.

183. Norwood S, McAuley C, et al. Prospective evaluation of the safety of enoxaperin prophylaxis for venous thromboembolism in patients with intracranial hemorrhagic injuries. *Arch Surg* 2002; 137:696–702.

184. Cipolle MD, Wojicik R, et al. The role of surveillance duplex scanning in preventing venous thromboembolism in trauma patients. *J Trauma* 2002; 52:453–62.

185. Shackford SR, Davis JW, Hollingsworth-Fridlund P, et al. Venous thromboembolism in patients with major trauma. *Am J Surg* 1990; 159:365–9.

186. Ruiz AJ, Hill SL, Berry RE. Heparin, deep venous thrombosis and trauma patients. *Am J Surg* 1991; 162:159–62.

187. Knudson MM, Collins JA, Goodman SB, McCory DW. Thromboembolism following multiple trauma. *J Trauma* 1992; 32:2–11.

188. O'Malley KF, Ross SE. Pulmonary embolism in major trauma patients. *J Trauma* 1990; 30:748–50.

189. Kudsk KA, Fabian TC, Baum S, et al. Silent deep venous thrombosis in immobilized multiple trauma patients. *Am J Surg* 1989; 158:515–9.

190. Rogers FB, Cipolle MD, et al. Practice Management for the Prevention of Venous Thromboembolism in Trauma Patients: The EAST Practice Management Guidelines Work Group. *J Trauma* 2002; pp. 142–64.

191. Conine TA, Sullivan T, Mackie T, Goodman M. Effect of serial casting for the prevention of equines in patients with acute head injury. *Arch Phys Med Rehabil* 1990; 71:310–2.

192. Imie PC, Eppinhous CE, Boughton AC. Efficacy of non-bivalved and bivalved serial casting on head injured patients in intensive care. *Physical Therapy* 1986; 66:748.

193. Keenan MA, Ure K, Smith CW, Jordan C. Hamstring release for knee flexion contracture in spastic adults. *Clin Orthop Rel Res* 1988; 236:221–6.

194. Garland DE, Bailey S, Rhoades ME. Orthopedic management of brain injured adults. Part II. *Clin Orthop Rel Res* 1978; 131:111–22.

195. Garland DE, Bailey S. Undetected injuries in head-injured adults. *Clin Orthop Rel Res* 1981; 155:162–5.

196. Garland DE, Keenan ME. Orthopedic strategies in the management of the adult head-injured patient. *Physical Therapy* 1983; 63:2004–9.

197. Garland DE, Dowling V. Forearm fractures in the head-injured adult. *Clin Orthop Rel Res* 1983; 176:190–6.

198. Stone L, Keenan MA. Peripheral nerve injuries in the adult with traumatic brain injury. *Clin Orthop Rel Res* 1988; 233:136–44.

199. Orcutt SA, Kramer WG, Howard MW, et al. Carpal tunnel syndrome secondary to wrist and finger flexor spasticity. *J Hand Surg* 1990; 15:940–4.

200. Philip PA, Philip M. Peripheral nerve injuries in children with traumatic brain injuries. *Brain Injury* 1992; 6:53–8.

201. Varghese G. Heterotopic ossification. In: Physical Medicine & Rehabilitation Clinics of North America. S Berrol (Ed.). *Philadelphia: Saunders*, 1992; 3:407–15.

202. Mysiw WJ, Tan J, Jackson RD. Heterotopic ossification: The utility of osteocalcin in diagnosis and management. *Am J Phys Med Rehabil* 1993; 72:184–7.

203. Garland DE, Razza BE, Waters RL. Forceful joint manipulation in head-injured adults with heterotopic ossification. *Clin Orthop Rel Res* 1982; 169:133–8.

VI

REHABILITATIVE CARE AND TREATMENT OF SPECIFIC POPULATIONS

20 TBI: A Pediatric Perspective

Andrew I. Sumich
Maureen R. Nelson
James T. McDeavitt

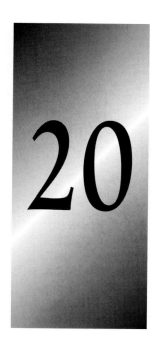erious illness in any child is a highly stressful event for all concerned: the child, parents, and family. Traumatic brain injury (TBI) can be particularly devastating. The injury commonly causes a variety of physical, emotional, cognitive and behavioral impairments. These impairments appear at a time of particular developmental vulnerability, and can significantly impact the child's ability to what children ordinarily do: grow, play, develop, learn, make friendships and gradually evolve into independent young adults. In an instant, parents' expectations for their child may be dramatically altered, and there is often no one in the health care system that can provide them with reliable information on recovery and prognosis.

Although many of the problems faced after brain injury in children occur in adults as well (e.g. seizures), children face a number of unique challenges in recovery. The following chapter will attempt to focus on those aspects of TBI which are unique to children.

EPIDEMIOLOGY

Traumatic brain injury is the most common cause of acquired disability in childhood, with an incidence of approximately 200/100,000 per year in the United States. Incidence has been further broken down to 185/100,000 children for ages 0 to 14 and 295/100,000 adolescents and young adults (ages 15 to 24) (1). The leading cause of TBI varies with age. Pedestrian injuries and falls affect younger children while adolescents and young adults are more commonly injured in motor vehicle collisions and assaults. This rise in incidence at age 15 correlates with increased motor vehicle operation and assault (1, 2). The prevalence of TBI is twice as high in boys as it is in girls. Other factors associated with a higher risk of TBI are poverty, living in congested residential areas and parental instability (3).

OUTCOMES

Of all children who sustain TBI, 95% survive (4); that number drops to 65% for those suffering severe TBI (5). Other studies have shown a biphasic association of age and survival after TBI. Highest mortality is in children less than 2 years of age with a gradual decline in mortality through age 12 and then a second peak in mortality at age 15 (6). With continued advancements in medical care, more and more children are surviving TBI. Survivor outcomes in pediatric TBI range from full recovery to severe physical and/or mental disabilities. It has been suggested that kids suffering TBI have better results in neurological and cognitive recovery compared with older groups. Using the Glasgow Outcome Scale (GOS), a study of 33 survivors showed good recovery for 27%, moderate disability for 55% and severe disability for 18% (7). Generally children and adolescents do better than those older than 21, however it is important to note that children under seven do worse than older children (8, 9). A study looking at longer-term outcome (an average of 23 year follow up) reported 32.7% of survivors with physical complaints and 17.6% with psychological or psychiatric complaints (10).

Communication and cognitive dysfunction seems to contribute most to dependency. A study of 42 children and young adults found 37% of respondents were independent while 49% were dependent in some area of living. Of communication and cognitive deficits, memory problems contributed the most to dependence. Younger age groups and shorter duration of coma are associated with better functional outcomes. It theorized that improved functional outcomes for younger patients are secondary to greater plasticity in the younger brain. Also of note, chronic seizure or epilepsy can lead to greater dependence while presence of early seizures is not predictive of functional outcome (11).

COGNITION AND PHARMACOLOGY

Cognitive deficits are a major contributor to disability following TBI, and this certainly holds true for the pediatric population. Cognitive impairments are manifest on many levels, including behavior, attention and memory (12). These changes probably are related to underlying alterations in cerebral neurochemistry. Brain injury results in a chain of neurochemical events beginning at the time of injury. Neurochemical changes have also been documented in chronic TBI.

Injury to a child's brain is particularly concerning because a child's brain is still developing. There are both immediate and long-term ramifications that result from pediatric brain injury. A child unable to learn new functional skills (physical and mental) as a result off a traumatic injury to the brain is severely disadvantaged as they progress to adulthood. Further complicating the issue is hidden deficits that may not be apparent immediately after injury. For example, one would not expect a three year hold, healthy or impaired, to display higher level thinking; therefore a deficit might not be recognized until years later (13).

Arousal and attention are commonly impaired after injury, which often interferes with the patients' ability to process new information and consequently interferes with the rehabilitation process (14). Pharmacological interventions often target increasing arousal and attention. Tricyclic antidepressants, dopamine, norepinephrine and serotonin up regulators are often used (15, 16, 17). Conversely, pharmacological agents can sometimes interfere with arousal and attention, particularly antiseizure and spasticity medications such as benzodiazepines and phenytoin.

Studies have shown a positive short-term effect of psychostimulants on behavior and cognitive functioning of adults with brain injury (18). While double blinded, placebo controlled, randomized studies of psychostimulants in the pediatric population are limited, there is some data involving methylphenidate. Methylphenidate presents perhaps the most intriguing possibility in the pediatric population because of its established use in attention deficit hyperactivity disorder. Williams et al. showed no significant difference between methylphenidate and placebo in terms of behavior, attention, memory and processing speed (19). However, the authors note some possible faults in study design including dosing, timing of intervention and length of intervention.

Many other drugs have also been used in the pediatric brain injured population, including tricyclic antidepressants, amantadine, atomoxetine and bromocriptine. Formal recommendations for pharmacotherapy in pediatric TBI are difficult to make because of the lack of solid evidence. White et al. point out that this is likely due to the lack of controlled studies, confounding effects of spontaneous recovery and imperfect outcome measures (20). While many drugs are used and often seem to have a clinical effect, further well designed clinical trials are needed.

POST-TRAUMATIC SEIZURES

Post-traumatic seizures are typically divided into three types depending on their timing in comparison to the trauma. Seizures occurring within minutes of trauma are referred to as immediate seizures. Early seizures, by definition occur within one week of trauma, while late seizures occur beyond the first week on injury. A person who suffers two or more late seizures can be diagnosed with post-traumatic epilepsy. It has been established in adults that post-traumatic seizures and epilepsy adversely affect recovery from TBI. An overall decrease in quality of life is seen in these patients as a result from inability to work, social isolation and less return to leisure activities (21).

Studies have shown that children suffering TBI have a 3% to 9% incidence of early post-traumatic seizures, which is higher than expected for adults. This being said, the risk for late seizures is lower in children compared to adults (24–27). Severity of brain injury correlates directly with the incidence of epilepsy. Further illustrating this point is the fact that the greatest predictor of post-traumatic epilepsy is severity of injury (21). Appleton found that the only specific risk factor that was clearly correlated with the development of post-traumatic epilepsy (PTE) was early seizure occurrence within the first week after injury. The drugs they chose to use for treatment of PTE were carbamazepine or lamotrigine (22).

The morbidity and mortality associated with post-traumatic seizures and epilepsy has resulted in an effort to find medications to reduce the risk of both. Phenytoin has commonly been used as anti-seizure therapy in all groups with TBI. Early seizures have been shown to be decreased with phenytoin therapy, however phenytoin has shown no reduction of post-traumatic epilepsy (23). In addition, anticonvulsants may actually impede recovery. Therefore, if no seizures are documented in the first week, antiseizure medications should be discontinued. In cases when early seizures are present one is faced with a clinical dilemma, both the seizures themselves and the treatment may actually negatively affect recovery (21).

Deep Venous Thrombosis/Pulmonary Embolus (DVT/PE)

Deep venous thrombosis and PE are seldom reported in pediatric literature and as a result there is limited information regarding thromboembolism and pediatric TBI. An incidence of < 5% has been reported in a general disabled pediatric population (28), further analysis showed one out of 185 children with closed head injury had a documented DVT (29). There are no current recommendations for screening for DVT in the pediatric population because of the low incidence. While DVT in children may present the classic with clinical signs and symptoms of leg swelling and pain, this is not always the case. A child may complain of only vague abdominal or inguinal pain. As a result, clinicians must maintain a high index of suspicion. General DVT/PE prophylactic anticoagulation is not currently recommended for prepubertal children (29).

PRECOCIOUS PUBERTY

Precocious puberty is defined as the onset of secondary characteristics before age 9 in boys and age 8 in girls (30). Onset of precocious puberty in healthy children can take a severe emotional toll on both the child and family. Social difficulties also arise. The occurrence of precocious puberty in the child with a brain injury only magnifies these difficulties.

One study of 33 children with TBI found 7 to develop precocious puberty (31). Severity of brain injury does correlate with incidence of precocious puberty. Girls seem to be more at risk to develop this problem than boys. Of note, however is the fact that precocious puberty is seen more often in girls in the general population. While the exact cause behind precocious puberty following TBI is unknown it does not diminish the importance of the issue. Shortened adult stature can result as a result of early closing epiphysis. Clinicians should consider luteinizing releasing hormone (LH-RH) agonist therapy for a temporary and reversible treatment if precocious puberty is suspected (32).

HETEROTOPIC OSSIFICATION

Heterotopic ossification (HO) is defined as ectopic bone formation that is seen in several medical conditions including central nervous system trauma, total hip replacement and burns. Incidence of HO in all TBI patients has been reported between 3% and 76% (33–35). In children and adolescents with TBI, incidence has previously been reported between 3%-20% (36, 37), depending on the methods used. An incidence of 22.5% was found using triple phase bone scan to screen all pediatric TBI patients, not just symptomatic children (38).

While there are no formal screening recommendations for HO, one must maintain a high index of suspicion. HO should be high on the differential when physical exam shows decreased range of motion, increased swelling or the patient complains of increased pain with joint movement. Further work up for HO should include triple phase bone scan and/or plain films.

The hips are the most common location for HO in children, followed by elbows, knees and shoulders (39). Several factors have been established as risk factors for HO. These include age older than 11 and coma lasting greater than 7 days. Multiple fractures have also been associated with increased incidence of HO. Perhaps the most concerning result of HO is that it has been shown to result in poorer functional outcomes (38).

Clinical findings often associated with HO include decreased range of motion (ROM), pain and swelling. DVT, infection and fracture can have similar presentations. In fact, there have been case reports of HO and DVT found simultaneously in pediatric patients (40). As in adults, the primary treatment of HO in children is ROM, both active-assisted and passive, as the mainstay. Etidronate has been shown to reduce the occurrence of HO in adults with severe head injury (41). A rachitic sydrome has been reported in a twelve year old boy with a brain injury and HO who was treated with etidronate. As a result, alternative treatment should be used in children (42). Nonsteroidal anti-inflammatory medications remain an option for treatment of HO in children. Indomethacin is often the NSAID of choice in treating HO. Pediatric dosing is recommended at 1–2 mg/kg/day divided in 2–4 doses, not to exceed 150–200 mg/day. Surgical removal of HO is rarely required and typically reserved for more severe cases, specifically when it interferes with positioning and personal care, which can lead to skin breakdown.

COGNITIVE/EDUCATION

Neuropsychological testing is done to understand patterns of cognitive problems and to obtain information on the general level of a child's impairment. Testing can estimate the child's pre-injury level of cognitive abilities by using some subtests that are less apt to decline with injury. Intellectual deficits are a relative factor depending on the child's pre-injury level of abilities. The pattern of cognitive assets and deficits that is found on this testing provides information for treatment approach in rehabilitation, as well as for school. It examine features such as whether someone is stronger at using verbal or visual learning and where memory strengths and weaknesses are, in order to formulate an effective treatment plan. Neuropsychological testing can also be performed to monitor a child's recovery pattern (43). The pattern of neuropsychological deficits depends on the developmental level at the time of injury as well as the hemisphere and site of lesion (44). Skills that are undeveloped at the time of injury may initially appear to be uninvolved, however as the brain becomes more mature, the impairment emerges (45). Children after TBI have been shown to have decrease in IQ, adaptive problem solving, memory and academic performance, along with psychomotor problem solving, compared to children without injury. The impairment on the testing is more severe in more severely injured children (46). IQ scores are minimally affected but testing shows decrease in speed and efficiency, more significantly with more involved children. Most of the children tested had few deficits from the TBI (46).

Bowen evaluated 22 children post -TBI and found no reliable association between neuroimaging data and cognitive measures, but found that children with more diffuse injury on scan did more poorly on the testing (47). Levin looked at 76 children with TBI and did find that the size of lesion on MRI was related to abnormalities in cognitive performance. He also found that cognitive impairment was more dramatically shown in children up to 10 years old than in teens (48).

Multiple studies have shown increased need for educational support and special education after TBI (49–53). One study of children with severe versus mild to moderate TBI showed significant effect in reading recognition, spelling and arithmetic scores in those with severe level, along with lower relative scores for teens than children in all levels of severity. This study also showed significant improvement from baseline to six months of injury but no change from six months to two years. They also found average achievement test scores at two years after TBI but 79% of the severely injured group were receiving special education or had failed a grade (54).

The effect of TBI on a child's language development has also been studied. In children there is more of an impact affecting linguistic abilities, where older children and teens have more of a disruption in higher order communication functions common due to the developmental level (55). More severely affected children have been shown to have more deficits in language skills (56).

One study examined pre-injury behavioral and learning characteristics of children, based on teacher assessment. There was a somewhat higher instance of premorbid behavioral problems in children with TBI. The TBI group also tended to include children of lower socioeconomic status (57). In those with behavioral difficulties after TBI, it is difficult to predict their prognosis. Behavioral evaluation can include many sources from throughout the environment. There is likely an interplay between cognitive deficits and behavioral difficulties (43).

Complex problem solving and abstract reasoning are high levels of cognitive processing. Difficulties with this affect new learning abilities and the ability to benefit from feedback and to solve problems. Being efficient in organizing activities in logical sequence can be impacted, as well as initiating and modifying behavior. This can lead to difficulties socially and in school (43).

Difficulty with executive function, in particular, reduced initiation and persistence, poor planning, poor organization and difficulty correcting errors are frequently seen post-TBI. This frequently leads to dissociation between a child's ability to verbally describe an activity versus an inability to actually perform the task. This may be related to deficits in speed of processing information. This may give the false appearance that a child is non-compliant with school requests (43).

FAMILY

A child incurring a TBI can have a significant impact on the whole family. The entire spectrum of family life can be impacted from emotional to financial. Parents have reported difficulty with maintaining work schedules, as well as financial difficulties, secondary to injury and care for the child post- injury. Children who are hospitalized for longer or who had multiple types of injuries had families who were most impacted (58). Approximately one third of families in one study reported that there was a deterioration in their family financial status since the child's injury and just under 30% reported that an adult lost a job, either through firing or quitting due to their child's care needs (59). The family medical leave act (FMLA) should decrease the number of firings due to a child's severe injury but will not eliminate them. Changes in housing, also, are sometimes required and can also have a financial impact (59). Siblings can also suffer adverse consequences. One study demonstrated that over 50% of families had siblings with behavior problems, withdrawal from their injured sibling, and increased fearfulness (59). Conversely, fifty percent of families described that siblings became more involved in their family after injury. They also described decrease in school performance and difficulty with peer interactions (59). McMahon found no statistically significant difference in depression, self-concept or behavior between siblings of children who had TBI and classmate controls. However, she did find that siblings of children with the most severe injuries did have a significantly lower self-perception, as well as, more symptoms of depression (60).

The importance of family needs and the percentage of needs that were unmet was a cause of significant amount of variability in family stress (61). Comparison of families with children with TBI versus other reasons for hospitalization has shown that parents of children with TBI are more likely to have unmet needs, including medical information, professional and community support, and a feeling of involvement in the child's care (62). One means of attempting to minimize the stress has been approaching the need for information by giving pamphlets about TBI (63). Snowdon described improving parental satisfaction by approaching the family's need for information, as well as, their need for social support (64). It has been described that the primary protection from a high level stress on the family and depression in family members of someone with TBI is a large amount of social support for the family (65). The number of medical problems was also found to be related to parental stress, with approximately one third of parents of children with TBI showing decreased psychological health (66). Social support was felt to be the biggest protector against psychological distress of families. If there was not adequate social support, caregiver distress was worsened with further time out from injury, cognitive dysfunction of the child, and unawareness of deficits by the child; but, if the social support was strong, these were not distressing factors (67).

The family also was found to have an impact on behavior and recovery of the children with TBI. Parental support and parental acute emotional reaction to the injury were predictive of the child's behavioral outcome in the first two years of TBI. This was believed to indicate the importance of the parents' coping on the child's development of behaviors (43). Psychosocial outcome in children post TBI has been described as more closely linked to pre-injury family function and behavior than to injury severity (68).

Coping strategies of the family have an impact on the stress of TBI in a child over the long-term period. Sixty percent of all families experience a change in their structure after TBI, showing changes in coping style, including cohesion and family roles (69).

It has been described that parents who are undergoing economic or personal stress more frequently respond punitively to their children. This may lead to the children then reacting with worse behavior in response (70). The stress of a TBI may adversely affect the parent-child interaction, which may then further exacerbate the child's behavior. Therefore, criticism by and conflict with the parents are seen more frequently with children with adjustment difficulty (71). High levels of parent-teen conflict have been shown to be related to higher risk of delinquency (70). Increase caregiver stress contributes to more negative interactions with their children (70).

In a study comparing children with TBI versus orthopedic injury, the group with severe TBI has similar levels of criticism and coldness as well as personal engagement and levels of conflict as did the group with orthopedic injuries (72). They did find that higher levels of criticism, coldness and conflict were associated with worse outcomes for those with a TBI (72). This study showed association between parenting conflict and criticism, with adjustment long- term in parent and patient. This suggests that decreasing conflict and criticism in the relationship may improve long term functioning on both sides (72).

SOCIAL/BEHAVIORAL

Success in social interactions is a key to positive outcomes in most areas of life. Social skills include the ability to understand another's feelings and the ability to interpret social cues and to predict and evaluate social/behavioral consequences (73). Social success is a combination of social skills, behaviors, and other factors such as athleticism and attractiveness (74). Social competence is felt to be a fundamental basis to developing friendships and to having positive evaluations from others (75). Impairment of social skills is correlated with poor social outcome (76).

It has been reported that the interrelationship of language, executive function and self-managing behavior may be the basis of social impairments associated with communication disorders (77). Chapman has demonstrated that traditional language tests underestimate communication difficulties in children with traumatic brain injury due to their difficulty with sequencing, developing resolutions, and obtaining the moral of a story, particularly if the frontal lobe is involved (78). These problems can have significant effects on the child's ability to interact in an acceptable manner with family, other children, and school personnel (79). Teenagers are at a key time for developing cognitive communication skills, to interpret implied meanings, particularly including sarcasm, negotiation, and complicated pragmatic cues. These skills may be compromised with a TBI during these years, thus compromising social abilities (80).

Cavell has described that social competence is measured at the following three levels: social skills, social performance on specific tasks, and social adjustment (74). Most testing examines social performance but not social skills. The latter includes the ability to perceive and interpret situations, decision skills that require the ability to determine expected outcomes of behavior, and, therefore, make decisions based on these, and enactment skills, which demonstrate the ability to generate a response (74).

Social skills frequently reported as impaired in adolescents with TBI include attentive listening behavior, perception of non-verbal cues, detection of sarcasm, sharing equal conversation burden, humility, and speaking at the listener's level (79). Turkstra studied normally developing teens and teens with TBI, looking at conversational skills. They examined the conversation skills of both, studying the emotions of anger, irritation, happiness, sadness and disgust, with consideration of the teens' self regulation of behavior as well as intelligence. They found no impact of gender, intelligence, or race on emotions or conversation ability. They did find that teens with TBI performed more poorly on identifying emotions, though their errors were similar to the control group of teens. On evaluating the accuracy of conversations, the teens with TBI had many more errors and with a pattern that was unlike the errors made by the control group of teens. They had the most difficulty with the ability to detect sarcasm and the response to sarcasm, and also had difficulty with identifying bragging and a response to bragging. They found no correlation between vocabulary and the ability to identify emotions or intent in conversation. The teens with TBI had significantly more difficulty overall with detecting and evaluating social behaviors. The fact that sarcasm and bragging were the most difficult areas of evaluation was interpreted to mean that there was greater difficulty in social inference, particularly with different explicit and implicit messages (76).

Social success depends on effective self-regulation of cognitive and social behavior (81). The surrounding environment and supportive behavior of others can exacerbate or improve self-regulatory impairment in those with a TBI. Interventions to address these deficits, therefore, need to be sensitive to the child's social context, and the child or teen's daily activities are key to address in attempting to improve the performance of executive function related abilities (81).

Social functioning is a critical predictor of quality of life (82). Children with TBI are more concerned about losing friends than about success in schoolwork, their health, their ability with sports, or getting in trouble at school (83). An intervention program for children with TBI, called "Building Friendships", was described with a team of child/parent peers and school staffs to meet periodically, set an action plan, and increase the number of social contacts for the students (84). Unfortunately, the program was not found to sustain itself once facilitators had stopped their involvement.

Social function is shown to improve during inpatient rehabilitation stay with children and teens with TBI, with those with the greatest deficits showing the greatest gains (85). Social function skills are shown to continue to improve after return from rehabilitation to home (86).

In a multicenter study of 65 children and teens, only 3% to 27% were reported as ready for age-expected participation at discharge in home, school, and community life, with social/behavioral deficits responsible for the majority of limitations (87). The Come Back Programme is a program for teens and young adults after TBI and after their initial rehabilitation program that had continued psychosocial deficits. The deficits reported were in independent living, employability, relationships, and contact with friends. In a follow up study one year or more after the completion of the program, there was no improvement seen in contact with family or leisure activities, however there was improvement in employability and independent living, but not back to the level of pre-injury (88). Their recommendations were for a second rehabilitation program, such as this, for psychosocial deficits as well as follow-up support and structural control for continued success (88). A program in New York worked with 80 individuals with TBI who had severe behavioral deficits at least two years post injury. This program's approach was long-term practice of participation-enhancing and disability-reducing strategies to result in automization and internalization of strategies to reduce the impairment (89). Critical components were described as intervention being in context with the person's life and teaching those directly involved with each life how to perform this intervention. They found with these customized supports that they had a cost-effective improvement in quality of life for the individual and their loved ones, and greater than 80% of those with significant behavioral disorders were returned to their home communities (89).

Behavioral changes and difficulties have been widely reported in children after a TBI. Stancin found that 89% of parents of children with TBI interviewed reported behavioral change post injury (90). A British study described two thirds of the children with TBI with significant maladaptive behaviors several years post injury (91). A French study showed a higher frequency of depressive tendencies in teens with TBI, as well as, behavioral problems and a lack of self-awareness of the behavioral problems (92). In a phone interview of parents of children and teens one year after TBI, 40% of the children were described as having behavioral problems (93).

Psychiatric disorders are sometimes described after TBI in children and teens. One study evaluating the first three months after TBI showed that in the short term, children with more severe injury, previous psychiatric disorder, family psychiatric history, dysfunctional family, or lower socioeconomic class had high risk of a new psychiatric disorder (94). In looking at psychiatric disorders one year post TBI in children and teens, attention deficit hyperactivity disorder and depressive disorders were the most common diagnoses described, both new onset and previous. For new diagnoses, which were reported in 48% of the children studied, 74% persisted. Internalized disorders are more likely to resolve than externalized disorders (95). Interestingly enough, this study attempted to exclude children with pre-injury psychiatric disorders but found 16 children with 20 previously undiagnosed disorders, primarily ADHD and anxiety disorders (95). Emotional distress may actually increase over time. Depression is commonly seen later as increases in cognition and self-awareness lead to recognition of deficits and, with that, depression (43).

Early agitation post-TBI may be a combination of an inability to filter out excessive stimulation, poor memory and cognitive limitations. This may manifest as combinations of old familiar memories intruding in current events and may appear to be psychiatric disturbances, but are in fact neuropsychologically based misperceptions (43).

In a broad ranging, greater than 25 year follow-up of 39 individuals in Finland who had TBI during the preschool years, it was reported that 59% of the children attended typical school, 21% attended a school for the physically disabled, and 18% attended a school for the mentally retarded. Only twenty three percent of adults worked full time in regular work environment with 26% working at a sheltered work place. With finding a large discrepancy between 59% reportedly having normal intelligence and normal school performance and only 23% in a regular full time work environment, it was interpreted to indicate that school performance or intelligence evaluation is not a guarantee for a good long-term prognosis (96).

CONCLUSION

The bromide that "children are not small adults" certainly holds true for pediatric brain injury. The unique emotional, social and developmental needs of children demand a holistic and comprehensive approach by a broad-based team. Families also require special care to help calm the inevitable turmoil created by a life-changing injury. This care is ideally provided by a team of specialists with experience in brain injury, and in the care of children.

References

1. Kraus J., Nourjah P. The epidemiology of uncomplicated brain injury. *J Trauma* 1988;28:1637–43.
2. MacKenzie E. J., Edelstein S. I., Flynn J. P. Trends in hospital discharge rates for head injury in Maryland, 1979–1988. *Am J Public Health.* 1990;80:217–19.
3. Klonoff H. Head injuries in children: Predisposing factors, accident conditions, accident proneness and sequelae. *Am J Public Health* 1971;61:2405–17.
4. Kraus J. F., Rock A., Hemyari P. Brain injuries among infants, children, adolescents, and young adults. *Am J Dis Child* 1990;144:684–91.
5. Berger M. S., Pitts L. H., Lovely M., et al. Outcome from severe head injury in children and adolescents. *J Neurosurgery* 1985;62:194–99.
6. Luerssen T. G., Klauber M. R., Marshall L. F. Outcome from head injury related to patient's age: A longitudinal prospective study of adult and pediatric head injury. *J Neurosurg* 1988;68:409–416.

7. Massagli T. L., Michaud L. J., Rivara F. P. Association Between Injury Indices and Outcome After Severe Traumatic Brain Injury in Children. *Arch Phys Med Rehabil* 1996;l77:125–132.
8. Kriel R. I., Krach L. E., Panser L. A. Closed head injury: comparison of children younger and older than 6 years of age. *Ped Neurol* 1989;5:296–300.
9. Johnston M. V., Gerring J. P. Head Trauma and its sequelae. *Pediatric Annals* 1992;21:362–8.
10. Klonoff H., Clark C., Klonoff P. S. Long-term outcome of head injuries: a 23 year follow up study of children with head injuries. *J of Neurology, Neurosurgery, and Psychiatry* 1993;56:410–415.
11. Eiben C. F., Anderson T. P., Lockman L., et al. Functional outcome of closed head injury in children and young adults. *Arch Phys Med Rehabil* 1984;65:168–70.
12. Hayes R. L., Jenkins L. W., Lyeth B. G. Neurochemical aspects of head injury: Role of excitatory neurotransmission. *J Head Trauma Rehabil* 1992;7:16–28.
13. Kreil R. L., Krach L. E., Pamser L. A. Closed head injury: Comparison of children younger and older than 6 years of age. *Pediatric Neurol* 1989;5:296–300.
14. Whyte J. Attention and arousal: basic science aspects. *Arch Phys Med Rehabil* 1992;73:940–9.
15. Wolf A. P. Gleckman A. D. Sinemet and brain injury: functional versus statistical change and suggestions for future research designs. *Brain Inj* 1995;9:487–93.
16. Ross E. D. Stewart R. M. Akinetic mutism from hypothalamic damage: successful treatment with dopamine agonists. *Neurology* 1981;31:1435–9.
17. Reinhard D. L. Whyte J. Sandel M. E. Improved arousal and initiation following tricyclic antidepressant use in severe brain injury. *Arch Phys Med Rehabil* 1996;77:80–3.
18. Gualtieri C. T., Evans R. W. Stimulant treatment for the neurobehavioral sequelae of traumatic brain injury. *Brain Injury.* 1988;2:273–290.
19. Williams S. E., Ris M. D., Ayyangar R., Schefft B. K., Berch D. Recovery in Pediatric Brain Injury: Is Psychostimulant Medication Beneficial. *J Head Trauma Rehabil* 1998;13:73–81.
20. Whyte J., Vaccaro M., Grieb-Nett P., Hart T. Psychostimulant use in the rehabilitation of individuals with traumatic brain injury. *J Head Trauma Rehabil* 2002;17:282–99.
21. Johnston M. V., Gerring J. P. Head trauma and its sequelae. *Pediatric Annals* 1992;21:362–8.
22. Appleton R. E. Demellweek C. Post-traumatic epilepsy in children requiring inpatient rehabilitation following head injury. *J Neurol Neurosurg Psychiatry* 2002;72:669–72.
23. Schierhout G. Roberts I. Prophylactic antiepileptic agents after head injury: a systematic review. *J Neurol Neurosurg Psychiatry* 1998;64:108–12.
24. Annegers J. F., Grabow J. D., Groover R. V., Laws E. R., Elveback L. R., Kurland L. T. Seizures after head trauma: a population study. *Neurology* 1980;30:683–689.
25. Salazar A. M., Jabbari B., Vance S. C., Grafman J., Amin D., Dillon J. D. Epilepsy after penetrating head injury. I. Clinical correlates: a report of the Vietnam Head Injury Study. *Neurology* 1985;3:1,1406–1414.
26. Hahn Y. S., Fuchs S., Flannery A. M., Barthel M. J., McLone D. G. Factors influencing post-traumatic seizures and post-traumatic epilepsy in children. *Neurosurgery* 1988;22:864–867.
27. Tenkin N. R., Kikmen S. S., Wilensky A. J., et al. A randomized, double blinded study of phenytoin for the prevention of post-traumatic seizures. *N Engl J Med* 1990;323:497.
28. Radecki R. T. Deep Vein Thrombosis in the Pediatric Disabled Patient. *Arch Phys Med Rehabil* 1988;69:743–744.
29. Radecki R. T., Gaebler-Spira D. Deep vein thrombosis in the disabled pediatric population. *Arch Phys Med Rehabil* 1994;75:248–50.
30. Maxwell M., Karacostas D., Ellenbogen R. G., Brzezinski A., Zervas N., Black P. Precocious puberty following head injury. *J Neurosurg* 1990;73:123–29.
31. Sockalosky J. J., Kriel R. L., Krach L. E., et al. Precocious puberty after traumatic brain injury. *J Pediatr* 1987;110:373-377.
32. Blendonohy P. M., Phillip P. A. Precocious puberty in children after traumatic brain injury. *Brain Injury* 1991;5:63–68.

33. Garland D. E., Blum C. E., Waters R. L. Periarticular heterotopic ossification in head injured adults. *J Bone Joint Surg* 1980; 1143–6.

34. Garland D. E. Clinical observations on fractures and heterotopic ossification in the spinal cord and traumatic brain injured populations. *Clin Ortho Rel Res* 1988;233:86–101.

35. Saxbon L., Najenson T., Tartakovsky M Becker E., Grosswasser Z. Widespread periarticular new-bone formation in long-term comatose patients. *J Bone Joint Surg* 1981;63:120–65.

36. Mital M. A., Garber J. E., Stinson J. T. Ectopic bone formation in children and adolescents with head injuries: Its management. *J Ped Ortho* 1987;7:83–90.

37. Hoffer M. M., Brink J. Orthopedic management of acquired cerebrospasticity in childhood. *Clin Orthop Rel Res* 1975;110:244–8.

38. Hurvitz E. A., Mandac B. R., Davidoff G., Johnson J. H., Nelson V. S. Risk factors for heterotopic ossification in children and adolescents with severe traumatic brain injury. *Arch Phys Med Rehabil* 1992;73:459–62.

39. Citta-Pietrolungo T. J., Alexander M. A., Steg N. L. Early detection of heterotopic ossification in young patients with traumatic brain injury. *Arch Phys Med Rehabil* 1992;73:258–62.

40. Sobus K. M., Sherman N., Alexander M. Coexistence of deep venous thrombosis and heterotopic ossification in the pediatric patient. *Arch Phys Med Rehabil* 1993;74:547–51.

41. Spielman G. Gennarelli T. A. Rogers C. R. Disodium etidronate: its role in preventing heterotopic ossification in severe head injury. *Arch Phys Med Rehabil* 1983;64:539–42.

42. Silverman S. L. Hurvitz E. A. Nelson V. S. Chiodo A. Rachitic syndrome after disodium etidronate therapy in an adolescent. *Arch Phys Med Rehabil* 1994;75:118–20.

43. Fraser RT and Clemmons D. C. Traumatic Brain injury Rehabilitation: Practical Vocational, *Neuropsychological and Psychotherapy Interventions.* CRC Press, New York, 2000.

44. Benz B., Ritz A., Kiesow S. Influence of age-related factors on long-term outcome after traumatic brain injury (TBI) in children: A review of recent literature and some preliminary findings. *Restor Neurol Neurosci* 1999;14:135–141.

45. Levin H. S., Eisenberg H. M., Wigg N. R., Kobayashi K. Memory and intellectual ability after head injury in children and adolescents. *Neurosurgery* 1982;11:668–673.

46. Jaffe K. M., Fay G. C., Polissar N. L., et al. Severity of pediatric traumatic brain injury and early neurobehavioral outcome: a cohort study. *Arch Phys Med Rehabil* 1992;73:540–547.

47. Bowen J. M., Clark E., Bigler E. D., et al. Childhood traumatic brain injury: neuropsychological status at the time of hospital discharge. *Dev Med Child Neurol* 1997;39:17–25.

48. Levin H. S., Culhane K. A., Mendelsohn D., et al. Cognition in relation to magnetic resonance imaging in head injured children and adolescents. *Arch Neurol* 1993;50:897–905.

49. Greenspan A. I., MacKenzie E. J. Functional outcome after pediatric head injury. *Pediatrics* 1994;94:425–432.

50. Berger E., Worgotter G., Oppolzer A. Neurological rehabilitation in children and adolescents. *Pediatr Rehabil* 1997;4:229–233.

51. Boyer M. G., Edwards P. Outcome 1 to 3 years after severe traumatic brain injury in children and adolescents. *Injury* 1991;22: 315–320.

52. Tomlin P., Clarke M., Robinson G., et al. Rehabilitation in severe head injury in children: outcome and provision of care. *Dev Med Child Neurol* 2002;44:828–837.

53. Hawley C. A., Ward A. B., Magnay A. R., et al. Children's brain injury: a postal follow up of 525 children from one health region in the U. K. *Brain Inj* 2002;16:969–985.

54. Ewing-Cobbs L., Fletcher J. M., Levin H. S., et al. Academic achievement and academic placement following traumatic brain injury in children and adolescents: a two-year longitudinal study. *J Clin Exp Neuropsychol* 1998;20:769–781.

55. Ewing-Cobbs L., Barnes M. Linguistic outcomes following traumatic brain injury in children. *Semin Pediatr Neurol* 2002;9:209–217.

56. Morse S., Haritou F., Ong K., et al. Early effects of traumatic brain injury on young children's language performance: a preliminary linguistic analysis. *Pediatr Rehabil* 1999;3:139–148.

57. Demellweek C., Baldwin T., Appleton R., et al. A prospective study and review of premorbid characteristics in children with traumatic brain injury. *Pediatr Rehabil* 2002;5:81–89.

58. Osberg J. S., Brooke M. M., Baryza M. J., et al. Impact of childhood brain injury on work and family finances. *Brain Inj* 1997;1;11–24.

59. Montgomery V., Oliver R., Reisner A., Fallat M. E. The effect of severe traumatic brain injury on the family. *J Trauma Inj Infect Crit Care* 2002;52(6):1121–1124.

60. McMahon M. A., Noll R. B., Michaud L. J., Johnson J. C. Sibling adjustment to pediatric traumatic brain injury: a case controlled pilot study. *J Head Trauma Rehabil* 2001;16:587–594.

61. Nabors N., Seacat J., Rosenthal M. Predictors of caregiver burden following traumatic brain injury. *Brain Inj* 2002;16(12): 1039–1050.

62. Armstrong K., Kerns K. A. The assessment of parent needs following pediatric traumatic brain injury. *Pediatr Rehabil* 2002; 5(3):149–160.

63. Morris K. C. Psychological distress in carers of head injured individuals: the provision of written information. *Brain Inj* 2001; 15(3):239–254.

64. Snowdon A. W., Kane D. J. Parental needs following the discharge of a hospitalized child. *Pediatr Nurs* 1995;21(5):425–428.

65. Harris J. K. J., Godfrey H. P. D., Partridge F. M., Knight R. G. Caregiver depression following traumatic brain injury: a consequence of adverse effects on family members? *Brain Inj* 2001; 15(3):223–238.

66. Hawley C. A., Ward A. B., Magnay A. R., Long J. Parental stress and burden following traumatic brain injury amongst children and adolescents. Brain Inj 2003;17(1):1–23.

67. Ergh T. C., Rapport L. J., Coleman R. D., Hanks R. A. Predictors of caregiver and family functioning following traumatic brain injury: social support moderates caregiver distress. *J Head Trauma Rehabil* 2002;17(2):155–174.

68. Anderson V. A., Catroppa C., Haritou F., et al. Predictors of acute child and family outcome following traumatic brain injury in children. *Pediatr Neurosurg* 2001;34(3):138–148.

69. Curtiss G., Klemz S., Vanderploeg R. D. Acute impact of severe traumatic brain injury on family structure and coping responses. *J Head Trauma Rehabil* 2000;15(5):1113–1122.

70. Patterson G. R., *Coercive Family Process.* Eugene, Oregon Castilia Publishing Co 1982.

71. Wamboldt M. Z., Wamboldt F. S. The role of the family in the onset and outcome of childhood disorders: Selected research findings. *J Am Acad Child Adolesc Psychiatry* 2000;39;1212– 1219.

72. Wade S. L., Taylor H. G., Drotar D., et al. Parent-Adolescent interactions after traumatic brain injury: their relationship to family adaptation and adolescent adjustment. *J Head Trauma Rehabil* 2003;18:164–176.

73. Schumaker J. B., Hazel J. S. Social skills assessment and training for the learning disabled: who's on first and what's on second? Part 1. *J Learning Dis* 1984;17:422–431.

74. Cavell T. Social adjustment, social performance, and social skills: a tricomponent model of social competence. *J Clin Child Psychol* 1990;19:111–122.

75. Windsor J. Language impairment and social competence. In: Fey M. E., Windsor J., Warren S. F., eds. Language Intervention: Preschool Through Elementary Years. Baltimore: Paul H Brooks Publishing;1995.

76. Turkstra L. S., McDonald S., DePompei R. Social information processing in Adolescents: Data from normally developing adolescents and preliminary data from their peers with traumatic brain injury. *J Head Trauma Rehabil* 2001;16(5):469–483.

77. Singer B. D., Bashir A. S. What are executive functions and self-regulation and what do they have to do with language learning disorders? *Language Speech Hearing Services Schools* 1999; 30:265–273.

78. Chapman S. B. Cognitive-communication abilities in children with closed head injury. *Am J Speech-Language Pathol* 1997;6: 50–58.

79. Turkstra L., McDonald S., Kaufman P. Assessment of pragmatic communication skills after adolescent traumatic brain injury. *Brain Inj* 1996;10:329–345.

80. Cohen S. Practical guidelines for teachers. In: Goldberg A., ed. Acquired Brain Injury in Adolescence. *Springfield*, Illinois: Charles C Thomas;1997.

81. Ylvisaker M., Feeney T. Executive functions: self-regulation, and learned optimism in pediatric rehabilitation: a review and implications for intervention. *Pediatr Rehabil* 2002;5(2):51–70.

82. Warschausky S., Kewman D., Kay J. Empirically supported psychological and behavioral therapies in pediatric rehabilitation of TB. I. *J Head Trauma Rehabil* 1999;14(4):373–383.

83. Bohnert A., Parker J., Warschausky S. Friendship adjustment in children following traumatic brain injury. *Dev Neuropsychol* 1997;13(4):477–486.

84. Glang A., Todis B., Cooley E., et al. Building social networks for children and adolescents with traumatic brain injury: a school based intervention. *J Head Trauma Rehabil* 1997;12(2):32–47.

85. Dumas H. M., Haley S. M., Rabin J. P. Short-term durability and improvement of function in traumatic brain injury: a pilot study using the Pediatric Evaluation of Disability Inventory (PEDI) classification levels. *Brain Inj* 2001;15(10):891–902.

86. Dumas H. M., Haley S. M., Ludlow L. H., Rabin J. P. Functional recovery in pediatric traumatic brain injury during inpatient rehabilitation. *Am J Phys Med Rehabil* 2002;81(9):661–669.

87. Bedell G. M., Haley S. M., Coster W. J., Smith K. W. Participation readiness at discharge from inpatient rehabilitation in children and adolescents with acquired brain injuries. *Pediatr Rehabil* 2002; 5(2):107–116.

88. DeKort A. C., Rulkens M. P., Ijzerman M. J., Maathuis CG. B. The Come Back Programme: a rehabilitation program for patients with brain injury with psychosocial problems despite previous rehabilitation. *Int J Rehabil Res* 2002;25(4):271–278.

89. Feeney T. J., Ylvisaker M., Rosen B. H., Greene P. Community supports for individuals with challenging behavior after brain injury: an analysis of the New York State Behavioral Resource Project. *J Head Trauma Rehabil* 2001;16(1):61–75.

90. Stancin T., Taylor H. G., Thompson G. H., et al. Acute psychosocial impact of pediatric orthopedic trauma, with and without accompanying brain injuries. *J Trauma-Inj Infect Crit Care.* 1998; 45(6):1031–1038.

91. Hawley C. A. Reported problems and their resolution following mild, moderate and severe traumatic brain injury amongst children and adolescents in the U. K. *Brain Inj* 2003;17(2):105–129.

92. Viguier D., Dellatolas G., Gasquet I., et al. A psychological assessment of adolescent and young adult inpatients after traumatic brain injury. *Brain Inj* 2001;15(3):263–271.

93. Greenspan A. I., MacKenzie E. J. Use and need for post-acute services following pediatric head injury. *Brain Inj* 2000;14(5): 417–429.

94. Max J. E., Smith W. L., Sato Y., et al. Traumatic brain injury in children and adolescents: psychiatric disorders in the first three months. *J Am Acad Child Adoles Psychiatry* 1997;36(1): 94–102.

95. Bloom D. R., Levin H. S., Ewing-Cobbs L., et al. Lifetime and novel psychiatric disorders after pediatric traumatic brain injury. *J Am Acad Adoles Psychiatry* 2001;40(5):572–579.

96. Koskiniemi M., Kyykka T., Nybo T., Jarho L. Long term outcome after severe brain injury in preschoolers is worse than expected. *Arch Pediatr Adoles Med* 1995;149:249–254.

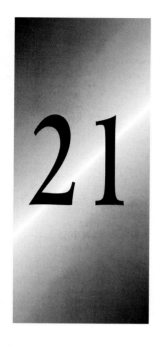

21 The Older Adult*

Jeffrey Englander
David X. Cifu
Trinh Tran

DEMOGRAPHICS OF AGING

The older adult or geriatric population includes all individuals aged 65 years and older. This chronological cutoff is arbitrary and more related to federal statutes (in the United States, Medicare and Social Security Administration Retirement) than scientific standards. Improvements in standards of living and health care have led to greater life expectancies, as well as increased survivability from injury and disease, resulting in a significant increase in the number of older adults. Currently, 12.4 percent (35 million people) of the U.S. population are aged 65 years and older. This percentage of older adults will rise to 21 percent (64 million people) of the population by the year 2050. In addition, those 85 years and older (the so-called *oldest old*) will increase from 1.4 percent (3.9 million people) to 5 percent (15 million) in that same time frame (1). For this chapter *older adults* are those aged 65 years and older, unless otherwise noted.

DISABILITY IN THE OLDER ADULT

More than 1.5 million (4.5%) older adults reside permanently in a nursing home and require functional assistance (1). According to the most recent data, more than ninety percent of all community dwelling (including assisted living) older adults have no reported deficits in everyday functional abilities (2). Interestingly however, 40% report having a "disability" on their 2000 census (3). The limitations reported by the 6 percent who do report deficits are walking (19%), bathing (10%), getting outside (10%), getting in and out of bed (8%), dressing (6%), toileting (4%), and self-feeding (2%). Unfortunately, only 10% of these individuals reporting limitations actually receive assistance with these functional activities. The need for functional assistance increases with increasing age, and nearly 40% of individuals 80 years and older require help (2, 4).

ETIOLOGY OF INJURY AND INJURY PREVENTION

Next to teenagers and young adults, older individuals have the next highest rate of hospitalization for TBI, with an annual rate of 121 per 100,000. It is the only age group where females and males have similar rates of injury. In the United States, Caucasians had 1 $\frac{1}{3}$ the incidence of

---

*This chapter is an updated version of the one that originally appeared in the book, *Rehabilitation of the Adult and Child with Traumatic Brain Injury, Third Edition*, edited by M. Rosenthal, E.R. Griffith, J.S. Kreutzer, and B. Pentland, published by F.A. Davis in 1999.

Asians, 1 ½ that of African-Americans and over 2 times that of Native Americans (5).

Unlike their younger cohorts, older adults sustain the majority of TBI's in domestic falls. Adults over 85 years old are 16.4 times more likely to sustain a TBI from a fall than those less than 65; 75–84 year olds are 7.6 times and 65–74 year olds are 3.1 times as likely. Moreover, the home discharge rates are 30% for those greater than 85, 41% for those 75–84, and 54% for those 65–74 compared to 86% for those less than 65 (6).

Risk factors for falls have been stratified into the following groups: 1) chronic, such as neurologic disease, sensory impairment, or musculoskeletal disease, particularly affecting the lower extremities; 2) short-term, such as episodic postural hypotension, acute illness, alcohol use, or medication effects; 3) activity-related, such as tripping while walking, climbing ladders, descending stairs or riding a bicycle; and 4) environmental, such as ill-fitting shoes or trousers, non-secure throw rugs, or poor lighting (8) These risk factors for falls also predispose the elderly to motor vehicle, pedestrian, and recreational accidents, any of which may result in TBI. The decrease in reaction time and walking pace commonly seen in the older adult additionally predisposes them to motor vehicle and pedestrian-motor vehicle accidents, respectively. Management of these risk factors includes scheduled, consistent, and competent primary physician care to minimize medical morbidities, regulate medications, and provide ongoing education. Additionally, focused rehabilitation interventions can be utilized to maximize physical abilities (gait, balance, strength), procure adaptive and assistive devices (canes, walkers, handicap parking stickers), and provide education. Finally, efforts to reduce violence against older adults are necessary to prevent this increasing cause of TBI.

MECHANISM AND PATHOLOGY OF INJURY

Severe trauma in individuals over age 70 is six times more likely to cause intracerebral lesions than severe chest, abdominal, or pelvic injury, a trend that begins at age 40 years (9). Falls tend to result in focal brain injuries, most commonly subdural hematomas (SDH) and/or focal cortical contusions, usually involving the frontal and temporal lobes. These contusions may occur in multiple foci that appear on computed tomography (CT) scan several days after injury (10). Individuals on anticoagulation therapy for cardioembolic risk prevention or with coagulopathy from other medical conditions will have a greater likelihood of intracranial hemorrhage after a fall. Immediate loss of consciousness implies some degree of diffuse axonal injury (DAI) that can also occur with falls and portends a worse prognosis.

Motor vehicle crashes that injure older adults are commonly low-speed collisions, unlike the high-speed collisions more typical of young adults. However, even these collisions can result in DAI in these individuals (11). Focal contusions and SDH's are also common in motor vehicle crashes.

Pedestrian-motor vehicle collisions in older adults frequently occur at crosswalks and in parking lots. They can result in DAI, focal contusions, and/or extra-axial lesions, most commonly SDH's. Individuals with these injuries are the most likely to have skeletal trauma, especially visceral injuries and pelvic and lower extremity fractures.

While assaults are a much more common cause of TBI in the middle-aged group, there is evidence that violent acts against elders are increasing, particularly in urban areas. These injuries invariably result in focal cortical contusions, skull fractures with SDH's and epidural hematomas (EDH), and intracranial bone and bullet fragments.

The injury severity profile of older individuals who survive their acute injuries and transition directly to acute rehabilitation differs from younger cohorts. In the NIDRR TBI National Data System (1989–2002, n = 3279: ≥65 years old = 259 subjects, <65 years old = 3020 subjects; all subjects are admitted to a model system emergency department within 24 hours of injury, are at least 16 years old, have acute trauma care followed immediately by acute inpatient rehabilitation), 71% have initial GCS 13–15 age ≥ 65 (27% < 65 years), 14% have GCS 9–12 (19% < 65 years), 7% have GCS 6–8 (28% < 65 years), and 8 % have GCS 3–5 (26% < 65 years). Time from injury to ability to follow commands is one day or less in 68% of those ≥ 65 years (39% < 65 years), 2–7 days in 17% (29% < 65 years), 8–31 days 25% (12% < 65 years) and greater than one month in only 2% (7% < 65 years). Computed tomography scans demonstrate no differences in degree of lateral shift or brainstem compression with regard to age group. Subdural hematomas occurred in 55% those ≥65 years (38% those <65 years) and EDHs in only 7% (11% < 65 years). Bone and or metal fragments from open head injuries occurred in 3.1% those ≥65 compared with 6.9% of those less than 65 years old. Subcortical contusions in basal ganglia, internal capsule, pons, brainstem or cerebellum occurred in 9.1% those ≥65 compared with 17.3% of those less than 65 years old. The number and frequency of cortical contusions, subarachnoid (SAH) and intraventricular hemorrhages was not more than 3% different between the older and younger age groups (12). These findings are reflective of the increased likelihood for older individuals to suffer falls and resultant focal cortical injury with less time in coma compared with the higher incidence of subcortical injury in younger inidivduals. They are also more likely to incur SDH due to relative brain atrophy and fragility of bridging veins than younger individuals.

MORTALITY

From 1989 to 1998, TBI-related deaths decreased in all age groups except those greater than 75 years, where the rate increased from 50 to 60.5 per 100,000. For that age group, falls, firearms and motor vehicles were the external causes, in that order of frequency, whereas for the 65–74 decade, firearms were the most frequent cause. Starting at age 55, mortality from firearm-related TBI was more common in Caucasians than African-Americans with the rate increasing every decade (13). An earlier CDC survey from 1980 to 1992, indicated that suicide was the third leading cause of traumatic death in those over age 65 after unintentional falls and motor vehicle crashes. Divorced and widowed men were in the highest risk group (14).

The largest group of older individuals with TBI studied in a neurosurgical population is from Rambam Medical Center in Haifa, Israel, consisting of 263 individuals. Mortality rate was 18%; however, many patients were transferred from other centers and had thus survived their initial injuries. The highest mortality group were those with subdural haematomas (33%), followed by contusions (27%), diffuse axonal injury (11%) and chronic subdural haematomas (3%) (15).

Smaller sample size studies from the early 1990s have indicated 80 % mortality and greater, with the great majority during the first 2 weeks of hospitalization. Subdural hematomas (SDH) requiring evacuation were the most common contributing cause of death. Cardiac, pulmonary and multi-system failure were more common in the older than younger individuals, but never exceeded 33% as the main etiology of death (16, 17). One research group proposed that it was futile to treat those over 80 years old with a GCS < 10, given the high degree of mortality and severe disability (18).

In clinical practice it may be difficult to limit the number and degree of interventions performed unless there are clear advanced directives giving relatives and health care providers guidance.

MORBIDITY

Multiple Trauma and Hypotension

Severe multiple trauma as measured by the Abbreviated Injury Severity (AIS) score is less common in older than in younger age groups. Hypotension and multiple trauma are closely associated. Severe multiple trauma without hypotension or hypoxia has not been associated with worse outcome as measured by the Glasgow Outcome Scale (GOS) (16).

Cerebrovascular events can occur as a result of hypotension in the peritraumatic period; strokes caused by thromboembolism, thrombosis, or ischemia from massive swelling are uncommon causes of peritraumatic stroke in older adults.

Fractures

In the NIDRR National Data System skull fractures occurred in 23% of those ≥65 years old compared to 37% under 65 years; lower extremity or pelvic fractures in 15% and 25%, upper extremity fractures in 12% and 13%, spine column fractures in 15% and 17% respectively. Combinations of TBI and spinal cord injury are 2–3 times more common among younger individuals (12).

Medical Complications

Respiratory failure requiring mechanical ventilation for more than 7 days occurs in 22% of those ≥65 years old compared to 40 % of those less than 65 years of age who go to acute rehabilitation. Gastrostomies or jejunostomies were prevalent in 23% and 35% respectively (12).

Acute anemia occurs in nearly all individuals who incur trauma. Older individuals have poor tolerance for blood loss. Anemia may effect energy level, tolerance for activity, appearance and overall sense of well being. Laboratory values may not reflect lowered hemoglobin levels until after rehydration occurs as a result of iatrogenic effects of diuretics, mannitol, and bedrest which can result in lowered intravascular volume and relative hemoconcentration. Coagulopathy requiring the use of fresh frozen plasma or platelets occurred in 7.4% of those over 65 and 7.3% less than 65 years old (12).

FACTORS AFFECTING OUTCOME

Age and acute injury recovery

Most of our knowledge about outcome of older adults with TBI comes from studies involving all age groups. These investigations report the positive associations between increasing age and mortality (19–24). Several studies have examined the functional outcomes of older adults who survive brain injury (11, 19, 25, 26, 28). The majority of these investigations demonstrate poorer prognosis for the older than the younger adult, with a correlation noted as young as 40 years of age.

Looking at acute hospital discharge data, the CDC reported increasing length of stay for each advancing age decade. Only 55% of older individuals were discharged home compared to over 78% for all other age groups. Thirty-five percent were discharged to another facility compared to less than 13% for all other age groups. Acute hospital discharge outcome as measured by Glasgow Outcome Scores indicated that only 57% of older individuals had "good recovery", 16% had moderate disability and 11% had severe disability; in all categories, older individuals had worse outcome (5).

An injury severity matched analysis of data from the NIDRR TBI Model Systems from 1989 to 1995 revealed that individuals aged 55 years and older had twice the rehabilitation lengths of stay and costs, half the rate of functional recovery, greater cognitive impairment at discharge, and twice the nursing home placement rate of individuals who were aged 50 years and younger. At discharge the level of physical impairment was comparable for the two groups (29). From 1995 to 2002, rehabilitation LOS averaged only 5 days longer in those individuals older than 55 years compared to those 15–55 years old, Disability Rating Scale (DRS) and Functional Independence Measure (FIM) indicated more disability, and discharge to a private residence was 80.8% compared to 94.3% (30)

Further analysis of this data set through 2002 without injury severity matching demonstrated that those ≥65 years old had mean acute care and rehabilitation length of stays of 20 and 30 days, respectively. This corresponded to mean acute care costs of $93,758 and inpatient rehabilitation costs of $43,306. Length of stay and costs did not differ appreciably in older versus younger age groups. The discharge rate to a private residence was 67% for those ≥65 years compared to 87% in those < 65. At one-year post TBI, 80% of those ≥65 years lived in private residences versus 92% of those < 65. Disability Rating Scale (DRS) scores were one point worse for the older adult group at rehabilitation discharge and at 1-year post TBI (12).

At acute rehabilitation discharge, the median DRS level of functioning subscale score was 3.0 for those ≥65, indicating requiring another person in the home, compared to 2.5 for those less than 65, indicating between needing a non-resident helper and a resident helper. Fourteen percent required placement in a skilled nursing facility (12).

Using two separate measures of independent functioning, the Disability Rating Scale (DRS) and Supervision Rating Scales (SRS), individuals ≥65 required and received higher degrees of supervision for their day to day care at one-year post TBI. On the DRS level of functioning scale, the median score for those ≥65 was 1.5, indicating between "independent in a special environment and requiring a non-resident helper, " while the median score for those less than 65 is 0.5, between "completely independent and independent in a special environment." On the SRS, the median score for those ≥65 was 4, indicating overnight and part-time daily supervision, compared to 2.0 for those less than 65, indicating unsupervised overnight but living with another person who is not always present (12).

This association between age and outcome is of course quite complex and appears to be associated with the severity of injury as measured by initial GCS, duration of coma, and duration of post-traumatic amnesia (PTA). The relationship between injury severity, particularly the GCS motor component, duration of coma or PTA and outcome that has been established in younger individuals probably applies to older individuals as well (6, 11, 17, 23, 31, 34, 35). Analyses from the Traumatic Coma Data Bank noted an association between those > 40 years old and both mortality and poorer functional outcome as measured by the GOS. The relationship was further strengthened when initial GCS motor score and evidence of midline shift or cisteral compression was noted on initial CT scans (36). No other published TBI datasets have focused on the potential impact of mechanism of injury, neuropathology, associated injuries, or premorbid conditions on outcome in older adults. Other factors that appear to have some impact on the association between age and outcome include: a history of acute or chronic alcohol intake, post-injury depression and/or agitation, and a variety of formal and informal social support factors (6, 11, 17, 23, 31, 32, 37, 39). In contrast, other studies have demonstrated that favorable outcomes are achievable in the older adult with similar costs (33).

Age and health after TBI

Individuals ≥55 years old living in the community who have experienced TBI within 4 years have more perceived health problems than age-matched controls. In a group of 49 individuals with TBI, prevalence of headache, thyroid problems, body temperature changes, skin and hair changes, headaches, speaking and understanding others, sensory changes, difficulty with movement and spasticity, sleeping problems, neck and back pain, were all greater than 30 age-matched controls (41).

REHABILITATION

Assessment

Medical   The rehabilitation approach to an older adult after TBI is similar to the general geriatric rehabilitation approach with some specific modifications. Clearly, an understanding of pre-injury activity levels, cognitive limitations, behavioral issues, and chronic medical conditions is vital. This information will assist in the assessment of the potential physiologic reserve present prior to acute injury, which can assist in the immediate determination of an individual's readiness and appropriateness for specific rehabilitation interventions (i.e., specificity, intensity, and goal setting for therapies). Direct communication with the individual's primary care physician (PCP) or geriatrician can help to better understand the level of pre-morbid abilities and limitations and facilitate their specific management strategies into the rehabilitation program. This step is of additional importance for patients in managed care networks, in which the PCP is often the gatekeeper for both current and future medical resource management.

An assessment of the acute medical and neurological status of the older adult with TBI must include a thorough evaluation of their medical systems, taking into account pre-morbid deficits. Screening of special senses (hearing, vision, touch) can provide useful information to the therapy treatment team on ways to optimally interact with the patient. While cerebrovascular, cardiovascular, metabolic and pulmonary diseases are common in this population, an appreciation of the clinical manifestations of these conditions will allow one to best structure the rehabilitation interventions. Joint and muscular abnormalities, especially pain, should be determined to help guide necessary management strategies and precautions. A thorough review of the patient's pre-injury and current medication routine is seminal in order to optimize treatments (e.g., pre-morbid medications may not have been restarted, numerous medications that are especially cognitive-impairing may no longer be necessary), define therapy parameters (e.g., anticoagulant use, antihypertensives), and prevent secondary conditions (e.g., antithrombotics are often underutilized in the frail older adult patient).

While serial brain-imaging studies are commonplace for patients with recent TBI, special attention should be paid to the presence of late or delayed bleeding and hydrocephalus. A follow-up imaging study, usually a CT scan, performed between 2 and 4 weeks post-injury can rule out these abnormalities, particularly if there has not been clinical improvement as expected. Indications for a MRI or dynamic imaging studies in the acute period after TBI would include unexplained clinical findings, such as brainstem pathology or a concomitant ischemic event. The patient's cognitive and behavioral status, diurnal variations in alertness, and ability to tolerate both physical and mental activities should be determined by examination and evaluation in the acutecare and rehabilitation settings. Formal neuropsychological evaluations have little role in this acute period, but may prove to be invaluable in the post-acute phase or rehabilitation.

Social Of equal importance is a comprehensive review of the social support network, which involves an understanding of both the formal and informal support systems available (37). Formal support systems include federal (Medicare, Social Security), state (Medicaid, Department of Rehabilitation Services, welfare, area agencies on aging), and local (adult day health programs, transportation, Meals on Wheels) resources. Informal supports include family, friends, and religious affiliations. Early involvement of family and friends in planning and implementing the rehabilitation program is vital. Older adults tend to have significant others who are either older, disabled, or deceased, thus they are more likely to have increased involvement of extended families in their systems of support. Daughters and female caregivers are more likely to play a major support role, particularly a physical or hands-on one, than sons are. It is essential to clearly understand the older adult's pre-morbid and/or present role in the social structure to which they expect to return. Additionally, one must consider advanced directives, congruence of patient and caregiver's goals, and religious and cultural factors.

Funding A working knowledge of the most common funding mechanisms available for post-TBI care of the older adults is extremely important. In the United States, for example, 98% of the older adults are primarily funded by a single source, Medicare. Similarly, in Canada, Australia, New Zealand, and most European countries, the government funds the overwhelming majority of rehabilitation care for the elderly. With Medicare, while physician (inpatient, outpatient, nursing home) fees and home-health and outpatient therapy are currently paid at 80% of "reasonable charges," inpatient and nursing home rehabilitation services have recently received a significant modification in reimbursement transitioning from the TEFRA to PPS (Prospective Payment System) model. The PPS reimbursement rate is adjusted if the patient is discharged to a skilled nursing facility. Secondary or co-payment insurance varies as greatly in coverage as standard commercial insurers, but rarely pays for extended rehabilitation services. Long term care or catastrophic insurance is increasingly available and provides reimbursement for subacute rehabilitation and custodial care within skilled nursing facilities (SNF).

Medicare is a federally sponsored program, so its coverage is uniform throughout the United States. Within *managed care Medicare health plans*, benefits vary depending on the plan chosen. Any individual who has paid into the federal tax system for 40 quarters (or was ever married to someone who has) and meets any of the following three criteria is eligible for Medicare part A at no cost: 1) age 65 years or older, 2) disabled and on Social Security Disability Insurance (SSDI) for more than 2 years, or 3) has end stage renal disease. Medicare part A reimburses for durable medical equipment, inpatient, and SNF rehabilitation services. Medicare part B, which is available to individuals on Medicare part A for a monthly fee, reimburses for physician services, home health and outpatient therapies.

Medicaid (e.g., Medi-Cal in California) is a state-sponsored and, therefore state-specific program to fund health insurance for the medically indigent, pregnant women, and children. Medicaid inpatient, outpatient, home health, nursing home, durable medical equipment, and physician benefits vary from state to state. Recently, numerous *managed care Medicaid* programs have become available that have further increased the diversity of covered services, in this case even within a state. At present, Medicaid pays for more than 85% of all custodial nursing home care in the United States. Older adults who continue to work or who have been disabled veterans, federal or railroad employees typically have different commercial or managed care insurance as their primary funding source.

Settings

Older adults with acute TBI should have access to rehabilitative services in the appropriate environment for their capabilities. Although most patients can benefit from some type and intensity of services, individuals who are most appropriate for 15 or more hours per week of interdisciplinary inpatient or day rehabilitation therapy programming are those who demonstrate the following characteristics: 1) an acute or new disability that is significantly below pre-morbid baseline; 2) a support system that will allow for return to a community residential setting; 3) the ability to tolerate, participate in, and improve with therapies, and 4) have appropriate funding to pay for services and after-care needs. See Table 21-1.

A return to the most familiar, pre-injury living environment is the first choice for discharge, but when not feasible an alternative reschedule (another family member's home, adult group home or assisted living) is a second option. Individuals who do not need or cannot tolerate inpatient or day rehabilitation services and can be managed in the community will often benefit from home health or outpatient therapy services. Skilled nursing facility-based subacute rehabilitation services are appropriate for older adults who are unable to tolerate the intensity of acute rehabilitation or cannot be otherwise managed at home. Common rehabilitation options are outlined in Table 21-1 (38–40, 42). In summary, the chosen rehabilitation pathway(s) will depend on medical and nursing acuity needs, endurance for therapeutic activities, formal and informal support systems, patient and family goals, and funding options.

MANAGEMENT OF THE OLDER INDIVIDUAL WITH TBI

Medical Issues

An assessment of rehabilitation issues should be initiated in the ICU. Early controlled mobilization in and out of bed minimizes the effects of prolonged bedrest, especially pressure sores, muscle contractures, spasticity, venous thromboembolism, cardiac deconditioning, atelectasis, aspiration pneumonia, constipation, urinary retention and infection, and sensory deprivation (43). Rest periods and up-down schedules may be required to gradually increase tolerance to activity. Improved participation and motivation can be facilitated by involving the individuals

with TBI and family in goal-setting and focusing on functional tasks that are similar to home routines.

Day-to-day medical management of the elderly individual recovering from acute trauma must be diligent and thorough. When a consistent team of rehabilitation professionals is working with an individual every day, changes in medical status and performance are more likely to be discovered earlier than by a smaller team of a physician, nurse, and family member. Newly identified problems must be evaluated efficiently and appropriate treatment instituted so that these problems interfere minimally with progress toward rehabilitation goals. If the identified problem is unlikely to resolve quickly, then the entire team must be informed so that the goals can be reformulated or the patient transferred to a different level of care.

Medication Management

More than 90% of the entire population aver age 65 takes at least one prescription medication daily; most take two or more. In addition, over-the-counter remedies are used ubiquitously (44). During the acute traumatic period, previously prescribed medications may be inappropriate, not feasible to administer, or unknown to the acute management team. Invariably, medications are used to treat or prevent conditions associated with acute trauma. Common medications include proton pump inhibitors or histamine-2 blocking agents to prevent stress ulceration, anticonvulsants to prevent seizures, sedatives and/ or hypnotics for agitation, antiarrhythmics for transient or chronic cardiac conduction events, narcotics and analgesics for pain control, aerosolized inhalers for respiratory problems, and antibiotics for diagnosed or presumed infection. Insulin is more likely to be used than oral hypoglycemic agents for blood sugar abnormalities in acute care settings.

Medication review with the acute treatment team is crucial as the individual is transitioned from emergent and acute care to rehabilitation settings. Families should be encouraged to bring in all medications that they find in the patient's home as well; they are likely to have been prescribed by multiple physicians. Nonessential medications should be tapered or discontinued as soon as feasible. Medications that must be continued should be prescribed in the simplest form—that is, the lowest frequency with the fewest pills, during typical waking hours and corresponding to routine activities for that person. Principles of drug absorption, distribution, metabolism, tissue sensitivity, excretion, interaction, and compliance should guide the physician's choice of medications for any given condition (43).

Pain

Acute pain from trauma is either nociceptive from visceral, bone and soft tissue damage or neuropathic from

TABLE 21-1

Levels of Care and Types of Rehabilitation Service Options for the Older Adult with Brain Injury

Level of Care	Therapy Intensity/ Frequency	Therapy Services	Reimbursement	Type of Setting	Duration of Program	Comments
Acute care services	5–6 days/wk; 0.5–2 hrs/day	Multidisciplinary (MD, N, PT, OT, SLP, RT, SW)	Medicare, Medicaid private insurance	Acute care hospital	3–21 days	After injury to prevent bedrest complications, allow comprehensive rehabilitation assessment
Acute inpatient Rehabilitation	6–7 days/week; 3–5 hrs/day	Interdisciplinary (MD, N, PT, OT, SW, TR, PSY, SLP, RT)	Medicare, Medicaid some private	Acute rehabilitation facility free-standing or attached to acute Hospital	7–35 days	After acute care or subacute care; specialization in rehabilitation medicine and therapy
Subacute care	3–5 days/ week; 0–2 Hrs/ day	Multidisciplinaray (MD, N, RT, PT, OT, SW, SLP)	Medicare, some private	Free-standing or attached to acute hospital	7–100 days	Specialize in respiratory care
Skilled Nursing Facility (SNF)	0–5 days/ week; 0–2 hrs/ day	Multidisciplinary	Medicare, Medicaid, some private	Free-standing	7–lifetime	If discharge to community setting not possible
Home health services	3 days/wk; 0.5–2 hr/day	Multidisciplinary (N, PT, OT, SLP, HHA, SW with MD order)	Medicare, Medicaid private	Patient's home	2–12 wk	Homebound for physical or cognitive reasons after acute/ subacute care, in-patient rehabilitation
Outpatient services	2–3 days/wk; 0.5–3 hr/day	Multidisciplinary (PT, OT, SLP, PSY, SW)	Medicare, Medicaid, private	Clinic	2–8 wk	Living in community with focused needs (language, mobility, ADL)
Day rehabilitation services	3–5 days/wk; 3–5 hr/day	Interdisciplinary (PT, OT, SLP, SW, PSY, TR)	Private insurance	After acute care hospital, inpatient rehab or day rehabilitation	4–8 wk	Sufficient endurance to travel and good informal support systems; may allow shorter acute hospital or inpatient rehab length of stay
Day care services	5 days/wk; 4–10 hr/day	Health care attendants; Outpatient therapies available for brief periods as needed	Medicaid (Partial)	Custodial care of community dwelling older adults who need supervision for safety or who need minor assistance	Indefinite	Cognitively-impaired individuals who are physically mobile and able to perform self-care ADL's with supervision–assist

Abbreviations: MD = physician; N = nursing; PT = physical therapy; OT = occupational therapy; SLP = speech and language pathology; SW = social work; TR = therapeutic recreation, HHA = home health aid; PSY = psychology; RT = respiratory therapy.

peripheral or central nervous system injury. In addition, older individuals are likely to have one or more chronic conditions, such as arthritis, osteoporosis, or peripheral vascular disease, that may contribute to their experience of pain. Comprehensive pain assessment tools are available and often need modification when individuals have cognitive impairments. The goal of pain management is improved function, mood, and sleep (45).

For nociceptive pain, analgesic medications and physical modalities are often necessary to facilitate mobility. Comfortable positioning, physical activity, heat, ice, ultrasound, and message are preferred first line non-medication interventions (46). If pain is occurring at predictable times of the day or with routine activities, then non-narcotic analgesic medications can be scheduled for these activities. Individuals may be incapable of asking for medications or knowing their schedules. Often just the anticipation of pain deters individuals from activities. The practice of scheduling pain medications allows for better overall pain control and facilitates the individual's performance of activities in the acute rehabilitation process. Acetaminophen requires no dosage adjustment in the elderly and has equal analgesic efficacy to non-steroidal anti-inflammatory medications (NSAIDs) (43, 47).

If there is concomitant inflammatory arthritis or heterotopic ossification, NSAIDs and disease modifying medications may be indicated, with appropriate monitoring for gastrointestinal, renal and cardiovascular toxicity (48, 49). Nociceptive pain that disturbs sleep may be addressed with bed positioning and non-narcotic analgesia at bedtime. Narcotic analgesics are more potent in older individuals and invariably cause constipation and lethargy; they should be reserved for pain refractory to the above approach.

Neuropathic pain caused by chronic pre-existing conditions, such as diabetes mellitus or alcoholism, will likely require long-term maintenance treatment. Pain from peripheral nerve, plexus injuries, or subcortical lesions may cause acute neuropathic pain. Tricyclic antidepressants and anticonvulsants are usually more effective than analgesic medications for both acute and chronic neuropathic pain syndromes. Cognitive and autonomic side effects, toxicity and drug interaction profiles will determine which of these medications will be most safe in the older individual.

Deep Venous Thrombosis and Pulmonary Embolism Risk

No standard of care yet exists for prophylaxis of deep venous thrombosis (DVT) after traumatic brain injury for any age group. In the acute hospital setting, DVT incidence was reported as high as 54% in those with "major TBI" (50). On admission to acute rehabilitation units the reported incidence ranges from 1.6–20% in various studies (50–53). Sequential compression devices (SCD's) with or without thigh-length antiembolism stockings are considered safe if they are initially applied within the first 2–3 days post-injury. Data support their use for DVT and pulmonary embolism (PE) prevention if they can be applied 23 hours per day (54, 55). This amount of SCD use is most feasible in acute care settings until the patient is mobilized out of bed for more than a few hours.

Low-dose unfractionated or low molecular weight subcutaneous heparin are often contraindicated with recent intracranial surgery or subdural hematoma. No consensus exists as to the exact time that post-injury prophylaxis is relatively less risky than recurrent intracranial hemorrhage or expansion of cerebral contusions. It is probably safe for individuals with DAI within a week post-injury (56–58). Although low molecular weight heparin may be superior to unfractionated heparin in high risk trauma cases, bleeding risk after severe TBI may preclude use of either agent. If DVT is suspected, duplex ultrasound is the least invasive but adequately sensitive test to detect symptomatic disease without confirmatory venography which carries more morbidity (58).

Seizure Risk

During acute care and inpatient rehabilitation the seizure frequency is 11% in those ≥65 years old and 12% in those <65 (12). Englander and colleagues followed individuals admitted to 4 trauma centers with TBI and intracerebral lesions for up to 2 years post injury. Individuals over 65 years old had 22.7% incidence of seizures compared with 18.7% between 16 and 64 tears old, which was not statistically significant (59). Most posttraumatic seizures (PTS) are focal or focal with generalization, rarely progressing to status epilepticus. If PTS occur within the first week post TBI or if an individual receives prophylactic medication during acute care, anticonvulsants can be stopped abruptly (phenytoin, fosphenytoin, carbamazepine, valproic acid, oxcarbazepine) or weaned (diazepam, lorazepam, barbiturates) to minimize risk of withdrawal symptoms without increasing the risk of subsequent seizures (60). For those with higher risk, such as those with penetrating injuries, intracerebral hematomas requiring surgery, or multiple contusions, the use of padded side rails or enclosure beds can protect the person from further injury, should seizures occur. The continued usage of anticonvulsant medication after 7 days post injury even in such higher-risk individuals is not recommended by the American Academy of Neurological Surgeons or the American Academy of Physical Medicine and Rehabilitation (60, 61).

If seizures occur in the absence of a correctable metabolic disturbance after the first week post TBI, then there is an 86% likelihood of recurrence (62). The choice of antiepileptic medication in older individuals is predicated on the same principles of choosing any medication for long-term usage: side effects, the degree of protein binding, drug interactions, cost, and compliance. Some of the newer antiepileptic drugs have fewer interactions, greater therapeutic windows, and do not require serum monitoring, such as oxcarbazepine and levitiracetam (63, 64).

Nutrition and Swallowing

Older individuals with TBI are just as likely as younger individuals to have neurogenic dysphagia and more likely to have some pre-injury gastrointestinal condition that effects eating or digestion, e.g., dental problems, gastroesophageal reflux. Dentures may no longer fit properly after they have been removed for even several days during acute care.

Reestablishment of adequate nutrition is important in facilitating health and optimal recovery. Determining an older individual's ideal body weight and eating habits is a start, although many older people have compromised nutritional baselines. Up to 20% of ambulatory older individuals have a measurable vitamin deficiency (43). Serum albumin levels less than 3 g/dl or cholesterol less than 160 mg/dl are indicators of inadequate nutrition. Low serum ferritin or iron levels are also common posttrauma; enteral formulas have variable amounts of iron, so supplemental iron is often necessary to replace iron stores even with normal hemoglobin levels. Full replacement of iron stores may take 3–6 months (65). Following weekly or biweekly weights can help monitor nutritional status; if this is not accurate or feasible, serial midarm circumference measurements are more accurate than skin fold thickness in older adults (66). Commonly used medications are associated with the side effect of decreased appetite, especially selective serotonin reuptake inhibitors (SSRI), NSAIDs, digoxin, L-dopa, and diuretics. Other medications and conditions can decrease psychomotor skills for self-feeding, such as antipsychotics, sedatives and the injury itself.

In order to avoid aspiration pneumonia, bedside evaluation of swallowing capabilities should be performed as soon as the patient is sufficiently alert. Further evaluation with videofluorscopic studies is best decided jointly by the physician along with the therapist who evaluates swallowing and those helping with feeding. These studies are most helpful when silent aspiration is suspected or when there is uncertainty regarding the best compensatory swallowing technique (67). Frequent monitoring for symptomatic aspiration by lung auscultation, listening for laryngeal pooling of food or liquids with breathing or spontaneous speech and coughing with proximity of eating and drinking are effective bedside monitoring techniques.

Until oral feeding can occur, appropriate enteral formulas are necessary. The smallest-gauge feeding tube should be used for optimal patient comfort. A gastrostomy may be preferable if prolonged enteral feeding is projected. Using formulas with fiber and starting with half-strength solutions are less likely to cause diarrhea. Lactobacillus supplements are often helpful in counteracting the tendency for loose bowel movements associated with recent or concurrent antibiotic therapy. Bolus feeding routines that correspond with eventual oral meal times makes transition to an eating routine easier and facilitates gastrocolic reflexes that aid in regular basel elimination.

Substance Abuse

After dementia and anxiety disorders, alcoholism is the third most common mental disorder among elderly men in the United States (68). In older adults alcoholism is closely associated with tobacco abuse, other drug dependence, hypertension, liver disease, and organic mental disorders such as delerium, dementia, and amnestic disorders (69). A substantial proportion of older individuals begin to have problem drinking after the age of 60; others have a life-long habit (70). Ascertaining the history of alcoholism and other substance abuse in TBI is a challenge in and of itself (71). The CAGE questionnaire is the one of the easiest and quickest clinical screening tools (72). Using the Center for Disease Control and Prevention (CDC) screening tool at one-year post injury, 19.7% of individuals ≥65 years old admitted to any alcohol use compared to 39.1% of younger individuals. Of those that drank, no one ≥65 admitted to drinking more than 5 drinks per day compared to 12.8% of younger individuals (12, 73).

Treatment of substance abuse in the older individual poses unique challenges. Most programs are designed for younger adults, and the group experience may be less relevant for the older individual. It is less likely for individuals of any age to live alone post-TBI, so caretakers or living partners must be educated on the consequences of ongoing substance use, such as increased risk for recurrent injury, lowered alcohol tolerance and seizure thresholds. It is advisable to make the discharge environment alcohol and substance-free. Co-dependency issues must be addressed and confronted directly. Hurt and colleagues recommend equally intense treatment of the older individual with alcoholism as the younger one. Follow-up of their cohort 2 to 11 years post-inpatient treatment showed that 25 percent were able to remain sober, 41 percent had returned to alcohol use, and 32 percent were dead, nearly one-half from alcohol-related causes (69).

Continence

Bladder Normal aging affects bladder function in the following ways: 1) prostate hypertrophy in men with relative bladder outlet obstruction and diminished capacity with symptoms of urinary frequency, hesitancy and/or diminished stream; 2) pelvic relaxation in women from uterine prolapse or cystocele resulting in intermittent stress incontinence; 3) decreased bladder capacity with urinary frequency; and 4) decreased capability to suppress bladder contractions at low volumes resulting in urgency (74). Individuals with TBI are typically incontinent with urinary frequency because of inability to sense bladder fullness and/or suppress the pontine micturition center (75). Increased frequency may be a symptom of urinary tract infection. Medications that commonly affect bladder emptying include those with anticholinergic side effects, calcium channel blockers, antihistamines and narcotics. Bowel impaction, prostatic hypertrophy, and peripheral neuropathy may cause relative obstruction or the tendency to retain urine, which may also lead to infection. Incontinence may also occur with normal bladder functioning if the individual has impaired mobility or self-care skills that prevent efficient use of a toilet or urinal. Assessment of pre-injury voiding patterns is helpful in discerning any underlying pathology, independent of the effects of the TBI.

The first step in re-assessing current bladder function is removal of the indwelling bladder catheter or diaper that invariably accompanies the individual with TBI from acute care or skilled nursing settings. Elimination of medications that interfere with bladder physiology as mentioned above permit adequate baseline performance. A timed voiding schedule using a bedside commode or toilet in sitting or standing position can then facilitate regular opportunities for bladder emptying. It is difficult for many able-bodied individuals to have adequate bladder emptying in bed. Measurement of the post void residual urine volume (PVR), either by portable bladder ultrasound or by one-time bladder catheterization, can quantify the degree of emptying. If the PVR is less than 50 cc, then further measurements are unnecessary; between 50–100 cc, it is advisable to perform several repeated measurements to insure that residual volumes do not put the individual at risk for infection. Larger PVRs greater than 30% of total bladder volume (spontaneous void plus PVR) may indicate mechanical outlet obstruction, poor detrusor contraction or incomplete sphincter relaxation. Common conditions associated with this pattern are prostatic hypertrophy, peripheral neuropathy, or cystocele. Alpha-receptor blockers such as alfuzocin, doxazocin, terazocin or tamulosin may aid in allowing the individual to relax the internal and external sphincters.

Timed voiding schedules and medication use can be re-evaluated as the individual's self-awareness, mobility and safety with toileting techniques improve. These interventions are often necessary for several weeks, but their usage can avoid the morbidity associated with diaper, indwelling or even condom catheter use.

Bowel Patients' bowel routines are typically disrupted during hospitalization for trauma and are a low priority in acute care settings. In older individuals, such disruption can become a preoccupation unless it is properly addressed. Fecal incontinence is prevalent in 68% of individuals with TBI on acute rehabilitation admission, 12.4% at rehabilitation discharge and 5.2% at one-year follow-up. Among other variables age is associated with incontinence at discharge and one-year post TBI (76).

Ascertaining a person's pre-injury bowel routine is the first step in establishing goals. Dietary changes, immobility and narcotic use for pain management are the most common causes for constipation is this population (43). However, until safe swallowing, mobility and routine gastrointestinal motility are re-established, interim measures are usually necessary.

For suspected fecal impaction which can present as loose incontinent stool leaking around the impacted area, one-time laxative, bowel stimulant and /or suppository often relieves the problem. Stool softeners or fiber may be advisable for some time because of ongoing therapeutic measures for pain management or iron replacement.

Diarrhea or loose stool is common with antibiotic usage and some enteral formulas. Infectious causes of diarrhea, especially *Clostridium difficile* should be treated. Fiber-containing enteral formulas or loctobacilles supplements can improve stool consistency. Bolus feedings encourage the gastrocolic reflex and more regular bowel evacuation patterns. Once an acceptable pattern has been established, interventions can be weaned serially to determine which if any are still necessary (77).

Sensory Health

Vision Normal aging is associated with changes in visual acuity and refractive power, decrements in extraocular motion, increases in intraocular pressure, decreased tear secretion, and decreased corneal and lens function (43). Most older individuals use corrective lenses for reading and many for distance vision as well. Corrective lenses are often lost or broken during the acute traumatic event and not used during acute hospitalization. Decreased visual function can add to perceptual deficits and confusional states. Easily correctable visual problems, especially the resumption of glaucoma medication or finding a useful pair of corrective lenses can aid the rehabilitation process.

Hearing Normal aging is associated with loss of sensitivity and signal distortion of higher frequencies, difficulty localizing signals needed for dual ear listening, and difficulty in understanding speech in unfavorable listening conditions. Life-long noise exposure, middle ear and vascular disease can also affect hearing. Presbycusis, affecting 60% of individuals over the age of 65, is a progressive sensorineural hearing loss separate from all of the above (43). With trauma, middle ear ossicles or cranial nerve VIII can be selectively damaged, especially with basilar skull fractures. The use of pre-injury prescribed hearing aids is challenging because the injured individual is often the only one familiar with their adjustment. Yet accurate communication is critical in helping individuals progress through their acute confusional state and communicate with caretakers and helping professionals. Until hearing aid use can be reestablished, written communication, direct eye contact to facilitate lip reading, gestural communication, and an environment without extraneous noise are helpful alternatives.

Smell Anosmia is probably the most frequent cranial nerve and sensory loss specifically associated with TBI (78, 79). It may result in decreased appetite while in the hospital. In the home environment it may impair the individual's ability to detect burning objects promptly. Presence of smoke detectors in the discharge environment is therefore part of the evaluation that should accompany home safety assessment with caregivers.

Taste Normal aging is accompanied by loss of lingual papillae, decreased saliva volume, and a relative decrement of taste acuity (43). It is relatively easy to test the basic elements of salty, bitter, sweet and sour tastes. It is best to have visitors bring in the patient's favorite foods when it is deemed safe for swallowing to fully ascertain whether the changes in taste or smell are going to affect the patient's appetite.

Touch, Vibration and Joint Position Sense Vibratory sense diminishes with age. Conditions associated with peripheral neuropathy are also more frequent in older individuals, although acute peripheral nerve, brachial and lumbosacral plexopathies are less frequent concomitant injuries in older adults. Reversible etiologies of peripheral neuropathy such as vitamin deficiencies, thyroid abnormalities, and neurotoxic medications should be identified and treated. Less reversible causes such as diabetes mellitus, alcoholism, uremia, HIV and syphilis are still worth identifying so that progressive neuropathy may be managed with better glucose control, alcohol abstinence or definitive treatment of the underlying condition. Compensation techniques, assistive devices for mobility and self-care, and adequate lighting may help the individual adapt to these impairments.

Behavior and Cognition

Dementia affects 3 to 11% of community-dwelling adults over age 65, 20 to 50% of those older than 85, and nearly 60% of centenarians. Traumatic brain injury is one of the multiple etiologies of dementia (80). Therefore, it is important to ascertain an inidividual's pre-injury motivation, behavior and mental capacity in order to have reasonable expectations for cognitive recovery from their TBI.

The typical recovery pattern for older adults with TBI is not appreciably different than younger individuals. It includes an initial period of diminished arousal, followed by hyperarousal and culminating in return to a new baseline level of arousal, that may differ from pre-injury function. Goldstein and Levin compared 22 individuals with TBI over age 50 living in the community with age, gender and education-matched controls and found that those with TBI had more difficulty with verbal and nonverbal learning, expressive language, executive functioning, and depression (81). The treatment team can influence a safe transition through the various levels of recovery by preventing secondary injury, treating concomitant symptoms and illnesses, targeting pharmacological interventions, and engineering the environment. Facilitating transition to the most familiar discharge setting and use of familiar calendars and memory aids can help with motivation and compensating for these deficits.

Attention

Decreased arousal and attention are common after DAI, hypoxic ischemic injury and dorsal lateral or deep frontal lobe injury. Hypoarousal is characterized by difficulty staying awake despite adequate sleep and appropriate stimulation. Hypoattention is characterized by inability to attend to conversation or self-care tasks with adequate alertness. Either deficit can interfere with progress in recovery. Management techniques include normalizing sleep-wake cycles, establishing routine up-down schedules, minimizing medications with sedating side effects, and control of distractions in the environment. Attention deficits can be treated safely in the older adult without concomitant coronary artery disease with methylphenidate; the short-acting preparation will yield results within several days (82). Carbidopa/levodopa may be useful if inattention is accompanied by bradykinesia and rigidity, with results apparent within 1–2 weeks of initiating therapy. Amantadine, modafenil, and SSRI's are usually safe medications but have longer onset of action (83).

Agitation

Restlessness and agitation occur in approximately one-third of individuals with moderate to severe TBI. They interfere with safety and participation in activities of daily living and especially rehabilitation programs (84, 85). The Agitated Behavior Scale and checklists that quantify specific behaviors are very useful for monitoring agitation over time (86, 87). Agitated individuals with TBI are more likely to have psychological adjustment difficulties, require supervision or institutional placement after discharge (88). Management strategies include behavioral plans, environmental modifications using cubicle or enclosure beds, structured therapy sessions with co-treatment, 1 to 1 attendant care, appropriate pain control, and medications for specific targeted behaviors (89). Commonly used medications include non-sedating anticonvulsants, tricyclic or heterocyclic antidepressants, amantadine, beta-blockers, and atypical antipsychotics. Benzodiazepines are generally thought to be safe medications, but can cause paradoxical agitation or increase levels of confusion and amnesia particularly when the sedative effect wanes (90).

Alteration in Mood and Sleep

Depression occurs in 20–70% of individuals during the first 2 years after TBI; studies do not stress that age is a risk factor for depression (91). In the general population, anxiety and major depression are less common in older than in younger individuals (92). Severity of injury and level of physical disability do not correlate with frequency or severity of depression (93).

Normalizing sleep-wake cycles is as important in managing mood disorders as it is in disorders of arousal and attention. Contributing factors to insomnia include interrupted sleep by hospital personnel or other patients, persistent effects of sedating medications, pain, and poor sleep hygiene. The latter can be addressed with a balanced activity schedule during the day, scheduled rest periods, minimizing nighttime disturbances, and having a daytime and evening routine (94). Low doses of eszopiclone, zolpidem or zaleplon can be useful for helping to initiate sleep for 3–4 weeks. If longer-term usage is anticipated, trazodone may be a better choice. Diphenhydramine and hydroxyzine are second-line agents, but should be used with caution because they may also cause urinary retention. Benzodiazepines frequently cause paradoxical reactions in the elderly, and tricyclic antidepressants are associated with postural hypotension and urinary retention that are poorly tolerated.

Psychological counseling is appropriate for the majority of individuals. Incorporating children and grandchildren into therapeutic and recreational activities can be most therapeutic. Early therapeutic outings to assess function in the home and community can enhance motivation. Methylphenidate is a short-acting agent that improves both arousal and attention and may assist in alleviating depressive symptoms. SSRI's are safe and common first-line antidepressant medications for older individuals because of their favorable side-effect profile. Onset of action is 3–6 weeks. Medication interactions and side-effect profiles are most important in this age group given concurrent morbidities (90).

Safety Judgment

Pre-morbid or newly acquired deficits in cognition, strength, balance and sensation often challenge an individual's safety in the discharge environment. Awareness and adjustment to these deficits determines the level of supervision needed at home (6). Prevention of future injury secondary to falls or wandering often requires added caretakers and resources in the discharge environment. See above section on Age and Outcome regarding supervision needs over time.

Competence and Capacity

The acute and chronic cognitve, behavioral and communication deficits described above may affect capabilities for self-determination for health care and financial decisions in anyone with a TBI. *Competence* is legal term pertaining to an individual's right to self-determination; *capacity* is a medical term that pertains to the physical and cognitive abilities to convey and carry out one's wishes. An interdisciplinary evaluation by an appropriate and interested physician, psychologist, occupational therapist and / or speech and language pathologist is recommended to provide a comprehensive assessment that includes topographical and verbal orientation, money management, communication and reasoning skills (95). Older individuals are more likely to have a pre-existing durable power of attorney than younger individuals. If available, health care and even financial decisions can be facilitated. If not, each state or province has different guidelines regarding who can help the individual with TBI make such decisions. Court-appointed temporary and permanent conservators may be necessary to facilitate ongoing medical and financial decisions.

Sexuality

As a consequence of common beliefs in our society, sexuality is often ignored in older adults. This tendency frequently persists in rehabilitation settings, particularly in the face of new disabilities. Sexuality encompasses a sense of self, the capacity to show affection, love and maintain relationships, and knowledge of the social context of sexual behavior and gender roles. In early stages of recovery from TBI, sexual comments may be less tolerated in older than younger individuals. Physiologic changes in vaginal mucosa, erectile and orgasmic performance often occur in normal aging. Changes in sexual desire in either direction can occur; there may be decreased interest and desire or an egocentric, impulsive, or disinhibited behavior pattern. Therefore, it is just as important to screen for sexual and relationship concerns in older individuals. Because of the multi-faceted nature of sexual relationships, techniques to enhance overall communication and interaction skills are most therapeutic (96). Sildenafil, tadalafil, and vardenafil, while effective for erectile dysfunction commonly encountered after TBI, is often contraindicated in older adults due to concomitant coronary artery disease and hypertension.

Self-Care

Standard rehabilitation principles to recover self-care abilities are just as effective in the older adult with TBI. They may have comparable difficulty being motivated to learn "splinter skills" that are a small portion of a task, such as range of motion exercises alone. More whole task oriented therapy is better accepted. Learning an individual's pre-injury habits and routines is vital to organizing relevant therapy. It is also important to secure some familiar clothing and grooming utensils, incorporating them into familiar daily routines in the hospital setting. Typical adaptive equipment recommendations include built-up or weighted utensils to accommodate upper body weakness, loss of dexterity and joint limitations; long-handled devices and reachers to accommodate difficulties with trunk balance and flexibility; bathroom safety aids (grab bars, tub or shower benches, hand-held shower heads, raised toilet seats or commode chairs) to compensate for decreased balance and strength. Home management skills, both physical performance as well as organization, are likely to require modification.

Mobility

Challenges to safe ambulation in the older adult include learning how to accommodate for alterations in vision, peripheral or central sensation, balance, strength, and overall endurance. Chronic arthritis, joint and muscle stiffness are more common in the elderly. Household mobility may be facilitated with a home evaluation by members of the rehabilitation team to assess architectural barriers (doorways, stairs, floor coverings), furniture arrangement, adequacy of natural and artificial lighting as well as training for caregivers in safe mobility practices in the discharge environment.

Community mobility goals include the ability to get from place to place with route-finding and bodily transport and negotiating different terrains such as pavement, grass, curbs and stairs. Public transportation for individuals with disabilities is becoming increasingly available throughout the world, with various levels of governmental support. Focusing on familiar routes and routines, then gradually progressing to finding one's way in new surroundings is a typical sequence for increasing community mobility skills.

Driving

Safe driving after a TBI must take into account the older adult's pre-injury capabilities and new impairments. Some jurisdictions require health care practitioners to report to public health authorities or the department of motor vehicles (DMV) physical or cognitive conditions that may alter one's driving safety. The DMV's response also varies by location, even within the same state. Some states or provinces may revoke a driver's license after being reported by a health care practitioner. Interviews and more rigorous testing procedures may be given to those with seizures, cognitive or motor deficits (97, 98). Comprehensive driving evaluations may be helpful, although third-party commercial or government insurance funding is rarely available, unless the disability is the result of a work or military service-related injury. Cognitive and physical testing may rule out an individual's inability to drive if there are no obvious deficits in strength, sensation or vision. No test replaces an actual on-the-road evaluation in order to insure driving safety (99, 100).

Recreation and Vocation

A thorough survey of an older adult's pre-injury recreational pursuits is necessary in order to explore options post-TBI. Sedentary activities can usually be resumed with minor modifications, if any. Socialization opportunities may have been the primary leisure activity and is appropriate afterwards, perhaps minus any accompanying substance use. Resumption of group activities in the rehabilitation setting and community settings is important to minimize feelings of isolation.

Return to work rates are poor for older adults after TBI. Realistic goals need to be established with appropriate supports in the work place. Often early retirement or part-time volunteer work is necessary when an individual cannot return to their workplace (101).

Case Example

AR is a 73-year-old married man who fell down a stairwell at a hotel party while on vacation, landing on his head. He lost consciousness at the scene, was initially unable to move his legs, and had significant scalp lacerations. In the ER, GCS was 12 and he began to move his legs. CT scan of his head revealed occipital and basilar skull fractures, multiple cerebral contusions, subdural and subarachnoid hemorrhages. None of these required surgical intervention. His associated injuries included right hemothorax and pulmonary contusions, grade 1 liver laceration, cervical 5–7 vertebral body fractures, thoracic, lumbar and sacral fractures, and bilateral pubic rami fractures. His past medical history included a cardiomyopathy, probably secondary to alcoholism, with 30 to 35% ejection fraction and an episode of ventricular tachycardia in the last year, gout, and colon cancer 10 years previously. He has an MBA, is retired as president of a construction company and has lived with his wife of 50 years in a 2-story home. His hobbies are playing tennis and traveling.

He was initially intubated for airway control and underwent tracheostomy, T3 – T12 laminectomies, rodding and bone graft; C3-7 posterior stabilization and lumbosacral stabilization. He was extubated and started following commands consistently 3 weeks post-injury. He required no intracranial surgery.

Four weeks post-injury he was transported to a hospital in his community via air ambulance. Occupational, physical and speech therapies were initiated. Within 2 days he needed to be mechanically ventilated again due to exacerbation of congestive heart failure and was gradually weaned from the ventilator over 2 weeks while his cardiac medications were re-adjusted.

At 6 weeks post injury he was admitted to acute rehabilitation, dependent in all areas of mobility and self-care at Rancho level 5. His speech was fluent and he was oriented to person, city, and that he was in the hospital because of a fall. Upper extremity strength was symmetrical and grade 3/5 strength at the shoulders, 4/5 at the elbows, wrists and hands with wasting of his interossei but good dexterity. Lower extremities were symmetrical except at the ankles with grade 1/5 strength at the hips, 2/5 at the knees and left ankle, 1/5 at the right ankle. Sensory exam showed a stocking distribution of loss to all modalities below the ankles. His tracheostomy was being plugged for most of the day.

He emerged from posttraumatic amnesia 2 months post-injury while watching Wimbledon tennis matches on TV, which aided his orientation to time and date. A nerve conduction study showed moderate severe peripheral polyneuropathy with an additional right peroneal nerve injury. He had near syncopal episodes whenever he removed his elastic support hose with SBP as low as 70 mm Hg. After $4\frac{1}{2}$ weeks of acute rehabilitation, he required extra time but was independent in eating, grooming, and using a urinal. He was supervised for donning a shirt and required less than 25% assistance for dressing and washing his lower body, transfers to unlevel surfaces using a sliding board. He could propel his wheelchair 100 feet before tiring and started walking using the parallel bars and a walker. He was discharged home with home health therapy for 3 weeks followed by outpatient therapy for 2 months. He progressed to using a front-wheeled walker or cane with a right ankle foot orthosis for household and short-distance ambulation. Within several months of discharge he was able to resume management of his financial affairs and even go on a cruise with his wife and friends. His most bothersome ongoing symptom is pain in his feet and legs from his polyneuropathy. One year later he still hopes to play tennis again.

AR had several poor prognostic signs, including previous symptomatic cardiomyopathy, multiple fractures requiring surgery and prolonged PTA. However, he received excellent medical and rehabilitative care, had good family support and the will to not just survive but make the most of his capabilities. His recovery illustrates how a coordinated system of care can produce favorable outcome despite many potential pitfalls.

TBI, Apolipoprotein E4 and Dementia

Apolipoprotein E4 (APOE-4) is a lipid transporter in the brain and cerebrospinal fluid (102). and is believed to play a role in the inflammatory response and neuronal repair following trauma. It is the product of a single gene and has been related to age-related cognitive impairment, decreased synapse-neuron ratio, increased susceptibility to neurotoxins, and hippocampal atrophy (103). Individuals with a history of TBI and apolipoprotein E4 (APOE 4) allele had 10 times the risk of developing Alzheimer's disease compared with 2 times the risk with APOE 4 alone and no increased risk with TBI alone (104). Nicoll and colleagues examined the brains of 90 individuals who died of severe TBI. All individuals homozygous for APOE 4 had beta amyloid placques (BAP); overall, 52% of those with BAP had at least one APOE 4 allele while only 16% of those with no BAP had APOE 4 (105). Teasdale and colleagues analyzed 89 individuals with TBI with and without apoE-4 allele. 57% of those with the allele versus 27% of those without had 6-month outcome of death, vegetative state or severe disability (106). The presence of APOE 4 alleles, especially in the homozygous condition appear to be associated with worse outcome after TBI. Individuals with APOE 4 allele also have associated poor outcome after spontaneous non-aneurymal intracerebral hemorrhage, amyloid angiopathy, and subarachnoid hemorrhage(103). Nearly all the above studies have been performed on individuals of western European genetic backgrounds and environments, so it is difficult to generalize the association across races and environments (107, 108).

AGING WITH TBI

Conflicting data exist in the literature regarding aging and TBI. Amongst the published studies, various issues were examined including: time of onset of Alzheimer's Disease (AD), long-term neuropsychological outcome, incidence and causes of mood disorders, re-hospitalization, morbidity, mortality, as well as psychosocial outcome and satisfaction with life.

Alzheimer's Disease

In a population-based cohort who acquired their TBI between 1935–1984, Nemetz et al found no greater incidence in the number of inidividuals with Alzheimer's disease, but a earlier onset, 10 years versus 18 years, suggesting that TBI may reduce the time of onset of dementia in those already at risk for Alheimer's disease (108).

Neuropsychological impairment

Increasing age is associated with greater neuropsychological impairment (e.g. diminished memory, slower processing speed), but it is unclear whether it is the case for aging with a brain injury.

Johnstone et al. studied 279 individuals with a TBI over a 4-year period. They used age-based normative data to determine the decline in cognition compared to pre-injury levels for different age groups. They found that neuropsychological impairments noted in older individuals with a TBI are typical of changes with normal aging (109). Millis and colleagues looked at neuropsychological recovery from 1 year to 5 years after injury. They studied 182 persons with mild to severe TBI. Digits forward and backward, logical memory I and II, token test, controlled oral word association test, symbol digit modalities test, trail making test, Rey auditory verbal learning test, visual form discrimination, block design, Wisconsin card sorting test, and grooved peg board were used as neuropsychological data. Improvement from 1 year after injury to 5 years was variable. On test measures, 22.2% improved, 15.2% declined and 62.2% were unchanged. Patients showing improvement were most likely to have changed on measures of cognitive speed, visual spatial construction, and verbal memory. Decline was most pronounced on measures requiring rapid performance and cognitive flexibility (110).

Mood Disorders

Little is known about the long-term risk of depression after TBI. Holsinger and colleagues compared the prevalence of depression 50 years after injury in 520 World War II veterans with and 1198 veterans without TBI. Head-injured veterans were more likely to report major depression in subsequent years and were more often currently depressed.

Lifetime prevalence of major depression in the head injured group was 18.5% versus 13.4% with no TBI. Current depression was detected in 11.2% of the veterans with brain injury versus 8.5% of those without (111). Thomsen found 20% incidence of psychotic behavior with onset 3 months to 6 years post injury; symptomatic memory problems in 75%, personality and emotional changes in 65%, concentration and mental slowness in 53% and loss of social contact in 68% of 40 individuals between 10–15 years post severeTBI (112).

Hospitalization

Regarding health issues after TBI, Marwitz and colleagues. investigated the incidence and etiology of rehospitalization 1 and 5 years after injury in 799 individuals. The annual incidence and of rehospitalization ranged from 22.9% 1 year after injury to 17.0% 5 years after injury. At 5 years after injury, general health maintenance was the most common reason for admission (36%) followed by seizures (18.7%), psychiatric (16%) and orthopedic (13.3%) etiologies (113).

Psychosocial Outcome

Corrigan JD and colleagues examined outcomes in the first 5 years after TBI. They studied 95 adults 6 months to 5 years after inpatient rehabilitation for a TBI. Their outcomes measures included the following: Functional Independence Measure (FIM), Sickness Impact Profile (SIP), Medical Outcome survey Short Form-36 (SF-36), Community Integration Questionnaire (CIQ) and Satisfaction with Life Scale (SWLS). Outcomes 5 years after discharge showed improvement with most change occurring within the first 2 years (114).

A study by Mazaux and colleagues followed 79 individuals with TBI by phone interview 9 years after injury to assess their late functional outcome and satisfaction with life. Sixty-five to 85% of individuals were independent in activities of daily living (ADL) whereas only 35–55% of persons with TBI were independent with social interaction. Most people were satisfied with their level of autonomy (67%), family life (66%) and financial status (41%). Dissatisfaction was expressed regarding leisure activities (36%), vocational adjustment (28%) and sexual function (32%) (115).

The TBI National Data Base has 178 subjects comprising a range of age 16 to 80 who have acute rehabilitation discharge, 1-year and 10-year follow-up data. Using a global functioning measure such as the DRS, there is evidence that individuals achieve overall improvement in capabilities and independence over time: scores improve from rehabilitation discharge (5.53, SD 2.87) to 1-year (2.93, SD 2.82) and 10-years (2.14, SD 2.65) post TBI. Competitive employment increases from 22.5 to 29.5% between 1 and 10-years post TBI, and there is also a trend towards retirement. Whether that is occurring for just age-related or medically-related reasons is not defined in the database. Return to school on at least a part-time basis is typical at 1-year post injury but not at 10 years. With this cohort there is also a bias with regards to their ability to be followed over time. Although there is no control group, the overall capabilities and employment demonstrated is less than the general population (12) (see Table 21-2). These and other data above indicate that improvement in social status and achievement can continue over time even as the basic neurological recovery has stabilized.

Mortality

Shavelle RM and collaborators examined causes of death more than one year after TBI. Mortality rate was elevated for circulatory diseases, respiratory diseases, choking/suffocation, and seizures. Mortality was higher between 1 and 5 years post-injury than after 5 years and was strongly related to reduced mobility. The markedly elevated mortality in those with reduced mobility is not

TABLE 21-2
Productive Activity Before and After TBI (12)

	PRE-INJURY	1 YEAR POST-INJURY	10 YEARS POST-INJURY
Competitive Employment	59.9%	22.5%	29.5%
Full-time student	9.0%	4.0%	0%
Part-time student	0.6%	5.8%	0.6%
Homemaker	1.1%	2.9%	2.9%
Retired (age)	4.5%	5.8%	29.5%
Unemployed	24.3%	53.8%	28.3%
Other	0.6%	5.2%	9.2%

surprising, as a sedentary lifestyle is known to be associated with increased mortality risk, especially because of diseases of the circulatory system (114).

CONCLUSION

Traumatic brain injury in the older adult occurs primarily as a result of falls, pedestrian versus motor vehicle collisions, and low- to moderate-speed motor vehicle crashes. The aging of the population in industrialized countries has resulted in an increasing incidence and prevalence of TBI in this age group and particularly among older women. Cerebral pathology in these injuries tends to be more focal with SDH's and contusions. Injuries from motor vehicle crashes also result in DAI. Severe injuries are less commonly survived, but individuals who do survive can have favorable functional outcomes.

Caring for the older individual with TBI requires employing a combination of the principles of geriatric medicine and brain injury rehabilitation, with close attention to the timing, setting and intensity of therapeutic interventions. Models of care need to adapt to the unique needs of the older adult.

Older individuals with TBI usually require more time to recover cognitively and physically than younger individuals. Removal or simplification of medication regimens is usually more efficacious than adding new ones. Therapeutic interventions must be tailored to the individual's and family's needs in their specific post-discharge environment with early training of caregivers and environmental modifications for safety (41, 77). Aging with TBI may progress more rapidly than aging without such injuries, particulary in some individuals with genetic predisposition. Most individuals improve gradually over time with regards to their physical and cognitive functioning,

frequency of rehospitalization and employment. However, as a group individuals with TBI have more medical and psychosocial challenges than those who were never injured.

Acknowledgements

Portions of this chapter were previously published by Jeffrey Englander and David X. Cifu, as "The Older Adult with Traumatic Brain Injury" in Rosenthal M, Griffith ER, Kreutzer JS and Pentland B (eds), *Rehabilitation of the Adult and Child with Traumatic Brain Injury*, 3rd edition. Philadelphia: FA Davis, 1999; 453–470, ISBN 0-8036-0391-6. Special thanks to Jerry Wright and Jenny Marwitz, MA for help with accessing the NIDRR TBI Model Systems Dataset and to Naomi McCarroll for manuscript preparation.

References

1. U.S. Census Bureau: The 65 years and over population: 2000. U.S. Department of Commerce, Washington, D.C., October 2000.
2. National Center for Health Statistics: National Health Interview Survey (NHIS). Department of Health and Human Services, Washington, D.C., March 2003.
3. U.S. Census Bureau: Profile of Selected Social Characteristics: 2000. U.S. Department of Commerce, Washington, D.C., October 2000.
4. Williams TF: *The aging process: biological and psychosocial considerations*. In Brody SJ, and Ruff, GE (eds): *Aging and Rehabilitation: Advances in State of the Art*. New York: Springer 1986, p. 13.
5. Langlois JA, Kegler SR, Butler JA, Gotsch KE et al. Traumatic brain injury-related hospital discharges: Results from a 14-state surveillance system, 1997. *MMWR* 2003; June 27, 2003;52 (SS04): 1–20.
6. Katz DI, Kehs GJ, Alexander MP. Prognosis and recovery from TBI: The influence of advancing age. *Neurology* 1990;40:276.
7. Public Health and Aging: Nonfatal Fall-related traumatic brain injury among older adults—California, 1996–1999. *MMWR* 2003; 52(13):276–278.
8. Tinetti MD, Speechley M. Prevention of falls in the elderly. *N Engl J Med* 1989;320:1055–9.
9. Gutman MB, Moulton RJ, Sullivan I, et al: Relative incidence of intracranial mass lesions and severe torso injury after accidental injury: Implications for triage and management. *J Trauma* 1991; 31:974–7.
10. Rakier A, Guilburd RJ, Soustiel JF, et al. Head injuries in the elderly. *Brain Inj* 1995;9:187–93.
11. Katz DI, Alexander MP. Traumatic brain injury: Predicting course of recovery and outcome for patients admitted to rehabilitation. *Arch Neurol* 1994;51:661–67.
12. Traumatic Brain Injury Model Systems National Data Center. TBI Model Systems Database. www.tbi.ndc.org
13. Adekoya N, Thurman DJ, White DD, Webb KW. Surveillance for traumatic brain injury deaths in the United States, 1989—1998. *MMWR* Surveillance Summary 2002;6 51(10):1–14.
14. Centers for Disease Control and Prevention. Suicide among older persons: United States, 1980–1992. *MMW*, 2002;51(SS 10):1–16
15. Rakier A, Guilburd JN, Soustie JF, Zaaroor M, Feinsod M. Head injuries in the elderly. *Brain Inj* 1996;9(2):187–193.
16. Chesnut RM, Marshall LF, Klauber MR, Blunt BA, Baldwin N, Eisenberg HM, Jane JA, Marmarou A, Foulkes MA. The role of secondary brain injury in dertermining outcome from severe head injury. *J Trauma* 1993;34(2):216–222.
17. Pennings JF, Bachulis BL, Simmons CT. Survival after severe brain injury in the aged. *Arch Surg* 1993;128:787–794.

18. Cagetti B, Cossu M, Pau A, Rivan C, Viale G. The outcome from acute subdural and epidural haematomas in very elderly patients. *British J Neurosurg* 1992;6:227–232.

19. Heiskanen H, and Sipponen P: Prognosis of severe brain injury. *Acta Neurol Scand* 1970;46:343–348.

20. Amacher AL, and Bybee DE. Toleration of head injury by the elderly. *Neurosurgery* 1979;20:954–58.

21. Sosin DN, Sacks JJ, and Smith SM. Head injury-associated deaths in the U.S. from 1979–1986. *JAMA* 1989;282:2251–55.

22. Morrison RG. Medical and public health aspects of boxing. *JAMA* 1986;255:2475–80.

23. Herneasniemi J. Outcome following head injuries in the aged. *Acta Neurochir (Wien)* 1979;49:67–79.

24. Jennett B, Teasdale G, Braakman R,et al. Predicting outcome in individual patients after severe head injury. *Lancet* 1976;1: 1031–34.

25. Braakman R, Gelpe GJ, Habbema JD, et al. Systematic selection of prognostic features in patients with severe head injury. *Neurosurgery* 1980;6:362–70.

26. Born JD, Albert A, Hans P, et al. Relative prognostic value of best motor response and brainstem reflexes in patients with severe head injury. *Neursurgery* 1985;16:595–601.

27. Choi S, Barnes TY, Bullock R, et al. Temporal profile of outcome in severe head injury. *J Neurosurg* 1994;81:169–73.

28. Luerssen T, Klauber M. and Marshall L. Outcome from head injury related to patient's age. *J Neurosurg* 1988;68:409–16.

29. Cifu DX, Kreutzer JS, Marwitz JH, Rosenthal M, Englander J. Medical and Functional Characteristics of Older Adults with Traumatic Brain Injury: A Multicenter Analysis. *Arch Phys Med Rehabil* 1996;77:883–8.

30. Frankel J, Marwithz J, Cifu DX et al. A follow-up study of older adults with traumatic brain injury: Taking into account decreasing length of stay. *Arch Phys Med Rehabil* 2006; 87: 57–62

31. Galbraith S. Head injuries in the elderly. *BMJ* 1987;294: 294–325,32.

32. Reeder K, Rosenthal M, Lichteberg P. et al: Impact of age on functional outcome following traumatic brain injury. *J Head Trauma Rehabil* 1996;11:22–31.

33. Saywell RM, Woods JR, Rappaport SA, et al. The value of age and severity as predictors of costs in geriatric head injury trauma patients. *J Am Geriatr Soc* 1989;37:625–30.

34. Carlsson CA, von Essen C, Losgren J. Clinical factors in severe head injuries. *J Neurosurg* 1968;29:242.

35. Galbraith S, et al. The relationship between alcohol and head injury and its effects on the conscious level. Br J Surg 1976;63:128.

36. 34a. Marshall, LF, Bowers-Marshall, S, Klauber, MR et al. A new classification of head injury based on computerized tomography. *J Neurosurg* 1991;75(suppl):S14–20.

37. Gershkoff AM, Cifu DX, and Means KM. Geriatric rehabilitation: Social, attitudinal and economic factors. *Arch Phys Med Rehabil* 1993;74:S402–05.

38. Walker WC, Kreutzer JS, Witol AD. Level of care options for the low-functioning brain injury survivor. *Brain Inj* 1996;10: 65–75.

39. Applegate WB, et al. Geriatric evaluation and management: Current status and future research directions. *J AM Geriatr Soc (suppl)* 1991;39(suppl):25

40. Rubenstein LZ, Stuck AE, Sui AL, et al: Impacts of geriatric evaluation and management programs on defined outcomes: Overview of the evidence. *J Am Geriatr Soc (suppl)* 1991;39:85–165.

41. Breed ST, Flanagan SR, Katson KR. The relationship between age and the self-report of health symptoms in persons with traumatic brain injury. *Arch Phys Med Rehabil* 2004;85(4 Suppl 2): S 61–7.

42. Stewart DG, and Cifu DX. Rehabilitation of the old, old stroke patient. *Journal of Back and Musculoskeletal Rehabilitation* 1994;4:135–.

43. Kane RL, Ouslander JG, Abrass IB. Essentials of Clinical Geriatrics, 4th edition. New York: McGraw-Hill, 1999;256–291.

44. Piranino AJ. Managing medication in the elderly. *Hospital Practice* 1995;June 15:59–64.

45. AGS Panel on Chronic Pain in Older Persons: The management of chronic pain in older persons. *J Am Geriatr Soc* 1998;46:635–651.

46. Basford JR. *Physical agents and biofeedback in* DeLisa JA, Currie DM, Gans BM, Gatens PF, Leonard JA, McPhee MC, *Rehabilitation Medicine: Principles and Practice.* Philadelphia: JB Lippincott, 1988;257–275.

47. Bradley J, Brandt K D, Katz BP. et al. Comparison of an anti-inflammatory dose of ibuprofen, an analgesic dose of ibuprofen and acetaminophen in the treatment of patients with osteoarthritis of the knee. *N Engl J Med*, 1991;325(2):87–91

48. Treatment Guidelines from the Medical Letter. Drugs for Rheumatoid Arthritis. Emmerson BT, January 2003;1(5).

49. Shehab D, Elgazzar AH, Collier BD, Heterotopic ossification. *J Nucl Med* 2002;43:346–353.

50. Geerts WH, Heit JA, Clagett CP, et al. Prospective study of venous thromboembolism after major trauma. *N Engl J Med* 1994;331: 1601–1606.

51. Lai JM, Yablon SA, Ivanhoe CB. Incidence and sequelae of symptomatic venous thrombembolic disease among patients with traumatic brain injury. *Brain Injury* 1997;11(5):331–334.

52. Meythaler JM, Devivo MJ, Hayne JB. Cost-effectiveness of routine screening for proximal deep venous thrombosis in acquired brain injury patients admitted to acute rehabilitation. *Arch Phys Med Rehabil* 1996;77:1–5.

53. Cifu DX, Kaelin DL, Wall BE. Deep venous thrombosis: incidence on admission to a brain injury rehabilitation program. *Arch Phys Med Rehabil* 1996;77:1182–1185.

54. Weinmann EE, Salzman EW. Deep-venous thrombosis. *N Engl J Med* 1994;331:1630–41.

55. Geerts WH, Heit JA, Clagett CP, et al. Prevention of Venous Thromboembolism. *Chest* 2001;119:132S–175S.

56. Hamilton MG, Hull RD, Pineo GF: Venous thromboembolism in neurosurgery and neruology patients: A review. *Neurosurgery* 1994;34:280–96.

57. Office of Medical Applications Research, NIG: Concensus conference: Prevention of venous thrombosis and pulmonary embolism. *JAMA* 1986;256:744.

58. Rogers FB, Cipolle MD, Velmahos G. et al. Practice management guidelines for the prevention of venous thromboembolism in trauma patients. *J Trauma* 2002;52(3):453–462.

59. Englander J, Bushnik T, Duong TT, Cifu DX, Wright, J, Hughes R, Bergman W. Analyzing risk factors for late posttraumatic seizures: a prospective, multi-center investigation. *Arch Phys Med Rehabil* 2003;84(3):365–373.

60. Brain Trauma Foundation and American Association of Neurological Surgeons, The role of antiseizure prophylaxis following head injury in Management and Prognosis of severe traumatic brain injury. *Brain Trauma foundation, Inc.;* 2000: 159–165.

61. Brain Injury Special Interest Group of the American Academy of Physical Medicine and Rehabilitation. Practice parameter: Antiepileptic drug treatment of posttruamatic seizures. *Arch Phys Med Rehabil* 1998;79:594–97.

62. Haltiner AM, Temkin NR, Dickmen SS. Risk of seizure recurrence after the first PTS. *Arch Phys Med Rehabil* 1997;78;835–840.

63. Sirven JI. Acute and chronic seizures in patients older than 60 years. *Mayo Clin Proc* 2001;76:175–183.

64. Treatment guidelines from the Medical Letter. *Drugs for epilepsy* 2003;1(9):57–64.

65. Schafer AL and Bunn HF. Anemias of iron deficiniency and iron overload in Braunwald E, Isselbacher KJ, Petersdorf RG, Wilson JD, Martin JB, Fauci AS (eds), Harrison's Priciples of Internal Medicine, 11th ed. New York: McGraw-Hill, 1987:1493–1498.

66. Morley JE and Miller DK, Malnutrition in the elderly. *Hosp Pract* (off ed): 1992;7:95–98, 101, 105–6, passim.

67. Groher MD and Picon-Nieto. *Evaluation of Communication and Swallowing Disorders in* Rosenthal M, Griffith ER, Kreutzer JS and Pentland B (eds), *Rehabilitation of the Adult and Child with Traumatic Brain Injury,* 3rd edition. Philadelphia: FA Davis 1999; 193–198.

68. Myers JK, Weisman MM, Tischler GL, et al. Six-month prevalence of psychiatric disorders in three communites: 1980–1982. *Arch Gen Psychiatry* 1984;41:959–67.

69. Hurt RD, Finlayson RE, Morse RM, Davis LJ. Alcoholism in elderly persons: medical aspects and prognosis of 216 inpatients. Mayo Clin Proc 1988;63:753–760

70. Council on Scientific Affairs, American Medical Association. *JAMA* 1996;275(10):797–801.

71. Corrigan JD, Bogner JA, Lamb-Hart GL. *Substance Abuse and Brain Injury* in Rosenthal M, Griffith ER, Kreutzer JS and Pentland B (eds), *Rehabilitation of the Adult and Child with Traumatic Brain Injury*, 3rd edition. Philadelphia: FA Davis, 1999;556–571.

72. Ewing JA, Detecting Alcoholism: The CAGE questionnaire. *JAMA* 1984;252(14):1905–1907.

73. Centers for Disease Control and Prevention, Behavioral Risk Factor Surveillance System User's Guide. Atlanta: U.S. Department of Health and Human Services, 1998. National Household Survey on Drug Abuse and Mental Health Services Administration, Office of Applied Studies.

74. Chutka DS, Fleming KC, Evans MP, et al. Urinary incontinence in the elderly population. *Mayo Clin Proc* 1996;71:93–101.

75. Opitz JL, Thorsteinsson G, Schutt AH, Barrett, Olson PK. *Neurogenic Bladder and Bowel.* In DeLisa JA, Currie DM, Gans BM, Gatens PF, Leonard JA, McPhee MC, *Rehabilitation Medicine: Prinicples and Practice*, 3rd edition Philadelphia: JB Lippincott, 1993:1073–1106.

76. Foxx-Orenstein A, Kolakowsky-Hayner S, Marwitz JH et al. Incidence, risk factors and outcomes of fecal incontinence after acute brain injury: findings from the traumatic brain injury model systems national database. *Arch Phys Med Rehabil* 2003;84:231–237.

77. Goodman H and Englander J. Traumatic brain injury in elderly indviduals. *Physical Medicine and Rehabilitation Clinics of North America* 1992;3:441–459.

78. Katz DI and Black SE. *Neurological and Neuroradiological Evaluation* in Rosenthal M, Griffith ER, Kreutzer JS and Pentland B(eds), *Rehabilitation of the Adult and Child with Traumatic Brain Injury*, 3rd edition. Philadelphia: FA Davis 1999;89–116.

79. Murphy C and Davidson TM. Geriatric issues: Special considerations. *J Head Trauma Rehabil* 1992;7(1):76–82.

80. Fleming KC, Adams AC, Petersen RC. Dementia: Diagnosis and evaluation. *Mayo Clin Proc* 1995;70:1093–1107.

81. Goldstein FC and Levin HS. Neurobehavioral outcome of traumatic brain injury in older adults: initial findings. *J Head Trauma Rehabil* 1995;10(1):57–73.

82. Kaelin D, Cifu DX, Matthies B. Methylphenidate effect on attention deficit in the acutely brain-injured adult. *Arch Phys Med Rehabil* 1996;77:6–9.

83. Cardenas DD and McLean, A. Psychopharmacologic Management of traumatic brain injury. *Physical Medicine and Rehabilitation Clinics of North America*, May 1992:272–290.

84. Sandel ME and Mysiw WJ. The agitated brain injured patient. Part 1: definitions, differential diagnosis and assessment. *Arch Phys Med Rehabil* 1996;77:617–623.

85. Mysiw WJ and Sandel ME. The agitated brain injured patient. Part 2: pathophysiology and treatment. *Arch Phys Med Rehabil* 1997;78:213–220.

86. Corrigan JD. Development of a scale for assesment of agitation following traumatic brain injury. *J Clin Exp Neuropsychol* 1989;11:261–77.

87. Santa Clara Valley Medical Center Rehabilitation Center. Behavior Management Guidelines, revised 2003.

88. Reyes RL, Bhattacharyya AK, Heller D. Traumatic head injury: restlessness and agitation as prognosticators of physical and psychological improvements in patients. *Arch Phys Med Rehabil* 1981;62:20–23.

89. Jacobs HE. Behavioral analysis, guidelines and brain injury rehabilitation: people, principles and procedure manual. Gaithersburg, MD: Aspen Publishing 1993.

90. Zafonte RD, Elovic E, Mysiw WJ, O'Dell M, Watanabe T. *Pharmacology in Traumatic BrainIinjury: Fundamentals and Treatment Strategies* in Rosenthal M, Griffith ER, Kreutzer JS and Pentland B(eds), *Rehabilitation of the Adult and Child with Traumatic Brain Injury*, 3rd edition. Philadelphia: FA Davis 1999;544–548.

91. Rosenthal M, Christensen BK, Ross TP. Depression following traumatic brain injury. *Arch Phys Med Rehabil* 1998;79:90–101.

92. Martin LM, Fleming KC, Evans JM. Recognition and management of anxiety anddepression in elderly patients. *Mayo Clin Proc* 1995;70:999–1006.

93. Alexander MP. Neuropsychiatric correlates of persistent post concussion syndrome. *J Head Trauma Rehabil* 1992;7:60–69.

94. Prinz PN, Vitiello MV, Raskind MA, Thorpy MJ. Geriatrics: Sleep disorders and aging. *N Engl J Med* 1990;323(8):520–526.

95. Callahan CD and Hagglund KJ. Comparing neuropsycholical and psychiatric evaluation of competency in rehabilitation. *Arch Phys Med Rehabil* 1995;76:909–912.

96. Herstein Gervasio A, Griffith ER. *Sexuality and Sexual Dysfunction* in Rosenthal M, Griffith ER, Kreutzer JS and Pentland B(eds), *Rehabilitation of the Adult and Child with Traumatic Iinjury*, 3rd edition. Philadelphia: FA Davis, 1999;479–502.

97. Klrumholz A. To drive or not to drive: The 3-month seizure-free interval for people with epilepsy. *Mayo Clin Proc* 2003;78:817–818.

98. Reuben DB and St. George P. Driving and dementia: California's approach to a medical and policy dilemma. *West J Med* 1996;164:111–121.

99. Hunt LA. Evaluation and retraining programs for older drivers. *Clin Geriatr Med* 1993;9:439–448.

100. Glaski T, Bruno RL, Ehle HT. Prediction of behind-the-wheel driving performance in patients with cerebral brain damage: a discriminant function analysis. *Am J Occup Ther* 1993;47:391–96.

101. Wehman P, West M, Johnson A, Cifu DX. *Vocational Rehabilitation for Individuals with Traumatic Brain Injury* in Rosenthal M, Griffith ER, Kreutzer JS and Pentland B (eds), *Rehabilitation of the Adult and Child with Traumatic Brain Injury*, 3rd edition. Philadelphia: FA Davis 1999;326–341.

102. Coleman M, Handler M, Martin C. Update on apolipoprotein E state of the art. *Hosp Phys* 1995:22–24.

103. Nathoo N, Chetty R, vanDellen JR, Barnett GH. Genetic vulnerability following traumatic brain injury: the role of apolipoprotein E. *J Clin Pathlo: Mol Pathol* 2003;56:132–136.

104. Mayeux R, Ottman R, Tang M, et al. Genetic susceptibility and head injury as risk factors for Alzheimer's disease among community-dwelling elderly persons and their first-degree relatives. *Ann Neurol* 1993;33:494–501.

105. Nicoll JA, Roberts GW, Graham DI. Apolipoprotein E e4 allele is associated with deposition amyloid B-protein following head injury. *Nat Med* 1995;1:135–137.

106. Teasdale GM, Nicoli JA, Murray G, et al. Association of apolipoprotein E polymorphysm with outcome after head injury. *Lancet* 1997;350:1069–1071.

107. Samatovicz RA. Genetics and brain injury. *J Head Trauma Rehabil* 2000;15(3):869–874.

108. Nametz PN, Leibson C, Naessens JM et al. Traumatic brain injury and time of onset of Alzheimer's Disease: A population-based study. Am J Epidemiol 1999;149:32–40.

109. Johnstone B, Childers MK, Hoerner J. The effects of normal aging on neuropsychological functioning following traumatic brain injury. Brain Injury 1998;12(7):569–76110.

110. Millis SR, Rosenthal M, Novack TA, et al. Long-term neuropsychological outcome after traumatic brain injury. J Head Trauma Rehabil.2001;16(4):343–55.

111. Holsinger T, Steffens DC, Phillips C et al. Head injury in adulthood and the risk of depression. Arch Gen Psychiatry. 2002; 59(1):23–4.

112. Thomsen IV, Late outcome and very severe blunt head trauma: a 10–15 year second follow-up. *J Neurol, Neurosurg, Psych* 1984; 47:260–268

113. Marwitz JH, Cifu DX, Englander J, High WM Jr. A multicenter analysis of rehospitalizations five years after brain injury. *J Head Trauma Rehabil* 2001, Aug;16(4):307–17.

114. Corrigan JD, Smith-Knapp K, Granger CV. Outcomes in the first 5 years after traumatic brain injury. *Arch Phys Med Rehabil* 1998;79:298–305.

115. Mazaux JM, Croze P, Quintard B, Rouxel L, Joseph PA, Richer E, Debelleix X, Barat M. Satisfaction with life and late psychosocial outcome after severe brain injury: a nine-year follow-up study in Aquitaine. *Acta Neurochir Suppl* 2002;79:49–51.

116. Shavelle, RM, Strauss D, Whyte J. Long-term causes of death after traumatic brain injury. *Am J Phys Med Rehabil* 2001 Jul;80(7):510–6.

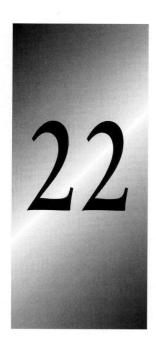

22 Mild TBI

Grant L. Iverson
Rael T. Lange
Michael Gaetz
Nathan D. Zasler

INTRODUCTION

Mild traumatic brain injuries are common. Bazarian and colleagues (1) reported that 56/100,000 people are evaluated in the emergency department each year for an *isolated* mild traumatic brain injury (MTBI). Sosin et al. (2), based on the National Health Interview Survey in 1991, estimated that 1.5 million Americans suffer a traumatic brain injury each year (i.e., 618/100,000), with the vast majority being mild in severity. This, of course, is much higher than previous estimates based on hospital admissions because most people who sustain a mild traumatic brain injury are not evaluated in the emergency department or admitted to the hospital (2). For example, mild injuries, such as concussions in sport, are very common. In a recent study, 30 percent of high school football players reported at least one previous concussion; 15 percent reported that they had experienced a concussion during the current football season (3).

For most people, MTBIs are self-limiting and generally follow a predictable course. Permanent cognitive, psychological, or psychosocial problems due to the biological effects of this injury are relatively uncommon in trauma patients and rare in athletes (see Refs. 4–9 for recent comprehensive reviews). Slow or incomplete recovery from MTBI is poorly understood, despite decades of research.

The purpose of this chapter is to provide a comprehensive overview of MTBI. The discussion is divided into the following 11 sections: (a) terminology, (b) pathoanatomy and pathophysiology, (c) S-100B as a marker for injury and predictor of outcome, (d) neuropsychological outcome, (e) early intervention, (f) return to work, (g) depression, (h) post-traumatic stress disorder, (i) risk for Alzheimer's disease, (j) persistent post-concussion syndrome, and (k) conclusions. This chapter does not provide a detailed review of concussions in sports or the differential diagnosis of the persistent post-concussion syndrome. Two chapters in this book are devoted to those topics.

TERMINOLOGY

There is no universally agreed-upon definition of MTBI. However, the most commonly used definitions are very similar. The maximum duration of unconsciousness, for example, has been 20, 30, or 60 min or less in various studies. The duration of post-traumatic amnesia has been 60 min or less in some studies, and less than 24 hr in others (see Ref. 10 for a review).

Some researchers have differentiated *complicated* from *uncomplicated* MTBI (11). A complicated MTBI is diagnosed if the person has a Glasgow Coma Scale (GCS) score of 13–15 but shows some brain abnormality (e.g., edema, hematoma, or contusion) on a CT-scan. Skull fractures were also considered characteristic of complicated injuries in Williams et al., but fractures have been investigated separately by other researchers. Williams and colleagues noted that patients with complicated MTBIs are more likely to have persistent cognitive and psychological symptoms, and their 6-month recovery pattern is more similar to persons with moderate head injuries. Complicated MTBIs are discussed in detail in the pathoanatomy/pathophysiology and the neuropsychological outcome sections of this chapter.

The uncomplicated MTBI is characterized by having no intracranial abnormality or skull fracture, with all other severity criteria in the mild range. Notably, there are several subtypes of injuries; the severity of injury, types of symptoms, and course of recovery can vary in relation to these subtypes. For example, it is assumed (although not well studied) that the person who is "dazed" and may have lost consciousness for a few seconds is much more likely to experience a rapid and complete recovery than a person who is unconscious for 20 min and has posttraumatic amnesia for 12 hr.

An interdisciplinary subcommittee published a definition of MTBI that was designed to clarify classification and improve cross-study comparisons. The definition was developed by the Mild Traumatic Brain Injury Committee of the Head Injury Interdisciplinary Special Interest Group of the American Congress of Rehabilitation Medicine (12). This definition is provided in Table 22-1.

This article was intended to provide a standard definition, established by consensus of a committee, to facilitate communication regarding MTBI in research and in clinical practice. The focus of the article was on how to determine whether an MTBI has occurred, by establishing injury severity criteria. The committee definition is widely cited in clinical practice and research. A major limitation to this definition, however, is the inclusion of a broad range of injury severity. This definition ranges from a *trivial* injury involving seconds of confusion, to a complicated MTBI involving 20–30 min of unconsciousness, several hours of post-traumatic amnesia, and a focal contusion.

In a report to the U.S. Congress in 2003, a working group provided the conceptual definition of MTBI set out in Table 22-2 (13). This Centers for Disease Control (CDC) working group also proposed limited criteria for identifying MTBI-related impairment, functional limitations, disability, and persistent symptoms in population-based surveys. These criteria are set out in Table 22-3.

The CDC working group acknowledged that this definition does not define subtypes of MTBIs within the

---

TABLE 22-1
ACRM (12) Definition of Mild Traumatic Brain Injury

A traumatically induced physiological disruption of brain function, as manifested by at least one of the following:

1. any loss of consciousness;
2. any loss of memory for events immediately before or after the accident;
3. any alteration in mental state at the time of the accident (e.g., feeling dazed, disoriented, or confused); and
4. focal neurological deficit(s) that may or may not be transient; but where the severity of the injury does not exceed the following:
   - loss of consciousness of approximately 30 min or less;
   - after 30 minutes, an initial Glasgow Coma Scale (GCS) of 13–15; and
   - posttraumatic amnesia (PTA) not greater than 24 hr.

Note: A better conjunction after point #3 should have been "or" as opposed to "and".

TABLE 22-2
National Center for Injury Prevention and Control (13) Conceptual Definition of MTBI

The conceptual definition of MTBI is an injury to the head as a result of blunt trauma or acceleration or deceleration forces that result in *one or more* of the conditions listed below.

Any period of observed or self-reported:

- Transient confusion, disorientation, or impaired consciousness;
- Dysfunction of memory around the time of injury;
- Loss of consciousness lasting less than 30 min.
- Observed signs of neurological or neuropsychological dysfunction, such as:
  - Seizures acutely following injury to the head;
  - Among infants and very young children: irritability, lethargy, or vomiting following head injury;
  - Symptoms among older children and adults such as headache, dizziness, irritability, fatigue or poor concentration, when identified soon after injury, can be used to support the diagnosis of mild TBI, but cannot be used to make the diagnosis in the absence of loss of consciousness or altered consciousness. Research may provide additional guidance in this area.

More severe brain injuries were excluded from the definition of MTBI and include *one or more* of the following conditions attributable to the injury:

- Loss of consciousness lasting longer than 30 minutes;
- Post-traumatic amnesia lasting longer than 24 hr;
- Penetrating craniocerebral injury.

spectrum of the injury, and that researchers might continue to establish the importance of subtypes. The working group noted that the presence of an intracranial abnormality was one injury characteristic that should routinely be reported when available.

TABLE 22-3

CDC Working Group Limited Criteria for Identifying MTBI-Related Impairment, Functional Limitation, Disability, and Persistent Symptoms in Population-Based Surveys [National Center For Injury Prevention and Control (13)]

Current symptoms reported consequent to MTBI not present before injury or those made worse in severity or frequency by the MTBI:

• Problems with memory
• Problems with concentration
• Problems with emotional control
• Headaches
• Fatigue
• Irritability
• Dizziness
• Blurred vision
• Seizures

Current limitations in functional status reported consequent to MTBI:

• Basic activities of daily living (e.g., personal care, ambulation, travel)
• Major activities (e.g., work, school, homemaking)
• Leisure and recreation
• Social integration
• Financial independence

The CDC working group cautioned that most of these symptoms and limitations in Table 22-3 are associated with many other conditions, not just MTBI. The working group expressed concern regarding the limitations associated with the lack of specificity of the symptoms and functional limitations, but thought that these problems could be partially mitigated by the careful selection of appropriate comparison groups, cautious interpretation of findings, and by evaluating pre- and post-injury symptom reporting.

Under the auspices of the European Federation of Neurological Sciences, a task force published a classification system for MTBI that could be used to guide initial *management decisions* for emergency physicians (e.g., whether or not to undergo brain CT scanning). The EFNS subclassifications (14) for MTBI are presented in Table 22-4.

In 2004, a comprehensive review of the literature on MTBI was published in a series of articles in the *Journal of Rehabilitation Medicine* (e.g., 5, 15–18). The WHO Collaborating Centre Task Force on Mild Traumatic Brain Injury provided the following definition.

> MTBI is an acute brain injury resulting from mechanical energy to the head from external physical forces. Operational criteria for clinical identification include: (i) one or more of the following: confusion or disorientation, loss of consciousness for 30 minutes or less, post-traumatic amnesia for less than 24 hours, and/or other transient neurological abnormalities such as focal signs, seizure, and intracranial lesion not requiring surgery; (ii) Glasgow Coma Scale score of 13–15 after 30 minutes post-injury or later upon presentation for healthcare. These manifestations of MTBI must not be due to drugs, alcohol, medications, caused by other injuries or treatment for other injuries (e.g. systemic

---

TABLE 22-4

EFNS Classification Guidelines (14) for the Acute Management of MTBI

Injury Severity Classification	Glasgow Coma Scale	Loss of Consciousness	Post-Traumatic Amnesia	Risk Factors
Category 0	15	None	None	None
Category 1	15	< 30 minutes	< 1 hour	None
Category 2	15	< 30 minutes	< 1 hour	Yes
Category 3	13–14	< 30 minutes	< 1 hour	Yes or No

Risk factors for intracranial complications following MTBI: (1) unclear or ambiguous accident history, (2) continued post-traumatic amnesia, (3) retrograde amnesia longer than 30 min, (4) trauma above the clavicles including clinical signs of skull fracture, (4) severe headache, (5) vomiting, (6) focal neurological deficit, (7) seizure, (8) age < 2 yr, (9) age > 60 yr, (10) coagulation disorders, (11) high-energy accident, (12) intoxication with alcohol/drugs.

Note: The subclassifications were proposed to facilitate initial management decisions. Category 0 was conceptualized as a head injury with no traumatic brain injury. "According to Advanced Trauma Life Support principles, a high-energy (vehicle) accident is defined as initial speed >64 km/h, major auto-deformity, intrusion into passenger compartment >30 cm, extrication time from vehicle >20 min, falls >6 m, roll over, auto-pedestrian accidents, or motorcycle crash >32 km/h or with separation of rider and bike (406, 407)" (p. 210).

injuries, facial injuries, or intubation), caused by other problems (e.g. psychological trauma, language barrier, or coexisting medical conditions) or caused by penetrating craniocerebral injury" (page 115; 10)

Without question, MTBIs can be characterized by damage to the structure and certainly the function of the brain. A minority of patients with MTBIs have visible abnormalities on CT or MRI conducted on the day-of-injury or within the first two weeks post injury. The mainstream definitions of MTBI include patients with these visible structural abnormalities. For the most part, however, the pathophysiology of MTBI is neurometabolic. The pathoanatomy and pathophysiology of MTBI are discussed in the next section.

PATHOANATOMY AND PATHOPHYSIOLOGY

MTBIs can be characterized by damage to the structure of the brain. Clinicians and researchers often emphasize that most patients with MTBIs have normal structural neuroimaging studies; this is certainly true. However, a substantial minority of patients have day-of-injury abnormalities visible on CT. Approximately 7 to 20 percent of consecutive patients presenting to the emergency room[1] with an MTBI have bleeding, bruising, or swelling on day-of-injury computed tomography (17, 19–24). Borg and colleagues conducted a comprehensive review of this literature and concluded that the estimated prevalence of CT abnormalities of patients seen in the hospital was 5 percent for those with GCS scores of 15 and 30 percent or more for those with GCS scores of 13 (17). Not surprisingly, patients with macroscopic abnormalities on their day-of-injury CT have microscopic damage or dysfunction as well, as reported in both the animal and human literature. For example, in animal (25) and human studies (26–28) there appear to be observable changes in the vicinity of brain contusions that are related to neuronal metabolic pathophysiology (most notably with N-acetylaspartate, creatine and phosphocreatine, glutamate, and lactate) and glial reactivity (e.g., choline and inositol).

Researchers have reported that some patients with normal CT scans show abnormalities on MRI (29–32) or single photon emission computed tomography (SPECT; 33–35). In some patients with mild or moderate TBIs, brain atrophy can be quantified on serial quantitative MRI over a interval of several months (36, 37). A careful MRI examination of Virchow–Robin spaces (i.e., extensions of the subpial space surrounding perforating arteries and emerging veins serving cerebral cortex—when enlarged, these have been linked to white matter injury) in noncomplicated (i.e., 23/24 with GCS of 15 and 20/24 with unremarkable MRI) MTBI might reveal trauma-related findings (38). Abnormalities on positron emission tomography (35, 39) and SPECT (40, 41) have been observed in some patients with persistent postconcussion syndromes. Of course, many patients with chronic complaints do not have abnormalities on functional imaging, such as fMRI (42). Notably, abnormal functional neuroimaging studies do not *diagnose* the presence of an MTBI; there is a large literature on functional imaging abnormalities in patients with diverse neurological or psychiatric problems.

In most people, MTBIs are not associated with macroscopic abnormalities on neuroimaging. Moreover, in animal studies the microscopic damage associated with the milder injuries is very sparse. The physiological changes following MTBI at the cellular level have been examined extensively over the past 20 years, through animal and in vitro modeling. Based on the animal literature, it is assumed that most of the pathophysiology of concussion renders neurons and neural systems *dysfunctional* but *not destroyed*.

Contrary to popular belief, mild (as well as moderate) traumatic brain injury does not result in "shearing" of axons. Axons stretch and twist without being sheared or torn (43–46), even after repeated stretch injuries (47). What was originally conceptualized as "shearing"[2] (48–50) is actually a gradual process where stretched and badly damaged axons swell and eventually separate (43). This process (in MTBI) occurs in a very small number of axons; the vast majority of axons that are initially affected recover over time. The cellular pathophysiology associated with traumatic brain injuries, of all severities, is described in the next section.

Pathophysiology

Advancements in neuroscience have changed our basic understanding of the pathophysiology of neuronal injury. It was once considered that excessive acceleration/deceleration forces caused shear strains on the brain that resulted in tearing or stretching of neurons at the time of

---

[1] Victims of serious assault, people who fall or are struck hard enough to fracture their skull, or people in high-velocity accidents are at increased risk for intracranial abnormalities (14), and these individuals are more likely to be seen in the emergency room. Note that at least 25 percent of people with MTBIs seek no medical attention and 14 percent are seen at their doctor's office or in clinics (2). Moreover, there is a low risk for observable intracranial abnormalities in athletic concussions, most athletes are not taken to the hospital, and a significant percentage of athletes with minor concussions don't even report the injury to their coaches or trainers (3). Therefore, the true incidence of structural lesions in *all people* with MTBIs is likely far less than these estimates.

---

[2] The original neuropathology studies were based on patients with severe TBIs who were rendered in a persistent vegetative state or with severe dementia.

injury (48, 51, 52). Further, it was considered that the brainstem was the focus of injury (53, 54). Taken together, these studies have led numerous clinicians and researchers to conclude that acceleration/deceleration injuries result in shear strains within the cranial vault, and these in turn lead to shearing of neurons and blood vessels occurring principally in the brainstem. Although no one doubts the existence of shearing strains as the primary pathophysiologic mechanism responsible for damage to axons, the pathophysiologic sequence that leads to traumatic injury to neurons is "a process, not an event" (Ref. 55, p. 163).

The Ommaya and Gennarelli (56) model of TBI suggested that acceleration/deceleration forces can cause mechanical strains that occur in a "centripetal sequence." Injuries of this nature occur when the head is propelled through space and is abruptly stopped by a solid object, such as the ground, or when the head is set into motion, such as when a car is struck from behind by another car. With mild forces, the sequence begins at the surface of the brain and then progressively affects deeper structures as forces become more severe.

Based on their original classification system, the authors postulated three critical predictions. First, when the degree of trauma is sufficient to produce LOC, cortex and subcortical white matter will be primarily affected, with damage to cortex and its associated white matter being more severe than that found in the rostral brainstem. Second, damage to the rostral brainstem will not occur without more severe damage occurring in the cortex and subcortical structures, because the mesencephalon is the last area to be affected by such centripetal forces Third, cognitive symptoms such as confusion and disturbance of memory can occur without LOC; however, the reverse cannot occur (i.e., LOC cannot occur without accompanying cognitive symptoms) (56). In addition to these critical predictions, the theory reinforced three important aspects of how TBI can occur and the potential effects that different acceleration/deceleration forces have on the brain. First, it reinforced the principle that the *direction* of force can determine severity of injury. Second, a continuum of injury exists whereby mild, moderate, and severe brain injuries caused by acceleration/deceleration forces are not discrete entities but occur on a continuum. This continuum occurs from the surface of the brain inward with increasing amounts of damage occurring at each level of depth as forces increase (49, 57). Third, acceleration/deceleration forces alone are sufficient to cause severe TBI, as supported by research in human trauma cases (58–61). Understanding the importance of acceleration/deceleration forces and their role in the pathophysiology of MTBI can be seen in the number of methods that are being developed to measure these forces in motor vehicles (62) and in athletes (63–66).

It is important to link the presence of acceleration/deceleration forces with the primary mechanism of injury in the neuron-axonal (and potentially dendritic) stretching. Recent studies have shown that axons of cultured human neurons have a remarkable capacity for stretch with no primary axotomy observed with strains below 65 percent of the length of the axon. In addition, axons exhibit the behavior of "delayed elasticity." In other words, stretch causes a temporary deformation of an axon that gradually returns to the original orientation and morphology even though internal damage was sustained (67). Once stretched, a pathophysiologic process begins that can lead to further structural change and metabolic dysfunction. First, strain on the axonal membrane causes an abnormal influx of Na^+ through mechanosensitive sodium channels, a reversal of the Na^+–Ca^{2+} exchangers, and activation of voltage-gated Ca^{2+} channels (68). This in turn causes selective proteolysis or a breakdown of Na^+ channels and progressively increasing levels of intra-axonal Ca^{2+} (69). The massive influx of Ca^{2+} leads to damage to the axonal cytoskeleton and initiates the pathophysiological process that follows.

Stretching of axons has functional and structural implications. In an animal model, stretch below four millimetres (mm) did not cause any morphological change in axons, a stretch of five mm produced changes in visual evoked potentials that were significantly different from controls, with a six mm stretch causing morphological change including retraction balls and axonal swellings (70). Therefore, a single acceleration/deceleration event might result in (a) no apparent change in structure or function, (b) functional or metabolic change, or (c) eventual structural change in the axon. These outcomes are dependent on the force applied to the brain.

Metabolic dysfunction that occurs in neurons following their exposure to acceleration/deceleration forces and blunt trauma has been recently reviewed (7, 71). Both reviews focus on compromised metabolic pathways that affect cellular energy production systems. Following axonal stretch, small ion species enter the axons at or near the nodes of Ranvier. This initiates metabolic dysfunction and when acceleration/deceleration forces are sufficiently high, will cause damage to the cytoskeleton and microtubules (this process will be described next) (43–46, 72–74). Immediately following this event, there is an indiscriminate release of neurotransmitters and uncontrolled ionic fluxes. The first of these are potassium (K^+) efflux and sustained calcium (Ca^{2+}) influx that activate pumps to restore cellular homeostasis. This will of course affect glucose utilization leading to dramatic increases in the local cerebral metabolic rates. Where this becomes problematic is when "hypermetabolism" occurs in the presence of decreased cerebral blood flow that can impact the functioning of ion pumps. In addition to increased glucose utilization, there may be impaired oxidative metabolism and diminished mitochondrial function. This can lead to the over-reliance on less efficient anaerobic metabolic pathways. The net effect can be elevated lactate and reduced intracellular magnesium levels (magnesium is a very important component for generation of adenosine-triphosphate [ATP-energy production], the initiation of protein synthesis, and the maintenance of the cellular membrane potential). Mitochondrial accumulations of Ca^{2+} can lead to metabolic dysfunction and eventually energy failure (7, 71).

Recently, animal experimentation has provided evidence that depressed mitochondrial functioning might be improved by treatment with hyperbaric oxygenation (75). (See Chapter 57 by McElligott and colleagues in this book for a discussion of this topic.) In humans, magnetic resonance spectroscopy has been useful in detecting additional metabolic changes that can occur following MTBI. N-acetylaspartate (NAA), a marker of neuronal axonal viability, total choline (Cho), a marker of membrane metabolism, total creatine (Cr), which reflects energy status, and lactate (Lac), an indicator of ischemia, were measured at 2–30 days following injury in 14 subjects with an average GCS score of 14.4 (range 13–15) and 10 of 14 with positive CT or MRI indicators of neurotrauma. Significant differences were found for the NAA/Cr ratio in parietal white matter, Cho/Cr ratio in occipital grey matter, and the NAA/Cho in four occipital lobe regions. All three ratios were different in temporal lobe compared to control. The ratios were consistent with decreased NAA and increased Cho found in severe TBI (26).

The sustained influx of Ca^{2+} has another important effect; the initiation of a pathophysiologic process of axonal injury. Axons contain numerous microscopic elements including microtubules and neurofilaments. Microtubules are thick cytoskeletal fibers and consist of long polar polymers constructed of protofilaments packed in a long tubular array. They are oriented longitudinally in relation to the axon and are associated with fast axonal transport (76). Neurofilaments are essentially the "bones" or cytoskeleton of the axon and are the most abundant intracellular structural element in axons (76). When acceleration/deceleration forces are sufficient, a massive influx of Ca^{2+} leads to damage to the axonal cytoskeleton and initiates the formation of axonal swellings. This process has been reviewed in detail by Gaetz (77) and will be summarized here.

The pathophysiologic events that lead to secondary axotomy associated with animal models of traumatic axonal injury (TAI)[3] occur within minutes of injury. Five minutes after a moderate injury, neurofilament networks appear dense or more tightly packed, and local mitochondrial abnormalities have been observed without any overt disruption of the overlying axolemma (74, 78). Within 30 minutes of a traumatic injury, scattered axons showed slight swelling, multiple swellings, and/or infolding of the axolemma. When this occurs, there can be focal neurofilament disarray and misalignment of the axon with local axolemmal infolding (74).

In the hours following injury, a gradual progression of axonal pathology occurs in the absence of local hemorrhage or damage in the surrounding tissue. Axonal swelling continues and focal aggregations of organelles occur (including mitochondria and neurotubules) with no physical tearing or shearing of the axon cylinder (43). Over a period of hours, this process leads to some axons having focal swellings with others in early stages of disconnection due to a disruption of axoplasmic transport (45). At three hr post-injury a further axonal change is observed including disconnection of the axon with continued expansion to form a mature reactive swelling. Some reactive axons display a proximal stump undergoing continued swelling due to increased accumulation of organelles capping an expanding neurofilamentous core (74). At four to six hr following brain injury, proximal and distal swellings are further enlarged, more complex, and are often separated by a thin strand of protein linking the two segments (43).[4] At 12–24 hr post-injury, Povlishock et al. (43) reported that swellings had progressed to resemble enlarged ball-like expansions with no continuity that could be identified between their proximal and distal axonal segments, suggesting an abrupt separation of the axon cylinder.

From 24 to 72 hr in animals, a further enlargement of cleanly separated axons was observed, with some showing what was assumed to be a regenerative attempt in the form of growth cones that protruded from reactive axonal swellings (45). At 24 hr in humans, the reactive swellings exhibit further change in their appearance and the process of axonal separation begins. From 30 hr to one week, grossly swollen axonal segments disconnected from one another are observable in humans (46, 73). At three to four days following injury, Povlishock and Becker (44) noted that the injury profiles differed from axon to axon. By 88 hr in humans, further progression of the reactive swellings had occurred with heterogeneity observed among the population of reactive axons (46).

At 5–7 days, various forms of reactive change were identified (44). This pattern continues until 9–14 days

---

[3]The term traumatic axonal injury has replaced diffuse axonal injury because the damage is to axons that tend to group in various areas of the brain and are therefore not considered truly "diffuse".

[4]This pathophysiologic process has been observed in humans following fatal motor vehicle accidents and *severe* brain injury (46, 73), although it appears to occur more slowly in humans. The degree to which this pathophysiological process occurs following MTBI, and the numbers and locations of cells involved, is unknown. Nonetheless, it very likely occurs in patients with MTBIs of the more serious nature, such as complicated MTBIs or MTBIs resulting from high speed motor vehicle accidents.

two conditions are predominant (44). In one group of cells, the degenerative response continued, displaying several retrogressive changes such as lobulation, increased electron density, and axolemmal/axoplasmic disruption, all of which were accompanied by focal macrophage accumulation. In another group of cells, a regenerative response was observed (44). At 17–30 days, regenerative or degenerative axonal changes predominated. Macrophages observed in the presence of degenerating axons actively phagocytosed the damaged swellings. Some of these pathophysiologic changes were observed by Oppenheimer (79) decades ago. Recently, Bigler (80) reported single case autopsy data showing "scattered macrophages in the white matter" in the frontal and temporal lobes in a patient with an MTBI who died from other causes several months post injury. This patient was in a high speed MVA, his vehicle was "demolished," he suffered cervical fractures due to projectiles, he had an initial GCS of 14, LOC of unknown duration, no significant post-traumatic amnesia, and a head CT that did not appear to show a trauma-related abnormality.

The changes observed in animal models and humans are consistent with a progressive series of neurophysiologic events initiated by acceleration/deceleration forces on the axon, and ending in some cases with a frank separation of proximal and distal axon segments. As Povlishock and Becker (44) stated, it had been long assumed that axonal shear or tensile force caused a physical disruption of the axon into a proximal and distal segment. These studies provide evidence contrary to the shearing hypothesis, and instead, suggest that even relatively low-intensity mechanical brain injury produces axonal change that is more subtle than that suggested previously (i.e., direct tearing of the axon).

Neuroscience has not only provided a new vantage point to consider the pathophysiology of injury, it has given us a better understanding about which neurons are vulnerable to injury. Early studies suggested that the brainstem was the primary site of injury (e.g., Refs 81, 82). However, recent studies point to cellular injury that does not specifically involve the brainstem, especially with injuries produced by mild to moderate forces. Various characteristics of neurons themselves appear to make them more susceptible to injury: when axons change direction, enter target nuclei, or when they decussate, they can be more easily damaged (45, 73, 79, 83, 84). Large caliber neurons are injured more often than smaller neurons that surround them (45). Of particular importance, injured axons are observed more often where a change in tissue density occurs, such as at the grey/white matter interface near cerebral cortex (49, 73, 84, 85), a finding supported by functional neurophysiology (86) and MRI. Because the cerebral cortex plays a substantial role in maintaining a distributed consciousness (87), trauma involving cortex and sub-cortical white matter will affect

consciousness because brainstem reticular cells will be suppressed due to a lack of input.

The features of cellular injury, dysfunction, and death have been described in detail in this section. It is important to appreciate that cell death is closely related to injury severity. Mild traumatic brain injuries, especially injuries on the milder end of the spectrum, are typically characterized by cellular dysfunction that is reversible. There is a continuum of injury, at the cellular level, ranging from completely and rapidly reversible cellular dysfunction, to slow but complete recovery, to slow and incomplete recovery, to cell death. Very mild concussions likely produce virtually no permanent damage to cells resulting in long-term symptoms or problems whereas severe traumatic brain injuries, especially those involving considerable forces, often produce widespread cellular death and dysfunction with clear functional consequences; complicated MTBIs and moderate TBIs likely fall in between.

S-100B AS A MARKER OF INJURY AND A PREDICTOR OF OUTCOME

Over the past decade, there has been an increased interest in the role of various biochemical markers for use as diagnostic and prognostic measures of brain damage in the first few days post-TBI (88, 89). Biochemical markers are of great interest because they may provide a more cost effective and efficient measurement of brain damage than can be assessed in the acute treatment phase. Clinicians typically rely on static imaging techniques such as CT and MRI to determine the extent of brain damage. However, CT scanning tends to have a low sensitivity to diffuse brain damage and the availability of MRI is limited in many settings dues to high costs (89). There is a growing body of research literature suggesting that the neuroprotein S-100B may be a reliable marker for brain damage (e.g., 88–95). S-100B is a calcium binding protein which is found in high concentrations in astroglial and Schwann cells, predominantly in the central nervous system. When these cells are structurally or ischemically damaged, it is believed that S-100B is rapidly released into the cerebrospinal fluid (CSF) and secondarily across the blood-CSF barrier into circulation (91). Measurements of S-100B are acquired from serum obtained from a standard blood sample (90). If the neuroprotein S-100B could be established as a reliable marker of brain damage, S-100B has the potential to serve as a cost-effective measure to (a) initially screen patients in the first hr post injury to detect brain damage, (b) monitor the occurrence of secondary complications during recovery, and (c) be used to predict future outcome (96).

Researchers have reported that the concentration level of S-100B is significantly higher in patients with MTBIs than in controls (91, 94, 97, 98). Unlike Glasgow

Coma Scale (GCS) scores, the presence of alcohol at the time of injury does not influence the serum concentrations of S-100B in patients with MTBIs or healthy controls (92, 98), even in injured patients with blood alcohol levels of 2.5 to 5 times (i.e., 250–500 mg/dl) the legal level of intoxication (91).

Researchers have reported that S-100B levels are associated with (a) the presence of brain abnormalities detected by CT scans (91, 95, 98, 99), (b) prediction of severe outcome 1 month post-injury as measured by the Extended Glasgow Outcome Scale (100), (c) the rate of failure to return to work 1 week post-injury in patients with very mild brain injuries (101), (d) injury severity as measured by the GCS and the Coma Remission scale (95, 97, 99, 102, 103), and (e) the presence of neuropsychological deficits 2 weeks and 6 months post-injury (95). However, not all studies have been as favorable. Some researchers have reported that S-100B levels taken directly after injury are *not* associated neuropsychological test results at 7 to 21 days post injury in an uncomplicated mild TBI sample (104) or with PCS symptom reporting 1-year following MTBI (105).

Although much of the research in this area does support a relationship between S-100B levels and outcome following MTBI, there are a number of limitations of using S-100B as a diagnostic marker for brain damage in this population. S-100B tends to be a sensitive marker for brain damage, but not a very specific marker. Various studies have examined the clinical value of S-100B levels to predict various outcomes from TBI such as abnormal CT scans (91, 97, 99, 103), abnormal MRI scans (106), severe disability as measured by the Extended Glasgow Outcome Scale scores (100), and return to work rates (101). A summary of the sensitivity, specificity, and predictive power values for S-100B to predict these outcomes is presented in Table 22-5. The results from these studies are remarkably consistent. Across all studies, sensitivity is high to very high (range = 80–100 percent) and specificity is moderate to high (range = 40.5–81 percent). However, positive predictive power (PPP) values are low to moderate (range = 21–40.5 percent). In contrast, negative predictive power (NPP) is very high (range = 95.1–100 percent).[5] Ideally, it is preferred for all four measures to be high. However, in these studies, only sensitivity and NPP have acceptable values. Nonetheless, these studies can provide some important information for prediction of outcome from MTBI using S-100B. These studies suggest that although S-100B *is not useful* for identifying individuals who are "at risk" of poor outcome from TBI (i.e., PPP), it *is useful* for identifying those individuals who are "*not* at risk" of poor outcome from TBI (i.e., NPP; individuals who will have a good outcome

post-injury). As a diagnostic tool, the practical implication of this finding is that S-100B measures will misidentify a significant portion of individuals "not at risk" (i.e., good outcome) as being "at risk" (i.e., poor outcome). That is, the test will be positive and they will falsely be labelled as being at risk for poor outcome. Theoretically, this could lead to unnecessary treatment or unnecessary worry for the patient. To our knowledge, there is no research that has compared the diagnostic accuracy of S-100B to current clinical decision rules.

Another limitation is the extracranial release of S-100B (105). Elevated S-100B levels have been found in trauma patients who *have not* sustained a head injury (107) and in healthy subjects involved in various sports (108–110). Anderson and colleagues found that S-100B levels measured immediately after admission to the emergency department were most elevated in trauma control subjects who had incurred bone fractures. However, patients with soft-tissue injuries and burns also had elevated S-100B levels that were 40 times greater than healthy controls[6] (107). Researchers examining athletes have found that the release of S-100B increases after various sporting activities compared to pre-activity levels (108–110). However, participation in certain sports results in the release of S-100B levels differently. Otto and colleagues found that competitive boxing resulted in the highest increase of S-100B, followed by jogging, running, 25km race, and sparring (108). Stalnacke and colleagues also found similar increases in S-100B levels in elite basketball, ice hockey, and soccer players (109, 110). Otto and colleagues hypothesised that the increase in S-100B after running activities may be the result from "brain tissue, axial vibration of the brain at each step" during the jogging and running action (108). This hypothesis, however, is purely speculative at this time. Although these studies do show that participation in various sports increases S-100B levels, the increase is lower than in patients who have sustained an MTBI (108, 111).

Methodological differences between studies make drawing any conclusions regarding the efficacy of S-100B as a useful marker for brain injury difficult. One major methodological difference relates to the time post-injury S-100B is measured. Measurement of S-100B greatly varies across studies ranging from as quickly as 44 minutes post-injury (93) to as long as 27 hr post-injury (95, 102). The majority of studies have measured S-100B within either 2 hr (97, 98, 100), 4 hr (99, 101, 103, 105), or 6 hr post-injury (94, 104, 112). This is an important issue because it is thought that S-100B levels rapidly increase in the circulation system within the first few minutes of injury, reaching a concentration peak within 20 min (91). S-100B is then eliminated quickly by renal

---

[5] See the table note in Table 22-5 for an explanation of these statistics.

[6] This study highlights the importance of comparing trauma controls to TBI in research studies.

TABLE 22-5

Summary of Sensitivity, Specificity and Predictive Power Values of S-100B Levels to Predict Outcome

First Author	N	Country	Setting	Sample Type	Time of Blood Sample	S-100B Criteria	Outcome	Sen.	Spec.	PPP	NPP
Stranjalis 2004	93	Greece	Hospital ED	MTBI (GCS = 15)	3 hr	0.15 µg/L	Failure to return to work 1 week post-injury (Yes/No)	80	74.4	37.5	95.1
Mussack 2002	20	Germany	Level 1 Trauma	Severe TBI (GCS 3–8)	M = 43.8 min (range 22.6–72.4 min)	0.76 ng/mL	"Unfavorable outcome" defined by GOS = 1–3	100	50	24.1	100
Biberthaler 2001	52	Germany	Level 1 Trauma	MTBI (GCS 13–15)	116 mins (SD = 18.8 mins)	0.1 ng/mL	Abnormal CT scan	100	40.5	40.5	100
Townend 2002	148	England	Hospital ED x 4	Mild-Severe TBI (88 percent GCS = 15)	M = 130 mins	0.32 µg/L	Severe disability at 1 month post-injury: GOSE < 5	93	72	33	99
Ingebrigtsen 2000	182	Norway Sweden Denmark	Hospital ED	MTBI (GCS = 13–15)	Within 3 hr	0.2 µg/L	Abnormal CT scan	90	65	13	99
Ingebrigtsen 1999	48	Norway Sweden Denmark	Hospital ED	MTBI	Within 6 hr	0.2 µg/L	Abnormal MRI scan	80	81	33	97
Romner 2000	278	Norway Sweden Denmark	Hospital ED	Mild-Severe TBI (91 percent MTBI)	M = 3.8 hr (range = 0.5 to 24 hr)	0.2 µg/L	Abnormal CT scan	92	66	21	99

Note: GOSE = Extended Glasgow Outcome Scale; GOS = Glasgow Outcome Scale; Sen = Sensitivity; Spec = Specificity; PPP = Positive predictive power; NPP = Negative predictive power.

For these studies, sensitivity, specificity, and predictive power statistics evaluate the ability of S-100B levels to predict; for example, abnormal CT and MRI scans, severe disability as measured by the GOSE, and return to work rates. Sensitivity is the true positive rate for a test/measure. It answers the question: knowing that the individual has a positive CT scan (for example), what percentage of these individuals will actually be correctly identified as having a positive CT scan using S-100B. Specificity is the true negative rate for a test/measure. It answers the question: knowing that that individual has a negative CT scan, what percentage of these individuals will actually be correctly identified as having a negative CT scan using S-100B. However, positive predictive power (PPP) and negative predictive power (NPP) are the statistics most suited as a diagnostic tool in a clinical setting (n = 1). These statistics provide us with information relating to how confident we can be, in terms of a percentage, that a given score on a test/measure actually predicts what the test is designed to predict. PPP statistics answer the question: knowing that the person has been classified as likely to have a positive CT scans based on S-100B, what is the probability that the person will actually have a positive CT scan. On the other hand, NPP statistics answers the question: knowing that the person has been identified as likely to have a negative CT scan using S-100B, what is the probability that the person will actually have a negative CT scan when scanned.

Sources: Strangalis 2004 (101); Mussack 2002 (91); Biberthaler 2001 (97); Townend 2002 (100); Ingebrigtsen 2000 (103); Ingebrigtsen 1999* (106).
*Data extracted from Ingebrigtsen and Romner (88).

metabolism and urinary excretion (113), with a number of studies demonstrating a significant decline in S-100B within the first few hours after injury (e.g., 95, 99, 102, 105). S-100B is estimated to have a biological half-life ranging from 30 to 113 min (91, 113, 114). To date, there is no consensus in the literature on the dynamics of S-100B after TBI (104) or when is the right time to measure it (105). There is a lack of knowledge regarding how quickly S-100B is released following injury and how quickly it is eliminated by the body (104). While current research shows promise for S-100B as a marker for brain damage, much more research will be required before this biochemical marker will be accepted as a reliable measure of brain injury. Future research must strive to understand the dynamics (i.e., time of release and elimination) of S-100B after TBI and employ trauma control subjects to determine whether S-100B levels are unique to TBI.

NEUROPSYCHOLOGICAL OUTCOME

Historically, some researchers and clinicians believed that loss of consciousness (LOC) was necessary for the *diagnosis* of MTBI. In the 1920s, Symonds (115) discussed the importance of traumatic LOC as an essential feature of concussion. He said that in

> the initial stage the patient is completely unconscious and in a state of flaccid paralysis. In a severe case the respiratory and cardiac functions may hardly continue. In a few minutes recovery begins; the visceral reflexes are the first to return, and vomiting is common at this stage. The other cerebral functions recover more gradually, and there may be a phase of some hr during which consciousness is clouded. Following this again there may be complaint of headache and giddiness, but at the end of twenty-four hr in an uncomplicated case of concussion recovery should be complete." (p. 829)

Of course, it has been recognized for many years that concussions can occur without LOC (e.g., 116). In fact, the vast majority of injuries in sports (117–119) and many injuries in medical trauma settings (e.g., 120–122) are not associated with LOC. The presence or duration of LOC is not always used as a criterion for MTBI in research studies (see Ref. 10 for a review).

The more interesting question is whether brief loss of consciousness is associated with worse outcome. Gennarelli and colleagues conducted an extraordinary series of primate studies (e.g., 123) illustrating that both the presence of diffuse axonal injury (i.e., traumatic axonal injury) and functional outcome are associated with duration of unconsciousness (i.e., coma). It is certainly well known that an *extended* period of unconsciousness/coma in humans is associated with poor long-term outcome. Repeated demonstrations in the literature of worse outcome

associated with more severe brain injuries—as defined by duration of coma—can understandably influence scientific beliefs regarding the importance of traumatic LOC in *very mild* injuries, such as those sustained in sports. There is no doubt, as a general rule, that patients with comas lasting 1–2 weeks have worse outcome than patients with comas lasting less than 24 hr (e.g., 124). However, this logic should not be assumed to hold true for MTBI. Researchers studying trauma patients have reported that there is no association between *brief* loss of consciousness and short-term neuropsychological outcome (e.g., 121, 125, 126) or vocational outcome (120). Some researchers examining *athletes* with concussions have reported an association between LOC and immediate or short-term outcome (e.g., 127–129), while others have not (e.g., 130, 131). However, athletes with concussions, as a rule, recover relatively quickly and fully (see the chapter by Collins, Iverson, Gaetz, and Lovell in this book for a review). Therefore, based on the literature to date, it would be a mistake to assume that brief LOC is a reliable predictor of worse short-, medium-, or long-term outcome in trauma patients.

Post-Traumatic Confusion and Amnesia

Post-traumatic amnesia (PTA) has been related to outcome in many (e.g., 132–136) but not all (e.g., 137) studies involving patients with moderate to severe traumatic brain injuries. By inference, mainly, it is often presumed that PTA is also a predictor of outcome following mild traumatic brain injury. However, the duration of PTA in mild cases is difficult to determine because, by definition, it is a relatively short period of time and it is rarely assessed prospectively. The accuracy of retrospective reports of PTA is questionable.

Post-traumatic amnesia lasting more than 30 min in patients with MTBIs has been associated with cerebral hypoperfusion on day-of-injury SPECT scans (33). The presence and duration of post-traumatic confusion/ amnesia has been associated with worse immediate outcome and slower recovery in athletes (128–130, 138, 139). Again, the literature regarding athletes is less relevant because they tend to recover quickly.[7] For trauma patients, there appears to be a relation between post-traumatic confusion/amnesia and short-term neuropsychological outcome (see the original data presented in Tables 22-7 and 22-8), but by three months post-injury this association may disappear (140). Some researchers have reported that duration of post-traumatic amnesia is related to one-year return to work rates, but this effect

---

[7]Athletes tend to be young, very healthy, highly motivated, and they usually don't have co-morbid conditions that might slow down recovery from MTBI or mimic the postconcussion syndrome in the post-acute period.

TABLE 22-6
Demographic and Injury Severity Variables by Post-Injury Confusion Groups

Variable	GOAT > 89 (N = 527)	GOAT < 90 (N = 227)
Age	26.0 (6.9)	26.1 (6.4)
Education	12.1 (1.8)	11.8 (2.0)
Gender	Male = 69.3 percent	Male = 72.7 percent
Race	Caucasian = 94.7 percent	Caucasian = 93.4 percent
	African-American = 3.3 percent	African-American = 5.5 percent
	Hispanic = 1.9 percent	Hispanic = 1.1 percent
Skull Fracture	18.0 percent	18.5 percent
Abnormal CT	12.5 percent	16.9 percent
GCS = 15	89.9 percent	73.6 percent
GCS = 14	10.1 percent	26.4 percent
Positive LOC	60.4 percent	65.7 percent
Negative or Equivocal LOC	39.6 percent	34.3 percent

GOAT = Galveston Orientation and Amnesia Test; GCS = Glasgow Coma Scale

TABLE 22-7
Neuropsychological Test Results for Persons With Versus Without Evidence of Post-Injury Confusion or Amnesia and Negative CT-Scans

Variable	GOAT > 89 (N = 175)		GOAT < 90 (N = 157)		P	Effect Size
	M	SD	M	SD		
Trails A	28.3	9.3	31.0	12.0	<.026	.25
Trails B	69.1	25.8	84.6	43.9	<.001	.43
COWAT	37.1	9.0	35.1	10.3	<.070	.21
WCST-64 Categories	3.6	1.4	3.4	1.5	<.422	.09
WCST-64 Perseverative Responses	9.9	7.3	10.0	7.4	<.929	.01
HVLT Total	24.3	3.9	22.1	4.7	<.001	.52
HVLT Delay	8.3	2.4	7.0	2.9	<.001	.47
Logical Memory I	23.6	6.3	21.8	6.7	<.024	.27
Logical Memory II	19.2	7.3	16.5	8.0	<.004	.36
Visual Reproduction I	33.5	4.9	32.0	5.9	<.018	.28
Visual Reproduction II	30.4	6.6	26.9	9.0	<.001	.44
Logical Memory Savings	80.4	20.1	72.2	24.4	<.004	1.12
Visual Reproduction Savings	90.3	14.6	82.4	22.0	<.001	.42
Digits Forward	8.8	1.8	7.8	2.0	<.001	.54
Digits Backward	6.5	2.2	5.8	2.3	<.006	.32

COWAT = Controlled Oral Word Association Test; WCST-64 = Wisconsin Card Sorting Test – 64; HVLT = Hopkins Verbal Learning Test. Effect Sizes (Cohen's d): small = .2, medium = .5, and large = .8.

was mostly due to the inclusion of patients with moderate TBIs and PTA greater than 24 hr (141).

Complicated MTBIs

Commonsense would suggest that patients with complicated MTBIs (i.e., bleeding, bruising, or swelling on their day-of-injury CT) would have worse short-, medium-, and long-term outcome than patients without obvious structural damage. Surprisingly, the literature is somewhat mixed on this issue. In most studies, patients with complicated MTBIs perform more poorly on neuropsychological tests in the initial days and weeks post injury (142–144), and they appear to have worse 6–12 month

TABLE 22-8
Neuropsychological Test Results for Patients with Abnormal CT-Scans

VARIABLE	GOAT > 89 (N = 25)		GOAT < 90 (N = 32)			
	M	SD	M	SD	P	EFFECT SIZE
Trails A	33.6	15.4	32.6	9.4	<.765	.08
Trails B	88.8	37.0	95.8	41.3	<.523	.18
COWAT	27.9	9.0	31.1	10.7	<.239	.33
WCST-64 Categories	3.5	1.3	2.8	1.7	<.064	.53
WCST-64 Perseverative Responses	11.6	8.5	16.7	17.1	<.169	.38
HVLT Total	22.3	4.5	20.2	4.5	<.167	.46
HVLT Delay	7.6	2.6	4.5	2.7	<.002	1.15
Logical Memory I	22.7	7.3	21.4	7.2	<.542	.18
Logical Memory II	17.0	8.1	11.6	8.4	<.028	.65
Visual Reproduction I	33.7	5.2	29.2	7.1	<.015	.71
Visual Reproduction II	30.9	5.1	21.5	9.6	<.001	1.23
Logical Memory Savings	70.4	26.0	51.8	30.8	<.030	.65
Visual Reproduction Savings	92.3	11.9	71.6	24.0	<.001	1.09
Digits Forward	7.9	1.9	7.9	2.1	<.972	.01
Digits Backward	5.7	2.0	5.8	1.8	<.845	.05

COWAT = Controlled Oral Word Association Test; WCST-64 = Wisconsin Card Sorting Test – 64; HVLT = Hopkins Verbal Learning Test. Effect Sizes (Cohen's d): small = .2, medium = .5, and large = .8.

(11, 30, 145) and 3–5 year (146) outcomes than patients with uncomplicated MTBIs. In contrast, some researchers have reported no differences (120) or equivocal differences associated with early structural abnormalities (36, 147). In a well-controlled prospective study, McCauley and colleagues reported that CT abnormalities were not associated with increased risk for postconcussion syndrome at 3 months post injury (148).

Original Research: Relation Between Post-Traumatic Confusion and Neuropsychological Outcome

There has been very little research that has examined the relation between post-traumatic amnesia and short-term neuropsychological outcome in trauma patients. We present here original data in a carefully defined sample of young adult trauma patients with mild traumatic brain injuries who completed neuropsychological testing within the first week post injury. Participants were selected from a large database (N = 1,695) of patients seen on the Trauma Service of Allegheny General Hospital in Pittsburgh, Pennsylvania between May of 1991 and June of 1994. The basic clinical pathway for any person with known or suspected brain injury, irrespective of severity, involved a GCS rating, skull x-ray, CT scan of the brain, and an assessment of post-traumatic amnesia with the Galveston Orientation and Amnesia Test (GOAT; 149).

To be included in this study, patients must have (a) had a GCS score of 14 or 15, (b) been under 40 years of age, and (c) been tested within *seven days post injury*. The total sample consisted of 484 patients who met these criteria. The average age of the total sample was 26.0 (SD = 6.7) years and their average education was 11.9 (SD = 1.9) years. Seventy-one percent were male and 29 percent were female. The mechanisms of injury for the patients were as follows: (i) motor vehicle accident without seatbelt = 47.5 percent, (ii) motor vehicle accident with seatbelt = 15.1 percent, (iii) falls = 10.1 percent, (iv) motorcycle with helmet = 7.6 percent, (v) struck by object = 6.2 percent, (vi) pedestrian = 4.3 percent, (vii) other = 4.1 percent, (viii) missing = 3.5 percent, and (ix) motorcycle with no helmet = 1.5 percent. Eighteen percent had GCS scores of 14 and 82 percent had scores of 15. The breakdown regarding loss of consciousness for the sample was 55.6 percent positive, 17.8 percent negative, 15.1 percent equivocal, and 11.6 percent missing. Skull fractures were present in 16.1 percent, absent in 72.3 percent, and missing in 11.6 percent of cases. The prevalence of intracranial abnormalities on day-of-injury CT was 11.8 percent. The remaining subjects had negative (68.6 percent) or missing (19.6 percent) results. Because 19.6 percent of the sample either did not undergo CT-scanning or their results were not coded into the database, it can be assumed that the actual prevalence of intracranial abnormalities was higher than 11.8 percent.

The patients underwent 35–45 minutes of neuropsychological testing. The tests administered are listed in Tables 22-7 and 22-8. Trails A and B are from the Halstead-Reitan Neuropsychological Battery (150). As tests of information processing speed, they require visual-motor tracking and sequencing. The Trails B test is more difficult because it requires set shifting (i.e., alternating between numbers and letters) during the sequencing task. Digit Span, Logical Memory, and Visual Reproduction were administered from the Wechsler Memory Scale-Revised (151). The ability to repeat a series of digits forward and backward is a measure of attention-concentration and mental control. The Logical Memory (LM) subtest is a memory test for stories. Two stories are read, one at a time, and the subject is asked to recall everything he or she can remember from the story. There is an immediate recall trial (Logical Memory I) and a 30-minute delayed recall trial (Logical Memory II). The LM percent retention score reflects the percentage of information retained after the delay interval (i.e., LMII/LMI). The Visual Reproduction subtest is a memory test for geometric designs. Each design is presented to the subject for 10 seconds, removed, and then the subject is instructed to draw it from memory. After 30 minutes the subject is asked to reproduce all of the previously presented designs (Visual Reproduction II; VRII). The Visual Reproduction retention score is derived by dividing VRII by VRI. The Controlled Oral Word Association Test (152) is a measure of lexical verbal fluency. Patients are given a letter of the alphabet (e.g., C, F, or L) and asked to orally-generate as many words that they can that begin with that letter.

The Wisconsin Card Sorting Test-64 (WCST-64; 153–154) is an abbreviated version on the WCST (155). The WCST contains two decks of 64 cards that the patient must sort on the basis of certain characteristics. This is a nonverbal problem-solving test. The WCST-64 employs only the first of the two decks (156). The Hopkins Verbal Learning Test (HVLT; 157) is a 12-item, three trial word list learning test. The original test has been modified to contain a delayed recall and recognition trial, and normative data are available (158).

The patients were sorted into two groups on the basis of their GOAT scores. Those with GOAT scores of 90 or more were viewed as having no obvious, sustained post-injury confusion. Those patients with scores below 90 were considered to have possible to probable post-injury confusion or amnesia. A score of 90 was the closest value to a median split, with 53 percent of the total sample in the higher group and 47 percent in the lower group. Demographic and injury severity characteristics of the two groups are presented in Table 22-6. The patients with lower GOAT scores had a greater proportion of subjects with GCS scores of 14 (X^2 (1) = 22.0, p < .001). The groups did not differ in their proportions of patients with skull fractures ($p < .90$), CT abnormalities ($p < .22$), or loss of consciousness ($p < .27$).

Descriptive statistics, mean comparisons, and effect sizes for the neuropsychological tests in the patients with *normal* CT-scans by group are presented in Table 22-7. The groups did not differ in age (t (482) = −.16, p < .88) or education (t (461) = 1.6, $p < .12$). The groups did not differ in gender ($p < .41$) or in race ($p < .49$), based on chi square analyses. The patients with high versus low GOAT scores were compared using parametric or nonparametric pairwise tests. Levene's test for equality of variances was used to determine whether the t-test was appropriate, or whether a nonparametric test should be used. The Kolmogorov-Smirnov procedure was used to determine whether the variables had non-normal distributions. Although the t-test is rather robust in regards to violations of general linear model assumptions (e.g., normally distributed variables and homogeneity of variance), nonparametric analyses (i.e., Mann-Whitney U tests) were conducted on most variables because heterogeneity of variance or non-normal distributions were present. The probability of Type 1 error increases when multiple statistical comparisons are conducted, so the reader should have the most confidence in findings that are below $p = .01$. Using this criterion, the patients with lower GOAT scores also scored significantly worse on Trails B, HVLT total and delayed recall scores, Logical Memory II and savings scores, Visual Reproduction II, and Digit Span Forward and Backward.

Descriptive statistics, mean comparisons, and effect sizes for the neuropsychological tests in the patients with *abnormal* CT-scans are presented in Table 22-8. The groups did not differ in age (t (55) = −.8, $p < .43$) or education (t (52) = .5, $p < .61$). The patients with high versus low GOAT scores were compared with parametric (i.e., independent t-tests) and nonparametric (i.e., Mann Whitney U) tests using the same procedures as reported for the patients with normal CT-scans. Although there were fewer significant findings, there was still a clear pattern of worse neuropsychological test performance in persons with lower GOAT scores. It should be noted that the significance values in Table 22-8, as compared to Table 22-7, are reduced as a function of sample size. By examining estimated effect sizes, it can be seen that variables with medium to large effect sizes, if stable, would be "more significant" if the sample sizes were increased.

In the present investigation, patients were sorted on the basis of their GOAT scores into high and low groups through an approximate median split. This is not a conventional method for examining GOAT scores. Rather, it is an attempt to estimate more subtle aspects of post-injury confusion as opposed to simply identifying frank PTA (i.e., GOAT scores below 75, which infrequently occur in people with MTBIs). The groups did not differ in age, education, gender, race, frequency of skull fracture, frequency of abnormal CT scans, or frequency of positive LOC. Not surprisingly, at admission, those with lower GOAT scores had lower GCS scores (i.e., a greater proportion had scores of 14). On the neuropsychological tests, significant differences emerged on several variables measuring aspects of concentration, processing speed, learning, verbal memory, and visual memory. This same methodology, when applied to similar groups but with loss of consciousness (LOC) as the independent variable, failed to reveal any significant differences on the neuropsychological tests (121, 125, 159). Therefore, when trauma patients are evaluated shortly after an MTBI, there is good evidence that post-traumatic confusion is related to worse short-term neuropsychological outcome and good evidence that brief traumatic LOC (e.g., less than 5 min) is *not* related to short-term neuropsychological outcome. Of course, these findings relate to short-term outcome (first few weeks post injury). To best understand long-term outcome, one should consider the results from several recent meta-analytic reviews of the literature.

Results From Meta-Analyses

A large number of prospective studies and several recent meta-analyses have greatly enhanced our understanding of the natural history of MTBI. Trauma patients and athletes often report extensive symptoms, and they perform more poorly on neuropsychological tests, in the initial days (118, 119, 128, 147, 160, 161) and up to the first month following the injury (e.g., 118, 140, 162, 163, 164). Due to natural recovery, neuropsychological decrements typically are not seen in athletes after 2–21 days (3, 118, 119, 160, 161, 165), and in trauma patients after 1–3 months (e.g., 140, 166, 167) or certainly a year (e.g., 124, 168–171) in prospective group studies. Several meta-analyses (4, 6, 8, 172) and recent reviews (5, 7, 173) of this literature are available and, as a rule, report very good neuropsychological outcome from MTBI.

Clinicians and researchers should carefully, deliberately, and critically read the literature relating to MTBI in trauma. Historically, the majority of studies over the decades have not been carefully controlled or prospective. It is essential to study the selection criteria and methods to appreciate the characteristics of the sample and the population to which that sample might generalize. Over the decades, there have been varying degrees of prevailing beliefs and themes that MTBIs (a) are minor injuries with no long-term consequences, (b) are serious injuries that frequently result in significant long-term consequences, or (c) are significant injuries that result in short-term consequences for most people and medium-term consequences for some. A person holding any particular belief or bias regarding MTBI can easily support that

view using select studies within the existing literature. It is getting increasingly difficult, however, to find good scientific evidence that MTBIs are associated with demonstrable cognitive deficits or symptoms that are due to the biological effects of the injury in more than a small minority[8] of patients who are more than 3 months post-injury.

Neuropsychological meta-analyses allow us to quantify the effects of certain injuries, conditions, or diseases on cognitive functioning. These aggregated estimates of effect size are important because they consider the literature as a whole and typically are based on hundreds, if not thousands, of subjects. The fact that clinical groups overlap substantially with the normal population, and with each other, is poorly understood amongst clinicians and researchers. Researchers, reporting the results from individual studies, emphasize the differences between groups that are statistically significant, and then write that group A could be "differentiated" from group B on the basis of these statistically significant findings. Small differences between groups can be statistically significant, but what is typically not reported is that the two groups are far more similar than they are dissimilar. Clearly, small statistically significant differences between groups might not have any practical, clinical, or real-world significance.

The distributions of neuropsychological test performance across diagnoses, circumstances, or conditions, based on meta-analytic reviews of the literature, are illustrated in Figure 22-1. The shaded line in the middle represents the average score for healthy normal adults (i.e., a z-score of zero). The upper and lower shaded lines represent the expected scores for 50 percent of healthy adults. Similarly, 80 percent of healthy adults are expected to score between the solid lines. As seen in the second column, 90 percent of normal adults are expected to score between the upper and lower "90." The ranges of scores for all of the clinical groups are based on the theoretical normal distribution. Deviations from normal (i.e., neuropsychological deficits) are based on the effect sizes reported in the meta-analyses, and for each clinical group one can see the spread of scores expected for 80 percent and 90 percent of that particular group.

In the third column, notice that athletes tested within the first 24 hr post-injury have a marked deviation from normal (effect size of −1.0), similar to the deviation seen in patients with moderate to severe traumatic brain injuries who are tested within the first six months post injury (effect size of −1.0). This illustrates the major adverse effect of concussion on neuropsychological functioning immediately after injury. However, after seven

---

[8]This "small minority' cannot be determined at this time but it is likely less than the 15-20 percent estimates in the past literature.

days (column 5), concussed athletes' neuropsychological functioning has essentially returned to normal[9] (as reported in this meta-analysis of the literature). Notice that there are relatively small deviations from normal in patients with MTBIs, and by 1–3 months post injury they cannot be distinguished from the general population. The effects of MTBI on neuropsychological functioning, after the acute recovery period, are considerably less than the effects of litigation, depression, or ADHD. A striking feature of Figure 22-1 is the substantial overlap in expected scores across the clinical groups. In other words, the overall neuropsychological test performances of people in these groups are much more similar than they are dissimilar.

Clearly, our ability to accurately detect cognitive and neurobehavioral decrements associated with an MTBI, through interview, rating scales, or neuropsychological testing, diminishes in tandem with the passage of time. This, of course, is due to recovery. Nonetheless, in clinical practice, we frequently see patients who do not return to their pre-injury level of functioning and who are highly symptomatic. These patients frequently are conceptualized as having poor outcome following an MTBI, and the MTBI is believed to be the direct and/or indirect cause of the poor outcome. These people are typically diagnosed with the controversial persistent postconcussion syndrome.

Differential diagnosis is very important in these cases. The clinician should try to identify and treat the underlying cause, or causes, of these symptoms and problems (which can be diverse, and include cranial and/or cranial adnexal injury, cervical injury, psychological problems and disorders, or pain disorders). Ideally, clinicians should try to *prevent* poor outcome in people who have suffered a MTBI. There is reasonably good evidence that early intervention, as simple as education and reassurance of a likely good outcome, can be effective for reducing symptoms and problems in most patients.

EARLY INTERVENTION

A number of intervention protocols designed to minimize persisting problems following MTBI have been described in the literature for some time (e.g., 174–176). In the early studies, researchers reported that simple intervention programs applied within the first 3 weeks post-injury can reduce the number and frequency of post-concussion symptoms (177) and increase return to work rates (178).

The content of early intervention programs varies, ranging from, at minimum, the provision of an educational brochure containing information regarding the effects of MTBI (e.g., Ref. 179) to a more comprehensive intervention program that couples educational material with various forms of treatment (e.g., access to a multi-disciplinary outpatient brain injury program; e.g., Ref. 180) and/or assessment (e.g., neuropsychological; e.g., 181)[10]. Providing educational information is a standard component in the majority of studies. Although the content of the educational sessions varies, these sessions typically aim to provide information regarding common symptoms, likely time course of recovery, reassurance of recovery, and suggested coping strategies following MTBI (e.g., Refs. 185–188). The mode of information dissemination ranges from the distribution of written information alone (e.g., 187) to providing written educational material and a discussion of its contents with a neuropsychologist (e.g., 180).

Research focusing on intervention following MTBI can be classified into three types of studies: (a) studies that treat MTBI patients with persistent symptoms many months post-injury, (b) studies that compare MTBI patients assigned to an intervention program versus a control group, and (c) studies that compare the efficacy of different types of intervention programs.[11] Two studies have evaluated the effectiveness of intervention programs for MTBI patients experiencing persistent problems. Ho and Bennet (189) reported that patients participating in a comprehensive brain injury treatment program had improved activities of daily living, neuropsychological test scores, and ratings on behavioral scales. Cicerone et al. (190) reported that 50 percent of patients who participated in a comprehensive brain injury program could be classified as having a good outcome (defined as resumption of pre-injury activities or other similar productive activity), improved scores on neuropsychological measures, and a reduced frequency of self-reported post-concussion symptoms following treatment. However, these two studies have been criticized by Paniak and colleagues for two reasons. First, they lack the inclusion of a control group that prevents ruling out explanations for improvement other than treatment. Second, they include patients who are first seen many months post-injury (and in some cases years), reducing the likelihood that patients are being treated for symptoms resulting from MTBI versus pre-existing disorders or co-morbid conditions (see 180 for a further discussion).

The majority of intervention studies compare patients assigned to a control group versus an intervention program within the first 1 to 3 weeks post-injury. In general,

---

[9]Please see the chapter by Collins, Iverson, Gaetz, and Lovell in this book for a comprehensive review of outcome from sport concussion.

[10]There are a few exceptions, with a handful of studies that have evaluated various interventions such as bed rest (182), hospital admission (183), and homeopathy (184).

[11]The first two types were conceptualized by Paniak et al. (180).

Z-SCORE	NORMAL	CONCUSSION: < 24 HR	CONCUSSION: 1–7 DAYS	CONCUSSION: > 7 DAYS	MTBI: 0–6 DAYS	MTBI: 7–30 DAYS	MTBI: 1–3 MONTHS	CANNABIS	LITIGATION	DEPRESSION	ADULT ADHD	MODERATE-SEVERE TBI: 0–6 MONTHS	MODERATE-SEVERE TBI: > 24 MONTHS	POOR EFFORT/ MALINGERING
1.6	90													
1.5														
1.4				90		90	90	90						
1.3			90		90				90	90				
1.2	80													
1.1				80		80	80	80			90			
1.0			80		80				80	80				
0.9											80	90		
0.8													80	
0.7												80		
0.6	50	90												
0.5														90
0.4														
0.3		80												80
0.2														
0.1														
0.0	Average													
-0.1		Average												
-0.2				Average			Average	Average						
-0.3														
-0.4			Average			Average								
-0.5					Average				Average	Average				
-0.6	50										Average			
-0.7													Average	
-0.8														
-0.9														
-1.0												Average		
-1.1														Average
-1.2	80													
-1.3			80	80										
-1.4					80	80	80	80						
-1.5														
-1.6	90													
-1.7				90						80				
-1.8			90					90	80		80			
-1.9					90	90	90							
-2.0									90				80	
-2.1										90				

FIGURE 22-1

Comparing the neuropsychological effects of MTBI to the normal population and other clinical groups: Distributions derived from meta-analyses.

Note: This figure illustrates, based on meta-analytic studies, the distributions of neuropsychological test performance across diagnoses, circumstances, or conditions. The shaded line in the middle represents the average score for healthy normal adults. 50 percent of healthy adults are expected to perform between the upper and lower shaded lines, and 80 percent of healthy adults are expected to perform between the solid lines. All groups are based on the theoretical normal distribution. The far left column represents z-scores (mean = 0, SD = 1). A z-score of -.67 falls at the 25th percentile and .67 falls at the 75th percentile. A z-score of -1.28 falls at the 10th percentile and 1.28 falls at the 80th percentile. A z-score of -1.64 falls at the 5th percentile and 1.64 falls at the 95th percentile. Deviations from the normal distribution are based on the effect sizes reported in the meta-analyses. For example, for MTBIs that are 1–3 months post injury, the effect size reported in the literature was .12. Therefore, the "Average" score for that group was dropped one position from the mean of zero, and the spread of scores was then centered around that average score. Effect sizes typically are expressed in pooled, weighted standard deviation units. However, across studies, there are some minor variations in the methods of calculation. By convention, effect sizes of .2 are considered small, .5 medium, and .8 large. This is from a statistical, not necessarily clinical, perspective. For this figure, the overall effect on cognitive or neuropsychological functioning is reported. Sport concussion < 24 hr, 1–7 days, and >7 days, all in Belanger & Vanderploeg (4); MTBI 0–6 days, 7–29 days, 30–89 days, moderate-severe TBI 0–6 months, >24 months, all in Schretlen & Shapiro (8); Cannabis (411); Depression (412); Litigation/financial incentives (339); ADHD (413); Depression (411); based on Full Scale IQ, 123 studies; Exaggeration/Malingering (414).

researchers have reported favorable outcomes. Patients participating in intervention programs consisting of educational materials plus various additional treatments and/or assessments (e.g., neuropsychological testing, meeting with a therapist, reassurance, access to a multidisciplinary team) report fewer post-concussion symptoms at 3 months post injury (181, 187) and at 6 months post injury (177, 185, 188) compared to patients who received standard hospital treatment. However, not all research as been as favorable. Some researchers have reported that early intervention programs using educational material alone and educational material plus access to a specialist outpatient brain injury team, did not result in reduced self-reported post-concussive symptoms in children 3 months post injury (179) and adults 6 months post injury (191).

Although the majority of the research in this area points towards the usefulness of early intervention programs, our understanding of the *type* of intervention required is limited. The intervention programs evaluated in the literature to date vary considerably, ranging from economical programs (e.g., distribution of written educational materials) to much more expensive programs (e.g., multidisciplinary brain injury programs). Few studies have attempted to evaluate different intervention programs. In one of the first studies of this kind, Alves, Macciocchi, and Barth (192) compared the outcome of patients provided with standard hospital treatment to two different intervention programs provided within the first week post-injury: (a) education only, and (b) education and reassurance. Alves and colleagues concluded that intervention assignment was not associated with the number or duration of self-reported post-concussive symptoms at 3, 6, or 12 months post-injury.

In a more recent study, Paniak and colleagues compared patients assigned to two different treatment modes: (a) single session (i.e., a brief, educational and reassurance oriented session) and (b) treatment as needed (i.e., including education, reassurance, psychological, personality, and neuropsychological testing and feedback, consultation with physical therapist, and access to multidisciplinary brain injury treatment program as needed). Paniak and colleagues concluded that the brief educational and reassurance oriented intervention was as effective as the more comprehensive and expensive treatment model. There was no difference between the two interventions in self-reported post-concussive symptoms at 3 months and 12 months post-injury (180, 186).

The research focusing on early intervention is promising. However, this research is certainly not without its methodological problems. Some of the more serious problems include (a) the differences in definition of MTBI used across studies, and (b) the high attrition rate of patients belonging to the "intervention" group. Nonetheless, the literature suggests that early intervention can be useful in this population by reducing the number of individuals who experience long term symptoms post-injury. In addition, and perhaps more importantly, research by Paniak and colleagues suggests that early intervention programs need not consist of complex multidisciplinary brain injury treatment programs, but may consist of a simple education session provided soon after injury. This is a conclusion echoed by Borg et al. (16) in their review of interventions for people with MTBIs. The effective use of simple education-oriented programs is supported in the literature (e.g., 181, 187). Future researchers are encouraged to (a) evaluate different treatment models in an effort to replicate the findings by Paniak and colleagues, (b) develop methods to minimize attrition rates, and (c) use "gold standard" definitions for selecting patients with MTBIs.

RETURN TO WORK

Vocational outcome following traumatic brain injury is important for individual patients and society as a whole (193–197). For many individuals, the inability to return to work can result in a number of economic, social, family, and interpersonal problems (198–200). In addition, the economic burden placed on society is of concern (e.g., long-term sickness benefits, unemployment benefits), particularly because many individuals who sustain a TBI tend to be young and have their whole working lives ahead of them (196).

Some researchers have reported that injury severity, as measured by post-traumatic amnesia, loss of consciousness, and/or Glasgow Coma Scale scores, is associated with the time in which individuals return to pre-injury employment following TBI (e.g., 194, 197, 201, 202). However, other studies have failed to support the relation between injury severity and post-injury employment status (e.g., 203–207).

Despite these inconsistencies, individuals who have sustained an MTBI have consistently higher return to work rates when compared to individuals who have sustained a moderate or severe TBI (e.g., 197, 198, 208–211). However, not all individuals who have sustained an MTBI return to work at the same rate. Within the spectrum of MTBI, those individuals with lesser injuries (e.g., GCS = 15; no LOC) tend to have a higher return to work rate compared to those with more significant injuries (e.g., GCS = 13–14; with LOC; e.g., 101, 212, 213).

Return to work rates following MTBI vary substantially in the research literature. Post-injury employment rates have ranged from (a) 25 percent to 100 percent within the first month post-injury (e.g., 101, 198, 200, 214), (b) 38 percent to 83 percent six to nine months post-injury (147, 198, 199, 212, 215, 216), (c) 47 percent to

83 percent one to two years post-injury (141, 198, 209, 211), and (d) 62 percent to 88 percent three or more years post-injury (193, 197, 208, 209, 213). The literature regarding return to work following MTBI is summarized in Table 22-9.

The variability in return to work rates is likely due to the many methodological differences between studies. The most problematic of these include (a) differences in definitions of return to work (e.g., return to pre-injury employment vs. return to meaningful activity), (b) variations in the definition of MTBI (e.g., inclusion of GCS = 15 only versus GCS = 13–15), (c) variations in the inclusion and exclusion of individuals who were unemployed or performing domestic duties pre-injury in the sample, and (d) the failure of some studies to take into account pre-injury employment status (e.g., return to full time vs. part time vs. unemployed). For a comprehensive discussion regarding return to work following TBI, the interested reader is referred to the chapter by West and colleagues in this book.

Under most circumstances, we should anticipate good recovery and return to work following an MTBI. Patients should be reassured, and health care providers can work with injured adults to address the difficulties they face with particular symptoms while they resume their normal daily activities (e.g., work or school). Unfortunately, some trauma patients transition from acute postconcussion symptoms and problems into a mild depression (or major depressive episode). In people who transition, it might not be possible to determine if their primary diagnosis is depression or postconcussion syndrome. Basic and clinical research is needed in this area. Although the neuropathophysiology might be difficult to describe, the condition might be amenable to pharmacological and psychological intervention.

DEPRESSION

Depression is common following traumatic brain injury of *all severities* (see 217 for a review). Prevalence estimates vary widely (e.g., from 11 percent to 77 percent; e.g., 218, 219, 220). In epidemiological studies, 11 percent to 21 percent of people with a history of TBI also have depression (e.g., 218, 221). In studies based on admissions to trauma centers or rehabilitation hospitals (222–227) or large samples of outpatients (228, 229) the rates of depression typically range from 14 percent to 42 percent. Recent well-controlled studies have concluded that depression occurs frequently in the first year post injury (224, 225), with rates decreasing over time (224, 230). Researchers have often reported that people who suffer traumatic brain injuries have higher rates of pre-injury psychiatric disorders (219, 231–233), such as depression and substance abuse.

Hibbard and colleagues (233) assessed 188 community-dwelling adults with *moderate to severe* traumatic brain injuries in a longitudinal cohort study. On average, the patients were evaluated 2.5 years post injury and then approximately 12 months later. The authors reported that 48 percent did not meet criteria for a major mood disorder at time one or time two, 29 percent were diagnosed with major depression at time one which resolved by time 2, 10 percent had late-onset depression (diagnosed at time 2 but not at time 1), and 14 percent had chronic depression (diagnosed at both time periods).

Depression is a heterogeneous condition. It can be a secondary or tertiary condition associated with traumatic brain injury, or it can be unrelated to the original brain injury. Researchers have speculated that depression can arise directly or indirectly from the biological consequences of the traumatic brain injury, it can be a psychological reaction to deficits and problems associated with having a brain injury, or both. A constant theme in the professional and scientific literature is that there are many methodological differences and scientific limitations across studies that make it very difficult to understand the prevalence, etiology, and natural history of depression in people with traumatic brain injuries. Moreover, most of the literature (as described in the previous paragraphs) relates to depression following *moderate or severe* traumatic brain injury. A review of prevalence studies relating to depression in people with MTBIs is presented in Table 22-10.

When patients report symptoms and problems many months after an injury, differential treatment often flows from differential diagnosis. Given the clear overlap between the symptoms of depression and postconcussion syndrome, some researchers have recommended treatment with antidepressants (e.g., 148, 234–236) or cognitive behavior therapy (e.g., 185, 237). Medications and psychotherapy would be an obvious choice, of course, if depression is simply mimicking the postconcussion syndrome. Those recommending cognitive behavior therapy have set forth a treatment protocol that is based on CBT principles but is tailored toward the postconcusison syndrome and belief systems relating to symptoms and brain damage.

Certainly, depression is relatively common in patients with traumatic brain injuries, although it is not necessarily more common in these patients than in patients with general trauma (227). The presence of depression in a person with a history of traumatic brain injury presents an obvious challenge if one attempts to diagnose a persistent postconcussion syndrome given the overlap in symptoms. Iverson (238) reported very high rates of possible *misdiagnosis* of persistent postconcussion syndrome in patients with depression. Participants were 64 physician-diagnosed inpatients or outpatients with depression who had independently-confirmed diagnoses on the Structured

TABLE 22-9

Summary of Return to Work Rates in the Research Literature

First Author	Setting	N	Country	Time Post-Injury	Percent RTW	MTBI Definition	RTW Definition	Pre-injury work status: Inclusion/Exclusion Criteria	Type of Study and Referrals
Stranjalis (2004)	HTC[1]	100	Greece	1 wk	84 percent	GCS = 15 PTA < 15 min LOC < 15 min	Return to work/activities	Included = students, homemakers, retired, and unemployed.	Consecutive[2] Prospective
Wrightson (1981)	HTC	66	New Zealand	1 wk	81.8 percent[3]	Described as "Minor HI" (however, 2 patients had PTA 18–36hrs). No GCS or LOC data reported.	Return to work i.e., no longer had to take days off work.	All patients in regular employment at the time of injury	Consecutive Prospective
Wrightson (1981)	HTC	66	New Zealand	2 wk	92.4 percent[3]	Described as "Minor HI" (however, 2 patients had PTA 18–36hrs). No GCS or LOC data reported.	Return to work i.e., no longer had to take days off work.	All patients in regular employment at the time of injury	Consecutive Prospective
Haboubi (2001)	RC	391	UK	2 wk	44 percent	GCS = 13–15	Return to regular employment	Included those only in regular employment	Consecutive Retrospective
Dikmen (1994)	LITC	213	USA	1 mth	25 percent	GCS = 13–15	Return to work irrespective of length of that employment	Excluded = students, homemakers, and retired; Included = Workers[4] (Employed & Unemployed).	Consecutive Prospective Longitudinal
Wrightson (1981)	HTC	66	New Zealand	1 mth	99 percent[3]	Described as "Minor HI" (however, 2 patients had PTA 18–36hrs). No GCS or LOC data reported.	Return to work i.e., no longer had to take days off work.	All patients in regular employment at the time of injury	Consecutive Prospective

Study	Type	N	Country	Follow-up	Percent	Criteria	Outcome measure	Inclusion/Exclusion	Sampling
van der Naalt (1999)	HTC	43	Netherlands	1 mth	39 percent	GCS = 13–14	Resumption of previous activities either partially or completely.	None	Consecutive Prospective
Stranjalis (2004)	HTC	100	Greece	1 mth	99 percent	GCS = 15 PTA < 15 min LOC < 15 min	Return to work/activities	Included = students, homemakers, retired, and unemployed.	Consecutive Prospective
Haboubi (2001)	RC	391	UK	6 wk	88 percent	GCS = 13–15	Return to regular employment	Included those only in regular employment	Consecutive Retrospective
van der Naalt (1999)	HTC	43	Nether-lands	3 mth	67 percent	GCS = 13–14	Resumption of previous activities either partially or completely.	None	Consecutive Prospective
Drake (2000)	NMC	121	USA	3 mth	53.7 percent	Described as "MTBI patients" but no specific criteria provided; LOC (M = 1.4 min, SD = 2.6 min); PTA (M = 3 hr, SD = 1.3 hr).	Return to full military duty defined by US Navy guidelines[5]	Included if in pre-injury active duty military status	Consecutive Prospective
Drake (2000)	NMC	121	USA	3 mth	100 percent	Described as "MTBI patients" but no specific criteria provided; LOC (M = 1.4 min, SD = 2.6 min); PTA (M = 3 hr, SD = 1.3 hr).	Return to full military duty defined by US Navy guidelines[5]	Included if in pre-injury active duty military status	Consecutive Prospective
McCullaugh (2001)	TTC	20	Canada	5 mth	37.5 percent	LOC < 20 mins PTA < 24 hr GSC 13–14	Return to previous work or studies	Excluded = retired, unemployed due to non-TBI injury; Included = employed, students, homemaker.	Consecutive Prospective
McCullaugh (2001)	TTC	37	Canada	5 mth	60 percent	LOC < 20 mins PTA < 24 hr GCS = 15	Return to previous work or studies	Excluded = retired, unemployed due to non-TBI injury; Included = employed, students, homemaker.	Consecutive Prospective

(continued)

TABLE 22-9 (continued)

First Author	Setting	N	Country	Time Post-Injury	Percent RTW	MTBI Definition	RTW Definition	Pre-injury Work Status: Inclusion/Exclusion Criteria	Type of Study and Referrals
Kraus (2005)	HTC	201	USA	6 mth	82.6 percent[6]	LOC < 30 mins GCS 13–15 PTA < 24 hr	No change in employment status post injury	Pre-injury work status not used to include/exclude patients.	Consecutive Prospective
Dikmen (1994)	LITC	213	USA	6 mth	63 percent	GCS = 13–15	Return to work irrespective of length of that employment	Excluded = students, homemakers, and retired; Included = Workers[4] (Employed & Unemployed).	Consecutive Prospective Longitudinal
van der Naalt (1999)	HTC	43	Nether-lands	6 mth	97 percent	GCS = 13–14	Resumption of previous activities either partially or completely.	None	Consecutive Prospective
Friedland (2001)	TTC	64	Canada	6–9 mth	44 percent	Initial GCS ≥ 13 PTA ≤ 24 hr LOC ≤ 30 min	Return to premorbid level or modified level.	Included all patients regardless of employment status.	Consecutive Prospective
Ruffolo (1999)	TTC	63	Canada	6–9 mth	42 percent[7]	GCS and LOC criteria used –LOC < 60 mins –GCS scores obtained but not reported.	Return to premorbid employment under usual or modified[8] conditions (paid or unpaid).	All working before the accident in paid or unpaid employment (e.g., students, volunteers, homemaker)	Consecutive Prospective
van der Naalt (1999)	HTC	43	Nether-lands	12 mth	100 percent	GCS = 13–14	Resumption of previous activities either partially or completely.	None	Consecutive Prospective
Dikmen (1994)	LITC	213	USA	12 mth	80 percent	GCS = 13–15	Return to work irrespective of length of that employment	Excluded = students, homemakers, and retired; Included = Workers[4] (Employed & Unemployed)	Consecutive Prospective Longitudinal
Dawson (2004)	TTC	38	Canada	1 yr	78.9 percent	GCS = 13–15	Return to productivity (i.e., paid employment and/or school)	Not described	Consecutive Prospective

Study	Abbrev.	N	Country	Follow-up	Percentage	Severity	Outcome	Inclusion/Exclusion	Design
van der Naalt (1999)	HTC	43	Nether-lands	1 yr	79 percent	GCS = 13–14	Resumed previous activities completely	None	Consecutive Prospective
Dikmen (1994)	LITC	213	USA	2 yr	83 percent	GCS = 13–15	Return to work irrespective of length of that employment	Excluded = students, homemakers, and retired; Included = Workers[4] (Employed & Unemployed)	Consecutive Prospective Longitudinal
Dawson (2004)	TTC	24	Canada	4 yr	79.2 percent	GCS = 13–15	Return to productivity (i.e., paid employment and/or school)	Not described	Consecutive Prospective
Vanderploeg (2003)	USVV	373	USA	8 yr	75.1 percent	Described as MTBI with no reported LOC – No specific criteria presented.	Return to full time employment	Vietnam veterans who (a) had at least 4 months of active duty, (b) served only one tour of duty, (c) achieved a military occupation subspecialty other than "trainee" of "duty soldier".	Consecutive Retrospective
Vanderploeg (2003)	USVV	253	USA	8 yr	81.8 percent	Described as MTBI + reported LOC – No specific criteria presented.	Return to full time employment	Vietnam veterans who (a) had at least 4 months of active duty, (b) served only one tour of duty, (c) achieved a military occupation subspecialty other than "trainee" of "duty soldier".	Retrospective Random selected sample

(continued)

TABLE 22-9 (continued)

First Author	Setting	N	Country	Time Post-Injury	Percent RTW	MTBI Definition	RTW Definition	Pre-Injury Work Status: Inclusion/Exclusion Criteria	Type of Study and Referrals
Asikainen (1996)	HOC	118	Finland	12 yr	61.9 percent	GCS = 13–15	Return to independent work only	No apparent exclusions based on work status	Retrospective Selected sample (patients with brain injury and post-injury problems in education and employment)
Asikainen (1996)	HOC	118	Finland	12 yr	72.9 percent	GCS = 13–15	Return to independent work or subsidized employment or education continuing	No apparent exclusions based on work status	Retrospective Selected sample (patients with brain injury and post-injury problems in education and employment)

Notes: [1]HTC = Hospital trauma center; RC = Rehabilitation clinic; LITC = Level 1 trauma center; NMC = U.S. Naval medical center; TTC = Tertiary trauma center; USVV = U.S. Vietnam veterans; HOC = Hospital outpatient clinic

[2]Consecutive = Consecutive referrals: Retrospective/Prospective = retrospective/prospective study design.

[3]A follow-up interview was obtained in 63 of the 66 patients 90 days post-injury regarding their condition on returning to work. Of these patients, 60 percent reported experiencing symptoms when they first returned to work and 46 percent reported that they were unable to do there work as well as usual.

[4]Workers were defined as individuals who defined themselves as "workers" regardless of whether they were employed or unemployed at the time of injury.

[5]Limited duty is a duty status within the military for individuals with ongoing medical problems; it has fewer responsibilities, some limitations, and decreased performance standards. Individuals are placed on limited duty for periods of six months, with the expectation of recovery and eventual return to full duty status" (p. 1106).

[6]It is not entirely clear whether this percentage includes individuals who were employed pre-injury, or also includes individuals who were retired, students, and unemployed.

[7]Of these patients, 12 percent returned to premorbid level of work and 30 percent returned to modified employment.

[8]Modified conditions was defined as "working shorter hr, performing lighter work, performing part of the job at home, or trading difficult tasks with other workers" (p. 393)

Sources: Asikainen, Kaste, & Sarna (208); Dawson, Levine, Schwartz, & Stuss (209); Dikmen, Temkin, Machamer, Holubkov, Fraser, & Winn (198); Drake, Gray, Yoder, Pramuka, & Llewellyn (216); Friedland & Dawson (215); Haboubi, Long, Koshy, & Ward (214); Kraus, Schaffer, Ayers, Stenehjem, Shen, & Afifi (199); McCullagh, Oucherlony, Protzner, Blair, & Feinstein (212); Ruffolo, Friedland, Dawson, Colantonio, & Lindsay (196); Stranjalis, Korfias, Papapetrou, Kouyialis, Boviatsis, Psachoulia, & Sakas (101); Uzzell, Langfitt, & Dolinskas (211); Vanderploeg, Curtiss, Duchnick, & Luis (213); van der Naalt, van Zomeren, Sluiter, & Minderhoud (141); Wrightson & Gronwall (200).

TABLE 22-10

Summary of Depression Prevalence Rates in MTBI

First Author	N	Country	Post-Injury Interval	Setting	Rate of Depression	MTBI Definition	Depression Definition	Type of Study/ Referrals
Goldstein (2001)	18	USA	2 months	Acute care neurosurgery services affiliated with University hospitals	33 percent	GCS 13 to 15 LOC < 20 min Normal CT or MRI	GDS > 10	Prospective Consecutive
Mooney (2001)	80	USA	Median = 25.5 weeks	Rehabilitation Program, University hospital	44 percent	ACRM criteria	DSM-IV criteria	Prospective Selected Sample (individuals who failed to recover as expected 3 months post injury)
Levin (2005)	129	USA	3 months	Level I trauma center	11.6 percent	GCS 13 to 15	SCID: DSM-IV	Prospective Consecutive
McCauley (2001)	95	USA	3 months	Level I trauma center	21.4 percent	GCS 13 to 15 LOC < 20 mins Normal CT	DSM-IV Major Depressive Disorder criteria	Prospective Consecutive
Levin (2001)	60	USA	3 months	Level I trauma center	18.3 percent	GCS 13 to 15 LOC < 20 mins Normal CT	DSM-IV Major Depressive Disorder criteria	Prospective Consecutive
Horner (2005)	524	USA	12 months	State hospital	21.3 percent	[1]Injury to the head ICD/AIS = 2	"Since your injury, has a doctor told you that you had depression?"	Retrospective Random Selection of TBI
Parker (1996)	33	USA	M = 20 months	Private Practice/ Compensation	36 percent	Dx of "Whiplash" from medical records or on self description- excluded if LOC > 5 minutes or presence of cerebral abnormalities.	DSM-III-R	Prospective Selected Sample

Note: GDS = Geriatric Depression Scale; ACRM = American Congress of Rehabilitation Medicine (LOC < 30 mins, initial GCS = 13–15, PTA < 24 hr). [1]"TBI was defined as an injury to the head associated with decreased consciousness, amnesia, neurological abnormalities, skull fracture, or intracranial lesion, in accordance with the Centre for Disease Control and Prevention" (p. 323), TBI severity was determined by translating ICD-9-CM codes to ICD/AIS scores using ICDMAP-90 software" (p.324) Sources: Goldstein, Levin, Goldman, Clark, & Altonen (169); Horner, Ferguson, Selassie, Labbate, Kniele, & Corrigan (221); Levin, McCauley, Josic, Boake, Brown, Goodman, & Merritt (408); Mooney & Speed (409); McCauley, Boake, Levin, Contant, & Song (148); Parker & Rosenblum (410).

Clinical Interview for DSM-IV. These patients completed the British Columbia Postconcussion Symptom Inventory-Short Form (239, 240), a 16-item measure designed to assess the frequency and severity of symptoms based on ICD-10 criteria for postconcussion syndrome. Specific endorsement rates of postconcussion-like symptoms ranged from 31 percent to 86 percent for symptoms rated mild or greater, and from 11 percent to 58 percent for symptoms rated moderate-to-severe. Approximately 9 out of 10 patients with depression met liberal self-report criteria for a postconcussion syndrome and more than 5 out of 10 met conservative criteria for the diagnosis (in the absence of a previous MTBI). Depression is also common in persons with chronic pain (241, 242), and it is associated with increased disability in these patients (243, 244). Chronic pain is a frequent co-morbidity with depression (245–247). Therefore, patients seen long after a mild traumatic brain injury who have chronic pain, depression, or both are very likely to meet diagnostic criteria for a persistent postconcussion syndrome, even if the problems associated with the mild traumatic brain injury have long-since resolved.

Post-Traumatic Stress Disorder

Post-traumatic stress disorder (PTSD; 248) occurs in some people who experience *intense fear, helplessness, or horror* during or immediately after experiencing or witnessing a traumatic event (except when "delayed"). Symptom onset typically occurs in the first few days (in fact the first 24 hr) in most people. The traumatic event is *persistently re-experienced* through (a) intrusive and distressing recollections of the event including visual images, thoughts, or perceptions; (b) distressing dreams (nightmares), (c) acting or feeling as if the traumatic event was happening again (e.g., dissociative flashbacks); (d) intense psychological distress when exposed to things (e.g., thoughts or external visual reminders) that symbolize or resemble an aspect of the event; or (e) physiological reactivity when exposed to things that symbolize or resemble an aspect of the traumatic event. In addition to the persistent re-experiencing, there is *persistent avoidance* of things associated with the traumatic event and a numbing of general responsiveness. Examples of avoidance and numbing of responsiveness include: (a) avoiding thoughts, feelings, or conversations associated with the event; (b) avoiding activities, places, or people that stimulate thoughts or memories of the event; (c) feeling detached or estranged from others; or (d) having a sense of a foreshortened future (e.g., not expecting to have a career, marriage, children, or a normal life span). In addition, the person has persistent symptoms of *increased arousal* such as (a) difficulty falling or staying asleep; (b) irritability or outbursts of anger; (c) difficulty concentrating; (d) hypervigilance; and (e) an exaggerated startle response. If a person meets criteria after one-month post event, PTSD is diagnosed.

Developing PTSD following a car accident is uncommon. Some estimates of the rate of this disorder in accident victims have been 9 percent (249), 12 percent (250), and 6.3 percent and 8.8 percent for men and women respectively (251). Essentially, 90 percent of people in car accidents do not develop PTSD. For comparison, less than 5 percent of individuals develop PTSD after a natural disaster (251). In a sample of survivors of the September 11, 2001 terrorist attack on the Pentagon, 14 percent had PTSD 7 months after the event (252). Sexual assault is associated with the highest incidence of PTSD, with estimates ranging from 46 percent to 80 percent (250, 251).

Patients with PTSD often report the same symptoms as patients who have sustained MTBIs. For example, in a sample of 128 patients with PTSD, 89 percent reported irritability, 56 percent reported memory problems, 92 percent reported concentration problems, and 90 percent reported difficulty sleeping (253). A controversial and confusing issue is whether a person who sustains a traumatic brain injury can develop PTSD. There are data to support the position that MTBI and PTSD typically are mutually exclusive (254–256), although researchers have put forward a compelling rationale for how, under certain circumstances, PTSD could emerge in a patient with a brain injury (257, 258). The conceptual question at the heart of the debate is whether a person with no memory for a traumatic event can develop PTSD. In other words, how can you be traumatized by an event you can't remember? How can you re-experience, through flashbacks, images, or dreams, an event you cannot remember? Some mechanisms might include islands of memory of traumatic events occurring outside of the amnestic gap (such as gaining awareness in the hospital with a tracheotomy in and on a ventilator), or so-called elaborative cognitions.

A recent, well-controlled study provides additional information to better understand this issue. Gil and colleagues prospectively studied 120 accident victims who sustained a mild traumatic brain injury and who were hospitalized for observation immediately after their trauma. They were assessed within the first 24 hr and at one week, three months, and six months. At 6 months post-injury, 14 percent met diagnostic criteria for PTSD. Predictors of PTSD at 6 months were (a) PSTD symptoms, depressive symptoms, and anxiety symptoms at one week post-injury, (b) history of psychiatric disorder, and (c) memory for the event. Of the patients with memory for the event, 13/55 (23 percent) had PTSD at 6 months post-injury, compared to only 4/65 (6 percent) who did not have memory for the event (259). Therefore, the literature to date suggests quite clearly that having no memory for the event likely protects the individual from developing PTSD.

Clinicians should be very cautious in diagnosing PTSD in a person who has sustained an MTBI if that person does not exhibit prominent symptoms in the initial days post injury. The onset of symptoms in PTSD generally is rapid. For example, the onset of PTSD symptoms in the survivors of the Oklahoma City bombing was swift, with 76 percent reporting symptoms on the day of the event (260). Delayed symptom onset is very uncommon. For example, there were no cases of delayed onset PTSD associated with the Oklahoma City bombing (261, 262) or a mass shooting incident (263, 264). Delayed onset PTSD, in the vast majority of studies, has been considered rare (e.g., 265–267). Therefore, if delayed onset phenomena appear, they might be a joint product of (a) insensitive diagnostic criteria and methods, (b) individual differences in avoidance behavior that masks other PTSD symptoms, (c) post-trauma stressors that exacerbate psychological distress, and/or (d) delayed compensation motivation (265, 268). As illustrated in the study by Gil and colleagues, patients with MTBIs are likely at increased risk for developing PTSD if (a) they have a psychiatric history, (b) they have memory for the event, and (c) they develop major symptoms within the first 24 hr or first week post injury (259).

RISK FOR ALZHEIMER'S DISEASE

There has been considerable research interest regarding whether mild, repetitive mild, moderate, or severe traumatic brain injuries increase a person's risk for developing Alzheimer's disease (AD). Before discussing this literature, it is important to consider the broader literature on risk for AD. Without question, the biggest risk factor for AD is age. Living longer greatly increases one's chance of developing the disease. Several meta-analytic studies have consistently found that the prevalence of AD around the world increases with age (e.g., 269–272). In an early meta-analysis of 22 studies, Jorm and colleagues (270) reported that the prevalence of AD doubled every 4.5 years; they reported the following prevalence rates stratified by age group: 65–69 years (1.4 percent), 70–74 years (2.8 percent), 75–79 years (5.6 percent), 80–84 years (11.1 percent), and 85 years or more (23.6 percent). Using the United States census data, Hebert and colleagues estimated that in 2000 4.5 million persons in the United States had AD, and by the year 2050 this figure will triple to 13.2 million due to the ageing population (273).

An overview of the recent literature reveals considerable scientific interest in many other potential risk factors, such as genetics (274), particularly the apolipoprotein E (ApoE) gene (275, 276); genetics and a high fat diet (277); oxidative stress, disturbed protein metabolism, and their interaction (278, 279); zinc metabolism (280); cerebrovascular disease and vascular risk factors (281, 282); cardiovascular disease, particularly in the subgroup with peripherial arterial disease (283); high cholesterol (284),

elevated plasma total homocysteine concentrations and low serum folate concentrations (285); midlife obesity (286); loss of microglial cell function (287); decreased melatonin (288); heavy metal exposure (289); and lack of exercise (290). The risk of AD appears to increase with the number of vascular risk factors (diabetes + hypertension + heart disease + current smoking), with diabetes and current smoking being the strongest risk factors in isolation or in clusters in a recent study (291). Mental health problems, such as a history of depression in adulthood (292), particularly for men (293), have been associated with an increased risk for AD. Even a man's height has been associated with risk for AD! Short men are at increased risk (presumably due to its association with childhood nutrition and other risk factors for dementia) (294). Watching too much television in middle-adulthood has been associated with an increased risk for AD, presumably as a marker for reduced participation in intellectually stimulating activities (295).

For the past 20 years there has been considerable interest in the relation between traumatic brain injury and the future development of AD. It has been suggested that traumatic brain injuries reduce "cognitive reserve," resulting in increased vulnerability to developing the disease (296). The animal literature has revealed evidence that some of the pathological features of AD arise shortly after traumatic brain injury (see 297 and 298 for reviews), and human autopsy studies also have supported these findings (299, 300). A number of studies have reported a relation between a history of traumatic brain injury and a current diagnosis of AD (e.g., 301–314), although several studies have failed to find this association (e.g., 315–323). Mortimer and colleagues conducted an important meta-analytic review of the literature published prior to 1991 (324). They reported that traumatic brain injuries were associated with a 1.82 relative risk (RR) (95 percent confidence interval = 1.26 to 2.67) for developing AD. The relative risk was significant for men (RR = 2.67, 95 percent CI = 1.64 to 4.41) but not women (RR = 0.85, 95 percent CI = 0.43 to 1.70). Fleminger and colleagues conducted a second meta-analytic review of the literature, published in 2003, and reported that the literature published since 1991 did *not* reveal a statistically significant increased risk for AD (325). However, the literature as a whole (i.e., the studies published before and after the Mortimer meta-analysis) did reveal an increased risk for AD associated with a history of TBI (Odds Ratio (OR) = 1.58, 95 percent CI = 1.21 to 2.06). Again, the increased risk was significant for men (OR = 2.26, 95 percent CI = 1.13 to 4.53) but not women (OR = 0.92, 95 percent CI = 0.53 to 1.59). Starkstein and Jorge (326) suggested that this increased risk in men and not women might simply reflect men getting more severe traumatic brain injuries. Jellinger, in his review of the literature, emphasized that epidemiological and autopsy studies have provided evidence of an association between *severe* traumatic brain injury and AD, but the relationship between AD and brain injury and apolipoprotein E status is still ambiguous (298). Overall, there are many conflicting results in this large literature spanning more than 20 years. Nonetheless, it is reasonable to conclude that patients who sustain *severe* TBIs are at a small increased risk for developing AD, as concluded by Starkstein and Jorge (326) and Jellinger (298).

> In conclusion, most prospective studies showed a significant, albeit weak, association between dementia and history of TBI. Some studies showed that a history of TBI may result in a relatively early onset of dementia, but this was not replicated by others. The association with the APOE-e4 allele status is conflicting as well, from one study showing a tenfold increase in the risk for dementia for individuals with both a history of TBI and APOE-e4, to another study showing an increased risk for dementia among those *without* an APOE-e4 allele. (p. 599; Ref. 326)

Given that (a) many studies have failed to find an association between history of TBI (of any severity) and AD, (b) the meta-analyses have only identified this association for men, (c) several studies have found a severity effect (i.e., risk is greater in patients with more severe brain injuries), and (d) the pathophysiology of MTBI, especially on the milder end of the spectrum of this injury, is temporary and reversible, it would be a mistake to assume, at this point in time, that patients with *MTBIs*, as a group, are at increased risk for AD. Several specific studies suggest that there is not a relationship between MTBI and risk for AD (e.g., 306, 310, 321).

PERSISTENT POST-CONCUSSION SYNDROME

There is a so-called "miserable minority" (327) of patients who appear to have poor long-term outcome following a mild traumatic brain injury (MTBI). The etiology of the so-called *persistent* postconcussion syndrome has never been agreed upon (see 7, 328–330 for reviews). For decades, researchers have questioned the validity of this diagnosis as a true syndrome or disease entity (e.g., 331–336). Others have noted that the syndrome is rare in prospective studies (e.g., 192, 333), and concerns regarding the role of financial compensation on symptom reporting have been expressed for many years (331, 337–340). Most researchers simply suggest that the etiology is due to the biological effects of the injury, psychological factors, psychosocial factors (broadly defined), chronic pain, or a combination of factors (171, 341–348). Ruff and colleagues (327, 330, 349) have stressed a multidimensional cumulative stressor conceptualization of the persistent post-concussion syndrome. Essentially, setbacks in several aspects of a person's life (physical, emotional, cognitive, psychosocial, vocational, financial, and recreational) serve as cumulative stressors that interact with personality and premorbid physical and mental health factors, resulting in the syndrome. This model stresses the complexity of the etiology and maintenance of the syndrome.

Experienced clinicians and researchers know that it is extraordinarily difficult to disentangle the many factors that can be related to self-reported symptoms in persons who have sustained remote MTBIs (328). This is a challenging and potentially contentious diagnosis, of course, because post-concussion-like symptoms are common in healthy subjects (240, 350–355), in patients with no history of brain injury, such as outpatients seen for psychological treatment (356), outpatients seen for minor medical problems (357), personal injury claimants (357, 358), patients with post-traumatic stress disorder (253), patients with orthopedic injuries (332), individuals with chronic pain (359–362) and patients with whiplash (363). Thus, the differential diagnosis of the persistent post-concussion syndrome is very challenging.

CONCLUSIONS

Mild traumatic brain injury, and the potential for incomplete recovery and poor psychosocial outcome, has been recognized as a public health problem (364–366). The pathophysiology of MTBI is predominately neurometabolic and reversible. However, this injury can be characterized by structural damage that is visible with static neuroimaging (e.g., CT or MRI; 17, 19–24) and cellular damage that is not visible through neuroimaging (80) in some people.

Despite decades of research, slow or incomplete recovery from MTBI is poorly understood. For a substantial majority of people, MTBIs are self-limiting and generally follow a predictable course. Permanent cognitive, psychological, or psychosocial problems due to the biological effects of this injury are relatively uncommon in trauma patients and rare in athletes (4, 6–9).

However, some people do not appear to recover completely following this injury; these individuals have been referred to as the "miserable minority" (173, 327, 328). Some have estimated that 10–20 percent of people with MTBIs will have incomplete recovery (e.g., 173, 367), although this figure is likely an over-estimate (7). When a person does not recover quickly, health care providers are very concerned about the possibility of a persistent postconcussion syndrome (328, 329, 341, 342, 345, 346), the development of depression (see 217 for a review), and/or a failure to return to work (101, 141, 147, 193, 197–200, 208, 209, 211–216). The underlying cause for poor outcome in a minority of patients is likely multifactorial, and could involve combinations of factors such as pre-existing personality characteristics, life stress, psychiatric conditions, or substance abuse problems (140, 330, 368); co-morbid conditions, such as chronic pain, depression, PTSD, life stress, or substance abuse (148, 359, 361, 362, 369–371); structural damage (macroscopic and microscopic) to the brain (11, 146); litigation (338, 340, 372); exaggeration or malingering (373–377); and symptom expectations, misattribution, and response bias (352, 370, 378–383).

Health care providers should try to prevent or reduce the severity of symptoms and problems that extend beyond a few weeks or months post injury. Early identification and intervention, with education and reassurance of the likelihood of a good outcome, to ameriolate anxiety and facilitate adjustment to transient impairment, is a recommended treatment for persons with MTBIs. Most researchers (177, 180, 181, 185–188) but not all (179, 191) have reported very favorable outcomes in studies on early intervention following MTBI.

Health care providers should be cautious when diagnosing someone with a persistent postconcussion syndrome, because this implies directly or indirectly that the person has "permanent brain damage." This can be a relief to some patients as an explanation for their perceived problems or it can have serious iatrogenic implications for other patients, a so-called "nocebo effect." This might promote a preoccupation with symptoms, fear of permanent brain damage, with hypochondriacal concern and adoption of a sick role (as per the ICD-10 diagnostic criteria for the postconcussion syndrome). For those with persistent problems, differential treatment often flows from differential diagnosis. Given the clear overlap between the symptoms of depression (and PTSD) and post-concussion syndrome, some researchers have recommended treatment with antidepressants (e.g., 148, 234–236) or cognitive behavior therapy (e.g., 185, 237). Those recommending cognitive behavior therapy have provided a treatment protocol that is based on CBT principles but is tailored toward the post-concussion syndrome and belief systems relating to symptoms and brain damage.

It will not be possible to significantly advance our understanding of poor outcome in people with MTBIs without multidisciplinary and multimodal research. This includes psychosocial and psychological research (e.g., symptom expectations and attributions), functional imaging studies, as well as differential diagnoses and specificity studies (e.g., direct comparisons with patients who have problems with depression, anxiety, substance abuse, or ADHD). Much more research is needed regarding the sensitivity and specificity of structural and functional neuroimaging techniques for trauma patients who have poor outcome from MTBI. Researchers should consider the broader neuroimaging literature in biological psychiatry.

This is because depression, chronic pain, PTSD, alcoholism, and ADHD are associated with abnormalities on SPECT (384, 385), PET (386–389), fMRI (387, 389–391), MR spectroscopy (392–396), and quantitative structural imaging (397–405). Therefore, trying to isolate imaging findings that are *specific* to the long-term effects of an MTBI should occur in the greater context of studying similar abnormalities associated with possible co-morbid conditions (e.g., depression, chronic pain, or substance abuse) or other mitigating factors.

The ability for patients with MTBIs to be properly diagnosed and treated will be greatly enhanced by three major and likely developments in the field of brain injury medicine. First, we need to develop and implement a system of standardized international terminology and classification for the condition. Second, we need to advance neurodiagnostic technology that facilitates the diagnosis of persistent cerebral functional impairment due to MTBI with high levels of sensitivity and specificity. Finally, we need to enhance our understanding of how pre-injury, injury, and post-injury vulnerability factors can affect functional outcome and can be accommodated for in the context of treatment planning. Although there is still much that we have to learn about the condition of MTBI, we have made significant progress and further progress will clearly lead to both better diagnostic accuracy and better neurological as well as functional outcomes.

References

1. Bazarian JJ, McClung J, Cheng YT, Flesher W, Schneider SM. Emergency department management of mild traumatic brain injury in the USA. *Emerg Med J* 2005;22:473–477.
2. Sosin DM, Sniezek JE, Thurman DJ. Incidence of mild and moderate brain injury in the United States, 1991. *Brain Inj* 1996;10:47–54.
3. McCrea M, Hammeke T, Olsen G, Leo P, Guskiewicz K. Unreported concussion in high school football players: implications for prevention. *Clin J Sport Med* 2004;14:13–17.
4. Belanger HG, Vanderploeg RD. The neuropsychological impact of sports-related concussion: A meta-analysis. *J Int Neuropsychol Soc* 2005;11:345–357.
5. Carroll LJ, Cassidy JD, Peloso PM, Borg J, von Holst H, Holm L, Paniak C, Pépin M. Prognosis for mild traumatic brain injury: Results of the WHO collaborating centre task force on mild traumatic brain injury. *J Rehabil Med* 2004;36:84–105.
6. Belanger HG, Curtiss G, Demery JA, Lebowitz BK, Vanderploeg RD. Factors moderating neuropsychological outcomes following mild traumatic brain injury: a meta-analysis. *J Int Neuropsychol Soc* 2005;11:215–227.
7. Iverson GL. Outcome from mild traumatic brain injury. *Curr Opin Psychiat* 2005;18:301–317.
8. Schretlen DJ, Shapiro AM. A quantitative review of the effects of traumatic brain injury on cognitive functioning. *Int Rev Psychiatry* 2003;15:341–349.
9. Rees PM. Contemporary issues in mild traumatic brain injury. *Arch Phys Med Rehabil* 2003;84:1885–1894.
10. Carroll LJ, Cassidy JD, Holm L, Kraus J, Coronado VG. Methodological issues and research recommendations for mild traumatic brain injury: the WHO Collaborating Centre Task Force on Mild Traumatic Brain Injury. *J Rehabil Med* 2004:113–125.
11. Williams DH, Levin HS, Eisenberg HM. Mild head injury classification. *Neurosurgery* 1990;27:422–428.

12. Mild Traumatic Brain Injury Committee ACoRM, Head Injury Interdisciplinary Special Interest Group. Definition of mild traumatic brain injury. *J Head Trauma Rehabil* 1993;8:86–87.

13. National Center for Injury Prevention and Control. *Report to Congress on Mild Traumatic Brain Injury in the United States: Steps to Prevent a Serious Public Health Problem.* Atlanta, GA: Centers for Disease Control and Prevention, 2003.

14. Vos PE, Battistin L, Birbamer G, Gerstenbrand F, Potapov A, Prevec T, Stepan Ch A, Traubner P, Twijnstra A, Vecsei L, von Wild K. EFNS guideline on mild traumatic brain injury: report of an EFNS task force. *Eur J Neurol* 2002;9:207–219.

15. Peloso PM, Carroll LJ, Cassidy JD, Borg J, von Holst H, Holm L, Yates D. Critical evaluation of the existing guidelines on mild traumatic brain injury. *J Rehabil Med* 2004:106–112.

16. Borg J, Holm L, Peloso PM, Cassidy JD, Carroll LJ, von Holst H, Paniak C, Yates D. Non-surgical intervention and cost for mild traumatic brain injury: results of the WHO Collaborating Centre Task Force on Mild Traumatic Brain Injury. *J Rehabil Med* 2004:76–83.

17. Borg J, Holm L, Cassidy JD, Peloso PM, Carroll LJ, von Holst H, Ericson K. Diagnostic procedures in mild traumatic brain injury: results of the WHO Collaborating Centre Task Force on Mild Traumatic Brain Injury. *J Rehabil Med* 2004:61–75.

18. Cassidy JD, Carroll LJ, Peloso PM, Borg J, von Holst H, Holm L, Kraus J, Coronado VG. Incidence, risk factors and prevention of mild traumatic brain injury: results of the WHO Collaborating Centre Task Force on Mild Traumatic Brain Injury. *J Rehabil Med* 2004:28–60.

19. French BN, Dublin AB. The value of computerized tomography in the management of 1000 consecutive head injuries. *Surg Neurol* 1977;7:171–183.

20. Iverson GL, Lovell MR, Smith S, Franzen MD. Prevalence of abnormal CT-scans following mild head injury. *Brain Inj* 2000;14:1057–1061.

21. Jeret JS, Mandell M, Anziska B, Lipitz M, Vilceus AP, Ware JA, Zesiewicz TA. Clinical predictors of abnormality disclosed by computed tomography after mild head trauma. *Neurosurgery* 1993;32:9–15;discussion 15–16.

22. Livingston DH, Loder PA, Koziol J, Hunt CD. The use of CT scanning to triage patients requiring admission following minimal head injury. *J Trauma* 1991;31:483–487;discussion 487–489.

23. Levin HS, Williams DH, Eisenberg HM, High WM, Jr., Guinto FC, Jr. Serial MRI and neurobehavioural findings after mild to moderate closed head injury. *J Neurol Neurosurg Psychiatry* 1992;55:255–262.

24. Tellier A, Della Malva LC, Cwinn A, Grahovac S, Morrish W, Brennan-Barnes M. Mild head injury: a misnomer. *Brain Inj* 1999;13:463–475.

25. Schuhmann MU, Stiller D, Skardelly M, Bernarding J, Klinge PM, Samii A, Samii M, Brinker T. Metabolic changes in the vicinity of brain contusions: a proton magnetic resonance spectroscopy and histology study. *J Neurotrauma* 2003;20:725–743.

26. Govindaraju V, Gauger GE, Manley GT, Ebel A, Meeker M, Maudsley AA. Volumetric proton spectroscopic imaging of mild traumatic brain injury. *AJNR Am J Neuroradiol* 2004;25: 730–737.

27. Garnett MR, Blamire AM, Corkill RG, Cadoux-Hudson TA, Rajagopalan B, Styles P. Early proton magnetic resonance spectroscopy in normal-appearing brain correlates with outcome in patients following traumatic brain injury. *Brain* 2000;123 (Pt 10):2046–2054.

28. Son BC, Park CK, Choi BG, Kim EN, Choe BY, Lee KS, Kim MC, Kang JK. Metabolic changes in pericontusional oedematous areas in mild head injury evaluated by 1H MRS. *Acta Neurochir Suppl* 2000;76:13–16.

29. Mittl RL, Grossman RI, Hiehle JF, Hurst RW, Kauder DR, Gennarelli TA, Alburger GW. Prevalence of MR evidence of diffuse axonal injury in patients with mild head injury and normal head CT findings. *AJNR Am J Neuroradiol* 1994;15:1583–1589.

30. van der Naalt J, Hew JM, van Zomeren AH, Sluiter WJ, Minderhoud JM. Computed tomography and magnetic resonance imaging in mild to moderate head injury: early and late imaging related to outcome. *Ann Neurol* 1999;46:70–78.

31. Voller B, Auff E, Schnider P, Aichner F. To do or not to do? Magnetic resonance imaging in mild traumatic brain injury. *Brain Inj* 2001;15:107–115.

32. Yokota H, Kurokawa A, Otsuka T, Kobayashi S, Nakazawa S. Significance of magnetic resonance imaging in acute head injury. *J Trauma* 1991;31:351–357.

33. Lorberboym M, Lampl Y, Gerzon I, Sadeh M. Brain SPECT evaluation of amnestic ED patients after mild head trauma. *Am J Emerg Med* 2002;20:310–313.

34. Audenaert K, Jansen HM, Otte A, Peremans K, Vervaet M, Crombez R, de Ridder L, van Heeringen C, Thirot J, Dierckx R, Korf J. Imaging of mild traumatic brain injury using 57Co and 99mTc HMPAO SPECT as compared to other diagnostic procedures. *Med Sci Monit* 2003;9:MT112–117.

35. Umile EM, Sandel ME, Alavi A, Terry CM, Plotkin RC. Dynamic imaging in mild traumatic brain injury: support for the theory of medial temporal vulnerability. *Arch Phys Med Rehabil* 2002; 83:1506–1513.

36. Hofman PA, Stapert SZ, van Kroonenburgh MJ, Jolles J, de Kruijk J, Wilmink JT. MR imaging, single-photon emission CT, and neurocognitive performance after mild traumatic brain injury. *AJNR Am J Neuroradiol* 2001;22:441–449.

37. MacKenzie JD, Siddiqi F, Babb JS, Bagley LJ, Mannon LJ, Sinson GP, Grossman RI. Brain atrophy in mild or moderate traumatic brain injury: a longitudinal quantitative analysis. *AJNR Am J Neuroradiol* 2002;23:1509–1515.

38. Inglese M, Bomsztyk E, Gonen O, Mannon LJ, Grossman RI, Rusinek H. Dilated perivascular spaces: hallmarks of mild traumatic brain injury. *AJNR Am J Neuroradiol* 2005;26: 719–724.

39. Chen SH, Kareken DA, Fastenau PS, Trexler LE, Hutchins GD. A study of persistent post-concussion symptoms in mild head trauma using positron emission tomography. *J Neurol Neurosurg Psychiatry* 2003;74:326–332.

40. Bonne O, Gilboa A, Louzoun Y, Kempf-Sherf O, Katz M, Fishman Y, Ben-Nahum Z, Krausz Y, Bocher M, Lester H, Chisin R, Lerer B. Cerebral blood flow in chronic symptomatic mild traumatic brain injury. *Psychiatry Res* 2003;124:141–152.

41. Abu-Judeh HH, Parker R, Singh M, el-Zeftawy H, Atay S, Kumar M, Naddaf S, Aleksic S, Abdel-Dayem HM. SPET brain perfusion imaging in mild traumatic brain injury without loss of consciousness and normal computed tomography. *Nucl Med Commun* 1999;20:505–510.

42. Perlstein WM, Cole MA, Demery JA, Seignourel PJ, Dixit NK, Larson MJ, Briggs RW. Parametric manipulation of working memory load in traumatic brain injury: behavioral and neural correlates. *J Int Neuropsychol Soc* 2004;10:724–741.

43. Povlishock JT, Becker DP, Cheng CL, Vaughan GW. Axonal change in minor head injury. *J Neuropathol Exp Neurol* 1983;42:225–242.

44. Povlishock JT, Becker DP. Fate of reactive axonal swellings induced by head injury. *Lab Invest* 1985;52:540–552.

45. Yaghmai A, Povlishock J. Traumatically induced reactive change as visualized through the use of monoclonal antibodies targeted to neurofilament subunits. *J Neuropathol Exp Neurol* 1992;51:158–176.

46. Christman CW, Grady MS, Walker SA, Holloway KL, Povlishock JT. Ultrastructural studies of diffuse axonal injury in humans. *J Neurotrauma* 1994;11:173–186.

47. Slemmer JE, Matser EJ, De Zeeuw CI, Weber JT. Repeated mild injury causes cumulative damage to hippocampal cells. *Brain* 2002;125:2699–2709.

48. Strich SJ. Shearing of nerve fibers as a cause of brain damage due to head injury. *Lancet* 1961;2:443–438.

49. Peerless SJ, Rewcastle NB. Shear injuries of the brain. *Can Med Assoc J* 1967;96:577–582.

50. Nevin NC. Neuropathological changes in the white matter following head injury. *J Neuropathol Exp Neurol* 1967;26: 77–84.

51. Holbourn AHS. Mechanics of head injury. *Lancet* 1943;2: 438–441.

52. Strich SJ. Diffuse degeneration of the cerebral white matter in severe dementia following head injury. *J Neurol Neurosurg Psychiatry* 1956;19:163–185.

53. Jane JA, Steward O, Gennarelli T. Axonal degeneration induced by experimental noninvasive minor head injury. *J Neurosurg* 1985;62:96–100.

54. Pilz P. Axonal injury in head injury. Acta Neurochir Suppl (Wien) 1983;32:119–123.

55. Gennarelli TA, Graham DI. Neuropathology of the head injuries. *Semin Clin Neuropsychiatry* 1998;3:160–175.

56. Ommaya AK, Gennarelli TA. Cerebral concussion and traumatic unconsciousness. Correlation of experimental and clinical observations of blunt head injuries. Brain 1974;97:633–654.

57. Povlishock JT, Hayes RL, Michel ME, McIntosh TK. Workshop on animal models of traumatic brain injury. *J Neurotrauma* 1994;11:723–732.

58. Duhaime AC, Christian CW, Rorke LB, Zimmerman RA. Nonaccidental head injury in infants—the "shaken-baby syndrome". *N Engl J Med* 1998;338:1822–1829.

59. Gieron MA, Korthals JK, Riggs CD. Diffuse axonal injury without direct head trauma and with delayed onset of coma. *Pediatr Neurol* 1998;19:382–384.

60. Henry GK, Gross HS, Herndon CA, Furst CJ. Nonimpact brain injury: neuropsychological and behavioral correlates with consideration of physiological findings. *Appl Neuropsychol* 2000;7: 65–75.

61. Varney NR, Varney RN. Some physics of automobile collisions with particular reference to brain injuries occuring without physical head trauma. *Appl Neuropsychol* 1995;2:47–62.

62. Olvey SE, Knox T, Cohn KA. The development of a method to measure head acceleration and motion in high-impact crashes. *Neurosurgery* 2004;54:672–677;discussion 677.

63. Crisco JJ, Chu JJ, Greenwald RM. An algorithm for estimating acceleration magnitude and impact location using multiple nonorthogonal single-axis accelerometers. *J Biomech Eng* 2004; 126:849–854.

64. Duma SM, Manoogian SJ, Bussone WR, Brolinson PG, Goforth MW, Donnenwerth JJ, Greenwald RM, Chu JJ, Crisco JJ. Analysis of real-time head accelerations in collegiate football players. *Clin J Sport Med* 2005;15:3–8.

65. Pellman EJ, Viano DC, Tucker AM, Casson IR. Concussion in professional football: location and direction of helmet impacts-Part 2. *Neurosurgery* 2003;53:1328–1340;discussion 1340–1341.

66. Withnall C, Shewchenko N, Gittens R, Dvorak J. Biomechanical investigation of head impacts in football. *Br J Sports Med* 2005;39 Suppl 1:i49–57.

67. Smith DH, Wolf JA, Lusardi TA, Lee VM, Meaney DF. High tolerance and delayed elastic response of cultured axons to dynamic stretch injury. *J Neurosci* 1999;19:4263–4269.

68. Wolf JA, Stys PK, Lusardi T, Meaney D, Smith DH. Traumatic axonal injury induces calcium influx modulated by tetrodotoxin-sensitive sodium channels. *J Neurosci* 2001;21:1923–1930.

69. Iwata A, Stys PK, Wolf JA, Chen XH, Taylor AG, Meaney DF, Smith DH. Traumatic axonal injury induces proteolytic cleavage of the voltage-gated sodium channels modulated by tetrodotoxin and protease inhibitors. *J Neurosci* 2004;24:4605–4613.

70. Bain AC, Raghupathi R, Meaney DF. Dynamic stretch correlates to both morphological abnormalities and electrophysiological impairment in a model of traumatic axonal injury. *J Neurotrauma* 2001;18:499–511.

71. Giza CC, Hovda DA. The pathophysiology of traumatic brain injury. In: Lovell MR, Echemendia RJ, Barth JT, Collins MW, editors. Traumatic Brain Injury in Sports. *Lisse: Swets & Zeitlinger*, 2004. p 45–70.

72. Erb DE, Povlishock JT. Neuroplasticity following traumatic brain injury: a study of GABAergic terminal loss and recovery in the cat dorsal lateral vestibular nucleus. *Exp Brain Res* 1991;83:253–267.

73. Grady MS, McLaughlin MR, Christman CW, Valadka AB, Fligner CL, Povlishock JT. The use of antibodies targeted against the neurofilament subunits for the detection of diffuse axonal injury in humans. *J Neuropathol Exp Neurol* 1993;52:143–152.

74. Pettus EH, Christman CW, Giebel ML, Povlishock JT. Traumatically induced altered membrane permeability: its relationship to traumatically induced reactive axonal change. *J Neurotrauma* 1994;11:507–522.

75. Daugherty WP, Levasseur JE, Sun D, Rockswold GL, Bullock MR. Effects of hyperbaric oxygen therapy on cerebral oxygenation and mitochondrial function following moderate lateral fluid-percussion injury in rats. *J Neurosurg* 2004;101:499–504.

76. Schwartz JH. Synthesis and trafficking of neural proteins. In: Kandel ER, Schwartz JH, Jessell TM, editors. Principles of neural science, 3rd ed. New York: Elsevier, 1991. p 49–65.

77. Gaetz M. The neurophysiology of brain injury. Clin Neurophysiol 2004;115:4–18.

78. Maxwell WL, Kansagra AM, Graham DI, Adams JH, Gennarelli TA. Freeze-fracture studies of reactive myelinated nerve fibres after diffuse axonal injury. *Acta Neuropathol (Berl)* 1988;76: 395–406.

79. Oppenheimer DR. Microscopic lesions in the brain following head injury. *J Neurol Neurosurg Psychiatry* 1968;31:299–306.

80. Bigler ED. Neuropsychological results and neuropathological findings at autopsy in a case of mild traumatic brain injury. *J Int Neuropsychol Soc* 2004;10:794–806.

81. Denny-Brown D, Russell W. Experimental cerebral concussion. *Brain* 1941;64:93–164.

82. Foltz EL, Schmidt RP. The role of the reticular formation in the coma of head injury. *J Neurosurg* 1956;13:145–154.

83. Adams H, Mitchell DE, Graham DI, Doyle D. Diffuse brain damage of immediate impact type. Its relationship to 'primary brainstem damage' in head injury. Brain 1977;100:489–502.

84. Povlishock JT. Pathobiology of traumatically induced axonal injury in animals and man. *Ann Emerg Med* 1993;22:980–986.

85. Gentry LR, Godersky JC, Thompson B, Dunn VD. Prospective comparative study of intermediate-field MR and CT in the evaluation of closed head trauma. *AJR Am J Roentgenol* 1988; 150:673–682.

86. Gaetz M, Bernstein DM. The current status of electrophysiologic procedures for the assessment of mild traumatic brain injury. *J Head Trauma Rehabil* 2001;16:386–405.

87. Picton TW, Stuss DT. Neurobiology of conscious experience. *Curr Opin Neurobiol* 1994;4:256–265.

88. Ingebrigtsen T, Romner B. Biochemical serum markers for brain damage: a short review with emphasis on clinical utility in mild head injury. *Restor Neurol Neurosci* 2003;21:171–176.

89. Ingebrigtsen T, Romner B. Biochemical serum markers of traumatic brain injury. *J Trauma* 2002;52:798–808.

90. Ingebrigtsen T, Romner B. Serial S-100 protein serum measurements related to early magnetic resonance imaging after minor head injury. Case report. *J Neurosurg* 1996;85:945–948.

91. Mussack T, Biberthaler P, Kanz KG, Heckl U, Gruber R, Linsenmaier U, Mutschler W, Jochum M. Immediate S-100B and neuron-specific enolase plasma measurements for rapid evaluation of primary brain damage in alcohol-intoxicated, minor head-injured patients. *Shock* 2002;18:395–400.

92. Biberthaler P, Mussack T, Wiedemann E, Kanz KG, Gilg T, Gippner-Steppert C, Jochum M. Influence of alcohol exposure on S-100b serum levels. *Acta Neurochir Suppl* 2000;76:177–179.

93. Mussack T, Biberthaler P, Kanz KG, Wiedemann E, Gippner-Steppert C, Mutschler W, Jochum M. Serum S-100B and interleukin-8 as predictive markers for comparative neurologic outcome analysis of patients after cardiac arrest and severe traumatic brain injury. *Crit Care Med* 2002;30:2669–2674.

94. de Kruijk JR, Leffers P, Menheere PP, Meerhoff S, Twijnstra A. S-100B and neuron-specific enolase in serum of mild traumatic brain injury patients. A comparison with health controls. *Acta Neurol Scand* 2001;103:175–179.

95. Herrmann M, Curio N, Jost S, Grubich C, Ebert AD, Fork ML, Synowitz H. Release of biochemical markers of damage to neuronal and glial brain tissue is associated with short and long term neuropsychological outcome after traumatic brain injury. *J Neurol Neurosurg Psychiatry* 2001;70:95–100.

96. Vos PE, Verbeek MM. Brain specific proteins in serum: do they reliably reflect brain damage? *Shock* 2002;18:481–482.

97. Biberthaler P, Mussack T, Wiedemann E, Kanz KG, Koelsch M, Gippner-Steppert C, Jochum M. Evaluation of S-100b as a specific marker for neuronal damage due to minor head trauma. *World J Surg* 2001;25:93–97.

98. Biberthaler P, Mussack T, Wiedemann E, Gilg T, Soyka M, Koller G, Pfeifer KJ, Linsenmaier U, Mutschler W, Gippner-Steppert C, Jochum M. Elevated serum levels of S-100B reflect the extent of

brain injury in alcohol intoxicated patients after mild head trauma. *Shock* 2001;16:97–101.

99. Romner B, Ingebrigtsen T, Kongstad P, Borgesen SE. Traumatic brain damage: serum S-100 protein measurements related to neuroradiological findings. *J Neurotrauma* 2000;17:641–647.

100. Townend WJ, Guy MJ, Pani MA, Martin B, Yates DW. Head injury outcome prediction in the emergency department: a role for protein S-100B? *J Neurol Neurosurg Psychiatry* 2002;73:542–546.

101. Stranjalis G, Korfias S, Papapetrou C, Kouyialis A, Boviatsis E, Psachoulia C, Sakas DE. Elevated serum S-100B protein as a predictor of failure to short-term return to work or activities after mild head injury. *J Neurotrauma* 2004;21:1070–1075.

102. Herrmann M, Curio N, Jost S, Wunderlich MT, Synowitz H, Wallesch CW. Protein S-100B and neuron specific enolase as early neurobiochemical markers of the severity of traumatic brain injury. *Restor Neurol Neurosci* 1999;14:109–114.

103. Ingebrigtsen T, Romner B, Marup-Jensen S, Dons M, Lundqvist C, Bellner J, Alling C, Borgesen SE. The clinical value of serum S-100 protein measurements in minor head injury: a Scandinavian multicentre study. *Brain Inj* 2000;14:1047–1055.

104. Stapert S, de Kruijk J, Houx P, Menheere P, Twijnstra A, Jolles J. S-100B concentration is not related to neurocognitive performance in the first month after mild traumatic brain injury. *Eur Neurol* 2005;53:22–26.

105. Stalnacke BM, Bjornstig U, Karlsson K, Sojka P. One-year follow-up of mild traumatic brain injury: post-concussion symptoms, disabilities and life satisfaction in relation to serum levels of S-100B and neurone-specific enolase in acute phase. *J Rehabil Med* 2005;37:300–305.

106. Ingebrigtsen T, Waterloo K, Jacobsen EA, Langbakk B, Romner B. Traumatic brain damage in minor head injury: relation of serum S-100 protein measurements to magnetic resonance imaging and neurobehavioral outcome. *Neurosurgery* 1999;45:468–475;discussion 475–466.

107. Anderson RE, Hansson LO, Nilsson O, Dijlai-Merzoug R, Settergren G. High serum S100B levels for trauma patients without head injuries. *Neurosurgery* 2001;48:1255–1258;discussion 1258–1260.

108. Otto M, Holthusen S, Bahn E, Sohnchen N, Wiltfang J, Geese R, Fischer A, Reimers CD. Boxing and running lead to a rise in serum levels of S-100B protein. *Int J Sports Med* 2000;21:551–555.

109. Stalnacke BM, Tegner Y, Sojka P. Playing ice hockey and basketball increases serum levels of S-100B in elite players: a pilot study. *Clin J Sport Med* 2003;13:292–302.

110. Stalnacke BM, Tegner Y, Sojka P. Playing soccer increases serum concentrations of the biochemical markers of brain damage S-100B and neuron-specific enolase in elite players: a pilot study. *Brain Inj* 2004;18:899–909.

111. Waterloo K, Ingebrigtsen T, Romner B. Neuropsychological function in patients with increased serum levels of protein S-100 after minor head injury. *Acta Neurochir (Wien)* 1997;139:26–31;discussion 31–22.

112. Akhtar JI, Spear RM, Senac MO, Peterson BM, Diaz SM. Detection of traumatic brain injury with magnetic resonance imaging and S-100B protein in children, despite normal computed tomography of the brain. *Pediatr Crit Care Med* 2003;4:322–326.

113. Ytrebo LM, Nedredal GI, Korvald C, Holm Nielsen OJ, Ingebrigtsen T, Romner B, Aarbakke J, Revhaug A. Renal elimination of protein S-100beta in pigs with acute encephalopathy. *Scand J Clin Lab Invest* 2001;61:217–225.

114. Jonsson H, Johnsson P, Hoglund P, Alling C, Blomquist S. Elimination of S100B and renal function after cardiac surgery. *J Cardiothorac Vasc Anesth* 2000;14:698–701.

115. Symonds CP. Observations on the differential diagnosis and treatment of cerebral states consequent upon head injuries. *Bmj* 1928;November 10:829–832.

116. Congress of Neurological Surgeons. Committee on head injury nomenclature: Glossary of head injury. *Clin Neurosurg* 1966;12:386–394.

117. Guskiewicz KM, Weaver NL, Padua DA, Garrett WE, Jr. Epidemiology of concussion in collegiate and high school football players. *Am J Sports Med* 2000;28:643–650.

118. Macciocchi SN, Barth JT, Alves W, Rimel RW, Jane JA. Neuropsychological functioning and recovery after mild head injury in collegiate athletes. *Neurosurgery* 1996;39:510–514.

119. McCrea M, Guskiewicz KM, Marshall SW, Barr W, Randolph C, Cantu RC, Onate JA, Yang J, Kelly JP. Acute effects and recovery time following concussion in collegiate football players: the NCAA Concussion Study. *JAMA* 2003;290:2556–2563.

120. Hanlon RE, Demery JA, Martinovich Z, Kelly JP. Effects of acute injury characteristics on neurophysical status and vocational outcome following mild traumatic brain injury. *Brain Inj* 1999;13:873–887.

121. Lovell MR, Iverson GL, Collins MW, McKeag D, Maroon JC. Does loss of consciousness predict neuropsychological decrements after concussion? *Clin J Sport Med* 1999;9:193–198.

122. Paniak C, MacDonald J, Toller-Lobe G, Durand A, Nagy J. A preliminary normative profile of mild traumatic brain injury diagnostic criteria. *J Clin Exp Neuropsychol* 1998;20:852–855.

123. Gennarelli TA, Thibault LE, Adams JH, Graham DI, Thompson CJ, Marcincin RP. Diffuse axonal injury and traumatic coma in the primate. *Ann Neurol* 1982;12:564–574.

124. Dikmen SS, Machamer JE, Winn R, Temkin NR. Neuropsychological outcome 1-year post head injury. *Neuropsychology* 1995;9:80–90.

125. Iverson GL, Lovell MR, Smith SS. Does brief loss of consciousness affect cognitive functioning after mild head injury? *Arch Clin Neuropsychol* 2000;15:643–648.

126. Leininger BE, Gramling SE, Farrell AD, Kreutzer JS, Peck EA, 3rd. Neuropsychological deficits in symptomatic minor head injury patients after concussion and mild concussion. *J Neurol Neurosurg Psychiatry* 1990;53:293–296.

127. Asplund CA, McKeag DB, Olsen CH. Sport-Related Concussion: Factors Associated With Prolonged Return to Play. *Clin J Sport Med* 2004;14:339–343.

128. McCrea M, Kelly JP, Randolph C, Cisler R, Berger L. Immediate neurocognitive effects of concussion. *Neurosurgery* 2002;50:1032–1040.

129. Pellman EJ, Viano DC, Casson IR, Arfken C, Powell J. Concussion in Professional Football: Injuries Involving 7 or More Days Out-Part 5. *Neurosurgery* 2004;55:1100–1119.

130. Collins MW, Iverson GL, Lovell MR, McKeag DB, Norwig J, Maroon J. On-field predictors of neuropsychological and symptom deficit following sports-related concussion. *Clin J Sport Med* 2003;13:222–229.

131. Guskiewicz KM, Ross SE, Marshall SW. Postural stability and neuropsychological deficits after concussion in collegiate athletes. *J Athl Train* 2001;36:263–273.

132. Brooks DN, Aughton ME, Bond MR, Jones P, Rizvi S. Cognitive sequelae in relationship to early indices of severity of brain damage after severe blunt head injury. *J Neurol Neurosurg Psychiatry* 1980;43:529–534.

133. Ellenberg JH, Levin HS, Saydjari C. Posttraumatic Amnesia as a predictor of outcome after severe closed head injury. Prospective assessment. *Arch Neurol* 1996;53:782–791.

134. Haslam C, Batchelor J, Fearnside MR, Haslam SA, Hawkins S, Kenway E. Post-coma disturbance and post-traumatic amnesia as nonlinear predictors of cognitive outcome following severe closed head injury: findings from the Westmead Head Injury Project. *Brain Inj* 1994;8:519–528.

135. Russell WR, Nathan PW. Traumatic amnesia. *Brain* 1946;69:280–301.

136. Wilson JT, Teasdale GM, Hadley DM, Wiedmann KD, Lang D. Post-traumatic amnesia: still a valuable yardstick. *J Neurol Neurosurg Psychiatry* 1994;57:198–201.

137. Alexandre A, Colombo F, Nertempi P, Benedetti A. Cognitive outcome and early indices of severity of head injury. *J Neurosurg* 1983;59:751–761.

138. Lovell MR, Collins MW, Iverson GL, Field M, Maroon JC, Cantu R, Podell K, Powell JW, Belza M, Fu FH. Recovery from mild concussion in high school athletes. *J Neurosurg* 2003;98: 296–301.

139. Collins MW, Field M, Lovell MR, Iverson G, Johnston KM, Maroon J, Fu FH. Relationship between postconcussion headache and neuropsychological test performance in high school athletes. *Am J Sports Med* 2003;31:168–173.

140. Ponsford J, Willmott C, Rothwell A, Cameron P, Kelly AM, Nelms R, Curran C, Ng K. Factors influencing outcome following mild traumatic brain injury in adults. *J Int Neuropsychol Soc* 2000;6:568–579.

141. van der Naalt J, van Zomeren AH, Sluiter WJ, Minderhoud JM. One year outcome in mild to moderate head injury: the predictive value of acute injury characteristics related to complaints and return to work. *J Neurol Neurosurg Psychiatry* 1999;66:207–213.

142. Borgaro SR, Prigatano GP, Kwasnica C, Rexer JL. Cognitive and affective sequelae in complicated and uncomplicated mild traumatic brain injury. *Brain Inj* 2003;17:189–198.

143. Iverson GL, Franzen MD, Lovell M, Smith S. Complicated versus uncomplicated mild head injury. *J Int Neuropsychol Soc* 1998;4:75.

144. Iverson GL, Franzen MD, Lovell MR. Normative comparisons for the controlled oral word association test following acute traumatic brain injury. *Clin Neuropsychol* 1999;13:437–441.

145. Wilson JTL, Hadley DM, Scott LC, Harper A. Neuropsychological significance of contusional lesions identified by MRI. In: Uzzell BP, Stonnington HH, editors. Recovery after Traumatic Brain Injury. Mahway, NJ: Lawrence Erlbaum Associates, 1996. p 29–50.

146. Temkin NR, Machamer JE, Dikmen SS. Correlates of functional status 3–5 years after traumatic brain injury with CT abnormalities. *J Neurotrauma* 2003;20:229–241.

147. Hughes DG, Jackson A, Mason DL, Berry E, Hollis S, Yates DW. Abnormalities on magnetic resonance imaging seen acutely following mild traumatic brain injury: correlation with neuropsychological tests and delayed recovery. *Neuroradiology* 2004;46:550–558.

148. McCauley SR, Boake C, Levin HS, Contant CF, Song JX. Postconcussional disorder following mild to moderate traumatic brain injury: anxiety, depression, and social support as risk factors and comorbidities. *J Clin Exp Neuropsychol* 2001;23: 792–808.

149. Levin HS, O'Donnell VM, Grossman RG. The Galveston Orientation and Amnesia Test. A practical scale to assess cognition after head injury. *J Nerv Ment Dis* 1979;167:675–684.

150. Reitan RM, Wolfson D. The Halstead-Reitan neuropsychological test battery: Theory and clinical interpretation, second edition. Tucson, AZ: Neuropsychology Press, 1993.

151. Wechsler D. Wechsler Memory Scale-Revised. San Antonio, TX: The Psychological Corporation, 1987.

152. Benton AL, Hamsher K, Sivan AB. Multilingual Aphasia Examination, Third Edition: A manual of instructions. Iowa City: University of Iowa Press, 1994.

153. Robinson LJ, Kester DB, Saykin AJ, Kaplan EF, Gur RC. Comparison of two short forms of the Wisconsin Card Sorting Test. *Arch Clin Neuropsychol* 1991;6:27–33.

154. Axelrod BN, Jiron CC, Henry RR. Performance of adults ages 20 to 90 on the abbreviated Wisconsin Card Sorting Test. *Clin Neurol* 1993;7:205–209.

155. Heaton RK, Chelune GJ, Talley JL, Kay GG, Curtiss G. Wisconsin card sorting test manual. Odessa, FL: Psychological Assessment Resources, 1993.

156. Kongs SK, Thompson LL, Iverson GL, Heaton RK. Wisconsin Card Sorting Test - 64 Card Version, Professional Manual. Odessa, FL: Psychological Assessment Resources, 2000.

157. Brandt J. The Hopkins Verbal Learning Test: Development of a new memory test with six equivalent forms. *Clin Neuropsychol* 1991;5:125–142.

158. Benedict RH, Schretlen D, Groninger L, Brandt J. Hopkins Verbal Learning Test - Revised: Normative data and analysis of interform and test-retest reliability. *Clin Neuropsychol* 1998;12: 43–55.

159. Iverson GL, Lovell MR, Smith S. Does brief loss of consciousness affect cognitive functioning after mild head injury? *J Int Neuropsychol Soc* 1997;3:75.

160. Bleiberg J, Cernich AN, Cameron K, Sun W, Peck K, Ecklund PJ, Reeves D, Uhorchak J, Sparling MB, Warden DL. Duration of cognitive impairment after sports concussion. *Neurosurgery* 2004;54:1073–1078;discussion 1078–1080.

161. Lovell MR, Collins MW, Iverson GL, Johnston KM, Bradley JP. Grade 1 or "ding" concussions in high school athletes. *Am J Sports Med* 2004;32:47–54.

162. Hugenholtz H, Stuss DT, Stethem LL, Richard MT. How long does it take to recover from a mild concussion? *Neurosurgery* 1988;22:853–858.

163. Levin HS, Mattis S, Ruff RM, Eisenberg HM, Marshall LF, Tabaddor K, High WM, Jr., Frankowski RF. Neurobehavioral outcome following minor head injury: a three-center study. *J Neurosurg* 1987;66:234–243.

164. Mathias JL, Beall JA, Bigler ED. Neuropsychological and information processing deficits following mild traumatic brain injury. *J Int Neuropsychol Soc* 2004;10:286–297.

165. Pellman EJ, Lovell MR, Viano DC, Casson IR, Tucker AM. Concussion in professional football: neuropsychological testing-part 6. *Neurosurgery* 2004;55:1290–1305.

166. Gentilini M, Nichelli P, Schoenhuber R, Bortolotti P, Tonelli L, Falasca A, Merli GA. Neuropsychological evaluation of mild head injury. *J Neurol Neurosurg Psychiatry* 1985;48:137–140.

167. Lahmeyer HW, Bellur SN. Cardiac regulation and depression. *J Psychiatry Res* 1987;21:1–6.

168. Dikmen S, Machamer J, Temkin N. Mild head injury: facts and artifacts. *J Clin Exp Neuropsychol* 2001;23:729–738.

169. Goldstein FC, Levin HS, Goldman WP, Clark AN, Altonen TK. Cognitive and neurobehavioral functioning after mild versus moderate traumatic brain injury in older adults. *J Int Neuropsychol Soc* 2001;7:373–383.

170. Fay GC, Jaffe KM, Polissar NL, Liao S, Martin KM, Shurtleff HA, Rivara JM, Winn HR. Mild pediatric traumatic brain injury: a cohort study. *Arch Phys Med Rehabil* 1993;74:895–901.

171. Bijur PE, Haslum M, Golding J. Cognitive and behavioral sequelae of mild head injury in children. *Pediatrics* 1990;86:337–344.

172. Binder LM. A review of mild head trauma. Part II: Clinical implications. *J Clin Exp Neuropsychol* 1997;19:432–457.

173. Ruff R. Two decades of advances in understanding of mild traumatic brain injury. *J Head Trauma Rehabil* 2005;20:5–18.

174. Gronwall D. Rehabilitation programs for patients with mild head injury: Components, problems, and evaluation. *J Head Trauma Rehabil* 1986;1:53–62.

175. Kay T. Neuropsychological treatment of mild traumatic brain injury. *J Head Trauma Rehabil* 1993;8:74–85.

176. Wrightson P. Management of disability and rehabilitation services after mild head injury. In: Levin HS, Eisenberg HM, Benton AL, editors. Mild head injury. New York, NY: Oxford University Press, 1989. p 245–256.

177. Minderhoud JM, Boelens ME, Huizenga J, Saan RJ. Treatment of minor head injuries. *Clin Neurol Neurosurg* 1980;82:127–140.

178. Relander M, Troupp H, Af Bjorkesten G. Controlled trial of treatment for cerebral concussion. *Br Med J* 1972;4:777–779.

179. Ponsford J, Willmott C, Rothwell A, Cameron P, Ayton G, Nelms R, Curran C, Ng KT. Cognitive and behavioral outcome following mild traumatic head injury in children. *J Head Trauma Rehabil* 1999;14:360–372.

180. Paniak C, Toller-Lobe G, Durand A, Nagy J. A randomized trial of two treatments for mild traumatic brain injury. *Brain Inj* 1998;12:1011–1023.

181. Ponsford J, Willmott C, Rothwell A, Cameron P, Ayton G, Nelms R, Curran C, Ng K. Impact of early intervention on outcome after mild traumatic brain injury in children. *Pediatrics* 2001;108: 1297–1303.

182. de Kruijk JR, Leffers P, Meerhoff S, Rutten J, Twijnstra A. Effectiveness of bed rest after mild traumatic brain injury: a randomised trial of no versus six days of bed rest. *J Neurol Neurosurg Psychiatry* 2002;73:167–172.

183. Lowdon IM, Briggs M, Cockin J. Post-concussional symptoms following minor head injury. *Injury* 1989;20:193–194.

184. Chapman EH, Weintraub RJ, Milburn MA, Pirozzi TO, Woo E. Homeopathic treatment of mild traumatic brain injury: A randomized, double-blind, placebo-controlled clinical trial. *J Head Trauma Rehabil* 1999;14:521–542.

185. Mittenberg W, Tremont G, Zielinski RE, Fichera S, Rayls KR. Cognitive-behavioral prevention of postconcussion syndrome. *Arch Clin Neuropsychol* 1996;11:139–145.

186. Paniak C, Toller-Lobe G, Reynolds S, Melnyk A, Nagy J. A randomized trial of two treatments for mild traumatic brain injury:1 year follow-up. *Brain Inj* 2000;14:219–226.

187. Ponsford J, Willmott C, Rothwell A, Cameron P, Kelly AM, Nelms R, Curran C. Impact of early intervention on outcome following mild head injury in adults. *J Neurol Neurosurg Psychiatry* 2002;73:330–332.

188. Wade DT, King NS, Wenden FJ, Crawford S, Caldwell FE. Routine follow up after head injury: a second randomised controlled trial. *J Neurol Neurosurg Psychiatry* 1998;65:177–183.

189. Ho MR, Bennett TL. Efficacy of neuropsychological rehabilitation for mild-moderate traumatic brain injury. *Arch Clin Neuropsychol* 1997;12:1–11.

190. Cicerone KD, Smith LC, Ellmo W, Mangel HR, Nelson P, Chase RF, Kalmar K. Neuropsychological rehabilitation of mild traumatic brain injury. *Brain Inj* 1996;10:277–286.

191. Wade DT, Crawford S, Wenden FJ, King NS, Moss NE. Does routine follow up after head injury help? A randomised controlled trial. *J Neurol Neurosurg Psychiatry* 1997;62:478–484.

192. Alves W, Macciocchi SN, Barth JT. Postconcussive symptoms after uncomplicated mild head injury. *J Head Trauma Rehabil* 1993;8:48–59.

193. Edna TH, Cappelen J. Return to work and social adjustment after traumatic head injury. *Acta Neurochir (Wien)* 1987;85:40–43.

194. Mazaux JM, Masson F, Levin HS, Alaoui P, Maurette P, Barat M. Long-term neuropsychological outcome and loss of social autonomy after traumatic brain injury. *Arch Phys Med Rehabil* 1997;78:1316–1320.

195. McMordie WR, Barker SL, Paolo TM. Return to work (RTW) after head injury. *Brain Inj* 1990;4:57–69.

196. Ruffolo CF, Friedland JF, Dawson DR, Colantonio A, Lindsay PH. Mild traumatic brain injury from motor vehicle accidents: factors associated with return to work. *Arch Phys Med Rehabil* 1999;80:392–398.

197. Stambrook M, Moore AD, Peters LC, Deviaene C, Hawryluk GA. Effects of mild, moderate and severe closed head injury on long-term vocational status. *Brain Inj* 1990;4:183–190.

198. Dikmen SS, Temkin NR, Machamer JE, Holubkov AL, Fraser RT, Winn HR. Employment following traumatic head injuries. *Arch Neurol* 1994;51:177–186.

199. Kraus J, Schaffer K, Ayers K, Stenehjem J, Shen H, Afifi AA. Physical complaints, medical service use, and social and employment changes following mild traumatic brain injury: a 6-month longitudinal study. *J Head Trauma Rehabil* 2005;20:239–256.

200. Wrightson P, Gronwall D. Time off work and symptoms after minor head injury. *Injury* 1981;12:445–454.

201. Cifu DX, Keyser-Marcus L, Lopez E, Wehman P, Kreutzer JS, Englander J, High W. Acute predictors of successful return to work 1 year after traumatic brain injury: a multicenter analysis. *Arch Phys Med Rehabil* 1997;78:125–131.

202. Ponsford JL, Olver JH, Curran C, Ng K. Prediction of employment status 2 years after traumatic brain injury. *Brain Inj* 1995;9:11–20.

203. Franulic A, Carbonell CG, Pinto P, Sepulveda I. Psychosocial adjustment and employment outcome 2, 5 and 10 years after TBI. *Brain Inj* 2004;18:119–129.

204. Keyser-Marcus LA, Bricout JC, Wehman P, Campbell LR, Cifu DX, Englander J, High W, Zafonte RD. Acute predictors of return to employment after traumatic brain injury: a longitudinal follow-up. *Arch Phys Med Rehabil* 2002;83:635–641.

205. Spikman JM, Timmerman ME, Zomeren van AH, Deelman BG. Recovery versus retest effects in attention after closed head injury. *J Clin Exp Neuropsychol* 1999;21:585–605.

206. Ip RY, Dornan J, Schentag C. Traumatic brain injury: factors predicting return to work or school. *Brain Inj* 1995;9:517–532.

207. Gollaher K, High W, Sherer M, Bergloff P, Boake C, Young ME, Ivanhoe C. Prediction of employment outcome one to three years following traumatic brain injury (TBI). *Brain Inj* 1998;12:255–263.

208. Asikainen I, Kaste M, Sarna S. Patients with traumatic brain injury referred to a rehabilitation and re-employment programme: social and professional outcome for 508 Finnish patients 5 or more years after injury. *Brain Inj* 1996;10:883–899.

209. Dawson DR, Levine B, Schwartz ML, Stuss DT. Acute predictors of real-world outcomes following traumatic brain injury: a prospective study. *Brain Inj* 2004;18:221–238.

210. Hawley CA, Ward AB, Magnay AR, Mychalkiw W. Return to school after brain injury. *Arch Dis Child* 2004;89:136–142.

211. Uzzell BP, Langfitt TW, Dolinskas CA. Influence of injury severity on quality of survival after head injury. *Surg Neurol* 1987;27:419–429.

212. McCullagh S, Oucherlony D, Protzner A, Blair N, Feinstein A. Prediction of neuropsychiatric outcome following mild trauma brain injury: an examination of the Glasgow Coma Scale. *Brain Inj* 2001;15:489–497.

213. Vanderploeg RD, Curtiss G, Duchnick JJ, Luis CA. Demographic, medical, and psychiatric factors in work and marital status after mild head injury. *J Head Trauma Rehabil* 2003;18:148–163.

214. Haboubi NH, Long J, Koshy M, Ward AB. Short-term sequelae of minor head injury (6 years experience of minor head injury clinic). *Disabil Rehabil* 2001;23:635–638.

215. Friedland JF, Dawson DR. Function after motor vehicle accidents: a prospective study of mild head injury and posttraumatic stress. *J Nerv Ment Dis* 2001;189:426–434.

216. Drake AI, Gray N, Yoder S, Pramuka M, Llewellyn M. Factors predicting return to work following mild traumatic brain injury: a discriminant analysis. *J Head Trauma Rehabil* 2000;15:1103–1112.

217. Moldover JE, Goldberg KB, Prout MF. Depression after traumatic brain injury: a review of evidence for clinical heterogeneity. *Neuropsychol Rev* 2004;14:143–154.

218. Silver JM, Kramer R, Greenwald S, Weissman M. The association between head injuries and psychiatric disorders: findings from the New Haven NIMH Epidemiologic Catchment Area Study. *Brain Inj* 2001;15:935–945.

219. Jorge RE, Robinson RG, Starkstein SE, Arndt SV. Depression and anxiety following traumatic brain injury. *J Neuropsychiatry Clin Neurosci* 1993;5:369–374.

220. Varney N, Martzke J, Roberts R. Major depression in patients with closed head injury. *Neuropsychology* 1987;1:7–8.

221. Horner MD, Ferguson PL, Selassie AW, Labbate LA, Kniele K, Corrigan JD. Patterns of alcohol use 1 year after traumatic brain injury: a population-based, epidemiological study. *J Int Neuropsychol Soc* 2005;11:322–330.

222. Bowen A, Neumann V, Conner M, Tennant A, Chamberlain MA. Mood disorders following traumatic brain injury: identifying the extent of the problem and the people at risk. *Brain Inj* 1998;12:177–190.

223. Deb S, Lyons I, Koutzoukis C, Ali I, McCarthy G. Rate of psychiatric illness 1 year after traumatic brain injury. *Am J Psychiatry* 1999;156:374–378.

224. Dikmen SS, Bombardier CH, Machamer JE, Fann JR, Temkin NR. Natural history of depression in traumatic brain injury. *Arch Phys Med Rehabil* 2004;85:1457–1464.

225. Jorge RE, Robinson RG, Moser D, Tateno A, Crespo-Facorro B, Arndt S. Major depression following traumatic brain injury. *Arch Gen Psychiatry* 2004;61:42–50.

226. Kersel DA, Marsh NV, Havill JH, Sleigh JW. Psychosocial functioning during the year following severe traumatic brain injury. *Brain Inj* 2001;15:683–696.

227. Levin HS, Brown SA, Song JX, McCauley SR, Boake C, Contant CF, Goodman H, Kotrla KJ. Depression and posttraumatic stress disorder at three months after mild to moderate traumatic brain injury. *J Clin Exp Neuropsychol* 2001;23:754–769.

228. Kreutzer JS, Seel RT, Gourley E. The prevalence and symptom rates of depression after traumatic brain injury: a comprehensive examination. *Brain Inj* 2001;15:563–576.

229. Seel RT, Kreutzer JS. Depression assessment after traumatic brain injury: An empirically based classification method. *J Phys Med Rehabil* 2003;84:1621–1628.

230. Ashman TA, Spielman LA, Hibbard MR, Silver JM, Chandna T, Gordon WA. Psychiatric challenges in the first 6 years after traumatic brain injury: cross-sequential analyses of Axis I disorders. *Arch Phys Med Rehabil* 2004;85:S36–42.

231. Chamelian L, Feinstein A. Outcome after mild to moderate traumatic brain injury: the role of dizziness. *Arch Phys Med Rehabil* 2004;85:1662–1666.

232. Federoff JP, Starkstein SE, Forrester AW, Geisler FH, Jorge RE, Arndt S, Robinson RG. Depression in patients with acute traumatic brain injury. *Am J Psychiatry* 1992;149:918–923.

233. Hibbard MR, Ashman TA, Spielman LA, Chun D, Charatz HJ, Melvin S. Relationship between depression and psychosocial functioning after traumatic brain injury. *Arch Phys Med Rehabil* 2004;85:S43–53.

234. Zafonte RD, Cullen N, Lexell J. Serotonin agents in the treatment of acquired brain injury. *J Head Trauma Rehabil* 2002;17:322–334.

235. Fann JR, Uomoto JM, Katon WJ. Cognitive improvement with treatment of depression following mild traumatic brain injury. *Psychosomatics* 2001;42:48–54.

236. Fann JR, Uomoto JM, Katon WJ. Sertraline in the treatment of major depression following mild traumatic brain injury. *J Neuropsychiatry Clin Neurosci* 2000;12:226–232.

237. Mittenberg W, Canyock EM, Condit D, Patton C. Treatment of post-concussion syndrome following mild head injury. *J Clin Exp Neuropsychol* 2001;23:829–836.

238. Iverson GL. Misdiagnosis of persistent postconcussion syndrome in patients with depression. *Arch Clin Neuropsychol* 2006;21:303–310.

239. Iverson GL, Gaetz M. Practical considerations for interpreting change following concussion. In: Lovell MR, Echemendia RJ, Barth J, Collins MW, editors. Traumatic brain injury in sports: An international neuropsychological perspective. Netherlands: Swets-Zeitlinger, 2004. p 323–356.

240. Iverson GL, Lange RT. Examination of "Postconcussion-Like" symptoms in a healthy sample. *Applied Neuropsychology* 2003;10:137–144.

241. Atkinson JH, Slater MA, Patterson TL, Grant I, Garfin SR. Prevalence, onset, and risk of psychiatric disorders in men with chronic low back pain: a controlled study. *Pain* 1991;45:111–121.

242. Campbell LC, Clauw DJ, Keefe FJ. Persistent pain and depression: a biopsychosocial perspective. *Biol Psychiatry* 2003;54:399–409.

243. Wilson KG, Eriksson MY, D'Eon JL, Mikail SF, Emery PC. Major depression and insomnia in chronic pain. *Clin J Pain* 2002;18:77–83.

244. Ericsson M, Poston WS, Linder J, Taylor JE, Haddock CK, Foreyt JP. Depression predicts disability in long-term chronic pain patients. *Disabil Rehabil* 2002;24:334–340.

245. Lahz S, Bryant RA. Incidence of chronic pain following traumatic brain injury. *Arch Phys Med Rehabil* 1996;77:889–891.

246. Beetar JT, Guilmette TJ, Sparadeo FR. Sleep and pain complaints in symptomatic traumatic brain injury and neurologic populations. *Arch Phys Med Rehabil* 1996;77:1298–1302.

247. Uomoto JM, Esselman PC. Traumatic brain injury and chronic pain: differential types and rates by head injury severity. *Arch Phys Med Rehabil* 1993;74:61–64.

248. American Psychiatric Association. Diagnostic and Statistical Manual of Mental Disorders. Fourth Edition. Text Revision. Washington, DC: American Psychiatric Association, 2000.

249. Blanchard EB, Hickling EJ. After the crash: Psychological assessment and treatment of survivors of motor vehicle accidents. Washington, DC: American Psychological Association, 1997.

250. Breslau N, Davis GC, Andreski P, Peterson E. Traumatic events and posttraumatic stress disorder in an urban population of young adults. *Arch Gen Psychiatry* 1991;48:216–222.

251. Kessler RC, Sonnega A, Bromet E, Hughes M, Nelson CB. Posttraumatic stress disorder in the National Comorbidity Survey. *Arch Gen Psychiatry* 1995;52:1048–1060.

252. Grieger TA, Fullerton CS, Ursano RJ. Posttraumatic stress disorder, alcohol use, and perceived safety after the terrorist attack on the pentagon. *Psychiatr Serv* 2003;54:1380–1382.

253. Foa EB, Cashman L, Jaycox L, Perry K. The validation of a self-report measure of posttraumatic stress disorder: The Posttraumatic Diagnostic Scale. *Psychol Assess* 1997;9:445–451.

254. Sbordone RJ, Liter JC. Mild traumatic brain injury does not produce post-traumatic stress disorder. *Brain Inj* 1995;9:405–412.

255. Klein E, Caspi Y, Gil S. The relation between memory of the traumatic event and PTSD: Evidence from studies of traumatic brain injury. *Can J Psychiatry* 2003;48:28–33.

256. Mayou R, Bryant B, Duthie R. Psychiatric consequences of road traffic accidents. *Bmj* 1993;307:647–651.

257. Bryant RA, Harvey AG. The influence of traumatic brain injury on acute stress disorder and post-traumatic stress disorder following motor vehicle accidents. *Brain Inj* 1999;13:15–22.

258. Harvey AG, Brewin CR, Jones C, Kopelman MD. Coexistence of posttraumatic stress disorder and traumatic brain injury: towards a resolution of the paradox. *J Int Neuropsychol Soc* 2003;9:663–676.

259. Gil S, Caspi Y, Ben-Ari IZ, Koren D, Klein E. Does memory of a traumatic event increase the risk for posttraumatic stress disorder in patients with traumatic brain injury? A prospective study. *Am J Psychiatry* 2005;162:963–969.

260. North CS, Nixon SJ, Shariat S, Mallonee S, McMillen JC, Spitznagel EL, Smith EM. Psychiatric disorders among survivors of the Oklahoma City bombing. *JAMA* 1999;282:755–762.

261. North CS. The course of post-traumatic stress disorder after the Oklahoma City bombing. *Mil Med* 2001;166:51–52.

262. North CS, Pfefferbaum B, Tivis L, Kawasaki A, Reddy C, Spitznagel EL. The course of posttraumatic stress disorder in a follow-up study of survivors of the Oklahoma City bombing. *Ann Clin Psychiatry* 2004;16:209–215.

263. North CS, Smith EM, Spitznagel EL. One-year follow-up of survivors of a mass shooting. *Am J Psychiatry* 1997;154:1696–1702.

264. North CS, McCutcheon V, Spitznagel EL, Smith EM. Three-year follow-up of survivors of a mass shooting episode. *J Urban Health* 2002;79:383–391.

265. Buckley TC, Blanchard EB, Hickling EJ. A prospective examination of delayed onset PTSD secondary to motor vehicle accidents. *J Abnorm Psychol* 1996;105:617–625.

266. Bryant RA, Harvey AG. Delayed-onset posttraumatic stress disorder: a prospective evaluation. *Aust N Z J Psychiatry* 2002;36:205–209.

267. Gray MJ, Bolton EE, Litz BT. A longitudinal analysis of PTSD symptom course: delayed-onset PTSD in Somalia peacekeepers. *J Consult Clin Psychol* 2004;72:909–913.

268. Ehlers A, Mayou RA, Bryant B. Psychological predictors of chronic posttraumatic stress disorder after motor vehicle accidents. *J Abnorm Psychol* 1998;107:508–519.

269. Corrada M, Brookmeyer R, Kawas C. Sources of variability in prevalence rates of Alzheimer's disease. *Int J Epidemiol* 1995;24:1000–1005.

270. Jorm AF, Korten AE, Henderson AS. The prevalence of dementia: a quantitative integration of the literature. *Acta Psychiatr Scand* 1987;76:465–479.

271. Hofman A, Rocca WA, Brayne C, Breteler MM, Clarke M, Cooper B, Copeland JR, Dartigues JF, da Silva Droux A, Hagnell O, et al. The prevalence of dementia in Europe: a collaborative study of 1980–1990 findings. Eurodem Prevalence Research Group. *Int J Epidemiol* 1991;20:736–748.

272. Rocca WA, Hofman A, Brayne C, Breteler MM, Clarke M, Copeland JR, Dartigues JF, Engedal K, Hagnell O, Heeren TJ, et al. Frequency and distribution of Alzheimer's disease in Europe: a collaborative study of 1980–1990 prevalence findings. The EURODEM-Prevalence Research Group. *Ann Neurol* 1991;30:381–390.

273. Hebert LE, Scherr PA, Bienias JL, Bennett DA, Evans DA. Alzheimer disease in the US population: prevalence estimates using the 2000 census. *Arch Neurol* 2003;60:1119–1122.

274. St George-Hyslop PH, Petit A. Molecular biology and genetics of Alzheimer's disease. *C R Biol* 2005;328:119–130.

275. Lahiri DK. Apolipoprotein E as a target for developing new therapeutics for Alzheimer's disease based on studies from protein, RNA, and regulatory region of the gene. *J Mol Neurosci* 2004;23:225–233.

276. Nielsen AS, Ravid R, Kamphorst W, Jorgensen OS. Apolipoprotein E epsilon 4 in an autopsy series of various dementing disorders. *J Alzheimers Dis* 2003;5:119–125.

277. Heininger K. A unifying hypothesis of Alzheimer's disease. III. Risk factors. *Hum Psychopharmacol* 2000;15:1–70.

278. Calabrese V, Butterfield DA, Stella AM. Nutritional antioxidants and the heme oxygenase pathway of stress tolerance: novel targets for neuroprotection in Alzheimer's disease. *Ital J Biochem* 2003;52:177–181.

279. Calabrese V, Scapagnini G, Colombrita C, Ravagna A, Pennisi G, Giuffrida Stella AM, Galli F, Butterfield DA. Redox regulation of heat shock protein expression in aging and neurodegenerative

disorders associated with oxidative stress: a nutritional approach. *Amino Acids* 2003;25:437–444.

280. Mocchegiani E, Bertoni-Freddari C, Marcellini F, Malavolta M. Brain, aging and neurodegeneration: role of zinc ion availability. *Prog Neurobiol* 2005;75:367–390.

281. Korf ES, Scheltens P, Barkhof F, de Leeuw FE. Blood Pressure, White Matter Lesions and Medial Temporal Lobe Atrophy: Closing the Gap between Vascular Pathology and Alzheimer's Disease? *Dement Geriatr Cogn Disord* 2005;20:331–337.

282. Decarli C. Vascular factors in dementia: an overview. J Neurol Sci 2004;226:19–23.

283. Newman AB, Fitzpatrick AL, Lopez O, Jackson S, Lyketsos C, Jagust W, Ives D, Dekosky ST, Kuller LH. Dementia and Alzheimer's disease incidence in relationship to cardiovascular disease in the Cardiovascular Health Study cohort. *J Am Geriatr Soc* 2005;53:1101–1107.

284. Sjogren M, Blennow K. The link between cholesterol and Alzheimer's disease. *World J Biol Psychiatry* 2005;6:85–97.

285. Ravaglia G, Forti P, Maioli F, Martelli M, Servadei L, Brunetti N, Porcellini E, Licastro F. Homocysteine and folate as risk factors for dementia and Alzheimer disease. *Am J Clin Nutr* 2005;82: 636–643.

286. Kivipelto M, Ngandu T, Fratiglioni L, Viitanen M, Kareholt I, Winblad B, Helkala EL, Tuomilehto J, Soininen H, Nissinen A. Obesity and vascular risk factors at midlife and the risk of dementia and Alzheimer disease. *Arch Neurol* 2005;62:1556–1560.

287. Streit WJ. Microglia and neuroprotection: implications for Alzheimer's disease. *Brain Res Brain Res Rev* 2005;48:234–239.

288. Srinivasan V, Pandi-Perumal SR, Maestroni GJ, Esquifino AI, Hardeland R, Cardinali DP. Role of melatonin in neurodegenerative diseases. *Neurotox Res* 2005;7:293–318.

289. Treiber C. Metals on the brain. *Sci Aging Knowledge Environ* 2005;2005:pe27.

290. Kiraly MA, Kiraly SJ. The effect of exercise on hippocampal integrity: review of recent research. *Int J Psychiatry Med* 2005; 35:75–89.

291. Luchsinger JA, Reitz C, Honig LS, Tang MX, Shea S, Mayeux R. Aggregation of vascular risk factors and risk of incident Alzheimer disease. *Neurology* 2005;65:545–551.

292. Andersen K, Lolk A, Kragh-Sorensen P, Petersen NE, Green A. Depression and the risk of Alzheimer disease. *Epidemiology* 2005;16:233–238.

293. Dal Forno G, Palermo MT, Donohue JE, Karagiozis H, Zonderman AB, Kawas CH. Depressive symptoms, sex, and risk for Alzheimer's disease. *Ann Neurol* 2005;57:381–387.

294. Beeri MS, Davidson M, Silverman JM, Noy S, Schmeidler J, Goldbourt U. Relationship between body height and dementia. *Am J Geriatr Psychiatry* 2005;13:116–123.

295. Lindstrom HA, Fritsch T, Petot G, Smyth KA, Chen CH, Debanne SM, Lerner AJ, Friedland RP. The relationships between television viewing in midlife and the development of Alzheimer's disease in a case-control study. *Brain Cogn* 2005;58:157–165.

296. Lye TC, Shores EA. Traumatic brain injury as a risk factor for Alzheimer's disease: a review. *Neuropsychol Rev* 2000;10: 115–129.

297. Szczygielski J, Mautes A, Steudel WI, Falkai P, Bayer TA, Wirths O. Traumatic brain injury: cause or risk of Alzheimer's disease? A review of experimental studies. *J Neural Transm* 2005;112:1547–1564.

298. Jellinger KA. Head injury and dementia. *Curr Opin Neurol* 2004;17:719–723.

299. Jellinger KA, Paulus W, Wrocklage C, Litvan I. Effects of closed traumatic brain injury and genetic factors on the development of Alzheimer's disease. *Eur J Neurol* 2001;8:707–710.

300. Jellinger KA, Paulus W, Wrocklage C, Litvan I. Traumatic brain injury as a risk factor for Alzheimer disease. Comparison of two retrospective autopsy cohorts with evaluation of ApoE genotype. *BMC Neurol* 2001;1:3.

301. Canadian Study of Health and Aging. The Canadian Study of Health and Aging: risk factors for Alzheimer's disease in Canada. *Neurology* 1994;44:2073–2080.

302. van Duijn CM, Tanja TA, Haaxma R, Schulte W, Saan RJ, Lameris AJ, Antonides-Hendriks G, Hofman A. Head trauma and the risk of Alzheimer's disease. *Am J Epidemiol* 1992;135:775–782.

303. Salib E, Hillier V. Head injury and the risk of Alzheimer's disease: a case control study. *Int J Geriatr Psychiatry* 1997;12: 363–368.

304. Graves AB, White KP, Koepsell TD, Reifler BV, van Belle G, Larson EB, Raskind M. The association between head trauma and Alzheimer's disease. *Am J Epidemiol* 1990;131:491–501.

305. O'Meara ES, Kukull WA, Sheppard L, Bowen JD, McCormick WC, Teri L, Pfanschmidt M, Thompson JD, Schellenberg GD, Larson EB. Head injury and risk of Alzheimer's disease by apolipoprotein E genotype. *Am J Epidemiol* 1997;146:373–384.

306. Plassman BL, Havlik RJ, Steffens DC, Helms MJ, Newman TN, Drosdick D, Phillips C, Gau BA, Welsh-Bohmer KA, Burke JR, Guralnik JM, Breitner JC. Documented head injury in early adulthood and risk of Alzheimer's disease and other dementias. *Neurology* 2000;55:1158–1166.

307. Chandra V, Philipose V, Bell PA, Lazaroff A, Schoenberg BS. Case-control study of late onset "probable Alzheimer's disease". *Neurology* 1987;37:1295–1300.

308. Guo Z, Cupples LA, Kurz A, Auerbach SH, Volicer L, Chui H, Green RC, Sadovnick AD, Duara R, DeCarli C, Johnson K, Go RC, Growdon JH, Haines JL, Kukull WA, Farrer LA. Head injury and the risk of AD in the MIRAGE study. *Neurology* 2000;54:1316–1323.

309. Luukinen H, Viramo P, Herala M, Kervinen K, Kesaniemi YA, Savola O, Winqvist S, Jokelainen J, Hillbom M. Fall-related brain injuries and the risk of dementia in elderly people: a population-based study. *Eur J Neurol* 2005;12:86–92.

310. Luukinen H, Viramo P, Koski K, Laippala P, Kivela SL. Head injuries and cognitive decline among older adults: a population-based study. *Neurology* 1999;52:557–562.

311. Rasmussen DX, Brandt J, Martin DB, Folstein MF. Head injury as a risk factor in Alzheimer's disease. *Brain Inj* 1995;9: 213–219.

312. Mayeux R, Ottman R, Tang MX, Noboa-Bauza L, Marder K, Gurland B, Stern Y. Genetic susceptibility and head injury as risk factors for Alzheimer's disease among community-dwelling elderly persons and their first-degree relatives. *Ann Neurol* 1993;33:494–501.

313. Schofield PW, Tang M, Marder K, Bell K, Dooneief G, Chun M, Sano M, Stern Y, Mayeux R. Alzheimer's disease after remote head injury: an incidence study. *J Neurol Neurosurg Psychiatry* 1997;62:119–124.

314. Mortimer JA, French LR, Hutton JT, Schuman LM. Head injury as a risk factor for Alzheimer's disease. *Neurology* 1985;35:264–267.

315. Amaducci LA, Fratiglioni L, Rocca WA, Fieschi C, Livrea P, Pedone D, Bracco L, Lippi A, Gandolfo C, Bino G, et al. Risk factors for clinically diagnosed Alzheimer's disease: a case-control study of an Italian population. *Neurology* 1986;36:922–931.

316. Ferini-Strambi L, Smirne S, Garancini P, Pinto P, Franceschi M. Clinical and epidemiological aspects of Alzheimer's disease with presenile onset: a case control study. *Neuroepidemiology* 1990;9:39–49.

317. Fratiglioni L, Ahlbom A, Viitanen M, Winblad B. Risk factors for late-onset Alzheimer's disease: a population-based, case-control study. *Ann Neurol* 1993;33:258–266.

318. Nemetz PN, Leibson C, Naessens JM, Beard M, Kokmen E, Annegers JF, Kurland LT. Traumatic brain injury and time to onset of Alzheimer's disease: a population-based study. *Am J Epidemiol* 1999;149:32–40.

319. Katzman R, Aronson M, Fuld P, Kawas C, Brown T, Morgenstern H, Frishman W, Gidez L, Eder H, Ooi WL. Development of dementing illnesses in an 80-year-old volunteer cohort. *Ann Neurol* 1989;25:317–324.

320. Li G, Shen YC, Li YT, Chen CH, Zhau YW, Silverman JM. A case-control study of Alzheimer's disease in China. *Neurology* 1992;42:1481–1488.

321. Mehta KM, Ott A, Kalmijn S, Slooter AJ, van Duijn CM, Hofman A, Breteler MM. Head trauma and risk of dementia and Alzheimer's disease: The Rotterdam Study. *Neurology* 1999;53: 1959–1962.

322. Chandra V, Kokmen E, Schoenberg BS, Beard CM. Head trauma with loss of consciousness as a risk factor for Alzheimer's disease. *Neurology* 1989;39:1576–1578.

323. Broe GA, Henderson AS, Creasey H, McCusker E, Korten AE, Jorm AF, Longley W, Anthony JC. A case-control study of Alzheimer's disease in Australia. *Neurology* 1990;40:1698–1707.

324. Mortimer JA, van Duijn CM, Chandra V, Fratiglioni L, Graves AB, Heyman A, Jorm AF, Kokmen E, Kondo K, Rocca WA, et al. Head trauma as a risk factor for Alzheimer's disease: a collaborative re-analysis of case-control studies. EURODEM Risk Factors Research Group. *Int J Epidemiol* 1991;20 Suppl 2:S28–35.

325. Fleminger S, Oliver DL, Lovestone S, Rabe-Hesketh S, Giora A. Head injury as a risk factor for Alzheimer's disease: the evidence 10 years on;a partial replication. *J Neurol Neurosurg Psychiatry* 2003;74:857–862.

326. Starkstein SE, Jorge R. Dementia after traumatic brain injury. *Int Psychogeriatr* 2005;17 Suppl 1:S93–107.

327. Ruff RM, Camenzuli L, Mueller J. Miserable minority: emotional risk factors that influence the outcome of a mild traumatic brain injury. *Brain Inj* 1996;10:551–565.

328. Wood RL. Understanding the 'miserable minority':a diasthesis-stress paradigm for post-concussional syndrome. *Brain Inj* 2004;18:1135–1153.

329. Ryan LM, Warden DL. Post concussion syndrome. Int Rev Psychiatry 2003;15:310–316.

330. Evered L, Ruff R, Baldo J, Isomura A. Emotional risk factors and postconcussional disorder. *Assessment* 2003;10:420–427.

331. Cook JB. The post-concussional syndrome and factors influencing recovery after minor head injury admitted to hospital. *Scand J Rehabil Med* 1972;4:27–30.

332. Mickeviciene D, Schrader H, Obelieniene D, Surkiene D, Kunickas R, Stovner LJ, Sand T. A controlled prospective inception cohort study on the post-concussion syndrome outside the medicolegal context. *Eur J Neurol* 2004;11:411–419.

333. Rutherford WH, Merrett JD, McDonald JR. Symptoms at one year following concussion from minor head injuries. *Injury* 1979;10:225–230.

334. Satz PS, Alfano MS, Light RF, Morgenstern HF, Zaucha KF, Asarnow RF, Newton S. Persistent Post-Concussive Syndrome: A proposed methodology and literature review to determine the effects, if any, of mild head and other bodily injury. *J Clin Exp Neuropsychol* 1999;21:620–628.

335. Mickeviciene D, Schrader H, Nestvold K, Surkiene D, Kunickas R, Stovner LJ, Sand T. A controlled historical cohort study on the post-concussion syndrome. *Eur J Neurol* 2002;9:581–587.

336. Lees-Haley PR, Fox DD, Courtney JC. A comparison of complaints by mild brain injury claimants and other claimants describing subjective experiences immediately following their injury. *Arch Clin Neuropsychol* 2001;16:689–695.

337. Miller H. Accident neurosis. *Bmj* 1961;1:919–925 & 992–998.

338. Reynolds S, Paniak C, Toller-Lobe G, Nagy J. A longitudinal study of compensation-seeking and return to work in a treated mild traumatic brain injury sample. *J Head Trauma Rehabil* 2003;18:139–147.

339. Binder LM, Rohling ML. Money matters: a meta-analytic review of the effects of financial incentives on recovery after closed-head injury. *Am J Psychiatry* 1996;153:7–10.

340. Paniak C, Reynolds S, Toller-Lobe G, Melnyk A, Nagy J, Schmidt D. A longitudinal study of the relationship between financial compensation and symptoms after treated mild traumatic brain injury. *J Clin Exp Neuropsychol* 2002;24:187–193.

341. Binder LM. Persisting symptoms after mild head injury: a review of the postconcussive syndrome. *J Clin Exp Neuropsychol* 1986;8:323–346.

342. Brown SJ, Fann JR, Grant I. Postconcussional disorder: time to acknowledge a common source of neurobehavioral morbidity. *J Neuropsychiatry Clin Neurosci* 1994;6:15–22.

343. Cicerone KD, Kalmar K. Persistent postconcussion syndrome: The structure of subjective complaints after mild traumatic brain injury. *J Head Trauma Rehabil* 1995;10:1–7.

344. Heilbronner RL. Factors associated with postconcussion syndrome: Neurological, psychological, or legal? *Trial Diplomacy J* 1993;16:161–167.

345. Youngjohn JR, Burrows L, Erdal K. Brain damage or compensation neurosis? The controversial post-concussion syndrome. *Clin Neuropsychol* 1995;9:112–123.

346. Lishman WA. Physiogenisis and psychogenisis in the 'post-concussional syndrome'. *Br J Psychiatry* 1986;153:460–469.

347. Mittenberg W, Strauman S. Diagnosis of mild head injury and the postconcussion syndrome. *J Head Trauma Rehabil* 2000;15:783–791.

348. Larrabee GJ. Neuropsychological outcome, post concussion symptoms, and forensic considerations in mild closed head trauma. *Semin Clin Neuropsychiatry* 1997;2:196–206.

349. Ruff RM, Richardson AM. Mild traumatic brian injury. In: Sweet JJ, editor. Forensic neuropsychology: Fundamentals and practice. Studies on neuropsychology, development, and cognition. *Bristol, PA: Swets & Zeitlinger*, 1999. p 315–338.

350. Gouvier WD, Uddo-Crane M, Brown LM. Base rates of post-concussion symptoms. *Arch Clin Neuropsychol* 1988;3:273–278.

351. Machulda MM, Bergquist TF, Ito V, Chew S. Relationship between stress, coping, and post concussion symptoms in a healthy adult population. *Arch Clin Neuropsychol* 1998;13:415–424.

352. Mittenberg W, DiGiulio DV, Perrin S, Bass AE. Symptoms following mild head injury: Expectation as aetiology. *J Neurol Neurosurg Psychiatry* 1992;55:200–204.

353. Trahan DE, Ross CE, Trahan SL. Relationships among postconcussional-type symptoms, depression, and anxiety in neurologically normal young adults and victims of brain injury. *Arch Clin Neuropsychol* 2001;16:435–445.

354. Sawchyn JM, Brulot MM, Strauss E. Note on the use of the Postconcussion Syndrome Checklist. *Arch Clin Neuropsychol* 2000;15:1–8.

355. Wong JL, Regennitter RP, Barrios F. Base rate and simulated symptoms of mild head injury among normals. *Arch Clin Neuropsychol* 1994;9:411–425.

356. Fox DD, Lees-Haley PR, Ernest K, Dolezal-Wood S. Post-concussive symptoms: Base rates and etiology in psychiatric patients. *Clin Neuropsychol* 1995;9:89–92.

357. Lees-Haley PR, Brown RS. Neuropsychological complain base rates of 170 personal injury claimants. *Arch Clin Neuropsychol* 1993;8:203–209.

358. Dunn JT, Lees-Haley PR, Brown RS, Williams CW, English LT. Neurotoxic complaint base rates of personal injury claimants: implications for neuropsychological assessment. *J Clin Psychol* 1995;51:577–584.

359. Smith-Seemiller L, Fow NR, Kant R, Franzen MD. Presence of post-concussion syndrome symptoms in patients with chronic pain vs mild traumatic brain injury. *Brain Inj* 2003;17:199–206.

360. Radanov BP, Dvorak J, Valach L. Cognitive deficits in patients after soft tissue injury of the cervical spine. *Spine* 1992;17:127–131.

361. Iverson GL, McCracken LM. 'Postconcussive' symptoms in persons with chronic pain. *Brain Inj* 1997;11:783–790.

362. Gasquoine PG. Postconcussional symptoms in chronic back pain. *Appl Neuropsychol* 2000;7:83–89.

363. Sullivan MJ, Hall E, Bartolacci R, Sullivan ME, Adams H. Perceived cognitive deficits, emotional distress and disability following whiplash injury. *Pain Res Manag* 2002;7:120–126.

364. Berube J. The Traumatic Brain Injury Act Amendments of 2000. *J Head Trauma Rehabil* 2001;16:210–213.

365. Center for Disease Control and Prevention. Traumatic brain injury in the United States: a report to Congress. Volume 2005, 2003.

366. National Institutes of Health. Rehabilitation of persons with traumatic brain injury. *NIH Consens Statement* 1998;16:1–41.

367. Alexander MP. Mild traumatic brain injury: pathophysiology, natural history, and clinical management. *Neurology* 1995;45:1253–1260.

368. Fenton G, McClelland R, Montgomery A, MacFlynn G, Rutherford W. The postconcussional syndrome: social antecedents and psychological sequelae. *Br J Psychiatry* 1993;162:493–497.

369. Karzmark P, Hall K, Englander J. Late-onset post-concussion symptoms after mild brain injury: the role of premorbid, injury-related, environmental, and personality factors. *Brain Inj* 1995;9:21–26.

370. Gunstad J, Suhr JA. Cognitive factors in Postconcussion Syndrome symptom report. *Arch Clin Neuropsychol* 2004;19:391–405.

371. Wilde EA, Bigler ED, Gandhi PV, Lowry CM, Blatter DD, Brooks J, Ryser DK. Alcohol abuse and traumatic brain injury: quantitative magnetic resonance imaging and neuropsychological outcome. *J Neurotrauma* 2004;21:137–147.

372. Feinstein A, Ouchterlony D, Somerville J, Jardine A. The effects of litigation on symptom expression: a prospective study following mild traumatic brain injury. *Med Sci Law* 2001;41:116–121.

373. Martin RC, Hayes JS, Gouvier WD. Differential vulnerability between postconcussion self-report and objective malingering tests in identifying simulated mild head injury. *J Clin Exp Neuropsychol* 1996;18:265–275.

374. Greiffenstein MF, Baker WJ, Gola T, Donders J, Miller L. The fake bad scale in atypical and severe closed head injury litigants. *J Clin Psychol* 2002;58:1591–1600.

375. Ross SR, Millis SR, Krukowski RA, Putnam SH, Adams KM. Detecting incomplete effort on the MMPI-2:an examination of the Fake-Bad Scale in mild head injury. *J Clin Exp Neuropsychol* 2004;26:115–124.

376. Larrabee GJ. Exaggerated MMPI-2 symptom report in personal injury litigants with malingered neurocognitive deficit. *Arch Clin Neuropsychol* 2003;18:673–686.

377. Mittenberg W, Patton C, Canyock EM, Condit DC. Base rates of malingering and symptom exaggeration. *J Clin Exp Neuropsychol* 2002;24:1094–1102.

378. Ferguson RJ, Mittenberg W, Barone DF, Schneider B. Postconcussion syndrome following sports-related head injury: expectation as etiology. *Neuropsychology* 1999;13:582–589.

379. Gunstad J, Suhr JA. Perception of illness: nonspecificity of postconcussion syndrome symptom expectation. *J Int Neuropsychol Soc* 2002;8:37–47.

380. Ferrari R, Obelieniene D, Russell AS, Darlington P, Gervais R, Green P. Symptom expectation after minor head injury. A comparative study between Canada and Lithuania. *Clin Neurol Neurosurg* 2001;103:184–190.

381. Gunstad J, Suhr JA. "Expectation as etiology" versus "the good old days":postconcussion syndrome symptom reporting in athletes, headache sufferers, and depressed individuals. *J Int Neuropsychol Soc* 2001;7:323–333.

382. Davis CH. Self-perception in mild traumatic brain injury. *Am J Phys Med Rehabil* 2002;81:609–621.

383. Lees-Haley PR, Williams CW, Zasler ND, Marguilies S, English LT, Stevens KB. Response bias in plaintiffs' histories. *Brain Inj* 1997;11:791–799.

384. Seedat S, Warwick J, van Heerden B, Hugo C, Zungu-Dirwayi N, Van Kradenburg J, Stein DJ. Single photon emission computed tomography in posttraumatic stress disorder before and after treatment with a selective serotonin reuptake inhibitor. *J Affect Disord* 2004;80:45–53.

385. Demir B, Ulug B, Lay Ergun E, Erbas B. Regional cerebral blood flow and neuropsychological functioning in early and late onset alcoholism. *Psychiatry Res* 2002;115:115–125.

386. Meyer JH, Houle S, Sagrati S, Carella A, Hussey DF, Ginovart N, Goulding V, Kennedy J, Wilson AA. Brain serotonin transporter binding potential measured with carbon 11-labeled DASB positron emission tomography: effects of major depressive episodes and severity of dysfunctional attitudes. *Arch Gen Psychiatry* 2004;61:1271–1279.

387. Peyron R, Laurent B, Garcia-Larrea L. Functional imaging of brain responses to pain. A review and meta-analysis (2000). *Neurophysiol Clin* 2000;30:263–288.

388. Wong DF, Maini A, Rousset OG, Brasic JR. Positron emission tomography—a tool for identifying the effects of alcohol dependence on the brain. *Alcohol Res Health* 2003;27:161–173.

389. Verne GN, Robinson ME, Price DD. Representations of pain in the brain. *Curr Rheumatol Rep* 2004;6:261–265.

390. Schulz KP, Fan J, Tang CY, Newcorn JH, Buchsbaum MS, Cheung AM, Halperin JM. Response inhibition in adolescents diagnosed with attention deficit hyperactivity disorder during childhood: an event-related FMRI study. *Am J Psychiatry* 2004;161:1650–1657.

391. Pfefferbaum A, Sullivan EV. Microstructural but not macrostructural disruption of white matter in women with chronic alcoholism. *Neuroimage* 2002;15:708–718.

392. Sanacora G, Gueorguieva R, Epperson CN, Wu YT, Appel M, Rothman DL, Krystal JH, Mason GF. Subtype-specific alterations of gamma-aminobutyric acid and glutamate in patients with major depression. *Arch Gen Psychiatry* 2004;61:705–713.

393. Lim MK, Suh CH, Kim HJ, Kim ST, Lee JS, Kang MH, Kim JH, Lee JH. Fire-related post-traumatic stress disorder: brain 1H-MR spectroscopic findings. *Korean J Radiol* 2003;4:79–84.

394. Hesslinger B, Thiel T, Tebartz van Elst L, Hennig J, Ebert D. Attention-deficit disorder in adults with or without hyperactivity: where is the difference? A study in humans using short echo (1)H-magnetic resonance spectroscopy. *Neurosci Lett* 2001;304:117–119.

395. Courvoisie H, Hooper SR, Fine C, Kwock L, Castillo M. Neurometabolic functioning and neuropsychological correlates in children with ADHD-H: preliminary findings. *J Neuropsychiatry Clin Neurosci* 2004;16:63–69.

396. Grachev ID, Ramachandran TS, Thomas PS, Szeverenyi NM, Fredrickson BE. Association between dorsolateral prefrontal N-acetyl aspartate and depression in chronic back pain: an in vivo proton magnetic resonance spectroscopy study. *J Neural Transm* 2003;110:287–312.

397. Apkarian AV, Sosa Y, Sonty S, Levy RM, Harden RN, Parrish TB, Gitelman DR. Chronic back pain is associated with decreased prefrontal and thalamic gray matter density. *J Neurosci* 2004;24:10410–10415.

398. Rosenbloom M, Sullivan EV, Pfefferbaum A. Using magnetic resonance imaging and diffusion tensor imaging to assess brain damage in alcoholics. *Alcohol Res Health* 2003;27:146–152.

399. Videbech P, Ravnkilde B. Hippocampal volume and depression: a meta-analysis of MRI studies. *Am J Psychiatry* 2004;161:1957–1966.

400. Campbell S, Marriott M, Nahmias C, MacQueen GM. Lower hippocampal volume in patients suffering from depression: a meta-analysis. *Am J Psychiatry* 2004;161:598–607.

401. Geuze E, Vermetten E, Bremner JD. MR-based in vivo hippocampal volumetrics:2. Findings in neuropsychiatric disorders. *Mol Psychiatry* 2004.

402. Lindauer RJ, Vlieger EJ, Jalink M, Olff M, Carlier IV, Majoie CB, den Heeten GJ, Gersons BP. Smaller hippocampal volume in Dutch police officers with posttraumatic stress disorder. *Biol Psychiatry* 2004;56:356–363.

403. Wignall EL, Dickson JM, Vaughan P, Farrow TF, Wilkinson ID, Hunter MD, Woodruff PW. Smaller hippocampal volume in patients with recent-onset posttraumatic stress disorder. *Biol Psychiatry* 2004;56:832–836.

404. Lacerda AL, Keshavan MS, Hardan AY, Yorbik O, Brambilla P, Sassi RB, Nicoletti M, Mallinger AG, Frank E, Kupfer DJ, Soares JC. Anatomic evaluation of the orbitofrontal cortex in major depressive disorder. *Biol Psychiatry* 2004;55:353–358.

405. Hesslinger B, Tebartz van Elst L, Thiel T, Haegele K, Hennig J, Ebert D. Frontoorbital volume reductions in adult patients with attention deficit hyperactivity disorder. *Neurosci Lett* 2002;328:319–321.

406. Bartlett J, Kett-White R, Mendelow AD, Miller JD, Pickard J, Teasdale G. Recommendations from the Society of British Neurological Surgeons. *Br J Neurosurg* 1998;12:349–352.

407. American College of Surgeons Committee on Trauma. Advanced trauma life support for doctors, 6th ed., 1997. 1–444 p.

408. Levin HS, McCauley SR, Josic CP, Boake C, Brown SA, Goodman HS, Merritt SG, Brundage SI. Predicting depression following mild traumatic brain injury. *Arch Gen Psychiatry* 2005;62:523–528.

409. Mooney G, Speed J. The association between mild traumatic brain injury and psychiatric conditions. *Brain Inj* 2001;15:865–877.

410. Parker RS, Rosenblum A. IQ loss and emotional dysfunctions after mild head injury incurred in a motor vehicle accident. *J Clin Psychol* 1996;52:32–43.

411. Grant I, Gonzalez R, Carey CL, Natarajan L, Wolfson T. Non-acute (residual) neurocognitive effects of cannabis use: a meta-analytic study. *J Int Neuropsychol Soc* 2003;9:679–689.

412. Christensen H, Griffiths K, Mackinnon A, Jacomb P. A quantitative review of cognitive deficits in depression and Alzheimer-type dementia. *J Int Neuropsychol Soc* 1997;3:631–651.

413. Frazier TW, Demaree HA, Youngstrom EA. Meta-analysis of intellectual and neuropsychological test performance in attention-deficit/hyperactivity disorder. *Neuropsychology* 2004; 18:543–555.

414. Vickery CD, Berry DT, Inman TH, Harris MJ, Orey SA. Detection of inadequate effort on neuropsychological testing: a meta-analytic review of selected procedures. *Arch Clin Neuropsychol* 2001;16:45–73.

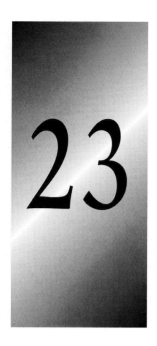

23 Post-Concussive Disorder

Grant L. Iverson
Nathan D. Zasler
Rael T. Lange

INTRODUCTION

A concussion, by definition, is a mild traumatic brain injury (MTBI). MTBIs are expected to be self-limiting and to follow a predictable course. Permanent cognitive, psychological, or psychosocial problems due to the biological effects of this injury are relatively uncommon in trauma patients and rare in athletes (1–6 and see chapters by Collins et al. and Iverson et al. in this book). However, some people do not appear to recover well following MTBI; these individuals have been referred to as the "miserable minority" (7, 8). When a person does not recover quickly, health care providers may be very concerned about the possibility of a persistent post-concussive disorder (9–14), the development of depression (see 15 for a review), and/or a failure to return to work (16–28), among other potential complications.

The post-concussive disorder is one of the most controversial syndromes/disorders in medicine and psychology. In medicine, we consider a syndrome a group of signs and symptoms that collectively indicate or characterize a disease, psychological disorder, or abnormal condition. The signs and symptoms of a syndrome are believed to have a common cause. It is widely believed that 10–20% of people who sustain an MTBI will develop a more persistent form of the syndrome (i.e., lasting one or more years). A 15% prevalence of poor outcome has been cited

frequently over the past 25 years based on the results from a prospective study in the mid 1970s by Rutherford and colleagues. These researchers followed consecutive admissions to the hospital for MTBIs and reported that 14.5% of patients had *at least one* symptom at one-year post-injury. However, fewer than 5% had multiple (four or more) symptoms. This figure is never cited. Moreover, the authors' concerns about the validity of the syndrome have been lost over the years, and only the "15%" figure has been retained.

> It is probably the multiplicity and the diversity of complaints which has given the term 'post-concussion syndrome' such widespread acceptance. However, of the 19 patients who complained, 6 had only 1 symptom and a further 7 had 2. The remaining 6 had between 4 and 9 symptoms. In a syndrome one expects groupings of inter-related symptoms. We found no such groupings either at 6 weeks or at 1 year (Ref. 29; p. 228).

The widely-cited estimate of 10–20% of patients suffering a long-term post-concussive disorder is both confusing and incorrect. It is confusing because there is often an assumption that if a person reports symptoms long after an MTBI, that the symptoms are causally-related to the biological effects of the injury (by logical inference, the symptoms are related to damage to the structure or function of the brain). It is incorrect because the constellation of symptoms comprising the post-concussive disorder likely occurs in far less than 10–20% of patients with remote MTBIs. Moreover, there are numerous potential underlying causes for these symptoms that are unrelated to traumatic brain damage.

If we consider *all* MTBIs, the percentage of people with poor long-term (e.g. greater than one year) outcome is likely very small (i.e., clearly less than 5%). This is because the definition of concussion, as it is generally defined, is so broad that a person simply needs to feel momentarily dazed, and unwell for a brief period of time, to meet criteria. A mild injury to the brain is common in daily life and in sports. Those injuries on the milder end of the "mild" spectrum, as a rule, do not result in biologically-based symptoms and problems that last beyond a few minutes, days, or weeks. For example, a substantial minority of amateur and professional athletes who sustain a concussion have no residual symptoms or problems after a few hours or a single day; and 90% of concussed university football players appeared recovered in 7 days (30). In a recent, large-scale prospective study with high school football players, approximately 90% were recovered within the first month post-injury (31). Although it is possible for an athlete to have a persistent post-concussive disorder, and we occasionally see these athletes in clinical practice, the incidence of this syndrome/disorder in athletes is extremely low (of course, far less than a 15% estimate of poor outcome at one-year post-injury).

The estimates that 10–20% of patients have poor outcome, and thus possibly a "persistent" post-concussive disorder, come from studies of trauma patients seen in the hospital, not athletes with MTBIs or civilians seen by their family doctors or in clinics. According to a US Census Bureau survey, more than 600 people per 100, 000 sustain a brain injury with loss of consciousness each year (32). Of these people, 35% are seen in the emergency room, 25% are hospitalized, 14% are seen in doctors' offices or clinics, and 25% seek no medical care. Historical prospective studies reporting poor outcome have been based on either the 25% of cases that are hospitalized or the 35% seen in emergency departments. In the past, these patient groups were broadly defined, in terms of injury severity, and likely included a subset of patients with complicated MTBIs or moderate TBIs. Researchers have reported that patients who agree to participate in prospective research on outcome from MTBI have more severe injuries than those who refuse participation (e.g., rate of CT abnormalities was 33% in participants and 6% in refusals; 33). Thus, the historical studies often began with a non-representative sample and then, due to attrition (severe in some studies), the final sample was highly non-representative. Moreover, in some studies patients were considered to have persistent problems if they endorsed a single symptom (e.g., headaches or concentration problems) at one-year post-injury! In a large scale prospective study, Alves and colleagues (34) reported that at one year post-injury single symptoms were commonly experienced but multiple symptoms were "extremely rare" (2–6% of subjects).

There are other data suggesting that the disorder, or at least some persistent symptoms, might occur in *more* than 10–20% of people at one-year post-injury (e.g., 35–37). In general, studies involving the "persistent post-concussive disorder" should be reviewed carefully from a methodological perspective to determine (a) the representativeness of the sample, and (b) the criteria used to "diagnose" the disorder. Is the sample comprised of patients and litigants long after an injury who are referred to a specialty clinic? What are the criteria for assuming continuing symptoms arising from the original injury? Does the person need to report one, two, three, or more symptoms? That is, can the condition be considered syndromal in the absence of a threshold number of symptoms and/or signs? If there are a specific number of symptoms and/or signs that need to be present to reach a threshold for diagnosing the disorder, which ones should they be? That is, are there symptoms/signs that should be more heavily weighted than others based on them being more likely to be a biological consequence of the MTBI rather than arising from other etiologic factors? For example, in a prospective study conducted in Lithuania, if the disorder was defined as endorsing three or more symptoms at one-year post-injury, 78% of patients with mild traumatic brain injuries met criteria. However, in the same study, 47% of trauma control subjects, with no history of head or brain injury, met criteria for the persistent post-concussive disorder using the three or more symptoms criteria (38). These authors reported that if a constellation of six core symptoms were necessary to meet criteria for the diagnosis, then after 3 months, only 1% of patients with MTBIs and 1.4% of trauma controls would meet criteria for diagnosis. At one-year post-injury, only 0.5% of patients with MTBIs and 0.005% of trauma controls had this symptom combination. Therefore, a researcher or clinician can draw radically different conclusions from different data presented in the same study.

Despite decades of research, the incidence, prevalence, and etiology of the post-concussive disorder have never been established in a manner that would meet evidence-based medicine criteria. We believe that the post-concussive disorder can arise following a mild traumatic brain injury as a direct or indirect consequence of this injury. The "true" disorder is very much influenced by psychological factors (e.g., see 39), with varying degrees of underlying neurological or neurophysiological problems. The disorder can also be misdiagnosed because the symptoms are non-specific. There are numerous diverse factors that can influence how people perceive and report their symptoms and functional problems long after a mild traumatic brain injury. The purpose of this chapter is to examine some of the more likely factors that may contribute to persistent and sometimes even permanent symptoms and problems following traumatic injuries that may (or may not) involve mild traumatic brain injury. The thesis of this chapter is that the post-concussive disorder is a non-specific cluster of symptoms that can be mimicked by a number of pre-existing or co-morbid conditions. The disorder, theoretically, also can occur in tandem with these conditions. Therefore, it is important to consider carefully the differential diagnosis of the disorder, in the hopes that differential diagnosis leads to differential treatment and rehabilitation, reduced patient suffering, and better functional outcomes. This chapter is divided into the following five sections: (a) diagnostic criteria, (b) differential diagnoses & co-morbidities, (c) iatrogenesis, (d) factors relating to the perception and reporting of symptoms, and (e) conclusions.

DIAGNOSTIC CRITERIA

There are two current sets of research criteria for the post-concussive disorder: the International Classification of Diseases, 10th edition (ICD-10), and the Diagnostic and Statistical Manual of Mental Disorders, Fourth Edition (DMS-IV). According to the ICD-10 (40), a person must have a history of "head trauma with a loss of consciousness" preceding the onset of symptoms by a period of up to 4 weeks and have at least three of six symptom categories. These include: (a) headaches, dizziness, general malaise, excessive fatigue, or noise intolerance, (b) irritability, emotional lability, depression, or anxiety, (c) subjective complaints of concentration or memory difficulty, (d) insomnia, (e) reduced tolerance to alcohol, and (f) preoccupation with these symptoms and fear of permanent brain damage.

> The syndrome occurs following head trauma (usually sufficiently severe to result in loss of consciousness) and includes a number of disparate symptoms such as headache, dizziness (usually lacking the features of true vertigo), fatigue, irritability, difficulty in concentrating and performing mental tasks, impairment of memory, insomnia, and reduced tolerance to stress, emotional excitement, or alcohol. These symptoms may be accompanied by feelings of depression or anxiety, resulting from some loss of self-esteem and fear of permanent brain damage. Such feelings enhance the original symptoms and a vicious circle results. Some patients become hypochondriacal, embark on a search for diagnosis and cure, and may adopt a permanent sick role. The etiology of these symptoms is not always clear, and both organic and psychological factors have been proposed to account them. The nosological status of this condition is thus somewhat uncertain. There

is little doubt, however, that this syndrome is common and distressing to the patient. Diagnostic Guidelines: At least three of the features described above should be present for a definite diagnosis. Careful evaluation with laboratory techniques (electroencephalography, brain stem evoked potentials, brain imaging, oculonystagmography) may yield objective evidence to substantiate the symptoms but results are often negative. The complaints are not necessarily associated with compensation motives (Ref. 40; section F07.2).

The specific research criteria for the Post-concussional Syndrome are set out in Table 23-1. Notice that the ICD-10 criteria do not require "objective" evidence of cognitive problems (in contrast to the DSM-IV criteria described later). The emphasis is on subjective cognitive complaints that are not, in fact, easy to document through neuropsychological testing. This, presumably, is to distinguish the diagnosis from the more serious injuries, conditions, and diseases affecting the brain that have more pronounced associated neurocognitive impairments. Also note that a person with "emotional changes, insomnia, and a pre-occupation with having brain damage" would meet diagnostic criteria for the syndrome. This definition incorrectly and implicitly "assumes" that numerous physical symptoms commonly considered secondary to MTBI are only associated with MTBI and do not have other etiologies, thereby implying a lack of need for adequate differential diagnosis of the cause of the various symptoms reported after traumatic injury.

The fourth edition of the *Diagnostic and Statistical Manual of Mental Disorders* (DSM-IV; 41) included research criteria for the Post-concussional Disorder (see 42, for an interesting discussion of the development and limitations of these criteria). According to these criteria, the individual must show objective evidence on neuropsychological testing of declines in some of his or her cognitive abilities, such as attention, concentration, learning, or memory. The person must also report three or more subjective symptoms from Category C, and these symptoms must be present for at least 3 months. The Category C symptoms are: (a) becoming fatigued easily, (b) disordered sleep, (c) headache, (d) vertigo or dizziness, (e) irritability or aggression on little or no provocation, (f) anxiety, depression, or affective liability, (g) changes in personality (e.g., social or sexual inappropriateness), and (h) apathy or lack of spontaneity. The DSM-IV includes the additional criteria: "The disturbance causes significant impairment in social or occupational functioning and represents a significant decline from a previous level of functioning."

> The essential feature is an acquired impairment in cognitive functioning, accompanied by specific neurobehavioral symptoms, that occurs as a consequence of closed head injury of sufficient severity to produce

---

TABLE 23-1

FO7.2 Post-Concussional Syndrome (Research criteria from the ICD-10)

Note: The nosological status of this syndrome is uncertain, and criterion A of the introduction to this rubric is not always ascertainable. However, for those undertaking research into this condition, the following criteria are recommended:

A. The general criteria of F07 must be met.
   (The general criteria for F07, Personality and Behavioral Disorders Due to Brain Disease, Damage and Dysfunction, are as follows: G1. Objective evidence (from physical and neurological examination and laboratory tests) and/or history, of cerebral disease, damage, or dysfunction. G2. Absence of clouding of consciousness and of significant memory deficit. G3. Absence of sufficient or suggestive evidence for an alternative causation of the personality orbehavior disorder that would justify its placement in section F6 (Other Mental Disorders Due to Brain Damage and Dysfunction and to Physical Disease).
B. History of head trauma with loss of consciousness, preceding the onset of symptoms by a period of up to four weeks (objective EEG, brain imaging, or oculonystagmographic evidence for brain damage may be lacking).
C. At least three of the following:
   (1) Complaints of unpleasant sensations and pains, such as headache, dizziness (usually lacking the features of true vertigo), general malaise and excessive fatigue, or noise intolerance.
   (2) Emotional changes, such as irritability, emotional lability, both easily provoked or exacerbated by emotional excitement or stress, or some degree of depression and/or anxiety.
   (3) Subjective complaints of difficulty in concentration and in performing mental tasks, and of memory complaints, without clear objective evidence (e.g. psychological tests) of marked impairment.
   (4) Insomnia.
   (5) Reduced tolerance to alcohol.
   (6) Preoccupation with the above symptoms and fear of permanent brain damage, to the extent of hypochondriacal over-valued ideas and adoption of a sick role.

---

a significant cerebral concussion. The manifestations of concussion include loss of consciousness, post-traumatic amnesia, and less commonly, post-traumatic onset of seizures. Specific approaches for defining this criterion need to be refined by further research. Although there is insufficient evidence to establish a definite threshold for the severity of the closed head injury, specific criteria have been suggested, for example, two of the following: 1) a period of unconsciousness lasting more than 5 minutes, 2) a period of post-traumatic amnesia that lasts more than 12 hours after the closed head injury, or 3) a new onset of seizures (or marked worsening of a pre-existing seizure disorder) that occurs within the first 6 months after the closed head injury (p. 760, DSM-IV-TR, Ref. 43).

Notice that the DSM-IV criteria require objective evidence of cognitive problems. The DSM-IV emphasizes that the "closed head injury" is sufficient to produce "a significant cerebral concussion." As is often the case in the literature, there is an intermingling of terminology that lacks precision in this definition. In some places "closed head injury" seems to imply cranial trauma and in other places it is used analogously with MTBI. The injury severity markers provided as examples included loss of consciousness (LOC) greater than five minutes, post-traumatic amnesia (PTA) greater than 12 hours, or the new onset of seizures. Clearly, it was the intent of the authors to differentiate the MTBI believed to underlie this

disorder from very mild concussions often experienced in day-to-day life. This definition implies that the disorder should be considered uncommon in people who do not have these more significant injury severity markers, although some researchers have reported that these markers are not reliable predictors of the disorder (e.g., 44, 45). Ruff and Jurica (44) reported that subjective complaints and neuropsychological test performance did not differ in a sample of post-acute patients with mild traumatic brain injuries, of different severities within the mild spectrum, as might be expected if the DSM-IV criteria were predictive of outcome.

When the ICD-10 and DSM-IV criteria are compared in the same set of patients, large diagnostic differences emerge (46, 47). This is because the DSM-IV criteria requires (a) neurocognitive impairment, and (b) impairment in important role functioning. The ICD-10 does not have these "impairment" criteria. Researchers have reported that consecutive patients with mild traumatic brain injuries, seen at a Level I trauma center and followed prospectively, have relatively low rates of diagnosis at three months post-injury using the DSM-IV criteria (i.e., 11% to 17%) compared to the ICD-10 criteria (54% to 64%) (46, 47).

Ruff (7) proposed four modifiers for the Post-concussional Disorder. These modifiers are as follows: (a) PCD with objective neuropathological features, (b) PCD with neurocognitive features, (c) PCD with psychopathological features, and (d) PCD with neurocognitive and psychopathological features. The PCD with objective neuropathological features classification identifies those patients with a combination of neuropsychological deficits and abnormalities identified on neuroimaging (i.e., those with "complicated" MTBIs). PCD with neurocognitive features is used if (a) a cluster of cognitive deficits consistent with MTBI are reliably documented on neuropsychological testing, (b) there is an absence of significant emotional overlay, and (c) there is an absence of positive neuroimaging. PCD with psychopathological features is used when (a) persistent emotional sequelae dominate the clinical picture (e.g., acute stress reaction, depression, panic attacks), (b) neuropsychological deficits are disproportionate with the duration of loss of consciousness or post-traumatic amnesia, and absence of neuroimaging findings, and (c) symptoms tend to persist or even worsen over time. PCD with neurocognitive and psychopathological features is used when there is a mixture of documented neurocognitive deficits and acquired emotional problems that demonstrate some improvements over time, and there is an absence of positive neuroimaging.

The most serious and obvious problem with the ICD-10 and the DSM-IV criteria for the post-concussive disorder is causally linking the subjective, self-reported symptoms to the original MTBI. In fact, the etiology of the so-called *persistent* post-concussive disorder has never been agreed upon (see 4, 12, and, 48 for reviews). For decades, researchers have questioned the validity of this diagnosis as a true syndrome or disease entity (e.g., 29, 38, 49–52). Others have noted that the syndrome is rare in prospective studies (e.g., 29, 34), and concerns regarding the role of financial compensation on symptom reporting have been expressed for many years (49, 53–56). Most researchers suggest that the etiology is due to the biological effects of the injury, psychological factors, psychosocial factors (broadly defined), chronic pain, or a combination of factors (9–11, 14, 39, 57–60). Ruff and colleagues (8, 48, 61) have stressed a multidimensional cumulative stressor conceptualization of the persistent post-concussive disorder. Essentially, setbacks in several aspects of a person's life (physical, emotional, cognitive, psychosocial, vocational, financial, and recreational) serve as cumulative stressors that interact with personality and premorbid physical and mental health factors, resulting in the disorder. This model stresses the complexity of the etiology and factors that might maintain the symptoms chronically. The model, as written, does not require "brain damage" as a pre-requisite for diagnosis. In addition to cumulative stressors, Wood (13) has described numerous factors that can mimic, reinforce, or perpetuate post-concussion or post-concussion-like symptom reporting.

The ICD-10 criteria explicitly recognize that the cause of the person's symptoms is not always clear. It has been documented repeatedly by researchers that the symptoms that comprise the diagnostic criteria are nonspecific and they occur frequently in healthy adults and in a variety of patient groups who have not suffered an MTBI (38, 62–77). Examples of the prevalence of these diagnostic criteria in healthy adults, patients with depression, and patients with fibromyalgia are provided in the next section.

Nonspecificity of ICD-10 & DSM-IV Diagnostic Criteria

In this section we provide information regarding the prevalence of the ICD-10 and DSM-IV diagnostic criteria in healthy adults and in patients with depression or fibromyalgia. These data illustrate (a) the nonspecificity of these criteria, and (b) how easy it is to misdiagnose a person with a post-concussive disorder. A post-concussion questionnaire, patterned after the ICD-10 criteria, was developed in the late 1990s and has been used in several studies (73, 78, 79).

The British Columbia Post-concussion Symptom Inventory (BC-PSI; see Appendix A & B) is a 16-item measure designed to assess the presence and severity of post-concussion symptoms (73, 78, 79). The test was based on ICD-10 (40) criteria for Post-concussional Syndrome, and requires the test taker to rate the frequency and intensity of 13 symptoms (i.e., headaches, dizziness or light-headedness, nausea or feeling sick, fatigue, sensitivity to noises, irritability, sadness, nervousness or tension, temper problems, poor concentration, memory problems, reading difficulty, and sleep disturbance), and the effect of three life problems on daily living (i.e., greater present versus past effects of alcohol consumption, worrying and dwelling on symptoms, and self-perception of brain damage).

Normative data for the BC-PSI are available for 158 healthy, community-dwelling, adults from the greater Vancouver metropolitan area. All subjects were working or going to school, and none had a current mental health problem. All were screened for depression and scored below 17 on the Beck Depression Inventory-Second Edition. As seen in Tables 23-2 and 23-3, most healthy adults endorse some symptoms. Approximately 32% of this sample obtained a total score of zero. However, 15% obtained a score of 10 or higher. Scores from 10–14 are considered unusually high and score above 15 are considered extremely high for healthy adults.

The BC-PSI has also been given to large samples of patients with depression or fibromyalgia. The patients with depression were referred by their psychiatrist or family physician (N = 64). All subjects were administered the Structured Clinical Interview for DSM-IV (SCID-I). The SCID-I is a semi-structured clinical interview used to establish DSM-IV Axis I diagnoses. The version of the SCID-I used in this study was the nonpatient research

TABLE 23-2

Frequencies, Percentages, and Cumulative Percentages of Total Scores in Healthy Adults: British Columbia Post-concussion Symptom Inventory

TOTAL SCORE	FREQUENCY	PERCENT	CUMULATIVE PERCENT
0	50	31.6	31.6
1	20	12.7	44.3
2	9	5.7	50.0
3	12	7.6	57.6
4	16	10.1	67.7
5	7	4.4	72.2
6	5	3.2	75.3
7	5	3.2	78.5
8	4	2.5	81.0
9	6	3.8	84.8
10	1	0.6	85.4
11	4	2.5	88.0
12	8	5.1	93.0
13	1	0.6	93.7
14	1	0.6	94.3
15	3	1.9	96.2
16	0	0.0	96.2
17	2	1.3	97.5
18	1	0.6	98.1
19	0	0.0	98.1
20	1	0.6	98.7
21	0	0.0	98.7
22	0	0.0	98.7
23	0	0.0	98.7
24	0	0.0	98.7
25	0	0.0	98.7
26	0	0.0	98.7
27	0	0.0	98.7
28	0	0.0	98.7
29	1	0.6	99.4
30	0	0.0	99.4
31	0	0.0	99.4
32	1	0.6	100.0

N = 158.

TABLE 23-3

Interpreting Total Scores in Healthy Adults: British Columbia Post-Concussion Symptom Inventory

TOTAL RAW SCORE	PERCENTILE RANKS	CLASSIFICATION
0	0 – 32%	Low
1 – 9	33 – 85%	Normal
10 – 14	86 – 95%	Unusually high
15+	96 – 100%	Extremely high

The community volunteers were from the Greater Vancouver area (N = 158). All were working or going to school, and none had current mental health problems. The sample was 41% male and 59% female. Their average age was 35.7 years (SD = 16.3). Their average education was 14.8 years (SD = 2.5). They should be considered a high functioning, well-educated sample of healthy adults. The internal consistency reliability (Cronbach's Alpha) for the items comprising the total score is r = .82.

majority of patients with depression or fibromyalgia. Headaches were reported by nearly 20% of healthy adults, 59% of patients with depression, and 72% of patients with fibromyalgia. Noise sensitivity was reported by 11% of healthy adults, 50% of patients with depression, and approximately 69% of patients with fibromyalgia. The ICD-10 diagnostic criteria also identify reduced tolerance to alcohol, fear of brain damage, and a preoccupation with symptoms and problems as characterizing the post-concussive disorder. The percentages of patients that endorsed these problems were as follows: (a) reduced tolerance for alcohol (depression = 39% and FM = 35%), (b) concern about having brain damage (depression = 28% and FM = 33%), and (c) worrying about or dwelling on their symptoms and problems (depression = 75%, FM = 85%).

Symptom endorsement for each group can be compared to the DSM-IV and ICD-10 diagnostic criteria. Six of the eight DSM-IV Category C symptoms are represented on the BC-PSI. For the depressed patients, the majority of subjects (85.9%) endorsed three or more DSM-IV Category C symptoms. Over half of the sample (53.1%) endorsed three or more of these symptoms at a clinically significant level (moderate-to-severe). Depressed patients' symptom endorsement also was compared to diagnostic criteria from the ICD-10. All diagnostic criteria from the ICD-10 are represented on the scale. These criteria are grouped into six categories. The specific rates of endorsement for the six mildly endorsed and moderately-severely endorsed symptom categories for the ICD-10 were as follows: (1) headaches, dizziness, general malaise and excessive fatigue, or noise intolerance = 92.2% and 65.6%; (2) irritability, emotional liability, depression, or anxiety = 87.5% and 68.8%; (3) subjective complaints of concentration or memory difficulty = 78.1% and 54.7%; (4) insomnia = 78.1% and 53.1%; (5) reduced

version 2.0, August 1998 revision (80). All patients had a SCID diagnosis of major depressive disorder (92%), dysthymic disorder (5%), or depressive disorder NOS (3%). The patients with fibromyalgia (N = 54) were recruited from two rheumatology practices and one outpatient hospital program. All patients were examined by a rheumatologist and were included in the study only if they met the American College of Rheumatology criteria for the syndrome (81). On average, the participants had 13.8 trigger points (SD = 2.1, Range = 11–18), and less than one control point (Range = 0 – 3).

As seen in Table 23-4, mild levels of symptom endorsement occur in a minority of healthy adults and a

TABLE 23-4

Percentages of Subjects Endorsing Symptoms at a Mild or Moderate-Severe Level (British Columbia Post-concussion Symptom Inventory.)

ITEMS	HEALTHY COMMUNITY VOLUNTEERS		PATIENTS WITH DEPRESSION		PATIENTS WITH FIBROMYALGIA	
	MILD	MODERATE-SEVERE	MILD	MODERATE-SEVERE	MILD	MODERATE-SEVERE
Headaches	19.6	3.2	59.4	28.1	72.2	37.0
Dizziness/light-headed	11.4	1.3	31.2	10.9	37.0	7.4
Nausea/feeling sick	13.3	0.0	40.6	10.9	35.2	18.5
Fatigue	27.8	5.1	85.6	57.8	96.3	79.6
Extra sensitive to noises	11.4	1.3	50.0	18.8	68.5	44.4
Irritable	21.5	5.1	76.6	35.9	53.7	25.9
Sadness	18.4	1.3	76.6	56.3	55.6	33.3
Nervous or tense	16.5	1.3	65.6	35.9	59.3	33.3
Temper problems	15.8	5.1	37.5	15.6	27.8	7.4
Poor concentration	16.5	3.2	78.1	46.9	75.9	44.4
Memory problems	13.3	3.8	70.3	42.2	74.1	44.4
Difficulty reading	8.2	1.9	40.6	23.4	48.1	24.1
Poor sleep	22.8	5.1	78.1	53.1	87.0	59.3

Healthy adults (N = 158), patients with depression (N = 64), and patients with fibromyalgia (N = 54). Patients with depression were diagnosed by their family physician or psychiatrist, and their diagnosis was confirmed using the SCID-I. Their average age was 41.1 years (SD = 12.5), and their average education was 14.6 years (SD = 3.2). Approximately 71% of the sample was female. The patients with fibromyalgia were mostly women (94%). Their average age was 51.4 years (SD = 12.8, Range = 17 – 75). Their average education was 13.5 years (SD = 2.4, Range = 7 – 20)

tolerance to alcohol = 35.9% and 12.5%; and (6) preoccupation with these symptoms and fear of permanent brain damage = 76.6% and 26.6%. The majority of the sample (89.1%) endorsed three or more ICD-10 Category C symptoms, with 57.8% endorsing these symptom categories at a clinically significant level.

The patients with fibromyalgia had similar results. The majority of subjects (81.5%) endorsed three or more DSM-IV Category C symptoms. Half of the sample (50.0%) endorsed three or more of these symptoms at a clinically significant level (moderate-to-severe). Their specific rates of endorsement for the six mildly endorsed and moderately-severely endorsed symptom categories for the ICD-10 were as follows: (1) headaches, dizziness, general malaise and excessive fatigue, or noise intolerance = 96.3% and 83.3%; (2) irritability, emotional liability, depression, or anxiety = 81.5% and 50.0%; (3) subjective complaints of concentration or memory difficulty = 77.8% and 53.7%; (4) insomnia = 87.0% and 59.3%; (5) reduced tolerance to alcohol = 35.8% and 33.3%; and (6) preoccupation with these symptoms and fear of permanent brain damage = 87.0% and 63.0%. The majority of the sample (94.3%) endorsed three or more ICD-10 Category C symptoms, with 66% endorsing these symptom categories at a clinically significant level.

What is clear from the data presented in this section is that (a) the diagnostic criteria for the post-concussive disorder are non-specific, and (b) patients with fibromyalgia who report problems with depression, chronic pain, or both are very likely to be diagnosed (or misdiagnosed) with the disorder. In fact, 9 out of 10 patients with depression or fibromyalgia report a symptom constellation that can meet criteria for a post-concussive disorder (in the absence of a traumatic injury to their head or brain). The rates at which the patients with depression and the patients with fibromyalgia met diagnostic criteria for the two classification systems were very similar because only the symptom criteria were applied. The additional DSM-IV criteria for measured neurocognitive impairment and impairment in real-world functioning were not applied. What is interesting, of course, is that when patients are followed prospectively out of the hospital and assessed at three months post-injury, a minority meet DSM-IV criteria (11–17%) and over half meet ICD-10 criteria (54–64%) (46, 47). However, as illustrated with this section of the chapter, if a person has depression (and no head or brain injury), he or she is 90% likely to meet ICD-10 criteria (if the head injury criterion is waived). The remainder of the chapter addresses the complexities of differential diagnoses.

DIFFERENTIAL DIAGNOSES AND CO-MORBIDITIES

There are many possible differential diagnoses, co-morbidities, and social-psychological factors that may *cause or maintain* the myriad of symptoms and problems reported by patients long after experiencing a mild injury to their head, brain, or both. These differential diagnoses or co-morbidities might be largely unrelated to the original MTBI. In practice, it is oftentimes difficult to disentangle the many factors that can be responsible for the symptoms following a remote MTBI or a craniocervical trauma with an MTBI. This is because the more chronic symptoms that are believed to be associated directly or indirectly to the remote injury are common in healthy subjects (62, 72–77), in patients with no history of brain injury, such as outpatients seen for psychological treatment (63) or minor medical problems (64), personal injury claimants (64, 65), patients with post-traumatic stress disorder (66), patients with orthopedic injuries (38), individuals with chronic pain (67–70), and patients with whiplash (71). Thus, the differential diagnosis of the persistent post-concussive disorder is very challenging. The most commonly encountered clinical conditions that might lead to a diagnosis of "post-concussive disorder" are traumatic cervical injuries due to whiplash-associated disorders; post-traumatic chronic pain, particularly headache (cephalalgia) and neck pain (cervicalgia); depression; and the anxiety spectrum disorders (including post-traumatic stress disorder). Each of these conditions might co-occur with an MTBI or they might occur independently from an MTBI. If they co-occur, the challenge is trying to determine if the person recovered from the MTBI and the ongoing symptoms and problems reported are more likely to relate to one of the co-morbid conditions. These conditions will be reviewed next.

Cervical Injuries and Whiplash-Associated Disorders

Cervical spine injuries are common, particularly following rear-end motor vehicle accidents (82). Most patients recover from these injuries in a few weeks. However, there are others who have longer-term problems related to numerous potential secondary complications. The diagnostic and treatment challenges are mainly relevant to this chronically-symptomatic group.

It is generally agreed that whiplash injury typically involves a flexion-extension movement, but torsional-rotational movement may also play a role. The presumed cause of the acute injury is mechanical strain with or without contusion of ligaments and muscles supporting the cervical spine. Safety belts appear to actually increase the risk for cervical injury and, to a lesser extent, thoracic vertebral fractures (83). Because most cervical acceleration/deceleration injuries are not exclusively in the sagittal plane, the pathomechanics can be complicated and this has important implications for what part of the neck might be damaged as a result of rotational injury. Structures that become more susceptible to injury when there is cervical rotation include the facet (zygapophyseal) joint capsules, alar ligament complex, and intervertebral discs (84). The forces involved in cervical injury include extension, flexion, lateral flexion, and shear. Shear forces typically are horizontal in nature. Cervical symptoms may be caused and maintained as a result of injury to multiple structures within the neck including intervertebral discs, muscles, ligaments, the atlantoaxial complex, cervical vertebra, zygapophyseal (facet) joints, and neurovascular structures (85). Imaging methods, particularly conventional radiography, do not visualize many of these types of lesions very well.

The most common acute symptoms following whiplash are neck pain, headache, and limitation in neck range of motion (82, 86, 87). Many other symptoms have been associated with this type of injury, including visual disturbances, dizziness, auditory disturbances, balance disorders, and cognitive dysfunction (85, 88).

Visual disturbances have been associated with whiplash and might be subjectively reported as "blurriness". Most commonly, this subjective impairment is associated with findings of decreased accommodative and convergence function (89, 90). Other problems, such as disturbances in saccadic eye movement, have also been reported (91).

Cervicogenic vertigo or dizziness is a complaint that often accompanies cervical whiplash injury and may be related to (a) problems with the afferent input from positional proprioceptors in the cervical and lumbar regions (92, 93), (b) over-excitation of the cervical sympathetic nerves (94), (c) compromise of vertebral artery blood flow (95, 96), and/or (d) cervical/lumbar hypertonicity (94). Non-cervicogenic causes of vertigo or dizziness include perilymphatic fistulas[1], post-traumatic endolymphatic hyprops[2] (e.g., Meniere's disease), and benign paroxysmal positional vertigo[3] (97–99). Some patients report general feelings of whooziness, giddiness, and/or imbalance. Stapley and colleagues hypothesized that this phenomena occurs as a result of neck muscle fatigue and associated increases in postural body sway (100). Balance disorders

---

[1] An abnormal communication between the fluid-filled perilymphatic space of the inner ear and the air-filled middle ear cavity.

[2] Increased hydraulic pressure within the inner ear's endolymphatic system that can cause hearing loss, episodic vertigo, tinnitus, and pressure sensation.

[3] Benign paroxysmal positional vertigo can occur following head trauma and might relate to a collection of debris in the inner ear. Symptoms include dizziness or vertigo, lightheadedness, imbalance, and nausea.

following whiplash are believed to be associated with (a) altered vestibular and/or proprioceptive input (101), (b) neck muscle fatigue (102), (c) joint position error (103), and/or (d) abnormal cervical afferent input (104).

Auditory symptoms, such as tinnitus, hyperacusis[4], and hearing loss (105, 106), may also occur following whiplash. There is controversy regarding the etiology of neuro-otological impairments of these types following cervical whiplash, but they clearly can occur in the absence of acquired brain injury. The cause of tinnitus has not been determined definitively, but it is possible that following whiplash cranio-cervical somatic dysfunction may modulate dorsal cochlear nucleus activity (107), and/or aberrant nociceptive input to the brainstem from upper cervical (e.g., atlas) and associated cervical myofascial dysfunction (108) may be the underlying cause(s). Temporomandibular joint dysfunction also might underlie tinnitus in some patients (109).

Neurocognitive complaints also are common following whiplash (110), and a substantial minority of patients remain symptomatic at one year post-injury (111, 112). These problems should be conceptualized as either perceived, self-reported symptoms or measured problems on neuropsychological tests. In a meta-analytic review of the literature, Kessels and colleagues (113) concluded that cognitive functioning, as measured by neuropsychological tests, can be adversely affected following whiplash. Not all studies, of course, report neuropsychological changes associated with whiplash injury (e.g., 114). The cause of cognitive complaints or measured cognitive decrements in a subset of patients with whiplash is unknown; researchers suggest they might be related to damage to the brain (110), somatization (114), distraction due to pain (115), or a combination of factors.

There are multiple potential causes of chronic pain following whiplash. Possible etiologies, singly or in combination, include myofascial dysfunction of the paracervical (anterior and posterior) and upper shoulder girdle musculature, C2-C3 facet joint pain, neuralgia of the greater and/or lesser occipital nerve, internal derangement of the temporo-mandibular joint, basilar artery migraine, and/or cervico-thoracic somatic dysfunction (116). Facial, neck, and shoulder dysesthesias (e.g., burning, pins and needles, itching sensation) can arise from the upper cranial nerves and their superficial branches (greater auricular nerve, superficial cervical nerve, and supraclavicular nerve), and the descending tract of the trigeminal nerve and/or its associated fibers (i.e., fibers 5, 7, 9, and 10). Knibestol and colleagues reported that some patients with whiplash have facial sensory changes in vibratory and temperature perception that might be related to damage to the central trigeminal system in the upper spinal cord segments and pontomedullary levels of the brainstem (117). Herren-Gerber

and colleagues reported that there is modulation of central hypersensitivity by nociceptive input following whiplash injury and that different mechanisms likely underlie hypersensitivity to pain (hyperalgesia) localized to areas around the pain site versus distant body areas (118). Chronic cervical facet joint pain can occur following whiplash. Dwyer and colleagues "mapped" characteristic patterns of cervical zygapophyseal joint pain in normal volunteers; this mapping may be useful for constructing pain charts (119).

The best initial treatment for cervicogenic pain is exercise and manual therapy. In more intractable cases, where facet involvement is suspected, interventional pain management through the use of local blocks and/or neuromodulation procedures is recommended (120, 121).

Cranial Trauma

Head injury can, of course, result in damage to the skull or its adjoining parts (i.e., the cranium or cranial adenexal structures). This damage might underlie some of the symptoms and problems reported by patients acutely and post-acutely without necessarily having concomitant brain injury (98).

Skull fractures are relatively uncommon in patients who sustain mild traumatic brain injuries. When they occur, they may be closed or compound and depressed or non-depressed. Basilar skull fractures, as opposed to linear skull fractures of the cranial vault, often have important clinical implications. If the dura mater is torn, the chance of a cerebrospinal fluid fistula is increased. A dural tear or basilar skull fracture will increase the patient's risk of meningitis. Cerebrospinal fluid leaks may occur through the nose (rhinorrhea) or ears (otorrhea) and may be missed in the acute setting. Approximately 4% of mild head injury patients may have an unsuspected temporal skull fracture (122).

Hearing loss can arise from damage to cranial adenexal structures. Longitudinal fractures are more commonly associated with conductive hearing loss due to either ossicular chain disruption or traumatic tympanic membrane tear and blood in the middle ear. Transverse temporal skull fractures often will be associated with either mixed or profound sensorineural hearing loss, hemotympanum, dizziness, and/or facial nerve injuries (123, 124). The conductive hearing loss associated with hemotympanum is typically temporary and resolves as the blood is re-absorbed. Progressive hearing loss following trauma should prompt further assessment for either perilymphatic fistula or endolymphatic hydrops (125). The most common type of ossicular dislocation associated with temporal skull fractures is the separation of the incudostapedial joint, with or without dislocation of the body of the incus from the articulation with the malleus head. Surgical correction can restore hearing.

---

[4] Hypersensitivity to sound.

Complaints of "dizziness" following head trauma and/or mild traumatic brain injury are extremely common. If these problems persist beyond the acute stage of recovery, thorough clinical evaluation is important. Neurodiagnostic evaluation of the dizzy patient might include: audiologic testing, a platform fistula test, electronystagmography, and/or posturography (99, 126). Labyrinthine concussion can result in transient auditory and vestibular symptoms without associated skull fracture. Sudden deafness following a blow to the cranium may be partially or completely reversible. Benign paroxysmal positional vertigo is the most common neuro-otologic problem following head trauma. Most patients demonstrate a paroxysmal positional nystagmus with rapid changes in position (127). Although, benign paroxysmal positional vertigo may have periodic exacerbations even after the symptoms have subsided, this is the exception rather than the rule. Vestibular suppressant medications may be used, but generally these agents should only be considered if symptoms are severe enough to dramatically compromise functional activities such as frequent falls or significant nausea and/or vomiting. Vestibular exercises may also be prescribed to hasten neurologic and functional recovery via several proposed physiologic mechanisms including central sensory substitution, rebalancing tonic activity, and physiologic habituation (128–132). Clinical researchers suggest that a three-pronged approach should be utilized as part of an organized vestibular rehabilitation program: (a) habituation exercises, (b) postural control exercises, and (c) general conditioning activities (133). Surgery may be considered as a last resort for intractable benign paroxysmal positional vertigo; it has been reported to be successful in more than 90% of cases (134).

The clinician should always consider the possibility of a post-traumatic endolymphatic hydrops (Meniere's syndrome) after cranial trauma when there is ipsilateral low-frequency hearing loss, tinnitus, and a sensation of fullness in the ear. Treatment of post-traumatic Meniere's disease may include vestibular suppressants if patients are symptomatic to the point that daily function is significantly adversely affected. Head movements and rapid changes in head position should be avoided. In the remission phase, Meniere's disease may be treated with medications including vestibular suppressants and/or diuretics as well as steroids, low pressure pulse generators (Meniett device), and surgical procedures (both destructive and non-destructive; 135, 136–138).

Post-traumatic perilymphatic fistula can occur following trauma as a result of rupture of the oval and less commonly the round window with subsequent communication between the inner ear and middle ear resulting in inappropriate stimulation of labyrinthine receptors (139). Unfortunately, there is no pathognomonic or characteristic electronystagmographic sign for the condition. Symptoms can include vertigo, fluctuating hearing loss (usually a late complication), tinnitus, chronic low grade nausea, endolymphatic hydrops, abnormal cervical muscle tone (myodystonia), and persistent or exertional headache (140). Patients quite frequently complain of aural fullness (141). Patients will often complain of nonspecific imbalance problems worsened by sudden turning, as well as disequilibrium with perceptually-complex external stimuli such as patterns and wide-field motion evidenced with escalator rides, revolving doors, and crowds (141, 142). The sensation while ambulating has been described as "walking on pillows" (135). The aforementioned experiences sometimes promote a mild agoraphobia. Although there is no definitive bedside clinical test for post-traumatic perilymphatic fistula, application of pressure to the tympanic membrane with a pneumatic otoscope (Hennebert's fistula test) or application of pressure over the tragus might produce worsening of vertigo or nystagmus. Both the aforementioned tests are suggestive but not diagnostic for a perilymphatic fistula. Some investigators believe that caloric hypoexcitability or unexcitability associated with even partial conservation of cochlear function is a very good indicator of the condition (143). Black, Lilly, and Nashner (144) described the platform fistula test utilizing posturography as a means of objectively diagnosing this clinical condition. The ability of posturographic testing to delineate perilymphatic fistulas has been questioned by one of the authors (NDZ) as well as others (145). However, further research is definitely indicated to clarify the role of this diagnostic modality. Early treatment measures include bedrest, head elevation, and avoidance of straining (135). The duration of bedrest is somewhat controversial although many clinicians advocate 5 to 10 days given the functional and physiologic implications of prolonged immobilization. Perilymphatic fistulas usually heal spontaneously. Exploratory tympanotomy is necessary to definitively establish the diagnosis, but is generally *not* recommended unless symptoms last longer than a month or if there is a progressive hearing loss. Chronic perilymphatic fistulas can be addressed surgically by "patching" the leaking oval/round window utilizing temporal aponeurosis or stapdedectomy with interposition (146). Recent work has shown that the presence of beta-2 transferrin may serve as a marker for perilymphatic fistula-related leaks (147, 148). Surgical treatment generally aids in control of vertigo much more so than the restoration of hearing (141, 143).

Tinnitus can occur following head trauma. It is important to note that tinnitus is a symptom not a disease entity, the etiology of which must be defined before it can be effectively treated. Audiologic battery testing is indicated in all post-head injury patients with complaints of tinnitus. Hearing aids, cochlear implants, tinnitus maskers, and hearing instruments have been used to decrease the subjective symptoms associated with this disorder. The protocol that is clearly the most well accepted is the Jastreboff tinnitus retraining program[5] (149). No drug has been FDA approved for treating tinnitus and current choices are at best controversial and poorly studied (150). Antidepressant medications, biofeedback, hypnosis, avoidance of stimulants including caffeine, and proper sleep hygiene have also been recommended because tinnitus can be exacerbated by stress and anxiety (151).

Olfactory and gustatory problems also can occur following injury to the cranium and/or brain. There are several million olfactory neurons located in the olfactory epithelium on the wall of the nasal cavity. Each of these neurons extends an axon to the olfactory bulb (on the surface of the brain, along the orbital-medial surface of the frontal lobe). The bulb neurons extend axons, via the olfactory tracts, to make contact with neurons located in the olfactory cortex. The primary olfactory cortex is located near the anteromedial part of the uncus on each side. Because the olfactory tract is attached to the outer aspect of the hemisphere, the impact of the skull's jagged interior[6] upon the uncus could damage the primary olfactory cortex or the terminal portion of the olfactory nerve or both. Costanzo and Zasler (153) listed the known and presumed mechanisms underlying olfactory impairment following head trauma or TBI as follows: (1) traumatic damage to the nasal epithelium; (2) shearing of the olfactory fila, arising from the nasal epithelium, prior to entering the olfactory bulbs, as a presumed consequence of movement of the brain relative to, and/or fracture of, the cribriform plate; and (3) contusions or edema effecting the olfactory bulb or the lateral or medial olfactory tracts. All of these mechanisms could cause impairment in the ability to detect odors. Isolated gustatory dysfunction is uncommon. Typically, peripheral injury involves the facial nerve (CN VII) because it is more prone to injury than the glossopharyngeal (CN IX) and vagus (CN X) nerves which are also involved in mediation of taste (153). Timely neuromedical and rehabilitative interventions (154) including comprehensive objective quantification of deficits through established "Chemosensory Clinics" can be helpful.

Visual problems can occur at a peripheral level and be unrelated to a brain injury. These deficits can be due

to disorders of the vitreous, both prefoveal and foveal, commonly associated with traction on the retina with resultant subjective symptoms of floating spots (so-called "floaters"; 155, 156). Retinal injury, including detachment, tear, and hemorrhage (157, 158), also causes visual symptoms. Approximately 20% of patients evaluated with mid-facial trauma were noted in one study to have accommodative and/or convergence insufficiency (159). A cursory assessment of the optic disc by the physician will obviously miss the types of subtle lesions responsible for many post-traumatic visual symptoms. It is therefore important to refer patients with visual complaints for appropriate diagnostic assessment as well as functionally oriented treatment. Professionals that may assist in these aforementioned areas include ophthalmology, neuro-ophthalmology, and neuro-optometry (See chapter in this text by Padula and colleagues).

Headache and neck pain are the most common physical complaints following concussion (mild brain injury) (See chapters in this text by Zasler, Martelli, et al. and Martelli, Zasler, et al. on Pain Management). Headaches, of course, are common in the general population as well (160, 161). Pre-existing headaches, post-traumatic headaches, or both might largely underlie a diverse set of symptoms and problems in people who have sustained an MTBI (as well as patients with whiplash-related problems or cranial-trauma related problems). Patients with problematic headaches, such as migraine or tension, often have comorbid depression (162–165). Elevated levels of psychological distress (i.e., symptoms of anxiety, depression, or both), that may or may not break threshold for diagnosing a psychiatric condition, have been reported in numerous studies involving patients with headache conditions (166–171).

When a patient presents with headaches long after an MTBI, it is difficult to determine whether (a) the original injury is the underlying cause of the headaches, and (b) to what extent other factors have caused, or are maintaining, the headaches. It is estimated that 4–5% of adults experience chronic daily headaches (172, 173). Medication overuse (i.e., drug rebound headache) is the most treatable cause of refractory headaches (174–179). Medication overuse might result from patients' attempt to treat their headaches or other bodily pain. Febrile or viral illnesses, general surgery, or a stressful life event appear to be the most common events that precede new daily persistent headaches (180).

When a person is involved in litigation, headaches typically are attributed to the tort (i.e., injury being litigated). Of course, headaches are common in daily life and people who are not involved in litigation attribute a variety of factors to the underlying cause of their headaches. Boardman and colleagues (181) conducted a large-scale survey study of adults in Great Britain. In this sample of 1, 871 adults who suffered from headaches in the past

---

[5] The authors know specialists in neuro-otology that strongly prefer to not take patients into a tinnitus retraining program while they are involved in litigation, given limited resources and less "subjective improvement" in patients involved in stressful, adversarial, protracted litigation.

[6] The upper border of the sphenoid bone is sharply angulated, like the edge of a shelf. In the center of the skull base, the sphenoid wings or ridges terminate in two bony projections called the anterior clinoid processes. They are adjacent and immediately anterior to the uncus on both sides and point posteriorly towards the foramen magnum. Therefore, with a violent forward movement of the brain relative to the skull, the anterior clinoid processes could produce contusions in the region of the uncus (152).

3 months, factors *perceived* (i.e., self-reported) to be related to their headaches were as follows: stress (71%), tiredness (65%), menstrual cycle (55%), having too much work to do (41%), drinking alcohol (33%), sleeping too long (21%), and not eating regularly (20%). The respondents also completed several psychological tests (e.g., measuring depression and anxiety) and questionnaires (measuring pain, disability, sleep problems, and alcohol and caffeine consumption). Headache occurrence was most strongly associated with anxiety and sleep problems.

Chronic Pain

Patients with chronic pain often complain of physical, cognitive, and psychological symptoms that closely resemble post-concussion-like symptoms (e.g., 68, 70, 114, 182–189). If chronic pain does not co-occur in patients who are slow to recover following an MTBI, then the similarity between chronic pain symptoms and post-concussion symptoms is not problematic. However, patients who sustain MTBIs in falls or motor vehicle accidents frequently have a comorbid chronic pain problem. Uomoto and Esselman (190) reported that 95% of patients with MTBI's reported the presence of at least one chronic pain symptom 24 months post-injury (e.g., headaches, neck/shoulder pain, or back pain). Thus, because chronic pain often accompanies MTBI, attributing post-concussion symptoms to brain injury in patients with comorbid pain is problematic.

McCracken and Iverson (185) reported that 54% of chronic pain patients from a university pain management center endorsed at least one subjective cognitive complaint (e.g., forgetfulness, minor accidents, difficulty finishing tasks, difficulty with attention). Roth et al. (187) found that 62% of chronic pain patients from a university hospital pain management program reported experiencing at least one subjective cognitive complaint as being a moderate to severe problem, and 28% of the patients endorsed 5 of 5 cognitive complaints as being a moderate to severe problem (i.e., trouble remembering, having to recheck things, difficulty making decisions, mind going blank, and trouble concentrating). Jamison, Sbrocco, and Parris (184) found that 54.5% of chronic pain patients from a university medical pain control center reported having moderate to extreme problems with both memory and concentration.

In a study comparing post-concussion-like symptoms to DSM-IV criteria for Post-concussional Disorder, Iverson and McCracken (68) examined 170 non-litigating, chronic pain patients with no history of head injury. On self-report inventories, 42% of these patients reported at least one cognitive complaint that had an impact on their health (i.e., attention, concentration, or memory). A large percentage (80.6%) of these patients endorsed three or more of the symptoms from Category C of the Post-concussional Disorder criteria in the DSM-IV (41). The percentage of these patients who would meet self report criteria for a Post-concussional Disorder was calculated by determining the number of patients who reported cognitive problems and three or more symptoms from Category C. Based on self report alone, 39% of the chronic pain patients met criteria for a Post-concussional Disorder (except, of course, they had no history of head injury).

Gasquoine (67) compared post-concussion-like symptom reporting in a small sample of 10 patients with MTBIs and 18 patients with chronic back pain. No differences between the MTBI group and chronic back pain group were found on any PCS symptoms, even on symptoms that were typically "head injury related" (e.g., headache, dizziness, recent memory, concentration). Smith-Seemiller and colleagues compared symptom reporting on the Rivermead Post-concussion Questionnaire in 32 patients with chronic complaints following an MTBI and 63 chronic pain patients. More than 80% of both groups met DSM-IV self-report symptom criteria for a Post-concussional Disorder. No differences between groups were found on the total post-concussion symptoms. However, on the subscales of the Rivermead Post-concussion Questionnaire, the MTBI patients endorsed more cognitive symptoms and fewer emotional symptoms compared to the chronic pain patients. There were no differences between groups on the somatic symptoms of the Rivermead. These authors cautioned, however, that there was a high base rate of patients undergoing litigation in the chronic pain sample that may have biased symptom reporting in this group (70).

Some researchers have suggested that the reporting of cognitive complaints in chronic pain patients may be associated with depression, anxiety, and fatigue (e.g., 185–187). Similarly, these complaints may be influenced by factors including the pain experience itself, comorbid psychiatric disorders, medication side effects, iatrogenic factors, and possible malingering. However, the influence of these factors is poorly understood. Given that (a) chronic pain conditions frequently accompany MTBI many months post-injury (190), (b) patients with chronic pain report identical symptoms as those attributed to a post-concussive disorder (e.g., 68, 70), (c) depression frequently co-occurs with chronic pain (191–195), and (d) patients with depression report very similar symptoms as those attributed to a post-concussive disorder (cf. the DSM-IV diagnostic criteria and associated features and Iverson (79)), it is not surprising that a person with chronic pain can be easily misdiagnosed as having a persistent post-concussive disorder, or chronic pain might be the predominant underlying cause of the disorder (See chapters in this text by Zasler, Martelli, et al. and Martelli, Zasler, et al. on Pain Management).

Depression, Anxiety, Stress, and Somatic Preoccupation

Depression is common following traumatic brain injuries of all severities (196, 197). Depression is also common in patients with chronic pain (191, 194), and it is associated with increased disability in these patients (193, 198). Depression is also common in trauma patients (199), and patients with chronic headaches (165, 200–202), post-traumatic stress disorder (66, 203–205), or substance abuse problems (206–210). Of course, depression is one of the most common mental health problems in the world, and people who suffer a single episode of major depression are at greatly increased risk for a future episode, with estimates of recurrence ranging from 50% to 80% (211–215). People who have had two or more episodes of depression are at extremely high risk for a future episode (43, page 372, 213, 216–218). Therefore, the underlying cause of depression, in any given person at any given time, can be very difficult, if not impossible, to determine. Depression represents the most challenging differential diagnosis for the post-concussive disorder (of course, depression might be the predominant etiology of the disorder for some patients). Many of the specific symptoms of depression, and other problems associated with this condition, are similar to the post-concussive disorder. The diagnostic criteria for major depression include the following symptoms: (a) diminished ability to think or concentrate, (b) indecisiveness, (c) fatigue or loss of energy, and (d) sleep problems (DSM-IV; 41; p. 327). In addition, major depression often is associated with irritability, excessive worry over one's health, and headaches (41; p. 323). Common lifestyle and psychosocial problems include strained social relationships, marital and family distress, occupational problems, academic problems, and substance abuse (41; p. 323). Therefore, it is extremely difficult to determine if a person's self-reported symptoms are due to depression, a persistent post-concussive disorder, or both because many of the symptoms are nearly identical in these conditions.

Patients with depression are expected to have cognitive complaints. Perceived cognitive impairment is a *cardinal feature* of depression (43). However, the relation between depression and cognitive difficulty goes much further. The co-occurrence of perceived cognitive problems and symptoms of depression has been demonstrated repeatedly in the literature in diverse groups of unselected community-dwelling adults (219–221) and specific clinical groups, such as patients with cancer (222), chronic fatigue syndrome (223), HIV (224, 225), major non-cardiac surgery (226), epilepsy (227, 228), chronic pain (185, 188), and sleep apnea (229). This is a consistent finding across different cultural and ethnic groups, including Chinese (230), French (231), Dutch (232), and African Americans (233). Therefore, broad and diverse research converges to illustrate clearly that the diagnosis of depression, or a depressive experience that does not meet criteria for a diagnosis, is likely to be accompanied by perceived cognitive problems.

The perceived cognitive problems reported by patients with depression have been illustrated more objectively through neuropsychological studies (234–247). However, there has never been a study showing that the cognitive effects of depression can be reliably differentiated from the cognitive effects of an MTBI. The problem for clinicians and researchers is that a person with depression is virtually guaranteed to meet diagnostic criteria for a post-concussive disorder, regardless of whether that person (a) has ever injured his brain, or (b) the past injury to his brain is causally-related to his current symptoms.

Another challenging differential diagnoses for the post-concussive disorder is Post-Traumatic Stress Disorder (PTSD). Patients with PTSD often report the same symptoms as patients who have sustained MTBIs. For example, in a sample of 128 patients with PTSD, 89% reported irritability, 56% reported memory problems, 92% reported concentration problems, and 90% reported difficulty sleeping (66). Therefore, it is easy to misdiagnose PTSD as a post-concussive disorder, and vice versa.

A controversial and confusing issue is whether a person who sustains a traumatic brain injury involving amnesia for the event can develop PTSD. There are data to support the position that TBI and PTSD typically are mutually exclusive (248–250), although researchers have put forward a compelling rationale for how, under certain circumstances, PTSD could emerge in a patient with a brain injury in the presence of amnesia (251, 252). The conceptual question at the heart of the debate is whether a person with no memory for a traumatic event can develop PTSD as a result of that traumatic event.

Gil and colleagues prospectively studied 120 accident victims who sustained an MTBI and who were hospitalized for observation immediately after their trauma. They were assessed within the first 24 hours and at one week, three months, and six months. At six months post-injury, 14% met diagnostic criteria for PTSD (notice that this prevalence rate is very similar to the rate of people believed to have the post-concussive disorder at 6–12 months post-injury). The statistical predictors of PTSD at 6 months were (a) PSTD symptoms, depressive symptoms, and anxiety symptoms at one week post-injury, (b) history of psychiatric disorder, and (c) memory for the event. Of the patients with memory for the event, 13/55 (23%) had PTSD at 6 months post-injury, compared to only 4/65 (6%) who did not have memory for the event (253). Therefore, the literature to date suggests quite clearly that having no memory for the event likely protects the individual from developing PTSD.

Therefore, a person who sustains an MTBI who has upsetting and traumatic memories of the accident, assault, or injury, and who has nightmares and sleep disturbance, might have PTSD, a post-concussive disorder, or both. It is extremely difficult to accurately diagnose both conditions in a patient, and the combination of the two is statistically uncommon. Therefore, it is more parsimonious to diagnose, and treat, the PTSD if it appears to be present and wait to see if the patient has ongoing residual problems that might relate to a brain injury following improvement or remission.

Symptoms of anxiety, stress, and somatic preoccupation also occur frequently in patients who are symptomatic beyond a few weeks post-injury. In a prospective study, Ponsford and colleagues reported that patients who were symptomatic at three months post-injury were likely to have high levels of stress and anxiety (254). As noted in the ICD-10 diagnostic criteria, symptoms following an MTBI "may be accompanied by feelings of depression or anxiety, resulting from some loss of self-esteem and fear of permanent brain damage. Such feelings enhance the original symptoms and a vicious circle results. Some patients become hypochondriacal, embark on a search for diagnosis and cure, and may adopt a permanent sick role" (40; section F07.2). Clinicians working with symptomatic patients are acutely aware that anxiety, and fear of permanent brain damage, can be prominent psychological features. Clinicians should take steps to reduce patients' subjective distress and guard against behavior that can be iatrogenic.

IATROGENESIS

An iatrogenic condition is a state of ill health or adverse effect caused by medical treatment, usually due to mistakes made in treatment (255). The word literally means "caused by a doctor" (*iatros* means physician in Greek), though such conditions can be the fault of therapists and/or pharmacists as well. This phenomenon is poorly researched in the field of rehabilitation, neurology, and neuropsychology, and there is no literature per se on the topic as related to MTBI. Nonetheless, it is a well-recognized issue in the field of brain injury rehabilitation.

> Professionals involved in rehabilitation have a clinical responsibility to patients with MTBI. To the extent that symptoms are ever iatrogenic, we provide a disservice to patients. To the extent that symptoms are neurologically, emotionally, environmentally, or motivationally based, we have a responsibility to understand and address these issues clinically to the best of our ability (Ref. 256, p. 57).

The tendency for medical, medical-legal, and rehabilitation professionals to diagnose "brain damage" or "diffuse axonal injury" as an explanation for persistent problems following a mild uncomplicated concussion (i.e., a "mild MTBI") can be iatrogenic. The authors have

seen, on numerous occasions, psychological harm resulting from telling people they have brain damage and they will need to cope and compensate for that damage, when in fact the probability of permanent brain damage was very low and the probability of a "treatable condition", such as depression, anxiety, sleep disturbance, and cumulative life stress, was high. Remember, if a person has chronic bodily pain, depression, or both, they are virtually guaranteed to meet self-report criteria for a post-concussive disorder regardless of whether they ever sustained a concussion. When a person is misdiagnosed as having presumed permanent brain damage it sends a strong, negative, prognostic message. It also might lead to (a) the person seeking support from brain injury associations, (b) the person receiving rehabilitation services normally designated for patients with moderate to severe brain injuries, and (c) the failure to provide effective treatment for the person's real underlying problems.

Roger Wood has noted that the early iatrogenic potential of general practitioners and hospital doctors may create insecurity and/or reinforce illness perceptions thereby instigating perceptions of disability and "illness behavior" due to both negative expectancies and the nocebo effect (see below) (13). Certainly, incorrect diagnosis may lead to treatment that is potentially both ineffective and possibly deleterious, physically and/or psychologically, to the patient. Oftentimes, misidentification and mislabeling of patients produces perpetuation of the actual impairment(s) and creates a more recalcitrant condition with a poorer prognosis (257). Parallel to experiences with pain patients, persons with MTBI may experience the negative ramifications of iatrogenesis in the context of over-investigation, particularly with unproven "neurodiagnostic" techniques, inappropriate information and advice, misdiagnosis, over-treatment, and inappropriate medication prescription (the latter which may produce further impairment and/or complications) (257). Iatrogenesis may not only have negative consequences on the patient but also on their family and/or significant other(s).

Physicians and other health care clinicians should be sensitized to the importance of avoiding iatrogenic complications. Some have considered iatrogenesis to be a "violation of moral norms, insufficient professionalism, negligence and indifference" (258). Others might argue that what sometimes appears to be iatrogenic illness may in fact be driven by unethical clinical practice, examiner bias, and/or examiner secondary gain. There are tremendous financial and professional pressures and incentives in the medical-legal setting, and it is widely believed that some experts adopt rather extreme, predictable, and polarized opinions that result in routine labeling of people as having long-term problems due to, presumably, permanent brain damage following a mild concussion. Better guidelines are clearly necessary to aide clinicians evaluating and treating persons with MTBI to avoid iatrogenesis. Moreover, everyone involved with patients conceptualized as having a post-concussive disorder should be aware of the numerous psychological factors that can cause or maintain the condition. These psychological factors are not only important for understanding the disorder, they represent obvious, typically overlooked, areas for treatment.

FACTORS RELATING TO THE PERCEPTION AND REPORTING OF SYMPTOMS

A diverse range of psychological factors can influence the perception and reporting of symptoms long after an MTBI. A person's psychological history, emotional response to injury, coping mechanisms, and psychosocial environment (e.g., work and family) are all factors that can influence the perception and reporting of symptoms and problems, as well as impact how the person functions in day-to-day life.

The experience of being ill can, in some ways, be rewarding for the patient. For example, the patient may get special privileges and extra attention from their spouse, family, coworkers, and friends. For many years, these issues have been studied in patients with chronic pain syndromes. Researchers have demonstrated that extra attention, changes in household responsibilities and routines, and the avoidance of undesirable activities all can *increase* patients' reporting of pain and disability. It is reasonable to think that some individuals with persistent symptoms and problems following an MTBI, similar to chronic pain patients, could derive reinforcement for disability behaviors. This is sometimes referred to as a *reinforced behavior pattern*.

The next section provides an overview of the role of personality characteristics and disorders in outcome from MTBI. The following sections relate to important social-psychological factors and influences on the etiology and maintenance of symptom experiencing and reporting in some patients.

Personality Characteristics and Disorders

Personality characteristics influence how people respond to illness, injury, or disease. Therefore, these characteristics are likely to be very important for understanding who is at risk for developing a persistent post-concussive disorder, and some of the psychological factors that maintain the disorder. At present, there is limited research available regarding the influence of personality styles as they might apply to the development, exacerbation, and maintenance of symptoms and problems following an MTBI.

As clinicians, it is very common to see a great deal of variation in individual response styles to life stressors and/or traumatic events. Although most people tend to be remarkably resilient to traumatic life events or injuries, some individuals are emotionally fragile and have relatively catastrophic reactions to seemingly small events. To most of us, it makes perfect intuitive sense that premorbid personality factors would influence individual response styles to life stressors and/or traumatic events.

In psychiatry and psychology, there is considerable interest in the role of personality characteristics in the etiology of mental health problems. This large literature, by extension, is relevant to understanding the post-concussive disorder, and the differential diagnosis of this disorder. Researchers frequently have reported that certain personality characteristics appear to be risk factors for major depression. People with high levels of neuroticism or negative affectivity, low self-esteem, and poor life coping skills are at increased risk for developing depression (259–263). These same personality characteristics, in addition to anger/hostility and narcissism, have been reported in numerous studies as risk factors for PTSD (264–267).

Kay and colleagues provided an elegant discussion of the role of personality styles and characteristics as they relate to the experience of symptoms and the recovery from MTBI (268). They proposed three personality factors that may influence the development and maintenance of symptoms following MTBI: (a) individual response style to trauma, (b) emotional significance of a particular event for each person, and (c) vulnerable personality styles.

First, individuals tend to respond to the acute symptoms in different ways. Some individuals tend to overemphasize cognitive and physical symptoms, whereas others tend to de-emphasize them. A certain symptom may be extremely debilitating for one person, yet another person may see this same symptom as simply slightly annoying. These response differences are not just determined by the differences in internal responses due to personality variables, but also by the environmental demands that challenge the person's ability to cope with that symptom. A laborer might be far less bothered by minor memory problems than a business-person, and an office worker might be only minimally concerned about mild balance problems compared to a roofer.

Second, there are differences in the emotional significance of a particular event for each person. Notwithstanding the emotional experience of the trauma itself, "for some persons the actual injury, the feelings evoked, and the response—or lack thereof—from others can trigger old, unresolved emotional issues. Often this takes the form of being vulnerable and unprotected, of not being responded to when hurt or sick, or of not being able to gain retribution when one has been wronged. Persons who grew up with significant holes in their emotional nurturing appear more at risk for responding in catastrophic ways to the emotional meaning of the injury" (p. 379–380) (268).

Third, based on their own clinical experience, Kay et al. proposed five different personality traits that they considered to be vulnerable to poor outcome following MTBI. These include: (a) overachievement, (b) dependency, (c) insecurity, (d) grandiosity, and (e) borderline personality characteristics (not disorder). Kay and colleagues explained the role of these traits as follows:

> The *overachiever*, who is often obsessive-compulsive and derives his or her sense of self from driven accomplishment, is at risk for a catastrophic reaction when subtle cognitive slippage takes the edge off his or her performance. The *dependent person* is susceptible to being paralyzed by his or her symptoms. The experience of decreased efficacy dips him or her below the critical threshold of ability to cope independently and results in a behavioral freezing up that can become self-perpetuating. The *insecure person*, while sharing some of the same dynamics of the dependent person, also has the tendency to focus in on and therefore magnify his or her symptoms, thus adding another dimension to perpetuating dysfunction. *Grandiose persons* get into trouble by being so unable to acknowledge their decrease in ability that they deny it to themselves and others and continue to blunder into situations that evoke failure. The crash of self-esteem, when it comes, is usually catastrophic. The person with *borderline personality characteristics* (not disorder), an individual who is often high-achieving but unable to relate to others, is a prime candidate for significant personality disorganization at all levels after MTBI (Ref. 268, p. 379).

These vulnerable personality traits have received support in the literature by some researchers and clinicians who have provided case studies to highlight the importance of these premorbid personality traits (8). Ruff and colleagues present case discussions of four patients who sustained a MTBI, who they characterized as (a) grandiosity and narcissistic features, (b) borderline traits with recurrent depression, (c) over-achiever with perfectionist tendencies, and (d) unmet dependency needs. In line with Kay et al., Ruff and colleagues concluded that "For the individuals we presented, the resistance to recovery appears to have had its basis in unmet needs and trauma from early childhood. As adults these individuals developed psychological defenses which enabled them to have some of their previously frustrated needs met, which preserved them a sense of self-esteem. However, their prior needs and insecurities were reactivated by the MTBI" (p. 562).

Hibbard and colleagues (269) examined the frequency of personality disorders before and after sustaining a traumatic brain injury. Participants were 100 patients seen at least one year following a TBI ranging from mild to severe. Using a modified SCID-II interview to reflect pre-injury characteristics, 24% of the sample was diagnosed with pre-injury personality disorders. The most common disorders were antisocial (15%) and obsessive-compulsive (6%) with incidence rates higher than community base rates reported in the literature. Higher rates of post-TBI personality disorders were found, with 66% of the sample meeting criteria for at least one personality disorder. The most common post-TBI disorders were borderline (26%), avoidant (26%), paranoid (17%), and obsessive-compulsive (24%). However, individuals with pre-TBI personality disorders were found to be at a greater risk of acquiring additional psychopathology post-TBI.

Evered and colleagues (48) examined the incidence and potential influences of emotional and personality problems in 129 patients with a history of MTBI and a presumed post-concussive disorder. The majority of patients (63.5%) met criteria for either Axis I and/or Axis II disorders, which is a rate of psychopathology that is higher than in the general public. The most common Axis II (i.e., personality) disorders were compulsive, histrionic, narcissistic, and dependent. This study clearly indicates that psychological problems, relating to personality and/or acute psychopathology, are prominent in patients with the presumed post-concussive disorder.

Greiffenstein and Baker (270) studied a unique sample of 23 patients involved in MTBI litigation (or disability evaluations) who had completed the MMPI prior to their injuries. They found that the majority of pre-injury MMPI profiles were abnormal in this group, with particular elevations on scales relating to physical symptoms, somatization, depression, and problems with thinking (i.e., Hs, D, Hy, and Sc scales; 83% to 87% of the sample had elevated scores on these scales). All 23 individuals had at least one elevated scale pre-injury, and 21 had two or more elevated scales pre-injury. Unexpectedly, when compared to their post-injury MMPI-2 profiles, their mean scores on the clinical scales pre-injury were actually *higher* than their mean scores post-injury. The highest mean scores post-injury were again the Hs, D, Hy, and Sc clinical scales (i.e., 74% to 100% of the sample with elevated scores on these scales). These findings suggest a very high prevalence of pre-injury psychopathology in this sample. However, the authors caution that there may have been a potential selection bias in this study towards sampling of patients (a) who were already abnormal, and (b) being worked up for past psychogenic contributions to medical complaints.

Although poorly understood, there is little doubt that personality characteristics influence the development and maintenance of the post-concussive disorder. These characteristics represent a large psychological component to the disorder. Other social-psychological factors, such as the nocebo effect, expectations, misattribution, the "good-old-days" bias, and diagnosis threat will be described in the next section.

Social-Psychological Factors

Without question, social-psychological factors can have an enormous impact on the development and maintenance of the post-concussive disorder. There have been a small number of fascinating studies in this area illustrating the importance of these factors.

Expectations and the Nocebo Effect. Approximately 15 years ago, Mittenberg and colleagues discussed "expectations" as a partial explanation to account for elevated symptom reporting in patients who sustained MTBIs (74). Symptom reporting was examined in 223 community volunteers and 100 patients referred for neuropsychological assessment following a brain injury. The injured patients were asked to report the presence or absence of current symptoms and symptoms pre-injury. Community volunteers reported current symptoms and the symptoms they would *expect* to experience after sustaining a brain injury. Two important results emerged: (a) the number of symptoms reported by patients post-injury was the same as the number of symptoms healthy controls would *expect* to experience after a brain injury, and (b) patients with brain injuries consistently *underestimated* the normal prevalence of PCS-like symptoms in their retrospective accounts (i.e., their pre-injury symptoms) compared with the base rate of PCS symptoms reported by normal controls (i.e., their current symptoms). To explain these findings, Mittenberg and colleagues proposed that for some people the presence of PCS symptoms following MTBI may be due to "the anticipation, widely held by individuals who have had no opportunity to observe or experience post-concussive symptoms, that PCS will occur following mild head injury" (p. 202). Following an injury, a patient may "reattribute benign emotional, physiological, and memory symptoms to their head injury" (p. 203) and disregard or inaccurately recall their pre-injury symptom experience. For example, an individual may attribute a headache post-accident to the injury rather than due to a stressful day at work (271). This explanation has been termed *expectation as etiology.* Other researchers have reported similar, although not identical, results (271, 272).

People might "expect" to experience certain symptoms and problems, and this expectation might partially underlie symptom reporting following an MTBI. However, Gunstad and Suhr (271) emphasized the importance of appreciating a more generalized expectation of negative outcome regardless of the event (e.g., accident, injury, illness, or disease), consistent with the "nocebo effect." The nocebo effect was introduced more than 40 years ago (273, 274) and research and discussion in this area has been ongoing (e.g., 275–281). The nocebo effect is the causation of sickness by the expectations of sickness and by associated emotional states. That is, the

sickness is, essentially, caused by expectation of sickness (282).

The nocebo effect in general, and expectations regarding symptoms and problems associated with MTBI in particular, likely represent significant psychological factors in the perception and reporting of symptoms in some patients. People's retrospective perception of their past functioning also can influence their perception of their current functioning. For example, a person might falsely perceive a bigger difference than is actually the case between their past and present functioning due to overestimating past abilities or under-estimating past problems. This has been termed the "good-old-days bias."

"Good-Old-Days" Bias. Researchers have reported that patients with back injuries, general trauma victims, as well as patients with head injury, overestimate the actual degree of change that has taken place post-injury by retrospectively recalling fewer pre-injury symptoms than the base rate of symptoms in controls (74, 271, 283–285). The *good-old-days* bias is a general response bias to view oneself as healthier in the past regardless of the presence or absence of brain injury and/or the experience of another negative event (e.g., an illness). The good-old-days bias seems to occur following a negative event (271, 284). As noted by Gunstad and Suhr (271), the "experience of any negative event, be it accident or illness, head injury or non-head-injury, may be required for one to focus on the past as 'better' than one's current state, for one to think about the 'good old days' prior to the negative event" (p. 330).

The tendency of people to recall past symptoms and functioning more favorably than is actually the case is further complicated by involvement in personal injury litigation. Researchers have reported that plaintiffs tend to exhibit a *response bias* in symptom recall compared to non-litigants. That is, personal injury claimants free from head trauma tend to report a lower pre-accident prevalence of cognitive, mental, and emotional symptoms in their daily lives compared to non-litigants (e.g., 286, 287). Specifically, in a preliminary study, Lees-Haley and colleagues reported that personal injury claimants reported "better" past levels of functioning in life in general, self-esteem, concentration, and memory than general medical patients who were asked to provide retrospective ratings. The personal injury litigants also reported less depression, anxiety, irritability, and fatigue (287). These findings were replicated in a large-scale, multi-site study (286). In addition, personal injury litigants rated their premorbid work or school status, marriage, and relationships with their children as better than controls. This response bias, combined with an expectation of certain symptoms following MTBI, can have a potent impact on symptom reporting.

Stereotype Threat and Diagnosis Threat. Psychological factors also are relevant to understanding neuropsychological test performance in people who are symptomatic long after an MTBI. For many years, researchers have been interested in the concept of *stereotype threat* to help explain performance differences between certain groups (e.g., 288–295). Research in this area is growing quickly (e.g., 296–301). The term *stereotype threat* was introduced by Steele (294) who defined this phenomenon as the "social-psychological threat that arises when one is in a situation or doing something for which a negative stereotype about one's group applies. This predicament threatens one with being negatively stereotyped, with being judged or treated stereotypically, or with the prospect of conforming to the stereotype" (294, p. 614).

Stereotype threat, as a theory and psychological factor, suggests that an individual's performance on a particular task can be negatively affected by the threat of an inferior and/or negative stereotype, such as men are superior to women in mathematics (288, 302). The adverse affect on performance is believed to be related to anxiety and/or a reduction of effort caused by the person's negative expectations (294, 303). Research has supported the influence of stereotype threat as a partial explanation for why (a) women perform more poorly than men on mathematics tests (293, 295, 298), (b) African Americans perform more poorly on selected items from the Graduate Record Examination than Caucasians (288), and (c) Caucasians perform more poorly than Asians on mathematics tests (289). Similarly, stereotype threat is also thought to partially explain (d) the presence of memory and cognitive decline in aging (291, 296, 297), and (e) differences in intellectual performance in students stereotyped as intellectually inferior versus superior (300).

Suhr and Gunstad (302, 304) have conducted two innovative studies relating to stereotype threat with university students who suffered past MTBIs. Suhr and Gunstad (304) hypothesized that in people with MTBI, "calling attention to a personal history of head injury and its potential effects on cognition might lead to worse cognitive performance than that seen in individuals with similar head injury history, but who do not have attention called to either the head injury history or the possible consequences of head injury" (p. 450). This hypothesis was called *diagnosis threat*. Suhr and Gunstad (304) examined the effect of diagnosis threat on cognitive performance in 36 undergraduate students with a self-reported history of MTBI. Participants were assigned either to a diagnosis threat condition or a neutral condition. All participants completed a brief neuropsychological test battery. Prior to participation, subjects in the diagnosis threat condition were provided with information highlighting their "diagnosis" of head injury and the expected cognitive deficits associated with head injury.

Participants in the diagnosis threat condition performed worse on measures of intellectual ability, immediate memory, and delayed memory, but not on measures of attention and psychomotor speed. Participants in the diagnosis threat condition rated themselves as putting forth less effort during testing, rated the tasks as more difficult, and felt they performed less well than participants in the neutral condition. In a follow-up replication study examining 53 undergraduate students with a history of self-reported MTBI, Suhr and Gunstad (302) reported that participants in the diagnosis threat condition performed worse on measures of memory, attention/working memory, and psychomotor speed. Contrary to the stereotype threat hypothesis however, differences in cognitive functioning between groups was not related to effort or anxiety.

The magnitude of the effect of diagnosis threat on neuropsychological test performance is not trivial. In fact, it's alarming. The results from the Suhr and Gunstad (302, 304) studies are presented with the results from several meta-analytic studies in Figure 23-1. Quite remarkably, the psychological effect of "diagnosis threat" has a large, adverse effect on neuropsychological test performance. Notice that the adverse effect of an MTBI on neuropsychological test performance, when measured beyond the acute recovery period, is very small and virtually undetectable in group studies. In contrast, the adverse effect of diagnosis threat, in university students, is comparable to the adverse effects of depression and litigation on neuropsychological test performance.

Litigation Stress, Exaggeration, and Malingering

Weissman (305) described aspects of litigation stress in the quote below. What is apparent from this quote is Weissman's belief that litigation produces negative effects on the plaintiff's mental state through multiple pathways, including greater susceptibility to stressors, attitude changes, motivational changes, and biases in self-reported problems.

> Involvement in litigation renders plaintiffs susceptible to stressors and to influences that may lead to increased impairment, biased reportage, and retarded recovery. Underlying personality patterns play a critical role in defining and shaping reactions to trauma, to the stress of litigation, and to treatment interventions. Protracted litigation creates conditions that promote mnemonic and attitudinal distortions, as well as conscious and unconscious motivations for secondary gain. (Ref. 305, p. 67).

Plaintiffs with acquired brain injuries or psychological problems find themselves in a very different health care environment compared to injured or emotionally distressed people not in litigation. For example, individuals other than the injured person have a vested interest in the assessment and rehabilitation of the plaintiff. As well, others have a vested interest in doubting the veracity of

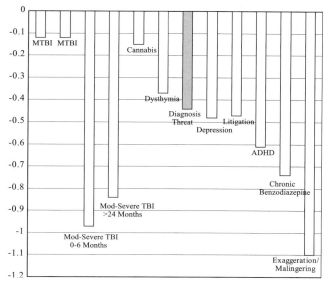

FIGURE 23-1

Effect sizes on overall neuropsychological functioning

Note: Effect sizes typically are expressed in pooled, weighted standard deviation units. However, across studies, there are some minor variations in the methods of calculation. By convention, effect sizes of .2 are considered small, .5 medium, and .8 large. This is from a statistical, not necessarily clinical, perspective. For this figure, the overall effect on cognitive or neuropsychological functioning is reported. The effect sizes are displayed in a negative direction to visually illustrate the "negative" or "adverse" effect on cognitive functioning. Effect sizes less than .3 should be considered very small and difficult to detect in individual patients because the patient and control groups largely overlap. First MTBI, moderate-severe TBI 0–6 months, >24 months, all in Schretlen & Shapiro (5), 39 studies, N = 1, 716 TBI, N = 1, 164 controls; second MTBI (338), 11 studies, N = 314 MTBI, N = 308 controls; Cannabis (339), long-term regular use, 11 studies, N = 623 users, N = 409 non or minimal users; Dysthymia, Depression, & Bipolar Disorder (340), 3 comparisons for dysthymia, 97 comparisons for depression, and 15 comparisons for bipolar disorder; Diagnosis Threat (302, 304), 2 studies, 23 comparisons; Litigation/financial incentives (55), 17 studies, N = 2, 353 total; ADHD (341), based on Full Scale IQ, 123 studies; Chronic benzodiazepine use (342), 13 studies, N = 384, 61 comparisons; Exaggeration/malingering (316), 32 studies published between 1985 and 1998, 41 independent comparisons

the patient's health problems. The effect of these vested interests can be seen in the skepticism frequently attached to diagnoses of post-concussive disorder, post-traumatic stress disorder, or major depression; outside the context of litigation, these diagnoses are accepted with less skepticism.

One result of these vested interests and skepticism is that plaintiffs with alleged post-concussive disorder or psychological problems will be subjected to more intensive, frequent, and possibly hostile assessment of their

health problems. Thus, an individual seeking relief for symptoms while in litigation will experience a very different health care environment than will the person seeking such relief outside the context of litigation. In fact, there might even be pressures to avoid effective treatments and remain off work in order to illustrate the damages resulting from the cause of action. Undoubtedly, protracted litigation can be very stressful, and a plaintiff who was once significantly injured but who has largely recovered might feel *entitled* to the compensation anticipated by his lawyer, thus feeling *justified* in his decision to grossly exaggerate his current disability.

Exaggeration and/or malingering is believed to be a serious problem in disability evaluations and personal injury litigation relating to MTBI and the post-concussive disorder (306, 307). Hundreds of studies and reviews relating to the detection of exaggerated symptoms, poor effort during neuropsychological testing, and malingering have been published in the past 15 years. It is virtually impossible for clinicians to keep up with the research in this area. Fortunately, there are many good reviews of this literature (e.g., 308–318). Specific guidelines and recommendations for identifying malingering in a neuropsychological evaluation have been available for several years (319), and have recently been published for pain-related disability evaluations (320).

Malingering is the intentional production of false or greatly exaggerated symptoms for the purpose of attaining some identifiable external reward (41). It is important, however, to differentiate malingering from symptom exaggeration (which as discussed below, may have many possible explanations), the latter being embellishment of a symptom or sign that has a true physiological or psychological basis. In the presence of litigation, an individual may exaggerate symptoms. The person might exaggerate memory problems, concentration difficulty, depression, anxiety, pain, dizziness, sleep disturbance, or personality change. During neuropsychological testing, a person who is malingering (or for that matter exaggerating) is more likely to deliberately under-perform by consciously making errors, by not putting forth full effort, and/or by amplifying/fabricating complaints.

Resnick (321) described three types of malingering, labeled "pure malingering," "partial malingering," and "false imputation." Pure malingering is characterized by a complete fabrication of symptoms. Partial malingering is defined by exaggerating actual symptoms or by reporting past symptoms as if they are continuing. False imputation refers to the deliberate misattribution of actual symptoms to the compensable event. Appreciating these types is important because mental health and legal professionals might have a simplistic view of malingering (i.e., only "pure malingering" is considered malingering).

Many lawyers and health care professionals adopt a rather extreme position regarding malingering. They assume that malingering represents total fabrication (fraud). An example would be the person who pretends to not be able to walk who is videotaped walking. Less blatant malingering is conceptualized differently, such as "exaggeration." Exaggeration is seen as common in personal injury litigation, and part of the function of the adversarial system is to illustrate to the trier of fact that exaggeration is present. Some professionals are tempted to believe that if a person has a well-documented psychiatric condition or visible brain damage on MRI that the person could not be malingering. However, it would be naïve to assume that a person with a psychiatric problem or the lingering effects of a traumatic brain injury could not malinger. That would be tantamount to concluding that people with these conditions are not capable of engaging in goal-directed behavior (e.g., exaggeration of symptoms to influence their litigation).

To conclude that a person might be malingering, the clinician must make an inference regarding a person's underlying motivation or reasons for providing poor effort during neuropsychological testing, exaggerating symptoms or problems, and/or fabricating symptoms and problems. As seen in Figure 23-2, there are many possible underlying motivations for exaggeration (singly or in combination). The "cry for help" euphemism implies that the person has serious psychological or psychiatric problems and is desperately seeking recognition of, and attention for, these problems. There is a long history of conceptualizing exaggeration as a cry for help in psychology and neuropsychology, whereas in psychiatry and general medicine clinicians are inclined to attribute exaggeration to "psychological factors," "psychiatric problems," or "non-organic factors." Second, in personal injury litigation, a person often feels angry about being injured and by perceived mistreatment from an insurance company. Some people feel justified in aggressively pursuing their litigation and feel entitled to generous compensation. Through a series of independent evaluations they might feel the need to exaggerate their symptoms or problems in order to be taken seriously, or to communicate how bad off they were in the past. There might be a number of secondary benefits relating to exaggerating one's problems, such as attention from family and friends, or avoidance of unpleasant activities. Third, some people with depression have an extremely negative view of themselves, the world, and their future. This negativistic thinking can manifest in exaggeration of symptoms and problems. Some people have a personality style that is prone to dramatizing and exaggerating their problems. Fourth, a person might deliberately exaggerate because he has a deep-seated psychological need to be perceived as sick and disabled. The motivation is not the litigation, per se, but to be seen and treated as a sick and disabled person. Under these circumstances, the person would be diagnosed with a factitious disorder. Finally, a person

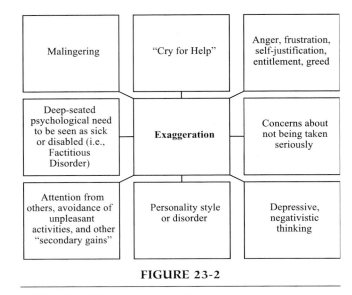

FIGURE 23-2

Possible reasons or motives for exaggeration

might deliberately exaggerate and/or under-perform during testing because he is trying to influence the outcome of his evaluations in order to influence the outcome of his litigation. This latter behavior is what we consider malingering.

In our experience, exaggeration is very common in people believed to have a persistent post-concussive disorder who are being evaluated in relation to a Worker's Compensation claim, disability evaluation, or personal injury litigation. Malingering is much less common than exaggeration, and it would be a mistake to assume, without careful deliberation, that the exaggeration reflects malingering.

CONCLUSIONS

There is no universally agreed upon etiology, pathophysiology, definition, or diagnostic criteria for the post-concussive disorder. Even the name of the syndrome/disorder varies in the literature (e.g., post-concussion syndrome, post-concussion disorder, and post-concussional disorder, to name a few). The disorder is assumed to be a direct and/or indirect consequence of an injury to the head or brain. However, a mild injury to the head or brain is not necessary (and often not sufficient) to produce the constellation of symptoms and problems that comprise this disorder. The symptoms and problems typically conceptualized as comprising the post-concussive disorder are non-specific; they can follow a mild injury to the brain or they can arise from other conditions, singly or in combination, such as chronic headaches, chronic bodily pain, depression, or post-traumatic stress disorder. These symptoms are also common in healthy, community-dwelling adults.

Following a mild traumatic brain injury, there is no doubt that most people experience a constellation of symptoms such as headaches, dizziness, fatigue, balance problems, sleep disturbance, difficulty thinking (e.g., concentration or memory), and/or emotional changes (e.g., irritability). These symptoms largely reflect the neurophysiology of concussion, which has been conceptualized as a multilayered neurometabolic cascade. The pathophysiology of this injury is largely reversible. However, under some circumstances people can have (a) macroscopic lesions, and/or (b) fairly widespread cellular damage or dysfunction (see the chapter by Iverson and colleagues in this book for a review).

Of course, not everyone experiences all symptoms, or symptoms to the same degree, but a core set of symptoms is commonly experienced. As a rule, these symptoms are at their worst in the first few days post-injury and they tend to get progressively better thereafter. This is illustrated in Figure 23-3. The data presented in Figure 23-3 represent a typical and common finding in the sport concussion literature and in clinical practice with concussed athletes. Athletes tend to report very high levels of symptoms and problems in the first few days post-injury, with relatively rapid resolution and recovery. Professional athletes seem to recover the fastest (322–325), followed by university athletes (30), and high school athletes (31, 326). This pattern reflects the reversible nature of the pathophysiology of mild concussions.

Trauma patients typically take longer to return to their baseline functioning. This is not surprising given that athletes tend to be young, healthy, highly motivated people with incentives to recover quickly and fully, and disincentives for having lingering problems. This creates a

very different psychological perspective on the injury. In contrast, trauma patients often are older, less healthy, and they get injured under unexpected circumstances such as motor vehicle accidents, assaults, or work-place accidents. MTBIs sustained under these circumstances can be psychologically traumatic, and they can also occur in tandem with other physical injuries. A trauma patient might have significant personality characteristics, life stressors or circumstances, and/or pre-existing mental health or medical problems that complicate the expected recovery from an MTBI. A person with poor coping skills and vulnerable personality characteristics who has co-occurring depression, chronic pain, PTSD, or a combination of problems is virtually guaranteed to endorse many "post-concussion-like" symptoms even if he or she has fully recovered from the injury. It is very easy to misdiagnose a person with a co-morbid condition as having a persistent post-concussive disorder (which carries the assumption of brain damage or dysfunction as the etiology of the symptoms).

Without a doubt, an MTBI is *not necessary* for producing the constellation of symptoms and problems that comprise the persistent post-concussive disorder. The disorder is not specific to an injury to the head, brain, or both. Therefore, this disorder should be considered a diagnosis of exclusion. The clinician should carefully study the history and progression of the symptoms and problems, and systematically attempt to rule out the most obvious differential diagnoses or competing explanations for the symptoms (see Table 23-5 and Figure 23-4). Once identified, the differential diagnosis should be treated.

In our view, it is very unlikely that the post-concussive disorder simply reflects a neurological problem arising from a mild traumatic brain injury. The *initial* pathophysiology is, without question, neurological. From the beginning, however, there is great variability in how people respond psychologically to being injured and to experiencing symptoms and problems. Injured adults are psychologically-susceptible to the nocebo effect (expecting a negative outcome following a negative event) and misattribution of symptoms, and health care providers can inadvertently reinforce these factors. Some people are very psychologically vulnerable to developing chronic problems following an injury to their head, brain, body, or "psyche," and the post-concussive disorder can be caused and maintained by factors that are entirely unrelated to permanent brain damage or dysfunction. In fact, in our view, the majority of people who appear to have the disorder (resulting from putative brain damage or dysfunction) actually have something else, such as depression or a combination of factors illustrated in Figure 23-4 (of course, a combination of factors might be the etiology for a post-concussive disorder).

People who sustain MTBIs characterized by structural damage on day-of-injury CT are, obviously, at

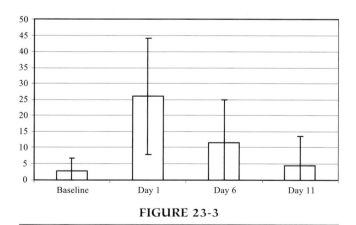

FIGURE 23-3

Total post-concussion symptom scores in concussed high school football players

Note: Total Post-Concussion Scale scores (mean and error lines equal one standard deviation) for 47 concussed high school football players tested preseason, within 4 days of injury (M = 1.7, SD = .9), within 8 days of injury (M = 5.5, SD = 1.4), and within 21 days of injury (M = 11.4, SD = 3.6)

TABLE 23-5
Normal and Unusual Outcomes from MTBI

2 WEEKS	2 WEEKS–3 MONTHS	3–6 MONTHS	6–12 MONTHS	1–3 YEARS
1. Recovery				
2. Symptoms/problems	Recovery			
3. Symptoms/problems	Partial recovery	Recovery		
4. Symptoms/problems	Partial recovery	Partial recovery	Recovery	
5. Symptoms/problems	Symptoms/problems	Partial recovery	Partial recovery	Recovery
6. Symptoms/problems	Symptoms/problems	Partial recovery	Partial recovery	Partial recovery
7. Symptoms/problems	Partial recovery	Worsening	Partial recovery	Recovery
8. Recovery	Worsening	Symptoms/problems	Partial recovery	Recovery
9. Symptoms/problems	Recovery	Worsening	Symptoms/problems	Symptoms/problems
10. Symptoms/problems	Symptoms/problems	Recovery	Worsening	Symptoms/problems
11. Symptoms/problems	Symptoms/problems	Recovery	Recovery	Symptoms/problems

Adapted with modifications from Iverson (4). The first four patterns represent the natural history of recovery from MTBI, in decreasing order of frequency. "Recovery" means few or no symptoms that are due to the biological effects of the original injury. The vast majority of concussed athletes and healthy adults with minor concussions in everyday life are represented by #1 (with very small numbers falling in patterns 2–11). The vast majority of trauma patients with *uncomplicated* MTBIs and no significant premorbid problems or comorbidities are represented by #1–3, with small numbers represented by pattern #4. The persistent post-concussive disorder is best illustrated by numbers 4–7 (psychological factors play a large role in maintaining symptom reporting). Numbers 8–11 represent patterns that frequently occur when a person is misdiagnosed with a persistent post-concussive disorder

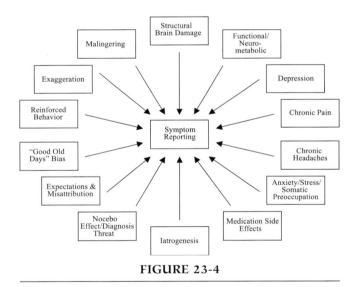

FIGURE 23-4

Possible factors influencing symptom reporting acutely, post-acutely, and long after a mild traumatic brain injury

increased risk for permanent brain damage (i.e., those with "complicated" MTBIs). However, most of these patients do not develop a persistent post-concussive disorder. When they do, it is likely that several factors depicted in Figure 23-4 are operative (including permanent brain damage). The antiquated notion of a binary distinction between "organic and psychological" contributes to the long-standing disagreements and polarized perspectives relating to the post-concussive disorder. As is increasingly being demonstrated in diverse fields of research, the "psychological" is often a link between biology and behavior. Do some people who appear to have the persistent post-concussive disorder have identifiable abnormalities on structural or functional neuroimaging? Of course they do. Does that mean that the abnormalities are the *predominant* underlying cause of the disorder? Of course not (but they might be major or minor contributors to the symptom presentation). Adopting a biopsychosocial perspective is the only reasonable way to have a comprehensive, unbiased understanding of this disorder.

In clinical and forensic practice, diagnosing someone with a persistent post-concussive disorder implies directly or indirectly that the person has "brain damage." This is a relief to a small number of patients seeking an explanation for their perceived problems. For many patients, however, it can have serious iatrogenic implications. The diagnosis can cause them to worry, dwell, and become focused on the belief that their brain is damaged. The diagnosis can be counter-therapeutic, reinforcing the misattribution of all symptoms to brain damage and leading to a sense of hopelessness regarding treatment and future improvement. According to the ICD-10 diagnostic criteria for the syndrome, one of the cardinal features is a preoccupation with symptoms and fear of brain damage with hypochondriacal concern and adoption of a sick role.

In our experience, the post-concussive disorder is over-diagnosed and frequently misdiagnosed. By over-diagnosed, we mean that there is often an assumption that a symptomatic person with a remote MTBI is suffering from brain damage that largely underlies the perceived and reported symptoms. This assumption of brain damage carries a very negative prognosis and tends to inhibit attempts at treatment. Although it might be true in some patients, for most people the original injury to the brain has *mostly* resolved and the disorder represents, in large part, an entrenched psychological disorder. By misdiagnosed, we mean that the person is actually suffering from something else, such as chronic pain, depression, or PTSD, which is misdiagnosed or co-diagnosed.

Of course, it is also possible that the diagnosis of post-concussive disorder can be missed. We have seen cases in the first three months post-injury where the treating clinician has diagnosed depression or PTSD when it seemed more likely that the patient was suffering from symptoms and problems arising predominately from the biological and psychological consequences of his or her MTBI.

So, what is the post-concussive disorder? The literature to date does not allow us to determine whether it is a single disorder, a spectrum disorder, or a group of disorders. The literature does not allow us to determine the degree to which abnormal brain physiology underlies some or all of the symptoms and problems associated with the disorder. There is no way to reliably differentiate the post-concussive disorder from depression, and it is possible that the disorder is a depression-spectrum disorder. In its "true" form, the post-concussive disorder arises as a direct *and* indirect consequence of mild injury to the brain (assuming it is not frankly misdiagnosed sometime long after an MTBI). When it manifests early and is maintained chronically the condition is almost always biopsychosocial. The "biological," the "psychological," and the "social" are all potentially treatable[7]. In our view, it is a mistake to conceptualize patients with the post-concussive disorder as if they are simply less "serious" versions of patients with severe traumatic brain injuries. These are distinct patient populations with distinct treatment and rehabilitation needs.

Ideally, clinicians and researchers should try to prevent the development of, or treat, the post-concussive disorder. There is evidence that early intervention, as simple as education and reassurance, is helpful for reducing the number and severity of symptoms experienced in the initial weeks and months post-injury (see the chapter by Iverson et al. for a review). This education, reassurance, and problem-solving should occur in the first two weeks post-injury.

When patients appear to have a *persistent* post-concussive disorder, differential treatment often flows from differential diagnosis. Given the clear overlap between the symptoms of depression and post-concussive disorder, some researchers have recommended treatment with anti-depressants (327–330) or cognitive behavior therapy (331, 332). Medications and psychotherapy would be an obvious choice, of course, if depression is simply mimicking the post-concussive disorder. Those recommending cognitive behavior therapy have set forth a treatment protocol that is based on those principles but is tailored toward the post-concussive disorder and belief systems relating to symptoms and brain damage.

We believe that the post-concussive disorder is *treatable* in the majority of patients. The first step is to identify whether a person really has it, or whether his or her symptoms and problems are more appropriately attributable to something else (thus, differential diagnosis leading to differential treatment). If the person is believed to be suffering from a post-concussive disorder, then general mental health and specific "symptomatic" treatment is indicated. Symptomatic treatment involves treating depression and anxiety, improving sleep, reducing stress, facilitating adaptive coping, helping the patient problem-solve life stressors, increasing exercise, and promoting a resumption to a more active and normal lifestyle.

Our research group (GLI) is in the process of piloting a new psychological treatment program for patients with persistent post-concussive disorder. This program arises from Contextual Behavior Therapy and Acceptance & Commitment Therapy (ACT; 333, 334). This approach has been successfully used with several clinical populations (e.g., depression, anxiety, stress, and substance abuse), as well as very difficult patients with chronic pain (335–337). Acceptance and Commitment Therapy is based on the idea that psychological suffering is usually caused by experiential avoidance, cognitive entanglement (i.e., "cognitive fusion"), and the resulting failure to take needed behavioral steps that are consistent with core values. This treatment approach takes the view that simply trying to change problematic thoughts and feelings as a means of coping might be relatively unhelpful. In contrast, powerful alternatives are available, including acceptance, mindfulness[8], cognitive defusion (learning to see thoughts as thoughts), value clarification, and committed values-based action. The treatment program includes components of traditional cognitive-behavioral therapy, and it includes psychoeducation

---

[7] Unfortunately, when treatment is offered it typically does not involve a broad-spectrum biopsychosocial approach, with an emphasis on identifying and addressing the diverse factors that underlie the ongoing symptoms and problems. Without this approach, the treatment is likely to be unsuccessful. Ineffective treatment contributes to the belief that the post-concussive disorder is "permanent."

[8] Mindfulness-based Cognitive Therapy, based largely on the work of Jon Kabat Zinn, includes simple breathing meditations and yoga stretches to help patients become more aware of the present moment, including getting in touch with moment-to-moment changes in the mind and the body. This therapy also includes basic education about depression, anxiety, and stress, and several exercises from cognitive therapy that show the links between thinking and feeling. The approach is closely linked to the Eastern insight meditation tradition that has been taught for two thousand years.

relating to the social-psychological factors that influence the perception and attribution of symptoms (e.g., nocebo effect, misattribution, and the "good-old-days" bias, as depicted in Figure 23-4).

To date, most attention in the literature has been devoted to describing characteristics or predictors of the post-concussive disorder, or debating its existence or etiology. It is our hope that researchers increasingly will turn their attention to treatment designed to reduce patient's suffering and improve their real-world functioning.

References

1. Belanger HG, Vanderploeg RD. The neuropsychological impact of sports-related concussion: A meta-analysis. *J Int Neuropsychol Soc* 2005;11:345–357.
2. Carroll LJ, Cassidy JD, Peloso PM, Borg J, von Holst H, Holm L, Paniak C, PÈpin M. Prognosis for mild traumatic brain injury: Results of the WHO collaborating centre task force on mild traumatic brain injury. *J Rehabil Med* 2004;36:84–105.
3. Belanger HG, Curtiss G, Demery JA, Lebowitz BK, Vanderploeg RD. Factors moderating neuropsychological outcomes following mild traumatic brain injury: a meta-analysis. *J Int Neuropsychol Soc* 2005;11:215–227.
4. Iverson GL. Outcome from mild traumatic brain injury. *Curr Opin Psychiat* 2005;18:301–317.
5. Schretlen DJ, Shapiro AM. A quantitative review of the effects of traumatic brain injury on cognitive functioning. *Int Rev Psychiatry* 2003;15:341–349.
6. Rees PM. Contemporary issues in mild traumatic brain injury. *Arch Phys Med Rehabil* 2003;84:1885–1894.
7. Ruff R. Two decades of advances in understanding of mild traumatic brain injury. *J Head Trauma Rehabil* 2005;20:5–18.
8. Ruff RM, Camenzuli L, Mueller J. Miserable minority: emotional risk factors that influence the outcome of a mild traumatic brain injury. *Brain Inj* 1996;10:551–565.
9. Binder LM. Persisting symptoms after mild head injury: a review of the post-concussive syndrome. *J Clin Exp Neuropsychol* 1986; 8:323–346.
10. Brown SJ, Fann JR, Grant I. Post-concussional disorder: time to acknowledge a common source of neurobehavioral morbidity. *J Neuropsychiatry Clin Neurosci* 1994;6:15–22.
11. Lishman WA. Physiogenisis and psychogenisis in the 'post-concussional syndrome'. *Br J Psychiatry* 1986;153:460–469.
12. Ryan LM, Warden DL. Post-concussion syndrome. *Int Rev Psychiatry* 2003;15:310–316.
13. Wood RL. Understanding the 'miserable minority': a diasthesis-stress paradigm for post-concussional syndrome. *Brain Inj* 2004;18: 1135–1153.
14. Youngjohn JR, Burrows L, Erdal K. Brain damage or compensation neurosis? The controversial post-concussion syndrome. *Clin Neuropsychol* 1995;9:112–123.
15. Moldover JE, Goldberg KB, Prout MF. Depression after traumatic brain injury: a review of evidence for clinical heterogeneity. *Neuropsychol Rev* 2004;14:143–154.
16. Asikainen I, Kaste M, Sarna S. Patients with traumatic brain injury referred to a rehabilitation and re-employment programme: social and professional outcome for 508 Finnish patients 5 or more years after injury. *Brain Inj* 1996;10:883–899.
17. Vanderploeg RD, Curtiss G, Duchnick JJ, Luis CA. Demographic, medical, and psychiatric factors in work and marital status after mild head injury. *J Head Trauma Rehabil* 2003;18:148–163.
18. Wrightson P, Gronwall D. Time off work and symptoms after minor head injury. *Injury* 1981;12:445–454.
19. Hughes DG, Jackson A, Mason DL, Berry E, Hollis S, Yates DW. Abnormalities on magnetic resonance imaging seen acutely following mild traumatic brain injury: correlation with neuropsychological tests and delayed recovery. *Neuroradiology* 2004;46: 550–558.
20. Kraus J, Schaffer K, Ayers K, Stenehjem J, Shen H, Afifi AA. Physical complaints, medical service use, and social and employment changes following mild traumatic brain injury: a 6-month longitudinal study. *J Head Trauma Rehabil* 2005;20:239–256.
21. McCullagh S, Oucherlony D, Protzner A, Blair N, Feinstein A. Prediction of neuropsychiatric outcome following mild trauma brain injury: an examination of the Glasgow Coma Scale. *Brain Inj* 2001;15:489–497.
22. Stranjalis G, Korfias S, Papapetrou C, Kouyialis A, Boviatsis E, Psachoulia C, Sakas DE. Elevated serum S-100B protein as a predictor of failure to short-term return to work or activities after mild head injury. *J Neurotrauma* 2004;21:1070–1075.
23. Dawson DR, Levine B, Schwartz ML, Stuss DT. Acute predictors of real-world outcomes following traumatic brain injury: a prospective study. *Brain Inj* 2004;18:221–238.
24. Dikmen SS, Temkin NR, Machamer JE, Holubkov AL, Fraser RT, Winn HR. Employment following traumatic head injuries. *Arch Neurol* 1994;51:177–186.
25. Drake AI, Gray N, Yoder S, Pramuka M, Llewellyn M. Factors predicting return to work following mild traumatic brain injury: a discriminant analysis. *J Head Trauma Rehabil* 2000;15: 1103–1112.
26. Edna TH, Cappelen J. Return to work and social adjustment after traumatic head injury. *Acta Neurochir (Wien)* 1987;85:40–43.
27. Friedland JF, Dawson DR. Function after motor vehicle accidents: a prospective study of mild head injury and post-traumatic stress. *J Nerv Ment Dis* 2001;189:426–434.
28. Haboubi NH, Long J, Koshy M, Ward AB. Short-term sequelae of minor head injury (6 years experience of minor head injury clinic). *Disabil Rehabil* 2001;23:635–638.
29. Rutherford WH, Merrett JD, McDonald JR. Symptoms at one year following concussion from minor head injuries. *Injury* 1979;10:225–230.
30. McCrea M, Guskiewicz KM, Marshall SW, Barr W, Randolph C, Cantu RC, Onate JA, Yang J, Kelly JP. Acute effects and recovery time following concussion in collegiate football players: the NCAA Concussion Study. *JAMA* 2003;290:2556–2563.
31. Collins MW, Lovell MR, Iverson GL, Ide T, Maroon J. Examining concussion rates and return to play in high school football players wearing newer helmet technology: a three year prospective cohort study. *Neurosurgery* in press.
32. Sosin DM, Sniezek JE, Thurman DJ. Incidence of mild and moderate brain injury in the United States, 1991. *Brain Inj* 1996;10:47–54.
33. McCullagh S, Feinstein A. Outcome after mild traumatic brain injury: an examination of recruitment bias. *J Neurol Neurosurg Psychiatry* 2003;74:39–43.
34. Alves W, Macciocchi SN, Barth JT. Post-concussive symptoms after uncomplicated mild head injury. *J Head Trauma Rehabil* 1993; 8:48–59.
35. de Kruijk JR, Leffers P, Meerhoff S, Rutten J, Twijnstra A. Effectiveness of bed rest after mild traumatic brain injury: a randomised trial of no versus six days of bed rest. *J Neurol Neurosurg Psychiatry* 2002;73:167–172.
36. Fee CR, Rutherford WH. A study of the effect of legal settlement on post-concussion symptoms. *Arch Emerg Med* 1988;5:12–17.
37. Stalnacke BM, Bjornstig U, Karlsson K, Sojka P. One-year follow-up of mild traumatic brain injury: post-concussion symptoms, disabilities and life satisfaction in relation to serum levels of S-100B and neurone-specific enolase in acute phase. *J Rehabil Med* 2005;37:300–305.
38. Mickeviciene D, Schrader H, Obelieniene D, Surkiene D, Kunickas R, Stovner LJ, Sand T. A controlled prospective inception cohort study on the post-concussion syndrome outside the medicolegal context. *Eur J Neurol* 2004;11:411–419.
39. Mittenberg W, Strauman S. Diagnosis of mild head injury and the post-concussion syndrome. *J Head Trauma Rehabil* 2000;15: 783–791.
40. World Health Organization. *International statistical classification of diseases and related health problems - 10th edition.* Geneva, Switzerland: World Health Organization, 1992.
41. American Psychiatric Association. *Diagnostic and Statistical Manual of Mental Disorders Fourth Edition.* Washington, DC: American Psychiatric Association, 1994.

42. Ruff RM, Grant I. Post-concussional disorder: Background to the DSM-IV and future considerations. In: Varney NR, Roberts RJ, editors. *The evaluation and treatment of mild traumatic brain injury.* Mahwah, NJ: Lawrence Erlbaum Associates, Inc., 1999. p 315–325.

43. American Psychiatric Association. *Diagnostic and Statistical Manual of Mental Disorders. Fourth Edition. Text Revision.* Washington, DC: American Psychiatric Association, 2000.

44. Ruff RM, Jurica P. In search of a unified definition for mild traumatic brain injury. *Brain Inj* 1999;13:943–952.

45. Sterr A, Herron K, Hayward C, Montaldi D. Are mild head injuries as mild as we think? Neurobehavioral concomitants of chronic post-concussion syndrome. *BMC Neurol* 2006;6:7.

46. McCauley SR, Boake C, Pedroza C, Brown SA, Levin HS, Goodman HS, Merritt SG. Post-concussional disorder: Are the DSM-IV criteria an improvement over the ICD-10? *J Nerv Ment Dis* 2005;193:540–550.

47. Boake C, McCauley SR, Levin HS, Contant CF, Song JX, Brown SA, Goodman HS, Brundage SI, Diaz-Marchan PJ, Merritt SG. Limited agreement between criteria-based diagnoses of post-concussional syndrome. *J Neuropsychiatry Clin Neurosci* 2004;16: 493–499.

48. Evered L, Ruff R, Baldo J, Isomura A. Emotional risk factors and post-concussional disorder. *Assessment* 2003;10:420–427.

49. Cook JB. The post-concussional syndrome and factors influencing recovery after minor head injury admitted to hospital. *Scand J Rehabil Med* 1972;4:27–30.

50. Satz PS, Alfano MS, Light RF, Morgenstern HF, Zaucha KF, Asarnow RF, Newton S. Persistent Post-Concussive Syndrome: A proposed methodology and literature review to determine the effects, if any, of mild head and other bodily injury. *J Clin Exp Neuropsychol* 1999;21:620–628.

51. Mickeviciene D, Schrader H, Nestvold K, Surkiene D, Kunickas R, Stovner LJ, Sand T. A controlled historical cohort study on the post-concussion syndrome. *Eur J Neurol* 2002;9:581–587.

52. Lees-Haley PR, Fox DD, Courtney JC. A comparison of complaints by mild brain injury claimants and other claimants describing subjective experiences immediately following their injury. *Arch Clin Neuropsychol* 2001;16:689–695.

53. Miller H. Accident neurosis. *Bmj* 1961;1:919–925 & 992–998.

54. Reynolds S, Paniak C, Toller-Lobe G, Nagy J. A longitudinal study of compensation-seeking and return to work in a treated mild traumatic brain injury sample. *J Head Trauma Rehabil* 2003;18: 139–147.

55. Binder LM, Rohling ML. Money matters: a meta-analytic review of the effects of financial incentives on recovery after closed-head injury. *Am J Psychiatry* 1996;153:7–10.

56. Paniak C, Reynolds S, Toller-Lobe G, Melnyk A, Nagy J, Schmidt D. A longitudinal study of the relationship between financial compensation and symptoms after treated mild traumatic brain injury. *J Clin Exp Neuropsychol* 2002;24:187–193.

57. Cicerone KD, Kalmar K. Persistent post-concussion syndrome: The structure of subjective complaints after mild traumatic brain injury. *J Head Trauma Rehabil* 1995;10:1–7.

58. Heilbronner RL. Factors associated with post-concussion syndrome: Neurological, psychological, or legal? *Trial Diplomacy J* 1993;16:161–167.

59. Larrabee GJ. Neuropsychological outcome, post-concussion symptoms, and forensic considerations in mild closed head trauma. *Semin Clin Neuropsychiatry* 1997;2:196–206.

60. Bijur PE, Haslum M, Golding J. Cognitive and behavioral sequelae of mild head injury in children. *Pediatrics* 1990;86:337–344.

61. Ruff RM, Richardson AM. Mild traumatic brian injury. In: Sweet JJ, editor. *Forensic neuropsychology: Fundamentals and practice. Studies on neuropsychology, development, and cognition.* Bristol, PA: Swets & Zeitlinger, 1999. p 315–338.

62. Gouvier WD, Uddo-Crane M, Brown LM. Base rates of post-concussional symptoms. *Arch Clin Neuropsychol* 1988;3:273–278.

63. Fox DD, Lees-Haley PR, Ernest K, Dolezal-Wood S. Post-concussive symptoms: Base rates and etiology in psychiatric patients. *Clin Neuropsychol* 1995;9:89–92.

64. Lees-Haley PR, Brown RS. Neuropsychological complain base rates of 170 personal injury claimants. *Arch Clin Neuropsychol* 1993;8:203–209.

65. Dunn JT, Lees-Haley PR, Brown RS, Williams CW, English LT. Neurotoxic complaint base rates of personal injury claimants: implications for neuropsychological assessment. *J Clin Psychol* 1995;51:577–584.

66. Foa EB, Cashman L, Jaycox L, Perry K. The validation of a self-report measure of post-traumatic stress disorder: The Post-traumatic Diagnostic Scale. *Psychol Assess* 1997;9:445–451.

67. Gasquoine PG. Post-concussional symptoms in chronic back pain. *Appl Neuropsychol* 2000;7:83–89.

68. Iverson GL, McCracken LM. 'Post-concussive' symptoms in persons with chronic pain. *Brain Inj* 1997;11:783–790.

69. Radanov BP, Dvorak J, Valach L. Cognitive deficits in patients after soft tissue injury of the cervical spine. *Spine* 1992;17:127–131.

70. Smith-Seemiller L, Fow NR, Kant R, Franzen MD. Presence of post-concussion syndrome symptoms in patients with chronic pain vs mild traumatic brain injury. *Brain Inj* 2003;17:199–206.

71. Sullivan MJ, Hall E, Bartolacci R, Sullivan ME, Adams H. Perceived cognitive deficits, emotional distress and disability following whiplash injury. *Pain Res Manag* 2002;7:120–126.

72. Machulda MM, Bergquist TF, Ito V, Chew S. Relationship between stress, coping, and post-concussion symptoms in a healthy adult population. *Arch Clin Neuropsychol* 1998;13:415–424.

73. Iverson GL, Lange RT. Examination of "Post-concussion-Like" symptoms in a healthy sample. *Appl Neuropsychol* 2003;10: 137–144.

74. Mittenberg W, DiGiulio DV, Perrin S, Bass AE. Symptoms following mild head injury: Expectation as aetiology. *J Neurol Neurosurg Psychiatry* 1992;55:200–204.

75. Trahan DE, Ross CE, Trahan SL. Relationships among postconcussional-type symptoms, depression, and anxiety in neurologically normal young adults and victims of brain injury. *Arch Clin Neuropsychol* 2001;16:435–445.

76. Sawchyn JM, Brulot MM, Strauss E. Note on the use of the Post-concussion Syndrome Checklist. *Arch Clin Neuropsychol* 2000;15:1–8.

77. Wong JL, Regennitter RP, Barrios F. Base rate and simulated symptoms of mild head injury among normals. *Arch Clin Neuropsychol* 1994;9:411–425.

78. Iverson GL, Gaetz M. Practical considerations for interpreting change following concussion. In: Lovell MR, Echemendia RJ, Barth J, Collins MW, editors. *Traumatic brain injury in sports: An international neuropsychological perspective.* Netherlands: Swets-Zeitlinger, 2004. p 323–356.

79. Iverson GL. Misdiagnosis of persistent post-concussion syndrome in patients with depression. *Arch Clin Neuropsychol* in press.

80. First MB, Spitzer RL, Gibbon M, Williams JBW. *Structured Clinical Interview for the DSM-IV Axis I Disorders - Non-Patient Edition (SCID-I/NP, Version 2.0 - 8/98 revision).* New York: Biometrics Research Department, New York State Psychiatric Institute, 1998.

81. Wolfe F, Smythe HA, Yunus MB, Bennett RM, Bombardier C, Goldenberg DL, Tugwell P, Campbell SM, Abeles M, Clark P. The American College of Rheumatology 1990 Criteria for the Classification of Fibromyalgia. Report of the Multicenter Criteria Committee. *Arthritis Rheum* 1990;33:160–172.

82. Pearce JM. Whiplash injury: a reappraisal. *J Neurol Neurosurg Psychiatry* 1989;52:1329–1331.

83. Teifke A, Degreif J, Geist M, Schild H, Strunk H, Schunk K. [The safety belt: effects on injury patterns of automobile passengers]. *Rofo* 1993;159:278–283.

84. Barnsley L, Lord S, Bogduk N. The pathophysiology of whiplash. In: Shapiro AP, editor. *Spine: State of the art reviews: Cervical flexion-extension/whiplash injuries.* Volume 7(3). Philadelphia: Hanley & Belfus, 1993. p 329–353.

85. Tollison CD, Satterthwaite, editors. Painful cervical trauma: *Diagnosis and rehabilitative treatment of neuromusculoskeletal injuries.* Baltimore: Williams & Wilkins, 1992.

86. Balla JI. Headache and cervical disorders: Report to the motor accidents board of Victoria on whiplash injuries. In: Hopkins A, editor. *Headache, problems in diagnosis and management.* London: Saunders, 1984. p 256–269.

87. Hildingsson C, Toolanen G. Outcome after soft-tissue injury of the cervical spine. A prospective study of 93 car-accident victims. *Acta Orthop Scand* 1990;61:357–359.

88. Croft AC. Soft tissue injuries: Long- and short-term effects. In: Foreman SM, Croft AC, editors. *Whiplash injuries: The cervical acceleration/deceleration syndrome, 3rd Ed.* Philidelphia, PA: Lippincott Williams & Wilkins, 2002. p 335–428.

89. Burke JP, Orton HP, West J, Strachan IM, Hockey MS, Ferguson DG. Whiplash and its effect on the visual system. *Graefes Arch Clin Exp Ophthalmol* 1992;230:335–339.

90. Brown S. Effect of whiplash injury on accommodation. *Clin Experiment Ophthalmol* 2003;31:424–429.

91. Mosimann UP, Muri RM, Felblinger J, Radanov BP. Saccadic eye movement disturbances in whiplash patients with persistent complaints. *Brain* 2000;123 (Pt 4):828–835.

92. Reicke N. Der vertebrogene schwindel. Aetiologie und differntialdiagnose. *Fortschr Med* 1978;96:1895–1902.

93. Hinoki M. Otoneurological observations on whiplash injuries to neck with special reference to the formation of equilibrial disorder. *Clinical Surgery (Toyko)* 1967;22:1683–1690.

94. Hinoki M. Vertigo due to whiplash injury: A Neurotological approach. *Acta Otolaryngologia (Stockh)* 1985;419 (Suppl.):9–29.

95. Sandstrom J. Cervical syndrome with vestibular symptoms. *Acta Otolaryngol* 1962;54:207–226.

96. Endo K, Ichimaru K, Komagata M, Yamamoto K. Cervical vertigo and dizziness after whiplash injury. *Eur Spine J* 2006.

97. Marzo SJ, Leonetti JP, Raffin MJ, Letarte P. Diagnosis and management of post-traumatic vertigo. *Laryngoscope* 2004;114:1720–1723.

98. Zasler ND. Neuromedical diagnosis and management of postconcussive disorders. In: Horn L, Zasler ND, editors. *Medical rehabilitation of traumatic brain injury*. Philadelphia, PA: Hanley & Belfus, Inc., 1996. p 133–170.

99. Ernst A, Basta D, Seidl RO, Todt I, Scherer H, Clarke A. Management of post-traumatic vertigo. *Otolaryngol Head Neck Surg* 2005;132:554–558.

100. Stapley PJ, Beretta MV, Toffola ED, Schieppati M. Neck muscle fatigue and postural control in patients with whiplash injury. *Clin Neurophysiol* 2006.

101. Madeleine P, Prietzel H, Svarrer H, Arendt-Nielsen L. Quantitative posturography in altered sensory conditions: a way to assess balance instability in patients with chronic whiplash injury. *Arch Phys Med Rehabil* 2004;85:432–438.

102. Gosselin G, Rassoulian H, Brown I. Effects of neck extensor muscles fatigue on balance. *Clin Biomech (Bristol, Avon)* 2004; 19: 473–479.

103. Treleaven J, Jull G, Lowchoy N. The relationship of cervical joint position error to balance and eye movement disturbances in persistent whiplash. *Man Ther* 2005.

104. Treleaven J, Jull G, Lowchoy N. Standing balance in persistent whiplash: a comparison between subjects with and without dizziness. *J Rehabil Med* 2005;37:224–229.

105. Tjell C, Tenenbaum A, Rosenhall U. Auditory function in whiplash-associated disorders. *Scand Audiol* 1999;28:203–209.

106. Claussen CF, Claussen E. Neurootological contributions to the diagnostic follow-up after whiplash injuries. *Acta Otolaryngol Suppl* 1995;520 Pt 1:53–56.

107. Levine RA. Somatic (craniocervical) tinnitus and the dorsal cochlear nucleus hypothesis. *Am J Otolaryngol* 1999;20:351–362.

108. Kaute BB. The Influence of Atlas Therapy on Tinnitus. *Int Tinnitus J* 1998;4:165–167.

109. Boniver R. Temporomandibular joint dysfunction in whiplash injuries: association with tinnitus and vertigo. *Int Tinnitus J* 2002;8:129–131.

110. Kischka U, Ettlin T, Heim S, Schmid G. Cerebral symptoms following whiplash injury. *Eur Neurol* 1991;31:136–140.

111. Ettlin TM, Kischka U, Reichmann S, Radii EW, Heim S, Wengen D, Benson DF. Cerebral symptoms after whiplash injury of the neck: a prospective clinical and neuropsychological study of whiplash injury. *J Neurol Neurosurg Psychiatry* 1992;55:943–948.

112. Radanov BP, Sturzenegger M, De Stefano G, Schnidrig A. Relationship between early somatic, radiological, cognitive and psychosocial findings and outcome during a one-year follow-up in 117 patients suffering from common whiplash. *Br J Rheumatol* 1994;33:442–448.

113. Kessels RP, Aleman A, Verhagen WI, van Luijtelaar EL. Cognitive functioning after whiplash injury: a meta-analysis. *J Int Neuropsychol Soc* 2000;6:271–278.

114. Guez M, Brannstrom R, Nyberg L, Toolanen G, Hildingsson C. Neuropsychological functioning and MMPI-2 profiles in chronic neck pain: a comparison of whiplash and non-traumatic groups. *J Clin Exp Neuropsychol* 2005;27:151–163.

115. Antepohl W, Kiviloog L, Andersson J, Gerdle B. Cognitive impairment in patients with chronic whiplash-associated disorder—a matched control study. *NeuroRehabilitation* 2003;18:307–315.

116. Teasell RW, Shapiro AP, editors. *Spine: State of the art reviews: Cervical flexion-extension/whiplash injuries*. Volume 7(3). Philadelphia: Hanley & Belfus, 1993.

117. Knibestol M, Hildingsson C, Toolanen G. Trigeminal sensory impairment after soft-tissue injury of the cervical spine. A quantitative evaluation of cutaneous thresholds for vibration and temperature. *Acta Neurol Scand* 1990;82:271–276.

118. Herren-Gerber R, Weiss S, Arendt-Nielsen L, Petersen-Felix S, Di Stefano G, Radanov BP, Curatolo M. Modulation of central hypersensitivity by nociceptive input in chronic pain after whiplash injury. *Pain Med* 2004;5:366–376.

119. Dwyer A, Aprill C, Bogduk N. Cervical zygapophyseal joint pain patterns. I: A study in normal volunteers. *Spine* 1990;15:453–457.

120. Malanga G, Peter J. Whiplash injuries. *Curr Pain Headache Rep* 2005;9:322–325.

121. Jensen S. Neck related causes of headache. *Aust Fam Physician* 2005;34:635–639.

122. Browning GG, Swan IR, Gatehouse S. Hearing loss in minor head injury. *Arch Otolaryngol* 1982;108:474–477.

123. Healy GB. Hearing loss and vertigo secondary to head injury. *N Engl J Med* 1982;306:1029–1031.

124. Williams GH, Giordano AM. Temporal bone trauma. In: Gudeman SK, editor. *Textbook of head injury*. Philadelphia: W. B. Saunders, 1989. p 367–377.

125. Lyos AT, Marsh MA, Jenkins HA, Coker NJ. Progressive hearing loss after transverse temporal bone fracture. *Arch Otolaryngol Head Neck Surg* 1995;121:795–799.

126. Rubin W. How do we use state of the art vestibular testing to diagnose and treat the dizzy patient? An overview of vestibular testing and balance system integration. *Neurol Clin* 1990;8: 225–234.

127. Zasler ND, Ochs AL. Oculovestibular dysfunction in symptomatic mild traumatic brain injury. *Archives of Physical Medicine and Rehabilitation* 1992;73:963.

128. Brandt T, Daroff RB. Physical therapy for benign paroxysmal positional vertigo. *Arch Otolaryngol* 1980;106:484–485.

129. Shepard NT, Telian SA, Smith-Wheelock M. Habituation and balance retraining therapy. A retrospective review. *Neurol Clin* 1990;8:459–475.

130. Shumway-Cook A, Horak FB. Rehabilitation strategies for patients with vestibular deficits. *Neurol Clin* 1990;8:441–457.

131. Badke MB, Shea TA, Miedaner JA, Grove CR. Outcomes after rehabilitation for adults with balance dysfunction. *Arch Phys Med Rehabil* 2004;85:227–233.

132. Cohen HS. Disability and rehabilitation in the dizzy patient. *Curr Opin Neurol* 2006;19:49–54.

133. Shepard NT, Telian SA. Programmatic vestibular rehabilitation. *Otolaryngol Head Neck Surg* 1995;112:173–182.

134. Gacek RR. Further observations on posterior ampullary nerve transection for positional vertigo. *Ann Otol Rhinol Laryngol* 1978;87:300–305.

135. Brandt T. *Vertigo: Its multisensory syndromes*. New York: Springer-verlag, 1991.

136. Kim HH, Wiet RJ, Battista RA. Trends in the diagnosis and the management of Meniere's disease: results of a survey. *Otolaryngol Head Neck Surg* 2005;132:722–726.

137. Gates GA. Treatment of Meniere's disease with the low-pressure pulse generator (Meniett device). *Expert Rev Med Devices* 2005;2:533–537.

138. Van de Heyning PH, Wuyts F, Boudewyns A. Surgical treatment of Meniere's disease. *Curr Opin Neurol* 2005;18:23–28.

139. Maitland CG. Perilymphatic fistula. *Curr Neurol Neurosci Rep* 2001;1:486–491.

140. Black FO, Lilly DJ, Peterka RJ, Shupert C, Hemenway WG, Pesznecker SC. The dynamic posturographic pressure test for the presumptive diagnosis of perilymph fistulas. *Neurol Clin* 1990;8: 361–374.

141. Bourgeois B, Ferron C, Bordure P, Beauvillain de Montreuil C, Legent F. [Exploratory tympanotomy for suspected traumatic perilymphatic fistula]. *Ann Otolaryngol Chir Cervicofac* 2005; 122:181–186.

142. Grimm RJ, Hemenway WG, Lebray PR, Black FO. The perilymph fistula syndrome defined in mild head trauma. *Acta Otolaryngol Suppl* 1989;464:1–40.

143. Legent F, Bordure P. [Post-traumatic perilymphatic fistulas]. *Bull Acad Natl Med* 1994;178:35–44; discussion 44–35.

144. Black FO, Lilly DJ, Nashner LM, Peterka RJ, Pesznecker SC. Quantitative diagnostic test for perilymph fistulas. *Otolaryngol Head Neck Surg* 1987;96:125–134.

145. Herdman S. Personal communication. 1991.

146. Baloh RW, Honrubia V. *Clinical neurophysiology of the vestibular system.* Philadelphia: F.A. Davis Company, 1990.

147. Michel O, Petereit H, Klemm E, Walther LE, Bachmann-Harildstad G. First clinical experience with beta-trace protein (prostaglandin D synthase) as a marker for perilymphatic fistula. *J Laryngol Otol* 2005;119:765–769.

148. Bluestone CD. Implications of beta-2 transferrin assay as a marker for perilymphatic versus cerebrospinal fluid labyrinthine fistula. *Am J Otol* 1999;20:701.

149. Jastreboff PJ, Jastreboff MM. Tinnitus retraining therapy for patients with tinnitus and decreased sound tolerance. *Otolaryngol Clin North Am* 2003;36:321–336.

150. Smith PF, Darlington CL. Drug treatments for subjective tinnitus: serendipitous discovery versus rational drug design. *Curr Opin Investig Drugs* 2005;6:712–716.

151. Marion MS, Cevette MJ. Tinnitus. *Mayo Clin Proc* 1991;66: 614–620.

152. Green P, Rohling ML, Iverson GL, Gervais RO. Relationships between olfactory discrimination and head injury severity. *Brain Inj* 2003;17:479–496.

153. Costanzo RM, Zasler ND. Epidemiology and pathophysiology of olfactory and gustatory dysfunction in head trauma. *Journal of Head Trauma Rehabilitation* 1992;7:15–24.

154. Zasler ND, McNeny MR, Heywood PG. Rehabilitative management of olfactory and gustatory dysfunction following brain injury. *Journal of Head Trauma Rehabilitation* 1992; 7:66–75.

155. Daily L. Whiplash injury as one cause of the foveolar splinter and macular wisps. *Arch Ophthalmol* 1979;97:360.

156. Cytowic R, Stump DA, Larned DC. Closed head trauma: Cognitive, somatic and ophthalmic sequelae in nonhospitalized patients. In: Whitaker HA, editor. *Neuropsychological studies of nonfocal brain damage.* New York: Springer-Verlag, 1988. p 226–264.

157. Carter JE, McCormick AQ. Whiplash shaking syndrome: retinal hemorrhages and computerized axial tomography of the brain. *Child Abuse Negl* 1983;7:279–286.

158. Kowal L. Ophthalmic manifestations of head injury. *Aust N Z J Ophthalmol* 1992;20:35–40.

159. al-Qurainy IA. Convergence insufficiency and failure of accommodation following midfacial trauma. *Br J Oral Maxillofac Surg* 1995;33:71–75.

160. Rasmussen BK. Epidemiology of headache. *Cephalalgia* 2001;21:774–777.

161. Rasmussen BK, Jensen R, Schroll M, Olesen J. Epidemiology of headache in a general population—a prevalence study. *J Clin Epidemiol* 1991;44:1147–1157.

162. Pine DS, Cohen P, Brook J. The association between major depression and headache: results of a longitudinal epidemiologic study in youth. *J Child Adolesc Psychopharmacol* 1996;6:153–164.

163. Mitsikostas DD, Thomas AM. Comorbidity of headache and depressive disorders. *Cephalalgia* 1999;19:211–217.

164. Zwart JA, Dyb G, Hagen K, Odegard KJ, Dahl AA, Bovim G, Stovner LJ. Depression and anxiety disorders associated with headache frequency. The Nord-Trondelag Health Study. *Eur J Neurol* 2003;10:147–152.

165. Breslau N, Lipton RB, Stewart WF, Schultz LR, Welch KM. Comorbidity of migraine and depression: investigating potential etiology and prognosis. *Neurology* 2003;60:1308–1312.

166. Magnusson JE, Becker WJ. Migraine frequency and intensity: relationship with disability and psychological factors. *Headache* 2003;43:1049–1059.

167. Wacogne C, Lacoste JP, Guillibert E, Hugues FC, Le Jeunne C. Stress, anxiety, depression and migraine. *Cephalalgia* 2003;23: 451–455.

168. Kowacs F, Socal MP, Ziomkowski SC, Borges-Neto VF, Toniolo DP, Francesconi CR, Chaves ML. Symptoms of depression and anxiety, and screening for mental disorders in migrainous patients. *Cephalalgia* 2003;23:79–89.

169. Venable VL, Carlson CR, Wilson J. The role of anger and depression in recurrent headache. *Headache* 2001;41:21–30.

170. Lipton RB, Hamelsky SW, Kolodner KB, Steiner TJ, Stewart WF. Migraine, quality of life, and depression: a population-based case-control study. *Neurology* 2000;55:629–635.

171. Holroyd KA, Stensland M, Lipchik GL, Hill KR, O'Donnell FS, Cordingley G. Psychosocial correlates and impact of chronic tension-type headaches. *Headache* 2000;40:3–16.

172. Castillo J, Munoz P, Guitera V, Pascual J. Epidemiology of chronic daily headache in the general population. *Headache* 1999;39:190–196.

173. Scher AI, Stewart WF, Liberman J, Lipton RB. Prevalence of frequent headache in a population sample. *Headache* 1998;38: 497–506.

174. Edmeads J. Analgesic-induced headaches: an unrecognized epidemic. *Headache* 1990;30:614–615.

175. Mathew NT. Transformed migraine, analgesic rebound, and other chronic daily headaches. *Neurol Clin* 1997;15:167–186.

176. Kudrow L. Paradoxical effects of frequent analgesic use. *Adv Neurol* 1982;33:335–341.

177. Warner JS. The outcome of treating patients with suspected rebound headache. *Headache* 2001;41:685–692.

178. Limmroth V, Katsarava Z, Fritsche G, Przywara S, Diener HC. Features of medication overuse headache following overuse of different acute headache drugs. *Neurology* 2002;59:1011–1014.

179. Mathew NT, Kurman R, Perez F. Drug induced refractory headache—clinical features and management. *Headache* 1990;30:634–638.

180. Li D, Rozen TD. The clinical characteristics of new daily persistent headache. *Cephalalgia* 2002;22:66–69.

181. Boardman HF, Thomas E, Millson DS, Croft PR. Psychological, sleep, lifestyle, and comorbid associations with headache. *Headache* 2005;45:657–669.

182. Parmelee PA, Smith B, Katz IR. Pain complaints and cognitive status among elderly institution residents. *J Am Geriatr Soc* 1993; 41:517–522.

183. Haldorsen T, Waterloo K, Dahl A, Mellgren SI, Davidsen PE, Molin PK. Symptoms and cognitive dysfunction in patients with the late whiplash syndrome. *Appl Neuropsychol* 2003;10: 170–175.

184. Jamison RN, Sbrocco T, Parris WC. The influence of problems with concentration and memory on emotional distress and daily activities in chronic pain patients. *Int J Psychiatry Med* 1988;18:183–191.

185. McCracken LM, Iverson GL. Predicting complaints of impaired cognitive functioning in patients with chronic pain. *Journal of Pain and Symptom Management* 2001;21:392–396.

186. Munoz M, Esteve R. Reports of memory functioning by patients with chronic pain. *Clin J Pain* 2005;21:287–291.

187. Roth RS, Geisser ME, Theisen-Goodvich M, Dixon PJ. Cognitive complaints are associated with depression, fatigue, female sex, and pain catastrophizing in patients with chronic pain. *Arch Phys Med Rehabil* 2005;86:1147–1154.

188. Schnurr RF, MacDonald MR. Memory complaints in chronic pain. *Clinical Journal of Pain* 1995;11:103–111.

189. Iverson GL, King RJ, Scott JG, Adams RL. Cognitive complaints in litigating patients with head injuries or chronic pain. *J Forensic Neuropsychol* 2001;2:19–30.

190. Uomoto JM, Esselman PC. Traumatic brain injury and chronic pain: differential types and rates by head injury severity. *Arch Phys Med Rehabil* 1993;74:61–64.

191. Atkinson JH, Slater MA, Patterson TL, Grant I, Garfin SR. Prevalence, onset, and risk of psychiatric disorders in men with chronic low back pain: a controlled study. *Pain* 1991;45:111–121.

192. Fishbain DA, Cutler R, Rosomoff HL, Rosomoff RS. Chronic pain-associated depression: antecedent or consequence of chronic pain? A review. *Clin J Pain* 1997;13:116–137.

193. Wilson KG, Eriksson MY, D'Eon JL, Mikail SF, Emery PC. Major depression and insomnia in chronic pain. *Clin J Pain* 2002;18:77–83.

194. Campbell LC, Clauw DJ, Keefe FJ. Persistent pain and depression: a biopsychosocial perspective. *Biol Psychiatry* 2003;54:399–409.

195. McWilliams LA, Cox BJ, Enns MW. Mood and anxiety disorders associated with chronic pain: an examination in a nationally representative sample. *Pain* 2003;106:127–133.

196. Kreutzer JS, Seel RT, Gourley E. The prevalence and symptom rates of depression after traumatic brain injury: a comprehensive examination. *Brain Inj* 2001;15:563–576.

197. Seel RT, Kreutzer JS, Rosenthal M, Hammond FM, Corrigan JD, Black K. Depression after traumatic brain injury: a National Institute on Disability and Rehabilitation Research Model Systems multicenter investigation. *Arch Phys Med Rehabil* 2003;84:177–184.

198. Ericsson M, Poston WS, Linder J, Taylor JE, Haddock CK, Foreyt JP. Depression predicts disability in long-term chronic pain patients. *Disabil Rehabil* 2002;24:334–340.

199. Levin HS, Brown SA, Song JX, McCauley SR, Boake C, Contant CF, Goodman H, Kotrla KJ. Depression and post-traumatic stress disorder at three months after mild to moderate traumatic brain injury. *J Clin Exp Neuropsychol* 2001;23:754–769.

200. Hung CI, Liu CY, Fuh JL, Juang YY, Wang SJ. Comorbid migraine is associated with a negative impact on quality of life in patients with major depression. *Cephalalgia* 2006;26:26–32.

201. Breslau N, Schultz LR, Stewart WF, Lipton RB, Lucia VC, Welch KM. Headache and major depression: is the association specific to migraine? *Neurology* 2000;54:308–313.

202. Sheftell FD, Atlas SJ. Migraine and psychiatric comorbidity: from theory and hypotheses to clinical application. *Headache* 2002;42:934–944.

203. Franklin CL, Zimmerman M. Post-traumatic stress disorder and major depressive disorder: investigating the role of overlapping symptoms in diagnostic comorbidity. *J Nerv Ment Dis* 2001;189:548–551.

204. Kessler RC, Sonnega A, Bromet E, Hughes M, Nelson CB. Post-traumatic stress disorder in the National Comorbidity Survey. *Arch Gen Psychiatry* 1995;52:1048–1060.

205. Shalev AY, Freedman S, Peri T, Brandes D, Sahar T, Orr SP, Pitman RK. Prospective study of post-traumatic stress disorder and depression following trauma. *Am J Psychiatry* 1998;155:630–637.

206. Nunes EV, Levin FR. Treatment of depression in patients with alcohol or other drug dependence: a meta-analysis. *JAMA* 2004;291:1887–1896.

207. Grothues J, Bischof G, Reinhardt S, Hapke U, Meyer C, John U, Rumpf HJ. Intention to change drinking behaviour in general practice patients with problematic drinking and comorbid depression or anxiety. *Alcohol Alcohol* 2005;40:394–400.

208. Frisher M, Crome I, Macleod J, Millson D, Croft P. Substance misuse and psychiatric illness: prospective observational study using the general practice research database. *J Epidemiol Community Health* 2005;59:847–850.

209. Grant BF, Stinson FS, Dawson DA, Chou SP, Dufour MC, Compton W, Pickering RP, Kaplan K. Prevalence and co-occurrence of substance use disorders and independent mood and anxiety disorders: results from the National Epidemiologic Survey on Alcohol and Related Conditions. *Arch Gen Psychiatry* 2004;61:807–816.

210. Brady KT, Verduin ML. Pharmacotherapy of comorbid mood, anxiety, and substance use disorders. *Subst Use Misuse* 2005;40:2021–2041, 2043–2028.

211. Pettit JW, Lewinsohn PM, Joiner TE, Jr. Propagation of major depressive disorder: Relationship between first episode symptoms and recurrence. *Psychiatry Res* 2006.

212. Mulder RT, Joyce PR, Frampton CM, Luty SE, Sullivan PF. Six months of treatment for depression: outcome and predictors of the course of illness. *Am J Psychiatry* 2006;163:95–100.

213. Bockting CL, Schene AH, Spinhoven P, Koeter MW, Wouters LF, Huyser J, Kamphuis JH. Preventing relapse/recurrence in recurrent depression with cognitive therapy: a randomized controlled trial. *J Consult Clin Psychol* 2005;73:647–657.

214. Keller MB, Lavori PW, Mueller TI, Endicott J, Coryell W, Hirschfeld RM, Shea T. Time to recovery, chronicity, and levels of psychopathology in major depression. A 5-year prospective follow-up of 431 subjects. *Arch Gen Psychiatry* 1992;49:809–816.

215. Frank E, Kupfer DJ, Perel JM, Cornes C, Jarrett DB, Mallinger AG, Thase ME, McEachran AB, Grochocinski VJ. Three-year outcomes for maintenance therapies in recurrent depression. *Arch Gen Psychiatry* 1990;47:1093–1099.

216. Kessing LV, Hansen MG, Andersen PK, Angst J. The predictive effect of episodes on the risk of recurrence in depressive and bipolar disorders - a life-long perspective. *Acta Psychiatr Scand* 2004;109:339–344.

217. Williams JM, Crane C, Barnhofer T, Van der Does AJ, Segal ZV. Recurrence of suicidal ideation across depressive episodes. *J Affect Disord* 2006.

218. Solomon DA, Keller MB, Leon AC, Mueller TI, Lavori PW, Shea MT, Coryell W, Warshaw M, Turvey C, Maser JD, Endicott J. Multiple recurrences of major depressive disorder. *Am J Psychiatry* 2000;157:229–233.

219. Ponds RW, Commissaris KJ, Jolles J. Prevalence and covariates of subjective forgetfulness in a normal population in The Netherlands. *International Journal of Aging and Human Development* 1997;45:207–221.

220. Cutler SJ, Grams AE. Correlates of self-reported everyday memory problems. *Journal of Gerontology* 1988;43:S82–90.

221. Bassett SS, Folstein MF. Memory complaint, memory performance, and psychiatric diagnosis: a community study. *Journal of Geriatric Psychiatry and Neurology* 1993;6:105–111.

222. Cull A, Hay C, Love SB, Mackie M, Smets E, Stewart M. What do cancer patients mean when they complain of concentration and memory problems? *British Journal of Cancer* 1996;74:1674–1679.

223. Wearden A, Appleby L. Cognitive performance and complaints of cognitive impairment in chronic fatigue syndrome (CFS). *Psychological Medicine* 1997;27:81–90.

224. van Gorp WG, Satz P, Hinkin C, Selnes O, Miller EN, McArthur J, Cohen B, Paz D. Metacognition in HIV-1 seropositive asymptomatic individuals: self-ratings versus objective neuropsychological performance. Multicenter AIDS Cohort Study (MACS). *Journal of Clinical and Experimental Neuropsychology* 1991;13:812–819.

225. Rourke SB, Halman MH, Bassel C. Neurocognitive complaints in HIV-infection and their relationship to depressive symptoms and neuropsychological functioning. *Journal of Clinical and Experimental Neuropsychology* 1999;21:737–756.

226. Dijkstra JB, Houx PJ, Jolles J. Cognition after major surgery in the elderly: test performance and complaints. *British Journal of Anaesthesiology* 1999;82:867–874.

227. Thompson PJ, Corcoran R. Everyday memory failures in people with epilepsy. *Epilepsia* 1992;33 Suppl 6:S18–20.

228. Sawrie SM, Martin RC, Kuzniecky R, Faught E, Morawetz R, Jamil F, Viikinsalo M, Gilliam F. Subjective versus objective memory change after temporal lobe epilepsy surgery. *Neurology* 1999;53:1511–1517.

229. Jennum P, Sjol A. Self-assessed cognitive function in snorers and sleep apneics. An epidemiological study of 1, 504 females and males aged 30–60 years: the Dan-MONICA II Study. *European Neurology* 1994;34:204–208.

230. Wang PN, Wang SJ, Fuh JL, Teng EL, Liu CY, Lin CH, Shyu HY, Lu SR, Chen CC, Liu HC. Subjective memory complaint in relation to cognitive performance and depression: a longitudinal study of a rural Chinese population. *Journal of the American Geriatrics Society* 2000;48:295–299.

231. Derouesne C, Lacomblez L, Thibault S, LePoncin M. Memory complaints in young and elderly subjects. *International Journal of Geriatric Psychiatry* 1999;14:291–301.

232. Comijs HC, Deeg DJ, Dik MG, Twisk JW, Jonker C. Memory complaints; the association with psycho-affective and health problems and the role of personality characteristics. A 6-year follow-up study. *Journal of Affective Disorders* 2002;72:157–165.

233. Bazargan M, Barbre AR. The effects of depression, health status, and stressful life-events on self-reported memory problems among aged blacks. *International Journal of Aging and Human Development* 1994;38:351–362.
234. Benoit G, Fortin L, Lemelin S, Laplante L, Thomas J, Everett J. Selective attention in major depression: clinical retardation and cognitive inhibition. *Can J Psychol* 1992;46:41–52.
235. Ellis HC. Focused attention and depressive deficits in memory. *J Exp Psychol Gen* 1991;120:310–312.
236. Lemelin S, Baruch P, Vincent A, Everett J, Vincent P. Distractibility and processing resource deficit in major depression. Evidence for two deficient attentional processing models. *J Nerv Ment Dis* 1997;185:542–548.
237. Ilsley JE, Moffoot AP, O'Carroll RE. An analysis of memory dysfunction in major depression. *J Affect Disord* 1995;35:1–9.
238. Sternberg DE, Jarvik ME. Memory functions in depression. *Arch Gen Psychiatry* 1976;33:219–224.
239. Weingartner H, Cohen RM, Murphy DL, Martello J, Gerdt C. Cognitive processes in depression. *Arch Gen Psychiatry* 1981;38:42–47.
240. Wolfe J, Granholm E, Butters N, Saunders E, Janowsky D. Verbal memory deficits associated with major affective disorders: a comparison of unipolar and bipolar patients. *J Affect Disord* 1987;13:83–92.
241. Austin MP, Mitchell P, Wilhelm K, Parker G, Hickie I, Brodaty H, Chan J, Eyers K, Milic M, Hadzi-Pavlovic D. Cognitive function in depression: a distinct pattern of frontal impairment in melancholia? *Psychol Med* 1999;29:73–85.
242. Degl'Innocenti A, Agren H, Backman L. Executive deficits in major depression. *Acta Psychiatr Scand* 1998;97:182–188.
243. Channon S. Executive dysfunction in depression: the Wisconsin Card Sorting Test. *J Affect Disord* 1996;39:107–114.
244. Channon S, Green PS. Executive function in depression: the role of performance strategies in aiding depressed and non-depressed participants. *J Neurol Neurosurg Psychiatry* 1999;66:162–171.
245. Merriam EP, Thase ME, Haas GL, Keshavan MS, Sweeney JA. Prefrontal cortical dysfunction in depression determined by Wisconsin Card Sorting Test performance. *Am J Psychiatry* 1999;156:780–782.
246. Zakzanis KK, Leach L, Kaplan E. On the nature and pattern of neurocognitive function in major depressive disorder. *Neuropsychiatry Neuropsychol Behav Neurol* 1998;11:111–119.
247. Rajkowska G, Miguel-Hidalgo JJ, Wei J, Dilley G, Pittman SD, Meltzer HY, Overholser JC, Roth BL, Stockmeier CA. Morphometric evidence for neuronal and glial prefrontal cell pathology in major depression. *Biol Psychiatry* 1999;45:1085–1098.
248. Sbordone RJ, Liter JC. Mild traumatic brain injury does not produce post-traumatic stress disorder. *Brain Inj* 1995;9:405–412.
249. Klein E, Caspi Y, Gil S. The relation between memory of the traumatic event and PTSD: Evidence from studies of traumatic brain injury. *Can J Psychiatry* 2003;48:28–33.
250. Mayou R, Bryant B, Duthie R. Psychiatric consequences of road traffic accidents. *Bmj* 1993;307:647–651.
251. Bryant RA, Harvey AG. The influence of traumatic brain injury on acute stress disorder and post-traumatic stress disorder following motor vehicle accidents. *Brain Inj* 1999;13:15–22.
252. Harvey AG, Brewin CR, Jones C, Kopelman MD. Coexistence of post-traumatic stress disorder and traumatic brain injury: towards a resolution of the paradox. *J Int Neuropsychol Soc* 2003;9:663–676.
253. Gil S, Caspi Y, Ben-Ari IZ, Koren D, Klein E. Does memory of a traumatic event increase the risk for post-traumatic stress disorder in patients with traumatic brain injury? A prospective study. *Am J Psychiatry* 2005;162:963–969.
254. Ponsford J, Willmott C, Rothwell A, Cameron P, Kelly AM, Nelms R, Curran C, Ng K. Factors influencing outcome following mild traumatic brain injury in adults. *J Int Neuropsychol Soc* 2000;6:568–579.
255. Ferguson RP. Iatrogenesis: 'the hidden and general dangers'. *Hosp Pract (Off Ed)* 1989;24:89–94.
256. Raskin SA, Mateer CA, editors. *Neuropsychological management of mild traumatic brain injury.* New York: Oxford University Press, 2000.
257. Kouyanou K, Pither CE, Rabe-Hesketh S, Wessely S. A comparative study of iatrogenesis, medication abuse, and psychiatric morbidity in chronic pain patients with and without medically explained symptoms. *Pain* 1998;76:417–426.
258. Rusakov VI. [The problem of iatrogenesis]. *Khirurgiia (Mosk)* 1998:45–48.
259. Kendler KS, Neale MC, Kessler RC, Heath AC, Eaves LJ. A longitudinal twin study of personality and major depression in women. *Arch Gen Psychiatry* 1993;50:853–862.
260. Ormel J, Oldehinkel AJ, Vollebergh W. Vulnerability before, during, and after a major depressive episode: a 3-wave population-based study. *Arch Gen Psychiatry* 2004;61:990–996.
261. Maier W, Lichtermann D, Minges J, Heun R. Personality traits in subjects at risk for unipolar major depression: a family study perspective. *J Affect Disord* 1992;24:153–163.
262. Van Os J, Jones PB. Early risk factors and adult person—environment relationships in affective disorder. *Psychol Med* 1999;29:1055–1067.
263. Hirschfeld RM, Klerman GL, Clayton PJ, Keller MB. Personality and depression. Empirical findings. *Arch Gen Psychiatry* 1983;40:993–998.
264. Bachar E, Hadar H, Shalev AY. Narcissistic vulnerability and the development of PTSD: a prospective study. *J Nerv Ment Dis* 2005;193:762–765.
265. Heinrichs M, Wagner D, Schoch W, Soravia LM, Hellhammer DH, Ehlert U. Predicting post-traumatic stress symptoms from pretraumatic risk factors: a 2-year prospective follow-up study in firefighters. *Am J Psychiatry* 2005;162:2276–2286.
266. Brewin CR, Andrews B, Valentine JD. Meta-analysis of risk factors for post-traumatic stress disorder in trauma-exposed adults. *J Consult Clin Psychol* 2000;68:748–766.
267. McNally RJ. Psychological mechanisms in acute response to trauma. *Biol Psychiatry* 2003;53:779–788.
268. Kay T, Newman B, Cavallo M, Ezrachi O, Resnick M. Toward and neuropsychological model of functional disability after mild traumatic brain injury. *Neuropsychology* 1992;6:371–384.
269. Hibbard MR, Bogdany J, Uysal S, Kepler K, Silver JM, Gordon WA, Haddad L. Axis II psychopathology in individuals with traumatic brain injury. *Brain Inj* 2000;14:45–61.
270. Greiffenstein FM, Baker JW. Comparison of premorbid and post-injury mmpi-2 profiles in late post-concussion claimants. *Clin Neuropsychol* 2001;15:162–170.
271. Gunstad J, Suhr JA. "Expectation as etiology" versus "the good old days": post-concussion syndrome symptom reporting in athletes, headache sufferers, and depressed individuals. *J Int Neuropsychol Soc* 2001;7:323–333.
272. Ferguson RJ, Mittenberg W, Barone DF, Schneider B. Post-concussion syndrome following sports-related head injury: expectation as etiology. *Neuropsychology* 1999;13:582–589.
273. Kennedy WP. The nocebo reaction. *Med Exp Int J Exp Med* 1961;95:203–205.
274. Luparello T, Lyons HA, Bleecker ER, McFadden ER, Jr. Influences of suggestion on airway reactivity in asthmatic subjects. *Psychosom Med* 1968;30:819–825.
275. Bootzin RR, Bailey ET. Understanding placebo, nocebo, and iatrogenic treatment effects. *J Clin Psychol* 2005;61:871–880.
276. Lancman ME, Asconape JJ, Craven WJ, Howard G, Penry JK. Predictive value of induction of psychogenic seizures by suggestion. *Ann Neurol* 1994;35:359–361.
277. Schweiger A, Parducci A. Nocebo: the psychologic induction of pain. *Pavlov J Biol Sci* 1981;16:140–143.
278. Benedetti F, Pollo A, Lopiano L, Lanotte M, Vighetti S, Rainero I. Conscious expectation and unconscious conditioning in analgesic, motor, and hormonal placebo/nocebo responses. *J Neurosci* 2003;23:4315–4323.
279. Benson H. The nocebo effect: History and physiology. *Prev Med* 1997;26:612–615.
280. Evans RW, Rogers MP. Headaches and the nocebo effect. *J Head Face Pain* 2003;43:1113–1115.
281. Speigel H. Nocebo: The power of suggestibility. *Prev Med* 1997;26:616–621.
282. Hahn RA. The nocebo phenomenon: concept, evidence, and implications for public health. *Prev Med* 1997;26:607–611.

283. Davis CH. Self-perception in mild traumatic brain injury. *Am J Phys Med Rehabil* 2002;81:609–621.

284. Gunstad J, Suhr JA. Cognitive factors in Post-concussion Syndrome symptom report. *Arch Clin Neuropsychol* 2004;19:391–405.

285. Hilsabeck RC, Gouvier WD, Bolter JF. Reconstructive memory bias in recall of neuropsychological symptomatology. *J Clin Exp Neuropsychol* 1998;20:328–338.

286. Lees-Haley PR, Williams CW, Zasler ND, Marguilies S, English LT, Stevens KB. Response bias in plaintiffs' histories. *Brain Inj* 1997;11:791–799.

287. Lees-Haley PR, Williams CW, English LT. Response bias in self-reported history of plaintiffs compared with nonlitigating patients. *Psychol Rep* 1996;79:811–818.

288. Steele CM, Aronson J. Stereotype threat and the intellectual test performance of African Americans. *J Pers Soc Psychol* 1995;69:797–811.

289. Aronson J, Lustina MJ, Good C. When white men can't do math: Necessary and sufficient factors in stereotype threat. *J Exp Soc Psychol* 1999;35:29–46.

290. Croizet JC, Claire T. Extending the concept of stereotype and threat to social class: The intellectual underperformance of students from low socioeconomic backgrounds. *Pers Soc Psychol Bull* 1998;24:588–594.

291. Levy B. Improving memory in old age through implicit self-stereotyping. *J Pers Soc Psychol* 1996;71:1092–1107.

292. Leyens JP, Desert M, Croizet JC. Stereotype treat: Are lower status and history of stigmatization preconditions of stereotype threat? *Pers Soc Psychol Bull* 2000;26:1189–1199.

293. Spencer SJ, Steele CM, Quinn DM. Stereotype threat adn women's math performance. *J Exp Soc Psychol* 1999;35:4–28.

294. Steele CM. A threat in the air. How stereotypes shape intellectual identity and performance. *Am Psychol* 1997;52:613–629.

295. Walsh M, Hickey C, Duffy J. Influence of item content and stereotype situation on gender differences in mathematical problem solving. *Sex Roles* 1999;41:219–240.

296. Chasteen AL, Bhattacharyya S, Horhota M, Tam R, Hasher L. How feelings of stereotype threat influence older adults' memory performance. *Exp Aging Res* 2005;31:235–260.

297. Hess TM, Auman C, Colcombe SJ, Rahhal TA. The impact of stereotype threat on age differences in memory performance. *J Gerontol B Psychol Sci Soc Sci* 2003;58:P3–11.

298. Johns M, Schmader T, Martens A. Knowing is half the battle: teaching stereotype threat as a means of improving women's math performance. *Psychol Sci* 2005;16:175–179.

299. Ben-Zeev T, Fein S, Inzlicht M. Arousal and stereotype treat. *J Exp Soc Psychol* 2005;41:174–181.

300. Croizet JC, Despres G, Gauzins ME, Huguet P, Leyens JP, Meot A. Stereotype threat undermines intellectual performance by triggering a disruptive mental load. *Pers Soc Psychol Bull* 2004;30:721–731.

301. Smith JL. Understanding the process of stereotype threat: A review of mediational variables and new performance goal directions. *Educ Psychol Rev* 2004;16:177–206.

302. Suhr JA, Gunstad J. Further exploration of the effect of "diagnosis threat" on cognitive performance in individuals with mild head injury. *J Int Neuropsychol Soc* 2005;11:23–29.

303. Suhr JA, Gunstad J. Post-concussive symptom report: the relative influence of head injury and depression. *J Clin Exp Neuropsychol* 2002;24:981–993.

304. Suhr JA, Gunstad J. "Diagnosis Threat": the effect of negative expectations on cognitive performance in head injury. *J Clin Exp Neuropsychol* 2002;24:448–457.

305. Weissman HN. Distortions and decptions in self presentation: Effects of protracted litigation on personal injury cases. *Behav Sci Law* 1990;8:67–74.

306. Larrabee GJ. Detection of malingering using atypical performance patterns on standard neuropsychological tests. *Clin Neuropsychol* 2003;17:410–425.

307. Mittenberg W, Patton C, Canyock EM, Condit DC. Base rates of malingering and symptom exaggeration. *J Clin Exp Neuropsychol* 2002;24:1094–1102.

308. Bianchini KJ, Mathias CW, Greve KW. Symptom validity testing: a critical review. *Clin Neuropsychol* 2001;15:19–45.

309. Hom J, Denney RL. *Detection of response bias in forensic neuropsychology.* New York: Haworth Medical Press, 2003.

310. Hayes JS, Hilsabeck RC, Gouvier WD. Malingering in traumatic brain injury: Current issues and caveats in assessment and classification. In: Varney NR, Roberts RJ, editors. *The evaluation and treatment of mild traumatic brain injury.* Mahwah, NJ: Lawrence Erlbaum Associates, 1999. p 249–290.

311. Iverson GL. Detecting malingering in civil forensic evaluations. In: Horton AM, Hartlage LC, editors. *Handbook of forensic neuropsychology.* New York: Springer, 2003.

312. Iverson GL, Binder LM. Detecting exaggeration and malingering in neuropsychological assessment. *J Head Trauma Rehabil* 2000;15:829–858.

313. Reynolds CR, editor. *Detection of malingering during head injury litigation.* New York: Plenum Press, 1998.

314. Rogers R. *Clinical assessment of malingering and deception (2nd. ed.).* New York: Guilford Press, 1997.

315. Sweet JJ. Malingering: Differential diagnosis. In: Sweet JJ, editor. *Forensic neuropsychology: Fundamentals and Practice.* Lisse: Swets & Zeitlinger, 1999.

316. Vickery CD, Berry DT, Inman TH, Harris MJ, Orey SA. Detection of inadequate effort on neuropsychological testing: a meta-analytic review of selected procedures. *Arch Clin Neuropsychol* 2001;16:45–73.

317. Millis SR, Volinsky CT. Assessment of response bias in mild head injury: beyond malingering tests. *J Clin Exp Neuropsychol* 2001;23:809–828.

318. Larrabee GJ. Assessment of malingering. In: Larrabee GJ, editor. *Forensic neuropsychology: A scientific approach.* New York: Oxford University Press, 2005. p 115–158.

319. Slick DJ, Sherman EM, Iverson GL. Diagnostic criteria for malingered neurocognitive dysfunction: proposed standards for clinical practice and research. *Clin Neuropsychol* 1999;13:545–561.

320. Bianchini KJ, Greve KW, Glynn G. On the diagnosis of malingered pain-related disability: lessons from cognitive malingering research. *Spine J* 2005;5:404–417.

321. Resnick PJ. Malingering of post-traumatic disorders. In: Rogers R, editor. *Clinical assessment of malingering and deception (2nd ed.).* New York: Guilford, 1997. p 130–152.

322. Pellman EJ, Viano DC, Casson IR, Arfken C, Powell J. Concussion in Professional Football: Injuries Involving 7 or More Days Out-Part 5. *Neurosurgery* 2004;55:1100–1119.

323. Pellman EJ, Viano DC, Casson IR, Arfken C, Feuer H. Concussion in professional football: players returning to the same game-part 7. *Neurosurgery* 2005;56:79–92.

324. Pellman EJ, Lovell MR, Viano DC, Casson IR, Tucker AM. Concussion in professional football: neuropsychological testing-part 6. *Neurosurgery* 2004;55:1290–1305.

325. Pellman EJ, Viano DC, Casson IR, Tucker AM, Waeckerle JF, Powell JW, Feuer H. Concussion in professional football: repeat injuries—part 4. *Neurosurgery* 2004;55:860–873; discussion 873–876.

326. Field M, Collins MW, Lovell MR, Maroon J. Does age play a role in recovery from sports-related concussion? A comparison of high school and collegiate athletes. *J Pediatr* 2003;142: 546–553.

327. McCauley SR, Boake C, Levin HS, Contant CF, Song JX. Post-concussional disorder following mild to moderate traumatic brain injury: anxiety, depression, and social support as risk factors and comorbidities. *J Clin Exp Neuropsychol* 2001;23: 792–808.

328. Zafonte RD, Cullen N, Lexell J. Serotonin agents in the treatment of acquired brain injury. *J Head Trauma Rehabil* 2002;17: 322–334.

329. Fann JR, Uomoto JM, Katon WJ. Sertraline in the treatment of major depression following mild traumatic brain injury. *J Neuropsychiatry Clin Neurosci* 2000;12:226–232.

330. Fann JR, Uomoto JM, Katon WJ. Cognitive improvement with treatment of depression following mild traumatic brain injury. *Psychosomatics* 2001;42:48–54.

331. Mittenberg W, Canyock EM, Condit D, Patton C. Treatment of post-concussion syndrome following mild head injury. *J Clin Exp Neuropsychol* 2001;23:829–836.

332. Mittenberg W, Tremont G, Zielinski RE, Fichera S, Rayls KR. Cognitive-behavioral prevention of post-concussion syndrome. *Arch Clin Neuropsychol* 1996;11:139–145.

333. Hayes SC, Follette VM, Linehan M, editors. Mindfulness and acceptance: Expanding the cognitive-behavioral tradition. New York: Guilford Press, 2004.

334. Hayes SC, Strosahl K, Wilson KG. *Acceptance and commitment therapy: An experiential approach to behavior change.* New York: Guilford Press, 1999.

335. McCracken LM, Vowles KE, Eccleston C. Acceptance-based treatment for persons with complex, long standing chronic pain: a preliminary analysis of treatment outcome in comparison to a waiting phase. *Behav Res Ther* 2005;43:1335–1346.

336. McCracken LM, Eccleston C. A prospective study of acceptance of pain and patient functioning with chronic pain. *Pain* 2005;118:164–169.

337. McCracken LM. *Contextual cognitive-behavioral thereapy for chronic pain. Progress in pain research and management, Volume 33.* Seattle, WA: IASP Press, 2005.

338. Binder LM, Rohling ML, Larrabee J. A review of mild head trauma. Part I: Meta-analytic review of neuropsychological studies. *J Clin Exp Neuropsychol* 1997;19:421–431.

339. Grant I, Gonzalez R, Carey CL, Natarajan L, Wolfson T. Non-acute (residual) neurocognitive effects of cannabis use: a meta-analytic study. *J Int Neuropsychol Soc* 2003;9:679–689.

340. Christensen H, Griffiths K, Mackinnon A, Jacomb P. A quantitative review of cognitive deficits in depression and Alzheimer-type dementia. *J Int Neuropsychol Soc* 1997;3:631–651.

341. Frazier TW, Demaree HA, Youngstrom EA. Meta-analysis of intellectual and neuropsychological test performance in attention-deficit/hyperactivity disorder. *Neuropsychology* 2004;18:543–555.

342. Barker MJ, Greenwood KM, Jackson M, Crowe SF. Cognitive effects of long-term benzodiazepine use: a meta-analysis. *CNS Drugs* 2004;18:37–48.

APPENDIX A
British Columbia Post-Concussion Symptom Inventory (BC-PSI)

BC-PSI

Name: _____   Date: _____

The following is a list of symptoms that you may have experienced. Please rate each symptom or problem in regards to how often it happens and how bad it is. *Consider your experience with these symptoms or problems over the past two weeks, including today.*

HOW OFTEN   **HOW BAD**

(Frequency)   *(Intensity)*
0 = Not at all   0 = Not at all
1 = 1–2 times   1 = Very mild problem
2 = Several times   2 = Mild Problem
3 = Often   3 = Moderate problem
4 = Very often   4 = Severe problem
5 = Constantly   5 = Very severe problem

SYMPTOMS & LIFE PROBLEMS	HOW OFTEN	HOW BAD
1. Headaches	_____	_____
2. Dizziness/light-headed	_____	_____
3. Nausea/feeling sick	_____	_____
4. Fatigue	_____	_____
5. Extra sensitive to noises	_____	_____
6. Irritable	_____	_____
7. Feeling Sad	_____	_____
8. Nervous or tense	_____	_____
9. Temper problems	_____	_____
10. Poor concentration	_____	_____
11. Memory problems	_____	_____
12. Difficulty reading	_____	_____
13. Poor sleep	_____	_____

14. Does alcohol affect you more than in the past?
    1   2   3   4   5
    Not at all   Somewhat   Very Much

15. Do you find yourself worrying and dwelling on the symptoms above?
    1   2   3   4   5
    Not at all   Somewhat   Very Much

16. Do you believe you have damage to your brain?
    1   2   3   4   5
    Not at all   Somewhat   Very Much

APPENDIX B
Scoring Template for the BC-PSI

SYMPTOM/PROBLEM	PRODUCT	ITEM SCORE	SYMPTOM CLASSIFICATION		
			NONE	MILD	MODERATE
Headaches					
Dizziness/light-headed					
Nausea/feeling sick					
Fatigue					
Extra sensitive to noises					
Irritable					
Sad					
Nervous or tense					
Temper problems					
Poor concentration					
Memory problems					
Difficulty reading					
Poor sleep					
Total Score	—		—	—	—

Step 1: Multiply the frequency rating by the severity rating and enter value in the "Product" column (e.g., 2 x 3 = 6).
Step 2: Convert product score to "Item Score" based on the following: Product = 0–1, Item score = 0; Product = 2–3, Item Score = 1; Product = 4–6, Item Score = 2; Product = 8–12, Item Score = 3; Product = 15+, Item Score = 4. Enter the Item scores into the grid. **Step 3:** Sum the Item Scores for the Total Score. **Step 4:** Place an "X" in the appropriate classification range for each symptom based on the following "Item Score" criteria: 0 = None, 1–2 = Mild, and 3+ = Moderate or greater. Total Scores: 0 = "Low", 1 – 9 = "Normal", 10 – 14 = "Unusually High", and 15+ = "Extremely High" relative to *healthy adults*.

24 Sport-Related Concussion

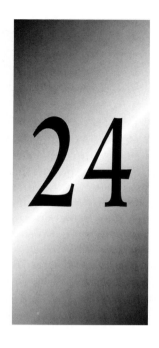

Michael W. Collins
Grant L. Iverson
Michael Gaetz
Mark R. Lovell

oncussion is a common injury in sport (1–11). Moreover, these injuries might be more prevalent than initially thought because some concussions may go unrecognized (12). Injuries without loss of consciousness (LOC) occur most frequently; in fact, approximately 90% of concussions in sport occur without LOC (13–15). Because most concussions lack the dramatic on-field nature of those with LOC, they are typically more difficult to detect and might be under-diagnosed by sports medicine practitioners (16). The importance of accurate diagnosis, management, and return-to-play decisions extends from the elite ranks of professional athletes to the child or adolescent athlete. This chapter, designed to be a comprehensive overview, is divided into the following eight sections: (a) definition of concussion, (b) pathophysiology, (c) injury severity markers (signs), (d) symptoms, (e) structural and functional neuroimaging, (f) neuropsychological outcome, (g) cumulative effects, (h) recovery time and return to play decision-making, and (i) conclusions.

DEFINITION OF CONCUSSION

There has not been a universally-accepted definition of concussion. Traditionally, the most widely accepted definition has been that proposed by the Committee on Head Injury Nomenclature of Neurological Surgeons in 1966 (17). That committee defined concussion as: "a clinical syndrome characterized by the immediate and transient post-traumatic impairment of neural function such as alteration of consciousness, disturbance of vision or equilibrium, etc., due to brain stem dysfunction."

More recently, many clinicians and researchers currently use the definition of concussion described by the American Academy of Neurology (AAN): "Concussion is a trauma-induced alteration in mental status that may or may not include a loss of consciousness" (18, p. 582). This definition was prompted by the belief of the AAN definition authors that previous definitions may be too limiting because the injury is not restricted to the brain stem and may involve other brain structures (e.g., cortical areas). This definition also served to emphasize the fact that concussion may occur with or without a loss of consciousness.

In 2001, and most recently in 2004, an International Symposium on Concussion in Sport was held where concussion experts from around the world met to discuss specific issues related to the injury. One major outcome of these symposia was the adoption of a global definition of concussion that improved upon previous definitions. The current definition is as follows: "Sports concussion is defined as a complex pathophysiological process affecting the brain, induced by traumatic biomechanical forces"

(19, p. 196). In addition to this definition, the features listed below were outlined.

1. "Concussion may be caused either by a direct blow to the head, face, neck, or elsewhere on the body with an "impulsive" force transmitted to the head.
2. Concussion typically results in the rapid onset of short-lived impairment of neurological function that resolves spontaneously.
3. Concussion may result in neuropathological changes, but the acute clinical symptoms largely reflect a functional disturbance rather than structural injury.
4. Concussion results in a graded set of clinical syndromes that may or may not involve loss of consciousness. Resolution of the clinical and cognitive symptoms typically follows a sequential course.
5. Concussion is typically associated with grossly normal structural neuroimaging studies." (19, p. 196)

PATHOPHYSIOLOGY

The pathoanatomy and pathophysiology of mild traumatic brain injury (MTBI) is reviewed, in detail, in the mild traumatic brain injury chapter in this book. In that chapter, it was described that brain injuries produced by acceleration/deceleration forces occur along a continuum of severity dependent upon the mechanical forces that caused them (20, 21). Concussion in athletes is typically produced by acceleration/deceleration forces (e.g., helmet to helmet contact in North American football or helmet to ice contact in ice hockey). Concussion can be considered an injury at the mild end of the MTBI continuum with LOC (when it occurs) and posttraumatic amnesia being considerably more brief in duration, and with low levels of axonal stretch. This limited axonal stretching can initiate a pathophysiologic process that leads to very limited cell death (largely dependent on the morphology of the cell) but in the vast majority of cells leads to a reversible series of metabolic events.

Giza and Hovda (22) describe the complex interwoven cellular and vascular changes that occur following concussion as a multilayered neurometabolic cascade. The primary mechanisms include ionic shifts, abnormal energy metabolism, diminished cerebral blood flow, and impaired neurotransmission. A brief summary of this process, derived from several sources (22, 23), is provided below.

Stretching of an axon results in an indiscriminate release of neurotransmitters and uncontrolled ionic fluxes. When ionic gradients are disrupted, cells respond by activating ion pumps in an attempt to restore the normal membrane potential. Pump activation increases glucose utilization. This contributes to dramatic increases in the local cerebral metabolic rate for glucose. This hypermetabolism occurs in tandem with decreased cerebral blood flow, which contributes to the disparity between glucose supply and demand. There also appears to be impaired oxidative metabolism and diminished mitochondrial function, resulting in the over-utilization of anaerobic energy pathways and elevated lactate as a by-product. Moreover, intracellular magnesium levels appear to decrease significantly and remain depressed for several days following injury. This is important because magnesium is essential for the generation of adenosine-triphosphate (ATP – energy production). Magnesium is also essential for the initiation of protein synthesis and the maintenance of the cellular membrane potential. A sustained influx of Ca^{2+} can result in mitochondrial accumulations of this ion contributing to metabolic dysfunction and energy failure. High intracellular Ca^{2+} levels, combined with stretch injury, can initiate an irreversible process of destruction of microtubules within axons.

Fortunately, the brain undergoes a dynamic restorative process in the initial days to weeks following a concussion. From a commonsense perspective, the ionic shifts, abnormal energy metabolism, diminished cerebral blood flow, and impaired neurotransmission believed to be associated with concussions in sports reinforces the importance of immediate rest following injury. Although not established empirically, it seems reasonable to assume that vigorous exercise or hard physical contact might exacerbate the pathophysiology described above.

INJURY SEVERITY MARKERS (SIGNS)

Appropriate acute care and management of the concussed athlete begins with a detailed and accurate assessment of the severity of the injury. As with any serious injury, the first priority is always to evaluate the athlete's level of consciousness and ABCs (airway, breathing, and circulation). The attending medical staff must always be prepared with an emergency action plan in the event that the evacuation of a critically head-or neck-injured athlete is necessary. This plan should be familiar to all staff, be well delineated, and frequently rehearsed.

Loss of Consciousness

Upon ruling out more severe injury via neurological and clinical examination, the acute evaluation continues with the assessment of concussion. First, the clinician should establish whether a loss of consciousness (LOC) has occurred. By definition, LOC represents a state of brief coma in which the eyes are typically closed and the athlete is unresponsive to external stimuli. LOC is relatively uncommon and reportedly occurs in less than 10% of concussive injuries in most (13–15), but not all (24) studies. Moreover, prolonged LOC (>1–2 minutes) in sport-related concussion occurs much less frequently. Athletes with LOC are typically unresponsive for only a brief period of time, sometimes only one to two seconds. This may at times make LOC difficult to identify because the response of medical personnel to injured athletes is beyond this time window.

Although many of the concussion grading and management scales rely heavily upon the presence or absence and duration of loss of consciousness, research on the relation between LOC and outcome is mixed. Large scale studies with trauma patients have not revealed a relation between LOC and neuropsychological outcome (e.g., 25, 26). Some researchers examining athletes with concussions have reported an association between LOC and immediate or short-term outcome (e.g., 24, 27, 28), while others have not (e.g., 29, 30).

Confusion

A more common form of mental status change following concussion involves confusion and amnesia. Confusion (i.e., disorientation), by definition, represents impaired awareness and orientation to surroundings, though memory systems are not necessarily directly affected. An athlete with post-injury confusion will typically appear stunned, dazed, or "glassy-eyed" on the sideline or playing field. Confusion is often manifested in athletes who do not remove themselves from play in the form of difficulty with appropriate play-calling, failure to correctly execute their positional assignment during play, or difficulty in communicating game information to teammates or coaches. Teammates are often the first to recognize that an athlete has been injured when the athlete shows these behaviors and has difficulty maintaining the flow of the game. On the sidelines, confused athletes may answer questions slowly or inappropriately, ask "what is going on" or "what happened," and may repeat himself or herself during evaluation. Some may be temporarily disoriented to time or place, and even, very rarely, to people they know well (e.g., not knowing coaches or teammates). To properly assess the presence of confusion, medical personnel can ask the athlete simple orientation questions such as the date, and names of the stadium, city, and opposing team. Please see Table 24-1 for a list of orientation questions extracted from the University of Pittsburgh Medical Center's Concussion Card.

Amnesia

Amnesia is emerging as perhaps the most important sign to carefully assess following concussion (after more serious injuries have been ruled out). Amnesia due to concussion may present as retrograde amnesia (difficulty with memory of events prior to the injury) or post-traumatic/anterograde amnesia (difficulty with memory for events

following the injury). Both forms of amnesia should be assessed thoroughly. Athletes who present with one or both types of amnesia may initially have difficulty recalling large spans of time before the injury, after the injury, or both. These larger periods of amnesia typically shrink as the injury becomes less acute. The presence and duration of amnesia, disorientation, or mental status disturbance has been associated with immediate outcome or slower recovery (24, 28, 29, 31, 32) in many, but not all studies (e.g., 30).

Post-traumatic amnesia and anterograde amnesia are synonymous terms that represent the duration of time between the head trauma (for example, an ice hockey player's forehead striking the boards) and the point at which the athlete reports a return of normal continuous memory functioning (e.g., remembering the athletic trainer asking the athlete orientation questions in the locker room). One method for assessing post-traumatic confusion and amnesia is provided in Table 24-1 (UPMC Concussion Card Mental Status Testing).

At times, especially during a sideline assessment, confusion and post-traumatic amnesia may be difficult to disentangle. It is important to remember that confusion is not necessarily associated with a loss of memory, whereas

---

TABLE 24-1
University of Pittsburgh Medical Centers'
Sideline Concussion Card: Acute (sideline
or on-field) Mental Status Testing

On-Field Cognitive Testing
Orientation (ask the athlete the following questions)
- What stadium is this?
- What city is this?
- Who is the opposing team?
- What month is it?
- What day is it?

Post-Traumatic Amnesia (ask the athlete to repeat the following words)
- Girl, dog, green

Retrograde Amnesia (ask the athlete the following questions)
- What happened in the prior quarter or half?
- What do you remember just prior to the hit?
- What was the score of the game prior to the hit?
- Do you remember the hit?

Concentration (ask the athlete to do the following)
- Repeat the days of the week backward, starting with today
- Repeat these numbers backward (63) (419)

Word list memory
- Ask the athlete to repeat the three words from earlier (girl, dog, green)

amnesia is only present with a loss of memory. This memory loss may span only a few seconds or minutes. It sometimes can span several hours, but rarely exceeds a day. A practitioner may be unable to differentiate confusion and amnesia until the athlete's confusion has resolved. Only then can memories surrounding the injury actually be discussed. Once the athlete is more lucid, the practitioner may gain additional insight into any existing post-traumatic amnesia by asking the athlete to recall the events that occurred immediately following the trauma (e.g., rising from the ground, walking/skating to sideline, memory for any part of the game played or observed after the injury, memory for the score of the contest, memory of the ride home, and so on). Post-traumatic amnesia is inferred by failure to remember events following the injury.

Retrograde amnesia is defined as the inability to recall events before the head trauma. Commonly used questions to assess retrograde amnesia are presented in Table 24-1. Medical personnel may ask for the athlete's memory of the actual injury (e.g., seeing a linebacker charge toward him with his helmet down, then falling backward and striking the back of his head to the ground). Then, additional questions can probe events that are increasingly remote from the injury (e.g., the score at the beginning of the first quarter, coming onto the field for stretching exercises, and getting dressed in the locker room). The length of retrograde amnesia will typically "shrink" over time. As recovery occurs, the period of retrograde amnesia may shrink from several minutes to a few seconds (in rare cases an athlete will have retrograde amnesia for hours or days). The presence and duration of retrograde amnesia has been associated with worse initial presentation and with slower recovery (27–29, 31).

SYMPTOMS

The initial signs and symptoms of concussion vary from athlete to athlete, depending on the biomechanical forces involved, specifically-affected brain areas, athletes' prior history of injury, and other factors. A summary of common on-field signs and symptoms of concussion is presented in Table 24-2. It is important to note that an athlete may present with as few as one symptom of injury or potentially a constellation of symptoms.

Headaches and dizziness are the most commonly reported symptoms of injury (9, 13). Moreover, headaches lasting more than three hours post injury (27), those present at seven days post injury (32), or those that are migraine-like (33) have been associated with slow recovery. However, the absence of headache does not rule out a concussion, highlighting the importance of a thorough assessment of all symptoms. Assessment of post-concussion headache may be complicated by the presence of musculoskeletal headaches and other pre-existing headache syndromes (e.g., migraine disorder or frequent stress headaches).

Most frequently, a "concussion headache" is described as a sensation of pressure in the skull that may be localized to one region of the head or may be generalized in nature. In some athletes (particularly athletes with a history of migraine), the headache may take the form of a vascular headache, may be unilateral, and is often described as throbbing or pulsating. The headache may not develop immediately after injury and may develop in the minutes, or even hours, following injury. Therefore, it is important to question the potentially concussed athlete regarding the development of symptoms beyond the first few minutes after injury. Post-concussion headache is often worsened with physical exertion. Thus, if the athlete complains of worsening headache during exertional testing or return to play, post-concussion headache should be suspected and conservative management is indicated. While headache following a concussion usually does not constitute a medical emergency, a severe or progressively severe headache, particularly when accompanied by vomiting or rapidly declining mental status, may signal a life-threatening situation such as a subdural hematoma or

---

TABLE 24-2

University of Pittsburgh Medical Center's Sideline Concussion Card: Signs and Symptoms of Concussion

Signs Observed by Staff	Symptoms Reported by Athlete
Loses consciousness	Feeling "foggy" or groggy
Forgets events prior to play (retrograde)	Change in sleep pattern (appears later)
Forgets events after hit (post-traumatic)	Feeling Fatigued
Appears to be dazed or stunned	Headache
Is confused about assignment	Nausea
Forgets plays	Balance problems or dizziness
Is unsure of game, score, or opponent	Double or fuzzy/blurry vision
Moves clumsily	Sensitivity to light or noise
Answers questions slowly	Feeling sluggish or slowed down
Shows behavior or personality change	Concentration or memory problems

intracranial bleed. This should prompt immediate transport to hospital and a CT scan of the brain.

In addition to headaches, many other symptoms may emerge as a result of concussive injury. For example, athletes will commonly experience blurred vision, changes in peripheral vision, or other visual disturbance. Moreover, an athlete may report increased fatigue, "feeling a step slow," or feeling sluggish. Fatigue is especially prominent in concussed athletes in the days following injury and this symptom may be as prominent as headache. Also, athletes may report cognitive changes, including problems with attention, concentration, short-term memory, learning, and multitasking. These symptoms sometimes become more noticeable after the athlete has returned to school or work.

Another frequently reported symptom which has gained recent research attention is a reported sensation of feeling "foggy" following concussion (34). In this study, a sample of concussed high school students who endorsed feeling "foggy" on a symptom inventory were compared to concussed high school athletes who did not endorse a sense of "fogginess." At one-week post injury, the foggy group demonstrated significantly slower reaction times, attenuated memory performance, and slower processing speed via computerized neurocognitive testing. In addition, the "foggy" athletes also endorsed a significantly higher number of other post-concussion symptoms when compared to the group who did not endorse fogginess.

Another commonly reported or observed symptom is that of emotional changes. Most often, athletes will report increased irritability, or having a "shorter fuse." However, other emotional changes may occur such as sadness/ depression, nervousness/ anxiety, or even (much less commonly) silliness or euphoria. Affect may be described by the athlete or parent as flattened or labile. Emotional changes may be very brief (e.g., a linebacker bursts into tears for 30 seconds on the sideline) or may be prolonged in the case of a more significant injury (athlete reports persistent depression).

STRUCTURAL AND FUNCTIONAL NEUROIMAGING

Given that concussion is largely a metabolic and not a structural injury, traditional neuroimaging techniques such as CT or MRI are almost always unremarkable following a single concussion. Despite this fact, these techniques are useful for ruling out more serious pathology (e.g., cerebral bleed or skull fracture) that occasionally occur in sports-related head injuries. Athletes most likely to show abnormalities on structural neuroimaging are boxers. This is not particularly surprising because historically damage could be seen with the naked eye at

autopsy (35). Studies on professional boxers, active and retired, have revealed the greatest number of CT abnormalities estimated to be between 25–50% (36–39). In these boxers, a cavum septum pellucidum was considered a CT sign of traumatic encephalopathy (40). CT abnormalities were correlated with the number of bouts fought (41) and were estimated to be less frequently observed in amateur boxers [between 0 and 20% had abnormalities (42–44)]. In addition to boxing, Sortland and Tysvaer (45) reported that approximately 33% of a sample of retired Norwegian international soccer players had widening of the lateral ventricles suggesting some form of generalized cerebral atrophy.

Magnetic resonance imaging (MRI) studies on boxers show a similar pattern of results as those using CT with the exception that MRI was able to detect subdural hematoma, white matter changes, and focal contusion not detected using CT (38, 46). MRI studies on young or amateur boxers consistently showed no change as a result of participation in their sport (42, 47, 48).

Recently, functional MRI (fMRI) and blood oxygen level dependent (BOLD) activity has been used to learn about the functional changes that can occur following concussion. One study compared symptomatic concussed athletes to a university student sample using a working memory task. Concussed athletes had areas of decreased activation compared to controls, such as the mid-dorsolateral prefrontal cortex. In addition, there was activation of regions beyond those of the control subjects in both temporal and parietal lobes (49). A prospective study on a small number of concussed athletes revealed differences from baseline brain activity using a number of cognitive tasks. Specifically, there was an increase in regions that were activated compared to baseline with greater signal intensity in these areas compared to baseline. Concussion induced differences in neural functioning were observed in the absence of behavioral deficits (50). These two small fMRI studies differed in methodology (between versus within subject designs) and in some of the results provided. There were two similarities: (a) Concussed athletes had a greater number of brain regions activated following concussion than did non-injured controls or the same athletes at baseline. This finding is consistent with recruitment of brain areas beyond those normally expected following concussion. (b) Both studies showed areas with greater levels of activation following concussion, however, Chen et al. reported a reduction in frontal lobe activity associated with working memory.

There are also few positron emission tomography (PET) and single photon emission computerized tomography (SPECT) studies on concussed athletes. The limited data on concussion in athletes suggests a pattern of frontal hypoactivation following injury. In amateur boxers, rCBF values were reported to be within the normal range while professional boxers had flow values that were below normal (51), especially in frontocentral regions (52). Other studies have revealed hypoperfusion in boxers (53). In general, there are differences in subjects and methodologies across studies that likely contribute to some of the discrepant findings. Nonetheless, there is some consistency across studies on blood flow following concussion suggesting hypoperfusion in the frontal lobes.

The electroencephalogram (EEG) has also been used to study concussion in athletes. Standard clinical EEG assessments revealed abnormalities associated with several years of involvement in boxing and soccer (e.g., 54–56). More recently, preliminary evidence for amplitude reductions across all standard frequency bands, especially during standing postures, were reported in 12 recently concussed athletes who were asymptomatic at the time of assessment (57). Similar reductions in gamma band activity were observed during a movement paradigm requiring a 50% maximal voluntary contraction (58).

In addition to EEG, there are a growing number of cognitive event-related potential (ERP) studies on concussed athletes. Although preliminary, the results suggest that these techniques may be of considerable benefit for the assessment of a single concussive event. One of the ERPs used in these studies was the N2/P3 or P300 response, a series of averaged EEG responses time-locked to a stimulus, with positive or negative peaks associated with different cognitive processes. P3 peak amplitude is believed to index allocation of attention (59, 60), while latency is related to stimulus evaluation and categorization time (61), transfer of information to consciousness and memory systems (60), and stimulus saliency (62).

Studies that used an auditory P3 paradigm have yielded mixed results. In one of these studies, five boxers were examined before and after a fight. Although several of the peaks showed no change in latency or amplitude, decreased amplitude was observed for the N2b peak (which precedes the P3 response) following the fights (63). Another study on amateur boxers reported no differences for auditory P3 latency or amplitude (64). In contrast, visual N2/P3 studies have yielded more consistent findings (65). In concussed athletes that were symptomatic, significant reductions in visual P3 amplitude were reported compared to recently concussed but asymptomatic athletes and never concussed athletes (66, 67). In addition, longer visual P3 peak latencies were correlated with self-reported attention and memory deficits in athletes with three or more concussions (68).

ERPs that precede movement have also been used experimentally to assess concussion in athletes. One of these studies showed negative results (68). Others have reported preliminary evidence for amplitude reductions using small numbers of concussed athletes in using a postural paradigm (69) and a movement paradigm requiring a 50% maximal voluntary contraction (58). Therefore, the electrophysiologic studies to date, while

experimental and preliminary, have revealed differences in brain function for some athletes with suspected cumulative effects, those who are symptomatic, and those with residual brain dysfunction beyond that indicated by self-reported symptoms.

NEUROPSYCHOLOGICAL OUTCOME

Many athletes with concussions have neurocognitive decrements as measured by traditional paper-pencil and computerized neuropsychological tests in the initial hours, days and potentially weeks post injury (15, 16, 24, 30, 70–76). In terms of group data, it has become a fairly robust finding that athletes tend to recover in terms of perceived symptoms and neuropsychological test performance within 2–14 days (1, 14, 15, 24, 77, 78).

In an NCAA prospective cohort study (14), 1,631 football players from 15 colleges completed preseason baseline testing during the 3 year study. Players with concussions (n = 94) and noninjured controls (n = 56) underwent assessment of symptoms, cognitive functioning, and postural stability immediately, 3 hours, and 1, 2, 3, 5, 7, and 90 days after injury. Concussed athletes' balance problems resolved within 3–5 days, self-reported postconcussion symptoms gradually resolved by day 7, and neurocognitive functioning improved within 5–7 days. By seven days post injury, 91% of athletes returned to personal baseline levels of symptom reporting.

Collins, Lovell, and Iverson recently have analyzed the results from a three-year, prospective, naturalistic, cohort study of high school football players. Participants were 2,141 high school athletes from Western Pennsylvania. During this 3-year study, 136 concussions were recorded and these athletes were carefully followed, clinically, until they were cleared to return to competition. The recovery rates were as follows: 1 week = 45%, 2 weeks = 73%, 3 weeks = 82%, 4 weeks = 91%, and 5 weeks = 97%. Thus, individual variability exists with recovery from sports concussion, especially in high school athletes, and the duration of symptoms can persist well beyond two weeks post injury.

Results from a six-year, prospective, National Football League concussion study have been published in a series of eight articles (9, 28, 78–83). A total of 887 concussions were recorded in 650 players during the study period. The time taken to return to play was as follows: (1) day of injury = 56.0%, (2) 1–6 days = 35.9%, (3) 7–14 days = 6.5%, and (4) more than 14 days = 1.6% (28). Those athletes who returned to play in the same game had fewer and briefer signs and symptoms of concussion, and they did not appear to have significantly increased risk for a second injury either in the same game or during the season (83).

A subset of concussed NFL players underwent baseline neuropsychological evaluations and then completed a second evaluation (N = 95) within a few days following their concussion (M = 1.4 days, SD = 1.3; (79)). The players did not show a single statistically significant decrement on any neuropsychological test when seen in the first few days post injury. These results, of course, are inconsistent with studies in both collegiate and high school athletes, where neurocognitive decrements are more pronounced. These results might reflect a selection bias (NFL athletes exhibit more rapid recovery, perhaps due to genetics/biological hardiness), or that age, and developmental factors may play a role in recovery from concussion. In fact, results from a recent study suggested that high school athletes might have slower recovery from concussive injury when compared to a matched collegiate sample (84).

In regards to cumulative effects, NFL athletes with a history of three or more concussions did not perform more poorly on neuropsychological testing than those with fewer than three (78). This finding, too, appears somewhat inconsistent with studies involving amateur athletes. Researchers have reported that three or more concussions in high school and university athletes are associated with small but measurable cumulative effects (34, 68, 85), and increased risk for future concussions (86, 87).

CUMULATIVE EFFECTS

Athletes, their families, coaches, athletic trainers, and sports medicine professionals are concerned about possible lingering effects, or permanent brain damage, resulting from multiple concussions. The literature on cumulative effects will be reviewed in detail in this section. When considering repeated subconcussive and concussive blows to the head, the most obvious athlete group to study is boxers. Few would debate that a *career* in boxing can result in obvious changes to the structure and function of the brain (38, 88–92). However, this may not be the case with amateur boxers. Professional boxing differs from amateur boxing in a number of ways: amateur boxers are typically not the elite in their weight-class, use headgear and larger gloves, and have fewer rounds per fight. Therefore, it is not surprising to observe differences between amateur and professional boxers, for example, on measures such as whole brain regional cerebral blood flow (rCBF) (51, 52).

Taken as a whole, studies on *amateur* boxers have offered mixed results regarding changes in brain structure and function. Significant changes in cerebral perfusion have been reported in amateur boxers compared to non-boxing athletic controls (53). On the other hand, a series of studies by Haglund and colleagues that compared high and low match amateur boxers versus athlete and non-athlete controls reported no differences on a mini-mental status

examination or platelet MAO activity (93), magnetic resonance imaging (MRI) or computed tomography (CT) (42), neuropsychologic testing (64), or auditory evoked or event-related potentials, with only slight or moderate electroencephalographic (EEG) deviations between high match boxers and athletic controls (94). Similarly, Porter (95) observed no statistical change in a group of 19 amateur boxers over a period of nine years using neuropsychological testing compared to non-boxing athletic controls.[1]

The literature on subconcussive blows to the head in other sports is also mixed. Some studies reported neuropsychological decrements (75) or temporary adverse effects immediately following repeatedly heading a soccer ball during practice (96). Other studies such as those associated with heading the soccer ball, tournament boxing,[2] or springboard diving generally suggest no statistically significant neuropsychological (6, 97–100) or balance effects (101).

Although the evidence regarding subconcussive effects is somewhat unclear, there is some evidence that a history of three or more concussions is associated with changes in cognitive neurophysiology (68), subjective symptoms (68, 102), and neuropsychological test performance (102). Furthermore, athletes with three or more concussions may be at increased risk of sustaining a future concussion (86), have worse on-field presentations of their next concussion (85), are more likely to have slowed recovery (86), and have greater acute changes in memory performance (102).

The literature regarding the persistent effects of two previous concussions is mixed. In regards to possible long-term effects, some researchers have reported significant findings (16, 103), others have not (68), and others reported equivocal results (e.g., 104). Further, no differences were observed on neuropsychological testing or symptom reporting for those with one versus two concussions (105). In a large-scale study, athletes with one or two previous concussions did not differ on neuropsychological testing or symptom reporting from athletes with no previous concussion on baseline, preseason testing (106). There is, however, preliminary evidence that athletes with two previous concussions have slower recovery times (86).

The studies indicating little or no change associated with subconcussive effects in boxers should be considered preliminary because they examine change over a short time frame (up to nine years) and do not take into account the possibility of long-term effects. This is important

---

[1] Sixty-six percent of the controls in this study were involved in some form of football with 28% reporting concussions.

[2] The study on boxers did not include those whose bout was stopped by the referee or those with epitaxis; boxers in these groups had increased simplex and choice reaction times compared to controls.

because the symptoms associated with chronic traumatic encephalopathy in boxers often show up later in life (107, 108). Similarly, the findings to date on three or more concussions should be considered preliminary – much additional research is needed because the aforementioned studies all have significant limitations in terms of methodology, generalizability, or both.

Pathophysiology of Cumulative Effects

Given that there is general agreement regarding the existence of some form of cumulative effects in some athletes, the question can be asked: What is the pathophysiologic basis of these injuries? Specifically, are the changes based in the functioning of previously injured neurons, genetic differences related to the susceptibility to cumulative effects, or some other form of measurable permanent change?

Researchers have reported that axons of cultured human neurons have a remarkable capacity for stretch with no primary axotomy observed with strains below 65% of the length of the axon. In addition, axons exhibit the behavior of "delayed elasticity". In other words, stretch causes a temporary deformation that gradually returns to the original orientation and morphology even though internal axonal damage was sustained (109). Once stretched, a pathophysiologic process begins that can lead to further structural change and metabolic dysfunction. First, strain on the axonal membrane causes an abnormal influx of Na^+ through mechanosensitive sodium channels, a reversal of the Na^+-Ca^{2+} exchangers, and activation of voltage gated Ca^{2+} channels (110). This in turn causes selective proteolysis or a breakdown of Na^+ channels and progressively increasing levels of intra-axonal Ca^{2+} (111). It is the massive influx of Ca^{2+} that leads to damage to the axonal cytoskeleton and initiates the formation of axonal swellings.

Using an animal optic nerve stretch model, it was determined that stretch below four mm did not cause any morphological change in axons, a stretch of five mm produced changes in visual evoked potentials that were significantly different from controls, with six mm stretch causing morphological change including retraction balls and axonal swellings (112). Therefore, there appears to be a progression following a single injury from no apparent change in structure or function, to functional change, to structural change in the axon based on the extent of stretch. However, researchers have reported that repetitive mild injuries using similar or *lower* levels of force than those used to produce single mild injuries caused a greater number of structural and functional changes. For example, when comparing animals that received two mild injuries (using lower levels of force) to those that sustained a single mild injury, the number of foci with injured axons in the frontal lobes was significantly

greater in the two injury group (113). In another study, two consecutive mild brain injuries three days apart produced a similar biochemical pattern as found in severe TBI while those separated by five days appeared as two distinct mild injuries (114). This study points out the possibility of a "critical window" where subsequent mild re-injury can lead to significant pathophysiological change. Further, repeated mild injuries have been shown to cause sublethal but significant biochemical markers of cellular injury and the production of neurites with a beaded and damaged appearance. In this study, it was noted that cells undergoing repeated injury resembled those that sustained a single injury produced with greater magnitudes of stretch (115).

Human studies on the pathophysiology of repeated mild injury are limited to case studies, usually in retired athletes with suspected permanent and significant brain damage (i.e., "chronic traumatic brain injury," "dementia pugilistica," or "punch-drunk syndrome"), a distinct clinical entity from Parkinsonism (116). Former athletes, usually boxers, with this serious condition often have slurred speech, ataxic gait, memory impairment, personality changes, and Parkinsonism. An autopsy on two boxers with repetitive brain injury related to participation in contact sport revealed neuronal cytoskeletal changes (117).

The preliminary evidence on cumulative effects has led some to ask whether athletes are at risk for developing dementia due to participation in their sport (118) and whether there is a genetic basis for cumulative effects (89)? These questions have evolved mostly from the sport of boxing. One of the more comprehensive studies on this topic assessed brain damage in 30 boxers with varying age and experience. All three boxers who exhibited evidence of severe brain damage or dysfunction had at least one copy of the APOE ε4 allele. This is compared with 50% of those with moderate damage, 25% of those with mild damage, and 18% of those with normal examinations. In addition, it was reported that there may be neuroprotective features associated with having the APOE ε2 allele (107). Kutner and colleagues reported that as a group, older players who had the APOE ε4 allele performed worse on cognitive testing than did all other players including those of the same age and younger players with the APOE ε4 allele (119).

Beyond studies on the genetic make-up of athletes, there is preliminary evidence that neuronal DNA itself can be altered following mild injuries in animals. Following MTBI in rats, cells with condensed nuclei, chromatin, and shrunken and round cell bodies were observed. On occasion these cells contained what appeared to be apoptotic cell bodies (120). Regarding cumulative effects, increased vulnerability of stretched neurons to a secondary insult (e.g., physical or biochemical) was associated with the production of reactive oxygen species (ROS) that were produced even when the stretch was sub-lethal. For example, the combination of mitochondrial ROS (superoxide) and nitric oxide (NO) into peroxynitrite leads to protein nitration, DNA degradation, and cell death. The DNA fragmentation seen in these cells was not considered apoptotic but was attributable to damage by reactive nitrogen species (121).

Second Impact Syndrome

Second impact syndrome is related to an *extraordinarily rare* cascade of events in which an athlete experiences a catastrophic brain injury following a seemingly mild concussion. In theory, sustaining a second brain injury during a period of increased vulnerability with unresolved metabolic dysfunction has been linked to second impact syndrome. The pathophysiologic basis for second impact syndrome is thought to be cerebrovascular congestion or a loss of cerebrovascular autoregulation leading to considerable brain swelling and edema (122, 123). It has been reported that relatively few athletes, approximately 35 or more in the years between 1980 and 1993, have succumbed to this syndrome (122). When it occurs, morbidity is 100% and mortality is reported to occur in up to 50% of cases (122). To date, most cases of second impact syndrome have been reported in children (e.g., 124) or adolescents (125, 126). Recent animal modeling has indicated that a single mTBI revealed transient and minimal impairment on a composite neuroscore test and minimal breach of the blood brain barrier. If a second mild injury was inflicted within 24-hours of the first injury, a marked breakdown of the blood brain barrier occurred leading to swelling and edema (127). This change in blood brain barrier integrity following a second concussive injury occurring shortly after the first may be a possible mechanism for the rapid swelling and edema formation that occurs in humans.

RECOVERY TIME AND RETURN TO PLAY DECISION-MAKING

Though significant individual variability exists in recovery from concussion, most group studies have indicated that a single concussion typically resolves in less than two weeks for most athletes (1, 14, 15, 24, 31, 77, 78). Current clinical experience and research has suggested that proper management of concussion should lead to a good prognosis in the vast majority of athletes. Most sports medicine researchers and professionals agree that returning an athlete to contact sport participation prior to complete recovery might increase the risk of poor outcome. Thus, the most important step a practitioner can take toward a positive prognosis is proper assessment and

management of concussion in the acute and follow-up stages of injury.

Concussion Grading Scales

Traditionally, return to play decisions were based partially on concussion grading scales that served to classify individual injuries according to severity and offer return to play guidelines. During the past thirty years, over twenty concussion management guidelines have been published with the intent of providing guidance and direction for the sports-medicine practitioner in making complex return to play decisions. The authors of each of these guidelines also provided an accompanying grading scale designed to reflect and characterize the severity of the injury. Although these guidelines have very likely resulted in improved care of the athlete, these multiple directives also created significant confusion and sparked almost continuous debate. A historical review of all past and current concussion guidelines is beyond the scope of this chapter, however, brief review of four of the more popular guidelines is provided in Table 24-3.

Cantu originally proposed his grading scale and management guidelines based on clinical experience (128). However, Cantu was careful to emphasize that these guidelines were intended to supplement rather than replace clinical judgment. The original Cantu guidelines allowed return to play the day of injury if the athlete was symptom free both at rest and following physical exertion. For athletes who experienced any loss of consciousness (e.g., grade 3 concussion), a restriction of contact for one month was recommended. Athletes who had suffered a Grade 2 concussion were allowed to return to play in two weeks, if asymptomatic for a period of 7 days.

The Colorado Guidelines (125) were published in 1991 following the death of a high school athlete due to presumed Second Impact Syndrome and were drafted under the auspices of the Colorado Medical Society. These guidelines allowed for same day return to play if symptoms cleared within 20 minutes of injury. For Grade 3 concussion, these guidelines recommended immediate transport to a hospital for further evaluation. These guidelines were later revised under the sponsorship of the American Academy of Neurology (18). The AAN guidelines allowed return to competition the same day of injury if the athlete's signs and symptoms cleared within 15 minutes of injury. Grade 2 concussion was managed in a manner similar to the Colorado Guidelines, with return to competition within one week, if asymptomatic.

More recently, Cantu has amended his guidelines to emphasize the duration of post-traumatic symptoms in grading the severity of the concussion and making return to play decisions (129). Grade 1 concussion was redefined by an absence of loss of consciousness, and post-concussion

TABLE 24-3
Recent Concussion Grading Scales

GUIDELINE	GRADE 1	GRADE 2	GRADE 3
Cantu (133)	1. No loss of consciousness 2. Posttraumatic amnesia last less than 30 minutes	1. Loss of consciousness lasts longer than 5 minutes OR 2. Posttraumatic amnesia lasts longer than 30 minutes	1. Loss of consciousness lasts longer than 5 minutes OR 2. Posttraumatic amnesia lasts longer than 24 hours
Colorado (125)	1. Confusion without amnesia 2. No loss of consciousness	1. Confusion with amnesia 2. No loss of consciousness	1. Loss of consciousness (of any duration)
AAN (18)	1. Transient confusion 2. No loss of consciousness 3. Concussion symptoms mental status changes resolve in less than 5 minutes	1. Transient confusion 2. No loss of consciousness 3. Concussion symptoms or mental status change lasts longer than 15 minutes	1. Loss of consciousness (brief or prolonged)
Cantu (129)	1. No loss of consciousness OR 2. Posttraumatic amnesia or signs/symptoms lasts longer than 30 minutes	1. Loss of consciousness lasts less than 1 minute OR 2. Posttraumatic amnesia lasts longer than 30 minutes but less than 24 hours	1. Loss of consciousness lasts more than 1 minute OR 2. Posttraumatic amnesia lasts longer than 24 hours OR 3. Post-concussion signs or symptoms last longer than 7 days

signs or symptoms lasting less than 30 minutes. Same day return to competition was allowed only if the athlete was completely asymptomatic following the injury.

The above mentioned management guidelines reached their peak popularity during the 1980's and 1990's. However, in the late 1990's, sports medicine practitioners and organizations began to question the scientific basis of these guidelines (130). This trend prompted the American Orthopaedic Society for Sports Medicine (AOSSM) to sponsor a workshop with the purpose of re-evaluating current guidelines and establishing practical alternatives (131). Although the AOSSM guidelines did not differ substantially from prior guidelines, this workshop started a trend away from the use of a numeric grading systems for determination of return to play following concussion (e.g., as developed by the Cantu, Colorado, and AAN guidelines). The AOSSM guidelines stressed more individualized management of injury, rather than applying general standards and protocols.

Current Return to Play Criteria

Currently, prevailing standards of care require an athlete to satisfy three conditions before returning to play. From the perspective of a sports medicine physician, the athlete should be asymptomatic at rest and during non-contact

exertion before return to play is indicated. Once asymptomatic at rest, the athlete is then progressed through increasing non-contact physical exertion, until he/she has demonstrated asymptomatic status with heavy non-contact physical exertion and non-contact sport-specific training. In addition, the athlete should demonstrate full recovery of cognitive function exhibited by his/her performance on a neuropsychological testing battery (if available).

Asymptomatic Status at Rest

Separately or in conjunction with administration of a neurocognitive test battery, the athlete should complete a symptom inventory (such as the Postconcusson Scale, see Table 24-4) or symptom interview both on the sideline (may be brief) and serially throughout recovery. Before progressing to any significant level of physical exertion, the athlete should report being asymptomatic at rest for at least 24 hours. If the athlete's report of asymptomatic status is suspected to be false, a careful discussion of the importance of reporting all symptoms should be initiated with the athlete. If there are others who present for evaluation with the athlete (e.g., parents, athletic trainers, or teammates), asking these third party informants about the athlete's previous or current symptom complaints might be helpful.

TABLE 24-4
Post-Concussion Scale

RATE YOUR SYMPTOMS OVER THE PAST 2 DAYS

SYMPTOM	NONE	MILD		MODERATE		SEVERE	
Headache	0	1	2	3	4	5	6
Nausea	0	1	2	3	4	5	6
Vomiting	0	1	2	3	4	5	6
Balance problems	0	1	2	3	4	5	6
Dizziness	0	1	2	3	4	5	6
Fatigue	0	1	2	3	4	5	6
Trouble falling asleep	0	1	2	3	4	5	6
Sleeping more than usual	0	1	2	3	4	5	6
Sleeping less than usual	0	1	2	3	4	5	6
Drowsiness	0	1	2	3	4	5	6
Sensitivity to light	0	1	2	3	4	5	6
Sensitivity to noise	0	1	2	3	4	5	6
Irritability	0	1	2	3	4	5	6
Sadness	0	1	2	3	4	5	6
Nervousness	0	1	2	3	4	5	6
Feeling more emotional	0	1	2	3	4	5	6
Numbness or tingling	0	1	2	3	4	5	6
Feeling slowed down	0	1	2	3	4	5	6
Feeling mentally "foggy"	0	1	2	3	4	5	6
Difficulty concentrating	0	1	2	3	4	5	6
Difficulty remembering	0	1	2	3	4	5	6
Visual problems	0	1	2	3	4	5	6

Asymptomatic Status with Physical Exertion

Once an athlete demonstrates asymptomatic status at rest, he or she should begin a graduated return to physical exertion prior to contact participation, because post-concussion difficulties might evolve with increased cerebral blood flow. The Vienna group and the Prague group have encouraged a graduated protocol (19, 132). Briefly, the protocol involves an athlete successfully moving through the following exertional steps in 24-hour periods: (1) light aerobic exercise (walking, stationary biking), (2) sport-specific training (ice skating in hockey, running in soccer- typically moderately exertional), and (3) non-contact training drills (usually heavily exertional). If the athlete's previously resolved post-concussion symptoms return at any point during the graded return to physical exertion, the athlete should return to the previous exertion level at which they were last asymptomatic.

Intact Neurocognitive Function (either compared to baseline or normative data)

Neurocognitive recovery can be considered achieved when the athlete's performance either returns to baseline levels or, in the absence of baseline, is consistent with premorbid estimates of functioning when the test data are compared to normative values (clinicians should utilize test batteries that have readily available athlete-specific norms).

Pre-season or baseline neuropsychological assessment can be very helpful for comparing post-injury functioning to "normal" functioning for the injured athlete. Some practitioners prefer to complete serial follow-up using computerized neuropsychological testing in order to gain insight into the extent and type of cognitive impairment created by the injury. The first test is often performed while the athlete remains symptomatic, then completed again once the athlete is asymptomatic to gauge progress and ensure a return to baseline or premorbid expectations of cognitive functioning. Other practitioners prefer to test the athlete when he/she is asymptomatic at rest and with heavy non-contact exertion, and prior to returning the athlete to any type of contact participation. This may maximize the chances that neuropsychological testing will only need to be performed once at follow-up.

Once the athlete is symptom free at rest and with physical exertion, as well as within expected levels on cognitive testing (if available), he/she may return to full-contact training, then to competition. Again, if any symptoms emerge with return to contact participation, the athlete should return to non-contact physical exertion.

CONCLUSIONS

This chapter was intended to be a comprehensive overview of concussion in sport, dealing with topics such as definitions, on-field/sideline presentation, pathophysiology, structural and functional imaging, neuropsychological outcome, cumulative effects, and return to play decision making. The pathophysiology of concussion has been conceptualized as a multilayered neurometabolic cascade (e.g., 22). The primary mechanisms include ionic shifts, abnormal energy metabolism, diminished cerebral blood flow, and impaired neurotransmission. Fortunately, the brain undergoes a dynamic restorative process in the initial days to weeks following a concussion. From a commonsense perspective, the ionic shifts, abnormal energy metabolism, diminished cerebral blood flow, and impaired neurotransmission believed to be associated with concussions in sports reinforces the importance of immediate rest following injury. Although not established empirically, it seems reasonable to assume that vigorous exercise or hard physical contact might exacerbate the pathophysiology described above.

Many athletes with concussions have neurocognitive decrements as measured by traditional paper-pencil and computerized neuropsychological tests in the initial hours, days, and potentially weeks post injury. In terms of group data, it has become a fairly robust finding that athletes tend to recover in terms of perceived symptoms and neuropsychological test performance within 2–14 days. However, individual variability exists in recovery rates, especially in high school athletes, and the duration of symptoms can persist well beyond two weeks post injury.

Researchers have reported that three or more concussions in high school and university athletes are associated with small but measurable cumulative effects, and increased risk for future concussions. The literature on subconcussive blows to the head, or the long-term effects of one or two previous concussions, is mixed. In general, there is insufficient evidence at this time to conclude that subconcussive blows or 1–2 previous concussions results in adverse long-term effects in the average athlete.

Ideally, athletes should satisfy three conditions before returning to play. The athlete should be asymptomatic at rest and during non-contact exertion. Once asymptomatic at rest, the athlete is then progressed through increasing non-contact physical exertion, until he/she has demonstrated asymptomatic status with heavy non-contact physical exertion and non-contact sport-specific training. In addition, the athlete should demonstrate full recovery of neurocognitive function exhibited by his/her performance on a neuropsychological testing battery (if available).

The management of sports-related concussion has evolved rapidly over the past decade and has been based on an explosion of laboratory and clinical research. Current prevailing models of assessing readiness for return to play following injury have been increasingly based on research studies rather than on panels of experts, which represented the zeitgeist in the 1980's and 1990's. Contemporary models of care have recognized the complexity of the recovery process following concussion and are beginning to consider the unique contribution of factors such as the athlete's age, developmental history, and past injury status in determining outcome. This recognition of the interplay between multiple variables is leading to the development of a much more sophisticated understanding of the recovery process; we anticipate that this will continue in the near future. Given the current trend towards research-based models of clinical care, we anticipate that concussion management will continue to grow and develop as our capacity for completing large-scale clinical research projects increases and we are able to meld this information with other advances in the neurosciences such as structural and functional neuroimaging and electrophysiological techniques.

References

1. Bleiberg J, Cernich AN, Cameron K et al. Duration of cognitive impairment after sports concussion. *Neurosurgery* 2004; 54: 1073–1078; discussion 1078–1080.
2. Hinton-Bayre AD, Geffen G, Friis P. Presentation and mechanisms of concussion in professional Rugby League Football. *J Sci Med Sport* 2004;7:400–404.
3. Koh JO, Cassidy JD. Incidence study of head blows and concussions in competition taekwondo. *Clin J Sport Med* 2004; 14: 72–79.
4. Koh JO, Cassidy JD, Watkinson EJ. Incidence of concussion in contact sports: a systematic review of the evidence. *Brain Inj* 2003;17:901–917.
5. Marshall SW, Spencer RJ. Concussion in Rugby: The Hidden Epidemic. *J Athl Train* 2001;36:334–338.
6. Rutherford A, Stephens R, Potter D. The neuropsychology of heading and head trauma in Association Football (soccer): a review. *Neuropsychol Rev* 2003;13:153–179.
7. Wennberg RA, Tator CH. National Hockey League reported concussions, 1986–87 to 2001–02. *Can J Neurol Sci* 2003; 30: 206–209.
8. Delaney JS. Head injuries presenting to emergency departments in the United States from 1990 to 1999 for ice hockey, soccer, and football. *Clin J Sport Med* 2004;14:80–87.
9. Pellman EJ, Powell JW, Viano DC et al. Concussion in professional football: epidemiological features of game injuries and review of the literature—part 3. *Neurosurgery* 2004;54:81–94; discussion 94–96.
10. Powell JW, Barber-Foss KD. Traumatic brain injury in high school athletes. *JAMA* 1999;282:958–963.
11. Schulz MR, Marshall SW, Mueller FO et al. Incidence and risk factors for concussion in high school athletes, North Carolina, 1996–1999. *Am J Epidemiol* 2004;160:937–944.
12. McCrea M, Hammeke T, Olsen G et al. Unreported concussion in high school football players: implications for prevention. *Clin J Sport Med* 2004;14:13–17.
13. Guskiewicz KM, Weaver NL, Padua DA et al. Epidemiology of concussion in collegiate and high school football players. *Am J Sports Med* 2000;28:643–650.
14. McCrea M, Guskiewicz KM, Marshall SW et al. Acute effects and recovery time following concussion in collegiate football players: the NCAA Concussion Study. *JAMA* 2003;290:2556–2563.

15. Macciocchi SN, Barth JT, Alves W et al. Neuropsychological functioning and recovery after mild head injury in collegiate athletes. *Neurosurgery* 1996;39:510–514.

16. Collins MW, Grindel SH, Lovell MR et al. Relationship between concussion and neuropsychological performance in college football players. *J Am Med Assoc* 1999;282:964–970.

17. Congress of Neurological Surgeons. Committee on head injury nomenclature: Glossary of head injury. *Clin Neurosurg* 1966;12:386–394.

18. American Academy of Neurology. Practice parameter: the management of concussion in sports (summary statement). Report of the Quality Standards Subcommittee. *Neurology* 1997;48:581–585.

19. McCrory P, Johnston K, Meeuwisse W et al. Summary and agreement statement of the 2nd International Conference on Concussion in Sport, Prague 2004. *Br J Sports Med* 2005;39:196–204.

20. Ommaya AK, Gennarelli TA. Cerebral concussion and traumatic unconsciousness. Correlation of experimental and clinical observations of blunt head injuries. *Brain* 1974;97:633–654.

21. Gaetz M. The neurophysiology of brain injury. *Clin Neurophysiol* 2004;115:4–18.

22. Giza CC, Hovda DA. The pathophysiology of traumatic brain injury. In: Lovell MR, Echemendia RJ, Barth JT, Collins MW, editors. *Traumatic Brain Injury in Sports.* Lisse: Swets & Zeitlinger, 2004. pp. 45–70.

23. Iverson GL. Outcome from mild traumatic brain injury. *Curr Opin Psychiat* 2005;18:301–317.

24. McCrea M, Kelly JP, Randolph C et al. Immediate neurocognitive effects of concussion. *Neurosurgery* 2002;50:1032–1040; discussion 1040–1032.

25. Iverson GL, Lovell MR, Smith SS. Does brief loss of consciousness affect cognitive functioning after mild head injury? *Arch Clin Neuropsychol* 2000;15:643–648.

26. Lovell MR, Iverson GL, Collins MW et al. Does loss of consciousness predict neuropsychological decrements after concussion? *Clin J Sport Med* 1999;9:193–198.

27. Asplund CA, McKeag DB, Olsen CH. Sport-Related Concussion: Factors Associated With Prolonged Return to Play. *Clin J Sport Med* 2004;14:339–343.

28. Pellman EJ, Viano DC, Casson IR et al. Concussion in Professional Football: Injuries Involving 7 or More Days Out-Part 5. *Neurosurgery* 2004;55:1100–1119.

29. Collins MW, Iverson GL, Lovell MR et al. On-field predictors of neuropsychological and symptom deficit following sports-related concussion. *Clin J Sport Med* 2003;13:222–229.

30. Guskiewicz KM, Ross SE, Marshall SW. Postural stability and neuropsychological deficits after concussion in collegiate athletes. *J Athl Train* 2001;36:263–273.

31. Lovell MR, Collins MW, Iverson GL et al. Recovery from mild concussion in high school athletes. *J Neurosurg* 2003;98:296–301.

32. Collins MW, Field M, Lovell MR et al. Relationship between postconcussion headache and neuropsychological test performance in high school athletes. *Am J Sports Med* 2003;31:168–173.

33. Mihalik JP, Stump JE, Collins MW et al. Posttraumatic migraine characteristics in athletes following sports-related concussion. *J Neurosurg* 2005;102:850–855.

34. Iverson GL, Gaetz M, Lovell MR et al. Relation between subjective fogginess and neuropsychological testing following concussion. *J Int Neuropsychol Soc* 2004;10:904–906.

35. Corsellis JA, Bruton CJ, Freeman-Browne D. The aftermath of boxing. *Psychol Med* 1973;3:270–303.

36. Casson IR, Siegel O, Sham R et al. Brain damage in modern boxers. *JAMA* 1984;251:2663–2667.

37. Casson IR, Sham R, Campbell EA et al. Neurological and CT evaluation of knocked-out boxers. *J Neurol Neurosurg Psychiatry* 1982;45:170–174.

38. Jordan BD, Zimmerman RD. Computed tomography and magnetic resonance imaging comparisons in boxers. *JAMA* 1990; 263:1670–1674.

39. Jordan BD, Jahre C, Hauser WA et al. CT of 338 active professional boxers. *Radiology* 1992;185:509–512.

40. Bogdanoff B, Natter HM. Incidence of cavum septum pellucidum in adults: a sign of boxer's encephalopathy. *Neurology* 1989; 39:991–992.

41. Ross RJ, Cole M, Thompson JS et al. Boxers—computed tomography, EEG, and neurological evaluation. *JAMA* 1983;249: 211–213.

42. Haglund Y, Bergstrand G. Does Swedish amateur boxing lead to chronic brain damage? 2. A retrospective study with CT and MRI. *Acta Neurol Scand* 1990;82:297–302.

43. McLatchie G, Brooks N, Galbraith S et al. Clinical neurological examination, neuropsychology, electroencephalography and computed tomographic head scanning in active amateur boxers. *J Neurol Neurosurg Psychiatry* 1987;50:96–99.

44. Sironi VA, Scotti G, Ravagnati L et al. CT-scan and EEG findings in professional pugilists: early detection of cerebral atrophy in young boxers. *J Neurosurg Sci* 1982;26:165–168.

45. Sortland O, Tysvaer AT. Brain damage in former association football players. An evaluation by cerebral computed tomography. *Neuroradiology* 1989;31:44–48.

46. Autti T, Sipila L, Autti H et al. Brain lesions in players of contact sports. *Lancet* 1997;349:1144.

47. Levin HS, Lippold SC, Goldman A et al. Neurobehavioral functioning and magnetic resonance imaging findings in young boxers. *J Neurosurg* 1987;67:657–667.

48. Jordan BD, Zimmerman RD. Magnetic resonance imaging in amateur boxers. *Arch Neurol* 1988;45:1207–1208.

49. Chen JK, Johnston KM, Frey S et al. Functional abnormalities in symptomatic concussed athletes: an fMRI study. *Neuroimage* 2004;22:68–82.

50. Jantzen KJ, Anderson B, Steinberg FL et al. A prospective functional MR imaging study of mild traumatic brain injury in college football players. *AJNR Am J Neuroradiol* 2004; 25: 738–745.

51. Rodriguez G, Ferrilo F, Montano V et al. Regional cerebral blood flow in boxers. *Lancet* 1983;Oct. 8:858.

52. Rodriguez G, Vitali P, Nobili F. Long-term effects of boxing and judo-choking techniques on brain function. *Ital J Neurol Sci* 1998;19:367–372.

53. Kemp PM, Houston AS, Macleod MA et al. Cerebral perfusion and psychometric testing in military amateur boxers and controls. *J Neurol Neurosurg Psychiatry* 1995;59:368–374.

54. Kaplan HA, Browder J. Observations on the clinical and brain wave patterns of professional boxers. *J Am Med Assoc* 1954; 156:1138–1144.

55. Kross R, Ohler K, Barolin GS. Cerebral trauma due to heading – Computerized EEG analysis of football players. *EEG-EMG* 1983;14:209–212.

56. Tysvaer AT, Storli OV. Soccer injuries to the brain. A neurologic and electroencephalographic study of active football players. *Am J Sports Med* 1989;17:573–578.

57. Thompson J, Sebastianelli W, Slobounov S. EEG and postural correlates of mild traumatic brain injury in athletes. *Neurosci Lett* 2005;377:158–163.

58. Slobounov S, Sebastianelli W, Simon R. Neurophysiological and behavioral concomitants of mild brain injury in collegiate athletes. *Clin Neurophysiol* 2002;113:185–193.

59. Duncan-Johnson CC, Donchin E. On quantifying surprise: the variation of event-related potentials with subjective probability. *Psychophysiol* 1977;14:456–467.

60. Picton TW. The P300 wave of the human event-related potential. *J Clin Neurophysiol* 1992;9:456–479.

61. Kutas M, McCarthy G, Donchin E. Augmenting mental chronometry: the P300 as a measure of stimulus evaluation time. *Science* 1977;197:792–795.

62. Polich J. Attention, probability, and task demands as determinants of P300 latency from auditory stimuli. *Electroencephalogr Clin Neurophysiol* 1986;63:251–259.

63. Breton F, Pincemaille Y, Tarriere C et al. Event-related potential assessment of attention and the orienting reaction in boxers before and after a fight. *Biol Psychol* 1991;31:57–71.

64. Murelius O, Haglund Y. Does Swedish amateur boxing lead to chronic brain damage? 4. A retrospective neuropsychological study. *Acta Neurol Scand* 1991;83:9–13.

65. Gaetz M, Bernstein DM. The current status of electrophysiologic procedures for the assessment of mild traumatic brain injury. *J Head Trauma Rehabil* 2001;16:386–405.

66. Dupuis F, Johnston KM, Lavoie ME et al. Concussion in athletes produce brain dysfunction as revealed by event-related potentials. *NeuroReport* 2000;11:4087–4092.

67. Lavoie ME, Dupuis F, Johnston KM et al. Visual p300 effects beyond symptoms in concussed college athletes. *J Clin Exp Neuropsychol* 2004;26:55–73.

68. Gaetz M, Goodman D, Weinberg H. Electrophysiological evidence for the cumulative effects of concussion. *Brain Inj* 2000; 14:1077–1088.

69. Slobounov S, Sebastianelli W, Moss R. Alteration of posture-related cortical potentials in mild traumatic brain injury. *Neurosci Lett* 2005;383:251–255.

70. Barr WB, McCrea M. Sensitivity and specificity of standardized neurocognitive testing immediately following sports concussion. *J Int Neuropsychol Soc* 2001;7:693–702.

71. Delaney JS, Lacroix VJ, Gagne C et al. Concussions among university football and soccer players: a pilot study. *Clin J Sport Med* 2001;11:234–240.

72. Erlanger D, Feldman D, Kutner K et al. Development and validation of a web-based neuropsychological test protocol for sports-related return-to-play decision-making. *Arch Clin Neuropsychol* 2003;18:293–316.

73. Erlanger D, Saliba E, Barth J et al. Monitoring resolution of postconcussion symptoms in athletes: Preliminary results of a web-based neuropsychological test protocol. *J Athl Train* 2001;36: 280–287.

74. Makdissi M, Collie A, Maruff P et al. Computerised cognitive assessment of concussed Australian Rules footballers. *Br J Sports Med* 2001;35:354–360.

75. Matser JT, Kessels AG, Lezak MD et al. A dose-response relation of headers and concussions with cognitive impairment in professional soccer players. *J Clin Exp Neuropsychol* 2001;23:770–774.

76. Warden DL, Bleiberg J, Cameron KL et al. Persistent prolongation of simple reaction time in sports concussion. *Neurology* 2001;57:524–526.

77. Lovell MR, Collins MW, Iverson GL et al. Grade 1 or "ding" concussions in high school athletes. *Am J Sports Med* 2004;32:47–54.

78. Pellman EJ, Lovell MR, Viano DC et al. Concussion in professional football: neuropsychological testing-part 6. *Neurosurgery* 2004;55:1290–1305.

79. Pellman EJ, Viano DC, Casson IR et al. Concussion in professional football: repeat injuries—part 4. *Neurosurgery* 2004;55:860–873; discussion 873–866.

80. Pellman EJ. Background on the National Football League's research on concussion in professional football. *Neurosurgery* 2003;53:797–798.

81. Pellman EJ, Viano DC, Tucker AM et al. Concussion in professional football: location and direction of helmet impacts-Part 2. *Neurosurgery* 2003;53:1328–1340; discussion 1340–1321.

82. Pellman EJ, Viano DC, Tucker AM et al. Concussion in professional football: reconstruction of game impacts and injuries. *Neurosurgery* 2003;53:799–812; discussion 812–814.

83. Pellman EJ, Viano DC, Casson IR et al. Concussion in professional football: players returning to the same game-part 7. *Neurosurgery* 2005;56:79–92.

84. Field M, Collins MW, Lovell MR et al. Does age play a role in recovery from sports-related concussion? A comparison of high school and collegiate athletes. *J Pediatr* 2003;142:546–553.

85. Collins MW, Lovell MR, Iverson GL et al. Cumulative effects of concussion in high school athletes. *Neurosurgery* 2002; 51:1175–1179; discussion 1180–1171.

86. Guskiewicz KM, McCrea M, Marshall SW et al. Cumulative effects associated with recurrent concussion in collegiate football players: the NCAA Concussion Study. *JAMA* 2003; 290: 2549–2555.

87. Zemper ED. Two-year prospective study of relative risk of a second cerebral concussion. *Am J Phys Med Rehabil* 2003;82: 653–659.

88. Zhang L, Ravdin LD, Relkin N et al. Increased diffusion in the brain of professional boxers: a preclinical sign of traumatic brain injury? *AJNR Am J Neuroradiol* 2003;24:52–57.

89. Rabadi MH, Jordan BD. The cumulative effect of repetitive concussion in sports. *Clin J Sport Med* 2001;11:194–198.

90. Dale GE, Leigh PN, Luthert P et al. Neurofibrillary tangles in dementia pugilistica are ubiquitinated. *J Neurol Neurosurg Psychiatry* 1991;54:116–118.

91. Roberts GW, Allsop D, Bruton C. The occult aftermath of boxing. *J Neurol Neurosurg Psychiatry* 1990;53:373–378.

92. Miele VJ, Carson L, Carr A et al. Acute on chronic subdural hematoma in a female boxer: a case report. *Med Sci Sports Exerc* 2004;36:1852–1855.

93. Haglund Y, Edman G, Murelius O et al. Does Swedish amateur boxing lead to chronic brain damage? 1. A retrospective medical, neurological and personality trait study. *Acta Neurol Scand* 1990;82:245–252.

94. Haglund Y, Persson HE. Does Swedish amateur boxing lead to chronic brain damage? 3. A retrospective clinical neurophysiological study. *Acta Neurol Scand* 1990;82:353–360.

95. Porter MD. A 9-year controlled prospective neuropsychologic assessment of amateur boxing. *Clin J Sport Med* 2003; 13:339–352.

96. Schmitt DM, Hertel J, Evans TA et al. Effect of an acute bout of soccer heading on postural control and self-reported concussion symptoms. *Int J Sports Med* 2004;25:326–331.

97. Moriarity J, Collie A, Olson D et al. A prospective controlled study of cognitive function during an amateur boxing tournament. *Neurology* 2004;62:1497–1502.

98. Putukian M, Echemendia RJ, Mackin S. The acute neuropsychological effects of heading in soccer: a pilot study. *Clin J Sport Med* 2000;10:104–109.

99. Zillmer EA. The neuropsychology of repeated 1- and 3-meter springboard diving among college athletes. *Appl Neuropsychol* 2003;10:23–30.

100. Straume-Naesheim TM, Andersen TE, Dvorak J et al. Effects of heading exposure and previous concussions on neuropsychological performance among Norwegian elite footballers. *Br J Sports Med* 2005;39 Suppl 1:i70–77.

101. Mangus BC, Wallmann HW, Ledford M. Analysis of postural stability in collegiate soccer players before and after an acute bout of heading multiple soccer balls. *Sports Biomech* 2004;3:209–220.

102. Iverson GL, Gaetz M, Lovell MR et al. Cumulative effects of concussion in amateur athletes. *Brain Inj* 2004;18:433–443.

103. Moser RS, Schatz P, Jordan BD. Prolonged effects of concussion in high school athletes. *Neurosurgery* 2005;57:300–306; discussion 300–306.

104. Moser RS, Schatz P. Enduring effects of concussion in youth athletes. *Arch Clin Neuropsychol* 2002;17:91–100.

105. Macciocchi SN, Barth JT, Littlefield L et al. Multiple Concussions and Neuropsychological Functioning in Collegiate Football Players. *J Athl Train* 2001;36:303–306.

106. Iverson GL, Brooks BL, Lovell MR et al. No cumulative effects for one or two previous concussions. *Br J Sports Med* in press.

107. Jordan BD, Relkin NR, Ravdin LD et al. Apolipoprotein E epsilon4 associated with chronic traumatic brain injury in boxing. *JAMA* 1997;278:136–140.

108. Omalu BI, DeKosky ST, Minster RL et al. Chronic traumatic encephalopathy in a National Football League player. *Neurosurgery* 2005;57:128–134; discussion 128–134.

109. Smith DH, Wolf JA, Lusardi TA et al. High tolerance and delayed elastic response of cultured axons to dynamic stretch injury. *J Neurosci* 1999;19:4263–4269.

110. Wolf JA, Stys PK, Lusardi T et al. Traumatic axonal injury induces calcium influx modulated by tetrodotoxin-sensitive sodium channels. *J Neurosci* 2001;21:1923–1930.

111. Iwata A, Stys PK, Wolf JA et al. Traumatic axonal injury induces proteolytic cleavage of the voltage-gated sodium channels modulated by tetrodotoxin and protease inhibitors. *J Neurosci* 2004;24:4605–4613.

112. Bain AC, Raghupathi R, Meaney DF. Dynamic stretch correlates to both morphological abnormalities and electrophysiological impairment in a model of traumatic axonal injury. *J Neurotrauma* 2001;18:499–511.

113. Raghupathi R, Mehr MF, Helfaer MA et al. Traumatic axonal injury is exacerbated following repetitive closed head injury in the neonatal pig. *J Neurotrauma* 2004;21:307–316.

114. Vagnozzi R, Signoretti S, Tavazzi B et al. Hypothesis of the postconcussive vulnerable brain: experimental evidence of its

metabolic occurrence. *Neurosurgery* 2005;57:164–171; discussion 164–171.

115. Slemmer JE, Matser EJ, De Zeeuw CI et al. Repeated mild injury causes cumulative damage to hippocampal cells. *Brain* 2002;125:2699–2709.

116. Davie CA, Pirtosek Z, Barker GJ et al. Magnetic resonance spectroscopic study of parkinsonism related to boxing. *J Neurol Neurosurg Psychiatry* 1995;58:688–691.

117. Geddes JF, Vowles GH, Nicoll JA et al. Neuronal cytoskeletal changes are an early consequence of repetitive head injury. *Acta Neuropathol (Berl)* 1999;98:171–178.

118. Spear J. Are professional footballers at risk of developing dementia? *Int J Geriatr Psychiatry* 1995;10:1011–1014.

119. Kutner KC, Erlanger DM, Tsai J et al. Lower cognitive performance of older football players possessing apolipoprotein E epsilon4. *Neurosurgery* 2000;47:651–657; discussion 657–658.

120. Raghupathi R, Conti AC, Graham DI et al. Mild traumatic brain injury induces apoptotic cell death in the cortex that is preceded by decreases in cellular Bcl-2 immunoreactivity. *Neuroscience* 2002;110:605–616.

121. Arundine M, Aarts M, Lau A et al. Vulnerability of central neurons to secondary insults after in vitro mechanical stretch. *J Neurosci* 2004;24:8106–8123.

122. Cantu RC. Second-impact syndrome. *Clin Sports Med* 1998;17:37–44.

123. Kelly JP, Rosenberg JH. Diagnosis and management of concussion in sports. *Neurology* 1997;48:575–580.

124. Bruce DA, Alavi A, Bilaniuk L et al. Diffuse cerebral swelling following head injuries in children: the syndrome of "malignant brain edema". *J Neurosurg* 1981;54:170–178.

125. Kelly JP, Nichols JS, Filley CM et al. Concussion in sports. Guidelines for the prevention of catastrophic outcome. *JAMA* 1991;266:2867–2869.

126. McQuillen JB, McQuillen EN, Morrow P. Trauma, sport, and malignant cerebral edema. *Am J Forensic Med Pathol* 1988;9:12–15.

127. Laurer HL, Bareyre FM, Lee VM et al. Mild head injury increasing the brain's vulnerability to a second concussive impact. *J Neurosurg* 2001;95:859–870.

128. Cantu RC. Cerebral concussion in sport. Management and prevention. *Sports Med* 1992;14:64–74.

129. Cantu RC. Posttraumatic Retrograde and Anterograde Amnesia: Pathophysiology and Implications in Grading and Safe Return to Play. *J Athl Train* 2001;36:244–248.

130. Collins MW, Lovell MR, McKeag DB. Current issues in managing sports-related concussion. *J Am Med Assoc* 1999;282:2283–2285.

131. Wojtys EM, Hovda D, Landry G et al. Current concepts. Concussion in sports. *Am J Sports Med* 1999;27:676–687.

132. Aubry M, Cantu R, Dvorak J et al. Summary and agreement statement of the First International Conference on Concussion in Sport, Vienna 2001. Recommendations for the improvement of safety and health of athletes who may suffer concussive injuries. *Br J Sports Med* 2002;36:6–10.

133. Cantu RC. Guidelines for return to contact sports after a cerebral concussion. *Physician Sportsmed* 1986;14:75–83.

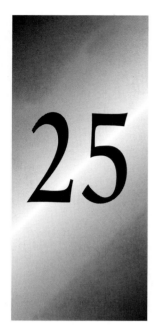

25 Assessment and Rehabilitative Management of Individuals with Disorders of Consciousness

Joseph T. Giacino
Douglas I. Katz
Nicholas Schiff

There has been a resurgence of interest and scientific inquiry concerning disorders of consciousness (DOC) over the last decade. American and European initiatives have led to the development of guidelines for assessment, prognosis and rehabilitation of individuals in coma and the vegetative state (VS) (1–3) and have contributed to the formulation of neurobehavioral criteria for the minimally conscious state (MCS) (4). These initiatives, coupled with the development of improved behavioral and neuroimaging assessment procedures, have fostered increasing consensus regarding conceptual and empirical approaches to understanding DOC.

This chapter will review and critique the major developments in this area that have influenced the clinical management of DOC. Following a review of the diagnostic criteria associated with coma, VS and MCS, new insights garnered from functional neuroimaging studies into the pathophysiology of these disorders will be discussed. Behavioral and radiologic assessment techniques developed specifically for this population will be discussed in relation to diagnostic and prognostic utility. Medical, environmental and neuromodulatory interventions designed to facilitate recovery of cognition will be reviewed and discussed relative to efficacy. Clinical predictors of outcome will be outlined, with particular attention to differences between individuals diagnosed with VS and MCS and general recommendations for clinical management will be outlined. Finally, ethical issues will be defined and future directions for research proposed.

DEFINITIONS AND DIAGNOSTIC CRITERIA

Numerous terms have been offered to characterize states of altered consciousness, many of which have not been operationalized (see table 25-1). Not surprisingly, estimates of misdiagnosis among disorders of consciousness range from 15% to 43% (5–7). In recognition of this problem, a multi-disciplinary group was assembled in 1995 through the auspices of the Aspen Neurobehavioral Conference to formulate a consensus statement regarding the diagnostic and prognostic criteria for coma, VS and MCS. The recommendations of the Aspen Group were subsequently endorsed by the American Academy of Physical Medicine and Rehabilitation, the American Association of Neurologic Surgeons, the American Congress of Rehabilitation Medicine, the Brain Injury Association of America. and the Child Neurology Society. The definition and diagnostic criteria for MCS, crafted by the Aspen Group, was published in 2002 in *Neurology*, the official journal of the American Academy of Neurology (4).

TABLE 25-1
Terms Used to Refer to Disorders of Consciousness

Akinetic mutism	Minimally responsive state
Apallic syndrome	Permanent vegetative state
Coma	Persistent vegetative state
Coma vigil	Post coma unawareness
Cognitive death	Prolonged coma
Decerebrate state	Prolonged post-traumatic
	unconsciousness
Low level	Vegetative state
Minimally conscious state	

Coma

Coma is a state of pathologic unconsciousness in which the eyes remain closed and the patient cannot be aroused (8). It is most often the result of severe, diffuse bihemispheric lesions of the cortex or underlying white matter, bilateral thalamic damage or paramedian tegmental lesions. The clinical criteria for diagnosing coma were described by Plum and Posner in 1982 (9) and remain well accepted. The defining feature of coma is the complete loss of spontaneous or stimulus-induced arousal. The eyes remain continuously closed despite the application of noxious stimuli and there are no sleep/wake cycles on EEG. On examination, there is no evidence of purposeful motor activity, no response to command and no indication of receptive or expressive language ability. Coma is a self-limiting state that typically resolves within two to four weeks in those who survive the initial injury.

Vegetative State (VS)

The vegetative state has been mired in controversy since it was first introduced by Jennett and Plum (10) more than 30 years ago. The term itself is controversial because it is considered to be pejorative by the lay public, and because clinicians have not been able to agree on the prognostic parameters associated with this diagnosis. VS is a condition in which awareness of self and environment is presumed to be absent and there is an inability to interact with others, although the capacity for spontaneous or stimulus-induced arousal is preserved (11). VS typically follows a period of coma but may also arise from developmental malformations or may represent the culmination of progressive degenerative or metabolic disorders. The neuropathologic substrate is usually determined by the cause of injury. Diffuse axonal injury is the most common finding in post-traumatic VS. Vascular causes of VS are often associated with paramedial thalamic damage and diffuse laminar cortical necrosis is frequently noted following anoxic brain injury. The diagnosis of VS is made when there is no evidence of sustained or reproducible, purposeful behavioral responses to visual, auditory, tactile or noxious stimuli, and no evidence of language comprehension or expression. Unlike coma, intermittent periods of wakefulness (i.e. eye opening) occur in VS and represent functional restoration of the reticular system.

The term *persistent* VS (PVS) remains controversial, in part, because it has been used inconsistently in the medical literature. The most current practice parameter on PVS published in 1995 by the American Academy of Neurology (1) stipulates that PVS can be diagnosed after one month following either traumatic or non-traumatic brain injury. After reviewing the published literature on PVS, the AAN introduced a new term, *permanent* VS, suggesting that this term be applied three months after non-traumatic brain injury, and after twelve months following traumatic injury. The distinction between persistent and permanent VS is intended to establish the point after which recovery of consciousness is highly improbable.

According to the AAN practice parameter, PVS is a diagnostic term and does not imply irreversibility. In view of the inconsistent application of PVS and the high rate of recovery of consciousness that occurs between three and twelve months post-injury in individuals who remain in VS longer than one month (12, 13), the Aspen Group recommended that the term PVS be abandoned. Instead, they proposed that when the diagnosis of VS is made, it should routinely be accompanied by a description of the injury and the length of time since onset as both of these factors provide prognostic information (14).

Minimally Conscious State (MCS)

MCS is a condition of severely altered consciousness in which there is minimal but definite behavioral evidence of self or environmental awareness (4). MCS usually represents a transitional state reflecting improvement in consciousness from coma or VS, or progressive decline as in neurodegenerative disease (e.g., Alzheimer's disease). The natural history and long term outcome have not been fully characterized, however, at least ten papers have been published on MCS since this condition was defined in 2002. The neuropathologic substrate of post-traumatic MCS was recently investigated in a post-mortem analysis completed by Jennett and colleagues (15) who found that the typical lesion profile consists of grade 2 or 3 diffuse axonal injury with multi-focal cortical contusions, sometimes accompanied by thalamic involvement. In comparison to patients diagnosed with VS, thalamic lesions were notably less prevalent in MCS (50%) relative to VS (80%). Based on these findings, MCS appears to be characterized by greater sparing of cortico-thalamic connections which may account for why patients in MCS retain some capacity for cognitive processing.

The diagnosis of MCS is based on clearly discernible evidence of one or more of the following behaviors: 1) simple command-following, 2) intelligible verbalization,

3) recognizable verbal or gestural "yes/no" responses (without regard to accuracy) or 4) movements or emotional responses that are triggered by relevant environmental stimuli and cannot be attributed to reflexive activity. Examples of the fourth criterion include a) smiling or crying following exposure to emotional (e.g., family photographs) but not neutral stimuli (e.g., photographs of objects), b) vocalizations or gestures that occur in direct response to specific linguistic prompts, c) accurate reaching toward objects placed within the immediate visual field, d) manipulation of objects placed in the hand and e) sustained visual fixation or pursuit eye movements.

In making the diagnosis of MCS, it is important to consider the frequency and complexity of the behavior observed. When there is evidence of rudimentary cognition only (e.g., inconsistent visual tracking), the diagnosis of MCS requires serial reassessment. At the opposite end of the MCS spectrum, patients who demonstrate consistent evidence of complex cognitively-mediated behavior (e.g., command following) fall at the upper limit of MCS.

Within the diagnostic category of MCS, there is a subgroup of patients whose behavior is difficult to characterize, both from a practical as well as theoretical standpoint. Some MCS patients infrequently initiate behavior or respond to environmental prompts, but on occasion, exhibit behaviors that infer complex cognitive processing (e.g., follow countermanding or go-no go commands). It is not unusual for these individuals to show marked fluctuations in behavioral responsiveness across examinations. We recently evaluated an individual who was able to provide reliable responses to a series of yes/no questions during the initial examination. On follow up examination conducted 24 hours later, responses to the same questions were inconsistent and unreliable. There is little agreement as to whether patients who infrequently engage in complex responses should be included in the MCS category. It is often difficult to determine whether the low rate of behavioral responsiveness observed in these individuals is primarily due to sensory limitations, motor dysfunction, abulia or fluctuations in level of consciousness.

Emergence from MCS

Emergence from MCS is signaled by the recovery of interactive communication or functional object use. In contradistinction to MCS, emergence from MCS requires *reliable and consistent* evidence of either communication or object use. Communication may occur through verbal responses, gestural means or augmentative devices. "Functional object use" requires discrimination among items presented (e.g., comb brought to head and toothbrush to mouth). Aphasia and apraxia must be ruled out as contributing or causative factors in patients who don't meet the criteria for reliable communication ability or functional object use.

The last ten years have witnessed movement toward achieving universally agreed upon terminology for disorders of consciousness. This is an essential step in assuring accurate diagnosis and promoting well-informed treatment decisions. Unless there is a common frame of reference to guide research and clinical practice, the difficulties inherent in evaluating and treating disorders of consciousness will prove insurmountable.

PATHOPHYSIOLOGY AND NEUROIMAGING

Neuropathology of VS and MCS

Traumatic and non-traumatic VS have distinct and identifiable pathologies. Adams et al. (16) studied 49 patients remaining in VS for at least one month until death and found that non-traumatic injuries included severe bilateral thalamic damage in all instances and, in the majority of cases, were associated with diffuse cortical damage. In contrast, traumatic etiologies associated with VS showed grade 2 and 3 diffuse axonal injuries and severe thalamic degeneration in almost all of patients who survived for 3 months before death. These pathological studies confirm the intuition that the chronic vegetative state is characterized by overwhelming cerebral damage. An important conclusion that is often overlooked is that the most consistent and severe pathologies arising from both types of injuries are in subcortical structures, particularly the thalamus. The cerebral cortex is generally spared in traumatic VS, with only about 10% of patients showing diffuse ischemic neocortical injury patterns; brainstem damage is uncommon in chronic VS patients emphasizing that VS is primarily a disorder of cerebral integration at the thalamocortical level.

No comprehensive study has evaluated specific anatomic pathologies associated with MCS. Jennett and colleagues (17) reported 65 autopsies of patients with traumatic brain injury leading either to VS or severe disability and found wide variation in underlying neuroanatomical substrates. This study included 12 patients with histories consistent with MCS at the time of death. Of note, two of the MCS patients demonstrated only focal brain injures, without DAI or focal thalamic infarction (a consistent finding in approximately half of the severely disabled patients). Further work to determine the pathological correlates of MCS is required.

Functional Neuroimaging Studies

Several new brain imaging techniques are providing important insight into the mechanisms of neurological disorders of consciousness. Functional MRI (fMRI) and functional positron emission tomography (^{15}O-PET) studies respectively correlate changes in blood oxygen level and cerebral blood flow with neuronal activation.

Precise correlational studies of single-unit and multi-unit neuronal recordings from brain regions simultaneously studied using fMRI techniques indicate that fMRI signal activations are tightly correlated with neuronal population activity (18). These findings support the use of both fMRI and ^{15}O-PET activations as a proxy for neuronal activation *per se*. Brain metabolism can also be quantified in neuroimaging studies using fluorodeoxyglucose positron emission tomography (FDG-PET) imaging, a measure of cerebral glucose metabolic rates. FDG-PET studies in patients with Parkinson's disease have correlated regional glucose metabolism with neuronal firing rates in cerebral structures (19). Direct measurements of cerebral metabolism and neuronal activity demonstrate a rough equivalence of metabolic rate and mean firing rate of population of neurons (20). Combined with traditional structural MRI imaging and EEG (or magnetoencephalography, MEG, recordings obtained from measurements of the brain magnetic field) these techniques offer an integrative view of the damaged brain.

Pet Studies   The clinical judgment of unconsciousness in PVS was first supported in imaging studies by fluorodeoxyglucose positron emission tomography (FDG-PET) studies that revealed overall cerebral metabolism to be reduced by 50% or more below normal levels in PVS patients (21–24). More recently, Schiff and colleagues used functional brain imaging techniques including fluoro-deoxyglucose-positron-emission tomography (FDG-PET), magnetoencephalography (MEG) and magnetic resonance imaging (MRI) were combined with clinical assessments (25, 26). These studies identified novel evidence of the modular organization of brain systems in three patients who retained small islands of cerebral metabolic activity that correlated with clinically identified behavioral fragments. In one case, a 42 year old male diagnosed with post-traumatic VS of seven years duration, repeatedly displayed selective emotional responses following exposure to specific environmental events. He exhibited pronounced eye and mouth-opening, pupillary dilatation and groaning when touched or presented with loud noise, giving the appearance of grave distress. Conversely, when exposed to soft music or his mother's soothing voice, he showed signs of sympathetic and behavioral relaxation. PET data indicated that the patient's global resting metabolic rate was approximately 30% of normal, however, the right putamen, caudate, orbitofrontal cortex, lateral and superior temporal cortex showed elevated metabolism up to nearly 50% of normal levels. When correlated with the behavioral findings, the PET results appeared to reflect partial preservation of the neural network responsible for receptive prosody.

Several investigators have employed ^{15}O-PET imaging techniques to the evaluate PVS patients. Laureys and colleagues have identified a marked loss of distributed network processing in the vegetative state (27–29). In their studies, elementary auditory and somatosensory stimuli were presented to PVS patients and normal control subjects and compared to baseline resting conditions in ^{15}O-PET subtraction paradigms; PVS patients demonstrated a loss of brain activations outside of primary sensory cortices for both types of stimuli. Cortical regions identified as 'hierarchically higher-order' multi-modal association areas active in the normal control subjects did not activate in the PVS patients. Laureys et al.'s findings are consistent with evidence of early sensory processing in PVS patients as measured by evoked potential studies and add important additional information about the integrity of cerebral information processing in PVS. Menon and colleagues (30) described a 26 year old woman in a persistent vegetative state (PVS) four months following an attack of acute disseminated encephalomyelitis that functionally impaired both cortical and subcortical (brainstem and thalamic) structures. Right occipital-temporal regions in this patient demonstrated selective activation of the right fusiform gyrus and extrastriate visual association areas with visual stimulation. These results were obtained in response to presentation of familiar faces and scrambled images. No other evidence of cortical processing was reported but the patient became increasingly responsive at 6 months and minimally expressive at 8 months into the course of her illness. Menon et al. interpreted this activity measured at four months as indicating a recovery of minimal awareness. However, such selective identification of relatively complex information processing may not alone index recovery of cognitive function or even potential for recovery (25, 31).

Only a few studies have addressed patterns of brain activation in MCS patients. Boly et al. (32) used the same ^{15}O-radiolabeled PET paradigms for auditory stimuli tested in PVS patients to examine responses in MCS compared to healthy control subjects. Both MCS and normal subjects showed activation of the bilateral superior temporal gyri (Brodmann areas 41, 42 and 22) compared to earlier studies in the PVS patients where activation was limited to bilateral Brodmann areas 41 and 42 (33). Laureys et al. showed more widespread activation of ^{15}O-radiolabeled PET responses for auditory stimuli with emotional valence (i.e., infant cries and patient's own name) than that for meaningless noise in an MCS patient (34).

fMRI Studies   Schiff et al. (35) presented fMRI studies of two MCS patients, one related to TBI and the other to a spontaneous intracranial hemorrhage who remained in MCS for more than 18 months. When these patients were passively exposed to audiotaped narratives provided by family members, widespread activation of the language network was observed on fMRI. However, an important dissociation was observed in MCS patients compared to normal controls., When the narratives were time-reversed so that the semantic content was no longer discernible, there was a marked reduction in the extent and magnitude of activation of language structures, unlike the normal controls who showed a slight increase in activation (see figure 25-1). For both patients studied, FDG-PET revealed marked reduction of resting metabolic rates to near VS levels. The low resting metabolic activity suggests that the MCS patients may suffer a severe deficit of 'baseline' brain activity proposed by Gusnard and colleagues (36) to account for high resting cerebral metabolic rates in the normal human brain. This suggests that patients in MCS may not be able to recruit "top-down" monitoring functions necessary for processing ambiguous or complex environmental information. It is important to note that although functional brain imaging may eventually provide useful correlates of the differences in MCS and PVS evident at the bedside, at present these studies cannot be used to advance diagnostic or prognostic distinctions.

Bekinschtein, Miklison, Sigman & Manes (37) recently reported evidence of emotion processing in an MCS patient who suffered a severe traumatic brain injury using functional magnetic resonance imaging (fMRI). When they played a recording of the patient's mother's voice, functional MRI demonstrated activation of the amygdala and the insula, subcortical structures related to emotion. Functional connectivity between the secondary auditory cortex and temporal and prefrontal cortices suggested some potential for higher order integrative processes necessary for conscious auditory perception in MCS patients.

CLINICAL ASSESSMENT

Prior to the last decade, procedures for evaluating individuals with disorders of consciousness were limited to the Glasgow Coma Scale (38) MRI and EEG studies. These procedures continue to be useful during the acute stage of recovery but represent relatively gross indicators of cerebral dysfunction. Specialized behavioral and neuroradiologic protocols have recently been developed in an attempt to provide a more specific means of monitoring recovery across the subacute and post-acute periods and to improve outcome prediction.

Bedside Examination

There are no standardized evaluation procedures for the clinical bedside examination of patients with impaired consciousness. Most clinicians rely on systematic evaluations of arousal and behavioral responses to various forms of stimulation. Nevertheless, frequent errors in diagnosis occur, (5, 6) either because of a misinterpretation of responses or examinations that are inadequate to detect minimal, inconsistent responsiveness.

The bedside neurological examination of patients with impaired consciousness should focus on two general areas, assessment of the integrity of the central nervous system, particularly brainstem pathways (e.g. pupilary responses, ocular movements, oculovestibular reflexes, breathing patterns) and the presence of higher level cortical functions (e.g. purposeful, voluntary behaviors). The examiner's task is to systematically elicit and distinguish behaviors that are reflexive or automatic, reliant on spinal or subcortical pathways, from those that are cortically-mediated and represent some level or awareness or purposeful intent.

Cognitive awareness or conscious intent may be difficult to interpret when responses are extremely inconsistent or simple. There is an inverse relationship between the dimensions of *complexity* and *consistency* when judging whether particular behaviors imply consciousness. When a behavior is more complex, such as a verbalization, fewer instances of the response are sufficient to demonstrate consciousness. When a behavior is less complex, such as a finger movement, more frequent occurrences are necessary to establish a link to stimulus awareness or conscious intention. For this reason, single bedside examinations are often inadequate to conclusively establish level of

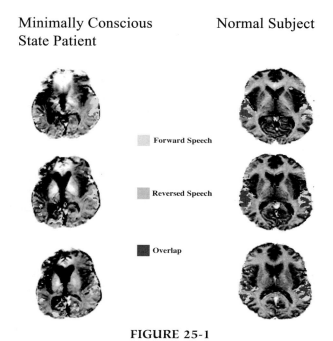

Minimally Conscious State Patient   Normal Subject

Forward Speech

Reversed Speech

Overlap

FIGURE 25-1

Images from fMRI studies of MCS patients and normal subjects. MCS patient shows widespread network activation for forward presentation of spoken narratives (yellow color), but time-reversed narratives produce only small regional activation of primary auditory cortex (red colored areas showing overlap for both stimulus types). In contrast, the normal subjects activate the entire network roughly equally for both stimulus conditions as seen in predominance of red colored regions for the normal subject

TABLE 25-2

A Systematic Approach to the Examination of Patients with Impaired Consciousness Includes the Following Steps

1. Brainstem integrity and other subcortical evaluation
   - Pupillary response, blink reflex to visual threat
   - Ocular movements, gaze deviations
   - Oculovestibular reflexes (oculocephalic ("doll's eyes") maneuvers, calorics)
   - Corneal response
   - Gag reflex
   - Breathing pattern
   - Decerebrate postures
   - Other posturing, reflexes and tone
2. Cortical functioning
   a. Observation of spontaneous activity
      - Purposeful, complex movements (involving cortically mediated isolated motor control) vs. posturing (decorticate or decerebrate) or reflex or stereotyped, patterned (subcortically mediated) movements
      - Spontaneous vocalizations or verbalizations
      - Eye movements (signs of fixation or tracking vs. nonspecific roving or no movement)
   b. Responses to stimulation or environment
      - Tracking or fixation to stimuli (try salient stimuli such as familiar pictures, faces, mirror)
      - Verbal stimulation (e.g. patient's name, commands, social greetings):
        Begin with simple commands sampling a variety of areas under different neural control, favoring those areas of potentially preserved movement.
        o Eye commands – e.g. 'look up', 'blink twice';
        o Limb commands – e.g. 'make a fist', 'show 2 fingers', 'raise your arm';
        o Oral commands – e.g. 'open mouth,' 'stick out tongue';
        o Axial or whole body commands – e.g. 'turn your head,' 'lean forward').
        o Ask patient to 'stop moving' or 'hold still' to distinguish from spontaneous repetitive movements.
      - Noxious stimulation
        o Look for localization or purposeful defensive maneuvers vs. reflexive or generalized, stereotyped movements or facial expressions.
      - Response in contingent relationship to environment or other stimuli
        o Look for intentional reach for or manipulation of objects on or around the patient (e.g. pulling at tubes, clothing, items placed in the hand)
        o Look for changes in facial expression contingent on stimuli such as familiar voices, particular conversation, pictures, music, etc.
        o Look for attempts at purposeful mobility in bed, chair, and even ambulation
        o Gestural behaviors indicating intentive communication (e.g. yes/no signals)
      - Confounding factors affecting arousal (e.g., centrally acting medications, concurrent illness, subclinical seizures);
      - The potential influence of aphasia, apraxia and other higher cortical disorders that may affect ability to respond to commands.

unconsciousness. Repeated assessments and use of standardized evaluations (see below) may be necessary for diagnostic accuracy. Table 25-2 presents a systematic approach to the neurological examination of patients with impaired consciousness.

There are several common problems that can lead to inaccurate diagnosis of consciousness in patients with impaired consciousness. These include:

- Attributing purposeful intent for responses that are reflexive or generalized to any form of stimulation;
- Inadequate evaluation to detect conscious behavior – e.g. insufficient sampling time, inadequate arousal, inappropriate choice of stimuli;

- Over- or underconsideration of family or other's observations of purposeful behavior (i.e., failure to recognize that family may be first to observe signs of consciousness or to overattribute purposeful intent);
- Simple, cortically mediated behaviors of uncertain cognitive significance; e.g. simple isolated limb movements;

The examiner should use strategies to account for some of these confounds and maximize the chance of detecting signs of conscious behavior. The clinician should:

1. *Assure optimal arousal.* There should be an adequate warm-up period, with verbal and tactile stimulation

to promote wakefulness. Deep pressure stimulation is often effective. Positioning is important and patients are usually more wakeful sitting up. The time of day, the patient's sleep-wake cycles and fatigue from activities preceding the neurological examination all have to be considered. Sedating medications should be avoided and treatable medical conditions should be addressed.

2. *Assure optimal environmental conditions.* Avoid distractions, provide adequate lighting, remove physical restrictions to movement and position stimuli to the patient's best advantage.

3. *Consider stimulus duration and rate.* Use a long enough presentation time and interstimulus interval to allow time for the patient to respond and to minimize perseveration. Recognize that as the interval between stimulus and response increases, the chance that a spurious response is mistakenly attributed to a stimulus also increases. Watch for signs of response fatigue.

4. *Avoid unnecessary complexity in command-following trials.* Use simple declarative language, one request at a time.

5. *Consider the patient's motor repertoire in choosing commands.* Use commands that incorporate motor responses that appear to be within the patient's capabilities, such as spontaneously observed movements.

6. *Distinguish purposeful from reflexive behavior.* When attempting to elicit movements to command, avoid responses that may represent common reflexive behaviors; e.g. squeeze hands, blink eyes.

7. *Evaluate a variety of potential responses and employ a range of different stimuli.* Attempt to elicit responses to a few different types of command – e.g. a limb command and an eye command. Look for other forms of purposeful behavior; e.g. manipulation of an object placed in the patients hand; social handshake; purposeful resistance to unpleasant stimulation.

8. *Assure adequate examination time and perform serial reassessments.* Quick bedside evaluations, such as typical morning rounds, are often not adequate in detecting responses in patients with DOC. Repeated reassessments are necessary to establish response consistency, validity of examination findings and accuracy of the diagnosis.

9. *Pay attention to observations of others.* Families, nurses, therapists, who are more familiar or spend more time with the patient, often observe behaviors associated with consciousness before they are observed by the physician. The physician's assessment should incorporate these observations.

Standardized Rating Scales

During the 1990's, advances in trauma care led to an increase in the number of survivors of severe brain injury.

Consequently, neurorehabilitation programs experienced an increase in the number of admissions involving patients with prolonged DOC. In light of these changes, neurorehabilitation specialists recognized the need for reliable assessment instruments that could detect subtle but potentially important clinical changes after the acute period of recovery. This resulted in a proliferation of standardized neurobehavioral assessment scales designed to gauge level of consciousness in unresponsive or poorly responsive patients. These instruments were intended to provide a comprehensive overview of neurobehavioral functions and, at the same time, to detect subtle changes in response frequency and complexity. The JFK Coma Recovery Scale (CRS) (39), the Western Neuro Sensory Stimulation Profile (WNSSP) (40), the Coma/Near Coma Scale (CNC) (41), the Sensory Modality Assessment Rehabilitation Technique (SMART) (42) and the Wessex Head Injury Matrix (43) represent examples of such measures. Although the validity and reliability of these instruments have been shown to be adequate (39–44), other important psychometric characteristics and their diagnostic and prognostic utility have not been well-studied.

The CRS was recently revised in an effort to improve differential diagnostic accuracy between VS and MCS (45). Interrater and test-retest reliability were found to be high for CRS-R total scores. Total scores were also significantly correlated with the Disability Rating Scale, providing evidence for concurrent validity. Analysis of internal consistency revealed moderate intercorrelations between the total CRS-R score and individual subscale scores suggesting that the scale is a reasonably homogenous measure of neurobehavioral function. There was also no evidence of ceiling or floor effects based on the distribution of scores. Regarding its clinical utility, the CRS-R reliably distinguished features of VS and MCS in a group of 80 patients with DOC, and identified 10 cases that were misdiagnosed as VS. Based on these findings, the CRS-R appears to meet minimal standards for measurement and evaluation tools designed for use in interdisciplinary medical rehabilitation.

Individualized Behavioral Assessment

The rigorous attention to methodologic consistency afforded by standardized measures does not allow case-specific questions to be addressed. For example, standardized procedures may not be able to differentiate between random movement and low frequency movement to command because the investigational technique is fixed and the number of observations restricted. For example, finger movement that occurs on two of four trials immediately after the command to "move your fingers" raises the possibility of verbal comprehension. However, if finger movement fails to occur during the next 20 trials administered, the probability that the two earlier responses represented evidence of verbal comprehension is diminished. Conversely, a patient may move his or her fingers following command on 10 consecutive trials but, if the same finger movement precedes the command, or persists well after the last command is administered, it is less likely that this response is an indication of verbal comprehension. To address this problem, DiPasquale and Whyte (46) developed an approach termed, "Individualized Quantitative Behavioral Assessment (IQBA)." IQBA applies principles of single subject research design to assess the cognitive and behavioral capacities of individuals with marked limitations in responsiveness. In this technique, clinical questions are individually tailored, stimuli and response criteria are operationally-defined and behavioral frequencies are analyzed statistically to determine whether the behavior of interest exceeds the rate predicted by chance. This approach has been successfully employed to investigate command-following, visual function, communication ability, emotional responses and drug efficacy (47).

Standardized and individualized procedures should be viewed as complementary as they serve different purposes. Standardized methods are designed to provide a broad overview of the integrity of sensory, motor and cognitive processes. When viewed *in toto*, these findings can help establish diagnosis, prognosis and lesion locus, and may inform the optimal approach to treatment. The inherent flexibility offered by the individualized approach provides an opportunity to control case-specific influences on behavior which contribute to diagnostic inaccuracy and erroneous judgements concerning consciousness.

TREATMENT INTERVENTIONS AND EFFECTIVENESS

The primary goal in treating individuals with disorders of consciousness is to restore basic functional competence. The degree to which this goal can be achieved is dependent upon multiple factors including arousal level, sensorimotor functions, communication ability, initiation and drive mechanisms and executive control processes. Treatment strategies, therefore, are usually designed to improve or augment one or more of these areas. Unfortunately, no treatment has definitively been shown to alter the natural course of recovery from coma, VS or MCS. This may be due, in part, to the lack of prospective, randomized controlled clinical trials (RCTs). RCTs represent the gold standard for testing treatment effectiveness, but are particularly difficult to organize because they require large sample sizes, tight control over exposure to related treatments and an extended period of follow up. Not surprisingly, most of the published research on treatment efficacy consists of uncontrolled case studies and case series.

Types of Treatment

Interventions available for individuals with disorders of consciousness can be grouped into three broad categories. Treatments that rely on *sensory stimulation (SS)* provide systematic exposure to a variety of environmental stimuli. The intent of SS is to improve arousal level and increase the frequency of purposeful behavior. Included within this category are environmental exposure strategies and structured sensory stimulation programs. *Physical management* strategies employ traditional rehabilitation techniques to promote physical health and prevent secondary complications. Interventions such as range of motion exercises, positioning schedules, bowel and bladder training, spasticity management and prevention of heterotopic ossification fall within this category. *Neuromodulation* protocols are designed to promote recovery by directly altering the neurophysiologic substrate presumed to be responsible for mediating consciousness. Pharmacologic interventions and deep brain stimulation represent examples of neuromodulatory approaches. Table 25-3 provides an overview of the treatments described above.

Treatment Efficacy

Treatment decisions should be guided by the strength of empirical evidence available for a particular intervention. A direct consequence of the lack of prospective RCTs on treatments for disorders of consciousness is that most existing efficacy studies have significant methodologic limitations that limit their interpretability and clinical application.

Research designs are often flawed and difficult to compare across studies. Diagnostic criteria are non-uniform, subject characteristics are inadequately reported, outcome measures are psychometrically weak or too insensitive to detect subtle but prognostically important changes over time and there is significant variation in the frequency and duration of the treatments employed. Nevertheless, the literature does provide some empirical information concerning the interventions used with this population.

Sensory Stimulation   In a recently completed evidence-based review, Giacino (48) found that the majority of published studies of SS represent class III and IV evidence (49) which is primarily comprised of case studies and retrospective data analyses (50–53). No class I prospective randomized controlled trials (RCT) were identified. A class II RCT, completed by Johnson, Roethig-Johnston and Richards, (54) provided multimodal SS to 14 patients in coma or VS within 24 hours of injury. Biochemical and physiologic markers were monitored before and after SS. On average, the treatment group received SS for 8 days and the placebo group was treated for 4 days. The authors reported that there was a significant stimulation effect

TABLE 25-3
Overview of Treatment Interventions Utilized in Disorders of Consciousness

TYPE OF INTERVENTION	RATIONALE	METHOD	INTENDED OUTCOME	EFFICACY STUDIES
Sensory Stimulation				
Environmental Exposure	Sensory enrichment prevents failure to thrive and loss of preserved functions	Exposure to naturally-occurring environmental stimuli/events (e.g. TV, music, group activities)	Activation of basic perceptual processes (e.g. visual scanning, sound localization)	No published studies
Structured Sensory Stimulation	Information processing efficiency is dependent upon proper calibration of stimulus intensity and response threshold	Administration of multi-modal sensory stimuli (e.g. auditory, visual, tactile, olfactory) titrated to existing sensory thresholds	Improve breadth and reliability of behavioral response repertoire	Hall, et al. (50) Wilson, et al. (51) Pierce, et al. (52) Wood, et al. (53) Johnson, et al. (54)
Physical Management				
	Health maintenance and physical re-conditioning maximize the likelihood and rate of recovery of spared neurologic functions	Implementation of range of motion exercises, positioning protocols, bowel/bladder schedules, skin care regimens, etc.	Prevention of aspiration, contractures, decubiti, malnourishment, heterotopic ossification, infection	Mackay, et al. (55) Timmons, et al. (57) Tanheco & Kaplan (58) Weber (59)
Neuromodulation				
Pharmacologic	Specific chemical agents may potentiate damaged neurotransmitter systems responsible for mediating attention and intention	Administration of cholinergic, dopaminergic, noradrenergic and serotonergic agonist medications	Improve arousal (i.e. wakefulness), alertness (i.e. vigilance) and intention (i.e. behavioral initiation)	Reinhard, et al. (61) Powell, et al. (62) Passler & Riggs (63) Meythaler, et al (64) Zafonte, et al. (65)
Deep Brain Stimulation	Electrophysiologic stimulation of the brain stem reticular system produces physiologic and behavioral changes associated with arousal	Chronic electrical stimulation of mesodiencephalic structures	Amelioration of arousal and/or cognitive deficits (e.g. neglect, memory disturbance) associated with disruption of thalamocortical circuits	Kanno, et al. (71) Tsubokawa, et al. (72) Schiff, et al. (73)

noted between groups at 6 days post-injury on only one of six biochemical markers. No difference was noted in biochemical or physiologic measures between survivors and deceased subjects. Of the remaining class III and IV studies (50–53), none were masked, approximately 50% provided inadequate subject and treatment descriptions and most lacked information necessary to determine the equivalence of the comparison group. In view of the dearth of methodologically sound studies involving SS, definitive conclusions regarding the effectiveness of this type of intervention cannot be drawn. Consequently, it is incumbent upon clinicians to clearly elucidate to family members, the high degree of clinical uncertainty associated with this form of treatment. To date, there have not been any published reports of harm associated with the use of SS.

Physical Management   Despite the universal acceptance and widespread use of physical management strategies employed to facilitate recovery of consciousness and function, no prospective RCTs have been conducted to date. Mackay, et al. (55) completed a retrospective study to assess the effectiveness of an organized inpatient rehabilitation protocol on length of stay and cognitive outcome. Retrospective chart reviews were completed on 38 individuals with severe TBI (initial GCS of 3 to 8) consecutively discharged from an inpatient rehabilitation facility. Seventeen individuals received an aggressive, formal program of multi-disciplinary rehabilitation during the acute hospitalization. Treatment methods were designed to promote physical recovery and prevent complications. The 21 remaining individuals did not receive any formal rehabilitative treatment. There were no statistically significant differences between the two groups on injury severity, brain stem reflexes, associated injuries or level of function on admission. Outcome data indicated that duration of coma and length of rehabilitation were approximately 66% shorter, discharge ratings on the Levels of Cognitive Functioning scale (LCFS) (56) were significantly higher and the percentage of home discharges was greater in the group that received the structured rehabilitation program. The generalizability of these findings is limited as they are based on a retrospective chart review and the authors provided only a cursory description of the treatment intervention.

Timmons, Gasquoine and Scibak (57) evaluated the degree of functional improvement noted in 47 patients who received interventions designed to promote health maintenance. All patients were admitted to rehabilitation at LCFS levels II to III within six months of injury. Since none of the patients reportedly showed functional communication, all were presumably in VS or MCS. Treatment consisted of interventions aimed at improving "physiologic integrity" and preventing complications. Procedures were administered by nursing staff and included hygiene procedures, positioning protocols, range of movement, pulmonary care and multisensory stimulation. By 12 months post-injury, 83% of the level III patients demonstrated functional improvement as compared to 31% of level II patients. Overall, 44% of the sample had regained functional communication, mobility or were able to use an upper extremity to perform activities of daily living. The authors suggested that amount of treatment influenced outcome since patients who did not improve received fewer hours of treatment than those who did (15 vs. 25 hours per week). This relationship did not appear to be related to length of time post-injury, however, the authors did not consider spontaneous recovery as a possible cause of the improvements noted.

Two additional case study reports describe functional improvement following introduction of physical management strategies. Tanheco and Kaplan (58) reported significant improvements in communication and self-care abilities in a 31 year-old woman with a six year history of eyes-closed coma resulting from a motor vehicle accident. The patient was admitted from a nursing home for inpatient rehabilitation after family members reportedly observed eye-opening, accurate head nods and occasional verbalizations. On admission, the patient was severely contracted with multiple decubiti, speech intelligibility was 10% to 25% and communication was compromised by vocal cord paralysis and limb contractures. Range of motion, stretching, serial casting and surgical releases were performed to facilitate motor function while breath control and single syllable vocabulary exercises were implemented to increase communication ability. An exercise regimen was begun to increase strength and endurance. After approximately six months of treatment, the patient was discharged home. By fourteen months, she was able to self-feed and groom with set up and could dress and transfer with moderate assistance. She was able to communicate bowel and bladder needs and rarely experienced incontinence. The decubiti healed and active range of movement improved enough to allow her to use her right upper extremity for pointing. This case is of interest given the late re-emergence of consciousness and degree of functional recovery that occurred after physically-based rehabilitation strategies were initiated.

Weber (59) monitored EEG responses in 3 patients (2 TBI, 1 anoxic) with GCS scores of eight or below during the first week post-injury in a neurologic intensive care unit. The treatment condition involved two 30 minute sessions of sensorimotor facilitation consisting of passive ranging, quick stretch exercises and joint traction. This was followed by proprioceptive and thermal stimulation accompanied by verbal requests for movement. Each patient served as their own control and received two 30-minute non-treatment sessions in an A-B-A-B design. EEG recordings were obtained before and after exposure to the treatment or non-treatment conditions. Data analyses revealed differential EEG responses by treatment condition. There were significant voltage fluctuations in the bandwidth of the damaged hemisphere that were associated with the patient's "awake" state. Significant voltage changes were not noted in the damaged hemisphere during the non-treatment condition. EEG tracings also suggested normalization of sleep following treatment exposure in all three patients. Unfortunately, follow up data was not collected so it is not known whether the reactive EEG changes presaged a favorable outcome.

Neuromodulation Neuromodulatory approaches to treatment of disorders of consciousness seek to alter the neurophysiologic disturbances that accompany severe brain injury. Pharmacologic intervention is the most widely used form of neuromodulation. Drug therapy has been utilized to improve arousal, promote behavioral initiation and persistence, stimulate speech and reduce agitation. The "workhorse" agents used in rehabilitation of individuals with disturbances in consciousness generally fall into three medication classes- psychostimulants, dopamine agonists and tricyclic anti-depressants. There is some evidence that stimulants and dopamine agonists are effective for improving arousal (i.e., wakefulness) and basic attentional functions (60). Significant improvements in behavioral initiation and response persistence have been noted following administration of amitriptyline (61), bromocriptine (62, 63) and amantadine (64, 65). Recovery of spontaneous speech (66, 67) and increases in verbal fluency (62) have also been tied to the use of bromocriptine in individuals diagnosed with MCS.

There are few controlled medication trials in patients with disorders of consciousness. Meythaler and colleagues (64) recently conducted one of the few prospective, randomized, controlled trials completed to date. These investigators administered amantadine hydrochloride (100 mg, bid) or placebo to 35 patients who were one to six weeks post-injury and had Disability Rating Scale scores between 15 and 22. A crossover design was used in which half the group received amantadine first, followed by placebo, while the other half received placebo first, followed by amantadine. Results indicated that cognitive and functional improvement was more rapid during the on-drug phase, regardless of whether subjects received AH or placebo first. At three and six month follow-up, there was no significant difference in DRS scores between treatment groups. Two important methodologic problems challenge the authors' conclusions, however. The group that received amantadine first was less severely disabled prior to treatment than the placebo group and may have achieved more favorable outcomes independent of treatment. Second, because a crossover design was used early in the course of recovery, the group that received amantadine first had improved substantially at the point of crossover, limiting their opportunity to improve to the same extent as the comparison group during the second phase of treatment. By the time the group treated with amantadine first reached crossover, the range of possible improvement on the DRS had narrowed from 15 points (during the active drug phase) to 5 points (during the placebo phase).

In a multicenter observational study of 124 patients with TBI, of all stimulants and dopaminergic agents administered, only amantadine was associated with better outcome (DRS scores) at 4 months post-injury (77). A subanalysis of those who received amantadine indicated that significant improvement in DRS scores occurred just after amantadine was initiated, suggesting that the medication influenced the improvement in functioning.

Passler and Riggs (63) investigated the effectiveness of another dopaminergic agent, bromocriptine (2.5 mg, bid), in improving functional outcome in a series of five patients in VS. In this study, bromocriptine was used in association with multidisciplinary rehabilitation interventions. The authors reported that physical and cognitive recovery at 12 months post-injury was greater in the bromocriptine-treated patients, relative to a group of historical controls. The strength of this study is limited by the small sample size, questionable comparability of the historical control group and failure to adequately address the influence of spontaneous recovery on outcome. It should be noted that a number of studies have reported adverse behavioral and cognitive side effects associated with the use of dopaminergic agents, including agitation, perseveration (68) and exacerbation of neglect (69).

Deep brain stimulation (DBS) is a neurosurgical procedure in which electrical pulses are delivered through electrodes implanted in brain stem or thalamic structures. This technique is derived from experimental findings in animals showing behavioral and EEG arousal responses in response to stimulation of the reticular system (70). One of the earliest clinical reports of DBS was described by Kanno and colleagues (71) and involved patients diagnosed with vegetative state. Clinical improvements were reported in three of the four patients treated and all four demonstrated improvements in EEG within two weeks of treatment. Improvements were noted in eye-opening, emotional expressiveness, verbal command-following and communication ability during the course of the trial. Tsubokawa and others (72) administered DBS to eight patients (TBI = 4, vascular = 3, anoxia = 1) who were reportedly in a vegetative state for more than six months. Stimulation was applied to sites in the mesencephalic reticular formation and non-specific thalamic nuclei. Behavioral changes associated with increased arousal, including opening of the eyes and mouth, vocalization and movement of the extremities, were observed in response to th stimulation. The behavioral changes coincided with desynchronization of the EEG and marked increases in regional cerebral blood flow and cerebral metabolic rates of oxygen and glucose. The authors noted that two of the eight patients recovered consciousness after 12 months post-injury.

Both of the DBS studies described above are compromised by significant methodologic flaws limiting their clinical applicability. Crude assessment and outcome measures were employed in both studies making it difficult to determine the accuracy of the patients' diagnoses as well as the nature and extent of the changes reported. Because neither study utilized a no-treatment control group, spontaneous recovery cannot be excluded to explain the improvement noted in some of the cases reported.

Schiff, Rezai and Plum (73) have recently proposed a re-designed protocol for DBS that focuses on activation of specific cortical fields via stimulation of carefully selected thalamic targets. In this approach, specific subdivisions of the intralaminar nuclei of the thalamus are stimulated to facilitate activation of damaged but still viable thalamocortical networks. This protocol is recommended for use with patients in MCS versus those in VS, given the that the former are more likely to have greater sparing of thalamocortical and corticocortical pathways relative to the latter, suggesting they may be better able to harness the stimulation effects.

There is a clear need for additional clinical trials of interventions designed to speed the pace of recovery from severe brain injury and improve functional outcome. Because relatively few rehabilitation centers offer services for patients with DOC, this can only be accomplished through multicenter collaborative studies. In the last year, a study of the effectiveness of amantadine hydrochloride, funded by the National Institute on Disability and Rehabilitation Research, was launched. This study involves eight rehabilitation centers in the U.S. and one in Germany. The primary aims are to determine if amantadine improves functional outcome during inpatient rehabilitation beyond the effects of a placebo, and whether amantadine-induced improvements persist following drug washout.

PROGNOSIS

Prognosis for patients with DOC has been analyzed with respect to three main outcome areas: recovery of consciousness, functional recovery and mortality. Outcome of VS and MCS are considered separately below. Most of the available information concerns patients in VS since MCS has only recently been operationally defined.

Outcome Following VS

Over 10 years ago, the Multi-Society Task Force on PVS (11) analyzed all available reports on outcome of VS and summarized prognosis for recovery of consciousness and functional recovery, based on the Glasgow Outcome Scale (74). The report included data on 434 adults and 106 children with traumatic brain injury, and 169 adults and 45 children with nontraumatic brain injury – primarily anoxic brain injury and stroke. Prognosis for recovery was substantially better for victims of traumatic brain injury than those who sustained nontraumatic injury. Of adults with traumatic brain injury who were unconscious at least 1 month, 33% recovered consciousness by 3 months post-injury, 46% by 6 month and 52% by 1 year. Approximately 35% of patients with TBI who were still unconsciousness at 3 months, regained consciousness by one year; if still unconscious for 6 months, 16% regained consciousness by 1 year. Of those adults with nontraumatic brain injuries unconscious for 1 month, only 11% recovered consciousness by 3 months and 15% by six months. No person with nontraumatic injury regained consciousness after 6 months post-injury.

Prognosis in children was only slightly more favorable. For those children with TBI who were unconscious at 1 month, 51% regained consciousness by 6 months and up to 62% of children with TBI recovered consciousness at one year after injury. After nontraumatic injury, recovery of consciousness occurred mainly within the first 3 months (11%), but a very small percentage (2%) regained consciousness between 6 and 12 months. Table 25-4 shows a summary of these outcome data.

The Task Force concluded that prognosis for recovery of consciousness was very poor 12 months after traumatic injuries and 3 months after nontraumatic brain injury for both adults and children. They suggested the term *permanent vegetative state* for patients who were still unconscious beyond these intervals after injury. Although unlikely, the chance of recovering consciousness is not absolutely lost. There are several reports of

TABLE 25-4

Prognosis and Functional Outcome According to the Glasgow Outcome Scale at 1 Year After Prolonged Unconsciousness in Adults with Traumatic Brain Injury (TBI) or Nontraumatic Brain Injury (nonTBI)

	TBI	NON-TBI
Unconscious at least 1 month:		
Death	33%	53%
VS	15%	32%
SD	28%	11%
MD	17%	3%
GR	7%	1%
Unconscious at least 3 months:		
Death	35%	46%
VS	30%	47%
SD	19%	6%
MD/GR	16%	1%
Unconscious at least 6 months:		
Death	32%	28%
VS	52%	72%
SD	12%	0%
MD/GR	4%	0%

(From: Multi-Society Task Force on PVS, 1994) (VS = vegetative state; SD = severe disability; MD = moderate disability; GR = good recovery).

later recovery of consciousness (11, 75) Childs and Mercer (75) pointed out that there is insufficient evidence in the Task Force study or any other studies to predict the incidence of late improvement. In fact, using the limited number of cases followed beyond 12 months in the Task Force report, they recalculated that the incidence of regaining consciousness after 12 months in that limited series of patients was 14%.

The Task Force report described functional outcome using the Glasgow Outcome Scale. By 12 months post-injury, more than one-half of the patients were *severely disabled*, nearly one-third were *moderately disabled* and a little more than an eighth achieved a *good recovery* level. Functional outcome was worse after nontraumatic injury; nearly three-quarters of those who regained consciousness were severely disabled at 12 months. Outcome for children was somewhat better at 12 months: one-half were severely disabled while most of the remainder achieved a good recovery. Older adults (>40 years old) tended towards a worse functional outcome, rarely improving beyond the level of severe disability.

According to the Task Force report, mortality is relatively high for patients in VS at least 1 month (82% at 3 years, and 95% at five years (11). Life expectancy improves the longer a patient in VS survives and younger patients have a greater chance for survival (76).

Although the Task Force analysis provides some general guidelines and probabilities for outcome after prolonged unconsciousness, outcome prediction for individuals with prolonged unconsciousness is difficult at best. A recent multicenter study of 124 patients with severely impaired consciousness (VS or MCS) of 1 month or more after TBI, examined a number of demographic, injury severity, functional and neuroimaging variables to predict outcome. Of all the variables tested, time from injury to initial rehabilitation evaluation, initial functional level in a rehabilitation facility and the rate of early functional recovery were highly predictive of both recovery of consciousness and functional outcome at 4 months post-injury (77).

Electrophysiologic studies may provide some information in determining prognosis after prolonged unconsciousness. Somatosensory evoked potential studies are useful in predicting permanent vegetative state after anoxic brain injury. Absence of the N20 potential in the presence of the earlier N14 potential is a very poor prognostic sign for recovery of consciousness (78). In general, the absence of cortical potentials indicates worse prognosis early in the course of recovery. The presence of the later cortical potentials does not necessarily carry a favorable prognosis. Cognitive event related potentials can provide additional prognostic information over SSEPs alone (79). A recent study by Fischer and others (80) demonstrated that if the cognitive evoked potential was present in patients with prolonged coma, the patient did not remain in a vegetative state. In that study, the best predictors for regaining wakefulness, though not necessarily consciousness, after coma of various etiologies were the presence of a pupilary reflex, followed by the presence of late auditory evoked potentials (N100) and middle-latency evoked potentials.

Structural neuroimaging (CT and MRI) is not very helpful in prognosticating outcome of impaired unconsciousness but there are some correlates with worse outcome. Kamplf and colleagues (81) found that location of brain lesions after trauma was a better predictor of recovery from prolonged unconsciousness than Glasgow Coma Scale scores, age and papillary abnormalities. Patients who did not recover consciousness by 12 months had a significantly higher frequency of corpus callosum, corona radiata and dorsolateral brainstem lesions than those that did regain consciousness. These locations are not specific for unconsciousness but are correlates of more severe grades of diffuse axonal injury (82).

Outcome Following MCS

Functional outcome appears to be substantially better for patients in MCS than those in VS when evaluated during a similar time post-injury. In a small series of patients with impaired consciousness followed for 4 months, Rappaport (41) reported improvement in 25% of a small group of patients with impaired consciousness noting that only

those in MCS (referred to as "near-coma") improved; none in VS improved in the follow-up period.

Although few prognostic studies of MCS have been completed, there is strong consensus that outcome from MCS following traumatic brain injury is highly variable, ranging from good recovery to severe disability on the Glasgow Outcome Scale (GOS) (74). The timeframe for establishing when MCS can be considered permanent is unclear as few empirical studies have addressed this particular subgroup.

Studies comparing functional outcome between individuals diagnosed with VS and MCS suggest that individuals in MCS show more rapid improvement, a longer period of recovery and significantly less functional disability at twelve months (77, 83, 84). Figure 25-2 depicts the results of a study conducted by Giacino & Kalmer (83) that investigated functional outcome on the Disability Rating Scale (DRS) (85) across the first year post-injury in patients diagnosed with VS or MCS. The VS and MCS groups were stratified further according to etiology of injury (i.e., traumatic or non-traumatic). Although both diagnostic groups presented with similar levels of disability at one month post-injury, outcome was significantly more favorable by twelve months in the MCS group, particularly after TBI. The differences in outcome became progressively more apparent at 3, 6 and 12 months post-injury. The probability of a more favorable outcome (moderate or no disability) by one year was much greater for the MCS group (38%) than the VS group (2%) and only occurred in those patients with TBI.

Giacino and Kalmar's findings have recently been replicated and extended by Lammi and colleagues (84) who followed 18 patients in traumatic MCS for two to five years after discharge from an inpatient brain injury

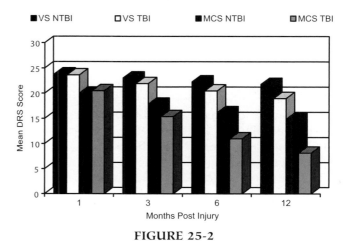

FIGURE 25-2

From "The vegetative and minimally conscious states: A comparison of clinical features and functional outcome," by J.T. Giacino and K. Kalmar, 1997, *Journal of Head Trauma Rehabilitation, 12(4)*, p. 42. Copyright 1997 by Aspen Publishers, Inc. Reprinted with permission

rehabilitation program located in Australia. The authors found that 15% of their sample had partial disability or less at follow-up while 20% fell in the extremely severe to vegetative category. In comparison, Giacino and Kalmar reported that 23% of their sample had no more than partial diability at 12 months with 17% classified as extremely severe to vegetative. In both samples, the most common outcome was moderate disability which occurred in approximately 50% of patients. Of particular importance, Lammi et al. also noted that duration of MCS was not correlated with DRS outcome and that 50% of their sample had regained independence in activities of daily living at follow-up. Both of these studies suggest a clear separation between MCS and VS in course of recovery and eventual functional outcome. Mortality following MCS appears to be similar to that of VS indicating that the presence of consciousness is not the critical factor predicting survival (86). Additional data concerning mortality after severe TBI is provided in the chapter by Shavelle, et al. in this volume.

RECOMMENDATIONS FOR A RATIONAL APPROACH TO CLINICAL MANAGEMENT

In the absence of empirically-established standards of care for clinical management of individuals with disorders of consciousness, clinicians should adhere to a core set of basic tenets to guide evaluation and treatment of patients with DOC. In that spirit, the following recommendations are proposed, not as a prescriptive mandate, but rather, as a self-study reference for brain injury rehabilitation programs that offer services to this population.

Assessment Strategies

Carefully-defined *inclusion criteria* should be developed for patients with DOC seeking admission to rehabilitation programs. This population has unique needs that may not be easily accommodated by traditional rehabilitative interventions. Specialized training is essential for staff members responsible for providing assessment and treatment services as few academic programs directly address the care of patients with DOC. Diagnosis, cause of injury, length of time post-onset, degree of medical stability, age, level of disability and adequacy of support system are factors that should be considered in admission decisions as each one can influence outcome. Creation of a local database is useful for monitoring these variables and may help identify admission and discharge trends, gauge program effectiveness and facilitate longitudinal research.

A *comprehensive neuromedical work up* should be obtained on admission. This should include a complete review of the history, comprehensive physical examination, neurologic assessment, neuroimaging studies (if recent scans are unavailable), nutritional assessment and review of current medications. Undetected or co-existing medical conditions such as post-traumatic epilepsy, hydrocephalus, late subdural hematoma, neuroendocrine dysfunction, nutritional deficiency, occult infection and drug toxicity must be excluded as potential causes of under-arousal and under-responsiveness (4).

A *well-defined assessment protocol* should be developed to monitor changes in neurologic, cognitive, physical and functional status. Standardized measures of neurobehavioral responsiveness (39–42, 44) and functional disability (85) should be utilized and supplemented with individualized assessment techniques (46), as needed. When conducting medication trials, outcome goals should be operationally-defined and objective measures employed to track progress. In most cases, patients should be serially reevaluated during the first three months post-injury to detect fluctuations in level of responsiveness. After the three month mark, assessment frequency should be determined by the patient's rate of change. Follow-up examinations should be completed at 12 months whenever possible as significant change is unlikely after this point.

There are no universally accepted *criteria for determining when rehabilitative treatment should be discontinued*. It is incumbent upon individual programs to determine local decision-making criteria to assure consistency across patients. There are four clinical factors that should be considered in the decision to discontinue treatment (48). The first two, cause of injury and length of time post-onset, represent important determinants of outcome, particularly when they are utilized in combination. As discussed earlier, the probability of recovering from VS after three months is significantly higher following traumatic versus non-traumatic brain injury (11, 83, 84). The patient's current level of neurobehavioral responsiveness is a third factor that should be taken into account as this reflects the extent of spared neural circuitry available to process sensoriperceptual input and mediate behavioral output. Response profiles dominated by reflexive brain stem activity offer little opportunity to promote higher-order cognitive processing given the loss of cortical connectivity. The fourth factor, rate of recovery, is perhaps the most important variable. Prior studies suggest that evidence of ongoing change is a favorable predictor of functional outcome, even in patient's who have not yet regained signs of consciousness (39, 77). The specific weight that should be assigned to each factor has not yet been elucidated. Additional research is needed before algorithms can be developed to guide treatment discontinuation decisions. This task should be viewed as an important objective in brain injury rehabilitation.

Treatment Strategies

Physical management interventions (e.g., range of motion, positioning, hygiene, etc.) should be considered a standard component of the rehabilitation regimen of patients with disorders of consciousness. While it is unknown whether these interventions can facilitate the pace or degree of neurophysiologic recovery, there are strong rational indications for their use, and little evidence that they are ineffective or unsafe. Steps should be taken to ensure that comfort is maintained and pain alleviated, particularly when intrusive medical and rehabilitative procedures are performed. Other interventions such as sensory stimulation and medication trials should be considered treatment *options* and should be construed as supplementary to the basic rehabilitative strategies described above.

Special emphasis should be placed on utilizing behavioral and pharmacologic strategies to promote arousal and facilitate neurogenic drive. Preserved cognitive function may be masked by deficiencies in these areas. Alternative or augmentative communication systems should be implemented in individuals diagnosed with MCS because sensory and neuromuscular impairments often accompany disturbances in consciousness (5, 6). Assisted communication systems should not be incorporated into long-term care plans until there has been an adequate period of assessment in which response consistency and reliability have been demonstrated.

Finally, a formal protocol for providing family/surrogate education and training should be developed. An explicit mechanism for allowing ongoing communication between caretakers and the rehabilitation team across the span of treatment is a pre-requisite for effective treatment. At a minimum, family conferences should be held shortly after admission and prior to discharge. The initial conference should include discussion of the preliminary assessment findings, particularly those that pertain to functional capacity and prognosis for further recovery. The treatment objectives recommended by the clinical team should be presented and integrated with the goals stipulated by the caretakers. Specific treatment methods should be outlined and accompanied by information regarding the efficacy of the proposed interventions and the anticipated outcome in each targeted area. A second meeting should be held prior to discharge to confirm or modify the initial diagnostic and prognostic impressions, clarify recommendations for clinical management and to establish a plan for follow-up assessment, as indicated.

ETHICAL CONSIDERATIONS

Neurorehabilitation specialists often encounter difficult ethical issues related to the clinical management of patients with DOC. While most clinicians have not received formal training in bioethics, it is important to have some awareness of the type of ethical questions that are likely to arise during the course of treatment. Comprehensive review of these issues is beyond the scope of this chapter but it is useful to summarize some of the questions clinicians can expect to be confronted with during acute and post-acute care of these patients. For additional discussion of ethical considerations, interested readers are referred to the chapter by Kothari, et al. in this text and the recent special issue of *Neurorehabilitation* on scientific advances and ethical dilemmas concerning life-sustaining treatments in VS (87).

- Is it appropriate to allocate resources to the treatment of patients with chronic disorders of consciousness at the same level as patient's who are fully conscious?
- At what point should rehabilitative treatment be considered futile?
- What services should be provided after VS and MCS are deemed permanent?
- Is it appropriate to withdraw artificial nutrition and hydration in non-terminal patients in permanent VS and MCS?
- Should artificial hydration and nutrition be discontinued in patients in VS and MCS before criteria for permanence are met?
- Should patients with disorders of consciousness be permitted to participate in clinical trials?

CONCLUSIONS AND FUTURE DIRECTIONS

Disorders of consciousness are arguably the most enigmatic conditions encountered in medical rehabilitation. Although progress has been made over the last decade in developing more reliable assessment methods, the psychometric integrity and clinical utility of these measures remain highly variable. Similarly, remarkably little is known about the neurophysiologic substrate underlying these disorders. These problems have been sustained, in part, by clinical nihilism – the belief that little effort should be invested in these patients because they cannot be helped. Recent initiatives to establish standards of care for evaluation and clinical management have begun to take hold and are expected to progress more rapidly in view of new insights gained from novel neurodiagnostic technologies.

At present, there are no treatment interventions that have been demonstrated to be effective in facilitating recovery of consciousness. Additional research is needed to 1) clarify the natural history of recovery from VS and MCS, 2) identify predictors of recovery of consciousness and cognition, 3) elucidate the pathophysiology underlying specific disorders and 4) develop treatments capable of altering outcome in patients with DOC. To accomplish these goals, it will be necessary to establish collaborative partnerships across rehabilitation centers and across disciplines. In the current healthcare climate, few rehabilitation centers can recruit patient samples large enough to carry out adequately powered clinical trials. Moreover, most centers do not have ready access to neuroscientists, biophysicists, neurosurgeons, neurologists and bioethicists, all of whom contribute uniquely to the study of patients with DOC.

References

1. American Academy of Neurology. Practice parameter: Assessment and management of persons in the persistent vegetative state. *Neurol* 1995;45:1015–1018.

2. American Congress of Rehabilitation Medicine. Recommendations for use of nomenclature pertinent to persons with severe alterations in consciousness. *Arch Phys Med Rehabil* 1995;76:205–209.

3. Andrews K. International working party on the management of the vegetative state: summary report. *Brain Injury* 1996;10(11):797–806.

4. Giacino J, Ashwal S, Childs N, Cranford R, Jennett B, Katz D, Kelly J, Rosenberg J, Whyte J, Zafonte R, Zasler N. The minimally conscious state: definition and diagnostic criteria. *Neurology* 2002;58:349–353.

5. Andrews K, Murphy L, Munday R, Littlewood C. Misdiagnosis of the vegetative state: Retrospective study in a rehabilitation unit. *BMJ* 1996;313:13–16.

6. Childs NL, Mercer WN, Childs HW. Accuracy of diagnosis of persistent vegetative state. *Neurol* 1993;43:1465–1467.

7. Tresch DD, Sims FH, Duthie EH, Goldstein, MD, Lane PS. Clinical characteristics of patients in the persistent vegetative state. *Arch Internal Med* 1991;151:930–932.

8. Medical Research Council, Brain Injuries Committee. A glossary of psychological terms commonly used in cases of head injury. In: *Medical Research Council War Memorandum #4 HMSO*, London, 1941.

9. Plum F, Posner J. *The diagnosis of stupor and coma, 3rd Edition* Philadelphia: F.A. Davis, 1982.

10. Jennett B, Plum F. Persistent vegetative state after brain damage: A syndrome in search of a name. *Lancet* 1972;1:734–737.

11. Multi-Society Task Force Report on PVS. Medical aspects of the persistent vegetative state. *NEJM* 1994;330:1499–1508, 1572–1579.

12. Choi SC, Barnes TY, Bullock R, Germanson TA, Marmarou A, Young HF. Temporal profile of outcomes in severe head injury. *J Neurosurg* 1994;81:169–173.

13. Dubroja I, Valent S, Miklic P, Kesak D. Outcome of post-traumatic unawareness persisting for more than a month. *J Neurosurg Psychiat* 1995;58:465–466.

14. Giacino JT, Zasler ND, Katz,DI, Kelly JP, Rosenberg JH, Filley CM. Development of practice guidelines for assessment and management of the vegetative and minimally conscious states. *J Head Trauma Rehabil* 1997;12(4):79–89.

15. Jennett B, Adams JH, Murray LS, Graham DI. Neuropathology in vegetative and severely disabled patients after head injury. *Neurology* 2001;56(4):486–490.

16. Adams JH, Graham DI, Jennett B. The neuropathology of the vegetative state after an acute brain insult. *Brain* 2000;123(7):1327–1338.

17. Jennett B, Adams JH, Murray LS, Graham DI. Neuropathology in vegetative and severely disabled patients after head injury. *Neurol* 2001;56(4):486–490.

18. Logothetis NK. The neural basis of the blood-oxygen-level-dependent functional magnetic resonance imaging signal. *Philos Trans R Soc Lond B Biol Sci* 2002;357(1424):1003–37

19. Eidelberg D, Moeller JR, Kazumata K, Antonini A, Sterio D, Dhawan V, Spetsieris P, Alterman R, Kelly PJ, Dogali M, Fazzini E, Beric A. Metabolic correlates of pallidal neuronal activity in Parkinson's disease. *Brain* 1997;120:1315–24.

20. Smith AJ, Blumenfeld H, Behar KL, Rothman DL, Shulman RG, Hyder F. Cerebral energetics and spiking frequency: the neurophysiological basis of fMRI. *Proc Natl Acad Sci USA* 2002;99(16):10765–70.

21. Levy DE, Sidtis JJ, Rottenberg DA, Jarden JO, Strother SC, Dhawan V, Ginos JZ, Tramo MJ, Evans AC, Plum F. Differences in cerebral blood flow and glucose utilization in vegetative versus locked-in patients. *Ann Neurol* 1987;22:673–82.

22. DeVolder AG, Goffinet AM, Bol A, Michel C, de Barsy T, Laterre C. Brain glucose metabolism in postanoxic stroke. *Arch Neurol* 1990;47:197–204.

23. Tomassino, C, Grana, C, Lucignani, G, Torri, G, Ferrucio, F. Regional metabolism of comatose and vegetative state patients. *J Neurosurg Anesthesiol* 1995;7:109–116.

24. Rudolf J, Ghaemi M, Ghaemi M, Haupt WF, Szelies B, Heiss WD. Cerebral glucose metabolism in acute and persistent vegetative state. *J Neurosurg Anesthesiol* 1999;11(1):17–24.

25. Schiff, N.D., Ribary, U, Plum, F, and Llinas, R. Words without mind. *J Cogn Neurosci* 1999;11(6):650–656.

26. Schiff N, Ribary U, Moreno D, Beattie B, Kronberg E, Blasberg R, Giacino J, McCagg C, Fins JJ, Llinas R, Plum F. Residual cerebral activity and behavioral fragments in the persistent vegetative state. *Brain* 2002;125:1210–1234.

27. Laureys S, Goldman S, Phillips C, Van Bogaert P, Aerts J, Luxen A, et al. Impaired effective cortical connectivity in vegetative state: preliminary investigation using PET. *Neuroimage* 1999;9:377–82.

28. Laureys S, Faymonville ME, Degueldre C, Fiore GD, Damas P, Lambermont B, Janssens N, Aerts J, Franck G, Luxen A, Moonen G, Lamy M, Maquet P. Auditory processing in the vegetative state. *Brain* 2000;123:1589–601.

29. Laureys S, Faymonville ME, Peigneux P, Damas P, Lambermont B, Del Fiore G, Degueldre C, Aerts J, Luxen A, Franck G, Lamy M, Moonen G, Maquet P. Cortical processing of noxious somatosensory stimuli in the persistent vegetative state. *Neuroimage* 2002;17(2):732–41.

30. Menon DK, Owen AM, Williams EJ, et al. Cortical processing in persistent vegetative state. *Lancet* 1998;352:1148–9

31. Schiff, N.D., and Plum, F. Cortical processing in the vegetative state. *Trends Cogn Sci* 1999;3(2):43–44.

32. Boly M, Faymonville ME, Peigneux P, Lambermont B, Damas P, Del Fiore G, Degueldre C, Franck G, Luxen A, Lamy M, Moonen G, Maquet P, Laureys S. (2004a) Auditory processing in severely brain injured patients: differences between the minimally conscious state and the persistent vegetative state. *Arch Neurol* 2004a;61(2):233–238.

33. Laureys S. Brain function in pathologic unconsciousness. Symposium conducted at the eighth annual conference of the Association for the Scientific Study of Consciousness. Antwerp, Belgium. June 24, 2004.

34. Laureys S, Perrin F, Faymonville ME, Schnakers C, Boly M, Bartsch V, Majerus S, Moonen G, Maquet P. Cerebral processing in the minimally conscious state. *Neurol* 2004;63(5):916–918.

35. Schiff, N, Rodriguez-Moreno, D, Kamal, A, Petrovich, N, Giacino, J, Plum, F and Hirsch, J. fMRI reveals large-scale network activation in minimally conscious patients. *Neurol* 2005;64:514–523.

36. Gusnard DA, Raichle ME, Raichle ME. Searching for a baseline: functional imaging and the resting human brain. *Nat Rev Neurosci* 2001;2(10):685–94.

37. Bekinschtein T, Leiguarda R, Armony J, Owen A, Carpintiero S, Niklison J, Olmos L, Sigman L, Manes F.J Emotion processing in the minimally conscious state. *J Neurol Neurosurg Psychiat* 2004;75(5):788.

38. Jennett B, Teasdale G, Aspects of coma after severe head injury. *Lancet* 1977;1 (8017):878–881.

39. Giacino JT, Deluca J, Kezmarsky MA, Cicerone KD, Monitoring rate of recovery to predict outcome in minimally responsive patients, *Arch Phys Med Rehabil*, 72, 897, 1991.

40. Ansell, B. J. and Keenan, J. E., The Western Neuro Sensory Stimulation Profile: A tool for assessing slow-to-recover head-injured patients. *Arch Phys Med Rehabil*, 70, 104, 1989.

41. Rappaport, M., Dougherty, A.M. and Kelting, D. L., Evaluation of coma and vegetative states, *Arch Phys Med Rehabil*, 73, 628, 1992.

42. Gill-Thwaites H, Munday R. The Sensory Modality Assessment Rehabilitation Technique (SMART): a valid and reliable assessment for the vegetative and minimally conscious state patient. *Brain Injury*. in press.

43. Horn S, Watson M, Wilson BA, McLellan DL. The development of new techniques in the assessment and monitoring of recovery from severe head injury: a preliminary report and case history. *Brain Injury*. 1992;6(4):321–325.

44. O'Dell MW, Jasin P, Lyons N, Stivers M, Meszaro F. Standardized assessment instruments for minimally-responsive, brain-injured patients. *NeuroRehabil* 1996;6:45–55.

45. Giacino JT, Kalmar K, Whyte J. The JFK Coma Recovery Scale-Revised: Measurement Characteristics and Diagnostic Utility. *Arch Phys Med Rehabil*, 2004;85(12):2020–2029.

46. DiPasquale, M. C. and Whyte, J., The use of quantitative data in treatment planning for minimally conscious patients, *J Head Trauma Rehabil*, 1996;11(6):9.

47. Whyte, J., Laborde, A. and Dipasquale, M. C., Assessment and treatment of the vegetative and minimally conscious patient, in *Rehabilitation of the Adult and Child with Traumatic Brain Injury* (3rd ed.), Rosenthal, M., Griffith, E.R., Kreutzer, J. and Pentland, B., Eds., F.A. Davis, Philadelphia, 435, 1999.

48. Giacino J. Sensory stimulation: theoretical perspectives and the evidence for effectiveness, *Neurorehabil* 1996;6:69–78.

49. Woolf, SH. Practice guidelines, a new reality in medicine. II. Methods of developing guidelines, *Arch Intern Med* 1992;152:946–952.

50. Hall, ME. MacDonald S, Young, GC. The effectiveness of directed multisensory stimulation versus non-directed stimulation in comatose CHI patients: Pilot study of a single subject design, *Brain Injury* 1992;6(5):435–445.

51. Wilson SL, Powell, GE, Elliott K, & Thwaites H. Sensory stimulation in prolonged coma: Four single case studies. *Brain Injury* 1991;4(5):393–400.

52. Pierce JP, Lyle DM., Quine S, Evans NJ, Morris J, Fearnside MR. The effectiveness of coma arousal intervention. *Brain Injury* 1990;4(2):191–197.

53. Wood RL, Winkowski TB, Miller JL, Tierney L, Goldman L. Evaluating sensory regulation as a method to improve awareness in patients with altered states of consciousness: a pilot study. *Brain Injury* 1992;6(5):411–418.

54. Johnson DA, Roethig-Johnston K, Richards D: Biochemical and physiological parameters of recovery in acute severe head injury: responses to multisensory stimulation. *Brain Injury* 1993;7(6):491–499.

55. Mackay LE, Bernstein BB, Chapman PE, Morgan AS, Milazzo LS. Early intervention in severe head injury: Long-term benefits of a formalized program. *Arch Phys Med Rehabil* 1992;73:635–641.

56. Hagan C, Malkmus D, Durham P. Levels of cognitive function. In: *Rehabilitation of the Head-Injured Adult: Comprehensive Physical Management*. Downey, CA, Professional Staff Association of Rancho Los Amigos Hospital, Inc, 1979.

57. Timmons , Gasquoine L, Scibak JW. Functional changes with rehabilitation of very severe traumatic brain injury survivors, *J Head Trauma Rehabil* 1987;2(3):64–67.

58. Tanheco J, Kaplan PE. Physical and surgical rehabilitation of patient after 6-year coma, *Arch Phys Med Rehabil* 1982; 63: 36–38.

59. Weber PL. Sensorimotor therapy: Its effect on electroencephalograms of acute comatose patients, *Arch Phys Med Rehabil* 1984;65:457–462.

60. Whyte J. Neurologic disorders of attention and arousal: Assessment and treatment. *Arch Phys Med Rehabil* 1992;73:1094–1103.

61. Reinhard DL, Whyte J, Sandel ME. Improved arousal and initiation following tricyclic antidepressant use in severe brain injury, *Arch Phys Med Rehabil* 1996;77:80–83.

62. Powell JH, Al-Adawi S, Morgan J, Greenwood RJ. Motivational deficits after brain injury: Effects of bromocriptine in 11 patients. *J Neurol Neurosurg Psychiat* 1996;60:416–421.

63. Passler MA, Riggs RV. Positive outcomes in traumatic brain injury- Vegetative state: Patients treated with bromocriptine. *Arch Phys Med Rehabil* 2001;82:11–315.

64. Meythaler JM, Brunner RC, Johnson A, Novack TA. Amantadine to improve neurorecovery in traumatic brain injury—associated diffuse axonal injury: a pilot double-blind randomized trial. *J Head Trauma Rehabil* 2002;17(4):300–313.

65. Zafonte R. Amantadine: A potential treatment for the minimally conscious state, *Brain Injury* 1998;12(7):617–621.

66. Campagnolo DI, Katz RT. Successful treatment of akinetic mutism with a post-synaptic dopamine agonist (abstract), *Arch Phys Med Rehabil* 1992;73:975.

67. Ross ED, Stewart M. Akinetic mutism from hypothalamic damage: Successful treatment with dopamine agonists, *Neurol* 1981;31:1435–1439.

68. Giacino JT, Rodriguez M, Cicerone KD Exacerbation of frontal release behaviors with use of amantadine following traumatic brain injury (abstract), *Arch Phys Med Rehabil* 1992;73:975.

69. Barrett AM. Adverse effect of dopamine agonist therapy in a patient with motor-intentional neglect, *Arch Phys Med Rehabil* 1999;80:600–603.

70. Moruzzi G, Magoun HW. Brain stem reticular formation and activation of the EEG, *EEG Clin Neurophysiol* 1949;1:455–473.

71. Kanno T, Kamei Y, Yokoyama T, Jain VK. Neurostimulation for patients in vegetative status. *PACE* 1987;10:207–208.Neurostimulation for patients in vegetative status, *PACE* 1987;10: 207–208.

72. Tsubokawa T, Yamamoto T, Katayama Y, Hirayama T, Maejima S, Moriya T. Deep brain stimulation in a persistent vegetative state: Follow up results and selection of candidates, *Brain Injury* 1990; 4(4):315–327.

73. Shiff ND, Rezai AR Plum FP. A neuromodulation strategy for rational therapy of complex brain injury states, *Neurol Res* 2000; 22:267–272.

74. Jennett B, Bond M. Assessment of outcome after severe brain damage: A practical scale. *Lancet* 1995;1(7905):480–484.

75. Childs NL, Mercer WN. Brief report: late improvement in consciousness after post-traumatic vegetative state. *N Engl J Med* 1996;334:24–25.

76. Strauss DJ, Shavelle RM, Ashwal S. Life Expectancy and median survival time in the permanent vegetative state. *Pediatric Neurol* 1999;21:626–631.

77. Whyte J, Katz D, Long D, DiPasquale M, Polansky M, Kalmar K, Giacino J, Childs N, Mercer W, Novak P, Maurer P, Eifert B. Predictors of Outcome in Prolonged Posttraumatic Disorders of Consciousness and Assessment of Medication Effects: A Multicenter Study. *Arch Phys Med Rehabil* 2005;86:453–462.

78. Zegers, De Beryl D, Brunko E. Prediction of chronic vegetative state with somatosensory evoked potentials. *Neurol* 1986;36:134.

79. Lew HL, Dikmen S, Slimp J, et al. Use of somatosensory-evoked potentials and cognitive event-related potentials in predicting outcomes of patients with severe traumatic brain injury. *Am J Phys Med Rehabil* 2003;82:53–61.

80. Fischer C, Luante J, Adeleine P, Morlet D: Predictive value of sensory and cognitive evoked potentials for awakening from coma. *Neurol* 2004;63:669–673.

81. Kampfl A, Schmutzhard E, Franz G, Pfausler B, Haring HP, Ullmer H, Felber F, Golaszewski, Aichner F. Prediction of recovery from post-traumatic vegetative state with cerebral magnetic-resonance imaging. *Lancet* 1998;351:1763–1767.

82. Adams JH, Doyle D, Ford I, Gennarelli TA, Graham DI, McLellan DR. Diffuse axonal injury in head injury: definition, diagnosis and grading. *Histopathol* 1989;15(1):49–59.

83. Giacino JT, Kalmar K. The vegetative and minimally conscious states: A comparison of clinical features and functional outcome. *J Head Trauma Rehabil* 1997;12(4):36–51.

84. Lammi MH, Smith VH, Tate RL, Taylor CM. The minimally conscious state and recovery potential: A follow-up study 2 to 5 years after traumatic brain injury. *Arch Phys Med Rehabil* 2005;86: 746–754.

85. Rappaport M, Hall K M, Hopkins K, Belleza T, Cope DN. Disability rating scale for severe head trauma: coma to community. *Arch Phys Med Rehabil* 1992;73:628–634.

86. Strauss DJ, Ashwal S, Day SM, Shavelle RM. Life expectancy of children in vegetative and minimally conscious states. *Pediatric Neurol* 2000;23:312–319.

87. Gigli GL, Zasler ND (eds.). Life-sustaining treatments in vegetative state: Scientific advances and ethical dilemmas. *Neurorehabil* 2004;19:273–391.

VII

NEUROLOGIC PROBLEMS

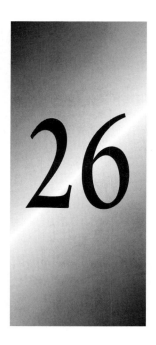

26 Post-Traumatic Seizures and Epilepsy

Stuart A. Yablon
Victor G. Dostrow

INTRODUCTION

Traumatic brain injuries (TBI) remain a leading cause of neurologic disability and death in the population of the United States and westernized nations. While the incidence of hospitalization for mild TBI in the United States has declined (1), the number of patients hospitalized for TBI remains significant, approximately 100/100,000 per year (1). Among the survivors of TBI, a sizable number remain with important medical and neurological sequelae, including seizures.

The relationship between TBI and subsequent development of post-traumatic seizure (PTS) disorders, including incidence, risk factors for initial occurrence and recurrence, and management, comprise the central themes of this review. Most cited studies address PTS among adults. Issues pertinent to diagnostic and therapeutic management of PTS in the patient with severe traumatic brain injury (TBI) are emphasized.

CLASSIFICATION OF POST-TRAUMATIC SEIZURES AND EPILEPSY

It is useful to review terms employed in the discussion of post-traumatic seizure disorders. These are defined in the Practice Parameter on the Antiepileptic Drug Treatment of Post-traumatic Seizures by the Brain Injury Special

Interest Group of the American Academy of Physical Medicine and Rehabilitation (2) (Table 1), and the Guidelines for Epidemiologic Studies on Epilepsy, by the Commission on Epilepsy and Prognosis of the International League Against Epilepsy (3). An *epileptic seizure* is a clinical manifestation presumed to result from an abnormal and excessive discharge of a set of neurons in the brain. The clinical manifestation consists of sudden and transitory abnormal phenomena, which may include alterations of consciousness, motor, sensory, autonomic, or psychic events, perceived by the patient or an observer (3). *Epilepsy* is a condition characterized by recurrent (two or more) epileptic seizures, unprovoked by any immediate identified cause (3).

Post-traumatic epilepsy (PTE) is a disorder characterized by recurrent late seizure episodes, not attributable to another obvious cause, in patients with TBI (2). Although PTE has commonly designated single or multiple seizures, including early seizures, the term should be reserved for recurrent, late PTS. Since most studies regarding seizures among patients with TBI do not address recurrence, the term post-traumatic seizures (rather than epilepsy) is preferred, since it encompasses both single and recurrent episodes. Thus, a *post-traumatic seizure* (PTS) refers to a single or recurrent seizure episode occurring after TBI (2). Post-traumatic seizures have been further classified into early (< 1 week after TBI) and late (>1 week after TBI) categories, primarily due to prevailing

443

opinion that they represent similar manifestations of different pathophysiologic processes (4). Classification of early seizures as those occurring within the first seven days after TBI has sparked some controversy (5), particularly with regard to long-term AED treatment decisions. There is little data to suggest that seizures that occur at day 8 or 14 have recurrence characteristics that justify classification as late seizures, and underlying mechanisms of seizure appearance are more likely to reflect acute pathophysiologic processes rather than those of chronic epilepsy.

The exclusion of "other obvious causes" is especially relevant to this patient population. Seizures occurring among patients with TBI may be the result of precipitants unrelated to mechanisms currently linked with post-traumatic epileptogenesis. Seizure precipitants have been defined as any endogenous or exogenous factor that promotes the occurrence of epileptic seizures (6). Examples of seizure precipitants among patients with TBI include hydrocephalus (7), sepsis (8), hypoxia (9), metabolic abnormalities (10) and mass-occupying lesions, including hemorrhage (11, 12). Among epileptic patients, more than 60% cite precipitants among recurrent seizures they experience. (6)

Drugs (13, 14), including alcohol (15, 16), prescribed psychotropic agents (14, 17–22), and recreational/illicit drugs (13, 23) warrant particular scrutiny as seizure precipitants among patients with TBI. In one study, for example, 19% of patients with severe TBI developed seizures attributed to tricyclic antidepressants (22). Antidepressants other than tricyclic agents are also implicated with seizure occurrence, including immediate (21) and sustained-release formulations of buproprion (17). While SSRIs are considered to have lower proconvulsant activity than other common antidepressants (24–26), several uncontrolled case studies of epileptic patients with depression have reported that SSRI administration increased seizure frequency (27, 28). Certain antipsychotic drugs, including newer atypical antipsychotic agents, particularly clozapine, may induce EEG abnormalities and seizures (18). Antibiotics, particularly imipenem (29) and quinolone agents (30), have been associated with seizures. Seizure risk is generally elevated among critically ill patients (31), however, and proper dose adjustment for renal clearance may mitigate much of the risk attributed to antibiotic administration (31, 32). Bromocriptine and amantadine, dopamine receptor agonists used to treat impaired arousal after TBI, have been implicated as seizure precipitants (33), although this association presently appears to be largely anecdotal. Recreational/illicit stimulants with well-known seizure-inducing properties include cocaine; however, few are probably aware that caffeine at high doses may also induce epileptic seizures (34). Amphetamine and related drugs rarely induce epileptic seizures at therapeutic doses (34). Moreover, methylphenidate and dextroamphetamine do

not appear to be associated with increased seizure risk among patients with TBI (33, 35).

Seizures and seizure disorders are classified according to their clinical and electroencephalographic characteristics, as developed by the Commission on Classification and Terminology of the International League Against Epilepsy (36, 37). Seizures have been divided into two categories, based primarily on pattern of onset. These include partial or focal seizures, and generalized seizures. Patients with nonpenetrating TBI frequently have sustained multiple foci of cerebral injury (38–40), and may manifest more than one type of seizure (4).

Generalized seizures denote those that are bilaterally symmetrical in origin without local onset (36). The most commonly recognized example is the grand mal, or tonic-clonic (GTC) seizure. Generalized-onset or secondarily generalized seizures (SGS) are reported in approximately half of the patients with PTS (41) and appear more frequently in patients with nonpenetrating TBI (42), and among children (43).

Partial or focal seizures originate in a localized area of one cerebral hemisphere. Partial seizures are further classified according to whether consciousness is maintained (simple partial [SPS]) or impaired (complex partial [CPS]) during the seizure. Characteristics of both vary, depending on the location of the seizure activity within the brain. Twelve percent of cases of CPS in the general population may be attributable to TBI (44). Partial-onset seizures are observed in slightly more than half of all patients with PTS, and appear more frequently in adults (4), and patients with early seizures (4, 42, 45), focal lesions on CT (46), penetrating TBI (PTBI) (42, 47), and nonpenetrating TBI of greater severity (46). Studies that incorporate videoelectroencephalography (VEEG) are more likely to detect subtle clinical signs that may indicate partial-onset PTS (48, 49).

The Working Group on Status Epilepticus (50) defines *status epilepticus* (SE) as more than 30 minutes of (1) continuous seizure activity or (2) two or more sequential seizures without full recovery of consciousness between seizures (50). More recent publications define SE as seizures that persist for shorter durations, (52, 51), based upon estimates of the duration necessary to cause injury to central nervous system neurons (51). This definition differs from those of other terms describing multiple seizure episodes, including serial seizures and acute repetitive seizures. *Serial seizures* are two or more seizures occurring over a relatively brief period (i.e., minutes to many hours), but with the patient regaining consciousness between the seizures (51). *Acute repetitive seizures* are clusters of seizures that appear to increase in frequency or severity over a short time. Acute repetitive seizures may become SE, but the frequency of this occurrence is unclear (53). Clinical manifestations of SE vary, and may include clinically obvious tonic-clonic movements, or small amplitude twitching movements of the eyes, face, or extremities (51). Some patients have no observable repetitive motor activity, and the detection of SE requires EEG. Further discussion regarding status epilepticus after TBI follows later in this review.

Nonepileptic seizures, (NES) often called pseudoseizures or psychogenic seizures, are terms used for episodic behavioral events which superficially resemble epileptic attacks but which are not associated with paroxysmal activity within the brain (54). NES may be psychogenic, or may include non-epileptic events such as syncopal episodes and cardiac events. NES are not uncommon in neurologic settings (55), and may coexist with epileptic seizures in patients with epilepsy (55, 56). The differentiation between nonepileptic and epileptic seizures cannot be made on the basis of clinical characteristics alone. Electroencephalographic monitoring (particularly with video) (56) is often helpful in establishing a diagnosis. Postictal prolactin (PRL) measurement (57) may provide additional diagnostic information if significant elevations are observed, suggesting that an epileptic seizure has occurred within one hour (58). The utility of this test to discriminate between epileptic seizures and NES has been questioned, however, as a subset of patients with video-electroencephalography (VEEG)-documented psychogenic NES have also been reported to experience an increase in PRL, particularly if the sample is obtained within 10–20 minutes of a suspected NES (58).

While recognized to occur among patients with TBI, relatively few studies address post-traumatic NES. Hudak et al reported that one-third of patients with moderate-to-severe TBI undergoing VEEG for diagnosis of epilepsy were found to have psychogenic NES (48). When non-diagnostic VEEG studies were excluded, patients with NES comprised 40% of the TBI sample (48). Barry et al. described the characteristics of 16 patients thought to have PTS, who actually had NES, as confirmed on VEEG monitoring. Patients with NES were characterized by injuries of much milder severity, although the disability associated with the NES was pronounced. The patients usually had manifestations of other conversion disorders as well, and psychiatric histories that predate the TBI (59).

Epilepsy has been classified into different epileptic syndromes, with two general divisions employed (3, 37). One division separates epilepsies characterized by generalized seizures from syndromes characterized by seizures of focal onset, termed localization-related epilepsies. The other division separates epilepsies of known etiology (secondary or symptomatic) from those that are idiopathic (primary) and those that are cryptogenic (seizures or epilepsy in which no known risk factor has been identified). Symptomatic epilepsies and syndromes are considered the consequence of a known or suspected disorder of the central nervous system, such as TBI (3, 37). Recurrent late post-traumatic seizures, or post-traumatic epilepsy, are a common and important type of remote symptomatic epilepsy (3), accounting for 20% of all symptomatic epilepsy in the general population (60). Symptomatic (or secondary) epilepsies comprise syndromes of great individual variability, based mainly on seizure type and anatomic localization.

MANIFESTATIONS OF POST-TRAUMATIC SEIZURES AND EPILEPSY

Seizures may present with a variety of manifestations, including cognitive, behavioral and affective changes that may not be attributed to an underlying epileptic disorder (61, 62). Patients with severe TBI may exhibit cognitive, behavioral, and affective sequelae that potentially confound attribution of episodic behavioral changes to an underlying epileptic disorder (48). The varied semiology of seizures that originate in the frontal or temporal lobes, and their associated ictal or postictal alteration of consciousness, justify their consideration in the differential diagnosis of any TBI patient with episodic (especially stereotypic) changes in mental status. Given the propensity of TBI contusion localization to the frontal and temporal lobes (40, 63), it is not surprising that these regions are the most frequent sites of origin for VEEG-verified partial-onset PTE (48). Presumed or pathologically-confirmed post-traumatic seizure foci, however, have been described in all major lobes of the brain (38, 48, 63–65).

Patients with frontal lobe epilepsy may exhibit complex, semipurposeful, complex motor automatisms such as kicking, screaming, and thrashing episodes (62). Frontal lobe interictal and postictal manifestations also include cognitive or affective symptoms, such as confusion, anger, hostility, and hallucinations (66, 67). Complex partial seizures of temporal lobe origin may also present with emotional symptoms such as fear or panic, followed by periods of postictal confusion and amnesia (37). Seizure-related aggression, however, is rare (68, 69). It is usually associated with postictal confusion, particularly while the patient is being restrained (69, 70). Conversely, reports of aggression are more frequent among epileptic patients, particularly with younger age, male gender, psychopathology, and prior brain injury (71), but aggression episodes are typically unrelated to seizure type, frequency, or age of onset (72). Conventional interictal scalp EEG are of limited diagnostic assistance in such cases. Electrographic manifestations of seizure activity in the orbitofrontal and mesial temporal regions of the brain may be difficult to recognize, and can be misleading (62) by showing no abnormality (37) at all. Table 26-1 shows the characteristics of localization-related epilepsies based upon the involved lobe of the brain (37, 67, 73–79).

TABLE 26-1
Characteristics of Localization-Related (partial-onset) Epilepsies

SITE OF ORIGIN	MANIFESTATIONS
Frontal	**Seizure types**: SPS, CPS, SGS, combinations; SE is frequent complication. Seizures often occur several times a day, and frequently during sleep. **Features**: Features strongly suggestive of frontal lobe epilepsies include: 1) Generally short seizures; 2) CPS often with minimal/no postictal confusion; 3) rapid secondary generalization; 4) prominent tonic/postural motor manifestations; 5) complex gestural automatisms at onset (frequent); 6) falling with bilateral discharge (frequent).
Cingulate	**Features**: CPS with complex gestural automatisms at onset; autonomic signs (common); changes in mood and affect (common); psychic/emotional auras, including fear and anger (frequent).
Orbitofrontal	**Features**: CPS with initial sudden, complex, bizarre motor and gestural automatisms that may be bilateral and mixed with staring, olfactory hallucinations/illusions and autonomic signs; psychoemotional auras are rare.
Dorsolateral	**Features**: Tonic (common) or clonic (less common) with versive eye and head movements and speech arrest. *Dorsolateral premotor cortex*-onset usually without aura, with tonic head/neck/eye movement or "pseudoabsence" (very brief lapse of consciousness <10 sec duration); *Prefrontal/Frontopolar*-psychic auras, visual illusions, or initial loss of consciousness followed by head and eye movements.
Motor Cortex	**Features**: SPS (most common) with manifestations reflecting the side and topography of the area involved: *Lower prerolandic area*-speech arrest, vocalization or dysphasia, contralateral tonic-clonic movements of the face, or swallowing. Generalization is frequent. *Rolandic area*-SPS without "march" (jacksonian seizures), particularly beginning in contralateral upper extremity. *Paracentral lobule*-tonic movements of the ipsilateral foot and contralateral leg, postictal paralysis (frequent).
Supplementary Motor Cortex	**Features**: Postural, focal tonic seizures, with vocalization, speech arrest, and fencing postures; usually no aura; may have autonomic symptoms.
Temporal	**Seizure types**: SPS, SGS, CPS, combinations. **Features**: Features strongly suggestive of temporal lobe epilepsies include: 1) SPS typically characterized by autonomic and/or psychic symptoms and certain sensory phenomena (e.g. olfactory and auditory), epigastric, often rising, sensation (most common); 2) CPS with onset of motor arrest or stare followed by oro-alimentary automatism (often), other automatisms frequently follow. Aura is common. Seizure duration typically >1 min, with postictal confusion/amnesia, and gradual recovery (common); 3) Interictal scalp EEG with no abnormality, slight or marked asymmetry of background activity, or temporal spikes, sharp waves, not always confined to the temporal region. Ictal scalp EEG onset may not precisely correlate with clinical onset.
Mesiobasal / Limbic	**Features**: CPS with visceromotor and behavioral symptoms, including rising epigastric discomfort, nausea, marked autonomic signs, and other symptoms, including belching, pallor, fullness/flushing of the face, respiratory changes, pupillary dilatation, fear, panic, and olfactory-gustatory hallucinations. Auditory symptoms do not occur. Interictal scalp EEG may be normal.
Lateral	**Features:** SPS with auditory hallucinations or illusions or dreamy states, visual misperceptions; or language disorders (dominant hemisphere). May progress to CPS with propagation to mesial temporal or extratemporal structures. The scalp EEG may show unilateral, bilateral midtemporal or posterior temporal spikes.
Occipital	**Seizure types:** SPS, SGS, CPS. CPS may occur with spread beyond the occipital lobe. **Features:** Usually visual manifestations, appearing in the visual field contralateral to the discharge (unless generalization occurs). Nonvisual symptoms have been reported, but most often reflect spread to other lobes. *Positive phenomena:* Visual hallucinations (most common), including sparks, flashes. Visual illusions have been reported, but probably reflect non-dominant parietal lobe involvement.

TABLE 26-1
(continued)

SITE OF ORIGIN	MANIFESTATIONS
	Negative phenomena: Ictal amaurosis, fleeting scotoma, hemianopsia. (well-recognized but less common).
Parietal	**Seizure types**: SPS (most common), SGS (especially with paracentral lobule), CPS.
	Features: Predominantly sensory with many characteristics, also some rotatory or postural motor phenomena may occur.
	Positive phenomena: Most common: (tingling, electric shock-like sensations, desire/sensation of movement in body part) usually involving hand, arm and/or face contralateral to seizure focus. Less common: intraabdominal sensation of sinking/nausea, particularly with inferior and lateral parietal lobe involvement. Rare: pain, visual phenomena occurring as formed hallucinations.
	Negative phenomena: numbness (common), disturbance in body image (a feeling that a body part is absent, asomatognosia [loss of awareness of a part or a half of the body, particularly with nondominant hemisphere involvement]), severe vertigo or spatial disorientation (inferior parietal lobe), receptive or conductive languages disturbances (dominant parietal lobe), lateralized genital sensation (paracentral parietal lobe).
Insula	**Seizure type**: SPS
	Features: Throat/laryngeal discomfort, paresthesias on contralateral (typical) side of body, dysarthria/aphonia, hypersalivation.

Ictal versus Postictal Focal Neurological Deficits

The presence of focal motor, sensory or language deficit of new-onset should alert the clinician to the possibility of a recent unwitnessed PTS. Todd's phenomenon/a are terms given to a heterogeneous group of focal signs of neurologic dysfunction that may follow a partial (9) or generalized tonic-clonic seizure (80). Todd's phenomena are recognized postictal manifestations of PTS (81). These do not reflect permanent structural damage, but rather represent transient *post*ictal disruption of function that typically resolves within 24 to 48 hours (9). Todd's phenomena should be differentiated from ictal paralysis, a "negative" *ictal* epileptic manifestation, (82).

Unclassified Phenomena (not considered to be post-traumatic seizures)

Transient behavioral changes, reminiscent of CPS (83–85), have been noted among TBI patients without concurrent seizures. In most reports, patients manifest interictal discharges on EEG, without the hypersynchronous EEG activity and stereotyped behaviors which characterize partial seizures and localization-related epilepsies (84, 85). When described among patients with TBI, these are usually reported among individuals with mild injury severity (84, 85). In these reports, many patients respond favorably to AEDs such as carbamazepine (CBZ) (85).

The resemblance of the behaviors to some CPS of temporal or frontal lobe origin, and favorable response to AEDs, tends to confuse clinical diagnosis. At present, the description of these behavioral abnormalities should not be considered diagnostic for epileptic seizures.

INCIDENCE OF POST-TRAUMATIC SEIZURES

Traumatic brain injuries are an important cause of epilepsy, accounting for 20% of symptomatic epilepsy observed in the general population, and 5% of all epilepsy (60). TBI is the leading cause of epilepsy in young adults (86). Many studies addressing the relationship between TBI and epilepsy derive from observations of veterans sustaining PTBI in battle (47, 87–99). Studies in civilian settings (4, 39, 41, 43, 46, 100–129) generally appeared later and reflect a larger patient population with nonpenetrating TBI, as opposed to PTBI. The observed results vary, reflecting differences in inclusion and exclusion criteria, methods for evaluation and description of seizure phenomena, attention to confounding variables, duration of follow up, and patient population studied (130). Nevertheless, these studies provide useful information regarding the incidence, risk factors, and natural history of PTS/PTE.

In summary, the overall incidence of late seizures in hospitalized patients following nonpenetrating TBI is approximately 4–7%, varying with the injury and patient characteristics (4, 102). Late seizures are observed less frequently among children (43, 102, 122). The incidence of PTS among patients with nonpenetrating TBI observed in the rehabilitation setting appears substantially higher than that reported in other civilian settings (103, 107, 108, 113, 118, 125, 127, 131), approximately 17%. This is probably a reflection of the increased severity of injury and concurrence of multiple risk factors encountered among inpatients in these settings (103, 113). In contrast, the incidence of seizures among adults after mild TBI is slightly greater than that observed in the general population (101, 102). PTS will be observed in approximately 35–65% of patients with PTBI (47, 88, 91, 92, 113). Discussion regarding the influence of specific risk factors upon the incidence of PTSz follows later in this chapter.

The incidence of early seizures is approximately 5% (4, 132) among all nonpenetrating TBI patients, and is higher in young children (4, 42, 43, 102, 104), among whom the incidence is approximately 10% (43, 102). However, continuous EEG monitoring of patients with severe TBI in the intensive care unit suggests that the incidence of early convulsive and nonconvulsive EPTS may be considerably higher than initially believed, approximately 22% (49). Immediate seizures, which make up 50–80% of EPTS (4, 42, 93, 122, 133), are particularly frequent among children with severe TBI (43, 102). EPTS are occasionally observed among children with mild TBI (4, 43), but are comparatively much less frequent among adults with mild TBI. Early seizures among these adults warrant investigation for an underlying intracranial hemorrhage. In a study of >4000 adults with mild TBI, an intracranial hemorrhage was found in almost half of the patients with EPTS (123).

The incidence of early seizures is approximately 10% (43, 102) among young children (4, 42, 43, 102). Immediate seizures, which make up 50–80% of EPTS (4, 42, 93, 122, 133), are particularly frequent among children with severe TBI (43, 102). Late seizures are observed less frequently among children (43, 104, 122) than adults.

NATURAL HISTORY OF POST-TRAUMATIC SEIZURES AND EPILEPSY

Onset

Approximately one-half to two-thirds of patients who suffer PTS will experience seizure onset within the first 12 months, and 75–80% by the end of the second year following injury (41, 46, 47, 92, 96, 97, 109). After five years, adults with mild TBI do not appear to have a significantly increased risk relative to the general population (101), However, patients with moderate or severe TBI and PTBI remain at increased risk after this postinjury duration (42, 46, 47, 101).

Recurrence

It is increasingly evident that seizure recurrence is a critical factor in determination of subsequent disability, and quality of life (135, 134). Greater seizure frequency significantly correlates with lower employment rates, which in one study ranged from 57% among patients seizure-free for 3 months, to 30% in patients with daily seizures. As seizure frequency increased, health care costs increased and measures of QOL declined (135).

Limited data exist regarding PTS recurrence. Earlier studies reported that about one-half of patients will experience a single PTS without recurrence (110, 122), and another quarter will suffer a total of 2–3 seizures (122). These reports addressed recurrence following early seizures. Recent studies addressing LPTS recurrence, however, suggests a more ominous prognosis (136, 137). Semah et al investigated the relationship between prognosis for seizure recurrence and the etiology of epilepsy. Among 50 patients with remote symptomatic epilepsy with history or radiographic evidence of TBI, only 30% of those with partial epilepsy experienced seizure free durations of >1y without recurrence (137). Haltiner and colleagues followed 63 adults with moderate or severe TBI, who developed LPTS during the course of participation in a randomized, placebo-controlled study of the effectiveness of phenytoin prophylaxis for prevention of LPTS (138). The cumulative incidence of recurrent late seizures was 86% by 2 years. However, 52% experienced at least 5 late seizures, and 37% had 10 or more late seizures within 2 years of the first late seizure (136).

Pohlmann-Eden (41) published results of a PTE study population derived from a tertiary referral epilepsy clinic. Fifty-seven patients with PTE were compared with 50 age and sex-matched control patients with severe TBI. Of all PTE patients, 35% became seizure-free (no seizures within the last 3 years), 3.5% without any treatment. Twenty-one percent experienced more than 1 seizure per week. The most important risk factors for poor seizure control were missile injuries, "combined seizure patterns," high seizure frequency, AED non-compliance and alcohol abuse (41).

In summary, recent evidence suggests that while patients with EPTS will experience a late seizure in 20–30% of cases, seizure onset after the first week is associated with a much higher likelihood of seizure recurrence (97, 136). Seizure frequency within the first year after injury may be predictive of future recurrence, particularly with PTBI (47). Persistent PTS may be more common in partial seizures, and less common in generalized seizures (47, 137). IPTS are generally believed to carry no increased risk of recurrence (4, 139). On the other hand, between one-fifth to one-third of patients with LPTS will experience frequent recurrences, apparently refractory to conventional AED therapy (41, 131, 136). Some of these patients may be helped with surgical intervention (38, 64, 140). TBI neuroimaging characteristics may be of value in predicting the appearance (113) and intractability (141) of PTE. Finally, few studies explicitly address rates of PTE remission, that is, disappearance of seizures (142). Early studies, derived mostly from PTBI populations, describe remission rates that range from 25–40%. Higher overall remission rates are reported in studies conducted after the development of effective AEDs (142).

Complications and Consequences of PTS

Potentially significant complications accompany seizures in the patient with TBI. Indeed, occurrence or recurrence of seizures is an important cause of non-elective rehospitalization (143) and death (144) among patients with severe TBI. Among patients with newly-diagnosed (145) or chronic remote symptomatic epilepsy, persistent seizures are associated with increased mortality, particularly among individuals with status epilepticus or generalized convulsions (146). Several studies have examined the sequelae of PTS (147–150). An appreciation of these potential consequences is useful when evaluating risk/benefit relationships for decisions regarding AED therapy.

Cognitive and Behavioral Function

As introduced earlier, manifestations of PTS include cognitive and behavioral dysfunction. Evidence of cognitive impairment may occur or persist during the interictal state, however, when the epileptic patient is not actively manifesting seizures (151–153). Similarly, persistent behavioral abnormalities and a significantly higher incidence of psychiatric-related hospitalizations have been noted among patients with PTS when compared with non-epileptic controls with PTBI (154). Mazzini et al (125) found that disinhibited behavior, irritability, and aggressive behavior were significantly more frequent and severe among rehabilitation inpatients with PTE, when compared with TBI patients without seizures.

Influence on Neurological Recovery

Animal studies suggest the existence of a complex relationship between post-traumatic seizures and neurological recovery (155). Specifically, depending on the severity of the seizure induced and time of presentation, seizures may inhibit, improve, or not affect functional recovery. In studies conducted with rodents, if "mild" subclinical kindled seizures occur early after brain damage, no delay is noted in somatosensory recovery. This suggests that brief infrequent PTS occurring during the early post-traumatic period did not adversely affect functional recovery. However, if more severe and widespread seizures are kindled within a 6-day critical period after brain lesion, a permanent impairment of functional recovery results. When these same seizures occur after this critical period, recovery of function proceeds unimpeded. It is important to note that contrasting results have been found using models of brain injury other than kindling models (155).

Outcome

Recurrent PTS may exert an adverse impact upon functional status among adults (156) and children (105) with TBI, independent of that attributable to the severity of injury. Among patients with PTBI in the Vietnam Head Injury Study, PTS were one of seven impairments which independently and cumulatively predicted employment status (156). PTS and increasing brain volume loss have been noted to exert independent and profound effects on cognitive performance among patients with restricted frontal lobe lesions due to PTBI (157).

However, studies among patients with nonpenetrating TBI less clearly discriminate the influence of seizures on functional prognosis (103, 104) and cognition (158) from those of injury. Haltiner (159) examined the relationship of LPTS to neuropsychological performance and aspects of psychosocial functioning. While patients with LPTS demonstrated greater impairment than those without seizures, after adjusting for injury severity, there were no significant differences in outcome at 1 year as a function of seizures. The authors concluded that poorer outcomes encountered among patients with PTS at 1 year postinjury reflect the severity of injury and not the effects of LPTS *per se*. Asikainen noted that patients with PTS had poorer outcome as measured by the Glasgow Outcome Scale (GOS), a gross global outcome measure, but no significant differences in employment outcome when compared with nonepileptic patients with TBI (104). Mazzini (125) also found that PTS correlated with significantly poorer outcome, as measured by the GOS, disability rating scale, functional independence measure, and subscales of the neurobehavioral rating scale at one year after severe TBI. In contrast, early seizures appear to have little influence on outcome (132, 160).

Status Epilepticus

Status epilepticus is the most clinically significant manifestation of PTS, and carries the greatest risk of adverse outcome. It may cause additional neurologic injury, potentially occurring within 10 minutes of seizure onset, according to some reports (161). One study employing continuous EEG monitoring suggests that early nonconvulsive SE may not be rare, occurring perhaps in as many as 6% of patients with severe TBI despite "therapeutic" levels of AED prophylaxis (49). Moreover, status epilepticus among patients early after TBI is associated with a very high mortality risk (49). Fortunately, *convulsive* SE remains an infrequent manifestation of PTS (122).

Additionally, SE is usually attributable to another cause, such as antiepileptic drug (AED) withdrawal, acute systemic or neurologic injury, such as anoxic encephalopathy or stroke (162), sepsis, metabolic derangements, or a combination of these conditions (8). Status epilepticus is more likely to be encountered as a PTS manifestation in children, (163). Deaths associated with SE are usually attributable to the disorder which precipitated it (164, 165).

Mortality

Mortality among patients with PTS remains consistently elevated in most reports (147, 149, 150, 166). However, the contribution of PTS to this increased mortality is unclear. Walker noted that men with PTS have a death rate somewhat exceeding that of comparable normal men. However, information supplied by relatives suggested that causes of death were not specific for men with TBI, and seemed to reflect those found in elderly people (149). In another related series of studies, deaths among PTBI patients with PTS appeared due to the sequelae of injury and unrelated to seizures. These patients approached the actuarial mortality norm for their peers after only 3 years (133, 148).

Sudden unexpected death in epilepsy (SUDEP) accounts for 18% of all deaths among patients treated in major epilepsy centers (167). Walczak and colleagues noted that occurrence of tonic-clonic seizures, treatment with more than two AEDs, and full-scale IQ less than 70 are independent risk factors for SUDEP. Tonic-clonic seizure frequency may be a risk factor, but only in women. The presence of cerebral structural lesions was not found to be a risk factor for SUDEP (167), and this phenomenon has not been described among patients with PTE.

In summary, sequelae associated with isolated LPTS are comparable to those found in any seizure. Isolated or infrequent late seizure episodes are generally associated with relatively little risk. Increasing frequency and severity of seizure disorders, including status epilepticus, carry greater associated risks of increased morbidity or mortality, and worsened cognitive and functional prognosis.

POST-TRAUMATIC EPILEPTOGENESIS

Epileptogenesis

Epileptogenesis refers to the dynamic process underlying the appearance and natural history of epilepsy (9). For decades, physicians treating patients with TBI have sought to prevent the appearance of PTS by interrupting the process of the development of seizures through the prophylactic administration of AEDs. However, the pathophysiologic mechanisms involved in acquired epileptogenesis are not well understood, though they clearly involve multiple pathways at the molecular and cellular level, as well as changes in neural networks that result in the appearance of spontaneous seizures (168). This limited understanding of the pathophysiology of acquired epileptogenesis has probably influenced the failures encountered with clinical trials of AED prophylaxis (169), discussed later in this chapter. Propelled by insights into the molecular genetics of epilepsy (170), the topic of acquired epileptogenesis is attracting increasing scientific investigation.

Aside from careful observations derived from clinical, electrographic, and neuroimaging studies among human subjects (171), much of what is known or postulated regarding acquired epileptogenesis has been derived from studying pathological specimens from surgical patients with epilepsy, as well as a large number of animal models of epilepsy (168, 171–174). These animal epilepsy models simulate human epilepsy, and provide a system for studying mechanisms that account for the characteristics of acquired epilepsy in humans (168). Such characteristics include the presence of a "latent" period between time of injury and recurrent seizure onset (171), as demonstrated in the kindling model of epilepsy, or the propensity for seizure occurrence with specific characteristics of TBI (175), as found in patients with hemorrhagic contusions and modeled in the ferric chloride model. Indeed, the presence of an unambiguous stimulus (TBI) for later appearance of epilepsy in patients with clearly identified risk factors has prompted great interest in post-traumatic epilepsy and epileptogenesis as an archetypal model for remote symptomatic epilepsy (176). The development of relevant animal models is important, as selection of AEDs for development for marketing worldwide are primarily based on results of preclinical animal model studies (169, 177). A number of these models suggest that many AEDs have antiepileptogenic potential (168). The theoretical and clinical implications of such models in the treatment of epilepsy, including post-traumatic epilepsy and epileptogenesis, have been reviewed elsewhere (155, 168, 171, 175, 177, 178). In the discussion that follows, animal models of epilepsy with historic relevance to post-traumatic epileptogenesis are followed by a review of more recent studies addressing this issue.

Ferric Chloride Model

Initially described by Willmore in 1978, the iron or ferric chloride model is the first considered to reflect mechanisms responsible for post-traumatic epilepsy in humans. Specifically, it is felt to model pathophysiologic processes resulting from a cortical contusion / focal neocortical injury. It is of theoretical interest because cortical deposits of hemosiderin may be important in the development of recurrent PTS (179). Patients with cerebral injuries characterized by contact of blood and cortical tissue manifest an increased incidence of PTS (180). Contusion or cortical laceration causes extravasation of red blood cells, with hemolysis and deposition of hemoglobin. Willmore demonstrated that recurrent focal epileptiform discharges could result from cortical injection of ferrous or ferric chloride (179). It is felt that the iron salts and hemoglobin in neural tissue may contribute to epileptogenesis by initiating lipid peroxidation, damaging cell membranes and inhibiting neuronal Na-K ATPase (174).

Kindling Models

The kindling model of epilepsy is arguably the most recognized animal model of epileptogenesis (173, 181). When initially described (182), brief trains of weak electrical stimulation were applied to susceptible areas of rodent brains, until a seizure was observed. When continued over a prolonged period of time, progressively less stimulation was required to induce the seizures, and spontaneous seizures eventually appeared. Once established, this enhanced sensitivity to electrical stimulation appears to be permanent for the life of the animal. Here, epileptogenesis is triggered by the kindling paradigm. The relevance of kindling to remote symptomatic epilepsy derives from the hypothesis that other stimuli, such as subclinical seizures or structural brain lesions, may trigger epileptogenesis (183).

Agents that retard or abort the kindling process are considered "antiepileptogenic," whereas those that merely suppress or block seizures in fully "kindled" animals are "anticonvulsant." Such studies have demonstrated that PHT (184) and CBZ (185, 186) have anticonvulsant effects but lack antiepileptogenic action. By contrast, studies that examined the effects of GABAergic drugs, including VPA, DZP, and PB, on kindling have shown that they demonstrate antiepileptogenic properties (168, 184, 187, 188). Among the newer AEDs, TGB and LEV show antiepileptogenic action (168) in kindling models. In contrast, TPM (168) and LTG show limited antiepileptogenic activity in kindling (189, 190, 191) and rodent status epilepticus models (192). Retardation of kindled seizures appears to outlast the period of exposure to antiepileptogenic drugs, suggesting that they were not simply masking seizure expression.

Several notable limitations exist with the kindling model. For example, the original kindling studies were performed on rats. Subsequently this phenomenon was demonstrated in rabbits, cats, and later, genetically-seizure-predisposed primates (184). Since neuroanatomical structural differences between species imply functional differences, it is not surprising that animal kindling models demonstrate significant phylogenetic variability in expression (193). Further, despite the efficacy of some compounds on the kindling model, none of them has had an indisputable antiepileptogenic action in animal models with spontaneous seizures (176) or in humans (168). Also, no disease-modifying effects have been described (192). Thus, the extent of this model's relevance to investigations of human PTE is considered controversial (181).

Recent Studies of Post-traumatic Epileptogenesis

Fluid Percussion Injury Model of Post-traumatic Epilepsy

In 2004, D'Ambrosio and colleagues described the results of a series of experiments that demonstrate, perhaps for the first time, reproduction of post-traumatic epilepsy induced by a single episode of lateral fluid percussion injury (194), a clinically-relevant model of nonpenetrating TBI (195). Prior studies of experimental TBI (including those incorporating fluid-percussion experimental injury [196]) describe acute seizures (197), and hippocampal hyperexcitability to electrical stimulation (196, 198) or exposure to proconvulsant agents (199). However, spontaneous chronic seizures, the hallmark of epilepsy, has not been described (194). Moreover, while neocortical epileptic foci commonly develop in humans following TBI (38), changes in neocortical excitability have not been studied in rat models of nonpenetrating TBI, which have focused on the hippocampus (194). To date, investigation of neocortical pathophysiology in PTE has been limited to two approaches: the first involves studying neocortical islands isolated by undercuts from the surrounding grey matter, and the second involves chronic neocortical implantation of ferrous chloride (179, 194). Both models bear limited resemblance to the human post-traumatic condition, however, as they lack its unique focal and diffuse mechanical and hemorrhagic components (194). These limitations, in turn, potentially influence the relevance of these models to mechanisms of human post-traumatic epileptogenesis and subsequent therapies that can be translated to human PTE (194).

The study's main findings demonstrate that a single episode of fluid percussion injury is sufficient to cause PTE in the rat. The characteristics of PTE appeared comparable to those of human PTE, as seizure manifestations emerged after a latent period, and were partial in onset after a focal injury. Moreover, epileptiform activity is first detected in the neocortex at the site of injury, which electrophysiologic studies demonstrate is chronically hyperexcitable after fluid percussion injury. Finally, postmortem pathological examination reveals that intense glial reactivity is observed at the site of injury. In summary, the clinical, electrophysiological, and structural changes of severe lateral fluid percussion injury appear to parallel changes seen after neocortical injury in human PTE (194).

Synaptic Plasticity

During recent years, a large (and increasing) number of studies demonstrate the ability of the brain to adapt to injury with changes in functional, and structural reorganization (198, 201, 202). These reorganizational changes, termed plasticity, may serve an adaptive role in development and recovery (200, 203), or a maladaptive role when they contribute to disorders such as epilepsy (203–206). Pathological studies of TBI reveal that compensatory collateral axonal sprouting occurs following brain injury (207) and may be a mechanism of importance in functional neurological recovery (200, 208). Under certain circumstances, however, collateral sprouting may give rise to the development of seizure foci (209) or the spread of epilepsy from a primary focus to synaptically-related brain regions (206). Additional excitatory synaptic contacts on cell somata could produce a marked increase in cell excitability, particularly if the new excitatory synapses replaced inhibitory ones (209). If the induced alterations in connectivity increase excitability, neural pathways could become progressively susceptible to epileptic events, and may contribute to the subsequent development of seizures (210).

While sprouting and subsequent formation of new synaptic connections has been proposed as a post-traumatic epileptogenic mechanism, it is not likely to be the only pathway to neuronal hyperexcitability (178). Postinjury development of neuronal hyperexcitability may be the result of three general types of plastic change: a) alterations in intrinsic membrane properties, b) changes in synaptic connectivitiy, and c) modifications of receptors and receptor subunits (178, 211). Direct axonal injury may render surviving neurons more excitable through alterations in intrinsic membrane properties. Loss of afferents can induce sprouting of axons, leading to hyperexcitability by increasing recurrent cortical pathways (178).

If the aforementioned models are important mechanisms common to both "adaptive plasticity" after TBI and "maladaptive plasticity" in PTS, potentially significant implications follow. Specifically, AEDs whose potential effects are exerted by preventing the development of compensatory excitatory neural pathways, i.e. a seizure focus, may concurrently retard neurological recovery through a similar mechanism of action (212). Moreover, since PTS occur among a minority of all patients with TBI, including severe TBI, AED therapy broadly directed against subclinical seizure activity among all TBI patients during recovery may be more detrimental to neurological and functional outcome than either seizures alone or initiation of AED therapy after seizure onset.

"ASYMPTOMATIC" MANAGEMENT OF POST-TRAMATIC SEIZURES & EPILEPSY: PREVENTION, PROPHYLAXIS & PRACTICE GUIDELINES

The term prophylaxis has been defined as "specific measures taken to prevent disease in an individual . . ."(213). In the context of PTS, the term applies to AED treatment administered to patients who have not manifested seizures. Several justifications can be proposed for prophylaxis of PTS. First, AEDs might prevent PTS at a time when they potentially pose the greatest risk of secondary injury, such as seizure-induced elevations in intracranial pressure (214). Second, seizure prevention may help avoid loss of employment, loss of driving privileges, or accidental injury (214). Third, there may exist concern over the medicolegal implications of negligent treatment if PTS appear. Finally, there exists the possibility that administration of AEDs may alter or arrest epileptogenesis. Thus far, however, animal and human studies fail to provide evidence that AED therapy prevents the development of the post-traumatic seizure focus (168), or alters the course of seizure recurrence aside from suppression of the seizure focus (177).

Identification of the "High-Risk" Patient

Methods have been proposed to improve identification of those patients at risk for PTS development, and therefore those most to gain from its prevention or potential recurrence. These include assessment of the clinical characteristics of the patient, the injury, as well as information yielded by neuroimaging and electrophysiologic assessment techniques (Table 26-2).

Patient Characteristics

Age, history of alcohol abuse, and family history represent the patient characteristics most frequently cited as factors influencing subsequent seizure risk. Patients with histories of alcohol abuse, particularly chronic alcoholism, demonstrate an increased risk of early (132) and late seizure development (93, 115, 117, 121, 122, 124, 216, 220) and recurrence (41) following TBI. Few data exist regarding PTS risk associated with low levels of alcohol use, either before or after TBI. Patient age appears to exert a strong influence on PTS risk (43, 102, 104, 122). Children demonstrate markedly lower risk for LPTS, and considerably higher risk for IPTS and EPTS, when compared with adult patients with comparable injury severity. Some studies suggest that age at onset of injury (64) or seizures (221) may influence susceptibility to seizures later in life.

Some authors note a modestly increased incidence of PTS among patients with nonpenetrating TBI and a family history of seizures (4, 93, 116, 216). This has not

TABLE 26-2
Risk Factors for Late Post-traumatic Seizures

RISK FACTOR	REFERENCE
Patient Characteristics	
Age	43, 102, 104, 122
Alcohol use	93, 115, 117, 121, 215
Family history	4, 93, 116, 216
APOE εallele	217
Injury Characteristics	
Bone/metal fragments	47, 88, 96,
Depressed skull fracture	4, 43, 94, 129
Focal contusions/injury	39, 46, 111, 113, 115, 218
Focal neurological deficits	4, 46, 47
Lesion location	46, 93, 157, 219
Dural penetration	47, 61, 93, 113, 219
Intracranial hemorrhage	43, 113, 117, 125, 218, 219
Injury severity	4, 47, 93, 97, 101, 102, 125, 219
Focal hypoperfusion	125
Other	
Early post-traumatic seizures	4, 47, 113, 115, 219

been consistently observed (47, 98, 222), suggesting that the influence of a family history of seizures appears weak when compared to the effects of extensive cerebral trauma (47). However, Diaz-Arrastia and colleagues recently noted that inheritance of the apolipoprotein (APOE) ???allele was significantly associated with development of late seizures, but not poorer outcome, after moderate and severe TBI (217). If such findings are replicated, genetic influence may ultimately be shown to have an important role in post-traumatic epileptogenesis.

Injury Characteristics

Certain injury characteristics demonstrate an increased likelihood of resulting in recurrent, late PTS. Virtually uniform agreement exists regarding observations of markedly increased seizure risk among patients with PTBI (41, 47, 88, 90, 91–93, 97). Blood appears to demonstrate an extremely irritating effect on cortical neurons, as demonstrated by increased seizure incidence among TBI patients with intracranial bleeding, (4, 41, 43, 47, 102, 112, 116, 117, 121, 124, 218, 219) particularly with subdural hematoma (113, 219). Increased extent of PTBI (47, 92, 166); and severity of nonpenetrating TBI (41, 43, 91, 100, 126, 128), as evidenced by prolonged duration of post-traumatic amnesia (4, 41, 93, 102, 112, 114, 127), prolonged duration to follow commands (219), lower GCS (4, 101, 102, 219) or impairment of consciousness (114, 117, 124, 127), are prominently associated with increased seizure risk.

General agreement exists regarding observations of increased PTS risk in patients with TBI characterized by focal neurologic deficits (4, 41, 47, 91, 95, 97, 108, 109, 117, 124), depressed skull fractures (4, 93, 94, 112, 129), cerebral contusions (39, 46, 100, 104, 109, 110, 115, 218), and retained bone or metal fragments (88, 89, 93, 97). Lesion location may affect incidence (46, 93, 95–100, 157, 219, 223), type (64), and possibly frequency (223) and treatment response (38) of PTS. The concurrent presence of multiple risk factors is consistently associated with increased seizure risk (4, 91, 117, 122, 124).

Late PTS rarely occur after mild TBI (101). Among adults, trivial blows to the head almost never result in seizures, but may occur in the presence of preexisting (224) or concurrent (123) brain lesions. In a recent multicenter study, 8% of patients with GCS scores in the mild range (13–15) developed late post-traumatic seizures within 24 months; all had CT-scan evidence of contusion or intracranial hemorrhage (113). Despite their rarity, PTS and even recurrent PTS *do* occur after mild TBI, but their presence in the adult patient should prompt an investigation for a precipitating cause, such as an intracranial mass lesion. Moreover, frequent LPTS after mild TBI should also prompt careful evaluation for NES (59).

Electroencephalography (EEG)

The utility of the interictal EEG as an objective predictor of subsequent PTS appears limited (115, 126, 225, 226). It is frequently abnormal in patients with TBI, both with and without PTS (46, 218, 227, 228), reflecting the severity of brain damage sustained (46, 226). Sleep-deprivation activation procedures similarly do not appear to differentiate between patients with and without PTS (229). The rare change of focal slow wave activity to focal spike discharges, particularly during the first month postinjury (100), or persistence of focal spike or sharp wave discharges may be suggestive of increased seizure risk (121, 225, 228). However, such discharges may be observed on the EEG of non-epileptic patients (218, 230). Conversely, a normal EEG may precede PTS onset (225–227, 231), though this finding is more frequently associated with a favorable prognosis (121, 218). EEG findings should be evaluated in context with other clinical risk factors when assessing the likelihood of PTS onset.

The EEG provides valuable information in focus localization, seizure persistence, and severity prognostication once PTS have been observed (89, 225, 232). In addition, the EEG may identify the presence of nonconvulsive seizures among patients with impaired consciousness, particularly early after severe TBI (49). The utility of the EEG in predicting PTS recurrence following a seizure-free period has not been established.

In the neurorehabilitation setting, we believe that the EEG is potentially helpful when considering the continuation of AED therapy in patients with a history of EPTS.

AED Prophylaxis Clinical Trials and Guidelines

Encouraged by animal studies suggesting that anticonvulsants may prevent the development of epileptic foci in animals, a number of studies have been published addressing the efficacy of AED prophylaxis in TBI. These studies have been extensively reviewed elsewhere (233), and their relevant findings and conclusions summarized here. These clinical trials and literature reviews have also served as a basis for practice management guidelines addressing AED prophylaxis of early and late seizures (2, 234).

Retrospective studies and nonrandomized open trials involving human subjects appeared first in the scientific literature (92, 115, 121, 133, 235–240) with generally favorable results (236–240). Decidedly unimpressive results were observed among prospective investigations (124, 138, 218, 220, 241–245) of chronic prophylaxis for late PTS. Indeed, published randomized, controlled prospective investigations almost uniformly fail to substantiate evidence of efficacy for CBZ (218), PHT (138, 241, 242, 244, 245), PB (124), or VPA prophylaxis (243) of late PTS. In four of these trials, the incidence of PTS was actually higher among the PHT-treated groups (138, 241, 244). Meta-analyses of these trials indicate that AED prophylaxis is not accompanied by a reduction in LPTS, (168, 242, 246–248), mortality, or neurological disability (246, 248).

In contrast, AED prophylaxis consistently reduces the incidence of early PTS (138, 218, 220, 249). As in some of the studies cited previously, however, there is no clinical evidence that AED prophylaxis of early seizures reduces the occurrence of LPTS, or has any effect on death or neurological disability (248). Most published trials lack sufficient numbers of patients with PTBI to conclude whether AED prophylaxis exerts a favorable or adverse influence on seizure incidence in this high-risk subset of TBI patients (250).

While disappointing, treatment failure among trials conducted thus far should not imply that future trials are similarly destined to fail. Different approaches are currently under investigation (251). These include: 1) the use of available AEDs that have not been previously studied for prophylaxis of PTE, such as $MgSO_4$; 2) different timing of administration (e.g. <12h postinjury) with presently-available AEDs (251); and 3) development and investigation of future AED's, preferably with demonstrated efficacy in a relevant animal model of human PTE.

Table 26-3 summarizes the practice management guidelines of four medical societies that have published guidelines pertinent to AED prophylaxis of PTS (2, 5, 234, 250). These include the Brain Injury Special Interest Group of the American Academy of Physical Medicine and Rehabilitation (BI-SIG) (2), the American Academy of Neurology (AAN) (5), the Brain Trauma Foundation ([BTF] in conjunction with the Joint Section on Neurotrauma and Critical Care) (234), and the Penetrating TBI Committee (250). The guidelines of the BI-SIG, AAN, and BTF are all very similar, and primarily address non-penetrating TBI in adults (2, 5). The guidelines of the Penetrating TBI Committee specifically

---

TABLE 26-3

Practice Management Guidelines for AED Prophylaxis of PTS

PATIENT POPULATION	SEIZURE TYPE	RECOMMENDATION	DEGREE OF CERTAINTY (252)
Nonpenetrating TBI (High-risk)	Late PTS (without EPTS)	Not recommended	Standard (2, 23) "Level B" (5)
Penetrating TBI	Late PTS (without EPTS)	Not recommended (2, 250) (No specific opinion for PTBI [5, 234])	Option (2, 250)
Penetrating TBI or high-risk nonpenetrating TBI	Early PTS	May be used	"Level A" (5) Option (2, 234)

Degree of Certainty-strength of recommendations: **Standards** refer to generally accepted principles for patient management that reflect a high degree of clinical certainty (i.e., based on class I evidence or, when circumstances preclude randomized clinical trials, overwhelming evidence from class II studies that directly addresses the question at hand or from decision analysis that directly addresses all the issues). **Guidelines** refer to recommendations for patient management that may identify a particular strategy or range of management strategies and that reflect moderate clinical certainty (i.e., based on class II evidence that directly addresses the issue, decision analysis that directly addresses the issue, or strong consensus of class III evidence). **Options** refer to strategies for patient management for which there is unclear clinical certainty (i.e., based on inconclusive or conflicting evidence or opinion) (252).

address prophylaxis with penetrating TBI, and conclude that AED prophylaxis for LPTS appears unjustified (250).

MANAGEMENT OF POST-TRAUMATIC SEIZURES AND EPILEPSY

It is beyond the practical scope of this review to critically examine the breadth of literature pertinent to the treatment of all patients with epilepsy, and the reader is referred to textbooks that serve this role (253, 254). Nevertheless, treatment issues that are particularly germane to patients with TBI and recurrent PTS will be briefly reviewed. In the discussion that follows, the authors' clinical experience will be incorporated into the literature review extrapolated from other epileptic populations when addressing symptomatic management of patients with PTS/PTE.

Diagnosis

An initial step in the management of suspected seizures is establishing whether or not a seizure disorder indeed exists (61). In light of the social, economic, and medical implications that accompany the diagnosis of an epileptic disorder, errors need to be avoided. In many cases, a diagnosis can be reliably made from clinical observations of seizure phenomena, particularly those noted by experienced staff in the hospital setting. Classification of the observed seizures is similarly important, as categorization can have significant prognostic and therapeutic implications.

There are situations, however, where the diverse or subtle clinical presentations of PTS complicate diagnosis. As noted earlier, epileptic manifestations (particularly those of CPS) may not be recognized in patients with significant cognitive and behavioral dysfunction. Alternatively, nonepileptic phenomena such as NES, myoclonus, or syncopal episodes may be mistaken for PTS. Clinical observations alone may thus be insufficient to render or rule out a diagnosis of PTS, prompting the use of other diagnostic options (48).

The EEG is the single most informative laboratory test for the diagnosis of epileptic disorders (255–257) and should be obtained in any patient with suspected PTS. The EEG may assist in assessing the likelihood of an underlying epileptic condition when correlated with the clinical diagnosis (258), or in localization of the seizure focus (255). Although interictal epileptiform activity is apparent in only approximately 50% of single awake recordings in adults with epilepsy, this proportion rises to approximately 80–85% if sleep is included. Two recordings obtained while the patient is awake will demonstrate epileptiform activity in 85% of individuals with epilepsy, and this rises to 92% of persons within four recordings (255). In patients who manifest only generalized seizures,

interictal discharges are bilateral, symmetrical and synchronous, generally of greatest amplitude over the frontal regions but sometimes located posteriorly. In patients with partial seizures, discharge topography will more or less closely correspond to that of the focus from which seizures arise. These focal interictal discharges may spread, producing secondarily generalized spike-and-slow-wave activity. If the generalization is rapid, the focal onset may be difficult to detect (255).

There exist limitations in the diagnostic sensitivity of the standard interictal EEG, however, and absence of EEG abnormalities does not exclude the presence of a seizure disorder (255). Postictal PRL measurement may be useful in some of these patients, as significant elevations in serum PRL levels reliably occur within 20–40 minutes following GTC seizures (259) and many CPS (259). PRL elevations are typically not observed after SPS (260), CPS of frontal lobe origin (261), or after 30 minutes in most patients with NES (57, 58, 260). Significant PRL elevation occurring after a possible PTS episode may help confirm clinical suspicion of an underlying epileptic disorder (262). Given the significant diurnal variation in serum PRL levels, however, it is often prudent to obtain a baseline value for comparison, drawn at the same time of day as the postictal specimen, within a few days.

When initial standard evaluations fail to resolve the clinical diagnosis, long-term EEG monitoring techniques, including ambulatory EEG monitoring (263, 264) and/or inpatient VEEG telemetry (255, 265) are effective and clinically valuable (48). Ambulatory EEG monitoring offers an intermediate-level option for recording while the patient conducts normal activities at home, work, or school (9, 263, 264). It is most useful for investigating the patient in a natural environment; for example, to test the claim that a patient has seizures at home which are not observed in hospital (255). A patient or observer log is maintained to identify the times and descriptions of behavioral episodes suspected of representing seizure activity (9). Ambulatory monitoring has been transformed by the recent development of recorders using solid-state memory or removable miniature digital discs (255). Ambulatory monitoring is usually performed without simultaneous video registration, however, and thus EEG telemetry with video monitoring provides the best opportunity to obtain an artifact-free ictal EEG while observing and evaluating associated clinical behavior (265). Concurrent computerized automatic seizure detection often identifies important events, particularly at night, that are not reported by the patient or nursing staff. Definitive diagnosis requires recorded examples of all seizure types experienced by the patient (255). Conversely, an absence of discharges during prolonged monitoring, particularly in a patient with frequent seizures, may serve to cast doubt on the diagnosis of epilepsy (255).

Hudak et al. recently described the utility of prolonged VEEG monitoring in the clinical management of paroxysmal behaviors in TBI survivors (48). In this retrospective record review, 127 patients with a documented history of moderate-to-severe brain injury preceding onset of frequent, disabling paroxysmal behaviors were evaluated in an epilepsy monitoring unit for management of medically intractable epilepsy. VEEG monitoring was conducted for an average of 4.6 days. AED administration was suspended during the assessment period. Monitoring was successful in establishing a diagnosis in 82% of the cases referred. Sixty-two percent of the evaluated patients had focal seizures, 6% had generalized seizures and 33% had psychogenic NES. The authors concluded that VEEG is a useful procedure in the evaluation of TBI survivors with paroxysmal behaviors suggestive of epilepsy, and that the yield of diagnoses that may alter treatment is substantial (48).

Treatment and Selection of the AED

While broad agreement exists regarding the appropriateness of AED treatment among patients who manifest two or more seizures, considerable debate remains concerning the benefits of treatment in reducing recurrence risk following a first seizure (266, 267). Overall, about 33 percent of patients with a first unprovoked seizure can be expected to have a second within the subsequent three to five years. This risk varies considerably, however, depending on clinical characteristics of the patient (268). Increased risk is observed among patients with remote symptomatic epilepsy (268, 269, 270). Approximately 44–48% percent of patients with a first remote symptomatic seizure will experience a second seizure in the next three to five years (268, 269). Of the patients with a second seizure, almost 87% will experience a third seizure at five years (268). Seizures occurring immediately following an acute precipitant or injury to the brain carry a lower risk of recurrence than a late seizure (271).

Treatment after first seizure has been advocated, though few randomized clinical trials have been conducted to establish the efficacy of this practice. One randomized multicenter clinical trial concluded that treatment of the first seizure with antiepileptic drugs leads to a significant reduction of relapse risk. The authors added, however, that the decision to start treatment in a patient with a first seizure must balance that patients risk of relapse, the benefits of avoiding the consequences of a second seizure, and the risk of AED toxicity (272).

Once a decision has been reached that pharmacological treatment of a patient with PTS is indicated, a primary goal is to attain control of seizures with one medication (9, 273). The decision of which specific agent to use will reflect the type of post-traumatic seizure, the route and frequency of drug administration, as well as the anticipated and realized adverse effects. Among patients with symptomatic localization-related epilepsy (273), including patients with TBI who manifest seizures of partial onset, extended release CBZ remains a commonly preferred drug (233, 273, 274). Patients with tonic-clonic seizures of generalized, secondarily generalized, or multifocal onset respond well to VPA (273–275). CBZ (275) and PHT (275, 276) are also effective anticonvulsants for GTC seizures. While generally effective for seizure control of tonic-clonic seizures (9, 276), the utility of PB is severely limited by prominent adverse effects on cognition and behavior (277), and is rarely used in current practice (278).

Anecdotal evidence suggests that neurologists and physiatrists increasingly employ newer "second generation" AEDs in symptomatic management of selected patients with PTE. Unfortunately, there currently exists little scientific data, specific to PTE, that support (or refute) the benefits of this practice. For example, a recent PUBMED literature search (September 2004), cross-referencing the terms "post-traumatic seizures" or "post-traumatic epilepsy" with key words of the newer AEDs, including "lamotrigine", "topirimate", "oxcarbazepine", "levetiracetam", or "tiagabine", failed to yield a single reference. Presently, extrapolation from scientific literature derived from other patient populations, particularly those with remote symptomatic epilepsy, and evolving clinical experience are all that exist to guide clinical practice with newer AEDs for patients with PTE.

Fortunately, two expert consensus panels recently address the use of the newer AEDs as initial monotherapy (273, 279), including patients with symptomatic localization-related epilepsy (SLRE) and symptomatic generalized epilepsy (SGE)(273). The Quality Standards and the Therapeutics and Technology Assessment Subcommittees of the American Academy of Neurology published a practice parameter summarizing an evidence-based assessment regarding the efficacy, tolerability, and safety of seven new AEDs in the management of new onset partial or generalized epilepsy, including GBP, LTG, TPM, TGB, OXC, LEV and ZNS (279). They found evidence that GBP, LTG, TPM, and OXC are effective as monotherapy in newly diagnosed adolescents and adults with either partial or mixed seizure disorders, but not generalized epilepsy syndromes. No specific guidelines were provided regarding AED use in remote symptomatic epilepsy or PTE (279). Karceski et al. employed an "expert consensus method" to survey epilepsy specialists (273) regarding AED preference in specific clinical scenarios. The survey revealed a preference for CBZ as the initial AED for management of symptomatic epilepsies. Besides CBZ, PHT, OXC and LTG were also cited as initial first line agents for SLRE manifested by simple partial seizures or complex partial seizures. For management of SLRE with secondarily generalized seizures, PHT, OXC, LTG, and VPA were identified as initial first line AEDs (273). A limitation of this consensus statement (273) is that it does not address the place of ZNS or LEV in the clinical armamentarium, as these agents were not in wide use at the time the survey data were obtained.

Adverse Effects of AED Therapy

Antiepileptic drugs commonly employed in the treatment of PTS may be associated with significant idiosyncratic and dose-related adverse drug reactions (279, 280, 281), requiring their discontinuation or substitution in as many as 20–30% of patients (282, 283). These include hematologic, dermatologic, hepatic, neurologic, endocrinologic, urologic, and teratogenic adverse effects (279, 284, 285). Transient or persistent leukopenia and thrombocytopenia may be observed in patients taking PHT and CBZ, though idiosyncratic aplastic anemia is extremely rare. Rashes are occasionally encountered with many AEDs and severe dermatologic reactions more rarely noted with LTG and PHT (279, 280). Hirsutism and gingival hyperplasia may be problematic in patients treated with PHT (280). Weight gain has been associated with VPA and GBP treatment, and weight loss reported with ZNS and TPM (275, 279). Mild and transient elevations of hepatic enzymes, up to two to three times normal in some cases, are reported to occur in patients receiving PHT, CBZ, and VPA, (286). Frequent and rigorous routine laboratory monitoring regimens, however, aside from baseline determination of hematologic and hepatic function or closer observation of noted abnormalities, are unjustified for most AEDs (with the notable exception of FBM). These typically do not provide meaningful protection from rare and potentially life-threatening manifestations (287, 288). Appropriate counseling for the patient, family, and/or caregivers regarding potential complications and symptoms that might herald an adverse event is far more useful and important (288).

Cognitive effects of AEDs warrant particular attention in the patient with TBI. Newer AEDs demonstrate superior cognitive adverse effect profiles and tolerability when compared with older agents (302, 303, 304). In contrast, older AEDs, particularly PB, PHT and CBZ, significantly impair memory performance in double-blind crossover trials among healthy adults (289). Patients with severe TBI already have significant cognitive impairment. Antiepileptic drugs may exert independent and additional adverse cognitive effects on the patient with TBI who is receiving chronic therapy (290). Among patients with severe TBI participating in the landmark prophylaxis trial of Temkin et al. (138), a significantly greater proportion (78%) of individuals treated with PHT demonstrated cognitive impairment sufficient to preclude testing at one month postinjury. This was observed in only 47% of corresponding patients treated with placebo (290).

Among older established AEDs, most studies demonstrate no comparative advantage in cognitive adverse effect profile between CBZ, PHT, or VPA, though few include subjects with TBI (291–294). Smith (294) found no significant difference on cognitive testing results among patients randomized to withdrawal from PHT and CBZ prophylaxis. Only 13 of the 82 studied patients sustained severe TBI, however, with the remainder receiving prophylaxis following craniotomy or mild/moderate TBI. There remains considerable evidence suggesting that PHT provides a relatively unfavorable cognitive side effect profile among patients with severe TBI (290, 291). Patients randomized to receive 6 months of VPA for prophylaxis of LPTS following severe TBI demonstrated no evidence of adverse cognitive effects when compared with those receiving 1 week of PHT (291). In contrast, an earlier study among comparably injured patients receiving PHT prophylaxis yielded unequivocal evidence of cognitive impairment among AED-treated patients (290).

While attention regarding adverse drug effects frequently focuses upon observable phenomena, such as lethargy, the influence of AED therapy upon the course of postinjury neurologic recovery also warrants consideration (295). Specifically, certain drugs, including AEDs, clearly impair recovery after brain injury in laboratory animals (296–298). Schallert et al. (298) demonstrated that diazepam administered to rats within 12 hours of neocortical damage delayed recovery indefinitely, whereas delayed administration of diazepam resulted in only transient reinstatement of neurologic deficit (298). Brailowsky observed that PHT increased the severity of cannula-induced cortical hemiplegia in rats, though motor impairment was not seen when administered to the animals after their hemiplegic syndrome had cleared (296). These findings suggest that AED administration with diazepam or PHT during certain critical periods following brain injury may exert a deleterious effect upon subsequent neurologic recovery.

In summary, dose-related and idiosyncratic adverse effects occur among a substantial subset of treated patients, particularly with older AEDs. Cognitive adverse effects may be particularly problematic, particularly with the older established agents, impacting upon long-term tolerability. The cited studies serve as a reminder that decisions regarding chronic AED treatment, and particularly prophylaxis, cannot be considered solely on the merits of effectiveness in seizure prevention. Rather, consideration must also be given to potentially significant adverse effects and toxicities of the AED regimen.

AED Substitution

Neurosurgeons and neurologists have preferred PHT for prophylaxis (299, 300) and symptomatic AED treatment, primarily because of its availability in parenteral forms that can be administered in the acute setting, where seizures are more likely to occur. Since the publication of prophylaxis guidelines (2, 5, 234), however, we have observed a clear trend towards less frequent use of AED prophylaxis. In addition, among patients receiving symptomatic AED treatment, PB use is rare, with PHT remaining the most commonly observed for use in acute care settings AED for initial symptomatic management. These patients are commonly maintained on the chosen AED until a satisfactory seizure-free duration has passed. AED substitution has previously been usually reserved for failure of seizure control or the manifestation of significant drug reactions (9). As mentioned earlier, selection of a newer AED as initial monotherapy is likely to improve tolerability, particularly with cognitive adverse effects, while maintaining comparable efficacy. For similar reasons, many neurorehabilitation specialists consider substitution of PHT monotherapy for other less cognitively-impairing medications, such as LTG, as clinical circumstances allow.

When substituting an AED for another drug, clinically effective levels of the latter AED should be attained prior to discontinuation of the former drug (9). Among the newer AEDs, serum levels are not commonly obtained, although these are available at reference laboratories. Once appropriate and effective doses of the new drug are achieved, a gradual taper of the former drug ensues. At one time, CBZ was the most common AED employed for substitution instead of PHT in our center. More recently, however, we use LTG as slow add-on therapy (usually added to PHT), followed by gradual withdrawal of PHT after maintenance of seizure control and effective doses of LTG (approximately 4–500mg /day). Our preference for LTG derives from a clearly favorable cognitive adverse effect profile, particularly when compared with either PHT or CBZ (301). Among patients requiring more rapid additional seizure control, LTG is not a therapeutic option, due to the increased danger of serious rash or Stevens-Johnson syndrome (305) associated with rapid dose increases. Instead, we employ VPA, as it is effective for both generalized and partial seizures (275), it demonstrates generally favorable tolerability among patients with TBI (291), and it is available in parenteral and once-daily oral formulations. VPA may also be a practical choice among patients with PTE that are also demonstrating post-traumatic mood lability and irritability. We are aware of colleagues that favor LEV as a preferred AED for substitution among patients with TBI, citing its ability to be rapidly titrated to effective dose range (306) as well as its tolerability. However, anecdotal reports of a lack of persistent antiepileptic effect, and documented psychiatric adverse effects (307), may limit the utility of this agent in some patients.

Duration of AED therapy

No clinical studies specifically address the duration of AED therapy for patients with recurrent LPTS. In general, it is reasonable to consider AED withdrawal from patients with epilepsy after a 2-year period free of seizures (308). Reported rates of relapse vary considerably, and reflect the type of seizure disorder being treated (9). The risk of seizure recurrence under a policy of slow AED withdrawal is still substantial when compared with a policy of continued treatment, particularly during the first year of withdrawal (309). Increased risk of recurrence has been reported among patients with a history of more frequent seizures, treatment with more than one AED, a history of GTC seizures (309), and abnormal or epileptiform discharges on pre-withdrawal EEGs (308, 310). Among patients for whom the risk of relapse after discontinuation appears low, the psychosocial benefits of discontinuation may be considerable (311). There is no consensus regarding the ideal period over which AEDs should be withdrawn in patients with recurrent seizures, although conservative recommendations advise a period of 12 months (9, 312). Worsening of seizures following PHT (313, 314) or CBZ (314) discontinuation is believed to reflect the loss of therapeutic drug effect rather than a withdrawal phenomenon. In contrast, withdrawal exacerbation of seizures is prominent with barbiturates (315) and benzodiazepines (316), and does not indicate that the drug was necessary for maintenance of seizure control (9).

Surgical Treatment of Post-traumatic Seizures

Recent studies are providing valuable insight into the natural course of history regarding post-traumatic seizure recurrence (136). These studies identify a subset of patients remaining refractory to treatment, even with multiple AEDs. The definition of "refractory" is debatable, and there is evidence that adding a 2nd or 3rd AED may facilitate seizure remission in about one-fifth of patients that remain with seizures while taking a single AED (317). Nevertheless, for those patients who continue to experience frequent seizures despite various AED monotherapy or polytherapy combinations, surgical treatment options are increasingly available, particularly in recent years (318).

Surgical Resection of Epileptic Focus

Advances in neuroimaging technology, coupled with results of recent landmark studies, have prompted a dramatic shift toward surgical treatment for certain types of medically-refractory epilepsy (217, 319). There is now growing sentiment among epilepsy specialists that surgical treatment for refractory epilepsy is seriously underutilized (319, 320). In the first randomized study comparing surgical and medical treatment for temporal lobe epilepsy,

58 percent of surgically treated patients were free of disabling seizures at one year, versus only 8 percent of those assigned to receive medical treatment (321). Significant improvements in outcome were observed in measures of quality of life as well as a trend with respect to social functioning (321). The Multicenter Study of Epilepsy Surgery similarly reported that resective surgery significantly reduced seizure recurrence after medial temporal (77% 1-year remission) and neocortical resection (56% 1-year remission) (322). In light of such findings, the American Academy of Neurology, in association with the American Epilepsy Society and the American Association of Neurological Surgeons, published a practice parameter supporting the benefits of anteromesial temporal lobe resection for disabling complex partial seizures. It further recommended referral of patients with these seizures to an epilepsy surgery center (319).

Surgical Excision of the Post-traumatic Seizure Focus

Surgical excision of the seizure focus also provides an important treatment option for carefully selected patients with refractory PTE. Favorable responses, including seizure freedom have been described among selected patients with PTE treated with resective surgery (38, 140, 323). Patients with unilateral post-traumatic frontal lesions who undergo complete resection of perilesional encephalomalacia/gliosis and adjacent electrophysiologically abnormal tissue respond particularly well to surgery (324, 325). The cumulative experience described in published studies, however, also highlight the challenges accompanying accurate identification of the seizure focus in patients with severe TBI, who often demonstrate bilateral and multifocal injury (38, 64). Marks described 25 patients with PTE treated in their tertiary epilepsy center, 21 of whom were treated surgically. Seventeen of these patients were felt to have mesial temporal lobe epilepsy, and another 8 patients were judged to have neocortical epilepsy. Of the 21 patients treated with surgery, only 9 (43%) had favorable outcomes, characteristically those with well-circumscribed hippocampal or neocortical focal lesions (64). Schuh and associates reported on 102 patients who underwent anterior temporal lobectomy. A history of TBI, alone or in combination with other factors, was significantly correlated with continued seizures after surgery (326).

Vagus Nerve Stimulation (VNS)

Vagus nerve stimulation (VNS) is an alternative to pharmacologic treatment of seizures in patients who have failed conventional pharmacotherapy, either due to lack of efficacy or adverse effects (327). The mechanism of action of VNS is not yet clear (328).

VNS is approved by the FDA for adjunctive treatment of intractable partial seizures in patients over 12 years old. Based on controlled, randomized trials, approximately 30% of these patients can be expected to have at least a 50% decrease in overall seizure frequency (329, 330). Efficacy in LPTS has not been specifically studied. Persistence of benefits has been demonstrated (331). While this technique is indeed invasive, no intracranial surgery is required, and surgical morbidity and mortality are limited. Adverse effects include hoarseness, cough and dysesthetic sensations in the throat (330).

While numbers of patients treated with this technique are limited compared to AED therapy, in 1999, the American Academy of Neurology Therapeutics and Technology Subcommittee classified VNS as safe and effective for intractable partial seizures, based on sufficient Class I evidence (332). At present, VNS is considered to be an appropriate therapy for patients with medically refractory epileptic seizures who are not optimal candidates for resective epilepsy surgery (327).

A potential advantage to the use of VNS in the context of LPTS is the relative absence of cognitive adverse effects. However the role of this technology in the treatment of epilepsy in the context of TBI remains to be delineated.

Consultation and Referral

Guidelines for the appropriate level of primary and specialty care of patients with seizures, including recommendations for referral to specialty centers, have been published (333). In summary, the first step for individuals experiencing an initial seizure or seizures is to consult their primary-care physician in their own community. The primary physician may then choose to begin a treatment program or refer the individual to a general neurologist for consultation. In any case, if seizures continue to occur after three months, a referral to a general neurologist is indicated. When the seizures are controlled, many patients appropriately return to the care of their primary physicians, with follow-up to the neurologist as needed. If seizure control is not achieved at the end of the first year of treatment, referral to a center that offers comprehensive diagnostic and treatment services to patients with intractable seizures is indicated (326).

CONCLUDING STATEMENTS

In light of the evidence previously discussed, our management approach for LPTS is presented. Patients with acute TBI who are transferred to the neurorehabilitation hospital setting receiving an AED for prophylaxis, and without reported early seizures, are gradually tapered from AEDs early in their hospital course. As mentioned previously, routine chronic AED prophylaxis of LPTS is unjustified, and with few exceptions* no AED therapy is provided unless late seizures are reported (2, 5). AED prophylaxis withdrawal in the hospital setting facilitates monitoring for the potentially varied manifestations of seizures. Since seizures tend to occur in the earlier postinjury period, this also helps insure the presence of trained personnel should a seizure be observed during or after AED withdrawal. We have observed that marked improvements in the cognitive status of patients frequently coincide with termination of AED prophylaxis.

If a possible late post-traumatic seizure is observed, either during the patient's hospitalization or after discharge, a search for an identifiable seizure precipitant takes place, and includes a neuroimaging study of the brain. If no obvious correctable seizure precipitant is identified, establishment of a diagnosis of seizure disorder ideally precedes initiation of AED therapy. Clinical description of the episode alone, provided by a family member or other witnesses, may be sufficiently convincing to initiate AED therapy. The patient and family are given instructions for keeping a "seizure logbook," and more frequent follow-up visits are often warranted. If a late PTS has been documented, we will typically proceed with selecting an AED for symptomatic seizure management. Most commonly, we choose between a CBZ-extended release formulation, VPA, or LTG. AED selection is influenced by the: 1) patient's cognitive and behavioral status; 2) type/manifestation of the seizure, (e.g., GTC status epilepticus versus SPS lip twitching); 3) perceived need for rapid achievement of a therapeutic dose, and 4) whether or not the patient has already been started on PHT or another AED in the emergency department. If the patient is receiving PHT and seizures are well-controlled, an alternative AED such as LTG is usually substituted at the earliest suitable point to minimize adverse side effects, particularly cognitive impairment.

For most physicians caring for patients with TBI in the rehabilitation setting, the issue of whether to institute prophylaxis of EPTS is usually moot. Nevertheless, postinjury prophylaxis of EPTS with PHT or FPT may be justified in patients with severe TBI belonging to high-risk groups. The patient is at their highest risk for seizure development, at a time when they can least afford to endure complications from a seizure. Prophylaxis may be continued for approximately 1 week if seizures are not observed, and then tapered gradually. Again, this should take place in a setting in which close observation can be provided. The risks incurred with such a short duration of treatment currently appear minimal, and acceptable.

Insufficient data exist to definitively guide AED therapy among patients whose only manifestation of a seizure disorder are EPTS. Most published reports exclude these patients from further study, thereby losing valuable information regarding the influence of continued AED therapy on LPTS recurrence risk. Issues to consider include onset (day 1 versus day 7 or later), severity (particularly status epilepticus), recurrence frequency, and clinical risk factors for recurrence. Factors favoring continuation of AED therapy would include later time of seizure onset, documented episodes of status epilepticus, persistent epileptiform activity or electrographic seizures on EEG, multiple seizure episodes throughout the first week of injury, and the presence of multiple risk factors suggestive of high risk for LPTS occurrence, such as penetrating TBI. In contrast, it may be reasonable to consider a monitored withdrawal of AED therapy in selected patients with isolated EPTS, particularly those with IPTS. Our experience suggests that most patients with nonpenetrating TBI and isolated EPTS will tolerate discontinuation of AED therapy without seizure recurrence (131, 334).

Major themes involving the symptomatic management of patients with PTS have been discussed above, and will not be repeated here. Still, important research questions remain, and involve a broad range of topics pertinent to the diagnosis and treatment of epileptic disorders. Investigation must be directed towards identifying laboratory models that reflect human response to prevention of an initial or recurrent PTS. Further study is needed to clarify the natural history of PTS, the prognostic implications of single or isolated seizures, and the effect of AED therapy upon recurrence risk. Future studies should address the comparative utility and adverse effects of symptomatic seizure treatment, including surgery, *upon adult and pediatric subjects with TBI*, and explore the potential effects of these therapies upon neurologic recovery and functional outcome.

Finally, assessment of each patient's risk and suitability for treatment must be made on an individual basis, guidelines or algorithms notwithstanding. Even with the publication of four guidelines (2, 5, 234, 250) addressing the issue of AED prophylaxis, discussion of issues related to PTS with the patient and family members is useful and important. Moreover, the clinician should be aware of the prevailing regional standards of care regarding symptomatic management. Lastly, in instances where questionable or repeated seizures occur, utilizing the assistance of neurological and neurosurgical consultants with

---

*Our exceptions to this general rule include: 1) history of episodes suggestive of EPTS, especially SE; 2) anticipated intracranial surgical procedure within the next 7–14 days; 3) EEG findings consistent with epileptiform activity and/or electrographic seizures; and 4) concurrent serious medical or neurological complications, such as sepsis or hydrocephalus awaiting shunt placement; and 5) patient history of severe alcohol or substance abuse with poor family/caregiver support. (Our experience has found that number of this latter group of patients have probably experienced undiagnosed seizures or epilepsy prior to their most recent TBI.)

specific interest in the unique management issues of this patient population can be invaluable.

Abbreviations: (For text and tables)

AED: Antiepileptic drug
APOE: Apolipoprotein E allele
CBZ: Carbamazepine
CPS: Complex partial seizure(s)
DZP: Diazepam
EPTS: Early post-traumatic seizure(s)
FBM: Felbamate
FPT: Fosphenytoin
GBP: Gabapentin
GCS: Glasgow Coma Scale
GOS: Glasgow Outcome Scale
GTC: Generalized tonic-clonic seizure(s)
IPTS: Immediate post-traumatic seizure(s)
LEV: Levetiracetam
LPTS: Late post-traumatic seizure(s)
LTG: Lamotrigine
NES: Nonepileptic seizures
OXC: Oxcarbazepine
PB: Phenobarbital
PHT: Phenytoin
PRL: Prolactin (serum level)
PTE: Post-traumatic epilepsy
PTBI: Penetrating traumatic brain injury
PTS: Post-traumatic seizure(s)
SE: Status epilepticus
SGE: Symptomatic generalized epilepsy
SGS: Partial onset seizure with secondary generalization
SLRE: Symptomatic localization-related epilepsy
SPS: Simple partial seizure(s)
SSRI: Selective serotonin reuptake inhibitor(s)
SUDEP: Sudden death in epilepsy
TBI: Traumatic brain injury
TGB: Tiagabine
TPM: Topiramate
VEEG: Video-electroencephalography
VNS: Vagus Nerve Stimulation
VPA: Valproate
ZNS: Zonisamide

Acknowledgements

We would like to acknowledge funding support provided through the Wilson Research Foundation, Jackson, Mississippi, and the National Institute on Disability and Rehabilitation Research, grants H133A020514 and H133A980035.

References

1. Thurman D, Guerrero J. Trends in hospitalization associated with traumatic brain injury. *JAMA.* 1999;282:954–7.

2. Brain Injury Special Interest Group of the American Academy of Physical Medicine and Rehabilitation. Practice parameter: antiepileptic drug treatment of post-traumatic seizures. *Arch Phys Med Rehabil* 1998;79:594–597.

3. Commission on Epidemiology and Prognosis, International League Against Epilepsy. Guidelines for epidemiologic studies on epilepsy. *Epilepsia* 1993;34:592–6.

4. Jennett B. *Epilepsy After Non-missile Head Injuries*, ed 2. William Heinemann, Chicago, 1975.

5. Chang BS, Lowenstein DH; Quality Standards Subcommittee of the American Academy of Neurology. Practice parameter: antiepileptic drug prophylaxis in severe traumatic brain injury: report of the Quality Standards Subcommittee of the American Academy of Neurology. *Neurology* 2003;60: 10–16.

6. Frucht MM, Quigg M, Schwaner C, Fountain NB. Distribution of seizure precipitants among epilepsy syndromes. *Epilepsia* 2000;41: 1534–9.

7. Mazzini L, Campini R, Angelino E, Rognone F, Pastore I, Oliveri G. Post-traumatic hydrocephalus: A clinical, neuroradiologic, neuropsychologic assessment of long-term outcome. *Arch Phys Med Rehabil* 2003;84: 1637–41.

8. Delanty N, French JA, Labar DR, Pedley TA, Rowan AJ. Status epilepticus arising *de novo* in hospitalized patients: an analysis of 41 patients. *Seizure* 2001;10: 116–9.

9. Engel J, Jr. (Ed). Seizures And Epilepsy. *Philadelphia, PA*: FA Davis;1990.

10. Messing RO, Simon RP. Seizures as a manifestation of systemic disease. *Neurol Clin* 1986;4: 563–84.

11. Hasan D, Schonck RSM, Avezaat CJJ, Tanghe HLJ, van Gijn J, van der Lugt PJM. Epileptic seizures after subarachnoid hemorrhage. *Ann Neurol* 1993;33: 286–91.

12. Jamjoon AB, Kane N, Sanderman D, Cummins B. *Epilepsy* related to traumatic extradural hematomas. BMJ 1991;302: 448.

13. Neiman J, Haapaniemi HM, Hillbom M. Neurological complications of drug abuse: pathophysiological mechanisms. *Eur J Neurol.* 2000;7:595–606.

14. Messing RO, Closson RG, Simon RP. Drug-induced seizures: A 10–year experience. *Neurology* 1984, 34: 1582–6.

15. Hauser A, Ng SKC, Brust JCM. Alcohol, seizures, and epilepsy. *Epilepsia* 1988;29 (suppl 2): S66–78.

16. Hillbom ME. Occurrence of cerebral seizures provoked by alcohol abuse. *Epilepsia* 1980;21: 459–66.

17. Bergmann F, Bleich S, Wischer S, Paulus W. Seizure and cardiac arrest during bupropion SR treatment. *J Clin Psychopharmacol* 2002;22: 630–1.

18. Centorrino F, Price BH, Tuttle M, Bahk WM, Hennen J, Albert MJ, Baldessarini RJ. EEG abnormalities during treatment with typical and atypical antipsychotics. *Am J Psychiatry* 2002;159: 109–15.

19. Gross A, Devinsky O, Westbrook LE, Wharton AH, Alper K. Psychotropic medication use in patients with epilepsy: Effect on seizure frequency. *J Neuropsych Clin Neurosci* 2000;12: 458–64.

20. Hedges DW, Jeppson KG. New-onset seizure associated with quetiapine and olanzapine. *Ann Pharmacother* 2002;36: 437–9.

21. Johnston JA, Lineberry CG, Ascher JA, Davidson J, Khayrallah MA, Feighner JP, Stark P. A 102–center prospective study of seizure in association with bupropion. *J Clin Psychiatry* 1991; 52:450–6.

22. Wroblewski BA, McColgan K, Smith K, Whyte J, Singer WD. The incidence of seizures during tricyclic antidepressant drug treatment in a brain-injured population. *J Clin Psychopharmacol* 1990;10: 124–8.

23. Smith PEM, McBride A. Illicit drugs and seizures. *Seizure* 1999;8: 441–3.

24. Favale E, Audenino D, Cocito L, Albano C. The anticonvulsant effect of citalopram as an indirect evidence of serotonergic impairment in human epileptogenesis. *Seizure* 2003;12: 316–8.

25. Hernandez EJ, Williams PA, Dudek FE. Effects of fluoxetine and TFMPP on spontaneous seizures in rats with pilocarpine-induced epilepsy. *Epilepsia* 2002;43: 1337–45.

26. Spigset O. Adverse reactions of selective serotonin reuptake inhibitors: reports from a spontaneous reporting system. *Drug Saf.* 1999;20:277–87.

27. Hargrave R, Martinez D, Bernstein AJ. Fluoxetine-induced seizures. *Psychosomatics* 1992;33:236–9.

28. Prasher VP. Seizures associated with fluoxetine therapy. *Seizure* 1993;2:315–7.

29. Calandra G, Lydick E, Carrigan J, Weiss L, Guess H. Factors predisposing to seizures in seriously ill infected patients receiving antibiotics: experience with imipenem/cilastin. *Am J Med* 1988; 84:911–8.

30. Tattevin P, Messiaen T, Pras V, Ronco P, Biour M. Confusion and general seizures following ciprofloxacin administration. *Nephrol Dial Transplant* 1998;13:2712–3.

31. Koppel BS, Hauser WA, Politis C, van Duin D, Daras M. Seizures in the critically ill: The role of imipenem. *Epilepsia* 2001;42: 1590–3.

32. Pestotnik SL, Classen DC, Evans RS, Stevens LE, Burke JP. Prospective surveillance of imipenem/cilastin use and associated seizures using a hospital information system. *Ann Pharmacother* 1993;27:497–501.

33. Wroblewski B. Epileptic potential of stimulants, dopaminergics, and antidepressants. *J Head Trauma Rehabil* 1992;7(3):109–11.

34. Zagnoni PG, Albano C. Psychostimulants and epilepsy. *Epilepsia* 2002;43 (Suppl 2):28–31.

35. Wroblewski BA, Leary JM, Phelan AM, Whyte J, Manning K. Methylphenidate and seizure frequency in brain injured patients with seizure disorders. *J Clin Psychiatry* 1992;53:86 9.

36. Commission on Classification and Terminology of the International League Against Epilepsy. Proposal for revised clinical and electroencephalographic classification of epileptic seizures. *Epilepsia* 1981;22:489–501.

37. Commission on Classification and Terminology of the International League Against Epilepsy. Proposal for revised classification of epilepsies and epileptic syndromes. *Epilepsia* 1989;30: 389–99.

38. Diaz-Arrastia R, Agostini MA, Frol AB, Mickey B, Fleckenstein J, Bigio E, Van Ness PC. Neurophysiologic and neuroradiologic features of intractable epilepsy after traumatic brain injury in adults. *Arch Neurol.* 2000;57:1611–6.

39. Eide PK, Tysnes OB. Early and late outcome in head injury patients with radiological evidence of brain damage. *Acta Neurol Scand* 1992;86:194–8.

40. Hardman JM. The pathology of traumatic brain injuries. Advances in *Neurology* 1979, 22:15–50.

41. Pohlmann-Eden B, Bruckmeir I. Predictors and dynamics of post-traumatic epilepsy. *Acta Neurol Scand* 1997: 95:257–262.

42. Pagni CA. Post-traumatic epilepsy. Incidence and prophylaxis. *Acta Neurochir Suppl (Wien)* 1990;50:38–47.

43. Hahn YS, Fuchs S, Flannery AM, Barthel MJ, McClone DG. Factors influencing post-traumatic seizures in children. *Neurosurgery* 1988;22:864–7.

44. Rocca WA, Sharbrough FW, Hauser WA, Annegers JF, Schoenberg BS. Risk factors for complex partial seizures: A population based case-control study. *Ann Neurol* 1987;21:22–31.

45. Locke GE, Molaie M, Biggers S, Leonard E. Risk factors for post-traumatic epilepsy [abstract]. *Epilepsia* 1991;32 (Suppl 3): S104–S105.

46. da Silva AM, Nunes B, Vaz AR, Mendonça D. Post-traumatic epilepsy in civilians: Clinical and electroencephalographic studies. *Acta Neurochir Suppl (Wien)* 1992;55:56–63.

47. Salazar AM, Jabbari B, Vance SC, Grafman J, Amin D, Dillon JD. Epilepsy after penetrating head injury: I. Clinical correlates. *Neurology* 1985;35:1406–14.

48. Hudak AM, Trivedi K, Harper CR, Booker K, Caesar RR, Agostini M, Van Ness PC, Diaz-Arrastia R. Evaluation of seizure-like episodes in survivors of moderate and severe traumatic brain injury. *J Head Trauma Rehabil.* 2004;19:290–5.

49. Vespa PM, Nuwer MR, Nenov V, Ronne-Engstrom E, Hovda DA, Bergsneider M, Kelly DF, Martin NA, Becker DP. Increased incidence and impact of nonconvulsive and convulsive seizures after traumatic brain injury as detected by continuous electroencephalographic monitoring. *J Neurosurg.* 1999;91: 750–60.

50. Working Group on Status Epilepticus. Treatment of convulsive status epilepticus. Recommendations of the Epilepsy Foundation of America's Working Group on Status Epilepticus. *JAMA* 1993;270:854–9.

51. Lowenstein DH, Alldredge BK. Status epilepticus. *N Engl J Med* 1998;338:970–6.

52. Waterhouse EJ. Status epilepticus. *Curr Treat Options Neurol* 2002;4:309–317.

53. Vining E. Gaining a perspective on childhood seizures. *N Engl J Med* 1998;338: 1916–18.

54. Holmes GL, Sackellares JC, McKiernan J, Ragland M, Dreifuss FE. Evaluation of childhood pseudoseizures using EEG telemetry and video tape monitoring. *J Pediatrics* 1980;97:554–8.

55. Betts T. Pseudoseizures: Seizures that are not epilepsy. *Lancet* 1990;336:163–4.

56. Leis AA. Psychogenic seizures. The *Neurologist* 1996;2: 141–9.

57. Pritchard PB III, Wannamaker BB, Sagel J, Daniel CM. Serum prolactin and cortisol levels in evaluation of pseudoepileptic seizures. *Ann Neurol* 1985;18:87–9.

58. Willert C, Spitzer C, Kusserow S, Runge U. Serum neuron-specific enolase, prolactin, and creatine kinase after epileptic and psychogenic non-epileptic seizures. *Acta Neurol Scand* 2004;109: 318–23.

59. Barry E, Krumholz A, Bergey GK, Chatha H, Alemayehu S, Grattan L. Nonepileptic post-traumatic seizures. *Epilepsia* 1998;39:427–31.

60. Hauser WA, Annegers JF, Kurland LT. Prevalence of epilepsy in Rochester, Minnesota: 1940–1980. *Epilepsia* 1991;32: 429–45.

61. Broglin D, Delgado-Escueta AV, Walsh GO, Bancaud J, Chauvel P. Clinical approach to the patient with seizures and epilepsies of frontal origin. *Adv Neurol* 1992;57:59–88.

62. Williamson PD, Spencer SS. Clinical and EEG features of complex partial seizures of extratemporal origin. *Epilepsia* 1986;27 (Suppl 2):S46–63.

63. Payan H, Toga M, Berard-Badier M. The pathology of post-traumatic epilepsies. *Epilepsia* 1970;11:81–94.

64. Marks DA, Kim J, Spencer DD, Spencer SS. Seizure localization following head injury in patients with uncontrolled epilepsy. *Neurology* 1995;45: 2051–7.

65. Oller L, Fossas P, Sanchez ME, Russi A. Versive seizures of probable occipital origin in a case of post-traumatic epilepsy. *Eur Neurol* 1985;24(5):355–9.

66. Adachi N, Onuma T, Nishiwaki S, Murauchi S, Akanuma N, Ishida S, Takei N. Inter-ictal and post-ictal psychoses in frontal lobe epilepsy: A retrospective comparison with psychoses in temporal lobe epilepsy. *Seizure* 2000;9:328–35.

67. Delgado-Escueta AV, Swartz BE, Walsh GO, Chauvel P, Bancaud J, Broglin D. Frontal lobe seizures and epilepsies in neurobehavioral disorders. *Adv Neurol* 1991;55:317–40.

68. Engel J, Jr. Neurobiology of behavior: Anatomic and physiological implications related to epilepsy. *Epilepsia* 1986;27 (Suppl 2): S3–13.

69. Treiman DM. Psychobiology of ictal aggression. In Smith D, Treiman D, Trimble M (eds): Advances in *Neurology*, Vol. 55, Raven Press, New York, 1991;341–56.

70. Devinsky O, Luciano D. Psychic phenomena in partial seizures. *Semin Neurol* 1991;11:100–9.

71. Mendez MF. Postictal violence and epilepsy. *Psychosomatics* 1998;39:478–80.

72. Bogdanovic MD, Mead SH, Duncan JS. Aggressive behaviour at a residential epilepsy centre. *Seizure* 2000;9:58–64.

73. Kotagal P, Arunkumar GS. Lateral frontal lobe seizures. *Epilepsia* 1998;39 (Suppl 4):S62–8.

74. Kotagal P, Arunkumar G, Hammel J, Mascha E. Complex partial seizures of frontal lobe onset statistical analysis of ictal semiology. *Seizure* 2003;12:268–81.

75. Wieser H-G. Ictal manifestations of temporal lobe epilepsy. *Adv Neurol* 1991;55:301–15.

76. Quesney LF. Clinical and EEG features of complex partial seizures of temporal lobe origin. *Epilepsia* 1986;27 (Suppl 2): S27–45.

77. Kuzniecky R. Symptomatic occipital lobe epilepsy. *Epilepsia* 1998;39 (Suppl 4):S24–31.

78. Kutsy RL. Focal extratemporal epilepsy: clinical features, EEG patterns, and approach. *J Neurol Sci* 1999;166:1–15.

79. Isnard J, Guénot M, Sindou M, Maugiére F. Clinical manifestations of insular lobe seizures: A stereo-electroencephalographic study. *Epilepsia* 2004;45:1079–90.

80. Rolak LA, Rutecki P, Ashizawa T, Harati Y. Clinical features of Todd's post-epileptic paralysis. *J Neurol Neurosurg Psychiatry* 1992;55:63–4.

81. Efron R. Post-epileptic paralysis: Theoretical critique and report of a case. *Brain* 1961;84:381–94.

82. Iriarte J, Urrestarazu E, Artieda J, Alegre M, Schlumberger E, Lazaro D, Viteri C. Ictal paralysis mimicking Todd's phenomenon. *Neurology* 2002;59:464–6.

83. Roberts RJ, Gorman LL, Lee GP, Hines ME, Richardson ED, Riggle TA, Varney NR. The phenomenology of multiple partial seizure-like symptoms without stereotyped spells: an epilepsy spectrum disorder? *Epilepsy Res* 1992;13:167–77.

84. Varney NR, Hines ME, Bailey C, Roberts RJ. Neuropsychiatric correlates of theta bursts in patients with closed head injury. *Brain Inj* 1992;6:499–508.

85. Verduyn WH, Hilt J, Roberts MA, Roberts RJ. Multiple partial seizure-like symptoms following 'minor' closed head injury. *Brain Inj* 1992;6:245–60.

86. Annegers JF. The epidemiology of epilepsy. In: Wyllie E, ed. *The Treatment of Epilepsy: Principles and Practice*. 2nd ed. Baltimore, Md: Williams & Wiliams;1996:165–72.

87. Ameen AA. Penetrating craniocerebral injuries: observations in the Iraqi-Iranian war. *Milit Med* 1987;152:76–9.

88. Ascroft PB. Traumatic epilepsy after gunshot wounds of the head. Br Med J 1941;1:739–44.

89. Askenasy JJM. Association of intracerebral bone fragments and epilepsy in missile head injuries. *Acta Neurol Scand* 1989;79: 47–52.

90. Brandvold B, Levi L, Feinsod M, George ED. Penetrating craniocerebral injuries in the Israeli involvement in the Lebanese conflict, 1982–1985. Analysis of a less aggressive surgical approach. *J Neurosurg* 1990, 72:15–21.

91. Caveness WF, Liss HR. Incidence of post-traumatic epilepsy. *Epilepsia* 1961;2:123–9.

92. Caveness WF, Meirowsky AM, Rish BL, Mohr JP, Kistler JP, Dillon JD, Weiss GH. The nature of post-traumatic epilepsy. *J Neurosurg* 1979;50:545–53.

93. Evans JH. Post-traumatic epilepsy. *Neurology* 1962;12:665–74.

94. Phillips G. Traumatic epilepsy after closed head injury. *J Neurol Neurosurg Psychiatry* 1954;17:1–10.

95. Russell WR, Whitty CWM: Studies in traumatic epilepsy: I. Factors influencing the incidence of epilepsy after brain wounds. *J Neurol Neurosurg Psychiatry* 1952;15:93–8.

96. Walker AE, Jablon S. A follow-up of head injured men of World War II. *J Neurosurg* 1959;16:600–10.

97. Walker AE, Jablon S. A follow-up study of head wounds in World War II. (Veterans Administration Medical Monograph), US Government Printing Office, *Washington D.C.*, 1961.

98. Watson CW. Incidence of epilepsy following cranial cerebral injury. II. Three year follow-up study. *AMA Arch Neurol Psychiatry* 1952;68:831–4.

99. Whitty CWM. Early traumatic epilepsy. *Brain* 1947;70: 416–39.

100. Angeleri F, Majkowski J, Cacchio G, Sobieszek A, D'Acunto S, Gesuita R, Bachleda A, Polonara G, Krolicki L, Signorino M, Salvolini U. Post-traumatic epilepsy risk factors: one-year prospective study after head injury. *Epilepsia* 1999 40:1222–30.

101. Annegers JF, Hauser WA, Coan SP, Rocca WA. A population-based study of seizures after traumatic brain injuries. *N Engl J Med* 1998;338:20–4.

102. Annegers JF, Grabow JD, Broover RV, Laws ER, Elveback LR, Kurland LT. Seizures after head trauma: A population study. *Neurology* 1980;30:683–9.

103. Armstrong KK, Saghal V, Block R, Armstrong KJ, Heinemann A. Rehabilitation outcomes in patients with post-traumatic epilepsy. *Arch Phys Med Rehabil* 1990;71:156–60.

104. Asikainen I, Kaste M, Sarna S. Early and late post-traumatic seizures in traumatic brain injury rehabilitation patients: brain injury factors causing late seizures and influence of seizures on long-term outcome. *Epilepsia* 1999;40:584–9.

105. Barlow KM, Spowart JJ, Minns RA. Early post-traumatic seizures in non-accidental head injury: relation to outcome. *Dev Med Child Neurol* 2000;42:591–4.

106. Black P, Shepard RH, Walker AE. Outcome of head trauma: Age and post-traumatic seizures. *Ciba Found Symp* 1975;34:215–9.

107. Bontke CF, Lehmkuhl LD, Englander J, Mann NR, Ragnarsson K, Zasler ND, Graves DE, Thoi LL, Chung CH. Medical complications and associated injuries of patients treated in TBI Model System programs. *J Head Trauma Rehabil* 1993;8:34–46.

108. Cohen M, Groswasser Z. Epilepsy in traumatic brain-injured patients [abstract]. *Epilepsia* 1991;32 (Suppl 1):S55.

109. da Silva AM, Vaz AR, Ribeiro I, Melo AR, Nunes B, Correia M. Controversies in post-traumatic epilepsy. *Acta Neurochir Suppl (Wien)* 1990;50:48–51.

110. De Santis A, Cappricci E, Granata G. Early post-traumatic seizures in adults. *J Neurosurg Sci* 1979;23:207–10.

111. De Santis A, Sganzerla E, Spagnoli D, Bello L, Tiberio F. Risk factors for late post-traumatic epilepsy. *Acta Neurochir Suppl (Wien)* 1992;55:64–7.

112. Desai BT, Whitman S, Coonley-Hoganson R, Coleman TE, Gabriel G, Dell J. Seizures and civilian head injuries. *Epilepsia* 1983;24:289–96.

113. Englander J, Bushnik T, Duong TT, Cifu DX, Zafonte R, Wright J, Hughes R, Bergman W. Analyzing risk factors for late post-traumatic seizures: a prospective, multicenter investigation. *Arch Phys Med Rehabil* 2003;84:365–73.

114. Guidice MA, Berchou RC. Post-traumatic epilepsy following head injury. *Brain Inj* 1987;1:61–4.

115. Heikinnen ER, Ronty HS, Tolonen U, Pyhtinen J. Development of post-traumatic epilepsy. *Stereotact Funct Neurosurg* 1990; 54–55:25–33.

116. Hendrick E, Harris L. Post-traumatic epilepsy in children. *J Trauma* 1968;8:547–55.

117. Japan Follow-up Group for Post-traumatic Epilepsy. The factors influencing post-traumatic epilepsy;multicentric cooperative study. *No Shinkei Geka* 1991;19:1151–9.

118. Kalisky Z, Morrison DP, Meyers CA, Von Laufen AV. Medical problems encountered during rehabilitation of patients with head injury. *Arch Phys Med Rehabil* 1985;66:25–9.

119. Kollevold T. Immediate and early cerebral seizures after head injuries, part I. *J Oslo City Hosp* 1976;26:99–114.

120. Kollevold T. Immediate and early cerebral seizures after head injuries, part II. *J Oslo City Hosp* 1977;27:89–99.

121. Kollevold T. Immediate and early cerebral seizures after head injuries, part III. *J Oslo City Hosp* 1978;28:78–86.

122. Kollevold T. Immediate and early cerebral seizures after head injuries, part IV. *J Oslo City Hosp* 1979;29:35–47.

123. Lee S-T, Lui T-N. Early seizures after mild closed head injury. *J Neurosurg* 1992;76:435–9.

124. Manaka S, Japan Follow-Up Research Group of Post-traumatic Epilepsy. Cooperative prospective study on post-traumatic epilepsy risk factors and the effect of prophylactic anticonvulsant. *Jpn J Psychiatry Neurol* 1992;46:311–5.

125. Mazzini L, Cossa FM, Angelino E, Campini R, Pastore I, Monaco F. Neuroradiologic and neuropsychological assessment of long-term outcome. *Epilepsia* 2003;44:569–74.

126. Paillas JE, Paillas N, Bureau M. Post-traumatic epilepsy. Introduction and clinical observations. *Epilepsia* 1970;5:16.

127. Sazbon L, Groswasser Z. Outcome in 134 patients with prolonged post-traumatic unawareness. Part 1: parameters determining late recovery of consciousness. *J Neurosurg* 1990, 72:75–80.

128. Thomsen IV. Late outcome of very severe blunt head trauma: A 10–15 year second follow-up. *J Neurol Neurosurg Psychiatry* 1984;47:260–8.

129. Wiederholt WC, Melton LJ III, Annegers JF, Grabow JD, Laws ER Jr, Ilstrup DM. Short-term outcomes of skull fracture: A population-based study of survival and neurologic complications. *Neurology* 1989;39:96–100.

130. Deymeer F, Leviton A. Post-traumatic seizures: An assessment of the epidemiologic literature. *Cent Nerv Syst Trauma* 1985;2:33–43.

131. Ng WK, Yablon SA, Dostrow VG. Risk of late post-traumatic seizure recurrence after withdrawal of antiepileptic drug therapy [abstract]. *Arch Phys Med Rehabil* 2000;81:1266–7.

132. Wiedemayer H, Triesch K, Schafer H, Stolke D. Early seizures following non-penetrating traumatic brain injury in adults: risk factors and clinical significance. *Brain Inj* 2002;16:323–30.

133. Rish B, Caveness W. Relation of prophylactic medication to the occurrence of early seizures following craniocerebral trauma. *J Neurosurg* 1973;38: 155–8.

134. Baker GA, Nashef L, van Hout BA. Current issues in the management of epilepsy: The impact of frequent seizures on cost of illness, quality of life, and mortality. *Epilepsia* 1997;38 (Suppl 1):S1–8.

135. van Hout B, Gagnon D, Souétre E, Ried S, Remy C, Baker G, Genton P, Vespignani H, McNulty P. Relationship between seizure frequency and costs and quality of life of outpatients with partial epilepsy in France, Germany, and the United Kingdom. *Epilepsia* 1997;38:1221–6.

136. Haltiner AM, Temkin NR, Dikmen SS. Risk of seizure recurrence after the first late post-traumatic seizure. *Arch Phys Med Rehabil* 1997;78:835–40.

137. Semah F, Picot M-C, Adam C, Broglin D, Arzimanoglou A, Bazin B, Cavalcanti D, Baulac. Is the underlying cause of epilepsy a major prognostic factor for recurrence? *Neurology* 1998;1256–62.

138. Temkin NR, Dikmen SS, Wilensky AJ, Keihm J, Chabal S, Winn HR. A randomized, double-blind study of phenytoin for the prevention of post-traumatic seizures. *N Engl J Med* 1990;323: 497–502.

139. McCrory PR, Bladin PF, Berkovic SF. Retrospective study of concussive convulsions in elite Australian rules and rugby league footballers: phenomenology, aetiology, and outcome. *BMJ* 1997; 314:171–4.

140. Jabbari B, Prokhorenko O, Khajavi K Mena H. Intractable epilepsy and mild brain injury: incidence, pathology and surgical outcome. *Brain Inj* 2002;16:463–7.

141. Kumar J, Gupta RK, Husain M, Vatsal DK, Chawla S, Rathore RKS, Pradhan S. Mgnetization transfer MR Imaging in patients with post-traumatic epilepsy. AJNR Am J Neuroradiol 2003;23:218–224

142. Frey LC. Epidemiology of post-traumatic epilepsy;a critical review. *Epilepsia* 2003;44 (Suppl 10):11–17.

143. Cifu DX, Kreutzer JS, Marwitz JH, Miller M, Hsu GM, Seel RT, Englander J, High WM Jr, Zafonte R. Etiology and incidence of rehospitalization after traumatic brain injury: a multicenter analysis. *Arch Phys Med Rehabil* 1999;80:85–90.

144. Shavelle RM, Strauss D, Whyte J, Day SM, Yu YL. Long-term causes of death after traumatic brain injury. *Am J Phys Med Rehabil* 2001;80:510–6.

145. Lindsten H, Nystrom L, Forsgren L. Mortality risk in an adult cohort with a newly diagnosed unprovoked epileptic seizure: A population-based study. Epilepsia 2000;41:1469–73.

146. Strauss DJ, Day SM, Shavelle RM, Wu YW. Remote symptomatic epilepsy. Does seizure severity increase mortality? *Neurology* 2003;60:395–9.

147. Corkin S, Sullivan EV, Carr FA. Prognostic factors for life expectancy after head injury. *Arch Neurol* 1984;41:975–7.

148. Rish BL, Dillon JD, Weiss GH. Mortality following penetrating craniocerebral injuries. *J Neurosurg* 1983;59:775–80.

149. Walker AE, Blumer D. The fate of World War II veterans with post-traumatic seizures. *Arch Neurol* 1989;46:23–6.

150. Weiss GH, Caveness WF, Eisiedel-Lechtape H, McNeel M. Life expectancy and causes of death in a group of head-injured veterans of World War I. *Arch Neurol* 1982;39:741–3.

151. Aarts JHP, Binnie CD, Smit AM, Wilkins AJ. Selective cognitive impairment during focal and generalized epileptiform EEG activity. *Brain* 1984;107:293–308.

152. Aldenkamp AP. Effect of seizures and epileptiform discharges on cognitive function. *Epilepsia* 1997;38 (Suppl 1):S52–5.

153. Binnie CD, Marston D. Cognitive correlates of interictal discharges. *Epilepsia* 1992;33 (Suppl 6):S11–17.

154. Swanson SJ, Rao SM, Grafman J, Salazar AM, Kraft J. The relationship between seizure subtype and interictal personality. Results from the *Vietnam Head Injury Study* 1995;118:91 103.

155. Hernandez TD, Naritoku DK. Seizures, epilepsy, and functional recovery after traumatic brain injury: a reappraisal. *Neurology* 1997;48:803–6.

156. Schwab K, Grafman J, Salazar AM, Kraft J. Residual impairments and work status 15 years after penetrating head injury: Report from the Vietnam Head Injury Study. *Neurology* 1993;43:95–103.

157. Grafman J, Jonas B, Salazar A. Epilepsy following penetrating head injury to the frontal lobes. In Chauvel P, Delgado, Advances in *Neurology*, Vol 57, Raven Press, New York 1992;369–78.

158. Dikmen S, Reitan RM. Neuropsychological performance in post-traumatic epilepsy. *Epilepsia* 1978;19:177–83.

159. Haltiner AM, Temkin NR, Winn HR, Dikmen SS. The impact of post-traumatic seizures on 1–year neuropsychological and psychosocial outcome of head injury. *J Int Neuropsychol Soc* 1996;2: 494–504.

160. Lee S-T, Lui T-N, Wong C-W, Yeh Y-S, Tzaan W-C. Early seizures after moderate closed head injury. *Acta Neurochir (Wien)* 1995; 137:151–4.

161. Lowenstein DH, Bleck T, MacDonald RL. It's time to revise the definition of status epilepticus. *Epilepsia* 1999;40:120–2.

162. Leppik IE. Status epilepticus. *Neurol Clin* 1986;4:633–43.

163. Kennedy CR, Freeman JM. Post-traumatic seizures and post-traumatic epilepsy in children. *J Head Trauma Rehabil* 1986;1(4): 66–73.

164. Hauser WA. Status epilepticus: Epidemiologic considerations. *Neurology* 1990;40 (suppl 2):9–13.

165. Leppik I. Status epilepticus: The next decade. *Neurology* 1990;40 (suppl 2):4–9.

166. Walker AE, Erculei F. Post-traumatic epilepsy 15 years later. *Epilepsia* 1970;11:17–26.

167. Walczak TS, Leppik IE, D'Amelio M, Rarick J, So E, Ahman P, Ruggles K, Cascino GD, Annegers JF, Hauser WA. Incidence and risk factors in sudden unexpected death in epilepsy: A prospective cohort study. *Neurology*. 2001;56:519–25.

168. Temkin NR, Jarell AD, Anderson GD. Antiepileptogenic agents: How close are we? *Drugs* 2001;61:1045–55.

169. Stables JP, Bertram EH, White HS, Coulter DA, Dichter MA, Jacobs MP, Loscher W, Lowenstein DH, Moshe SL, Noebels JL, Davis M. Models for epilepsy and epileptogenesis: Report from the NIH Workshop, Bethesda, Maryland. *Epilepsia* 2002;43: 1410–20.

170. Chang BS, Lowenstein DH. Epilepsy. *N Engl J Med* 2003;349: 1257–66.

171. Herman ST. Epilepsy after brain insult: targeting epileptogenesis. *Neurology* 2002;59 (9 Suppl 5):S21–6.

172. Pitkänen A. Drug-mediated neuroprotection and antiepileptogenesis. *Neurology* 2002;59:S27–33.

173. Sato M, Racine RJ, McIntyre DC. Kindling: basic mechanisms and clinical validity. *Electroenceph Clin Neurophysiol* 1990;76: 459–72.

174. Willmore LJ. Post-traumatic epilepsy: Cellular mechanisms and implications for treatment. *Epilepsia* 1990;31 (Suppl 3):S67–73.

175. White HS. Animal models of epilepsy. *Neurology* 2002;59: S7–14.

176. Löscher W. Animal models of epilepsy for the development of antiepileptogenic and disease-modifying drugs. A comparison of the pharmacology of kindling and post-status epilepticus models of temporal lobe epilepsy. *Epilepsy Res* 2002;50:105–23.

177. Schmidt D, Rogawski MA. New strategies for the identification of drugs to prevent the development or progression of epilepsy. *Epilepsy Res* 2002;50:71–8.

178. Jacobs KM, Graber KD, Kharazia VN, Parada I, Prince DA. Postlesional epilepsy: the ultimate brain plasticity. *Epilepsia* 2000;41 (Suppl 6): S153–61.

179. Willmore LJ, Sypert GW, Munson JB. Recurrent seizures induced by cortical iron injection: a model of post-traumatic epilepsy. *Ann Neurol* 1978;4:329–36.

180. D'Alessandro R, Ferrara R, Benassi G, Lenzi PL, Sabattini L. Computed tomographic scans in post-traumatic epilepsy. *Arch Neurol* 1988;45:42–3.

181. Goldensohn ES. The relevance of secondary epileptogenesis to the treatment of epilepsy: Kindling and the mirror focus. *Epilepsia* 1984;25: Suppl 2:S156–73.

182. Goddard BV. Development of epileptic seizures through brain stimulation at low intensity. *Nature* 1967;214:1020–1.

183. Cavalheiro EA, Leite JP, Bortolotto ZA, Turski WA, Ikonomidou C, Turski L. Long-term effects of pilocarpine in rats: Structural damage of the brain triggers kindling and spontaneous recurrent seizures. *Epilepsia* 1991;32:778–82.

184. Schmutz M, Klebs K, Baltzer V. Inhibition or enhancement of kindling evolution by antiepileptics. *J Neural Transm* 1988;72: 245–57.

185. Albertson TE, Joy RM, Stark LG. Carbamazepine: a pharmacological study in the kindling model of epilepsy. *Neuropharmacology* 1984;23:1117–23.

186. Wada JA, Sato M, Wake A, Green JR, Troupin AS. Prophylactic effects of phenytoin, phenobarbital, and carbamazepine examined in kindling cat preparations. *Arch Neurol* 1976;33:426–34.

187. Silver JM, Shin C, McNamara JO. Antiepileptogenic effects of conventional anticonvulsants in the kindling model of epilepsy. *Ann Neurol* 1991;29:356–63.

188. Wada JA. Pharmacological prophylaxis in the kindling model of epilepsy. *Arch Neurol* 1977;34:389–95.

189. Postma T, Krupp E, Li X-L, Post RM, Weiss SRB. Lamotrigine treatment during amygdala-kindled seizure development fails to inhibit seizures and diminishes subsequent anticonvulsant efficacy. *Epilepsy* 2000;41:1514–21.

190. Stratton S, Large CH, Cox B, Davies G, Hagan RM. Effect of lamotrigine and levetiracetam on seizure development in a rat amygdala kindling model. *Epilepsy Res* 2003;53:95–106.

191. Otsuki K, Morimoto K, Sato K, Yamada N, Kuroda S. Effects of lamotrigine and conventional antiepileptic drugs on amygdala- and hippocampal-kindled seizures in rats. *Epilepsy Res* 1998;31: 101–112.

192. Nissinen J, Large CH, Stratton SC, Pitkänen A. Effect of lamotrigine treatment on epileptogenesis: an experimental study in rat. *Epilepsy Res* 2004;58:119–32.

193. Wada JA. Erosion of kindled epileptogenesis and kindling-induced long-term seizure suppressive effect in primates. In Wada JA (ed): *Kindling 4*; Plenum Press, New York, 1990;383–5.

194. D'Ambrosio R, Fairbanks JP, Fender JS, Born DE, Doyle DL, Miller JW. Post-traumatic epilepsy following fluid percussion injury in the rat. *Brain* 2004;127:304–14.

195. Laurer HL, McIntosh T. Experimental models of brain trauma. *Curr Opin Neurol* 1999;12:715–21

196. Santhakumar V, Ratzliff AD, Jeng J, Toth Z, Soltesz I. Long-term hyperexcitability in the hippocampus after experimental head trauma. *Ann Neurol* 2001;50:708–17.

197. Nilsson P, Ronne-Engström E, Flink R, Ungerstedt U, Carlson H, Hillered L. Epileptic seizure activity in the acute phase following cortical impact trauma in rat. *Brain Res* 1994;637: 227–32.

198. Lowenstein DH, Thomas MJ, Smith DH, McIntosh TK. Selective vulnerability of dentate hilar neurons following traumatic brain injury: a potential mechanistic link between head trauma and disorders of the hippocampus. *J Neurosci* 1992;12:4846–53.

199. Golarai G, Greenwood AC, Feeney DM, Connor JA. Physiological and structural evidence for hippocampal involvement in persistent seizure susceptibility after traumatic brain injury. *J Neurosci* 2001;21:8523–37.

200. Albensi B, Janigro D. Traumatic brain injury and its effects on synaptic plasticity. *Brain Inj* 2003;17:653–6.

201. Levin HS. Neuroplasticity following non-penetrating traumatic brain injury. *Brain Inj* 2003;8:665–74.

202. Seitz RJ, Huang Y, Knorr U, Tellman L, Herzog H, Freund HJ. Large-scale plasticity of the human motor cortex. *Neuroreport* 1995;6:742–4.

203. Schwartzkroin PA. Mechanisms of brain plasticity: from normal brain function to pathology. *Int Rev Neurobiol* 2001;45:1–15.

204. Salin P, Tseng GF, Hoffman S, Parada I, Prince DA. Axonal sprouting in layer V pyramidal neurons of chronically injured cerebral cortex. *J Neurosci* 1995;15:8234–45.

205. Sankar R, Shin D, Liu H, Wasterlain C, Mazarati A. Epileptogenesis during development: injury, circuit recruitment, and plasticity. *Epilepsia.* 2002;43 Suppl 5:47–53.

206. Teyler TJ, Morgan SL, Russell RN, Woodside BL. Synaptic plasticity and secondary epileptogenesis. *Int Rev Neurobiol* 2001;45: 253–67.

207. Tsukahara N. Synaptic plasticity in the mammalian central nervous system. *Annu Rev Neurosci* 1981;4:351–79.

208. Gage RH, Bjorklund A, Stenevi U. Reinnervation of the partially deafferented hippocampus by compensatory collateral sprouting from spared cholinergic and noradrenergic afferents. *Brain Res* 1983;268:27–37.

209. Prince DA, Connors BW. Mechanisms of epileptogenesis in cortical structures. *Ann Neurol* 1984;16(Suppl):S59–64.

210. Sutula T, Xiao-Xian H, Cavazos J, Scott G. Synaptic reorganization in the hippocampus induced by abnormal functional activity. *Science* 1988;239:1147–50.

211. Coulter DA. Epilepsy-associated plasticity in gamma-aminobutyric acid receptor expression, function, and inhibitory synaptic properties. *Int Rev Neurobiol* 2001;45:237–52.

212. Montanez S, Kline AE, Gasser TA, Hernandez TD. Phenobarbital administration directed against kindled seizures delays functional recovery following brain insult. *Brain Res* 2000;860: 29–40.

213. *International Dictionary of Medicine and Biology.* John Wiley & Sons, Inc. 1986;2316.

214. Deutschmann CS, Haines SJ. Anticonvulsant prophylaxis in neurological surgery. *Neurosurgery* 1985;17:510–7.

215. Hauser WA, Tabaddor K, Factor PR, Finer C. Seizures and head injury in an urban community. *Neurology (Cleveland)* 1984;34: 746–51.

216. Caveness WF. Onset and cessation of fits following craniocerebral trauma. *J Neurosurg* 1963;20:570–583.

217. Diaz-Arrastia R, Gong Y, Fair S, Scott KD, Garcia MC, Carlile MC, Agostini MA, Van Ness PC. Increased risk of late post-traumatic seizures associated with inheritance of APOE εallele. *Arch Neurol* 2003;60:818–22.

218. Glötzner FL, Haubitz I, Miltner F, Kapp G, Pflughaupt KW. Epilepsy prophylaxis with carbamazepine in severe brain injuries. *Neurochirurgia* 1983, 26:66–79.

219. Temkin NR. Risk factors for post-traumatic seizures. *Epilepsia* 2003;44 (Suppl 10):18–20.

220. Pechadre JC, Lauxerois M, Colnet G, Commun C, Dimicoli C, Bonnard M, Gibert J, Chabannes J. Prevention de L'epilepsie post-traumatique tardive par phenytoine dans les traumatismes craniens graves. Suivi durant 2 ans. *Presse Med* 1991;20: 841–5.

221. Koh S, Storey TW, Santos TC, Mian QY, Cole AJ. Early-life seizures in rats increase susceptibility to seizure-induced brain injury in adulthood. *Neurology* 1999;53:915–921.

222. Schaumann BA, Annegers JF, Johnson SB, Moore KJ, Lubozynski MF, Salinsky MC. Family history of seizures in post-traumatic and alcohol-associated seizure disorders. *Epilepsia* 1994;35:48–52.

223. Salazar AM, Amin D, Vance SC, Grafman J, Schlesselman S, Buck D. Epilepsy after penetrating head injury: Effects of lesion location. In Wolf P, Dam M, Janz D, Dreifuss FE (eds.): Advances in *Epilepsy*, Vol 16, Raven Press, New York, 1987;753–7.

224. Clear D, Chadwick DW. Seizures provoked by blows to the head. *Epilepsia.* 2000;41:243–4.

225. Courjon J. A longitudinal electro-clinical study of 80 cases of post-traumatic epilepsy observed from the time of the original trauma. *Epilepsia* 1970;11:29–36.

226. Jennett B, van de Sande. EEG prediction of post-traumatic epilepsy. *Epilepsia* 1975;16:251–6.

227. Blackwood D, McQueen JK, Harris P, Townsend HRA, Brezinova V, Kalbag R, Betty M, Strong A, Johnson A. A clinical trial of phenytoin prophylaxis of epilepsy following head injury: Preliminary report. In Dam M, Gram L, Penry JK: Advances in Epileptology: *XIIth Epilepsy* International Symposium. Raven Press, New York, 1981;521–5.

228. Scherzer E, Wessely P. EEG in post-traumatic epilepsy. *Eur Neurol* 1978;17:38–42.

229. Thomaides TN, Kerezoudi EP, Chaudhuri KR, Cheropoulos C. Study of EEGs following 24–hour sleep deprivation in patients with post-traumatic epilepsy. *Eur Neurol* 1992;32:79–82.

230. Zivin L, Ajmone-Marsan C. Incidence and prognostic significance of "epileptiform" activity in the EEG of non-epileptic subjects. *Brain* 1968;91:751–8.

231. Reisner T, Zeiler K, Wessely P. The value of CT and EEG in cases of post-traumatic epilepsy. *J Neurol* 1979;221: 93–100.

232. Jabbari B, Vengrow MI, Salazar AM, Harper MG, Smutok MA, Amin D. Clinical and radiological correlates of EEG in the

late phase of head injury: a study of 515 Vietnam veterans. *Electroenceph Clin Neurophysiol* 1986, 64:285–93.

233. Yablon SA. Post-traumatic seizures. *Arch Phys Med Rehabil* 1993;74:983–1001.

234. Bullock R, Chestnut RM, Clifton GL, Ghajar J, Marion DW. Narayan RK. Newell DW, Pitts LH, Rosner MJ, Walters BC, Wilberger JE. Role of antiseizure prophylaxis following head injury. *J Neurotrauma* 2000;17:49–53.

235. Murri L, Arrigo A, Bonuccelli U, Rossi G, Parenti G. Phenobarbital in the prophylaxis of late post-traumatic seizures. Ital *J Neurol Sci* 1992;13:755–60.

236. Murri L, Parenti G, Bonnucelli. Phenobarbital prophylaxis of post-traumatic epilepsy. Ital *J Neurol Sci* 1980;1:225–30.

237. Price DJ. The efficiency of sodium valproate as the only anticonvulsant administered to neurosurgical patients. In Parsonage MJ, Caldwell ADS (eds): *The place of sodium valproate in the treatment of epilepsy.* Academic Press, London, 1980;23–34.

238. Servit Z, Musil F. Prophylactic treatment of post-traumatic epilepsy: results of a long-term follow-up in Czechoslovakia. *Epilepsia* 1981;22:315–20.

239. Wohns RNW, Wyler AR. Prophylactic phentoin in severe head injuries. *J Neurosurg* 1979;57:507–9.

240. Young B, Rapp R, Brooks W, Madauss W, Norton JA. Post-traumatic epilepsy prophylaxis. *Epilepsia* 1979;20:671–81.

241. McQueen JK, Blackwood DHR, Harris P, Kalbag RM, Johnson AL. Low risk of late post-traumatic seizures following severe head injury: implications for clinical trials of prophylaxis. *J Neurol Neurosurg Psychiatry* 1983;46:899–904.

242. Temkin NR, Dikmen SS, Winn HR. Post-traumatic seizures. *Neurosurg Clin* 1991;2:425–35.

243. Temkin NR, Dikmen SS, Anderson GD, Wilensky AJ, Holmes MD, Cohen W, Newell DW, Nelson P, Awan A, Winn HR. Valproate therapy for prevention of post-traumatic seizures: a randomized trial. *J Neurosurg* 1999;91:593–600.

244. Young B, Rapp RP, Norton JA, Haack D, Tibbs PA, Bean JR. Failure of prophylactically administered phenytoin to prevent late post-traumatic seizures. *J Neurosurg* 1983;58:236–41.

245. Young B, Rapp RP, Norton JA, Haack D, Walsh JW. Failure of prophylactically administered phenytoin to prevent post-traumatic seizures in children. *Child's Brain* 1983;10:185 92.

246. Beghi E. Overview of studies to prevent post-traumatic epilepsy. *Epilepsia* 2003;44 (Suppl 10):21–6.

247. Schierhout G, Roberts I. Anti-epileptic drugs for preventing seizures following acute traumatic brain injury. *Cochrane Database Syst Rev* 2001;(4):CD000173.

248. Schierhout G, Roberts I. Prophylactic antiepileptic agents after head injury: a systematic review. *J Neurol Neurosurg Psychiatry* 1998;64:108–12.

249. Young B, Rapp RP, Norton JA, Haack D, Tibbs PA, Bean JR. Failure of prophylactically administered phenytoin to prevent early post-traumatic seizures. *J Neurosurg* 1983;58:231–5.

250. No authors listed. Antiseizure prophylaxis for penetrating brain injury. *J Trauma* 2001;51 (2 Suppl):S41–3.

251. Benardo LS. Prevention of epilepsy after head trauma: Do we need new drugs or a new approach? *Epilepsia* 2003;44 (Suppl 10):27–33.

252. Quality Standards Subcommittee of the American Academy of Neurology. Practice parameters: Assessment and management of patients in the persistent vegetative state. (Summary statement) *Neurology* 1995;45:1015–1018.

253. Engel J, Jr., Pedley TA (Eds). *Epilepsy: A Comprehensive Textbook.* Lippincott Williams & Wilkins. 1st Ed. 1998.

254. Wyllie E, ed. *The Treatment of Epilepsy: Principles and Practice.* 3rd ed. Lippincott Williams & Wilkins;2001.

255. Binnie CD, Stefan H. Modern electroencephalography: its role in epilepsy management. *Clin Neurophys* 1999;110:1671–97.

256. Blume WT. Current trends in electroencephalography. *Curr Opin Neurol* 2001;14:193–197.

257. Chadwick D. Diagnosis of epilepsy. *Lancet* 1990;336:291–5.

258. van Donselaar CA, Schimsheimer RJ, Geerts AT, Declerck AC. Value of the electroencephalogram in adult patients with untreated idiopathic first seizures. *Arch Neurol* 1992;49:231–7.

259. Dana-Haeri J, Trimble MR, Oxley J. Prolactin and gonadotropin change following generalized and partial seizures. *J Neurol Neurosurg Psychiatry* 1983;46:331–5.

260. Laxer KD, Mullooly JP, Howell B. Prolactin changes after seizures classified by EEG monitoring. *Neurology* 1985;35:31–5.

261. Meierkord H, Shorvon S, Lightman S, Trimble MB. Comparison of the effects of frontal and temporal lobe seizures on prolactin levels. *Arch Neurol* 1992;49:225–30.

262. Hammond FM, Yablon SA, Bontke CA. Potential role of serum prolactin measurement in the diagnosis of late post-traumatic seizures. A case report. *Am J Phys Med Rehabil* 1996;75:304–6.

263. Ebersole JS, Leroy RF. An evaluation of ambulatory, casette EEG monitoring: II. Detection of interictal abnormalities. *Neurology* 1983;33:8–18.

264. Ebersole JS, Leroy RF. Evaluation of ambulatory casette EEG monitoring: III. Diagnostic accuracy compared to intensive inpatient EEG monitoring. *Neurology* 1983;33:853 60.

265. American Academy of Neurology, Therapeutics and Technology Assessment Subcommittee. Assessment: Intensive EEG/video monitoring for epilepsy. *Neurology* 1989;39:1101–2.

266. Hauser WA. Should people be treated after a first seizure? *Arch Neurol* 1986;1287–8.

267. Treiman DM. Current treatment strategies in selected situations in epilepsy. *Epilepsia* 1993;34 (Suppl 5):S17–23.

268. Hauser WA, Rich SS, Lee JRJ, Annegers JF, Anderson VE. Risk of recurrent seizures after two unprovoked seizures. *N Engl J Med* 1998;338:429–34.

269. Hauser WA, Rich SS, Annegers JF, Anderson VE. Seizure recurrence after a 1st unprovoked seizure: An extended follow-up. *Neurology* 1990;40:1163–70.

270. Lindsten H, Stenlund H, Forsgren L. Seizure recurrence in adults after a newly diagnosed unprovoked epileptic seizure. *Acta Neurol Scand* 2001;104:202–7.

271. Hart YM, Sander JWAS, Johnson AL, Shorvon SD. National General Practice Study of Epilepsy: Recurrence after a first seizure. *Lancet* 1990;336:1271–4.

272. First Seizure Trial Group. Randomized clinical trial on the efficacy of antiepileptic drugs in reducing the risk of relapse after a first unprovoked tonic-clonic seizure. *Neurology* 1993;43: 478–83.

273. Karceski S, Morrell M, Carpenter D. The expert consensus guideline series: Treatment of epilepsy. *Epilepsy Behav* 2001;2:A1–50.

274. Pellock JM. Who should receive prophylactic antiepileptic drug following head injury? *Brain Inj* 1989;3:107–8.

275. Mattson RH, Cramer JA, Collins JF, Department of Veterans Affairs Epilepsy Cooperative Study No. 264 Group. A comparison of valproate with carbamazepine for the treatment of complex partial seizures and secondarily generalized tonic-clonic seizures in adults. *N Engl J Med* 1992;327:765–71.

276. Mattson RH, Cramer JA, Collins JF, Smith DB, Delgado-Escueta AV, Browne TR, Williamson PD, Treiman DM, McNamara JO, McCutchen DB, Homan RW, Crill WE, Lubozynski MF, Rosenthal NP, Mayersdorf A. Comparison of carbamazepine, phenobarbital, phenytoin, and primidone in partial and secondarily generalized tonic-clonic seizures. *N Eng J Med* 1985;313: 145–51.

277. Farwell JR, Lee YJ, Hirtz DG, Sulzbacher SI, Ellenberg JH, Nelson KB. Phenobarbital for febrile seizures-effects on intelligence and on seizure recurrence. *N Engl J Med* 1990;322:364–9.

278. Feely M. Drug treatment of epilepsy. *BMJ* 1999;318:106–9.

279. French JA, Kanner AM, Bautista J, Abou-Khalil B, Browne T, Harden CL, Theodore WH, Bazil C, Stern J, Schachter SC, Bergen D, Hirtz D, Montouris GD, Nespeca M, Gidal B, Marks WJ Jr, Turk WR, Fischer JH, Bourgeois B, Wilner A, Faught RE Jr, Sachdeo RC, Beydoun A, Glauser TA;Therapeutics and Technology Assessment Subcommittee of the American Academy of Neurology;Quality Standards Subcommittee of the American Academy of Neurology;American Epilepsy Society. Efficacy and tolerability of the new antiepileptic drugs I: treatment of new onset epilepsy: report of the Therapeutics and Technology Assessment Subcommittee and Quality Standards Subcommittee of the American Academy of Neurology and the American Epilepsy Society. *Neurology* 2004;62:1252–60.

280. Collaborative Group for Epidemiology of Epilepsy. Adverse reactions to antiepileptic drugs: A follow-up study of 355 patients with chronic antiepileptic drug treatment. *Epilepsia* 1988, 29: 787–93.

281. Collaborative Group for Epidemiology of Epilepsy. Adverse reactions to antiepileptic drugs: A multicenter survey of clinical practice. *Epilepsia* 1986;27:323–30.

282. Homan RW, Miller B, Veterans Administration Epilepsy Cooperative Study Group. Causes of treatment failure with epileptic drugs vary over time. *Neurology* 1987, 37:1620–3.

283. Smith DB, Mattson RH, Cramer JA, Collins JF, Novelly RA, Craft B, Veterans Administration Epilepsy Cooperative Study Group. Results of a nationwide Veterans Administration cooperative study comparing the efficacy and toxicity of carbamazepine, phenobarbital, phenytoin, and primidone. *Epilepsia* 1987;28 (Suppl 3):S50–8.

284. Meythaler JM, Yablon SA. Antiepileptic drugs. *Phys Med Rehabil Clin N Am* 1999;10:275–300.

285. Scolnik D, Nulman I, Rovet J, Gladstone D, Czuchta D, Gardner HA, Gladstone R, Ashby P, Weksberg R, Einarson T, Koren G. Neurodevelopment of children exposed in utero to phenytoin and carbamazepine monotherapy. *JAMA* 1994;271:767–70.

286. Porter RJ, Kelley KR. Antiepileptic drugs and mild liver function elevation. *JAMA* 1985;253:1791–2.

287. Camfield C, Camfield P, Smith E, Tibbles JAR. Asymptomatic children with epilepsy: little benefit from screening for anticonvulsant-induced liver, blood, or renal damage. *Neurology* 1986, 36:838–41.

288. Pellock JM, Willmore LJ. A rational guide to routine blood monitoring in patients receiving antiepileptic drugs. *Neurology* 1991;41:961–4.

289. Meador KJ, Loring DW, Abney OL, Allen ME, Moore EE, Zamrini EY, King DW. Effects of carbamazepine and phenytoin on EEG and memory in healthy adults. *Epilepsia* 1993;34:153–7.

290. Dikmen SS, Temkin NR, Miller B, Machamer J, Winn HR. Neurobehavioral effects of phenytoin prophylaxis of post-traumatic seizures. *JAMA* 1991;265:1271–7.

291. Dikmen SS, Machamer JE, Winn HR, Anderson GD, Temkin NR. Neuropsychological effects of valproate in traumatic brain injury: a randomized trial. *Neurology*. 2000;54:895–902.

292. Massagli TL. Neurobehavioral effects of phenytoin, carbamazepine, and valproic acid: Implications for use in traumatic brain injury. *Arch Phys Med Rehabil* 1991;72:219–26.

293. Kirschner KL, Sahgal V, Armstrong KJ, Bloch R. A comparative study of the cognitive effects of phenytoin and carbamazepine in patients with blunt head injury. *J Neuro Rehab* 1991;5:169–74.

294. Smith KR Jr, Goulding PM, Wilderman D, Goldfader PR, Holterman-Hommes P, Wei F. Neurobehavioral effects of phenytoin and carbamazepine in patients recovering from trauma: A comparative study. *Arch Neurol* 1994;51:653–60.

295. Goldstein LB. Prescribing of potentially harmful drugs to patients admitted to hospital after head injury. *J Neurol Neurosurg Psychiatry* 1995;58:753–55.

296. Brailowsky S, Knight RT, Efron R. Phenytoin increases the severity of cortical hemiplegia in rats. *Brain Res* 1986;376:71–7.

297. Feeney DM, Gonzalez A, Law WA. Amphetamine, haloperidol, and experience interact to affect rate of recovery after motor cortex injury. *Science* 1982;217:855–7.

298. Schallert T, Hernandez TD, Barth TM. Recovery of function after brain damage: Severe and chronic disruption by diazepam. *Brain Res* 1986;379:104–11.

299. Dauch WA, Schutze M, Guttinger M, Bauer BL. Post-traumatic seizure prevention—results of a survey of 127 neurosurgery clinics. *Zentralbl Neurochir* 1996;57:190–5.

300. Rapport RL II, Penry JK. A survey of attitudes toward the pharmacological prophylaxis of post-traumatic epilepsy. *J Neurosurg* 1973;38:159–66.

301. Gillham R, Kane K, Bryant-Comstock L, Brodie MJ. A double-blind comparison of lamotrigine and carbamazepine in newly-diagnosed epilepsy with health-related quality of life as an outcome measure. *Seizure* 2000;9:375–9.

302. Brodie MJ, Richen A, Yuen AWC, for the UK Lamotrigine/Carbamazepine Monotherapy Trial Group. Double-blind comparison of lamotrigine and carbamazepine in newly diagnosed epilepsy. *Lancet* 1995;345:476–479.

303. Gilliam F, Vazquez B, Sackellares JC, Chang GY, Messenheimer J, Nyberg J, Risner ME, Rudd GD. An active-control trial of lamotrigine monotherapy for partial seizures. *Neurology* 1998;51:1018–1025.

304. Steiner TJ, Dellaportas CI, Findley LJ. Lamotrigine monotherapy in newly diagnosed untreated epilepsy. *Epilepsia* 1999;40:601–607.

305. Messenheimer JA. Rash in adult and pediatric patients treated with lamotrigine. *Can J Neurol Sci* 1998;25:S14–S18.

306. LaRoche SM, Helmers SL. The new antiepileptic drugs: Clinical applications. *JAMA* 2004;291:615–20.

307. White JR, Walczak TS, Leppik IE, Rarick J, Tran T, Beniak TE, Matchinsky DJ, Gumnit RJ. Discontinuation of levetiracetam because of behavioral side effects: A case-control study. *Neurology* 2003;61:1218–21.

308. Callaghan N, Garrett A, Goggin T. Withdrawal of anticonvulsant drugs in patients free of seizures for two years: A prospective study. *N Engl J Med* 1988;318:942–6.

309. Medical Research Council Antiepileptic Withdrawal Study Group. Randomised study of antiepileptic drug withdrawal in patients in remission. *Lancet* 1991;337:1175–80.

310. Gherpelli JLD, Kok F, dal Forno S, Elkis LC, Lefevre BHW, Diament AJ. Discontinuing medication in epileptic children: A study of risk factors related to recurrence. *Epilepsia* 1992;33:681–6.

311. Jacoby A, Johnson A, Chadwick D, Medical Research Council Antiepileptic Drug Withdrawal Study Group. Psychosocial outcomes of antiepileptic drug discontinuation. *Epilepsia* 1992;33:1123–31.

312. Schmidt D. Withdrawal of antiepileptic drugs. In Wolf P, Dam M, Janz D, Dreifuss FE (eds.): Advances in *Epilepsy*, Vol 16, Raven Press, New York, 1987;373–7.

313. Bromfield EB, Dambrosia J, Devinsky O, Nice FJ, Theodore WH. Phenytoin withdrawal and seizure frequency. *Neurology* 1989;39:905–9.

314. Marks DA, Katz A, Scheyer R, Spencer SS. Clinical and electrographic effects of acute anticonvulsant withdrawal in epileptic patients. *Neurology* 1991;41:508–12.

315. Theodore WH, Porter RJ, Raubertas RF. Seizures during barbiturate withdrawal: Relation to blood level. *Ann Neurol* 1987;22:644–7.

316. Vining EPG. Use of barbiturates and benzodiazepines in treatment of epilepsy. *Neurol Clin* 1986;4:617–32.

317. Stephen LJ, Brodie MJ. Seizure freedom with more than one antiepileptic drug. *Seizure* 2002;11:349–52.

318. Diaz-Arrastia R, Agostini MA, Van Ness PC. Evolving treament epilepsy. *JAMA* 2002;287:2917–20.

319. Engel J Jr., Wiebe S, French J, Sperling M, Williamson P, Spencer D, Gumnit R, Zahn C, Westbrook E, Enos B. Quality Standards Subcommittee of the American Academy of Neurology; American Epilepsy Society; American Association of Neurological Surgeons. Practice parameter: Temporal lobe and localized neocortical resections for epilepsy. *Neurology* 2003;60:538–47.

320. Engel J Jr. Finally, a randomized, controlled trial of epilepsy surgery. *N Engl J Med* 2001;345:165–7.

321. Wiebe S, Blume WT, Girvin JP, Eliasziw M;Effectiveness and Efficiency of Surgery for Temporal Lobe Epilepsy Study Group. A randomized, controlled trial of surgery for temporal-lobe epilepsy. *N Engl J Med* 2001;345:311–8.

322. Spencer SS, Bert AT, Vickrey BG, Sperling MR, Bazil CW, Shinnar S, Langfitt JT, Walczak TS, Pacia SV, Ebrahimi N, Frobish D;Multicenter Study of Epilepsy Surgery. Initial outcomes in the multicenter study of epilepsy surgery. *Neurology* 2003;61:1680–5.

323. Doyle WK, Devinsky O, Perrine K, Pacia S, Vasquez B, Luciano D. Surgical management of post-traumatic epilepsy who underwent surgical management. *Epilepsia* 1996;37 (Suppl 5):185.

324. Hosking PG. Surgery for frontal lobe epilepsy. *Seizure* 2003;12:160–66.

325. Kazemi NJ, So EL, Mosewich RK, O'Brien TJ, Cascino GD, Trenerry MR, Sharbrough FW. Resection of frontal encephalomalacias for intractable epilepsy: Outcome and prognostic factors. *Epilepsia* 1997;38:670–7.

326. Schuh LA, Henry TR, Fromes G, Blaivas M, Ross DA, Drury I. Influence of head trauma on outcome following anterior temporal lobectomy. *Arch Neurol* 1998;55:1325–8

327. Salinsky MC. Vagus nerve stimulation as treatment for epileptic seizures. *Curr Treat Options Neurol* 2003;5:110–20.

328. Vonck K, Van Laere K, Dedeurwaerdere S, Caemaert J, De Reuck J, Boon P. The mechanism of action of vagus nerve stimulation for refractory epilepsy: the current status. *J Clin Neurophysiol* 2001, 18:394–401.

329. Handforth A, DeGiorgio CM, Schachter S, Uthman BM, Naritoku DK, Tecoma ES, Henry TR, Collins SD, Vaughn BV, Gilmartin RC, Labar DR, Morris GL 3rd, Salinsky MC, Osorio I, Ristanovic RK, Labiner DM, Jones JC, Murphy JV, Ney GC, Wheless JW. Vagus nerve stimulation therapy for partial-onset seizures;a randomized active-control trial. *Neurology* 1998, 51:48–55.

330. The Vagus Nerve Stimulation Study Group. A randomized controlled trial of chronic vagus nerve stimulation for treatment of medically intractable seizures. *Neurology* 1995, 45:224–230.

331. Morris GL, Mueller WM. Long-term treatment with vagus nerve stimulation in patients with refractory epilepsy. The Vagus Nerve Stimulation Study Group E01–E05. *Neurology* 1999;53:1731–5.

332. Fisher RS, Handforth A. Reassessment: vagus nerve stimulation for epilepsy: a report of the Therapeutics and Technology Assessment Subcommittee of the American Academy of Neurology. *Neurology.* 1999;53:666–9.

333. National Association of Epilepsy Centers. Patient referral to specialty epilepsy care. Epilepsia 1990;31 (Suppl 1):S10–11.

334. McCarthy AD, Barletta AP, Lux WE, Bleiberg J. Withdrawal of anticonvulsants in a head injury rehabilitation setting [abstract]. *Arch Phys Med Rehabil* 1991;72:818.

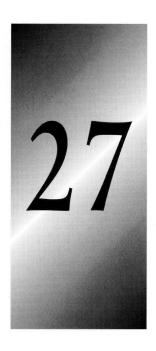

27 Movement Disorders After TBI

Joachim K. Krauss
Joseph Jankovic

Trauma to the central and peripheral nervous system is an important etiologic factor in a variety of movement disorders. While it is widely accepted that traumatic brain injury may result in both transient and persistent movement disorders (1, 2), their occurrence after peripheral injury still has not become generally appreciated (3, 4). Kinetic tremors and dystonia are the best investigated posttraumatic movement disorders after severe brain injury (5–7), but many other types of hypokinetic and hyperkinetic movement disorders have been reported as sequelae of injury to the central nervous system. The manifestation of movement disorders after moderate or mild brain injury has been less well documented. The association between brain injury and Parkinson's disease (PD) is the subject of ongoing research (8, 9). Trauma as a cause for the development of movement disorders has multifaceted implications regarding medical and psychological, but also legal aspects (10–12). In some cases of posttraumatic movement disorders a definite cause-and-effect relationship is difficult to establish. This is partly due to associated cirumstances, including medicolegal factors, but also because the appearance of movement disorders may be delayed and cause-and-effect relationships may not be recognized.

Posttraumatic movement disorders can lead to marked disability in the affected individual. Reviews on this subject have concentrated more on phenomenological aspects and medical treatment options (1, 2, 13), and less on neurorehabilitation and neurosurgical options (14). Contemporary functional stereotactic surgery may provide long-term symptomatic and functional benefits in many patients with movement disorders who do not benefit sufficiently from medical treatment (15). Radiofrequency lesioning of the thalamus and pallidum was the method of choice for years for patients with disabling tremor or parkinsonism and levodopa-induced dyskinesias, but in patients with diffuse axonal injury (DAI) ablative procedures, particularly when performed bilaterally, have been frequently associated with complications such as increased dysarthria or gait disturbance. Deep brain stimulation (DBS) is used increasingly as an option in such patients. In this chapter, we review the current understanding of the role of central trauma in the development of movement disorders, their diagnosis and treatment including neurosurgical options.

MOVEMENT DISORDERS AND BRAIN INJURY

Phenomenologic Classification of Movement Disorders

Movement disorders in the following context are understood as phenomenological entities manifested either by slowness and poverty of movement, that is hypokinesia, by excessive, abnormal involuntary movements, that is hyperkinesia, or by other signs and symptoms that can not easily be grouped under these two categories. Note, that the term *movement disorder* is not synonymous with *motor disorder* covering also paresis, spasticity and ataxia which will not be discussed in this chapter. Also, the hypertonic postures seen in comatose patients with decorticate and decerebrate rigidity after severe head injury will not be the subject of this review. Most frequently, movement disorders are associated with dysfunction of the thalamus or the basal ganglia and their circuitry. Therefore, such disorders have also been summarized as *extrapyramidal disorders*, previously. This term, however, is not considered useful anymore, since the arbitrary concept of a pyramidal versus an extrapyramidal motor system does not adequately reflect the complexity of the organization of the motor system. In the past few years, much progress has been made in the understanding of the functional neuroanatomy, the neurochemistry, and the neurophysiology of the basal ganglia and their circuitry. These advances have had an extraordinary impact on new pharmacological treatments and the reevaluation of surgical approaches.

Many different classifications of movement disorders exist. The International Classification of Diseases Tenth Revison: Neurological Adaptation, a result of collaboration between the World Health Organization and the Movement Disorder Society has provided a classification which can be periodically revised and up-dated, and which can serve as a basis for international communication, research, and education (16). *Tremor* has been defined as a rhythmic, oscillatory movement, and it can be further divided according to the position, posture, or motor activity necessary to make it manifest (17). *Rest tremor* is seen when the body part is in complete repose. Maintenance of a posture such as holding the arms outstretched reveals *postural tremor*, whereas moving the body part from one position to another (e.g. the finger-to-nose maneuver) brings on *kinetic tremor* (termed *intention tremor* when tremor occurs only shortly before the goal of the movement is reached). *Dystonia* is characterized by involuntary, sustained, patterned muscle contractions of opposing muscles resulting in repetitive twisting movements or abnormal postures (18). Dystonic movement disorders often are misdiagnosed or they are not even recognized because the full spectrum of phenomenology has not been appreciated. Dystonia may be accompanied by tremor or rapid jerking movements. It may be present at rest, but it is usually exacerbated or elicited by voluntary activity (action dystonia). According to its distribution dystonia can be classified as focal, segmental, generalized or as hemidystonia. The term *athetosis* is used when phasic writhing dystonic movements of the extremities prevail in patients with secondary generalized dystonia. In *chorea*, rapid unpredictable movements spreading from one muscle group to the other prevail, predominantly affecting the distal limbs. *Ballism* has been defined as continuous, non patterned, purposeless movements involving chiefly proximal portions of limbs (19). It usually presents as hemiballism and is related most frequently to lesions of the contralateral subthalamic nucleus. Experimental data suggest that chorea and ballism are parts of a continuum of movement disorders (20). Ballism, thus, can be considered a form of forceful, flinging, high-amplitude, coarse chorea. *Tics* are usually rapid jerklike movements or involuntarily produced sounds and words occurring out of a background of normal activity. Both motor and vocal tics may be categorized as simple or complex. Tics are differentiated from other movement disorders also with regard to their particular features such as the presence of premonitory feelings or sensations, variability, temporary suppressibility, and distractibility. *Myoclonus* is defined as a sudden, brief, shocklike involuntary movement that may be caused by both active muscle contraction (positive myoclonus) and inhibition of ongoing muscle activity (negative myoclonus). *Hyperekplexia* is characterized by exaggerated startle responses to sudden unexpected stimuli. *Stereotypy* is an involuntary, patterned, repetitive, continuous, coordinated, purposeless or ritualistic movement, posture, or utterance which may either be simple or complex, such as self-caressing. *Akathisia* refers to a sense of restlessness and the feeling of a need to move. *Paroxysmal dyskinesias* occur intermittently with bouts of sudden-onset, short-lived involuntary movements which may be dystonic or choreic. *Parkinsonism* is characterized by a combination of bradykinesia, rigidity, rest tremor, and postural instability. *Bradykinesia*, slowness of movement, is the clinical hallmark of hypokinetic movement disorders.

Epidemiology of Movement Disorders Related to Brain Injury

Most posttraumatic movement disorders are due to severe brain injury. There are only few epidemiologic studies that have investigated the relative incidence of posttraumatic movement disorders. These studies yielded a wide variability ranging from 13% to 66% of patients who suffered severe brain injury (21–25). In a study on severe pediatric brain injury in Poland "extrapyramidal syndromes" were described in 18 out of 100 (18%) children (25). In another study, from Japan, 33 of 57 (58%) patients who were in a persistent vegetative state secondary to severe brain injury in motor vehicle accidents had "involuntary movements" (23). In this group palatal myoclonus and dystonia were observed most frequently. In another study of severe pediatric closed head injury, 4 out of 31 children were described to develop a "basal ganglia syndrome" (21). Exceedingly high rates of posttraumatic tremors were found in a questionnaire-based survey, screening severely head-injured children for the presence of "significant tremor" (22). Tremors were reported in 66% of the responders to the survey (131 of 199 children). Taking into account that tremors might not have been present in cases that did not return the questionnaires the frequency of tremor in this pediatric population still was as high as at least 45%. We have analyzed the frequency of posttraumatic movement disorders in survivors of severe head injury who were admitted to a multidisciplinary trauma unit over a period of 5 years (24). This study included 398 consecutively admitted patients with a Glasgow Coma Score (GCS) of 8 or less. Follow-up was available on 221 of the 264 survivors. Overall, posttraumatic movement disorders were found in 22.6% (50 of 221 patients); they were only transient in 10.4% (23 of 50 patients), but were still present at the time of the investigation at a mean follow-up of 3.9 years in 12.2% (27 of 50 patients) (Table 27-1). Tremors were the most frequent movement disorders. Only in 5.4% of all patients, however, were the movement disorders considered disabling. The presence of generalized edema on the CT scan at admission was significantly associated with the occurrence of movement disorders. Similar associations were detected for focal cerebral lesions, but not for subdural or epidural hematomas.

The absolute number of severe head injuries has decreased in most industrialized countries during the last two decades. Also, the management of head injury has improved considerably. It is still unclear whether these factors will translate into a lower frequency and a difference in the severity of movement disorders secondary to craniocerebral injury in the future. Different movement disorders may co-occur in a patient subsequent to severe head injury. In the study on the frequency of posttraumatic movement disorders in survivors of severe head injury mentioned above, 50 patients had a total of 59 phenomenologically distinct movement disorders (24). Treating one component with medication or surgery will not necessarily have an impact on the other. Furthermore, the co-existence of spastic hemiparesis or quadriparesis is observed frequently. In the individual patient, it may be difficult to distinguish dystonia from accompanying spasticity. It is pivotal to appreciate co-existing neurologic deficits in these patients in order to determine whether or not surgical treatment directed specifically to the movement disorder will make an impact in the patient's overall functional disability.

Systematic study of the frequency of posttraumatic movement disorders after moderate or mild brain injury is sparse. Such associations have been documented, however, by numerous anecdotal case reports or case series. In a survey of 519 patients who suffered head injury with a GCS between 9 and 15 upon admisson to the hospital, 158 patients were available for a detailed follow-up study (26). In 16 of these 158 patients (10.1%) we diagnosed a posttraumatic movement disorder. Overall, movement disorders were transient in 7.6% (12 patients) and persisted only in a minority of 2.6% (4 patients). With regard to possible bias by selection of the sample group, the frequency of posttraumatic movement disorders could be even lower. Movement disorders which occurred in this series are listed in Table 27-2. Postural/ intention tremor phenomenologically similar to enhanced physiological or essential tremor was the most frequent finding. Movement disorders were not disabling and did not require medical therapy in any instance in this series. Patients suffering from "minor" brain injury, that is those with a GCS of 15, developed movement disorders less frequently than those with GCS scores ranging from 9 to 14, the difference being statistically significant.

General Pathomechanisms in Movement Disorders After Brain Injury

Movement disorders after trauma often have a delayed onset, sometimes up to months or years post-injury. In exceptional cases a delay of more than 20 years has been reported (27). In most patients with movement disorders

---

TABLE 27-1
Frequency of Movement Disorders Secondary to Severe Brain Injury

	TRANSIENT	PERSISTENT
Low frequency intention tremor (2.5 – 4 Hz)	1.4 %	0.9 %
Postural/ kinetic tremor (2.5 – 4 Hz)	–	3.2 %
Postural/ intention tremor (>4 Hz)	4.1 %	3.6 %
Unclassified tremor	4.5 %	1.4 %
Focal dystonia	0.5 %	1.8 %
Hemidystonia	–	0.9 %
Hemidystonia + contralateral focal dystonia	–	0.9 %
Hemidystonia + cervical dystonia	–	0.5 %
Stereotypies	–	0.9 %
Myoclonus	–	0.5 %
Parkinsonism	–	0.9 %
Paroxysmal hypnogenic dyskinesias	–	0.5 %
Hyperekplexia (exaggerated startle)	–	0.5 %

The percentages refer to a cohort of 221 patients (Glasgow Coma Scores between 3 and 8 at the time of trauma) with long-term follow-up at a mean of 3.9 years. Several patients had more than one movement disorder. (*from (24) with permission*).

TABLE 27-2

Frequency of Movement Disorders Secondary to Moderate or Mild Brain Injury

	TRANSIENT	PERSISTENT
Postural/ intention tremor (>4 Hz)	8.2 %	1.3 %
Hyperekplexia (exaggerated startle)	–	0.6 %
Cervical myoclonic twitches	–	0.6 %

The percentages refer to a cohort of 158 patients (Glasgow Coma Scores between 9 and 15 at the time of trauma) with long-term follow-up at a mean of 5.2 years. One patient had both a transient and a persistent movement disorder (*from (26) with permission*).

secondary to brain injury structural lesions will be seen with modern imaging techniques. The pathomechanisms resulting in a posttraumatic movement disorder are only partially understood. It is likely that both primary and secondary lesions are responsible for their development. Primary damage involves focal contusions particularly to the basal ganglia and their pathways, DAI with preferential lesions of the superior cerebellar peduncles, and ischemia or hemorrhage due to injury of penetrating arteries associated with rotational forces of the trauma (28, 29). Secondary damage caused by hypoxia, hypotension and increased intracranial pressure may also contribute to the extent of the lesion and the subsequent development of movement disorders. Sequential imaging analyses of the lesions that result in

posttraumatic movement disorders have only rarely been performed (30). Figure 27-1 shows serial CT scans and the development of a thalamic lesion causing focal dystonia. Other factors that might be involved in the pathophysiology of posttraumatic movement disorders include the release of toxic cytokines, other neurotoxins, oxidative stress associated with the deposition of hemosiderin and iron facilitating the production of free radicals and other metabolic effects (31–34). The sequelae of mechanical injury have been studied also at cellular and molecular levels (35, 36). Genetic factors may influence the rate and extent of recovery after severe brain injury (37, 38). The balance between neurodegeneration and restorative neuroplasticity may determine whether a lesion results in permanent damage or in subsequent recovery (39, 40). Restorative processes themselves, however, could also contribute to the development of a posttraumatic movement disorder. Neuroplastic phenomena including aberrant sprouting, ephaptic transmission and alterations of neurotransmitter sensitivity could be responsible for the delay of onset of movement disorders (41).

DIAGNOSIS OF POSTTRAUMATIC MOVEMENT DISORDERS

Tremor

The most common posttraumatic movement disorder is tremor. High-amplitude postural and kinetic tremors which may interfere with any motor function are the most disabling tremors (42, 43). Often, the tremor is present

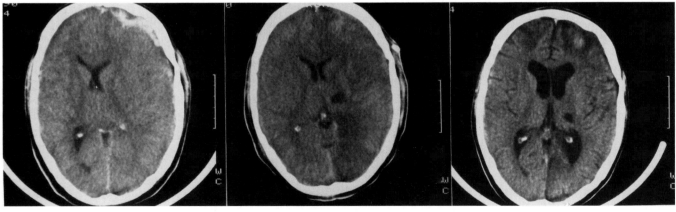

FIGURE 27-1

Serial CT scans of a patient who sustained severe head injury at age 23 and suffered from posttraumatic dystonia of his right hand showing the development of a left thalamic lesion thought to be responsible for his focal dystonia. The scan obtained immediately after head injury shows a left frontal subdural hematoma and generalized brain edema (**left**); there is less midline shift 10 days after trauma, but a hypodense lesion in the left thalamus is now visible (**middle**); five weeks later the thalamic lesion is clearly demarcated (**right**). (*from (30) with permission*)

during the whole range of a movement and increases in amplitude towards reaching the goal. The frequency of these coarse tremors, in general, ranges between 2.5 and 4 Hz and the amplitudes can be larger than 10 cm. The rhythmic oscillatory movements may be interrupted by irregular jerking movements leading to a "myoclonic" appearance (44) and may even resemble "hemiballistic" movements (45). Tremor may be present also at rest. Such slow posttraumatic tremors have been categorized as "midbrain", "rubral" or "Holmes" tremors or "myorhythmias" (17, 42, 46, 47). In a series of 35 patients with severe posttraumatic tremor the kinetic component of the tremor was the most prominent feature (48). Bilateral tremor was evident in 10 patients. Commonly, posttraumatic tremor affects predominantly or exclusively the upper extremity. Persistent posttraumatic kinetic tremors are usually secondary to severe closed head injury (48, 49). The most frequent cause is automobile accident with a history of deceleration trauma of the car driver. Kinetic tremors have also been described to occur in pedestrians who were strucked by cars and suffered closed head injury. The mean age at trauma was 11 years with a range from 3 to 29 years in one series (48). Most patients are comatose for weeks and often exhibit transient apallic syndromes or akinetic mutism during recovery. The delay between the trauma and the manifestation of the tremor is variable, ranging between 4 weeks up to a year. Commonly, the tremors are associated with ataxia of the affected limb. Tremor almost never is an isolated symptom. Psychological/cognitive alterations were found in 91% of patients, dysarthria in 86%, oculomotor nerve deficits in 69%, truncal ataxia in 91%, and residual hemiparesis or tetraparesis in 91% at a mean of 7 years after brain injury (48).

The history of deceleration trauma and the associated clinical findings indicate that the majority of patients with posttraumatic tremor suffer DAI. This is also supported by neuroradiological findings. In a series of 19 patients with posttraumatic kinetic tremor there was evidence of DAI in 18 patients according to late-phase MR studies revealing corpus callosal atrophy, ventriculomegaly, subcortical lesions and brainstem lesions (50). Lesions of the dentatothalamic pathways were found in 22 out of 25 instances (50). Lesions affecting the predecussational course of the dentatothalamic pathway will result in ipsilateral tremor (Fig. 27-2), while postdecussational lesions are responsible for contralateral tremor (Fig. 27-3). Two of three patients with an accompanying parkinsonian-like rest tremor had lesions involving the substantia nigra (Fig. 27-4). Tremor at rest may be present in patients with lesions of the dentatothalamic pathways without any evidence of contralateral nigrostriatal lesions. Traumatic lesions of the red nucleus and adjacent 3rd nerve nucleus may cause ipsilateral ptosis and limitation of ocular adduction and contralateral postural and

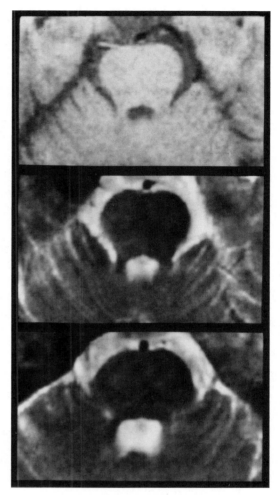

FIGURE 27-2

Axial magnetic resonance imaging studies at 2.0 T in a 27-year-old man with right-sided postural and kinetic tremor 22 years after a traffic accident. T1-weighted images **(upper)** show a small *ipsilateral* hypointense signal alteration of the right brachium conjunctivum adjacent to the fourth ventricle, that is predecussational. Heavily T2-weighted RARE images demonstrate a corresponding apparently larger hypointense lesion **(middle and lower)**. *(from (50) with permission)*

rest tremor (Benedikt's or Claude's syndrome) (51). Isolated cases of thalamic lesions have been reported to cause tremor. In both, cerebellar and thalamic tremors the crescendo appearance with goal-directed movements may be the result of amplification of the tremor in reverberating circuits secondary to impaired thalamic relay. The pathophysiologic mechanisms how lesions of the dentatothalamic pathways result in the delayed appearance of tremor have not been fully elucidated (52). It is well known that such lesions trigger both orthograde and retrograde fiber degeneration. Magnetic resonance spectroscopic techniques suggest transsynaptic changes in the development of posttraumatic tremor (53). Transsynaptic

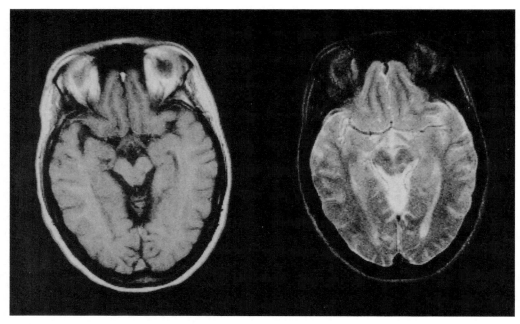

FIGURE 27-3

Magnetic resonance imaging studies at 1.0 T in a 30-year-old woman with right-sided postural and kinetic tremor 12 years after having sustained severe head injury. **The axial** scans reveal a small ***contralateral*** postdecussational lesion not extending to the substantia nigra. (*from (50) with permission*)

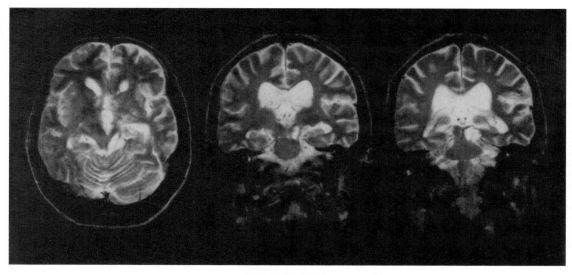

FIGURE 27-4

Magnetic resonance imaging studies at 2.0 T in a 37-year-old man with right-sided parkinsonian tremor at rest, postural and kinetic tremor 33 years after severe head injury. The axial **(left)** and coronal **(middle and right)** scans show a ***contralateral*** postdecussational lesion extending into the substantia nigra. (*from (50) with permission*)

neuronal degeneration could also involve the inferior olives, although palatal myoclonus, a well known symptom in olivary degeneration, is not commonly observed in posttraumatic tremor. Finally, the disinhibition of thalamic rhythmic network oscillations and modifications of long-loop reflexes could be relevant. Marked decrease in 18F-dopa uptake in the contralateral striatum without significant changes in the D2-specific binding was found in patients with posttraumatic 'midbrain' tremor who improved with levodopa therapy (54). In another patient with posttraumatic tremor who had a complete contralateral loss of the nigrostriatal pathway after midbrain injury as shown by missing [123J]FP-CIT uptake in the contralateral striatum, it was thought that concurrent lesioning of the subthalamic nucleus had prevented the occurrence of parkinsonism (55).

Dystonia

Hemidystonia is the most typical presentation of posttraumatic dystonia (6, 7, 56–58) (Fig. 27-5). In patient series with symptomatic hemidystonia from different etiologies head injury accounted for 7% to 9% of the cases (59, 60). Rare manifestations of craniocerebral trauma include cervical dystonia, segmental axial dystonia and spasmodic dysphonia (6, 61, 62). The presence of the DYT1 mutation does not seem to increase the risk of secondary dystonia, and the latter is not associated with the DYT1

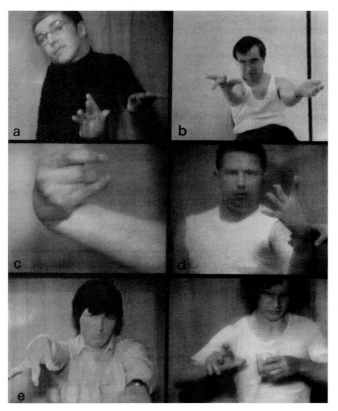

FIGURE 27-5

Clinical presentation of patients with posttraumatic dystonia. **A**: patient with right-sided hemidystonia and cervical dystonia, before thalamotomy. **B**: same patient at long-term follow-up after left-sided thalamotomy. **C**: dystonic posture of right hand. **D**: left-sided dystonia with superimposed athetotic movements. **E**: right-sided hemidystonia. **F**: typical increase of dystonia upon intended movement. (*from (6) with permission*)

mutation (63). The DYT1 mutation is found more frequently among dystonic patients with Ashkenazi Jewish origin, and it is characterized by a 3 base-pair deletion in a gene coding for an ATP-binding protein, termed torsinA.

Several patiens with posttraumatic hemidystonia were described over the decades since the first report by Austregesilio in 1928 (64). Nevertheless, posttraumatic dystonia is probably underreported. There is a predominance of men which, however, most likely reflects the male preponderance among patients suffering craniocerebral trauma. Age at the time of trauma varies, but almost all patients with only few exceptions were in their infancy or adolescence. It is possible that the delay of onset of dystonia after static brain lesions is associated with the age at trauma. Patients with hemidystonia secondary to brain damage before the age of 7 years had a longer latency between the lesion and the manifestation of dystonia than adults who suffered structural cerebral damage (41). Most patients suffer severe brain injury, but occasional cases of hemidystonia and cervical dystonia were reported after moderate or mild head injury (65). Posttraumatic hemidystonia frequently is preceded by or associated with ipsilateral hemiparesis. The delay between trauma and appearance of hemidystonia is variable and may be as short as one day but may take as long as 6 years (41, 60, 66). In a series of patients with posttraumatic hemidystonia the mean latency between injury and the onset of dystonia was 20 months (6). The natural history of hemidystonia seems to be initial progression with spread over months to years, followed by eventual stabilisation (67).

Posttraumatic dystonia is associated most frequently with basal ganglia or thalamic lesions. Pathoanatomical correlations are similar to those reported for other causes of secondary dystonia (59, 60, 67). Figure 27-6 illustrates typical early magnetic resonance imaging findings in a 19-year-old patient who later developed right hemidystonia. In one series, 7 of 8 patients with posttraumatic hemidystonia had lesions involving the contralateral caudate or putamen (6) (Fig. 27-7). Cases of pallidal lesions resulting in dystonia are rare (68, 69) (Fig. 27-8). Occasionally, hemidystonia or focal dystonia, in particular, hand dystonia, is associated with thalamic lesions (30). A contralateral mesencephalic lesion was found in a patient with hemidystonia plus torticollis (6) (Fig. 27-9). Patients with posttraumatic kinetic tremor due to mesencephalic lesions or to lesions of the superior cerebellar peduncles may also have mild dystonic postures (48).

Primary as well as secondary factors are likely to contribute to the basal ganglia lesions in posttraumatic dystonia. Some of the caudatoputaminal lesions in posttraumatic hemidystonia correspond to vascular territorries, in particular to the anterior (and more rarely posterior) group of the lateral lenticulostriate branches of the middle cerebral artery. Stretch of these vessels by rotating forces may either result in hemorrhage or in ischemia secondary to lesions of

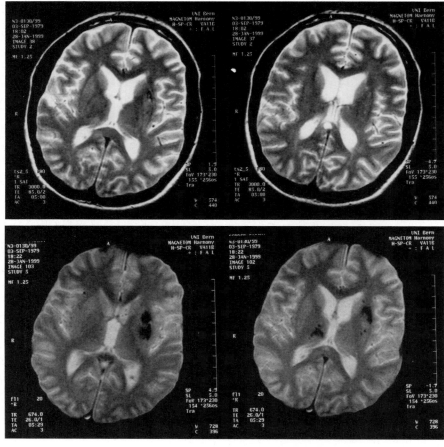

FIGURE 27-6

Magnetic resonance imaging studies of a 19-year-old man two months after suffering severe closed head injury with an initial Glasgow Coma Score of 4. Later on, right hemidystonia and cervical dystonia developed. **Upper row**: Axial Turbospin-Echo 3000/85 scans show poorly defined lesions of the left putamen. **Lower row**: Axial T2 FLASH 674/26 sequences which are more susceptible to hemosiderin better demonstrate the extent of the hypointense lesions in the putamen and reveal other small lesions in addition. *(from (14) with permission)*

the intima (70). This mechanism is probably also responsible for the fact that in patients with dystonia due to brain injury as compared to patients with other secondary dystonia, caudotoputaminal lesions are much more frequent than thalamic lesions (59). In general, the prognosis of traumatic basal ganglia hematoma is poor. In a recent series, only 6 of 34 patients (16%) made a favorable recovery (28). Rarely, blunt or penetrating carotid artery injuries have been described to result in ischemic cerebral lesions with subsequent development of dystonia (71, 72). Secondary damage to the basal ganglia is also possible. Many patients with posttraumatic dystonia were reported to have hematoma contralateral to the hemidystonia as well. Hypoxia is known to result in damage following "topistic" patterns, i.e. damage of specific nuclei or to neuronal subpopulations such as selective striatal vulnerability, for example (73).

Deranged function of both the direct and the indirect striatopallidal pathways is thought to underlie the development of dystonia. Regional cerebral blood flow studies in acquired hemidystonia secondary to basal ganglia or thalamic lesions have shown frontal overactivity on movement indicating that dystonia ultimately is due to thalamofrontal disinhibition secondary to disruption of the normal inhibitory control by the basal ganglia (74). It is puzzling that isolated lesions of the globus pallidus internus in healthy people can result in dystonia, but lesioning or stimulation of the same structure in dystonic people can alleviate dystonia. This observation, nevertheless, emphasizes that disturbed pallidal discharge and subsequent deranged pallidothalamic output is responsible for secondary dystonia (75).

Ballism and Chorea

Overall, ballism is a rare movement disorder. There have been occasional descriptions of hemiballism and hemichorea

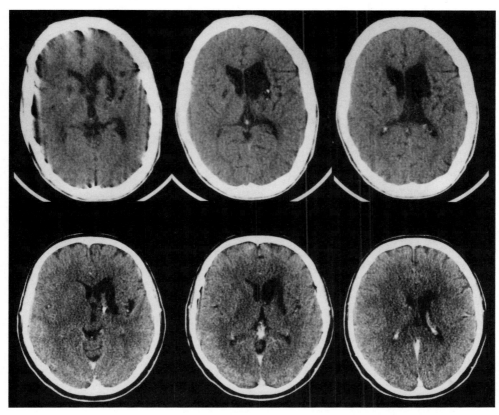

FIGURE 27-7

CT scans of a 21-year old man who sustaind a severe closed head injury at age 7 and subsequently developed *bilateral* hemidystonia. On the left side there is a lesion of the caudate, anterior internal capsule and putamen corresponding to supply of lateral lenticulostriate branches of middle cerebral artery and small lesions of the ventrolateral thalamus; on the right side there is a lesion of anterior putamen **(upper)**. CT scans showing a caudatoputaminal lesion in a 50-year old woman who sustained a moderate brain injury at age 9 and who developed contralateral hemidystonia 4 years thereafter **(lower)**. *(from (6) with permission)*

secondary to craniocerebral trauma (19, 68, 76, 77). While some reports appear to describe true hemiballism, the categorization of the movement disorder remains somewhat unclear in other instances (45, 78). Often, the term "violent" movement disorder has been wrongly used to assign the diagnosis of hemiballism in patients with large amplitude hyperkinesia including tremors with superimposed irregular myoclonic jerks. Posttraumatic hemiballism is associated with severe closed head injury. It may occur with a delay of weeks or months when patients recover from coma. Histopathological examination revealed subthalamic nucleus atrophy in a patient with a traumatic pallidal lesion who developed hemiballism at 2 years postinjury (68). In another patient with posttraumatic hemiballism, no structural abnormalities were found with conventional imaging studies but single photon emission computed tomography (SPECT) revealed a subthalamic lesion (79).

Choreatic movement disorders may be caused by epidural or subdural hematomas in the rare case (80). Chronic subdural hematomas may present with contralateral, ipsilateral or bilateral choreatic movements (81, 82).

Paroxysmal Dyskinesias

The pathophysiology of paroxysmal dyskinesias remains unclear. It has been assumed that they present a certain type of subcortical epilepsy or reflex epilepsy. They are also thought to be associated with dysfunction of sensory processing at the level of the basal ganglia or the thalamus. There have been several reports on paroxysmal dyskinesias secondary to brain injury (83–90). Imaging findings have been inconclusive. In single cases putaminal lesions were found (83). Positron emission tomographic scan studies showed abnormal metabolism in the

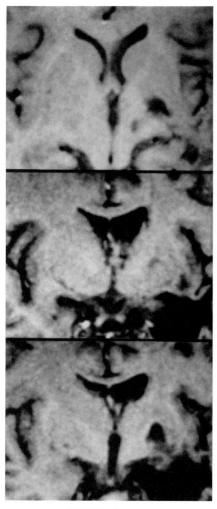

FIGURE 27-8

Magnetic resonance imaging studies in a 32-year-old man with postttraumatic hemidystonia after severe head injury at age 7. The axial scan through the lower part of basal ganglia **(upper)** shows the posttraumatic pallidal lesion extending to posterior putamen and a small lesion in the subthalamic region after stereotactic surgery which provided partial relief of the hemidystonia for more than 16 years. The coronal scans **(middle and lower)** more clearly show the additional lesion to the putamen. *(from (6) with permission)*

contralateral basal ganglia during an attack of paroxsymal posttraumatic hemidystonia (87).

Tics and Tourettism

Adult-onset disorders with both motor tics and vocalizations secondary to a known cause have been referred to as "tourettism" to contrast it with the more common idiopathic Tourette's syndrome (91). Posttraumatic tics and tourettism following head trauma have been described in few patients (92–96). Since tics are relatively common, the coincidental occurrence of tics after head trauma must

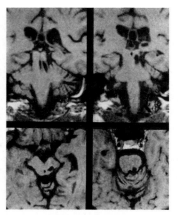

FIGURE 27-9

Magnetic resonance scans of a 28-year-old man with right-sided hemidystonia and cervical dystonia. The coronal images show a longish pontomesencephalic tegmental lesion on the left side **(upper row)**. The axial scans demonstrate more clearly the lesion also affecting the dentatothalamic pathway thought to be responsible for the additional tremor in this case **(lower row)**. *(from (6) with permission)*

always deserve special consideration. A causative role of trauma is favored in patients with evidence of other posttraumatic sequelae, and a negative history of motor tics prior to head injury. A history of well documented trauma to the head is mandatory. The older age at onset of patients with posttraumatic tourettism is notable, in contrast to Tourette's syndrome. We studied the characteristics in 6 patients with tics secondary to craniocerebral trauma (93). All patients were male and the mean age at the time of the trauma was 28 years. Craniocerebral injury was moderate or mild in 5 patients, and neuroimaging studies did not reveal basal ganglia lesions. In another patient who had tics and marked obsessive-compulsive behavior secondary to severe brain injury, extensive periventricular and subcortical leukencephalopathy was detected by magnetic resonance imaging studies (93) (Fig. 27-10). Preexisting tics may exacerbate after head injury (13). Secondary, including posttraumatic tic disorders were recently reviewed (97).

Other Posttraumatic Hyperkinesias

Various other hyperkinetic movement disorders, often in the frame of case reports, were reported after craniocerebral trauma including instances of myoclonus, opsoclonus, palatal myoclonus, stereotypies, akathisia, and galloping tongue (98–105).

Posttraumatic Parkinsonism and Parkinson's Disease

Parkinsonism after Single Head Injury   Although the concept of posttraumatic parkinsonism was well accepted in

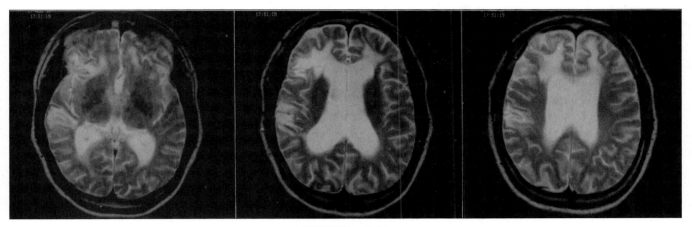

FIGURE 27-10

Magnetic resonance imaging studies of a 33-year-old man with posttraumatic tics and obsessive-compulsive behavior 12 years after he sustained a series of two severe head injuries. There is panventricular dilatation, cortical atrophy, and extensive periventricular and subcortical leukencephalopathy, particularly of the frontal and the right temporoparietal white matter. There are no focal basal ganglia lesions. (*from (91) with permission*)

the first part of the 20th century, review of cases in the literature raises doubts that most are truly examples of parkinsonism resulting from trauma (106, 107). The causal relationship in most cases has been largely speculative and the interpretation complicated by medicolegal issues. In some cases, the initial injury actually seemed to have resulted from, rather than caused, motor impairment. Posttraumatic parkinsonism, in general, is secondary to severe closed head injury (108, 109). Occasionally, parkinsonism has been described to be associated with lesions of the substantia nigra (110, 111). Direct lesions to the substantia nigra have been reported secondary to injuries by knives, screwdrivers, shell splinters or gunshots, and usually present with hemiparkinsonism (112–114). The parkinsonian syndrome is dominated by akinetic-rigid symptoms. Other movement disorders and pyramidal dysfunction may be present. We have recently studied a young man who suffered acute flexion-extension injury playing American football, followed by 3-week coma attributed to bilateral hemisphere hemorrhage, who is left with residual, levodopa-responsive parkinsonism, without any evidence of damage to the substantia nigra on imaging studies.

There have been several reports of parkinsonism secondary to chronic subdural hematoma (115). Parkinsonian symptoms become evident within weeks after trivial head injury. The clinical picture is dominated by hypomimia, bradykinesia and tremor. Other neurological signs and symptoms are usually present, although some instances of pure parkinsonism have been described (115, 116). Diagnostic evaluations appear to be delayed and initial misinterpretations are common. Favorable outcome is achieved in most instances after drainage of

the hematoma with complete or almost complete remission of parkinsonism. Chronic subdural hematomas may also cause deterioration of preexisting parkinsonian syndromes (115). Also, acute subdural hematomas when associated with brainstem compression and reduced fluorodopa uptake in the contralateral putamen can induce a hemiparkinsonian syndrome (117).

Parkinsonism after Repeated Head Injury   Boxing is the most frequent cause for parkinsonism associated with repeated head trauma (118–122). Obvious tremors, bradykinesia and hypophonia in Muhammed Ali has helped to draw the public attention to this problem. Although cumulative brain injury occurs also in other professional sports (123), only exceptional instances of parkinsonism have been reported (122). "Pugilistic" parkinsonism (PP) or "punch-drunk" syndrome is a chronic encephalopathy which results from the cumulative effects of subclinical concussions secondary to rotational acceleration traumas by direct blows to the head. Usually, PP appears with a delay of several years after ending an active boxing career (124). The frequency of PP has been estimated to range between 20% to 50% of professional boxers. The severity of PP correlates with the length of the boxing career and the number of bouts (125). Clinically, a variable spectrum of signs and symptoms can be present including behavioral changes, dementia, and corticospinal and cerebellar symptoms. Another frequent finding is marked dysarthria or hypophonia. In contrast to posttraumatic parkinsonism secondary to a single severe head injury, tremor at rest is a relatively frequent feature of PP. In addition to extensive nigral damage, dysfunction of striatal dopaminergic terminals has been suggested. Proton magnetic resonance spectroscopy studies have demonstrated a significant reduction in the concentration of N-acetylaspartate in the lenticular nuclei of PP patients as compared to controls and PD patients (126). PET studies showed uniform nigrostriatal involvement but relative sparing of caudate function in PP (122). Neuropathological studies have revealed depigmentation of the substantia nigra but an absence of Lewy bodies, the histological hallmark for PD. While the number of fatalities has decreased steadily over the years due to preventive measures in the ring it remains to be seen whether this will result also in a decrease of PP among boxers (127). There has been controversy as to the development of chronic encephalopathy in amateur boxing. Most studies do not show clinical evidence of chronic encephalopathy (128). In one study finger-tapping performance was worse in some amateur boxers as compared to other athletes (129). It has been shown recently that high-exposure professional boxers with an apolipoprotein epsilon4 allele have significantly greater scores on a scale measuring chronic encephalopathy than those without the allele (130). Thus, genetic susceptibility to the effects of repeated head trauma is likely.

Parkinson's Disease and Head Trauma In his original *Essay on the Shaking Palsy* James Parkinson suggested that the disease that now bears his name might result from trauma to the medulla. Head trauma as a possible risk factor for PD has been the subject of controversy for years (8, 9, 131–134). It has been shown that head trauma sustained in motor vehicle accidents can exacerbate parkinsonism transiently in patients with PD, however, without resulting in increased persistent disability or acceleration of the clinical course of the disease (135). Several studies have found a higher frequency of head injury in patients with PD (136, 137). Usually, the history of head trauma dates back to 20 or 30 years prior to onset of PD and, therefore, any cause-and-effect relationship is difficult to establish. With regard to head injury and other possible environmental factors it has been suggested that PD might be the consequence of clinically silent exposure in early or middle life with symptoms becoming manifest only later when there is a further decline of dopaminergic neurons with advancing age. Some studies suggested that susceptibility to trauma is more important than the severity of trauma itself. Several studies which have shown a positive association between head injury and trauma suffer from methodological flaws. The major problem with retrospective case control studies is recall bias. Unfortunately, there is a paucity of cohort studies which might be better suited to answer the inherent questions. One cohort study did not detect a significant increase in standardized morbidity ratios for PD in adults with head injury (138).

However, this study had a 30% probability of not detecting a hypothetical twofold relative risk. In a recent case-control study, subjects who experienced a mild head trauma with only amnesia had no increased risk for PD; however, subjects who had a mild head trauma with loss of consciousness or a more severe trauma had a much higher odds ratio (9). Since head trauma, overall, was considered rather a relatively rare event, the population attributable risk was estimated to be at 5%.

TREATMENT OF POSTTRAUMATIC MOVEMENT DISORDERS

Rehabilitation of patients with posttraumatic movement disorders must consider both associated neurological and psychosocial dysfunction resulting from brain injury and the specific movement disorders. The physical disability of patients with severe kinetic tremors can be extreme because they are neither able to reach or to manage an object when the syndrome is fully expressed. Their disabilities should be treated according to the standard principles of rehabilitation care. It is important to anticipate and prevent potential obstacles for reintegration, to identify and offer strategies to manage present disabilities, and to develop adaptive and coping skills to achieve more independance. Physical therapy is helpful to prevent contractures in the most severely affected cases with dystonia.

Tremor after Severe Brain Injury

Medical Treatment It is difficult to predict the prognosis of posttraumatic tremor in the initial period after its manifestation. It may lessen or resolve spontaneously within 1 year after its onset. The majority of patients, however, have persistent violent shaking movements. Posttraumatic tremor, then, is notoriously difficult to treat. Only few patients have been reported to respond favorably to medical treatment. Drugs reported to improve posttraumatic tremor include glutethimide, isoniazid, L-tryptophan, propranolol, benzodiazepines, carbamazepine, levodopa/carbidopa and anticholinergics (53, 139–141). Botulinum toxin injections may be helpful to relief the tremor temporarily but the high dosages administered to both proximal and distal arm muscles limit the usefulness of this treatment (142).

Surgical Treatment The largest surgical experience for posttraumatic tremor comes from ablative functional stereotactic surgery with radiofrequency lesioning in the ventrolateral thalamus and the subthalamic region, which can effectively abate posttraumatic tremor (45, 48, 143–160) (Fig. 27-11). The data of a total of 128 patients who underwent ablative stereotactic surgery as documented in

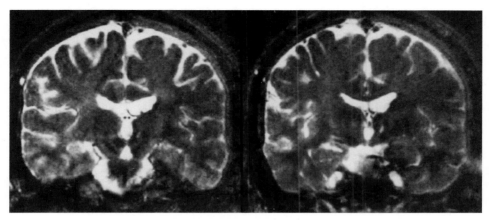

FIGURE 27-11

Magnetic resonance imaging studies obtained 3 years after combined ablative stereotactic surgery in the ventrolateral thalamus and zona incerta for treatment of posttraumatic tremor of the right arm. The coronal scans demonstrate the location of the small left stereotactic lesion and its topography in relation to adjacent nuclei. *(from (48) with permission)*

the literature are shown in Table 27-3. Persistent improvement on long-term follow-up has been observed in 88% of patients with the tremor being absent or markedly reduced in 65% in one study (48). Tremor at rest usually is completely abolished but the most striking improvement is the reduction of postural and kinetic tremor. Also, valuable gain in functional disability has been achieved. Functional improvement was more striking in patients who had severe incapacitating tremor but comparatively less other neurological or mental deficits. There is a marked risk for adverse effects, however, in this vulnerable group of patients. Immediate postoperative side effects have been reported to occur in 50% to 90% of patients and persistent side effects are being observed in up to 63%. Most frequently, such side effects consist chiefly of aggravation of preoperative symptoms such as dysarthria or gait disturbance. There is a trend for patients with left-sided surgery to present more frequently with increased dysarthria than patients who have right-sided procedures. Surprisingly, single patients may benefit from marked amelioration of their dysarthria after radiofrequency lesioning (48). On long-term follow-up, it has been observed that there may be an increase in dystonic postures despite improvement of tremor, or new dystonic symptoms may become manifest. It is unclear whether this is related to the surgical procedure or whether this may present delayed-onset dystonia (41). The high frequency of side effects is remarkably different from that observed after thalamotomy for other types of tremor, for example, essential tremor. The size of the lesions necessary to control severe kinetic tremors has been debated. It has been stated that larger lesions should be made in such cases to achieve long-term relief (154). On the other hand, with regard to the propensity of these patients for postoperative morbidity, small lesions in the basal ventrolateral thalamus and the subthalamic region involving the zona incerta might be more advantageous. Gamma knife Vim thalamotomy has been reported also to result in modest improvement in posttraumatic tremor (161), but delayed effects of radiation may limit this procedure.

There is relatively little experience with thalamic deep brain stimulation (DBS) for treatment of posttraumatic tremor (162–167). Similar to other kinetic tremors due to stroke or multiple sclerosis (168), DBS has been found to be less effective than in parkinsonian tremor or essential tremor (Table 27-4). Occasionally, thalamic DBS was described as completely ineffective (166). In other instances, however, patients achieved variable symptomatic and functional benefit. It appears that DBS may be less effective in control of tremor but is associated with less side effects than radiofrequency lesioning in this special group of patients. Long-term follow-up data is very limited. There have been divergent opinions what should be considered the ideal thalamic target for DBS to treat proximal kinetic tremors. Nguyen et al. suggested that proximal contacts in the Vim would be most beneficial (165), whereas others think that stimulation of a target located more anteriorly is important (167). Kitagawa et al. recently demonstrated that stimulation of the subthalamic area can be effective in patients with proximal tremors (169). Electrodes placed in the zona incerta were most effective to control contralateral tremor. We recommend to wait at least one year after onset of posttraumatic tremor before surgery is considered. Further studies are clearly necessary to establish the role of DBS in posttraumatic tremor. We prefer DBS over thalamotomy in these patients regarding the high occurrence of side effects, presently.

TABLE 27-3

Functional Stereotactic Surgery for Posttraumatic Tremor: Lesioning Procedures

AUTHOR(S) AND YEAR	TARGET	CASES	IMMEDIATE IMPROVEMENT	LONG-TERM FOLLOW-UP	LAST FOLLOW-UP, MEAN YRS (RANGE)	SYMPTOMATIC IMPROVEMENT (%)	FUNCTIONAL IMPROVEMENT (%)	PERSISTENT SIDE EFFECTS
Cooper, 1960	VL	2	2	1	1.3	1/1	1/1	NA
Spiegel et al., 1963	STR	1	1	1	NA	0/1	NA	NA
Fox and Kurtzke, 1966	VL	1	1	1	0.5	1/1	1/1	0/1
Samra et al., 1970	VL	5	5	NA	NA	5/5 (100)	NA	NA
Van Manen, 1974*	VL	2	2	2	7	1/2	NA	1/2
Eiras and García, 1980	GP, Vop	1	1	1	2.5	1/1	1/1	0/1
Andrew et al., 1982	VL	8	8	NA	NA	8/8 (100)	8/8 (100)	5/8 (63)
Kandel, 1982*	VL, STR, GP	10	NA	NA	NA	NA	NA	NA
Niizuma et al., 1982*	Vim, Sub-Vim	3	3	NA	NA	NA	NA	NA
Ohye et al., 1982	Vim	8	8	NA	NA	NA	NA	1/8 (13)
Hirai et al., 1983	VL	5	4	NA	NA	NA	NA	0/5
Bullard and Nashold, 1984	VL	7	7	7	1.5 (0.2 to 3)	7/7 (100)	6/7 (86)	3/7 (43)
Bullard and Nashold, 1988**	VL	10	10	8	1.3 (0.2 to 3)	8/8 (100)	7/8 (90)	4/8 (50)
Iwadate et al., 1989	VL	3	2	NA	NA	2/3 (66)	NA	NA
Richardson, 1989	VL	1	1	NA	NA	1/1	NA	NA
Goldman and Kelly, 1992	VL	4	4	4	3 (1.4 to 4.5)	3/4 (75)	3/4 (75)	0/4 (0)
Marks, 1993	Vim	7	6	NA	NA	6/7 (86)	NA	1/7 (14)
Taira et al., 1993	Vop, Vim	3	1	NA	3		0.5	1/3 (33)
NA	2/3 (66)							
Krauss et al., 1994	VL, Zi	35	35	32	10.5 (0.5 to 24)	28/32 (88)	26/29 (90)	12/32 (38)
Jankovic et al., 1995	Vim	6	6	6	4	6/6 (100)	3/6 (50)	3/6 (50)
Shahzadi et al., 1995*	Vim	11	11	NA	NA	NA	NA	6/11 (55)
Louis et al., 1996	VL	2	2	2	0.3 and 4	2/2	NA	NA
Total		128	113/118 (96%)	68 (53 %)		81/92 (88 %)	56/65 (86 %)	38/103(37%)

Target: GP = globus pallidus; STR = subthalamic region; Vim = (nucleus) ventralis intermedius (thalami); VL = ventrolateral thalamus; Vop = (nucleus) ventrooralis posterior (thalami); Zi = zona incerta.
  NA = not available.
 * Series with tremors of different etiologies, usually cerebellar-type tremors. Specific data for posttraumatic tremor not always available.
 ** The series of Bullard & Nashold from 1988 includes the patients in the series from 1984.
 (from (14) with permission).

TABLE 27-4

Functional Stereotactic Surgery for Posttrauamtic Tremor: Deep Brain Stimulation

AUTHOR(S) AND YEAR	TARGET	CASES	IMMEDIATE IMPROVEMENT	LONG-TERM FOLLOW-UP	LAST FOLLOW-UP, YEARS	SYMPTOMATIC IMPROVEMENT	FUNCTIONAL IMPROVEMENT	PERSISTENT SIDE EFFECTS
Andy, 1983	CM-PF, Zi	1	1	NA	NA	1/1	1/1	0/1
Broggi et al., 1993	Vim	1	1	1	0.8	1/1	1/1	0/1
Nguyen and Degos,1993	Vim	1	1	1	1	1/1	1/1	0/1
Benabid et al.. 1996*	Vim	X/7	NA	NA	NA	"inconsistently, less significantly, or not improved"	"significant improvement observed in the quality of daily living"	NA
Standhart et al., 1998	Vim	1	0	NA	NA	0/1	NA	NA
Nobbe, 2000**	Vop	1	1	1	0.5	1/1	1/1	0/1
Krauss, 2000**	Vop/Vim	1	1	1	1.5	1/1	1/1	0/1
Vesper et al., 2000	Vop/Vim	4	4	4	0.5	4/4	4/4	NA

Target: CM-PF = centrum medianum – (nucleus) parafascicularis (thalami); Zi = zona incerta.
NA = not available.
* Series with tremors of different etiologies, usually cerebellar-type tremors. Specific data for posttraumatic tremor not always available.
**Unpublished data.
(from (14) with permission).

Tremor After Moderate and Mild Brain Injury

The postural and intention tremors that may occur after mild and moderate head injury usually do not require therapy and subside spontaneously (26). In some patients tremor persists and head tremor can also develop. In those cases medical therapy with clonazepam, propranolol or primidone, or botulinum toxin injections may provide relief (170, 171).

Dystonia

Medical Treatment   In patients with posttraumatic dystonia, spontaneous remission is unusual, although some improvement can be seen particularly in patients with thalamic lesions. Medical treatment is usually ineffective. Occasionally, there is a mild response to anticholinergic drugs. Botulinum toxin injections are the treatment of first choice in patients with posttraumatic torticollis and other focal dystonias (18, 142).

Surgical Treatment   The prognosis is favorable in the rare cases of dystonia related to subdural hematoma after drainage of the hematoma (172–174). Functional stereotactic surgery is a treatment option in patients with disabling hemidystonia or segmental dystonia (6, 175). Targets include ventrolateral thalamus, the subthalamic region, the pulvinar and the globus pallidus internus. Improvement of dystonia in the early postoperative period has been described in most instances. Experience with long-term follow-up, however, is limited (Fig. 27-9). At a mean follow-up of 18 years after thalamic radiofrequency lesioning, 3 of 6 patients with posttraumatic hemidystonia still benefited from some improvement of their hemidystonia (6). Recently, pallidal surgery has been reintroduced for treatment of dystonia (176). In contrast to thalamotomy, the improvement after pallidotomy may be delayed by several weeks or months. It is unclear at this time whether thalamic or pallidal targets should be preferred in patients with secondary dystonia (177). In a series of patients with various forms of dystonia, the response to pallidal surgery for dystonia was dependent on etiology (178). Patients with secondary dystonia who had extensive structural cerebral lesions had no improvement after pallidal surgery, whereas patients with primary dystonia, particularly those with DYT1 dystonia, had striking benefit and patients with secondary dystonia without structural lesions had mild benefit. Villemure and colleagues reported on two dystonia patients with secondary dystonia who did not improve with pallidal surgery but benefited with thalamic targets (179). In a recent study, on the other hand, no difference in outcome between pallidal or thalamic targets was seen in patients with secondary dystonia (180). Overall, patients with secondary dystonia experienced more modest improvement as compared to patients with primary dystonia regardless of the target used. The response of posttraumatic dystonia to pallidotomy appears to be difficult to predict. We did not observe improvement of posttraumatic hemidystonia after pallidotomy in a young patient despite his imaging studies did not show structural brain lesions. In contrast, bilateral pallidotomy was reported to result in marked improvement in a patient with generalized posttraumatic dystonia (181).

DBS has been used in only few patients with hemidystonia secondary to craniocerebral trauma. Marked improvement of dystonic movements and postures has been described in a 16-year-old boy with a thalamic lesion who underwent stimulation of the ventroposterolateral thalamus over 8 months (182). We have followed a patient for 6 years who continues to show consistent improvement of posttraumatic dystonia of the left arm with stimulation of the contralateral globus pallidus internus (183) (Fig. 27-12). Chronic intrathecal baclofen administered via implanted pumps may provide useful improvement in patients with more generalized dystonia or accompanying spasticity (184–186).

Ballism and Chorea

In contrast to vascular hemiballism, posttraumatic hemiballism seems to be more persistent with less tendency for spontaneous improvement. Patients who do not respond adequately to conservative treatment, such as tetrabenazine, a monoamine depleting drug, can benefit from functional stereotactic surgery (187). Due to the rarity of posttraumatic hemiballism, however, experience is very limited. Targets in the contralateral pallidum or thalamus are useful.

In chorea associated with chronic subdural hematoma, the prognosis usually is favorable after drainage of the hematoma.

Paroxysmal Dyskinesias

Posttraumatic paroxysmal dyskinesias often respond favorably to anticonvulsive medication, in particular kinesigenic dyskinesias (90). Thalamic stimulation has been shown to be beneficial in a patient with paroxysmal non-kinesigenic dyskinesia (188).

Posttraumatic Parkinsonism

Patients with substantia nigra lesions may benefit from levodopa therapy (111). Medical treatment of posttraumatic parkinsonism, in general, is similar to that for idiopathic PD (189). There are no data available for the specific outcome of functional stereotactic surgery in patients with parkinsonism secondary to brain injury.

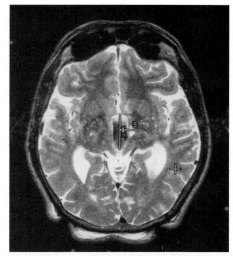

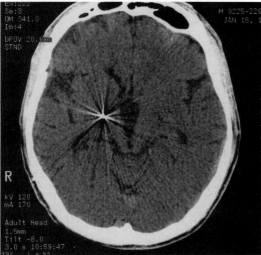

FIGURE 27-12

A: Stereotactic T2-weighted axial magnetic resonance scan of a 24-year-old man who sustained severe closed head injury at age 15 and who subsequently developed left-sided low-frequency tremor and hemidystonia. The tremor was successfully relieved by a right-sided thalamotomy; hemidystonia, however, increased over the years. This MR image was used for target calculation to implant an electrode in the posteroventral lateral globus pallidus internus (sides are reversed). B: Axial CT scan 4 years later demonstrating the position of the electrode in the pallidal target providing relief of dystonic posture and phasic movements and dystonia-associated pain. *(from (180) with permission)*

CONCLUSIONS

Traumatic brain injury can result in a variety of movement disorders. The mediation of the effects of trauma and the pathophysiology of the development of post-traumatic movement disorders require further study.

Proper identification of such movement disorders is pivotal for rehabilitation. Functional stereotactic neurosurgery should be considered in patients with disabling movement disorders refractory to medical treatment.

References

1. Jankovic J: Post-traumatic movement disorders: central and peripheral mechanisms. *Neurology* 1994;44:2006–2014.
2. Goetz CG, Pappert EJ: Trauma and movement disorders. *Neurol Clin* 1992;10:907–919.
3. Jankovic J: Can peripheral trauma induce dystonia and other movement disorders? Yes! *Mov Disord* 2001;16:7–12.
4. Weiner WJ: Can peripheral trauma induce dystonia? No! *Mov Disord* 2001;16:13–22.
5. Curran TG, Lang AE: Trauma and tremor, in Findley LJ, Koller WC (eds): *Handbook of tremor disorders*. New York, Basel, Hong Kong, Marcel Dekker, 1995, pp 411–428.
6. Krauss JK, Mohadjer M, Braus DF, Wakhloo AK, Nobbe F, Mundinger F: Dystonia following head trauma - a report of nine patients and review of the literature. *Mov Disord* 1992;7:263–272.
7. Lee MS, Rinne JO, Ceballos-Baumann A, Thompson PD, Marsden CD: Dystonia after head trauma. *Neurology* 1994;44:1374–1378.
8. Ben-Shlomo Y: How far are we in understanding the cause of Parkinson's disease? *J Neurol Neurosurg Psychiatry* 1996;61:4–16.
9. Bower JH, Maraganore DM, Peterson BJ, McDonnell SK, Ahlskog JE, Rocca WA. Head trauma preceding PD: A case-control study. *Neurology* 2003;60:1610–1615.
10. Lang A, Fahn S: Movement disorder of RSD. *Neurology* 1990;40:1476–1477.
11. Monday K, Jankovic J: Psychogenic myoclonus. *Neurology* 1993;43:349–352.
12. Scarano VR, Jankovic J: Post-traumatic movement disorders: effect of the legal system on outcome. *J Forensic Sci* 1998;43:334–339.
13. Koller WC, Wong GF, Lang A: Posttraumatic movement disorders: a review. *Mov Disord* 1989;4:20–36.
14. Krauss JK, Jankovic J. Head injury and posttraumatic movement disorders. *Neurosurgery* 2002;50:927–940.
15. Krauss JK, Jankovic J, Grossman RG (eds.). *Surgery for Parkinson's disease and movement disorders*. Lippincott Williams & Wilkins, 2001.
16. Jankovic J. International classification of diseases. Tenth revision: neurological adaptation (ICD-10 NA) extrapyramidal and movement disorders. *Mov Disord* 1995;10:533–540.
17. Deuschl G, Bain P, Brin M: Consensus statement of the Movement Disorder Society on Tremor. *Mov Disord* 13, Suppl 1998;3:2–23.
18. Jankovic J, Fahn S: Dystonic disorders, in Jankovic J, Tolosa E (eds): *Parkinson's Disease and Movement Disorders*, 4th edition. Philadelphia, Lippincott, Williams and Wilkins, 2002, pp 331–357.
19. Krauss JK, Borremans JJ, Nobbe F, Mundinger F: Ballism not related to vascular disease: a report of 16 patients and review of the literature. *Park Rel Disord* 1996;2:35–45.
20. Dewey RB Jr, Jankovic J: Hemiballism-hemichorea: clinical and pharmacologic findings in 21 patients. *Arch Neurol* 1989;46:862–867.
21. Costeff H, Groswasser Z, Goldstein R: Long-term follow-up review of 31 children with severe closed head trauma. *J Neurosurg* 1990;73:684–687.
22. Johnson SLJ, Hall DMB: Post-traumatic tremor in head injured children. *Arch Dis Child* 1992;67:227–228.
23. Kono M, Oka N, Horie T, Sanada T, Shimazaki K, Okimura Y, Nagai M, Yamaura A: Involuntary movements after severe head injury. *Proc. of the Xth International Congress of Neurological Surgery.* Acapulco, Mexico, October 17–22, p. 391, 1993 (Abstract).
24. Krauss JK, Traenkle R, Kopp KH: Posttraumatic movement disorders in survivors of severe head injury. *Neurology* 1996;47:1488–1492.

25. Szelozynska K, Znamirowski R: Zespól pozapiramidowy w pourazowych niedowl adach pol owiczych u dzieci [Extrapyramidal syndrome in post-traumatic hemiparesis in children]. *Neur Neurochir Pol* 1974;8:167–170.

26. Krauss JK, Traenkle R, Kopp KH: Movement disorders secondary to moderate and mild head injury. *Mov Disord* 1997;12:428–431.

27. Krack P, Deuschl G, Kaps M, Warnke P, Schneider S, Traupe H: Delayed onset of "rubral tremor" 23 years after brainstem trauma. *Mov Disord* 1994;9:240–242.

28. Boto GR, Lobato RD, Rivas JJ, Gomez PA, de la Lama A, Lagares A: Basal ganglia hematomas in severely head injured patients: clinicoradiological analysis of 37 cases. *J Neurosurg* 2001;94:224–232,

29. Kampfl A, Franz G, Aichner F, Pfausler B, Haring HP, Felber S, Luz G, Schocke M, Schmutzhard E: The persistent vegetative state after closed head injury: clinica and magnetic resonance imaging findings in 42 patients. *J Neurosurg* 1998;88:809–816.

30. Traenkle R, Krauss JK: Posttraumatische fokale Dystonie nach kontralateraler Thalamusläsion. *Nervenarzt* 1997;68:521–524.

31. Baker AJ, Moulton RJ, MacMillan VH, Shedden PM: Excitatory amino acids in cerebrospinal fluid following traumatic brain injury in humans. *J Neurosurg* 1993;79:369–372.

32. Bullock R, Zauner A, Woodward JJ, Myseros J, Choi SC, Ward JD, Marmarou A, Young HF: Factors affecting excitatory amino acid release following severe human head injury. *J Neurosurg* 1998;89:507–518.

33. Halliwell B: Oxidants and the central nervous system: some fundamental questions. Is oxidant damage relevant to Parkinson's disease, Alzheimer's disease, traumatic injury or stroke? *Acta Neurol Scand Suppl* 1989;126:23–33.

34. Muizelaar JP, Marmarou A, Young HF, Choi SC, Wolf A, Schneider RL, Kontos HA: Improving the outcome of severe head injury with the oxygen radical scavenger polyethylene glycol-conjugated superoxide dismutase: a phase II trial. *J Neurosurg* 1993;78:375–382.

35. Bullock MR, Lyeth BG, Muizelaar JP: Current status of neuroprotection trials for traumatic brain injury: lessons from animal models and clinical studies. *Neurosurgery* 1999;45:207–220.

36. Hodge CJ, Boakye M: Biological plasticity: the future of science in neurosurgery. *Neurosurgery* 2001;48:2–16.

37. Teasdale GM, Graham DI: Craniocerebral trauma: protection and retrieval of the neuronal population after injury. *Neurosurgery* 1998;43:723–738.

38. Teasdale GM, Nicoll JA, Murray G, Fiddes M: Association of apolipoprotein E polymorphism with outcome after head injury. *Lancet* 1997;350:1069–1071.

39. Boyeson MG, Jones JL, Harmon RL: Sparing of motor function after cortical injury. A new perspective on underlying mechanisms. *Arch Neurol* 1994;51:405–414.

40. Carr LJ, Harrison LM, Evans Al, Stephens JA: Patterns of central motor reorganization in hemiplegic cerebral palsy. *Brain* 1993;116:1223–1247.

41. Scott BL, Jankovic J: Delayed-onset progressive movement disorders after static brain lesions. *Neurology* 1996;46:68–74.

42. Kremer M, Russell WR, Smyth GE: A mid-brain syndrome following head injury. *J Neurol Neurosurg Psychiatry* 1947;10:49–60.

43. Samie MR, Selhorst JB, Koller WC: Post-traumatic midbrain tremors. *Neurology* 1990;40:62–66.

44. Obeso JA, Narbona J: Post-traumatic tremor and myoclonic jerking. *J Neurol Neurosurg Psychiatry* 46:788,1993.

45. Bullard DE, Nashold BS Jr: Stereotaxic thalamotomy for treatment of posttraumatic movement disorders. *J Neurosurg* 1984;61:316–321.

46. Friedman JH: "Rubral" tremor induced by a neuroleptic drug. *Mov Disord* 1991;7:281–282.

47. Masucci EF, Kurtzke JF, Saini N: Myorhythmia: a widespread movement disorder. clinicopathological correlations. *Brain* 1984;107:53–79.

48. Krauss JK, Mohadjer M, Nobbe F, Mundinger F: The treatment of posttraumatic tremor by stereotactic surgery. *J Neurosurg* 80:810–819, 1994.

49. Louis ED, Lynch T, Ford B, Greene P, Bressman SB, Fahn S: Delayed-onset cerebellar syndrome. *Arch Neurol* 1996;53:450–454.

50. Krauss JK, Wakhloo AK, Nobbe F, Tränkle R, Mundinger F, Seeger W: MR pathological correlations of severe posttraumatic tremor. *Neurol Res* 1995;17:409–416.

51. Seo SW, Heo JH, Lee KY, Shin WC, Chang DI, Kim SM, Heo K: Localization of Claude's syndrome. *Neurology* 2001;57:2304–2307.

52. Elble RJ: Animal models of action tremor. *Mov Disord* 1998; 13 (Suppl 3):35–39.

53. Newmark J, Richards TL: Delayed unilateral post-traumatic tremor: localization studies using single-proton computed tomographic and magnetic resonance spectroscopy techniques. *Mil Med* 1999;164:59–64.

54. Remy P, de Recondo A, Defer G, Loc'h C, Amarenco P, Plante-Bordeneuve V, Dao-Castellana MH, Bendriem B, Crouzel C, Clanet M, Rondot P, Samson Y: Peduncular 'rubral' tremor and dopaminergic denervation: a PET study. *Neurology* 1995;45:472–477.

55. Zijlmans J, Booij J, Valk J, Lees A, Horstink M. Posttraumatic tremor without parkinsonism in a patient with complete contralateral loss of the nigrostriatal pathway. *Mov Disord* 2002;7:1086–1088.

56. Burke RE, Fahn S, Gold AP: Delayed-onset dystonia in patients with "static" encephalopathy. *J Neurol Neurosurg Psychiatry* 1980;43:789–797.

57. Mauro AJ, Fahn S, Russman B: Hemidystonia following "minor" head trauma. *Trans Am Neurol Assoc* 1980;105:229–231.

58. Messimy R, Diebler C, Metzger J: Dystonie de torsion du membre superieur gauche probablement consecutive a un traumatisme cranien. *Rev Neurol* 1977;133:199–206.

59. Marsden CD, Obeso JA, Zarranz JJ, Lang AE: The anatomical basis of sympomatic hemidystonia. *Brain* 1985;108:463–483.

60. Pettigrew LC, Jankovic J: Hemidystonia: a report of 22 patients and a review of the literature. *J Neurol Neurosurg Psychiatry* 1985;48:650–657.

61. Jabbari B, Paul J, Scherokman B, Van Dam B: Posttraumatic segmental axial dystonia. *Mov Disord* 1992;7:78–81.

62. Lee MS, Lee SB, Kim WC: Spasmodic dysphonia associated with a left ventrolateral putaminal lesion. *Neurology* 1996;47:827–828.

63. Bressman SB, de Leon D, Raymond D, Greene PE, Brin MF, Fahn S, Ozelius LJ, Breakefield XO, Kramer PL, Risch NJ: Secondary dystonia and the DYT1 gene. *Neurology* 1997;48:1571–1577.

64. Austregesilo A, Marques A: Dystonies. *Rev Neurol* 1928;2:562–575.

65. Brett EM, Hoare RD, Sheehy MP, Marsden CD: Progressive hemidystonia due to focal basal ganglia lesion after mild head trauma. *J Neurol Neurosurg Psychiatry* 1981;44:460.

66. Silver JK, Lux WE: Early onset dystonia following traumatic brain injury. *Arch Phys Med Rehabil* 1994;75:885–888.

67. Chuang C, Fahn S, Frucht SJ. The natural history and treatment of acquired hemidystonia: report of 33 cases and review of the literature. *J Neurol Neurosurg Psychiatry* 2002;72:59–67.

68. King, RB, Fuller C, Collins GH: Delayed onset of hemidystonia and hemiballismus following head injury: a clinicopathological correlation. *J Neurosurg* 2001;94:309–314.

69. Münchau A, Mathen D, Cox T, Quinn NP, Marsden CD, Bhatia KP: Unilateral lesions of the globus pallidus: report of four patients presenting with focal or segmental dystonia. *J Neurol Neurosurg Psychiatry* 2000;69:494–498.

70. Maki Y, Akimoto H, Enomoto T: Injuries of basal ganglia following head trauma in children. *Child's Brain* 1980;7:113–123.

71. Andrew J, Fowler CJ, Harrison MJG, Kendall BE: Posttraumatic tremor due to vascular injury and its treatment by stereotactic thalamotomy. *J Neurol Neurosurg Psychiatry* 1982;45:560–562.

72. Krauss JK, Jankovic J: Hemidystonia secondary to carotid artery gunshot injury. *Child's Nerv Syst* 1997;13:285–288.

73. Hawker K, Lang AE: Hypoxic-ischemic damage of the basal ganglia. *Mov Disord* 1990;5:219–224.

74. Ceballos-Baumann AO, Passingham RE, Marsden CD, Brooks DJ: Motor reorganization in aquired hemidystonia. *Ann Neurol* 1995;37:746–757.

75. Sanghera M, Grossman RG, Kalhorn CG, Hamilton WJ, Ondo W, Jankovic J:Basal ganglia neuronal discharge in primary and secondary dystonia in patients undergoing pallidotomy. *Neurosurgery* 2003;52:1358–1373.

76. Levesque MF, Markham C, Nakasato N: MR-guided ventral intermediate thalamotomy for posttraumatic hemiballismus. Stereotact *Funct Neurosurg* 1992;58:88 (Abstract).

77. Naddeo M, Bioliho P, Zappi D: L'hemiballisme post-traumatique. *Neurochirurgie* 1983;29:285–287.

78. Bullard DE, Nashold BS: Posttraumatic movement disorders, in Lunsford LD (ed.): *Modern Stereotactic Neurosurgery*. Boston, Martinus Nijhoff, 1988, pp 341–352.

79. Kant R, Zeiler D: Hemiballismus following closed head injury. *Brain Inj* 1996;10:155–158.

80. Adler JR, Winston KR: Chorea as a manifestation of epidural hematoma. *J Neurosurg* 1984;60:856–857.

81. Kotagal S, Shutter E, Horenstein S: Chorea as a manifestation of bilateral subdural hematoma in an elderly man. *Arch Neurol* 38:195,1981.

82. Yoshikawa M, Yamamoto M, Shibata K, Ohta K, Kamite Y, Takahashi M, Shimizu Y, Ohba S, Kuwabara S, Uozumi T: Hemichorea associated with ipsilateral chronic subdural hematoma. *Neurol Med Chir* (Tokyo) 1992;32:769–772.

83. Biary N, Singh B, Bahou Y, Al Deeb M, Sharif H: Posttraumatic paroxysmal nocturnal hemidystonia. *Mov Disord* 1994;9:98–99.

84. Chandra V, Spunt AL, Rusinowitz MS: Treatment of post-traumatic choreoathetosis with sodium valproate. *J Neurol Neurosurg Psychiatry* 1983;46:963.

85. Demirkiran M, Jankovic J: Paroxysmal dyskinesias: clinical features and classification. *Ann Neurol* 1995;38:571–579.

86. Drake ME, Jackson RD, Miller CA: Paroxysmal choreoathetosis after head injury. *J Neurol Neurosurg Psychiatry* 1986;49: 837–838.

87. Perlmutter JS, Raichle ME: Pure hemidystonia with basal ganglion abnormalities on positron emission tomography. *Ann Neurol* 1984;15:228–233.

88. Richardson JC, Howes JL, Celinski MJ, Allman RG: Kinesigenic choreoathetosis due to brain injury. *Can J Neurol Sci* 1987;14: 626–628.

89. Robin JJ: Paroxysmal choreoathetosis following head unjury. *Ann Neurol* 1977;2:447–448.

90. Blakeley J, Jankovic J: Secondary paroxysmal dyskinesias. *Mov Disord* 2002;17:726–734.

91. Jankovic J, Kwak C: Tics in other neurological disorders, in Kurlan R (ed): *Handbook of Tourette's syndrome and related tic and behavioral disorders*. New York, Basel, Hong Kong, Marcel Dekker,2004, in press.

92. Fahn S: A case of post-traumatic tic syndrome, in Friedhoff AJ, Chase TN (eds): *Gilles de la Tourette Syndrome*. New York, Raven Press, 1982, pp 349–350.

93. Krauss JK, Jankovic J: Tics secondary to craniocerebral trauma. *Mov Disord* 1997;12:776–782.

94. Siemers E, Pascuzzi R: Posttraumatic tic disorder. *Mov Disord* 1990;5:183.

95. Singer S, Sanchez-Ramos J, Weiner WJ: A case of post-traumatic tic disorder. *Mov Disord* 1989;4:342–344.

96. Majumdar A, Appleton RE. Delayed and severe but transient Tourette syndrome after head injury. *Pediatr Neurol* 2002;27: 314–317.

97. Kwak C, Jankovic J: Tourettism and dystonia after subcortical stroke. *Mov Disord* 2002;17:821–825.

98. Deuschl G, Mischke G, Schenk E, Schulte-Mönting J, Lücking CH: Symptomatic and essential rhythmic palatal myoclonus. *Brain* 1990;113:1645–1672.

99. Hallett M, Chadwick D, Marsden CD: Cortical reflex myoclonus. *Neurology* 1979;29:1107–1125.

100. Keane JR: Galloping tongue: post-traumatic, episodic, rhythmic movements. *Neurology* 1984;34:251–252.

101. Obeso JA, Artieda J, Rothwell JC, Day B, Thompson P, Marsden CD: The treatment of severe action myoclonus. *Brain* 1989; 112:765–777.

102. Starosta-Rubinstein S, Bjork RJ, Snyder BD, Tulloch JW: Posttraumatic intention myoclonus. *Surg Neurol* 1983;20:131–132.

103. Stewart JT: Akathisia following traumatic brain injury: treatment with bromocriptine. *J Neurol Neurosurg Psychiatry* 1989;52: 1200–1201.

104. Troupin AS, Kamm RF: Lingual myoclonus. *Dis Nerv Sys* 1974; 35:378–380.

105. Turazzi S, Alexandre A, Bricolo A, Rizzuto N: Opsoclonus and palatal myoclonus during prolonged post-traumatic coma. *Eur Neurol* 1977;15:257–263.

106. Grimberg L: Paralysis agitans and trauma. *J Nerv Ment Dis* 1934;79:14–42.

107. Lindenberg R: Die Schädigungsmechanismen der Substantia nigra bei Hirntraumen und das Problem des posttraumatischen Parkinsonismus. *Dtsch Zeitschr Nervenheilk* 1964;185:637–663.

108. Doder M, Jahanshahi M, Turjanski N, Moseley IF, Lees AJ: Parkinson's syndrome after closed head injury: a single case report. *J Neurol Neurosurg Psychiatry* 1999;66:380–385.

109. Giroud M, Vincent MC, Thierry A, Binnert D, Marin A, Dumas R: Parkinsonian syndrome caused by traumatic hematomas in the basal ganglia. *Neurochirurgie* 1988;34:61–63.

110. Bhatt M, Desai J, Mankodi A, Elias M, Wadia N: Posttraumatic akinetic-rigid syndrome resembling Parkinson's disease: a report on three patients. *Movement Disorders* 2000;15:313–317.

111. Nayernouri T: Posttraumatic parkinsonism. *Surg Neurol* 1985;24:263–264.

112. Krauss JK, Traenkle R, Raabe A: Tremor and dystonia after penetrating diencephalic-mesencephalic trauma. *Park Rel Disord* 1997;3:117–119.

113. Morsier de G: Parkinsonisme consecutife a une lesion traumatique du nojau rouge et du locus niger. *Psychiat Neurol* 1960; 139:60–64.

114. Rondot P, Bathien N, De Recondo J, Gueguen B, Fredy D, De Recondo A, Samson Y: Dystonia-parkinsonism syndrome from a bullet injury in the midbrain. *J Neurol Neurosurg Psychiatry* 1994;57:658.

115. Wiest RG, Burgunder JM, Krauss JK: Chronic subdural hematomas and parkinsonian syndromes. *Acta Neurochir* 1999; 141:753–757.

116. Peppard RF, Byrne E, Nye D: Chronic subdural haematomas presenting with parkinsonian signs. *Clin Exp Neurol* 1986;22:19–23.

117. Turjanski N, Pentland B, Lees AJ, Brooks DJ: Parkinsonism associated with acute intracranial hematomas: an ^{18}F dopa positron-emission tomography study. *Mov Disord* 1997;12:1035–1038.

118. Friedman JH: Progressive parkinsonism in boxers. *South Med J* 1989;82:543–546.

119. Mawdsley C, Ferguson FR: Neurological disease in boxers. *Lancet* 1963;2:795–801.

120. Roberts AH. *Brain damage in boxers*. London: Pitman Medical Scientific Publishing,1969.

121. Roberts GW, Allsop D, Bruton C: The occult aftermath of boxing. *J Neurol Neurosurg Psychiatry* 1990;53:373–378.

122. Turjanski N, Lees AJ, Brooks DJ: Dopaminergic function in patients with posttraumatic parkinsonism: An ^{18}F-dopa PET study. *Neurology* 1997;49:183–189.

123. Bailes JE, Cantu RC: Head injury in athletes. *Neurosurgery* 2001; 48:26–46.

124. Corsellis JAN: Observations on the pathology of insidious dementia following head injury. *J Ment Sci* 1959;105:714–720.

125. Lampert PW, Hardman JM: Morphological changes in brains of boxers. *JAMA* 1984;251:2676–2679.

126. Davie CA, Pirtosek Z, Barker GJ, Kingsley DPE, Miller DH. Lees AJ: Magnetic resonance spectroscopic study of parkinsonism related to boxing. *J Neurol Neurosurg Psychiatry* 1995;58: 688–691.

127. Ryan AJ: Intracranial injuries resulting from boxing. *Clin Sports Med* 1998;17:155–168.

128. Butler RJ, Forsythe WI, Beverly DW, Adams LM: A prospective controlled investigation of the cognitive effects of amateur boxing. *J Neurol Neurosurg Psychiatry* 1993;56:1055–1061.

129. Haglund Y, Eriksson E: Does amateur boxing lead to chronic brain damage? A review of some recent investigations. *Am J Sports Med* 1993;21:97–109.

130. Jordan BD, Relkin NR, Ravdin LD, Jacobs AR, Bennett A, Gandy S: Apolipoprotein E epsilon4 associated with chronic traumatic brain injury in boxing. *JAMA* 1997;278:136–140.

131. Factor SA, Weiner WJ: Prior history of head trauma in Parkinson's disease. *Mov Disord* 1991;3:30–36.

132. Hubble JP, Cao T, Hassanein RE, Neuberger JS, Koller WC: Risk factors for Parkinson's disease. *Neurology* 1993;43:1693–1697.

133. Stern MB: Head trauma as a risk factor for Parkinson's disease. *Mov Disord* 1991;6:95–97.

134. Ward CD, Duvoisin RC, Ince SE, Nutt JD, Eldridge R, Calne DB: Parkinson's disease in 65 pairs of twins and in a set of quadraplets. *Neurology* 1983;33:815–824.

135. Goetz CG, Stebbins GT: Effects of head trauma from motor vehicle accidents on Parkinson's disease. *Ann Neurol* 1991;29:191–193.

136. Godwin-Austen RB, Lee P, Marmot MG, Stern GM: Smoking and Parkinson's disease. *J Neurol Neurosurg Psychiatry* 1982;45: 577–581.

137. Tanner CM, Chen B, Wang WZ, Peng ML, Liu ZL, Liang XL, Kao LC, Gilley DW, Schoenberg BS: Environmental factors in the etiology of Parkinson's disease. *Can J Neurol Sci* 1987; 14 (Suppl): 419–423.

138. Williams DB, Annegers JF, Kokmen E, O'Brien PC, Kurland LT: Brain injury and neurologic sequelae: a cohort study of dementia, parkinsonism, and amyotrophic lateral sclerosis. *Neurology* 1991;41:1554–1557.

139. Ellison PH: Propranolol for severe post-head injury action tremor. *Neurology* 1978;28:197–199.

140. Harmon RL, Long DF, Shirtz J: Treatment of post-traumatic midbrain resting-kinetic tremor with combined levodopa/carbidopa and carbamazepine. *Brain Inj* 1991;5:213–218.

141. Jacob PC, Chand RP: Posttraumatic rubral tremor responsive to clonazepam. *Mov Disord* 1998;13:977–978.

142. Jankovic J, Brin M: Therapeutic uses of botulinum toxin. *N Engl J Med* 1991;324:1186–1194.

143. Andrew J, Fowler CJ, Harrison MJG: Tremor after head injury and its treatment by stereotaxic surgery. *J Neurol Neurosurg Psychiatry* 1982;45:815–819.

144. Cooper IS: Neurosurgical alleviation of intention tremor of multiple sclerosis and cerebellar disease. *N Engl J Med* 1960;263: 441–444.

145. Eiras J, Cosamalon JG. Síndrome mioclónico posttraumático: Effectividad de las lesiones talámicas sobre las mioclonías de acción. *Arch Neurobiol* 1980;43:17–28.

146. Fox JL, Kurtzke JF. Trauma-induced intention tremor relieved by stereotaxic thalamotomy. *Arch Neurol* 1966;15:247–251.

147. Goldman MS, Kelly PJ. Symptomatic and functional outcome of stereotactic ventralis lateralis thalamotomy for intention tremor. *J Neurosurg* 1992;77:223–229.

148. Hirai T, Miyazaki M, Nakajima H, Shibazaki T, Ohye C. The correlation between tremor characterisics and the predicted volume of effective lesions in stereotaxic nucleus ventralis intermedius thalamotomy. *Brain* 1983;106:1001–1018.

149. Iwadate Y, Saeki N, Namba H, Odaki M, Oka N, Yamaura A. Post-traumatic intention tremor - clinical features and findings. *Neurosurg Rev* 1989;12 (Suppl 1):500–507.

150. Jankovic J, Cardoso F, Grossman RG, Hamilton WJ: Outcome after stereotactic thalamotomy for parkinsonian, essential, and other types of tremor. *Neurosurgery* 1995;37:680–687.

151. Kandel EI. Treatment of hemihyperkinesias by stereotactic operations on basal ganglia. *Appl Neurophysiol* 1982;45:225–229.

152. Marks PV: Stereotactic surgery for post-traumatic cerebellar syndrome: an analysis of seven cases. *Stereotact Funct Neurosurg* 1993;60:157–167.

153. Niizuma H, Kwak R, Ohyama H, Ikeda S, Ohtsuki T, Suzuki J, Saso S: Stereotactic thalamotomy for postapoplectic and post-traumatic involuntary movements. *Appl Neurophysiol* 1982;45: 295–298.

154. Ohye C, Hirai T, Miyazaki M, Shibazaki T, Nakajima H: VIM thalamotomy for the treatment of various kinds of tremor. *Appl Neurophysiol* 1982;45:275–280.

155. Richardson RR: Rehabilitative neurosurgery: posttraumatic syndromes. *Stereotact Funct Neurosurg* 1989;53:105–112.

156. Samra K, Waltz JM, Riklan M, Koslow M, Cooper IS: Relief of intention tremor by thalamic surgery. *J Neurol Neurosurg Psychiatry* 1970;33:7–15.

157. Shahzadi D, Tasker RR, Lozano A: Thalamotomy for essential and cerebellar tremor. *Stereotact Funct Neurosurg* 1995;65:11–17.

158. Spiegel EA, Wycis HT, Szekely EG, Adams J, Flanagan M, Baird HW: Campotomy in various extrapyramidal disorders. *J Neurosurg* 1963;20:871–884.

159. Taira T, Speelman JD, Bosch DA: Trajectory angle in stereotactic thalamotomy. *Stereotact Funct Neurosurg* 1993;61:24–31.

160. Van Manen J: Stereotaxic operations in cases of hereditary and intention tremor. *Acta Neurochirur Suppl* 1974;21:49–55.

161. Young RF, Jacques S, Mark R, Kopyov O, Copcutt B, Posewitz A, Li F: Gamma knife thalamotomy for treatment of tremor: long-term results. *J Neurosurg* 2000;93:128–135.

162. Andy OJ: Thalamic stimulation for control of movement disorders. *Appl Neurophysiol* 1983;46:107–111.

163. Benabid AL, Pollak P, Gao D, Hoffmann D, Limousin P, Gay E, Payen I, Benazzouz A: Chronic electrical stimulation of the ventralis intermedius nucleus of the thalamus as a treatment of movement disorders. *J Neurosurg* 1996;84:203–214.

164. Broggi G, Brock S, Franzini A, Geminiani G: A case of post-traumatic tremor treated by chronic stimulation of the thalamus. *Mov Disord* 1993;8:206–208.

165. Nguyen JP, Degos JD: Thalamic stimulation and proximal tremor. A specific target in the nucleus ventrointermedius thalami. *Arch Neurol* 1993;50:498–500.

166. Standhart H, Pinter MM, Volc D, Alesch F: Chronic eletrical stimulation of the nucleus ventralis intermedius of the thalamus for the treatment of tremor. *Mov Disord* 13, Suppl 3:141, 1998.

167. Vesper J, Funk T, Kern BC, Wagner F, Kestenbach U, Jahnke U, Straschill M, Brock M: Thalamic deep brain stimulation: present state of the art. *Neurosurgery Quarterly* 2000;10: 252–260.

168. Krauss JK, Simpson RK Jr, Ondo WG, Pohle T, Burgunder JM, Jankovic J: Concepts and methods in chronic thalamic stimulation for treatment of tremor: technique and application. *Neurosurgery* 2001;48:535–541.

169. Kitagawa M, Murata J, Kikuchi S, Sawamura Y, Saito H, Sasaki H, Tashiro K: Deep brain stimulation of subthalamic area for severe proximal tremor. *Neurology* 2000;55:114–116.

170. Biary N, Cleeves L, Findley L, Koller WC: Post-traumatic tremor. *Neurology* 1989;39:103–106.

171. Jankovic J, Schwartz K: Botulinum toxin treatment of tremors. *Neurology* 1991;41:1185–1188.

172. Dressler D, Schönle PW: Bilateral limb dystonia due to chronic subdural hematoma. *Eur Neurol* 1990;30:211–213.

173. Eaton JM: Hemidystonia due to subdural hematoma. *Neurology* 38:507,1988.

174. Nobbe FA, Krauss JK: Subdural hematoma as a cause of contralateral dystonia. *Clin Neurol Neurosurg* 1997;99:37–39.

175. Cardoso F, Jankovic J, Grossman RG, Hamilton WJ: Outcome after stereotactic thalamotomy for dystonia and hemiballismus. *Neurosurgery* 1995;36:501–507.

176. Ondo WG, Desaloms JM, Jankovic J, Grossman RG: Pallidotomy for generalized dystonia. *Mov Disord* 1998;13:693–698.

177. Ondo WG, Krauss JK: Surgical therapies for dystonia, in Brin MF, Comella C, Jankovic J (eds): *Dystonia Monograph.* Philadelphia, Lippincott, Williams and Wilkins, 2003 in press.

178. Alkhani A, Farooq K, Lang AE, Hutchison WD, Dostrovsky J: The response to pallidal surgery for dystonia is dependent on the etiology. *Neurosurgery* 47:504,2000.

179. Villemure JG, Vingerhoets F, Temperli P, Pollo C, Ghika J: Dystonia: pallidal or thalamic target? *Acta Neurochir* 142:1194, 2000.

180. Yoshor D, Hamilton WJ, Ondo W, Jankovic J, Grossman RG: Comparison of thalamotomy and pallidotomy for the treatment of dystonia. *Neurosurgery* 2001;48:818–826.

181. Teive H, Sa D, Grande CV, Fustes OJH, Antoniuk A, Werneck LC: Bilateral simultaneous globus pallidus internus pallidotomy for generalized posttraumatic dystonia. *Mov Disord* 13, Suppl 2:33 (Abstract),1998.

182. Sellal F, Hirsch E, Barth P, Blond S, Marescaux C: A case of symptomatic hemidystonia improved by ventroposterolateral thalamic electrostimulation. *Mov Disord* 1993;8:515–518.

183. Loher TJ, Hasdemir M, Burgunder JM, Krauss JK: Long-term follow-up of chronic globus pallidus internus stimulation for posttraumatic hemidystonia. *J Neurosurg* 2000;92:457–460.

184. Meythaler JM, Guin-Renfroe S, Grabb P, Hadley MN: Long-term continuously infused intrathecal baclofen for spastic-dystonic

hypertonia in traumatic brain injury: 1-year experience. *Arch Phys Med Rehabil* 1999;80:13–19.

185. Penn RD, Gianino JM, York MM: Intrathecal baclofen for motor disorders. *Mov Disord* 1995;10:675–677.

186. Hou JG, Ondo W, Jankovic J: Intrathecal baclofen for dystonia. *Mov Disord* 2001;16:1201–1202.

187. Krauss JK, Mundinger F: Functional stereotactic surgery for hemiballism. *J Neurosurg* 1996;85:278–286.

188. Loher TJ, Krauss JK, Burgunder JM, Taub E, Siegfried J: Chronic thalamic stimulation for treatment of dystonic paroxysmal nonkinesigenic dyskinesia. *Neurology* 2001;56:268–270.

189. Jankovic J: Therapeutic strategies in Parkinson's disease, in Jankovic J, Tolosa E (eds): *Parkinson's Disease and Movement Disorders*, 4th edition. Philadelphia, Lippincott, Williams and Wilkins, 2002, pp 116–151.

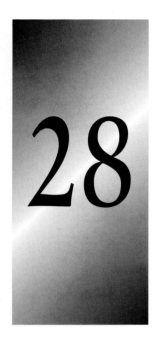

28 Balance and Dizziness

Neil T. Shepard
Richard A. Clendaniel
Michael Ruckenstein

INTRODUCTION AND OVERVIEW

While a large number of different etiologies can be the cause for complaints of dizziness (representing a wide variety of specific symptoms) and imbalance, traumatic brain injury (TBI) ranks among those of significant complexity and difficult to rehabilitate. Patients diagnosed with TBI often present with dizziness complaints in the midst of a wide variety of other symptoms, as is evidenced by the diversity of discussion in this text. Experience in treating this group of patients for imbalance and other dizziness complaints shows that the time course of recovery is significantly longer than patients with similar damage to the peripheral or central balance system, yet for reasons other than TBI. To date, as a group those with TBI diagnoses do poorer overall in treatment formats of Vestibular and Balance rehabilitation therapy than other groups with peripheral vestibular injuries, not of a head injury origin. The assumption used to explain these differences in time and level of recovery during group comparisons, is that there are co-morbidities of a central nervous system origin, not distinguished by traditional diagnostics that cause the interference with recovery. Additionally, there are known disorders that can develop secondary to a TBI that are known to limit and slow down recovery of balance and dizziness complaints such as post-traumatic stress syndrome and other psychiatric conditions, or development

of post-traumatic migraine or seizure disorders, all discussed elsewhere in this text.

The purpose of this chapter is to provide an introductory review of the potential sources of complaints of vertigo, lightheadedness and imbalance that can result from a traumatic brain injury. Additionally, the chapter will review the various direct treatment options for these resulting conditions, the principle one being that of Vestibular and Balance Rehabilitation Therapy (VBRT).

For reference it will be useful to start with a brief overview of the elements of the balance system and its normal functioning.

No single structure subserves balance function. Rather, the system consists of multiple sensory inputs from the vestibular end organs, the visual system, and the somatosensory/proprioceptive systems. The input information is then integrated at the level of the brain stem and cerebellum with significant influence from the cerebral cortex, including the frontal, parietal, and occipital lobes. The integrated input information results in various stereotypic responses for eye movement, postural control, and perception of movement and orientation in space. Only a brief overview of the major elements of the input and output structures and their basic physiological functioning will be provided here, other literature providing detailed descriptions is available (1–5).

When considering the function of the balance system, it is helpful to view it in light of the major functional purposes that the system attempts to accomplish. One can view these purposes as three distinct areas:

- Perceptions of orientation relative to gravity, the direction and speed of movement and when a change in the attitude of movement occurs.
- Maintenance of clear visual imaging of the seen world with the head in motion, target in motion or both in relative motion.
- Ability to maintain static and dynamic upright stance, and to perform volitional movements ranging from routine ambulation to complicated sequences involved in sports, dance etc. There are two areas that sub serve this last purpose (6):
  - Balance-correction responses allowing for automatic responses to unexpected perturbations of the body's center of gravity.
  - Balance-stabilizing responses allow for the volitional control of the movement of the center of gravity of the body.

Ocular Motor Control and Perceptions of Motion

The membranous labyrinth is housed within the bony labyrinth in the petrous portion of the temporal bone, where it is secured by connective tissue and is bathed in perilymph. Endolymph is contained within the membranous structure, where the specialized sensory neuroepithelium is located. The vestibular apparatus consists of two groups of specialized sensory receptors: (a) the three semicircular canals—lateral (or horizontal), posterior, and superior, and (b) the two otolithic organs—the utricular macula and the saccular macula, both located in the vestibule. The canals and otolith organs are organized into functional pairs. The two members of each pair are in parallel planes of orientation and function in a 'push / pull' manner. Therefore, if one member of the pair is stimulated by a head movement, the other member is inhibited in its neural activity. The function of the semi-circular canals is to be responsive to angular acceleration and deceleration of the head. The otolith organs are responsive to linear acceleration and deceleration, which includes the force of gravity.

Contiguous with the vestibular portion of the membranous labyrinth is that of the auditory structure, the cochlea. Also housed with in the petrous portion of the temporal bone the cochlea shares the same perilymph and endolymph fluids with the vestibular end-organ. It is these structures, the vestibular and auditory portions of the labyrinth, their innervating neural elements (VIIIth cranial nerve, auditory and vestibular divisions) and the motor and sensory nerves for facial expression and taste (VIIth cranial nerve that traverses through this portion of the temporal bone) which are in harms way from temporal bone fractures following head injuries.

Acceleration or deceleration movement of the head, producing stimulation of one or more of the receptors on one side with corresponding reduction of neural stimulation (inhibition) on the other side, results in asymmetrical neural input from the vestibular nerves. This asymmetrical input is interpreted by the central nervous system as either angular or linear movement. In addition, the asymmetry resulting from action of the semicircular canals causes a compensatory reflexive eye movement in the plane of the canals being stimulated. This compensatory reflex movement of the eye is called the vestibulo-ocular reflex (VOR), and is opposite to the direction of acceleration. It is the VOR from the semi-circular canals or the otolith organs that is the basis for the primary function of the vestibular end-organ, stabilization of the visual scene while the head is in motion (1, 2, 5). While there is top down control of the peripheral vestibular and auditory systems, this is especially true for the vestibular mechanism. This control is dominated in the brain stem and cerebellum, but cerebral influence can be easily demonstrated (1, 2).

Postural and Motor System Control

The cerebral cortex influences lower motor centers via projections through two pathways. The first are long fibers of the corticospinal tract (the pyramidal system), which plays a major role in the control of fine, isolated, versatile movements that set the basis for skill acquisition. The second pathway for cerebral cortex projections is the extra-pyramidal system. These extra-pyramidal pathways provide the mechanisms for large gross movement patterns that are primarily reflexive and constitute major postural adjustments. The pyramidal and extra-pyramidal systems are not independent but must function in a coordinated fashion. The skilled movements of the pyramidal system that are non-postural in nature typically require that a coordinated postural adjustment accompany the smooth skilled movement such as picking up an object from directly in front of the subject while standing. This requires a shift in the overall position of the center of gravity just prior to the arm reach and the grasping of the object by the hand.

Three tracts originate from, or are heavily contributed to via, the vestibular nuclei: the medial and lateral vestibulospinal tracts, and the reticulospinal tract. Given the projections from the medial vestibular nucleus to both the ascending and descending portions of the medial longitudinal fasiculus (MLF) in the medial vestibulospinal tract, this tract may play a major role in the cervical-vestibulo-ocular reflexes, coordinating eye-head movements. Similarly, by examining the inputs to the various areas in the vestibular nucleus and the pathways from those areas to the lateral vestibulospinal and reticulospinal tracts, it is suggested that these have greater influence on the coordination of head and upper body movement with the lower limbs. It is clear that both the central and peripheral structures participate in the tasks of postural control and ambulation. The organization of this cooperative effort, and its normal functioning during routine daily activities is beyond the scope of this chapter, but available from other sources (7–9).

Central Vestibular Compensation Process

The vestibular system is the only special sensory system in which unilateral loss of function can seriously threaten the long-term survival or well-being of an organism. In humans, injury to the central or peripheral system may result in considerable disability. Fortunately, most disease processes involving the vestibular labyrinth are self-limited, and spontaneous functional recovery can be expected. This is due to the remarkable ability of the central nervous system to recover after a labyrinthine injury, a process known as vestibular compensation. Failure to recover from a peripheral labyrinthine insult may be due to ongoing fluctuating condition in the vestibular end-organ itself or to failure of central vestibular compensation. Being alert to this critical distinction and its clinical implications is crucial for successful management of the dizzy patient (10, 11). The underlying foundations for this process will be discussed in detail in the second half of the chapter.

SOURCES OF BALANCE AND DIZZINESS COMPLAINTS AFTER A TBI EVENT

Combinations of specific disorders resulting from a head injury can occur, but for the purposes of this discussion the most common entities will be considered individually. For all of the disorders of the peripheral or central systems, the temporal course of the symptoms (length of spells or events if symptoms are not continuous), and the nature of the symptom onset being spontaneous or provoked by head or visual motion and whether hearing loss is involved with the symptoms are the key features of the history. The history, as with other patients complaining of dizziness or imbalance, is the single most important evaluation tool for the investigation of the cause of the complaints. For each of the encapsulated description disorders below these features will be reported.

Disorders of Peripheral Vestibular Origin

Post-traumatic injury to the peripheral vestibular system can occur in isolation or in association with a hearing loss. In cases where clear indications for peripheral vestibular involvement is lacking, but suspected, the presence of a documented post injury hearing loss adds significantly to the argument for peripheral dysfunction.

Benign Paroxysmal Positional Vertigo This is considered one of the most common causes for complaints of dizziness (vertigo) and imbalance, and the most common source for dizziness post head trauma. It is characterized by brief spells (typically <1 minute) of vertigo, falling or lightheadedness provoked by a movement of the head. In the most common form of this disorder, the provocative movements are in the saggital plane. The provoked symptoms are very frequently accompanied by complaints of general imbalance during daily routines. The character of the disorder is to have it resolve spontaneously and then recur. The length of time for symptoms can vary from as short as a single day to greater than 1 year. Resolution length has equally as large a variance. This is a disorder of the inner ear where the semi-circular canals, which are not sensitive to the pull of gravity, have an altered mechanics that make them sensitive to gravity. This occurs secondary to suspected displacement of crystal structures from the otoliths into the semi-circular canal system. Hearing loss is not a typical feature associated with this disorder, but certainly could occur given head trauma as the precipitating source. Treatments are highly successful and typically consist of head maneuvers referred to as 'canalith repositioning procedures' during which the crystal structures are repositioned out of the involved canal (see below) (12–17).

Labyrinthine Concussion This disorder is characterized by hearing loss and vertigo both of sudden onset following a head trauma. The symptoms typically improve over days and in many cases some recovery of hearing may occur. Usually the symptoms of continuous vertigo resolve into being present only when provoked by head movements in any direction. It is thought that the violent movement of the fluids and tissues with in the inner ear can cause tearing of tissues and / or set up a series of events where metabolically the cells undergo deterioration and death. This condition occurs in the absence of a documented fracture of the temporal bone (18). Secondary to the typical long-term symptoms of head movement provoked brief spells (seconds to minutes <5) these patients are good candidates for management with vestibular and balance rehabilitation therapy. Suppressive medication is many times needed at the initiation of this condition to control the sudden onset of vertigo and associated neurovegetative symptoms (19, 20).

A long term consequence of damage to the vestibular labyrinth, independent of the etiology, is the development of spontaneous spells of vertigo lasting minutes to hours. In some cases these can be associated with fluctuant or progressive hearing loss in a format classic for Meniere's disease. However, this is considered a secondary Meniere's resulting from the previous trauma. When it takes the form of only the spells of vertigo without associated auditory symptoms the older term is that of post-traumatic endolymphatic hydrops. If the symptoms involve only the spontaneous events, vestibular and balance rehabilitation therapy is typically not applicable and the treatment options are the same as those used in cases of Meniere's of idiopathic origin (21).

Temporal Bone Fractures   Both blunt and penetrating trauma to the temporal bone can lead to damage to the ear or VIIIth nerve complex. These injuries may result in a conductive hearing loss secondary to trauma to the external and/or middle ears, or a sensorineural hearing loss secondary to labyrinthine or VIIIth nerve trauma. Vertigo and subsequent imbalance may occur as an isolated symptom, or may be associated with a sensorineural hearing loss.

Approximately 75% of head injuries occur in motor vehicle accidents, with approximately 20% of these patients displaying some symptoms related to temporal bone trauma (22, 23). Thus, motor vehicle accidents are the most common cause of blunt trauma to the temporal bone (45%) with falls (20%), altercations (10%), and athletic injuries (10%) accounting for the majority of the remaining injuries.

Penetrating trauma is a less common cause of temporal bone injury, with etiologic agents for this form of injury ranging from bullets and knives to pencils and cotton swabs.

Temporal bone fractures elicited by blunt trauma have classically been defined by the relationship of the axis of the fracture line to the long axis of the temporal bone. Thus, longitudinal fractures, course along the external auditory canal, through the tegmen of the middle ear, and then pass anterior to the labyrinth to terminate in one of the foramina (lacerum or spinosum).

Transverse fractures run perpendicular to the long axis of the temporal bone, traversing the petrous bone between the foramen magnum and the foramen spinosum or lacerum, typically disrupting either the bony labyrinth or internal auditory canal. More recent data indicate that most temporal bone fractures possess properties of both longitudinal and transverse fractures, and are thus classified as mixed or oblique fractures. Projectiles may involve any or all components of the temporal bone, depending on their trajectory. More benign penetrating objects (e.g. pencils, cotton swabs), may elicit neurovestibular symptoms by disrupting the interface between the stapes and the labyrinth, creating a perilymph fistula (see below).

Trauma to the external canal manifests with bloody otorrhea and severe pain. A traumatic tympanic membrane perforation will have a similar presentation, with hearing loss always being present. Disruption of the ossicular chain most commonly involves the incus and results in a persistent conductive hearing loss. Disruption of the stapes may result in a conductive, mixed, or profound hearing loss (see perilymphatic fistula below).

The hallmark of a labyrinthine injury secondary to blunt or penetrating trauma is the presence of vertigo and hearing loss. In cases of severe head injury, in which the patient has been comatose for a period of time, the symptom of vertigo may be supplanted by the complaint of imbalance. Fractures that approximate a longitudinal course do not cause a direct disruption of the inner ear or VIIIth nerve. However, patients may suffer both sensorineural hearing loss and vertigo secondary to what has been referred to as *a labyrinthine concussion* (see above). In this situation, the vertigo is typically acute and self-limited, and the hearing loss is, at least partially, reversible. In contrast, fractures that traverse the otic capsule or internal auditory canal will cause profound hearing loss and vertigo.

Signs on physical examination indicative of inner ear trauma include tuning fork tests that lateralize to the unaffected ear and spontaneous nystagmus consistent with either an irritative (toward the affected ear) or paretic (away from the affected ear) lesion.

Audiometric assessment will define the nature of the hearing loss (conductive, sensorineural, mixed) and vestibular testing will document a vestibular injury. High resolution CT scan of the temporal bone is indicated to define the nature of the fracture and the structures involved.

External canal trauma should not be manipulated at initial presentation, as a traumatic dural or brain exposure may be present. Once CT scan has ruled-out these complications, the ear should be gently microdebrided and attempt made to reposition any avulsed pieces of skin. A post-traumatic ear canal stenosis may occur which will require surgical repair, both to improve hearing and prevent cholesteatoma formation secondary to the presence of squamous epithelium trapped medial to the stenosis. Tympanic membrane perforations should be managed conservatively as the rate of spontaneous healing is close to 100%. Disruption of the incus will require an ossiculoplasty once the primary healing process is completed (6 weeks to 3 months).

Other than for a perilymph fistula (see below), no specific treatment exits for blunt or penetrating inner ear trauma. Vestibular suppressants can be used for acute vertigo control, if not otherwise contraindicated by the patient's overall medical status. Hearing aid amplification may be useful in patients with partial sensorineural hearing loss, and vestibular rehabilitation therapy is indicated in those patients with a slow recovery from their vestibular loss.

The majority of patients sustaining temporal bone injuries develop little or no inner ear dysfunction. Patients who do sustain a noncompensated vestibular loss generally respond well to vestibular rehabilitation therapy. Benign paroxysmal positional vertigo (BPPV) is a common sequela of head injury and is in fact, the most common form of post-traumatic vertigo. Any patient complaining of

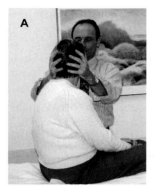 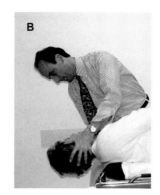

FIGURE 28-1

The left Dix-Hallpike Test. (A) The patient sits with legs extended on the table and cervical spine rotated 45 degrees to the left. The examiner places his hands on either side of the patient's head, with his right fore-arm behind the patient's left shoulder. (B) The patient is quickly brought into supine and the cervical spine extended approximately 10 degrees. The examiner observes the patient for nystagmus and symptoms

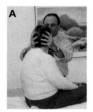 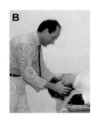 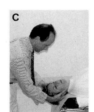

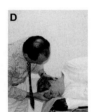 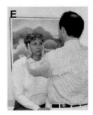

FIGURE 28-2

The Canalith Repositioning Maneuver for left-sided BPPV. (A) The starting position is identical to the initial position in the Dix-Hallpike test, with the cervical spine rotated 45 degrees to the left. (B) The patient is brought into supine and the cervical spine is extended approximately 10 degrees (45 degrees of left cervical rotation is maintained). (C) The cervical spine is rotated 90 degrees to the right to end up in 45 degrees rotation to the right. (D) The patient is rotated onto their right side, maintaining the cervical rotation to the right. The cervical spine is brought out of extension, and is laterally flexed to the right. (E) The patient is brought into sitting. As the patients rises from right side lying to sitting, the cervical rotation to the right is maintained

vertigo after a head trauma should have a Dix–Hallpike maneuver performed in the office (see Figure 28-1). If the diagnosis of BPPV is confirmed, then an canalith repositioning maneuver (see Figure 28-2) should be performed.

This therapeutic maneuver is highly efficacious and greatly appreciated by the patient.

Perilymphatic Fistula A Perilymph Fistula (PLF) occurs when the boundary between the middle and inner ear has been violated, allowing egress of perilymph and inner ear dysfunction. The topic of PLF remains controversial, particularly with respect to the spontaneous variety.

Perilymph fistulae are proposed to occur via three possible mechanisms. Congenital inner ear anomalies involving the otic capsule may result in dehiscences in the labyrinth that allow communication between the middle ear and the labyrinthine fluids. These are typically children who present with severe to profound hearing loss and recurrent meningitis or CSF leak (24).

More relevant to this discussion is the development of a PLF due to disruption of the oval (or less commonly, round) window secondary to external trauma. This trauma may be iatrogenic (e.g. post-stapes surgery) or secondary to blunt or penetrating trauma. Barotrauma and acoustic trauma have been proposed to create fistula via the transmission of rapid pressure changes to the round and oval windows (so called "implosive trauma") (25). However, as indicated above, these forms of trauma rarely result in a frank PLF.

Most of the controversy pertaining to PLF surrounds the spontaneous variety. This is proposed to occur through leaks through congenital dehiscences in the otic capsule, typically occurring in the regions of the oval and/or round windows. The leak through these dehiscences was thought to be precipitated by an increase in intracranial pressure being transmitted to the inner ear ("explosive trauma") (25). The validity of the concept of a spontaneous perilymph fistula has been critically scrutinized by otologists over the past two decades with a consensus emerging amongst most authorities that spontaneous fistulae rarely, if ever, occur (26–28).

A wide gamut of symptomatology has been ascribed to the PLF. Currently, most otologists would consider the diagnosis of a fistula when a patient presents with a sudden sensorineural hearing loss associated with tinnitus and vertigo, occurring immediately subsequent to a traumatic insult. Fluctuations in hearing may support the diagnosis if they appear provoked by pressure fluctuations or straining.

Despite intense effort no valid and accurate diagnostic test for PLF exists. A fistula test, in which a pressure change is applied to the inner ear via a pneumatic otoscope or tympanometer, may be considered positive if it evokes symptoms and nystagmus. However, this test is nonspecific and may also be positive in Meniere's disease and otosyphilis. Audiovestibular testing, including electrocochleography, do not reveal any pathognomonic findings. Detection of fluorocein in the middle ear subsequent to intravenous or intrathecal injection has not proven to be clinically useful. Similarly, the detection of beta2 transferrin in the middle ear has not proven to be an accurate method of identifying a PLF (29).

Most authorities agree that the only manner in which the presence of a PLF can be confirmed is by direct observation of the leakage (30). Based on recent results, it would appear that the most accurate way of performing this exploration is by using endoscopes passed through a myringotomy incision (31, 32). This technique appears to avoid false positive results that occur secondary to pooling of fluid, such as anesthetic injection, during the raising of tympanomeatal flap.

Bed rest, head elevation, and avoidance of straining are the initial treatments employed when a PLF is suspected. If symptoms of fluctuations of hearing and/or vertigo persist for 2–3 days while on this treatment regimen, a middle ear exploration and patching of the fistula site (oval and/or round window) should be considered.

In one study, 68% of patients with identifiable fistulae at the time of exploration improved after patching of the fistula (30). The majority of these patients had undergone previous stapes surgery. In patients who sustain a frank stapes subluxation subsequent to an external trauma, the prognosis is more guarded for recovery of auditory function.

Central Nervous System Causes for Balance and Dizziness

There are multiple sources of injury and secondary disorders to head trauma that can originate in the central nervous system and manifest in symptoms of balance and dizziness. Both post-traumatic seizures and post-traumatic stress syndrome / anxiety disorders can be direct causes for complaints of symptoms ranging from vertigo to vague lightheadedness and imbalance. Mechanisms, investigation and treatment for these entities are considered elsewhere in this text and will not be repeated herein. It is important to realize that there can be dramatic effects of psychological disorders that develop with long term disorders and are expressed in the complaints of dizziness (33–35).

Direct trauma to the brain stem and / or cerebellum will result in complaints of imbalance with standing and walking and occasional complaints of true vertigo. The pathophysiology of injuries of this nature is addressed in another chapter in this text. The nature of the signs and symptoms will vary depending on the location of the lesion with in the central nervous system (36). Lesions within the brain stem and cerebellum have typical ocular motor abnormalities that can be recognized during the office or laboratory examinations of these patients (see discussion below). Given that these are typically stationary lesions vestibular and balance rehabilitation therapy will comprise a major portion of the treatment plan.

These are usually not spontaneous events of symptoms but are more likely to be continuous sensations of disorientation, and imbalance with gait (37).

Post-traumatic migraine headaches, as with nontraumatic migraines, can have dizziness as an aura for the migraine event. This can occur with or without the pain phase of the migraine event. When the events of dizziness are not temporally related to actual headaches this entity can be quite difficult to diagnosis as it has to be a diagnosis of exclusion. Symptoms from migraine associated dizziness can be spontaneous spells of true vertigo to vague complaints of increased sensitivity to motion sickness and anything in between. Recognition of this is typically accomplished by having a history that the head aches being experienced meet the criteria for migraine, or pre-trauma the patient had a migraine history. Once diagnosed these are treated by direct treatment of the head aches (38, 39). In some cases the patient can be assisted with the use of vestibular and balance therapy as long as there is simultaneous focused treatment on the underlying migraine disorder.

In addition to the above descriptions of the direct effects of the central nervous system lesions producing symptoms of dizziness and imbalance, all of the above can have an indirect effect as well. In patients with combined peripheral and central lesions, the presence of the central lesion in the brain stem and / or cerebellum may not be causing direct symptoms of dizziness or imbalance but could cause disruptions in the natural central system compensation process. This would have the effect of slowing or preventing the compensation process from reducing the symptoms from the peripheral vestibular insult. This disruption in the compensation process can also occur from psychological difficulties, migraines or seizure disorders. In these instances direct treatment for the other disorders would be necessary in order to allow for as full a compensation process as possible.

OVERVIEW OF ASSESSMENT TOOLS AND THEIR USE IN DIAGNOSIS AND TREATMENT

Even though a head injury with TBI may be the precipitating event that results in complaints of imbalance and dizziness, one must proceed in the evaluation of those complaints in a systematic manner to uncover the source of the symptoms. Therefore, the evaluation is not different from what would be performed for a patient presenting without a known antecedent event. In considering the evaluation of the patient with complaints of vertigo, lightheadedness, imbalance or combinations of these descriptors, one must look beyond just the peripheral and central vestibular system with its ocular motor connections. The various pathways involved in postural control, only part of which have direct or indirect vestibular input should be kept in mind during an evaluation. The event that produced the head injury could easily have caused injury to any of these postural control pathways independent of the resultant TBI. Additionally, significant variations in symptoms and test findings can be generated by migraine disorders (37, 38) and / or anxiety disorders (33–35), yet these are diagnosed primarily by history requiring a specific line of questioning.

The evaluation of the dizzy patient should proceed being guided by what information is needed to make initial and subsequent management decisions. When various tests are reviewed, and correlated with high level activities of daily living, virtually no significant relationships exist for the chronic dizzy patient. Tests considered extent and site-of-lesion studies, Electronystagmography (ENG), Rotational chair and specific protocols in postural control assessment (5, 40), give results that are unable to be used to predict symptom type, magnitude or the level of disability of an individual patient. Conversely, patient complaints can not be used to predict the outcomes of these tests (41–44). In a limited manner more functionally oriented evaluation tools, computerized dynamic posturography (CDP), dynamic visual acuity testing (45) provide for some correlation between results, patient symptoms and functional limitations. Add to the testing specific or general health inventories like the Dizziness Handicap Inventory (41) and predictive assessment of disability is improved but remains significantly limited. It is hypothesized that the reason for this dichotomy in test results versus functional disability and symptom complaints is the inability of the tests to adequately characterize the status of the central vestibular compensation process (5, 46). It is the exception, not the rule that vestibular and balance laboratory tests return results that would drive management of the dizzy patient. It would be extremely rare that these studies return a diagnosis. Therefore, the routine use of these tools to determine how to proceed with the management of a dizzy patient is a false line of reasoning and not productive in the majority of the patients. In general the laboratory studies are productive in determination of extent and site-of-lesion within the peripheral and central vestibular system and the functional limitations in static and dynamic postural control (44). The use of this information is in the confirmation of the suspected site-of-lesion and diagnosis derived from patient history and direct physical office vestibular evaluation.

To summarize the above discussion, the following are required elements to management decisions for the chronic dizzy patient; detailed neurotologic history, office vestibular and physical examination, and formal audiometric testing given the inescapable anatomical relationship between the auditory and vestibular peripheral systems. The following are considered important, however less likely to directly drive the management in the typical case; laboratory vestibular and balance-function studies, neuroradiographic evaluations and serological tests. It is important to realize that there will be patients for whom unexpected findings on any one of these latter studies will either alter the complete course of the management or add dimensions to the management not originally considered. But for the majority of patients the vestibular and balance tests will be confirmatory in nature.

The following discussion will be a very brief overview of the major elements available for assessment. A recent comprehensive summary of the evaluation of the dizzy patient and detailed descriptions are found elsewhere for the interested reader (5, 9, 40, 44, 47).

Neurotologic History

Given the various tools for assessment, the history is the single most important factor in determining the course of management, and therefore requires discussion. The differentiation between the various peripheral vestibular disorders, that can result from a head injury, is particularly dependent upon historical information and the conclusions that the physician draws from the interview. Most vestibular disorders cannot be distinguished from one another simply by vestibular testing or other diagnostic interventions. Failure to properly discriminate these disorders on historical grounds may lead to improper management by the physician. In addition, balance function study results are best interpreted in light of a proper clinical history.

It is very important to question the patient regarding the association of a hearing loss or other auditory symptoms with the onset of vertigo. A complete audiometric assessment should be performed early in the evaluation. The presence of an associated sensorineural hearing loss, whether stable, progressive, or fluctuating, is the single strongest incriminating factor in identifying a pathologic labyrinth. The presence of other otologic symptoms such as aural fullness and tinnitus may also be helpful in lateralization. The features in the history will be the primary determiners of the initial choice for treatment (see Management Options sections below).

Office Examination

A variety of test procedures may be used in the office setting to assess the balance-disorder patient. These, like the laboratory studies, assist in the identification of the extent and site of the lesion. These straight-forward clinical tests are essentially variations of the related laboratory studies, but have less ability to quantify the outcomes. The theoretical basis behind many of these tests is well founded in the physiological considerations discussed above and in the references provided. Due to the subjective nature of these tools, the validity and reliability of these tests are reduced compared to the formal laboratory studies.

It is important that the person evaluating the dizzy patient be aware that simple tools do exist which provide for an effective evaluation. In the majority of patients this evaluation produces the same impressions as the extensive laboratory studies discussed below. These tools are, however, not as sensitive to mild anomalies as the laboratory studies. A recent summary of these techniques is available in the literature (9).

Laboratory Studies

Electronystamography (ENG)   Traditional ENG, using electrodes placed around the eyes or infrared video techniques for eye movement recordings, is a process that estimates the position of the eye as a function of time. Since the primary purpose of the vestibular apparatus is to control eye movements, the movements of the eyes may be used to examine the activity of the peripheral vestibular end organs and their central vestibulo-ocular pathways. The ENG evaluation is a series of sub-tests performed to assess portions of the peripheral and central vestibular systems. It is important to understand that peripheral vestibular system assessment with ENG is significantly limited, typically reflecting function of the horizontal semicircular canal with restricted information from vertical canals and otolith organs. With the use of computerized ENG systems, which afford significant visual stimulus control and quantitative analysis, evaluation of the central vestibulo-ocular pathways can be quite thorough.

Rotary Chair   Rotary chair testing has been used to expand the evaluation of the peripheral vestibular system. As with the ENG findings, the rotational chair evaluation can assist in site-of-lesion determination, counseling the patient and confirmation of clinical suspicion of diagnosis and lesion site, but is not likely to significantly alter or impact on the course of patient management, excepting the bilateral peripheral weakness patient.

As with the ENG, electrode or video techniques are used to monitor and record the outcome measure of interest, jerk nystagmus, that is generated in response to the angular acceleration stimulus produce by the circular movements of the chair.

Postural Control Assessment   Just as all patients that are being evaluated in the laboratory need tests for peripheral and central vestibulo-ocular pathway involvement, they also require some assessment of postural control ability. There are several different general approaches to formal postural control testing, each with specific technical equipment requirements and goals for the testing (5, 48). Briefly, the most common equipment detects vertical and horizontal forces from the feet by two independent force plates upon which the subject stands. Three principle testing protocols are used in patient evaluation, the Sensory Organization Test (SOT), the Motor Control Test (MCT) and Postural Evoked Responses (PER). These allow for assessment ranging from strictly functional (not site-of-lesion) with the SOT to site and limited pathology specific results with PER. Because of the functional assessment using SOT, postural control assessment is useful in the development and monitoring of vestibular and balance rehabilitation management option discussed below.

OVERVIEW OF TREATMENT OPTIONS

The options for management of the dizzy and balance-disordered patient fall into the major categories of medication, surgery, dietary changes and vestibular and balance rehabilitation therapy (VBRT), or combinations of these techniques (5). In general it will be the rare patient with dizziness secondary to head injury that is going to be managed with medication alone. The most common use of medications in this arena would be short term or 'as needed' use of vestibular suppressant medications for acute symptom control at the onset or with recurrent spontaneous events of vertigo lasting hours. Other than migraine and psychological disorders there is little call for use of chronic medication. Of the medications most commonly used for vestibular suppression the primary classes are those of antihistamines (Meclizine & Promethazine), anticholinergics (Scopolamine), phenothiazine (Prochlorperazine) and benzodiazepines (Diazepam, Lorazepam & Clonazepam). There are other classes and other specific medications within these listed drug classes that have been used for the control of acute vertigo and the vegetative symptoms that accompany the sensation of vertigo. It is important to remember that use of these medications should be on a short term basis and only 'as needed' when possible. These classes of medications have an effect that can significantly slow the natural compensation process and the effectiveness of VBRT (17).

Surgical intervention for this group of patients is used even less frequent than medication. The patients for whom surgery may be considered are those discussed above associated with temporal-bone injuries and perilymphatic fistulas. The treatment option that would be the most common is VBRT. This option will be discussed in detail below.

The major feature that drives an initial decision as to the use of medication / surgery versus VBRT is the evidence that the peripheral or central vestibular lesion is unstable (varying over time), as opposed to an uncompensated stable lesion. This distinction comes dominantly from the patient's presenting symptoms. Therefore, the patient should be asked to describe the progression of symptoms over time, along with the nature and duration of typical spells. Specifically, one wishes to know if the symptoms are continuous or occur in discrete episodes. If the symptoms are episodic, it is extremely important to distinguish whether they are spontaneous or motion-provoked. If the symptoms are brief and predictably produced by head movements or body position changes, the patient most likely has a stable lesion, but has not yet completed central nervous system compensation. Those who describe these symptoms sometimes also note a chronic underlying sense of disequilibrium or lightheadedness. The chronic symptoms may be quite troublesome, but any intense vertigo should be primarily motion-provoked. These patients are suitable candidates for vestibular rehabilitation. It is important to point out that historical information is essential in deciding who might benefit from rehabilitation therapy.

If the episodic spells described by the patient are longer periods of intense vertigo that occur spontaneously and without warning, this is probably a progressive or unstable peripheral dysfunction. One must also suspect a progressive lesion if the vertigo is accompanied by fluctuating or progressive sensorineural hearing loss. Such patients are managed with medical therapy, and if this fails, they constitute the best candidates for surgical intervention. Such patients are not candidates for vestibular rehabilitation, except as an adjunctive modality. For the chronic patient, including those with known head trauma event, the primary effort is to determine why they have not had the natural central compensation process run to completion.

When dealing with the TBI patient group, VBRT is many times used as one component of a comprehensive traumatic brain injury rehabilitation program involving physical, occupational, speech and cognitive therapy aspects.

VESTIBULAR AND BALANCE REHABILITATION THERAPY PROGRAMS

As indicated above, VBRT is the most frequently used management option for patients with balance and dizziness complaints from head injury, or other causes. Therefore, the remainder of this chapter will be a detailed discussion of this technique.

Since traumatic brain injury can lead to damage of the vestibular system from peripheral to central structures, as well as cause other CNS damage, the types of exercises used to treat the dizziness and imbalance can be quite comprehensive. The aims of the following sections of this chapter are to 1) review the rational behind vestibular and balance rehabilitation therapy (VBRT), 2) identify the types of problems that can be treated with VBRT, 3) describe the various types of exercises used in VBRT, 4) discuss modifications of treatment programs for individuals with traumatic brain injury, and 5) describe the outcomes to date.

The use of exercise for the treatment of individuals with vestibular dysfunction is not new. In the 1940's Sir Terrence Cawthorne, an otolaryngologist, and F. S. Cooksey, a physiotherapist, devised a series of exercises for the treatment of individuals with unilateral vestibular paresis and post-concussion syndrome (49–51). Cawthorne and Cooksey realized that head movements often provoked an individual's symptoms of dizziness. They also observed that patients who were active recovered faster and hypothesized that head movements must be important in the recovery of function. Their initial exercise program consisted of a variety of eye, head, and body movements to habituate the dizziness. Since the development of those exercises, several other approaches to the treatment of patients with complaints of vertigo and dysequilibrium have been described. These exercises generally fall under four different categories, exercises to promote habituation, exercises to promote adaptation, exercises to promote substitution, and exercises designed to treat benign paroxysmal positioning vertigo. Any of these exercise approaches may be indicated in an individual with dizziness secondary to traumatic brain injury. The challenge to those treating these individuals is to identify the nature of the cause of the dizziness and to design the appropriate treatment programs.

Habituation exercises, like those described initially by Cawthorne and Cooksey, are based on the principle that repeated exposure to a noxious, or provocative, stimulus (in this case movements) will lead to a reduction in the body's response to that stimulus.

The exercises to induce adaptation of the vestibular system, while similar to the approaches mentioned above, reflect our increased knowledge of the function and adaptation of the vestibular system. Adaptation exercises are designed to promote long term (plastic) changes in the neuronal response of the vestibular system to a given head movement, with the goals of decreasing retinal slip, improving postural stability, and decreasing symptoms. These exercises are typically used in individuals with an uncompensated unilateral vestibular loss. The treatment approach for individuals with unilateral vestibular hypofunction differs in both theory and practice from the approach for individuals with bilateral vestibular loss. For individuals with bilateral vestibular loss, exercises to promote the substitution of alternative strategies for gaze stability and postural control are appropriate.

Finally, the exercises to treat BPPV are based upon the hypothesis that there are crystalline structures, which are consistent with degenerating otoconia from the otolithic membrane (52). These crystals cause an abnormal mechanical stimulation of the vestibular system with changes in head position relative to gravity. These exercises, while simplistic in the current arena of high tech medicine, are very effective in alleviating the signs and symptoms of BPPV. Benign Paroxysmal Positioning

Vertigo can occur in conjunction unilateral vestibular loss, central vestibular disorders, and in some cases with bilateral vestibular loss. Consequently, the treatment of BPPV is often combined with other exercise approaches to treat the identified problems. Determination of the appropriate exercise program rests on the findings of the clinical examination and available vestibular function tests.

Who Is an Appropriate Candidate for Vestibular Rehabilitation?

Generally, individuals with stable vestibular function and symptoms provoked by head motion (either self-motion or motion in the environment) or environmental situations (e.g. absence of visual cues, altered somatosensory cues) will benefit from vestibular rehabilitation. Individuals with vestibular function that fluctuates, as in Meniere's disease, or those who have true spontaneous episodic bouts of dizziness, typically will not benefit from vestibular rehabilitation.

Treatment of Individuals with Benign Paroxysmal Positioning Vertigo

Benign Paroxysmal Positioning Vertigo (BPPV) can affect any of the three semicircular canals, although the most commonly encountered presentation is that of posterior canal BPPV (53). In addition, the BPPV is thought to be caused by one of two mechanisms, cupulolithiasis (54) or canalithiasis (55, 56). In canalithiasis, the otoconia are mobile in the long arm of the semicircular canal; in cupulolithiasis, the otoconia are adherent to the cupula. The effect, in both cases, is to make the involved canal sensitive to the pull of gravity. The presentation of the two types of BPPV differs, as do the treatments for each condition. The methods used to determine the involved canal and the nature of the BPPV as well as a comprehensive review of the various treatment techniques are beyond the scope of this chapter. The interested reader is referred to the following articles for review (57, 58). Identification and treatment of posterior canal canalithiasis, the most common form of BPPV encountered in the clinic, will be reviewed here. The test for BPPV is the Dix-Hallpike maneuver (59). To perform this test, the patient sits with their legs extended on the examination table, their cervical spine is rotated approximately 45° to one side, their head is supported in the examiner's hands, and they are quickly brought into supine, with the cervical spine extended 10° to 20° and the head hanging off the table (see Figure 28-1). The patient is held in this position for up to 60 seconds, and the eye movements and the patient's symptoms are monitored. In a patient without BPPV, this test will produce no vertigo and no nystagmus. In a patient with BPPV, the Dix-Hallpike test will provoke both vertigo and a mixed vertical-torsional nystagmus.

The fast phase (beat) of the vertical component of the nystagmus will be upwards (relative to the patient). Torsional eye movements are rotations of the eye around the line of sight axis, and the direction of the nystagmus is named for the movement of the superior pole of the eye (again relative to the patient) during the fast phase of the nystagmus. The torsional component of the nystagmus will beat towards the involved ear, which is generally the dependent ear in the Dix-Hallpike maneuver. The nystagmus and vertigo will be present less than 2 minutes, and will generally persist for 30 seconds or less. The observed nystagmus and vertigo are due to an abnormal stimulation of the posterior semicircular canal, presumably due to movement of the otoconia away from the cupula. On arising to sitting, there is often a recurrence of the vertigo and a reversal of the nystagmus. This reversal of the nystagmus is due to the otoconia now moving back towards the cupula of the semicircular canal.

Treatment of this form of BPPV is straightforward. John Epley (60) first described a series of positioning maneuvers designed to move the offending otoconia out of the involved canal. Others have modified his procedure by altering some of the movements, changing the time in each position, and not using a mastoid vibrator during the treatment. This modified procedure is typically referred to as the canalith repositioning maneuver (CRM) or canalith repositioning procedure (CRP) (57, 61, 62). For the following description of the maneuver, we will assume that the patient has left-sided, posterior canal canalithiasis. If the patient had right-sided, posterior canal canalithiasis, the direction of the rotations would be reversed. To begin the CRM, the patient is long sitting on a treatment table, with the cervical spine rotated 45° to the affected side (Fig. 28-2A). The patient, whose head is supported by the examiner, is then brought into supine, and the cervical spine is extended 10° or 20° (Fig. 28-2B), and this position is maintained for 30 seconds to 2 minutes. The patient's neck is then extended further (if possible) and then rotated 90°, so that the final position is 45° rotation to the right(Fig 28-2C). This position is maintained for 30 seconds to 2 minutes. The patient then rolls onto the right side, maintaining the same degree of cervical rotation. During this rotation of the body, the cervical spine is brought into neutral with respect to flexion and extension and laterally flexed to the right, to bring the head down toward the treatment table (Fig. 28-2D). This position is maintained for 30 seconds to 2 minutes. The patient is finally brought to into sitting from the side lying position, maintaining the cervical rotation until the patient is upright (Fig. 28-2E). The time spent in each position varies among practitioners. Epley (60, 63) suggested that each position be held for 1.5 times the duration of the nystagmus observed in the Dix-Hallpike test. Post-treatment instructions to the patient also vary among practitioners. Some suggest that the patient remain upright for 24 hours post-treatment; while others will retest the patient to determine the efficacy of the treatment. If one elects to re-assess the patient after the initial treatment, then one should repeat the treatment even if the post-test is negative. The treatment is repeated to avoid the possibility of having the otoconia move back into the affected semicircular canal during the re-assessment. Following successful treatment, patients are generally instructed to perform the CRM or Brandt-Daroff exercises at home in an attempt to prevent a recurrence of the BPPV.

Treatment of Gaze Instability

One of the primary functions of the vestibular system is to generate compensatory eye movements to a given head movement, the vestibulo-ocular reflex (VOR). The VOR, when functioning appropriately, allows the individual to maintain the object of interest on the fovea, thereby preserving visual clarity. If the vestibular system is not functioning appropriately, the eye movements generated in response to head movement will not be sufficient to keep the object of interest on the fovea. The resulting movement of the image on the retina, retinal slip, will lead to a degradation of visual acuity. In individuals with remaining vestibular function (for example those with a unilateral vestibular deficit), the exercises are designed to foster adaptation of the remaining vestibular signals to generate the appropriate eye movement responses. For those individuals without vestibular function (for example those with bilateral vestibular loss) there is no remaining vestibular signal to adapt. Consequently, the exercises for these individuals are designed to promote the use of alternative strategies to promote gaze stability during head movements. The two general exercise approaches and the rationale behind the exercises will be explained separately.

Exercises to Enhance Vestibular Adaptation The rehabilitation of individuals with unilateral peripheral vestibular hypofunction or loss (UVH) is based upon the plasticity inherent within the vestibular system. The ability of the vestibular system to modify its behavior during development, as well as in disease states, has been well documented (for a review see review by du Lac and colleagues (64)). In the case of an insufficient VOR, due to vestibular hypofunction, the vestibular system will not generate sufficient eye movements in response to head movements. This will cause the visual image to move across the retina. This retinal slip in the presence of head movements appears to be an effective stimulus for inducing adaptation of the VOR (65). For patients with remaining vestibular function, the exercises used in the treatment of gaze stability deficits are designed to generate these error signals and thereby foster adaptation of the vestibular system (66). The goals of this aspect of the rehabilitation program are to 1) improve

visual acuity during head movements, 2) improve visual-vestibular interactions during head movements, and 3) decrease the individual's sensitivity to head movements.

As a consequence of the error signal produced by the exercises, performance of the exercise is frequently associated with symptoms of dizziness or nausea. The patient must be aware that provocation of their symptoms is a necessary part of the rehabilitation process. If there is no symptom provocation with the exercises, then the patient is not challenging the vestibular system and adaptation will not occur. The first exercise to address the gaze instability issue is often called x1 (times one) viewing, since the eye velocity must equal the inverse of the head velocity to maintain visual fixation (Fig. 28-3A). To perform the exercise, the patient fixates on a visual target (a small letter or number) located on a plain visual background, approximately 3 feet away. The patient then rotates his/her head, maintaining fixation on the visual target throughout the head rotation. The image should remain in focus and stable in space. The amount of head rotation should be approximately 30°–45° to either side of midline. The patient should avoid maximum deviation of the eyes as visual acuity decreases in these positions and end gaze nystagmus should be avoided. Cervical range of motion limitations and glasses, especially bifocals, may limit the degree of head rotation. Head rotation, both horizontal and vertical, should be performed as rapidly as the individual can tolerate, with the restriction that the visual target must remain in focus and stationary. Oscillopsia will develop if the velocity of the head rotation exceeds the capacity of the VOR. The exercise should be performed continuously for 1 (initially) to 2 minutes. The duration should be progressed gradually to avoid severe exacerbation of the symptoms or provocation of cervical pain. As the individual improves, the velocity of head rotation can be increased. Altering the postural demands or the visual conditions will vary the stimulus context. If the patient has difficulty with independent stance, then the exercise can be performed initially while sitting. Having the patient stand with a wide base of support on a firm surface increases the postural demand. This condition forces the CNS to utilize somatosensory and visual cues to maintain balance in the presence of fluctuating vestibular signals. As the patient improves, they begin to perform the exercise with a narrower base of support, which is a more challenging position. This gradual reduction in the base of support is continued until the patient can perform the exercise in tandem stance. The exercise can also be performed on a foam cushion to perturb the somatosensory signals. This progression in postural demands occurs over the course of several weeks. On any given day the patient will perform the x1 viewing exercise under only one postural condition.

Since adaptation of the vestibular system is context specific, (67) the context of the visual stimulus should vary to reflect the different visual conditions that an individual normally encounters. The influence of the optokinetic system (parafoveal visual stimuli) on gaze stability can be incorporated into the exercise program by placing the visual target within a "full-field" visual stimulus such as a checkerboard. When the visual target is at the same depth as the full-field visual stimulus, then the optokinetic system will assist the VOR in generating the appropriate compensatory eye movements. If the visual target is in front of the full-field visual stimulus, then the optokinetic system will actually generate anti-compensatory eye movements, since the visual world behind the object of interest appears to move in the same direction as the head movement. Since both of these stimulus conditions are encountered in normal activities, both conditions are incorporated into the rehabilitation program.

When the object of interest is near, the translation of the eyes relative to the visual target is greater than when the target is at a distance. The neural circuitry controlling the VOR normally takes target distance into account when generating the compensatory eye movements. Therefore the x1 viewing exercises are also performed with larger visual targets at a distance (8–15 feet). Again these exercises are performed in standing, with the feet positioned to challenge postural stability. The head is rotated as quickly as possible for 2 minutes, with the restriction that the visual target must remain in focus and stationary.

Gaze stability during head movements requires not only normal functioning of the VOR, but also interaction with other visual systems, such as the smooth pursuit system. To encourage this interaction, the x1 viewing exercise is modified. The individual is again challenged to maintain clear and stable vision during head movements; however, rather than use a stationary target, the individual holds the target and moves it in the direction opposite to the head movement (Fig. 28-3B). If the target moves at the same speed as the head but in the opposite direction, then the eyes have to move at twice the head velocity to maintain clear vision. Consequently this exercise is often referred to as times two (x2) viewing. This exercise can be performed in sitting, if necessary, and progressed to standing with a progressively decreasing base of support. The exercise can be performed with both a simple visual target as well as a target located in a complex visual background.

Exercises to Foster the Substitution of Alternative Strategies for Gaze Stability Bilateral vestibular hypofunction (BVH) may result in major or complete loss of bilateral vestibular function. Therefore, the exercises are designed to enhance the remaining function of the vestibular system and to foster substitution for the loss of vestibular function with alternative strategies to maintain gaze stability (66). In the absence of vestibular signals, these individuals must use cervical inputs and knowledge of upcoming head movements (pre-planning) to generate the compensatory eye movements (see Table 28-1).

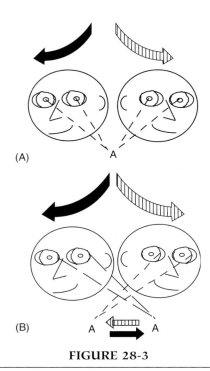

FIGURE 28-3

Exercises to induce adaptation of the vestibule-ocular reflex. (A) x1 viewing exercise. The patient views a stationary target, which should be a letter, number or word (in this case the letter A), while he turns his head back and forth. The speed of the rotation is increased to the point where faster movements would induce oscillopsia. Both horizontal and vertical rotations are performed. (B) x2 viewing exercise. The patient views a target that moves in the opposite direction of the head movement, while he turns his head back and forth. As with the x1 viewing exercise, the target should be a letter, number or word (in this case the letter A). The speed of the rotation is increased to the point where faster movements would induce oscillopsia. Both horizontal and vertical head rotations and target movements are performed

The cervical-ocular reflex (COR) normally contributes less than 15% to the generation of compensatory eye movements for low frequency head rotations (66). Following bilateral vestibular loss, the COR can account for up to 25% of the compensatory eye movements for both low and high frequency head rotations (68). The x1 viewing exercise described in the previous section can be used to increase the gain of the COR and to enhance the remaining function of the VOR. Generally, these exercises will be conducted at lower velocities than in individuals with unilateral vestibular hypofunction. When these exercises are performed actively, the CNS can also use foreknowledge of the upcoming movement to generate a compensatory eye movement. If performed passively, then the preplanning information is lost and the eye movements must be generated by the COR.

Another exercise which may improve the response of the COR, but also uses the central nervous system's

---

TABLE 28-1
Exercises to Promote Alternative Strategies for Gaze Stability

---

1. X1 viewing exercises
2. Active eye-head movements between two targets:
   Horizontal targets: Look directly at one target being sure that your head is also lined up with the target. Look at the other target with your eyes and then turn your head to the target. Be sure to keep the target in focus during the head movement. Repeat in the opposite direction.
   Vary the speed of the head movement, but always keep the targets in focus.
   Note: Place the two targets close enough together that when you are looking directly at one, you can see the other with your peripheral vision. Practice for 2–5 minutes, resting if necessary. This exercise can also be performed with two vertically placed targets.

3. Visualization of imaginary targets:
   Look at a target directly in front of you. Close your eyes and turn your head slightly, imagining that you are still looking directly at the target. Open your eyes and check to see if you have been able to keep your eyes on the target. Repeat in the opposite direction. Be as accurate as possible.
   Vary the speed and the amount (stopping point) of head rotation.
   Practice for 2–5 minutes, resting if necessary.
   Note: This exercise can be performed actively or passively while looking at a near target (within 2 feet) or at a distant target (across the room); it can also be performed vertically.

---

knowledge of upcoming movements, is the visualization of a remembered target location during head rotation. In this exercise the patient fixates a visual target, closes his eyes, and rotates his head in one direction. While turning his head, the patient attempts to keep his eyes on the target location. When the patient stops the head rotation, he opens his eyes and looks at the visual target. If his gaze is accurate, he will be looking directly at the target. If his compensatory eye movements are insufficient, his eyes will have moved with his head and he will have to make a corrective saccade to view the target. This exercise should be performed with both horizontal and vertical head movements. The visual target should be placed at different eccentric positions and different distances relative to the patient. The degree and speed of the rotation should be varied to force the patient to attend to all sensory cues.

Difficult tasks for individuals with BVH are gaze shifts that require both eye and head movements. Normally this task is accomplished by a patterned response. Initially, there is a saccade that is directed toward the object of interest. A head movement towards the target begins shortly after the saccade. While both the eye and head are moving towards the target, the VOR must be suppressed. When the eye reaches the desired location, the head is typically still turning. At this point the VOR must be used to keep the eyes on target during the remaining head movement. For patients with BVH, this head movement would cause the eyes to move beyond the intended object of interest and visual acuity would diminish. Individuals with BVH typically adopt one of two strategies to minimize this visual disturbance (68). One

strategy is to make a hypometric saccade and allow the head movement to carry the eyes onto the object of interest. A second approach is to make an accurate initial saccade, followed by a corrective backward saccade that is triggered by the head movement. Both of these strategies will minimize the amount of time that the visual image is not on the fovea. We do not attempt to teach one strategy or the other. We simply have the patient perform an activity that will encourage adoption of one of these strategies. For instance, two targets are placed at eye level, arm's length away, and slightly greater than shoulder width apart. The patient starts with her head rotated to the right, directly facing the target. The patient then shifts her gaze to the target on the left. The patient is told to move both her head and her eyes so that she is looking directly at the target. She is instructed to perform this as quickly as possible, but to keep the target in focus. The movement is then repeated in the opposite direction.

Treatment of Motion Sensitivity

Symptom provocation due to either head movements or visual motion is a common finding in individuals with vestibular dysfunction, and these findings are very common in individuals with dizziness secondary to TBI. Patients with sensitivity to head movements will describe increased symptoms associated with either head movements in general or rather specific movements. Patients with visual motion sensitivity will note increased symptoms when they are in busy visual environments such as crowds, department / grocery stores, or in traffic. The determination of head motion or visual motion sensitivity can often be made through the patient interview. One method of determining head motion sensitivity is through a series of rapid positioning maneuvers designed to elicit symptoms (69). These movements incorporate horizontal, vertical, and diagonal head movements with the head in different orientations relative to gravity. The symptom severity and duration in each of these movements is noted and used to determine a "Motion Sensitivity Quotient". The results of this test can be used to identify patterns of motion that provoke symptoms and to track changes in the patient's motion sensitivity. The general approach to the treatment of motion sensitivity is that of habituation, defined here as the long-term reduction of the response to a noxious stimulus (specific movement), brought about by repeated exposure to the provocative stimulus. The motion-provoked symptoms in patients with vestibular dysfunction is thought to be due to the sensory mismatch among the vestibular, visual, and somatosensory systems, which is brought about by movement. Repeated exposure to these movements is thought to lead to central adaptation and reorganization of the inputs to decrease the sensory mismatch and decrease the symptoms (70).

Exercises to Decrease Head Motion Sensitivity   The x1 viewing exercises, since they involve head movements can be used as a habituation exercise. So in some individuals with head motion sensitivity, who have normal visual acuity during head movements, performance of the x1 viewing exercise can lead to a reduction in their symptoms. For other individuals, however, performing the x1 viewing exercise may be too symptom provoking, or may not reduce all of their symptoms. In these cases habituation exercises may be used to reduce the motion sensitivity. These exercises are generally of greater amplitude and velocity than the x1 viewing exercises. However, the amplitude and velocity of the head movement is adjusted

to the patient's condition. The exercises are designed to provoke symptoms, but following completion of the each exercise session, the symptoms should return to baseline levels within 15 to 30 minutes. The selection of the exercises and movement patterns may be based on either the patient's description of provocative movements or on the results of the motion sensitivity examination. Examples of these exercises are presented in Table 28-2. Typically up to 4 specific movements are selected for each exercise session. Generally, one pattern of movement (horizontal, vertical, or diagonal) is chosen for the exercise program and then the program progressed over time. Caution should be taken with the exercises that have patients move from a "heart low" to "heart high" position if there are concerns about orthostatic hypotension.

Exercises to Decrease Visual Motion Sensitivity   A number of the previously described exercises can be used to try and decrease visual motion sensitivity. Performance of the x1 viewing exercise with the visual target located in front of a complex visual background can be used as an effective exercise to decrease visual motion sensitivity. As noted above, this exercise will induce movement of the visual background in an anti-compensatory fashion relative to the head movement. The habituation exercises described above (particularly the horizontal and vertical head movement exercises), if performed with eyes open, facing a visual scene with lots of color and contrast, can also be used as an exercise to decrease the visual motion sensitivity. If the combination of visual motion and head motion is too symptom provoking, then another exercise, which does not involve head movement, may be used. In this case, the patient performs a visual following task, with the object of interest located in front of a busy visual background. The exercise is similar to the x1 viewing

---

TABLE 28-2
Exercises to Decrease Motion Sensitivity

1. While sitting, turn your head quickly from right to left 5 times. Look in the direction you are turning. Wait for your symptoms to subside. Repeat 3 times.
2. While sitting, alternate looking up at the ceiling and down at the floor quickly 5 times. Look in the direction you are moving your head. Wait for your symptoms to subside. Repeat 3 times.
3. Sit on the edge of your bed. Turn your head about 45 degrees to the left. Now quickly lie on your right side. Wait for any symptoms to pass. Keeping your head turned, quickly sit up. Again, wait for the symptoms to pass. Now turn your head approx. 45 degrees to the right. Quickly lie on your left side. Wait for the symptoms to pass. Quickly sit upright. Wait for the symptoms to pass. Repeat 5 times.
4. Lie on your back. Quickly roll to the right side. Wait for symptoms to pass. Return to your back. Quickly roll to the left side. Wait for symptoms to pass. Return to your back. Repeat 5 times.
5. While sitting in a chair, bend your head forward about halfway toward your knees. Now quickly sit upright. Wait for the symptoms to pass. Repeat 5 times. (*Note*: this can be done tipping the head to right or left knee instead of straight down if that movement is more provocative)
6. Stand in a corner with your back to the wall. Now make a quick turn so that you are facing the wall. Stop and wait for symptoms to pass. Now make a turn in the opposite direction so that your back is again facing the wall. Repeat 5 times.

exercise; however, the patient keeps their head still and moves the visual target from side to side (or up and down). Since the smooth pursuit system is limited in frequency and velocity, the movement of the target will be relatively slow. Again, the patient's task is to keep the visual target in focus during the movement. Like the x1 viewing exercise, this exercise is performed for 2 minutes at a time.

Another approach to this problem is to immerse patients in the environments that provoke their symptoms. Patients are encouraged to walk through grocery stores, department stores, shopping malls, or crowds (provided these environments provoke symptoms). They can grade the intensity of the exercise in several ways. One, they can control their exposure by limiting the time they are in the particular environment. They can often adjust the intensity of the visual motion by selecting different times of the day to perform this exercise. Early in the morning there are generally fewer people in the stores than later in the day or evening. As their symptoms decrease, they are encouraged to walk for longer periods of time and at times when the stores are more crowded.

Treatment of Postural Instability

Another function of the vestibular system is to help maintain postural stability, or postural control. Postural control is defined as the ability to maintain the center of gravity over the base of support within a given sensory environment. Postural control requires the ability to perceive sensory information (somatosensory, visual, and vestibular), to centrally weight and select the appropriate sensory information, and to generate a suitable motor response to maintain stability. The selection of the appropriate motor response is based upon the available sensory information, biomechanical constraints, environmental contexts, and prior experience. Vestibular, visual, and somatosensory cues are all used to detect movement of the body and to trigger appropriate postural responses. If the vestibular system is not functioning appropriately, then the individual will have difficulty maintaining their balance when visual or somatosensory cues are altered or absent (e.g. at night, walking on uneven or compliant surfaces). In individuals with remaining vestibular function (for example those with a unilateral vestibular deficit), the exercises are designed to foster adaptation of the remaining vestibular signals to generate the appropriate postural responses. Unlike the VOR, the signal utilized for modification of the vestibulo-spinal reflexes (VSR) is not known. Presumably a similar visual-somatosensory-vestibular error signal is needed (71). Exercises used in the treatment of UVH are designed to generate these error signals and thereby foster adaptation of the vestibular system (66). For those individuals without vestibular function (for example those with bilateral vestibular loss) there is no remaining vestibular signal to adapt. Consequently, the exercises for these individuals are designed to promote the use of alternative strategies to promote postural stability. The two general exercise approaches and the rationale behind the exercises will be explained separately.

Exercises to Improve Static and Dynamic Postural Stability in Patients with Remaining Vestibular Function Exercises to promote static and dynamic postural stability in various sensory environments involve the manipulation of visual, vestibular and somatosensory cues to force the individual to utilize vestibular cues for postural stability (see Table 28-3). Single, progressing to multiple, sensory modalities are manipulated to increase the difficulty of the postural control task. Varied sensory conditions may include: 1) somatosensory changes (firm, conforming, level, uneven, and moving surfaces), 2) visual changes (eyes open with foveal, full field, or moving visual stimuli, or eyes closed), and 3) vestibular changes (different head orientations and head rotation). The exercises are also progressed from static to dynamic activities.

The initial exercise to improve standing balance progresses from standing with minimal external support to standing without assistance. Once the individual can stand independently (usually within 2 to 3 days from the onset of the UVH), they perform the exercise with a decreasing base of support to increase the task difficulty. This exercise sequence may be performed with the arms outstretched to facilitate stability. As the individual's balance improves, the exercise is performed with the arms at the side or folded across the chest to increase the difficulty of the task. Sensory cues can be modified to increase the difficulty of the task. Visual cues for postural stability can be removed by having the individual perform the exercise with their eyes closed. Having the individual stand on 4-inch thick, medium density foam, or pillows while assuming the various stance positions can alter somatosensory cues. Obviously, visual and somatosensory can be altered simultaneously by having the individual perform the exercise with eyes closed while standing on the compliant surface. This sequence of standing balance exercises can be repeated while standing on inclines. The exercises can also be repeated with the head tilted in various directions to alter the otolith inputs.

Exercises for improving dynamic postural stability involve progressively more difficult head and trunk movements while moving through space. Initially, the individual works on simple weight shifting activities, holding the end range position for three to five seconds, and independent ambulation. The progression from assisted to independent ambulation is usually very rapid. Providing there are no underlying orthopedic or other neurological problems, the patients are generally able to walk independently within several days of the initiation of ambulation. Typically these individuals avoid head rotation

TABLE 28-3

Exercises to Improve Static and Dynamic Postural Stability

The purpose of these exercises is to develop strategies for performing daily activities even when deprived of visual, somatosensory, or normal vestibular inputs. The activities are designed to help you develop confidence and establish functional limits. On all of these exercises, precautions should be taken to prevent *falls*.

1. Stand with your feet shoulder width apart with both hands helping you keep your balance by touching a wall (or countertop). Take your hands off the wall for longer & longer periods of time while keeping your balance. Try moving your feet closer together. Practice for 5 minutes.
2. Stand with your feet shoulder-width apart, eyes open, looking straight ahead at a target on the wall. Progressively narrow your base of support (move your feet one inch at a time) from feet apart, to feet together, to a semi-heel-to-toe position, to heel-to-toe (one foot in front of the other), to heel-to-toe onto to on "tip-toes."

   Do the exercises first with arms outstretched, then with arms close to your body, and then with arms folded across your chest.

   Hold each position for 15 seconds, and then move to the next most difficult position.
3. Repeat exercise #2 with head bent forward 30 degrees and then bent back 30 degrees.
4. Repeat exercise #2 with eyes closed, at first intermittently and then continuously, while making an effort to mentally visualize your surroundings.
5. Repeat exercise #2 and/or #4 while standing on a foam pillow.
6. Stand with your feet a comfortable distance apart and eyes open. Now sway forward and back so that weight shifts from your toes to your heels. Make sure there is no jack-knifing at the hips. Practice this for a minute or so. Now stop and close your eyes and stand as still and steady as possible. To progress this activity: Practice the swaying activity with eyes closed, practice with narrow base of support, and practice on compliant surfaces.
7. Walk close to a wall with your hand available for balancing. Walk with a narrower base of support. Finally, walk heel-to-toe. Do this with eyes open / closed. Practice for 2 minutes.
8. Walk close to a wall and turn your head to the right and left as you walk. Try to focus on different objects as you walk. Gradually turn your head further & faster. Practice for 2 minutes.
9. Practice turning around while you walk. At first, turn in a large circle but gradually make smaller and smaller turns. Be sure to turn in both directions.
10. Take 5 steps and turn around to the right (180°) and keep walking. Take 5 more steps, turn left (180°) and keep walking. Repeat 5 times, rest, and repeat the entire sequence.
11. Walk outside on an uneven surface or walk inside on a compliant surface.
12. Climb up your stairs without using your arms. Practice for 2 minutes.
13. Practice walking in a grocery store. To make it more difficult:
    – try to walk without a grocery cart,
    – go when there are few people there, then when it is crowded,
    – increase the number of aisles you walk through.
14. Practice walking in a shopping mall:
    – first when it is not crowded, then
    – when it is crowded, but walk with the flow of the crowd, then when it is
    – crowded, but walk against the flow of the crowd.
15. Participate in golf, tennis, dance, racquetball, etc.

The following balance exercises are performed at home with a partner:
   While standing, kick a ball between you.
   Practice batting a nerf ball.
   Play a game of catch. Progress in the following manner:
      Start with just an easy game keeping the ball in the midline.
      Then throw to either side.
      Take a step to the side to catch the ball. Your partner should let you know to which side he will be throwing the ball.
      To further progress throw randomly from one side to another.
      Catch the ball without taking a step as the ball is thrown to either side.

All of the activities listed above can be performed on a compliant surface.

during ambulation and assume a wide base of support while walking. Once they are able to walk independently, low frequency, small amplitude head rotations with concurrent gaze shifts are incorporated into the exercise program. To avoid excessive symptom provocation and marked gait ataxia, the individual performs the head rotation – gaze shift every 5th step. This may be performed with both horizontal and vertical head movements. This exercise forces the individual to adapt to the head rotations and prevents them from using visual fixation for postural stability. As recovery proceeds, the amplitude and peak velocity of the head rotation can be increased. To decrease the base of support, the patients walk with a progressively narrower base of support, ultimately walking heel to toe (tandem gait). Patients can also walk with the head tilted in either the frontal or sagittal planes to alter the otolith inputs. Patients are also encouraged to walk outdoors, which poses two distinct sensorimotor challenges. One, the support surface will change, which necessitates rapid postural adjustments. Two, visual cues for postural stability are at a greater distance than those indoors. This change in visual cues often causes increased dysequilibrium because the normal degree of postural sway results in smaller movements of visual images across the retina. This is an analogous situation to the normal experience of height vertigo.

The exercises described above challenge an individual's ability to move linearly. Another set of exercises is designed to rehabilitate the ability to rotate. This exercise involves walking approximately ten feet and turning around 180°. This is then repeated with rotation in the opposite direction. As the individual's balance improves, the radius of the turn is gradually decreased. This exercise can ultimately be performed with an abrupt rotation, or standing pivot. This exercise can also be performed with the eyes closed. A further extension of the exercise for the advanced stages of the rehabilitation process is rapid rotation combined with higher velocity linear movements. Examples include dance steps or shifting from a forehand to backhand in any of the racquet sports.

A more rigorous exercise to improve dynamic postural stability is hopping on one foot. Caution must be used with this exercise, or any exercise, which involves jarring movements to the head, post-surgery. There must be adequate time to allow for healing of the involved tissues before these strenuous exercises can be attempted. The difficulty of this exercise can be increased by eye closure. One of the final exercises used in the rehabilitation of dynamic postural stability is an obstacle course, where the individual walks over various surfaces, rotates, side-steps, and goes through a series of position changes (sit to stand, bending over, reaching, etc.). Lastly individuals are encouraged to resume their normal activities, especially those activities that involve postural changes and head movements, such as dancing, racquet sports, and golf.

Exercises to Improve Static and Dynamic Postural Stability in Patients without Vestibular Function The exercises to improve static and dynamic postural stability are similar to the exercises described for patients with remaining vestibular function (Table 28-2). Unlike the individuals with compensated unilateral vestibular lesions, those with bilateral vestibular hypofunction will have varying degrees of difficulty maintaining their balance when both visual and somatosensory cues are perturbed. Consequently, the exercises may need to be modified to allow the utilization of one sensory cue or to decrease the task complexity by widening the base of support.

The initial postural stability exercises for patients with BVH are simple standing balance exercises, with the goal of developing independent stance. As the patient is able to stand is able to stand without assistance, the exercise is made more challenging by progressively decreasing the base of support, until balance cannot be maintained. As with the static postural stability exercises for individuals with UVH, these exercises can be performed initially with the arms outstretched, then at the side, and finally folded across the chest. In these exercises both visual and somatosensory cues are available to the patient.

Individuals with BVH tend to initially rely solely on visual cues but gradually utilize somatosensory cues for postural stability (72). If the examination of the patient reveals that they are not using somatosensory cues for postural stability, then the standing balance exercises can be performed with the eyes closed. Eye closure may need to be intermittent at first but is progressed until the patient can perform the exercise for 30 seconds. It is often helpful in the beginning stages of this exercise to have the individuals visualize their surroundings when their eyes are closed. In addition, active weight shifting with eyes closed increases somatosensory awareness and awareness of the supporting surface. Should the unlikely situation arise where an individual is attending to somatosensory and not visual cues, the postural stability exercises can be performed with eyes open while standing on a compliant surface, such as a foam pad, to perturb the somatosensory inputs. Altering visual and somatosensory input to optimally challenge the individual should only be performed with the necessary safety measures to prevent falls.

The role of cervical input in the maintenance of postural stability is questionable. Bles et al (73). reported that static cervical positions did not contribute to postural stability in BVH. In light of these findings, the static postural exercises performed with head tilts may challenge the balance system by changing the visual frame of reference. The role of dynamic cervical input is not known at this time. Individuals with BVH have difficulty maintaining balance with head rotation during ambulation. This degradation of balance may be due to the loss of a stable visual frame of reference. However, their ability to walk and turn their head does improve with practice.

Patients with BVH also tend to walk with a wide base of support. Having these patients walk with a decreased step width, ultimately ambulating heel to toe, can challenge their dynamic postural stability. Changes in direction, as described for the patients with UVH, are also a challenge for the individual with BVH. An obstacle course or functional tasks that require positional changes, movement, and changing visual or somatosensory cues are also beneficial by forcing the patient to adapt to changing environmental conditions and to shift between the available sensory cues.

Patients should be instructed in behavioral and environmental modifications to optimize function and reduce the risk of falling. Environmental modifications may include: adequate lighting (including emergency lighting in case of a power failure), removal of thick carpeting and area (or throw) rugs, non-skid floors, pathways clear of obstructions, stable tables and chairs, reorganization of cabinets and shelves to minimize bending and reaching, and stairs with railings. Behavioral modifications may include: learning to plan movements, avoiding hurried movements, sitting to work, visual fixation on distant objects for stability, light touch on objects for balance, restricting rapid head movements and walking in crowds. Frequently, individuals with BVH are unable to drive due to oscillopsia. For those that have adequate visual acuity during head movements, many are unable to drive at night due to reduced visual cues. While assistive devices may not be needed around the home or during the day, the devices may be needed for safety concerns at night, in unfamiliar environments, and on uneven surfaces. For some individuals, an assistive device is necessary as an outward sign that there is a physical problem. Since there are no outward signs of a vestibular deficit, the individual is concerned that their staggering may be perceived as inebriation.

Exercise Guidelines for Individuals with TBI

Confounding orthopaedic and neurological factors often complicates treatment of vestibular deficits in patients with traumatic brain injury. First, the exercise programs described above will provoke the patient's symptoms. The exercises, if conducted appropriately, will generate an error signal in the CNS, which is thought to provoke symptoms of vertigo, dizziness or dysequilibrium. Depending upon the individual's symptoms, cognitive level, and degree of agitation, the symptom provocation may not be tolerated well. In those individuals with marked dizziness, motion sensitivity and agitation, the x1 viewing exercises may simply provoke too many symptoms. In these cases, it is recommended that the initial course of vestibular rehabilitation be simple habituation exercises, performed to tolerance. Once the habituation exercises have decreased the motion sensitivity, then x1 viewing exercises, if needed, may be initiated.

As the patient's status improves and their agitation decreases, the intensity of the exercises (either habituation or adaptation exercises) can be increased. With this increase, patients are told to expect greater symptom provocation and that provocation of their symptoms is actually beneficial to their recovery. A general guideline is that symptoms may be provoked for 15 to 30 minutes following the exercises. If the increased symptoms persist longer, the speed, duration, or context of the stimulus should be reduced. If the exercises are performed in a manner that does not challenge the system or provoke the symptoms, then the error signal will not be generated. Consequently, there will be no stimulus for adaptation. Similarly, the use of CNS depressants (such as meclizine or benzodiazepines) to treat the symptoms of vertigo and dysequilibrium are thought to retard the adaptation process.

The exercises may need to be modified due to other aspects of their injury. If for example, the patient suffers diplopia on lateral gaze to one side due to lateral rectus muscle palsy from the injury, then the x1 viewing exercise is modified to avoid lateral gaze to the affected side. Similarly, static and dynamic postural stability exercises may need to be modified due to muscle weakness, spasticity, or lower extremity fractures. Clinical judgment is required to adapt the basic exercise programs described above to meet the needs of the individual patient.

Vestibular and Balance Rehabilitation Therapy Outcomes

At this point, there have been no comprehensive studies examining vestibular and balance rehabilitation therapy outcomes inpatients with TBI. There are, however, numerous studies that have demonstrated the efficacy of VBRT programs in different populations of patients with vestibular disorders (54, 74, 75–77). Herdman and colleagues (74) demonstrated that, following acoustic neuroma resection, patients that underwent vestibular adaptation exercises demonstrated improvements in dysequilibrium, ataxia, and static postural stability as compared to individuals that had undergone a sham exercise program. Horak and colleagues (54) reported that individuals with chronic vestibular dysfunction treated with vestibular rehabilitation exercises developed improved motion sensitivity measures and static postural stability measures when compared to similar individuals treated with either condition exercises or vestibular suppressant medication. Similar results have been shown in patients with bilateral vestibular loss (76). Shepard and colleagues (75) reported that patients that underwent a customized VBRT program had greater improvements than those that received a generic VBRT program. Are the exercises always effective? No, but reports suggest that the exercise approach is successful in reducing symptoms and improving function up to 85% of the time (75, 78).

References

1. Baloh & Honrubia. *Clinical Neurophysiology of the Vestibular System*. Edition F.A. Davis Company, 1990
2. Leigh & Zee. *The Neurology of Eye Movements*. Edition 3. F.A. Davis Company, 1999.
3. Harada, Y. *The Vestibular Organs – SEM atlas of the inner ear*. Kugler & Ghedini Publications, Amsterdam, Berkeley, Milano, 1998.
4. Nashner LM (1993a) Practical biomechanics and physiology of balance. In Jacobson GP, Newman CW, Kartush JM, eds. *Handbook of Balance Function Testing*. St. Louis: Mosby–Year Book, Inc; 280–307.
5. Shepard, N.T. & Telian, S. A: *Practical Management of the Balance Disorder Patient*. Singular Publishing Group, Inc., 1996.
6. Allum JHJ, Shepard NT (1999) An overview of the clinical use of dynamic posturography in the differential diagnosis of balance disorders. *J of Vestibular Research* 9:223–252.
7. Woollacott MH, Shumway-Cook A. *Development of posture and gait across the life span*. Columbia: University of South Carolina Press 1989.
8. Bronstein, Brandt & Woolacott. *Clinical Disorders of Balance and Gait*. Oxford University Press & Arnold, 1996.
9. Shepard, N.T. & Solomon, D. *Practical Issues in the Management of the Dizzy and Balance Disorder Patient* The Otolaryngologic Clinics of North America, WB Saunders Co, Vol 33, # 3, June 2000.
10. Curthoys IS, Halmagyi GM (1995) Vestibular compensation: A review of the oculomotor, neural, and clinical consequences of unilateral vestibular loss. *J Vestib Res* 5:67–107.
11. Vidal PP, De Waele C, Vibert N, Muhlethaler M (1998) Vestibular compensation revisited. *Otolaryngology-Head and Neck Surgery* 119:34–42.
12. Brandt T, Daroff RB: Physical therapy for benign paroxysmal positional vertigo. *Arch Otolaryngol* 1980;106:484–485.
13. Epley JM: The canalith repositioning procedure for treatment of benign paroxysmal positional vertigo. *Otolaryngol Head Neck Surg* 1992;107:399–404.
14. Brandt T, Steddin S: Current view of the mechanism of benign paroxysmal positioning vertigo: Cupulolithiasis or canalolithiasis? *J Vestib Res* 1993;3:373–382.
15. Brandt T. Benign paroxysmal positioning vertigo. *Adv Otorhinolaryngol* 1999;55:169–194.
16. Herdman SJ, Tusa RJ, Zee DS et al: Single treatment approaches to benign paroxysmal positional vertigo. *Arch Otolaryngol* 1993;119:450–454.
17. Herdman, S.J. *Vestibular Rehabilitation*. 2nd ed. F.A. Davis Co, 1999.
18. Hasso AN, Ledington JA: Traumatic injuries of the temporal bone. *Otolaryngologic Clinics of North America* 1988;21:295–316.
19. Cannon CR, Jahrsdoerfer RA: Temporal bone fractures. Review of 90 cases. *Archives of Otolaryngology* 1983;109:285–288.
20. Schuknecht HF. *Pathology of the ear*. Cambridge: Harvard University Press, 1974:295–298.
21. Ruckenstein MJ. Vertigo and Dysequilibrium with Associated Hearing Loss. In: Shepard NT, Solomon D, eds. *The otolaryngologic clinics of north america*. Philadelphia: WB Saunders Co, 2000;33 (3):535–562.
22. Cannon CR, Jahrsdoerfer RA: Temporal bone fractures. Review of 90 cases. *Archives of Otolaryngology* 1983;109:285–288.
23. Hasso AN, Ledington JA: Traumatic injuries of the temporal bone. *Otolaryngologic Clinics of North America* 1988;21:295–316.
24. Phelps PD: Congenital cerebrospinal fluid fistulae of the petrous temporal bone. *Clinical Otolaryngology & Allied Sciences* 1986;11:79–92.
25. Goodhill V: Sudden deafness and round window rupture. *Laryngoscope* 1971;81:1462–1474.
26. Friedland DR, Wackym PA: A Critical Appraisal of Spontaneous Perilymphatic Fistulas of the Inner Ear. *American Journal of Otology* 1999;20:261–279.
27. Hughes GB, Barna BP, Kinney SE, Calabrese LH, Nalepa NL: Predictive value of laboratory tests in "autoimmune" inner ear disease: preliminary report. *Laryngoscope* 1986;96:502–505.
28. Shea JJ: The myth of spontaneous perilymph fistula [editorial] [see comments]. *Otolaryngology - Head & Neck Surgery* 1992;107:613–616.
29. Buchman CA, Luxford WM, Hirsch BE, Fucci MJ, Kelly RH: Beta-2 transferrin Assay in the Identification of Perilymph. *American Journal of Otology* 1999;20:174–178.
30. Rizer FM, House JW: Perilymph fistulas: the House Ear Clinic experience. *Otolaryngology - Head & Neck Surgery* 1991;104:239–243.
31. Poe DS, Bottrill ID: Comparison of endoscopic and surgical explorations for perilymphatic fistulas. *American Journal of Otology* 1994;15:735–738.
32. Poe DS, Rebeiz EE, Pankratov MM: Evaluation of perilymphatic fistulas by middle ear endoscopy. *American Journal of Otology* 13:529–533, 1992.
33. Staab JP. Diagnosis and treatment of phychologic symptoms and psychiatric disorders in patients with dizziness and imbalance. In: Shepard NT, Solomon D, eds. *The otolaryngologic clinics of north america*. Philadelphia: WB Saunders Co, 2000;33 (3):617–636.
34. Tusa RJ. Psychological problems and the dizzy patient. In: Herdman SJ, ed. *Vestibular rehabilitation*. Philadelphia: FA Davis Co, 2000:316–330.
35. Yardley L. Overview of psychologic effects of chronic dizziness and balance disorders. In: Shepard NT, Solomon D, eds. *The otolaryngologic clinics of north america*. Philadelphia: WB Saunders Co, 2000;33 (3):603–616.
36. Brandt T, Dietrich M. Assessment and management of central vestibular disorders. In: Herdman SJ, ed. *Vestibular rehabilitation*. Philadelphia: FA Davis Co, 2000:264–297.
37. Schumway-Cook A. Vestibular rehabilitation of the patient with traumatic brain injury. In: Herdman SJ, ed. *Vestibular rehabilitation*. Philadelphia: FA Davis Co, 2000:476–493.
38. Tusa RJ. Diagnosis and management of Neuro-otological disorders due to migraine. In: Herdman SJ, ed. *Vestibular rehabilitation*. Philadelphia: FA Davis Co, 2000:298–315.
39. Neuhauser H, Leopold M, von Brevern M, et al. The interrelations of migraine, vertigo and migrainous vertigo. *Neurology* 2001;56:436–441.
40. Jacobson GP, Newman CW, Kartush JM eds. *Handbook of Balance Function Testing*. St. Louis MO: Mosby–Year Book, Inc. 1993.
41. Jacobson GP, Newman CW. The development of the dizziness handicap inventory. *Arch Otolaryngol Head Neck Surg* 1990;116:424–427.
42. Jacobson GP, Newman CW, Hunter Left, Balzer G. Balance function test correlates of the dizziness handicap inventory. *J Am Acad Audiol* 1991;2:253–260.
43. Robertson DD, Ireland DJ. Dizziness handicap inventory correlates of computerized dynamic Posturography. *Oolaryngol Head and Neck Surg* 1995;24:118–124.
44. Shepard, N.T.: Management of the Patient with Chronic Complaints of Dizziness: *An Overview of Laboratory Studies*. NeuroCom Publication, Clackamas, Oregon, April 2003.
45. Herdman SJ, Tusa RJ, Blatt P, et al. Computerized dynamic visual acuity test in the assessment of vestibular deficits. *Am J Otol* 1998;19:790.
46. Zee DS. Vestibular Adaptation. In: Herdman SJ, ed. *Vestibular rehabilitation*. Philadelphia: FA Davis Co, 2000:77–90.
47. Shepard, N.T.; Solomon, D.; Ruckenstein, M.; Staab, J.: Evaluation of the Vestibular (Balance) System. In Ballenger, J.J.; Snow, J.B. (eds) *Otorhinolaryngology Head and Neck Surgery, 16th Edition*. Singular Publishing Group, Inc, San Diego, CA, 2003.
48. Allum, J.H.J.; Shepard, N.T.: An overview of the clinical use of dynamic posturography in the differential diagnosis of balance disorders. *J of Vestibular Research* 199;9:223–252.
49. Cawthorne T. The physiological basis for head exercises. *J Chart Soc Physiother* 1944:106–107.
50. Hecker HC, Haug CO and Herndon JW. Treatment of the vertiginous patient using Cawthorne's vestibular exercises. *Laryngoscope* 1974;84:2065–2072.
51. McCabe BF. Labyrinthine exercises in the treatment of diseases characterized by vertigo: their physiologic basis and methodology. *Laryngoscope* 1970;80:1429–1433.

52. Welling DB, Parnes LS, OBrien B, Bakaletz L, Brackmann DE and Hinojosa R. Particulate matter in the posterior semicircular canal. *Laryngoscope* 1997;107:90–94.

53. Korres S, Balatsouras DG, Kaberos A, Economou C, Kandiloros D and Ferekidis E. Occurrence of semicircular canal involvement in benign paroxysmal positional vertigo. *Otol Neurotol* 2002; 23:926–932.

54. Schuknecht HF. Cupulolithiasis. *Arch Otolaryngol* 1969;90: 765–778.

55. Parnes LS and McClure JA. Free-floating endolymph particles: a new operative finding during posterior semicircular canal occlusion. *Laryngoscope* 1992;102:988–992.

56. Moriarty B, Rutka J and Hawke M. The incidence and distribution of cupular deposits in the labyrinth. *Laryngoscope* 1992;102:56–59.

57. Herdman SJ, Tusa RJ, Zee DS, Proctor LR and Mattox DE. Single treatment approaches to benign paroxysmal positional vertigo. *Arch Otolaryngol Head Neck Surg* 1993;119:450–454.

58. Parnes LS, Agrawal SK and Atlas J. Diagnosis and management of benign paroxysmal positional vertigo (BPPV). *CMAJ* 2003;169:681–693.

59. Dix M and Hallpike C. The pathology, symptomatology and diagnosis of certain common disorders of the vestibular systems. *Ann Otol Rhinol Laryngol* 1952;61:987.

60. Epley JM. The canalith repositioning procedure: for treatment of benign paroxysmal positional vertigo. *Otolaryngol Head Neck Surg* 1992;107:399–404.

61. Parnes LS and Price-Jones RG. Particle repositioning maneuver for benign paroxysmal positional vertigo. *Ann Otol Rhinol Laryngol* 1993;102:325–331.

62. Wolf JS, Boyev KP, Manokey BJ and Mattox DE. Success of the modified Epley maneuver in treating benign paroxysmal positional vertigo. *Laryngoscope* 1999;109:900–903.

63. Epley JM. Positional vertigo related to semicircular canalithiasis. *Otolaryngol Head Neck Surg* 1995;112:154–161.

64. du Lac S, Raymond JL, Sejnowski TJ and Lisberger SG. Learning and memory in the vestibulo-ocular reflex. *Ann Rev Neurosci* 1995;18:409–441.

65. Gauthier GM and Robinson DA. Adaptation of the human vestibuloocular reflex to magnifying lenses. *Brain Res* 1975;92: 331–335.

66. Herdman SJ. Exercise strategies for vestibular disorders. *Ear Nose Throat J* 1989;68:961–964.

67. Shelhamer M, Robinson DA and Tan HS. Context-specific adaptation of the gain of the vestibulo-ocular reflex in humans. *J Vestib Res* 1992;2:89–96.

68. Kasai T and Zee DS. Eye-head coordination in labyrinthine-defective human beings. *Brain Research* 1978;144:123–141.

69. Smith-Wheelock M, Shepard NT, Telian SA. Physical therapy program for vestibular rehabilitation. *Am J Otol* 1991;12:218–225.

70. Norre ME and Deweerdt W. Treatment of Vertigo Based on Habituation. 1. Physio-Pathological Basis. *Journal of Laryngology and Otology* 1980;94:689–696.

71. Gonshor A and Jones GM. Postural adaptation to prolonged optical reversal of vision in man. *Brain Res* 1980;192:239–248.

72. Bles W, de Jong JMBV and de Wit G. Compensation for vestibular defects examined by the use of a tilting room. *Acta Otolaryngol (Stockh)* 1983;95:576–579.

73. Bles W, de Jong JMBV and Rasmussens JJ. Postural and oculomotor signs in labyrinthine defective subjects. *Acta Otolaryngol (Stockh)* 1984;406:101–104.

74. Herdman SJ, Clendaniel RA, Mattox DE, Holliday MJ and Niparko JK. Vestibular adaptation exercises and recovery: acute stage after acoustic neuroma resection. *Otolaryngol Head Neck Surg* 1995;113:77–87.

75. Shepard NT and Telian SA. Programmatic vestibular rehabilitation. *Otalaryngol Head Neck Surg* 1995;112:173–182.

76. Krebs DE, Gill-Body KM, Riley PO and Parker SW. Double-blind, placebo-controlled trial of rehabilitation for bilateral vestibular hypofunction: preliminary report. *Otolaryngol Head Neck Surg* 1993;109:735–741.

77. Yardley L, Beech S, Zander L, Evans T and Weinman J. A randomized controlled trial of exercise therapy for dizziness and vertigo in primary care. *Br J Gen Pract* 1998;48:1136–1140.

78. Krebs DE, Gill-Body KM, Parker SW, Ramirez JV and Wernick-Robinson M. Vestibular rehabilitation: useful but not universally so. *Otolaryngol Head Neck Surg* 2003;128:240–250.

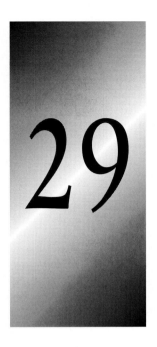

29 Evaluating and Treating Visual Dysfunction

William V. Padula

Lezheng Wu

Vincent Vicci

John Thomas

Christine Nelson

Daniel Gottlieb

Penelope Suter

Thomas Politzer

Raquel Benabib

INTRODUCTION

Complaints concerning vision are common following a traumatic brain injury (1). A traumatic brain injury can cause a wide variety of symptoms related to vision such as headaches, diplopia, vertigo, asthenopia, inability to focus, movement of print when reading, difficulty with tracking and fixations, and photophobia. Persons experiencing these types of visual problems frequently will have other medical sequela related to the TBI.

Epidemiological studies of vision problems relating to traumatic brain injury have been sparse in both literature and research. However, a limited number of studies demonstrate that vision dysfunction is common following a TBI and can affect any part of the visual process (2).

In one study, the most common complaint was blurred vision (46%) followed by diplopia (30%) and headaches (13%). Thirty-five percent of the subjects displayed a visual field defect of which the most common was a compression of peripheral fields followed by homonymous hemianopsia. Thirty-three percent of the subjects experienced cranial nerve palsies of which third nerve palsy (exotropia) was the most common. Ninety-five percent of these subjects had normal funduscopic findings while of those with abnormal funduscopic evaluations, twenty-six percent demonstrated optic nerve abnormality.

Binocular dysfunction is highly prevalent (3) following a TBI and relate to many of the symptoms regarding vision that a person may experience (4). Often, exotropia (an eye deviated outward) or exophoria (tendency for the eyes to deviate) occur following a TBI either through direct cranial trauma or whiplash (5, 6).

Following a TBI, visual sensory deficits can be caused by areas other than the stria of the occipital lobe which is often noted as the primary visual cortex (7). The extent and impact of a TBI on overall sensory function can be quite profound but due to the true nature and primary influence of visual processing, no interference can be as significant as that of the visual system following a

TBI. Mechanisms for sensory deficits require awareness and recognition of the problem by the affected person without which, there is a significant potential for interference in the overall rehabilitation process (8).

The use of vision to lead and guide motor function is often compromised following a brain injury (9) affecting visual perception and visual motor dysfunctions. New evidence has emerged demonstrating that neuromotor function also contributes to spatial awareness and affects egocentric concepts of visual midline (10) beyond the role of acuity. Visual midline is the perceived lateral and anterior-posterior visual concept of egocentric position relative to sensory-motor concepts. The influence of homonymous hemianopsia will also directly affect the perception of visual midline, posture, and balance.

Use of visual evoked potentials (VEPs) have disclosed that dysfunction in visual processing may be a cause of many of the conditions of strabismus following TBI (11). Researchers have also documented through VEP patterns that there are many visual abnormalities significantly related to the clinical disability of persons with TBI (12). The result of such research are leading many to begin questioning the traditional examination methods of examining persons with a TBI relative to diagnosing binocular dysfunction or to assess visual processing of the bimodal system of vision.

Recent studies (11, 13) involving visual evoked potentials (VEPs) have directed consideration that binocular dysfunction and visual midline shift are due to dysfunction of visual processing and not necessarily due to muscle or cranial nerve palsy following TBI. Until recently, research involving the bimodal process of vision had not been considered clinically relevant at the same level as binocular function. In particular, dysfunction of binocularity had been looked at primarily as the cause related to the symptoms. Understanding the true nature of the bimodal visual process may now give the documentation necessary to understand the nature of binocular function in relationship to cortical and subcortical mechanisms that organize vision and sensory motor information. In turn, the visual evoked potential may now give the researcher as well as the clinician the means to join in the study of process related to clinical function. In addition, it may also provide new means of understanding the significant interferences caused by TBI related to a wide variety of visual symptoms following a TBI.

It is common for persons to experience vertigo, dizziness, and other balance disorders following a TBI (14). While studies have emphasized the vestibular system as the primary mechanism for maintaining stability of the visual field, new information regarding the role of the pretectum and superior colliculus offers insight into vision stabilizing the retinal image and establishing peripheral fusion. In addition, the superior colliculus also mediates visual processing affecting posture, movement, and orientation to positional space (15). A new model of processing related to the sensorimotor feedback loop providing a feedforward system to other higher areas of cortical function has been proposed and gives real insight into the role of the motor system affecting sensory perception and stability (16).

VISION: A BIMODAL PROCESS

Seventy percent of all sensory processing in the entire body is directly affected by information coming from the two eyes (17). These visual influences are directed to the midbrain and the majority extend themselves to the occipital cortex for purposes of seeing (15). As a dominant system in the sighted person, vision is often taken for granted. Fortunately, we do not have to think about the process of using vision as we automatically employ vision in our daily activities. The important dynamics of visual processing are masked behind our intense attention and concentration to the accomplishment of the task at hand. For example, the task of writing involves vision but we do not think about where we are looking when we move the pen on the page. Nor do we think of how we see print as we read. Do we see each individual letter on the page or do we see more globally and embrace whole words and phrases?

Trevarthen (18) and Liebowitz and Post (19) have disclosed that there are two modes of visual processing; the focal process and the ambient process. The focal process delivers information for the purpose of attention, concentration, and higher cognitive processing. Information is sent primarily to the occipital cortex for the purpose of seeing detail. This is the portion of the system which enables us to attend to a task or concentrate. If we had only the focal process, the world we see would break apart into a mosaic of fragments. We would see only the lines, shadows, and shapes on a person's face and although we would see clearly, we would not be able to recognize the inter-relationship of all of these details. We would not be able to recognize the person's face as a familiar gestalt.

Approximately twenty percent of fibers from the peripheral retinas of both eyes are delivered to the midbrain (20). Here, the visual process matches information gathered from the kinesthetic, proprioceptive, tactile, and vestibular systems. This function has been labeled the sensory-motor feedback loop (21). It serves to organize spatial information about balance, movement, and orientation in space. The visual process is very much involved in movement and postural control. The superior colliculus, a critical area in the midbrain system, receives fibers from the optic tract via the superior brachium, occipital cortex via the optic radiations through the lateral geniculate, and from the spinotectal tract connecting it with sensory motor information from the spinal cord and medulla. It is in the midbrain that sensorimotor matching concepts of midline, body awareness, posture, and orientation are established. Once this is accomplished, a feedforward phenomenon occurs. Information is relayed from the midbrain to the occipital cortex where it is used to preprogram the higher seeing area as to how to organize or look at incoming visual information. This is first done spatially and has been termed the ambient visual process. Following this, focalization on detail will occur. In this manner, the occipital cortex will organize information spatially before it looks at the detail. In other words, it is as if we know where to look before we completely identify the target. Spatial information from this midbrain ambient visual system is also used in other processing levels at the occipital cortex for purposes of bringing together detail information relative to spatial boundaries. In particular, the binocular coordination cells that receive information imaging from both the right and left eye have the primary purpose of beginning to integrate or fuse the two separate images together as one. It is the spatial information from the ambient visual process delivered by the superior colliculus that becomes the binding format of the fusion process (22).

In fetal development, the eye is created from endoderm, mesoderm, and neuroectoderm. Of importance is the fact that neuroectoderm also develops the cortex which allows for recognition that the eyeball is neurologically an end result in part of developing brain tissue. The eyeball is richly endowed with nerve fibers that feed all aspects of the cortex as well as relaying information to midbrain structures. Nerve fibers emanating from the macula or central portion of the eye will align centrally in the optic nerve and optic tract directing themselves to localize in central areas of the visual occipital cortex. Peripheral retinal nerve fibers orient themselves in the optic nerve and optic tract around the central fibers and align themselves in peripheral areas of the occipital cortex.

While the central image from the macula occupies the major portion of our cortical attention and concentration for perception and cognitive processing, how we organize and process visual information is not a simple phenomenon. The dorsal ganglion of the lateral geniculate body seems to function as an integrating center in addition to its role as a relay and distribution center. Therefore the lateral geniculate is important to the relay of visual information to portions of the brain other than the occipital cortex.

It has also been demonstrated that 20% of the peripheral retinal nerve fibers relay information through axons to the thalamus or midbrain for spatial match with kinesthetic, proprioceptive, and vestibular information being received from other sensory-motor systems. The developmental purpose is to organize spatial information to orient higher sensorimotor experiences affecting posture, movement, and balance. Once this has been established, information from the thalamus is sent to higher cortical functions (16). The occipital cortex is not an exception to this process. It receives spatial information in order to organize the detail information processed.

Ganglion cells from the retina emanate through the optic chiasm to the optic tract where they reach three major destinations: 1) the lateral geniculate body for relay to the visual cortex, 2) the pretectal nucleus (pupillary constriction), and 3) the superior colliculus which becomes related to posture, movement, and orientation to positional space (15).

In order to shift the position of the eyes from one point to another, we must spatially orient to the next destination before shifting the eyes (aiming the fovea) to look at detail (23). The ambient process is critical for anticipating change. Without this process, visual information becomes isolated details and there is difficulty shifting visual regard and attention. Also, there is a lack of awareness of body position in a spatial context caused by a shift in visual midline. Due to a mismatch between the ambient visual process, the kinesthetic, proprioceptive, the vestibular input system and the ambient visual process, the concept of visual midline will shift. As will be discussed later in this chapter, if the visual midline shifts, it will reinforce and/or cause postural imbalances.

The ambient process is not a conscious process as is the focal system. We orient this portion of the visual system to monitor and manipulate the spatial environment. The ambient visual process works to integrate sensory-motor information. Without the ambient visual process, an individual would experience fragmented vision as well as difficulty with organizing posture and movement. The bimodal process, however, in many ways has been ignored and/or misunderstood clinically (24).

Ganglion cells traveling from the retinas can be categorized based both on physiology and function into three types; P-cells (parvocellular), M-cells (magnocellular), and K-cells (koniocellular). These cells provide information similar to that which was discussed previously regarding the focal and ambient process. The M-cells and P-cells provide a physiological substrate for the ambient and focal processes. M-cells transmit visual information about shape and movement rapidly, but without detail. P-cells transmit the detail information contained in shapes and are much slower. These cells emanate from the retina through two major brain pathways; the retino-geniculo-cortical pathway and the retino-tectal pathway. The retino-geniculo-cortical pathway contains both P-cells and M-cells and is the most recent in evolution providing a mechanism for focal processing in the cortex. The retino-tectal pathway is mainly derived from M-cells and is more primitive and provides a basis for spatial information particularly related to spatial orientation prior to focalization. For example, a saccadic eye movement (via the ambient pathway) first requires spatial orientation to establish the direction and trajectory of the eye movement prior to the focalization response. The retino-tectal pathway is most critical in early development of the child and some functions are taken over later in development by the retino-geniculo-cortical pathway (25). However, the midbrain ambient system remains important for spatial orientation and balance. It can be demonstrated clinically that children and adults with oculomotor dysfunction and aspects of dyslexia affecting reading ability demonstrate improvement with pursuit tracking and saccadic fixations as well as with the ability to track a line of print with sensory motor support such as by physically pointing at words.

The P-cell subsystem has been related to the focal visual process whereas the retino-tectal projection of the M-cell subsystem is a substrate for the ambient visual process. Neurons in the retino-tectal pathway are almost completely myelinated at birth whereas those of the retino-geniculo-cortical pathway are not. It is also of interest to know that the superior colliculus has essentially a normal adult organization and neuronal activity at birth whereas the occipital cortex does not (26). These authors have emphasized that while cerebral cortical processes have taken over much of the visual motor functioning, massive innervations still remain between cortical and midbrain structures.

Through development, experience is established to couple and bring balance between the ambient and focal visual process as well as the M-cell and P-cell subsystems. While balance between the spatial (ambient) and detail (focal) visual processing systems provide a means by which organization of time and space become a normal process for humans, injury as a result of a TBI can affect the balance between the systems. A decoupling of the focal and ambient visual process including the magno-parvo cellular systems is suggested as a basis for interference with function and performance. M-cells have larger diameter axons and have demonstrated to be more susceptible to damage in conditions such as ischemia and glaucoma.

More specifically, the decoupling of cerebral blood flow (CBF) and cerebral glucose metabolism (CMGL) has been described. This decoupling is described in terms of ischemia-hyperemia resulting in metabolic imbalances which derange neuronal energy production and cell membrane permeability ultimately causing potential cytoxicity (27) even in a minor whiplash accident. This can be the basis of visual problems following TBI.

A patient with mild TBI is most frequently under-diagnosed or misdiagnosed relative to visual impairments (28, 29). The walking wounded with a negative CT scan or MRI is a potentially classic case of an injured person whose symptoms are frequently dismissed as exaggerated and/or psychosomatic in origin. The many individuals who suffer significant visual symptoms following a brain injury potentially suffer equally from discrimination without identification of the causative factors (29).

The basis of the dysfunction of the visual process is related to the traumatic force imposed upon the central nervous system whether through blunt trauma or inertial acceleration or angular acceleration trauma of whiplash (hyperextension/hyperflexion). This can affect potassium adflux and secondary calcium influx. It is the influx of calcium ions that activate cellular proteate enzymes triggering cytoskeletal disruption and simultaneous neurotransmitter hypercholinergic activity.

It is hypothesized to be the cytotoxic response that initiates cytoskeletal collapse and ultimately deafferentation that is etiologic to the symptoms of post-trauma vision syndrome. In turn, the lifelong established engrams that provided the automaticity of controls affecting the very complex sensory motor components that subserve the visual process become eroded resulting in degradation of our dominant sensory perception, our dominant guidance system: visual information processing (30).

POST-TRAUMA VISION SYNDROME (PTVS)

Following a TBI, visual symptoms may occur (31) such as diplopia, seeing words and print appearing to move, difficulty shifting gaze, difficulty adapting to environments where there is movement in the periphery (such as in a store), and photophobia (Table 29-1). Characteristically, an examination of the visual system may demonstrate binocular dysfunction such as strabismus, convergence insufficiency, divergence excess, oculomotor dysfunction, and accommodative insufficiency. Some researchers have reported that diplopia, reduced acuities, and poor accommodation are prevalent among those with traumatic brain injuries (28). Others have reported intermittent diplopia present in certain positions of gaze (31). Soden and Cohen (32) as well as Nelson and Benabib (21) have correlated postural adaptation of the body with compensation for vision dysfunction and diplopia produced in certain positions of gaze. In addition, these researchers have found secondary contracture and/or muscle spasms due to poor body posture. A high prevalence of exotropia and exophoria have been reported for persons who have suffered even a mild traumatic brain injury (4, 5, 33).

Studies of binocularity have recognized dysfunction of oculomotor, convergence, and accommodations. A high prevalence of exotropia (5, 6, 34) is evidenced in the literature. While symptoms and characteristics are logically related to the visual dysfunction attributed to nerve palsy (35), the mechanism for the cause of the binocular dysfunctions appear to be more complexly related to the affect of the trauma on the bimodal visual processing systems as related by more recent studies

---

TABLE 29-1
Post-Trauma Vision Syndrome

Common characteristics and symptoms associated with post-trauma vision syndrome characteristics:

- Exotropia or high exotropia
- Accommodative dysfunction
- Convergence insufficiency
- Low blink rate
- Spatial disorientation
- Poor fixations and pursuits
- Unstable ambient vision

Symptoms:

- Possible diplopia
- Objects appear to move
- Poor concentration and attention
- Staring behavior
- Poor visual memory
- Photophobia (glare sensitivity)
- Asthenopic symptoms
- Associated neuro-motor difficulties
  - Balance and coordination
  - Posture

---

on visual evoked potentials (11, 13). In this study, the researchers demonstrated that changes in amplitude under binocular testing were found to correlate statistically with an experimental population (persons with TBI) compared to a control group of which the experimental group of subjects also experienced symptoms and demonstrated characteristics as discussed in the previous paragraph. An increase in amplitudes was produced following treatment with base-in prism and binasal occlusion for the experimental group of subjects. A decrease in amplitudes was found for those in the control group. Changes were also reported in amplitudes and latencies following a TBI.

The researchers have explained that following a TBI, there appears to be interference in the ambient (spatial) organization of the visual field which as a result, affects the focalization process (36). As mentioned previously in this chapter, the spatial match of information between the ambient and sensory motor process can provide a feedforward (37) to the higher cortical processes including the occipital cortex of which the binocular integration cells require the spatial information to bind and establish peripheral vision fusion. A decrease in amplitude of the binocular visual evoked potential as demonstrated by the study emphasizes the role of the ambient visual process in providing this spatial binding for the fusion process. In turn, the decrease in the amplitude provides evidence of the lack of ambient vision feedforward support for higher binocular fusion prior to the focal visual process establishing awareness of detail.

The result of the dysfunction of ambient visual processing becomes characteristic of the binocular dysfunctions such as convergence insufficiency, accommodative insufficiency, exophoria, and may even be the basis for post-traumatic exotropia (38).

The characteristics of dysfunction of the binocular vision process as well as commonly measured comitant and noncomitant strabismus may be more a function of disruption related to ambient and focal visual processing than of specific neuronal interferences. Other studies have demonstrated that lesions in the superior colliculus can produce disturbances of convergence ability (39).

The dysfunction and lack of support through ambient visual processing leaves the person compromised in the attempt to use the focal visual process which isolates detail and does not serve the need for anticipation of change (23). For example, following a TBI, persons will often have to work harder at near vision tasks. The research provides evidence that the ambient process being compromised also interferes with the anticipatory spatial role to provide for release of fixation and detail as well as for change. In turn, the visual process becomes focally bound, isolating to detail rather than utilizing the ambient visual process for release from detail and the anticipation of spatial organization that affects continuity and sequence of visual performance.

This research also demonstrates that the structure of binasal occluders (vertical boundaries in the nasal portion of the visual field) in addition to base-in prism (prism affecting spatial organization), rebalances the ambient visual process. In turn, a reduction in symptoms was noted in these subjects corresponding to implementation of this mode of treatment. Specifically, subjects reported a significant reduction in symptoms (11) as previously mentioned.

The effects of dysfunction between ambient and focal processing as related to common characteristics of binocular dysfunction as frequently seen following a TBI are more common than previously recognized. Binocular dysfunction such as convergence insufficiency is a frequently misdiagnosed condition following a traumatic brain injury. Convergence insufficiency should always be considered in the diagnosis of patients with head trauma.

The dysfunction relative to focal and ambient visual processing has been termed post-trauma vision syndrome (PTVS). Persons who suffer from post-trauma vision syndrome will often have clear sight and their eyes will be healthy. Upon being referred for a routine eye examination, if the examiner is not familiar with PTVS, the examiner will often report that there is nothing wrong with the person's eyes and the symptoms appear to be more psychological in nature. Many persons will spend years suffering from this condition unless it is diagnosed and treated appropriately. Needless to say, this can be the cause of additional inappropriate referral and treatment at a high cost to families and third party reimbursement systems. Appropriate treatment will not only reduce symptoms, but directly affect attention, concentration, and cognitive processing while preventing secondary emotional complications. The methods of evaluation and treatment through neuro-optometric rehabilitation and neuro-ophthalmological evaluation will be discussed later in this chapter.

VISUAL MIDLINE SHIFT SYNDROME (VMSS)

Postural orientation is vital for daily function for both adults and children. Postural adaptation that begins in the early stages of development provides a means for the infant to organize space for balance, spatial orientation, and ambulation. For functioning adults and children, anti-gravity alignments are initiated with limbs and/or with head movements. The vestibular system contributes a balance response necessary when the center of gravity has shifted while the cerebellar and midbrain structures through ambient/sensory motor support contribute to the desired qualities of smoothness and coordination for motor planning.

The ambient visual process is primary in the establishment of postural orientation related to boundaries by orienting boundaries in the vertical and horizontal planes with spatial information from sensory motor systems. Early in development, this establishes concepts of visual midline that provide experience for postural orientation (20). Established in relationship with multi-sensory motor cooperation, the ambient visual process together with sensory motor match, feedforwards information to diverse areas of the cerebral cortex including the occipital cortex. This vital component enables anticipation for postural adaptation and movement (37).

Following a TBI, a person may be left with hemiplegia or hemiparesis. The loss of neurological and motor function has traditionally been thought to be the sole cause for the inability to weight-bear on the affected side. Also, in cases of visual field loss such as with homonymous hemianopsia, it has been observed that individuals will begin to lean away from the side of visual field loss even if they do not have a hemiparesis.

Prior to the consideration of vision as a bimodal process, discussion has been centered on a lack of visual cognition and attention leading to neglect (40, 41). These authors have identified the phenomenon where people have limited or no attention to a specific side of their body as well as correlating field of vision. Right hemisphere damage often produces the characteristic left field neglect (42, 43). The spatial component of vision has been primarily considered related to the relationship of magnocellular function with right hemisphere involvement. The complete concept of the ambient process related to

midbrain and sensory-motor interaction should also be considered.

Relative to the concept of the bimodal process of vision, inattention is a focal processing phenomenon. The authors of this chapter offer the possibility that the focal visual processing dysfunction of inattention is secondary to the spatial ambient visual processing disorder that is more directly associated with the affect on sensory-motor processing from the TBI.

Studies (10) have demonstrated that the visual midline will shift relative to a hemiparesis and/or homonymous hemianopsia. This may be observed by passing an object in front of a person's face and asking them to report when the object appears to be directly in front of their nose. In the case of a visual field loss such as a homonymous hemianopsia, the person will often report the target in front of their nose when it is directed to the side away from the visual field loss. An interesting observation occurs when working with patients with hemiparesis or hemiplegia. The person will also project the concept of midline in the majority of cases by leaning away from the neurologically affected side. The shift affects weight-bearing on the affected side in most cases and in turn, interferes with aspects of physical rehabilitation. The shifting of perceived visual midline away from the affected side is a compensatory mechanism and essentially reinforces the neglect of visual space caused by the hemiparesis and/or hemianopsia.

The shifting of the visual midline is caused by a distortion (compression and expansion) of the ambient visual process. The midline can shift laterally and/or in the anterior/posterior axis. The perceived visual midline will usually shift away from the affected side. This has been termed visual midline shift syndrome.

NEURO-OPHTHALMOLOGY

Progress and overall rehabilitation for a person who has suffered a TBI are often interfered with due to visual problems that are sometimes ignored or misdiagnosed (2).

The provision of skilled neuro-ophthalmological services can positively affect the rehabilitation outcome. Referrals for neuro-ophthalmological evaluations are often initiated by physicians or rehabilitation professionals and optometrists practicing neuro-optometric rehabilitation who recognize visual interference with daily living skills and/or perceptual motor function.

The literature lacks good demographic studies on the prevalence of neuro-ophthalmological problems in TBI. Sabates reports that of 181 consecutive patients referred with visual complaints following head trauma, the most common etiology was motor vehicle accident in 57% of the cases. For direct trauma to the head, 15% were represented and 13% were related to injuries sustained from a fall. He also reports that in over 88% of the eyes tested, acuity of 20/20 was reported. Of this population, 33% suffered cranial nerve palsy.

NEURO-OPTOMETRIC REHABILITATION

Neuro-optometric rehabilitation represents a new and evolving specialty within the profession of optometry devoted to clinical assessment and rehabilitative treatment of visual binocular/processing disorders following a traumatic brain injury. While there is overlap in the assessment between ophthalmological/neuro-ophthalmological and neuro-optometric rehabilitation, the latter emphasizes rehabilitation of visual processing disorders. The fields of ophthalmology and optometry work in conjunction with individuals who have suffered visual and ocular-visual problems following a TBI.

Neuro-optometric rehabilitation is defined as:

> Neuro-optometric rehabilitation is an individualized treatment regimen for patients with visual deficits as a direct result of physical disabilities, traumatic and/or acquired brain injuries. Neuro-optometric therapy is a process for the rehabilitation of visual/perceptual/motor disorders. It includes but is not limited to acquired strabismus, diplopia, binocular dysfunction, convergence, and/or accommodation, paresis/paralysis, oculomotor dysfunction, visual spatial dysfunction, visual perceptual and cognitive deficits, and traumatic visual acuity loss.
>
> Patients of all ages who experience neurological insults can benefit from neuro-optometric rehabilitation. Visual problems caused by traumatic brain injury, cerebrovascular accident, cerebral palsy, multiple sclerosis, etc. may interfere with performance causing the person to be identified as learning disabled or as having attention deficit disorder.
>
> The visual dysfunctions can manifest themselves as psychological sequela such as anxiety and panic disorders as well as spatial dysfunctions affecting balance and posture. A neuro-optometric treatment plan improves specific acquired vision dysfunction determined by standard diagnostic criteria. Treatment regimens encompass medially necessary noncompensatory lenses and prisms with and without occlusion and other appropriate rehabilitation strategies (23).

The role of the ophthalmologist is to provide excellence of care relative to treatment of disease and trauma affecting the eye orbit and neurology affecting visual function. The ophthalmologist can and should be involved in treatment for acute care as well as long term ophthalmological needs for the person who has suffered a TBI.

The optometrist practicing neuro-optometric rehabilitation can affect visual processing disorders such as PTVS, VMSS, and other binocular spatial disorders causing diplopia, vertigo, etc. as rehabilitation is established. The neuro-optometric rehabilitation assessment includes a careful review of medical and rehabilitative records as well as establishing a history based on visual and spatial dysfunction.

Evaluation and History

The neuro-ophthalmological and neuro-optometric rehabilitation assessment requires a complete history and differentiation of symptoms and characteristics from pre-morbid conditions. The symptoms must be assessed relative to the medical history and a complete review of medical records and medications is imperative. It is important to reconstruct the event relative to the history in order to assess injury and lesions relative to inertial force and impact. Understanding the pre-event medical history is necessary relative to determining the nature of injuries.

Oculomotor and Binocular Function Assessment An oculomotor evaluation is performed to determine cranial nerve function. One of the most debilitating visual conditions following a TBI is diplopia. Strabismus can often occur following lesions affecting cranial nerve 3 (oculomotor nerve), 4 (trochlear nerve), or 6 (abducens nerve). These lesions can occur from blunt head trauma affecting origin, insertion, and or innervation of the extraocular muscles, trauma to brain stem, midbrain or cortex, vestibular trauma, and/or trauma affecting orbital structure and orbital space occupying lesions (21, 39). Often, as is the case, CT scans and MRI are unable to detect lesions related to these specific oculomotor neurons. The authors have previously suggested a dysfunction of the ambient visual process and the lack of feedforward support for peripheral fusion lock.

The inability to provide spatial information will cause a highly focalized nature of vision. In turn, the visual world becomes fragmented. This causes increased concentration on detail and yields increased fragmentation of the visual world. The result can be diplopia that will be characterized and measured by strabismus (exotropia, esotropia, hypertropia, hypotropia). When an individual has diplopia, the spatial reference by which to use vision to lead posture, balance, and motor function is compromised. In turn, it can affect cognitive-perceptual processing due to the distracting influence of physiological stress. In one study (2), the second most common symptom was that 30% of the subjects experienced diplopia following a TBI.

The most common result of lesions of the cranial nerve following a TBI is third nerve palsy. A third nerve palsy is associated with exotropia as well as ptosis and mydriasis of the pupil on the affected side with complete compromise. In most cases, the affect is incomplete causing variations from decompensated exophoria to intermittent exotropia. Diplopia depends on visual fatigue and chronic development of suppression. Vertical palsies resulting from the affect of cranial nerve 4 will produce hyperphoria and hypertropia as well as decompensation in specific gaze direction and head tilt. Sixth cranial nerve palsy interferes with abduction of the related eye, causing esotropia.

A variety of cranial nerve and binocular function tests are designed to provoke oculomotor failure causing decompensation of binocularity. These tests are described as follows:

1. Cover Test: The examiner will perform this test with the patient first fixating on a distant target (ten feet or beyond) and then at a near target (40 cm). The Alternate Cover Test is done by passing a cover alternately from one eye to the other and observing the movement of the eye emerging from under the cover. A heterophoria can be elicited. If observed, the examiner will perform a Cover Test by covering and uncovering each eye to discern from a tropia.

2. Krimsky Test: This is similar to the Cover Test, however, compensating prism is introduced to neutralize the motion of the phoria or tropia to determined the extent of deviation.

3. Bielchowsky's Head Tilting test: Cranial nerve and oculomotor function is analyzed by having the patient hold fixation in primary gaze while the examiner rotates the patients head first to the left and then to the right testing 3rd and 6th nerve function. The patient's head is moved in extension and flexion and tilted first to the right shoulder and then to the left shoulder to evaluate 4th nerve palsy affecting over and under-compensating oblique muscles.

4. Lancaster Red/Green Test: The patient is given glasses in which the OD has a red lens and the OS has a green lens. The examiner holds a red flashlight and the patient holds a green flashlight. The examiner shines the red flashlight on a screen and moves it into the nine cardinal gazes of fixation while asking the patient to superimpose their projected green light on the red light. Any deviation in a particular gaze direction will be noted and related to an underactive, overactive, or restricted ocular muscle.

5. Red Lens Test: The examiner holds a red lens before one of the patient's eyes and the patient is asked to fixate on a penlight. If the patient reports seeing two lights, the test is positive for diplopia at the respective working distance.

6. Worth Four Dot Test: The patient is given red/green glasses to wear while looking at the projection of four dots that form a diamond. The top dot is red, the inferior dot is white, and the lateral dots are both green. If the patient is binocular, four dots will be seen. If binocularity is compromised and the patient reports seeing five dots, diplopia has been elicited. If two or three dots are observed, a corresponding suppression is present.

7. Maddox Rod Test: The examiner holds a cylinder before one of the patient's eyes while the patient observes a penlight. The eye behind the cylinder will see a vertical or horizontal line of light depending on how the cylinder is positioned. If the line is reported to either the left or right side of the light, a heterophoria or tropia is present at the respective working distance. If the line appears above or below the light, a vertical deviation has been elicited.

Binocular dysfunctions often present as convergence insufficiency or strabismus of which exotropia is the most common following a TBI. This can cause diplopia. The diplopia can be masked by intermittent suppression or accompanying field loss (i.e. homonymous hemianopsia). Any interference with binocularity will affect stereopsis and depth perception. In addition, oculomotor disturbances will affect pursuit tracking, saccades, and fixations.

For those experiencing blurred vision at near, accommodative insufficiency or accommodative spasms have been found as an interfering mechanism causing the related symptoms. Studies have also related binocularity with the neurological correlates such as cranial nerve palsies (35).

The term divergence paralysis was first described by Parinaud in 1883. Relative to TBI, the literature emphasizes the third nerve palsy as being the cause of the majority of those with exotropia following a TBI (34). Other types of neurological disorders affecting binocularity are sixth nerve palsies causing esotropia and fourth nerve palsies affecting vertical imbalances.

Sensory motor and binocular analysis should be performed to evaluate oculomotor function. Assessment should use quantity of function to analyze any limitations of oculomotor movements as well as quality of function (assessing fixation losses and difficulties encountered with pursuit tracking or saccadic fixations into particular fields). This may relate to oculomotor palsies. The assessment of convergence and accommodation quantitatively as well as qualitatively will enable the clinician to begin to understand levels of visual stress in performing visual skill activity (23).

The refractive sequence will objectively and subjectively analyze refractive error as well as variations in refractions which may relate to an unstable nature of accommodation and/or subluxation of the accommodative lens following trauma to the eye or head. Careful analysis of eye muscle balance through phoria, vergence, and duction testing will provide the clinician with an understanding of states of eye muscle balance and muscle reserves related to dysfunction of ambient and focal processing. More specifically, a dysfunction of the ambient visual process will cause a lack of spatial support, thus affecting phoria, duction, and/or vergence measurements causing PTVS. In the most severe condition, exotropia can be produced, which is also known as third nerve palsy.

Surgical intervention has been used to affect oculomotor paresis. However, the success from surgery can be compromised if there is interference with the ambient spatial feedforward to binocular cortical cells (23).

The use of botulinum toxin has been found effective in reducing over action and muscle spasticity in affecting general muscle tone in the body as well as in cases of oculomotor spasm (45).

Pupillary assessment can offer an understanding of interruption of afferent and efferent sensory pathways (46). Defects in pupillary function can cause variations in response such as with the Marcus-Gunn pupil (47). Dilation of the consensual response indicates asymmetry in the conduction of afferent sensory fibers anterior to the chiasm and it differentiates a unilateral occurrence.

Wernicke's hemianopic pupil is another method by which to differentiate homonymous hemianopsia of tract lesions from the homonymous hemianopic lesions occurring in optic radiation dysfunction. The pupil sign demonstrates an inappropriate or impaired reaction in both pupils when light is specifically delivered to the amourotic half of either retina (47). Parinaud's syndrome can occur following a TBI and is characterized by displaced pupils, ptosis, nystagmus, oculomotor palsies (limitation of supraduction), papilledema, as well as producing symptoms of vertigo and ataxia (48). Papilledema and optic nerve atrophy are also characteristics that should be carefully evaluated through direct and indirect ophthalmoscopy (48).

PSYCHOPHYSIOLOGICAL TESTING

Evaluation of visual function is important to identify lesions for the purpose of diagnosis and prognosis of treatment in visual problems following a TBI. Two kinds of examinations, psychophysiological and electrophysiological, allow assessment of the disorders in the entire length of the visual pathway. The following is a description of psychophysiological testing.

Visual Acuity

Acuities should be functionally based and objectively based. The assessment of visual acuity should be performed both monocularly and binocularly. The standard Snellen Acuity Test can be performed at six meters and forty centimeters. However, other types of tests may be more appropriate if there is vision impairment present.

Tests such as the Feinbloom charts and the Sloan Acuity Charts may offer more precise measurements.

Behavioral assessment and functional variations should be noted such as a monocular acuity that is better than a binocular acuity. Often, interferences with contrast sensitivity following post-trauma vision syndrome will affect acuity in varying environmental conditions (49).

Visual acuity and visual field assessments are routinely psychophysiological tests. However, motion perception is also one of the elementary visual phenomena, especially in the affect from neurological trauma.

Visual Field Also important is a careful assessment of the visual field (50, 51). Visual field is an island or hill of vision in a sea of darkness (Figure 29-1). When visual defects occur, the corresponding part of the island is lost. The field of vision at any particular sensitivity level is changed.

Abnormalities of any point along the visual pathway affect the visual field, often in a pattern characteristic of a particular disorder process or location. The visual field defects in the visual pathway correlate with the lesion sites and field defects. Homonymous refers to a defect present in both eyes with the same laterality, while heteronymous refers to visual loss that usually respects the vertical meridian. Congruous fields are symmetric in both eyes. The lesions of upper or lower occipital banks produce quadrantanopia defects, while lesions within the temporal and parietal lobes cause field defects that tend not to respect the horizontal meridian.

More sensitive and precise evaluation of visual field can be obtained by automated and computerized threshold perimeter or kinetic testing of Goldmann perimeter. In many instances, the computerized threshold perimetry is a more reproducible test for patients with defects on optic neuropathies, chiasmal disturbances and so on. Computerized threshold perimeter performs static threshold

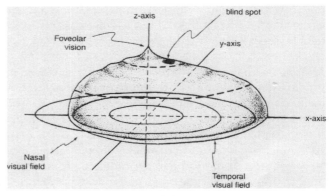

FIGURE 29-1

Visual field is an island or hill of vision in a sea of darkness (57)

measurement. New statistical software empowers the user with additional means of refining the assessment and representation of visual field.

The Goldmann perimeter allows interaction with the examiner and may be more appropriate for patients with neurological impairments. It is a substantially more sophisticated method of field assessment. Kinetic perimetry is usually the preferred method. It involves moving the target from a non-seeing area into a seeing area. A contour map of the island of vision can thus be established by using targets of varying size and brightness. Computerized perimetry is currently the more popular test method in visual field testing.

The visual field must be tested for each eye separately. The visual field is a dynamic area that changes according to a large number of variables. It should always keep in mind that all modalities for visual field evaluation are subjective and depend on the patient's level of alertness, cooperation, ability to fixate centrally, and response rapidity.

Visual field assessment should include standard objective instrument measurements of threshold visual fields when possible, but persons with traumatic brain injury may not be able to sustain attention and organization for a purposeful evaluation in automated field tests. Confrontation visual field assessment which will include holding the person's gaze while presenting objects in the peripheral field are effective as well as a saccadic confrontation visual field assessment. The latter can be used effectively for individuals who cannot hold fixation and are peripherally distractible.

The methods for this form of testing are to provide stimuli or targets in various portions of the field. The examiner observes the functional behavior of the patient as they shift their eyes via saccadic movements into the various visual fields. This may be performed monocularly as well as binocularly.

Homonymous deficits often will relate to spatial problems affecting posture and balance. Visual field neglect is a condition in which there is no hemianopsia, but spatial information in the affected field (usually the left visual field) is ignored (24). Dysfunction caused by field loss will be discussed later in this chapter.

Motion Perception   Motion perception is as elementary a visual perception as form or color senses (52). It includes three-dimension stereo-sense, location, and layer sense. The projected pathway of motion perception is from retinal sensory cells through ganglion cells, lateral geniculate body of thalamus to striate cortex. The abnormalities of motion perception have been seen in optic neuropathy and glaucoma and it was also reported that motion perception decreased or diminished in cerebral traumatic patients with normal visual acuity or color perception.

Three methods for evaluating motion perception are used: 1) using the motion stimuli of the random dots; 2) using the stimuli of sinusoidal grating strips; and 3) using bar target stimuli. The bar targets projected on a monitor can be observed clearly and distinguished easily by subjects. The size and density of bar targets as well as variations in direction of the bars and flickers can be controlled (vertical, horizontal, and oblique).

ELECTROPHYSIOLOGICAL TESTING

Most electrophysiological tests are evoked responses for which adjusting stimulus conditions and techniques of recording makes possible a representation of the sequence of events along the visual pathway (53–55). Besides international standards of ERG, PERG, EOG, and VEP, it is necessary that each laboratory should have its own normal data to evaluate patient's response recording because the amplitude and implicit time of wave may vary among laboratories.

Visual Evoked Response (VEP)

Visual evoked response is a measure of the electrical activity through the visual cortex. Certain conditions are required for VEP measurement: visual stimulus, scalp electrodes, amplifier, averaging system, and recording equipment. The electrodes are positioned in the midline at the occipital and posterior frontal region. An electrode placed on the ear provides a ground.

VEP is response to stimulation by flashes or pattern stimuli with alternating checkerboard or stripes on a monitor. The flash VEP is applied in the persons with very poor vision. A full field Ganzfeld stimulator is used for flash stimuli. The pattern stimulus is preferable when the eye is optically correctable, since the occipital cortex is more sensitive to sharp edges and contrast, while it is relatively insensitive to diffuse light.

The VEP is characterized by the waves N, P, N, and P. The amplitude and implicit time of the wave depends on the check size, contrast, and frequencies of the stimulus. The temporal aspect (latency) of the VEP is more reliable with the significance in clinical application of acuity and focalization, however, the amplitude of VEP under binocular assessment has more relevance to ambient spatial relationships.

The VEP traditionally has been used to confirm the diagnosis of neuropathy in the visual system. It assesses disorder of optic nerve fibers, estimates visual acuity in nonverbal and verbal persons, evaluates potentials for reasonable visual acuity in some kinds of patients, and detects and locates visual field. In some cases, the VEP is even more sensitive for detecting compressive lesions than subjective perimetry.

Multifocal Visual Electrophysiology

Multifocal Electroretinogram (mfERG)

Multifocal Evoked Response (mfVEP) In 1992, Sutter and his co-workers reported presenting pseudorandomly multifocal stimulation together with retinal or cortical scaling of the size of the stimulated areas. They were able to stimulate numerous locations of the visual field simultaneously and to extract individual responses from each of them. The electrode permitted the recording of reliable responses from numerous retinal locations such as areas 61, 103, 241 loci of the visual field. This work establishes the multifocal electroretinogram (mfERG) and multifocal visual evoked response (mfVEP) with field topographic mapping of ERG or VEP components.

The mfERG or mfVEP is based on the Wiener kernel expansion and uses deterministic pseudorandom binary m-sequence stimulation. It permits computation of the signal by cross-correlation of the response evoked by m-sequence stimulation with m-sequence itself. Therefore, it is very effective for mapping.

The technique allows computation of the first order or higher order kernel which characterizes the nonlinear interaction between visual events. The amplitude of the averaged quadratic VEPs is in proportion to visual field losses. The mfERG or mfVEP is a powerful method for the investigation of brain activity and mechanisms of human visual perception.

Electrophysiological analysis through use of binocular visual evoked potentials assesses the relationship of support for focal processing by the ambient (spatial) system (10).

The visual evoked potential should be performed with habitual corrective lenses. A P100 cross-pattern reversal analysis is performed. Following the initial response, two diopters of base-in prism in conjunction with binasal occlusion should be introduced before both eyes in addition to the corrective lenses. The amplitude and latency of the P100 should be compared. An amplitude increase following the introduction of base-in prism with binasal occlusion is seen as a test positive for PTVS (11).

Electro-Oculogram (EOG) The EOG technique of recording eye movement is widely available and reliable. Since the eye acts as a dipole, the electrical current changes are caused between the cornea and posterior pole of the eyeball when the eye is moving in different directions. The EOG is performed by placing four cutaneous electrodes are placed on the canthal regions of both eyes. An electrode placed on the ear serves as the ground. The potential is recorded when alternate fixations or target movement is performed. Changes in illumination, skin resistance, and speed of the target will affect the results of the EOG. The EOG can yield reasonable recordings of horizontal movements, however, vertical movements may be affected by eyelid blinks and nonlinearities.

Observation of eye movements by the clinicians provides a simple qualitative assessment and in most cases is able to identify most abnormalities. Therefore, the EOG is used to distinguish the affects of specific ocular modalities and to determine the presence or absence of improved motor function during therapy for visual pathways.

NEURO-MOTOR ASSESSMENT

The neuro-motor assessment can be performed to evaluate the role of the ambient visual process in establishing concepts of visual midline and how it affects posture, balance, and movement. Concerning posture, dysfunction of the ambient visual process will also affect seating position and posture.

The visual midline test may be performed in those individuals that can respond actively (10). Observation of the patient in a seated position as well as during ambulation should be performed to evaluate the correlation of the visual midline shift test to tendencies to drift to one side and/or lean forward or backward during ambulation. Lateral shift of the visual midline will often cause a lean or drift during ambulation. An anterior shift can cause a lean or flexion forward. In more severe cases of the anterior shift of visual midline, toe-walking will develop in an attempt to compensate for the imbalance. A posterior shift of visual midline will cause an extension posture and tendency to lean backward in retropulsion.

VISUAL-VESTIBULAR INTEGRATION DYSFUNCTION

There are numerous treatises that discuss the anatomy, physiology, and treatment of the separate visual, vestibular, and sensory motor systems, however, until recently, few were able to discuss the functional integration and relationships that exist between these three systems. Dizziness, vertigo, and imbalance are common symptoms following a TBI and often indicate miscommunication between these systems. Inner-ear disorder of the vestibular system is a common diagnosis, however, the relationship to the visual process is often overlooked or misinterpreted.

Coordinated movement involves a complex interaction between sensory afferents from the visual system, somatosensory system, and the vestibular system. In particular, the semicircular canals and utricle/saccule respond to rotational and linear/gravitational information and is transmitted via the vestibule-cochlear nerve through the ascending and descending axon branches of the brainstem vestibular nuclei. At times, vision supercedes or enhances vestibular input. The vestibulo-ocular reflex (which maintains foveal fixation during head movements), the vestibulospinal pathways (which are responsible for postural control under static and dynamic circumstances), and the vestibulocerebellar pathways (allowing for modulation of motor output via the flocculonodular lobe of the cerebellum) are all integrated at this level of the brainstem.

The vestibular nuclei accept information from the visual system relative to the ambient visual process to support movement and visual interaction of the environment. The subset of the ambient process, the magnocellular system, provides information about perception of contrast and movement involving short wavelength and low and middle spatial frequency input. This affects awareness of depth perception, motion detection, and alterations in brightness. The parvocellular system is mostly responsible for detail discrimination, color perception, and identification of patterns or shapes.

An important differential between magnocellular and parvocellular processing is that the former is responsive to the onset and offset of receptive stimuli, whereas the latter is responsive to longer stimulus duration. Parvocellular input projects to the occipital lobes along the retinal-geniculate-cortical pathway and then may send axons to the temporal brain region. It is the ambient process inclusive of the magnocellular system that supports posture, balance, and spatial orientation. Information synapsing in the occipital lobe will proceed to temporal and parietal lobes for higher level processing while the information from the superior colliculus will integrate with head and body postural reflexes flowing through the vestibulospinal and vestibulocerebellar tracts.

The vestibulo-visual relationship supports a stabilization of vision during movement of the head, neck, or body. Diplopia is the most frequently considered symptom of disruption in this interaction in addition to other interferences with binocularity.

The significance of the vestibulo-oculo-cervical triad is the quality and organization of somatosensory input (20) which occurs in the thalamus and is transmitted to the cerebellum and primary somatosensory cortex within the parietal lobe. Multisensory integration and conscious perception occur as this information is projected into the secondary and association cortices of the frontal, temporal, and parietal lobes where the perception of dizziness, vertigo, or imbalance may be the result.

A complete medical history with careful analysis of the visual process and vestibular system is necessary for diagnosis and prognosis. Too often, functional vestibular rehabilitation for vertigo and dizziness is begun before the relationship to visual processing problems is determined. Under the age of fifty, TBI is the most common cause of dizziness and vertigo from a direct head trauma and whiplash.

Differential diagnosis for dizziness without vestibular dysfunction includes PTVS, hyperventilation, dehydration,

orthostatic hypotension, vasovagal syndrome, arteriosclerosis, osteoarthritis, and central nervous system disorders. A Group II Disorder such as aortic, carotid, vertebrobasilar, subclavian, and cerebral artery insufficiency should be ruled out.

Once a Group II disorder has been ruled out, vestibular anomalies such as vestibular neuritis (acute labyrinthitis), benign paroxysmal positional vertigo (BPPV), nucleo-reticular vestibular syndrome, Meniere's Disease, Perilymphatic Hypertension, and Perilymphatic Fistula should be ruled out.

Since destabilization of the ambient process following trauma has been clinically found to cause vertigo and dizziness which are symptoms of PTVS. By treating PTVS, stability is created in ambient visual processing, thereby increasing the efficiency of matching information with vestibular, kinesthetic, and proprioceptive processes. This, in turn, frequently reduces or eliminates symptoms of vertigo and dizziness.

VISUAL FIELD DYSFUNCTION

A visual field loss is relative to the area of cortical lesion or optic nerve insult. Field defects that occur beyond the optic chiasm will always cause a homonymous hemianopsia not necessarily congruous (56). Depending upon the area of the cortex affected, geniculate lesions are often not suspected and are rarely diagnosed. However, in the case of a homonymous hemianopsia involving primarily the central visual field sparing the peripheral field, the geniculate body should be considered as the source.

Temporal lobe lesions will often produce an incongruous superior quadrantopsia with a sloping margin. In addition to field loss, parietal lobe lesions cause a lack of awareness of the field loss. It can be differentiated by confrontation visual field assessment when the clinician presents simultaneous targets in opposite fields. The parietal lobe lesion will cause an extinction phenomenon yielding a person to be aware of only one target at a time. If the target is moving in both fields, often the extinction phenomenon will not occur. The target must be stationary in order to demonstrate the possibility of a parietal lobe lesion. The common defect is an inferior homonymous quadrantopsia.

Occipital lobe lesions are characterized mostly by their congruous nature. These can encompass the entire hemianopic field or portions thereof depending on the specific location of the lesion. Riddoch's phenomenon described in 1917, involves the inability to see stationary objects presented on the affected side but could see objects that were moving. Recent research related to focal and ambient visual processing suggests that the ambient visual process is a survival system that particularly responds to movement in the peripheral vision. Perhaps an additional interpretation from the original one would be that areas of the lesion are being circumvented when feedforward occurs from the ambient visual process. However, when stationary targets are presented to those with PTVS in conjunction with a field loss, it will cause them to over-focalize on the sensory component of the target they are looking at. This over-focalization and lack of an ambient feedforward response can possibly cause a condition related to field neglect and/or extinction phenomenon.

Like visual field loss, visuospatial neglect may manifest as a complete loss of visual perception on the side affected or as a relative loss where less is perceived in the neglected field particularly when there are competing stimuli in the opposite hemifield (57). With appropriate treatment, the functional effect of the hemianopsia and/or neglect can be minimized. Patients with visual field loss who do not receive training, rarely use adaptive search strategies (58). Training the patient to scan into the area of loss, in some cases, creates incomplete recovery of visual field (59–62). Zihl and von Cramon (63) have reported extensive field recovery taking place only during periods of appropriate treatment. Patients with visuospatial neglect require additional training to gain skills for compensation for many activities of daily living.

A homonymous hemianopsia can be functionally very debilitating to the patient in rehabilitation. Not only does it represent a complete loss of visual field, but it also affects concepts of midline. The concept of visual midline shift syndrome is an important one to understand relative to visual motor rehabilitation for any person following a TBI, but particularly for those who have suffered a homonymous hemianopsia. When the visual midline shifts and the individual begins to lean in the direction of the midline, the sensory stimulation from the proprioceptive, kinesthetic, and vestibular system will reinforce the lack of weight bearing on the paretic side. In turn, this also reinforces the development of spatial neglect.

To counter the compressions and expansions that distort spatial perception following TBI, prisms can be effectively used. A prism is a wedge of glass or plastic. Optically when one looks through a prism, the image of what is being looked at appears to be shifted toward the apex or thin edge of the prism and away from the base or thick edge. The shift in image occurs because the prism expands space on one side and compresses space on the other. The prism expands and compresses in a three dimensional manner, but for the purpose of this discussion let us consider it only two dimensionally. The prism can be used to alter the distortion of space caused by a visual midline shift if placed in the appropriate direction before each eye. This is termed a yoked prism system. The amount of prism can be varied depending upon the amount of distortion in the visual process. Yoked prisms are an effective means by which to shift the concept of visual midline, but also should be used in conjunction

with other methods of field enhancement or to increase awareness in the affected homonymous hemianopic field.

An enhanced sector prism system is used to affect homonymous hemianopsia by increasing awareness of peripheral visual fields on a sensory level, whereas the yoked prism is used to affect VMSS sensory motor level. The enhanced sector prism system (mounted binocularly or monocularly) is positioned to the side of the line of sight in a spectacle frame with the base end of the prism positioned temporally in the direction of the hemianopic field. When looking into the prism(s), the image will be shifted toward the apex enabling the individual to see objects to the side they would normally not be able to see unless they took a significant eye and head turn in the direction of the hemianopic field. Many individuals with a homonymous hemianopsia frequently bump their head and body on objects that they did not see. This causes numerous bruises as well as the possibility of more significant injuries.

The experienced clinician will recognize that individuals who have a visual midline shift syndrome as well as a homonymous hemianopsia will often have difficulty adapting to the use and succeeding with an enhanced sector prism system because the midline reinforces the spatial neglect. Therefore, treatment with yoked prisms for VMSS is necessary prior to or in conjunction with an enhanced sector prism system. By addressing the issue of VMSS, the success of rehabilitation with an enhanced sector prism system will be increased. The combination of yoked prism in the carrier lenses as well as the sector field prism positioned appropriately laterally to the line of sight can be an effective combination. Rehabilitation with yoked prisms to treat visual midline shift syndrome will directly affect field neglect as well as VMSS. Training can then be established to utilize the enhanced sector prism systems (49, 64). In other cases of visual loss including trauma with constricted visual fields, single or multiple prisms are used mounted laterally on each lens (65).

Sector prism systems used to increase a patient's peripheral awareness can be made out of Fresnel press-on prisms (66). Peli (67) reported that the press-on sectoral prisms when applied to the upper and lower part of the spectacle lens causes a refractive exotropia and thus improves simultaneous awareness and greater obstacle avoidance. However, due to the poor optical quality of the press-on Fresnel prisms, sometimes patients experience a decrease in acuity, or have problems with reflections or distortions which negatively affect the patient's acceptance and success (66). Gottlieb, et al. (65) found that press-on prisms sometimes even decreased a patient's tendency to scan into their field of neglect due to their dislike of looking through these prisms and hence amplified avoidance of this area.

Complex visual loss is no longer an insurmountable obstacle in the way of effective rehabilitation and recovery

of function. Using technology along with proven rehabilitation strategies can aid in meeting the goals of the
patient and rehabilitation team.

Literature reinforces that enhanced sector prism systems yield fewer mishaps of bumping into objects or people and their fear of collisions notably decrease (68, 69).
The primary result of this improved function is an increase
in safety and secondarily a decreased risk for insult and
injury (70). In the long term, a patient may experience
some recovery of vision in the hemianopic field (49).
In a study by Gottlieb, Freeman, and Williams in 1992,
27 of the 34 patients who had been fitted with enhanced
sector prism systems to use them full or part time over
the next 2.5 years. The prism used in this study increased
the patient's peripheral field awareness an average of
13.25 degrees.

VISUAL PHENOMENA ASSOCIATED WITH TBI

Visual phenomena following a TBI can be quite diverse.
Sometimes these phenomena are bizarre and assumed to
be of psychological nature. Some of these symptoms will
be visual hallucinations, flashing lights, palinopsia, variations in homonymous field defects, and scintillating sco-
tomas. It has been reported that visual hallucinations can
be associated with temporal and parietal lobe lesions. Following a TBI, individuals may report hallucinations that
take several forms. Some individuals will experience movement of the visual field. Sometimes, the entire visual field
will appear to shift or move as they move their eyes or
body. Others will report seeing movement in their peripheral vision but when they turn to look, they find only stationary objects. Another common hallucination is seeing
things or persons in the periphery and/or central vision.
Some patients report seeing snakes dropping from the ceiling or wriggling across the floor. Others will perceive
strange type of creatures appearing to move and shift.

Many of these phenomena are reported by persons
who have PTVS. It has been found clinically that treatment for post-trauma vision syndrome will often stop the
perceived hallucinations (23). Although it has been noted
in literature that parietal and temporal lobe lesions as
well as occipital lobe lesions can be the cause of these hallucinations, it has also been suggested that some of the
hallucinations may be due to psychiatric disorders. It is
not uncommon for persons following a TBI who are
experiencing hallucinations to be placed on psychotropic
medications. It is the author's experience that many of
the hallucinations will persist even though these medications are being used.

One possible explanation for the existence of hallucinations following TBI is that when there is dysfunction to the ambient visual process, the ability to stabilize

the retinal image is compromised. The superior colliculus
is responsible to a great extent for providing the spatial
matched information for ambient and sensory motor
processes to the occipital cortex but more specifically, to
provide a stabilization of the peripheral retina. When the
ambient visual process is compromised, the visual processing system that remains, the focal process, isolates to
detail but does not have a spatial grounding to stabilize
the retinal image.

It has been noted clinically that persons experiencing PTVS will perceive words on a page or objects in the
field appear to move when they perform movements of
their eyes such as saccadic fixations. Saccadic fixations in
a field of vertical lines will produce a shimmering movement of the vertical lines. The lines will appear to move
in various manners similar to the movement of a snake.
It is hypothesized that at least some of the hallucinations
experienced following a traumatic brain injury are due to
the unstable nature of the ambient visual process in PTVS.
The interpretation of 'snakes' and other objects appearing to move are perceived movement of vertical and horizontal lines in their environment due to the unstable
nature of the peripheral retina related to the compromise
of the ambient visual process. It has been found clinically
that by treating individuals for PTVS, the hallucinations
will often cease within hours to days.

BINOCULAR INTERVENTION

Treatment for diplopia varies depending upon the philosophy of the treating doctor as well as the rehabilitation program. Some do not recommend any treatment
and choose to wait to determine if time will be the healing factor. Others recommend patching of the deviating
eye to eliminate the diplopia, whereas others recommend
patching of the fixating eye in order to stimulate fixation
in the eye that is deviating. The lack of any treatment
approach and often an inappropriate treatment regimen
for a person in a state of diplopia can and will interfere
with all aspects of rehabilitation.

The visual process is the dominant and primary sensory motor system affecting all aspects of posture, movement, balance, as well as cognitive-perceptual function.
Vision works to reinforce all that we do. If vision is dysfunctional, it will interfere with all performance.

Failure to eliminate diplopia can directly affect the
outcome of rehabilitation which financially is being
undertaken at tremendous costs by insurance programs
as well as individual funding from families and relatives.
Therefore, in view of the limited amount of time for rehabilitation and the extraordinary amount of money that
is often spent to rehabilitate the person, it is logical to
attempt to rehabilitate the condition causing diplopia
through treatment of PTVS, compensating prism, and/or

vision therapy. It has been suggested that surgical intervention, while possible, is at best a challenge for treating diplopia following a traumatic brain injury (44).

Pathophysiology of Injuries Contributing to Diplopia

Injury to the visual system can be diffuse and/or focal and can localize to any, or a combination of the ocular structures, cortical areas, midbrain, or nerve nuclei. Brain injuries affecting vision typically occur via axonal shearing, hemorrhage, infarct, inflammation, and/or compression. Ophthalmoplegias (cranial nerve palsies) may completely, or partially involve any single or all three of the nerves controlling ocular motility.

The third nerve controls the medial, superior and inferior rectus muscles, inferior oblique, ciliary body, levator, and papillary sphincter muscles. Clinically, a complete acquired CNIII palsy will present with ptosis, hypoexotropia, dilated and fixed pupil, paralysis of accommodation and limitation of gaze on the affected side. Partial involvement can be any combination of, but not all of the above. Spontaneous recovery, if any, is usually within six months.

The sixth nerve controls the lateral rectus muscle. Clinically, the patient will have an esotropia in primary gaze that increases as they attempt to look towards the affected side. There is a limitation of gaze to abduction of the affected eye. Spontaneous recovery, if any, is usually within six months.

The fourth nerve controls the superior oblique muscle. Clinically, the patient will present with their head tilted to the contra-lateral side in an effort to offset cyclical, or torsional movement of their eyes. Spontaneous recovery, if any, usually occurs within six months.

Vision Rehabilitation

Vision Therapy. Vision therapy (also referred to as vision training or orthoptics) is a clinical approach to treat a variety of visual disorders including certain strabismic conditions. The practice of vision therapy uses a variety of non-surgical procedures to modify the visual process affecting function. By first evaluating the bimodal processing of vision, the doctor will establish a plan of treatment designed to affect balance between the focal and ambient visual processes as well as the ability to match information with sensory motor systems. The goal is to improve the visual process and affect binocularity, spatial organization, balance, movement, etc.

Vision therapy will typically involve a series of treatments. During treatment sessions, individually planned activities are conducted under optometric supervision. The specific procedures and necessary instrumentation are determined by the individual patient's needs and the nature and severity of the diagnosed problems. Vision therapy techniques employ the use of lenses, prisms, computers, biofeedback, stereoscopic devices, and a variety of other instruments and techniques designed to affect the visual process.

Prism Rehabilitation As mentioned previously regarding VMSS and visual field loss, prisms are ophthalmic tools that refract light while also compressing and expanding it. Prisms are used clinically in a therapeutic manner to reestablish balance of ambient and focal visual relationships causing visual dysfunction or in a compensatory manner to offset the affects of a binocular imbalance.

In binocular and strabismic dysfunctions, use of prism can reduce symptoms, improve function, and hasten recovery. In these situations, prescription of therapeutic prism (an amount, type, and orientation of prism to reduce or neutralize the binocular/vision dysfunction or to stimulate visual function and fusion) can help reduce or eliminate symptoms and aid treatment. To affect spatial imbalance caused by ambient and focal dysfunction (see PTVS and VMSS), yoked prisms are prescribed.

There are times, patients, and situations when remediation of a visual problem is not possible or feasible. In these situations, prescription of compensatory prism (an amount, type, and orientation of prism to reduce pr neutralize the binocular strabismic dysfunction) can help reduce or eliminate diplopia.

Patching. Patching has frequently been used to eliminate diplopia (21, 71). While effectively eliminating diplopia, patching renders the patient monocular. The chief problems of monocular vision are loss of stereopsis, reduction of peripheral visual field, and VMSS (10, 21, 72).

Monocular vision reduces the field of vision by approximately 25%, decreases stereoscopic vision, decreases visual acuity (due to lack of binocular summation), and impairs spatial orientation. Monocular versus binocular individuals will have a disadvantage in visual motor skills, exteroception of form and color, and appreciation of the dynamic relationship of the body to the environment which facilitates control of manipulation, reaching, and balance (44).

Problems arising from acquired monocular vision will manifest as difficulties in eye hand coordination, clumsiness, bumping into objects and/or people, ascending or descending stairs or curbs, crossing the street, driving, various sports and other activities of daily living which require stereopsis and peripheral vision (72).

In the case of diplopia following TBI, a standard recommendation in acute care facilities and rehabilitation hospitals is to patch one eye. As discussed previously in the section about VMSS, this will cause and/or reinforce a shift in concept of visual midline affecting posture and balance as well as having an adverse affect on physical/occupational therapy.

Patching can be performed but should be done with respect to the ambient visual process. A central occlusion patch can be placed on the deviating eye. For example, if there is a left exotropia, vertical adhesive tape can be placed in front of the deviating eye so that it is built from the nasal portion of the eyeglass frame out to just block the center of the pupil or line of sight. In this way, diplopia will be eliminated when the person looks directly at something, but the peripheral field of the deviating eye is respected by not covering it. In turn, it allows the ambient visual process of both eyes to begin to match information with other sensory motor systems. This will support visual midline concept for posture, balance, and ambulation.

Another method involves use of a partial and selective occlusion. The spot patch is a procedure that eliminates diplopia without compromising peripheral vision (73). It is a small, usually round or oval patch made of adhesive tape, blurring film, or other filters. It is placed on the lens of glasses and directly in the line of sight of one eye. The diameter is generally about one centimeter, but will vary on the individual angular subtense required for the particular strabismus, ophthalmoplegia, or gaze palsy. Final size and placement is determined by evaluating different sizes and shapes to arrive at the smallest one which effectively eliminates the diplopia. If there is a paresis, the spot patch should be placed in front of the affected eye.

By eliminating diplopia through central occlusion, the ambient process becomes more effective and supportive. The spot patch is indicated in cases of intractable diplopia where other methods of treatment are either not viable, have failed, or are contraindicated. Examples of such cases include refractory, third nerve ophthalmoplegia, sixth nerve palsy, and inter-nuclear ophthalmoplegia. Central occlusion is effective if the diplopia is constant and the patient exhibits relief and improved general function as a result of eliminating the diplopia.

Determining size, shape, and placement of a central occlusion patch requires measuring the diplopic field, determining limitation of ocular motility, and measuring the angle of strabismic deviation.

CONCLUSION

Rehabilitation of a person with a traumatic brain injury requires applying the science of understanding neurological dysfunctions as they pertain to interference with motor, sensory, and cognitive processes. Until recently, if a person suffered visual dysfunction in the way of binocular, spatial perception, and/or perceptual motor dysfunction, rehabilitation treatment was limited to patching of the deviating eye causing diplopia or primarily hospital based occupational and physical therapy.

Recent research has demonstrated that often traumatic brain injury affects visual processing which can cause or relate to the performance dysfunction as well as binocular problems. Neuro-ophthalmology has provided an important means of intervention for neurological problems affecting the visual system. Diagnostic assessment through use of electro-physiology analysis in addition to the state of the art assessment through MRI and CT scan enables a neuro-ophthalmologist to function as a critical member of a multi-disciplinary team serving the person with a TBI. A careful evaluation of cranial nerve function and abnormalities is essential for establishing the diagnosis as well as determining appropriate neuro-medical recommendations for treatment. A range of options are available such as utilizing medications, botulinus toxin, and surgery.

Experience has shown that skilled optometrists familiar with the practice of neuro-optometric rehabilitation can be an important contributing member to the rehabilitation team. The skills of the optometrist are in applying the new science and understanding of the bimodal process of vision to the art of visual rehabilitation. The neuro-optometric rehabilitation evaluation involves the careful analysis of binocularity and spatial and perceptual motor function related to dysfunction between the ambient and focal visual processes by utilizing a variety of techniques incorporating lenses, prisms, and sectoral occlusion. The optometrist can affect performance and function at the appropriate critical stages of rehabilitation not being provided in rehabilitation hospitals and long-term care programs. This does not exclude individuals who are still suffering from binocular and spatial-motor disorders after being released from such programs. Neuro-optometric rehabilitation has been found effective in improving binocularity as well as visual spatial-motor dysfunctions affecting balance and posture by treating PTVS and VMSS years after the neurological insult has occurred.

The role of the neuro-ophthalmologist as well as the optometrist practicing neuro-optometric rehabilitation are important in advancing overall rehabilitation for a person with a TBI. The neuro-ophthalmologist and optometrist will provide critical insights into neurological dysfunction as well as the means by which to rehabilitate the high incidence and prevalence of visual dysfunction affecting performance following a traumatic brain injury.

References

1. Hellerstein LF, Fishman B. Vision Therapy and Occupational Therapy an Integrated Approach. *J of Behavioral Optometry* 1990;1:122–126.
2. Sabates N, Gouce M, Farris B. Neuro-Ophthalmologic Findings in Closed Head Trauma. *J of Clinical Neuro-Ophthalmology* 1991;11:273–277.
3. Gianutsos R, Glosser D, Elbaum J, Vrounen G. Visual Interception in Brain-Injured Adults: Multifaceted Measures. *Research Phys Med Rehab* 1983;64:456–461.
4. Hart C. Disturbances of Fusion Following Head Injury. *Proceedings of the Royal Society of Med* 1964;62.

5. Carroll R. Acute Loss of Fusional Convergence Following Head Trauma. *Archives of Ophthalmology* 1984;88:57–59.
6. Stanworth A. Defects of Ocular Movement and Fusion after Head Injury. *British J of Ophthalmology* 1974;58:266–271.
7. Sergent J. Interference from Unilateral Brain Damage about Normal Hemispheric Functions in Visual Pattern Recognition. *Psychological Bulletin* 1984;96:99–115.
8. Gianutsos R, Ramsey G, Perlin R. Rehabilitation Optometric Services for Survivors of Acquired Brain Injury. *Archive of Phys Med Rehab* 1988;69:573–588.
9. Zolltan B. Visual, Visual Perceptual and Perceptual-Motor Deficits in Brain Injured Adults. *Traumatic Brain Injury* 1992;3:337–355.
10. Padula W, Argyris S. Post-Trauma Vision Syndrome and Visual Midline Shift Syndrome. *J NeuroRehab* 1996;6:165–171.
11. Padula W, Argyris S, Ray J. Visual Evoked Potentials (VEP) Evaluating Treatment for Post-Trauma Syndrome (PTVS) in Patients with Traumatic Brain Injury (TBI). *Brain Injury* 1994;8:125–133.
12. Rapport M, Herrero-Backe C, Winterfield K, Rapport ML, Hemuerle A. Visual Evoked Potential Pattern Abnormalities and Disability in Severe Traumatic Brain Injured Patients. *J Head Trauma* 1989;4:45–52.
13. Sarno S, Erasmus G, Lippert M, Lipp B, Schlaegel W. Electrophysiological Correlates of Visual Impairment after Traumatic Brain Injury. *Vision Research* 2000;40:3029–3038.
14. Catz A, Ron S, Soliz P, Korczyn A. Vestibulo-Ocular Reflex Suppression Following Hemispheric Stroke. *Scand J Rehab Med* 1993;25:149–152.
15. Wolfe E. *Anatomy of the Eye and Orbit* Philadelphia:Saunders Co, 1968.
16. Benabib R, Nelson C. Efficiency in Visual Skills and Postural Control:Dynamic Interaction. *Occupational Therapy Practice* 1991; 3:57–68.
17. Gesell A, Ieg F, Bullis F. *Vision: It's Development in Infant and Child* Santa Ana CA: Optometric Extension Program Publishers, 1998.
18. Trevarthen CB, Sperry R. Perceptual Unity of the Ambient Visual Field in Human Commissurotomy Patients. *Brain* 1973;96:547–70.
19. Liebowitz H, Post R, Beck JJ (ed.). *The Two Modes of Visual Processing Concept and Some Implications in Organization and Representation in Perception* New Jersey, 1982.
20. Moore J. *Brain Atlas and Functional Systems* Rockville MD: American Occupational Therapy Assoc, 1993.
21. Borish I. *Paralytic Strabismus Clinical Refraction, 3rd Edition* Chicago IL: The Professional Press Inc, 1975.
22. Nashold B, Seaber J. Defects of Ocular Motility after Stereo Tactic Midbrain Lesions in Man. *Arch of Ophthalomolgy* 1972;88: 245–248.
23. Padula W. *Neuro-Optometric Rehabilitation* Santa Ana CA: Optometric Extension Program Publishers, 2000.
24. Streff J. Visual Rehabilitation of Hemianopic Head Trauma Patients Emphasizing Ambient Pathways. *Neuro Rehab* 1996;6: 173–181.
25. Posner M, Raickle M. *Images of Mind* New York: Scientific American Library, 1994.
26. Eubank T, Ooi T. Improving Visually Guided Action Perceptual Through Use of Prisms. *Inst of American Optometric Assoc* 2001;7227.
27. Cartwright R, Seth R. *Brain Injury Source* 2001;3:32–45.
28. Gianutsos R, Ramsey G. Enabling Rehabilitation Optometrists to Survivors of Acquired Brain Injury. *Inst of Vision Rehab* 1998;2: 37–58.
29. Horn L, Zasler N. The Neuromedical Diagnosis and Management of Post-Concussive Disorders. *J Phys Med and Rehab: State of Art Reviews* 1992;6.
30. Suter P. *Rehabilitation and Management of Visual Dysfunction Following Traumatic BrainInjury* Boca Raton FL: CRC Press Inc, 1995.
31. Rook J. *Whiplash Injuries* Butterworth/Heinemann, 2003.
32. Soden R, Cohen A. An Optometric Approach to the Treatment of Noncomitant Deviation. *J American Optometric Assoc* 1983; 54:451–454.
33. Rutkowski P, Bureau H. Divergence Paralysis Following Head Trauma. *J American Ophthalmology* 1982;73:660–662.
34. Weed H. Divergence Paralysis Due to Head Injury. *Transcript, American Academy Ophthalmology*;1934;39:189.
35. Neger R. The Evolution of Diplopia in Head Trauma. *J Head Trauma Rehab* 1989;4:27–34.
36. Streff J. The Use of Binasal Occluded Treatment for Patients with Head Trauma. *Neuro-Opt Rehab Assoc Newsletter* 1992;2.
37. Brooks V. *The Neural Basis of Motor Control* New York: Oxford University Press, 1986.
38. Politzer T. *Vision Function, Examination, and Rehabilitation in Patients Suffering from Traumatic Brain Injury. Minor Traumatic Brain Injury, Diagnosis and Treatment* Boca Raton FL: CRC Press, 2000.
39. Cogan D. *Neurology of Ocular Muscles, 2nd Edition* Thomas, 1955.
40. Warren M. A Hierarchical Model for Evaluation and Treatment of Visual Perceptual Dysfunction in Adult Acquired Brain Injury, Part 1. *American J of Occupational Therapy* 1993;47:46–66.
41. Shaw J. Rehabilitation of Neuropsychological Disorders: A Practical Guide for Rehabilitation Professionals. *Psychology Press* 2001.
42. Cherney L, Halper A. Unilateral Visual Neglect in Right Hemisphere Stroke: A Longitudinal Study. *Brain Injury* 2001;15(7): 585–592.
43. Landis T. Disruption of Space Perception due to Cortical Lesions. *Spatial Vision* 2000;13(2, 3):179–191.
44. von Noorden G. *Etiology of Heterophoria and Heterotropia. Binocular Vision and Ocular Motility, 4th Edition* St Louis MO: CV Mosley Co, 1990.
45. Zasler, Nathan. *Brain Injury Source*;1998;2 (4).
46. Moses R. *Adler's Physiology of the Eye* St. Louis, MO: CV Mosley Co, 1970.
47. Harley R. *Pediatric Ophthalmology* Philadelphia PA: WB Saunders Co, 1975.
48. Gieraets W. *Ocular Syndromes* Philadelphia PA: Lea & Febiger, 1976.
49. Gottlieb DD, Fuhr A, Hatch WV, Wright KD. Neuro-Optometric Facilitation of Vision Recovery After Acquired Brain Injury. *NeuroRehabilitation* 1998;197–199.
50. Parrish RK. *Atlas of Ophthalmology* Boston MA: Butterworth Heinman, 2000.
51. Mesulam M. Spatial Attention and Neglect: Parietal, Frontal and Cingulated Contributions to the Mental Representation and Intentional Targeting of Salient Extra Personal Events. *Philosophical Transactions of the Royal Society of London, Series B: Biological Sciences* 1999;29:1325–46.
52. Wang JD, Wu DZ, Fltzke, FW. The Test of Motion Perception of the Normal Chinese Subjects. *Chinese Medical Journal* 1998;111(3):275–277.
53. Klistorner A, Graham S, Grigg J, Billsou F. Multifocal Topographic Visual Evoked Potential: Improving Objective Detection of Local Visual Field Defects. *Ophthalmology Visual Science* 1998;39(6):937–950.
54. Miller N, Newman, N. *Clinical Neuro-Ophthalmology, 5th Edition* Baltimore MD: The Essentials, 1999.
55. Forrester J, Dick A, Mcnamin P, Lee W. *The Eye, 2nd Edition* Edinburgh: WB Saunders, 2002.
56. Silverstone D, Hirsh J. *Automated Visual Field Testing: Techniques of Examination and Interpretation* Norwalk CT: Appleton-Century-Crofts, 1986.
57. Liu GT, Volpe NJ, Galetta SL. *Neuro-Ophthalmology, Diagnosis and Management* WB Saunders, 2001.
58. Kerkoff G, Munsinger U, Haof E, Meier E. Neurovisual Rehabilitation in Cerebral Blindness. *Archive of Neurology* 1994;51: 474–481.
59. Zilh J, von Cramon D. Recovery of Visual Functions in Patients with Cerebral Blindness: Effect of Specific Practice with Saccadic Localization. *Exp Brain Research* 1981;44:159–169.
60. Zilh J, von Cramon D. Restitution of Visual Field in Patients with Damage to the Geniculostraite Visual Pathway. *Human Neurobiology* 1982;1:5–8.
61. Zilh J, von Cramon D. Visual Field Recovery from Scotoma Patients with Post Geniculate Damage. *Brain* 1985;108:335–365.
62. Zilh J, von Cramon. Visual Field Rehabilitation in the Cortically Blind. *J Neural Neurosurgery Psychiatry* 1986;49:965–967.

63. Zilh J, von Cramon. Restitution of Visual Function in Patients with Cerebral Blindness. *J Neural Neurosurgery Psychiatry* 1979; 42:312–322.

64. Hellerstein LF, Fishman B. Vision Therapy and Occupational Therapy an Integrated Approach. *J Behavioral Optometry* 1990; 1(5):122–126.

65. Gottlieb DD, Allen CH, Eikenberry J, Woodruff SI, Johnson M. *Living With Vision Loss – Independence, Driving and Low Vision Solutions* St. Barthelemy Press Ltd, 1996.

66. Lee AG, Perez AM. Improving Awareness of Peripheral Visual Field Using Sectoral Prism. *J American Optometric Assoc* 1999; 70:624–8.

67. Peli E. Field Expansion of Homonymous Hemianopsia by Optically Induced Peripheral Exotropia. *Optometry and Vision Science* 2000;77:453–464.

68. Park W. Post-Trauma Vision Syndrome: Prescribing Prism for the Brain Injury Patient. *Primary Care Optometry News* 1998; 31–32.

69. Windsor RL, Windsor L. Low Vision Rehabilitation. *The Rehabilitation Professional* 2001;9(2):37–45.

70. Snowden S. Treating the Older Patient Geriatric Optometry. *The Southern J Optometry* 1997;15(1):7–10.

71. Griffin J. *Management of Horror Fusional Binocular Anomalies Procedure for Vision, 2nd Edition* Chicago IL: The Professional Press Inc, 1978.

72. Brady F. *A Singular View: The Art of Seeing with One Eye, 2nd Edition* Ordell NJ: Medical Economics Co, 1979.

73. Politzer T. Case Studies of a New Approach Using Partial and Selective Occlusion for the Clinical Treatment of Diplopia. *Neuro Rehab* 1996;6:213–217.

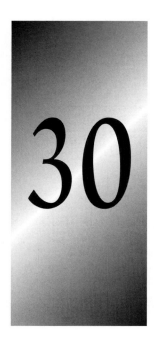

30 Cranial Nerve Disorders

Flora M. Hammond
Brent E. Masel

INTRODUCTION

Cranial nerves provide motor and sensory innervation to the head and neck, and are termed such owing to the fact that they emerge from the cranium. Injury to the cranial nerves is common with traumatic brain injury (TBI). In this chapter the anatomy, pathway, function, injury incidence, mechanism of injury, examination, treatment, and prognosis will be discussed for each of the cranial nerves. Introductory information about cranial nerves and their injury is briefly reviewed before discussing each nerve individually.

The true incidence of cranial nerve injuries is difficult to estimate. The olfactory nerve (cranial nerve I) is reported to be the most often injured, followed next in frequency by the facial and vestibulocochlear nerves, less commonly the optic and oculomotor nerves, and rarely the trigeminal and lower cranial nerves (1). Cranial nerve palsies may occur with TBI for several reasons, including acceleration-deceleration, shearing forces, skull fracture, intracranial hemorrhage, intracranial mass lesion, uncal herniation, infarct, or vascular occlusion. These circumstances may cause insults to the nerves through such mechanisms as compression, traction, transection, or ischemia. Central injury may occur from brainstem or cerebral damage; peripheral injury results from fracture or local injury. Cranial nerves are particularly at risk for injury as they traverse over bony protuberances and

through bony canals, or by direct injury from basilar skull fracture. The cranial nerves most susceptible to injury due to fracture are: olfactory, optic, oculomotor, trochlear, facial, auditory, and trigeminal (first two branches). The site of cranial fractures should indicate to the clinician the possibility of cranial nerve injury.

Injury to the cranial nerves may result in significant consequences to the individual with TBI, which may be further compounded by the deficits caused by cortical injury. Resulting impairments in sensation (sight, hearing, smell, taste) and motor function (facial expression, mastication, swallowing, speech) may impact such things as appetite, safety, interpersonal communication, and cosmesis.

Cranial nerves pass through the brainstem, and thus, abnormality in these nerves may serve as a reflection of injury severity. For example, pupillary, oculovestiluar, and oculocaloric reflexes have been shown to be strong prognostic indicators of mortality (2–6) and persistent cognitive disability (7).

Diagnosis is generally based on physical examination. Table 30-1 lists the examination tests and supplies for each cranial nerve. In the presence of altered consciousness examination may be difficult and incomplete. Thus, as one recovers from TBI those aspects of the examination that were previously not possible will need to be performed. A good cranial nerve examination can help identify important problems, and direct treatment. Electromyography and nerve conduction studies may aid the clinician in lesion

TABLE 30-1
Cranial Nerve Function and Examination

Nerve	Function	Test	Supplies
Olfactory (I)	Smell	Evaluate patency of the nasal passages. Then, determine if the person can detect familiar, non-noxiuos smells with eyes closed. Giving the person choices may help overcome word finding problems.	Odors or smelling card
Optic (II)	Visual acuity; visual fields	Have patient identify # of fingers held in visual fields and read up close and far away	Snelling visual acuity card
Oculomotor (III)	Pupillary reaction; lid retraction; and eye movement	Shine light in each eye to assess pupil reaction; note lid function; test eye movement for upward, downward, & medial gaze	Penlight
Trochlear (IV)	Intorsion and downward eye movement	Have patient follow finger to move eye downward	
Trigeminal (V)	Facial sensation; corneal sensation; chewing function	Test facial sensation for all three divisions; test corneal reflex; hold mouth open against resistance; clench teeth	
Abducens (VI)	Lateral eye movement	Have patient move eyes form side to side,	
Facial (VII)	Facial motor function; lid closure; taste sensation (anterior)	lateral gaze Smile, wrinkle forehead, wink, puff cheeks, close eye tight, identify tastes with anterior tongue	
Acoustic (VIII)	Hearing; balance	Test hearing; assess for nystagmus; finger to nose & heel to knee; Dix-Hallpike; vesitbulo-ocular reflex; Rhomberg; Sharpened Rhomberg; Fucada Stepping Test; Caloric Stimulation Test	
Glossopharyngeal (IX)	Swallowing; voice	Say "ah"; swallow; test gag reflex	Tongue depressor
Vagus (X)	Gag reflex	Tested above via gag reflex	Tongue depressor
Spinal (XI)	Neck strength	Resist head rotation, shoulder shrugs	
Hypoglossal (XII)	Tongue movement & strength	Stick out tongue; resist tongue movement with tongue depressor	Tongue depressor

localization and prognostication. A range of treatment approaches exist for cranial nerve deficits. With many of the nerve injuries measures should be instituted to avoid secondary injury.

The cranial nerves carry up to six modalities as defined in Table 30-2: general sensory, visceral sensory, special sensory, somatic motor, branchial motor, and visceral motor. The modalites served by each cranial nerve are indicated by color in Figure 1 and are summarized below:

Sensory Pathways Three neurons make up the cranial nerve sensory pathways: primary, secondary, and tertiary. The cell bodies of the primary neuron of cranial nerves are located in ganglia outside of the central nervous system. The secondary neuron cell bodies (sensory nuclei) lie in the brainstem and project to the thalamus. From the thalamus the tertiary neuron projects to the sensory cortex. The sensory loss resulting from a cranial nerve injury depends on the lesion location. Peripheral nerve lesions result in a loss of all sensations supplied by that nerve, where as central nerve injury to the sensory pathway depends on the part

injured. Damage in the thalamus causes contralateral patchy hemianesthesia and hemianalgesia.

Somatic and Branchial Motor Pathways The cranial nerves carrying motor functions are: III, IV, V, VI, VII, IX, X, XI, XII. Two neurons, the upper and lower motor neurons, compose the cranial nerve motor pathways. The upper motor neuron originates in the cerebral cortex and projects to the corticobulbar tract for synapse with the lower motor neuron. Most project bilaterally to contact lower motor neurons on both sides. Lesions to upper motor lesions are evidenced by paresis/paralysis, increased muscle tone, and hyperreflexia. The cell body of lower motor neurons reside in the brainstem and project peripherally. Lower motor neuron lesions cause paresis/paralysis, loss of muscle tone and muscle stretch reflexes, rapid atrophy, and fasciculations.

Visceral Motor Pathways The cranial nerves that perform parasympathetic efferent functions include: III, VII, IX, and X. Three neurons compose the visceral motor

TABLE 30-2
Components of Cranial Nerves

MODALITY	CRANIAL NERVES	FUNCTION
General sensory	V, VII, IX, X	Touch, pain, temperature, pressure, vibration, proprioception
Visceral sensory	IX, X	Sensory input (except pain) from viscera (carotid body and sinus, pharynx, larynx, thoracic, abdominal viscera)
Special sensory	I, II, VII, VIII, IX	Smell, vision, taste, hearing, balance
Somatic motor	III, IV, VI, XII	Motor function of muscles developed from the somites (extraocular eye muscles and tongue muscles except palatoglossus)
Branchial motor	V, VII, IX, X, XI	Motor function of muscles that develop from the branchial arches (muscles of mastication, tensors tympani, veli palatine, facial expression, stylopharyngeus, pharynx, sternomastoid, and trapezius)
Visceral motor	III, VII, IX, X	Motor function of viscera, including glands and smooth muscle (ciliary and constrictor pupillae muscles; lacrimal, submandibular, and sublingual glands; oral and nasal mucosa; parotid gland; carotid body vasculature; smooth muscles of pharynx, larynx, thoracic and abdominal viscera; cardiac muscle)

pathways to regulate smooth muscle, cardiac muscle, and secretory cells: first-order, second-order, and third-order neurons. The first order neurons originate from the hypothalamus and higher centers and project to parasympathetic nuclei in the brainstem. From the nuclei the second-order neurons project to ganglia that lie out of the central nervous system. The third-order neurons in turn project peripherally to their targets.

OLFACTORY NERVE (CRANIAL NERVE I)

Cranial nerve I provides the special sensory function of smell. The central axons of the bipolar olfactory neurons pass through the cribiform plate of the ethmoid bone, synapsing in the olfactory bulbs to relay sensations of smell to the brain. From here projections travel to the entorhinal cortex, hypothalamus, and the dorsal medial thalamic nucleus and then to the orbitofrontal cortex.

Cranial nerve I lesions may result in alteration of smell. Olfactory nerve injury may also alter the sense of taste because flavor perception results from a combination of smell, taste, and stored memories. Altered smell and taste may impact safety, appetite/weight control, confusion, behavior, daily activities, avocational and vocational pursuits.

The following are terms used to describe the nature and extent of the altered olfactory sensation:

- Dysnosmia = impaired sense of smell.
- Anosmia = complete loss of smell.
- Hyposmia = partial loss of smell.
- Parosmia = sensation of smell in the absence of stimulus.

- Cacosmia = awareness of a disagreeable or unusually offensive order that does not exist; may be part of an aura prior to seizure onset.

As many as 2 million people in the United States experience some type of olfactory dysfunction, causes of which include head trauma, upper respiratory infections, tumors of the anterior cranial fossa, and exposure to toxic chemicals or infections. It is difficult to estimate the true incidence of olfactory nerve injury in association with TBI due to the inability to examine cranial nerve I function in the unresponsive patient, and also the inconsistent seeking of medical attention after mild TBI. Olfactory nerve injury is reported to occur in 7% of all patients with TBI (8–11). The incidence is higher following moderate and severe TBI than mild TBI. Costanzo and Becker (12) report 19.4% with moderate TBI and 24.5% with severe. Injury to the olfactory nerve is the only cranial nerve commonly associated with mild TBI. This is because the fine nerve filaments of the olfactory nerve are particularly at risk for injury, even in mild TBI, as the fibers run through the cribriform plate of the ethmoid bone to reach the olfactory bulb. There should be a high index of suspicion for olfactory nerve injury in the following cases: cerebral spinal fluid rhinorrhea, frontal and occipital blows, frontal vault fractures. It is reported that 40% of those with CSF rhinorrhea after TBI experience anosmia.

Cranial nerve I injury may occur from damage to the olfactory nerves in the nasal mucosa, damage to the nerves as they cross the cribriform plate, or intracranial lesions affecting the olfactory bulbs. The olfactory filaments are particularly vulnerable to injury, as they may be sheared during the rotation of the brain or injured by cribiform plate fractures. The olfactory bulbs may be

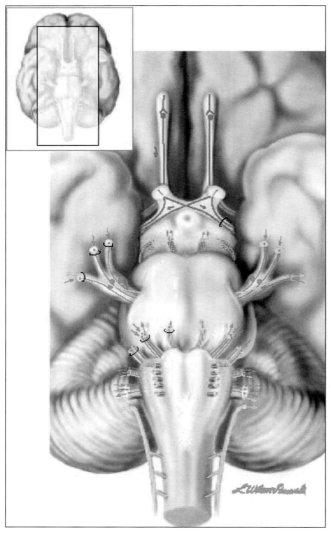

FIGURE 30-1

Basal view cranial nerves exiting the brain and brainstem. The components of the cranial nerves are indicated by color: aqua = general sensory; purple = visceral sensory; green = special sensory; pink = somatic motor; yellow = branchial motor; blue = visceral motor. (see color plate)

compressed by hemorrhage, edema, contusion, or abrasion by the cribiform plate. Olfactory structures also can be injured during craniotomies involving the anterior cranial base or from subarachnoid hemorrhage, which may disrupt the fine fibers of the olfactory nerve. Delayed onset of olfactory nerve dysfunction may be the consequence of scarring or gliosis of the tissues in the cribiform plate. Other causes of olfactory sensory abnormality should also be considered, such as nasal obstruction, injury to the nasal passages, acute viral respiratory infections, rhinitis sicca, allergic sinusitis, chronic polyposis, depression, medications, and seizures. Partial complex

epilepsy with a mesial temporal focus classically includes an aura of foul-smelling odors that occur before seizure onset. Olfactory hallucinations from uncinate fits do not imply actual olfactory nerve involvement. Paranasal sinus endoscopy may lead to violation of the cribiform plate with associated olfactory nerve injury, and also potential infectious complications.

Report of impaired smell may be the first signal of olfactory nerve injury. Because olfactory nerve function is not often evaluated in an emergency situation, the dysfunction may not be detected until weeks after the injury when the patient complains of changes in taste or smell. To examine cranial nerve I function, first evaluate the patency of both nasal passages. Then, determine if the person can detect odor in each nostril by testing with a familiar substance and an empty bottle. Stimulants such as organic solvents, camphor, peppermint, or ammonia should be avoided as they may also stimulate cranial nerve V (13). Next smell discrimination can be tested with the patient choosing between a series of common odors, such as coffee, lemon, and soap. Providing choices is a helpful way of limiting the influence of word finding problems on testing. Several different scratch and sniff cards are available to make testing more convenient. The University of Pennsylvania Smell Identification Test (UPSIT) is one useful tool, consisting of 40 items which evaluate olfactory and trigeminal nerve function in the nasal cavity. Central hyposmia may manifest as abnormalities in odor recognition rather than odor detection.

Olfactory encephalography establishes the presence of alpha rhythm, and its disappearance with odor perception. Ethmoid tomography may be used to determine if a basal skull fracture is present. Positron emission tomography (PET) and functional MRI are promising modalities to assist in making the diagnosis of different types of hyposmia (central vs peripheral), as well as in delineation of the role of limbic structures as sites of odor recognition, memory, and integration of multisensory inputs. Thorough evaluation of patients who have anosmia includes imaging of the anterior cranial structures. Patients experiencing parosmia should be evaluated for seizure activity on electroencephalography.

Unfortunately, there are no established effective treatments for this condition (1), while nontraumatic causes and seizure may be amenable to treatment. Early recovery may occur due to resolution of edema or pressure; while later recovery is contributable to neurofibril regrowth and central adaptation (14). Many regain the sense of smell within 2 years, but for some this remains a permanent problem. Costanzo & Becker (12) observed 33% recovery, 27% worsening, and 40% no change. Although it is a generally annoying development, parosmia may be the first evidence of functional return. When recovery occurs, it is usually noticed within the first 6 months and complete by 12 months post-injury (13).

However, late recoveries, up to 5 years, have been reported (8). For safety purposes, individuals with altered sensation should be aware of potential risks associated with the lack of smell (eg, inability to detect dangers such as smoke, spoiled foods, toxins), reminded to install smoke alarms on all floors of their home.

OPTIC NERVE (CRANIAL NERVE II)

The optic nerve, a fiber tract of the brain containing one million axons, provides the special sense of sight. This nerve receives its input from the rods and cones (first order neurons) which pass the signal to the ganglion cell layer of the retina (secondary sensory neurons). The long axons of the ganglion cells penetrate the lamina cribrosa as the optic nerve, which passes posteriorly through the optic canal. At the optic chiasm, where fibers from the nasal halves of the retina cross, the optic tract is formed, containing fibers from the ipsilateral halves of the retina. The optic tract continues posteriorly to the lateral geniculate bodies, where a third synaptic relay occurs. At this point, a small number of axons leave the optic tract and project to the pretectal midbrain to form the afferent loop of the Edinger-Westphal nucleus. From the lateral geniculate body, the optic tract continues posteriorly as the optic radiations, which project to the occipital lobe. Throughout their projection to the occipital lobe, the neurons maintain a highly topographic orientation of the retinal image.

Optic nerve injury occurs in up to 5% of patients with TBI (9). Optic nerve palsy may occur with injury to the globe, causing damage to the intraorbital portion of the nerve within the optic canal (15). In the orbit, the nerve is redundant and cushioned by fat. It is, therefore, not liable to indirect injury. However, the nerve is strongly tethered to bone intermittently throughout the canal. It is therefore subject to shearing forces as the brain and orbital contents are free to move, while the nerve is not (16). Injury to the optic nerve occurs most frequently in the intracanalicular portion of the nerve (17). Injury to the intracranial portion is less common.

Injury to the optic nerve typically occurs in one of two ways: 1) primary lesions causing hemorrhages in the nerve, dura and sheath spaces, tears in the nerve or chiasm, and, rarely, contusion necrosis; or, 2) secondary lesions from circulatory events subsequent to the initial injury causing edematous swelling of the nerve, necrosis from circulatory failure or local compression, and infarction related to vascular obstruction. Because the optic nerve is a direct extension of the brain, any injury to the optic nerve axons which do not regenerate is permanent.

Immediate monocular blindness occurs with great frequency in optic nerve injuries, especially in the intracanalicular portion of the nerve. Monocular blindness may be partial, and the extent of partial blindness should be documented immediately and followed closely for deterioration. The treatment of traumatic optic neuropathy is controversial. Although some studies have shown that steroids and/or optic canal decompression to be of benefit (18–20), other studies have shown that irrespective of timing post injury, neither treatment improved visual outcome (21, 22). Complete monocular blindness with preservation of normal pupillary reflexes is usually a sign of malingering or other types of functional (non-organic) disorders.

Visual field defects are due to injury to the optic nerve or its tracts posterior to the bulbar portion. These defects are quadrantanopias or hemianopias of varying degrees. When such defects are due to causes other than direct pressure from a mass lesion, surgical intervention is rarely helpful. Some visual field deficits may be helped by special optics that allow the patient to "see" in the affected field (15, 23). Careful evaluation by a neuro-opthalmologist or neuro-optometrist is warranted, and training in the use of such lenses is often necessary. Visual training may improve the visual spatial disorders for those with visual neglect (24). It is also important for the clinician to recognize non-physiologic visual field deficits.

Non-nerve-related injury also may affect visual function. Trauma to the cornea may cause visual blurring and scotomata. Visual blurring may be caused by vitreous tears, traumatically induced cataracts, retinal hemorrhage, or retinal detachment. Injury to the cornea or contents of the anterior chamber (including the lens) may cause monocular diplopia (25). If eyeglasses are of no benefit, surgery may be necessary to correct blurring caused by either corneal or lens problems. Visual blurring also may be caused by Torsions's syndrome (intrabulbar hemorrhage). The hemorrhage may resorb spontaneously over time or may require surgical removal for complete restoration of vision. The potential presence of occiptial seizures should also be considered (26).

Examination includes testing visual acuity, visual fields, pupillary reactivity, and direct visualization by ophthalmoscope. These tests are reviewed briefly:

Pupillary Reactivity to Light Light is shown into each eye and pupillary constriction (or lack of response) observed. It is also helpful to test for an afferent pupillary defect using the swing eye-to-eye test. If there is an afferent lesion involving the optic nerve, light shone into the affected eye fails to produce a response in either eye (contrast that with an efferent defect as described with cranial nerve III injury in the following section). This test may be difficult to assess due to altered level of consciousness.

Vision Acuity This can be performed by testing the ability to read a visual acuity card or newsprint. Unfortunately, this is often unable to be performed in patients who are minimally responsive, confused, or aphasic.

Saccadic responses to optokinetic stimuli may be checked to provide evidence of residual visual acuity function. The presence of an accommodation reflex can also provide evidence of visual fixation. Visual-evoked potentials may also help establish the integrity of the optic nerve and its cortical pathways.

Visual Fields   This entails asking the person to count fingers or identify a small object along the periphery of the vision. Each eye should be tested separately. Confrontation using a red-colored object is preferred. Evidence of visual inattention may be detected using a test of double, simultaneous extinction by presenting the test stimulus to bilateral visual fields at the same time. Tangent screen testing can provide visual field maps of deficits. Deficits may not be detected if the person is not able to fixate.

Direct Visualization by Ophthalmoscope   This may be helpful in identifying papilloedema (a hallmark of increased intracranial pressure), anterior chamber hemorrhage, and retinal detachment.

OCULOMOTOR NERVE (CRANIAL NERVE III)

The oculomotor nerve provides somatic motor and visceral motor functions. The nucleus of the oculomotor nerve arises in the paramedian midbrain ventral to the aqueduct of Sylvius near the superior colliculus. Mainly uncrossed fibers course anteriorly through the red nucleus and inner side of the substantia nigra, emerging on the medial side of the cerebral peduncles near the pontomedullary junction at the midline, penetrating the dura at the cavernous sinus. It travels along the lateral wall of the cavernous sinus, adjacent to the trochlear nerve, and superior to the abducens. Parasympathetic fibers from the Edinger-Westphal nucleus, which lies superior and dorsal to the oculomotor nucleus, course in close proximity to the oculomotor nerve through the cavernous sinus. The oculomotor nerve emerges through the superior orbital fissure to innervate the internal, superior and inferior rectus muscles, the inferior oblique muscle, and levator palpebrae muscle. The parasympathetic nerve fibers that travel with the oculomotor nerve innervate the sphincter muscle of the iris and to the ciliary muscle, which controls the shape of the lens during accommodation.

A palsy of this nerve can be caused by brain disorders (such as a head injury, tumor, or an aneurysm in an artery supplying the brain) or by diabetes. Injury may occur along its course: at the orbit, cavernous sinus, or an intracranial locus. This nerve is often injured at the point it exits through the dura, or from compression caused by uncal herniation due to increased intracranial pressure.

Isolated oculomotor nerve palsies due solely to TBI are not unusual, occurring in 17% of patients in one

study (27). Another study showed that persons with complete oculomotor palsy have a high incidence of traumatic subarachnoid hemorrhage (71%) or skull fractures (57%) (28). An orbital blowout fracture may produce clinical findings suggesting an oculomotor palsy; however, the simultaneous finding of infraorbital numbness argues against the diagnosis of an oculomotor nerve palsy (8).

Oculomotor nerve palsy causes a characteristic clinical picture: Divergent strabismus, since the eye is turned out by the intact lateral rectus muscle and slightly depressed by the intact superior oblique muscle. The eye may only be moved laterally. The affected eye turns outward when the unaffected eye looks straight ahead, producing double vision. The affected eye can move only to the middle when looking inward and cannot look upward and downward. There is ptosis of the eyelid, absent accommodation and in cases of complete palsy, a dilated and fixed ipsilateral pupil.

Examination involves tracking an object in the six cardinal positions, convergence on near targets, pursuit movements, saccades, pupillary reaction, and eyelid elevation. Clinical testing of oculomotor function in the conscious patient is not difficult. The examiners observes difficulty in moving the eye inward, or upward and downward, with preserved outward movement suggesting third nerve dysfunction (often with pupillary dilatation and ptosis).

In the unconscious patient, oculomotor testing is not possible, and thus, information is gathered during the performance of such tests as the doll's eye maneuver and pupillary light testing. Such tests must be performed serially, especially in the acutely injured patient, to ensure that an expanding lesion, uncal herniation, and/or hemorrhage is not overlooked. A blown pupil serves as a warning sign of herniation because of the nerves location medial to the temporal lobe at the edge of the tentorium. Dilation and fixation of both pupils indicates deep coma and possibly brain death.

Each eye is tested separately for pupillary reaction to light. With an efferent defect involving CN III, light shone into either eye fails to produce a response in the affected eye while light shone in the affected eye produces constriction of the opposite pupil. Pupillary dilation on one side is characteristic of cranial nerve III palsy, and is commonly accompanied by ptosis and lateral eye deviation (due to unopposed abducen's function). The swinging flashlight test (moving light rapidly from one eye to the next) may be helpful. The normal response to this test is constriction in the illuminated eye. A Marcus Gunn sign is present when there is dilation of the pupil of the abnormal eye after light is shone briefly into it.

The diagnosis is based on the results of neurologic examination as described above and computed tomography (CT) or magnetic resonance imaging (MRI). A spinal tap (lumbar puncture) is performed only if hemorrhage is supected and CT does not detect blood. Cerebral angiography is performed when a hemorrhage due to an aneurysm is suspected or when the pupil is affected but no head injury has occurred.

Return of function may begin within 2–3 months of injury, but generally remains incomplete. The chances for complete recovery are poor (28), with 40% reported to experience complete recovery (25). However, the majority fortunately experience functional recovery, which generally occurs within 6–12 months of injury.

Occlusive therapy (patching) will resolve the diplopia while the patch is on, but produces no long-term effects. Pleoptics (eye exercises) also have not been proven to be very effective (29). Strabismus surgery should not be undertaken until maximum visual acuity has been restored. Surgery should be delayed 6–9 months post injury, as one-third of patients will recover spontaneously (30). The procedure is empirical and consistent results cannot be guaranteed. Nevertheless, one large study showed successful alignment in 81% of adults who underwent strabismus surgery (31). This correction only improves the cosmetic deformity, however, and does nothing to improve the underlying cause.

TROCHLEAR NERVE (CRANIAL NERVE IV)

The trochlear nerve is the smallest of all the cranial nerves. It is somatic motor and innervates only one muscle, the superior oblique muscle. The trochlear nucleus is located in the lower midbrain and projects dorsally to cross the midline and eventually emerges from the dorsal aspect of the midbrain immediately caudal to the inferior colliculus. The trochlear nerve then traverses the lateral aspect of the cavernous sinus and enters the orbit through superior orbital fissure to innervate the *contralateral* superior oblique muscle. Injury of the trochlear nerve may result from trauma, ischemia, infarction, hemorrhage, aneurysm, cavernous sinus thrombosis, inflammation, meningitis, or tumor. TBI is the most common cause. The trochlear nerve is particularly liable to traumatic injury in that it has the longest course of any cranial nerve within the skull. Trochlear nerve injury is reported to occur in 0.2–1.4% of individuals with TBI (25).

Usually, the diagnosis is suspected in a person who, after a head injury, complains of vertical diplopia and cannot turn the affected eye inward and downward. The affected eye is typically observed to be rotated outward. The individual may also have a compensatory head tilt away from the affected side. In this position, unaffected muscles are employed and the vertical diplopia can often be eliminated. The double vision is commonly precipitated when walking down stairs.

What causes the vertical diplopia? With the superior oblique muscle paralyzed on one side, the antagonist inferior oblique extorts and slightly elevates the involved eye. Consequently, the visual fields are projected onto different areas of the right and left retinae resulting in the perception of two different images.

The superior oblique muscle performs two major functions: intorsion and downward gaze. Intorsion is difficult to detect on examination. Watching for movement of the conjuctival vessel may prove useful in this effort. Downward gaze is easier to detect. Thus, cranial nerve IV is generally tested by having the person adduct the involved eye and attempt to gaze downward. Individuals with trochlear nerve palsy are unable to look downward when the eye is adducted. Adduction of the eye prior to testing downward gaze is important because movement of the superior oblique muscle depends on the starting position of the eye.

Further examination may be pursued with CT scan or MRI imaging. Treatment depends on the cause of the palsy. Eye exercises may help. Sometimes surgery is necessary to eliminate double vision.

TRIGEMINAL NERVE (CRANIAL NERVE V)

The trigeminal nerve provides general sensory and branchial motor modalities. The nerve arises from the ventrolateral pons with a large sensory and small motor root. The two roots extend forward to the tip of the petrous bone, where the sensory portion merges with the gasserian (semilunar) ganglion and then forms the three divisions of the trigeminal nerve. The motor portion travels along the inferior aspect of the ganglion and becomes part of the mandibular division.

The motor fibers exit through the foramen ovale to innervate the muscles of mastication: the masseter, temporalis, and medial and lateral pterygoid muscles. The fibers also innervate several smaller muscles: the tensor tympani and tensor veli palatini via the otic ganglion, and the mylohyoid and anterior belly of the digastric via the mylohyoid nerve.

The ophthalmic division (V-1) exits through the cavernous sinus and then the superior orbital fissure to supply sensation from the forehead, conjunctiva and cornea, as well as the mucosa of the nose, frontal, sphenoid and ethmoid sinuses, and the lacrimal duct. The maxillary division (V-2) also travels through the cavernous sinus and exits the foramen rotundum to supply sensation from the skin of the mid-face, the mucosa of the anterior nasopharynx, the upper portion of the hard and soft palate, the gums of the upper jaw and the upper teeth. The sensory portion of the mandibular division (V-3) supplies sensation from the lower face, the mucosa of the lower jaw, floor of the mouth, lower teeth and gum. It supplies general sensation (but not taste) from the anterior two-thirds of the tongue.

The incidence of trigeminal nerve injury from TBI is 1.4–2% (8). The supraorbital nerve, from V-1 and the infraorbital nerve, from V-2 can be injured exiting the skull as the result of direct trauma such as blow out fractures of the orbit. Such injuries tend to occur in motor vehicle accidents, unprotected falls, golfing and baseball injures. The peripheral branches can also be injured by a superficial blow to the face. Numbness typically follows the distribution of the nerve.

The roots and/or the gasserian ganglion may be damaged in transverse skull fractures (32), but are rare in blunt head trauma (8). Penetrating wounds involving the gasserian ganglion are also rare but may cause severe dysesthesias and trigeminal neuralgia-type pain.

Clinical testing of the trigeminal nerve involves testing of all three divisions for sensation along all of the peripheral pathways. The examiner should look for sensory sparing at the angle of the jaw which is supplied by the upper cervical roots. Testing of corneal sensation involves a crossed reflex, and involves a motor response from the facial nerve. Thus, touching one cornea lightly with a wisp of cotton normally evokes a prompt closure of both eyelids. The masseters are amongst the most powerful muscles in the body, and subtle weakness may be difficult to detect. Pterygoid weakness is easier to detect, and the examiner may note jaw deviation toward the affected muscles on jaw opening.

Decreased corneal sensation may lead to corneal abrasions and drying as indicated by marked scleral injection. Treatment includes frequent eye irrigation and use of a lubricating gel with patching of the affected eye, especially at night. If irritation continues, lateral or complete tarsorrhaphy becomes the treatment of choice to avoid corneal ulceration and the development of corneal opacities.

Although injuries to the gasserian ganglion causing dysesthetic pain are rare, as with any peripheral nerve, stretch injuries tend to damage the nerves at fixed attachments at points of sharp angulation (8). Patients with trigeminal injuries may therefore complain of dysesthesias and symptoms of trigeminal neuralgia. Patients may respond to various anticonvulsants including: carbamazepine, gabapentin, lamotrigine, zonisamide, oxcarbazepine and levetiracetam (33).

ABDUCENS NERVE (CRANIAL NERVE VI)

The abducens nerve is somatic motor. The nerve originates at the abducens nucleus in the pons; exits the ventral pons near the midline at the pontomedullary junction; pierces the dura lateral to the dorsum sellae of the sphenoid bone; continues forward between the dura and the petrous temporal bone; takes a deep right angle turn; traverses the cavernous sinus and enters the orbit through superior orbital fissure to innervate the lateral rectus muscle. Within the cavernous sinus the 6th nerve is situated lateral to the internal carotid artery and medial to cranial nerves III, IV, V_1 and V_2. The cranial nerves III, IV, V_1 and V_2 travel through the dural wall, while the 6th nerve does not travel through the dura but is free within the cavernous sinus. Cranial nerve VI palsies are the most commonly reported ocular motor palsies, owing to its long intracranial course (34). This nerve has the longest intracranial course of all the cranial nerves.

Abducens nerve palsy may result from TBI, tumor, diabetes, hypertension, multiple sclerosis, meningitis, blockage of an artery supplying the nerve, aneurysm, surgery, increased pressure within the skull, orbit fractures, hydrocephalus/shunt malfunction. Injury to the Abducen's nerve in association with TBI is reported to occur in 0.4–4.1% (25).

Cranial nerve VI is often associated with injury to other cranial nerves depending on where along its course the abducens nerve is injured. Injury at the abducens nucleus is invariably associated with ispilateral fascial nerve palsy as fascicles of fascial nerve loops around the six nerve nucleus. Cranial nerves nerves III, IV, V_1 and V_2 may also be damaged when the injury occurs within the cavernous sinus due to their close proximity. When injured as the nerve passes through the superior orbital fissure, cranial nerves III, IV, and V_1 may be affected as they also pass through the fissure.

The lateral rectus muscle serves to move the eye laterally away from the midline (abduction). The affected eye cannot fully turn outward and may be turned inward when the person looks straight ahead. Double vision results when the person looks toward the side of the affected eye. Coordinated movements of the medial and lateral rectus muscles are required for horizontal movements. If both eyes cannot align on the same target the visual fields will be projected to different areas of the right and left retinae, resulting in the perception of two images.

These patients have an esotropia that is worsened by lateral gaze, and will often turn their heads laterally toward the paretic side to compensate. To test the abducens nerve function specifically, the patient is instructed to move the eyes through the full extent of the horizontal plane while the examiner looks for deficiency in lateral gaze.

Usually, doctors can easily identify an abducens nerve palsy, but the cause is less obvious. In the case of TBI, the cause is often apparent, but not necessarily the location. Depending on the history and presentation further work up may be needed. CT scan or MRI may be warranted to exclude tumors. A spinal tap (lumbar puncture) may be useful if meningitis is suspected. Injury to the nucleus of the nerve causes complete lack of ispilateral gaze; injury to the nerve after it comes off the brainstem results in inability to look to the side.

Treatment depends on the cause of the palsy. When the cause is treated, the palsy usually resolves. Abducens nerve palsy following TBI generally resolves over time.

FACIAL NERVE (CRANIAL NERVE VII)

Four modalities are carried by the facial nerve: general sensory (tactile sensation to parts of the external ear, auditory canal, and external tympanic membrane), special sensory (taste sensation to anterior two-thirds of the tongue), branchial motor (muscles of facial expression), and visceral motor (lacriminal glands and mucous membranes of mouth and nose; submandibular and sublingual salivary glands). The sensory components originate in the geniculate ganglion, the branchial motor in the main motor nucleus (pons), and the visceral motor in the superior salivatory nucleus (pons). The facial nerve exits the lower pons laterally and passes through the internal auditory meatus into the middle ear (where the chorda tympani branch arises to carry taste fibers); then enters the facial canal and exits the cranium through the stylomastoid foramen. In the parotid gland the facial nerve divides into its terminal branches.

The main function of each of the two seventh cranial nerves is ipsilateral facial movement including forehead wrinkle, eyelid closure, and movement of half of the face. A message is sent from the motor strip of the cerebral cortex crossing over to stimulate the contralateral seventh cranial nerve.

Injury to the facial nerve is the second most common, one-third as common as olfactory nerve palsy (1). Facial nerve injury most commonly occurs within its passage through the temporal bone, though it may occur at any point (13). Facial nerve injury due to TBI is most commonly peripheral, in association with temporal bone fractures. Temporal bone fractures are most commonly longitudinal accounting for 90% of all temporal bone fractures (14). Transverse fractures of the petrous bone result in immediate and complete CN VII paralysis in 30 to 50% of cases due to tearing of the nerve (13, 14). The facial nerve and vestibulocochlear nerve (CN VIII) course through the petrous bone in close proximity, and thus transverse petrous bone fractures may injure one or both of these nerves. Fractures near the internal auditory meatus usually involve both nerves resulting in ipsilateral facial weakness (i.e., the forehead musculature is involved as well as the face), ageusia in the anterior two-thirds of the tongue, and ipsilateral deafness. Temporal bone fractures further along its course may result in ipsilateral facial weakness (1).

Longitudinal fracture may result in a delay of CN VII paralysis from 2 to 3 days and up to 2 weeks. Delayed facial weakness, especially in patients with hemotympanum, is indicative of facial nerve swelling in the facial canal. In this setting, corticosteroids should be initiated, otolaryngology consulted, and facial nerve decompression considered (1). The nerve is usually intact, and typically recovers within 6–8 weeks (13, 14).

Facial nerve palsy may occur from injury anywhere along its course from the cortex to the innervation site. Forehead wrinkle is the one clinical feature that can differentiate the cause of facial weakness. Owing to the bilateral innervation of the upper face by the two cerebral hemispheres, upper motor neuron lesions (lesions above the level of the motor nucleus of cranial nerve VII) only cause contralateral paralysis of the face below the eyes. This occurs because the part of the nucleus that innervates the frontalis and orbicularis muscles continues to receive input from the ipsilateral hemisphere, allowing these muscles to continue functioning. On the other hand, lower motor neuron VII lesions (damage to the facial nucleus or its axons along its course after leaving the nucleus) cause ipsilateral paralysis of the entire face on one side with flattening of the forehead and inability to close the eye. Pontine lesions involving the facial nucleus cause complete ipsilateral facial paralysis along with contralateral hemiparesis (resulting from damage to the descending corticospinal fibers from the motor cortex before crossing over in the medulla), and are often accompanied by lateral rectus muscle paralysis (due to proximity of abducens nucleus to the facial nucleus).

Lesions within the fallopian canal may be localized to one of the three major segments (mastoid, tympanic, and labyrinthine) based on the presentation. Loss of taste on the ipsilateral anterior two-thirds of the tongue indicates damage of the mastoid segment (which branches into the chorda tympani). Injury to the tympanic segment which serves the stapedius muscle to dampen sound waves may cause hyperacusis (sounds appear excessively loud) and loss of the stapedius reflex, as well as loss of ipsilateral taste. Impaired ipsilateral tear production (in addition to the above findings) indicates damage to the labyrinthine segment from which the greater superficial petrosal nerve originates.

Comprehensive examination of the facial nerve involves testing the five main functions of this nerve: facial expression, taste, external ear sensation, stapedius muscle function and lacrimal and salivary gland function. First, facial expression in conversation should be observed, followed by requesting performance of specific facial actions: wrinkle forehead by raising eyebrows (frontalis), close eyes tightly (orbicularis oris), press lips firmly together (buccinator and orbicularis oris), smile, and clench jaw (platysma). An enlarged palpebral fissure may be a subtle sign of facial nerve injury. Taste may be tested by using a cotton swab moistened in a sugary or salty solution. The cotton is applied to one side of the protruded tongue, taste identified, cotton applied to other side to test for side-to-side differences; mouth rinsed with water; test repeated with the other solution. This test may be facilitated by using pre-written choices of sweet, sour, bitter, salty to which the person may point. Pain and light touch sensation is tested at the small strip of skin supplied by the facial nerve at the posteriomedial surface of the auricle, although abnormality is rarely detectable. Stapedius muscle function may be tested by having the person compare the loudness of sudden clapping behind each ear. Lacrimal and salivatory function may be assessed by asking about dry eyes, dry mouth and need for drinking water to swallow food. Lacrimal function may be formally tested using the Schirmer's test where a 5 mm by 25 mm piece of filter paper is inserted into the lower conjunctival sac for 5 minutes with less than 10 mm moisuture indicating abnormal function. Because of the close proximity to cranial nerve VIII, balance and hearing should also be assessed when cranial nerve VII is found to be damaged.

Electromyography and nerve conduction studies may be helpful in providing prognostic information. In cases of complete facial nerve disruption rehabilitative surgical techniques may be helpful, such as microsurgical cranial nerve XII crossover to the cranial nerve VII. Nerve-muscle pedicle grafts from the contralateral side may offer more rapid return of nerve function without compromising neck function (35).

Misguided nerve regeneration of the salivary and lacrimal fibers may result in "crocodile tears" (tearing instead of salivation upon eating).

Inadequate lid closure may result in drying of the cornea (exposure keratitis). The problem may be further compounded by accompanying loss of corneal sensation (trigeminal nerve) (13). A topical lubricant should be used frequently to protect the eye from dryness. Additional protection may be provided by taping the lid closed with eye pad, although this is not fool proof. In severe cases, tarsorrhaphy (operation to close eye lid) may be required for protection.

VESTIBULOCOCHLEAR NERVE (CRANIAL NERVE VIII)

Cranial nerve VIII provides special sensory functions of hearing and equilibrium/balance. Disorders of the VIII nerve may result in vertigo, tinnitus, and/or deafness. The vestibular nerve originates at the vestibular ganglion and the cochlear nerve at the spiral ganglion. In the internal auditory meatus the vestibular and cochlear nerves join and enter the brainstem at the cerebellopontine angle. Because the vestibulocochlear nerve is actually two distinct nerves that course together in close proximity through the internal auditory meatus and across the cerebellopontine angle, these two nerves are usually injured simultaneously. Once synapsing at their nuclei the nerves

take different courses, and thus, are less likely to both be injured as they run more proximally. The vestibular nuclei project through the thalamus to the somatosensory cortex providing conscious awareness of head position and balance. The cochlear nerve is represented bilaterally via fibers from the ventral cochlear nuclei.

Trauma may cause sensory and conductive types of hearing loss. *Sensory hearing loss* is caused by disruption of the transmission of auditory pathway impulses. Projections from the cochlea run bilaterally. Thus, unilateral central nervous system injury alone should not cause hearing loss. *Conductive hearing loss* results from disruption of sound transmission from damage to the tympanic membrane, ossicles, or cochlea. Hearing loss associated with TBI is more commonly sensorineural than conductive (36). Sensorineural hearing loss is reported to occur with TBI at an incidence of 85%, and 71% in the absence of temporal bone fracture (36).

Vestibulocochlear nerve injury is common with temporal bone fractures. Of all temporal bone fractures, 80–90% are longitudinal and 10–20% transverse (13). The type of temporal bone fracture, transverse or longitudinal, provides a clue as to the injury and type of hearing loss that might result. *Transverse fractures*, which tend to result from frontal or occipital blow, have been reported to result in sensorineural hearing loss in 100% of cases (37). Such injury is thought not to be amenable to surgery (13). On the other hand, *longitudinal fractures* (which occur from temporal or parietal forces) tend to result in conductive hearing loss or mixed conductive and sensorineural hearing loss (37). The incidence of sensorineural or mixed hearing loss in association with longitudinal fracture is 88%. Conductive hearing loss associated with temporal bone fractures occurs due to either ossicular chain disruption or tympanic membrane tear (13). Spontaneous recovery is reported in 80% of patients with conductive hearing loss occurring with temporal bone fractures (38). When conductive hearing loss fails to recover spontaneously, surgery should be considered. Surgical repair is associated with excellent results for all types of conductive hearing loss (37). Disruption at the incudostapedial joint occurs in 82% of cases, fracture of the stapedial arch in 30%, and malleus fracture in 11% (39). In 75% of cases of ossicular chain disruption the posterior auditory wall is also fractured (13). Although, conductive hearing loss is more common with longitudinal fractures, sensorineural or mixed hearing loss may also occur with this type of injury.

Patient examination and hospital record review may reveal important findings often associated with cranial nerve VIII injury by looking for battle's sign, mastoid fracture, otorrhea, bleeding from the ear, and hemotympanum. Hemorrhage from the ear is a common sign of longitudinal temporal bone fracture. Visualization of the tempanic membrane can be helpful to reveal tears.

Cranial nerve VIII is tested through testing eye movements, postural responses, and hearing. These assessments and how they guide lesion localization are discussed in brief detail below.

Vestibular dysfunction may manifest clinically with vertigo, nystagmus, and/or ataxia. Vertigo, the sensation of the room spinning, is a specific symptom of vestibular dysfunction. When the eyes are open, patients see the environment move; and when the eyes closed, patients feel like they are turning or whirling in space. Abnormalities in vestibular testing can be associated with lesions in the vestibular apparatus of the inner ear, the vestibular portion of CN VIII, the vestibular nuclei in the brainstem, the cerebellum, or pathways in the brainstem (such as the medial longitudinal fasciculus) that connect the vestibular and oculomotor systems. It is through observations of nystagmus and responses to provocative tests that a clinician can narrow down the origin of the problem. Thus, nystagmus elicited with extraocular movement testing, cold water caloric response testing, Dix-Hallpike Maneuver, or a rotating chair test (Ba'ra'ny Test) are key diagnostic tests in the diagnosis of vestibular pathway injury. Accompanying signs and symptoms may also provide clues to distinguish peripheral and vestibular lesions. Peripheral vestibular lesions may be accompanied by ipsilateral hearing loss and tinnitus; while central lesions may be associated with motor and sensory disturbances of the limbs, dysarthria, dysphagia or diplopia, indicating additional cranial nerve injuries.

Nystagmus Nystagmus is the movement of the eye in response to stimulation of the vestibular labyrinth, retrocochlear pathways, or central vestibulo-ocular pathways. To test for nystagmus, the patient is asked to follow the examiner's finger with the eyes while the examiner's finger moves through horizontal and vertical gaze. There are two components to nystagmus: slow and fast. The slow component is caused by vestibular stimulation and is mediated through the three-neuron arc from the semicircular canals to the extraocular muscles. The fast component returns eyes to the resting position and requires a functioning cerebral cortex. As a result, the fast component will not be present in coma or under general anesthesia. If nystagmus is present, record the directions of the fast-phase and slow-down phases. Nystagmus is described clinically in terms of the direction of the *fast corrective* phase, not the direction of gaze. Nystagmus is a particularly important finding because it is generally not as performance dependent as balance and coordination tests. Electronystagmography (ENG) may be used to quantify the nystagmus and provide information on the suppressive potential of visual fixation. However, ENG is not required for the diagnosis and may be considerably uncomfortable for the patient to endure.

Vertigo The vertigo presentation and the type of nystagmus present are important as they can help differentiate central (CNS) from peripheral (vestibular) origin. These characteristic features are described here. *Peripheral vertigo*, commonly presenting with vertigo and emesis, is usually characterized by horizontal nystagmus with a rotary component. The fast component points away from the affected side. Duration of peripheral nystagmus is generally minutes to weeks. Some of the causes of peripheral vertigo include: benign positional vertigo, labyrinthitis, vestibular neuronitis, motion sickness, Meniere's disease, peripheral vestibulopathy, acoustic neuroma, and perilymphatic fistula. *Central vertigo* may have more insidious onset and produce mild symptoms. Central nystagmus can occur in any direction, and dissociation of movements between the eyes is possible. In central nystagmus there is no relation between the direction of the nystagmus and the location of the lesion. In general, the following types of nystagmus are central in origin: vertical nystagmus, active nystagmus without vertigo, direction changing/unipositional nystagmus, gaze paretic nystagmus, nystagmus with disconjugate eye movement, and failure of fixed suppression. Vertical nystagmus is always central in location. Central nystagmus is generally longer in duration and may be present for years. Some of the processes that present with central vertigo are: dysfunction of the vestibular portion of CN VIII, upper and lower brainstem lesions, basilar artery migraines, vertebrobasilar ischemia or infarctions, multiple sclerosis, acute cerebellar lesions (hemorrhage or infarction), cerebellopontine tumors, seizures and spinocerebellar degeneration. Metabolic causes of vertigo may be appropriate to consider which include drug toxicity, hypoglycemia, and hypothyroidism. The response to provocative tests, as described below, may also help provide such distinction. Most causes of dizziness can be determined by a complete patient history and physical examination including some of the observations described here.

Nylen-Ba'ra'ny or Dix-Hallpike Positional Testing This test can help distinguish peripheral from central causes of vertigo. The patient sits on the examining table, rotates the head 45 degrees with one ear down, and the examiner supports the patient's head as the patient lays back with the head extending over the edge of the table. The patient is asked to keep their eyes open and report any sensations of vertigo, while the examiner looks for nystagmus. The maneuver is then performed with the opposite ear down. The position change causes maximal stimulation of the posterior semicircular canal of the ear that is down, and of the anterior semicircular canal of the ear that is up. With *peripheral lesions*, there is usually a few second delay in the onset of nystagmus and vertigo, which then fades away within approximately 1 minute. The nystagmus is horizontal or rotatory and does not change directions (just as with peripheral nystagmus described in the above paragraph). If the same maneuver is repeated, there is often adaptation, so that the nystagmus and vertigo are briefer and less intense each time. In *central lesions*, the nystagmus and vertigo generally begin immediately, and do not adapt. Nystagmus that persists while in this position but is not present while sitting is indicative of a central vestibular lesion.

Vestibulo-Ocular Reflex (VOR) This is a simple test that can be performed at the bedside and is used to determine whether or not the vertigo is vestibular in origin. Through the VOR, rapid movement of the head produces an equal and opposite movement of the eyes. This test would only be preformed when there is no suspicion of spinal column instability. The patient fixates on a target while the physician quickly moves the patient's head approximately 15°. When the VOR is intact, the eyes will remain focused immediately on the target after the head is thrust. If the patient must make corrective eye movement to see the target, the VOR is decreased. Corrective eye movements (saccade) with left and right head thrust indicate vestibular dysfunction on the left and right sides, respectively.

Head-Shaking Nystagmus This is nystagmus that appears after vigorous horizontal head shaking for about 15 seconds, at a frequency of approximately 2 Hz. Head-shaking nystagmus occurs when there are differences in the peripheral vestibular input reaching the central velocity storage mechanism of the brainstem. Thus, a positive head-shake test is suggestive of a peripheral lesion.

Walking with Sudden Turns Test This test produces veering toward the side of cerebellar or labyrinthine disease. To perform this test the patient should pivot on given points on the floor.

Fucada Stepping Test This test is performed by asking the patient to march in place with eyes closed for 50 steps at normal walking speed. The examiner makes note of distance and angle of displacement from starting to final standing point, angle of rotation, body sway, changes in head position relative to the body, position of the arms in horizontal or vertical directions. The final standing position is regarded as abnormal if there is more than 30° of body rotation or more than 50 cm of displacement from the starting point. Individuals with unilateral vestibular pathology often turn excessively. The test is not specific to vestibular dysfunction, but may provide a supportive finding taking other findings into account.

Caloric Stimulation Testing For individuals in a low neurologic functioning state, assessment of the vestibular system through the above tests is not possible. In such patients, caloric stimulation testing may be particularly helpful for this purpose. This test is performed with the head of the bed placed at 30 degrees to have the horizontal semicircular canal in a vertical plane. The external auditory canal is then irrigated with 30 degree Celsius water over thirty minutes while direction of eye deviation and nystagmus are observed. With the intact vestibular system, the eyes tonically deviate to the side of cold irrigation, and then followed after an approximate 20 second latent period by nystagmus to the opposite side that generally lasts 1.5 to 2 minutes. The procedure is repeated using 44 degree Celsius water. With warm water irrigation the nystagmus is normally to the side of the irrigation. The normal nystagmus response to caloric testing follows the mnemonic COWS (Cold Opposite Warm Same). When there is dysfunction in the vestibular pathway this response may be reduced or absent.

Hearing loss can be caused by lesions in the acoustic and mechanical elements of the ear, the neural elements of the cochlea, or the acoustic nerve (CN VIII). There are three general types of deafness: conductive, sensorineural, and central. Conductive hearing loss results from a defect in the mechanism by which sound is transformed and conducted to the cochlea as occurs with disorders of the external or middle ear. Sensorineural hearing loss results from disease of the cochlea or of the cochlear division of the eighth cranial nerve. Central hearing loss is caused by lesions of the cochlear nuclei and their connections with the primary receptive areas for hearing in the temporal lobes.

After the hearing pathways enter the brainstem, they cross over at multiple levels and ascend bilaterally to the thalamus and auditory cortex. Therefore, clinically significant unilateral hearing loss is invariably caused by peripheral neural or mechanical lesions. On the other hand, the bilaterality of the CNS connections prevents unilateral central injury from causing significant hearing loss.

Hearing may be assessed at the beside by seeing if the patient can hear the examiners fingers rubbed together outside of the auditory canal. Similarly, the patient may be asked to cover one ear while the examiner whispers in the other ear and has the patient repeat what is heard. Testing on the two sides is compared. If hearing impairment is detected the cause may be localized and differentiated as sensorineural or conductive using the Rinne and Weber's Tests.

Rinne Test For the Rinne Test, a 512 Hertz tuning fork is placed over the mastoid process (bone conduction) until the patient indicates that the ringing sound is no longer heard, and then the tuning fork is placed a few centimeters from the external auditory canal (air conduction). In this second position of air conduction, sound is normally conducted through the external and middle ear to the cochlea. Normally, the tone is heard better by air conduction, and thus, with normal hearing the ringing should be heard again in the second position. Not being able to hear the sound again by air conduction implies conductive hearing loss. That is, the problem is in the external or middle ear. With conductive hearing loss, bone conduction is heard as it bypasses problems in the external or middle ear. Rinne Test findings in sensorineural hearing loss are the same as with normal hearing, air conduction is greater than bone conduction in both ears, except hearing is decreased in the affected ear.

Weber Test The Weber Test is performed by placing the tuning fork over the middle of the forehead transmitting sound via bone to the cochlea and bypassing the middle ear mechanism. Normally the sound is heard equally on both sides. In sensorineural hearing loss the ringing is not as loud on the affected side, while in conductive hearing loss the ringing is heard louder on the affected side. You can replicate this increase in sound on the side of conduction block by covering and uncovering one ear with the cup of your hand while humming.

Formal audiometry may be helpful to detect and quantify hearing loss, differentiate sensorineural from conductive loss, and guide treatment decisions. In the lower neurologic functioning individual with TBI, brainstem auditory evoked potentials can be used to test the intactness of the auditory pathway. This may be particularly important in helping guide therapy towards more visual stimuli in trying to elicit reactions. Hearing loss may pose significant obstacles to the patient and treatment team in rehabilitation and community integration that should be considered in the rehabilitation program.

Treatment of cranial nerve VIII injuries can best be discussed in terms of the 2 main problems of vestibular and hearing impairment. Treatment of vestibular dysfunction is based on the vestibular system's capacity to habituate to stimuli (13). To decrease the vestibular sensitivity, labyrinthine exercises are used that incorporate equilibrium and righting reflexes (40). Referral to a physical therapists knowledgeable in the diagnosis and treatment of dizziness related to TBI can be a valuable component in the management of this disorder. Medications commonly used for vestibular problems (such as meclazine or dimenhydrinate) are generally not helpful and are discouraged due to potential sedation, cognitive side effects, and prevention of central adaptation (13).

Significant unilateral hearing loss may be improved using a CROS (contralateral routing of signal) type hearing aid which transfers sound to the intact ear (13). Surgical correction is an important consideration for conductive hearing loss that fails to recover spontaneously. For the management of tinnitus, masking sound devices and biofeedback have both been successful in some cases (13) and may be worth consideration.

GLOSSOPHARYNGEAL NERVE (CRANIAL NERVE IX)

The glossopharyngeal nerve serves general, visceral and special sensory functions, as well as branchial and visceral motor functions. This nerve exits from the jugular foramen in close proximity to the last three cranial nerves; therefore, lesions, especially traumatic ones, tend to affect some or all of those nerves. The glossopharyngeal nerve provides general cutaneous function and taste to the posterior one-third of the tongue, and sensation to the soft palate, pharynx, faucil tonsils, tragus of the ear and nasopharynx. Its tympanic branch supplies sensation to the tympanic membrane, eustachian tube and mastoid area. Chemo and baroreceptors are also carried by the glossopharyngeal nerve from the carotid body and carotid sinus. Its motor fibers innervate the stylopharyngeus muscle and, along with the vagus nerve, the pharyngeal constrictor muscles. Parasympathetic secretory and vasodilatory fibers innervate the parotid gland.

The incidence of glossopharyngeal dysfunction following trauma is 0.5-.1.6% (8). Symptoms include loss of taste over the posterior one-third of the tongue, deviation of the uvula toward the contralateral side, decreased salivation and slight dysphagia. Examination includes testing oropharyngeal sensation and gag reflex. Loss of sensation to the posterior palate with a subsequent absent gag reflex may place the patient at risk for aspiration. Treatment for an isolated glossopharyngeal nerve injury is symptomatic, as the symptoms are usually minimal. However, injury to the glossopharyngeal nerve usually involves the vagus as well, and thus, may result in severe laryngeal and pharyngeal dysfunction. Treatment of such injuries is covered below.

VAGUS (CRANIAL NERVE X)

The vagus nerve arises from the lateral medulla, leaving the skull through the jugular foramen with the glossopharyngeal and accessory nerves. It contains motor, sensory and parasympathetic fibers. The vagus nerve supplies motor fibers to all the striated muscles of the pharynx and soft palate except the tensor veli palatini and stylopharyngeus. Through the superior and recurrent laryngeal nerves, the vagus supplies all of the striated muscles of the larynx. Parasympathetic motor fibers supply the smooth muscle of the trachea, bronchi, esophagus and gastrointestinal tract, and cause gastrin release from the antral mucosa. It also sends inhibitory fibers to the heart muscle, slowing the heart rate and reducing the amplitude of the heart beat. Sensory fibers innervate the pharyngeal plexus, larynx, and thoracoabdominal viscera.

The incidence of vagal involvement in TBI is .05 to .16% (8), usually as the result of blunt trauma associated with occipital condyle fractures. Bilateral vagal disruption is fatal.

To examine vagus nerve function test palate elevation and gag reflex. Injury to the vagus nerve, especially the superior and recurrent laryngeal nerves, may result in: paralysis of the palate with loss of the gag reflex, dysphagia, and aphonia with unilateral paralysis of the vocal fold. Alternative feeding techniques should be identified for those at risk for aspiration. Pharyngeal exercises may improve dysarthria in individuals with mild dysfunction (40). Glottic incompetence can be treated by procedures that augment vocal cord bulk, such as the injection of Teflon, Gelfoam or fat. More aggressive surgical procedures such thyroplasty and arytenoids adduction have been reported beneficial to those with high vagal lesions (41).

SPINAL ACCESSORY (CRANIAL NERVE XI)

The spinal accessory nerve is a pure motor nerve with two parts. The cranial part (accessory vagal nerve) arises from the medulla, exits the skull via the jugular foramen, and in conjunction with the vagus nerve, supplies all the intrinsic muscles of the larynx except the cricothyroid. The spinal part (accessory spinal nerve) arises from anterior horn cells of the first through sixth cervical cord segments. The fibers form a trunk that ascends and enters the foramen magnum, where it joins the accessory vagal nerve before exiting the jugular foramen. After joining with the vagus nerve, the fibers split off to descend in the neck to supply the sternocleidomastoid muscle and the upper half of the trapezius.

Trauma, especially from missiles, is the most common cause of spinal accessory nerve dysfunction. Symptoms include the inability to turn the head to the opposite side, and ipsilateral shoulder drooping, resulting in shoulder dysfunction and pain.

Examination includes testing trapezius function on shoulder shrug, sternocleidomastoid on contralateral head turning, and flaring of the scapula. Aggressive physical therapy should be initiated as soon as possible. Surgical repair of the accessory nerve after sectioning may be possible in some patients.

HYPOGLOSSAL (CRANIAL NERVE XII)

The hypoglossal nerve serves somatic motor function. It emerges from the medulla, and leaves the skull via the hypoglossal canal. It innervates the ipsilateral intrinsic tongue musculature as well as the hyoglossus, styloglossus, genioglossus and geniohyoid muscles. It is responsible for tongue protrusion to the opposite side.

Injury to the hypoglossal nerve causes dysarthria and dysphagia . Injury to the hypoglossal nerve alone most often occurs with penetrating wounds to the neck and submental region. Ipsilateral atrophy and tongue fasciculations are noted on examination. Upon protrusion, the tongue deviates toward the lesion by the unopposed, contralateral muscles. With a supranuclear (central) lesion, however, the tongue will deviate opposite the lesion due to contralateral innervation of the brainstem.

Examination of hypoglossal nerve function involves noting tongue protrusion. The tongue deviates to the side of the lesion. Exercises for the treatment of dysarthria may help to improve tongue coordination and strength. Treatment of hypoglossal nerve injuries due to penetrating wounds is surgical, and the nerve tends to recover quite well.

References

1. Weiner WJ, Goetz CG (eds.). *Neurology for the non-neurologist. 2nd Edition* Philadelphia: J.B. Lippencott Company, 1989.
2. Zafonte RD, Hammond FM, Peterson J: Predicting outcome in the slow to respond traumatically brain-injured patient: Acute and subacute parameters. *NeuroRehabilitation* 1996;6:19–32.
3. Braakman R Jennet WB, Minderhoud JM: Prognosis of post-traumatic vegetative state. *Acta neuochir* 1988;95:49–52.
4. Levati A, Farina M, Vecchi G, Rossanda M. Marrubini MB: Prognosis of severe head injuries. *J Neurosurg* 1982;57:779–783.
5. Narayan RK, Greenburg RP, Miller JD, Enas GG, Choi SC, Kishore PR, Selhorst JB, Lutz HA 3rd, Becker DP: Improved confidence of outcome prediction in severe head injury. A comparative analysis of the clinical examination, multimodality evoked potentials, CT scanning, and intracranial pressure. *Journal of Neurosurgery* 1981;54(6):751–62.
6. Braakman R, Gelpke GJ, Habbema JD, Maas AI, Minderhoud JM: Systematic selection of prognostic features in patients with severe head injury. *Neurosurgery* 190;6(4):362–70.
7. Alexandre A. Colombo F. Nertempi P. Benedetti A. Cognitive outcome and early indices of severity of head injury. *Journal of Neurosurgery* 1983;59(5):751–61.
8. Keane JR, Baloh RW. Post-traumatic cranial neuropathies. Neurolic Clinics 1992;10:849–867.
9. Rovit RL, Murali R: Injuries to the cranial nerves. In Cooper, PR (ed): *Head Injury*, 3rd Edition. Baltimore, Williams and Wilkins, 1993.
10. Jennett B, Teasdale G (eds). *Management of Head Injuries*. Philadelphia, F.A. Davis Company 1981, pp. 272–278.
11. Summer D: On testing the sense of smell. *Lancet* 1962;2:895–903.
12. Costanzo RM, Becker DFP. Sense of smell and taste disorders in head injury and neurosurgery patients. In Meiselman HL, Rivlin RS (eds): *Clinical management of taste and smell*. New York, Macmillan Publishing Co., 1986, pp. 565–578.
13. Berrol S. Cranial nerve dysfunction. *Physical Medicine and Rehabilitation: State of the Art Reviews*. 1989;3(1): 85–93, Philadelphia, Hanley & Belfus, Inc.
14. Horn LJ, Zasler ND (eds). Thomas MD, Zasler ND: Sensory-Perceptual Disorders After Traumatic Brain Injury. 499–514. In *Medical Rehabilitation of Traumatic Brain Injury*. 1996; Philadelphia, Hanley & Belfus, Inc.
15. Padula WV: Neuro-optometric rehabilitation for persons with a TBI or CVA. *Journal of Optometric Vision Development* 23:4–8,1992.
16. Glaser RA: *Neuro-opthalmology*. Baltimore, Harper and Row, 1978, p. 126.
17. Canavero S: Dynamic reverberation. A unified mechanism for central and phantom pain. *Neurosurgery Clinics of North America* 1994;42(3):203–207.
18. Awerbuch GI, Sandyk R: Mexiletine for thalamic pain syndrome. *International Journal of Neuroscience* 55:129–133,1990.

19. Spoor TC, McHenry JG. Management of traumatic optic neuropathy. *Journal of Craniomaxillofacial Trauma.* Spring;2(1): 14–26;discussion 27. 1996.

20. Li KK, Teknos TN, Lai A, Lauretano A, Terrell J, Joseph MP. Extracranial optic nerve decompression: a 10-year review of 92 patients. *Journal of Craniofacial Surgery.* 1999;Sept;10(5):454–9.

21. Levin LA, Beck RW, Joseph MP, Seiff S, Kraker R. The treatment of traumatic optic neuropathy: the International Optic Nerve Trauma Study. *Ophthalmology.* 1999;July;106(7):1268–77.

22. Steinsapir KD: Traumatic optic neuropathy. *Current opinion in ophthalmology.* 1999;10(5):340–342.

23. Padula WV, Shapiro JB: Head injury and the post-trauma vision syndrome. *RE:view* 24:153–158,1993.

24. Kerkhoff G. Rehabilitation of Visuospatial Cognition and Visual Exploration in Neglect: a Cross-over Study. *Restorative Neurology and Neuroscience.* 12(1):27–40.1998.

25. Keane JR: Neuro-ophthalmic signs and symptoms of hysteria. *Neurology* 32:757–762,1982.

26. Obyan A, Zafonte R, Hammond F: Occipital Status Epilepticus: An Unusual Cause of Post-traumatic Blindness. *Arch Phys Med Rehabil* 1995;76(11):1085.

27. Sabates NR, Gonce MA, Farris BK: Neuro-ophthalmological findings in closed head trauma. *Journal of Clinical Neuro-ophthalmology* 11:273–277,1991.

28. Tokuno T, Nakazawa K, Yoshida S, Matsumoto S, Shingu T, Sato S, Bar S, Yamamoto T: Primary oculomotor nerve palsy due to head injury:analysis of 10 cases. *No Shinkei Geka.* Jun;23(6): 497–501.1995.

29. Vaughn D, Asbury T: *General Ophthalmology,* Los Altos, California, Lange Medical Publications, 1974, p 182.

30. Lagreze WA:Neuro-ophthalmology of trauma. *Current opinion in ophthalmology.* 9(6):33–39,1998.

31. Beauchamp GR,Black BC,Coats Dk, Enzenauer RW, Hutchinson AK, Saunders RA, Simon JW, Stager DR, Stager Dr, Jr, Wilson ME, Zobal-Ratner J, Felius J. The management of strabismus in adults-I. clinical characteristics and treatment. *Journal of the American Academy of Pediatric Ophthalmology and Pediatrics.* August; 7(4):233–40.2003.

32. Dacey RG, Jane JA: Craniocerebral Trauma. In Baker AB, Baker IH (eds): *Clinical Neurology,* revised. Philadelphia, Harper and Row, 1987, pp1–61.

33. Backonja MM: Use of anticonvulsants for treatment of neuropathic pain. *Neurology* 59:S14–17, 2002.

34. *Rosen's Emergency Medicine: Concepts and Clinical Practice,* 4th ed., Copyright © 1998 Mosby-Year Book, Inc.; pp 1278.

35. Kay PP, Kinney SE, Levine H, Tucker HM. Rehabilitation of facial paralysis in children. *Arch Otolaryngol* 1983;109:642–647.

36. Podoshin L, Fradis M: Hearing loss after head injury. *Arch Otolaryngol* 1975;101:15–18.

37. Sismanis A. Post-concussive neuro-otological disorders. Physical Medicine and Rehabilitation: State of the *Art Reviews.* 1992; 6(1):79–88.

38. Tos N: Prognosis of hearing loss in temporal bone fractures. *Laryngol Otol* 1971;85:1147–1159.

39. Hough TFD. Restoration of hearing loss after head trauma. *Ann Otol Rhinol Laryngol* 1969;210–226.

40. Tangeman PT, Wheeler J: Inner ear concussion syndrome: vestibular implications and physical therapy treatment. *Top Acute Care Rehabil* 1986;1:72–73.

41. Yorkston KM, Beukelman DR, Strand EA, Bell KR: *Management of Motor Speech Disorders,* 2nd ed. Austin Tx, Pro-ed, 1999.

42. Eibling DE, Boyd EM:Rehabilitation of lower cranial nerve deficits. *Otolaryngologic clinics of North America* 30:865–875, 1997.

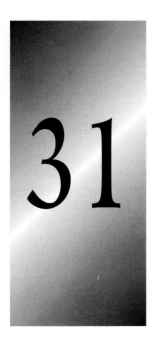

31 Fatigue: Assessment and Treatment

Jonathan L. Fellus
Elie P. Elovic

atigue is a commonly reported symptom following Traumatic brain injury (TBI), yet it is both poorly understood and challenging to treat. The word symptom is used in contradistinction to diagnosis because fatigue in general and specifically in TBI is so problematic to define and operationalize. Since TBI is a descriptive term for a heterogeneous collection of injuries to the brain that can result in physical, behavioral, cognitive or emotional dysfunction, it has been particularly vexing to determine the origin of and how to best characterize post-traumatic fatigue (PTF). As a result, the determination of its incidence has been problematic. Some attempts to quantify its incidence in TBI have placed the range between 21 and 73 % (1, 2, 3). PTF affects not only an individual's emotional well being but may also affect potential functional recovery from brain injury. Kreutzer, Seel, & Gourley (4) reported an incidence of 46% among persons in an outpatient TBI clinic and suggested that further information needs to be gathered regarding prognostication and the efficacy of treatment alternatives. However because of its multifaceted nature, the overall burden of fatigue in this population is not precisely known. However, individuals with TBI clearly suffer from fatigue with resultant diminished functioning in multiple spheres of cognition, quality of life and activities of daily living. This

functional limitation is especially problematic because the inability to sustain purposeful, goal-directed mental effort is a key requirement for independent functioning. Clinicians who attend to persons with TBI often possess few diagnostic or therapeutic resources to offer accurate assessment and treatment. Recently, however, a number of new and sophisticated neuro-imaging tools and techniques have helped to begin unraveling the underlying pathophysiology of PTF and should soon reveal more about treatment. The following discussion will review the available knowledge concerning fatigue in the TBI population. Our intent is to simultaneously educate and increase readers' interest and understanding of fatigue; to promote research in this critical area leading to productive, multi-disciplinary efforts addressing the problem of fatigue; and to facilitate the development of treatment protocols through the identification of possible fatigue generating mechanisms. Meanwhile, the state of the art approach to managing PTF is offered.

For the following discussion, TBI will be defined using the well established definition advanced by the TBI Model Systems Task Force: "damage to brain tissue caused by an external mechanical force, as evidenced by loss of consciousness, post-traumatic amnesia, skull fracture, or objective neurological findings that can be reasonably attributed to TBI on physical examination or mental status examination" (5).

DEFINITION

Prior to embarking on a further discussion of PTF, we develop a working definition for it. It is important to recognize that no universally accepted definition or broad consensus on a conceptual framework of fatigue in general exists. Nevertheless, discussions in the fatigue literature make a distinction between *central* fatigue, which results from dysfunction of supratentorial structures involved in mentation, versus *peripheral* fatigue, which is of a more purely physical, metabolic or muscular origin. Clearly, it is the *central* type that is of greatest interest with regard to those with isolated TBI. Beyond this dichotomy, the debate over PTF or fatigue in general has moved beyond the idea of fatigue as a unitary concept and towards a belief that fatigue is multifaceted (6, 7) with components likely arising from distinct mechanisms and brain networks (8).

Lezak's reductionist, "fatigue needs no definition" (9), may be the battle cry of the lumpers in this debate; however, such a pronouncement does little to advance our understanding of this phenomenon and for the development of effective treatment strategies. On the other end of the spectrum, Chauduri and Behan (10) carefully define PTF as " . . . the failure to initiate and/or sustain attentional tasks and physical activities requiring self motivation (as opposed to external stimulation) . . ." and they lay out an elegant clinico-anatomic, pathophysiological explication of why fatigue follows acquired brain injury. Clinical experience echoes their definition in that fatigue impacts upon cognitive function (11) and the ability to perform instrumental activities of daily living.

Historically, various surrogates, markers, synonyms and clinical imitators of fatigue have been pursued in the literature, leading the casual reader astray from a purer characterization of the fatigue that follows TBI. Yet almost paradoxically, the more focused and penetrating the research on the essence of fatigue becomes, the less singular a phenomenon it appears to be. Thus, even as one measures, correlates and localizes the fundamental components of fatigue, the syndrome or symptom cannot merely be appreciated in isolation. Rather, fatigue must be appreciated in its full context, across various domains and with the understanding that the fatigue experience is not static or constant. Ultimately, the clinical picture of PTF that emerges is colored and textured by a multitude of primary and secondary, even tertiary factors that reliably engender the principle aspects of fatigue for persons with TBI. The current discussion hopes to elucidate the most likely generators of PTF and critique the current literature as well as propose an operational definition based on the most appropriate measurement tools for its assessment.

EPIDEMIOLOGY

Currently employed methods of surveillance for disease burden due to TBI do not collect information beyond that of the total number of emergency room visits and the total number of hospitalizations. Moreover, the vast majority of TBI's are deemed *mild* and the CDC has labeled this variant the "silent epidemic" because many such cases never receive medical attention. Consequently the magnitude of the problem of fatigue among all TBI survivors or that subset "permanently disabled" is not directly known. Disappointingly even databases developed through the comprehensive Traumatic Brain Injury Model Systems are simply silent with respect to surveillance of PTF or its consequences. Thus, TBI stands as a persistent public health burden that, despite primary prevention successes, will likely continue to grow because of the increasing sophistication and effectiveness of contemporary emergency care, further resulting in a growing *prevalence* of TBI-associated problems such as fatigue. In the vast majority of studies, PTF is evaluated predominantly by self-report—in other words, subjectively. A number of investigators over the last several decades have attempted to identify the incidence or prevalence of fatigue in the TBI population, but these studies have not always been adequately controlled for such common confounds as anxiety and depression. Lezak (9) identified fatigue as one of the "subtle" sequelae of brain damage, along with distractibility and perplexity, and compared the incidence of fatigue between those patients seen in consultation, (i.e. relatively briefly), with those enrolled in detailed, longitudinal research protocols. Forty-two percent of 50 subjects reported fatigue if examined once and 60% if examined more often. Among the group in research studies (n = 46) the reporting of fatigue reached an astounding 98%. This study exposes how a methodological flaw can seriously compromise the estimated incidence of PTF. The marked discrepancy suggests that thoroughness of assessment is essential and that without such an approach, patients are at risk for having their fatigue go unrecognized especially as TBI severity increases and with it, cognitive dysfunction such as memory and self awareness.

Middleboe (1) analyzed a cohort of 51 patients with mild TBI and noted that 21% reported fatigue one year post injury. Olver (3) studied a longer follow-up period for 254 patients at 2 years and 103 at 5 years. The majority of these patients had suffered a severe injury as reflected by a mean Glasgow Coma Score of 5.1. Fatigue was reported by 68% at two years and 73% at 5 years. Masson (12) studied a group of 231 adults five years after injury. The sample was stratified with respect to TBI severity and in addition, a lower limb injury cohort was used for comparison. Among the four groups, 30.6% of limb injured, 35.1% of mild TBI, 32.4% of moderate TBI and 57.7% of severe TBI subjects endorsed fatigue suggesting an association between severity of brain injury and fatigue incidence. Hillier (2) examined a cohort of 67 primarily severely brain injured patients and noted a fatigue self-report rate of 37% five years post-TBI. This number may be artificially low in light of the under self-reporting noted by Lezak especially since the overwhelming majority of patients in this study were severely injured (73%) and likely to have disabling cognitive impairments. Kreutzer et al. (4) examined the epidemiology of depression in a cohort of 722 TBI outpatients on average 2.5 years after injury and with a mean duration of unconsciousness of 10 days. The self-report of fatigue in this severely injured group was 46% and fatigue was the most frequently reported problem.

From these type of epidemiological studies based on self report, PTF ranges from 2 to 98 percent (13). What remains unclear from these reports is how fatigue impacts upon mentation or on function. Limited formal neuropsychological evidence exists to elucidate the effect of PTF on cognitive performance. In addition, it is not clear what the natural history of fatigue is, or what the associations are between fatigue and a multitude of TBI-specific factors such as length of coma, duration of posttraumatic amnesia and mechanism of injury. Finally, it is unknown how the incidence and magnitude of fatigue interrelate, affect, and are affected by other common TBI sequelae.

ASSESSMENT

To date there is no single measurement instrument that has been validated to study PTF. Nevertheless, it is important to begin the process by assessing the *impact* of PTF. Efforts at the assessment of PTF have been complicated by its multifaceted nature. Many measures that are commonly used rely on subjective reporting. Some of the more commonly employed scales used in neurological populations are the Fatigue Severity Scale (FSS) (14), Fatigue Impact Scale (FIS) (15) and the Modified Fatigue Impact Scale (MFIS). The FSS (14) is assessed by having participants rate 9 different questions rating one's fatigue from 1 (low) to 7 (high). The FSS is the average of these 9 values. The FIS (15) is a 40-item questionnaire that the person rates from 0, no problems, to 4, severe problems. These items are grouped into three separate functional categories—physical, cognitive and psychosocial. The MFIS is a 21-item derivative of the FIS that is more commonly used in the multiple sclerosis population.

In an effort to delineate both subjective and objective assessment of fatigue Lachapelle (16) evaluated thirty subjects with TBI a mean of 44.3 months after injury and compared them to an age and gender matched healthy control group. The study purported to parse fatigue into objective and subjective components; the paradigm for objective fatigue was a continuous thumb-pressing task. Over time, normal and TBI groups demonstrated a decline in the number of repetitions per unit of time, however the difference was statistically insignificant. The subjective evaluation of fatigue was quantified by visual analogue, the FSS and FIS scales. Despite the statistical parity on the objective measure, TBI patients demonstrated significantly greater subjective fatigue scores on the FSS and FIS versus normal controls. Likewise, Walker (13) looked at the measures of quadriceps strength and physical endurance to test those complaining of PTF versus normals and found no statistical difference. Researchers trying to characterize peripheral fatigue note the significant impact upon challenging physical actions facing those with brain trauma, such as mobility, ADLs and sustaining endurance for a given task. Brain trauma often involves lesions of central pathways governing simple and complex motor function, for instance resulting in hemiplegia, spasticity, ataxia or the upper motor neuron syndrome with various well-known positive and negative signs and static and dynamic disturbances. Given the working definition of peripheral fatigue as "any reduction of maximal force output"(17), it is easily appreciated how impaired motor and sensory (modulation) centers translate into increased energy demands and reduced efficiency of ambulation, for example, quickly resulting in a fatigued individual. Thus, while we have seen above how some effort is made to distinguish *central* from *peripheral* fatigue in theory, there remains such overlap that no specific study targeting this distinction has yet been published. We are therefore left with the crude assessment tools currently available, leaving us sliding either way on a slippery slope because even purely *peripheral* fatigue must necessarily be perceived by and processed within the context of the *central* nervous system. It should thus not be surprising that so frequent a dichotomy exists between what is measured and what is perceived.

MECHANISMS

The biological "substrate" of fatigue in normal individuals is not known. Furthermore, the study of PTF is made more difficult by the fact that in our clinical experience this symptom does not occur in isolation but rather is part of a broader array of signs and symptoms post injury. Functional neuroimaging reflects yet another level of inquiry into the morphology of the fatigued brain, attempting to correlate anatomy with task-specific activity.

Anatomical

Given the heterogeneity and variety of lesions from TBI, a discussion of the source of fatigue should begin with a consideration of the underlying neuroanatomy associated with known pathophysiological mechanisms. For instance, TBI may include focal or diffuse, hemorrhagic or non-hemorrhagic, coup and contrecoup, contusional, and compressive (epi- and subdural) as well as numerous secondary and clinically superimposed causes of CNS tissue damage. Because natural traumatic forces never injure the brain in exactly the same way, the various neural circuits that support optimal cognition are differentially impaired. This leads to different degrees of cognitive dysfunction from individual to individual, further permutated by the occurrence of damage within the context of each brain's unique set of premorbid strengths and weaknesses. From a strictly statistical standpoint, the generally fatigued brain may yield a potentially infinite number of specific patterns of underperformance.

The multiple structures subserving arousal are known collectively as the ascending reticular activating system (ARAS), emanating from the brainstem and represented in each of its three divisions by the following nuclei:

> Medulla: raphe and reticularis ventralis (serotonergic)

> Pons: parabrachialis (cholinergic), locus ceruleus (noradrenergic), reticularis pontis oralis and caudalis and the gigantocellularis

> Midbrain: pedunculopontine tegmental (PPT) and laterodorsal tegmental (LDT) nucleus (cholinergic); raphe (serotonergic) and ventral tegmental area or VTA (dopaminergic)

The outputs from these structures coalesce into two pathways, the ventral and dorsal pathways of the RAS. The ventral pathway terminates in the subthalamus and posterior hypothalamus, which in turn send histaminergic fibers to a broad array of cortical end points. In addition, the ventral pathway contains a projection via the MFB to the septal nucleus and basal forebrain, which in turn send a broad array of cholinergic fibers to the cortex. The dorsal pathway projects to the interlaminar nucleus of the thalamus from which, in turn, glutaminergic tracts emerge to project across a variety of cortical and striatocortical endpoints (18).

The ARAS is a fundamental structure maintaining arousal as a prelude to alertness and bilateral injures in the brainstem nuclei result in loss of consciousness (19). This system, however, is a part of a larger and more complex system, which maintains sensory attention and tonic arousal. When there is sufficient diffuse damage (DAI) to tracts or pathways mediating general arousal, immediate unconsciousness continues over a period of variable duration depending on the extent of damage (see Chapter 8 in this book). Therefore, a frequent and major component of TBI is a disruption in the neuro-anatomical structures maintaining arousal through shearing of

axonal connections. DAI thus results in insufficient amounts of neurotransmitters normally released by more caudal structures reaching their targets, yielding an unstable platform from which to launch desired cognitive processes and behaviors, including fundamental elements subserving cognition such as attention and processing speed.

Basal Ganglia

In a recent review article, the investigators Chauduri and Behan (10) offer the hypothesis that the basal ganglia (BG) are the neuroanatomical site at which fatigue is generated following neurological injury. Specifically, they identify the disruption of two "loops", the striato-cortical fibers and the striato-thalamo-cortical fibers, as the mechanism responsible for central fatigue. Such critical pathways have been carefully delineated over the last two decades and now reveal influential and tight connections between the striatum of BG and a key component of limbic signaling, the archistriatum or amygdala. The limbic system clearly provides a route by which unconscious, spontaneous, emotionally driven motivational forces may exert influence on the motor system, thereby altering the chances that goal-directed behaviors get initiated and sustained.

In bilateral BG damage, a lack of drive, initiation and motivation is often encountered. Termed *abulia* when severe, it may be misinterpreted or overlooked altogether when more mild and is usually identified as mere apathy by rehabilitation team members. A dopaminergic pathway called the mesencephalofrontal activating system (MFAS) projects from the VTA of the midbrain to frontal regions, especially cingulate gyrus, and drives internal states towards motivated behavior. Thus, under normal circumstances, initiation and sequential performance of a task require an internally driven mechanism integrated at the level of the BG to prepare the emotive, motor and sensory apparatus responsible for the next and subsequent set of responses. Disruption of these algorithms of the sequential task processing mechanism would have the effect of not only delaying initiation, but also preventing the seamless, well-timed execution of the target task (10).

Although direct support for their theory is lacking, if it is placed within the context of the ARAS as the "substrate" for maintaining alertness, then fatigue may represent a decrease in this normal state of alertness. How this occurs is not known; however, Whyte et al. (20) have demonstrated how difficulty sustaining arousal and attention post-TBI affects cognition. They compared a cohort of 26 TBI patients with normal controls using a visual vigilance task. The results revealed "severe TBI does result in difficulties maintaining stable performance over time in an attention demanding task, independent of specific distracting events." While there was no formal assessment of fatigue in the TBI cohort in this study, the authors hypothesize that this inability to sustain performance reflects declining arousal or increasingly frequent lapses of attention. In a separate paper, Whyte drew a distinction between the tonic and phasic arousal. The former term is used to describe baseline alertness and wakefulness, while the latter refers to the arousal that is demonstrated in response to stimuli or as demanded by a distinct task. This runs parallel to the concept of the ARAS as not only mediating tonic activation and arousal but also playing an important role in the ability to phasically turn on cortical tissue in an efficient manner to perform upon demand.

This concept is also reflected by Heilman and Valenstein's (21) assertion that "brain regions . . . are essentially silent unless and until activated by release of the appropriate transmitter . . ." Thus, PTF may be conceptualized as an inability not only to activate but also to efficiently sustain and recruit cortical tissue subserving cognitive tasks.

Riese et al. (22) attempted to study the impact of central (mental) fatigue on cognition. These investigators studied eight young severely injured TBI patients more than nine months post injury. All of the patients studied had suffered not only severe but also diffuse injury and in fact one inclusion criterion was "no documented focal lesions". Fatigue was not assessed via self report. Rather, the authors assessed the ability to sustain workload via a "continuous dynamic divided attention task". The study findings revealed no difference between control and TBI subject groups in terms of the effect of "task load" on performance but an increased amount of mental effort was required among the TBI cohort for maintaining the task. The finding of increased mental effort among the TBI cohort was corroborated through both subjective and physiological indicators of distress. It is conceivable that this increased effort may correlate with perceived fatigue.

Neuroimaging

A recent fMRI study by Christodoulou et al. (23) examining working memory may offer one possible explanation for the findings in both the Whyte and Riese studies. This fMRI study examined the differences in cortical activation in seven controls versus nine TBI subjects while performing the mPASAT, a progressively more difficult computation task commonly used to assess working memory. Impairments in working memory among TBI subjects resulted not surprisingly in a higher incidence of error on the mPASAT test but interestingly, fMRI scanning further revealed a more regionally dispersed and more lateralized pattern of cerebral activation. In a related case report by Hillary et al. (24), the TBI participant completed the working memory task in the fMRI both pre and post treatment

with stimulant medication (methylphenidate and modafinil). Performance improvement was observed with stimulant medication, which also resulted in decreased cerebral activation on fMRI that correlated with the patient's self-report of greater ease in performing the task.

This increased level of cortical activation for a given task likely reflects not only inefficiency in 'phasic' recruitment of cortical assets but also suggests that the inefficiency results in increased metabolic demands as visualized on the fMRI images. The increased amount of cortex required per task in TBI versus normal controls is accompanied by the perception of greater mental effort as well.

Therefore, informed speculation leads us to identify motor coordination centers (basal ganglia), executive and motor planning areas (frontal circuits) and internal motivational apparati (hypothalamus and related limbic structures) as the main arbiters of fatigue-associated behavior. When one or more of these systems is affected, individuals routinely fail to complete the execution of incremental or serial tasks that demand sustained motivation and attention.

Functional

In seeking an all-inclusive, unifying theory of the mechanism of PTF, we cannot ignore the contribution of several, clinically encountered factors. Clinicians will certainly recognize the recurring theme of one symptom or system dysfunction reflexively exacerbating another component of the index disease. For example, mood disturbances will impact upon sleep/wake cycles which, when disturbed, tend to amplify mood disorders. Pain, (frequently encountered with comorbid multi- or craniocervical trauma), puts the individual at higher risk for mood and sleep disturbance; and conversely, those with dysfunctional mood or sleep are more apt to experience magnified pain (25–27). It is easy to appreciate how these interactions pose a mounting burden that cumulatively impedes optimal cognitive function. Perhaps, at its simplest mechanistic level, PTF represents and reflects the final common pathway's *product* of neural processing, impaired by some combination of primary damage and secondary or tertiary factors impeding cohesive, efficient and coordinated cognitive output.

OTHER COMPONENTS OF THE FATIGUE EXPERIENCE

In addition to primary neurological injury, there are many other factors that can impact both the functional and subjective reporting of fatigue in populations other than TBI. Since they are also found in TBI, such factors can also likely impact PTF. The following sections discuss these issues.

Psychology/Psychiatry

Depression commonly manifests as disturbances in sleep and appetite, decreased concentration, loss of interest, fatigue, and suicidal behaviors—all of which may often be found following TBI. At least two thirds of those studied describe fatigue, low energy or listlessness, making this one of the most common somatic complaints of depression (28, 29). Kreutzer (4) and Seel et al. (30) also found fatigue to be the most common symptom endorsed by depressed individuals with TBI. Statistically, depression predicts fatigue and fatigue predicts depression in the general population.

The neurobiological dysfunction in depression consistently involves 5-HT and NE systems and the limbic-hypothalamic-pituitary-adrenal (LHPA) axis (31), again demonstrating tremendous overlap with impairments following TBI (see endocrinology section below). Many attentional and cognitive deficits seen in depression are thought to be mediated by the prefrontal cortex, which receives significant NE and 5-HT input (32). Functional neuroimaging studies have recently elucidated frontal cortical-limbic pathways critical to modulation of depression and anxiety (33, 34). Given the frequency with which frontal damage occurs in TBI, one should commonly expect psychological dysfunction with its additive burden upon cognition, especially with what is known about how these internally distracting disease states interfere with cognition in those without TBI.

Biochemical

TBI results in a cascade of events that includes biochemical and cellular derangements. The ability to make sense of these changes is limited by the complexity of neurochemical processing in the brain. At the biochemical level, it is well known that amino acid levels are altered by TBI. Aquilani et al. (35) noted that levels of tyrosine and essential amino acids are decreased after TBI and that there is a persistent decline even upon discharge from acute rehabilitation. Two especially important amino acids for CNS function are tyrosine, a precursor to brain catecholamines, and tryptophan, an essential amino acid and precursor to serotonin. The neurotransmitter serotonin has been implicated in fatigue. The relationship between TBI disruptions in neurochemistry and the sensation of fatigue is suggested by Dwyer and Browning (36) who noted that m-chlorophenylpiperazine (m-CPP), a 5HT1A agonist, induces fatigue in an animal model, and that exercise training over a prolonged period diminished the response to this agent. Bloomstrand (37) concluded that exercise-related fatigue in the CNS was correlated to 5HT because elevated levels impaired performance whereas decreased levels improved running in an animal model. One known mechanism of tryptophan regulation provides further support for its role in central fatigue, namely that, through competitive binding for CNS transport proteins, branched-chain amino acids (BCAA) have an inverse relationship with tryptophan levels. During exercise, the ratio of tryptophan to BCAA increases and, as shown by Blomstrand (38), giving BCAA reduces perceived exertion and mental fatigue and improves cognitive performance *after* exercise.

Agents commonly used in the clinical treatment of fatigue, such as the psychostimulants methylphenidate, dextroamphetamine, pemoline and amantadine act via the dopamine neurotransmitter whereas those currently used to treat depression elevate levels of 5HT. Additional neurotransmitters to consider include histamine, which has an arousing effect on the CNS and histaminergic fibers project diffusely to cortex as discussed above with respect to the ARAS. Clinically, pharmaceuticals with an antihistaminergic mechanism of action induce sedation and fatigue. The novel agent modafinil acts, as one of its known mechanisms, as a histamine agonist. The ARAS is known to utilize cholinergic, histaminergic, glutaminergic and serotoninergic neurotransmission (18).

Endocrine

In populations other than TBI with endocrine abnormalities, especially anterior pituitary dysfunction, a wide variety of symptoms including fatigue are reported. (39–41). Of course, no one hormonal abnormality is correlated exclusively with fatigue and there are numerous other symptoms that are manifested as a result. However in other populations, the association between endocrine dysfunction and fatigue has been particularly well documented in regards to thyroid, growth hormone (GH) and cortisol deficiencies. Deficiencies in GH has been associated with decreased bone mineral densities, (42) aerobic capacity, muscle strength, lower quality of life and cognitive impairments, in addition to increased fatigue (43, 44).

Treating these deficits has been shown to be helpful in other populations. In particular, treatment of GH insufficiency has been shown to increase lean body mass and reduce body fat (45), increase exercise tolerance (46), improve quadriceps strength (47), increase energy and mood (48), increase activity and alertness (49) and an individual's sense of well being and quality of life (50).

The importance of this issue is of course dependent on the overall incidence of endocrine dysfunction associated with TBI. It has been known for nearly one hundred years that brain injury may produce endocrine dysfunction but until recently was considered a relatively rare event (51). Escamilla and Lisser (52) reported an incidence of only 0.7% (4 of 595 TBI subjects) manifesting endocrine dysfunction while Kalisky et al. (53) reported an incidence of only 4% and Edwards and Clark (54) reported a small percentage of TBI cases were associated with hypopituitarism. However, more recently, the magnitude of the problem has become more evident. Benvenga et al. (55) documented 367 cases of head trauma associated with hypopituitarism. Among these patients, 15% were not diagnosed with pituitary dysfunction till greater than 5 years after injury.

In the past few years, posttraumatic endocrine dysfunction has been studied in a prospective manner. As a result of this work the scientific and medical communities are becoming more aware of the issue of posttraumatic endocrinopathy. Kelley et al. (56) reported that 8 of 22 individuals with TBI had endocrine abnormalities when they underwent provocative testing. Lieberman et al. (51) studied 70 patients with TBI in a postacute brain injury program and identified endocrine abnormalities in 59% of subjects: GHD in 14%, hypothyroidism in 21% and low morning basal cortisol in 45%.

These studies in TBI however only identified the presence of endocrine abnormalities. The relationship between endocrine abnormalities and fatigue in the individual with TBI is an area that is currently under study. In pilot work Doppalapudi et al. (57) have demonstrated an inverse relationship between fatigue and Insulin Growth Factor 1 (IGF1) in persons with TBI. IGF1 is commonly used as a screening measure for GH deficiency because of their correlation. In addition we have noted a direct correlation with a.m. cortisol and subjective reporting of fatigue. While still preliminary, the relationship between endocrinopathy and PTF is exciting as this may potentially lead to an effective treatment.

Sleep

In general, disturbances of sleep may be characterized as insomnia (deficient sleep initiation or maintenance), hypersomnia (excessive sleep or what is referred to as excessive daytime sleepiness—EDS), and altered sleep-wake cycles (circadian pattern disarray). Sleep disturbances following TBI range in frequency from 36% to 70% (58,59). Several key CNS loci regulate sleep patterns, including brainstem, basal forebrain and hypothalamic nuclei—all areas commonly disrupted in brain trauma. Serotonin and acetylcholine are the two common substances involved. The comprehensive study of posttraumatic sleep disorders is complicated by the frequently encountered comorbidities of depression, anxiety, substance abuse, chronic pain and medication use, all of which independently exert negative influences upon normal sleep. Also not to be overlooked is whether one may implicate a prior (perhaps undiagnosed) sleep disorder as the proximate cause of the brain injury itself. For instance, falling asleep while driving is not uncommon, especially in persons with sleep apnea.

Controversy exists over whether severity of TBI is directly correlated with increased prevalence of insomnia.

Clinchot et al. (60) and Fitchenberg (61) showed an *inverse* relationship and Cohen (62) noted increased prevalence with increasing TBI severity. Some researchers have postulated that the reason for this counterintuitive finding lies in the fact that the severely brain injured likely underreport and the milder brain injured are more aware of their problems and therefore over report or perhaps overly attribute their fatigue to poor sleep. Clinchot et al. (60) examined 100 TBI patients during inpatient rehabilitation and followed them up again one year later. These authors reported that 50% of TBI subjects complained of difficulty sleeping. Of this sub-group 64% admitted waking up too early, 25% experienced increased sleep time, and 45% reported difficulty falling asleep. In this same cohort of 100 patients, 63% reported significant problems with fatigue. Interestingly, 80% of those admitting to sleeping difficulty also admitted to fatigue as a problem. Cohen et al. (62) have pointed to a temporally differentiated sleep disruption pattern whereby difficulty initiating or maintaining sleep tends to occur soon after TBI and excessive daytime sleeping (EDS) tends to occur more often over the months and years following TBI. Controversy also exists over whether TBI may cause a secondary narcolepsy (see Chapter 32 in this book on sleep disorders).

Several varieties of disturbed sleep-wake cycles are seen—the delayed, advanced and disorganized types—with very little literature available specific to the TBI population. Schreiber et al. (63) described sleep-wake disturbance in 15 persons with mild TBI and without history of apnea syndrome, neurological or psychiatric illness. Using polysomnography and actigraphy (activity detection device), more than half were found to have delayed-phase and the rest disorganized type.

Thus, the brain injured population experiences disruption in normal sleep physiology. Specific abnormalities discovered include reductions in REM sleep, sleep spindles, vertex sharp waves and K complexes. These electroencephalographic findings point to an overall decrease in total sleep time, a disappearance of the deeper stages of sleep as well as more frequent awakening (64). Conversely, it has been also found that as cognition improves, so too does REM sleep architecture. There also appears to be an association between cognition and sleep architecture among TBI patients across time so that as the former improves, so too does the latter (65). In addition, it has been well described in the normal, non-TBI injured population, that as sleep time declines and sleep quality worsens there is a decline in cognitive performance as well as an increase in fatigue (66).

Overall, while sleep disturbance after TBI is common, there is little work directly relating this disturbance with fatigue. However, it is likely that the relationship between sleep and fatigue observed in other populations applies to persons with TBI. While these findings are perhaps predictable, unfortunately even in the normal population we do not know the mechanism whereby sleep reduces the self-perception of fatigue and enhances cognitive performance.

MANAGEMENT OF PTF

As is the case for most medical conditions in general and neurological conditions in particular, complete cure remains elusive. Nevertheless, it remains critical to start on the road to cure by addressing the fundamentals, relying upon the interdisciplinary treatment team when available. Routine performance of a home exercise program not only optimizes cardiovascular health and physical well being but secondarily enhances important emotional and immune system functioning, which in turn may play important roles in the fatigue experience. Classic rehabilitation practice includes instructing the fatigued individual in compensatory strategies to conserve "energy" and can be tailored to one's specific functional requirements as they intersect with the particular areas of cognitive functional deficit. The instruction may be as simple as the admonition to *pace* oneself. Psycho-education frequently comprises teaching the person with PTF (and involved caregiver) how the clinical sequelae of focal and diffuse injuries alter the brain's ability to successfully perform certain tasks that consistently engender fatigue. Therefore, clients may learn how to prioritize activities to meet the goals of daily functioning. When efforts fall short, personal expectations may need to be reconciled with actual abilities and performance (see below). Attempts should be made to counsel those with PTF about dietary habits, with the goal of both weight reduction (given the frequency of post-TBI weight gain) and energy efficiency. At a minimum, obtaining a sleep history should lead to counseling about basic sleep hygiene (see Chapter 32 in this book). When appropriate, more in-depth investigation with polysomnography may reveal a treatable sleep disorder at the root of PTF. As alluded to in the endocrine section, serum hormonal screening may reveal a remediable imbalance although too few studies exist to predict how much success may be expected from a neuropharmacoendocrinologic intervention.

Formal psychiatric care or psychological counseling may be needed to minimize the influence of psychological distress upon cognition and fatigue behavior, through treatment of anxiety and depressive states. Pharmacological management by a professional knowledgeable in TBI leads to the best choice aimed at neutralizing internally distracting states while often parsimoniously addressing other sequelae of TBI such as headache, irritability, perseveration and sleep disturbance. Practically, our bias is to use the most activating of antidepressants such as fluoxetine, bupropion (whose putative dopaminergic action may also address abulic features), venlafaxine at higher (more noradrenergic) doses, protriptyline and the latest agent, duloxetine, with a novel mechanism of selective noradrenergic and serotonergic reuptake inhibition.

Once modifiable factors have been addressed and conservative measures fail, the first practical pharmacological approach to PTF is to substitute for or eliminate those agents that cause fatigue itself or potentiate any of the common components of PTF. One of the most common obstacles to optimizing efficient cognitive function is the often inappropriately prolonged use of anticonvulsants (67–69) (see Chapter 26 in this book). If posttraumatic epilepsy exists, the least sedating and cognitively debilitating choice of drug must be pursued. Some literature even suggests that one anticonvulsant, lamotrigine, may even be *activating*. Commonly used gastric promotility, anti-spasticity, psychoactive and antihypertensive agents may also hamper optimal cognitive and behavioral (e.g. motivational) function (70).

Regarding clinical use of drugs targeting fatigue, most of the information and experience comes from their use for sequelae other than PTF and from the treatment of fatigue in other disease states. Thus, amantadine has been used sometimes with dramatic effect in TBI to improve various facets of the fatigue experience (e.g. arousal, abulia) and long ago showed efficacy in treating the fatigue associated with MS (71, 72). Numerous papers have reported on the use of methylphenidate, dextroamphetamine, and amantadine to treat cognitive deficits secondary to brain injury and fatigue in other populations. Brietbart and associates (73) demonstrated the benefit of methylphenidate and pemoline in HIV-related fatigue, whereas Wagner and Rabkin (74) reported a similar benefit of dextroamphetamine. Emonson and Vanderbeek (75) reported that dextroamphetamine was also useful for flight crews flying during Desert Shield.

The "classic" stimulants enjoy widespread use in TBI but few, if any, well-designed and powered studies have specifically named PTF as the dependent variable despite the intuitive connection. Until such studies become available, dosing remains mostly symptomatic, aimed at improving function and quality of life. We use short-acting methylphenidate (MP) and dextroamphetamine (DAA), dosed in accordance with their relatively short half-lives, to coincide with therapy sessions or periods of important activity. Long-acting preparations clearly have many advantages but cost remains a major drawback. While these drugs (including *pemoline*) enhance catecholaminergic activity in general, a newer agent, *atomexitine* is noradrenergic-selective. With this class of stimulant drugs, clinicians should heed the typical cautions (though not seen clinically to a significant degree) (76) to monitor blood pressure and heart rate at a minimum.

The novel wake-promoting agent *modafinil* is known to less-likely cause psychomotor agitation than the classic stimulants, reflecting animal studies showing activation of more subcortical, particularly hypothalamic regions. Originally approved for the treatment of narcolepsy and, more recently, for shift work sleep disorder and under-treated sleep apnea, it does not activate dopaminergic pathways but seems to exert at least part of its action through histaminergic stimulation. Modafinil has been reported to be useful in various populations with neurological disorder including stroke, MS, depression, Parkinson disease and schizophrenia (77). It has also been shown to reduce the fatigue associated with certain medications possessing a sedative side effect.

While its use, too, is often cost-prohibitive, modafinil together with atomexitine have the distinct advantage of being less *scheduled*, making prescription refills possible and theoretically reducing the risk of medication abuse, which is of particular concern in the largest TBI demographic.

It remains unclear whether treatment with such medications actively ameliorates dysfunction at the level of the supposed fatigue generator, at the behavioral or output level, at the perceptual level; or simply mitigates one to several of the secondary inputs to the ultimate fatigue experience. Given this lack of hard data, the therapeutic relationship may be enhanced through the suggestion that rational trials of complementary or alternative remedies (nostrums?) may, so long as they are not patently harmful, be beneficial. Examples in this category include piracetam (a non-FDA-approved nootropic widely used outside of but obtainable from certain compounding pharmacies in the US), acupuncture and various herbal preparations.

Chapter 57 in this book is dedicated to the pharmacological properties of herbal medication and the readers are referred to that section for an in depth discussion of the material. However, as these agents are becoming more widely used by the medical community (78) and being recommended for the treatment of fatigue (79) a brief discussion is warranted.

Ginkgo Biloba (80) has been suggested as a treatment for many different conditions in numerous populations with suggested doses ranging from 120 to 240 mg a day. Some evidence of its efficacy in the treatment of Chronic Fatigue Syndrome has been demonstrated (81). Ginseng is a complex alternative medication that consists of many compounds and has been suggested to exert its effect through activity on nitric oxide (82). Work by Sorensen and Sonne (83) demonstrated that a dose of 400 mg resulted in improved reaction time. Acetyl-L-carnitine in doses of 1500mg twice a day has been suggested to be beneficial in energy issues and cognitive function post TBI (84). In animal studies it has been shown to be active in the cholinergic system (85) as well as having a neuroprotective effect

on brain cells (86). Citicholine (CDP-choline), which readily crosses the blood brain barrier, dissociates to the acetylcholine precursor choline (84). It has a demonstrated neuroprotective effect and has been widely used in Europe and Asia in the treatment of patients with stroke and TBI. A study by Leon-Carrion demonstrated an improvement in both attention and vigilance (87), with suggested dosing ranging from 1–3 grams per day (84).

FUTURE DIRECTIONS

The cause of PTF has not been demonstrated to uniquely follow from damage to one particular anatomic locus. The work of Christodoulou et al. (23) and Hillary et al. (24) suggests that neuroimaging may at sometime in the future be better able to correlate deficits in function with morphology. In addition, as neuropharmacological interventions improve and the potential to target medications to specific abnormalities becomes more developed, better treatment outcomes may be obtained. The potential for the use of imaging modalities to select pharmacologic interventions and to predict effectiveness is an exciting prospect. In addition, improved management of endocrine abnormalities, cognitive deficits, mood and sleep disorders may also lead to improved treatment outcomes.

Additional efforts to establish the relationship between fatigue and well known TBI-related deficits, particularly arousal, attention, vigilance, and memory will be critical. The future holds tremendous promise in uncovering the mechanisms of fatigue generation after TBI through a combination of neuroimaging, pharmaceutical interventions and traditional neuropsychological test batteries.

Finally, individuals with TBI have numerous medical issues that differentiate them from other patients who have fatigue. Improvements in the treatment of spasticity, endocrine abnormality, sleep disturbance and mood disorder are just some of the areas where better medical management may make a substantial difference in the nebulous area of the treatment of fatigue associated with TBI.

References

1. Middleboe T, Andersen HS, Birket-Smith M, Friis ML. Minor head injury: impact on general health after 1 year. A prospective follow-up study. *Acta Neurol Scand* 1992;85:5–9.
2. Hillier SL, Sharpe MH, Metzer J. Outcomes 5 years post-traumatic brain injury (with further reference to neurophysical impairment and disability). *Brain Inj* 1997;11(9):661–675.
3. Olver JH, Ponsford JL, Curran CA. Outcome following traumatic brain injury: a comparison between 2 and 5 years after injury. *Brain Inj* 1996;10:841–848.
4. Kreutzer JS, Seel RT, Gourley E. The prevalence and symptom rates of depression after traumatic brain injury: a comprehensive examination. *Brain Inj* 2001;15(7):563–76.
5. Harrison-Felix C, Zafonte R, Mann N, Dijkers M, Englander J, Kreutzer J. Brain injury as a result of violence: preliminary findings from the traumatic brain injury model systems. *Arch Phys Med Rehabil* 1998;79(7):730–737.

6. Brassington JC and Marsh NV. Neuropsychological aspects of multiple sclerosis. *Neuropsychology Rev* 1998;8:43–77.

7. Elkins LE, Krupp LB, and Scherl W. The measurement of fatigue and contributing neuropsychiatric factors. *Sem Clin Neuropsychiatry* 2000;5:58–61.

8. Iriarte J, Subira ML, and Castro P. Modalities of fatigue in multiple sclerosis: correlation with clinical and biological factors. *Mult Sclerosis* 2000;6:124–130.

9. Lezak MD (ed.). *Neuropsychological Assessment, 3rd Edition* New York: Oxford University Press 1995.

10. Chaudhuri A & Behan PO. Fatigue and basal ganglia. *J Neurol Sci* 2000;17:34–42.

11. Deluca J (ed.). *Fatigue as a Window to the Brain.* Cambridge: MIT Press, 2005.

12. Masson F, Maurette P, Salmi LR, et al. Prevalence of impairments 5 years after a head injury, and their relationship with disabilities and outcome. *Brain Inj* 1996;10:487–497.

13. Walker GC, Cardenas DD, Guthrie MR, McLean A Jr & Brooke MM. Fatigue and depression in brain-injured patients correlated with quadriceps strength and endurance. *Arch Phys Med Rehabil* 1991;72:469–472.

14. Krupp LB, LaRocca NG, Muir-Nash J, Steinberg AD. The fatigue severity scale. Application to patients with multiple sclerosis and systemic lupus erythematosus. *Arch Neurol* 1989;46:1121–1123.

15. Fisk JD, Pontefract A, Ritvo PG, Archibald CJ, Murray TJ. The impact of fatigue on patients with multiple sclerosis. *Can J Neurol Sci* 1994;21:9–14.

16. LaChapelle L, Finlayson MA. An evaluation of subjective and objective measures of fatigue in patients with brain injury and healthy controls. *Brain Inj* 1998;12(8):649–59.

17. Krupp LB and Pollina DA. Mechanisms and management of fatigue in progressive neurological disorders. *Curr Opinions Neurol* 1996;9:456–460.

18. Carpenter MB. *Core Text of Neuroanatomy. 3rd edn.* Baltimore: Williams & Wilkins 1985.

19. Plum F, Posner JB. *The Diagnosis of Stupor and Coma, 3rd ed.* Philadelphia: F.A. Davis Company 1980.

20. Whyte J, Polansky M, Fleming M, Coslett HB, Cavalucci C. Sustained arousal and attention after traumatic brain injury. *Neuropsychologia* 1995;Jul 33 (7):797–813.

21. Heilman KM, Valenstein E (ed.). *Clinical Neuropsychology,* 4th edn Oxford: Oxford University Press, 2003.

22. Riese H, Hoedemaeker M, Brouwer WH, Mulder LJM, Cremer R, Veldman JBP. Mental fatigue after very severe closed head injury: Sustained performance, mental effort, and distress at two levels of workload in a driving simulator. *Neuropsychol Rehabil* 1999;9:189–205.

23. Christodoulou C, Deluca J, Ricker JH, et al. Functional magnetic resonance imaging of working memory impairment after traumatic brain injury. *J Neurol Neurosurg Psych* 2001;71:161–168.

24. Hillary F, Elovic E, Ricker J. Stimulant induced improvement in brain efficiency as documented by functional magnetic resonance imaging: A case report. *Am J Phys Med Rehabil* 2003; 82(3):240.

25. Covington EC. Depression and chronic fatigue in the patient with chronic pain. *Prim Care* 1991;18:341–358.

26. Manu P, Matthews DA, Lane TJ, et al. Depression among patients with a chief complaint of chronic fatigue. *J Affect Disord* 1989;Sep 17(2):165–172.

27. Wessely S, Powell R. Fatigue syndromes: a comparison of chronic "postviral" fatigue with neuromuscular and affective disorders. *J Neurol Neurosurg Psychiatry* 1989;Aug 52(8):940–948.

28. Tylee A. Depression in the community: physician and patient perspective. *J Clin Psychiatry* 1999;60 Suppl 7:12–16.

29. Maurice-Tison S, Verdoux H, Gay B, Perez P, Salamon R & Bourgeois ML. How to improve recognition and diagnosis of depressive syndromes using international diagnostic criteria. *Brit J Gen Prac* 1998;48:1245–1246.

30. Seel RT and Kreutzer JS. Depression assessment after traumatic brain injury: an empirically based classification method. *Arch Phys Med Rehabil* 2003;84(11):1621–8.

31. Holsboer F. Implications of altered limbic-hypothalamic-pituitary-adrenocortical (LHPA)-function for neurobiology of depression. *Acta Psych Scand* 1988;Supplement 341:72–111.

32. Drevets WC. Functional anatomical abnormalities in limbic and prefrontal cortical structures in major depression. *Prog Brain Res* 2000;126:413–431.

33. Liotti M, Mayberg HS, Brannan SK, McGinnis S, Jerabek P, Fox PT. Differential limbic—cortical correlates of sadness and anxiety in healthy subjects: implications for affective disorders. *Biol Psychiatry* 2000;Jul 48(1):30–42.

34. Brody AL, Barsom MW, Bota RG, Saxena S. Prefrontal-subcortical and limbic circuit mediation of major depressive disorder. *Semin Clin Neuropsychiatry* 2001;6:102–112.

35. Aquilani R, Iadarola P, Boschi F, Pistarini C, Arcidiaco P, Contardi A. Reduced plasma levels of tyrosine, precursor of brain catecholamines, and of essential amino acids in patients with severe traumatic brain injury after rehabilitation. *Arch Phys Med Rehabil* 2003 Sep;84(9):1258–1265.

36. Dwyer D and Browning J. Endurance training in Wistar rats decreases receptor sensitivity to a serotonin agonist. *Acta Physiol Scand* 2000;170(3):211–6.

37. Blomstrand E. Amino acids and central fatigue. *Am Acids* 2001;20:25–34.

38. Blomstrand E, Hassmen P and Newsholme EA. Effect of branched-chain amino acid supplementation on mental performance. *Acta Physiol Scan* 1991;143:225–226.

39. Elovic EP. Anterior pituitary dysfunction after traumatic brain injury, Part I. *J Head Trauma Rehabil* 2003;18:541–543.

40. Elovic EP. Anterior Pituitary Dysfunction After Traumatic Brain Injury Part 2. *J Head Trauma Rehabil* 2004;19:184–187.

41. Larsen PR, Kronenberg HM, Melmed S & Polonsky KS. *Williams Textbook of Endocrinology, 10th ed.* Philadelphia: Saunders 2003.

42. Colao A, Di Somma C, Pivonello R, Loche S, Aimaretti G, Cerbone G, Faggiano A, Comeli G, Ghigo E, Lombardi G. Bone loss is correlated to the severity of growth hormone deficiency in adult patients with hypopituitarism. *J Clin Endocr Metab* 1999;84:1919–1924.

43. Deijen JB, de Boer H, Blok GJ, van der Veen EA. Cognitive impairments and mood disturbances in growth hormone deficient men. *Psychoneuroendocrinology* 1996;21:313–322.

44. Simpson H, Savine R, Sonksen P, et al. Growth hormone replacement therapy for adults: into the new millennium. *Growth Hormones and IGF Res* 2002;12:1–33.

45. Newman CB, Kleinberg DL. Adult growth hormone deficiency. *Endocrinologist* 1998;8:178–186.

46. Jørgensen JOL, Thiesen L, Müller J, Ovesem P, Skakkebæk N & Christiansen JS. Three years of growth hormone treatment in growth hormone-deficient adults: near normalization of body composition and physical performance. *Eur J Endocrin* 1994;130:224–8.

47. Jørgensen JO, Pedersen SA, Thuesen L, Jørgensen J, Moller J, Muller J et al. Long-term growth hormone treatment in growth hormone deficient adults *Acta Endocrinol* (Copenh) 1991;125(5):449–453

48. Gibney J, Wallace JD, Spinks T, Schnorr L, Ranican A, Cuneo RC, et al. The effects of 10 years of recombinant human growth hormone (GH) in adult GH-deficient patients. *J Clin Endocrin Metab* 1999;84:2596–2602.

49. Burman P, Broman JE, Hetta J et al. Quality of life in adults with growth hormone (GH) deficiency: response to treatment with recombinant human GH in a placebo-controlled 21-month trial. *J Clin Endocr Metab* 1995;80:3585–3590.

50. Carroll PV, Christ ER, Bengtsson BA, et al. Growth hormone deficiency in adulthood and the effects of growth hormone replacement: a review. Growth Hormone Research Society Scientific Committee. *J Clin Endocr Metab* 1998;83:382–395.

51. Lieberman SA, Oberoi AL, Gilkison CR, Masel BE & Urban RJ. Prevalence of neuroendocrine dysfunction in patients recovering from traumatic brain injury. *J Clin Endocrin Metab* 2001;86:2752–2756.

52. Escamilla RF, Lisser H. Simmonds disease. *J Clin Endocrin* 1942;2:65–96.

53. Kalisky Z, Morrison DP, Meyers CA, Von Laufen A. Medical problems encountered during rehabilitation of patients with head injury. *Arch Phys Med Rehabil* 1985;66:25–29.

54. Edwards OM & Clark JD. Post-traumatic hypopituitarism. Six cases and a review of the literature. *Medicine* 1986;65:281–290.

55. Benvenga S, Campenni A, Ruggeri R, Trimarchi F. Clinical review 113: Hypopituitarism secondary to head trauma. *J Clin Endocr Metabolism* 2000;85:1353–1361.

56. Kelly DF, Gonzalo IT, Cohan P, Berman N, Swerdloff R, Wang C. Hypopituitarism following traumatic brain injury and aneurysmal subarachnoid hemorrhage: a preliminary report. *J Neurosurg* 2000;93:743–752.

57. Doppalapudi, HS, Miller, M. Millis, S. Fellus, JL, Masel, BE, Urban, RJ, Elovic and EP. The Relation between Fatigue and Endocrine Abnormalities in an Outpatient Traumatic Brain Injury Sample: A Preliminary Report. *Arch Phys Med Rehabil* (in press).

58. McLean A, Dikmen S, Temkin NR. Psychosocial functioning at one month after head injury. *Neurosurg* 1984;14:393–399.

59. Keshavan MS, Channabasavanna SM & Reddy GN. Post traumatic psychiatric disturbances: Patterns and predictions of outcome. *Brit J Psychiatry* 1981;138:157–160.

60. Clinchot DM, Bogner J, Mysiew WJ, et al. Defining sleep disturbance after brain injury. *Am J Phys Med Rehabil* 2003;77(4): 291–295.

61. Fichtenberg NL, Putnam SH, Mann NR, Zafonte RD, Millard AE. Insomnia screening in postacute traumatic brain injury: utility and validity of the Pittsburgh Sleep Quality Index. *Am J Phys Med Rehabil* 2001;80:339–345.

62. Cohen M, Oksenberg A, Snir D, Stern MJ, Groswasser Z. Temporally related changes of sleep complaints in traumatic brain injured patients. *J Neurol Neurosurg Psych* 1992;55:313–315.

63. Schreiber S, Klag E, Gross Y, Segman RH, Pick CG. Beneficial effect of risperidone on sleep disturbance and psychosis following traumatic brain injury. *Inter Clin Psychopharm* 1998;13: 273–275.

64. Busek P & Faber J. The influence of traumatic brain lesion on sleep architecture. *Sbovník Lékarsky* 2000;101:233–239.

65. Ron S, Algom D, Hary D, Cohen M. Time-related changes in the distribution of sleep stages in brain injured patients. *Electroencephalographic Clin Neurophysiol* 1980;48:432–441.

66. Roth T, Costa E Silva JA, Chase MH. Sleep and cognitive (memory) function: research and clinical perspectives. *Sleep Med* 2001; 2(5):379–87.

67. Temkin NR, Dikmen SS, Wilensky AJ, Keihm J, Chabal S, Winn HR. A randomized, double blind study of phenytoin for the prevention of post-traumatic seizures. *New Eng J Med* 1990;323(8): 497–502.

68. Brain Injury Special Interest Group (BISIG) of the American Academy of Physical Medicine and Rehabilitation. Practice Parameter: antiepileptic drug treatment of posttraumatic seizures. *Arch Phys Med Rehabil* 1998;79:594–597.

69. Chang BS, Lowenstein DH. Practice Parameter: Antiepileptic drug prophylaxis in severe traumatic brain injury: Report of the Quality Standards Subcommittee of the American Academy of Neurology, *Neurology* 2003;60:10–16.

70. Goldstein LB. Rehabilitation and recovery after stroke. *Curr Treat Options Neurol* 2000;2:319–328.

71. Krupp LB, Coyle PK, Doscher C, et al. Fatigue therapy in multiple sclerosis: results of a double-blind, randomized, parallel trial of amantadine, pemoline, and placebo. *Neurol* 1995;45: 1956–1961.

72. Cohen RA & Fisher M. Amantadine treatment of fatigue associated with multiple sclerosis. *Arch Neurol* 1989;46(6):676–80.

73. Breitbart W, Rosenfeld B, Kaim M, Funesti-Esch J. A randomized, double-blind, placebo-controlled trial of psychostimulants for the treatment of fatigue in ambulatory patients with human immunodeficiency virus disease. *Arch Int Med* 2001;12:161(3),411–420.

74. Wagner GJ & Rabkin R. Effects of dextroamphetamine on depression and fatigue in men with HIV: a double blind, placebo-controlled trial. *J Clin Psychiatry* 2000;61(6):436–40.

75. Emonson DL & Vanderbeek RD. The use of amphetamines in U.S. Air Force tactical operations during Desert Shield. *Space Environ Med* 1995;66(3):260–263

76. Burke DT, Glenn MB, Vesali F, Schneide JC, Burke J, Ahangar B, Goldstein R. Effects of Methylphenidate on heart rate and blood pressure among inpatients with acquired brain injury. *Am J Phys Med Rehabil* 2004;82(7):493–497.

77. Rammohan KW, Rosenberg JH, Lynn DJ, Blumenfeld AM, Pollak CP, Nagaraja HN. Efficacy and safety of modafinil (Provigil) for the treatment of fatigue in multiple sclerosis: a two centre phase 2 study. *J Neurol Neurosurg Psychiatry* 2003;72(2):179–83.

78. Eisenberg DM, Davis RB, Ettner SL, et al. Trends in alternative medicine use in the United States, 1990–1997: results of a follow-up national survey. *JAMA* 1998 Nov 11;280(18):1569–1575.

79. Diamond BJ, Shiflett SC, Feiwel N, et al. Ginkgo biloba extract: mechanisms and clinical indications. *Arch Phys Med Rehabil* 2000 May;81(5):668–678.

80. Elovic EP, Zafonte RD. Ginkgo biloba: applications in traumatic brain injury. *J Head Trauma Rehabil* 2001 Dec;16(6):603–607.

81. Logan AC, Wong C. Chronic fatigue syndrome: oxidative stress and dietary modifications. *Altern Med Rev* 2001 Oct;6(5): 450–459.

82. Gillis CN. Panax ginseng pharmacology: a nitric oxide link? *Biochem Pharmacol* 1997 Jul 1;54(1):1–8.

83. Sorensen H, Sonne J. A double masked study on the effects of ginseng on cognitive function. *Curr Ther Res* 1996;57:959–968.

84. Brown RB, Gerbarg PL. Alternative Treatments. In: Silver JM, McAllister TW, Yudofsky SC, (eds.) Textbook of Traumatic Brain Injury. Washington, D.C.: *American Psychiatric Press*, 2005: 679–696.

85. Pettegrew JW, Levine J, McClure RJ. Acetyl-L-carnitine physical-chemical, metabolic, and therapeutic properties: relevance for its mode of action in Alzheimer's disease and geriatric depression. *Mol Psychiatry* 2000 Nov;5(6):616–632.

86. Calvani M, Rigoni-Martelli E. Attenuation by acetyl-L-carnitine of neurological damage and biochemical derangement following brain ischemia and reperfusion. *Int J Tissue React* 1999;21(1):1–6.

87. Leon-Carrion J, Dominguez-Roldan JM, Murillo-Cabezas F, del RD-M, Munoz-Sanchez MA. The role of citicholine in neuropsychological training after traumatic brain injury. *NeuroRehabilitation* 2000;14(1):33–40.

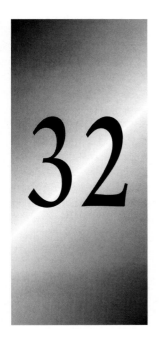

32

Sleep Disturbances: Epidemiology, Assessment, and Treatment

Lora L. Thaxton
Amish R. Patel

SLEEP DISTURBANCES IN TBI: EPIDEMIOLOGY, ASSESSMENT, AND TREATMENT

Objectives: Sleep disturbances in people with traumatic brain injuries, although quite common remains a problematic management issue for caregivers. This chapter will review the epidemiology of sleep disturbances in this population, sleep architecture, sleep neurophysiology, the biochemical pharmacology of sleep, assessment measures and treatment, both nonpharmacologic and pharmacologic. This information will hopefully assist in the decision-making processes of caregivers managing individuals with traumatic brain injury and sleep disturbances.

EPIDEMIOLOGY

Sleep disturbances occur commonly in patients whom have suffered a traumatic brain injury. The patients may experience sleep disturbances during all stages of recovery. Occurrence rates for sleep disturbances following recent TBI range from 36% (1–3) to 81.2% for hospitalized patients, and 72.7% for discharged patients (4). Disorders of initiating and maintaining sleep (DIMS) were more common among hospitalized patients with recent brain injury. Disorders of excessive somnolence (DOES) were more common in post acute injured patients (4). The total

cost for treatment of insomnia in the U.S. taking into account lost productivity and insomnia-related accidents, may exceed $100 billion per year (5). Patients whom have suffered a brain injury usually will experience difficulties in many realms of their lives including personal, professional, social, and avocational. Insomnia and sleep disturbances may compound these difficulties due to the fact that disordered sleep can have adverse behavioral and cognitive consequences. Insomnia in the absence of brain injury has been associated with increased absences from work (6), increased health care costs/utilization, and social disability (7). Mahmood et al. (206) hypothesized that TBI patients may experience sleep-related cognitive deficits even without meeting the formal diagnosis of insomnia.

DEFINITIONS OF INSOMNIA

Primary insomnia is sleeplessness that is not attributable to a medical, psychiatric, or environmental cause.

Secondary insomnia, more commonly diagnosed, is the result of an underlying medical, psychiatric, or environmental condition. Acute insomnia refers to the onset of sleep difficulties caused by emotional or physical discomforts. Acute insomnia could be considered a subset of secondary insomnia.

Sleep-onset insomnia refers to an extended time from going to bed until falling asleep. Circadian rhythm disorders are considered a subset of sleep-onset insomnias (8).

CLASSIFICATION OF SLEEP DISORDERS

The International Classification of Sleep Disorders categorizes sleep disturbances as dyssomnias or disorders that result in insomnia or excessive sleepiness; parasomnias or disorders of arousal, partial arousal, or sleep stage transition; and sleep disorders associated with medical or psychiatric disorders (9). An extensive review of the medical conditions that can cause insomnia is beyond the scope of this chapter. However, medical conditions should be considered in patients with sleep difficulties. Table 32-1 includes the most common disorders in each category.

Sleep related breathing disorders are commonly divided into 3 categories: obstructive sleep apnea (OSA), central sleep apnea (CSA), and mixed sleep apnea (11). Obstructive sleep apnea is characterized by periodic apnea

and asphyxia from upper airway obstruction or collapse in the pharynx that continues despite continued respiratory effort. Central sleep apnea is defined as the lack of airflow accompanied by the lack of respiratory effort. Mixed apneas have components of both obstructive and central apneas (11). Symptoms related to sleep apnea include excessive daytime sleepiness and cognitive difficulties such as impaired memory, loss of judgment, inability to concentrate, irritability, and depression. These symptoms are often present in TBI patients in the absence of sleep apnea making clinical diagnosis difficult (200). Secondary cardiovascular morbidity associated with sleep-related breathing disorders includes systemic and pulmonary hypertension, cardiac arrythmias, cor pulmonale, stroke, and sudden death (12). Other factors that may be present in the TBI population contributing to fatigue and excessive daytime sleepiness include: electrolyte disturbances, hydrocephalus, occult infection, seizures and endocrine disorders (200).

Webster et al. (200) is one of the first studies of sleep apnea in the traumatic brain injured population.

Restless legs syndrome (RLS) is characterized by unpleasant sensations in the legs or feet that are temporarily relieved by moving the limbs. Symptoms increase in the evening, especially when a person is lying down and remaining still. The dysesthesias cause difficulty falling asleep and are often accompanied by periodic limb movements (13).

Periodic limb movement disorder (PLMD), is characterized by bilateral repeated, rhythmic, small-amplitude jerking, or twitching movements in the lower extremities, and less frequently, in the arms. These movements occur every 20 to 90 seconds and lead to arousals usually not perceived by the patient. The patient complains of not feeling rested. The bed partner often reports these movements. This condition is more common in older individuals (14).

TREATMENT OF SPECIFIC DYSSOMNIAS OBSTRUCTIVE SLEEP APNEA

The treatment of Obstructive Sleep Apnea partly depends upon the severity of the sleep-disordered breathing. The severity of OSA is defined arbitrarily and differs among centers. The apnea-hypoapnea index (AHI) has been used to grade severity of apnea. AHI of 5 to 20/hour is mild apnea; 20 to 60/ hour is moderate apnea; and greater than 60 is severe apnea (137).

Patients with mild apnea have a wider variety of options, while those with moderate to severe apnea should be treated with nasal continuous positive airway pressure (CPAP) (137, 138). CPAP works by splinting the upper airway and preventing soft tissues from collapsing resulting in improvements in apneas and normalizing oxygen saturation (138). The most common side effects of CPAP are dry mouth, rhinitis, and sinus congestion

---

TABLE 32-1

Dyssomnias
Intrinsic sleep disorders arising from bodily malfunctions:
Psychophysiological insomnia
Obstructive sleep apnea
Central sleep apnea
Restless legs syndrome (RLS)
Periodic limb movement disorder (PLMD)

Parasomnias
Group of disorders of arousal, partial arousal, and sleep-stage transition:
Sleep-walking (somnambulism)
Sleep talking (somniloquy)
Sleep terrors
Nightmares
Teeth grinding (bruxism)
REM sleep behavior disorder (RBD)
Enuresis

Medical and psychiatric
Anxiety
Chronic pain
Alcoholism
Parkinsonism
Dementia/delirium
Depression
Gastroesophageal reflux
Chronic obstructive pulmonary disease
Asthma
Atherosclerotic cardiovascular disease
Diabetes mellitus
Thyroid disease (10)

(138). These can be treated effectively with humidification, antihistamines or nasal steroids. Unfortunately, compliance is a major problem.

Dental devices act by moving the tongue or mandible forward. They can be effective with an AHI of less than 40/hour (139). Dental devices are appropriate first line therapy in mild OSA and can be used as an alternative if the patient does not improve with CPAP (139).

Correction of the upper airway is generally recommended only for patients in whom CPAP has failed, patients who refused to consider CPAP, or those who have very mild OSA (AHI less than 10/hour) (140). The resection of the uvula and soft palate known as uvulopalatopharyngoplasty (UPPP) is effective in about 40% of patients (140). Predicting which patients will benefit from this procedure is impossible. Tracheostomy is another surgical technique that is effective by passing the obstruction. This procedure is indicated for very severe OSA especially when the patient does not tolerate CPAP or has cor pulmonale (140).

RESTLESS LEG SYNDROME

Patients with Restless Leg Syndrome (RLS) who are sensitive to caffeine, alcohol, or nicotine should avoid these substances (141). Some patients may benefit from different physical modalities, such as hot or cold baths, whirlpool baths, limb massage, vibratory or electrical stimulation of the feet and toes before bedtime (141). Supplementation to correct vitamin deficiencies, electrolytes, or iron may improve symptoms in some patients. Patients with prominent varicose veins in the legs may benefit from TED hose.

Continuous pharmacologic treatment should be considered if patients complain of RLS symptoms at least three nights each week (142). Dopaminergic agents are first line treatment. Levadopa with carbidopa has been shown to improve sensory symptoms and periodic leg movements of sleep (PLMS) in primary RLS and in secondary RLS due to uremia (143). Other dopamine agonists such as Pramipexole, Pergolide, Ropinirole hydrochloride, have been used to treat RLS. Benzodiazepines such as Clonazepam have been shown to ease sensory symptoms and PLMS in RLS (143). Opioids have been used also successfully in decreasing symptoms of RLS (144). Gabapentin is indicated for patients whose symptoms include pain, and/or neuropathy (144).

NARCOLEPSY

Nonpharmacologic treatment consists of sleep hygiene. Most patients improve if they maintain a regular sleep schedule usually 7.5 to 8 hours of sleep per night (145). Patients with narcolepsy should avoid heavy meals and alcohol (146). A well-designed exercise program can be beneficial and stimulating (147). Encourage children to participate in after-school activities and sports. School personnel should have the child with narcolepsy refrain from activities if he or she appears drowsy.

Pharmacologic treatment of narcolepsy involves central nervous system stimulants to increase wakefulness, vigilance, and performance, and depressants to reduce cataplectic attacks. Modafinil, an alpha 1-agonist, has been used for several years in Europe to treat narcolepsy and was approved in the United States in 1999 (148). The mechanism of action is not well understood, but it does not appear to alter levels of dopamine or norepinephrine (148). Methylphenidate, the most frequently used stimulant, has been shown to improve sleep tendency in a dose-related fashion (148). Pemoline, the initial drug of choice in children younger than seven with narcolepsy, is a less potent amphetamine that also improves excess daytime sleepiness (EDS) and has relatively little effect on blood pressure (149, 150). Antidepressants such as clomipramine and fluoxetine have been shown to reduce the frequency of cataplexy in narcolepsy.

TREATMENT OF PARASOMNIAS
SLEEP WALKING AND SLEEP TERRORS

Sleepwalking and sleep terrors, especially in children, usually do not necessitate treatment, other than by identifying and minimizing risk factors. Risk factors include: sleep deprivation, pregnancy, menstruation, and specific medications, including psychotropic drugs (eg, lithium carbonate and agents with anticholinergic effects) (151,152). Reports of polysomnographically confirmed cases indicate that most adult cases are not causally related to a psychiatric disorder, although stress can have a contributory role (153). However, in cases involving sleep-related injury (usually in adults), pharmacotherapy is necessary and can be lifesaving. Long-term nightly treatment with a benzodiazepine has been found to be safe and remarkably effective in adults with sleepwalking, sleep terrors, and other parasomnias; the incidences of side effects and misuse or abuse are low (154). Clonazepam (Klonopin), 0.25 to 1.5 mg taken 1 hour before sleep onset, is usually effective. Alprazolam (Xanax), diazepam (Valium), imipramine hydrochloride (Tofranil), and paroxetine hydrochloride (Paxil) also may be used. Use of self-hypnosis techniques can be effective in milder cases in both adults and children. Sleepwalking and sleep terrors are not usually controlled without the treatment of a concurrent psychiatric disorder (152, 153).

REM SLEEP BEHAVIOR DISORDER

Clonazepam (0.5 to 1.5 mg taken at bedtime) is remarkably effective in controlling both the behavioral and the dream-disordered components of REM sleep behavior disorder. The long-term efficacy and safety of this regimen have been established (154). In addition, maximizing the safety of the sleeping environment should always be encouraged.

NOCTURNAL SLEEP-RELATED EATING DISORDERS

Treatment of sleep-related eating is directed at controlling the underlying sleep disorder (155). For cases related to sleepwalking and restless legs syndrome with periodic limb movements, monotherapy or combined therapy with dopaminergic agents (levodopa with carbidopa [Sinemet]), benzodiazepines (clonazepam), and opiates (codeine) can be effective. Fluoxetine hydrochloride (Prozac) and bupropion hydrochloride (Wellbutrin) can also be effective as adjunctive treatments.

BRUXISM

Psychotherapy has been used to treat bruxism. The belief that bruxism is linked to stress and other emotional and psychological factors gives rise to a variety of psychotherapeutic approaches (156). For instance, calmness and self-confidence, may be fostered by listening to progressive relaxation, visual imagery, or autosuggestion tapes just before going to sleep (157). Another psychological approach to stress reduction resorts to instrumentation. During bruxism, the relevant muscles are active, and this increased activity or tenseness can in turn be measured with an electromyograph (EMG: electro = eletric; myo = muscle; graph = record). During treatment sessions at home or the laboratory, the patient sits or reclines comfortably. One or more pairs of recording electrodes are then attached to the surface of the skin, in close contact to appropriate muscles (e.g., masseter muscles). These electrodes transmit information about the level of muscle activity to a computer monitor. The patient is instructed to consciously lower that level below a threshold line (also visible on the screen). Gradually, by becoming alert to the presence of muscle tension, patients may develop techniques for reducing that tension, and hence, bruxism.

One problem with this approach is the expense of the machinery and expert guidance. Another problem is that muscles can be tense for a variety of reasons, and not simply because patients grind or clench. An unpleasant recollection, for instance, may result in a high reading, although it may have nothing to do with bruxism. Moreover, as in the case of many other psychotherapeutic approaches, the training takes place in the daytime, when the patient is awake and when his behavior is under conscious control.

It is not at all clear that such learning is transferable to the unconscious, sleeping brain.

The main problem is the lack of evidence that EMG feedback benefits the patient. In one study, for example, subjects undergoing this treatment for two weeks, along with a program of listening to relaxation tapes, seemed to brux no less than control subjects (who received no treatment) while they were receiving this treatment, or six months after treatment ceased (158).

Another controversial approach is the so-called masked negative practice, a scholarly variation of the folk principle of reverse psychology. Here the patient is told to voluntarily clench the jaw for five seconds, relax it for five seconds, and repeat this procedure five times in succession, six different times a day, for a duration of two weeks (159). Alternatively, the duration of the clenching period may be individually tailored to each patient, with each clench continuing to the point of discomfort (158). This technique involves little or no cost and it does not interfere with the patient's sleep. But, by itself, this approach damages the teeth and may aggravate other bruxism symptoms (160). Notwithstanding early enthusiastic clinical reports, at the moment the evidence for the effectiveness of this approach is meager at best. Pierce and Gales study shows that subjects undergoing this treatment performed no better than controls, while they were receiving the treatment or six months after treatment ceased (158).

Splints are by far the most common treatment regimen for bruxism. Much current research on the treatment of bruxism has been centered on the use of such dental appliances. Many other researchers insist, in fact, that the splint only provides a measure of protection for the teeth, and, in the case of grinders, a moderation of the sound. Some patients find the splint uncomfortable to wear, remove it during sleep, and it may negatively affect one's bite, cause tooth decay, and lead to degenerative joint disease of the temporomandibular joint (161).

In the treatment of bruxism, sleep feedback may involve electromyographic (EMG)-activated alarm (162). Bruxism involves tensing of certain facial muscles. This tensing causes an increase in electrical activity of the muscles, which can in turn be recorded by an electromyograph. The electrodes of this instrument are placed on the facial area where these muscles are located. When the tenseness exceeds a certain predetermined level, the alarm goes off. The loudspeaker can be free standing, or, to prevent waking others, connected to earphones that the patient wears during sleep. This approach is sensible and is fairly unobtrusive, the patient needs not insert anything into the mouth, but needs only attach electrodes externally to the face. On the other hand, this procedure may fail to correct any bruxing behavior, which is associated with muscle tension lower than the predetermined intensity or duration threshold (158, 162). Another obvious problem is that muscle tension may occur in the absence of bruxism.

SLEEP OVERVIEW

The words sleep and somnolence are derived from the Latin word somnus; the German words sleps, slaf, or schlaf; and the Greek word hypnos (15). Hippocrates suggested a humoral mechanism for sleep; sleep was induced by the retreat of blood and warmth into the inner body. Aristotle thought sleep was related to food and heat (15).

Loomis, an American physiologist, and colleagues made the discovery of different stages of sleep reflected in EEG changes in 1937 (16). Aserinsky and Kleitman discovered rapid eye movement (REM) in the 1950's at the University of Chicago (17).

A comprehensive review of sleep architecture is beyond the scope of this chapter. A brief overview is provided.

Sleep is divided into two stages based on behavioral and physiologic characteristics: rapid eye movement (REM) and non-rapid eye movement (NREM).

REM sleep accounts for approximately 20–25% of total sleep time after the age of two years (18). REM sleep is further divided into 2 stages: tonic and phasic. A desynchronized EEG, hypotonia or atonia of major muscle groups, and depression of monosynaptic and polysynaptic reflexes characterizes the tonic phase. The phasic tone is discontinuous and marked by bursts of REM (with rapid eye movements both horizontal and vertical), myoclonic twitches of the limbs and face, and autonomic lability with irregularities of heart rate and respiration with variable blood pressure (19). PGO (ponto-geniculo-occipital) spikes also occur that are not normally seen on polysomnography. PGO activity is a phasic feature of REM sleep, generated in the pons and projected through the lateral geniculate body and other thalamic nuclei to the occipital cortex. It is of 2 types: Type I PGO activity is independent of eye movements, and Type II occurs simultaneously with eye movements (18). Dreams and fragmented images have been associated with PGO spike activity (18).

During REM sleep the brain is very active metabolically, physiologically, and psychologically. This is a result of central activation because the brain neither depends on external stimuli nor expresses a motor output in response to the activation (65). Some authors believe that REM sleep is important to particular brain metabolic processes because of this central activation (65).

NREM sleep accounts for 75–80% of sleep time in adults. It is divided into 4 stages based on EEG criteria. Stage I equals 3–8% of sleep time; Stage II equals approximately 45–55%, Stage III and IV combined equals 15–20% and are described as slow-wave sleep (SWS) (20). Table 32-2 summarizes the distinct differences in the 4 stages.

K complexes are composed of an initial sharp component followed by a slow component. Sleep spindles are episodically occurring rhythmical complexes occurring

---

TABLE 32-2
Distinct Differences in NREM Sleep Stages

STAGE 1
  Low voltage
  Mixed frequency EEG
STAGE 2
  K complexes
  Sleep spindles
STAGE 3
  Arousal threshold high
  Delta waves = 20–50%
STAGE 4
  Delta waves = >50%
  (19,30)

---

with frequency of 7–14 cycles per second . They are grouped in sequences lasting 1–2 seconds and can occur alone or can be superimposed on K complexes. They usually arise from gamma-aminobutyric acid (GABA)-ergic neurons in the reticular thalamic nucleus. On scalp recordings , spindles occur maximally over the frontal and vertex areas (18). Sleep spindles may also be found in Stage 3 and 4 NREM sleep or even in REM sleep. They are most characteristic of Stage 2 NREM sleep (19).

Delta waves are high voltage waves (greater than or equal to 75 microvolts), with a frequency range of .5–4 hertz (19,30). Thalamocortical cells are most capable of generating delta or slow waves, but other areas such as the anterior hypothalamus, preoptic region, and basal forebrain are also involved (18).

ONTOGENY OF SLEEP

Newborns spend about 2/3 of their life sleeping. When they fall asleep they immediately go into REM sleep that is accompanied by restless movements of the arms and legs. At 3 months of age, the REM-NREM cycle is established. Polyphasic sleep progresses to biphasic sleep in preschool kids, and moves to monophasic sleep in adulthood (20). REM sleep patterns remain stable in adults. However, the pattern of REM sleep seen in the young adult with progressively longer periods is not seen in the elderly. Their REM sleep is more equally distributed over the course of the night (21). The proportion of REM sleep tends to decline with deterioration in cognitive function and with specific organic mental disorders (22,23).

PHYLOGENY OF SLEEP

Many studies have been performed to determine if other mammals have sleep stages. The purpose of these studies is to understand the physiologic and anatomic correlates of sleep as you ascend the ladder of phylogeny. Tobler (24) concluded that sleep is homeostatically regulated, in a strikingly similar manner, in a broad range of mammals.

Mammals can be long or short sleepers. Small animals that have a high metabolic rate; also have a shorter life span and sleep longer than larger animals with slower metabolic rates (25). Smaller animals also have a shorter REM-NREM cycle. Both vertebrates and invertebrates display sleep and wakefulness (26). Birds show EEG activity of sleep but their REM-NREM cycles are very short (27).

SLEEP NEUROPHYSIOLOGY

Effector neurons are the neurons directly leading to the production of different REM sleep components. Most of the physiologic events of REM sleep have effector neurons located in the brain stem reticular formation, with important neurons concentrated in the pontine reticular formation (PRF). As REM sleep stages are approaching the PRF neurons undergo depolarization and once reach threshold will generate action potentials. Their discharge rate increases as REM sleep is approached and the high level of discharge is maintained throughout REM sleep (28). Neurons in the midbrain reticular formation, originally described as the ascending reticular activating system, are especially important for EEG activation (28). It is also thought that cholinergic neurons (by excitation of the brain stem reticular neurons), and monoaminergic neurons (using serotonin and norepinephrine) contribute to EEG activation (28). Cholinergic compounds have excitatory actions on approximately 80% of PRF neurons, including those that are important in REM sleep (29).

The laterodorsal tegmental nucleus (LDT) and the pedunculopontine tegmental nucleus (PPT), are two nuclei at the pons-midbrain junction where cholinergic projections arise in the brain stem. Their rostral projections are important for EEG activation of both REM sleep and waking.

BIOCHEMICAL PHARMACOLOGY OF WAKEFULNESS

Wakefulness is maintained by the tonic activity of neurons distributed throughout the brainstem reticular formation with projections to the thalamus, hypothalamus and the basal forebrain (31). The dopaminergic and noradrenergic neurons of the ponto mesencephalic tegmentum, the posterior hypothalamic histaminergic neurons, and the cholinergic neurons of the basal forebrain, are the major neurotransmitter systems that appear to regulate wakefulness (31).

Stimulants both increase wakefulness and decrease REM sleep. Withdrawing stimulants in chronic users both

increases total sleep and REM sleep (32). The stimulating effects of amphetamines (33) and cocaine (34) on sleep are suggestive of a role for dopamine in promoting wakefulness. There is no clear-cut role for dopamine in the sleep-wake cycles. Single cell recordings of dopaminergic neurons in the substantia nigra show only minor changes in the sleep-wake cycle (35).

Noradrenergic neurons (found in the locus ceruleus) also have no clear-cut role for sleep-wake cycles. These cells have a state dependent firing rate, a high firing rate during wakefulness that decreases over NREM sleep until they are virtually silent during REM sleep (36).

Histamine has arousing effects and antihistamines have sleep-inducing effects (37–39). An ascending histaminergic pathway from the posterior hypothalamus innervates the cortex, striatum, hippocampus, and amygdala of the forebrain with cell bodies originating in the posterior hypothalamus and midbrain regions (40, 41). Studies suggest that neurons in the ventrolateral pre-optic area (VLPO) of the anterior hypothalamus are involved in the generation of NREM sleep (42). A descending histaminergic pathway extends from the posterior hypothalamus to the mesopontine tegmentum (40,43) where they intermingle with other neuronal projections that play a role in the generation of wakefulness and REM sleep (44, 45). Administrations of substances that impair histamine transmission or synthesis increase NREM, whereas enhancement increases quiet wakefulness (46–48). The role of the H1 and H2 systems is of increasing NREM sleep, and also suggested modulation of the balance between wakefulness and NREM sleep (49).

Cholinergic mechanisms play a clear role in maintaining arousal at both cortical and subcortical sites (50–53). Acetylcholine is released from the hippocampus and the cerebral cortex during REM sleep (54). 5-HT is probably not involved in NREM sleep but rather in the regulation of the stages of sleep. Jouvet et el, postulated that 5-HT, released by axonal nerve endings in the basal hypothalamus as a neurotransmitter during waking, might act as a neurohormone and induce the synthesis or liberation of hypnogenic factors that would be secondarily responsible for NREM and REM sleep (55).

PHARMACOLOGY OF SLEEP

There are certain substances found within the nervous system that are felt to affect sleep. Since the role of these substances is not well understood, they are discussed separately in the following section.

Delta Sleep-Inducing Peptide (DSIP) is an isolate that is obtained from the blood of rabbits, when in an electrically induced sleep state that induces NREM sleep in recipient rabbits when given by intracerebroventricular infusion (56). These effects are seen with infusions in cats and rats when given IV or subcutaneously (57). Intravenous infusions of DSIP in humans increased total sleep time regardless of administration times (58–61).

Blood plasma levels of DSIP exhibited a circadian rhythm in both humans and rats with a peak in the late afternoon and a trough in the early morning (62, 63). Not only does DSIP effect sleep but also has many physiologic activities. Graf and colleagues (64) have proposed that in addition to sleep facilitation, DSIP may also exert a chronopharmologic action as a natural programming substance by inducing changes in cerebral neurotransmitters and plasma proteins.

Sleep-promoting substances uridine and SPS-B are both implicated in the more frequent occurrence of NREM and REM sleep episodes with normal sleep-waking behavior (65).

Muramyl peptides are proposed to induce sleep, which in turn enhances immunoreaction, serving a recuperative function in the mammalian body. A muramyl tripeptide isolated from humans is an active somnogen (66–69). Muramyl peptides are peptidoglycans that form the backbone of bacterial cell walls and exert profound pyrogenic and immunostimulatory activities in the mammalian body (70–72).

Krueger et al. (67) proposed that sleep has a reciprocal relationship with the immune system. Sleep is enhanced by certain immune modulators, and may enhance certain aspects of immune regulation. Interleukin-1 belongs to a family of polypeptides that mediate a variety of host-defense functions and possess pyrogenic activity. It is liberated by macrophages to activate T lymphocytes and induce fever by acting on hypothalamic cells. IL-1 and other immune modulators have been found to be elevated in humans during sleep (73). This peak in plasma levels occurs during SWS shortly after sleep onset (73).

A naturally occurring peptide isolated from the pineal gland, arginine vasotocin, modifies conditioned behavior, inhibits gonadotropin release, and possibly enhances NREM sleep (65).

Caffeine shortens REM latency and decreases sleep, particularly NREM sleep, presumably through it's blockade of adenosine receptors. Adenosine is a naturally occurring purine nucleoside that causes sedation and inhibits neuronal firing activity (74). Extracellular concentrations of adenosine decrease with sleep. It is suggested that the duration and depth of sleep are increased by elevated concentrations of adenosine after waking (65).

The prostaglandin-dependent humoral theory of sleep regulation was developed by Ueno et al. (75,76) and Matsumura et al. (77). Two different prostaglandins: PGD2 and PGE2 have been shown to work reciprocally to affect sleep. When PGD2 increases, PGE2 decreases sleep time in a dose-dependent manner (75–77). Reciprocal activities of the PGD2 and PGE2 in or near the pre-optic area and posterior hypothalamus may regulate the state of vigilance (78).

Melatonin is a major hormone secretion of the pineal gland in mammals. The synthesis and release is timed by one or more biological clocks but occurs only in humans after dark. Melatonin is purported to have sleep-inducing properties (79) in cats, rats, young chickens, and humans (81–85). Its physiological actions include a phase-shifting effect on circadian rhythms, increased sleepiness when administered during daytime hours, and vasoconstriction (13). It can also be used for the treatment of jet lag and delayed sleep-phase syndrome (80). Melatonin secretion at night generally decreases as normal and pathologic aging occurs. Whether this natural process is associated with poor sleep is unknown, despite claims by numerous authors that exogenous melatonin restores natural sleep (65). It is unlikely that melatonin has any direct effects on sleep regulation secondary to the high doses needed, however it may affect sleep indirectly by altering the phase of the circadian pacemaker (86).

GABA has a role in sleep induction through the use of benzodiazepine medications, which enhance GABAergic inhibitory transmission (87). They also aid sleep through anxiolytic and muscle relaxation mechanisms.

ASSESSMENT OF SLEEP DISTURBANCES

Patients need to be asked specific questions about their sleeping habits and difficulties at each visit. It is very helpful for both physician and patient, to have the patient keep a sleep diary for a specific period of time. A period of 2 weeks to 1 month has been suggested by various authors. The patient is to record a night-to-night history of their sleeping schedule and perception of sleep quality. This information may enable the clinician to identify modifiable causes for the sleep difficulties.

Table 32-3 provides a concise representation of the approach to sleep disturbances.

INSOMNIA QUESTIONNAIRES

Various questionnaires have been developed to aid in the diagnosis of insomnia within the general population. Recently published examples include the Epworth

---

TABLE 32-3
Approach to Sleep Disturbance

- Comprehensive evaluation of insomnia
- Sleep hygiene measures
- Environmental alterations
- Behavioral/cognitive therapies
- Pharmacological treatment

Sleepiness Scale (88), The Sleep Disorders Questionnaire (89), and the Pittsburgh Sleep Quality Index (90). The difficulty lies in correlating these questionnaires to patients who have suffered a traumatic brain injury. Few formal measures were found to be validated in a population characterized with TBI. Other helpful questionnaires when evaluating patients with TBI who report sleep difficulties include:

The Beck Depression Inventory (91) and the Multidimensional Pain Inventory (MPI) (92). The Beck Depression Inventory consists of 21 items, each of which requires the respondent to rate the presence or absence of a specific sign of mood disturbance on a 4-point scale. It provides information on the cognitive, affective, and somatic aspects of depression (91).

The MPI consists of 61 items that requires patients to rate the magnitude of various pain-related problems on a 7-point scale. It evaluates an individual's experience of pain from a psychosocial perspective and contains measures of self-perceived pain intensity and pain interference with functional activities (92).

The Sleep Disorders Questionnaire has 43 questions related to various medical conditions and symptoms as reported by the patient and the family members that are applicable in the past six months. It is very helpful to not only assess actual symptoms related to insomnia, but also the patient's perception of those symptoms.

The Epworth Sleepiness Scale evaluates daytime alertness by asking the patient to rate the likelihood of dozing or falling asleep in eight different situations, such as conversing with another person, riding in a car, resting after lunch, and reading a book. It uses a 4-point scale and has been shown to possess good sensitivity and specificity to sleep apnea, narcolepsy, and hypersomnia (88).

The Multiple Sleep Latency Test (MLST) can be ordered to determine the severity of sleepiness and give an indication of the presence or absence of the early onset of REM sleep (93). It is the only scientifically validated objective test of excessive sleepiness and is used to establish a diagnosis of specific sleep disorders or to determine the severity of sleepiness. This test is indicated for all patients suspected of narcolepsy to confirm diagnosis and severity of sleepiness; patients with mild to moderate obstructive sleep apnea syndrome who complain of moderate to severe sleepiness; in evaluation of patients suspected of having idiopathic hypersomnia, periodic limb movement disorder or when the cause of excessive sleepiness is unknown (166, 168). The MSLT is indicated in the evaluation of the complaint of insomnia when the presence of moderate to severe excessive sleepiness is suspected, and is useful in assessing the response to treatment following effective therapy for disorders that cause sleepiness to ensure occupational safety (167).

The MLST consists of five 20-minute nap opportunities, with each nap separated by 2 hours. The patient lies in a dark room and attempts to sleep. The time before sleep is recorded for each nap, and the mean latency for all 5 naps is determined. Patients with a mean sleep latency of < 5 minutes are considered to have pathological sleepiness and those who fall asleep between 5–10 minutes are considered normal. Sleep is staged during the naps. If REM sleep occurs during 2 or more naps, the test is consistent with a diagnosis of narcolepsy, if other causes of sleep-onset rapid movements have been excluded (94).

The Pittsburgh Sleep Quality Index (PSQI) examines sleep quality and disturbances for a 1-month period. Patients provide specific sleep-related information including: usual bed time, rising time, minutes to fall asleep, and hours of actual sleep each night. They also rate a variety of sleep-related factors on a 4-point scale including: subjective sleep quality, use of sleep medications, daytime alertness and mood, and sleep disturbances such as nighttime awakenings, respiratory distress, physical discomfort, and disturbing dreams (90). Poor sleepers and insomniacs are readily identified by the PSQI and it is well suited for research examining general sleep patterns and problems (90). The PSQI was demonstrated to be a valid and useful screening tool for assessing insomnia and sleep difficulties among patients with postacute TBI (95). Steele et al. (192) have studied the effect of TBI on the timing of sleep but have concluded that the Morningness-Eveningness Questionnaire (MEQ) may not be suitable for use in a cognitively impaired patient population.

OBJECTIVE SLEEP TESTING MEASURES ACTIGRAPHY

Actigraphy is a method utilizing a portable device, to study sleep-wake patterns and circadian rhythms by assessing movement, most commonly at the wrist. Actigraphy is reliable and valid for detecting sleep in normal healthy populations, but less reliable in disturbed sleep (163). Actigraphy is not indicated for the routine diagnosis, assessment of severity, or management of any of the sleep disorders, including the insomnias, obstructive sleep apnea syndrome and periodic limb movement disorder (163). Actigraphy may be a useful adjunct to modified portable sleep apnea testing when determining the rest activity pattern during the testing period (164). Actigraphy is an effective means of demonstrating multi day human rest-activity patterns and may be used to estimate sleep-wake patterns in the occasional clinical situations where a sleep log or diary cannot provide similar information (165). Actigraphy may also be useful in characterizing and monitoring circadian rhythm patterns or disturbances in the elderly and nursing home patients with or without dementia; newborns, infants, children, and adolescents; hypertensive individuals; depressed or schizophrenic patients; and individuals in inaccessible situations (space flight) (163).

POLYSOMNOGRAPHY

Polysomnography (PSN), is routinely indicated for the diagnosis of sleep-related breathing disorders; for continuous positive airway pressure titration in patients with sleep-related breathing disorders; for documenting the presence of obstructive sleep apnea in patients prior to laser-assisted uvulopalatopharyngoplasty; with a multiple sleep latency test in evaluation of suspected narcolepsy; or when there is a strong clinical suspicion of periodic limb movement disorder (169, 170). Diagnosis of narcolepsy and posttraumatic hypersomnia requires a MSLT after a relatively normal night's sleep as documented by nocturnal PSN (201). Guilleminault et al. (193) found a MSLT score <10 in 82.6% and sleep disordered breathing in 32% of patients with head or neck trauma. PSN is not indicated for the diagnosis of circadian rhythm sleep disorders or to establish a diagnosis of depression (170). Masel et al. (202) concluded that due to patients inability to perceive their hypersomnolence, a sleep laboratory evaluation should be considered part of their medical management.

NONPHARMACOLOGIC MEASURES FOR TREATING SLEEP DISTURBANCE

Nonpharmacologic measures should be attempted in all patient populations, not only those with TBI and should be undertaken as quickly as possible once insomnia and sleeping difficulties have been identified. Sleep hygiene refers to health practices and environmental influences on sleep. The following suggestions should be of benefit to all patient populations affected:

- Awake at the same time daily.
- Limit total daily caffeine consumption and discontinue consumption 4 to 6 hours before retiring.
- Nicotine is a stimulant and should be avoided in all forms.
- Do not eat heavily close to bedtime.
- Sleep may be enhanced by performing a regular exercise program in the late afternoon or early evening at least 3 hours before bedtime.
- Move the clock out of view from the bed.
- Maintain the sleeping environment as comfortable as possible, minimize noise, light, and excessive temperatures (13).

STIMULUS CONTROL INSTRUCTIONS

A set of techniques to establish sleep/wake patterns, cues for sleeping, and reduction of associations with activities that interfere with sleep:

- Lie down when feeling sleepy.

- If having difficulty with sleep, leave the bedroom. Return to bed when sleepy. The goal is to develop a positive association between the bedroom and sleep.
- Use the bedroom only for sleep and sexual activity.
- Awake at the same time each day.
- No napping (10).

SLEEP RESTRICTION

The goal of this treatment measure is to increase the percentage of time in bed asleep. The patient limits the amount of time spent in bed to the actual time that is spent sleeping. The type of treatment often results in a mild sleep deprivation state initially that should promote more rapid sleep onset and more efficient, restorative sleep. The rising time should remain constant and the bedtime altered to maintain a regular sleep/wake rhythm. For example, if a patient only reports sleeping 4 hours a night but arises at 5 AM daily, then he should stay up until 1 AM. Each night they will go to bed 15 minutes earlier. This procedure is followed over several weeks until the desired sleep duration is achieved. This type of treatment is modified for older patients by allowing them to take an afternoon nap (13).

ENVIRONMENTAL MEASURES CHRONOTHERAPY

Chronotherapy is a treatment measure developed primarily for circadian rhythm disorders in which the individual's sleep/wake cycle is out of phase with the bedtime (96). This treatment is very effective for patients with delayed sleep phase syndrome, who exhibit difficulty falling asleep at night and report feeling tired in the morning when awakened. The patient's bedtime is delayed by daily increments of 3 hours until sleep onset coincides with the desired bedtime (97).

BRIGHT LIGHT THERAPY

This treatment has also been used for a number of circadian rhythm disorders. Research has shown that properly timed exposure to bright light (7000–12,000 lux) for 2–3 days can shift the phase of the sleep rhythm (98). As a frame of reference, typical indoor room light is <500 lux; a few minutes after dawn, sunlight produces about 2500 lux; and at noon, sunlight is ~100,000 range (99). It is also important to have periods of darkness without bright light (98).

CRANIAL ELECTROTHERAPY STIMULATION

CES (Cranial Electrotherapy Stimulation) is a process, which utilizes minute electrical stimulation for therapeutic treatment of anxiety, depression, and insomnia (184).

Applied through electrodes to the area between the mastoids and the jaw, the sensation felt by the individual is normally one of relaxation (184). If there is high stress or anxiety just prior to treatment, the individual may go to sleep while using CES, particularly if sitting in a reclining position (184). Sleep at the time of application is not required to benefit from CES, although individuals frequently report an improvement in the quality of their night time sleep (184). As with a number of medications, the mechanism of action of CES is not fully understood. Research has led to the hypothesis that CES has a mild effect on the hypothalamic area of the brain (185, 186). Researchers also have noticed rapid increases in serotonin, also associated with relaxation and calmness, and decreases in cortisol, one of the primary stress-related biochemicals (186,187). Interestingly, CES also increases levels of norepinephrine and dopamine, both associated with alertness and feelings of pleasure (187). No negative effects or major contraindications have been found from the use of CES to date, either in the US or other parts of the world.

BEHAVIORAL AND COGNITIVE THERAPIES

Cognitive therapy involves identifying dysfunctional beliefs and attitudes about sleep and replacing them with more adaptive substitutes (13). The primary goal is to change the patients' view of the sleep problem from one of a victim, to one in which they are capable of developing adaptive coping skills. These changes in their way of thinking often helps to decrease the anxiety the patient experiences, thereby facilitating sleep. Paradoxical intention is the approach that instructs the patient who has difficulty falling asleep to stay awake as long as possible. Multiple studies have evaluated this technique with mixed results regarding its effectiveness (97).

RELAXATION THERAPY, MEDITATION, AND BIOFEEDBACK

Many patients are anxious and have high levels of arousal that interfere with their ability to fall asleep. The goal of this treatment is to allow the patient to relax and fall asleep more easily. These therapies are useful for both sleep-onset and sleep-maintenance insomnia problems (97).

SLEEP DIFFICULTIES SPECIFICALLY RELATED TO TBI

The emergence of insomnia after TBI concerns treatment providers, because as Zafonte et al (101) have noted, disordered sleep can have adverse behavioral and cognitive consequences. Patients with TBI are prone to depression, particularly the mild TBI patient. Strong correlation exists between insomnia and depression in the non-TBI population. Insomnia is a common feature of depression. Both Beetar et al (103) and Fichtenberg et al. (102) find as association between insomnia and milder brain injury. It is not surprising that there is an association between insomnia and depression in the post-acute TBI patient. This follows the course of recovery after TBI. During the acute stage, dysregulation of sleep seems to be a function of the diffuse disruption of cerebral functioning in the wake of both direct physical damage to the brain and secondary neuropathological events. Sleep abnormalities are more likely to occur in patients with lesions in the pontine tegmentum located in the midpontine region (100). As brain functioning becomes reorganized and some degree of neurological stability is reestablished, sleep can be expected to normalize in the absence of damage to neural sleep structures (104). Insomnia is linked to both depression and mild brain injuries. The determinants of insomnia and depression may differ from the acute and the post-acute stage. Neurological factors may play a role in the early recovery process, and psychosocial factors may contribute later (104). When assessing insomnia in the brain-injured population, it is imperative to diagnose depression, as well as other psychiatric and emotional disturbances.

Changes in sleep patterns in patients that have suffered a traumatic brain injury are fairly common. Reports have shown decreased REM and slow wave sleep, as well as an increase in the number of times an individual awakens during sleep (105). Brain injury is believed to contribute to a shortening of the total sleep time and the disappearance of deep sleep (106). Sleep complaints of patients with brain injury are found to correlate with the presence of fatigue, higher Glasgow Coma Scale scores, better immediate memory, a positive substance abuse history, older age, and female gender (107). Sleep complaints are common in patients with recent injury, and those sustaining injury 2–3 years previously (105). Disorders in initiating or maintaining sleep (DIMS) occur more often in patients with recent injury, and disorders of excessive somnolence (DOES) occur more often in those patients with injuries sustained 2–3 years prior (105). TBI may also result in sleep apnea, which can have obvious effects on sleep maintenance (103).

ALTERNATIVE/COMPLEMENTARY MEDICINE TECHNIQUES

Various methods of alternative/complementary medicine may be helpful in facilitation of sleep including: acupuncture, aerobic exercise, massage, ultrasound, cranial electrical stimulation, and reflexology. Every patient must be questioned about the presence of pain and it's interference with sleep. Aggressive evaluation, intervention and treatment of pain in both TBI and non-TBI patients is warranted. Treatment of the patient's pain may facilitate sleep.

MELATONIN

Melatonin is a hormone synthesized in the pineal gland and, to a lesser extent, in the retina. Melatonins excretion, which peaks after dark, follows a day/night rhythm not only in humans but also in all species studied, and is responsible for sleep induction. Physiological concentrations of melatonin can stimulate the release of opioid peptides by activated T-helper lymphocytes (180). These melatonin-induced-immuno-opioids (MIIO) mediate the immunoenhancing and anti-stress effects of melatonin and cross-react immunologically with anti-beta-endorphin and anti-met-enkephalin antisera (180). Studies have also shown the hypnotic effect ascribed to melatonin is exerted through its effect on the thermoregulatory mechanism(181). Those authors believe that by lowering core body temperature, melatonin reduces arousal and increases sleep propensity (181). Melatonin has also been shown to accelerated sleep initiation, improved sleep maintenance, decreased sleep stage 1 and increased sleep stage 2 (182). The influence of exogenous melatonin on the sleep-wake cycle was investigated. Sleep onset time and wake time were significantly earlier when using melatonin than during placebo (183). Contraindications for the use of melatonin include: heart disease, atherosclerosis and stroke secondary to vascular constriction effects. It may also negatively affect fertility (195). Fluexetine decreases melatonin levels; TCA's and fluoxamine increase melatonin concentrations (195).

Research shows that a number of natural sleep aids may benefit anyone involved in the pursuit of a good night's rest. Valerian, kava kava, hops, passionflower have all been shown to improve sleep quality. The German government and European community sanction these herbs for the treatment of insomnia.

The active chemical constituents of valerian are primarily the valepotriates, which possess sedative activity (171). The valepotriates weakly bind GABA-A receptors. Sedation in the central nervous system is primarily controlled through these receptors. Because valerian weakly binds these receptors, its sedative actions do not result in dependence and potential addiction (171). Numerous human sleep studies have demonstrated that valerian produces a significant improvement in sleep quality, and an increase in deep REM sleep (dream phase) without producing the side effects of sleep drugs (172).

Kava kava is recognized for the ability to produce relaxation without the loss of mental sharpness (173). The active constituents of Kava consist of a group of lactones similar in structure to gamma-butyrolactone, (GBL)

a precursor to gamma hydroxybutyrate (GHB) (173). GHB produces sleepiness and depresses the dopaminergic pathway when given in high doses (173). Numerous clinical and experimental studies have documented the relaxing, sleep-promoting and anti-anxiety actions of kava extracts that contain high levels of Kava lactones. In a 1991 double-blind, placebo-controlled four-week study of patients suffering from anxiety, a group receiving kava lactone extract three times daily showed reduction in anxiety after just one week and were significantly improved at the end of the study (173). The kava group experienced a significant reduction in menopausal symptoms, anxiety and depression compared to the control group (173). A study compared the effects of a kava lactone to oxazepam (a benzodiazepine drug) in patients suffering from anxiety for four weeks. Each substance reduced symptoms of anxiety equally (174). The kava lactone produced no negative side effects and oxazepam produced side effects such as drowsiness, dizziness, headaches and vertigo (174).

Passionflower was listed in the National Formulary from 1916 to 1936 and approved as a sedative and OTC sleep drug (175). Italian researchers tested Passionflower alone and in combinations with other sedative herbs (175). They observed a synergistic effect of sedative activity from the herbal combinations. Studies have shown that oral administration and injections of passionflower into rats prolonged sleeping time, protected animals from convulsive chemicals and relaxed their muscles (175).

Hops are extensively used in botanical formulas for the treatment of insomnia because they influence relaxation in the central nervous system (176). They are recommended by herbalists to ease tension and anxiety, and may be used when tension leads to restlessness. Studies have demonstrated equivalent efficacy and tolerability of a hop-valerian preparation compared with a benzodiazepine preparation in patients suffering from sleep disorders (176). The researchers concluded that a hop-valerian preparation in the appropriate dose is a sensible alternative to benzodiazepines for the treatment of non-chronic and non-psychiatric sleep disorders (177).

Chamomile is derived from the flower heads of either of two annual plants: German chamomile (Matricaria recutita), or Roman chamomile (Chamaemelum nobile) (178). Chamomile is a popular folk remedy for digestive problems, fever, menstrual discomfort, stomachache, and anxiety. It is used to treat insomnia in children because it is a very mild relaxant and has a pleasant taste (178). Flavonoids such as apigenin as well as a distinctive blue essential oil (azulene) derived from chamomile have been found to reduce inflammation and encourage the healing of wounds (179). Apigenin may also be responsible for chamomile's anti-anxiety and sedative effects, via action on central benzodiazepine drug receptors (179). Both oral and topical chamomile products are considered nontoxic and gentle enough for use in children or pregnant and lactating women (178).

PHARMACOLOGIC TREATMENT FOR SLEEP DISTURBANCES

All psychosocial and physical aspects must be taken into consideration when prescribing medications to patients with traumatic brain injury. Every patient's unique and individual circumstances will affect medication choices.

ANTIHISTAMINES

Antihistamines are frequently purchased over-the-counter to produce or enhance sleep. When utilized by patients that have sustained a traumatic brain injury, they may produce negative cognitive effects by means of their anticholinergic actions (101). Furthermore, in studies by Roth et al. (114) and Nicholson (115, 116), it was shown that traditional antihistamines produced increased daytime sleepiness, most clearly apparent at the usual nadir in the circadian cycle of alertness. In these studies, however, antihistamines such as loratadine (in doses of 10 and 40 mg), terfenadine, and astemizole were not associated with these undesired side effects.

ANTIEPILEPTICS

Drowsiness and lethargy are often reported side effects of anticonvulsant medications. Caregivers using these medication(s) in patients with traumatic brain injury must keep in mind the potential undesired side effects on sleep and arousal that may be produced (101). Phenytoin administration long-term produces a decrease in sleep onset latency, a transient increase in SWS, and possibly a transient reduction in REM sleep (109, 117, 118). Carbamazepine produces a decrease in stage I sleep, an increase in SWS, and an increase in total sleep continuity (101, 109). Sodium valproate tends to increase total sleep time by decreasing total awakenings (119).

Gabitril (tiagabine) a newer, well-tolerated anticonvulsant , is rapidly absorbed after oral administration, has an elimination half-life of seven to nine hours (120).

Tiagabine significantly increased sleep efficiency by increasing SWS, caused by changes in stages 3 and 4, especially during the second and third two-hour intervals of the sleep period (121). The promotion of deep sleep was further corroborated by elevations in slow-wave activity within non-REM sleep. Tiagibine had demonstrated no effect upon sleep onset latency or total time spent in bed (121).

Pregabalin is a gamma-aminobutyric acid (GABA) analogue that binds to calcium channels, not GABA receptors, and modulates calcium influx, resulting in antiepileptic, analgesic, and anxiolytic activity. (122, 123). It has shown greater potency than gabapentin in pain and seizure disorders (124).

Pregabalin has shown increased duration of nonrapid eye movement sleep, decreased rapid eye movement sleep, and did not affect sleep onset latency (125).

ANTIDEPRESSANTS

Antidepressant medications may impact sleep patterns both directly (by means of suppression of REM sleep and prolongation of REM latency) (126) and indirectly (e.g., by their effect on the underlying depression and its associated sleep disturbances (109). Monoamine oxidase inhibitors cause the greatest suppression of REM sleep, perhaps therapeutic in that regard, because the depressed patient may be experiencing excessive REM sleep (127). The tricyclic antidepressant drugs and selective serotonin reuptake inhibitors also lead to varying degrees of REM sleep suppression. According to Arew (128), the primary indication for tricyclic antidepressants in treating insomnia is the patient whose sleep problems are secondary to depression. Nefazodone and Remeron, newer generation antidepressants unrelated to the SSRIs, tricyclics, and monoamine oxidase inhibitors, improve sleep initiation secondary to sedating side effects. Exact mechanism is unknown; however, it is presumed to be by means of serotonergic mechanisms (101). A newer agent, mirtazapine has serotonin blocking properties and has been shown to improve sleep architecture and efficiency (208).

SEDATIVE/HYPNOTICS

Historically, the benzodiazepine class of medications has been most commonly prescribed for insomnia and has demonstrated efficacy in short-term treatment (108).

The hypnotic agents act by means of gamma-aminobutyric acid (GABA) transmission through modulation of chloride channels to decrease phasic interruptions of sleep and increase total sleep time (101). Activation of the benzodiazepine receptor leads to an increase in GABA. This class of medications can produce a variety of side effects including physical dependence, sedation, and impairment of motor and cognitive abilities. This class is typically used for 4 weeks. Long-term use can have the potential for habituation and withdrawal symptoms. More effective long-term management of insomnia is attained if these medications are used in conjunction with behavioral therapy techniques (112). Agents with a shorter half-life should be prescribed first, since they are eliminated from the system by morning, decreasing the likelihood of residual daytime effects. These agents may improve sleep during the first part of the night, but can lead to withdrawal-like syndromes, with REM sleep rebound and sleep fragmentation during the latter part of the night (109). Sedative and hypnotic medications can also worsen sleep apnea syndromes (109).

Zolpidem (Ambien), although not a true benzodiazepine, is often included with the class because the site of action is the benzodiazepine receptor site (110). Most hypnotic agents bind to three omega receptors; zolpidem has an affinity for the omega 1-receptor (101). It also seems to preserve stage 3 and 4 sleep and produces only minor inconsistent changes in REM sleep (111). Ambien, enhances the brain's major inhibitory neurotransmitter, gamma aminobutyric acid (GABA). GABA receptors are located in the cerebellum and cerebral cortex, but not in the spinal cord or peripheral tissues (188). Ambien in vitro preferentially binds to a subunit of the GABA receptor (also called the benzodiazepine receptor) (188, 190). Although Ambien binds to the benzodiazepine receptor, it is an imidazopyridine with chemical structure unrelated to benzodiazepines or barbiturates (189, 190). While these drugs share some of the pharmacologic properties of benzodiazepines, they differ in binding to receptor cells in the GABA complex, producing sedative, muscle relaxant, anti-convulsant and anxiolytic effects. Imidazopyridines selectively bind to just the receptor cells responsible for sedation, thereby producing less side effects and less potential for addiction (188,189).

The longer acting agents flurazepam (Dalmane) and quazepam (Doral) can cause daytime sleepiness but are less likely to produce rebound insomnia (108). Benzodiazepines are preferred to barbiturates and other agents such as chloral hydrate. Chloral hydrate is often used in TBI patients, because it affords rapid sleep induction without increasing the seizure threshold (109). It is not recommended for treatment of insomnia in the general population because of the narrow therapeutic ratio, rapid development of tolerance, systemic toxicity, potential for abuse, and the possibility of severe clinical complications of withdrawal (13). Sonata is a hypnotic agent with a chemical structure unrelated to the benzodiazepines, barbiturates, and other drugs with hypnotic properties. It has been shown to decrease the time to sleep onset. It has not been shown to increase total sleep time or decrease the number of awakenings (113). Eszopiclone, a new non-narcotic, non-benzodiazepine hypnotic, is indicated for improved sleep maintenance. It is the first and only hypnotic agent at publication approved for long-term use with no tolerance observed in a 6-month trial (209).

ANTIPSYCHOTICS

This class of medications, have both direct effects on sleep and the ability to promote sleep by attenuating symptoms that interfere with sleep, such as psychosis and agitation. As a group, they increase daytime somnolence, total sleep time, REM percentage of total sleep, and sleep continuity. The antipsychotic drugs also lead to decreased sleep latency and percentages of sleep in stages 1 and 2 (129–133).

LITHIUM

Chesnik and Mendels have pointed out that lithium has multiple effects on sleep/wake patterns (134). It increases the percentage of stage 2 and SWS, the REM latency, and the total sleep time. The obvious assumption follows that it also increases daytime somnolence, a hypothesis that has proven true in most clinical cases (135).

OPIATES

Opiates promote feelings of peacefulness, drowsiness, and pain-relief that lead to the impression they are promoting sleep. There is noted psychomotor slowing. The strong analgesic properties may permit sleep in people who would otherwise be unable to do so, such as those with chronic pain syndromes or restless legs syndrome (109). Although not borne out by polysomnographic changes in sleep, narcoleptic patients treated with codeine report better sleep (136). Patients who have suffered acute traumatic brain injury often have associated fractures and injuries. They may derive sleep benefits from treatment of their pain using opiates.

Table 32-4 organizes the medications by class and their documented effects on sleep.

CONCLUSION

Insomnia and sleep disturbances are common complaints of both the general patient population as well as the brain injured populations. The architecture of sleep, assessment of sleep disturbances and insomnia, and treatment methods; both nonpharmacologic and pharmacologic have been reviewed. Prescription medications affecting the sleep cycles were reviewed in detail, and common effects compared and contrasted.

Once a sleep disturbance has been identified and investigated, a plan of care is formulated. The least-invasive techniques should be utilized initially and followed by prescription sleep aids if the symptoms fail to resolve. All psychosocial and physical aspects must be taken into consideration when prescribing medications for patients with TBI. It has been suggested that serotonergic agonists (trazodone, doxepin, amitriptyline) be used for sleep initiation problems. Sleep maintenance problems may be more efficiently handled with catecholaminergic agonists (nortriptyline) (137).

TABLE 32-4
Medications by Class and Their Effects on Sleep

MEDICATION TYPE	DRUG	INCREASES OR POSITIVE EFFECTS ON SLEEP
Antihistamine	H1 antagonists: Diphenhydramine Loratadine Terfenadine	Daytime somnolence
Antiepileptics	Clonazepam Valproate sodium Carbamazepine Phenytoin Tiagabine Pregabalin	Stage 4% Daytime somnolence Daytime somnolence Sleep continuity in epileptics SWS% (transient) Sleep efficiency SWS Enhancement of slow EEG components Nonrapid eye movement sleep Pain-relief Somnolence Anxiolytic
Antidepressant	Selective serotonin reuptake inhibitors: Fluvoxamine Fluoxetine Tricyclic antidepressants: Doxepin Clomipramine Desipramine Nortriptyline Amitriptyline Imipramine Serotonergic agent: Trazodone Nefazodone Remeron	Sleep latency REM latency Total sleep time Stage 2% Daytime somnolence REM latency Daytime somnolence Sleep continuity SWS% REM latency Sleep initiation Sleep continuity Sleep initiation
Sedative/Hypnotic	Benzodiazepines: Triazolam Temazepam Quazepam Nitrazepam Midazolam Lormetazepam Flurazepam Zolpidem Barbiturates: Amobarbital Secobarbital Phenobarbital Pentobarbital Chloral hydrate Sonata	 Total sleep time Sleep continuity Stage 2% REM latency Sleep continuity SWS% Daytime somnolence Total sleep time Sleep continuity Stage 2% REM latency Total sleep time Sleep induction Sleep initiation

TABLE 32-4 (continued)

MEDICATION TYPE	DRUG	INCREASES OR POSITIVE EFFECTS ON SLEEP
Antipsychotic	Haloperidol, trifluoperazine, loxapine, chlorpromazine	Sleep continuity Daytime somnolence Total sleep time REM%
Lithium		Daytime somnolence Total sleep time SWS% Stage 2% REM latency
Opiate	Morphine, codeine, heroin	Pain-relief Daytime somnolence

Comprehensive evaluation and interpretation of the patient's symptoms combined with the information in this chapter should allow formulation of a safe and effective treatment plan for sleep difficulties in patients with traumatic brain injury.

ACKNOWLEDGMENT

Special thanks to Steven Mayo for his invaluable assistance with literature review in the preparation of writing and revising this chapter.

References

1. Chesnut RM, Carney N, Maynard H, Patterson P, Mann NC, Helfand M. *Rehabilitation for traumatic brain injury.* Evidence report/technology assessment no 2. Rockville (MD): Department of Health and Human Services; Feb 1999. Agency for Health Care Policy and Research Publication No. 99-E006.
2. Max W, Mackenzie EJ, Rice, CP. Head injuries: cost and consequences. *J Head Trauma Rehab* 1991;6(2): 76–91.
3. McLean, A., Dikmen, S., Temkin, N. R. *et al.: Psychosocial functioning at one month after head injury. Neurosurgery* 14: 393–399, 1984.
4. Cohen, M., Okenber, A., Snir, D. et al.: Temporally related changes of sleep complaints in traumatic brain injured patients. *Journal of Neurology, Neurosurgery, & Psychiatry* 55: 313–315, 1992.
5. Stoller MK. Economic effects of insomnia. *Clin Ther.* 1994;16: 873–897.
6. Kupperman M, Lubeck DP. Mazonson PD, et al. Sleep problems and their correlates in a working population. *J Gen Intern Med.* 1995: 10:25–32.
7. Simon GE, Vonkorff M. Prevalence, burden, and treatment of insomnia in primary care. *Am J Psychiatry.* 1997;154: 1417–1423.
8. Regestein QR, Monk TH. Delayed sleep phase syndrome: A review of its clinical aspects. *Am J Psychiatry.* 1995;152:602–608.
9. Diagnostic Classification Steering Committee. American Sleep Disorders Association *The International Classification of Sleep Disorders.* Lawrence. KS: Allen Press: 1990.
10. Thaxton L. Myers MA. Sleep Disturbances and their Management in Patients with Brain Injury. *J Head Trauma Rehab* 2002, 17(4): 335–348.
11. Breznitz EA, Goldberg R, Kosinski RM. Epidemiology of obstructive sleep apnea. *Epidemiol Rev* 1994;16:210–27.
12. Hudgel DW. Treatment of obstructive sleep apnea. A review, *Chest* 1996;109: 1346–58.
13. Walsh, JK, Benca Rin, et al. Insomnia: assessment and management in primary care. *AM Family Physician* 1995;59(11).
14. Hening WA, Walters AS, Choknoverty S. Motor functions and dysfxn of sleep. In: Chokroverty S. ed. *Sleep disorders Medicine: Basic Science, Technical Considerations and Clinical Aspects.* Boston: Butterworth- Heinemann; 1994: 255–294.
15. Borbely A. *Secrets of Sleep.* New York: Basic Books, 1984.
16. Loomis AL, Harvey EN, Hobart GA. Cerebral states during sleep as studied by human brain potentials. *J Exp Physiol* 1937; 21:127.
17. Aserinsky E, Kleitman N. Regular occurring periods of eye motility and concomitant phenomena during sleep. *Science* 1953; 118:273.
18. Comella CL, Walter AS. Hening WA. Sleep and wakefulness. In: Goetz CG, Pappert EJ, eds: *Textbook of Clinical Neurology.* Philidelphia: WB Saunder, 1999: 17–29.
19. McCarley RW. Neurophysiology of Sleep: Basic mechanisms underlying control of wakefulness and sleep. In: *Sleep Disorders Medicine: basic science, technical considerations and clinical aspects.* Boston: Butterworth Hienemann; 1994: 17–36
20. Chokroverty S. An Overview of Sleep . In: *Sleep disorders medicine: basic science, technical considerations, and clinical aspects.* Boston: Butterworth Heinemann: 1999: 8–9.
21. Bliwise DL. Sleep in normal aging and dementia. *Sleep.* 1993;16: 40–81.
22. Fowles DG. A profile of older Americans 1988. Washington DC: American Association of Retired Persons: 1989.
23. Reynolds CF, Kupfer DJ, Taska LS. Et al. EEG Sleep in elderly depressed demented and healthy subjects. *Biol Psychiatry.* 1985; 20: 431–442.
24. Tobler I. Is sleep fundamentally different between mammalian species? *Behavior Brain Res* 1995;69: 35.
25. Zepelin H, Rechtschaffen A. Mammalian sleep, longitivity and energy metabolism. *Brain Behav Evol* 1974;10: 425.
26. Hartse Km. Sleep in Insects and Non-mammalian Vertebrates. In MH Kryger, T Roth, WC Dement (eds) *Principles and Practice of Sleep Medicine* (2nd ed). Philadelphia: Saunders, 1994;95.
27. Amlaner CJ JR, Ball NJ. Avian Sleep. In MH Kryger, T Roth, WC Dement (eds), *Principles and Practice of Sleep Medicine* (2nd ed). Philadelphia: Saunders, 1994;81.

28. McCarley RW Sleep Neurophysiology: Basic Mechanisms Underlying Control of Wakefulness and Sleep. In: *Sleep Disorders Medicine* Boston Butterworth-Heineman 1999: 24–7.

29. Stevens DR, McCarley RW, Green RW. 5HT and 5HT2 receptors hyperpolarize and depolarize separate population of medial pontine neurons in vitro. *Neuroscience* 1992;47: 545.

30. Rechtschaffen A, Kales AA. A Manuel of Standardized Terminology, Techniques and Scoring system for Sleep Stages of Human Subjects. Los Angeles: UCLA Brain Information Service/Brain Research Institute 1968.

31. Jones BE. Paradoxical sleep and its chemical/structural substrates in the Brain. *Neuroscience* 1991;40:637.

32. Watson R, Hartmann E, Schildkraut J. Amphetamine withdrawal: affective state sleep patterns and MHPG excretion. *Am J Psychiatry* 1972;129:39.

33. Gillin JC, van Kammen DP, Graves J et al. Differential effects of D- and L-amphetamine on the sleep of depressed pts. *Life Sci* 1975;17: 1233.

34. Post RM, Gillin JC, Goodwin FK, et al. The effect of orally administrated cocaine on sleep of depressed patients. *Psychopharmacology* 1974;37:59.

35. Miller JD, Farber K, Gatz P et al. Activity of mesencephalic dopamine and non-dopamine neurons across stages of sleep and waking in the rat. *Brain Res* 1983;273:133.

36. Aston-Jones G. Bloom FE. Norepinephrine-containing locus coeruleus neurons in behaving rats exhibit pronounced responses to non-noxious environmental stimuli. *J Neurosci* 1981;1: 887.

37. Monnier M. Sauer R, Hatt AM. The activating effects of histamine on the central nervous system. *Int Rev Neurobiol* 1970;12: 265.

38. Nicholson AN, Pascoe PA, Stone BM. Histaminergic systems and sleep: studies in man with Histamine H1 and H2 receptor antagonists. *Neuropharmocology* 1985;24: 245.

39. Monti JM. Involvement of histamine in the control of the waking state. *Life Sci* 1993;53:1331

40. Inagaki N, Yamatodani A, Ando-Yamamoto M; et al. Organization of histaminergic fibers in the rat brain. *J Comp Neurol* 1988;273:283.

41. Lin JS, Luppi PH, Salvert D, et al. Histamine-containing neurons in the cat hypothalamus. *C R Acad Sci* 1986;303:371.

42. Sherin JE, Shiromani PJ, McCarley RW, et al. Activation of ventrolateral preoptic neurons during sleep. *Science* 1996;271:216

43. Lin JS, Kitahama K, Fort P, et al. Histminergic system in the cat hypothalamus with reference to type B Monamine Oxidas. *J Comp Neurol* 1993;330:405.

44. Jouvet M. The role of monoamines and acetylcholine containing neurons in the regulation of the sleep-waking cycle. *Eng physiol* 1972;64:166.

45. Lin JS, Hou Y, Sakai K et al. Histaminergic descending inputs to the mesopontine tegmuntum and their role in the control of cortical activation and wakefulness in the cat. *J Neurosc* 1996;16: 1523.

46. Lin JS, Sakai K, Jouvet M. Evidence for histaminergic arousal mechanisms in the hypothalamus of cats. *Neuropharmacology* 1988;27: 111.

47. Lin JS, Sakai K, Vanni-Mercier G, et al. Involvement of histaminergic neurons in arousal mechanisms demonstrated with H3-receptor ligands in the cat. *Brain Res* 1990;523: 325.

48. Monti JM, Jantos H, Boussard M, et al. Effects of selective activation or blockade of the histamine H3 receptor on sleep and wakefulness. *Eur J Pharmacol* 1991;205:283.

49. Nicholson AN. Histaminergic Systems: Daytime Alertness and Nocternal Sleep. In A Wauguier, JM Gaillard, JM Monti, et al. (eds) *Sleep: Neurotransmitters and Neuromodulators*, New York: Raven, 1985: 211.

50. Vanderwolf CH, Robinson TE. Reticulo-cortical activity and behavior: a critique of the arousal theory and new synthesis. *Behav Brain Sci* 1981;4:459.

51. Buzsaki G, Bickford RG. Ponomareff G. et al. Nucleus basalis and thalamic control of neocortical activity in the freely moving rat. *J Neurosci* 1988;8:4007.

52. Steriade M, Datla S, Pare D, et al. Neuronal activities in brainstem cholinergic nuclei related to tonic activation patterns in thala cortical systems. *J Neurosci* 1990;10:2541.

53. Steriade M, Dossi RC, Nunez A. Network modulation of a slow intrinsic oscillation of cat thalamocortical neurons implicated in sleep delta waves: Cortically induced synchronization and brainstem cholinergic suppression. *J Neurosci* 1991;11:3200.

54. Jasper H. Tessier J. Acetylcholine liberation from cerebral cortex during paradoxical (REM) sleep. *Science* 1971;172:601.

55. Jouvet M, Buda C, Cespuglio R. et al. Hypogenic effects of some Hypothalamo-pituitary peptides. In: W E Bunney JR. E Costa, SG Potkin (eds) *Clinical Neuropharmacology*. (Vol 9, Suppl 4) New York: Raven, 1986:465.

56. Monnier M, Hosli L. Dialysis of sleep and waking factors in blood of rabbit. *Science* 1964;146:796.

57. Inoue S. *Biology of Sleep Substances*. Boca Raton; FL: CRC, 1989.

58. Schneider-Helmert D, Gniess F, Monnier M, et al. Acute and delayed effects of DSIP (delta sleep-inducing peptide) on human sleep behavior. *Int J. Clin Pharmacol Ther Toxicol* 1981; 19:341.

59. Schneider-Helmert D, Schoenenberger GA. Effects of DSIP in man. Multifunctional psychophysiological properties besides induction of natural sleep. *Neuropsycholobiology* 1983;9: 197.

60. Blois R, Monnier M, Tissot R, et al. Effects of DSIP on Diurnal and Nocturnal Sleep in Man. In WP Koella (ed) *Sleep* 1980, Basal: Karger, 1981;301.

61. Schneider-Helert D, Gniess F. Schoenenberger GA. Effect of DSIP Applications in Healthy and Insomniac Adults. In UP Koella (ed), *Sleep* 1980. Basel: Karger, 1981: 417.

62. Fischman HJ, Kastin AJ, Graf M. Circadian variation of DSIP-like material in rat plasma. *Life Sci* 1984;35: 2079.

63. Kato N, Nagaki S, Takahashi Y, et al. DSIP-Like Materials in Rat Brain Human Cerebrospinal fluid, and plasma as determined by enzyme Immunoassay. In S Inoue, AA Borbely (eds). *Endogenous Sleep Substances and Sleep Regulation*. Tokyo: Japanese Scientific Society Press, 1985;141.

64. Graf MV, Christen H, Schoenenberger GA. DSIP/DSIP-P and circadian motor activity of rats under continuous light. *Peptides* 1982; 3: 623.

65. Zoltoski RK, de Jesus Cabeza R, Gillin, JC. Biochemical Pharmacology of Sleep. In: *Sleep Disorders Medicine: basic science, technical considerations and clinical aspects*. Boston Butterworth-Heinemann: 1999:63–94

66. Krueger JM. Muramyl peptide enhancement of slow-wave sleep. Methods Find Exp *Clin Pharmacol* 1986;8:105

67. Krueger JM, Walter J, Levin C. Factor S and Related Somnogens: An Immune theory for Slow Wave Sleep. In DJ McGinty, R Drucker-Colin, A Morrison, et al. (eds.), *Brain Mechanisms of Sleep*. New York: Raven, 1987;253.

68. Krueger JM, Toth LA, Cady AB, et al. Immunomodulation and Sleep. In S Inoue, D Schneider-Helmert (eds), *Sleep Peptides: Basic and Clinical Approaches*. Berlin: Springer, 1988;95.

69. Krueger JM, Karnovsky ML. Sleep and immune response. *Ann NY Acad Sci* 1987;496:510.

70. Adam A, Lederer E. Muramyl peptides: immunomodulators, sleep factors and vitamins. *Med Res Rev* 1984;4: 111.

71. Karnovsky ML. Muramyl peptides in mammalian tissues and their effects at the cellular level. *Fed Proc* 1986;45:2556.

72. Werner GH, Floch F, Migliore-Samour D, et al. Immunomodulating peptides. *Experientia* 1986;42:521.

73. Moldofsky H, Lue FA, Eisen J, et al. The relationship of interlukin-1 and immune functions to sleep in humans. *Psychosom Med* 1986;48:309.

74. Karacan I, Thornby JI, Anch AM, Dose-related sleep disturbances induced by coffee and caffeine. *Clin Pharmacol Ther* 1976;20:682.

75. Ueno R, Hayaishi O, Osama H, et al. Prostaglandin D2 Regulates Physiological Sleep. In S Inoue, AA Borbely (eds), *Endogenous Sleep Substances and Sleep Regulations*. Tokyo: Japanese Scientific Society Press, 1985;193.

76. Ueno R, Honda K, Inoue S, et al. Prostaglandin D2, a cerebral sleep-inducing substance in rats. *Proc Natl Acad Sci* USA 1983; 80:1735.

77. Matsumura H, Honda K, Goh Y, et al. Awaking effect of prostaglandin E2 in freely moving rats. *Brain Res* 1989;481:242.

78. Hayaishi O. Molecular mechanisms of sleep-wake regulation: roles of prostaglandins D2 and E2, *FASEB J* 1991;5: 2575.

79. Practice parameters for the use of polysomnography in the evaluation of insomnia. Standards of Practice Committee of the American Sleep Disorders Association. *Sleep.* 1995;18:55–57.

80. Skidmore-Roth L. *Mosby's Handbook of Herbs and Natural Supplements* St Louis: Mosby 2001.

81. Marczynski TJ, Yamaguchi N, Ling GM, et al. Sleep induced by the administration of melatonin (5-methoxy-N-acetyltryptamine) to the hypothalamus in unrestrained cats. *Experientia* 1964: 20:435.

82. Hishikawa Y, Cramer H, Kuhlo W. Natural and melatonin-induced sleep in young chickens—a behavioral and electrographic study. *Exp Brain Res* 1969;7:84.

83. Anton-Tay F, Diaz JL, Fernandez-Guardiola. On the effect of melatonin on human brain. Its possible therapeutic implications. *Life Sci* 1971;10: 841.

84. Cramer H, Rudolph J, Consbruch U, et al. On the effects of melatonin on sleep and behavior in man. *Adv Biochem Psychopharmacol* 1974;11:187.

85. Holmes SW, Sugden D. Effects of melatonin on sleep and neurochemistry in the rat. *Br J Pharmacol* 1982;76: 95.

86. Lewy AJ, Ahmed S, Sack RL. Phase shifting the human circadian clock using melatonin. *Behav Brain Res* 1995;73:131.

87. Mendelson WB, Canin M, Cook JM, et al. A benzodiazepine receptor antagonist decreases sleep and reverses the hypnotic actions of flurazepam. *Science* 1983;219: 414.

88. Johns MW. Reliability and factor analysis of the Epworth Sleepiness Scale. *Sleep.* 1992;15: 376–381.

89. Douglas A, Bornstein R, Nino-Murica G. Et al. The Sleep Disorders Questionnaire: creation and multivariate structure of DSQ. *Sleep.* 1994;17: 160–167.

90. Buysse DJ, Reynolds CF, Monk TH. Berman SR. Kupfer DJ. The Pittsburg Sleep Quality Index: A new instrument for psychiatric practice and research. *Psychiatry Res* 1989;28:193–213.

91. Beck AT: Beck Depression Inventory. San Antonio, TX, The Psychological Corporation, 1987.

92. Kerns RD, Turk DC, Rudy TE; The West Haven-Yale Multidimensional Pain Inventory (WHYMPI). *Pain* 1985;23:345–56.

93. Carskadon ME et al. Guidelines for the Multiple Sleep Latency Test (MLST) a standard measurement of sleepiness. *Sleep.* 986;9:519+.

94. American Sleep Disorders Association: The clinical use of the multiple sleep latency test. *Sleep* 1992;15:268–276.

95. Fichtenberg NL, Putnam SH, Mann NR, Zafonte RD, Millard AE. Insomnia screening in postacute traumatic brain injury: utility and validity of The Pittsburgh Sleep Quality Index. *AM J Phys Med Rehabilitation.* 2001;80:339–345.

96. Czeisler CA, Richardson GS, Coleman RM. et al. Chronotherapy: resetting the circadian clocks of patients with delayed sleep phase insomnia. *Sleep.* 1981;4:1–21.

97. Bootzin RR, Perlis ML. Nonpharmacholologic treatments of insomnia. *J Clin Psychiatry.* 1992;53:6 (Suppl) 37–41.

98. Czeisler CA, Kronauer RE, Allen JS, et al. Bright light induction of strong (type 0) resetting of the human circadian pacemaker. *Science.* 1989:244:1328–1333.

99. Terman M. Light therapy. In: Kryger MH, Roth T, Dement WC, eds. *Principles and Practices of Sleep Medicine.* Philadelphia: W.B. Saunders; 1989:717–722.

100. Markland ON, Dyken ML. Sleep abnormalities in patients with brain stem lesions. *Neurology.* 1976;26:769–776.

101. Zafonte RD, Mann NR, Fitchenberg NL. Sleep disturbance in traumatic brain injury: pharmacological options. *NeuroRehabilitation.* 1996;7:189–195

102. Fitchenberg NL, et al. Factors associated with insomnia among post-acute traumatic brain injury survivors. *Brain Injury.* 2000; 14:659–667.

103. Beetar JD, Guilmette TJ, Sparadeo FR. Sleep and pain complaints in symptomatic traumatic brain injury and neurologic populations. *Arch Phys Med Rehabil.* 1996;77:1298–1302

104. Ron S, Algom D, Hary D, et al. Time-related changes in the distribution of sleep stage in brain injured patients. *Electroencephalogr Clin Neurophysiol.* 1980;48:432–441.

105. Cohen M, Oksenberg A, Snir D, Stern MJ, Groswasser Z. Temporally related changes of sleep complaints in traumatic brain injured patients. *J Neurol Neurosurg Psychiatry.* 1992; 55:313–315.

106. Harda M, Minami R, Haltori F, et al. Sleep in brain-damaged patients an all night sleep study of 105 cases. *Kumamoto Med J.* 1976;29:110–127.

107. Clinchot DM, Bogner J. Mysiw WJ, Fugate L, Corrigan J. Defining sleep disturbance after brain injury. *Am J Phys Med Rehabil.* 1998;77:291–295.

108. Nowel PD, Mazundar S, Buysse DJ, Dew MA, Reynolds CF, Kupfer DJ. Benzodiazepines and zolpidem for chronic insomnia: a meta analysis of treatment efficacy. *JAMA.* 1997;278: 2170–2177.

109. Obermeyer WH, Benca RM. Sleep apnea. Part II Effects of drugs on sleep. *Otolaryngol Clin North Am.* 1999;32(2):289–302.

110. Eddy M, Walbroehl GS. Insomnia. *Am Fam Physician.* 1999; 59(7):1911–1918.

111. Greenblatt D. New hypnotic agents. *Am J Med.* 1990; 88(suppl):185–245.

112. Holbrook AM, Crowther R, Lotter A, et al. The role of benzodiazepines in the treatment of insomnia. *CMAJ.* 2000;162:25–33.

113. *Physicians Desk Reference (PDR).* 54th edition. Montvale, NJ: Medical Economics. 2000.

114. Roth T, Roehrs T, Koshorek G, Sicklesteel J, Zorick F. Sedative effects of antihistamines. *J Allergy Clin Immunol.* 1987; 80:94–98.

115. Nicholson AN. Antihistamines and sedation. (Abstract). *Lancet.* 1983;2:211.

116. Nicholson AN. New antihistamines free of sedative side effects. *Trends Pharmacol Spinal Cord Injury.* 1987;8:247.

117. Roder-Wanner U, Noachtar S, Wolf P. Response of polygraphic sleep to phenytoin treatment for epilepsy: a longitudinal study of immediate, short and long-term effects (Abstract). *Acta Neurol Scand.* 1987;76:157.

118. Wolf P, Roder-Wanner U, Brede M. Influence of the agent Phenobarbital and phenytoin medication on the polygraphic sleep of patients with epilepsy (Abstract). *Epilepsia.* 1984;25:467.

119. Trimble M, Thompson P. Anticonvulsant drugs, cognitive function, and behavior. *Epilepsia.* 1983;24:556–563.

120. Leach JP, Brodie MJ. Tiagabine. *Lancet.* 1998;351:203–7.

121. Mathias S, et al. The GABA uptake inhibitor tiagabine promotes slow wave sleep in normal elderly subjects. *Neurobiology of Aging.* 2001;22: 247–253.

122. Pande Atul C. et al. Pregabalin in Generalized Anxiety Disorder: A Placebo-controlled trial. *Am J Psychiatry* March 2003; 160:533–540.

123. Bialer M, Johannessen SI, Kupferberg HJ et al. Progress report on new antiepileptic drugs: a summary on the fifth Eilat conference (EILAT V). *Epilepsy Res* 2001;43:11–58.

124. Willmore LJ: Clinical pharmacology of new antiepileptic drugs. *Neurology* 2000;55 (Suppl 3):S17–24.

125. Kubota T, Fang J, Meltzer LT. et al. Pregabalin enhances non-rapid eye movement sleep. *J Pharmacol Exp Ther* 2001; 299(3):1095–1105.

126. Vogle GW, Buffenstine A, Minter K et al. Drug effects on REM sleep and on endogenous depression (Abstract) *Neurosci Biobhav Rev.* 1990;14:49.

127. Kupfer D, Spider D, Colbe P. Sleep and treatment for endogenous depression. *Am J Psychiatry.* 1981;138:429–434.

128. Arew JC. Tricyclic antidepressants in the treatment of insomnia. *J Clin Psychiatry.* 1983;44:25–28.

129. Adam K, Oswald I. The hypnotic effects of an antihistamine: promethazine (Abstract). *Br J Clin Pharmacol.* 1986;22:715.

130. Branchey MH, Brebbia Dr, Cooper TB. et al. Effects of loxapine on the sleep of chronic schizophrenics. (Abstract). *Psychopharmacology.* (Berl). 1979;62:201.

131. Feinberg I, Wender PH, Koresko RL, et al. Differential effects of chlorpromazine and Phenobarbital on EEG sleep patters. *J Psychiatr Res.* 1969;7:101.

132. Kaplan J, Dawson S, Vaughan T, et al. Effect of prolonged chlorpromazine administration on the sleep of chronic schizophrenics. *Arch Gen Psychiatry.* 1974;31:62.

133. McDaniel W. Serotonin syndrome: early management with cyproheptadine. *Ann Pharmacother.* 2001;35:870–873.

134. Chesnik DA, Mendels J. Longitudinal study of the effects of lithium carbonate on the sleep of hospitalized depressed patients. *Biol Psychiatry* 1974;9:117.

135. Kuper DJ, Reynolds CF 3rd, Weiss BL et al. Lithium carbonate and sleep in affective disorder: further consideration. *Arch Gen Psychiatry* 1974;30:79.

136. Fry JM, Pressman MP, Diphillipo MA, et al. Treatment of narcolepsy with codeine (Abstract) *Sleep.* 1986;9:269.

137. American Thoracic Society: Indications and standards for use of nasal continuous positive airway pressure (CPAP) in sleep apnea syndromes. *Am J Respir Crit Care Med* 1994;150: 1738–45

138. Engleman HM, Martin SE, Deary IJ, Douglas NJ: Effect of continous positive airway pressure treatment on daytime function in sleep apnea/hypoapnea syndrome. *Lancet* 1994 Mar 5; 343:572–5.

139. Schmidt-Nowara W, Lowe A, Wiegand L, et al: Oral appliances for the treatment of snoring and obstructive sleep apnea: a review. *Sleep* 1995 Jul; 18(6): 501–10

140. Sher AE, Schechtman KB, Piccirillo JF: The efficacy of surgical modifications of the upper airway in adults with obstructive sleep apnea syndrome. *Sleep* 1996 Feb; 19 (2): 156–77

141. Allen RP, Earley CJ: Restless Legs Syndrome. *Journal of Clinical Neurophysiology* 2001;18(2): 128–147

142. Restless Legs syndrome: Detection and management in primary care. National Heart, Lung, and Blood Institute Working Group on Restless Legs Syndrome. *Am Fam Phys* 2000 Jul 1;62(1): 108–14

143. Trenkwalder C, Walters AS, Hening W: Periodic limb movements and restless legs syndrome. *Neurol Clin* 1996 Aug; 14(3): 629–50

144. Evidente VG, Adler CH: How to help patients with restless legs syndrome. Discerning the indescribable and relaxing the restless. *Postgrad Med* 1999 Mar; 105(3): 59–61, 65–6, 73–4.

145. Rogers AE, Aldrich MS, Lin X: A comparison of three different sleep schedules for reducing daytime sleepiness in narcolepsy. *Sleep* 2001 Jun 15;24(4): 385–91.

146. Fry JM, Treatment modalities for Narcolepsy. *Neurology* 1998; 50(2 Suppl 1): 43–48

147. Guilleminault C, Pelayo R. Narcolepsy in prepubertal children. *Ann Neurol* 1998 Jan; 43(1): 135–42

148. U.S. Modafinil in Narcolepsy Study Group: Randomized trial of modafinil for the treatment of pathological somnolence in narcolepsy. *Annal of Neurology* 1998;43: 88–97.

149. Wise M. Childhood narcolepsy. *Neurology* 1998;50(2 Suppl 1): 37–41

150. Han F, Chen E, Wei H. Childhood Narcolepsy in North China. *Sleep* 2001 May 1;24(3): 321–4

151. Hublin C, Kaprio J, Partinen M, et al. Prevalence and genetics of sleepwalking: a population-based twin study. *Neurology* 1997;48(1):177–81

152. Lloredo MD, Currier MB, Norman SE, et al. Night terrors in adults: phenomenology and relationship to psychopathology. *J Clin Psychiatry* 1992;53(11):392–4

153. Schenck CH, Milner DM, Hurwitz TD, et al. A polysomnographic and clinical report on sleep-related injury in 100 adult patients. *Am J Psychiatry* 1989;146(9):1166–73

154. Schenck CH, Mahowald MW. Long-term, nightly benzodiazepine treatment of injurious parasomnias and other disorders of disrupted nocturnal sleep in 170 adults. *Am J Med* 1996; 100(3):333–7

155. Schenck CH, Hurwitz TD, O'Connor KA, et al. Additional categories of sleep-related eating disorders and the current status of treatment. *Sleep* 1993;16(5):457–66

156. Murray B. A psychologist investigates what sets people's teeth on edge. 1998. *APA Monitor Online,* 29 (6).

157. Horowitz L. G. Freedom from Teeth Grinding and Night Clenching. Rockport: *Tetrahedron,* 1989.

158. Pierce C J, Gale EN. A comparison of different treatments for nocturnal bruxism. *Journal of Dental Research,* 1988;67:597–601.

159. Thompson BH, Blount BW, Krumholtz TS. Treatment approaches to bruxism. *American Family Physician,* 1994;49:1617–22.

160. Feehan M, Marsh N. The reduction of bruxism using contingent EMG audible biofeedback: A case study *Journal of Behavioural Therapy and Experimental Psychiatry.* 1989;20:179–183.

161. Messing SG. Splint Therapy. In A. S. Kaplan & L. A. Assael. *Temporomandibular Disorders.* Philadelphia: Saunders. 1992 pp. 395–454.

162. Cassisi JE, Mcglynn FD, Belles DR. EMG-activated feedback alarms for the treatment of nocturnal bruxism: current status and future directions. *Biofeedback & Self Regulation,* 1987;12: 13–30.

163. Sadeh A, Hauri PJ, Kripke D, Lavre P. The role of actigraphy in evaluation of sleep disorders. *Sleep* 1995;18:288–302.

164. Pilsworth SN, King MA, Smith IE. A Comparison between measurements of sleep efficiency and sleep latency measured by polysomnography and wrist actigraphy. *Sleep* 2001;24 supplement, abstract # 171.

165. Kushida CA, Chang A, et al. Comparison of actinographic, polysomnographic and subjective assessment of sleep parameters in sleep-disordered patients. *Sleep Medicine* 2001;2:389–396.

166. Aguire M, Broughton R. Complex event-related potentials (P300 and CNV) and MSLT in the assessment of excessive daytime sleepiness in narcolepsy-cataplexy. *Electroencephalogr Clin Neurophsyiol* 1987;67:298–316.

167. Poceta JS, Ho S, Jeong D, Mitler MM. The Maintenance of wakefulness test in obstructive sleep apnea syndrome. *Sleep* 1990; 19;268.

168. Carskadon MA, Dement WC. The Multiple Sleep Latency Test: What does it mean? *Sleep* 1982;5:567–72.

169. Polysomnography Task Force, Clesson AL, Chairman. American Sleep Disorders Association. The Indications for polysomnography. *Sleep* 1997;20:423–487.

170. American Sleep Disorders Association. Practice parameters for the use of polysomnography of insomnia. *Sleep* 1995;18:55–7

171. Brown D. Valerian: A possible substitute for benzodiazepines? *Quart Rev Nat Med. Winter Quarter.* 1993; pp. 17–18.

172. Dressing H, Riesman D, et al. Are Valerian/Mellisa combinations of equal value to bezodiazeopine? *Therapiewoch.* 1992;42:726–36.

173. Kinzler E, Kromer J, & Lehmann E. Clinical efficacy of a kava extract in patients with anxiety syndrome: Double-blind placebo-controlled study over four weeks. *Arzneimittel-Forsch.*1991;41: 584–88.

174. Lindenberg D, Pitule-Schodel H. D, l-kavain in comparison with oxazepam in anxiety disorders. A double-blind study of clinical effectiveness. *Forschr Med.* 1990;108: pgs 49–50, 53–54.

175. Speroni E, Minghetti A. Neuropharmacological Activity of Extracts from Passiflora incarnata. *Planta Medica.*1988;54: 488–491.

176. Schmitz M, Jackel M. Comparative study for assessing quality of life of patients with exogenous sleep disorders (temporary sleep onset and sleep interruption disorders) treated with a hops-valarian preparation and a benzodiazepine drug . *Wien Med Wochenschr.* 1998;148(13):291–8.

177. de la Motte S, et al. "Double-blind comparison of an apple pectin-chamomile extract preparation with placebo in children with diarrhea," *Arzneimittelforschung* 1997;47(11):1247–9.

178. Viola H, et al., "Apigenin, a component of Matricaria recutita flowers, is a central benzodiazepine receptors-ligand with anxiolytic effects," *Planta Medica* 1995;61(3):213–16.

179. Yamada K, et al., "Effect of inhalation of chamomile oil vapour on plasma ACTH level in ovariectomized-rat under restriction stress," *Biol Pharm Bull* 1996;19(9):1244–6

180. Touitou Y, Arendt J, Pevet P, Melatonin and the Pineal gland – From basic science to clinical application, *Proceedings of the International Symposium on Melatonin and the Pineal Gland,* 295–302, Elsevier Science Publ., 1993: pgs 295–302.

181. Dawson D, Encel N. Melatonin and sleep in humans, *J. Pineal Res.*1993;15 (1): 1–12.

182. Waldhauser F, Weiszenbacher G, Tatzer E, Gisinger B, Waldhauser M, Schemper M & Frisch H. Alterations in nocturnal serum melatonin levels in humans with growth and aging. *Journal of Clinical Endocrinology and Metabolism,* 1988;66(3): 648–652.

183. Dahlitz M, Alverez B, Vignau J, English J, Arendt J and Parkes JD. Delayed sleep phase syndrome response to melatonin. *Lancet* 1991;337:1121–1124.

184. McKenzie RE, Costello RM. Electrosleep (Electrical Transcranial Stimulation) in the Treatment of Anxiety, Depression and Sleep

Disturbance in Chronic Alcoholics, *J Altered States of Consciousness, 1976;2(2):185–195.*

185. Schmitt R, Capo BS, Boyd E. Cranial Electrotherapy Stimulation as a Treatment for Anxiety in Chemically Dependent Persons, Alcoholism, *Clinical and Experimental Research,* 1986; 10(2):158–160.

186. Madden RE, Kirsch DL. Low Intensity Transcranial Electrostimulation Improves Human Learning of a Psychomotor Task. *American Journal of Electromedicine,* 1987;4(2):41–45.

187. Smith RB, Day E. The Effects of Cerebral Electrotherapy on Short-Term Memory Impairment in Alcoholic Patients, *The International Journal of the Addictions,* 1977;12(4):575–582.

188. Holm KJ, Goa KL. Zolpidem: an update of its pharmacology, therapeutic efficacy and tolerability in the treatment of insomnia. *Drugs.* 2000;59(4): 865–889.

189. Maarek L, Cramer P, Attali P, Coquelin JP, Morselli PL. The safety and efficacy of Zolpidem in insomniac patients: a long-term open study in general practice. *J Int Med Res.* 1992;20(2): 162–170.

190. Scharf MB, Roth T, Vogel GW, Walsh JK. A multicenter, placebo-controlled study evaluating zolpidem in the treatment of chronic insomnia. *J Clin Psychiatry.* 1994;55(5):192–199.

191. Nagtegaal JE, Kerkhof GA, Smits MG, Swart AC, van der Meer YG. Traumatic brain injury-associated delayed sleep phase syndrome. *Funct. Neurol.* 1997 Nov–Dec;12(6):345–8.

192. Steele DL, Rajaratnam SM, Redman JR, Ponsford JL. The effect of traumatic brain injury on the timing of sleep. *Chronobiol Int.* 2005;22(1):89–105.

193. Guilleminault C, Yuen KM, Gulevich MG, Karadeniz D, Leger D, Philip P. Hypersomnia after head-neck trauma: a medicolegal dilemma. *Neurology.* 2000 Feb 8;54 (3):653–9.

194. Richter KJ, Cowan DW, Kaschalk SM. Sleep and pain complaints in TBI. *Arch Phys Med Rehabil.* 1997 Apr;78(4):451.

195. Rao V, Rollings P. Sleep Disturbances Following Traumatic Brain Injury. *Curr Treat Options Neurol.* 2002 Jan;4(1):77–87.

196. Perlis ML, Artiola L, Giles DE. Sleep complaints in chronic post-concussion syndrome. *Percept Mot Skills.* 1997 Apr;84(2): 595–9.

197. Schreiber S, Klag E, Gross Y, Segman RH, Pick CG. Beneficial effect of risperidone on sleep disturbance and psychosis following

traumatic brain injury. *Int Clin Psychopharmacol.* 1998 Nov; 13 (6):273–5.

198. Quinto C, Gellido C, Chokroverty S, Masdeu J. Posttraumatic delayed sleep phase syndrome. *Neurology.* 2000 Jan 11;54(1): 250–2.

199. Tobe EH, Schneider JS, Mrozik T, Lidsky TI. Persisting insomnia following traumatic brain injury. *J Neuropsychiatry Clin Neurosci.* 1999 Fall; 11(4):504–6.

200. Webster JB, Bell KR, Hussey JD, Natale TK, Lakshminarayan S. Sleep apnea in adults with traumatic brain injury: a preliminary investigation. *Arch Phys Med Rehabil.* 2001 Mar;82(3): 316–21.

201. Castriotta RJ, Lai JM. Sleep disorders associated with traumatic brain injury. *Arch Phys Med Rehabil.* 2001 Oct; 82 (10): 1403–6.

202. Masel BE, Scheibel RS, Kimbark T, Kuna ST. Excessive daytime sleepiness in adults with brain injuries. *Arch Phys Med Rehabil.* 2001 Nov; 82(11):1526–32.

203. Fichtenberg NL, Zafonte RD, Putnam S, Mann NR, Millard AE. Insomnia in a post-acute brain injury sample. *Brain Inj.* 2002 Mar; 16(3):197–206.

204. Li Pi Shan RS, Ashworth NL. Comparison of lorazepam and zopiclone for insomnia in patients with stroke and brain injury: a randomized, crossover, double-blinded trial. *Am J Phys Med Rehabil.* 2004 Jun; 83(6):421–7.

205. Ouellet MC, Morin CM. Cognitive behavioral therapy for insomnia associated with traumatic brain injury: a single-case study. *Arch J Phys Med Rehab.* 2004 Aug; 85(8):1298–302.

206. Mahmood O, Rapport LJ, Hanks RA, Fichtenberg NL. Neuropsychological performance and sleep disturbance following traumatic brain injury. *J Head Trauma Rehabil.* 2004 Sep-Oct; 19(5):378–90.

207. Kowatch RA. Sleep and head injury. *Psychiatr Med.* 1989;7(1): 37–41.

208. Ouellet MC, Savard J, Morin CM. Insomnia following traumatic brain injury: a review. *Neurorehabil Neural Repair.* 2004 Dec; 18(4):187–98.

209. Krystal AD, Walsh JK, Laska E, et al. Sustained efficacy of eszopiclone over 6 months of nightly treatment: results of a randomized, double-blind, placebo-controlled study in adults with chronic insomnia. *Sleep.* 2003;26:793–799.

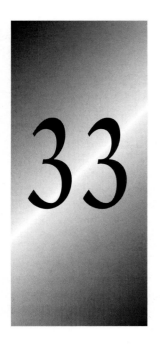

33

Diagnosis and Management of Late Intracranial Complications of TBI

David F. Long

INTRODUCTION

Purpose and Overview

Purpose Although many patients show excellent progress during rehabilitation from traumatic brain injury (TBI), intracranial complications occur frequently and can result in an adverse outcome. In many instances, prompt and accurate diagnosis of these complications can either be life-saving or can dramatically improve the extent of recovery which takes place.

Overview Complications addressed in this chapter include central nervous system (CNS) infections and the conditions predisposing to them, hydrocephalus and shunt management, and late post-traumatic vascular and mass lesions.

Specific Chapter Sections

Infection and Risk of Infection The potential risk of serious CNS infection changes the management of some patients even before an infection occurs. Topics discussed in this section include compound depressed skull fractures, penetrating injuries, basilar skull fractures, cerebrospinal fistulae, and pneumocephalus. CNS infections themselves are then discussed including meningitis, brain abscess and subdural empyema. Because specific management options,

especially antibiotic selection, are frequently subject to change, the general approach to diagnosis and management is emphasized in this section. A section on craniectomy and cranioplasty has also been added in view of the increasing recognition of the effects of these procedures on neurologic recovery.

Hydrocephalus and Shunts Hydrocephalus is probably the most difficult common complication to diagnose and manage during the rehabilitation of patients with TBI. Not only is it a challenge to identify which patients will benefit from a shunt, but management often becomes even more complicated after shunting. In order to optimally manage these patients, physicians need to understand the different types of shunts and their physiology, as well as common shunt complications. Programmable shunts and other recent innovations are now routinely available, and offer an opportunity for intervention to improve outcome during rehabilitation without requiring further surgery.

Vascular and Late Mass Lesions Although vascular lesions such as post-traumatic aneurysm and carotid cavernous fistula are relatively uncommon, physicians treating patients with TBI need to be aware of these complications in order to recognize and treat them promptly when they do occur. Finally, late mass lesions such as chronic subdural hematoma and hygroma, late presenting epidural hematoma, and delayed post-traumatic intracerebral hemorrhage are discussed.

CONDITIONS INVOLVING RISK OF INFECTION

Skull Fractures and Penetrating Injuries

Depressed Skull Fractures   Depressed skull fractures are generally considered significant if the fragment is depressed below the inner table of the skull by more than the thickness of the skull (1). Tangential skull radiographic views show these fractures most effectively. Compound depressed skull fractures are distinguished from simple depressed skull fractures by the presence of an overlying open wound or laceration, and are therefore associated with a substantial increased risk of infection. This infection risk includes subdural empyema and brain abscess, which are otherwise uncommon following closed head injury. These compound fractures account for up to 85% of depressed skull fractures (1). Both simple and complex depressed skull fractures are often elevated for cosmetic reasons and in the hope of preventing epilepsy. Compound depressed skull fractures are debrided to reduce the risk of infection. Prophylactic antibiotics are often administered to patients with compound depressed skull fractures, although this remains controversial (2–5).

Penetrating Injuries   Gunshot wounds confer a high risk of infection for several reasons. In contrast with higher velocity military missile wounds, the bullet is retained inside the skull in about 70% of civilian gunshot wounds. The retained bullet becomes a nidus for infection, and retained bone fragments are an even greater problem increasing the risk of infection by a factor of 10 (6). Focal necrosis of tissue in the path of the bullet is also believed to be crucial in the possible development of brain abscess. For these reasons, surgical debridement has been emphasized. In contrast to cerebrospinal fluid (CSF) rhinorrhea, in which antibiotic prophylaxis remains controversial, 87% of 966 neurosurgeons reported that they use antibiotic prophylaxis in patients with gunshot wounds (7). Post-traumatic brain abscess is most common after missile injury. Other types of penetrating injury also associated with increased infection risk include knife wounds in young adults and accidental trans-orbital accidents in children, such as with pencils or wires.

Basilar Skull Fractures   The base of the skull is comprised of five bones: the sphenoid, ethmoid (including cribriform plate), frontal, temporal (petrous and squamous), and occipital bones (1). Clues to likely basilar skull fracture include CSF leaks, pneumocephalus, hemotympanum,

Battle's sign (ecchymosis in the mastoid region), hearing impairment, peripheral facial nerve weakness, periorbital ecchymosis, fracture of the frontal sinus, and anosmia (8). Because the dura is closely adherent to the bones of the skull base, basilar fractures are frequently associated with dural tears; the resultant fistulous connection between brain and sinuses or ear provides a possible route of entry for infection. Antibiotic prophylaxis after basilar skull fracture has been controversial. A recent meta-analysis of 12 studies with a total of 1241 patients with basilar skull fracture did not find a statistically significant decrease in meningitis in patients treated with antibiotic prophylaxis (9).

Cerebrospinal Fluid Fistula

Cerebrospinal Fluid Rhinorrhea   CSF rhinorrhea is a definite indication of a fistulous tract from the intracranial compartment through the dura and skull base. It is therefore important to determine whether CSF rhinorrhea is present in brain injured patients. CSF rhinorrhea is typically a watery discharge with a salty taste, which does not cause nasal excoriation or stiffen bed linen (10). It may be unilateral, may increase with leaning over or prone positioning, and may be associated with a dull constant headache from low intracranial pressure (10, 11). Differential diagnosis includes vasomotor rhinitis, which is typically bilateral with sneezing and lacrimation, and pseudo-CSF rhinorrhea after surgery in the region of the pericarotid sympathetic plexus (12), with nasal stuffiness and hypersecretion, facial flushing, and absent ipsilateral lacrimation.

Glucose strips or tape are notoriously unreliable for diagnosis of CSF rhinorrhea with false-positive rates as high as 75% (13). Quantitative glucose determinations are somewhat more reliable for clear nasal fluid collected in a test tube, but not reliable when fluid is bloody. The definitive test is the beta-2 transferrin assay, which is sensitive and specific for CSF (14, 15). This form of transferrin is not normally found in serum, tears, saliva, or nasal secretions.

Common fistula sites causing CSF rhinorrhea include the ethmoid/cribriform plate region, posterior frontal sinus, roof of the orbit, and sphenoid sinus regions. When rhinorrhea is unilateral, it accurately predicts the site of the dural tear and fracture in 95% of cases. However, only one-half of patients with bilateral rhinorrhea have bilateral dural tears (1). Fractures are particularly common into the ethmoidal air cells just lateral and posterior to the cribriform plate (Figure 33-1)(10), and injury in this area is characteristically associated with anosmia (1). Rhinorrhea into the ethmoid air cells sometimes stimulates fibroblastic proliferation that may grow to close the underlying defect (10). In contrast, dural tears of the posterior wall of the frontal sinus do not tend to heal, and typically cause persistent rhinorrhea requiring surgery. Frontal sinus fracture can be associated with

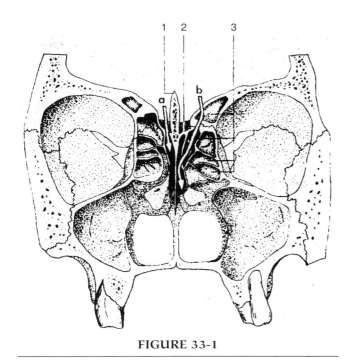

FIGURE 33-1

(a) Fracture in cribriform plate, (b) Fracture through ethmoidal cells, which is the more usual type. (1) crista galli, (2) cribriform plate, (3) ethmoidal cells. (From MacGee EE: Cerebrospinal fluid fistula. In Vinken PT, Bruyn GW (eds): Handbook of Clinical Neurology, vol. 24. New York, Elsevier, 1976, with permission.)

anesthesia of the supraorbital nerves, subconjunctival ecchymosis, palpable depression over the frontal sinus region, and air in the orbit. A leak into the sphenoid sinus is particularly likely to cause profuse rhinorrhea (16).

Several diagnostic techniques are used to localize the site of a CSF leak. Radioisotope cisternography, with radioisotope injected into the CSF and measured in pledgets placed in the nose is not as precise as newer methods for pinpointing the exact location of the leak, but can be useful for lateralization of a slow or intermittent leak (17). Special MRI techniques, using images with heavy T2 weighting may highlight CSF sufficiently to show the leak (17, 18). CT cisternography, with CT scan after injection of a contrast dye, is effective in patients with an active leak but may fail to visualize intermittent leaks, and is an invasive technique. Intrathecal fluorescein with endoscopic visualization has been reported as a very effective means of precisely identifying slow leaks, especially as part of an endoscopic surgical repair procedure (17, 18). Although a high incidence of side effects was initially reported with intrathecal fluorescein, including transient paraparesis and seizures(19), others have used the technique more recently and encountered little difficulty (17, 18).

CSF Fistula and Meningitis Risk   CSF rhinorrhea implies a 10-fold increase in the risk of subsequent meningitis (20).

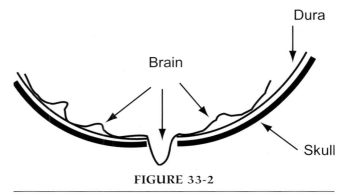

FIGURE 33-2

Fistula with brain tissue protruding through dura and skull. Even in the absence of active CSF fluid leakage, this presents a significant risk for eventual development of meningitis. Over time the plug of brain tissue may shrink somewhat with changes in brain compliance and provide route of entry for infection

However even when rhinorrhea resolves, as it does in 85% of cases within 1 week (21), there is now strong evidence of a very high (30–40% or more) risk of late meningitis (8, 17, 18, 22) In one series of 44 patients with meningitis, over one-half of the episodes occurred more than 1 year after injury (8), and cases have been reported many years later. Such late occurrences of meningitis underscore the importance of taking an aggressive approach to ensure closure of dural tears acutely and of considering a possible fistula when patients with a prior TBI present with meningitis. Rhinorrhea has also presented years after the original trauma in multiple cases (22, 23, 24, 25). Coughing, sneezing, hard work, or inverted posture may facilitate opening of the leak. Computed tomography (CT) or magnetic resonance imaging (MRI) may show evidence of encephalocele (brain protrusion through a skull defect) without clinical signs of basal fracture or CSF leak. In some late presenting cases brain tissue has been trapped in the dural defect, apparently making a temporary seal but preventing dural closure (23)(Figure 33-2). In cases presenting years after the injury the cerebral plug may become inadequate with brain atrophy or change in cerebral compliance.

Endoscopic extracranial techniques can now repair 90% of fistulae without requiring craniotomy (17). This avoids additional brain trauma and often preserves smell, which is typically lost with intracranial repair. Large defects or those associated with mass lesions may still require craniotomy. Lumbar drainage has often been used postoperatively after definitive dural repair, but it is not usually recommended as sole treatment (21, 22, 26).

Although prophylactic antibiotic use in patients with CSF rhinorrhea remains highly controversial, there is more support for prophylaxis in patients with rhinorrhea than in patients with basilar skull fracture alone (1, 9, 10, 20, 27, 28). One meta-analysis study found a statistically significant benefit by pooling studies which showed a similar trend but individually lacked sufficient numbers to achieve statistical significance (27), while another meta-analysis came to the opposite conclusion (9).

Cerebrospinal Fluid Otorrhea   Otorrhea occurs when petrous temporal bone fracture and dural tear are combined with tympanic membrane tear. The exact incidence of temporal bone fracture is uncertain since as many as 60% of these fractures may be missed with routine CT imaging (29). However they are believed to constitute over one third of basilar skull fractures (29). Otorrhea has been estimated to occur in approximately 7% of all patients with basilar skull fractures (30), or approximately 20–25% of those with temporal bone fractures (1). Petrous temporal bone fractures are divided into longitudinal and transverse types. Both types are associated with otorrhea. Longitudinal fractures run in the anteroposterior direction and are five times more common. Longitudinal fractures often are associated with torn tympanic membrane, ossicular disruption, and delayed transient impairment of the facial nerve. Transverse fractures run at right angles to the petrous axis and are associated with injury to the inner ear and eighth nerve, and immediate lasting injury to the facial nerve. Unlike CSF rhinorrhea, CSF otorrhea almost always resolves spontaneously in less than 1 week (1, 23). In the few cases that persist, the reported rate of cessation after a single surgical procedure is 98% (1).

Pneumocephalus   Pneumocephalus is defined as gas within the cranial cavity. In TBI this is usually air, with the exception being gas produced in a brain abscess by anaerobic infection. Air may be present in any of the intracranial compartments, but frontal subdural or intracerebral air were most common in a series of 295 patients (31). Pneumocephalus occurs in 15% of patients with a fistula (22), and concurrent rhinorrhea is reported in 30–50% (31).

Two major mechanisms for posttraumatic pneumocephalus have been proposed, the inverted bottle mechanism and the ball-valve mechanism. Relatively early pneumocephalus in patients with rhinorrrhea or otorrhea is consistent with the inverted bottle mechanism. It is similar to what happens when one drinks or pours from a bottle; as CSF escapes from the cranium, eventually air must enter to allow more CSF to exit. On the other hand, in the ball-valve mechanism, air is forced into the cranium with pressure, as by a cough or sneeze, and then cannot exit because the meninges or cerebral tissue tamponades the leak. The delayed build-up of intracranial air from this recurrent one-way valve mechanism fits the peak incidence of pneumocephalus at 1–3 months post injury.

The term "tension pneumocephalus" is used when intracranial air acts as a mass lesion, compressing the

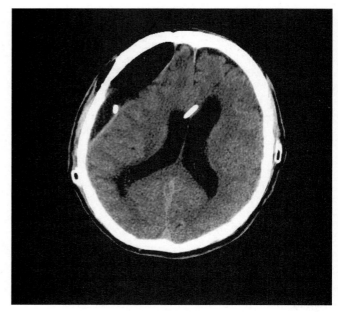

FIGURE 33-3

CT scan showing sizeable right-sided extra-axial pneumocephalus. Patient initially had TBI with subdural hematoma, later hydrocephalus and recurrent right subdural hygroma treated with ventriculoperitoneal shunt and shunt into subdural space on right, followed by subsequent postoperative development of pneumocephalus. In this film, some fluid is now seen inferiorly in the subdural space surrounding the catheter, in addition to the air superiorly. Catheter is also seen entering the right lateral ventricle. Despite the mild mass effect seen, both the subdural air and fluid eventually resolved from this point with conservative management

underlying brain and causing headache, motor paresis, meningeal signs, and even psychosis. Sometimes this type of picture is seen postoperatively, such as after evacuation of a subdural hematoma (Fig. 33-3).

Tension pneumocephalus has been described to present with severe progressive unilateral headache as much as four years after original brain injury (32). Although this late presentation is not common, it underscores the importance of considering this diagnosis in the comprehensive assessment of the post-traumatic headache patient.

One bedside finding, the "bruit hydro-aerique (31)," or cranial succession splash, is pathognomonic for pneumocephalus. It is heard by auscultation of the head during head movement and is sometimes also described subjectively by the patient. Although reported in only 7% of patients with pneumocephalus, it is likely that many examiners have not looked for it.

Definitive treatment for pneumocephalus entails repair of the underlying dural tear and fistula. In some obtunded patients with tension pneumocephalus, the air collection is tapped via a burr hole as an initial temporizing measure (31).

INFECTIOUS COMPLICATIONS

Meningitis

Presentation and Approach to Management Trauma to the head is the most common cause of meningitis in adults (33). The classical symptoms of meningitis are well known, including headache, fever, stiff neck, and confusion. However, typical features may be lacking in 20% of patients, particularly the very young, the very old, and the immunosuppressed (34). Focal signs are typically absent in meningitis, and their presence warrants obtaining a CT scan to rule out abscess, empyema, or other mass lesion. Lumbar puncture characteristically reveals CSF pleocytosis (predominantly polymorphonuclear cells) with lowered glucose (less than one-third the blood glucose in three fourths of patients). Identification of the causative organism in the cerebrospinal fluid generally guides specific antibiotic selection, along with general principles such as ability of the antibiotic to cross the blood brain barrier, effectiveness in purulent fluid, and ability to exert a bacteriocidal effect (35, 36). Due to the changing development of drug resistant strains, availability of newer antibiotics, and the need for treatment to be tailored to the specifics of each case, only some broad guidelines are offered here, and the reader is advised to check updated resources for best management of each case.

Common Organisms and Management Streptococcus pneumoniae are by far the most common causative organisms causing post-traumatic meningitis, accounting for over 80% of some series (33). Whereas penicillin was previously the mainstay of treatment for these pneumococci, with the emergence of resistant strains, the use of third generation cephalosporins (such as cefotaxime, ceftazidime, or ceftriaxone) is now often suggested, sometimes accompanied by vancomycin and rifampin (35). Hemophilis is important in young children, and third generation cephalosporins have also been advocated. (35) Patients with penetrating injuries are more likely to have Staphylococcus aureus or gram-negative meningitis (20). Staphylococcus aureus can be treated with nafcillin or oxacillin, or vancomycin for resistant organisms. Adult meningitis during the first few days after nonpenetrating injury is almost always pneumococcal. Gram-negative infections usually present later, necessitating broader-spectrum coverage in late presenting meningitis. Shunt-related infections warrant special mention, because they often are indolent clinically and usually caused by Staphylococcus epidermidis. Shunt removal is generally necessitated along with vancomycin intravenously, or even intrathecally for refractory cases (see hydrocephalus section for further discussion)(37, 38). Broad spectrum coverage of posttraumatic meningitis with a combination of agents, such as vancomycin plus ceftazidime, can sometimes be instituted when diagnostic results from cerebrospinal fluid are not available (37).

Subdural Empyema

Risk Factors and Presentation Subdural empyema is most common in males under age 20, and is actually more often secondary to paranasal or ear infections than trauma (16, 20). Post-traumatic subdural empyema is usually secondary to septic compound skull fracture, comprising 77% of a series of 53 cases of post-traumatic subdural empyema. (39) Presentation is acute and fulminant with fever, headache, and obtundation (20). Periorbital swelling (40) or tenderness over the sinuses or mastoid may provide additional clues. Focal signs and seizures are common(16, 34).

Evaluation and Management CT scans show an extraaxial collection with medial membrane enhancement (41). MRI scans typically shows low signal on Tl-weighted imaging and high signal on T2-weighted images(42). Lumbar puncture is contraindicated. Multiple organisms are usually present, including streptococci. When only one organism is cultured, it is most often Staphylococcus. In addition to appropriate antibiotics, either burr hole drainage or craniotomy is recommended (20, 34, 40, 42, 43). Although success has frequently been reported with burr holes (34, 40), large size, midline shift, parafalcine or posterior fossa location, and loculation have been identified as factors favoring craniotomy (43).

Brain Abscess

Risk Factors and Clinical Presentation Trauma is a less common cause of brain abscess, compared with spread from sinusitis or middle ear infection, or hematogenous spread from pulmonary or dental infection. In fact, only approximately 10% of brain abscesses are secondary to TBI or neurosurgical procedure. Among patients with TBI, brain abscess is three times as likely after gunshot wounds, and eight times as likely with wound complications, such as hematomas, fluid collections, wound infection and cerebrospinal fistula (44). Brain abscess is rarely seen as a complication of basal fracture alone (45). Classically the presentation of brain abscess peaks at about 2–3 weeks after injury, but the mean time of presentation was actually more than 3 months post injury in one series of 36 patients (46). Presentation is frequently with signs of increased intracranial pressure rather than with acute febrile illness. In one series headache was present in 90% and vomiting in 65% (47), while as many as half of patients are afebrile at presentation (45, 47). Focal signs occur in 50–75%, with changes in mental status notable in one half of patients, and seizures in one-third (45). Table 33-1 contrasts key features of meningitis, subdural empyema, and brain abscess.

TABLE 33-1
Distinguishing Features of Different Types of Intracranial Infection

	MENINGITIS	SUBDURAL EMPYEMA	BRAIN ABSCESS	SHUNT INFECTION
Predisposing condition	Basal fistula	Penetrating injury, Compound depressed fracture, Paranasal sinus/ear	Penetrating injury, Compound depressed fracture, Paranasal sinus/ear, Hematogenous	Recent shunt or shunt revision (70% within 2 months)
Organisms	*Pneumococci* (early) Gram negatives (late) *Staphylococci* (late)	Mixed/*Streptococci Staphylococci* Gram negatives	Polymicrobial/ anaerobic *Staphylococci*	*Staphylococcus epidermidis*
Presentation	Acute Headache, nuchal rigidity, mental status change	Acute fulminant Periorbital swelling Sinus tenderness Increased ICP, Seizures, focal signs	Subacute/ progressive Increased ICP Focal signs	Indolent Malaise, nausea irritability
Fever	Yes	Yes	Only 50%	Low-grade
WBC	Elevated	Elevated	Often normal	Often normal
CT/MRI	Negative or meningeal enhancement	Extra-axial – medial rim enhancement	Intra-axial ring enhancement, especially late; MRI T2 capsule low signal	Often nondiagnostic
Lumbar puncture	Increased WBC, decreased glucose	Contraindicated (Increased WBC, normal glucose)	Contraindicated (Often negative)	LP not reliable Must tap shunt for diagnosis
Management	Antibiotics	Antibiotics Burr hole/craniotomy	Antibiotics Debridement Stereotaxic aspiration	Antibiotics, Steroids Remove shunt

Key: ICP = intracranial pressure, WBC = white blood count, LP = lumbar puncture.

Abscess Stages and Imaging Stages of abscess formation have been recognized pathologically and correlated with CT and MRI scan findings (45). Early on the term cerebritis is used because of the presence of inflammatory cells in a perivascular location. CT scan at this stage shows low density with little enhancement, which may be solid. MRI during cerebritis is more sensitive (34) and shows uniform signal with indistinct margins (47). Later in cerebritis both the necrotic center and surrounding edema may reach maximal size, fibroblasts and macrophages are found at the periphery, and CT scan may show a thin rim of enhancement and increasing edema. Next a capsule of collagen and reticulin begins to develop; this forms more slowly on the ventricular side of the abscess. CT scan now shows a ring-enhancing capsule (less medially) and a low-density center. MRI scan shows the capsule as low signal on T2-weighted images (47). Diffusion weighted MRI has been effective in distinguishing brain abscess from other mass lesions, such as brain tumors. On diffusion weighted MRI the central core of a brain abscess is hyperintense, whereas tumors such as glioblastoma or metastasis are typically hypointense centrally (48).

Organisms and Treatment Most brain abscesses are polymicrobial and include anaerobes. Gas on CT scan may help in early differentiation from tumor and suggests anaerobic organisms. Staphylococci are found in about 10% of brain abscesses and are more frequent after trauma (45). Lumbar puncture is contraindicated in brain abscess and usually not diagnostically helpful if performed inadvertently. Therefore, choice of antibiotic reflects the anticipated polymicrobial etiology supplemented by information from aspiration of the abscess. For example, in the absence of specific culture information, a combination of a third generation cephalosporin, nafcillin or vancomycin for Staph, and metronidazole for anaerobes might be utilized. As an abscess heals, the capsule becomes more isodense on serial CT scans. Steroids are frequently used effectively in brain abscess to decrease edema, but may delay encapsulization of the abscess and make monitoring of response to therapy more difficult. Surgical management of brain abscess includes excision or CT-guided stereotactic aspiration (49, 50). Indications to the stereotactic approach include surgically inaccessible location, cerebritis stage, or poor neurologic or general medical condition. Excision is useful for removal of foreign material and necessary for posterior fossa lesions. Adverse prognostic factors in brain abscess include young or old age; large, deep abscess; coma; or rupture into the ventricular system. Mortality from brain abscess in

Vietnam was 54%, and survival was worse with gram-negative organisms. However, good recovery can occur, and 30% or less of survivors are reported to have significant residual hemiparesis.

CRANIECTOMY AND CRANIOPLASTY

Craniectomy and Cranioplasty

Role of Cranioplasty in the Recovery Process Craniectomy (skull flap left out) is performed acutely in many patients with either uncontrollable intracranial pressure or with penetrating or contaminated wounds. Traditionally cranioplasty (replacement of bone flap or prosthesis) was often delayed six months or longer to minimize risks of infection or complication (16, 51, 52), and the procedure was considered more cosmetic and protective than therapeutic. However, it now appears that many patients with craniectomy develop the so called "syndrome of the trephined" (53), and can show considerable neurologic and functional improvement with early performance of cranioplasty. The deficits shown to improve upon performance of cranioplasty have included headaches, apathy, hemiparesis (54), midbrain syndrome with eye movement disorder (55), tremor, gait, and cognitive function (53). Patients exhibiting the syndrome of the trephined have been described to show the "sinking skin flap syndrome", where the craniectomy flap tends to be markedly ingoing (53). This is particularly likely to occur in patients with concurrent shunts for hydrocephalus (56), and because craniectomy changes the brain compliance it may actually play a role in inducing hydrocephalus (53, 56).

In those patients where marked clinical improvement occurs with cranioplasty, the improvement has correlated with cerebral blood flow improvements of up to 30% as well as improved distribution of flow. Based upon measurements of transcranial cerebral oximetry and of ratios of phosphocreatine to inorganic phosphate (sensitive to rate of oxygen depletion), it has been suggested that cranioplasty induces more energy efficient mitochondrial function (53). The practical impact of these studies is the desirability of performing cranioplasty earlier, particularly in patients with markedly ingoing skull defects or ventriculoperitoneal shunts.

Cranioplasty Alternatives Cranioplasty can be performed with the patient's own bone flap, which can be frozen and stored (57), or stored in the patient's abdomen (58). Alternatively multiple materials can be used to create a cranioplasty flap, including titanium mesh (59), hydroxyapatite, and polymethylmethacrylate (60), and computerized techniques can be used to generate a custom made cranioplasty prosthesis (61). For patients with shunts and depressed skull flaps, it has been suggested to clip the shunt

temporarily to reexpand the brain prior to cranioplasty to minimize dead space at the time of surgery (62).

HYDROCEPHALUS

Overview

Importance After TBI Hydrocephalus is the most common treatable neurosurgical complication during rehabilitation of traumatic brain injury (TBI)(63), and its treatment can sometimes have a dramatic impact on rehabilitation and outcome. One recent study estimated an incidence of post-traumatic hydrocephalus at 45% in patients with severe TBI (64). However, differentiation of dynamic hydrocephalus from central atrophy or ex vacuo ventricular dilation remains problematic(65), and the physiology relevant to the decision process in managing these patients is complex. Practical management after a shunt includes prevention and treatment of other complications such as overdrainage and subdural hematoma, and the introduction of programmable shunts now offers additional opportunity for the physician to intervene medically during rehabilitation. Therefore the pathophysiology and clinical presentation of hydrocephalus, noninvasive and invasive diagnostic studies, shunt types including newer valve innovations, and shunt complications will be reviewed in some detail.

Types and Variants Hydrocephalus is divided into communicating and noncommunicating types(66). In communicating hydrocephalus, the different portions of the ventricular system are interconnected, and fluid may exit the ventricular system freely to the cisterns and subarachnoid space, whereas in noncommunicating (obstructive) hydrocephalus CSF flow is obstructed either between the ventricles or in exiting the ventricular system.

Post-traumatic hydrocephalus is communicating in the vast majority of cases, and enlargement characteristically involves all components of the ventricular system. Blood products, protein, or fibrosis typically interfere with circulation of cerebrospinal fluid and its absorption into the bloodstream through the arachnoid granulations (67).

When only selected portions of the ventricular system are enlarged, noncommunicating hydrocephalus should be considered. For example, large lateral and third ventricles with a small fourth ventricle in a patient with a large head circumference is generally attributable to aqueductal stenosis (66, 68), a congenital condition which may become decompensated by TBI. Lumbar puncture is contraindicated in these patients. Endoscopic third ventriculostomy can effectively bypass the aqueductal obstruction without requiring a shunt in some cases (69). The procedure involves placing hole in the floor of the 3rd ventricle creating a connection with the adjacent cistern.

Focal ventricular enlargement frequently occurs on an atrophic or porencephalic basis in brain areas that have sustained known damage. Less often, trapping of an isolated portion of the ventricular system may produce focal enlargement with signs of increased intracranial pressure or focal deficits (70–73). Occasional cases of multiloculated hydrocephalus are encountered, usually secondary to meningitis, ventriculitis, or intraventricular hemorrhage (74). The multiple irregular intraventricular septations of the enlarged ventricular system can be effectively treated with fenestration by intraventricular endoscopy (74–76).

Pathophysiology of Chronic Communicating Hydrocephalus Including Normal Pressure Hydrocephalus (NPH)

Pascal's Law Pascal's law of hydraulic systems states that F = P x A, where F is the force against the ventricular wall, P is the intraventricular pressure, and A is the area of the ventricular wall (77). This formula implies that when the area of the ventricular wall is large, a substantial expanding force may be generated from within the ventricle without the necessity of high pressure. For example, if a certain degree of ventricular enlargement initially results from increased pressure, ongoing enlargement may take place, even though pressures are no longer elevated (78).

Decreased Parenchymal Pressure and Compliance Rather than the absolute intraventricular pressure, the difference between the intraventricular pressure and that of the surrounding tissue determines ventricular size (77, 79). This concept may be understood more clearly by considering that the size of a balloon is determined not only by the pressure inside the balloon, but by the pressure of the air inside relative to the air outside the balloon. Changes in the viscoelastic properties of brain parenchyma with related decrease in parenchymal pressure therefore probably contribute significantly to the development of hydrocephalus, since it is the difference between cerebrospinal fluid pressure and intraparenchymal pressure which determines ventricular size (80). A gradient of reduced blood flow has been documented in the periventricular white matter of patients with NPH, as well as altered blood flow autoregulation which likely contributes to watershed ischemia (81). Damage to myelin and axons has also been described when hydrocephalus is longstanding (82). These factors are probably among those that contribute to the decreased elasticity or compliance of the brain parenchyma which is felt to be important in the development of NPH.

Pulsatile CSF Flow Disturbances of pulsatile CSF flow may be more important than blockage of CSF absorption in causing chronic communicating hydrocephalus (83). According to the Monro-Kellie doctrine, the volume of the intracranial contents including brain, blood, and CSF is constant (84). This means that arterial blood inflow during systole is accompanied by both outflow of venous blood and shifting of CSF into the spinal compartment (84). Furthermore CSF movement is not simple unidirectional flow but complex, and the basal cisterns probably play an important role in dynamic compliance. When intracranial compliance is decreased, restricted arterial pulsation and increased pulse pressure in brain capillaries have been postulated to play a causative role in chronic hydrocephalus (85).

Clinical Presentation of Hydrocephalus

Acute Hydrocephalus Early post injury acute hydrocephalus can present with symptoms of increased intracranial pressure including headache, nausea, vomiting, and lethargy or decreasing mental status. Associated signs can include a tense bulging craniectomy flap, papilledema, and Cushing's triad of hypertension, bradycardia, and hypoventilation.

Normal-Pressure Hydrocephalus NPH is well known to present with the clinical triad of dementia, gait ataxia, and urinary incontinence. Of the three, gait impairment is the most important diagnostically and most likely to respond to shunting. The classic gait disturbance is short stepping, wide based, with a "magnetic" difficulty in lifting the feet, and characteristic of frontal or subcortical rather than cerebellar dysfunction (86, 87). The cognitive difficulties in NPH are apt to include long latency responses, decreased attention, and poor initiation rather than deficits such as aphasia or agnosia. In patients with TBI, the presentation of hydrocephalus is not limited to the classic triad of normal pressure hydrocephalus, and should be considered in any patient who worsens or fails to progress adequately. A pretectal syndrome (88) or akinetic mutism are additional clinical syndromes that should particularly raise suspicion for hydrocephalus. Patients with meningitis or intracranial hemorrhage, especially subarachnoid or intraventricular hemorrhage, are particularly at risk for development of hydrocephalus.

Computed Tomography (CT) and Magnetic Resonance Imaging (MRI)

Ventriculomegaly CT and MRI scans have been invaluable in providing information about ventriculomegaly, and multiple methods have been devised for measuring ventricular size, calculating ventricle to brain ratios, and assessing shunt function (89–93). However, ventricular size alone has not been a reliable predictor of whether a patient has shunt responsive hydrocephalus rather than cerebral atrophy (94). In fact, ventriculomegaly has been reported in as many as 72% of patients with severe TBI (95), and it is now recognized that the extent of ventriculomegaly can be correlated with severity of diffuse axonal injury and outcome, complicating assessment for hydrocephalus in patients already known to have severe TBI (96–98). Ventricular configurations favoring dynamic hydrocephalus include enlargement of temporal horns, convex shape of the frontal horns, widening of the frontal horn radius, and frontal horn location closer to midline narrowing the "ventricular angle" (70).

Sulcal Absence and Periventricular Lucency Ex-vacuo ventricular dilatation or cerebral atrophy typically involves sulcal prominence. Small or absent sulci on a CT scan in combination with ventriculomegaly are predictors of a good response to shunting, although the presence of sulci does not preclude a positive response (94). Periventricular lucency has been a valuable predictor of a good response to shunting, especially when lucencies have been seen in multiple periventricular locations (see Figure 33-4) (94, 99). In hydrocephalus, fluid seeps across the ependymal lining of the ventricle and causes interstitial edema. This transependymal fluid is seen as lucency on CT and as smooth increased T2 signal on MRI. Contusion, infarction, or demyelination in the periventricular white matter can be difficult to distinguish from transependymal fluid, but are usually more irregular and asymmetric (100).

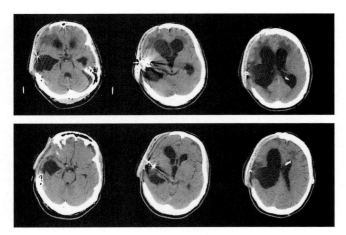

FIGURE 33-4

Hydrocephalus pre- and post shunting. In the pre-shunt scans (top) note marked periventricular lucency in the white matter consistant with transependymal fluid in addition to ventricular enlargement. There is also artifact from aneurysm clip and right hemispheric encephalomalacia, maximal in the right temporal lobe. Post shunt scans show persisting encephalomalacia of the right hemisphere including the right lateral ventricle and right temporal horn. Shunt is now seen entering the left lateral ventricle which has now normalized (including left temporal horn), and periventricular lucency has largely resolved. Surprisingly a CSF tap test (see text) had actually been negative in this patient, but after performance of ventriculoperitoneal shunt there was nonetheless marked clinical improvement

Additional MRI Findings MRI provides more anatomic detail about the configuration of the ventricular system than CT, including imaging of structures such as the Sylvian aqueduct and foramen of Monro. More rapid flow through the Sylvian aqueduct can be detected as decreased signal or "flow void" in the aqueduct in patients with hydrocephalus due to decreased compliance of the ventricular wall of the 3rd ventricle during systole (70, 101, 102). A series of linear measurements on MRI, essentially reflecting size and configuration of the third ventricle, can be used to distinguish obstructive hydrocephalus from atrophy, but the effectiveness of this approach in chronic communicating hydrocephalus in TBI has not been assessed (103).

SPECT Scans SPECT scans may be helpful in differentiating hydrocephalus from atrophy (64). Subcortical low flow improved in follow up SPECT after shunting in 10 of 11 patients who improved clinically but did not in 3 clinically unimproved patients(104). In a series of eight patients showing clinical improvement after a shunt, a "high percentage" showed improvement of previous temporal lobe hypoperfusion (64).

Invasive Testing

Cisternography Radioisotope cisternography had long been a mainstay in the diagnosis of hydrocephalus. After lumbar injection of radioisotope, pooling in the ventricles rather than progression of uptake over the convexity was taken as indicative of normal pressure hydrocephalus. However, cisternogram findings may really be more of a dilution and concentration process than a true measurement of CSF flow (84), and cisternography does not improve the diagnostic accuracy of combined clinical and CT criteria (105). Cisternography based predictions were the same in 43% of patients, better in 24%, and worse in 33% (105).

Lumbar Infusion Studies Infusion of fluid via a lumbar or ventricular catheter with measurement of drainage at designated pressures allows calculation of the outflow resistance, a measure of the difficulty of CSF absorption (94). If the outflow resistance is low, significant volumes of CSF can be readily absorbed and a shunt is not likely to help. On the other hand, increased outflow resistance means CSF is not readily absorbed. It is related to decreased compliance of the system, and is predictive of a positive response to shunting(68, 94, 106–110). Of interest, ventricular size does not correlate well with either outflow resistance or response to shunting (84, 106). Infusion studies have relatively low risk compared with the long-term morbidity of a shunt (107, 108). Unfortunately, despite their reported value and frequent use in Europe, these studies are infrequently performed in many U.S. hospitals. The suggestion of a one-stage "test and shunt if needed" procedure may make infusion studies more practicable (68).

CSF Tap Test and CSF Drainage Trial   A lumbar puncture with the removal of 50 ml of CSF has been widely advocated as a CSF tap test (99, 103, 112–116) If the patient shows an improvement in neurologic status after lumbar puncture, the test is viewed as positive. However, a lack of response does not preclude response to a shunt, because shunting produces more sustained ventricular decompression (67, 86). Therefore, the CSF tap test is most useful to identify patients who otherwise might not be shunted; a strong candidate would be shunted even in the face of a negative tap test. A more prolonged CSF drainage trial with a spinal catheter for 3 to 5 days has been shown to have both greater sensitivity and predictive value of shunt success than a simple tap test alone. (111, 112).

Combined Studies   A recent patient series had both lumbar infusion testing and CSF tap tests (114). The two tests agreed in only 45% of patients, with use of both tests recommended, since each test identified patients missed by the other test. When the tap test was positive, 94% of patients had a good response to shunting, but if the test were used alone, 58% of positive shunt responders would have been missed. The lumbar infusion test was only 80% predictive of success, but false negatives were 16%. In another series, perfusion weighted MRI or SPECT were performed before and 1 day after CSF tap tests (115). Nine patients were both clinically improved and had improved blood flow after the tap, and all responded well to shunting. In addition, six patients who were not clinically improved by the tap test, but did have improved blood flow on perfusion weighted MRI or SPECT after the tap test also showed good response to shunting.

Approach to Shunt Decision Making.

Establishing the Diagnosis and Therapeutic Expectations Table 33-2 reviews multiple considerations relevant to identifying dynamic hydrocephalus. The combination of the clinical course and findings, CT and MRI appearance, and in some cases SPECT and CSF tap test (and lumbar infusion testing if available) may help establish the diagnosis. Patients with TBI are likely to show only a partial response to shunting, because deficits from hydrocephalus are superimposed on deficits from the original TBI. This should be clearly explained to family members before pursuing shunting, to prevent or minimize any unrealistic expectations. However, given the potential significant benefit to patient outcome, an aggressive approach to identification and treatment of hydrocephalus is warranted for the severe TBI patient.

Treatment

Treatment Without a Shunt   The definitive treatment of hydrocephalus is surgical, usually the placement of a shunt. Treatment with carbonic anhydrase inhibitors, such as acetazolamide or furosemide (116), or with serial lumbar punctures is only a temporizing measure. Similarly, external ventricular drainage may be used on a temporary basis, particularly for obstructive mass effect or

---

TABLE 33-2
Factors Distinguishing Dynamic Hydrocephalus from Ex Vacuo Ventricular Dilatation

FEATURE OR TEST	DYNAMIC HYDROCEPHALUS	EX VACUO VENTRICULAR DILATATION
Antecedent history	Hemorrhage, esp IVH or SAH	Anoxia or diffuse axonal injury
Clinical deficits	NPH triad (dementia, gait impair, urinary incontinence), pretectal syndrome (loss of upgaze), akinetic mutism	Consistent with location and severity of injury
Clinical course	Worsening, intermittent, or static	Chronic slow improvement
Skull flap (craniectomy)	Bulging (increased ICP) or increasing prominence	Depressed, ingoing
Ventriculomegaly pattern	Temporal horns, 3rd ventricle, convex frontal horns	Diffuse enlargement, porencephalic dilatation in areas of focal injury
Sulci, fissures, cisterns	Decreased	Increased
Periventricular abnormality	Smooth periventricular signal on T2 MR or lucency on CT (transependymal fluid)	Absent, or frontal contusions or periventricular infarct
SPECT	Periventricular low flow	Normal or Alzheimer's pattern
CSF tap test	Positive or no response	No response
Lumbar/ventricular infusion studies	Increased outflow resistance (poor CSF absorption)	Normal (lower) outflow resistance (good CSF absorption)

Key: IVH = intraventricular hemorrhage, SAH = subarachnoid hemorrhage, NPH = normal pressure hydrocephalus, ICP = intracranial pressure, CSF = cerebrospinal fluid.

while excessive blood products are likely to clog a shunt, but conversion to a shunt is needed for treatment of persisting hydrocephalus. Third ventriculostomy, where a connection is endoscopically created between the floor of the third ventricle and the underlying cistern, is the one exception of a definitive treatment for hydrocephalus not requiring placement of a shunt. It is most commonly used to treat aqueductal stenosis (117), where the procedure can bypass the obstruction at the Sylvian aqueduct (83). More recently there has been renewed interest in the procedure for other forms of hydrocephalus as well, mainly because of the potential to improve intracranial compliance without diverting fluid from the CSF compartment (85, 118).

Shunt Types Ventriculoperitoneal shunts are used most commonly for post-traumatic hydrocephalus, but ventriculoatrial, ventriculopleural, and lumboperitoneal shunts are useful in certain circumstances. Ventriculoatrial shunts are used more frequently in children with obstructive hydrocephalus. Occasionally ventriculopleural shunts may be substituted in cases with abdominal infection, very high CSF protein, or rarely to drain very low pressure hydrocephalus to the negative pressure of the pleural space (119). Ventriculopleural shunts characteristically cause a small pleural effusion that disappears with shunt malfunction (66). Pleural shunts are avoided in younger children because of the likelihood of symptomatic hydrothorax with a smaller pleural cavity (75). Lumboperitoneal shunts are not commonly seen, but can be used for communicating but not obstructive forms of hydrocephalus. Lumboperitoneal shunts have also been used for pseudotumor cerebri, when ventriculoperitoneal shunt placement may be difficult because of small ventricular size (66). Placement of a lumboperitoneal shunt often obliterates the basal cisterns on CT scan of the head, and the return of previously obliterated cisterns is a reliable indicator of shunt malfunction (120). Although usually asymptomatic, cerebellar tonsillar herniation (iatrogenic Chiari malformation) has been described in as many as 70% of patients with lumboperitoneal shunts (121).

Shunt Valves and Components The basic components of a ventriculoperitoneal shunt are the ventricular catheter, valve, and distal tubing. A reservoir may be added proximal to the valve to facilitate access to the ventricular system. Virtually all shunt systems have some type of one-way valve to allow forward flow down the shunt when the pressure gradient exceeds a threshold range and to prevent back flow from the peritoneum. Therapy staff often ask whether a shunt contraindicates inverted position; because of the one-way valve, this is not a problem. Detailed diagrams on a variety of different past and present valve systems and components are available (122). Basic valve types include slit valves, cruciate valves, mitre valves, diaphragm valves,

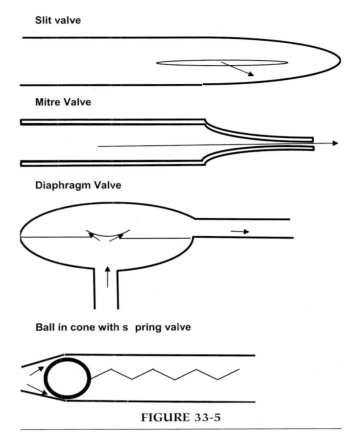

Slit valve

Mitre Valve

Diaphragm Valve

Ball in cone with s pring valve

FIGURE 33-5

Common shunt valve types

and ball/spring valves (see Figure 33-5) (122–124). Slit valves open and allow CSF flow when sufficient pressure develops within the tubing; setting is determined by tube thickness. Cruciate valves are similar but have two perpendicular slits instead of one horizontal slit.

Sometimes two slit or cruciate valves are housed in one unit with a pumping chamber between them. Although most shunt systems feature a valve mechanism located over the skull, it is also possible to have a slit valve in the distal tubing instead. The leaflets of a mitre valve act as springs to regulate CSF flow (123). Diaphragm valves allow movement of a diaphragm from its seat or pin as determined by CSF pressure. Reservoirs or flushing chambers are added to many shunt systems. They allow manual pumping of the shunt and potential access to sample CSF or to inject into the shunt system. It is important to know the specifics of a shunt system before injecting into it, because some shunt components (especially older components such as the Spitz-Holter valve, Coe-Schulte second bubble, or Hakim-Cordis valve) may be damaged by needle perforations (125). Most modern shunts, however, have a portion that can be injected without damage. Flushing chambers may be of either single bubble or double-bubble design (see Figure 33-6). If the chamber is proximal to all valves, compression of a

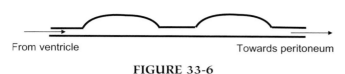

FIGURE 33-6

Double bubble reservoir

single bubble may send fluid both down the shunt and back into the ventricle. If the chamber is between valves, compression may push fluid only in the forward direction. Compression of the distal bubble of a double-bubble shunt after occluding the proximal bubble may also force fluid in the forward direction. A similar result may be obtained in some single-chamber devices by occlusive digital compression of areas of proximal tubing before compression of the flushing chamber. Alternatively, compression of distal bubble or tubing before digital compression of the proximal chamber may force retrograde flow into the ventricle (e.g., intrathecal administration of antibiotics). Of course, access to the ventricle is possible only when a chamber is proximal to all valves.

Shunt valves are also specified by the approximate pressure necessary for opening and forwarding CSF flow, and are commonly divided into low, medium, and high pressure valves (122, 123). Such valve settings are approximate and function differently depending on the compliance of the ventricular system, especially given that CSF flow is pulsatile in nature (126). In general, because of Pascal's law ($F = P \times A$), larger ventricles require a lower pressure for adequate decompression (86). However, valve pressure settings have poor correlation with actual intracranial pressure, which also varies widely among patients with the same valve, and within the same patient with different head of bed positioning (127). When patients do not respond to a shunt, conversion to a shunt of lower pressure occasionally results in clinical improvement (128). Because of the obvious undesirability of reoperation to place a valve with a different pressure, programmable valves have been developed which allow changing the effective opening pressure of the valve noninvasively at the bedside with an external magnet (see further discussion below).

Shunt Complications

Frequency of Shunt Complications   The overall incidence of shunt complications is high. Shunt complications include shunt failure, infection, seizures, subdural hematoma, and overdrainage. In 356 adult patients over an 18-year interval, the incidence of revision was 29% (129). In a series of 1, 179 patients shunted for hydrocephalus (only 312 patients over age 5 years), the probability of shunt malfunction after 12 years was 81% (130).

Shunt Failure   Shunt failure may present with irritability, confusion, lethargy, and headache unrelieved by position change. However, shunt failure may also present in a more fulminant manner than the original hydrocephalus, requiring prompt treatment (131). Proximal occlusion of the ventricular catheter is the most common source of blockage, usually accounting for at least 30% of cases of shunt dysfunction (131). Ventricular overdrainage may predispose to proximal occlusion by abutting the catheter tip against the ventricular wall (130). Distal shunt obstruction can be caused by encystment and loculation of the peritoneal contents around the distal catheter tip (72, 75). Abdominal pain, palpable pseudocyst, and ultrasound or abdominal CT may establish the diagnosis. Disconnections of shunt components have accounted for as much as 15% of shunt revisions and often are shown by a shunt series of plain radiographs (132).

Bedside palpation of the shunt sometimes gives a clue to shunt malfunction; excessive resistance to digital compression of the shunt chamber suggests possible distal occlusion, whereas inadequate refill suggests proximal occlusion. Unfortunately, palpation was neither sensitive nor reliable for determining shunt malfunction in a consecutive series of 200 patients (133). CT scans are helpful in demonstrating increase in ventricular size in many cases of shunt malfunction.

Definitive information about shunt blockage can be obtained by performing a shuntagram, where a needle is inserted into the safely perforable portion of the shunt, a pressure recording is done, and the progression of isotope or contrast is followed down the catheter and into the peritoneum (134, 135). With distal obstruction, pressure may be elevated with rapid ventricular filling but lack of distal flow. With proximal occlusion, the distal catheter fills, but pressure is low with slow disappearance of tracer and lack of ventricular filling (135).

Shunt Infection   Shunt infection has been described in 7–29% of cases. Most infections are acquired at the time of surgery, and 70% present within the first 2 months (136). Staphylococcus epidermidis is most common, accounting for approximately one-half of infections, followed by Staphylococcus aureus and gram-negative organisms (137). Presentation is typically insidious with low-grade fever, malaise, irritability, and nausea; meningeal irritation is usually not present (137, 138). Erythema over the shunt site, however, is a highly specific sign (136–138).

Diagnosis should be established by performing a shunt tap, not by doing a lumbar puncture. Tapping the shunt leads to accurate diagnosis in 95% of cases, whereas lumbar puncture is positive in only 7–26% of cases (136). Diagnosis is based on culture results, because CSF protein and glucose may be normal and cell count may not be much greater with shunt infection than with shunt alone.

Treatment needs to be individualized to the clinical situation, but in general, the highest overall response rate (96%) has been reported with shunt removal or externalization combined with antibiotics (136). Staph epidermidis is the most common organism causing shunt infection, and sometimes can be difficult to eradicate; intravenous vancomycin, intrathecal vancomycin or a regimen of both vancomycin and rifampin are sometimes used (139).

Seizures The prevalence of seizures after shunting has ranged from 5–48% (72), but in patients with posttraumatic hydrocephalus seizures may also result from the original TBI.

Overdrainage Overdrainage by shunts is a major clinical problem, causing acute and chronic clinical symptoms, and fostering both proximal shunt obstruction and development of postoperative subdural collections. It has been the driving force behind the development of antisiphon devices, programmable valves, and gravitational shunts. Intraventricular pressure normally becomes slightly subatmospheric when we stand. However, after placement of a shunt, orthostatic intraventricular pressure becomes markedly low (124), reflecting the additional negative hydrostatic pressure from the distal tubing (Figure 33-7). This may cause excessive siphoning of CSF and a low pressure syndrome of orthostatic headache, dizziness, nausea and vomiting, lethargy, and diplopia (131, 140–142).

Some patients with chronically overdraining shunts develop the slit-ventricle syndrome (131, 140, 141). Such patients develop severe nonpostural headaches in the face of persistently small ventricles. Slight increase in ventricular size at the time of clinical symptoms and sluggish shunt refill suggest intermittent proximal shunt malfunction with ventricular collapse against the catheter. Such symptoms develop an average of 4.5 years after shunting and are analogous to pseudotumor cerebri in the tendency toward elevated pressures with small stiff ventricles (140, 141).

Chronic Subdural Hematoma Chronic subdural hematomas and hygromas are recognized complications of shunting, occurring in 4.5–28% of patients, and are particularly likely when ventricles are extremely large preoperatively (72). Normally intracranial pulsatile flow and upright posture both shift CSF within the cranium and to the lumbar region, but CSF remains within the CSF compartment; however with shunting CSF exits to the peritoneum, and this can result in an underfilled CSF compartment (84, 118). Since the volume in the cranium is fixed, a loss of fluid in the ventricular compartment may result in creation of increased potential subdural space leading to development of subdural hygroma and hematoma (142, 143). Furthermore, with upright posture, low intraventricular pressures caused by standing are thought to predispose to tearing and leakage from bridging veins. The occurrence of subdural hematoma may require tying off the shunt or turning up the valve

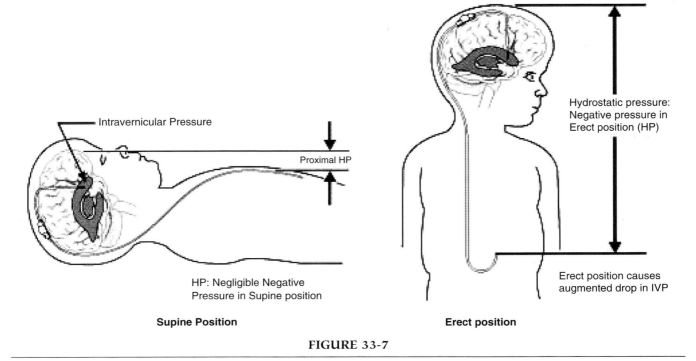

Supine Position — Intravernicular Pressure — Proximal HP — HP: Negligible Negative Pressure in Supine position

Erect position — Hydrostatic pressure: Negative pressure in Erect position (HP) — Erect position causes augmented drop in IVP

FIGURE 33-7

Positional changes in hydrostatic pressure

pressure setting if the patient has a programmable valve (72, 86, 143). Not all subdural collections are clinically significant; with MRI even very small fluid collections can be imaged (70). Post shunt meningeal fibrosis, with collagenous material in the subdural space, is distinguished from subdural fluid by its dramatic enhancement with gadolinium (70).

Antisiphon Devices, Programmable Valves, and Gravitational Valves

Antisiphon Devices Problems related to overdrainage have led to the development of several special shunt components. Antisiphon devices have been developed with diaphragms that close to counteract negative standing hydrostatic pressures (124, 144). Successful prevention of the dramatic negative standing intracranial pressure has been documented (145). A less useful device is the valve with an on/off occluder bubble following the flushing chamber. Originally designed in hopes of preventing subdural development by transient occlusion, it is not used frequently today. Fortunately palpation or radiographs can determine whether the occluder has inadvertently been compressed (124). Several newer valves have been designed to assist with CSF overdrainage. The Orbis-sigma valve is a flow regulated valve, with variable resistance with three stages of flow. It initially functions like a standard low pressure valve but shows increased resistance with larger flow rates; it also has a decreased resistance safety valve to deal with higher pressures. The delta valve is similar to an antisiphon device in combination with a standard valve, but has been engineered to minimize the area of the valve diaphragm responsive to pressure effects of fluid in the distal tubing. This design was intended to increase physiologic resistance to flow in the upright position selectively (146).

Programmable Valves A revolutionary development in shunting for hydrocephalus has been the development of programmable valves which can have their opening pressure changed at the bedside by use of an external magnet (83, 122, 147–153). The Codman Hakim and PS Medical Strata valves (see Figure 33-8) are available in the USA, and the Sophy valve is also available in Europe.

The opening pressure of the Codman Hakim valve can be adjusted in increments of 10 mm H_2O anywhere from 30 to 200, using a small bedside electromagnet. The Codman Hakim valve has a ruby ball and spring mechanism; the valve's spring tension is controlled by rotation of its spiral Cam with steps, which can in turn be adjusted by placing a small electromagnet over the shunt mechanism and dialing up the new pressure. When reprogramming the shunt, extreme care should be taken in precisely locating the active shunt mechanism by palpation, and carefully centering the electromagnetic programmer over it; otherwise the valve may program to a completely wrong setting. In cases where palpation is difficult, precise localization of the active shunt mechanism can be facilitated by a preliminary Xray with temporary placement of a radiopaque marker (beebee), which can then be removed prior to programming once the proper spot is identified. After programming the valve, one must confirm that the valve was correctly set by obtaining an Xray (see Figure 33-9); the setting can be difficult to see on Xray, and requires that the beam to pass first directly perpendicular to the shunt mechanism, then through the head, then to the Xray plate. A small dot on the right side of the device indicates proper orientation of film and placement of shunt (right hand rule); if it appears in the left, either the film was taken with the device against the Xray plate or the shunt is implanted upside down There is a procedure for programming an upside down shunt, and the reader is advised to check with the

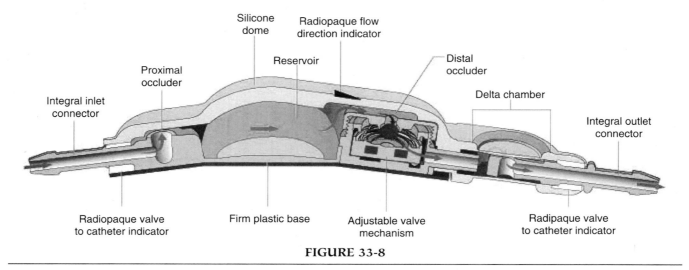

FIGURE 33-8

Medtronics PS Medical Strata (programmable) valve

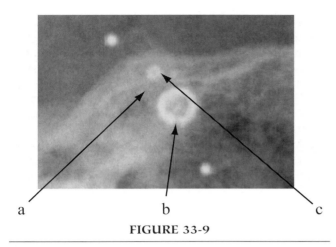

a   b   c

FIGURE 33-9

Xray of Codman Hakim Programmable Shunt mechanism.

 a. Points toward the location of the ruby ball and it's seat.
 b. Points to the notch in the circle, which is the cam rotor determining shunt pressure setting. Shunt setting is determined by the location of this notch.
 c. This is the right hand marker indicating film is done correctly for reading.

Note: the small circles at the top and bottom are small beebees used by examiner to help confirm location of active shunt mechanism.

manufacturer in this instance. The Xray appearance is then compared with the settings template to identify the setting.

Patients with programmable valves can have MRI scans, but must have an Xray to the check valve setting and may need reprogramming afterwards; valve settings were changed by MRI in 26.8 % of patients (147). Valve settings may also be changed by any very large magnets in the environment, and even by "filliping" of the shunt (abrupt manual manipulation such as flicking it with a finger)(154).

Valve pressure settings can be lowered for inadequate response to shunting, or raised for symptoms of overdrainage. Shunt settings should never be raised more than 30 mm at one time. Orthostatic headaches from overdrainage are particularly responsive to reprogramming of the valve, with headaches improving in 71% of patients (148). In some patients who develop subdural hematoma after shunting, surgical drainage of the subdural can be avoided by turning up the opening pressure of the valve(148). In two recent series reprogramming was performed in 41- 64% of patients with programmable valves at least once, and some had multiple adjustments (147-151). Based on the assumption that an adjustment of 50 mm or more would have warranted surgically changing the valve if it were not programmable, a cost benefit analysis of 541 programmable valves indicated

that the increased cost of the programmable valve was outweighed by the cost savings in avoiding additional surgeries (149). The possible benefit of reprogramming shunt valves during rehabilitation has only just begun to be explored. In one study of 114 patients, adjustments were deemed necessary in 13% of patients, and changes of 20–70 mm in steps correlated with significant functional improvement as scored on the Barthel index (151).

The PS Medical Strata valve has five settings which can be adjusted at bedside with magnetic tools. It has a ruby ball in cone with circular spring design, and includes an antisiphon component of the type found in the delta valve. Although is less flexible with regards to valve pressure settings (only 5 instead of 18 settings), the adjustment tools are easy to use, and the shunt setting can be confirmed at the bedside, making confirmatory Xray optional. One interesting aspect is that the relative positions of the Strata's delta chamber and the ventricular tip of the catheter can substantially effect the amount of antisiphon effect of the Strata system (83, 122, 153).

Gravitational Shunts Overdrainage of shunts has been particularly problematic because of the negative intraventricular pressures generated in the upright position by the column of fluid in the distal shunt tubing and the related siphon effects. In order to address this problem in a specific manner, gravitational shunts are designed with a higher opening pressure in the upright position than supine. The one used most extensively has been the Miethke Dual Switch Valve (113, 155–157). This is actually two valves in one, ingeniously designed so that the lower pressure valve opens in the supine position but is mechanically closed off by a ball in the vertical position, forcing flow through the higher pressure half of the valve when upright. A related invention is the Shunt Assistant valve (157, 158), essentially a gravitational antisiphon device which can be put in series with another valve, such as the Codman Hakim programmable valve. In the vertical position a tantalum sphere compresses a sealing ball to substantially increase the orthostatic opening pressure of the valve system specifically. At least 185 patients with normal pressure hydrocephalus have been carefully diagnosed and treated with either Meithke Dual switch valves or a combination of the Codman Hakim Programmable valves combined with the Shunt Assistant valve. Good or excellent outcome was described in 70% of patients and the incidence of overdrainage was only 4% (157). Of great interest, the patients with greatest favorable clinical response to shunting had minimal or no significant change in ventricular size post shunting (156, 157). It has been suggested that part of the reason for favorable outcome in this patient group may have been the avoidance of complications of overdrainage so commonly seen after implantation of more conventional shunt systems.

VASCULAR COMPLICATIONS

Traumatic Aneurysm

Intracranial Traumatic Aneurysms Traumatic intracranial aneurysms are rare; they comprise less than 1% of all intracranial aneurysms (159–161) and are more common after missile injuries than closed head injury. In missile injuries direct contact of missile or bone fragments with the artery is common, whereas in blunt injuries up to 40 % of case do not have associated fracture (161). Traumatic aneurysms can be classified as true, false, mixed, or dissecting types, but false aneurysms are the most common (162–164). In true aneurysms, the adventitial wall is preserved, whereas in false aneurysms all elements of the vascular wall are disrupted and blood is contained only by the surrounding arachnoid, hematoma, or brain parenchyma. Mixed aneurysms have a combination of true and false elements. In dissecting aneurysms, blood channels within the vessel wall, effectively narrowing or occluding the vessel itself.

Common clinical presentations of traumatic intracranial aneurysms include seizures, focal neurological deficits, altered consciousness, and severe persistent headache (159, 161). Traumatic intracranial aneurysms are highly unstable and prone to rupture (162, 163); in fact, although the time interval from injury to rupture varies from days to years, 90% bleed within 3 weeks of injury (160, 163). The most common locations for traumatic aneurysms are the distal middle cerebral branches, distal anterior cerebral artery, and proximal carotid and vertebral arteries (161). Traumatic petrous and cavernous carotid aneurysms are often associated with basilar skull fracture, while supraclinoid carotid aneurysms are sometimes associated with orbital or anterior clinoid process fractures (161). Epistaxis, pharyngeal mass, and delayed cranial nerve palsy have also been described with aneurysms near the skull base (161, 165), and traumatic aneurysms should be suspected in patients with delayed subarachnoid or intracerebral hemorrhage. Although angiography remains the definitive test for diagnosis, it is now recognized that the combination of Magnetic Resonance Angiography (MRA) with perfusion weighted Magnetic Resonance Imaging (MRI) can be a very useful screening tool, especially given the difficulty of clinically identifying patients with these aneurysms (161).

Treatment of traumatic intracranial aneurysms can be problematic since they are typically false aneurysms and therefore cannot be clipped (162–164). Because the parent vessel often must be sacrificed, extracranial to intracranial distal revascularization procedures are sometimes performed at the time of definitive treatment (161).

Recently developed endovascular approaches have often been useful, including detachable balloons, detachable coils to the occlude the parent vessel, or stents to exclude the aneurysm from the circulation while maintaining the patency of the parent vessel (161).

Cervical Arterial Trauma Including Dissection Traumatic injury to the cervical internal carotid or vertebral arteries may be seen after penetrating injuries, or after hyperextension and flexion neck injuries, as in motor vehicle accidents; many patients with blunt injuries show little or no overt external neck trauma (161). The incidence of injury to the carotid artery in patients with TBI has been estimated at 0.5% (161). When carotid injury occurs, mortality is estimated at 20–40% and neurologic deficits are seen in 80% of survivors. Presentation is typically that of infarction in the distribution of the involved vessel, either secondary to thrombosis, embolism or dissection. For example, after carotid artery trauma hemiparesis and hemisensory loss occur, but onset of these symptoms exceeds 10 hours from initial injury in half of cases, and is sometimes delayed for up to 48 hours (161). Acute headache can be a very important clue to the early diagnosis of arterial dissection, occurring in 60% of cases of carotid dissection, and slightly less often with vertebral artery dissection, where the headache tends to be occipital (166). Other important clues to possible cervical carotid injury include mandibular fracture, neck pain, pulsatile tinnitus, visual changes, lower cranial nerve palsies, and ipsilateral Horner's syndrome(161). Revascularization or direct repair is sometimes attempted for carotid dissection, but only if it can be done within 4 hours of onset in a conscious patient(162). Otherwise management is medical, with consideration of antiplatelet or anticoagulation therapy depending on clinical course and associated injuries. Anticoagulation with heparin or coumadin has been the traditional management when not contraindicated, but lacks a strong evidence base (166).

Carotid Cavernous Fistula

Types and Presentation Traumatic carotid cavernous fistulas are typically direct fistulas from the internal carotid artery. Classified as type A, with fast flow and high pressure, they contrast with spontaneous carotid cavernous fistulas (types B, C, and D), which have low pressure and slow flow and typically receive dural blood supply (167, 168). The cavernous sinus is anatomically unique in that a large artery passes through a large venous space; for this reason a tear in the arterial wall alone can create an arteriovenous fistula without any additional venous anomaly (169). Visual impairment is a major presenting symptom and concern for further visual loss is a frequent management concern in patients with carotid cavernous fistula. Additional presenting signs of carotid cavernous fistula include supraorbital bruit, exophthalmus, orbital congestion, oculomotor palsies, and trigeminal nerve involvement (167, 170, 171). Pulsatile exophthalmus is seen in carotid cavernous fistula but also has been described in a patient with orbital encephalocele and hydrocephalus (172). Pulsatile tinnitus may result from arteriovenous fistulas and malformations or from altered jugular venous flow (173–177). Onset of carotid cavernous fistula is often delayed; 43.5% are diagnosed over 1 month after trauma(170). Angiography is the definitive diagnostic test.

Treatment Spontaneous closure of a carotid cavernous fistula has been described in some patients; it is much more likely with a spontaneous low-flow fistula than with the traumatic high-flow fistula. Patients have been trained in intermittent manual compression of the cervical carotid artery with the contralateral hand. Although the success rate is lower with direct fistulas, 17% of patients had successful closure with this technique (178). The definitive treatment of traumatic carotid cavernous fistula has become the endovascular placement of detachable balloons(168, 179, 180). Successful fistula closure was accomplished by the detachable balloon technique in 92 of 95 cases of traumatic carotid cavernous fistula, with preservation of the internal carotid artery in over 70% of cases (168).

LATE INTRACRANIAL MASS LESIONS

Subdural Hematoma and Hygroma

Differences Between Acute and Chronic Subdural Hematoma Subdural hematoma is the most common late-presenting mass lesion. Although acute, subacute (3–20 days), and chronic (3 weeks or more) subdural hematomas are distinguished by time of detection after injury, it is important to recognize that chronic subdural hematoma is a different pathophysiologic process than acute subdural hematoma, not simply an older blood clot (181–185). As a result, differences are also seen in the epidemiology, clinical presentation, prognosis, and treatment techniques (73, 182, 184) (Table 33-3). The incidence of chronic subdural hematoma peaks in the seventh and eighth decades, and only 60–65% of patients have known TBI (184, 186) Male predominance (70–90%) and parietal location (91%) are characteristic(181, 184). Headaches are a cardinal symptom (184, 187), sometimes following a symptom-free interval. Three major clinical presentations include hemiparesis (40%), personality or intellectual change (30%), and signs of increased intracranial pressure, including papilledema (20%)(181). In contrast with acute subdural hematoma, seizures are relatively uncommon with chronic subdural hematoma (4–7%), and ongoing anticonvulsant prophylaxis is not routinely required (188), although some authorities have recommended it in the immediate postoperative period(187). Transient episodes of aphasia or sensorimotor disturbance have also been described with chronic subdural hematomas, mimicking either transient ischemic attacks or seizures, and resolving after the immediate postoperative period following surgical drainage (189, 190).

Scan Findings in Subdural Hematoma CT scans characteristically show decreased density in chronic subdural hematoma. However, the isodense appearance characteristic of subacute subdural hematoma may last longer than 1 month in some instances (191). In questionable cases, contrast enhancement helps to identify isodense subdural collections(192). In other cases, a layer of isodensity or increased density is seen below a hypodense layer; this sedimentation level likely reflects interval rebleeding (192, 193). Isodensity at the medial margin

TABLE 33-3
Differences Between Acute and Chronic Subdural Hematoma

FEATURE	ACUTE SUBDURAL HEMATOMA	CHRONIC SUBDURAL HEMATOMA
Age Peak	30–49 years	60–70 years
Known TBI	Virtually all	60–65%
Clinical Presentation	Acute mental status change, focal signs, seizures, increased intracranial pressure	Personality or chronic mental status change, headache, hemiparesis, increased intracranial pressure
Composition	Blood clot	Fluid, membrane
Pathophysiology	Venous bleeding especially from torn bridging veins	Initial subdural hygroma or initial venous bleeding, inflammatory process with leaky macrocapillaries, disordered hemostatic mechanism
Treatment	Craniotomy	Burr holes, twist drill craniostomy, or craniotomy

of a fluid collection also may represent fresher bleeding (192). Compared with CT scan density, the factors determining signal intensity on MRI are much more complex. Whereas acute subdural hematoma shows increased CT density, subacute and chronic subdural hematoma have increased signal on MRI (29, 187, 194). Subacute subdural hematoma is seen as a hyperintense collection on T1-weighted images, largely because of the presence of methemoglobin. Chronic subdural hematoma presents with more variable signal intensity on T1-weighted images but consistently shows increased signal intensity on T2-weighted images (29, 187, 194). In addition, fluid collections that are homogeneous on CT sometimes show hypointense septations and mixed intensities on MRI. In some instances, a sedimentation level of a hyperintense (fluid) upper layer and hypointense (more cellular) lower layer is seen. Such findings are consistent with the conceptualization of subdural hematoma as an ongoing process with interval rebleeding rather than a static collection of blood. As described below, an outer membrane is characteristic in chronic subdural collections; this membrane enhances significantly with gadolinium on T1-weighted imaging in many cases (29). Although CT and MRI are the definitive tests for diagnosing subdural collections, abnormalities also are seen in the electroencephalogram (EEG) and in testing of cerebral blood flow. In addition to delta slowing on the side of a subdural collection, ipsilateral suppression of voltage is seen on EEG in 25% of patients(184, 186). Diffuse reductions in cerebral blood flow preoperatively often show a recovery 1 month postoperatively (195).

Pathology of Chronic Subdural Hematoma   On pathologic examination, the fluid of chronic subdural hematoma shows a range of color and appearance, including brown-black, dark red, amber-brown, and almost clear and watery (184, 194). Coagulated masses of blood and fibrin are sometimes present. A thicker outer membrane attached to the dura and thinner inner membrane bordering on the arachnoid are characteristic (184). Enlarged ectatic capillaries, often called giant capillaries or sinusoids, are prominent on the outer membrane and associated with inflammatory cells, fibroblasts, and hemosiderin-laden macrophages (184). With age, the outer membrane also may become calcified.

Subdural Hygroma   Subdural hygroma has been described as a subdural collection of cerebrospinal fluid, often with a modified composition (196). The distinction between subdural hygroma and chronic subdural hematoma has often been unclear in the literature, partly because subdural fluid composition varies, sometimes exhibiting xanthochromia or containing blood products. Also the term hygroma has sometimes been used to describe low density extraaxial collections on CT scan without mass effect (196), even when identification of cortical veins lateral to the collection on MRI might more correctly identify it as subarachnoid fluid associated with atrophy (29). It has been proposed that a tear in the arachnoid may acutely allow CSF into the subdural space, and rare surgical documentation of this process has been provided (196). More often the development of subdural hygroma may be more gradual, and in these cases subdural hygroma formation requires separation of the dura-arachnoid interface and sufficient potential subdural space (143, 197–199). Low intracranial pressure (such as orthostatic negative pressures with a shunt), an underfilled CSF compartment, and atrophy are factors in creating sufficient subdural space (84, 118, 142, 143). Many patients have slight cranial asymmetry in the occipital region, with one side flatter than the other. In the supine position the cranium tends to turn slightly to the flattened side, and subdural hygromas tend to form frontally to the opposite side, or bilaterally in patients with a more symmetrical cranium (143, 197). The time course of hygroma development, enlargement, and in most instances resolution can be plotted.

Pathophysiology of Chronic Subdural Hematoma   Recent work has significantly clarified our understanding of the relationship beteen subdural hygroma and chronic subdural hematoma, and the pathophysiology of their development. Chronic subdural hematomas occasionally develop from acute subdural hematomas, but more often chronic subdural hematomas develop from subdural hygromas (143). When hygromas do not resolve, a neomembrane forms from dural border cells, followed by leakage of blood from the fragile giant capillaries in the outer membrane induced by the inflammatory process (182, 200, 201). A disordered local hemostatic mechanism has been identified in fluid from chronic subdural hematoma (182, 183) with both excessive activation of the clotting system and the fibrinolytic system. Chronic subdural collections can sometimes show increasing density on CT scans for a period of weeks to months (143). The size of a chronic subdural collection may resolve spontaneously if absorption exceeds rebleeding, or alternatively the collection may continue to enlarge (143).

Approach to Chronic Subdural Hygroma or Hematoma Management   Management of the patient with chronic subdural hygroma or chronic subdural hematoma is largely a matter of clinical judgement. Decreasing size of the collection, stability of the neurologic exam, and a lack of mass effect or compression on the underlying brain on CT or MRI scan are all factors which mitigate in favor of observation and serial scanning. While there is no set time interval for repeat scanning, in the absence of clinical worsening and depending somewhat on the size and appearance of the collection, a period of 2 to 4 weeks can often be utilized. Alternatively, clinical worsening, the appearance of significant mass effect or midline shift on CT or MRI scan, or serial enlargement or substantial increase in CT density consistent with significant interval rebleeding would likely necessitate a surgical approach. It has often been the author's practice to obtain neurosurgical input early on, even when the immediate management is almost certainly conservative, so that a neurosurgical plan is in place and can be enacted quickly if circumstances warrant shifting to a more aggressive approach.

Surgery for Chronic Subdural Hematoma Surgical removal of a certain critical mass of fluid, containing degradation products from the subdural space may be important in interrupting the vicious cycle of disordered hemostasis and facilitating the recovery from chronic subdural hematoma (182, 183). Successful surgery, therefore, may reduce the residual volume to a degree that allows further resorption rather than fully removing the blood clot. Twist drill trephination or burr holes are the first line treatments for chronic subdural hematoma (181, 184, 202–204). Occasionally the presence of sizable clots or loculation may necessitate craniotomy, as is commonly done for acute subdural hematoma (182, 205). Postoperative drainage has been advocated to assist with brain reexpansion (182, 202). The hematoma cavity is commonly washed out with saline, and it has been suggested that continuous irrigation (to remove coagulation degradation products) may decrease the duration of drainage or frequency of recurrence(206, 207). Persisting subdural fluid was described postoperatively in 78% of patients, but had returned to normal by 40 days postoperatively in 27 of 32 cases, leading to the suggestion that reoperation should be avoided until at least 3 weeks postoperatively unless marked clinical deterioration occurs (208). Because of the active inflammation in the dural border cell layer and associated inflammatory cytokine production, postoperative anti-inflammatory medication/steroids have been suggested by some (182, 204). The overall prognosis from chronic subdural hematoma is much more favorable than the prognosis for acute subdural hematoma (184), although the residual deficits in the areas of personality and memory may be problematic (207). Patients with even severe neurologic deficits preoperatively may have successful outcomes (181), although the extent of preoperative deficit has been a useful predictor of outcome in some series(207).

Epidural Hematoma

Presentation Although epidural hematoma is usually considered the most acute posttraumatic mass lesion, it presents more than 5 days after injury in 10% of cases (209) and may present as late as the second or third week after injury (210). Although epidural hematoma most often presents in the temporal fossa (57–83% of cases) due to injury to the middle meningeal artery, delayed presentation is more common with extratemporal location, especially frontal or posterior fossa lesions (209, 211). Clouding or decreased level of consciousness is considered the most important sign of epidural hematoma (209). Onset is slowest with frontal lesions, and symptoms may be vague. Unilateral exophthalmus is an unusual sign that has been described with subfrontal epidural hematoma (211).

Posterior Fossa Epidural Hematoma Posterior fossa epidural hematomas are unique among epidural hematomas in that they are of venous rather than arterial origin. An occipital bone fracture is seen in 84.2% of cases and characteristically crosses the venous sinus, causing this venous bleeding (212). The venous origin helps explain why a slower clinical presentation may occur. A lucid interval is common, and progressive decrease in the level of consciousness is characteristic. Battle's sign is often seen, and neck stiffness, occipital headache, and vomiting may be prominent. Symptoms and signs of increased intracranial pressure as well as brainstem, cranial nerve, and cerebellar dysfunction are common (212, 213). Posterior fossa epidurals are not common; they are seen in only 0.3% of patients with TBI (212). However, they have the highest mortality rate (209) and are notoriously difficult to diagnose (211).

Intracerebral Hemorrhage

Delayed traumatic intracerebral hemorrhage is defined as an intracerebral hematoma that is not visualized on initial CT but is seen on a follow-up study. It occurs in 5.6–7.4% of patients with severe TBI (214). Time of onset is typically about 24 hours after original injury (214), and 80% of cases occur within 48 hours of injury (187). Cardinal signs of delayed traumatic intracerebral hemorrhage include decreased level of consciousness, focal signs, or seizures (215). Factors postulated to play a role in the pathogenesis include dysregulation of blood flow, coagulation disorders, and removal of tamponade effect by evacuation of another mass lesion, such as an epidural or subdural hematoma. Outcome is worse with temporal lobe location, which shows an increased incidence of herniation (216).

SUMMARY AND FUTURE DIRECTIONS

Risks and Infections

Risks Conditions associated with increased risk of infection have been discussed including skull fractures and penetrating injuries, and cerebrospinal fluid (CSF) fistula. With the exception of penetrating wounds, where antibiotic prophylaxis is almost universal, the approach to prophylaxis remains controversial. A large well controlled study would be helpful to resolve the indications for antibiotic prophylaxis. It appears that the ongoing presence of a fistulous connection between the atmosphere or sinuses and the intracranial compartment (through the skull and dura) implies a very substantial risk for development of meningitis, even in the absence of overt CSF drainage, and sometimes even years after injury. Therefore an aggressive approach to identification and closure of a CSF fistula is warranted. Glucose testing is not reliable in suspected CSF rhinorrhea, but assessment of beta-2 transferrin assay is reliable.

Cranioplasty was often delayed in the past partly because of concerns of complications including infection if performed early. However it has recently become clear that some patients with craniectomy exhibit the syndrome of the trephined with a markedly ingoing flap in the area of missing bone. These patients not only tolerate having cranioplasty performed earlier, but sometimes actually show significant neurologic improvement after cranioplasty is performed.

Infections Meningitis typically pursues a fulminant course. The exception is infection of a ventriculoperitoneal shunt, which tends to pursue a very indolent course without overt signs of acute infection. Shunt infection can only reliably be diagnosed by tapping the shunt, not by lumbar puncture, and Staphylococcus epidermitis is the most common organism and in this setting is usually real rather than a contaminent.

Subdural empyema and brain abscess are rare complications of TBI except with compound depressed skull fracture, CSF fistula or penetrating wounds. Subdural empyema typically presents with acute signs of infection, while brain abscess often presents as a mass lesion without evidence of acute infection. Lumbar puncture is contraindicated for both, while newer imaging modalities such as diffusion weighted MRI are proving useful in establishing the diagnosis in some cases.

Hydrocephalus

Diagnosis Ventriculomegaly is common after severe TBI, but it remains difficult to distinguish dynamic hydrocephalus from ex-vacuo ventricular dilatation. Both the CSF tap test and lumbar infusion studies, possibly combined with SPECT studies, appear to have utility in sorting difficult cases. Further research on CSF drainage trials and lumbar infusion testing in TBI patients with possible hydrocephalus would be valuable, and might spur increased routine use of these studies.

Shunts The mechanisms, complications and innovations in shunt technology have been reviewed at length. Programmable shunts may offer significant promise specifically for the patient with post-traumatic hydrocephalus, given the frequency of communicating hydrocephalus without high pressure, difficulty in predicting appropriate pressure settings, and uncertain magnitude of clinical response. However further research demonstrating proven superiority over standard shunts in this population is still needed, especially as use of these shunts is complex and can be labor intensive on the part of the physicians managing them. Overdrainage has been a major complication with ventriculoperitoneal shunts, and the recent development of shunt systems which effectively drain at a higher opening pressure standing than supine could be a major advance.

Late vascular and mass lesions

Vascular Complications Traumatic intracranial aneurysms are uncommon, but are often false aneurysms and extremely prone to rupture. Clinical features to aid diagnosis are discussed, and MRA and perfusion weighted MRI may be helpful for screening. Endovascular approaches including coils and stents have recently changed management considerably. Carotid cavernous fistula is the most common post-traumatic arteriovenous malformation, and often presents with visual symptoms along with localizing signs of cavernous sinus involvement. Endovascular approaches with balloons have proven effective. Trauma to the cervical carotid and vertebral arteries can induce thrombosis or dissection. Presentation with severe head and neck pain can be a diagnostic clue prior to development of cerebral infarction, and anticoagulation is often utilized.

Late Mass Lesions Subdural hygroma and chronic subdural hematoma are frequently encountered, whereas delayed epidural and intracerebral hematomas are less commonly seen. Posterior fossa epidural hematoma is of venous origin, typically in association with occipital fracture, and a rare but serious complication. Chronic subdural hematoma is a clinically distinct entity from acute subdural hematoma, both in terms of epidemiology and management. It now appears that many chronic subdural hematomas develop from a subdural hygroma. The approach to management of chronic subdural collections is discussed at length.

References

1. Cooper PR. Skull fracture and traumatic cerebrospinal fluid fistulas. In Cooper PR (ed). *Head Injury*, 3rd ed. Baltimore, Williams & Wilkins, 1993, pp 115–136.
2. Dunn LT, Foy PM. Anticonvulsant and antibiotic prophylaxis in head injury. *Ann R Coll Surg Engl* 1994;76(3):147–9.
3. Al-Haddad SA, Kirollos R. A 5-year study of the outcome of surgically treated depressed skull fractures. *Ann R Coll Surg Engl* 2002;84(3):196–200.

4. Ali B, Ghosh A. Antibiotics in compound depressed skull fractures. *Emerg Med J* 2002;19(6):552–3.

5. Mendelow AD, Campbell D, Tsementzis SA, Cowie RA, Harris P, Durie TB, Gillingham FJ. Prophylactic antimicrobial management of compound depressed skull fracture. *J R Coll Surg Edinb* 1983;28(2):80–3.

6. Roy R, Cooper PR. Penetrating injuries of the skull and brain. In Braakman R (ed). *Handbook of Clinical Neurology*, Amsterdam, Elsevier. 1990;13:299–315.

7. Kaufman HH. The acute care of patients with gunshot wounds to the head. *Neurotrauma Med Rep* 1990;4:1–2.

8. Laun A. Traumatic cerebrospinal fluid fistulas in the anterior and middle cranial fossae. *Acta Neurochir* 1982;60:215–222.

9. Villalobos T, Arango C, Kubilis P, Rathore M. Antibiotic prophylaxis after basilar skull fractures:a meta-analysis. *Clin Infect Dis* 1998;27(2):364–9.

10. MacGee E. Cerebrospinal fluid fistula. In Vinken PJ, Bruyn GW (eds). *The Handbook of Clinical Neurology*, Amsterdam, Elsevier. 1976;24(183–199).

11. Frederiks JAM:Post-traumatic CSF hypotension. In Vinken PJ, Bruyn GW (eds). *Handbook of Clinical Neurology*, New York, Elsevier. 1976;24:255–259.

12. Cusimano MD, Sekhar LN. Pseudo-cerebrospinal fluid rhinorrhea. *J Neurosurg* 1994;8:26–30.

13. Wakhloo AK, VanVelthoven V, Schumacher M, et al. Evaluation of MR imaging, digital subtraction cisternography, and CT cisternography in diagnosing CSF fistula. *Acta Neurochir* 1991; 111:119–127.

14. Ryall RG, Peacock MK, Simpson DA Usefulness of beta-2 transferrin assay in the detection of cerebrospinal fluid leaks following head injury*J Neurosurg* 1992;77(5):737–9.

15. Zaret DL, Morrison N, Gulbranson R, et al. Immunofixation to quantity B2-transferrin cerebrospinal fluid to detect leakage of cerebrospinal fluid from skull injury. *Clin Chem* 1992;38: 1909–1912.

16. Miller JD:Infection after head injury. In Vinken PJ, Bruyn GW (eds): *Handbook of Clinical Neurology*, Amsterdam, Elsevier 1976;24:215–230.

17. Schlosser RJ, Bolger WE. Nasal Cerebrospinal Fluid Leaks. *J Otolaryngol* 2002;31(Supp1):S28–S37.

18. Swift AC, Foy P. Advances in the management of CSF rhinorrhea. *Hosp Med* 2002;63(1):28–32.

19. Mosely JI, Curtin CA, Stern WE. Spectrum of complications in the use of intrathecal fluorescein. *J Neurosurg* 1978;48:765–7.

20. Tunkel AR, Scheld WM. Acute infectious complications of head trauma. In Braakman R (ed). *Handbook of Clinical Neurology*, Amsterdam, Elsevier 1990;13:317–326.

21. Shapiro SA, Scully T:Closed continuous drainage of cerebrospinal fluid via a lumbar subarachnoid catheter for treatment or prevention of cranial spinal cerebrospinal fluid fistula. *Neurosurgery* 1992;30:241–245.

22. Probst CH. Neurosurgical treatment of traumatic frontobasal CSF fistulae in 300 patients (1967–1989). *Acta Neurochir* 1990; 106:37–47.

23. Okada J, Tsuda T, Takasugi S, et al. Unusually late onset of cerebro-spinal fluid rhinorrhea after head trauma. *Surg Neurol* 1991; 35:213–217.

24. Sindou M, Guyotat-Pelissou I, Chidiac A, et al. Transcutaneous pressure adjustable valve for the treatment of hydrocephalus and arachnoid cysts in adults. *Acta Neurochir* 1993;121:135–139.

25. Salca HC, Danaila L. Onset of uncomplicated cerebrospinal fluid fistula 27 years after head injury:case report. *Surg Neurol* 1997; 47(2):132–3.

26. McCormack B, Cooper PR, Perksy M, et al. Extracranial repair of cerebrospinal fluid fistulas:Technique and results in 37 patients. *Neurosurgery*1990;27:412–417.

27. Brodie HA. Prophylactic antibiotics for Posttraumatic Cerebrospinal Fluid Fistula. *Arch Otolaryngol Head Neck Surg* 1997; 123:749–52.

28. Friedman JA, Ebersold MJ, Quast LM. Post-Traumatic Cerebrospinal Fluid Leakage. *World J Surg* 2001;25:1062–6.

29. Gean AD. *Imaging of Head Trauma*. Raven Press, NY 1994 pp. 56, 577.

30. Jennett B, Teasdale G *Management of Head Injuries* F.A.Davis, Phila 1982;p. 203.

31. Markham JW. Pneumocephalus. In Vinken PJ, Bruyn GW (eds). *Handbook of Clinical Neurology*, New York, Elsevier, 1976;24: 201–213.

32. Zasler ND. Posttraumatic Tension Pneumocephalus. *J Head Trauma Rehabil* 1999;14(1):81–4.

33. Hand WL, Sanford JP. Posttraumatic bacterial meningitis. *Ann Intern Med* 1970;72:869–874.

34. Anderson M. Management of cerebral infection. *J.Neurol Neurosurg Psychiatry* 1993;56:1243–1258.

35. Chowdhury MH, Tunkel AR. Antibacterial Agents in Infections of the Central Nervous System. *Infect Dis Clin NA* 2000;14(2): 391–408.

36. Kearney BP, Aweeka FT. The Penetration of Anti-infectives into the central nervous system. *Neurologic Clinics* 1999;17(4): 883–900.

37. Hasbun R, Aronin SI, Quagliarello VJ. Treatment of Bacterial Meningitis. *Comp Ther* 1999;25(2):73–81.

38. Luer MS, Hatton J. Vancomycin administration into the cerebrospinal fluid:a review. *Ann Pharmacother* 1993;27(7–8): 912–21.

39. Nathoo N, Nadvi SS, Van Dellen JR. Traumatic cranial empyemas:a review of 55 patients. *Br J Neurosurg* 2000;14(4):326–30.

40. Bok APL, Peter JC. Subdural empyema:Burrholes or craniectomy? *J Neurosurg* 1993;78:574–578.

41. Weisberg L. Subdural empyema. *Arch Neurol* 1986;43: 497–500.

42. Feverman T, Wackym PA, Gade GF, et al. Craniotomy improves outcomes in subdural empyema. Surg Neurol 1989;32:105–110.

43. Pathak A, Sharma BS, Mathuriya SN, et al. Controversies in the management of subdural empyema. *Acta Neurochir* (Wien) 1990; 102:25–32.

44. Clark CW, Muhlbauer MS, Lowrey R, et al. Complications of intracranial pressure monitoring in trauma patients. *Neurosurgery* 1989;25:20–24.

45. Malavi A, Dinubile MJ. Brain abscess. In Harris AA (ed). *Handbook of Clinical Neurology*. Amsterdam, Elsevier 1988; 8: 143–166.

46. Patir R, Sood S, Bhatia R. Post-traumatic brain abscess:experience of 36 patients. *Br J Neurosurgery* 1995;9:29–35.

47. Yang S, Zhao C:Review of 140 patients with brain abscess. *Surg Neurol* 199339:290–296.

48. Guzman R, Barth A, Lovblad KO, El-Koussy M, Weis J, Schroth G, Seiler R. Use of diffusion weighted magnetic resonance imaging in differentiating purulent brain processes from cystic brain tumors *J Neurosurg* 2002 97:1101–1107.

49. Miller ES, Dias PS, Uttley D, et al:CT scanning in the management of intracranial abscess:A review of 100 cases. *Br J Neurosurg* 19882:439–446.

50. Stapleton SR, Bell BA, Uttley D, et al. Sterotactic aspiration of brain abscesses:Is this the treatment of choice. *Acta Neurochir* (Wien) 1993;121:15–19.

51. Rish BL, Dillon JD, Meirowksy AM, et al. Cranioplasty:A review of 1030 cases of penetrating head injury. *Neurosurgery* 1979; 4:381–385.

52. Bullitt E, Lehman RAW. Osteomyelitis of the skull. *Surg Neurol* 1979;11:163–166.

53. Dujovny M, Agner C, Aviles A. Syndrome of the trephined:theory and facts. *Crit. Rev. Neurosurg* 1999;9(5):271–278.

54. Muramatsu H, Nathan RD, Shimura T, Teramoto A. Recovery of stroke hemiplegia through neurosurgical intervention in the chronic stage. *Neurorehabilitation* 2000;15(3):157–66.

55. Gottlob I, Simonsz-Toth B, Heilbronner R. Midbrain syndrome with eye movement disorder:dramatic improvement after cranioplasty. *Strabismus* 2002;10(4):271–7.

56. Czosnyka M, Copeman J, Czosnyka Z, McConnell R, Dickinson C, Pickard JD. Post-traumatic hydrocephalus:influence of craniectomy on the CSF circulation. *J Neurol Neurosurg Psychiatry* 2000; 68:246–7.

57. Nagayama K, Yoshikawa G, Somekawa K, Kohno M, Segawa H, Sano K, Shiokawa Y, Saito I. Cranioplasty using the patient's autogenous bone preserved by freezing - an examination of post operative infection rates *No shinkei Geka* 2002;30(2):165–9.

58. Flannery T, McConnell RS. Cranioplasty:why throw the bone flap out? *Br J Neurosurg* 2001;15(6):518–20.

59. Ducic Y. Titanium Mesh and hydroxyapetite cement cranioplasty: a report of 20 cases. *Oral maxillofacial Surg* 2002;60(3): 272–6.

60. Moreira-Gonzalez, Jackson IT, Miyawaki T, Barakat K. Clinical Outcome in cranioplasty:critical review in long term follow up. *J Craniofac Surg* 2003;14(2):144–53.

61. Agner C, Dujovny M, Park H. Delayed Minimally Invasive cranioplasty. *Minimally Invasive Neurosurg* 2003;46(3):186–90.

62. Liao C, Kao M. Cranioplasty for patients with severe depressed skull bone defect after cerebrospinal fluid shunting. *J Clin Neurosci* 2002;9(5):553.

63. Cope DN, Date ES, Mar EY. Serial computerized tomographic evaluations in traumatic head injury. *Arch Phys Med Rehabil* 1988;69:483–486.

64. Mazzini L, Campini R, Angelino E, Rognone F, Pastore I, Oliveri G. Posttraumatic Hydrocephalus:A Clinical, Neuroradiologic, and Neuropsychologic Assessment of long-term outcome. *Arch Phys Med Rehabil* 2003;84:1637–41.

65. Long D. Issues in behavioral neurology and brain injury. In Ellis DW, Christensen AL (eds). *Neuropsychological treatment after brain injury*. Boston, Kluwer, 1989, pp 39–90.

66. Milborat TH:*Pediatric Neurosurgery*. Philadelphia, F.A. Davis, 1978;pp91–135.

67. Salmon JH:Surgical treatment of severe posttraumatic encephalopathy. *Surg Gynecol Obstet* 1971;133:634–636.

68. Lundar T, Nornes H. Determination of ventricular fluid outflow resistance in patients with ventriculomegaly. *J Neurol Neurosurg Psychiatry* 1990;63:896–898.

69. Nishiyama K, Mori H, Tanaka R. Changes in cerebrospinal fluid hydrodynamics following endoscopic third ventriculostomy for shunt–dependent noncommunicating hydrocephalus. *J Neurosurg* 2003;98(5):1027–31.

70. Barkovich AJ, Edwards MSB. Applications of neuroimaging in hydrocephalus. *Pediatr Neurosurg* 1992;18:65–83.

71. Boyar B, Ildan F, Begdatoglv H, et al. Unilateral hydrocephalus resulting from occlusion of foramen of Monro:A new procedure in the treatment: Stereotactic fenestration of the septum pellucidum. *Surg Neurol* 1993;39:110–114.

72. Scott RM. The Treatment and prevention of shunt complications. In Scott RM (ed): *Hydrocephalus*. Baltimore, Williams & Wilkins, 1990, pp 115–122.

73. Seelig GM, Becker DP, Miller JD, et al. Traumatic acute subdural hematoma. *N Engl J Med* 1981;304:1511–1518.

74. Nida TY, Haines SJ. Multiloculated hydrocephalus:Craniotomy and fenestration of intraventricular septations.*J Neurosurg* 1993; 781:70–76.

75. Epstein F:How to keep shunts functioning or "the impossible dream." *Clin Neurosurg* 1985;32:608–631.

76. Nowoslawska E, Polis L, Kaniewska D, Mikolajczyk W, Krawczyk J, Szymanski W, Zakrewski K, Podciechowska J. Effectiveness of neuroendoscopic procedures in the treatment of complex compartmentalized hydrocephalus in children. *Child's Nerv Syst* 2003;19(9):659–65.

77. Zander E, Foroglou G:Posttraumatic hydrocephalus. In Vinken PJ, Bruyn GW (eds). *Handbook of Clinical Neurology*. New York, Elsevier 1976;24:231–253.

78. Friedland RP. "Normal"-pressure hydrocephalus and the saga of the treatable dementias. *JAMA* 1989;262:2577–2581.

79. Conner ES, Foley L, Black PM. Experimental normal-pressure hydrocephalus is accompanied by increased transmantle pressure. *J Neurosurg* 1984;61:322–327.

80. Hakim CA, Hakim R, Hakim S. Normal-pressure hydrocephalus. *Neurosurg Clin NA* 2001;12(4):761–73.

81. Momjian S, Owler BK, Czosnyka Z, Czosnyka M, Pena A, Pickard JD. Pattern of white matter regional cerebral blood flow and autoregulation in normal pressure hydrocephalus. *Brain* 2004;127(Pt 5):965–72.

82. Del Bigio MR. Pathophysiologic Consequences of Hydrocephalus. *Neurosurg Clin NA* 2001;12(4):639–660.

83. Scott RM, Madsen JR. Shunt technology:Contemporary Concepts and Prospects. *Clin Neurosurg* 2002;5 (14):256–267.

84. Bergsneider M. Evolving Concepts of Cerebrospinal Fluid Physiology. *Neurosurg Clin NA* 2001;12(4):631–638.

85. Greitz D. Radiological assessment of hydrocephalus:new theories and implications for therapy. *Neurosurg Rev* 2004;27(3): 145–65.

86. Black PM. The normal pressure hydrocephalus syndrome. In Scott RM (ed). *Hydrocephalus*. Baltimore, Williams & Wilkins, 1990, pp. 109–144.

87. Sudarsky L, Simon S. Gait disorder in late life hydrocephalus. *Arch Neurol* 1987;44:263–267.

88. Keane JR:The pretectal syndrome:206 patients. *Neurology* 1990; 40:684–690.

89. Pakkenberg B;Boesen J;Albeck M;Gjerris F. Unbiased and efficient estimation of total ventricular volume of the brain obtained from CT-scans by a stereological method. *Neuroradiology* 1989; 31(5):413–7.

90. Hamano K;Iwasaki N;Takeya T;Takita H. A comparative study of linear measurement of the brain and three-dimensional measurement of brain volume using CT scans. *Pediatr Radiol* 1993; 23(3):165–8.

91. O'Hayon BB, Drake JM, Ossip MG, Tuli S, Clarke M. Frontal and Occipital Horn Ratio:A Linear Estimate of Ventricular Size for Multiple Imaging Modalities in Pediatric Hydrocephalus. *Pediatr Neurosurg* 1998;29:245–9.

92. Mesawala AH, Avellino AM, Ellenbogen RG. The Diagonal Ventricular Dimension:A Method for Predicting Shunt Malfunction on the basis of Changes in Ventricular Size. *Neurosurgery* 2002; 50:1246–1252.

93. Jamous M, Sood S, Kumar R, Ham S. Frontal and occipital horn width ratio for the evaluation of small and asymmetrical ventricles. *Pediatr Neurosurg* 2003;39(1):17–21.

94. Borgensen SE, Gjerris F. The predictive value of conductance to outflow of CSF in normal pressure hydrocephalus. *Brain* 1982; 105:65–86.

95. Levin HS, Meyers CA, Grossman RG, et al. Ventricular enlargement after closed head injury. *Arch Neurol* 1981;38:623–629.

96. Bigler ED, Kurth SA, Blatter D, Abildskov T. Day-of-injury CT as an index to pre-injury brain morphology:degree of post-injury degenerative changes identified by CT and MR neuroimaging. *Brain Injury* 1993;7(2):125–34.

97. Bigler, E.D., Burr, R., Gale, S., Norman, M.A., Kurth, S.M., Blatter, D.D., & Abildskov, T. Day of injury CT scan as an index to pre-injury brain morphology. *Brain Injury* 1994;8(3): 231–238.

98. Blatter DD, Bigler ED, Gale SD, Johnson SC, Anderson CV, Burnett BM, Ryser D, MacNamara SE, Bailey BJ. MR-based brain and cerebrospinal fluid measurement after traumatic brain injury:Correlation with neuropsychological outcome. *American Journal of Neuroradiology* 1997;18:1–10.

99. Poca MA, Mataro M, Del Mar Matarin M, Arikan F, Junque C, Sahuquillo J. Is the placement of shunts in patients with idiopathic normal-pressure hydrocephalus worth the risk? Results of a study based on continuous monitoring of intracranial pressure. *J Neurosurg* 2004;100(5):855–66.

100. Gerard G, Weisberg LA:Magnetic resonance imaging in adult white matter disorders and hydrocephalus. *Semin Neurol* 1986; 6:17–23.

101. Bradley WG Jr. Diagnostic tools in hydrocephalus. *Neurosurg Clin NA* 2001;12(4):661–84.

102. Stollman AL, George AE, Pinto RS, et al. Periventricular high signal lesions and signal void on magnetic resonance imaging in hydrocephalus. *Acta Radiol* 1986;Supp 369:388–391.

103. Segev Y, Metser U, Beni-Adani L, Elran C, Reider-Grosswasser I, Constantini, S. Morphometric Study of Midsagittal MR Imaging Plane in Cases of Hydrocephalus and Atrophy and in Normal Brains. *Am J Neuroradiol* 2001;22:1674–1679.

104. Waldemar G, Schmidt JF, Delecluse F, et al. High resolution SPECT with 99m Tc-d, 1-HMPAO in normal pressure hydrocephalus before and after shunt operation. *J Neurol Neurosurg Psychiat* 1993;56:655–664.

105. Vanneste J, Augustijn P, Davies GAG, et al. Normal-pressure hydrocephalus:Is cisternography still useful in selecting patients for a shunt? *Arch Neurol* 1992;49:366–370.

106. Borgesen SE, Gjerris F. Relationships between intracranial pressure, ventricular size, and resistance to CSF outflow. *J Neurosurg* 1987;67:535–539.

107. Marmarou A, Foda MA, Bandoh K, Yoshihara M, Yamamoto T, Tsuji O, Zasler N, Ward JD, Young HF. Posttraumatic ventriculomegaly: hydrocephalus or atrophy? A new approach for diagnosis using CSF dynamics. *J Neurosurg* 1996;85(6):1026–35.

108. Morgan MK, Johnston IH, Spittaler PJ, et al. A ventricular infusion technique for the evaluation of treated and untreated hydrocephalus. *Neuro-surgery* 1991;29:832–837.

109. Sahuquillo J, Rubin E, Codina A, et al. Reappraisal of the intracranial pressure and cerebrospinal fluid dynamics in patients with so-called "normal pressure hydrocephalus" syndrome. *Acta Neurochir* 1991;112:50–61.

110. Tans JTJ, Poortvliet DCJ. Relationship between compliance and resistance to outflow of CSF in adult hydrocephalus. *J Neurosurg* 1989;71:59–62.

111. McGirt MJ, Woodworth G, Coon AL, Thomas G, Williams MA, Rigamonti D. Diagnosis, treatment, and analysis of long-term outcomes in idiopathic normal-pressure hydrocephalus. *Neurosurgery*, 2005;57(4):699–705.

112. Marmarou A, Bergsneider M, Klinge P, Relkin N, Black PM. The value of supplemental prognostic tests for the preoperative assessment of idiopathic normal-pressure hydrocephalus. *Neurosurgery*, 2005;57(Suppl 3):S17–28.

113. Meier U, Miethke C. Predictors of outcome in patients with normal-pressure hydrocephalus. *J Clin Neurosci* 2003;10(4):453–9.

114. Kahlon B, Sundbarg G, Rehncrona S. Comparison between the lumbar infusion and CSF tap tests to predict outcome after shunt surgery in suspected normal pressure hydrocephalus. *J Neurol Neurosurg Psychiatry* 2002;73(6):721–6.

115. Hertel F, Walter C, Schmitt M, Morsdorf M, Jammers W, Busch HP, Bettag M. Is a combination of Tc-SPECT or perfusion weighted magnetic resonance imaging with spinal tap test helpful in the diagnosis of normal pressure hydrocephalus? *J Neurol Neurosurg Psychiatry* 2003;74(4):479–84.

116. Gilmore HE. Medical treatment of hydrocephalus. In Scott RM (ed). *Hydrocephalus.* Baltimore, Williams & Wilkins, 1990, pp 37–46.

117. Oi S, Shimoda M, Shibata M et al. Pathophysiology of long-standing overt ventriculomegaly in adults. *J Neurosurg* 2000; 92:933–940.

118. de Jong DA, Delwel EJ, Avezaat CJJ. Hydrostatic and Hemodynamic Considerations in Shunted Normal Pressure Hydrocephalus. *Acta Neurochir* (Wien) 2000 142:241–7.

119. Owler BK, Jacobson EE, and Johnston IH. Low Pressure Hydrocephalus:Issues of diagnosis and treatment in 5 cases. *Br J Neurosurg* 2001;15:353–359.

120. Chuang S, Hochhauser L, Fritz C, et al. Lumboperitoneal shunt malfunction. *Acta Radiol* 1986;Suppl 369:645–648.

121. Chumas PD, Armstrong DC, Drake JM, et al. Tonsillar herniation: The rule rather than the exception after lumboperitoneal shunting in the pediatric population. *J Neurosurg* 1993; 78:568–573.

122. Drake JM, Sainte-Rose C. *The Shunt Book.* Blackwell Scientific, Cambridge, Mass. 1995·228pp.

123. Post EM:Currently available shunt systems:A review. *Neurosurgery*1985;16:257–260.

124. Portnoy HD, Schulte RR, Fox JL, et al. Anti-siphon and reversible occlusion valves for shunting in hydrocephalus and preventing post-shunt subdural hematomas. *J Neurosurg* 1973;38:729–738.

125. Shurtleff DB. Characteristics of the various CSF shunt systems. *Clin Pediatr*1978;17:154–160.

126. 187. Watts C, Keith HD. Testing the hydrocephalus shunt valve. *Childs Brain* 1983;10:217–228.

127. *Cook SW, Bergsneider M. Why valve opening pressure plays a relatively minor role in the postural ICP response to ventricular shunts in normal pressure hydrocephalus:modeling and implications. *Acta Neurochir* 2002;Suppl. 81:15–7.

128. Seliger, GM, Katz DI, Seliger M, et al. Late improvement in closed head injury with a low-pressure valve shunt. *Brain Inj* 1992; 6:71–73.

129. Puca A, Anile C, Maira G, et al. Cerebrospinal fluid shunting for hydrocephalus in the adult:Factors related to shunt revision. *Neurosurgery*1991;29:822–826.

130. Sainte-Rose L, Piatt JH, Renier D, et al. Mechanical complications in shunts. *Pediatr Neurosurg* 1991;17:2–9.

131. Rekate HL. Shunt revision:Complications and their prevention. *Pediatr Neurosurg*1991–1992;17:155–162.

132. Aldrich EF, Harmann P. Disconnection as a cause of ventriculoperitoneal shunt malfunction in multicomponent shunt systems. *Pediatr Neurosurg* 1990–1991;16:309–312.

133. Piatt JH. Physical examination of patients with cerebrospinal fluid shunts:Is there useful information in pumping the shunt? *Pediatrics* 1992;89:470–473.

134. Hayden PW, Rudd TG, Shurtleff DB, et al. Combined pressure-radionuclide evaluation of suspected cerebrospinal fluid shunt malfunction:A seven year clinical experience. *Pediatrics* 1980; 66:679–684.

135. Uvebrant P, Sixt R, Bjure J, et al. Evaluation of cerebrospinal fluid shunt function in hydrocephalic children using 99m Tc-DTPA. *Childs Nerv Syst*1992;8:76–80.

136. Klein DM:The treatment of shunt infections. In Scott RM (ed). *Hydrocephalus.*Baltimore, Williams and Wilkins, 1990, pp. 87–98.

137. Schoenbaum SC, Gardner P, Shillito J. Infections of cerebrospinal fluid shunts:Epidemiology, clinical manifestations, and therapy. *J Infect Dis*1975;131:543–552.

138. Quintaliani R, Cooper BW:Central nervous system infections due to staphylococci. In Harris AA (ed). *Handbook of Clinical Neurology*, Amsterdam, Elsevier, 1988;8:71–76.

139. Chapman PH, Borges LF. Shunt infections:Prevention and treatment. *Clin Neurosurg* 1985;32:652–664.

140. Foltz EL: Hydrocephalus:Slit ventricles, shunt obstructions, and third ventricle shunts:A clinical study. *Surg Neurol* 1993;40: 119–124.

141. Wisoff JH, Epstein FJ. Diagnosis and treatment of the slit ventricle syndrome. In Scott RM (ed). *Hydrocephalus.* Baltimore, Williams and Wilkins, 1990, pp. 79–86.

142. Kelley GR, Johnson PL. Sinking brain syndrome:craniotomy can precipitate brainstem herniation in CSF hypovolemia. *Neurology* 2004;62(1):157.

143. Lee KS. Natural history of chronic subdural haematoma. *Brain Injury* 2004;18(4):351–8.

144. Foltz EL, Blanks J, Meyer R, et al.: Shunted hydrocephalus: Normal upright ICP by CSF gravity-flow control. *Surg Neurol* 1993;39:210–217.

145. Chapman PH, Cosman ER, Arnold MA, et al. The relationship between ventricular fluid pressure and body position in normal subjects and subjects with shunts: A telemetric study. *Neurosurgery* 1990;26:181–189.

146. Watson DA. The delta valve: A physiologic shunt system. Presented at the Consensus Conference on Pediatric Neurosurg. Assisi, Italy, 1992.

147. Zemack G, Romner B. Seven Years of clinical experience with the programmable Codman Hakim valve:a retrospective study of 583 patients. *J Neurosurg* 2000;92:941–948.

148. Kay AD, Fisher AJ, O'Kane C et al. A clinical audit of the Hakim programmable valve in patients with complex hydrocephalus. *Br J Neurosurg* 2000;14:535–542.

149. Zemack G, Romner B. Do adjustable shunt valves pressure our budget? A retrospective analysis of 541 implanted Codman Hakim programmable valves. *Br J Neurosurg* 2001;15:221–227.

150. Yamashita N, Kamiya K , Yamada K. Experience with the programmable valve shunt system. *J Neurosurg* 1999;91:26–31.

151. Muramatsu H, Koike K, Teramoto A. Ventriculoperitoneal Shunt dysfunction During Rehabilitation; Prevalence and Countermeasures. *Am J Phys Med Rehabil* 2002;81:517–578.

152. Pollack IF, Albright AL, Adelson PD and the Hakim-Medos Investigator Group. A Randomized Controlled Study of a Programmable Shunt Valve versus a Conventional Valve for Patients with Hydrocephalus *Neurosurgery* 1999;45:1399–1411.

153. PS Medical Strata Valve:The Adjustable Delta Valve. *Medtronic Technical Bulletin.*2001 Medtronic Neurosurgery, Goleta, California.

154. Miwa K, Kondo H, and Sakai N. Pressure changes observed in Codman-Medos programmable valves following magnetic exposure and filliping. *Child's Nerv Syst* 2001;17:150–153.

155. Meier U, Kintzel D. Clinical experiences with different valve systems in patients with normal-pressure hydrocephalus:evaluation of the Miethke dual-switch valve. *Child's Nerv Syst* 2002;18(6–7):288–94.

156. Meier U, Kiefer M, Sprung C. Evaluation of the Miethke dual-switch valve in patients with normal pressure hydrocephalus. *Surg Neurol* 2004;61(2):119–27;discussion 127–8.

157. Kiefer M, Eymann R, Meier U. Five Years Experience with Gravitational Shunts in Chronic Hydrocephalus of Adults. *Acta Neurochir*2002;144:755–767.

158. Tokoro K, Suzuki S, Chiba Y, Tsuda M. Shunt assistant valve:bench test investigations and clinical performance.*Child's Nerv Syst* 2002;18:492–9.

159. Tureyen K. Traumatic intracranial aneurysm after blunt trauma. *Brit J Neurosurg* 2001;15(5)429–31.

160. Kumar M, Kitchen ND. Infective and Traumatic Aneurysms. *Neurosurg Clin NA* 1998;9(3):577–586.

161. Burke JP, Marion DW. Cerebral Revascularization in Trauma and Carotid Occlusion. *Neurosurg Clin NA* 2001;36(3):595–611.

162. Batjer HH, Giller CA, Kopitnik TA, et al. Intracranial and cervical vascular injuries. In Cooper PR (ed). *Head Injury,* 3rd ed. Baltimore, Williams and Wilkins, 1993, pp. 373–404.

163. Flores JS, Vaquero J, Sola RG, et al. Traumatic false aneurysms of the middle meningeal artery. *Neurosurgery* 1986;18:200–203.

164. Wortzman D, Tucker WS, Gershater R, et al. Traumatic aneurysm in the posterior fossa. *Surg Neurol* 1980;13:329–332.

165. Matricali B. Internal carotid artery aneurysms. In Samii M, Brihaye J (eds). *Traumatology of the Skull Base.* New York, Springer Verlag, 1983, pp 196–200.

166. Rothrock JF. Headaches due to vascular disorders. *Neurol Clin NA*2004;22:21–37.

167. Bonafe A, Maneife C. Traumatic carotid-cavernous sinus fistulas. In Braakman R (ed). *Handbook of Clinical Neurology,* Amsterdam, Elsevier, 1990;13:345–366.

168. Debrun GM, Vinuela P, Fox AJ, et al.: Indications for treatment and classification of 132 carotid-cavernous Fistulas. *Neurosurgery* 1988;22:285- 289.

169. Phatouros CC, Meyers PM, Dowd CF, Halbach VV, Malck AM, Higashida RT. Carotid Artery Cavernous Fistulas. *Neurosurg Clin NA* 2000;11(1):67–84.

170. Dubov WE, Bach JR. Delayed presentation of carotid cavernous sinus fistula in a patient with traumatic brain injury. *Am J Phys Med Rehabil* 1991;70:178–180.

171. Miyachi S, Negoro M, Handa T, et al. Dural carotid cavernous sinus fistula presenting as isolated oculomotor nerve palsy. *Surg Neurol* 1993;39:105–109.

172. Koehler PJ, Blauw G. Late posttraumatic nonvascular pulsating eye. *Acta Neurochir* 1992;116:62–64.

173. Buckwalter JA, Sasaki CT, Virapongse C, et al. Pulsatile tinnitus arising from jugular megabulb deformity: A treatment rationale. Laryngoscope 1983;93:1534–1539.

174. Hentzer E. Objective tinnitus of the vascular type. *Acta Otolaryngol* 1968;66:273–281.

175. Hvidegaard T, Brask T. Objective venous tinnitus. *J Laryngol Otol* 1984;98:189–191.

176. Rovillard R, Leclerc J, Savary P, et al. Pulsatile tinnitus: A dehiscent jugular vein. Laryngoscope 1985;95:188–189.

177. Vallis RC, Martin FW. Extracranial arteriovenous malformation presenting as objective tinnitus. *J Laryngol Otol* 1984;98: 1139–1142.

178. Higashida RT, Hieshima GB, Halbach W, et al. Closure of carotid cavernous sinus fistulae by external compression of the carotid artery and jugular vein. *Acta Radiol* 1986;Suppl 369:580–583.

179. Batjer HH, Purdy PD, Neiman M, et al. Subtemporal transdural use of detachable balloons for traumatic carotid-cavernous fistulas. *Neurosurgery*1988;22:290–296.

180. Brosnahan D, McFadzean RM, Teasdale E, et al. Neuro-ophthalmic features of carotid cavernous fistulas and their treatment by endoarterial balloon embolization. *J Neurol Neurosurg Psychiatry* 1992;55:553–556.

181. Cameron MM. Chronic subdural hematoma:A review of 114 cases. *J Neurol Neurosurg Psychiatry* 1978;41:834–839.

182. Drapkin AJ. Chronic subdural hematoma:Pathophysiological basis for treatment. *Br J Neurosurg* 1991;5:467–473.

183. Kawakami Y, Chikama M, Tamiya T, et al. Coagulation and fibrinolysis in chronic subdural hematoma. *Neurosurgery* 1989;25:25–29.

184. Loew F, Kivelitz R:Chronic subdural hematomas. In Vinken PJ, Bruyn GW (eds): *Handbook of Clinical Neurology*, New York, Elsevier, 1976;24:297–327.

185. Stone JL, Rifai MHS, Lang RGR, et al. Subdural hematomas. Acute subdural hematoma:Progress in definition, clinical pathology and therapy. *Surg Neurol* 1983;19:216–231.

186. Feldman RG, Pincus JH, McEntee WJ, et al. Cerebrovascular accident or subdural fluid collection? Arch Intern Med 1963;112:204–214.

187. Cooper PR. Posttraumatic intracranial mass lesions. In Cooper PR (ed). *Head Injury*, 3rd ed. Baltimore, Williams & Wilkins, 1993, pp 275–330.

188. Rubin G, Rappaport ZH:Epilepsy in chronic subdural haematoma. *Acta Neurochir* 1993;123:39–42.

189. Kaminski HJ, Hlavin ML, Likavec MJ, Schmidley JW. Transient Neurologic Deficit Caused by chronic subdural hematoma. *Am J Med* 1992;92(6):698–700.

190. Rahimi AR, Poorkay M. Subdural hematomas and isolated transient aphasia. *J Am Med Dir Assoc* 2000 1(3):129–31.

191. Kirn KS, Hemmati M, Weinberg PE, et al. Computed tomography in isodense subdural hematoma. *Radiology* 1978;128:71–74.

192. Tsai FY, Huprich JE. Further experience with contrast enhanced CT in head trauma. *Neuroradiology* 1978;16:314–317.

193. Kao MCK:Sedimentation level in chronic subdural hematoma visible on computerized tomography. *J Neurosurg* 1983;58:246–251.

194. Hosoda K, Tamaki N, Masumura M, et al. Magnetic resonance images of chronic subdural hematomas. *J Neurosurg* 1987;67:677–683.

195. Ishikawa T, Kawamura SH, et al. Uncoupling between CBF and oxygen metabolism in a patient with chronic subdural hematoma: Case report. *J Neurol Neurosurg Psychiatry* 1992;55:401–403.

196. St. John JN, Dila C. Traumatic subdural hygroma in adults. *Neurosurgery* 1981;9:621–626.

197. Lee KS, Bae WK, Yoon SM, Doh JW, Bae HG, Yun IG. Location of the traumatic subdural hygroma:role of gravity and cranial morphology. *Brain Injury* 2000 14(4):355–61.

198. Lee KS, Bae WK, Doh JW, Bae HG, Yun IG. Origin of chronic subdural hematoma and relation to traumatic subdural lesions. *Brain Injury* 1998;12(11):901–910.

199. Lee KS, Bae WK, Bae HG, Yun, IG. The fate of traumatic subdural hygroma in Serial Computed Tomographic Scans. *J Korean Med Soc* 2000 15:560–8.

200. Yamashima T, Yamamoto S, Friede RL, et al. The role of endothelial gap junctions in the enlargement of chronic subdural hematomas. *J Neurosurg* 1983;59:298–303.

201. Yamoshima T, Yamamoto S. How do vessels proliferate in the capsule of a chronic subdural hematoma. *Neurosurgery* 1984;15:672–678.

202. Kotwica Z, Brzezinski J. Chronic subdural haematoma treated by burr holes and closed system drainage:Personal experience in 131 patients. *Br J Neurosurg* 1991;5:461–465.

203. Weigel R, Schmiedek P, Krauss JK. Outcome of contemporary surgery for chronic subdural hematoma:Evidence based review. *J Neurol Neurosurg Psychiatry* 2003;74:937–43.

204. Frati A, Salvati M, Mainiero F, Ippoliti F, Rocchi G, Raco A, Caroli E, Cantore G, Delfini R. Inflammation markers and risk factors for recurrence in 35 patients with a posttraumatic chronic subdural hematoma: a prospective study. *J Neurosurg* 2004;100(1):24–32.

205. Mohamed EEH. Management of chronic subdural haematoma. *Br J Neurosurg* 1991;5:525–526.

206. Ram Z, Hadani M, SaharA, et al. Continuous irrigation-drainage of the subdural space for the treatment of chronic subdural haematoma: A prospective clinical trail. *Acta Neurochir* 1993;120:40–43.

207. Robinson RG:Chronic subdural hematoma:Surgical management in 133 patients. *J Neurosurg* 1984;61:263–268.

208. Markwalder TM, Steinsiepek F, Rohner M, et al. The course of chronic subdural hematomas after burr-hole craniostomy and closed-system drainage. *J Neurosurg* 1981;55:390–396.

209. Jamieson KG, Yelland JDN. Extradural hematoma. *J Neurosurg* 1968;29:13–23.

210. Illingworth R, Shawdon H: Conservative management of intracranial extradural haematoma presenting late. *J Neurol Neurosurg Psychiatry* 1983;46:558–560.

211. Hirsh LF: Chronic epidural hematomas. *Neurosurgery* 1980; 6:508–512.

212. Hooper RS: Extradural hemorrhages of the posterior fossa. *Br J Surg* 1954;42:19–26.

213. Roda JM, Gimenez D, Perez-Higueras A, et al. Posterior fossa epidural hematomas:A review and synthesis. *Surg Neurol* 1983; 19:419–424.

214. Mertol T, Buner M, Acar V, et al. Delayed traumatic intracerebral hematoma. *Br J Neurosurg* 1991;6:491–498.

215. Cooper PR. Delayed Traumatic Intracerebral Hemorrhage. *Neurosurg Clin NA* 1992 3(3):659.

216. Andrews BT, Chiles BW, Olsen WL, Pitts LH. The effect of intracerebral hematoma location on the risk of brain stem compression and on clinical outcome. *J Neurosurg* 1988;69:518–522.

VIII

NEUROMUSCULOSKELETAL PROBLEMS

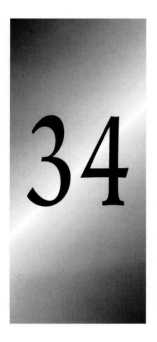

34

Complications Associated with Immobility after TBI

Kathleen R. Bell

INTRODUCTION

Immobilization of the human body has long been known to affect physiology in ways detrimental to normal function, even in the time of Hippocrates (1). Despite this knowledge, prolonged bedrest was used for many years in the treatment of medical disorders. However, studies emanating from the manned space program since the 1960's defining the effects of a gravity-free environment have clarified many of these effects in healthy humans. Most of the studies performed on animals, however, rely on hindlimb suspension models of immobilization and many studies on humans rely on the head down tilt position in bed to mimic microgravity. None of these conditions precisely reproduces the conditions of prolonged bedrest in a medical situation. Nonetheless, general principles regarding the effect of inactivity on the body can be derived from these experiments. As an additional complicating factor in severe traumatic brain injury (TBI), the effects of immobilization may be prolonged and worsened by a number of disorders stemming from the brain injury itself such as posturing, spasticity, dysautonomia, endocrine abnormalities, and other body system injuries. Thus the importance of prevention and prompt management of these disorders is highlighted in addition to early mobilization of the patient with TBI.

Prolonged bedrest brings about reduced function in multiple body systems simultaneously. For example, deconditioning is a diagnosis in its own right (2). Deconditioning results from reduced functional capacity of both the musculoskeletal and cardiovascular systems; changes to one system are unlikely to be significant without accompanying decrements in the other system. The effects of deconditioning can be studied in young, healthy experimental subjects, eliminating the effects of pathology. The effects of mobilization and exercise on this group emphasizes the importance of early mobilization for those with illness or injury (2).

This chapter seeks to address those general aspects of immobility that may be seen in any situation where prolonged bedrest occurs and to discuss the impact of traumatic brain injury on related causal factors and treatment (Table 34-1). There are very few studies that actually examine the specific effects of immobility on persons recovering from TBI (or any other illness or injury) so associations and recommendations are made derived from literature on healthy individuals or those with other disorders.

EFFECTS OF IMMOBILITY ON THE PERSON WITH TRAUMATIC BRAIN INJURY

Musculoskeletal System

Significant changes occur in the musculoskeletal system in the first 4–6 weeks of immobilization affecting all

TABLE 34-1

A Summary of the Effects of Immobility on Organ Systems with Associated TBI-Related Physiological Stressors

ORGAN SYSTEMS	POSSIBLE EFFECTS	TBI RELATED DISORDERS
Musculoskeletal	Muscle weakness, osteopenia, muscle and joint contracture	Spasticity and other movement related disorders, paresis, associated trauma
Respiratory	Hypoventilation, pooling of secretions	Tracheostomy, altered immune function
Cardiovascular/Hematologic	Deconditioning, postural hypotension, thromboembolic disorders	Autonomic instability, hyperhidrosis, paresis, fluid and metabolic disorders
Dermatological	Pressure ulcers	Paresis, catabolism, dysphagia
Neurological/Psychological	Sensory deprivation, balance disorder	Special senses disturbances, cognitive impairment, vertigo
Metabolic/Neuroendocrine	Volume contraction, hypercalcemia	Sodium disorders, hyperhidrosis, paresis
Gastrointestinal and Urologic	Constipation, reflux, and urinary stasis	Dysphagia and impaired cognition requiring enteral feeding

components of the system, including up to 40% loss of muscle strength, decrements in bone density, and shortening of collagen-containing tissues. These changes are the results of a lack of the usual weight-bearing forces acting in the vertical position and the decrease in muscular contraction especially in the postural muscles (3). While these types of changes occur in even healthy young people, the effects are magnified in populations such as the elderly with baseline alterations in muscle strength and bone density. One concern is whether persons subjected to prolonged periods of bedrest will be at higher risk of osteoporosis as they age if stores are not recovered (3). As we will see, persons with TBI are likely to be more profoundly affected as well, because of associated conditions.

Bone Density Loss   Bone is constantly undergoing alteration and remodeling during normal activities. The activity of osteoclasts that reabsorb mineralized bone matrix and osteoblasts which are responsible for the synthesis and mineralization of bone is governed by mechanical stresses and systemic stimuli. Participants in the regulation of bone density include mechanical stresses, hormones, growth factors, and cytokines. In addition to osteoclasts and osteoblasts, chondroprogenitor cells may become either chondrocytes covering the joint surface of bone or growth plate chondrocytes that are the basis for metaphyseal bone formation. These cells form bone modeling units (BMUs) whose activity is altered by physical activity or immobility, nutrition, aging, and illness (4). Specifically, skeletal muscle activity at least partially regulates bone density maintenance via growth factors (e.g., IGF-1) even during periods of disuse (5).

Chronic illness or prolonged recovery from trauma such as that seen in TBI is most likely associated with the

growth hormone/IGF-1 axis, along with impaired thyroid and gonadal function (4, 6). Immobilization specifically is associated with a moderate decrease in bone resorption but an even larger decrease in mineralization of bone matrix (7, 8). A negative calcium balance occurs within a week of bedrest, and 20 weeks of bedrest in healthy, young men results in a 60% increase in urinary calcium. Fecal calcium loss also occurs in conjunction with reduced intestinal absorption (3). There is decreased bone mineral density in the lumbar spine, femoral neck, tibia, and calcaneus but not the radius noted in young men on 4 months of bedrest (9). There are no significant changes in serum parathyroid hormone or in serum 1,25-dihydroxyvitamin D during bedrest in healthy men, but persons with spinal cord injury have been shown to have decreased levels of both (10). In persons with TBI, an additional factor to consider in factoring the degree of bone loss is the frequent presence of hemiplegia or other patterns of paralysis. Data from persons recovering from stroke and other neurologic disorders offer some insight although not directly applicable to the brain-injured population because of the differences in average age and degree of paralysis and immobility. Bone loss early after stroke appears to be primarily due to increased bone resorption while later bone loss is more clearly related to the degree of paresis and vitamin D levels (11). 1,25-dihydroxyvitamin D production appears to be inhibited (12). Nearly all fractures after falls occur on the hemiparetic side in stroke patients (13). Bone mineral density was significantly lower in both femurs in stroke patient who were non-ambulatory after stroke. The difference in bone loss only on the hemiparetic side between the non-ambulatory and ambulatory patients was also significant. Most of the loss occurred within the first seven months after stroke (14). Bone density loss in the limbs is even more striking after spinal cord injury; however, vertebral bone density is not significantly compromised because of continued weight-bearing in the seated position (15).

Recovery of bone mineral density after loss is quite slow for longer periods of immobilization. Although dogs recover to baseline in 12 weeks after 12 weeks of immobilization, for longer periods of immobility, bone did not recover even after 7 months (16). Calcaneal bone density deficits have been noted in astronauts even 5 years after space flight (3, 17). There are few studies of reversing or minimizing bone loss after neurologic insults. Vitamin D and calcium supplementation have been demonstrated to be helpful in preventing fracture in elderly patients but caution should be used after stroke in the presence of hypercalcemia (18, 19). Etidronate which inhibits bone resorption has been studied in spinal cord injury and stroke and may be effective in preventing bone resorption (20, 21). Clenbuterol, a beta-2-agonist, has been tested to prevent muscle and bone loss in rats with a significant prevention of muscle atrophy and accompanying lessening of bone mass loss (22).

Muscle Weakness and Atrophy There is no doubt that muscle strength and size are affected after prolonged bedrest. As might be predicted, the weight-bearing muscles of the lower limb are affected to a greater degree than the muscles of the arm (23). There are even more local differences in the degree of muscle atrophy. The knee extensors lose more mass than do the knee flexors (24). There are a number of possible mechanisms that result in muscle weakness and atrophy that are further discussed below.

Protein Breakdown By the fifth day of bedrest, there is a significant increase in the urinary excretion of nitrogen, peaking in the second week of bedrest. This reflects protein degradation and is an early marker of muscle atrophy (25–27). The cross sectional area of muscles is reduced 7–14% in 4–6 weeks of immobilization, especially in muscles responsible for resisting gravity such as the knee extensors (28, 29). Lower limb muscles are affected more than upper limb muscles.

Decreased Protein Synthesis Shortly after a limb is immobilized, decreases in total RNA and protein synthesis can be seen in muscles (30). Some alterations in pretranslational and translational mechanisms for protein production begin within six hours of immobilization, reflected in decreased alpha-actin and cytochrome c protein synthesis and decreased cytochrome c mRNA in rats (31–33).

Regrowth after inactivity-induced atrophy involves a number of mechanisms including 1) increased protein synthesis, 2) continued elevations of protein degradation, 3) increased proliferation of muscle precursor cells, 4) and increases in myonuclear number (myonuclei per 100 myofibers) (30). Unfortunately, muscle regrowth after atrophy is not always complete, especially in the elderly (34, 35). As a clinical example, muscle wasting in 64-year-old patients after total hip arthroplasty persisted 5 months postoperatively (36). This limited regrowth may be due to low satellite cell numbers and lower levels of growth factors (such as IGF-1) (30).

Disruption of Antioxidants in Skeletal Muscle In pathological conditions, such as post-trauma catabolism, other mechanisms may be at play in the volume of muscle loss during bedrest and immobilization. Typically, antioxidant protein and scavenger protection protect skeletal muscle against oxidative stress. However, during hindlimb unloading in rats, there has been demonstrated large shifts in superoxide dismutase activity with impaired antioxidant activity (decreased catalase, glutathione peroxidase, and nonenzymatic antioxidant scavenging capacity) (37–39). This disruption of protection can result in muscle fiber damage and loss that, when combined with a state of protein loss after severe trauma, is accelerated.

There is disagreement between animal and human experiments on which muscle fibers appear to be most affected by this loss of volume induced by immobilization. Generally, in animals, slow-twitch fibers are predominantly affected. In humans, however, fast-twitch fibers appear to be most affected. It is possible that this may be somewhat misleading as the relative sizes of slow- and fast-twitch muscle are different in rats and humans (3).

There is some evidence that some of this muscle atrophy and loss of oxidative capacity can be prevented by isometric exercise during the period of immobilization (40, 41). Isometric exercises appear to be more effective in slow tonic muscles like the soleus as compared to the fast-twitch muscles such as the gastrocnemius (40). In addition to having a salutary effect on bone density, clenbuterol also appears to reduce muscle degeneration in dystrophic or denervated muscle (42). In addition, there is some evidence that oral creatine supplementation enhances the muscle hypertrophy response to exercise after a period of immobilization (43).

Not unexpectedly, these findings suggesting protein breakdown and a loss of muscle mass would lead one to predict an accompanying decrease in muscle strength. Microgravity studies have demonstrated that 30 days of bed rest will result in an 18–20% decrease in knee extensor strength (44, 45).

Endurance is also decreased after prolonged immobility. Decrements up to 17% are noted in torque production in limbs unloaded for 4 weeks; this does not recover to baseline even after 7 weeks of recovery (46). These findings may be due to changes in muscle oxidative enzymes as well as decreased oxygen delivery to muscle after disuse (3).

Part of the loss of muscle strength observed after prolonged bed rest is the result of decreased efficiency in motor neuron recruitment. While electromyographic activity is reduced by half in muscles that are shortened, there does not appear to be a relationship between the electrical activation of muscle and the relative decrease in muscle mass (47). However, there is evidence for reduced motor neuron activation after immobilization and a subsequent need for increased neuronal activation to produce the same degree of muscle force output (48–50). These neuromuscular inefficiencies can be totally reversed with training after the cessation of bedrest (49). This type of data also supports the notion of early movement and weight-bearing, as much of the muscle loss seen in the first 2 weeks of bedrest can be easily restored.

Joint Contractures   There are a number of changes in connective tissue and muscle during immobilization of a limb that can result in a loss of passive range of motion in a joint. For instance, studies have demonstrated reductions in both the length and diameter of muscle fibers and in muscle extensibility (51–53). Additionally, there is an increase in intramuscular connective tissue and reduced capillary density in muscle (54, 55). In addition to these muscle changes, there is a significant increase in endomysial and perimysial connective tissue. More fibers are deposited perpendicularly to the adjacent muscle fibers. The network of collagen fibers become indistinguishable from each other (56).

Patients with TBI have an assortment of risk factors associated with their injuries that may contribute to the formation of joint contractures. Spasticity and rigidity may be extremely difficult to control in the acute stages of TBI. In examining the patient with TBI for contractures, it is important to assess the contribution of dynamic (spasticity dependent) aspects of joint movement limitation. It may be useful to perform a peripheral nerve block for this purpose. In later stages of TBI, postural control, especially of the axial skeleton, may lead to contractures of the neck and spine that are challenging to address. Weakness and prolonged maintenance of any posture will also contribute to joint contracture. Other general risk factors include age, edema, and diabetes mellitus. Reported incidence of ankle plantar flexion contractures in persons with acute moderate to severe TBI has ranged from 16–76%, depending on the definition of contracture (57, 58).

Prevention of joint contracture depends on the maintenance of proper joint position with the use of splints, adequate treatment of spasticity, and active and passive range of motion exercises to the joint several times daily. Standing is the optimal method of maintaining ankle range of motion and prone lying is very helpful to prevent hip flexion contractures. Serial casting is one option to treat mild to moderate equinovarus deformities of the ankle and contractures of the upper limb (59, 60). Short changing intervals of 1–4 days were more effective than intervals of 5–7 days in restoring range of motion (60).

Respiratory System

Many patients with severe TBI have tracheostomies for assisted ventilation and respiratory toilet in the acute stages. In addition, impaired alertness will result in a decreased drive for deep inspiration. Therefore, TBI patients are already at risk for pulmonary complications during their rehabilitation. Prolonged bedrest adds to that risk. Simulated weightlessness with a head-down tilt in healthy individuals demonstrates that the functional residual capacity of the lungs falls by 33% during this period with insignificant changes in lung tissue volume. Diffusing capacity decreases gradually to 4–5% below baseline values. Pulmonary blood flow also decreases by 16% (61). All of these changes result in higher risk for atelectasis and pulmonary infection. Treatment consists of early mobilization of the patient and aggressive pulmonary toilet with suction and the use of equipment such as the in-exsufflator to assist in the management of secretions.

Cardiovascular System

Research on cardiovascular effects of immobility is drawn both from microgravity experiments during space flight and from experiments utilizing a head-down tilt position to mimic weightlessness. Obviously, these studies seek to maximize the effects of bedrest. Normal head-up positioning of patients in bed after TBI will mitigate the severity of cardiovascular effects.

Reduction of Cardiopulmonary Functional Capacity and Postural Hypotension   Functional efficiency of the heart depends on both intravascular volume (hydrostatic forces) and coordinated filling and emptying of the ventricles (hydrodynamic forces). Normally, arterial pressures and certain levels of intravascular volume interact to maintain adequate body and cerebral perfusion in the face of gravity. However, when the body is placed horizontally for a prolonged period of time, about a liter of fluid is relocated from the legs to the chest area. Initially, this increases diastolic filling and increases the stroke volume of each cardiac contraction (i.e., the Frank-Starling mechanism). However, baroreceptor responses eventually result in a diuresis and loss of plasma volume within 24–48 hours (62). When a normal upright position is resumed, there is a sudden decrease in both ventricular filling and stroke volume that results in orthostatic symptoms (63). Cardiovascular baroreflex responses become attenuated without the challenges of baroceptor unloading that comes from upright standing (64). Other factors may include disordered sympathetic activation in combination with hypovolemia and diminished baroreceptor reflexes (65). Particularly interesting in the context of TBI is the involvement of brain autonomic nuclei such as the paraventricular nucleus of the hypothalamus that includes basal and reflex control of the sympathetic nervous system vasopressin and oxytocin release and secretion of corticotrophin releasing factor (66).

Other changes in cardiac function have been noted. After immobilization, the maximal oxygen uptake (vO_{2max}) is reduced and the heart rate is increased in response to submaximal exercise (67). This equates to a loss in aerobic capacity of 0.9% per day over thirty days of bedrest (2). The heart rate during prolonged bedrest is higher for the same oxygen requirement (68). Part of this is related to the fluid changes noted above; these effects are much less during supine submaximal exercise (67). The heart rate is probably increased due to increased beta-adrenergic receptor sensitivity (68).

Simple replacement of volume does not abolish the orthostatic response (69). It appears that there are some alterations to the ventricles themselves during a period of prolonged bedrest leaving them less distensible (70). This appears to be an effect on cardiac muscle similar to the loss of muscle volume seen in skeletal muscle during prolonged immobilization (63). Actual muscle contractile properties seem to be preserved (71). The effects on stroke volume and cardiac output after prolonged bedrest will persist for at least a month (71). These effects are partially masked by an increase in peripheral volume and retention of sodium and, at least initially, an increase in sympathetic nerve activity (72).

Other peripheral mechanisms also come into play during prolonged bedrest. Deconditioning causes a reduction in red blood cell mass by 5–25% that may compromise blood oxygen-carrying capacity. However, the hematocrit generally remains stable during bedrest. Therefore, the effect of reduced blood cell mass is still unclear (68). As noted elsewhere in this chapter, there is a significant decrease in resting blood flow to the leg muscles and a reduction in capillarization. This is correlated with fatigability in calf muscles (73, 74) (See Figure 34-1 (68)). Interestingly, the role of the nervous system as another contributor to orthostatic intolerance has been recently promulgated. A subset of neurons in the paraventricular nucleus may be part of the puzzle in determining sympathetic nervous system excitation in response to blood volume and baroreflexes (66).

Reversing these effects requires not only the upright position and adequate fluid volume but also exercise that induces arterial baroreceptor loading (64). In animals, daily standing for only 1 hour per day prevented depression of myocardial contractility (75).

Thrombogenesis Thromboembolic disease is a well described risk in the setting of immobilization. In the

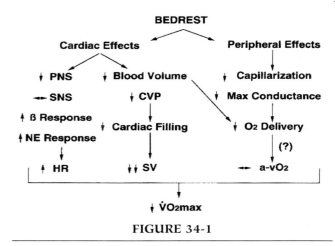

FIGURE 34-1

Model of cardiovascular mechanisms controlling maximal oxygen uptake during bed rest. (Permission requested:Convertino VA. Cardiovascular consequences of bed rest: effect on maximal oxygen uptake. *Med Sci Sports Exerc* 1997;29(2): 191–196.)

brain injured patient, this risk remains present with significant complicating factors for diagnosis and treatment. Often after significant trauma, each of the factors of Virchow's triad (stasis, endothelial damage and hypercoagulable state) is present on admission to the emergency room. In the TBI patient, one sequela of the injury may be hemiparesis which contributes to stasis in a more discrete and prolonged manner. Patients with TBI may also present with bleeding in the subdural or subarachnoid space, limiting the choice of treatment modalities. The TBI patient may also be impulsive and have considerable fall risk which may limit pharmacologic prophylaxis and treatment options. Identification and treatment of venous thromboembolism is therefore of increased complexity but of great necessity in the traumatic brain injured population (76).

Initial traumatic injury inherently carries with it risk for hypercoagulability when multiple organ systems are involved and bleeding is present at one or more sites. When bleeding occurs, the body initiates the coagulation cascade, a response that may be prolonged when blood remains present acting as a nidus for continued production of coagulation factors. In traumatic brain injury, bleeding may occur at any site in the body due to concomitant trauma, but is of particular concern in the subarachnoid or subdural space. The patient may require prolonged monitoring to ensure resorption or neurosurgical intervention to reduce mass effect due to bleeding, contributing to further stasis. A functional limitation of TBI may be hemiparesis or bilateral weakness which may persist following the acute period of immobility after trauma. Thrombi are noted to occur most frequently in the paralyzed limb of hemiparetic patients and more likely to occur in the proximal segment of the limb placing them at higher risk for propagation (77). In a similar setting, DVT risk has been found to be comparable following brain tumor surgery as in the orthopaedic hip replacement population (78). The traumatic brain injury patient is also likely to have suffered endothelial damage with the initial inciting injury.

Identification of thromboembolism may be suspected clinically by the presence of a warm, edematous and painful limb. Unfortunately, the affected limb often exhibits no signs at all of thrombophlebitis therefore physical exam is unreliable for venous thrombosis diagnosis (79). The venous duplex exam is the mainstay of diagnosis. Testing carries high accuracy, is non-invasive and often readily available at the bedside (80). If pulmonary embolism (PE) is suspected by clinic findings of decreased oxygen saturation, tachypnea and pleuritic chest pain, studies to assist in diagnosis for PE should be employed as well as the above mentioned venous duplex to identify the potential source of the embolus. The D-dimer assay, spiral computerized tomography (CT) and ventilation-perfusion studies are all well accepted means to assist in diagnosis of pulmonary embolism. In the TBI patient, there are noted limitations to the use of these means of diagnosis. Following trauma, it is anticipated that D-dimer levels will be unspecifically high and therefore are not as helpful in diagnosis. Using D-dimer levels has not been shown to be useful in predicting deep venous thrombosis after acute TBI (81). However, a low D-dimer level may assist to rule out a pulmonary embolism if this be the goal. A ventilation-perfusion scan may be limited by any other concomitant pulmonary conditions such as pneumonia, secretions or atelectasis. The spiral CT is the most readily available tool for reliable diagnosis, albeit at a higher initial cost.

Treatment for identified thromboembolism is primarily pharmacologic by using unfractionated or regular heparin. Heparin acts initially by enhancing antithrombin III activity. In high doses, heparin also acts to inhibit prothrombin and platelet aggregation. This constitutes its efficacy in meeting the key treatment goals for PE and thromboembolism by inducing a hypocoagulable state and decreased potential for clot propagation (79). However, the TBI patient may have co-morbidities limiting the use of anticoagulation in their pharmacologic regimen. In the setting of TBI, the patient may have suffered a subarachnoid or subdural hemorrhage making anticoagulation undesirable. Further, impulsivity and significant fall risk may instill hesitation for use of anticoagulation in this population. In this setting, the use of retrievable inferior vena cava filters is increasing as a means to disrupt the clot pathway to decrease risk of pulmonary embolism. These filters are generally used in patients in whom recurrent PE has occurred despite treatment with anticoagulants or those in whom anticoagulant therapy is contraindicated (82). A review of multiple case series has indicated that these filters are successfully removed in 91% of cases; 9% of filters could not

be removed because of large trapped thrombus (83). It is important to note that these filters are associated with a 2-fold increase in the incidence of recurrent deep venous thrombosis. If it is safe to anticoagulate a patient, they should remain on therapeutic anticoagulation even with a filter in place for the recommended length of time (84).

Prophylaxis of thromboembolism to decrease the risk of a potential pulmonary embolism is the single most effective means of decreasing morbidity and mortality from venous embolic disease. Often patients are placed on mechanical and pharmacologic means of prophylaxis. The mainstays of mechanical means, compression stockings and sequential compression devices, may be appropriate in the TBI patient when in bed; however their use may be limited as they may interfere with ambulation and the rehabilitation process. The TBI patient may be appropriate for heparin or unfractionated heparin therapy if no contraindications exist. However, in the setting of intracranial hemorrhage, inferior vena cava filters may assist in limiting pulmonary embolism if intiated as a means of prophylaxis acutely after injury.

Integumentary System

Pressure ulcers are a well-known complication of bedrest, particularly when complicated by paresis of any kind. Pressure ulcers are associated with increased mortality, morbidity, length of stay, and cost of treatment (85, 86). While TBI patients have not been specifically examined, immobility and decreased body weight are both independent risk factors for the development of pressure sores (87). After acute TBI, inadequate tissue perfusion because of unrelieved pressure at bony prominences is chiefly responsible for the development of pressure ulcers (88, 89). Pressure wounds heal best when kept moist with occlusive dressings. Other methods used to improve healing have included serial casting in patients with spasticity; the casts are thought to reduce friction associated with repetitive movements.

Neurological Systems

Effects of Bedrest on Cognitive and Psychiatric Function
Confinement to bed has been associated with a number of undesirable psychological and cognitive effects. Much of the data has come from studies on healthy young men as part of the space program research projects. These studies have used a 6-degree head-down tilt that more closely reproduces microgravity conditions than normal bedrest. Nonetheless, these studies have some application to medically-driven bedrest. These studies have noted enhanced levels of depression and emotional distress. In addition, impairments in overall cognitive capabilities have been described as well with self-reported confusion and depressed scores on cognitive testing (90, 91).

An additional area that may be affected by prolonged immobilization in bed is sleep. Chronic insomnia can be perpetuated by increased time spent in bed (92). Studies on elderly hospitalized patients on bedrest in poorly lit rooms have demonstrated that patients report poor sleep quality and that phase shifts for sleep are noted (93). Although these conditions have not been evaluated in patients with brain injury, it is reasonable to assume that worsening of confusion and sleep disorder can result from prolonged bed rest.

Balance Disorder and Incoordination Neuromuscular changes associated with inefficient recruitment of motor neurons may be partly responsible for the findings of increased postural sway, gait changes, and impaired kinesthetic sense after prolonged space travel (3, 94, 95). These changes in response to immobilization and bedrest may occur at multiple levels of the nervous system (96). For instance, it has been demonstrated that training can enlarge the size of the cortical area involved in the task. Conversely, it appears that there are reduced cortical responses after immobilization of a joint that are proportional to the length of time of immobilization. The amplitude of motor evoked potentials decreases after joint splinting during motor imagery tasks but not motor activation tasks (97). Other changes have been noted in the motor strategies used to perform a static muscle contraction after immobilization; some people were noted to produce a bursting pattern with reduced EMG amplitude in contrast to the pre-immobilization pattern of progressive increase in the amplitude of EMG activity (98, 99). The organization of neurons to provide maximal voluntary contraction appears to be diminished after 6 weeks of immobilization of a limb; peak force produced voluntarily during a maximum contraction was lower than that produced by electrical stimulation (100). Although the specific effects of immobilization on sensory inputs on control of movement have not been studied, there is evidence that sensory feedback such as vibration can evoke a cross-training effect and increase the power production capability of muscles (49,101).

Endocrine and Metabolic System

There is no literature that directly addresses the influence of bedrest on the endocrine system or metabolism after TBI. A few points, however, may be interesting to review with an emphasis on how these factors may be affected by conditions after TBI such as hyperhydrosis (resulting in volume loss) and intrinsic damage to the pituitary-adrenal axis. Growth hormone resistance has been observed in chronic illness and/or malnutrition resulting from resistance at the hepatic growth hormone receptor leading to impaired hepatic IGF-1 generation and decreased growth hormone bioactivity. Growth hormone and thyroid hormone have synergistic actions and potentiate the effects of each other on normal skeletal growth while acting on osteoblasts to stimulate bone remodeling. Involvement of growth hormone/IGF-1 and thyroid hormones can result in decreased skeletal growth, low bone mass, and low serum concentration of osteocalcin (4). Prolonged immobilization can be seen as a physiological stress and, as such, has been associated with elevated corticosterone levels and decreased plasma ACTH levels (102).

Hypercalcemia has been noted to be a particular problem in young adolescents who are immobilized for prolonged periods of time, particularly after spinal cord injury. However, there has been noted suppression of the parathyroid—1,25-dihydroxyvitamin D axis resulting in calcium loss as well as increased serum phosporus and an elevated phosphorus renal threshold (103). Additionally, losses of magnesium in both feces and urine during immobilization in rats have been observed, resulting in a negative magnesium balance despite replacement (104). Nitrogen loss has been studied for many years; urinary nitrogen excretion peaks in the second week of bedrest at 20–43% above baseline (25).

Volume-regulating systems are affected by head-down bedrest (HDBR) and likely, by extension but to a lesser degree, to bedrest. Sodium and chloride are excreted as volume is lost, reflected by weight loss. Potassium excretion is delayed but then is elevated for the duration of HDBR experiments. An elevation in plasma renin activity accompanied these changes as well as a decrease in autonomic responses, with a shift towards sympathetic control (105). A high sodium diet does not seem to stabilize this loss of plasma volume (106).

Gastrointestinal and Urologic Systems

Constipation and Abnormal Absorption. Intestinal absorption in generally is decreased during the period of bedrest (3). More specifically, calcium absorption decreases from 31% to 24% of dietary intake over 17 weeks of bedrest (107). However, bone resorption accounts for a large proportion of the hypercalciuria seen after prolonged bedrest.

Gastroesophageal Reflux After severe traumatic brain injury, there are many issues that interfere with normal ingestion and digestion of food. Both neurologically based and cognitively based dysphagia predispose the patient to aspiration and almost always result in the use of parenteral feeding via a gastric or jejunal feeding tube. There has been little study of gastroesophageal reflux in patients on bedrest and none on patients with TBI or stroke, but it seems likely that the combination of dysphagia, tube feeding and related gastroparesis, and bedrest would increase the risk. One study of all patients admitted to a hospital via the emergency department found that, while symptoms of reflux were reduced in the whole population, those on bedrest or who received non-steroidal anti-inflammatory drugs had increased risk of reflux-like symptoms (108). Patients with prolonged nasogastric tube feeding have demonstrated increased rates of esophageal damage (108).

Urinary stasis The recumbent position is associated with a reduced urinary flow rate and, although the difference in post-void residuals does not reach the level of significance, there is a trend toward higher volumes in recumbent voiding (109).

PREVENTION OF COMPLICATIONS

In general, it can be said that any mobilization is beneficial in ameliorating the effects of prolonged bedrest. From the limited work done on the effects of exercise during prolonged bedrest, it is apparent that both isotonic and isokinetic exercises help to maintain cardiac functional capacity (peak vO$_2$), and help to preserve the red cell volume and positive body water balance. However, these two types of exercise had varying effects on quality of sleep and mental concentration (isotonic exercise surprisingly seemed to impair both) and had no effect on orthostatic tolerance when the experimental subjects were remobilized (110).

Remobilization after prolonged bedrest of the elderly patient with TBI should be done cautiously because the effects on bone density will be magnified in this population. Exercise directed at the weight-bearing trunk and lower limbs should be approached in a graduated basis.

Adequate hydration and nutrition are extremely important in maintaining bone, skin, and muscle integrity during rehabilitation after TBI, especially while the patient is on bedrest. Hydration is often difficult to maintain in patients with spasticity, dysautonomia, and hyperhydrosis. Range of motion and good positioning of the limbs, trunk and head are essential in preventing contractures and preserving the ability of the patient to utilize neurological recovery effectively at a later date.

References

1. Chadwick J, Mann WN. *The Medical Works of Hippocrates.* Oxford: Blackwell; 1950.
2. Convertino VA, Bloomfield SA, Greenleaf JE. An overview of the issues:physiological effects of bed rest and restricted physical activity. *Med Sci Sports Exerc* 1997;29(2):187–90.
3. Bloomfield SA. Changes in musculoskeletal structure and function with prolonged bed rest. *Med Sci Sports Exerc* 1997;29(2):197–206.
4. Daci E, van Cromphaut S, Bouillon R. Mechanisms influencing bone metabolism in chronic illness. *Horm Res* 2002;58 Suppl 1:44–51.
5. Alzghoul MB, Gerrard D, Watkins BA, Hannon K. Ectopic expression of IGF-I and Shh by skeletal muscle inhibits disuse-mediated skeletal muscle atrophy and bone osteopenia in vivo. *Faseb J* 2004;18(1):221–3.
6. Zdanowicz MM, Teichberg S. Effects of insulin-like growth factor-1/binding protein-3 complex on muscle atrophy in rats. *Exp Biol Med* (Maywood) 2003;228(8):891–7.
7. Schneider VS, Hulley SB, Donaldson CL, et al. Prevention of bone mineral changes induced by bed rest:modification by static compression, simulated weight bearing, combined supplementation of oral calcium and phosphate, calcitonin injections, oscillating compression, the oral diphosphonate disodium etidronate, and lower body negative pressure(Final Report). San Francisco, CA:Public Health Hospital NASA CR-141453;1974. Report No.ntis nO. n75–13331/1ST.
8. Vico L, Chappard D, Alexandre C, et al. Effects of a 120-day period of bed-rest on bone mass and bone cell activities in man:attempts at countermeasure. *Bone Miner* 1987;2:383–394.
9. LeBlanc A, Schneider VS, Evans HJ, Engelbretson DA, Krebs JM. Bone mineral loss and recovery after 17 weeks of bed rest. *J Bone Miner Res* 1990;5:843–850.
10. Bloomfield SA, Girten BE, Weisbrode SE. Effects of vigorous exercise training and beta-agonist administration on bone response to hindlimb suspension. *J Appl Physiol* 1997;83(1):172–8.
11. Sato Y, Kuno H, Kaji M, Ohshima Y, Asoh T, Oizumi K. Increased bone resorption during the first year after stroke. *Stroke* 1998;29(7):1373–7.
12. Sato Y, Oizumi K, Kuno H, Kaji M. Effect of immobilization upon renal synthesis of 1, 25-dihydroxyvitamin D in disabled elderly stroke patients. *Bone* 1999;24(3):271–5.
13. Chiu KY, Pun WK, Luk KD, Chow SP. A prospective study on hip fractures in patients with previous cerebrovascular accidents. *Injury* 1992;23(5):297–9.
14. Jorgensen L, Jacobsen BK, Wilsgaard T, Magnus JH. Walking after stroke:does it matter? Changes in bone mineral density within the first 12 months after stroke. A longitudinal study. *Osteoporos Int* 2000;11(5):381–7.
15. Biering-Sorensen F, Bohr HH, Schaadt OP. Longitudinal study of bone mineral content in the lumbar spine, the forearm and the lower extremities after spinal cord injury. *Eur J Clin Invest* 1990;20(3):330–5.
16. Jaworski ZF, Uhthoff HK. Reversibility of nontraumatic disuse osteoporosis during its active phase. *Bone* 1986;7(6):431–9.
17. Tilton FE, Degioanni JJC, Schneider VS. Long-term follow-up of Skylab bone demineralization. *Aviat Space Environ Med* 1980;51:1209–1213.
18. Dawson-Hughes B, Harris SS, Krall EA, Dallal GE. Effect of calcium and vitamin D supplementation on bone density in men and women 65 years of age or older. *N Engl J Med* 1997;337(10):670–6.
19. Tilyard MW, Spears GF, Thomson J, Dovey S. Treatment of postmenopausal osteoporosis with calcitriol or calcium. *N Engl J Med* 1992;326(6):357–62.
20. Storm T, Steiniche T, Thamsborg G, Melsen F. Changes in bone histomorphometry after long-term treatment with intermittent, cyclic etidronate for postmenopausal osteoporosis. *J Bone Miner Res* 1993;8(2):199–208.
21. Grigoriev AI, Morukov BV, Oganov VS, Rakhmanov AS. Effect of exercise and bisphosphonate on mineral balance and bone density during 360 day antiorthostatic hypokinesia. *J Bone Miner Res* 1992;7 (Suppl. 2):S449–S455.
22. Zeman RJ, Hirschman A, Hirschman ML, Guo G, Etlinger JD. Clenbuterol, a beta 2-receptor agonist, reduces net bone loss in denervated hindlimbs. *Am J Physiol* 1991;261(2 Pt 1):E285–9.
23. LeBlanc AD, Schneider VS, Evans HJ, Pientok C, Rowe R, Spector R. Regional changes in muscle mass following 17 weeks of bed rest. *J Appl Physiol* 1992;73(5):2172–8.
24. Miles MP, Clarkson PM, Bean M, Ambach K, Mulroy J, Vincent K. Muscle function at the wrist following 9 d of immobilization and suspension. *Med Sci Sports Exerc* 1994;26(5):615–23.
25. Deitrick JE, Whedon GD, Shorr E. Effects of immobilization upon various metabolic and physiologic functions of normal men. *Am J Med* 1948;4:3–36.
26. Goldspink DF, Morton AJ, Loughna P, Goldspink G. The effect of hypokinesia and hypodynamia on protein turnover and the growth of four skeletal muscles of the rat. *Pflugers Arch* 1986;407(3):333–40.

27. Thomason DB, Booth FW. Influence of performance on gene expression in skeletal muscle:effects of forced inactivity. *Adv Myochem* 1989;2:79–82.

28. Berg HE, Dudley GA, Haggmark T, Ohlsen H, Tesch PA. Effects of lower limb unloading on skeletal muscle mass and function in humans. *J Appl Physiol* 1991;70(4):1882–5.

29. Hather BM, Adams GR, Tesch PA, Dudley GA. Skeletal muscle responses to lower limb suspension in humans. *J Appl Physiol* 1992;72:1493–1498.

30. Machida S, Booth FW. Regrowth of skeletal muscle atrophied from inactivity. *Med Sci Sports Exerc* 2004;36(1):52–9.

31. Morrison PR, Muller GW, Booth FW. Actin synthesis rate and mRNA level increase during early recovery of atrophied muscle. *Am J Physiol* 1987;253(2 Pt 1):C205–9.

32. Morrison PR, Montgomery JA, Wong TS, Booth FW. Cytochrome c protein-synthesis rates and mRNA contents during atrophy and recovery in skeletal muscle. *Biochem J* 1987;241(1):257–63.

33. Watson PA, Stein JP, Booth FW. Changes in actin synthesis and alpha-actin-mRNA content in rat muscle during immobilization. *Am J Physiol* 1984;247(1 Pt 1):C39–44.

34. Chakravarthy MV, Davis BS, Booth FW. IGF-I restores satellite cell proliferative potential in immobilized old skeletal muscle. *J Appl Physiol* 2000;89(4):1365–79.

35. Zarzhevsky N, Menashe O, Carmeli E, Stein H, Reznick AZ. Capacity for recovery and possible mechanisms in immobilization atrophy of young and old animals. *Ann N Y Acad Sci* 2001;928: 212–25.

36. Reardon K, Galea M, Dennett X, Choong P, Byrne E. Quadriceps muscle wasting persists 5 months after total hip arthroplasty for osteoarthritis of the hip:a pilot study. *Intern Med J* 2001;31:7–14.

37. Girten B, Oloff C, Plato P, Eveland E, Merola AJ, Kazarian L. Skeletal muscle antioxidant enzyme levels in rats after simulated weightlessness, exercise and dobutamine. *Physiologist* 1989; 32(1 Suppl): S59–60.

38. Lawler JM, Song W, Demaree SR. Hindlimb unloading increases oxidative stress and disrupts antioxidant capacity in skeletal muscle. *Free Radic Biol Med* 2003;35(1):9–16.

39. Kondo H, Nakagaki I, Sasaki S, Hori S, Itokawa Y. Mechanism of oxidative stress in skeletal muscle atrophied by immobilization. *Am J Physiol* 1993c;265(6 Pt 1):E839–44.

40. Hurst JE, Fitts RH. Hindlimb unloading-induced muscle atrophy and loss of function:protective effect of isometric exercise. *J Appl Physiol* 2003;95(4):1405–17.

41. Motobe M, Murase N, Osada T, Homma T, Ueda C, Nagasawa T, et al. Noninvasive monitoring of deterioration in skeletal muscle function with forearm cast immobilization and the prevention of deterioration. *Dyn Med* 2004;3(1):2.

42. Zeman RJ, Peng H, Danon MJ, Etlinger JD. Clenbuterol reduces degeneration of exercised or aged dystrophic (mdx) muscle. *Muscle Nerve* 2000;23(4):521–8.

43. Hespel P, Op't Eijnde B, Van Leemputte M, Urso B, Greenhaff PL, Labarque V, et al. Oral creatine supplementation facilitates the rehabilitation of disuse atrophy and alters the expression of muscle myogenic factors in humans. *J Physiol* 2001;536(Pt 2):625–33.

44. Dudley GA, Duvoisin MR, Convertino VA, Buchanan P. Alterations of the in vivo torque-velocity relationship of human skeletal muscle following 30 days exposure to simulated microgravity. *Aviat Space Environ Med* 1989;60(659–663).

45. Adams GR, Caiozzo VJ, Baldwin KM. Skeletal muscle unweighting:spaceflight and ground-based models. *J Appl Physiol* 2003; 95(6):2185–201.

46. Tesch PA, Berg HE, Haggmark T, Ohlsen H, Dudley GA. Muscle strength and endurance following lowerlimb suspension in man. *Physiologist* 1991;34:S104-S106.

47. Fournier M, Roy RR, Perham H, Simard CP, Edgerton VR. Is limb immobilization a model of muscle disuse? *Exp Neurol* 1983;80(1):147–56.

48. Kozlovskaya IB, Grigoryeva LS, Gevlich GI. Comparative analysis of effects of weightlessness and its models on velocity and strength properties and tone of human skeletal muscles. *Kosm Biol Aviakosm Med* 1984;18:22–26.

49. Sale DG, McComas AJ, MacDougall JD, Upton AR. Neuromuscular adaptation in human thenar muscles following strength training and immobilization. *J Appl Physiol* 1982;53(2):419–24.

50. Deschenes MR, Britt AA, Chandler WC. A comparison of the effects of unloading in young adult and aged skeletal muscle. *Med Sci Sports Exerc* 2001;33(9):1477–83.

51. Tabary JC, Tabary C, Tardieu C, Tardieu G, Goldspink G. Physiological and structural changes in the cat's soleus muscle due to immobilization at different lengths by plaster casts. *J Physiol* 1972;224(1):231–44.

52. Williams PE, Goldspink G. Changes in sarcomere length and physiological properties in immobilized muscle. *J Anat* 1978;127(3): 459–68.

53. Kannus P, Jozsa L, Kvist M, Lehto M, Jarvinen M. The effect of immobilization on myotendinous junction:an ultrastructural, histochemical and immunohistochemical study. *Acta Physiol Scand* 1992;144(3):387–94.

54. Booth FW. Regrowth of atrophied skeletal muscle in adult rats after ending immobilization. *J Appl Physiol* 1978;44(2):225–30.

55. Kvist M, Hurme T, Kannus P, Jarvinen T, Maunu VM, Jozsa L, et al. Vascular density at the myotendinous junction of the rat gastrocnemius muscle after immobilization and remobilization. *Am J Sports Med* 1995;23(3):359–64.

56. Jarvinen TA, Jozsa L, Kannus P, Jarvinen TL, Jarvinen M. Organization and distribution of intramuscular connective tissue in normal and immobilized skeletal muscles. An immunohistochemical, polarization and scanning electron microscopic study. *J Muscle Res Cell Motil* 2002;23(3):245–54.

57. Yarkony GM, Sahgal V. Contractures. A major complication of craniocerebral trauma. *Clin Orthop* 1987;(219):93–6.

58. Singer BJ, Jegasothy GM, Singer KP, Allison GT, Dunne JW. Incidence of ankle contracture after moderate to severe acquired brain injury. *Arch Phys Med Rehabil* 2004;85(9):1465–9.

59. Singer BJ, Jegasothy GM, Singer KP, Allison GT. Evaluation of serial casting to correct equinovarus deformity of the ankle after acquired brain injury in adults. *Arch Phys Med Rehabil* 2003; 84(4):483–91.

60. Pohl M, Ruckriem S, Mehrholz J, Ritschel C, Strik H, Pause MR. Effectiveness of serial casting in patients with severe cerebral spasticity:a comparison study. *Arch Phys Med Rehabil* 2002;83(6): 784–90.

61. Schulz H, Hillebrecht A, Karemaker JM, ten Harkel AD, Beck L, Baisch F, et al. Cardiopulmonary function during 10 days of head-down tilt bedrest. *Acta Physiol Scand* (Suppl 1992);604: 23–32.

62. Perhonen MA, Zuckerman JH, Levine BD. Deterioration of left ventricular chamber performance after bed rest: "Cardiovascular deconditioning" or hypovolemia? *Circulation* 2001;103(14): 1851–7.

63. Levine BD, Zuckerman JH, Pawelczyk JA. Cardiac atrophy after bed-rest deconditioning:a nonneural mechanism for orthostatic intolerance. *Circulation* 1997;96(2):517–25.

64. Convertino VA. Effects of exercise and inactivity on intravascular volume and cardiovascular control mechanisms. *Acta Astronaut* 1992;27:123–9.

65. Kamiya A, Michikami D, Fu Q, Iwase S, Hayano J, Kawada T, et al. Pathophysiology of orthostatic hypotension after bed rest: paradoxical sympathetic withdrawal. *Am J Physiol Heart Circ Physiol* 2003;285(3):H1158–67.

66. Mueller PJ, Cunningham JT, Patel KP, Hasser EM. Proposed role of the paraventricular nucleus in cardiovascular deconditioning. *Acta Physiol Scand* 2003;177(1):27–35.

67. Convertino VA, Hung J, Goldwater D, DeBusic FR. Cardiovascular responses to exercise in middle-aged men after 10 days of bed rest. *Circulation* 1982;65:134–140.

68. Convertino VA. Cardiovascular consequences of bed rest: effect on maximal oxygen uptake. *Med Sci Sports Exerc* 1997;29(2): 191–196.

69. Gaffney FA, Buckey JC, Lane LD. The effects of a 10-day period of head-down tilt on the cardiovascular responses to intravenous saline loading. *Acta Physiol Scand* 1992;144(121–130).

70. Saltin B, Blomqvist G, Mitchell JH, Johnson RLJ, Wildentahl K, Chapman CB. Response to exercise after bed rest and training. A longitudinal study of adaptive changes in oxygen transport and body composition. *Circulation* 1968;38(Suppl 7):1–78.

71. Sundblad P, Spaak J, Linnarsson D. Cardiovascular responses to upright and supine exercise in humans after 6 weeks of head-down tilt (-6 degrees). *Eur J Appl Physiol* 2000;83(4 -5):303–9.

72. Johansen JB, Gharib C, Allevard DL, Siguodo D, Christensen NJ, Drummers C, et al. Haematocrit, plasma volume and noradrenaline in humans during simulated weightlessness for 42 days. *Clin Physiol* 1997;17:203–210.

73. Convertino VA, Doerr DF, Mathes KL, Stein SL, Buchanan P. Changes in volume, muscle compartment, and compliance of the lower extremities in man following 30 days of exposure to simulated microgravity. *Aviat Space Environ Med* 1989;60:653–658.

74. Greenleaf JE, Kozlowski S. Physiological consequences of reduced physical activity during bed rest. *Med Sci Sports Exerc* 1982;14: 477–480.

75. Sun B, Yu ZB, Zhang LF. [Daily 1 h standing can prevent depression of myocardial contractility in simulated weightless rats]. *Space Med Med Eng* (Beijing) 2001;14(6):405–9.

76. Yablon SA, Rock WA, Jr., Nick TG, Sherer M, McGrath CM, Goodson KH. Deep vein thrombosis: prevalence and risk factors in rehabilitation admissions with brain injury. *Neurology* 2004;63(3): 485–91.

77. Turpie AG. Prophylaxis of venous thromboembolism in stroke patients. *Semin Thromb Hemost* 1997;23(2):155–7.

78. Carman TL, Kanner AA, Barnett GH, Deitcher SR. Prevention of thromboembolism after neurosurgery for brain and spinal tumors. *South Med J* 2003;96(1):17–22.

79. Rogers FB. Venous thromboembolism in trauma patients. *Surg Clin North Am* 1995;75(2):279–91.

80. Hamilton MG, Hull RD, Pineo GF. Venous thromboembolism in neurosurgery and neurology patients:a review. *Neurosurgery* 1994;34(2):280–96;discussion 296.

81. Meythaler JM, Fisher WS, Rue LW, Johnson A, Davis L, Brunner RC. Screening for venous thromboembolism in traumatic brain injury:limitations of D-dimer assay. *Arch Phys Med Rehabil* 2003;84(2):285–90.

82. Stein PD, Kayali F, Olson RE. Twenty-one-year trends in the use of inferior vena cava filters. *Arch Intern Med* 2004a;164: 1541–1545.

83. Stein PD, Alnas M, Skaf E, Kayali F, Siddiqui T, Olson RE, et al. Outcome and complications of retrievable inferior vena cava filters. *Am J Cardiol* 2004b;94:1090–1093.

84. Streiff MB. Vena caval filters:a review for intensive care specialists. *J Intensive Care Med* 2003;18(2):59–79.

85. Allman RM, Laprade CA, Noel LB, Walker JM, Moorer CA, Dear MR, et al. Pressure sores among hospitalized patients. *Ann Intern Med* 1986;105(3):337–42.

86. Allman RM, Goode PS, Burst N, Bartolucci AA, Thomas DR. Pressure ulcers, hospital complications, and disease severity: impact on hospital costs and length of stay. *Adv Wound Care* 1999;12(1): 22–30.

87. Allman RM, Goode PS, Patrick MM, Burst N, Bartolucci AA. Pressure ulcer risk factors among hospitalized patients with activity limitation. *JAMA* 1995;273(11):865–70.

88. Wywialowski EF. Tissue perfusion as a key underlying concept of pressure ulcer development and treatment. *J Vasc Nurs* 1999; 17(1):12–6.

89. Curry K, Casady L. The relationship between extended periods of immobility and decubitus ulcer formation in the acutely spinal cord-injured individual. *J Neurosci Nurs* 1992;24(4):185–9.

90. Ishizaki Y, Ishizaki T, Fukuoka H, Kim CS, Fujita M, Maegawa Y, et al. Changes in mood status and neurotic levels during a 20-day bed rest. *Acta Astronaut* 2002;50(7):453–9.

91. Gouvier WD, Pinkston JB, Lovejoy JC, Smith SR, Bray GA, Santa Maria MP, et al. Neuropsychological and emotional changes during simulated microgravity:effects of triiodothyronine alendronate, and testosterone. *Arch Clin Neuropsychol* 2004; 19(2):153–63.

92. Spielman AJ, Saskin P, Thorpy MJ. Treatment of chronic insomnia by restriction of time in bed. *Sleep* 1987;10(1):45–56.

93. Monk TH, Buysse DJ, Billy BD, Kennedy KS, Kupfer DJ. The effects on human sleep and circadian rhythms of 17 days of continuous bedrest in the absence of daylight. *Sleep* 1997;20(10): 858–64.

94. Chekirda IF, Bogdashevskiy RB, Yeremin AV, Kolosov IA. Coordination structure of walking of Soyuz-9 crew members before and after flight. *Kosm Biol Med* 1971;5:48–52.

95. Purakhin Y, N., Kakurin LI, Georgiyevskiy VS, Petukhov BN, Mikhaylov VM. Regulation of vertical posture after flight on the "Soyuz-6" to "Soyuz-8" ships and 120-day hypokinesia. *Kosm Biol Med* 1972;6:47–53.

96. Duchateau J, Enoka RM. Neural adaptations with chronic activity patterns in able-bodied humans. *Am J Phys Med Rehabil* 2002;81(11 Suppl):S17–27.

97. Kaneko F, Murakami T, Onari K, Kurumadani H, Kawaguchi K. Decreased cortical excitability during motor imagery after disuse of an upper limb in humans. *Clin Neurophysiol* 2003;114(12): 2397–403.

98. Semmler JG, Kutzscher DV, Enoka RM. Gender differences in the fatigability of human skeletal muscle. *J Neurophysiol* 1999; 82(6):3590–3.

99. Semmler JG, Kutzscher DV, Enoka RM. Limb immobilization alters muscle activation patterns during a fatiguing isometric contraction. *Muscle Nerve* 2000;23(9):1381–92.

100. Duchateau J, Hainaut K. Electrical and mechanical changes in immobilized human muscle. *J Appl Physiol* 1987;62(6):2168–73.

101. Bosco C, Cardinale M, Tsarpela O. Influence of vibration on mechanical power and electromyogram activity in human arm flexor muscles. *Eur J Appl Physiol* 1999;79(306–311).

102. Hauger RL, Millan MA, Lorang M, Harwood JP, Aguilera G. Corticotropin-releasing factor receptors and pituitary adrenal responses during immobilization stress. *Endocrinology* 1988; 123(1):396–405.

103. Mechanick JI, Brett EM. Endocrine and metabolic issues in the management of the chronically critically ill patient. *Crit Care Clin* 2002;18(3):619–41, viii.

104. Zorbas YG, Yaroshenko YY, Kuznetsov NK, Verentsov GE. Daily magnesium supplementation effect on magnesium deficiency in rats during prolonged restriction of motor activity. *Metabolism* 1998;47(8):903–7.

105. Grenon SM, Sheynberg N, Hurwitz S, Xiao G, Ramsdell CD, Ehrman MD, et al. Renal, endocrine, and cardiovascular responses to bed rest in male subjects on a constant diet. *J Investig Med* 2004;52(2):117–28.

106. Williams WJ, Schneider SM, Gretebeck RJ, Lane HW, Stuart CA, Whitson PA. Effect of dietary sodium on fluid/electrolyte regulation during bed rest. *Aviat Space Environ Med* 2003;74(1): 37–46.

107. LeBlanc A, Schneider V, Spector E, Evans H, Rowe R, Lane H, et al. Calcium absorption, endogenous excretion, and endocrine changes during and after long-term bed rest. *Bone* 1995;16(4(Suppl)): 301S-304S.

108. Newton M, Kamm MA, Quigley T, Burnham WR. Symptomatic gastroesophageal reflux in acutely hospitalized patients. *Dig Dis Sci* 1999;44(1):140–8.

109. Riehmann M, Bayer WH, Drinka PJ, Schultz S, Krause P, Rhodes PR, et al. Position-related changes in voiding dynamics in men. *Urology* 1998;52(4):625–30.

110. Greenleaf JE. Intensive exercise training during bed rest attenuates deconditioning. *Med Sci Sports Exerc* 1997b;29(2):207–15.

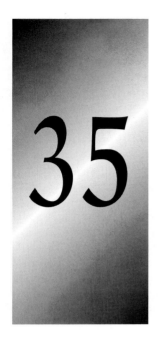

35 Assessing and Treating Muscle Overactivity in the Upper Motoneuron Syndrome

Nathaniel H. Mayer
Alberto Esquenazi
Mary Ann E. Keenan

INTRODUCTION

A lesion of the corticospinal tract produces an *upper motoneuron* syndrome (UMNS) (1, 2). Since the 19th century days of Hughlings Jackson, clinicians have classified UMN phenomena as positive or negative signs. Negative signs signified loss of voluntary motor behaviors (e.g. force production or dexterity of movement) that reflected *phenomena of underactivity or absence.* In contrast, positive signs such as increased stretch reflexes, spasms or co-contraction signified *muscle overactivity or phenomena of presence,* whether entirely new or merely enhanced beyond their normal presence. "Spasticity" was often used as a collective term for positive signs but, strictly speaking, spasticity is only one of many positive signs seen in UMNS (3).

In this chapter, we use "muscle overactivity" as a collective term for positive signs in UMNS because it captures the dynamic quality of excessive muscle contraction that is characteristic of the positive signs of the UMNS. The issue is not semantics. The pathophysiology of positive signs varies and so will their treatment. For example, co-contraction, likely of supraspinal origin, will differ in its treatment from clonus, a phenomenon of the segmental stretch reflex loop.

Studies have suggested that UMN muscles stiffen and develop contracture after being subjected to prolonged overactivity (4–6). Some have argued that such viscoelastic and plastic changes, termed *rheologic* changes, can be more dysfunctional for the patient than many of the classic positive and negative signs (7). We agree with this perspective because we view the ubiquitous presence of stiffness and contracture, commonly responsible for disability in UMNS, as a third sign of UMNS. Negative signs represent the broad issue of impaired voluntary control and, when control is absent, muscle overactivity creates unbalanced forces across joints that restrain range of motion and promote stiffness and contracture. In our view, clinical problems seen in UMNS result from a combination of impaired production and control of movement ('negative signs'), various forms of muscle overactivity ('positive signs') and a third sign of muscle stiffness and contracture (rheologic change). Moreover Herman has shown that muscle overactivity can be influenced by the stiffness characteristics of muscle. He studied 220 hemiplegic patients, divided into four clinical groups based on stretch reflex activity and physical extensibility of the calf muscles (4). Groups varied from an early hypotonic stage (group I) to a late "burned out" stage (group IV) that was characterized by increased tissue stiffness, lost range of motion and fixed contracture. For Group IV, Herman found reduced tissue extensibility to be linked with reduced tonic stretch reflexes. Increased resistance to passive stretch was due to changes in the physical stiffness of the triceps surae muscle. Patients with calf muscle contracture typically walk with difficulty. From a therapeutic perspective, treatment of contracture is very different from treatment of negative signs of muscle underactivity and positive signs of muscle overactivity.

POSITIVE SIGNS: 1. SPASTICITY

Spasticity is a term linked to stretch reflexes (8). It has a specific definition with respect to stretch reflexes but it has often been used confusingly as a collective term for all positive signs, many of which are not based on stretch reflexes. Strictly speaking, the term "spasticity" refers to an increase in excitability of muscle stretch reflexes, both phasic and tonic, that is present in most patients with an UMN lesion (9). Clinically, the defining characteristic of spasticity is excessive resistance of muscle to passive stretch. It is the nature of that resistance to increase as the examiner increases the velocity of stretch (10). Faster rates of stretch result in a sudden increase in resistance felt by the examiner after stretch has commenced. The afferent-efferent character of the stretch reflex was first identified in Sherrington's seminal studies (11, 12) on the cat's myotatic reflex which provided strong physiological underpinnings for later clinical descriptions of spasticity. The clinical character of spastic stretch reflexes is succinctly described by Peter Nathan (8): "Spasticity is a condition in which the stretch reflexes that are normally latent become obvious. The tendon reflexes have a lowered threshold to tap, the response of the tapped muscle is increased, and usually muscles besides the tapped one respond; tonic stretch reflexes are affected in the same way." The quick whack of a tendon tap resembles an engineering impulse function and the resulting brevity of the jerk response aptly classifies it as a *phasic* reflex, based on its phasic (transient) output response. In contrast, longer duration passive stretch of a spastic muscle induces sustained tension for the duration of stretch and reflects underlying stretch reflex activity of the *tonic* type. Resistance perceived by the examiner is elevated in the spastic state and varies with the velocity of stretch. If resistance develops suddenly during rapid passive stretching, the act of passive stretch may be interrupted for an instant and the examiner will feel a "spastic catch" phenomenon. Clonus develops under similar circumstances.

Physiologically, afferent information regarding stretch of the muscle and its muscle spindle is signaled to the central nervous system by group Ia and group II afferents. However, there has been no evidence to suggest that spindle afferent activity is increased in spastic patients (13). Rather, the central excitatory state of the cord appears to be high (14). A number of theories of spasticity emphasize the concept of signal "mishandling" at the level of the spinal cord. For example, Delwaide points out that the normal mechanism of pre-synaptic inhibition in the spinal

cord is altered for patients with hyperreflexia (15). Ia afferent activity from the muscle spindle is normally adjusted at a pre-motoneuronal level depending on supraspinal facilitatory influences and preeding Ia discharges. In spasticity, according to Delwaide, the interneuron responsible for pre-synaptic inhibition becomes less active due to a reduction of supraspinal facilitatory influences. Accordingly, the stretch reflex of the patient with hyperreflexia is no longer subject to tonic inhibitory control by the mechanism of pre-synaptic inhibition . Instead, all proprioceptive afferent impulses are able to gain direct access to alpha motor neurons and hyperreflexia results. Other theories of signal "mishandling" at the level of the spinal cord include Veale, Mark and Rees' work on Renshaw system disinhibition (16) and Jankowska's work on abnormal handling of group II afferent activity from the muscle spindle by a specific interneuronal system in the spinal cord (17). What is common to these theories is an enhanced central excitatory state that promotes exaggerated motor responses to ordinary cord input.

Lance characterized spasticity as an increase in velocity-dependent *tonic* stretch reflexes along with exaggerated (*phasic*) tendon jerk responses (18). The term "phasic" means time varying. "Tonic" has a time invariant quality, though time scales are always relative. However, the literature's use of 'phasic' and 'tonic' can be confusing because some authors describe the input stimulus as 'phasic' or 'tonic' while others describe the output response as 'phasic' or 'tonic'. *Tonic* stretch reflexes discussed by Lance referred to the output response of a muscle group that was being stretched at different rates of stretch. The output jerk response of a tendon tap was an example of a *phasic* stretch reflex. At the bedside, phasic stretch reflexes are tested by tendon taps while tonic stretch reflexes are tested by passively stretching a muscle group through the full (available) range of motion, repeating this manouver a number of times in order to vary the velocity of stretch for each repetition. When a patient is spastic, resistance to stretch experienced by the examiner will increase as the rate of stretch is increased. Physiologically, an increase in electromyographic (EMG) activity generated by the stretched muscle is observed, producing tension that opposes the stretching force of the examiner. Figure 35-1 illustrates stretch reflex activity in a patient with traumatic brain injury (TBI) undergoing passive stretch of the elbow flexors at different rates of stretch. Although the examiner, as he stretches, feels a unitary resistance, the reader can see that different muscles may respond differently to the same input stretch. The reader may infer that differential muscle responses may have different treatment requirements.

Stretch reflex activity of antagonist muscles may also be triggered during voluntary movement when a shortening contraction produced by agonist muscles on one side of a joint is necessarily accompanied by lengthening (stretching) of antagonist muscles on the other side of the joint. Paretic patients often move slowly so that velocity of stretch during voluntary effort is low enough to minimize spastic reactivity in antagonist muscles. In this regard, co-contraction is a phenomenon that can be confused with spasticity. Co-contraction is characterized by *simultaneous* activation of agonist and antagonist muscles during voluntary movement (19). Spasticity depends on muscle stretch and its onset occurs after movement has begun after some stretch displacement has already taken place. Simultaneous activation of agonists and antagonists is more easily observed on EMG records. (Figure 35-2)

2. CLONUS

Clonus is a low frequency rhythmic oscillation in one or more limb segments. (Figure 35-3) Clonus is generated by rapid stretch and hold of a muscle group. It may also be triggered by a patient who unintentionally stretches a

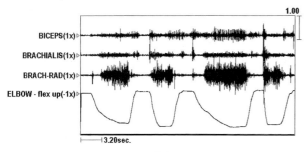

FIGURE 35-1

Passive stretch of elbow flexors performed by an examiner at different rates of stretch in a patient with TBI and UMN. As the velocity of stretch increases, more EMG is generated. Note, however, that different muscles respond differently to the same input

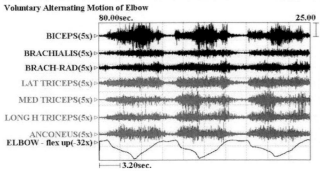

FIGURE 35-2

Co-contraction of elbow flexors and extensors during voluntary alternating movements at the elbow. The patient complained of fatigue and she felt as if she were "fighting herself" when she made these movements

muscle group during limb positioning (e.g. by mechanically stretching the calf when placing the foot on a wheelchair's footpedal). Clonus may be triggered during voluntary movement, for example, during a reaching effort when voluntary elbow extension triggers clonus in elbow flexors. Electromyographically, clonus is characterized by repetitive, rhythmic bursts of short duration electrical activity. Clonus occurs at typical frequencies of 6 to 8 Hz. Clonus can appear synchronously in one or more muscles. Clonus can also alternate between agonist and antagonist muscles. Figure 35-4 shows a patient with hemiparesis who was

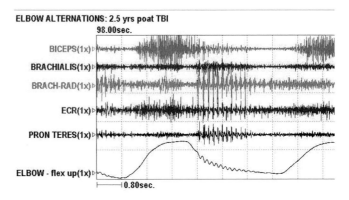

FIGURE 35-3

Illustration of clonus during extension phase of voluntary alternating movements of the elbow. Clonus is a low-frequency rhythmic oscillation, approximately 6-8 Hz, in one or more limb segments. This patient illustrates clonic bursts of EMG in brachioradialis, extensor carpi radialis, and pronator teres. The displacement trace reveals clonic oscillations of the elbow 'sitting atop' the extension phase of the movement

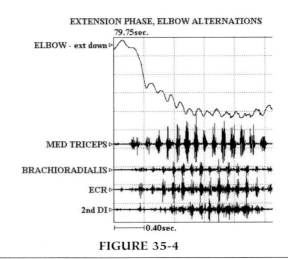

FIGURE 35-4

A patient with hemiparesis (gunshot wound of the brain) extends his elbow. Alternating bursts of clonic EMG activity are seen between medial triceps and brachio-radialis. Spread of activity to distal muscles (e.g., first dorsal interosseous) is also observed

asked to extend his elbow. Bursts of EMG can be seen to alternate between medial triceps and brachioradialis. In addition, spread of activity to more distal muscles (extensor carpi radialis and 1st dorsal interosseous) is also observed. Clonus may be sustained or unsustained and it can be stopped by re-positioning clonic muscles at shorter lengths. Clonus is usually associated with other hyperexcitable phasic stretch reflexes. In addition to rapid stretch, various cutaneous stimuli, especially cold or noxious stimuli, may give rise to ipsilateral or even contralateral clonus (20). Clonus may represent auto-oscillation of a hyperexcitable stretch reflex loop (21). Rack et al. viewed clonus as a self-sustaining oscillation of the stretch reflex pathway but they felt that the frequency of clonus was determined by physical parameters such as load rather than central neurological mechanisms (22). Dimitrijevic et al. were of the opinion that a central oscillator produced clonus (23). Therapeutically, dantrolene sodium, an agent that acts directly on skeletal muscle and muscle spindle fibers, is particularly effective for damping the low frequency ('low tone') oscillations of clonus. Unfortunately, it is not very effective in 'high tone' situations such as the high frequency drive of decerebrate rigidity after TBI.

3. CO-CONTRACTION

Co-contraction is another form of muscle over-activity seen in UMN that may be described as simultaneous activation of agonist and antagonist muscles during voluntary movement. Co-contraction can be activated and deactivated at a cortical level and is related to the switching mechanism of reciprocal inhibition in the cord (24). Abnormalities of Ia reciprocal inhibition have been reported for patients with UMN and co-contraction in such patients may represent an impairment of supraspinal control of reciprocal inhibition (25–27). Co-contraction may occur during isometric effort so that it is not necessarily related to muscle stretch. Figure 35-5 illustrates co-contraction during forward reach by an adult with UMNS. Simultaneous activation of flexors and extensors of the elbow is observed in the record. The movement trace reveals slow, unsmooth extension. Though co-contraction can be a normal mechanism to provide joint stability, in this case, the patient's elbow flexors appear to be exerting an unwanted restraining action because the patient struggled to extend his elbow clinically during reaching. Figure 35-5 reveals that brachioradialis and biceps activity occurred at the very onset of movement, indicating that early activity in these muscles was not stretch induced but was likely linked to the supraspinal reach "command". A key feature of co-contraction is that it is generated by simultaneous motor drive to agonist and antagonists during voluntary effort (28). When a co-contracting antagonist, undergoing stretch, develops superimposed spasticity, the combination has been called spastic co-contraction.

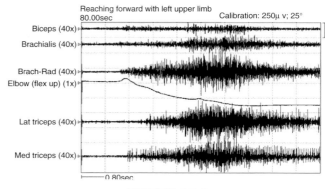

FIGURE 35-5

Co-contraction during forward reach by an adult with UMNS. Simultaneous activation of flexors and extensors of the elbow is observed in the record. The movement trace reveals a slow, nonsmooth extension trajectory (flexors restrain extensors)

Clinically, patients with co-contraction make slow, effortful movements. Speed of 'back' and 'forth' or alternating movement is often asymmetrical. For example, when a patient is asked to alternately flex and extend a limb, co-contraction of flexors during extension phase may prolong extension phase compared with flexion phase. We typically test for antagonist restraint by asking the patient to perform voluntary alternating movements about a joint for the full available range. Normally, alternating 'back' and 'forth' movements are symmetrical in time ('back' duration = 'forth' duration) and amplitude (endpoints or 'back' and 'forth' movements are at full range, respectively). Patients with restraining co-contraction, however, exhibit temporal and range asymmetries. Therapeutically, co-contracting antagonist muscles may respond to a weakening strategy (chemodenervation, tendon lengthenings). Among central muscle relaxants, only tizanidine has been described as having a potential effect on Ia reciprocal inhibition (29).

4. FLEXOR AND EXTENSOR SPASMS

According to Lance, a characteristic feature of UMN, both physiologic and clinical, is release of flexor reflex afferents (30). The flexor reflex, a polysynaptic reflex that results in flexor muscle contraction, is elicited by afferent stimuli collectively known as flexor reflex afferents. Among others, these afferents include exteroceptive cutaneous receptors responding to touch, temperature and pressure, nociceptors responding to painful stimuli, secondary endings from muscle spindles (group II afferents) and free nerve endings scattered ubiquitously over muscles that generate slowly conducting afferent activity in group III and IV axons. The polysynaptic flexor reflex has a prolonged latency (more than twice that of a monosynaptic tendon jerk) due to slow afferent conduction to the cord and also to central delay. In the cord, flexor reflex afferent activity travels up and down to synapse in the internuncial pool, a system of spinal interneurons that is influenced by inputs coming from peripheral as well as central sources including the brainstem. Compared to segmental stretch reflexes, the time course of polysynaptic flexor reflexes is slower and, unlike segmental stretch reflexes, flexor reflexes represent coordinated activity of motoneuron pools spanning many segments, resulting in muscle contraction across several joints, sometimes bilaterally. By typically recruiting flexor muscles across several joints, the flexor reflex is an example of an interjoint reflex that has tissue protective value such as enabling quick withdrawal from a noxious stimulus. Extensor reflexes are also polysynaptic and interjoint in nature and may serve certain support functions. Flexor and extensor reflexes may be core substrate for more complex coordinated patterns such as locomotor stepping generators.

After UMN, particularly after spinal cord lesions, release of inhibitory descending influences makes reflexes such as the flexor reflex more pronounced. When complaints are traced to flexor and extensor spasms, it is likely that spasms represent disinhibited flexor and extensor reflexes. A variety of overt stimuli can trigger flexor and extensor spasms or they may be set off by covert stimuli such as a full bladder, a stool distended bowel, a tight diaper, unseen skin ischemia from sitting or lying in one position too long and other unobserved or masked sensory sources.

Clinically, flexor reflexes can range from the familiar toe response of the Babinski sign to a mass flexor reflex characterized by intense, often painful interjoint flexion with spread to the abdominals. Patients may call them a muscle spasm but they mean whole limb involvement rather than focal spasm of a single muscle group. In UMN lesions, the elicitation threshold of the flexor reflex is reduced, the intensity of muscle contraction for the same stimulus input is increased and interjoint components of the reflex are often expanded (i.e. more muscles and more joints are recruited). Drugs such as baclofen and diazepam can inhibit polysynaptic activity in the cord and reduce the frequency and intensity of flexor spasms (but in TBI they may sedate (baclofen and diazepam) or affect memory (diazepam)). Excessive flexor withdrawal on ground contact can impair stance phase of gait for patients with TBI. Excessive flexion during swing phase can mimic steppage and impair advancement or subsequent foot placement on the floor.

5. SPASTIC DYSTONIA

The term 'spastic dystonia' originated with Denny-Brown (31). He examined postural reactions of monkeys after cerebral cortex ablations. Lesions were independent of,

or in addition to, damage to the pyramidal tract. When the bodies of animals with cortical ablations were held in different positions, their limbs developed fixed positions or postures. For all postures, any attempt by the examiner to pull the limb away from its fixed position was met by an increasing resistance of spring-like quality. The limb would 'fly' back to its original posture when released. Denny-Brown called this fixed attitude *dystonia*, meaning that the fixed limb posture was maintained by *active muscle contraction*. The continuous nature of muscle contraction that maintained cortical dystonia was present without the monkey making limb or body movements elsewhere and the dystonia did not depend on afferent input from the limb, since it persisted even after the relevant dorsal roots were cut. Moreover, EMG recordings of dystonic monkey muscles revealed sustained or tonic EMG activity and Denny-Brown thought that dystonia of this kind represented release of motor mechanisms that had direct access to alpha motoneurons. What seems clear, therefore, is that these dystonic postures were mediated efferently from above and had nothing to do with spinal reflex activity. However, what is not clear to these authors is the exact meaning of the term: 'spastic dystonia'. Denny-Brown himself pointed out that there were dystonic monkeys without spastic features such as increased tendon jerk reflexes. Nevertheless, he indicated that dystonia may occur in the presence of spasticity (enhanced phasic and tonic stretch reflexes) He referred to such a combination as "spastic dystonia". Many clinicians seem to use the term 'spastic dystonia' when they see a UMN patient with fixed limb postures (e.g. flexed elbow, clenched fist) in the absence of obvious stretch or voluntary effort. It is not clear, however, just from visual observation that a fixed posture is driven by sustained, supraspinal efferent activity-a necessary requirement of the term 'spastic dystonia'. We prefer to use the term when such a patient has tonic muscle activity, demonstrated by EMG, that maintains the limb in a fixed posture in the absence of phasic stretch or voluntary effort. Spastic dystonia is primarily due to abnormal supraspinal drive, characterized by an inability to inhibit muscle activity despite efforts to do so. Gracies et al. state that spastic dystonic muscles are sensitive to the degree of tonic stretch imposed on them (32). Figures 35-6 and 35-7 show a patient with right hemiparesis due to a brain gunshot wound who was asked to stand quietly 'at rest'. EMG recordings showed tonic activity in biceps and occasional activity in brachioradialis. Flexion posture of the elbow was persistent, the patient was not making a voluntary effort to hold the position nor was he undergoing phasic (time varying) stretch. Clinically, the patient had signs of spasticity. One might describe this patient as having 'spastic dystonia'. In Denny-Brown's sense of mechanism for this phenomenon, tonic biceps activity comes from supraspinal drive of alpha motoneurons. This is not so easy

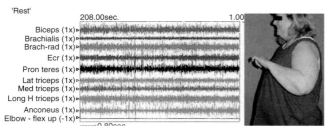

FIGURE 35-6

Spastic dystonia. This patient with an upper motoneuron syndrome and left hemiparesis was asked to stand quietly "at rest." The flexed posture of the elbow was persistent, and the patient readily acknowledged that she was not making any voluntary effort to hold this position. Persistent elbow flexion was her chief complaint. An EMG record during "rest" revealed persistent activity in many muscles about the elbow and forearm

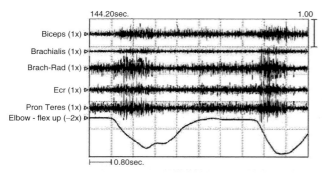

FIGURE 35-7

Passive stretch of the elbow flexors of the patient in Figure 35-6 revealed that her dystonic activity was stretch-sensitive. According to Denny-Brown, the dystonic phenomenon (activity at rest) is of supraspinal origin and is mediated efferently, not afferently. However, the presence of stretch sensitivity suggests that some patients may also have a component of spasticity

to prove, yet its assertion has therapeutic implications. For example, one would not expect central agents such as diazepam and baclofen, known to suppress spinal reflex activity, to be very useful for treating 'spastic dystonia'. Focal chemodenervation by botulinum toxin, neurolysis by phenol or direct contraction inhibition by dantrolene would seem to have stronger therapeutic rationales.

EMG equipment, if available, can help identify persistent muscle activity that may be consistent with a dystonic form of muscle overactivity. Without such study, clinical assumptions about the mechanism of a limb posture may be risky. A net balance of force created by passive tissue stiffness may be sufficient to maintain limb posture. Contracture can hold a limb in fixed position

as can heterotopic ossification. Finally, associated reactions can generate limb muscle activity that ends in postures reflecting a net balance of muscle forces acting across various joints.

6. ASSOCIATED REACTIONS

Associated reactions were first described by Walshe in 1923 as 'released postural reactions deprived of voluntary control' (33). 'Synkinesis' is a term used by Bourbonnais more recently (34). An associated reaction refers to involuntary activity in one limb that is associated with a voluntary movement effort made by other limbs. Associated reactions may be due to disinhibited spread of voluntary motor activity into a limb affected by a UMN lesion. Figure 35-8 shows a patient with left hemiparesis due to a brain gunshot wound attempting to readjust his sitting position by pushing down on the wheelchair's armrest with his right arm. The patient was unable to use the left upper extremity in this task because voluntary control was severely impaired. Dynamic EMG of elbow musculature during this activity revealed high EMG recruitment in flexor and extensor muscles about the elbow (figure 35-9). Despite elbow extensor activity, the photograph reveals *flexed* elbow posturing indicating that a net balance of muscle forces about the elbow favored flexion. The intensity of an associated reaction may depend upon how much voluntary effort is made. Dewald and Rymer thought that impaired descending supraspinal commands were involved in generating associated reactions (35). They hypothesized that unaffected bulbospinal motor pathways may have taken over the role of damaged UMN tracts during the transmission of descending voluntary commands.

Assuming that associated reactions are supraspinal in origin, one would not expect efficacy from central relaxants such as baclofen and diazepam. Depending on the contractile intensity of an associated reaction, dantrolene sodium, an inhibitor of muscle contraction, might have some therapeutic value. Tizanidine has known effects at spinal levels, but it may also act supraspinally by influencing activity in descending coeruleospinal pathways. Reports of depressed neuronal activity in the locus coeruleus by alpha-2 adrenergic agonist drugs have emphasized their impact on cord mediated reflexes such as flexor reflexes but not on supraspinally mediated behaviors such as associated reactions (36). The authors are not aware of reports regarding tizanidine and associated reactions in man.

The 'real life' impact of spasticity, strictly defined, may be less than advertised when one reflects on how often patients and caregivers might actually stretch spastic muscles at rates that would elicit intense spastic responses. We have commonly observed patients and

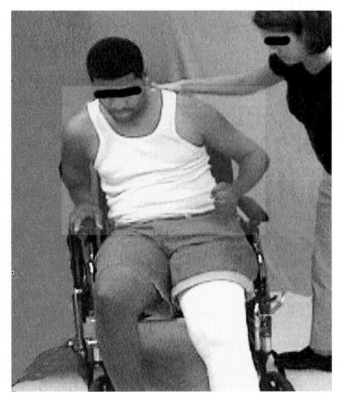

FIGURE 35-8

An "associated reaction" refers to involuntary activity in one limb that is associated with a voluntary movement effort made in other limbs. This figure illustrates an associated reaction in the left arm of a patient with left hemiparesis (gunshot wound of brain) who is readjusting his sitting position in the wheelchair by volitionally pushing down on the armrest with his right arm. The patient was unable to use the left upper extremity in this task because voluntary motor control was severely impaired on the left

caregivers performing limb manipulations at slow rates of stretch in order to avoid or minimize rate sensitive spastic resistance. In addition, what frequently passes for dynamic spastic resistance may be, in large measure, an increase in static stiffness due to intrinsic changes in the physical properties of muscle tissue. By contrast, frequent occurrence of associated reactions may be unavoidable in 'real life' situations because voluntary movement made by 'uninvolved' limbs happen all the time. High intensity voluntary efforts required during transfers, gait and activities of daily living might be expected to promote associated reactions as a high frequency form of muscle overactivity. For patients with UMN, it is conceivable that the everyday potential for generating associated reactions may contribute to the development of muscle stiffness and contracture more than spasticity does. More studies along this line would help.

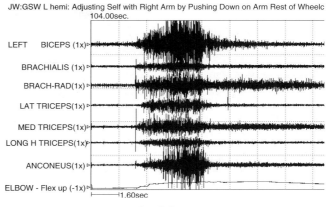

JW:GSW L hemi: Adjusting Self with Right Arm by Pushing Down on Arm Rest of Wheelc
104.00sec.

LEFT   BICEPS (1x)

BRACHIALIS (1x)

BRACH-RAD(1x)

LAT TRICEPS(1x)

MED TRICEPS(1x)

LONG H TRICEPS(1x)

ANCONEUS(1x)

ELBOW - Flex up (-1x)

1.60sec

FIGURE 35-9

Dynamic EMG study of elbow musculature in the patient of Figure 35-8 was performed during the same manouver of readjusting position in the wheelchair. Findings revealed high EMG recruitment for flexor *and* extensor muscles about the elbow. Despite elbow extensor EMG activity, the photograph in Figure 35-8 reveals *flexed* elbow posturing indicating that, despite extensor muscle contraction, a net balance of muscle forces about the elbow favored flexion posturing. The intensity of a limb's associated reaction may depend on the magnitude of voluntary effort made by the patient elsewhere

7. MUSCLE STIFFNESS AND CONTRACTURE

Muscle contracture refers to physical shortening of muscle length and it is often accompanied by fixed shortening of other soft tissues such as fascia, nerves, blood vessels and skin. Muscle *contracture*, an invariant physical state of fixed shortening, should not be confused with muscle *contraction*, a dynamic, variable state of internal shortening produced by sliding action of actin and myosin filaments within a muscle fiber. The development of contracture is promoted by a number of processes that start when an acute UMN lesion occurs: paresis impairs cycles of shortening and lengthening of agonist and antagonist muscles promoted by everyday muscle usage, the force of gravity generates positional effects on limb segments and joints, positional effects are created by a net balance of static rheologic forces across joints, and, as preferential muscle overactivity develops in particular muscle groups, a net balance of dynamic contractile forces promotes positional effects leading to contracture. Contracture implies that even if one blocked all muscle *contraction* by local or general anesthesia, physical shortening of muscle would still remain. Since central muscle relaxants such as tizanidine and baclofen, peripheral agents such as dantrolene, chemodenervation/neurolytic agents such as botulinum toxin/phenol affect dynamic muscle contraction only, a clinical picture dominated by contracture will not respond to these types of interventions. Physical and surgical methods are necessary to undo contracture.

TABLE 35-1

Common Patterns of Upper Motoneuron Dysfunction, Potential Muscles Involved and the Authors'
Botulinum Toxin Dose Ranges

The Adducted/Internally Rotated Shoulder	Flexed Hip
Flexed Elbow	Scissoring Thigh(s)
Pronated Forearm	Stiff Knee
Bent Wrist	Flexed Knee
Clenched Fist	Equinovarus Foot with Curl or Claw Toes
Thumb-in-Palm	Valgus Foot
Intrinsic Plus Hand	Hitchhiker's Hyperextended Great Toe

CLINICAL PATTERN	POTENTIAL MUSCLES INVOLVED	BOTOX ® A DOSE units/visit	# INJECTION SITES
Upper Limb			
Adducted/Internally	Pectoralis major	60–120	3
Rotated Shoulder	Latissimus dorsi	80–160	4
	Teres major	25–50	1
	Subscapularis	20–50	1
Flexed Elbow	Brachioradialis	40–80	2
	Biceps	60–120	4
	Brachialis	30–60	2
Pronated Forearm	Pronator teres	25–50	1
	Pronator quadratus	20–40	1
Flexed Wrist	Flexor carpi radialis	30–60	2
	Palmaris longus	30–40	1
	Flexor carpi ulnaris	20–30	1
	Extrinsic finger flxors	40–80	4
Thumb-in-Palm	Flexor pollicis longus	20–30	1
	Flexor pollicis brevis	10–15	1
	Adductor pollicis	10–15	1
Clenched Fist	Various muscle slips FDP	40–80	4
	Various muscle slips FDS	40–80	4
Intrinsic Plus Hand	Dorsal Interossei	40	4
	Lumbricales	40	4
Lower Limb			
Flexed Hip	Iliacus	50–100	1
	Rectus femoris	75–150	3
Flexed Knee	Medial hamstrings	50–150	2
	Lateral hamstrings	50–150	2
Adducted Thighs	Adductor longus	50–100	2
	Adductor magnus	50–100	2
Stiff (extended) Knee	Rectus femoris	50–150	3
	Vastus lateralis	25–50	1
	Vastus medialis	25–50	1
	Vastus intermedius	25–50	1
Equinovarus Foot	Medial gastrocnemius	25–75	2
	Lateral gasdtrocnemius	25–75	2
	Soleus	25–75	1
	Tibialis posterior	25–75	1
	Tibialis anterior	25–75	2
	Flexor digitorum longus	20–50	1
	Extensor hallucis longus	20–50	1
Hitchhiker's (Striatal) Toe	Extensor hallucis longus	20–50	1

After a UMN lesion, paralyzed muscles immobilized for long periods in a shortened position became shortened and stiffer. When muscle overactivity develops in these shortened muscles, tension is generated at shorter lengths. A lack of voluntary contraction in the antagonists of these shortened muscles prevents their natural re-extension, leading to a continuation of the process of stiffness and fixation. In the upper limb, for example, muscles that typically shorten include shoulder adductors and internal rotators, elbow flexors, forearm pronators, wrist, finger and thumb flexors and thumb adductors. However, other patterns are possible and observed. Familiar UMN patterns of deformity develop in both the upper and lower limbs (Table 35-1) (figures 35-10 and 35-11). The position of a given joint results from a net balance of static and dynamic muscle forces acting across one or more joints. Literature support of this idea comes from many studies. Herman described changes in the rheologic properties of spastic muscles in a large number of hemiplegic patients (4). Patients with contracture often had *reduced* reflex activity, yet resistance to passive stretch was high because muscle tissue had become physically more stiff. His study indicated that a description of muscle tone must consider the complex interaction between rheologic and reflex properties of muscle because stretch reflex properties of spastic muscle may be influenced considerably by alterations in the physical properties of muscle. Along similar lines, Dietz et al. (5) (stroke, cerebral palsy) and Thilmann et al. (37) have argued that hypertonia might not be related to exaggerated reflexes but rather to changes in soft tissues. Hufschmidt and Mauritz (38) proposed that abnormal cross-bridge connections could contribute to the resistance of passive movement and that these changes would very likely occur in muscles subjected to prolonged positioning. Akeson (39) demonstrated in animals that immobility led to stiffness associated with water loss and collagen deposition and Gossman (40), Herbert (41), Carey and Burghardt (42) have suggested that immobility imposed on a patient by the negative signs of UMN can result in soft tissue contracture. Other animal studies have suggested that when muscles are immobilized in a shortened position, some sarcomeres are lost and others become shorter and stiffer (Tabary (43); Williams and Goldspink (44); Witzmann (45)). Soft tissues other than muscle become less compliant in chronically shortened positions. It is for this reason that surgery for a severe contracture should not corrected for more than about half the lost range for fear of snapping nerves and occluding blood vessels. These soft tissues will require gradual physical stretching techniques postoperatively to achieve reversal of the second half of the range. Special surgical intervention for skin contracture may also be required.

Human biopsy studies of muscle with contracture have shown shorter fiber lengths for patients with cerebral

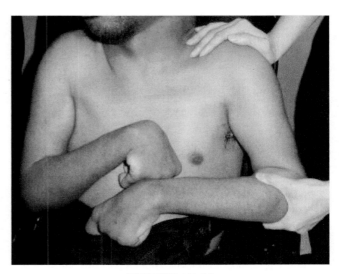

FIGURE 35-10

A familiar UMN pattern of upper limb deformity: adducted/internally rotated shoulder; flexed elbow; pronated forearm; bent wrist; clenched fist; thumb-in-palm. The position of a given joint results from a net balance of static and dynamic muscle forces acting across one or more joints that are promoted by a variety of UMN phenomena that are triggered frequently, likely every day (e.g., spasticity, co-contraction, flexor and extensor spasms, associated reactions)

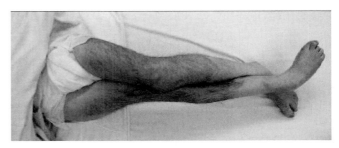

FIGURE 35-11

A familiar UMN pattern of lower limb deformity: flexed hip, adducted (scissoring thighs); flexed knee; stiff knee; equinovarus foot

palsy compared to normal (46). Shorter fiber lengths would have fewer sarcomeres in series. When antagonist muscle fibers with fewer sarcomeres are stretched during normal agonist concentric contraction, stretched sarcomeres become longer, compared with sarcomeres of normal fibers. During stretch, these longer than normal sarcomeres are thought to be the main reason that many patients with cerebral palsy have excessive passive tension in their muscles. A similar process might conceivably account for elevated passive tension in adults with UMN lesions. A different finding was recently described by Friden and Lieber (47) who found that single fibers taken from spastic subjects with cerebral palsy developed passive tension at significantly shorter sarcomere lengths than fibers taken from subjects without spasticity. Patient fibers were almost twice as stiff as controls and resting sarcomere lengths were shorter. Friden and Lieber found that the force borne by spastic fibers was similar to normal fibers, even though the cross-sectional area of spastic fibers was less than one third of normal fibers. Greater stress resulted when spastic fibers were passively stretched. Their study suggested that sarcomeres in subjects with cerebral palsy do not have to be stretched beyond normal lengths to develop excessive passive tension. From this perspective, their study challenged the assumption that tendon lengthenings or even stretching exercises that aim to allow a muscle to relax to normal sarcomere lengths will lessen passive tension to normal levels. Their study challenges the current theoretical framework which suggests that when muscle-tendon length is adjusted appropriately, sarcomeres will operate over a more normal range of lengths and there will be a reduction in passive tension and an increase in active force potential. Their study of chronic spastic muscle fibers (during childhood development) points to a process of considerable intrinsic structural remodeling of muscle tissue components that may not be easily reversed by current surgical or physical manipulations.

GENERAL COMMENTS ON THE APPROACH TO EVALUATION

Clinical Aspects of Evaluation   In broad terms, evaluation of muscle overactivity focuses on three issues: (1) identifying the clinical pattern of motor dysfunction; (2) identifying the patient's ability to control muscles involved in the clinical pattern; and (3) identifying the role of muscle stiffness and contracture as it relates to the functional problem. In Table 15-1, we identify fourteen common patterns of motor dysfunction, organized by joint or limb segment, that are typically found in patients with TBI who have upper motor neuron lesions. For each pattern, a number of muscles may be involved in motor dysfunction. Evaluation focuses on the characteristics of these muscles in terms of their voluntary or selective control, type of muscle overactivity, rheologic stiffness and contracture. Does the patient have voluntary control over a given muscle? What is the nature of a muscle's overactivity? (e.g. Is the muscle spastic? Does the muscle co-contract? Is it dystonic? Is it part of an associated reaction?) Does the muscle have increased stiffness when slowly stretched? Is contracture present? There are two or more muscles that cross each axis of most limb joints and each muscle can vary in its UMN characteristics. Since each muscle may contribute to movement of its joint, information about each muscle's contribution is useful to the assessment as a whole. We use dynamic electromyography to identify the characteristics

of muscle overactivity and voluntary control during upper and lower limb movements. We use anesthetic nerve blocks to identify properties of stiffness and contracture in particular muscle groups.

Technology Aspects of Evaluation   Laboratory measurement of upper and lower extremity motion is a cornerstone of modern analysis of muscle overactivity and impaired voluntary control of movement. Gait and motor control analysis of movement is capable of measuring specific contributions of muscles to movement by means of multichannel electromyography (dynamic EMG). Dynamic EMG is measured simultaneous with joint motion (kinematics) and ground reaction forces (kinetics). Force platforms enable the measurement of ground reaction forces during walking and standing and permit force vector analysis. Computations based on photo marker systems allow collection of three-dimensional quantitative motion data that provide information regarding range, direction, velocity and acceleration of limb movements. Clinical correlations and interpretations are significantly enhanced by slow-motion video that provides frame-by-frame display of walking and other limb movements. Measurement of passive movement responses combined with pre- and post-nerve block data allow for clinical interpretations of tone and contracture. What is abundantly clear, especially after TBI, is that clinical examination alone may be insufficient to identify voluntary and muscle overactivity characteristics of the many muscles impaired by UMN. Combined with clinical information, laboratory measurements provide the degree of detail necessary to generate practical hypotheses about findings that lead directly to the formulation of rational treatment interventions.

Considerations Related to Time Course of Motor Recovery   Evaluation and treatment will also depend on a clinician's expectation for motor recovery. We arbitrarily divide neurological recovery into two periods: an early period during which neurological motor recovery may be expected and a late period when motor recovery for all practical purposes has ended. In our experience, practical UMN motor recovery after head injury winds down significantly between six and twelve months after injury. Functional recovery is a different story. Even if many years have elapsed after a head injury, interventions aimed at improving function can produce practical changes. For example, a non-ambulatory patient whose base of support is severely compromised by equinovarus deformity during stance phase may regain ambulation through neuro-orthopaedic re-balancing of muscles crossing the ankle joint that change the base of support. Functional recovery may occur at any time after head injury provided that compensatory interventions are feasible and the patient has sufficient motor control to take advantage of the changes in biomechanical conditions.

Clinical Commentary on Treatment Perspectives Before 1980, little heed was given to cognitive, behavioral and psychosocial aspects of head injury. Patients with severe disability after TBI were not considered candidates for rehabilitation. Those with lesser disability who were admitted to a rehabilitation center were given physical rehabilitation, based on approaches used for patients with stroke and spinal cord injury. The pendulum shifted in the next decades toward cognitive and behavioral aspects of TBI as professionals began to recognize that families were more vulnerable to the burdensome effects of impaired behavior and cognition than they were to the effects of physical impairment (48). With a relatively reduced emphasis on physical rehabilitation, treatment of muscle overactivity was approached less aggressively. Drugs used in spinal cord injury and multiple sclerosis such as diazepam, baclofen and dantrolene were looked upon cautiously because of their sedating, fatiguing and weakening side effects. Surgery was typically based on inferences made from physical examination alone and was considered an option of last resort, often focused on reduction of severe deformity rather than increasing functional performance. Surgeons were not well acquainted with cognitive and behavioral issues that might affect their pre-operative decisions and post-operative care. Rehabilitation staff who dealt with cognitive and behavioral issues generally thought that surgery was an aggressive choice of last resort. Many nonsurgical physicians thought so too — especially since the experience of local surgeons with an interest in neurological problems varied greatly.

We believe that good conservative and surgical methods are available for improving function of patients with muscle overactivity. Psychosocial considerations and time course of motor recovery are important in the planning process. Most importantly, we emphasize focal analysis of muscles, joint by joint, that exhibit positive and negative signs of UMN because UMN pathology is highly variable. When TBI produces UMNS, the degree of voluntary function that remains varies greatly from muscle to muscle, even in the same limb segment. Factors related to poor production and regulation of movement need to be distinguished from those that reflect different forms of muscle overactivity along with rheologic changes. These distinctions may be based on physical examination alone but technology-based evaluations provide increasingly useful and objective support to complement clinical analysis. Treatment of motor dysfunction associated with UMNS is linked not only to muscle overactivity but also to concepts of voluntary production and control of movement along with rheologic change.

PATTERNS OF UMN MOTOR DYSFUNCTION

The varied forms of muscle overactivity in UMN lead to familiar postures of upper and lower extremity joints by virtue of a net balance of contractile and rheologic forces generated in time. Many common patterns have been presented in Table 35-1. We now expand them in bullet format below. The remainder of the chapter adds discussion of central muscle relaxants, chemodenervation and neurolysis. Finally, a special section on neuro-orthopaedics allows the reader to gain greater familiarity with this approach through details of the operative techniques it employs.

The Adducted, Internally Rotated, Flexion Restricted Shoulder

Description, Functional Consequences and Penalties

- S&S (signs and symptoms): shoulder adducted and internally rotated; some patients have hyperextension as their main problem; painful passive stretching of adductors is a common complaint
- PF (passive function): axillary redness, maceration and skin breakdown may be present; restriction of access to axilla for washing and hygiene is problematic for caregivers and patients
- AF (active function): some shoulder adductors are also shoulder extensors so, depending on the net balance of shoulder muscle forces, impaired voluntary flexion, abduction and rotation of the shoulder can make whole limb actions such as reaching, pushing, stabilizing and otherwise placing the hand in space problematic; difficulty raising the arm and placing the hand behind and on top of the head is common

Differential Diagnosis and Diagnostic Work Up

- Muscles that may contribute: adduction &/or internal rotation: pectoralis major (PM), teres major (TM), latissimus dorsi (LD), anterior deltoid (AD), subscapularis (SC); hyperextension or flexion restricting: long head of triceps (LHT), teres major, latissimus dorsi, posterior deltoid (PD)
- Taut tendons of PM, TM and LD palpable in the axilla; resistance to passive abduction, external rotation and extension of shoulder is typically high and often painful
- Restricted motion from capsulular tightness needs to be distinguished from increased muscle resistance; examine passive internal and external rotation with humerus at side of thorax and with humerus abducted
- Single voluntary movements: when passive exceeds active range for abduction, abductor weakness or adductor over-activity is suggested; when passive exceeds active flexion range, flexor weakness or extensor over-activity is suggested; when passive

exceeds active external rotation range, external rotator weakness or internal rotator over-activity is suggested
- Alternating (to and fro) movements: if voluntary abduction is slower than adduction, voluntary flexion is slower than extension, voluntary external rotation is slower than flexion, then weakness of abductors, flexors, external rotators and/or over-activity of adductors, extensors, internal rotators may be present
- With so many muscles potentially weak or overactive, dynamic EMG helps supplement clinical exam
- Radiographs should be obtained to rule out restricted motion caused by heterotopic ossification
- Local anesthetic blocks may clarify sources of restriction (muscles, over-activity, contracture): motor point blocks for PM, TM, LHT AD, PD; thoracodorsal nerve block for LD; access to SC is very difficult

Findings and Treatment Options

- Unmasked voluntary shoulder flexion and/or abduction and/or external rotation after diagnostic blocks improves prospects for placing the hand in space, especially for reaching
- Consider chemodenervation with botulinum toxin and/or neurolysis with phenol
- Use of phenol for large muscles (e.g. LD, PM) offsets the need to use large doses of botulinum toxin in such muscles, thereby preserving the use of toxin for many smaller, more distal muscles; PM, TM, LHT, AD, PD are amenable to both chemodenervation and neurolysis
- Limited change in range of motion after local block suggests muscle contracture and/or capsular tightness
- Drugs for pain and blocks for over-activity may help an aggressive range program for focal contracture

The Flexed Elbow Deformity

Description, Functional Consequences and Penalties

- S&S: riding up during standing and walking; fist and fingers may contact throat or face; pain on passive stretching
- PF: reddened, macerated elbow crease, skin breakdown; caregiver has difficulty with dressing, bathing; impact on balance during gait
- AF: restrained elbow extension during forward reaching; bringing objects to and from body is impaired

Differential Diagnosis and Diagnostic Work Up

- Muscles that may contribute to this deformity include: biceps, brachialis, brachioradialis and pronator teres and extensor carpi radialis

- Resting posture: elbow flexed, forearm more often pronated than supinated; ECR and PT may contribute when wrist is flexed, forearm pronated; an acutely flexed elbow can lead to stretch injury of ulnar nerve
- Very slow passive stretch establishes the available range of motion and the likely presence of contracture (fixed shortening)(Figure 35-12). Changing the velocity of stretch from slow to fast helps identify presence of spasticity. Ashworth test for spasticity: take joint through fully available passsive extension in about one second. Brachioradialis and biceps contractions, when present, are easily observed. Much more difficult to ascertain brachialis contribution. Dynamic EMG is useful
- When "single" joint voluntary extension movements fall short of the available passive range of motion, flexor overactivity is likely but extensor weakness and changes in physical stiffness of flexors must be considered
- When patient is able to do alternating voluntary movements of flexion and extension, timing and amplitude asymmetries can be identified. When extension movements are visibly longer in time than flexion movements, overactivity of flexors is likely, but extensor weakness and flexor stiffness may be factors. Amplitude asymmetries have similar implications. In addition, contracture may be present
- An effort to move the limb as a whole as in reaching for an object or pushing a door may exhibit flexor or extensor synergy (pattern overlay), either partly or fully. Pattern overlay, a centrally generated phenomenon, may be less amenable to relief by peripheral interventions

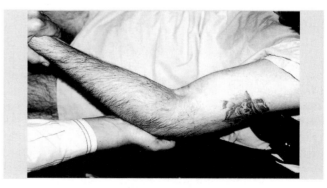

FIGURE 35-12

Example of an elbow flexion contracture. Very slow passive stretch establishes the available range of motion and the likely presence of contracture (fixed shortening). Contracture is a physical phenomenon and requires physical methods of treatment such as aggressive stretching, serial casting or surgical lengthening

- Radiographs are obtained when bony block and heterotopic ossification is suspected
- Musculocutaneous nerve block in the axillary region can help differentiate role of muscle over-activity versus contracture of biceps and brachialis. A separate motor point block of brachioradialis is required to determine its role. Flexor blocks may unmask voluntary extension

Findings and Treatment Options

- If range of motion improves completely after nerve blocks, muscle over-activity without contracture is likely the cause of the posturing
- An x-ray positive formH.O. establishes a mechanical block as likely source of motion impairment. Underlying motor control may be established using dynamic EMG (even if motion is not present) because the patient can produce alternating voluntary recruitment patterns in flexors and extensors respectively if they have good motor control
- Partial improvement in range or no improvement suggests contracture
- Serial casting may be considered, preceded by local anesthetic block or phenol block if a dynamic component has been established by maneuvers described above
- In the early period of recovery, serial casting, phenol blocks of musculocutaneous nerve and motor point of brachioradialis may be considered. Botulinum toxin is useful for biceps, brachioradialis and brachialis, even pronator teres and ECR can be elbow flexors by reverse origin and insertion
- Treating elbow muscular should be accompanied by treatment of shoulder, wrist and finger muscles, as necessary, as the limb should be thought of as a whole

The Pronated Forearm

Description, Functional Consequences and Penalties

- S&S: forearm pronates excessively at alltimes; passive stretching may be painful
- PF: may be difficult to passively supinate palm for washing, fingernail clipping due to tight pronators
- AF: impaired voluntary underhand reaching; patient has difficulty orienting hand to objects

Differential Diagnosis and Diagnostic Work Up

- Muscles that may contribute: pronator teres (PT) and pronator quadratus (PQ)

- Resting posture: forearm is pronated, elbow typically flexed by flexor muscles including pronator teres
- Very slow passive stretch establishes the available range of motion and the likely presence of pronator contracture. Since PT crosses the axis of rotation of the elbow, an extended elbow may increase tension in pronator teres. Stretching the pronators by passive supination at different velocities helps identify presence of spasticity. Tension in PT is clinically palpable but PQ is not palpable. Dynamic EMG is useful (Figure 35-13)
- When voluntary supination movement falls short of the available passive range, pronator over-activity is likely but supinator weakness and changes in physical stiffness of pronators must be considered
- When a patient is able to do alternating voluntary pronation and supination movements, timing and amplitude asymmetries can be identified. When supination movements are visibly longer in time than pronation movements, over-activity of pronators is likely, but supinator weakness and pronator stiffness may be factors. Amplitude asymmetries may also suggest pronator contracture
- Radiographs are obtained to rule out bony block, especially if forearm fractures have occurred
- MP blocks of PT and PQ (through the interosseous membrane) can be performed to distinguish between intense muscle over-activity and contracture but not usual to do so

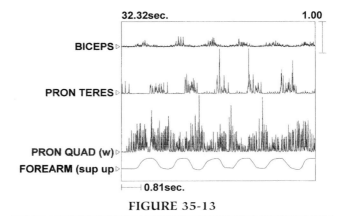

FIGURE 35-13

Dynamic EMG study of pronation/supination of the forearm. This patient with TBI complained of difficult reaching underhand. The record shows good reciprocal innervation of biceps and pronator teres.When the biceps is active as a forearm supinator, pronator teres is inactive. When the pronator teres is active as a forearm pronator, the biceps is inactive. The same cannot be said of pronator quadratus, which is active during pronation *as well as* supination. These findings are consistent with co-contraction phenomenon in pronator quadratus but not pronator teres. Treatment implication: focal chemodenervation or surgery should be aimed at pronator quadratus, not pronator teres

- Dynamic EMG helps identify patterns of weakness in supinators and overactivity in pronators

Findings and Treatment Options

- When dynamic EMG suggests overactivity in PT and/or PQ and contracture is mild or absent, consider chemodenervation with botulinum toxin
- When contracture is present, chemodenervation combined with serial casting can be used but casts must go above elbow and include the wrist
- When neurological recovery is no longer expected, consider surgical lengthening of PT and PQ

The Flexed Wrist Deformity

Description, Functional Consequences and Penalties

- S&S: wrist flexed excessively; passive stretching may be painful; pressure in carpal tunnel may lead to carpal tunnel syndrome
- PF: redness and possible skin breakdown in wrist crease; may create difficulty for caregivers during dressing
- AF: impaired wrist extension during reaching; ulnar deviation may be present

Differential Diagnosis and Diagnostic Work Up

- Muscles that may contribute: flexor carpi ulnaris (FCR), palamaris longus (PL), flexor carpi ulnaris (FCU), flexor digitorum sublimis and profundus, extensor carpi ulnaris (ECU) (consider when ulnar deviation is present), wrist extensors (weak)
- Wrist range examined with elbow extended to maximize flexor stretch (& simulate what would occur during a full reach)
- Since extrinsic finger flexors as well as wrist flexors can provide stretch activated flexion forces across the wrist, their respective contributions are sorted out by passive extension of the wrist with fingers held flexed by the examiner and with fingers held extended
- Passive stretch: bowstringing of FCR is common, PL often involved as is FCU; resistance to stretch is enhanced by holding elbow in maximum available extension; passive abduction with wrist in neutral reveals stretch activity in ulnar deviators (FCU and ECU); when resistance to passive extension of the wrist is enhanced by simultaneous finger extension, extrinsic finger flexor spasticity also contributes to the wrist flexion deformity
- Dynamic EMG is helpful in identifying whether wrist flexor overactivity and/or wrist extensor

under-activity is present during reaching and whether overactivity is present in superficial or deep finger flexors or in both
- When selective voluntary extension of the wrist falls short of the available passive range of motion, flexor over-activity is likely but extensor weakness and flexor physical stiffness may be factors
- When a patient is able to do alternating voluntary flexion and extension, timing and amplitude asymmetries can be identified. When extension movements are visibly longer in time than flexion movements, over-activity of flexors is likely, but extensor weakness and flexor stiffness may be factors. Amplitude asymmetries have similar implications. In addition, contracture may limit extension amplitude
- Motor point block of FCU and/or ECU can help sort their contributions to ulnar deviation

Findings and Treatment Options

- Consider chemodenervation with botulinum toxin for overactive wrist flexors and finger flexors without significant contracture
- When contracture and overactivity are both important limiters of range, chemodenervation and serial casting are considered. When chemodenervation is used, some delay before cast application may be necessary to allow for chemodenervation to take hold. Alternatively, proximal median nerve infiltration with local anesthetic can block not only most of the major wrist flexors but also most of the extrinsic finger flexors. Proximal ulnar nerve block can be added, if needed
- When additional neurological recovery is not expected, consider surgical tendon lengthenings and carpal tunnel release as indicated

The Clenched Fist Deformity

Description, Functional Consequences and Penalties

- S&S: fingers clenched into the palm, wrist most often flexed but some patients have an extended wrist that will exacerbate finger flexion by tenodesis: malodor and maceration are common; skin breakdown occurs when fingernails dig into the palm
- PF: washing, and maintaining a dry, clean palm, donning splints and gloves, filing and painting fingernails all pose problems for patients with a clenched fist and for their caregivers (Figure 35-14)
- AF: impaired finger extension during reaching; individual fingers or groups of fingers may be flexed; flexed index and long fingers impair object acquisition by web space on radial side of hand (Figure 35-15)

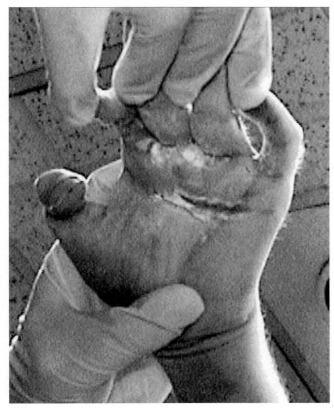

FIGURE 35-14

An example of passive dysfunction of the hand reflected by poor cleanliness and hygiene of the hand. A clenched fist reduces access to the palm for cleaning and leads to moisture retention, malodor, and tissue maceration

Differential Diagnosis and Diagnostic Work Up

- Muscles that may contribute: flexor digitorum sublimis (FDS), flexor digitorum profundus (FDP): intrinsic overactivity may be masked by strength of extrinsics; extensor digitorum communis (EDC) (weakness)
- Resting position: When FDP is overactive, fingernails are not easily seen as they dig into the palm; when FDS but not FDP is involved, the distal interphalangeal joint (DIP) is extended, the fingernails are visible and the proximal interphalangeal joint (PIP) is flexed
- Passive stretch: we examine with elbow relatively extended and wrist in neutral (when possible) so as not to be fighting overly tight wrist flexors; finger flexor tension is reduced by flexing the wrist and this allows assessment of intrinsic musculature (interossei and lumbricales) as well as finger joints for contracture; though many examine the group of extrinsic finger flexors as a whole, we prefer to examine FDS and FDP for each finger individually,

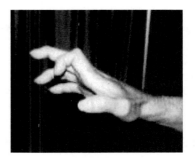

FIGURE 35-15

This photo reveals that individual fingers can be differentially involved in the clenched fist deformity. The flexed index finger and flexed thumb of this patient narrowed the web space opening on the radial side and limited the size of objects that could be acquired by the hand. Focal chemodenervation applied solely to the muscle slip of flexor digitorum of the index finger and to flexor pollicis longus is indicated

keeping in mind that FDP flexes the DIP joint while FDS flexes the PIP joint

- Dynamic EMG with wire electrodes helps distinguish behavior of FDS and FDP during voluntary tasks such as reaching. Dynamic EMG is also useful in determining intrinsic muscle behavior, especially when the stronger extrinsics dominate the clinical picture; wire electrode recordings reveal voluntary behavior of EDC
- When selective voluntary extension of the fingers falls short of the available passive range, flexor overactivity and weakness of extensor digitorum communis are likely. Contracture of finger flexors is also common
- When a patient is able to do alternating voluntary flexion and extension, timing and amplitude asymmetries can be identified. When extension movements are visibly longer in time than flexion movements, overactivity of flexors is likely, but extensor digitorum communis weakness is typical and flexor stiffness may be a factor. Amplitude asymmetries have similar implications. In addition, contracture may limit extension amplitude

Findings and Treatment Options

- Consider chemodenervation with botulinum toxin for overactive finger flexors without significant contracture.
- When contracture and muscle overactivity limit range, chemodenervation followed by aggressive ranging and serial splinting may be considered.
- FDS can be chemodenervated separately from FDP. Individual muscle slips of FDS and FDP can be identified by electrical stimulation through the injecting

hypodermic needle. We use electrical stimulation to guide chemodenervation of FDS and FDP because EMG guidance is less certain for these deep muscles.

- When additional neurological recovery is not expected, consider tendon lengthenings. A superficialis to profundus transfer is considered for a nonfunctional hand with major hygiene problems.

The Thumb-in-Palm Deformity

Description, Functional Consequences and Penalties

- S&S: thumb flexed into the palm at rest or with effort (Figure 35-16); thumbnail digs into skin
- PF: impaired access to palm for washing, donning gloves; psychologically bothersome appearance
- AF: impaired 3 jaw chuck, key pinch, other types of grasp; small web space limits size of objects that can be acquired by the radial side of the hand

Differential Diagnosis and Diagnostic Work Up

- Muscles that may contribute: flexor pollicis longus, and brevis, adductor pollicis, 1st dorsal interosseous
- Thumb range, tone examined with wrist extended and flexed; thumb intrinsics examined with wrist flexed
- Flexion of distal interphalangeal joint (DIP) suggests FPL involvement; carpometacarpophalangeal joint flexion with a flexed wrist points to potential involvement of FPB; a narrowed web space and adducted thumb suggests potential involvement of AP and/or 1st DI
- Voluntary thumb extension is tested with the wrist flexed in order to minimize FPL tightness
- Ulnar nerve block in Guyon's canal eliminates overactivity in AP and 1st DI, opening the web space
- If the web space remains narrow, muscle contracture is suggested; examine for skin contracture as well

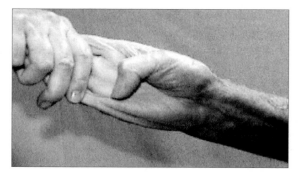

FIGURE 35-16

Example of a thumb-in-palm deformity. Flexor pollicis longus is clearly involved. Flexor pollicis brevis must also be considered because of flexion of the metacarpophalangeal joint

- Median nerve block in carpal tunnel eliminates median innervated intrinsics of the thenar eminence
- Dynamic EMG of thumb intrinsics and extrinsics may be useful in localizing muscle overactivity

Findings and Treatment Options

- If diagnostic block of ulnar nerve in Guyon's canal opens the web space, muscle overactivity without contracture is the likely cause of an adducted thumb
- Consider botulinum toxin for muscle overactivity without contracture
- If web space remains tight after block, muscle contracture is likely; examine for joint contracture as well
- During early recovery, stretching exercises, dynamic splinting, serial casting may be considered
- If FPL is overactive, consider botulinum toxin injection; stretch FPL contracture after toxin injection
- When further neurological recovery is not expected, skin, muscle and joint contractures may be handled surgically
- When thumb flexion is weak, fusion of the DIP joint may enhance pinch power; when thumb flexion is adequate, thumb extension by an orthosis with elastic properties is theoretically desirable but often difficult to fabricate
- Chemical or surgical relief of the thumb-in-palm (TIP) deformity can enhance 'hand as a holder' function i.e. the insertion of objects into the TIP hand for useful holding (without manipulation)

The Flexed Hip Deformity

Description, Functional Consequences And Penalties

- Flexed hip deformity during stance phases with forward flexed trunk. (Figure 35-5)
- Other findings include compensatory knee flexion during stance phase and relative leg length discrepancy with increased energy consumption. Limited hip extension with shortening of the contralateral step length. Hyperlordosis in an attempt to keep upright posture.

Differential Diagnosis and Diagnostic Work Up

- Muscles, which can contribute to this deformity, include the iliopsoas, rectus femoris and in some cases the hip adductors and pectineus.
- Hip range of motion should be examined with the Thomas test reducing spine motion. The Eli test will help elucidate the contribution of the rectus femoris to the deformity.
- The hip flexion may be caused as a compensation for equinus deformity and will be evident only during

walking but not confirmed by passive range of motion examination of the hip. Involvement of the rectus femoris may be clinically elucidated by observation of gait with knee extension and hip flexion occurring always together.

- Dynamic EMG is helpful in clarifying the contribution of rectus femoris vs. hip adductors and iliopsoas.
- Radiographs should be obtained to rule out bony deformity of the hip.
- Obturator nerve block or a motor branch block to the rectus femoris with local anesthetic can help differentiate the role of the hip adductors vs. iliopsoas or rectus femoris vs. iliopsoas.
- Increase stance phase hip extension following a diagnostic block helps to determine contribution from other muscles.
- Persistent hip flexion post block will point to the iliopsoas as the deforming force.
- Hip adduction deformity may be present in conjunction with flexion.

Findings and Treatment Options

- If a temporary nerve or motor branch block results in increased hip extension, muscle overactivity without contracture of the hip adductors or rectus femoris is the likely cause of the deformity.
- If the hip flexion persists and no radiographic evidence of bony involvement is evident, iliopsoas is the source of the deficit.
- Botulinum toxin could then be injected into the iliacus followed by stretching. If there is no change in the hip range of motion a contracture is determined.
- In the early period of recovery, stretching and botulinum toxin to control hip flexion is considered.
- If EMG studies or blocks demonstrate static origin to the deformity or sufficient time has elapsed for further neurological recovery, surgical intervention should be considered.
- Stretching of the hip flexors and strengthening of the hip extensors should be undertaken.

The Adducted Hip Deformity

Description, Functional Consequences And Penalties

- Adducted hip deformity during swing phase with narrow base of support. (Figure 35-17)
- Other findings may include associated hip flexion and relative leg length discrepancy with decrease stability in stance phase. Limited hip extension with shortening of the contralateral step length and difficulty with limb advancement in swing phase.

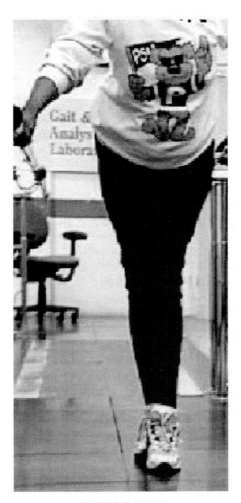

FIGURE 35-17

The consequence of an adducted hip is a narrow base of support

DIFFERENTIAL DIAGNOSIS AND DIAGNOSTIC WORK UP

- Muscles, which can contribute to this deformity, include the adductor magnus, adductor brevis and adductor longus, in some cases the iliopsoas and pectineus may be involved.
- Hip range of motion with hips in flexion and extension should be examined.
- Limitation in hip extension may be secondary to the limitation in hip abduction.
- Dynamic EMG is helpful in clarifying the contribution of the adductor magnus, adductor brevis and adductor longus and the lack of activation of the gluteus medius.
- Radiographs should be obtained to rule out bony deformity of the hip.
- Diagnostic Obturator nerve block with local anesthetic can help differentiate muscle overactivity from contracture.

- Increase hip abduction with widening of the base of support following a diagnostic block helps to differentiate muscle overactivity from contracture.
- Persistent hip flexion post block will point to the pectineus or iliopsoas as deforming forces.
- Hip flexion deformity may be present in conjunction with adduction.

Findings and Treatment Options

- If a temporary nerve block results in increased hip abduction, spasticity without contracture of the hip adductors is the likely cause of the deformity.
- If the hip adduction persists and no radiographic evidence of boney involvement is evident a contracture is the likely source of the deformity.
- Phenol or botulinum toxin can be used to achieve longer term relief of over-activity in the early period of recovery, stretching of the hip adductors and strengthening of the abductors should follow these interventions.
- If over-activity is severe, obturator neurectomy can be entertained.
- If blocks demonstrate a static origin of the deformity or neurological recovery has lapsed, hip adductor tenotomy should be considered.
- Stretching of the hip flexors and strengthening of the hip extensors should be undertaken.

The Stiff Knee Deformity

Description, Functional Consequences And Penalties

- Stiff knee deformity during swing phase with impairment of limb clearance. (Figure 35-3)
- Limited limb advancement in swing phase.
- Other findings include pelvic hick and trunk lean during stance phase and relative leg length discrepancy with increased energy consumption. Ipsilateral circumduction and contralateral vaulting as compensatory mechanisms in swing phase.

Differential Diagnosis and Diagnostic Work Up

- Muscles, which can contribute to this deformity, include the quadriceps, hamstrings, iliopsoas and gastrocnemius.
- Knee range of motion should be examined with the hip extended and flexed.
- The knee extension caused by the quadriceps is often noted by inspection during ambulation. Hip extension reduces the stiff knee deformity.
- Dynamic EMG is helpful in differentiating the contribution of muscles such as the vastii from the rectus femoris.

- Radiographs should be obtained to rule out bony deformity at the knee or hip.
- Femoral nerve motor branch block in the anterior thigh with local anesthetic can help differentiate the role of overactive knee extensors vs. hip extensors.
- Increase swing phase knee flexion following a diagnostic block helps to determine ambulatory potential.
- Persistent knee extension post femoral motor branch block will point to the hip extensors or ankle plantarflexors as the deforming force.
- Ankle plantarflexion deformity may be present in conjunction with stiff knee.

Findings and Treatment Options

- If a temporary diagnostic femoral nerve motor branch block results in increased knee flexion, spasticity without contracture is the likely cause of the deformity.
- If the knee extension persists hip extensors may be the cause of the deformity.
- If EMG studies or blocks demonstrate dynamic origin to the deformity, botulinum toxin injection or motor branch block with phenol should be considered.
- Botulinum toxin injection of the hip extensors should be considered.
- Stretching of the knee extensors and strengthening of the knee flexors should be undertaken.
- Surgery in the form of a transfer of the rectus to the gracilis and lengthening of the vastii is considered in late recovery.

The Flexed Knee Deformity

Description, Functional Consequences And Penalties

- Flexed knee deformity during stance phase with knee instability with weight bearing. (Figure 35-2)
- Limited knee extension in the terminal swing phase
- Other findings include pelvic drop and trunk lean during stance phase and relative leg length discrepancy with increased energy consumption. Limited knee extension with shortening of the step length.

Differential Diagnosis and Diagnostic Work Up

- Muscles, which can contribute to this deformity, include the hamstrings, gracilis, gastrocnemius and adductor longus.
- Knee range of motion should be examined with the hip extended and flexed.
- The knee flexion caused by the hamstrings is often noted by inspection during ambulation. Hip extension reduces the flexed attitude of the knee.
- Dynamic EMG is helpful in clarifying the contribution of muscles such as the medial vs. lateral hamstrings or the adductor longus.

- Radiographs should be obtained to rule out bony deformity at the knee.
- Sciatic nerve motor branch block in the gluteal fold with local anesthetic can help differentiate the role of dynamic spasticity with respect to contracture in this deformity.
- Increase stance and swing phase knee extension following a diagnostic block helps to determine ambulatory potential.
- Persistent knee flexion post sciatic nerve block will point to the hip adductors as the deforming force.
- Hip adduction deformity may be present in conjunction with flexion.

Findings and Treatment Options

- If a temporary diagnostic sciatic nerve motor branch block results in increased knee extension, spasticity without contracture is the likely cause of the deformity.
- If the knee flexion persists hip adduction may be he cause of the deficit.
- If there is no significant change in the knee range of motion after a sciatic nerve block, a static deformity i.e., knee contracture is determined.
- In the early period of recovery, orthotic management to control knee flexion is considered.
- If EMG studies or blocks demonstrate dynamic origin to the deformity, Botulinum toxin injection or motor branch block with phenol should be considered.
- Stretching of the knee flexors and strengthening of the knee extensors should be undertaken.
- Surgery in the form of distal hamstrings lengthening is considered for a static deformity in late recovery.
- A capsular release is considered if knee flexion is present while under general anesthesia.

The Equinovarus Foot Deformity

Description, Functional Consequences and Penalties

- Abnormal base of support during stance phase with weight bearing applied to the lateral border of the foot with pain and ankle instability with antalgic gait pattern.
- Equinovarus posturing in swing phase
- Other findings include hyperextension at the knee with recurvatum thrust (Figure 35-18), impaired forward progression of the center of gravity and relative leg length discrepancy with increased energy consumption.

Differential Diagnosis and Diagnostic Work Up

- Muscles, which can contribute to this deformity, include the gastrocnemius, soleus, tibialis anterior,

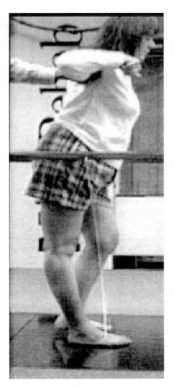

FIGURE 35-18

This patient has plantarflexor overactivity and contracture leading to hyperextension at the knee with recurvatum thrust and impaired forward progression of the body over the stance phase limb

tibialis posterior, extensor hallucis longus, extensor digitorum, flexor digitorum and foot intrinsics (Figure 35-19).
- Ankle range of motion should be examined with the knee extended and flexed.
- The inversion pull of tibialis anterior is often noted by inspection during ambulation. Hind foot inversion is often generated by spastic tibialis posterior.
- Dynamic EMG is helpful in clarifying the contribution of muscles such as the tibialis posterior and anterior.
- Radiographs should be obtained to rule out bony deformity at the ankle.
- Tibial nerve block in the popliteal fossa with local anesthetic can help differentiate the role of dynamic spasticity with respect to contracture in this deformity.
- An improved base of support following a diagnostic block helps to determine ambulatory potential.
- Persistent ankle inversion post tibial nerve block will point to the tibialis anterior as the deforming force.
- Curled toes may be associated with the equinovarus deformity and worsened by increase ankle dorsiflexion.

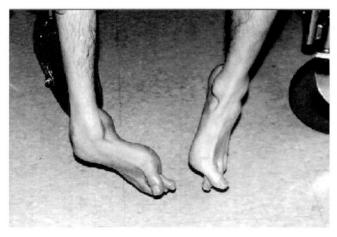

FIGURE 35-19

Two feet with equinovarus deformities in the same patient. As confirmed electromyographically, left foot varus was attributable to tibialis anterior overactivity. Right foot varus was driven by tibialis posterior overactivity. Note bilateral great toe hyperextension, variously termed: striatal toe or hitchhiker's toe

Findings and Treatment Options

- If a temporary diagnostic tibial nerve block results in increased ankle dorsiflexion, spasticity without contracture is the likely cause of the deformity.
- If varus persists in swing phase, the most likely cause is tibialis anterior and/or extensor hallucis longus.
- If there is no significant change in the range of motion after a tibial nerve block, a static deformity i.e., contracture is determined.
- In the early period of recovery, orthotic management to control equinus is considered, with appropriate components to control ankle inversion and toe flexion.
- If EMG studies or blocks demonstrate dynamic origin to the deformity, Botulinum toxin injection or percutaneous motor point blocks with phenol should be considered.
- Stretching of the ankle plantar flexors and strengthening of the ankle dorsiflexors should be undertaken.
- Surgery in the form of tendo Achilles lengthening or intramuscular lengthening is considered for a static deformity in late recovery.
- A SPLATT (Split Anterior Tibialis Tendon Transfer) is considered if ankle inversion is present during swing phase and is caused by tibialis anterior. If inversion is caused preferentially by tibialis posterior, a lengthening of this muscle is indicated.

Concepts in Pharmacological Intervention

Pharmacological reduction of muscle overactivity may be beneficial in selected clinical problems. However, drug treatment of overactivity is often a trade off against side effects. Three drugs, dantrolene sodium, baclofen and diazepam are commonly used to treat spasticity. Their use in TBI must be considered carefully because the side effect of sedation, though typically different for each drug, can be problematic for patients with arousal or cognitive dysfunction. It is ironic and sobering that patients with TBI, who often need help for muscle overactivity more than most, are also among the most sensitive to the side effects of these agents with respect to functions such as attention and cognition.

Dantrolene Sodium   Dantrolene sodium exerts its effect directly on skeletal muscle fibers. Physiologically, a neural signal to a muscle triggers a motor unit action potential that causes release of calcium from sarcoplasm storage sites within the muscle fiber itself. Calcium ions initiate cross-bridging of myofilaments and build-up of contractile tension. By inhibiting release of calcium from the sarcoplasmic reticulum, dantrolene sodium reduces the force of muscle contraction and, thereby, has the potential for reducing tension in overactive muscles. It should be noted that tendon jerk respones and electrically induced twitch tensions of muscle are reduced much more effectively than tetanic stimulation or sustained volitional contraction. In the latter conditions, the amount of calcium released into the sarcoplasmic reticulum over the course of continued stimulation of muscle by nerve activity (whether through volition or through electrical stimulation) tends to accumulate and overcome the inhibitory effects of the drug. This latter observation is important in understanding the utility and limitations of dantrolene sodium as a clinical agent. Dantrolene sodium may be useful in treating short duration, low frequency spastic phenomena such as clonus or brief spasms (49) (Figure 35-4). Phasic, small tension overactivity rather than tonic, large tension overactivity is favored for treatment with dantrolene sodium. Patients with TBI who have severe overactivity are not typically responsive to dantrolene sodium. Though its influence on treating spasticity is peripheral, dantrolene sodium apparently has a number of side effects that are central in nature and it can be sedating to patients with arousal dysfunction. Nevertheless, it may be a reasonable choice for mild to moderate overactivity, especially for clonus or other phasic behaviors involving many different muscles. Clonus often remits at a dose level of 50 mg q.i.d. though doses of up to 400 mg a day may be used. Cases of hepatotoxicity have been reported and liver function tests should be monitored, especially in those at risk for liver toxicity for other reasons.

Diazepam   This agent, centrally acting and highly sedating, increases the central inhibitory effects of gamma amino-butyric acid (GABA) (50). Diazepam appears to bind to receptors located at GABA-ergic synapses and increases GABA-induced inhibition at those sites. Antispastic characteristics of diazepam appear to arise from GABA-related inhibitory effects on alpha motor neuron activity in the spinal cord. Since diazepam also exerts sedative effects in the brain, some of its muscle relaxant properties may be due to diazepam's ability to produce a more generalized state of sedation. Although it is often successful in reducing spasticity of skeletal muscle, the primary problem with diazepam is sedation. Diazepam is not a suitable drug for persons with TBI who have attention or cognitive dysfunction. For patients who have persistent phasic flexor spasms that disturb activities of daily living or nighttime sleep, small doses of diazepam may be effective in reducing the frequency and intensity of these spasms with tolerable sedation.

Baclofen   This drug, a derivative of GABA, appears to act as a GABA agonist inhibiting transmission at specific synapses within the spinal cord (51). When used as an antispastic agent, baclofen ultimately appears to have an inhibitory effect on alpha motor neuron activity. It is unclear whether this inhibition is presynaptic (through inhibition of other excitatory neurons that synapse with the alpha motor neuron), or whether it is postsynaptic on the alpha motor neuron itself. Nevertheless, the net result of baclofen's action is to inhibit the firing pattern of the alpha motor neuron pool in the spinal cord with subsequent reduction of muscle overactivity in skeletal muscles.

Clinical research studies using baclofen for overactivity have primarily addressed the problems of patients with multiple sclerosis or spinal cord injury (52). Baclofen has been effective in these populations, especially when the clinical problem has related to flexor spasms. Oral baclofen is generally initiated at 10 mg a day in divided doses and increased to 80 mg or more as needed. Such high doses will invariably lead to side effects in many patients that can overshadow any benefits. In patients with TBI who are in a persistent vegetative state and are not expected to recover, high doses may be considered since cognitive and arousal function are not an issue. Nevertheless, on the remote possibility that the patient might be making some recovery, it might be wise to taper the drug periodically and observe.

Oral baclofen has been little studied in spasticity of cerebral origin (53). Meythaler et al. performed a retrospective review of 35 adult patients with acquired brain injury before and after starting treatment with oral baclofen. Twenty two patients had TBI and were found to have a change in Ashworth grade and deep tendon reflexes in the lower limbs. For the upper limbs, no significant change in Ashworth grade or deep tendon reflexes and spasm frequency didn't change in upper or lower limbs. The average dosage at follow-up was 57 mg baclofen (range: 15–120 mg/day). For the group as a whole, a 17% incidence of somnolence limited the maximum daily

dosage. The authors speculated that the lack of effect of oral baclofen on Ashworth scores and tendon reflexes may have been related to their observation that systemic delivery may have profound central side effects at brain level before it reaches adequate concentrations at cervical cord level necessary for affecting upper limb spasticity. Drowsiness, confusion and memory impairment are known side effects of oral baclofen and can be particularly troublesome for patients with TBI who already have impairments of arousal, attention and cognition (52, 54). A potential method for reducing central side effects is the intrathecal delivery of baclofen (ITB)(55), an approach for controlling hypertonia in ABI that has more extensive literature than oral ingestion. A drug pump is implanted subcutaneously to infuse baclofen into the lumbar subarachnoid space. Compared with oral administration, the pump allows much smaller doses of baclofen to be used (56–58). Side effects are reduced and effectiveness in refractory cases is enhanced (53). The pump has an eighteen milliliter reservoir, connected to an intrathecal catheter, that is refilled periodically by percutaneous puncture. The rate of baclofen infusion is adjusted by an external computer. The most common adverse effects of ITB include hypotonia, drowsiness, dizziness, nausea, vomiting, hypotension and headache (59, 60). Life-threatening complications associated with overdose or withdrawal have occurred, linked to mechanical failure or human error. (61–64) Intrathecal overdose can cause coma and respiratory depression. Sudden withdrawal of the drug (e.g. by unrecognized pump failure) can cause an exaggeration of spasticity along with hallucinations and seizures. The system is expensive and potentially hazardous when technical problems arise. However, the pump system may be useful for patients who have regional muscle over-activity distributed across many lower extremity muscle groups, especially bilateral hip flexor, adductor and hamstrings groups. Most studies with ITB (as with oral baclofen) have focused on the evaluation of stretch reflexes and spasms and active function has not been systematically investigated (53, 65). In a pilot study, Francisco and Boake reported an improvement in walking speed in 10 patients with poststroke spastic hemiplegia after ITB in combination with physical therapy.

Tizanidine   Tizanidine has muscle relaxant properties, acting as an agonist at alpha-2 adrenergic receptor sites both spinally and supraspinally. Placebo-controlled studies have shown that tizanidine reduces muscle response to passive stretch in both the spinal and cerebral forms of spasticity including patients with TBI (66–68). Tizanidine does not appear to confer functional changes (67, 69). Adverse effects have included hypotension, sedation, generalized fatigue, falls, dry mouth, reduced renal clearance and the potential for hepatotoxicity and hypotension (70). Sedation, a particular problem for patients with TBI, is the commonest adverse effect, occurring in almost 50% of patients who use it (71). The amount of tizanidine that a clinician can use for patients with TBI is necesserily curtailed by its side effects, particularly drowsiness. Hence, its therapeutic effect for muscle overactivity is often limited. In addition to spastic stretch reflexes, tizanidine has been shown to have a physiologic effect on co-contraction, a common positive sign of UMN activity that hampers voluntary movement (29).

Botulinum Neurotoxin (BoNT)

Pharmacological management of muscle over-activity often requires a balance between acceptable reduction in over-activity and acceptable side effects. From this perspective, botulinum neurotoxin (BoNT) is an excellent therapeutic agent because of its focal action without significant side effects. A number of double-blind, placebo-controlled studies have reported significant reductions in muscle tone for patients with acquired brain injury, primarily stroke (72–74). Yablon et al. performed an open-label study of 21 patients with TBI who had severe wrist and finger flexor spasticity (75). Improvements were seen in range of motion at the wrist and in the modified Ashworth scale. There were no significant side effects. Brashear, Gordon, Elovic et al. performed a large scale multi-center trial that was a randomized, double-blind, placebo-controlled study of BoNT A in persons with spasticity of the wrist and finger flexors after a stroke (76). The study assessed efficacy and safety of BoNT A in 126 subjects who received a one-time injection of 200 to 240 units. The primary outcome measure was self-reported disability in four areas: personal hygiene, dressing, pain and limb position at six weeks. At base line, each subject selected one of these areas as the principal target of treatment. Based on Ashworth scores, they found significantly greater improvement in subjects treated with BoNT A in wrist and finger flexor tone at all follow-up visits through 12 weeks than did subjects who received placebo. In addition, subjects treated with BoNT A had greater improvement in the principal target of treatment at weeks 4, 6, 8 and 12. There were no major adverse events associated with injection of the neurotoxin. Brashear, Zafonte, Corcoran et al. demonstrated inter- and intrarater reliability for the the Disability Assessment Scale as well as for the Ashworth Scale applied to elbow, wrist, finger and thumb flexors of poststroke patients (77). Brashear et al. have reported results of an open-label, single-treatment session using BoNT B (MyoBloc; Elan) in 10 patients with upper limb spasticity (elbow, wrist, fingers) (78). Improvements in Ashworth scores as well as global assessment changes by investigators and patients were obtained. Nine of 10 subjects reported dry mouth at week 4 of the study with resolution by week 12. No changes were seen on functional measures.

BONT type A (BoNT A) is injected directly into affected muscle groups, usually under electromyographic or electrical stimulation guidance, causing reversible, dose-dependent muscle relaxation by blocking acetylcholine release at the neuromuscular junction (Figures 35-20 and 35-21). The purpose of toxin injection is to reduce force generated by UMN muscle over-activity in order to create a more favorable net balance of forces acting across joints (Figures 35-22 and 35-23). When target muscles are identified, the toxin's localized inhibitory effect makes it a very useful agent for carrying out focal strategies for managing muscle over-activity. A reduction in excessive tension can lead to improvement in passive and active range of motion and allows for more successful stretching of dynamically and statically tight musculature. More subtly, and more importantly, a patient's improved control over movement and posture may allow for compensatory behaviors during functional activities that rely on active as opposed to passive movement. A reduction in muscle over-activity in one muscle group may have consequences for tone in other muscle groups of the limb through a reduction in the overall effort required to perform movement and/or possibly through changes in sensory information going to the central nervous system from that limb.

In contrast to phenol or alcohol, exposure to the toxin causes reversible denervation atrophy without fibrosis. There are seven serologically distinct toxins produced by *Clostridium botulinum* that are potent

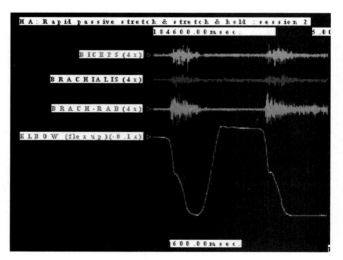

FIGURE 35-20

Prior to injection of BoNT A: Rapid passive stretch of elbow flexors followed by rapid passive stretch and hold in a patient with TBI and hemiparesis reveals spastic reactivity in all three elbow flexors during dynamic stretch. Tonic activity is also seen in brachioradialis during static stretch ("hold" phase). Bottom movement trace shows a "spastic catch" midway during displacement

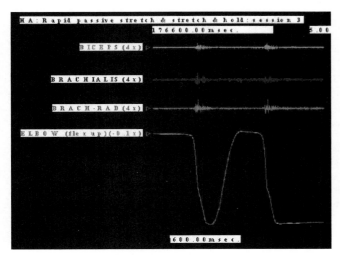

FIGURE 35-21

Biceps was injected with 120 units BoNT A (Botox®); brachioradialis was injected with 80 units. The figure is a 22-day follow-up study: Note marked reduction in stretch reflex activity and absence of "spastic catch" in the movement trace. as reflected in EMG of all flexors during stretch. BoNT A inhibits muscle contraction by blocking acetylcholine release at the neuromuscular junction

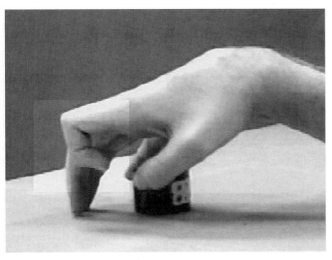

FIGURE 35-22

Flexed index finger during reach to grasp in a 22-year-old woman two years after TBI. Muscle overactivity on the radial side of the hand impairs access of objects into the webspace of the hand

neuroparalytic agents and these are designated as BoNT A, B, C, D, E, F and G. Only two types (A and B) are available for therapeutic human use. BoNT type A is synthesized as single chain polypeptides with a molecular mass of approximately 150 kDa. Neurotoxin activation

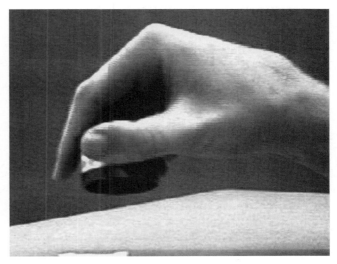

FIGURE 35-23

Twenty-two days after injection of 20 units BoNT A (Botox®) into isolated muscle fascicles of flexor digitorum profundus and flexor digitorum sublimis of the index finger. Access to the webspace was improved and objects were more easily grasped

requires a two-step modification in the structure of the protein. In the first step, the parent chain is cleaved. The result is the formation of a heavy chain tethered by a disulfide bond to a light chain that is associated with one atom of zinc. The second activation step, disulfide reduction requires internalization by the target cell. The toxin must enter the endplate zone to exert its effect. The process is partially dependent on nerve stimulation and independent of Ca^{2+} concentration. A commercial form of BoNT A in the United States (US) is Botox® [Allergan] which is currently approved by the US Food & Drug Administration (FDA) for the treatment of blepharospasm, facial spasm, strabismus, cervical dystonia and torticollis and certain cosmetic uses. BoNT B is branded as MyoBloc [Solstice] and is approved for the treatment of cervical dystonia in the US. Dysport is a different (non-interchangeable) version of BoNT A that is available in Europe and elsewhere but not the US. In Europe and Canada, BoNT A is also approved for the management of spasticity secondary to cerebral palsy and stroke.

Patients may begin to experience benefits three to seven days after injection. The duration of action in the management of muscle overactivity is about three to four months, after which re-injection is indicated. Reported adverse effects have included excessive weakness of injected muscles, pain at injection site, local irritation, headache, fatigue and flu-like symptoms. No anaphylactic response has ever been reported due to BoNT A injection. Treatment success, in part, depends on the skill of the injector. Muscle selection, injection technique and dose must be individualized. (see Table 35-1)

Nerve Blocks   Nerve and motor point blocks are very useful in targeting specific muscles or muscle groups for diagnostic and therapeutic maneuvers. The purpose of the nerve or motor point block is to reduce force produced by a contracting spastic muscle or muscle group. A reduction in spastic tension can lead to improvement in passive and active range of motion and allows for more successful stretching of tight musculature. More subtly, and more importantly too, a patient's improved control over movement and posture may allow for compensatory behaviors during functional activities. A reduction in spastic activity in one muscle or muscle group may have consequences for tone in other muscle groups of the limb through a reduction in the overall effort required to perform movement and/or through changes in sensory information going to the central nervous system from that limb. Finally, the application of external devices such as braces, casts, even shoes, can be facilitated by nerve and motor point blocks.

Blocks may be classified broadly as diagnostic or therapeutic in nature. Diagnostic blocks are typically performed with short acting local anesthetics such as lidocaine or bupivacaine. These quick acting, short duration agents allow the examiner to evaluate factors described above such as passive range of motion, muscle stiffness unrelated to overactivity, changes in active range of motion when dynamic resistance is blocked, and enhanced motor control during functional movements. For example, a patient with overactive adductors causing scissoring during gait may be prone to fall because of the narrow base of support. A temporary block of the obturator nerve with 2% lidocaine will allow the examiner to observe whether the base of support widens and stability improves. The key to understanding the use of a diagnostic nerve block is that it be used to test a hypothesis. In the given example, the hypothesis behind the obturator nerve block is that the base of support was narrowed by excessive adduction of the leg caused by spastic adductors. It was further postulated that a wider base of support would lead to greater stability during dynamic gait. After the nerve block is performed with a quick-acting local anesthetic, the patient is ambulated in order to test the hypotheses about widening the base of support and improving stability during ambulation. If improved ambulation results, then more permanent (i.e. less reversible) types of intervention may be contemplated with a greater sense of outcome prediction. Therefore, the prediction of a likely outcome for an intervetnion is an important feature of temporary nerve or motor point blocks. In the given example, it is possible that the base of support might not widen. For example, a severe adductor contracture will not remit after a nerve block. However, this information is useful in designing the next step in the treatment program. Similarly, it is possible that the nerve block may be physiologically successful, spasticity

of the adductors are blocked, and the base of support widens. Yet the overall gait pattern is only partially improved because instability was coming from other sources of neuromuscular neurological impairment. Again, this kind of information can lead to further diagnostic testing of other hypotheses relevant to why the patient has an ambulation dysfunction.

Therapeutic nerve and motor point blocks are primarily performed with aqueous solutions of phenol. When it is injected in or near a nerve bundle, phenol denatures protein in the myelin sheath or cell membrane of axons with which it makes contact. When administered in the operating room under direct nerve visualization, phenol is instilled directly into the nerve bundle in a glycerin solution to minimize leakage. Related to this technique, the desired motor nerves are identified by electrical stimulation prior to injection, mixed nerves with sensory and motor fibers are avoided because of consequent dysesthesias, and the duration of effect is often six months or more because the injection of the nerve is so direct. An aqueous solution of phenol, on the other hand, is the medium used for percutaneous injection in the laboratory or at the bedside and the location of the nerve is approximated by an electrical stimulation technique which typically results in variable contact of phenol with axons (Figure 35-24). This variability is a key factor in the duration of effectiveness of a percutaneous phenol nerve or motor point block. As Glenn has indicated, a peripheral

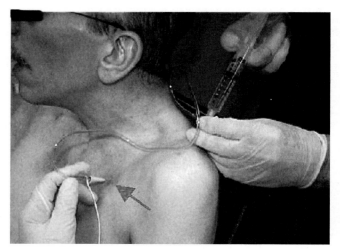

FIGURE 35-24

Phenol injection into a motor point of pectoralis major. A motor point is defined electrophysiologically rather than by anatomy. It is the most distal location of a motor nerve at which electrical current produces a visible or palpable contraction of muscle. The hypodermic needle in the photo is insulated on the outside and has a conductive core on the inside. When connected to an electrical stimulator, the needle is used to find a motor point and, when found, to inject phenol into the region of the motor point

nerve block is more likely to last longer than a block of a motor point [a motor nerve branch located much closer to a muscle than the more proximal peripheral nerve]. Phenol neurolysis of peripheral nerve may result in Wallerian degeneration. Re-innervation probably takes longer for the proximally blocked peripheral nerve because it has a longer distance for axoplasm to advance in order to reach muscle compared with the re-innervation distance of nerve blocked at the more distal motor point. The smaller size of the nerve involved in a motor point block may also make it harder to localize percutanously. In addition, if a mixed sensory-motor nerve is selected for phenolization [typically in a low level patient where there is less concern about consequent dysesthesia], a reduction in afferent drive of spasticity may add to the effectiveness of the block as well. It is our impression that a motor point block with phenol can influence over-activity for three to five months. Nevertheless, reports on duration effectiveness in the literature have varied over a vary broad range from several days to three years. The reader should glean from this that phenol blocks are a temporizing measure and are most effectively used in the period of expectant neurological recovery. The rationale for the other injectable agents such as alcohol and botulinum toxin, is in our view, essentially the same.

The strategy of performing a block is as follows: a surface stimulator is used to locate the selected peripheral verve or motor point. The skin is then prepared with an antiseptic iodine solution, swabbed with alcohol and subcutaneously anesthetized with lidocaine prior to insertion of the teflon coated, 22 gauge injecting needle (see Figure 35-24). The electrically conductive inner core of the tip of the needle is used to pass current to the tissues. As the needle is advanced closer to the nerve, less current is required to produce similar amounts of muscle contraction. When a minimal current producing a visible or palpable muscle contraction is reached, we typically inject 3–5cc of aqueous phenol in concentration of 7%. When injecting multiple nerves or motor points, we usually do not exceed a total volume of 15cc and we generally avoid injecting patients taking anticoagulants where the risk of systemic absorption of phenol is greater. [In very large quantities, systemically absorbed phenol can cause seizures, central nervous system depression and cardiovascular collapse]. The essence of the technique is in the clinical manipulation of needle advancement towards the nerve. Depth of penetration and directional orientation of the needle tip require a steady hand, competent knowledge of anatomy and a good assistant. Morbidity is typically benign. Local irritation at the site of the block is treated symptomatically with ice, compression or mild analgesics. We avoid mixed sensory-motor nerves so as not to induce painful dysesthesias and we will substitute motor point blocks that involve motor branches only. The injection technique is a good temporizing measure during the period of expectant neurological recovery and facilitates serial casting, range of motion exercises, passive ADL functions and active movements and function as well.

Borg-Stein et al. have made an initial comparison of phenol and botulinum toxin injections (79). They indicated that a reduction in over-activity after phenol motor point block tends to diminish after several months, but may last as long as several years. The effect of botulinum toxin appears to last for about three to four months with a more complete return to baseline than is generally seen after phenol injection. Botulinum toxin is not associated with dysesthesia, but neither is motor point block with phenol. Only injection of phenol into a mixed sensory/motor nerve may produce such an effect. The cost of the toxin compared with the cost of phenol is large and the cost will escalate if multiple injections are required to titrate a desired clinical effect. Second, it is not clear how to control the titration process for an overactive muscle that also has volitional capacity. An ideal agent would eliminate a muscle's over-activity while preserving its voluntary capacity. Third, the technique for injecting deeper muscles with toxin requires electrical stimulation to verify the muscle's identity. This requires searching skill akin to the skill of advancing toward a motor nerve using the phenol technique. For deep muscles, EMG guidance does not really specify which muscle is being injected. Such a technique may be useful in dystonia, but is riskier in UMN muscle over-activity. Phenol has local anesthetic properties so that one can see an immediate result after injection (Figures 35-25 and 35-26). Botulinum toxin effects are variably seen after 5–14 days. On the whole, injecting botulinum toxin into a single superficial muscle under EMG guidance is quicker than injecting

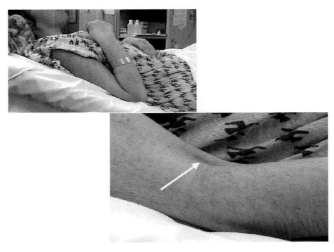

FIGURE 35-25

Phenol has local anesthetic properties so that one can see an immediate result after injection. In this photo, a prominent biceps tendon is observed when the biceps is stretched

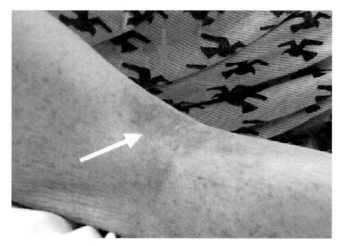

FIGURE 35-26

This photo was taken 5 minutes after phenol block of the musculocutaneous nerve was performed with 4 cc of 7% aqueous phenol. The biceps tendon is no longer prominent because the local anesthetic effect of phenol has eliminated stretch reflex activity in the biceps (and brachialis). Beginnings of the longer-term denaturation effect of phenol is not expected for 48-72 hours after phenol injection

phenol but more individual muscles are injected with the toxin so that total work time may turn out to be a wash. To inject phenol, we typically utilize an assistant. Botulinum toxin can be managed entirely by the physician. Finally, BoNT and phenol can be used together in situations where large proximal muscles receive phenol blocks and smaller distal muscles receive toxin. Since the current upper range of toxin use is 600 units, large muscles would absorb most if not all of the prescribed toxin leaving little left over for many smaller distal muscles. Hence, phenol applied to proximal musculature spares toxin for use elsewhere.

Special Section on Neuro-Orthopaedic Principles, Selected Procedures and Post-Operative Rehabilitation for UMN Muscle Overactivity After TBI

Neuro-orthopaedic Principles and Perspective Six or more months after TBI, when the patient is neurologically stable and a majority of motor recovery has occurred, decisions can be made regarding neuro-orthopaedic surgery to correct limb deformities and rebalance muscle forces. It is at this time that a neuro-orthopaedic surgeon can make the greatest contribution to a patient's functional recovery. When evaluating patients with brain injury, questions commonly arise regarding \indications for surgery, cost, expected outcome, and practicality of this approach. These issues should be considered on an individual basis for each patient. We have delineated

general principles that serve as our guidelines for decision making.

Operate Early — Before Deformities Are Severe and Fixed Orthopaedic surgery is a powerful rehabilitation tool. It is often the only treatment that will correct a limb deformity or improve function. Surgery should not be considered a treatment of last resort when "conservative" measures have failed. The choice of treatment technique, surgical or non-surgical, should be predicated on which one will provide the most optimal result.

Better Underlying Motor Control Means Better Function for the Extremity Orthopaedic surgery cannot impart control to a muscle. Lengthening a spastic muscle can improve its function by improving joint range of motion, by diminishing unwanted force generated by muscle overactivity, unmasking volitional strength of agonists when antagonists are modified by lengthening and uncovering any latent motor control that was present. Successful surgery depends on a careful evaluation preoperatively to determine the amount of volitional control present in each individual muscle that is affecting limb posture and movement.

Distinguish Between the Function of the Extremity and the Function of the Individual We think of active function and passive function of the extremity. These terms refer to the expected outcomes for a limb but do not indicate the outcome for the person as a whole. Surgical releases of an arm contractured in a flexed and internally rotated position in a hemiplegic patient often allows the person to become independent in dressing even though the arm itself does not have volitional movement.

Consider the Cost of Not Correcting Limb Deformities Allowing limb deformities to occur or persist is detrimental to well being and quality of life of the person with brain injury. Likewise, the cost of laboratory based motor control evaluation using dynamic electromyography (EMG); video and motion analysis is relatively modest for the benefits it provides. Dynamic EMG is a one-time expense. The cost of performing an incorrect surgical procedure that fails to correct or worsens a limb deformity is much greater. The cost of performing a surgical procedure is likewise limited when compared to a lifetime of attendant care, spasticity medications, repeated blocks, orthotics to control limb position, complications such as skin ulceration and infection and lost productivity for the patient and caregivers.

Perspective on Neuro-Orthopaedic Treatment of Muscle Overactivity Treatment of muscle overactivity is most effective when functional problems are formulated in focal rather than diffuse terms. For example, a patient may have muscle overactivity across all joints of the upper

IX

MEDICAL MANAGEMENT ISSUES

36 Gastrointestinal and Nutritional Issues

Donald F. Kirby
Linda Creasey
Souheil G. Abou-Assi

Depending on the extent of neurological injury, the spectrum of gastrointestinal and nutritional ramifications can be vast. Often the patient who has suffered a traumatic brain injury (TBI) or a spinal cord injury (SCI) is well nourished prior to the injury; however, hypermetabolism resulting from an injury can quickly deplete nutritional stores, especially protein, resulting in a nitrogen death (1).

Many other gastrointestinal (GI) and nutritional problems are common and predictable. Knowledge of their occurrence and protocols for their prevention can help limit their impact on patients. This chapter discusses the GI and nutritional problems that can befall the patient with TBI in the acute and chronic phases of injury. Patients with SCI in addition to TBI may complicate the overall care, and the care of patients with SCI will generally not be discussed in this chapter. However, older references may not have delineated between the two patient populations of TBI with and without SCI. Thus, we will attempt to highlight some of the short comings in our present knowledge of patients with TBI.

Although Drew et al. reported on the rapid nutritional deterioration after craniotomy in 1947, it was not until 1975 that hypermetabolism was correlated with TBI (2, 3). It was noted that many patients tolerated gastric feeding poorly and widely regarded that hyperosmolar parenteral solutions could worsen cerebral edema (4). Thus, many patients succumbed to their neurological illness or injury, not so much from the initial insult, but from the lack of subsequent feeding during the hospitalization. Furthermore, it was not until 1983 that Rapp and colleagues showed that there was a higher survival rate in patients feed early by total parenteral nutrition (TPN) rather than by attempts at intragastric feeding (5). This was an important conceptual advance since it dispelled the myth that the hyperosmolar TPN solutions would exacerbate cerebral edema, and thereby increase morbidity and mortality.

The actual molecular and cytokine reactions to TBI are beyond the scope of this chapter. However, certain GI or nutritional problems may be associated with changes in hormonal actions that are important to recognize. These will be highlighted with their physiologic consequences.

BACKGROUND

The interrelationships of gastrointestinal and nutritional reactions to TBI were not appreciated for many years.

GASTROINTESTINAL COMPLICATIONS

Gastrointestinal complications should be separated into conditions that are associated with acute injury and later events. There will also be some differences when there is also an associated spinal cord injury.

Gastritis/Erosions/Ulcers

Depending upon the severity of the neurological damage, there appears to be an increased incidence of acute GI erosive lesions in the stomach. A prospective study by Kamada et al. demonstrated a higher rate of gastroduodenal lesions (6). Up to 75% of patients had lesions that were mostly in the stomach (78%). Erosive gastritis was the most common lesion and was often found in the first week after the injury. The use of steroids did not seem to affect the incidence of gastritis. However, it should be noted that this study was performed prior to the commonplace usage of H_2-receptor antagonist blockers or proton pump inhibitors and the advent of early enteral feeding, all of which may ameliorate this type of injury.

The risk of gastric ulceration from TBI has also been well described and may be the result of another mechanism unrelated to the high incidence of stress gastritis previously mentioned. It has been reported that there is gastric acid hypersecretion which can be the direct result of the elevated serum gastrin levels that have been seen in patients with head injury (7). While gastric ulceration is well known after traumatic injuries, those associated with brain injury have been noted to be potentially quite severe and may progress to perforation. These have been referred to as Cushing's ulcers (8). Since gastric acid hypersecretion can be controlled with either H_2-receptor antagonist blockers or proton pump inhibitors, initial care protocols for the patient with TBI should include one of these classes of medications to control intragastric pH. Table 36-1 lists commonly used protocols; note that these may not be specifically approved by the Food and Drug Administration (FDA), but rather what is commonly used in clinical practice (9–14).

Delayed gastric emptying

Delayed gastric emptying or gastroparesis can occur either with isolated head injury, as previously mentioned, or with cervical spinal cord injuries (15,16). This has ramifications for both nutrition and general care as some patients may experience severe gastric stasis or dilatation that may require nasogastric decompression. Ileus is variably present, but appears more commonly in patients with spinal cord pathology (17). Since the enteric nervous system and smooth muscle layers are still intact, promotility agents should be useful. Unfortunately due to concerns over cardiovascular side effects, cisapride has been removed from the market for common usage. Although it is still available under strict protocol for compassionate usage

TABLE 36-1
Control of Intragastric pH in Prevention of Stress Gastritis/Erosions/Ulcers*

ROUTE	MEDICATION	USUAL PROTOCOL
Histamine-2-Receptor Antagonists (H_2RA)		
IV	Cimetidine** (Tagamet)	300 mg bolus, 50 mg/ hr continuous infusion; Creatinine Clearance (CrCl) < 30ml/min reduce dose by 50%
	Famotidine (Pepcid)	20 mg bolus, 40 mg every 24 hours continuous infusion (or 20 mg every 12 hours) (CrCl) < 50ml/min reduce dose by 50% or increase interval to every 36–48 hours
	Ranitidine (Zantac)	50 mg bolus, 150–200 mg every 24 hours continuous infusion (or 50 mg every 8 hours) (CrCl) < 50ml/min 50mg every 18–24 hours, give more frequently every 12 hours, as necessary
Proton Pump Inhibitors (PPI)		
Enteral	Lansoprazole suspension (Prevacid)	30 mg every 12 hours
Enteral	Omeprazole suspension (Prilosec)	40 mg bolus, repeat 40 mg dose in 6 hours, then 20 mg daily (or 40 mg/ day or 20 mg every 12 hours)
	Pantoprazole IV (Protonix)	40 mg every 12 hours (some centers bolus with 80 mg initially)

*Table created from references 9–14. Trade name in parentheses.
**Currently the only FDA-approved agent for stress ulcer prophylaxis, often not preferred clinically as the first line H_2RA due to drug interactions

as an investigational limited access study drug which requires an Institutional Review Board protocol and approval, it is less likely to be used in the initial care of the TBI/SCI patient. With further study it may have been preferred over metoclopramide due to its lack of CNS side effects, but limited data exists in patients with TBI (18). Metoclopramide is presently the only FDA-approved promotility agent. Unfortunately, its use may be limited by its potential for CNS side effects due to its central dopaminergic blocking activitiy. The drug should not be used in epileptics since the severity and frequency of seizures may be increased. Also, patients that are receiving medications that can increase the risk of extrapyramidal side effects should avoid this medication. Published experience with metoclopramide in TBI is limited and consists mostly of case reports (19).

Erythromycin is a macrolide antibiotic that is structurally similar to the GI hormone motilin. It has been used very effectively as a promotility agent, but as an off-label use and not as a FDA-approved indication. There are currently no known trials of its use for this indication in patients with TBI.

Domperidone is another promotility agent that is available outside the United States. It has not been approved for sale in the U.S., but can often be obtained from pharmacies in Canada or Mexico or even as a compounded, unapproved medication from some pharmacies in America. Thus, inpatient use is unlikely, but it may be useful in carefully selected outpatients.

Diarrhea and Constipation

Diarrhea is not a common finding in patients with TBI. Thus, patients who have diarrhea should be investigated like any other patient who presents with this symptom. Table 36-2 lists some of the key elements in investigating the cause of diarrhea. If the patient is hospitalized and/or has recently, up to six weeks, received antibiotics, then the standard workup should include stool for white blood cells, investigation for ova and parasites, and stool cultures that include testing for *Clostridia difficle*. Flexible sigmoidoscopy or colonoscopy may be required in some patients.

Other causes of diarrhea must also be considered. The administration of liquid versions of medications may contain sorbitol, which even in modest amounts can cause diarrhea. Antacids may contain magnesium and other medications, like lactulose, are commonly used. Many other drugs may have diarrhea as a side effect, and medication profiles should be reviewed carefully for potential clues.

Diarrhea is the most common complication of enteral tube feeding; however, reports have varied in the incidence from 2.3–68% (20–22). Differences in definitions by various investigators make many studies difficult

---

TABLE 36-2
Diarrhea

QUESTIONS TO CONSIDER

How is "diarrhea" being defined?
Is there a new fever?
Has the patient received antibiotics in the past 6 weeks?
Is the patient being tube fed?
What medications are being given to the patient, especially liquid meds?
Does the patient have diabetes mellitus?
Are there any GI complications that could lead to diarrhea?
Does the patient have a malabsorptive disorder?
Is the diarrhea "secretory" or "osmotic"?
Is there visible or occult blood in the stool?
Is there a history of inflammatory bowel disease, radiation therapy or ischemic bowel?
Is there a pre-existing motility disorder?

STANDARD WORKUP – VARIES WITH THE CLINICAL SITUATION*

Complete Blood Count (CBC), Erythrocyte Sedimentation Rate (ESR)
Serum chemistries
Thyroid studies
Giardia antigen*
Clostridia difficle toxin*
Stool cultures, including *Shigella, Salmonella, Yersinia* and *Clostridia difficle*
Stool for ova & parasites
Stool examination for blood

MORE INVOLVED WORK-UP

Gastrointestinal Consultation
Intake & Output measurements
Endoscopic procedures
Radiologic investigations
Stool for osmolarity

---

to compare or interpret. It may be that the actual genesis of diarrhea in these patients is multifactorial. Etiologies can include concurrent use of antibiotics or diarrhea-inducing medications, formula composition, rate of infusion, altered bacterial flora, enteral formula contamination, and hypoalbuminemia (23, 24). Additionally, it appears that the more critically ill patients seem to experience a higher incidence of tube feeding-related diarrhea (22). Initiation of feedings at slower rates until tolerance is seen can help limit this problem.

Blood in the stool must also concern the clinician to look for inflammatory causes or ischemic bowel. Occult blood in the stool is a nonspecific finding, but may require a more throughout investigation and gastrointestinal consultation. Etiologies are numerous and are beyond the scope of this review.

Constipation can be a much more serious problem in the TBI/SCI patients. Patients who have spinal cord lesions above the fifth thoracic root can experience autonomic dysreflexia which can be a life threatening event. Either bladder distention or fecal impaction can precipitate this abnormal autonomic reflex that can lead to tachycardia and severe hypertension (25). Treatment must be prompt since subarachnoid hemorrhage, stroke or seizures can occur. These patients should be managed with prevention of constipation and routine bladder catheterization to avoid this complication.

Gallbladder Disease

Acute acalculous cholecystitis is an often unrecognized and a potentially fatal complication that may develop among patients hospitalized for trauma. The cause, although not yet clearly defined, is believed to be multifactorial, resulting from bile stasis, ischemia, bacterial infection, sepsis, narcotics (opiates) that induce sphincter of Oddi spasticity and the activation of factor XII (26). Mortality rates of 10–75% have been reported. That high mortality is attributed to the fact that the gallbladder disease (i.e., necrosis, gangrene, or perforation) is frequently advanced by time of diagnosis. The symptoms and signs are not much different from those of cholecystitis with stones, the most common being right upper quadrant pain, fever, and leukocytosis. However, in the posttraumatic neurosurgical patient, obtundation or neurological deficits can make these valuable physical findings hard to detect (26, 27). Most reports showed that symptoms usually begin between 1–4 weeks after the trauma. The most important factor in early diagnosis of this condition is the clinician's awareness of abnormal laboratory findings and any unexplained deterioration of a previously improving posttraumatic course. Suggestive laboratory findings include elevated serum bilirubin, alkaline phosphatase, liver enzymes and leukocytosis; suggestive physical findings consist of fever, vomiting, abdominal distention, ileus, and in some cases palpable right upper quadrant mass (28, 29).

Ultrasonography is the investigation of first choice and strongly recommended whenever acalculous cholecystitis is suspected. Additional radiologic studies should include plain abdominal X-ray, which is useful predominantly to exclude a perforated viscus, bowel ischemia, or renal stones. Another advantage of ultrasonography includes its ability to examine the liver, pancreas, kidneys, and bile ducts in addition to the gallbladder (30, 31). Ultrasonographic features suggestive of acalculous cholecystitis may include the following: 1) absence of gallstones or sludge; 2) thickening of the gallbladder wall (>5 mm)

with pericholecystic fluid; 3) a positive Murphy's sign induced by the ultrasound probe; 4) failure to visualize the gallbladder; 5) emphysematous cholecystitis with gas bubbles arising in the fundus of the gallbladder (champagne sign); and, 6) frank perforation of the gallbladder with associated abscess formation.

On the other hand, in a retrospective study Puc and coworkers questioned the utility of ultrasonography and found that abdominal ultrasound was sensitive only in 30% and specific in 93% of 62 trauma patients who underwent cholecystectomy for suspected acute acalculous cholecystitis (32). In stable patients in whom the diagnosis is unclear after ultrasonography, radioisotope HIDA scan may be useful. HIDA is an iminodiacetic acid derivative, which is given by intravenous injection, taken up by hepatocytes, and excreted into bile with concentration in the gallbladder. Failure to opacify the gallbladder is indicative of cystic duct obstruction or necrosis with very high sensitivity up to 100% and 90% specificity. Leakage into the pericholecystic space suggests perforation. HIDA should not be recommended in critically ill patients in whom a delay in therapy can be potentially fatal (30, 33). Treatment should be instituted promptly, intravenous broad spectrum antibiotics should be started, and emergent cholecystectomy is now believed to be the treatment of choice. Although cholecystostomy has been advocated, it should be only reserved for the sickest patients not tolerating surgery (26, 27, 34). In a series reported by DuPriest et al, a gangrenous gallbladder was found in 52% of cases (35).

Pancreatitis

Elevations of serum amylase and lipase have been described in patients in the neurointensive care setting. Hyperamylasemia has been observed in 19–41% of patients with severe head injury and in 45–60% of patients with intracranial bleeding from head trauma with no clinical signs or symptoms of pancreatitis (36, 37). However, making the diagnosis of acute pancreatitis can be difficult in this patient population. These patients often suffer from altered mental status or require therapeutic sedation +/or paralysis to reduce intracranial pressure, so the clinical information obtained from the physical examination may not always be accurate. In addition, it is not clear whether this enzyme elevation is due to head trauma itself, intracranial bleeding, or some nonspecific intracranial event. Proposed causes include vagal stimulation, altered modulation of the central control of pancreatic enzyme release, and release of cholecystokinin from the brain (36, 37). To investigate the role of intracranial events in patients with TBI, Justice et al. prospectively studied 38 patients admitted to their neurointensive care unit with traumatic intracranial bleeding for elevations of pancreatic enzymes (38). Twenty-five patients (66%) had elevated lipase enzyme activity, and 17 of the 25 also had elevated amylase without any evidence of clinical pancreatitis. Most lipase elevations occurred earlier than those of amylase, and there was significant interaction between lipase elevation and decreasing Glasgow Coma Score (GCS), indicative of increasing severity of intracranial bleeding (38). Similar findings were seen in a retrospective study by Liu and coworkers of 75 patients with TBI from Cook County Hospital where none of the patients with elevated serum lipase and amylase had any clinical or radiographic evidence of pancreatitis (37). In summary, because of the lack of their diagnostic value, routine pancreatic enzyme monitoring should not be performed in this patient population unless it is clinically indicated, and physician awareness of the association between intracranial bleeding with elevation of pancreatic enzyme of no significance can save the patient needless cost and manipulation.

Other Less Frequent GI Problems

There are several other GI problems that occur in the patients with TBI and/or SCI, but they are less common than the other problems already discussed. The first two of these can be considered extensions of the altered bowel function that can occur with constipation and less commonly with TBI unless the patient is at a low level of function. Over time, diverticulosis can occur in these patients and lead to the usual complications of this disease; diverticulitis and/or diverticular hemorrhage (17). In the chronic SCI patient, this may be particularly problematic as the abdominal presentation may be altered and even delayed, leading to an acute abdomen in cases of diverticulitis. A diverticular bleed may be minor or cause hemodynamic compromise and potentially be life threatening. This argues for the adherence of a good bowel program to try and minimize the occurrence of these potential complications.

The superior mesenteric artery (SMA) syndrome has been reported in patients with neurological diseases. The syndrome occurs when the SMA that naturally crosses over the duodenum obstructs the duodenum, usually due to a more acute angle than usual. This can lead to dilatation of the proximal duodenum and stomach (39, 40). Multiple precipitating factors can be seen in TBI/SCI patients including weight loss, prolonged bed rest, loss of tone in the abdominal wall musculature and previous abdominal surgery.

Once SMA syndrome is considered, a radiological study is usually confirmatory. The diagnosis can be made by an upper GI series, computed abdominal tomography or rarely angiography. Management can include removal or reversal of a precipitating factor, nasogastric decompression as well as intravenous hydration. Occasionally, patients are tube feed for a short period of time while patients, who are very thin, gain weight.

COMPLICATIONS OF BRAIN INJURY WITH NUTRITIONAL SIGNIFICANCE

Several other problems can be seen in patients with TBI that can have an impact on the patient's nutritional condition. These include the following: hyperglycemia, syndrome of inappropriate antidiuretic hormone (SIADH), cerebral salt wasting, seizures and the use of barbiturates.

Hyperglycemia

TBI is associated with an acute sympathoadrenomedullary response characterized by increased blood levels of norepinephrine, epinephrine, and dopamine. Catecholamines levels reflect the severity of head injury and appear to predict the neurological outcome in both the acute and chronic phases of TBI. This increase in circulating catecholamines seems to contribute to intracranial hypertension, hyperdynamic cardiovascular response, increase in brain oxygen requirements, and the rise in serum glucose levels (41, 42). Rosner et al. showed that hyperglycemia occurred within minutes of experimental head injury in cats (43). In this animal model, hyperglycemia was related to severity of injury and was thought to be caused by catecholamine release. Similar results were also seen in rats (44). In another study in humans, Young et al. found that at the time of hospital admission 48% of 59 brain-injured patients had a blood glucose concentration >200 mg/dL (45). Patients with peak 24-hour admission glucose greater than 200 mg/dL had worse neurologic outcome at 18 days, 3 months and 1 year than those with glucose levels less than or equal to 200 mg/dL. In a larger study of 169 patients who underwent surgery because of a traumatic intracranial hematoma, Lam and colleagues reported that glucose concentration at the time of hospital admission depended on the initial GCS (46). Patients with a best day-1 score of < 8 had an admission serum glucose of 192 ± 7mg/dL, compared with only 130 ± 8 mg/dL in patients with a score of 12 to 15. Patients who subsequently remained in a vegetative state or died had significantly higher glucose levels both on admission and postoperatively than patients with good outcome or moderate disability. Among the more severely injured patients (GCS score < 8), a serum glucose level greater than 200 mg/dL postoperatively was associated with a significantly worse outcome (p < 0.01) (46).

In summary, hyperglycemia is a common metabolic derangement seen early after both experimental and human TBI and is a significant predictor of poor outcome. It is thought that high glucose levels enhance ischemia-mediated cell damage, probably through lactate accumulation (47). When hyperglycemia is over 150 mg/dL, it is advisable to treat it with insulin. It has been shown that maintaining blood glucose at or below 110 mg/dL reduces morbidity and mortality in critically ill patients in a surgical intensive care unit (48). However, more studies are needed to see if this can positively affect the neurologic outcome in patients with TBI.

Syndrome of Inappropriate Secretion of Antidiuretic Hormone (SIADH)

The syndrome of inappropriate antidiuretic hormone secretion (SIADH) should be suspected in any patient with TBI with hyponatremia (<135 mEq/L), hypoosmolality (<280 mOsm/L), a urine osmolality greater than that of plasma, a urine sodium concentration that is usually above 25 mEq/L, normal acid-base and potassium balance, and frequently a low plasma uric acid concentration. An inappropriate elevation in ADH release will produce hyponatremia by interfering with urinary dilution, thereby preventing the excretion of ingested water (49). In a review of 1808 patients with craniocerebral injuries, Doczi et al. reported that 84 patients (4.6%) developed SIADH. The prevalence varied depending on the severity of their head injury as follows: SIADH occurred in 0.6% of patients with mild **head** injury, 10.6% of those with moderate **head** injury, and 4.7% of the severe ones (II-10).

In another study of 109 patients with severe **head** injury with GCS <7, 33% of the patients had SIADH. The authors proposed to subdivide SIADH into two clinical forms: an early syndrome (5% of the patients) that becomes apparent towards the second day and is significantly associated with lesions at the base of the skull; and a delayed syndrome, which is more common occurring at the end of the first week where the cause could be due to different factors linked to intensive care procedures (51). Patients with this syndrome are generally responsive to fluid restriction, but this should be performed with extreme caution given the importance of maintaining normovolemia in patients with TBI (52). If serum sodium level falls below 140 mEq/L, the maintenance intravenous infusion should be changed to normal saline. For hyponatremia below 130 mEq/L, intravenous urea is safe and rapidly effective in correcting this problem. Urea is a potent osmotic diuretic and significantly increases sodium reabsorption at the kidney. The usual dose is forty grams of urea in 150 ml of normal saline, to be given over 2 hours and can be repeated every 8 hours. On average the serum sodium levels will rise 6 and 10 mEq/L after 24 and 48 hours of initiating therapy. Infusion of hypertonic saline is also effective, but generally takes longer than urea in correcting the hyponatremia and requires close monitoring of urine electrolytes (53). When tube feeding is done with patients with SIADH, formulas that are calorie dense (2 Kcal/cc) are generally used to limit the total volume delivered to the patient. Feeding tubes are then flushed with small amounts of normal saline rather than water.

Cerebral Salt Wasting (CSW)

A less common syndrome than SIADH has been described in patients with brain injury (particularly subarachnoid hemorrhage) that mimics all of the findings in the SIADH, except that salt wasting is the primary defect with the ensuing volume depletion leading to a secondary rise in ADH release. The major distinction from SIADH is the volume status of the patient. In patients with CSW, the extracellular volume is contracted and the patient often appears dehydrated, whereas in SIADH a clinical picture of fluid overload is often seen. In addition to salt-wasting, affected patients also may have hypouricemia due to increased urinary uric acid excretion. The course of hypouricemia after therapy of hyponatremia may be helpful in distinguishing cerebral salt-wasting from SIADH. There is a suggestion that, after the correction of hyponatremia with fluid restriction, cerebral salt wasting is more likely to be present if hypouricemia continues in combination with an elevated fractional excretion of urate (>10 percent) (49, 54).

The etiology of this putative syndrome is unclear. Preliminary studies supported the possible role of a circulating factor that impairs renal tubular function in many patients with intracranial disease. It had been proposed that a natriuretic hormone was released from the brain in response to certain types of injury; candidates included atrial natriuretic peptide, brain natriuretic peptide, and endogenous ouabain (55).

With the different pathogenesis, patients with CSW are treated differently from those with the SIADH. The objectives of the treatment are volume replacement and maintenance of a positive salt balance. Intravenous hydration with normal saline (0.9% NaCl), hypertonic saline (3% NaCl), or oral salt may be used alone or in combination, depending on the severity of hyponatremia and the ability of the patient to tolerate enteral administration. If the patient can tolerate oral intake, then 2–3 gm of NaCl are given 2–3 times daily or via a feeding tube, as appropriate. Volume status in response to treatment is best evaluated by daily weight and central venous pressure or pulmonary artery wedge pressure measurements (54, 56).

Seizures

Three kinds of seizures can complicate the care of patients with severe brain injury, and these are distinguished by the time interval following trauma: 1) impact seizures, appearing within 24 hours; 2) early seizures, occurring within 1 week; and, 3) late seizures, observed from day 8 through to 2 years, but frequently later. The seizure type also varies with time period after brain injury, with a relatively high proportion of generalized seizures at an early stage and a progressively larger prevalence of partial seizures later (57, 58).

In a randomized trial of patients sustaining moderate or severe brain injuries, including patients with depressed skull fractures, Temkin and co-workers confirmed the effectiveness of prophylactic administration of phenytoin in significantly reducing the risk of seizures during the first week after injury (59). Routine administration of phenytoin for 7 days after sustaining a depressed skull fracture is supported by this study. In addition, other studies have shown that pharmacological control of early seizures with phenytoin, phenobarbital, valproic acid, and/or carbamazepine is effective. Anticonvulsants should be administered parenterally first, if possible, (phenobarbital 200 mg/day, phenytoin 500 to 750 mg/day, valproic acid 30 mg/kg/day, or carbamazepine 300 to 600 mg/day orally, since it is not available in intramuscular/intravenous formulations) and then switched to the oral route as soon as feasible. The enteral route is preferred due to cost and irritation to the veins from intravenous phenytoin. It should be noted that topiramate and valproic acid have been shown to cause diarrhea. Gastrointestinal function should be monitored, and treatment for diarrhea should be instituted to prevent skin breakdown for these patients (60, 61). Routine blood monitoring of anticonvulsants concentrations should also be performed when necessary for appropriate agents, and it is advisable to keep drug concentrations in the higher end of the therapeutic range (57, 62).

On the other hand, the efficacy of anticonvulsant therapy in reducing the incidence of late epilepsy remains unproven. Therefore, no acceptable effective prophylactic strategies are in place to inhibit late epileptogenesis following severe brain trauma. However, according to some authors, the decision to institute long-term prophylactic anticonvulsants can be justified in high-risk patients where the incidence of late seizures is over 20%. Such individuals would include those with the combination of post-traumatic amnesia of over 24 hours duration, seizures occurring during the first week after injury, and dural laceration or intracranial hematoma (63, 64).

It is important when providing nutrition for these sick patients at risk for post-traumatic seizures to look carefully at the factors that can lower their seizure threshold and try to address them promptly, and these include low anticonvulsant levels, electrolyte derangements (particularly low serum sodium, magnesium or calcium levels), hypoglycemia, hypoxemia, alcohol withdrawal and meningitis. It is important to recall that enteral feedings can decrease phenytoin availability by as much as 70%, and tube feedings should be held for 1 to 2 hours before and after phenytoin administration (65). This strategy has not always been effective, and serum levels of phenytoin are important to monitor. Increasing enteral doses of phenytoin may be required or even intravenous phenytoin to keep levels in the appropriate ranges (66, 67).

Barbiturates

It is estimated that 10–15% of patients admitted with severe brain injury will ultimately manifest medically and surgically intractable elevated intracranial pressure (ICP) with an associated mortality of 84 to 100%. High dose barbiturates have been known since the 1930s to have ICP-lowering effects. However, their risks are well known, and complications have limited their applications to the most extreme of clinical situations (68). Barbiturates appear to exert their cerebral protective and ICP lowering effects through several distinct mechanisms: alterations in vascular tone, suppression of metabolism, and inhibition of free radical mediated lipid peroxidation. Pentobarbital is usually administered in an initial dose of 5 to 10 mg/Kg, given as a bolus dose of 50 mg initially, until the EEG shows burst suppression. Further intermittent intravenous doses can then be administered to maintain blood levels between 3.0 and 4.5 mg/dL. Pentobarbital usage is associated with a 20% decrease in the energy expenditure as measured by the Harris-Benedict equation (69).

Several studies showed that high dose barbiturate therapy was efficacious in lowering ICP and decreasing mortality in the setting of uncontrollable ICP refractory to all other conventional medical and surgical ICP-lowering treatments. When this therapy is used, consideration should be given to monitoring arteriovenous oxygen saturation as some patients may develop oligemic cerebral hypoxia (68, 70, 71). On the other hand, utilization of barbiturates for the prophylactic treatment of ICP was not shown to be effective and is not indicated. In a randomized controlled trial of 53 severely head-injured patients, Ward et al. showed no difference between the prophylactic barbiturate-induced coma group and the control, in the incidence of elevated ICP, the duration of ICP elevation, or the response of ICP elevations to treatment (72). Also, there were more complications seen in the treated group; arterial hypotension occurred in 14 patients (54%) in the treated group and only in two patients (7%) in the untreated group.

GOALS OF NUTRITION THERAPY

The first important goal of nutrition therapy is to decrease the incidence of mortality associated with previously mentioned difficulties in feeding patients with TBI. These patients exhibit hypermetabolism, increased protein breakdown and turnover (73). Nutritional assessment is complicated by rapid volume shifts and fluid accumulation. Alterations in gut motility can also complicate the usual attempts to enterally feed patients.

Fortunately, most new patients with TBI/SCI are usually adequately nourished prior to their injury. The complex physiologic response to injury creates difficulty in estimating calorie and protein needs, since these patients are often hypermetabolic (74). The hypermetabolic response can be prolonged and is usually inversely correlated with patient's GCS. Thus, the more severely brain-injured patients have a higher measured resting energy expenditure (MREE) (75). Caloric estimation is often calculated by the Harris-Benedict (HBE) equation; however, this formula has been shown to significantly underestimate energy expenditure in nearly 70% of critically ill patients (76). When available, indirect calorimetry is a better means of estimating the resting energy expenditure. Makk and colleagues showed that predictive formulas, like the HBE, could only correctly estimate the measured values obtained by indirect calorimetry in about 56% of traumatic brain injured patients (77).

It is commonly believed that the protein losses in patients with TBI come from immobility and the mobilization of protein to meet increased protein needs. However, data from trauma patients have shown that there is both increased protein synthesis and catabolism (78). The amount of nitrogen loss is associated with increased hormone levels that are associated with hypermetabolism, epinephrine, norepinephrine and glucagon (79). Immobility may exacerbate nitrogen losses, but steroid administration appears to have little effect (80). Trials that have attempted to correct negative nitrogen balance in the acute injury setting have had mixed results. Provision of high protein can help decrease nitrogen losses, but high nitrogen excretion is not eliminated by just simply increasing caloric intake (81). Recommendations for provision of protein in these patients will be discussed in more detail later. While patients are in critical condition in an Intensive Care Unit (ICU), it is more important to provide "some" nutrition rather than trying to meet 100% of a patient's estimated nutritional needs. Once out of the ICU setting, the nutritional focus should be to provide sufficient calories for growth and repair of body stores and proper weight attainment depending on the patient's functional capacity. The provision of protein is important to decrease the amount of cannibalization of muscles as a source of protein, since there is no distinct storage form for protein as there is for lipids, adipose tissue, or carbohydrate, glycogen in liver and muscle.

NUTRITION ASSESSMENT AND REQUIREMENTS

Predicting the nutritional needs of a patient with TBI is not a simple task because no single test can predict nutrition status. In the recovery from a brain injury, nutrition status will not remain static, and therefore will require periodic reassessment and adjustments that are made depending on current weight and functional capability.

As most patients are either comatose or confused and unable to provide accurate information, family members or caregivers should be contacted as part of an initial subjective global assessment.

Subjective Global Assessment

Subjective global assessment is well documented in the literature as a valid measure of nutritional status in hospitalized patients (82). It consists of 5 key areas from the medical history: 1) amount of weight loss over the previous six months; 2) usual dietary intake and if abnormal, length of time of abnormal intake; 3) gastrointestinal symptomatology (e.g, nausea, vomiting, diarrhea); 4) previous functional capacity (i.e., bedridden or independent); and, 5) metabolic demands of current disease state(s). A physical examination should also be completed to assess for muscle wasting, ascites, and edema. These factors should give an overall assessment of the patient's prior status and ability to utilize nutrients (82).

In response to brain injury, the systemic inflammatory process characterized by the previously discussed hormonal response, causes a shift from anabolism to catabolism (83). Hepatic glucose production leads to hyperglycemia in response to counterregulatory hormones. Despite exogenous insulin, resistance at the peripheral tissues makes glucose control difficult. Elevations in epinephrine and glucagon also increase lipolysis, which offers an additional fuel source. However, current data suggests that few lipids are oxidized and utilized for fuel (84). Therefore, protein is the major source of fuel following brain injury. Although the demand increases for acute-phase protein production by the liver, the liver is unable to keep up with urinary losses of nitrogen as protein is also used for gluconeogenesis. These losses contribute to further tissue breakdown and loss of muscle stores (83).

Severity of injury directly correlates with the degree of substrate mobilization. Therefore, the lower the GCS, the more significant the protein mobilization and calorie expenditure (85). Increased intracranial pressure is also associated with an increase in caloric expenditure (86).

In addition to severity of injury and intracranial pressure, motor activity, infection, fever, level of sedation, level of consciousness, and other trauma can also affect caloric expenditure. Ideally, indirect calorimetry is helpful in guiding nutritional care to assure adequate calories to allow protein synthesis and avoid overfeeding.

Calculating Protein and Calorie Requirements

As indirect calorimetry may not always be available, several formulas have been published to estimate calorie needs. Estimated caloric requirements can vary from 140% to 200% above the normal. Studies have shown that this hypermetabolism can last from weeks up to one year post-injury (78). Current practice guidelines recommend to provide 40–50 non-protein kcal/kg/day for patients with a GCS < 5 and 30–35 non-protein kcal/kg/day for patients with a GCS 8–12 (87, 88). As severe brain injury is correlated with significant stress, one must be prudent not to provide large amounts of carbohydrate as this may exacerbate hyperglycemia and potentially complicate ventilator weaning (89).

As many brain injuries do not occur in isolation, it is important to note if a spinal cord injury is present. As caloric expenditure decreases in correlation with the degree of muscle immobility, this will alter feeding regimens. Estimated caloric needs for spinal cord injury can be as low as 28 kcal/Kg for paraplegia and 23 kcal/kg for quadraplegia (78).

Despite adequate calories, excessive nitrogen losses have been noted in brain injury patients. Urinary nitrogen losses of up to 30 g/day have been documented in the acute course of injury. Nitrogen loss is well associated with epinephrine and glucagons levels (80). In addition, immobility can account for 25% of nitrogen losses (90).

Patients with TBI require 1.5–2 g of protein/Kg of usual body weight daily. Despite providing adequate calories and protein, positive nitrogen balance is often unachievable in the early weeks after injury and may be difficult to achieve until the patient stabilizes medically (88).

Weight Loss Expectations

A secondary effect from hypermetabolism and hypercatabolism is weight loss. Loss of <10% of usual body weight is not considered significant. However, severe weight loss of up to 40% of usual body weight correlates with mortality. On average, patients lose 15.6 ± .9 pounds during their acute hospitalization despite the provision of adequate nutrition support (75). If the patient also has a spinal cord injury, another 5–10% weight loss is expected due to muscle loss from immobility dependent on paraplegia or quadraplegia.

ENTERAL VS. PARENTERAL NUTRITION SUPPORT

The use of enteral and parenteral nutrition has undergone significant changes over the past three decades. Initial fears about the use of hyperosmolar solutions in patients with TBI have been replaced with the aggressive use of TPN, but now attempts to use the GI tract as early as possible are commonplace.

Gastric Feeding vs. Intestinal Feeding

The decision about what form of nutrition support to choose for a new patient with a TBI/SCI is an important one, and it should be addressed shortly after the initial injury. As previously shown, delays in providing nutrition

increase the risk of mortality or at least could prolong rehabilitation time (5). For patients with TBI, the main question will be if there is an associated abdominal injury that requires laparotomy? If so, then a surgeon may place a jejunal feeding tube at the time of surgery, thereby providing small bowel access. This concept has been popular at many trauma centers around the country, and more importantly, early enteral feeding may limit the progression to multiple organ failure (91–95). For isolated brain injury, facial fractures and spinal injury must be detected and stabilized before decisions regarding enteral nutrition can be made. These issues are important because they guide clinical decisions regarding the initial blind passage of nasoenteric tubes and the possible use of either radiologic or endoscopic enteral access options.

Although providing parenteral nutrition may be easier than obtaining adequate enteral access, enteral nutrition has a decreased incidence of complications and cost compared to parenteral nutrition with no significant differences in measured nutritional parameters (91,93). Also, provision of fuel substrates to the intestine can stimulate gut immune function and limit deterioration of the intestinal mucosa with bacterial translocation and its potential for contributing to sepsis (96, 97). It is known that attempts at bolus feeding (BF) in patients with TBI are associated with a high incidence of intolerance (98). It is believed that elevations in intracranial pressure delay gastric emptying. Also, BF can also be associated with gastric emptying delays. Recently, Rhoney and coworkers showed in a brain-injured population that continuous gastric feeding was significantly better tolerated than BF (99). Prokinetic agents were not found to be helpful, and medications such as propofol and sucralfate were associated with feeding intolerance.

Klodell and colleagues showed that after early PEG placement that intragastric feeding was well tolerated in their patients with TBI. Five of the 118 patients did experience aspiration, but there was no evidence of intolerance prior to the aspiration (100).

In a related study, Neumann and DeLegge compared gastric versus small bowel feeding in an intensive care setting (101). They were also able to show that the gastric route was highly successful in feeding ICU patients without a marked increase in complications.

It is becoming clearer that attempts at enteral therapy should be made before using parenteral nutrition. Protocols for feeding should be developed for individual intensive care areas that stress the available resources for that unit. Careful attention must be made so that pulmonary aspiration is limited. Taylor et al. showed that enhanced enteral nutrition (started feeding rate at estimated needs the first day of feeding) appeared to enhance neurological recovery, as well as postinjury inflammatory responses and incidence of major complications (102).

Our group has shown that it is possible to obtain early enteral access in patients with TBI/SCI (103–106). Our present protocol is to attempt gastric feeding, if it is deemed safe and feasible. Otherwise, endoscopic or fluoroscopic tube placement is performed as soon as it can be arranged. In this way, patients are fed as quickly as possible.

When to Use Parenteral Nutrition

If the gut is nonfunctioning or safe enteral access cannot be achieved, then it is appropriate to fall back on the use of parenteral nutrition. Central venous access is necessary to infuse the hyperosmolar solutions, but the solutions are not dangerous, as previously believed. More importantly, it is crucial to be diligent over electrolyte changes and glucose levels. It is known that hyperglycemia over 220 mg/dl is associated with changes in the immune system so that attention to this detail is potentially critical in limiting infections associated with the use of parenteral nutrition (107).

Another common pitfall for the clinician is the concept that nutrition support must be "all or none." If the patient's nutritional needs cannot be met by enteral means alone, then it is acceptable to supplement this with intravenous nutrition to help approximate a patient's needs. Although overlap of enteral and parenteral nutrition is more common during the transition from parenteral to enteral therapy, there is no reason not try to reach a patient's requirements by whatever combination yields results safely.

Choosing an Appropriate Formula

Depending on calorie and protein needs, the clinician will need to utilize either a 1 kcal/cc high protein formula or a 2 kcal/cc formula. It has been our experience, that most 2 kcal/cc formulas do not meet estimated protein requirements for this population. Therefore, most patients will initially require use of a protein supplement to meet needs. A calorie dense formula may also be warranted in instances of fluid restriction for control of the syndrome of inappropriate antidiuretic hormone (SIADH).

The use of fiber must be considered in light of the medical plan of care. Fiber is avoided in cases where paralytics or pressors are being used as they may aggravate constipation from either reduced peristalsis or reduced gut perfusion. Once these medications are discontinued, fiber should be a part of the bowel regimen. This is especially important for patients with TBI that are likely to have long-term immobility or in patients with associated SCI.

Monitoring the Effectiveness of the Care Plan

Daily assessment is critical in the intensive care unit to respond to changes in medical status. At a minimum, daily assessment should include an assessment of laboratory values, gastrointestinal function, tolerance to feedings, fluid balance, and medication changes. If intracranial pressure monitoring is present, it is helpful to know how frequently it is drained as this may correlate with feeding tolerance. As feeding intolerance is noted, alternative recommendations should be noted. Weekly, a prealbumin and weight should be monitored for assessment of overall nutritional status.

Once medically stable and transferred to a non-intensive care unit, feeding tolerance should be monitored daily. Laboratory values may be checked more infrequently as long as not medically indicated, and the patient continues to tolerate feedings. Weights and prealbumins remain important indicators in this population to monitor overall status and needs. As time progresses, a patient's metabolism may slow, requiring a change in feeding regimen in order to achieve weight maintenance or loss. Prealbumin is useful in determining if calories and protein intake are adequate to prevent skin breakdown, while continuing to decrease overall calories. Feedback from physical and occupational therapists regarding mobility and skin breakdown is also helpful in estimating ongoing calorie and protein needs.

Micronutrient Supplementation

Vitamins and minerals should be supplemented if feeding volumes or oral intake does not meet the recommended dietary allowances. Antioxidants are felt to play a protective role in the recovery after brain injury. No significant changes in vitamin E levels have been observed in a recent study after brain injury. Therefore, it is felt that there is no benefit for additional supplementation (108).

Ascorbic acid is also known for its antioxidant properties. Polidori and coworkers demonstrated that ascorbic acid levels decreased during the first week after brain injury likely as a result of oxidative stress. These levels were inversely related to the GCS score and the major diameter of the lesion. Further studies are needed to see if vitamin C supplementation would be beneficial (109).

Zinc deficiency has been observed on admission and through the first two weeks of hospitalization (110). Adequate zinc status is necessary to minimize neuroimmune cell death in animal models. In addition, zinc supplementation has been utilized to treat deficiency and the severe protein turnover in patients with TBI (111). Daily supplementation of 12 mg of zinc is recommended (112). Losses can be substantial if patients have diarrhea or associated traumatic injury with enterocutaneous fistulas that drain significant amounts of fluid.

IMMUNE ENHANCING NUTRITIONAL SUPPORT ISSUES

The Role of Arginine

Arginine is a conditionally essential amino acid. Under normal circumstances it is synthesized endogenously from

L-citrulline. However, during stressful periods such as growth, illness, or metabolic stress, endogenous synthesis is unable to meet the increasing body demands, and a dietary source is required. On administration of pharmacologic doses, arginine stimulates the pituitary growth hormone, insulin-like growth factor, prolactin, insulin and other hormones, resulting in net positive effect on wound healing and immune functions (113). It is also a precursor for growth substances like putrescine, spermine, and spermidine. Importantly, arginine is a precursor for nitrates, nitrites, and nitric oxide. Nitric oxide is particularly important as a vasodilator, but it also participates in immunologic reactions, including the ability of macrophages to kill tumor cells and bacteria. These and other functions of arginine are still being evaluated, but it is clear that supplementation of arginine can have a generally positive effect on immune system functions and wound healing in humans and animal (114,115). Numerous studies have demonstrated suppression of T-cell mediated immune function after major surgery or trauma. Daly et al. studied the effect of 30 g per day of arginine on patients undergoing elective surgeries compared to an isonitrogenous placebo (116). T-cell mediated immune function was evaluated preoperatively and 1, 4, and 7 days postoperatively. Patients who received arginine demonstrated a quicker return to normal T-cell function measured by *in vitro* mitogen proliferation assays. This study also revealed increases in the CD_4 phenotype, which further suggests that supplemental level of arginine helps T-cell levels to recover faster (116).

The Role of Glutamine

Glutamine is also considered a conditionally essential amino acid. Of interest, it is the most abundant amino acid in the body. One of glutamine's major roles is as an oxidative fuel for rapidly replicating cells including gastrointestinal mucosal cells, enterocytes and colonocytes, as well as immune cells, lymphocytes and macrophages (113). Furthermore, glutamine appears to convey a protective or restorative influence on the GI tract, which may decrease translocation of enteric bacteria across the mucosal barrier. Perhaps the most compelling evidence for the immunomodulatory effects of glutamine comes from Ziegler et al. who studied 45 bone marrow transplant patients receiving either TPN supplemented with glutamine or an isonitrogenous, isocaloric control. Patients who received glutamine in their TPN demonstrated decreased incidence of infection and shorter hospital stay compared to the control group (117).

Unfortunately, the chemical structure of glutamine is relatively unstable in solution, unless the glutamine is bound to protein. Until recently, enteral formulas supplemented with glutamine were available only in powder form. Also, new technology using glutamine hydrolysate formulas and glutamine dipeptide has lead to the development of high glutamine liquid formulas that are compatible with TPN. It is important to note that there are no studies available that currently assess the direct effect of either glutamine or arginine in patients with TBI.

Are Immune Enhancing Formulas Indicated in This Population?

There is sparse information available discussing immune enhancing diets and brain injury. The first study was published in abstract form, patients with severe closed head injury defined as GCS <8 with evidence of brain injury on imaging were randomized to an immune-modulated diet rich in glutamine, arginine, fish oil and nucleotides (11 patients), Impact (Novartis Nutrition, Minneapolis, MN) or standard diet (9 patients), both via feeding tube (118). Patients were followed prospectively up to one week. In their findings, the infection rate was significantly lower in the enhanced diet group (9.1% vs 100%, p<0.0001), also there was significant improvement in the total lymphocyte count and percent of CD_4 count in the study group (118). However, this study generated several areas of concerns as follows: the study is only available in abstract form, and also the sample size was too small to provide significant statistical analysis. The next paper addressing the use of immune enhancing formulas compared two immune diets; Crucial (Nestle Nutrition, Deerfield, IL) and Impact (119). This study involved multiple trauma patients, but 9 of 13 patients had severe closed head injury. This prospective study consisted of 13 patients randomized to receive enterally either Crucial or Impact. The randomized diet was given for seven days with study measurements obtained at study entry and day 7. The feedings goals were calculated based on protein delivery of 1.5 g/Kg body weight. Feedings were started at 30 ml per hour and advanced 20 ml per hour every 4 to 8 hours until goal was met. The exact study conclusion was very difficult to interpret. The authors concluded that patients receiving Crucial had normalization of IL-1 release from peripheral monocytes incubated with lipopolysaccharide (LPS) *in vitro*, but no alteration was noted with Impact (119). This limited study did not lead to any concrete conclusions regarding these diets in patients with TBI.

The most recent study dealing with immune enhancing diets in head injury compared early enteral feeding to late enteral feeding with Impact in a prospective, randomized fashion. The early group received enteral feeding <72 hours after admission and the late group received feeding upon resolution of the ileus from their head injury. The overall conclusion was that there was no significant difference between the two studied groups, but there was trend for higher mortality in the late group (4 of 15) (120).

Based on the available studies, very few conclusions on the use of immune modulated formulas in patients with TBI can be made. The single best conclusion is that these diets seem to be well tolerated. Further clinical investigations are needed in this area, involving larger number of patients, to be studied in a randomized, prospective blinded way, comparing the immune enhancing diets to an isonitrogenous control.

REHABILITATION ISSUES

Once the patient stabilizes and transfers to the rehabilitation service, the team's goals are to normalize the patient's care in a safe environment and provide education for post-discharge placement. The major nutritional issues are dysphagia, maintaining a realistic body weight, and bowel regimens.

Dysphagia

The treatment of dysphagia requires a team effort between the speech-language pathologists, physiatrist, nursing staff, and dietitian. The overall goal is to find the least restrictive diet that promotes safe swallowing and maintains nutritional status. Patients who have been found to be at the highest risk for oropharyngeal dysphagia include the following: those with an admitting GCS of 3–5, a Ranchos Los Amigos Scale of Cognitive Functioning at Level II, a CT scan which demonstrated midline shift or brain pathology requiring an emergency craniotomy, or ventilation time greater than or equal to 15 days (121). Patients who remain lethargic and have a GCS less than 12 should not be considered for oral intake without a swallowing evaluation.

Typical swallowing disorders include oral preparatory problems, oral transit disorders, delayed pharyngeal swallow and pharyngeal neuromuscular abnormalities. A modified barium swallow or flexible endoscopic evaluation of a swallow are two useful tests to identify safe consistencies for oral intake and patients at risk for silent aspiration (122).

In addition to evaluating a functional swallow, patients must be assessed for readiness to feed. Barriers to feeding include cognitive and motor planning behaviors, such as impulsivity, distractability, inability to stay on task, poor sequencing skills, lack of initiation, and inability to motor plan self-feeding. For patients exhibiting these behaviors it is imperative to provide an environment for feeding that is free of distractions and yet can provide a safe level of supervision and assistance (123). For further review of dysphagia issues, please refer to Chapter 47 entitled "Evaluation and Treatment of Swallowing Problems After TBI."

The National Dysphagia Diet was instituted in April 2002 to standardize food consistencies and terminology throughout the health care continuum. Liquids can be given as thin, nectar-like, honey-like, and spoon-thick. Of concern, is that the thicker the liquid is made, the less fluid is usually consumed by the patient. Many of these patients will require an additional source for hydration either by intravenous fluids or by a feeding tube (124).

Solid food consistency can be determined by the speech language pathologist. These textures may vary from a blended smooth texture (called pureed), to a ground moist consistency (called mechanically altered), to a general diet. Dry foods are generally eliminated as they are difficult to maneuver in the oral phase with decreased tongue movement and/or difficult to propel with disco-ordination in the pharyngeal phase of the swallow.

Once a patient is advanced to oral intake, nutrition support regimens should be reevaluated. A dietitian is helpful in evaluating adequacy of oral intake and assisting in making recommendations for the weaning of nutrition support. Feeding schedules should either be nocturnal or after a meal to encourage oral intake. Calorie counts are often useful in weaning a patient from tube feeding. According to the Nutrition Practice Guidelines for Dysphagia of the American Dietetic Association, tube feedings should be discontinued when patients can consume 80% or greater of their estimated nutritional needs consistently.

Maintenance of Realistic Body Weight

The hypercatabolism of brain injury that drives weight loss generally stops and plateaus at three months post-injury. Information regarding mobility and progress in therapies and activities of daily living are useful in reassessing calorie needs. The more muscle groups utilized, the more muscle that is spared from disuse (125). Many patients have increased calorie needs during rehabilitation due to the calories spent during the work process of therapy. This increase can be 30–60% higher than control groups. Assistive devices can ease this increase (126).

Weekly weights are very useful in monitoring for weight gain or loss. As medical status normalizes, calorie demands decrease. Of utmost importance for patients and their families is to realize that if they have limited mobility or paresis, calorie needs are likely lower than normal. Indirect calorimetry was performed on non-ambulatory tube fed adults with neurologic disabilities. This study demonstrated an approximate 25% decrease in caloric needs for patients with fixed upper extremity contractures (127). Weight gain is also the result of altered food intake patterns. Some patients experience hyperphagia, which is compounded by a poor memory of when they last ate. Brain injured patients are noted to consume larger meals and more calories per day than controls. This occurs without regard to pre-meal stomach contents. Also, social factors are not an indicator of meal size (128).

These are important considerations in regards to planning a diet for weight loss or weight maintenance.

Behavior strategies should be employed that will limit access to food and get individuals into a set schedule of eating. Memory boards or diaries may be helpful in reminding individuals of the time and content of their last meal. Individuals should be discouraged from automatically eating because they think they are hungry.

Patients should be encouraged to follow a low-fat well-balanced diet. The food guide pyramid is a starting resource for diet planning. In addition, they should consult a registered dietitian or recognized weight management center (e.g. Weight Watchers) for assistance with individualized dietary meal plans. A registered dietitian can also provide the caregivers' support and assist in monitoring the effectiveness of the weight loss plan.

Obesity and decreased mobility can precipitate pressure sore development in the chronic care setting (129, 130). Therefore, all brain injury patients with limited mobility should receive periodic routine skin assessments If skin breakdown is noted, a further nutritional assessment is warranted.

Malnutrition can delay wound healing. It is important that deficiencies of protein, vitamins and minerals be repleted to allow for tissue growth and repair. Frequently, a deficiency is not clinically noted; however, it has become practice to provide daily supplementation of vitamins (131, 132). In patients without significant liver or renal disease, a daily multivitamin and an additional 500 mg of ascorbic acid are recommended. Vitamin A and zinc should also be given if pressure sores do not heal or progress in staging (133). Clinicians should review dietary habits with patients to also ensure adequate calories and increased protein for wound healing (134).

Bowel Regimens

For non-ambulatory patients and especially those with a spinal cord injury, bowel programs are an essential part of their medical management. The chronic patient should eat a high fiber diet of at least 30 grams per day. Good sources of fiber include whole grains, bran products, leafy greens and raw vegetables (135).

WITHDRAWAL OF FEEDINGS

It is beyond the scope of this chapter to delve in to all of the medical, legal, religious, and emotional issues that concern the potential withdrawal of nutrition support. Many states in the U.S. as well as many countries worldwide deal with end of life issues differently. Most importantly we, as health care professionals, must be advocates for the patient who may not be able to voice an opinion, and we must seek guidance as to their possible wishes from family and/or other loved ones.

CONCLUSIONS

Care of patients with TBI can be complex, yet rewarding. The gastrointestinal and nutritional ramifications of an individual's disease may be straightforward or require a specialist's input. Time should be taken to review the potential needs of each patient and care plans should be created and implemented. Further understanding of the underlying disease will improve the delivery of comprehensive care to these afflicted patients. The next few decades will likely see marked advances in both.

References

1. Cahill GF Jr. Starvation in man. *N Engl J Med* 1970;282:668–675.
2. Drew JH, Koop CE, Grigger RP. A nutritional study of neurosurgical patients. *J Neurosurg* 1947;4:7–15.
3. Haider W, Lackner F, Schlick W, et al. Metabolic changes in the course of severe brain damage. *Eur J Int Care Med* 1975;1:19–26.
4. White R. Aspects and problems of total parenteral alimentation in the neurosurgery patient. In Manni C, Magalini SI, Scrascia E (eds): *Total Parenteral Alimentation*. pp208–214. Amsterdam, Excerpta Medica, 1976.
5. Rapp RP, Young AB, Twyman DL, et al. The favorable effect of early parenteral feeding on survival in head-injured patients. *J Neurosurg* 1983;58:906–912.
6. Kamada T, Fusamoto H, Kawano S, et al. Acute gastroduodenal lesions in head injury: An endoscopic study. *Am J Gastroenterol* 1977;68:249–253.
7. Idjadi F, Robbins R, Stahl WM, Essiet G. Prospective study of gastric secretion in stressed patients with intracranial injury. *J Trauma* 1971;11:681–688.
8. Cushing H. Peptic ulcers and interbrain. *Surg Gynecol Obstet* 1932;55:1–34.
9. Larson C, Cavuto NJ, Flockhart DA, et al. Bioavailability and efficacy of omeprazole given orally and by nasogastric tube. *Dig Dis Sci* 1996;41:475–479.
10. Chun AH, Shi HH, Achari R, et al. Lansoprazole administration of the contents of a capsule dosage formulation through a nasogastric tube. *Clin Ther* 1996;18:833–842.
11. Balaban DH, Duckworth CW, Peura DA. Nasogastric omeprazole: Effects on gastric pH in critically ill patients. *Am J Gastroenterol* 1997;92:79–83.
12. Pisegna JR. Switching between intravenous and oral pantoprazole. *J Clin Gastroenterol* 2001;32:27–32.
13. Morris J, Karlstadt R, Blatcher D, et al. Intermittent intravenous pantoprazole rapidly achieves and maintains gastric pH >4 compared with continuous infusion H_2-receptor antagonist in intensive care unit patients. *Crit Care Med* 2001;29(suppl 12):485, 147A.
14. Cook DJ, Reeve BK, Guyatt GH, et al. Stress ulcer prophylaxis in critically ill patients: Resolving discordant meta-analyses. *JAMA* 1996;275:308–314.
15. McArthur CJ, McLaren IM, Critchley JA, Oh TE. Gastric emptying following brain injury: Effects of choice of sedation and intracranial pressure. *Intensive Care Med* 1995;21:573–576.
16. Segal JL, Milne N, Brunnemann SR. Gastric emptying is impaired in patients with spinal cord injury. *Am J Gastroenterol* 1995; 90:466–470.
17. Gore RM, Mintzer RA, Calenoff L. Gastrointestinal complications of spinal cord injury. *Spine* 1981;6:538–544.
18. Altmayer T, O'Dell MW, Jones M, et al. Cisapride as a treatment for gastroparesis on traumatic brain injury. *Arch Phys Med Rehabil* 1996;77:1091–1094.
19. Jackson MD, Davidoff G. Gastroparesis following traumatic brain injury and response to metoclopramide therapy. *Arch Phys Med Rehabil* 1989;70:553–555.
20. Cataldi-Betcher EL, Seltzer MH, Slocum BA, Jones KW. Complications occurring during enteral nutrition support: A prospective study. *JPEN* 1983;7:546–552.

21. Kelly TWJ, Patrick MR, Hillman KM. Study of diarrhea in critically ill patients. *Crit Care Med* 1983;11:7–9.

22. Edes TE, Walk BE, Austin JL. Diarrhea in tube-fed patients: Feeding formula not necessarily the cause. *Am J Med* 1990;88:91–93.

23. Broom J, Jones K. Causes and prevention of diarrhea in patients receiving enteral support. *J Hum Nutr* 1981;35:123–127.

24. Eisenberg PG. Causes of diarrhea in tube-fed patients: A comprehensive approach to diagnosis and management. *Nutr Clin Prac* 1993;8:119–123.

25. McGuire TJ, Kumar V. Autonomic dysreflexia in the spinal cord-injured: What the physician should know about this medical emergency. *Postgrad Med* 1986;80:81–84, 89.

26. Branch C, Albertson D, Kelly D. Post-traumatic acalculous cholecystitis on a neurosurgical service. *Neurosurgery* 1983;12:98–101.

27. Okada Y, Tanabe R. Postraumatic acute cholecystitis: Relationship to the initial trauma. *Am J Forensic Med Pathol* 1987;8:164–168.

28. Orlando R, Gleason E, Drezner A. Acute acalculous cholecystitis in the critically ill patient. *Am Surg* 1983;145:472–476.

29. Ganuza F, La Banda F, Montalvo R. Acute acalculous cholecystitis in patients with acute traumatic spinal cord injury. *Spinal Cord* 1997;35:124–128.

30. Klliafas S, Ziegler DW, Flancbaum L, Choban PS. Acute acalculous cholecystitis: Incidence, risk factors, diagnosis, and outcome. *Am Surg* 1998;64:471–475.

31. Molenat F, Boussuges A, Valantin V, Sainty JM. Gallbladder abnormalities in medical ICU patients: An ultrasonographic study. *Intensive Care Med* 1996;22:356–361.

32. Puc M, Tran H, Wry P, Ross S. Ultrasound is not a useful screening tool for acute acalculous cholecystitis in critically ill trauma patients. *Am Surg* 2002;68:65–69.

33. Westlake PJ, Hershfield NB, Kelly JK. Chronic right upper quadrant pain without gallstones: Does HIDA scan predict outcome after cholecystectomy? *Am J Gastroenterol* 1990;85:986–991.

34. Heruti R, Bar-On Z, Gofrit O. Acute acalculous cholecystitis as a complication of spinal cord injury. *Arch Phys Rehabil* 1994;75:822–824.

35. DuPriest RW, Khaneja SC, Cowley RA. Acute cholecystitis complicating trauma. *Ann Surg* 1979;189:84–89.

36. Bouwman D, Altshuler J, Weaver D. Hyperamylasemia: A result of intracranial bleeding. *Surgery* 1983;94:318-323.

37. Liu K, Atten M, Lichtor T, Cho M, et al. Serum amylase and lipase elevation is associated with intracranial events. *Am Surg* 2001;67:215–220.

38. Justice A, Dibenedetto R, Stanford E. Significance of elevated pancreatic enzymes in intracranial bleeding. *South Med J* 1994;87:889–893.

39. Wilson-Storey D, MacKinlay GA. The superior mesenteric artery syndrome. *J R Coll Surg Edinb* 1986;31:175–178.

40. Hines JR, Gore RM, Ballantyne GH. Superior mesenteric artery syndrome: Diagnostic criteria and therapeutic approaches. *Am J Surg* 1984;148:630–632.

41. Flakoll P, Wentzel L, Hyman S. Protein and glucose metabolism during isolated closed- head injury. *Am J Physiol* 1995;269:E636–E641.

42. De Salles A, Muizelaar J, Young H. Hyperglycemia, cerebrospinal fluid lactic acidosis, and cerebral blood flow in severely head-injured patients. *Neurosurg* 1987;21:45–50.

43. Rosner M, Newsome H, Becker DP. Mechanical brain injury: The sympathoadrenal response. *J Neurosurg* 1984;61:76–86.

44. Cherian L, Goodman J, Robertson C. Hyperglycemia increases brain injury caused by secondary ischemia after cortical impact injury in rats. *Crit Care Med* 1997;25:1378–1383.

45. Young B, Ott L, Dempsey R, et al. Relationship between admission hyperglycemia and neurologic outcome of severely brain-injured patients. *Ann Surg* 1989;210:466–472.

46. Lam A, Winn R, Cullen B, Sundling N. Hyperglycemia and neurological outcome in patients with head injury. *J Neurosurg* 1991;75:545–551.

47. Rovlias A, Kotsou S. The influence of hyperglycemia on neurological outcome in patients with severe head injury. *Neurosurg* 2000;46:335–343.

48. den Berghe GV, Wouters P, Weekers F, et al. Intensive insulin therapy in critically ill patients. *N Engl J Med* 2001;345:1359–1367.

49. Yuan XQ, Wade CE. Neuroendocrine abnormalities in patients with traumatic brain injury. *Front Neuroendocrinol* 1991;12:209–30.

50. Doczi T, Tarjanyi J, Huszka E, Kiss J. Syndrome of inappropriate secretion of antidiuretic hormone (SIADH) after head injury. *Neurosurg* 1982;10:685–688.

51. Born J, Hans P, Smitz S, et al. Syndrome of inappropriate secretion of antidiuretic hormone after severe head injury. *Surg Neurol* 1985;23:383–387.

52. Wijdicks EF, Vermeulen M, Hijdra A. Hyponatremia and cerebral infarction in patients with ruptured intracranial aneurysms: Is fluid restriction harmful? *Ann Neurol* 1985;17:137–140.

53. Decaux G, Brimioulle S, Genette F, Mockel J. Treatment of the syndrome of inappropriate secretion of antidiuretic hormone by urea. *Am J Med* 1980;69:99–102.

54. Harrigan M. Cerebral salt wasting syndrome. *Crit Care Clin* 2001;17:125–138.

55. Harrigan M. Cerebral salt wasting syndrome: A Review. *Neurosurg* 1996;38:152–160.

56. Zafonte R, Mann N. Cerebral salt wasting syndrome in brain injury patients: A potential cause of hyponatremia. *Arch Phys Med Rehabil* 1997;78:540–542.

57. Iudice A, Murri L. Pharmacological prophylaxis of post-traumatic epilepsy. *Drugs* 2000;59:1091–1099.

58. Diaz-Arrastia R, Agostini M, Frol A. Neurophysiologic and neuroradiologic features of intractable epilepsy after traumatic brain injury in adults. *Arch Neurol* 2000;57:1611–1616.

59. Tempkin N, Dikmen S, Wilensky A. A randomized, double blind study of phenytoin for the prevention of post-traumatic seizures. *N Engl J Med* 1990;323:497–502.

60. Ricacoba MR,Salas PX. Efficacy and tolerability of long-term topiramate in drug resistant epilepsy in adults. *Rev Neurol* 2002;34:101–105.

61. Veerman, MW. Excipients in valproic acid syrup may cause diarrhea: A case report. *DICP* 1990;24:832–833.

62. Claasen J, Peery M, Kreiter M. Predictors and clinical impact of epilepsy after subarachnoid hemorrhage. *Neurology* 2003;60:208–214.

63. Jennett B, Miller J, Braakman R. Epilepsy after non-missile depressed skull fracture. *J Neurosurg* 1974;41:208–216.

64. Westbrook L, Devinsky O, Geocadin R. Nonepileptic seizures after head injury. *Epilepsia* 1998;39:978–982.

65. Bauer LA. Interference of oral phenytoin absorption by continuous infusion nasogastric feedings. *Neurology* 1982;32:570–572.

66. Ozuna J, Friel P. Effects of enteral tube feedings on serum phenytoin levels. *J Neurosurg Nurs* 1984;16:289–291.

67. Holtz L, Milton J, Sturek JK. Compatibility of medications with enteral feedings. *JPEN* 1987;11:183–186.

68. The Brain Trauma Foundation. Use of Barbiturates in the control of intracranial hypertension. *J Neurotraum* 2000;17:527–530.

69. Dempsey DT, Guenter P, Mullen J, et al. Energy expenditure in acute trauma to the head with and without barbiturate therapy. *Surg Gynecol Obstet* 1985;160:128–160.

70. Dereeper E, Berre J, Vandesteene A. Barbiturate coma for intracranial hypertension: Clinical observations. *J Crit Care* 2002;17:58–62.

71. Lee M, Deppe S, Sipperly E. The efficacy of barbiturate coma in the management of uncontrolled intracranial hypertension following neurosurgical trauma. *J Neurotraum* 1994;11:325–331.

72. Ward J, Becker D, Miller D. Failure of prophylactic barbiturate coma in the treatment of severe head injury. *J Neurosurg* 1985;62:383–388.

73. Young B, Ott L, Haack E, et al. Effect of total parenteral nutrition upon intracranial pressure in severe head injury. *J Neurosurg* 1987;67:76–80.

74. Young B, Ott L, Norton J, et al. Metabolic and nutritional sequelae in the non-steroid treated head injury patient. *Neurosurgery* 1985;17:784–791.

75. Clifton GL, Robertson CS, Grossman RG, et al. The metabolic response to head injury. *J Neurosurg* 1986;60:89–98.

76. Robertson CS, Clifton GL, Grossman RG. Oxygen utilization and cardiovascular function in head-injured patients. *J Neurosurg* 1984;63:714–718.

77. Makk LJK, McClave SJ, Creech PW, et al. Clinical application of the metabolic cart to the delivery of parenteral nutrition. *Crit Care Med* 1987;13:818–829.

78. Sunderland PM, Heilbrun MP. Estimating energy expenditure in traumatic brain injury: Comparison of indirect calorimetry with predictive formulas. *Neurosurgery* 1992;31:246–253.

79. Birkhahn RH, Long CL, Fitkin D, et al. Effects of major skeletal trauma on whole body protein. *Surgery* 1980;88:294–300.

80. Chiolero R, Schultz Y, Lemerchand T, et al. Hormonal and metabolic changes following severe head injury and noncranial injury. *JPEN* 1992;13:5–12.

81. Ott L, Schmidt J, Young B, et al. Comparison administration of two standard intravenous amino acid formulas to severely brain-injured patients. *Drug Intell Clin Pharm* 1988;22:763–768.

82. Detsky AS, McLaughlin JR, Baker JP, et al. What is subjective global assessment of nutritional status? *JPEN* 1987;11:8–13.

83. Chiolero R, Revelly J, Tappy L. Energy metabolism in sepsis and injury. *Nutrition* 1997;13(suppl):45S–51S.

84. Clifton GL, Robertson CS, Choi SC. Assessment of nutritional requirements of head-injured patients. *J Neurosurg* 1986; 64: 895–901.

85. Robertson CS, Clifton GL, Grossman RG, et al. Oxygen utilization and cardiovascular function in head injury patients. *J Neurosurg* 1985;15:307–9.

86. Bucci MN, Dechert RD, Arnoldi DK, et al. Elevated intracranial pressure associated with hypermetabolism in isolated head injury. *Acta Neurochir (Wien)* 1988;93:133–4.

87. Varella L, Jastemski C. Neurological Impairment. In: Gottschlich M (ed). The Science and Practice of Nutrition Support: *A Core Based Curriculum.* 2001, Dubuque, Kendall Hunt Publishing Company, pp421–444.

88. Clifton GL, Ziegler M, Grossman RG. Circulating catecholamines and sympathetic activity after head injury. *Neurosurgery* 1991;8:10–14.

89. Ott L, Young B. Neurosurgery. In: Zaloga GP (ed). *Nutrition in Critical Care.* St. Louis: Mosby Year Book; 1994: pp. 691–706.

90. Young B, Ott L. The neurosurgical patient. In: Rombeau JL, Caldwell MD (eds). *Clinical Nutrition: Parenteral Nutrition* (2nd ed.). Philadelphia: W.B. Saunders Company, 1993:585–596.

91. Moore EE, Jones TN. Benefits of immediate jejunostomy feeding after major abdominal trauma: A prospective, randomized study. *J Trauma* 1986;26:874–880.

92. Adams S, Dellinger EP, Wertz MJ, et al. Enteral versus parenteral nutritional support following laparotomy for trauma: A randomized prospective trial. *J Trauma* 1986;26:883–890.

93. Moore FA, Moore EE, Jones TN, et al. TEN versus TPN following major abdominal trauma: Reduced septic morbidity. *J Trauma* 1989;29:916–922.

94. Kudsk KA, Croce MA, Fabian TC, et al. Enteral versus parenteral feeding: Effects on septic morbidity after blunt and penetrating abdominal trauma. *Ann Surg* 1992;215:503–511.

95. Moore FA, Feliciano DV, Andrassy RJ, et al. Early enteral feeding, compared with parenteral, reduces postoperative septic complications: The results of a meta-analysis. *Ann Surg* 1992;216: 172–183.

96. Alverdy J, Chi HS, Sheldon GF. The effect of parenteral nutrition on gastrointestinal immunity: The importance of enteral stimulation. *Ann Surg* 1985;202:681–684.

97. Deitch EA, Winterton J, Li M, Berg R. The gut as a portal of entry for bacteremia: Role of protein malnutrition. *Ann Surg* 1987; 205:681–692.

98. Clifton GL, Robertson CS, Contant CF. Enteral hyperalimentation in head injury. *J Neurosurg* 1985;62:186–193.

99. Rhoney DH, Parker D Jr, Formea CM, et al. Tolerability of bolus versus continuous gastric feeding in brain-injured patients. *Neurol Res* 2002;24:613–620.

100. Klodell CT, Carroll M, Carrillo EH, Spain DA. Routine intragastric feeding following traumatic brain injury is safe and well tolerated. *Am J Surg* 2000;179:168–171.

101. Neumann DA, DeLegge MH. Gastric versus small-bowel tube feeding in the intensive care unit: A prospective comparison of efficacy. *Crit Care Med* 2002;30:1436–1438.

102. Taylor SJ, Fettes SB, Jewkes C, Nelson RJ. Prospective, randomized, controlled trial to determine the effect of early enhanced enteral nutrition on clinical outcome in mechanically ventilated patients suffering head injury. *Crit Care Med* 1999;27: 2525–2531.

103. Kirby DF, Clifton GL, Turner H, et al. Early enteral nutrition after brain injury by percutaneous endoscopic gastrojejunostomy. *JPEN* 1991;15:298–302.

104. Duckworth PF Jr, Kirby, DF, McHenry L Jr, et al. Percutaneous endoscopic gastrojejunostomy (PEG/J) made easy: A new over-the-wire technique. *Gastrointest Endosc* 1994;40:350–353.

105. DeLegge MH, Duckworth PF Jr, McHenry L Jr, et al. *Percutaneous endoscopic gastrojejunostomy: A dual center safety and efficacy trial.* 1995;19:239–243.

106. Patrick PG, Marulendra S, Kirby DF, DeLegge MH. Endoscopic nasogastric/jejunal feeding tube placement in critically ill patients. *Gastrointest Endosc* 1997;45:72–76.

107. Hennessey PJ, Black CT, Andrassy RJ. Nonenzymatic glycosylation of immunoglobulin G impairs complement fixation. *JPEN* 1991;15:60–64.

108. Paolin A, Nardin L, Gaetani P, et al. Oxidative damage after severe head injury and its relationship to neurological outcome. *Neurosurgery* 2002;4:949–950.

109. Polidori MC, Mecocci P, Frei B. Plasma vitamin C levels are decreased and brain damage in patients with intracranial hemorrhage or head trauma. *Stroke* 2001;32:898–902.

110. Ott L, Young B, McClain C. The metabolic response to brain injury. *JPEN* 1987;11:488–493.

111. Yeiser EC, Vanlandingham JW, Levenson CW. Moderate zinc deficiency increases cell death after brain injury in the rat. *Nutr Neurosci* 2002;5:345–52.

112. Evans NJ, Compher CW. Nutrition and the Neurologically impaired patient. In: Torosian MH (ed). *Nutrition for the Hospitalized Patient.* New York: Marcel Dekker 1995, pp. 567–589.

113. Wesley AJ. Immunoenhancement via enteral nutrition. *Arch Surg* 1993;128:1242–1245.

114. Kirk SJ, Hurson M, Regan MC. Arginine stimulates wound healing and immune function in elderly human beings. *Surgery* 1993;114:155–160.

115. Barbul A, Sisto DA, Wasserkrug HL, Efron G. Arginine stimulates lymphocyte immune response in healthy human beings. *Surgery* 1981;90:244–251.

116. Daly JM, Reynolds J, Thom A. Immune and metabolic effects of arginine in the surgical patients. *Ann Surg* 1988;208:512–522.

117. Ziegler TR, Young LS, Benfell K. Clinical and metabolic efficacy of glutamine-supplemented parenteral nutrition after bone marrow transplantation. *Ann Intern Med* 1992;116:821–828.

118. Chendrasekhar A, Fagerli JC, Prabhakar G. Evaluation of an enhanced diet in patients with severe closed head injury. *Crit Care Med* 1997;25:A80.

119. Jeevanandam M, Shahbazian LM, Peterson SR. Proinflammatory cytokine production by mitogen-stimulated peripheral blood mononuclear cells in trauma patients fed immune-enhancing enteral diets. *Nutrition* 1999;15:842–847.

120. Minard G, Kudsk KA, Melton S. Early versus delayed feeding with an immune-enhancing diet in patients with severe head injuries. *JPEN* 2000;24:145–149.

121. Mackay LE. Factors affecting oral feeding with severe traumatic brain injury. *J Head Trauma Rehabil* 1999;14:435–447.

122. Logemann J. Treatment for aspiration related to dysphagia: An overview. *Dysphagia* 1986;1:34–38.

123. Jacobsson, C. Outcomes of individualized interventions in patients with severe eating difficulties. *Clin Nurs Res* 1997;6: 25–44.

124. Finestone, HM. Quantifying fluid intake in dysphagic stroke patients: A preliminary comparision of oral and nonoral strategies. *Arch Phys Med Rehabil* 2001;82:1744–1746.

125. Janssen I. Low relative skeletal muscle mass in older persons is associated with functional impairment and physical disability. *J Am Geriatr Soc* 2002;50:889–896.

126. Gonzalez EG, Edelstein JE. Energy expenditure during ambulation. In: Gonzalez EG, Myers SJ, Edelstein JE, Lieberman JS, Downey JA (eds). *Downey and Darling's Physiological Basis of Rehabilitation Medicine.* pp 417–448. Boston: Butterworth-Heinemann. 2001. 3rd ed.; pp. 210–250.

127. Dickerson, RN. Effect of upper extremity posturing on measured resting energy expenditure on non-ambulatory tube-fed patients with severe neurodevelopemental disabilities. *JPEN* 2002; 26:278–284.

128. Henson MB, DeCastro JM, Stringer AY, et al. Food intake by brain-injured humans who are in the chronic phase of recovery. *Brain Inj* 1993;7:169–178.

129. Daniel RK, Priest DL, Wheatly DC. Etiologic factors in pressure sores: An experimental model. *Arch Phys Med Rehabil* 1981; 62:492–498.

130. Andersen KE, Jensen O, Kvorning SA, et.al. Prevention of pressure sores by identifying patients at risk. *BMJ* 1982;284: 1370.

131. A.S.P.E.N. Board of Directors. Guidelines for use of parenteral and enteral nutrition in adult and pediatric patients. *JPEN* 2002;26(supplement):51–52, 65–67, 76–78, 88–89.

132. Salomon HK, McKnight LA. Management of a patient with severe burn injury and significant stress-induced weight loss: A case study. *Support Line* 1999;21(4):11–20.

133. Flanigan KH. Nutritional aspects of wound healing. *Adv Wound Care* 1997;10:48–52.

134. Guralnik JM, Harris TB, White LR, et al. Occurrence and predictors of pressure sores in the National Health and Nutrition Examination Survey follow-up. *J Am Geratr Soc* 1988;36: 807–812.

135. Cameron K, Nyulasi I, Colier G, et al. Assessment of the effect of increased dietary fiber intake on bowel function in patients with spinal cord injury. *Spinal Cord* 1996;34:277–283.

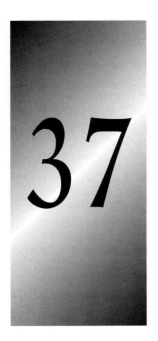

37 Sexuality, Reproduction, and Neuroendocrine Disorders Following TBI

M. Elizabeth Sandel
Richard Delmonico
Mary Jean Kotch

INTRODUCTION

Our understanding of human sexuality has evolved over the last century to a greater appreciation of the biological, cultural and psychological factors that underpin sexual behavior. Freud's groundbreaking and controversial theories on psychosexual development and sexuality were based on the understanding that sexuality is a primary component of human development and functioning. Although some of Freud's beliefs about sexual development have been questioned, his understanding of the importance of sexuality in human life has been an important contribution to medicine, science, and the social sciences.

Biologists and ethnologists have studied animal models of sexual physiology and functioning, and these models have been important in advancing our understanding of human sexual behavior. These approaches have informed us that there is a wide range of variability in the expression of sexual and reproductive behaviors across species. In addition, anatomists and physiologists have further advanced our understanding of human reproduction and human sexuality.

Social and cultural beliefs have also contributed to our evolving understanding of sexual behavior. Sociologists and anthropologists have studied broad variations in human behavior across cultures. Behaviors considered deviant in one culture might be accepted practices in another. Gender, sex roles, and sexual orientation are prime examples of differences that may be heavily influenced by cultural and political forces. Human sexual behavior is based upon a complex interaction of biological, psychological, and cultural factors. Unfortunately, most of sexology research over the last few decades has focused on males and on heterosexual populations, although this bias is gradually being recognized and funding of research in the area has been more comprehensive in recent years. Research focused on women with traumatic brain injury is also sparse (1).

A traumatic brain injury (TBI) profoundly affects every aspect of an individual's functioning. These injuries have an impact on physical, cognitive, emotional, behavioral, and social functioning. Physical disabilities may be caused by anatomic or physiologic changes as a result of the injury. Cognitive disabilities commonly include problems with concentration, learning, memory, information processing, language, problem-solving, reasoning, planning, and organizational skills. Emotional difficulties are not only limited to psychological disorders such as depression, but also difficulties that affect behavior and personality. Behavioral problems can include impulsivity, poor initiation, perseverative behaviors, and other frontal lobe disturbances. Interpersonal skills problems may significantly influence social and occupational functioning. The complexity of all of these factors and their interrelationships creates a number of methodological challenges for research in the area of sexuality and TBI.

SEXUAL RESPONSE MODELS AND SEXUAL DYSFUNCTION

According to the Masters and Johnson model of the 1960's, the sexual response cycle consists of four phases: excitement, plateau, orgasm, and resolution (2). A simplified model, described by Kaplan (3), included only desire, excitement, and orgasm. More recently described models take into account new perspectives and new research, suggesting that the genital focus of previous models and the linear sequence inherent to these models inaccurately reflects the cyclical nature of the interactions within the mind and between the mind and body during intimacy and sexual activity. Sexuality for women, and also for men, includes an interaction of personal factors such as self-image and desire for connection, but must also be seen within the context of family, interpersonal relationships, society and culture. Life stressors, including financial and health issues, also contribute to the sexual and intimate interactions between couples (4, 5).

An alternative sexual response cycle model described by Basson (6) takes into account other aspects of sexuality and intimacy: the desire to express affection and to share pleasure, a sense of being attracted to and attractive to another, and a sense of commitment. This model emphasizes that sexual experiences may begin with a non-sexual state of mind, and take place within a much larger context of cognition and behavior, acknowledging the importance of the aspects of intimacy that contribute to both the non-sexual and the sexual state of mind. These factors include communication, respect, trust, vulnerability, and fear of loss.

Definitions of Sexual Dysfunction

Sexual desire disorders include sexual aversion and hypoactive sexual desire. Sexual arousal disorders result in poor lubrication in women and erectile disorders in both men (penile) and women (clitoral). Orgasmic disorders include anorgasmia in men and women and premature ejaculation in men. Sexual pain disorders include dyspareunia and vaginismus. An international consensus development conference on female sexual dysfunction resulted in an expansion of these classifications.

The existing classification system for sexual dysfunction, based on the World Health Organization (WHO) International Classifcation of Disease-10 (7) and the Diagnostic and Statistical Manual of Mental Disorders (8), has been challenged by an interdisciplinary consensus conference panel, consisting of 19 experts in female sexual dysfunction. The former classifications were expanded to include psychogenic and organic causes of desire, arousal, orgasm, and sexual pain disorders. A personal distress criterion has been added; this criterion specifies that a condition is considered a disorder only if

it creates distress for the woman experiencing the condition. As noted by Sipski (9), patients with traumatic brain injuries may lack awareness and appreciation of "personal distress." Definitions of sexual arousal and hypoactive sexual desire disorders were developed in this new classification system, and a category of noncoital sexual pain disorder was added (10).

Many psychological and biological factors influence the processing of sexual, sensual, or erotic stimuli. Psychological factors include past experiences (positive, affirming, negative, or traumatizing) and responses to the present sexual context. Inadequate or impaired emotional development may also influence openness to sexual experience, and result in lack of sexual arousal or even dysphoric arousal. Emotional intimacy and physical satisfaction with the sexual experience may not necessarily include orgasmic release. Biological factors that affect the processing of sexual stimuli include depression, medications that impair sexual function, fatigue, sleep disturbance, substance use, other medical conditions, and neuroendocrine factors.

Individuals may also experience anxiety about intimacy, sexual performance, or consequences of sexual activity. This anxiety may be a primary or secondary factor in the development of sexual dysfunction. Anxiety may interfere with any stage of the sexual response cycle and commonly plays a role in arousal conditions such as premature ejaculation, erectile dysfunction, and arousal dysfunction in women.

Studies suggest that sexual dysfunction is more prevalent in women than in men in the United States and a number of other countries. Prevalence data is dependent on the assessment techniques, which are variable (4). The Massachusetts Women's Health Study (11,12) documented decreased sexual desire among married women, those with psychological symptoms, cigarette smokers, and those in the perimenopausal state. However, of note, in healthy women, the prevalence of sexual dysfunction actually appears to decline with age, and frequency of sexual intercourse is not related to menopausal status. (11–13)

There may be differences in sexual desire and drive between men and women, although this is still an area of considerable controversy (14). Male sex drive may be more urgent, less distractible, more goal-oriented, and more focused on intercourse; female sex drive may be more diffuse, more distractible, more receptive, and more motivated by a desire for affection and emotional connection. Female desire may be more contextual, more aroused by words than images, more emotional than biological, more sensual than genital, more flexible and mutable. Men report more sexual fantasies and thoughts and experience more spontaneous sexual desire, report having more desire for more sexual partners, masturbate at younger ages and with greater frequency, and become aware of their sexual drive earlier than women. Men also show a greater preference for sexual variety and novelty, have more favorable attitudes towards their genitals, and report higher and more consistent levels of desire across their lifetime (15, 16). To what extent these differences are culturally driven, or influenced by societal roles, teachings and expectations, is poorly understood (14–16).

Most studies of sexuality to date have focused on heterosexual populations. The research related to sexuality within gay, lesbian, and transgender populations suggests that even more complexity is inherent in the study of human sexuality than has been formerly appreciated. As these topics are discussed and researched more widely, our understanding of human sexuality is evolving towards a greater awareness of how societal and cultural influences shape the understanding and expression of sexuality. This may in fact lead to more openness, acceptance, diversity of expression, and greater sexual health for all.

NEUROLOGICAL SYSTEMS AND SEXUALITY

The neurological aspects of sexuality include widespread and complex relationships among the neuroanatomic, neurochemical, neurophysiological, and neuropsychological systems that govern behavior, including what we define as emotional, physical, sensory, and cognitive components. The resulting sexual behaviors can be described more concretely as motivation, desire, arousal, genital responses, and orgasm.

Our understanding of the brain-behavior relationships that are the basis for human sexuality is primarily derived from animal studies, and therefore our conclusions must be tentative. The inter-relationships among the systems that contribute to these concrete behaviors are not completely understood. However, the peripheral nervous system, including motor, sensory and autonomic neurons, and subcortical and cortical systems, contribute to sexual interest and responsiveness through an elaborate network. Lesions at any level may influence this behavior, although the actual effects of such lesions in humans are not fully established. Central nervous system control of sexual function is similarly organized in men and women (17).

Chemical Messengers

Neurotransmitters play a critical role in the physiological basis of sexual behaviors and sexual response. Spinal cord centers are under the control of brain regions that exert both excitatory and inhibitory influences. Sexual desire has been linked to activity of dopaminergic systems, including the mesolimbic and mesocortical systems. Serotonin may have an inhibiting effect on sexual function. Hypothalamic spinal pathways using oxytocin as a neurotransmitter have also been identified. Nitric oxide, crucial for sexual function at the genital level, may also be an important central nervous system messenger. Receptors for gonadal hormones include neurons in the midbrain, hypothalamus, and amygdala. The supraspinal sites involved in the sexual response network have both extensive interconnections and receive genital sensory input. There does not appear to be a strict division between reflexive and psychogenic responses given this organizational structure (17).

Spinal Systems

A coordinated system of sympathetic, parasympathetic, and somatic spinal outflow tracts are the basis for human sexual response. The spinal cord is "necessary and sufficient" to produce sexual responsiveness (17). Genital innervation is somatic as well as autonomic (i.e., parasympathetic and sympathetic). Somatic sensory afferents, synapsing in the sacral spinal cord, induce local sexual responses and project sensory information to cortical regions, resulting in sexual awareness and sexual excitation. Parasympathetic innervation originating at the sacral level, organized in the pelvic nerves, supply the neuronal inputs and outputs responsible for the initiation and maintenance of the erectile response. Erections are observed after lesions of sacral cord segments and pelvic nerves and the psychogenic erections in paraplegics with conus or cauda equina lesions may occur because of other non-cerebral proerectile pathways operating via the hypogastric nerves (18). Psychogenic mechanisms of arousal may also be transmitted in sympathetic pathways. Sympathetic neurons from the thoracic cord, contained in the hypogastric plexus, provide efferent and afferent innervations to the internal genitalia; this system provides the neurological basis for emission. Ejaculation is a result of sympathetic outflow from T11-L2 segments including the sympathetic chain, the hypogastric plexus, and pelvic and pudendal nerve systems (19).

In women, these neurological connections are also the basis for sexual responses, including arousal, lubrication, and female ejaculation. Parasympathetic activity causes clitoral erection, engorgement of the labia, and vaginal lubrication. Orgasmic sympathetic activity results in contraction of pelvic structures including uterus, fallopian tubes, paraurethral glands, and pelvic floor muscles (20).

The Brainstem and Related Structures

Brainstem centers that contribute to human sexual responses include the reticular activating systems of the pons and midbrain. These pathways, which provide input for initiation and maintenance of arousal and alertness, connect with limbic and other frontal structures, many of which play a role in sexual and sexually related behaviors, including affective responses. Brainstem regions connect with diencephalic structures and limbic and paralimbic structures including the hippocampus, septal complex, cingulate gyrus, amygdala, and hypothalamus. Stimulation of these structures produces erection, and in some cases pre-orgasmic sensations of pleasure. Lesions of the piriform cortex, which is inter-connected with the olfactory cortex, produce hypersexual responses in animals. The role of the basal ganglia in sexual function is not clear, although stimulation may result in species-specific sexual behaviors (21).

Subcortical Systems

The primary areas of the hypothalamus that contribute to sexual response are the paraventricular nucleus, tuberal region, medial preoptic area, and the dorsal hypothalamic area. These hypothalamic regions are likely involved in both sexual desire and sexual response. The basal hypothalamus is influenced by tissue levels of testosterone, dihydrotestosterone, and estradiol. The preoptic area has high concentrations of androgen and estrogen receptors, and the enzyme that converts androgens to estrogens. Manipulating androgens and androgen receptors in this region affects sexual behavior. Lesions in the medial preoptic area of the hypothalamus reduce or eliminate sexual behavior. This area receives neuronal inputs from other brain regions such as the olfactory system and the cerebral cortex, including the visual cortex (17, 19, 22).

The dorsomedial nucleus of the hypothalamus, when stimulated, produces ejaculation. This nucleus may receive input from the medial preoptic area and probably from other brain and body regions. The ventromedial nucleus of the hypothalamus appears to play a role in female sexual behaviors. This nucleus is also strongly influenced by sex hormones, in particular estrogen and progesterone. The hypothalamus receives some of its information in the form of neuronal messages, but other information arrives in the form of chemical messages, including gonadal steriods. In addition, the hypothalamus synthesizes and secretes hormones of its own, many of which exert influences over sex and reproduction (22).

The pituitary hormones play a crucial role in the sexual and reproductive activity of humans. Gonadotropin-releasing hormone stimulates the release of follicle-stimulation hormone (FSH) and luteinizing hormone (LH) regulates the menstrual cycle in women and testosterone secretion in men. Males with hypothalamo-pituitary disorders have decreased or absent sexual desire, and often this is the first symptom to appear. In females with hypothalamo-pituitary disorders, two-thirds notice absence or a considerable decrease in sexual desire; lubrication and anorgasmia are also very common (23).

Cortical Systems

The Kluver-Bucy syndrome results from injury or ablation to the anterior temporal poles, and the syndrome includes hypersexual and exploratory behaviors, and hyperorality (24, 25). Temporal lobe seizures may be manifested by genital sensation and other sexual phenomena, with hypersexual or hyposexual behavior during both ictal and interictal periods. Endocrine disturbances, which are common in both men and women with temporal lobe epilepsy, result in decreased libido, impotence, menstrual disturbances, and reproductive disorders (26–28).

The frontal lobes are clearly involved in the regulation of sexual behaviors. Injury to the orbitofrontal regions (limbic and paralimbic lesions) may produce hypersexual responses. Socially inappropriate behaviors are displayed more often than sexual behaviors. In the case of dorsolateral frontal injury, when attention and initiation impairments are primary, libido or sexual assertiveness may be impaired (29). Injury to these areas may also lead to an inability to fantasize (30). The role of the olfactory system is unclear, but recent research indicates that anosomia may not significantly affect sexual function. The hypothalamus is a crucial structure in the elaboration of the human sexual response. The supraoptic nucleus of the hypothalamus synthesizes oxytocin, a hormone involved in lactation, birthing, and orgasm. Naloxone, an opiate antagonist, prevents the release of oxytocin, suggesting that the release at orgasm is controlled, at least in part, by the endorphin system (31, 32).

SEXUAL DYSFUNCTION AFTER BRAIN INJURY

For the person with a disabling disease, condition, or injury, questions of sexuality are complex. Because of multiple, interrelated impairments that coexist after traumatic brain injury, questions concerning the specific etiologies of sexual dysfunction remain unanswered. How do we understand the impact of the pathophysiologic processes on the individual? What alterations in sexual desire, drive, arousal, or sexual responses are due to organic factors, and what can be attributed to secondary factors, such as cognitive, emotional, behavioral, and communication impairments or mobility deficits that result from the disease, condition, or injury?

Although much of the literature about TBI focuses on psychosocial consequences, no well-designed studies have established clear links between both the various impairments that frequently occur and the sexual dysfunction. Are impairments such as communication or cognitive deficits more important in interpersonal relationships than physical deficits? What roles do depression or other psychological conditions play? What are the effects of medication? What interpersonal and relationship issues contribute to sexual dysfunction? What are the anatomic correlates of sexual dysfunction?

The impact of TBI on relationships within the family and on mood and affective states of significant others and spouses has been explored in a large number of studies both in the United States and abroad. Thomsen's study (33) of 50 severely injured Danish patients demonstrated that family members were more disturbed by intellectual than physical deficits. The relationships were better between single adult patients and mothers than between patients and spouses. In Rosenbaum and Najenson's study (34) of brain-injured veterans in Israel, wives endorsed with high frequency the statement "dislikes physical contact with husband." The spouse's mood was associated with decreased levels of sexual activity. Lezak (35) emphasized that emotional adjustment for family members, including spouses, occurred only after detachment and acceptance of the permanence of deficits. This adjustment culminated in divorce, separation, and long-term placements for some partners. Bond (36) noted that the level of sexual activity among partners was not related to severity as measured by the duration of post-traumatic amnesia or level of cognitive or physical impairment.

Sexual function and marital adjustment were studied in a small group of married couples (37). Frequency of intercourse declined for all couples, but to a greater degree for couples in which the husband was brain-injured; orgasm in female spouses also showed a significant decline. Kreuter and associates (38) examined quality of relationships in 92 persons with TBI from 1 to 20 years post injury. They found that 58% had a stable partner relationship at the time of the study and of these 55% were established after the injury. In a larger study, sexual functioning, mood, and quality of life were examined in 322 individuals with TBI and a non-TBI sample of 264 individuals without disability (39). This study found that men with TBI were less sexually active and fewer were involved in a relationship when compared with non-disabled controls. Interestingly, there were no significant differences between women with and without TBI on these same variables.

Kreuter, Dahloff and associates (40) also examined sexual adjustment following TBI. In a group of subjects who were sexually active prior to their injury, 30% of the men experienced erectile dysfunction and fewer ejaculations. Although 59% reported no changes in orgasm, 40% experienced orgasm difficulties. "Dissatisfaction with the frequency of sexual activity" was found in 56% of the subjects. This study found that approximately one third of respondents had no intimate partner following the injury. However, they found that sexual dissatisfaction in individuals with partners was related to decreased interest, low self-esteem, partners' decreased interest (willingness to engage in sexual activity), "physical unattractiveness," and decreased sexual ability.

Kosteljanetz and associates (41) noted a correlation between intellectual impairment and sexual dysfunction in a group of 19 mildly injured patients. Although some studies (34) indicate no relationship between locus of lesion and sexual dysfunction, medial basal-frontal injury or diencephalic injury was associated with hypersexuality and limbic injury with changes in sexual orientation in a population of 8 patients (42) Kreutzer and Zasler (43) studied a population of 21 brain-injured men and noted declines in sex drive, erectile function, and frequency of intercourse. Although one third of the married subjects reported their relationship as worse post-injury, 40% rated their relationships as good or very good when compared to their pre-injury relationship status. The authors found no correlation between affect and sexual behavior.

Although Zasler (44) found no association between affect and sexual dysfunction, a larger study (45) using measures of anxiety and depression for both partners found a significant level of psychiatric dysfunction. In addition, as time since injury increased, males with TBI became more sexually dissatisfied and sexual communication became more problematic for their partners. Age and time since injury were related to measures of psychosexual dysfunction, but severity of injury was not. TBI subjects in another study reported significant levels of anxiety and depression and found significant correlations between sexual adjustment and measures of psychosocial adjustment (38, 40).

The negative impact of pre-injury and/or post-injury substance use on physical, cognitive, and psychosocial functioning is clearly documented in the literature The rates of pre-injury and post-injury substance abuse in individuals with TBI are substantial. Approximately 16% to 66% have chronic pre-injury problem drinking and 10% to 50% continue to experience post-injury problems with alcohol (46–48). Problems include a higher incidence of medical and psychological complications during TBI recovery, poorer cognitive recovery, poorer long-term outcome, and exacerbation of cognitive and behavioral deficits. Most substances of abuse have been shown to adversely affect sexual functioning at some stage in the sexual response cycle in non-TBI subjects, and have a substantial negative impact on sexual functioning in individuals with TBI who use substances (49).

Given that most injuries occur in individuals between the ages of 15 and 25, limitations in the person's pre-injury sexual experience can influence post-injury sexual functioning. Individuals with limited sexual experience and knowledge often have significant deficits and experience in establishing and maintaining intimate relationships. These relationship deficits can greatly reduce their ability to meet people who may become potential intimate partners. In individuals who have an intimate relationship at the time of injury, cognitive, emotional, behavioral, physical impairments, and substance abuse post-injury can clearly have a negative effect on the quality of the relationship as well as the sexual functioning of partners. For individuals who have limited relationship skills prior to their injury, these problems are amplified.

The impact of TBI on the sexual response cycle has also been closely examined. In general, problems may occur at any stage (desire, excitement or arousal, orgasm, and resolution). Sexual difficulties are found in a number of areas including decreased frequency of intercourse, decreased desire, impaired arousal, and orgasmic dysfunction (40,41,45) Aloni and Katz (50) reviewed the existing literature on the effects of TBI and the sexual response cycle. Although significantly more individuals with TBI experience decreased desire, some report increased desire. Kreuter et al. (40) examined 65 men and 27 women with TBI and found decreased desire, erectile dysfunction, and orgasmic dysfunction in many of their subjects. However, 59% of their sample reported no change in orgasm post-injury and 50% noted no change in frequency of sexual intercourse post-injury.

A study by Sandel and associates (51) examined sexual functioning in a group of male and female outpatients with severe traumatic brain injuries (average length of post-traumatic amnesia was 54 days). Sexual function was consistently lower than in the normal population but significantly only on the (1) orgasm and (2) drive and desire subscales of the Derogatis Interview of Sexual Function (52). Location of injury was relevant; patients with frontal lesions and right hemisphere lesions reported higher sexual satisfaction and higher function. No correlations were found with cognitive measures or clinical examination. Subjects with more recent injuries and subjects with right hemisphere injuries reported greater levels of arousal.

Hibbard et al. (39) examined sexual response cycle difficulties as well as other aspects of sexual function in both male and female subjects with TBI and without TBI. Men with TBI experienced significantly more difficulties on self-ratings of sexual energy, drive, ability to initiate sexual activity, ability to experience orgasm, and the ability to maintain an erection. Women with TBI experienced significantly more difficulties than women without TBI on self-ratings of sexual energy, drive, ability to initiate sexual activity, arousal, pain during sex, ability to masturbate, ability to experience orgasm, and with vaginal lubrication. This study found significant difficulties in both men and women with TBI in sexual positioning, sensation, and body image variables. Clearly, the findings noted above are dependent on many factors that include cognitive, emotional, interpersonal, physical, and physiological functioning.

The etiologies of sexual dysfunction in TBI are certainly multiple. Sexual dysfunction following TBI may be due to one or more factors, including injury to specific brain regions, neurochemical changes related to this pathology, endocrinologic abnormalities, medications, secondary medical conditions, physical limitations, cognitive deficits, emotional difficulties, behavioral deficits, and interpersonal difficulties.

DISABILITY AND SEXUALITY

Individuals with disabilities are a diverse group of people, representing a range of sexual expression and orientation, just as is the case in the population of individuals without disabilities. Providers often incorrectly assume that individuals with disability are sexually inactive or neglect to consider the issue of sexuality. In a recent study (53), 94% of the subjects with physical disabilities were found to be sexually active, a rate matching that of non-disabled individuals.

The paucity of information and biases that exist in the medical and scientific literature include myths that individuals with disabilities are asexual, lack sexual desire or attractiveness, are incapable of healthy sexual function, and lack the social and/or problem-solving skills necessary for sexual functioning. In addition, women with disabilities are viewed as less affected sexually than men with disabilities. These myths are not based on scientific data and have been perpetuated by a general lack of knowledge about disability and sexual functioning, although they may still guide healthcare professionals' behavior (54, 55).

The result of this general lack of awareness or bias is that individuals with disabilities may not receive adequate screening, education, or treatment for sexual dysfunction or reproductive health (55). Women with physical disabilities encounter serious barriers to receiving general, as well as reproductive health care, and have difficulty locating physicians who were knowledgeable about the disability to assist them in managing their pregnancy (53).

For individuals with disabilities, the associated features of the disabling condition may adversely influence the assessment and treatment of sexual dysfunction. Incontinence may have a serious impact in their sexual functioning (56). Intellectual or cognitive disabilities may present as an invisible disability. For this reason, healthcare professionals may not recognize the ways in which the disabling condition may affect sexuality and intimacy. Deficits in cognitive and social skills may have a serious effect on self-esteem, and contribute to difficulties establishing and maintaining relationships. An individual with a traumatic brain injury may lack insight, judgment, self-awareness, and perception of others needs or social cues. In other cases, the patient may not initiate conversation with the healthcare provider regarding issues related to sexuality. Individuals with TBI who have attention, memory, and judgment deficits may experience difficulties identifying and describing their symptoms. Conditions can be neglected or misdiagnosed.

For persons with TBI, a combination of cognitive and behavioral deficits may place them at increased risk of exposure to sexually transmitted diseases. Given the risk and potentially serious impact of sexually transmitted diseases and sexual victimization in persons with disabilities, it is extremely important for healthcare providers to be knowledgeable about sexuality and sexual functioning and to be prepared to open the discussion in the clinical setting. Professionals should perform a careful and comprehensive history and physical that includes information about all aspects of sexuality and sexual functioning as outlined in subsequent sections of this chapter.

Cultural and religious beliefs and values can impact how open the patient will be to discussing sexuality and to accepting information. For example, in many Latino, Asian and Native American cultures, women are not permitted to talk about their sexuality (57). Cultural awareness and sensitivity are essential during any clinical encounter.

LESBIAN, GAY, BISEXUAL, AND TRANSGENDER AND INTERSEX INDIVIDUALS

Lesbian, gay, bisexual, transgender, and intersex (LGBTI) issues in individuals with TBI have received little attention in the literature. Given the diversity among the lesbian, gay, bisexual, transgender and intersex members of society, combined with stigmatization, negative attitudes, and the political climate, population estimates are difficult to obtain. Prevalence estimates range from 5.5% to 20.8% depending on the definition (57).

Sexual prejudice has led to homophobic, heterosexist attitudes and heterosexual-centric attitudes in many areas of our culture including healthcare (57–59). Having a disability and being in a sexual minority places one at risk for discriminatory behavior for multiple reasons. Individuals who are LGBT with TBI may not receive an optimal level of medical care or rehabilitation. For example, lesbian and gay sexuality issues may not be appropriately addressed in sexuality education, examinations, or treatment (59). Intersex or abnormal sexual differentiation conditions and their effects are often poorly understood by medical professionals.

Sexual dysfunction may not be accurately identified due to a lack of knowledge or discomfort among healthcare professionals. Professionals lacking specific knowledge about LGBT issues or holding certain biases may make incorrect conclusions or diagnoses based on inadequate information, especially if the patient feels threatened or lacks trust in the provider. The stress of sexual orientation disclosure and a fear about including partners in the treatment program may result in inadequate or inappropriate recommendations. Concerns regarding confidentiality may limit the amount of information the LGBT individual and partner will disclose, particularly in an interdisciplinary setting, where a team of healthcare providers are providing care.

The incidence of traumatic brain injury in adolescents and early adulthood is significant. During this stage of development there is a developing awareness of sexuality and TBI "can terminate such exploration" (60). Building a trusting and open relationship with LGBT adolescent patients and using a non-judgmental communication style will both facilitate discussion and identify if the adolescent should receive counseling to facilitate exploration of sexual orientation.

NEUROENDOCRINE DYSFUNCTION AFTER BRAIN INJURY

Introduction

Neuroendocrine disorders occur at a frequency that varies according to research methodologies but is not insignificant. In fact, more recent studies suggest incidence and prevalence rates that are higher than previously reported. Neuroendocrine dysfunction after TBI may include temperature lability, appetite disturbances, hypothalamic and pituitary disorders, disorders of fluid regulation, hypertension, and immunologic disorders. The neuroendocrine system mediates hormonal and neuronal responses to stress, and therefore, a disruption in this system can have widespread effects. Neuroendocrine disorders after TBI are a consequence of specific injury to centers of regulation of physiological functions, represented in many different brain regions, but most frequently the hypothalamic-pituitary axis. Alterations in antidiuretic hormone (ADH), cortisol, growth hormone (GH), thyroxine, follicle stimulating hormone (FSH), luteinizing hormone (LH), prolactin, glucagon, and somatostatin have been reported (61–63).

The most recognized pituitary hormone abnormality after TBI is a result of effects (which are not well-understood) on the posterior pituitary, resulting in disordered production of vasopressin (also termed antidiurectic hormone or ADH). ADH is released from the posterior pituitary gland in response to hyperosmolarity, hypovolemia, nausea, and other factors and then acts on the renal distal tubule and collecting duct to increase water resorption. Diabetes insipidus (DI) results in excessive urination in conjuction with hypernatremia and hyperosmolarity. The syndrome of inappropriate secretion of antidiuretic hormone (SIADH), associated with hyponatremia, may occur as well. The other major hormonal abnormalities that occur after TBI are the result of anterior pituitary dysfunction.

Until recently, anterior pituitary dysfunction following TBI was considered uncommon, although in the 1980's, Horn reported 28% of TBI patients in a rehabilitation setting had abnormal endocrinologic studies and 12% required treatment (61, 62). More recent studies have shown anterior pituitary damage to be fairly common following TBI. Dysfunction of the anterior pituitary gland may lead to a compromise in growth hormone (GH), thyroid, glucocorticoid, sex hormone (testosterone in men/estrogen in women), and prolactin production. The clinical presentation of this syndrome varies widely, depending on the particular neuroendocrine axes that are involved, and the severity and rapidity of pituitary damage. Depending on which anterior pituitary hormones are missing, the presentation might range from subclinical disease to marked muscle dysfunction or cardiovascular collapse. Anterior pituitary dysfunction often accompanies posterior pituitary dysfunction (64). Immediate hormonal replacement is recommended for patients with panhypopituitarism, adrenal insufficiency, hypothyroidism, and diabetes insipidus. Replacement therapy includes adrenal and thyroid replacement, anti-diuretic hormone, and if necessary, gonadal and growth hormone replacement. In the case of growth hormone deficiency, retesting is recommended prior to a determination of replacement.

Incidence of Hypopituitarism

What is not clear from research to date are: 1) the implications of deficiencies for each of the axes, 2) the time frames for when these deficiencies develop, 3) the permanency of the deficiencies, 4) appropriate ways of testing for GH.

Two studies (41, 65) indicate that posttraumatic hypopituitarism with permanent hypogonadotrophic hypogonadism is a rare complication of TBI. More recent studies question this finding, at least for patients with severe brain injury. The prevalence of post-traumatic hypopituitarism was initially reported over 50 years ago as less than 1%. However, in a more recent study of men with severe head injury, 88% had subnormal testosterone levels at 7–10 days after TBI; 3–6 months later, 24% of a smaller sample still had low testosterone levels with loss of libido and impotence (66). A recent review also suggests the prevalence may be much higher (67). A total of 367 cases (from 1942–1998) were reviewed; the highest prevalence of disorders within the category of hypopituitarism was hypogonadism, hypothyroidism, (over 90% of the sample) and adrenal insufficiency (about 50%). Diabetes insipidus was present in about 30%, and growth hormone deficiency in about 25% of the sample.

Risk factors for hypopituitarism in TBI include moderate to severe head injury (Glasgow Coma Scale of 10 or less), diffuse brain swelling, and a hypotensive/hypoxic episode (although the latter has not been observed in every study). Some degree of hypopituitarism appears to exist in about 40% of patients with moderate to severe head injury, with growth hormone and gonadotropin deficiencies occurring at the highest frequency (68). In a study of 70 adults with traumatic brain injury, 21.7% had evidence of growth hormone deficiency, and 87% had both TSH and free T4 below the mid-normal level. Basal morning cortisol was below normal in 45.7% of subjects.

Hypogonadism and hyperprolactinemia were uncommon in this study population (69).

Recent recommendations at the Global Experts Consensus Panel in Philadelphia included guidelines for assessment of hypopituitarism after traumatic brain injury (70). Patients with moderate and severe TBI should undergo baseline hormonal evaluation at 3 months and 12 months after discharge from the ICU. Adrenal insufficiency and diabetes insipidus should be considered in patients with symptoms. The hormonal screening should include 0900 AM serum cortisol, fT3, fT4, TSH, FSH, LH, testosterone in men and E2 in women, prolactin, and IGF-I. In patients with polyuria or diuresis, urine density, sodium, and plasma osmolality should also be evaluated. Low IGF-I levels strongly predict severe growth hormone deficiency (in the absence of malnutrition). Normal IGF-I levels may be found in patients with growth hormone deficiency; therefore, provocative tests are necessary in patients with another identified pituitary hormone deficit. If IGF-I levels are below the 25th percentile of age related normal limits, provocative testing is recommended.

CLINICAL EVALUATION OF NEUROENDOCRINE DISORDERS

Posterior Pituitary Dysfunction

The syndrome of inappropriate antidiuretic hormone secretion (SIADH) is more common than diabetes insipidus (DI). In the case of SIADH, patients are usually symptomatic only when the sodium serum level drops below 125 mEq/L. Symptoms include nausea, fatigue, muscle cramps, and eventually psychosis, seizures, and coma can develop. The workup should include urine and serum osmolalities, and the diagnosis is made on the basis of a finding of inappropriately high urine osmolality in the face of a low serum osmolality. For SIADH, when levels fall below 125 mEq/L, fluid restriction (500–1000 mL/day) is usually sufficient to correct the abnormality, but caution should be taken in elderly patients (71). Furosemide, with replacement of sodium and potassium, is an alternative to demeclocycline, which should not be used in children or in any patient with hepatic disease (72).

DI may occur in mild, moderate and severe TBI. The usual onset post-trauma is 10 days. Facial and basilar skull fractures may be a risk factor, even in the presence of a relatively mild TBI (73). Polyuria and polydipsia are clinical symptoms that may be overlooked in the hospital setting. A high serum sodium level may not be present if the patient has access to water replacement. The best test is a water deprivation test, but an alternative is a spot check of plasma and urine osmolalities, and employ a nomogram to identify the abnormality (73, 74). Hyponatremia may occur as a consequence of cerebral salt-wasting syndrome or inappropriate secretion of ADH. In the former, water and sodium are not conserved; in the latter, water is conserved. For cerebral salt-wasting, fludrocortisone acetate may be an effective treatment (71).

Anterior Pituitary Dysfunction

Patients with hypothyroidism have cold intolerance, constipation, fatigue, and may have myxedema and bradycardia in later stages; TSH is low. In one study of TBI patients, 21.7% had abnormal T4 and TSH (69).

In the case of hypogonadism, libido is reduced, and impotence, menstrual abnormalities, infertility, breast and testicular atrophy may be present; an AM free testosterone, and estradiol in females and a prolactin level are diagnostic.

Growth hormone (GH) deficiency may present with fatigue, decreased muscle mass, exercise intolerance, and truncal obesity; a GH stimulation test may be diagnostic. Cognitive deficits, including impaired judgment, problem solving, concentration, and memory may be present. In one study of TBI patients, 15% had an abnormal glucagon stimulation test (69).

Patients with adrenal insufficiency from decreased ACTH (Addison's disease) present with weakness, fatigue, weight loss, hypoglycemia, postural hypotension, and occasionally nausea and vomiting and abdominal pain. AM cortisol levels are low, and adrenal insufficiency is based on deficient plasma cortisol response to ACTH stimulation. In TBI, the incidence of low cortisol levels may be as higher than previously recognized (67). An acute phase reaction, with the finding of low cortisol levels two hours after injury has been reported in a series of 400 patients with trauma, including severe brain injury (75). Disturbed sleep may be a manifestation of a more common phenomenon in TBI patients, i.e. dysfunctional cortisol diurnal rhythm (61, 62, 72).

Precocious Puberty

Sexual/reproductive effects of brain injury in children can be identified as either hypogonadotropic hypogonadism or precocious puberty. Klachko and associates (76) reported the case of a 39-year-old man with hypopituitarism due to a severe brain injury at age 4 years. Shaul (77) reported accelerated growth of pubic hair and estrogenization of the vaginal mucosa occurring within 5 months of a brain injury. Two other cases (girls, ages 3 and 5), were described after traumatic brain injury; both exhibited breast development, pubic hair, and changes in vaginal mucosa consistent with estrogenization (78). The neuroendocrinologic mechanism is postulated to be destruction of inhibitory neuronal pathways into the hypothalamus, with premature activation of gonadotropin-releasing hormone from the arcuate nucleus

GENDER DIFFERENCES IN OUTCOME: PROGESTERONE AND ESTROGEN

Studies suggest that female patients with traumatic brain injury may recover better than males. Laboratory studies in animals suggest that either progesterone or estrogen or both may be protective or even facilitate regeneration (79, 80). The effect in humans seems to depend on the presence of functioning ovaries (81).

Progesterone and estrogen have widespread effects on brain metabolism. Progesterone may be protective during the injury cascade, may correlate with reduced levels of edema, and may increase neuronal survival. The mechanisms postulated for these effects may be through interactions with cytokines, excitotoxicity, apoptosis, GABA, or other factors. Estrogen may also have a neuroprotective or neuroregenerative effect. Ovarectomized female rats with estrogen replacement have improved survival following traumatic brain injury. The mechanism may be cerebral blood flow preservation, with microvascular effects involving a combination of endothelial nitric oxide synthase induction and an antioxidant effect (80).

SEIZURE DISORDERS AND NEUROENDOCRINE DYSFUNCTION

Temporal lobe seizures usually arise from limbic structures, such as the amygdala, that exert a modulatory influence on the hypothlalamic regulation of the pituitary. Limbic and brainstem structures contain neurons with high concentrations of gonadal hormone receptors. Approximately 20% of patients with post-traumatic epilepsy have temporal lobe seizures (82). Up to 58% of men with temporal lobe seizure disorders are impotent or hyposexual, and up to 40% of women have menstrual irregularities or reproductive dysfunction, including polycystic ovarian syndrome, premature menopause, hypogonadotropic hypogonadism, and anovulatory cycles (26–28). Estrogens lower the seizure threshold, and frequency of seizures often increases in females at the time of menses and during pregnancy. Temporal lobe epilepsy has effects on the hypohalamic-pituitary-gonadal axis through effects on dopamine. Because dopamine is a prolactin-inhibitory hormone within this system, decreases in dopamine result in hyperprolactinemia.

Hypogonadotropic hypogonadism, accompanied by amenorrhea in patients with temporal lobe seizures, is associated with low levels of luteinizing hormone (LH). Because no hypothalamic disorder has been identified, this abnormality may be due to limbic discharges that result in altered secretion of gonadotropin-releasing hormone (26). Premature menopause also occurs. In polycystic ovarian syndrome, which also is associated with temporal lobe seizures, LH and prolactin are elevated, whereas follicle-stimulating hormone (FSH) is depressed (28). Men with temporal lobe epilepsy and hypogonadism, unlike those with isolated hypogonadism, may have no improvement in libido or potency when parenteral testosterone is given; however, initial treatment of the epilepsy, followed by neuroendocrine treatment (bromocriptine or pergolide for hyperprolactinemia and testosterone for hypogonadism), is sometimes effective (27).

COMPREHENSIVE EVALUATION

Medical History

Evaluation of the patient begins with a careful history including past illnesses, surgeries, and sexual activity and function (18). Many diseases and chronic conditions can influence sexual function (83). Whenever possible and with consent, information should be obtained from the current partner. Cultural aspects should be considered and sensitivity to cultural differences is essential. Questions should focus on the following areas: (1) a review of neurologic, cardiovascular, endocrine, andurologic medical and surgical history; (2) preinjury and postinjury sexual functioning; (3) sexual orientation (4) history of victimization, including sexual assault, domestic violence; (5) substance use and abuse history: (6) current medication; (7) safe sex practices; and (8) reproductive history and contraceptive practices.

The history should define the patient's expectations in regard to sexual activity and functioning, and through the course of the evaluation, information gaps and misconceptions will become apparent. Dependency patterns, lack of self-esteem, and perceptions of unattractiveness should be identified. Education can be provided during the course of the history-taking session and written materials should be provided (84–86). The examiner must be comfortable discussing all aspects of sexuality, including alternative forms of sexual expression and alternative lifestyles (60). A nonjudgmental style is essential; staff training that focuses on attitudinal issues as well as education is recommended for physicians (87).

In regard to sexual functioning, the following areas should be further explored: 1) sexual desire; 2) sensory experience, as related to sexual arousal, and including a history of painful experiences during sexual activity; 3) sexual response including patterns of erections (penile or clitoral) and vaginal lubrication, 4) ejaculation (including forceful ejaculation of fluids from the urethra during orgasm in women); and 5) orgasmic sensations and experiences.

Psychological Evaluation

A comprehensive evaluation of sexual functioning includes a psychological evaluation. Establishing rapport with the client or with the couple is essential when discussing sexual issues. A widely used approach in the field of sexuality is the PLISSIT model (88). This approach emphasizes the importance of giving the client permission to discuss uncomfortable sexual issues. It also highlights the importance of helping the client feel comfortable discussing sexuality and intimacy, and other related issues. It is important for clinicians to remember that sexuality and relationship issues are often very difficult for clients and their partners to discuss. The more comfortable they feel during the interview, the more specific and useful the assessment will be. Establishing the etiology of the sexual difficulty provides the basis for the development of an appropriate treatment plan. It is often more comfortable for clients if the interview begins with a review of the medical history, demographic information, marital/relationship and family history and then gradually begins to focus on emotional, relationship, intimacy, sexuality, and sexual dysfunction issues (89).

Although there are many different formats for organizing and conceptualizing information, the Multiaxial Problem-Oriented System for Sexual Dysfunctions (90) is a useful guide. This approach assists the clinician in classifying sexual problems across a number of domains: desire, arousal, orgasm, coital pain, and frequency dissatisfaction. Another category labeled "Qualifying Information" includes sexual practices such as fetishism, exhibitionism, as well as other problems that may interfere with sexual functioning such as substance abuse and severe psychopathology. In addition, problems are classified as lifelong vs. not lifelong to more clearly identify individuals who have a history of relatively normal functioning followed by a period of sexual dysfunction. The circumstances under which the problems occur (global or all situations vs. specific situations) are also documented. This model provides the clinician with a framework in which to conceptualize the individual's sexual dysfunction as the basis for a problem-focused treatment plan. The DSM-IV utilizes a similar model; subtypes of conditions are used to more clearly define the onset of sexual dysfunction (life-long vs. acquired), context (generalized vs. situational) and presumed etiology (psychological vs. combined factors) (8).

The sexual assessment and history should focus on identifying the sexual difficulties and how they function within the individual or the couple's relationship. LoPiccolo and Heiman (91) provide an outline for the interview and suggest using open-ended questions and including information about the client and the primary partner (if one exists) in all domains. It should include information about the client/couple's life situation, adolescent and sexual development, attitudes, and values and beliefs toward sex (both past and current). Information about current behavior, including relationship issues, communication, displays of affection, intimacy, and sexual orientation, should also be obtained. The clinician must determine specific information about the nature of the sexual difficulty including onset, frequency, circumstances, treatment attempted, and both the client and partner's responses to the problem.

The history must include information about previous psychological problems and treatment, as well as history of physical, emotional, and/or sexual abuse. Current psychological symptoms must be examined, including anxiety, depressive or mood, adjustment, psychotic behavior, personality disorders, and use and abuse of substances. In addition, it is important to obtain information about coping strategies, interpersonal communication skills, sexuality-specific anxieties (e.g. performance anxiety) and social support. Although most of this information can be obtained through an interview, some psychological assessment instruments such as the Beck Depression Inventory–2 (92), the Minnesota Multiphasic Personality Inventory–2 (93) the Millon Clinical Multiaxial Inventory–3 (94) may be helpful. When psychological disorders are identified, they must be treated because they are often significant contributing factors to sexual and relationship difficulties.

The cognitive difficulties experienced by survivors of TBI are well documented in the literature. Problems with attention, speed of processing, learning, memory, and problem-solving/reasoning skills are common and can clearly impact the sexual problem(s) and relationship. If the cognitive issues have not recently been assessed, a neuropsychological evaluation may be helpful. The neuropsychological evaluation may clarify the nature of the deficits as well as compensatory strategies to lessen their impact on the person's functioning. The impact of these deficits can then be incorporated into the treatment plan for the sexual dysfunction.

Questionnaires

A number of questionnaires have been developed to assess sexuality in more detail than the usual history-taking session. The Derogatis Interview of Sexual Functioning (52) collects information by self-report in the five domains of fantasy, arousal, experience, orgasm, and drive and desire. A general sexual satisfaction score is obtained as well as a total score.

The Golombok-Rust Inventory of Sexual Satisfaction (GRISS) (95) is a 28 item self-report scale, provides male and female scores (two versions) in the categories of vaginismus, anorgasmia, impotence, premature ejaculation, non-sensuality, avoidance, dissatisfaction, infrequency, and non-communication, as well as a total score. This scale examines sexual functioning within the context of a relationship.

Kreutzer and Zasler (43) developed an 11-item Psychosexual Assessment Questionnaire. The items are grouped into 3 domains: sexual behavior; affect and

self-esteem; and relationship issues with a focus on changes in functioning following a TBI.

Another scale originally developed for use in spinal cord injury, but modified and used in TBI, is the Sexual Interest and Satisfaction Scale (SIS) (96). This scale examines sexual desire, satisfaction with sex before and after injury, and ability to satisfy a partner.

For the woman with a history of sexual dysfunction, a number of instruments have recently been developed. These include the Female Sexual Function Index (FSFI) (97), the Female Sexual Distress Scale (FSDS) (98), and the Sexual Function Questionnaire (SFQ) (99).

Physical Examination

A neurological and general physical examination should be completed, with a focused assessment to identify impairments that may influence communication, positioning, movement, oral ability, and sensory awareness. Aphasias, dysarthrias, aprosodias, and deficits in attention and concentration or memory should be noted. Facial scars, oral and facial movement and visual and hearing impairments should be identified. Range of motion, especially in the proximal lower extremities, must be evaluated, along with movement of the limbs and trunk. Sensation is a crucial aspect of the examination. The genitalia, rectum, and the breasts should be examined. The bulbocavernosus muscles can be palpated in the male, and tested for voluntary and reflex contraction. Anal sphincter tone should be assessed. The cremasteric reflex (L1) and the bulbocavernosus and anal reflex (S2–5) should also be evaluated. In women, a Papanicolaou smear and pelvic examination are essential (44).

Medication Review

A thorough review of all medications is necessary. The most common cause of impotence in the general patient population is medication. Drug-related effects on sexual function are usually reversible after discontinuation of the drug. Frequently implicated are (1) antihypertensive agents, (2) antipsychotic drugs, (3) antidepressants, (4) anxiolytics, (5) sedatives; and (6) hormonal agents (including contraceptives and tamoxifen).

The most frequent adverse reactions with selective serotonic reuptake inhibitors (SSRIs) are decreased desire, anorgasmia, and ejaculatory delay (100). Impotence is less frequently reported with SSRIs than non-selective monoamine reuptake inhibitors. Trazadone has the highest number of reports of priapism of the antidepressants, and has also been implicated in persistent sexual arousal syndrome in women. High-dose sildenafil may be effective in reducing ejaculatory latency (101).

Antihypertensive drugs may affect sexual function (libido and sexual response) through vascular or neurologic effects. Alpha- and beta-adrenoreceptor blocking agents can cause ejaculatory failure. Antipsychotic agents may cause priapism, ejaculatory failure, and painful retrograde or spontaneous ejaculations (102).

In addition to the above medications, large number of other agents have been implicated: baclofen, cimetidine, clofibrate, cyproterone, digoxin, estrogen, indomethacin, lithium, metoclopramide, naproxen, phenoxybenzamine, prazosin, and progesterone, to name a few (103).

Laboratory Tests

Screening tests for sexual dysfunction include sedimentation rate, blood cell count, fasting blood sugar, serum lipids, urinalysis, hepatic function, kidney and thyroid function studies, prolactin and testosterone levels (in both men and women).

Hypopituitarism may be manifested by low levels of growth hormone, thyroxine or cortisol or by hypogonadism. In men, low sperm count, low serum levels of testosterone, and low levels of LH and FSH characterize hypogonadism. Because protein-bound testosterone may be increased by thyroid hormone therapy or cirrhosis and decreased by hypothyroidism or obesity, free testosterone levels or sex steroid-binding globulin may give a more accurate picture. In women, low serum levels of estradiol and low serum levels of LH and FSH characterize hypogonadism. Hypogonadism may be caused by primary gonadal failure, as well as secondary failure at a central level. Klinefelter syndrome, for example, which has an incidence of 1 in 500 men, may be an unrelated cause of low testosterone in a patient with brain injury. The gonadotropin-releasing hormone test is useful in distinguishing hypothalamic from pituitary causes of hypogonadism, although it is not infallible. The clomiphene citrate-provocative test is also used to evaluate the gonadal axis. Single determinations of any of the above levels may not be accurate reflections of function (104).

Neurophysiologic and Vascular Evaluation

Spontaneous nocturnal penile tumescence and rigidity can be measured in the sleep laboratory using strain gauges, visual inspection, and other measures and is the most accurate technique for measuring erectile function. Rigidometers for evaluation at home have also been utilized (105–107). If no major vascular problem is present, intracorporeal injection (papaverine, papaverine/phentolamine, or prostaglandin E1) can be used as a diagnostic tool (108). If intracorporeal injection testing of penile tumescence is suggestive of a vascular etiology of sexual dysfunction, penile blood pressure using a Doppler method can helpful to further evaluate (109).

Neurophysiological and vascular studies may further elucidate the pathophysiological underpinnings of the disorder. Somatic sensory, somatic motor, autonomic, and visceral sensory testing are available in some centers to further evaluate sexual dysfunction. These tests include dorsal penile nerve conduction studies, pudendal somatosensory evoked potential tests, pudendal motor latency, bulbocavernosus and anal reflex latency measurements, and electromyography (corpus cavernosum and somatic), cystometry, and anorectal manometry.

For women, magnetic resonance imaging (MRI) technology and vaginal photo-plethysmograph devices are used for objective measurement of sexual response. Vaginal photoplethysmograph devices measure blood flow or engorgement following response to visual sexual stimulation (4, 110, 111).

PHARMACOTHERAPY

The following review of the literature focuses on medications that may have potential benefit, as there are no well-controlled studies in patients with brain injury. Clearly much more research is needed to understand the types of sexual disorders that occur in women, both disabled and non-disabled, and effective treatments for these disorders.

Women's sexuality has not been adequately addressed in research to date, but progress is being made. Recently the Diagnostic and Statistical Manual of Mental Disorders-IV (DSM-IV) classifications of female sexual dysfunction have been expanded to include psychogenic and organic causes of desire, arousal, orgasm, and sexual pain disorders that cause personal distress (8). The United States Food and Drug Administration Guidance paper10 details the recommendations for the clinical development of pharmacologic interventions for female sexual dysfunction. Major pharmaceutical companies are now developing agents for female sexual disorders and or post-menopausal symptoms. These include dopaminergic agonists and related substances, melanocortin-stimulating hormones, adrenoceptor antagonists, nitric oxide delivery systems, prostaglandins, and androgens (4).

Phosphodiesterase Inhibitors

For men, major progress has been achieved in the development of medications for erectile dysfunction by the introduction of phosphodiesterase 5 inhibitors, and these agents have been utilized in a variety of populations with success (112–116). Phosphodiesterase enzymes are ubiquitous throughout the body and participate in a variety of functions. PDE5 is the predominant enzyme in the corpus cavernosum, and plays a significant role in penile erection. Sildenafil, tadalafil, and vardenafil are all potent inhibitors of PDE5. This class of medications is the most effective oral agents for the treatment of erectile dysfunction (117). These medications have led to a significant decrease in the use of other methods of treatment for erectile dysfunction. Side effects include flushing, headache, dyspepsia, and visual disturbances (112). These medications interact with nitrates, and should not be given to patients on nitrates (118). Improved sexual function and sexual satisfaction appears to be well maintained over years following the initiation of treatment (119).

Antidepressant-associated (SSRI) or antipsychotic-associated sexual dysfunction may be effectively treated with sildenafil or other agents of this class (120, 121).

Prostaglandin E1

These agents are utilized topically for men with erectile dysfunction to maximize genital smooth muscle relaxation (122). Topical alprostadil (prostaglandin E1) has been recommended for men with erectile dysfunction, and appears to be well tolerated, with the most common adverse side effect being urogenital pain (123). Sildenafil combined with alprostadil administered via the intraurethal or intracavernous route was effective in some men with erectile dysfunction who failed other monotherapy. (Steers, 2003) Topical administration of alprostadil has been utilized in the study of women with sexual arousal and orgasmic disorders and ultrasound studies document clitoral cavernosal arterial changes that may be helpful in diagnosis of underlying pathology, but is not recommended as an intervention at this time (124).

Dopaminergic Agents

Dopaminergic agents may be efficacious in the treatment of erectile dysfunction, and may be an alternative to treatment with phosphodiesterase inhibitors. Because dopaminergic systems may be particularly vulnerable to traumatic brain injury (especially mesocortical and mesolimbic systems), sexual dysfunction may be associated with decreases in dopaminergic activity. L-dopa was investigated following the observation that patients with Parkinson's disease who were treated with the drug reported increased sexual activity (125).

Apomorphine (a D2 greater than D1 dopamine receptor nonselective short-acting agonist) decreases secretion of prolactin, stimulates production of growth hormone, and induces erections. Apomorphine may act on neurons located within the paraventricular nucleus and the medial preoptic area of the hypothalamus (126). A MRI study (placebo-controlled) demonstrated frontal limbic area activity after administration of apomorphine (127). A PET study has demonstrated cerebral activity in the right prefrontal cortex (128). Used in research to establish potential efficacy of longer-acting agents (129,130) the drug is now licensed in some countries, for the treatment of erectile dysfunction, in a sublingual formulation. Side effects are nausea, dizziness, diaphoresis, syncope, and hypotension. The rug interacts with nitrates, increasing the risk of hypotension. Apomorphine combined with phentolamine was effective in one study and this combination may prove to be an alternative to phosphodiesterase inhibitors (131).

Hormonal Agents

O'Carroll and associates reviewed the results of investigations of hypoactive sexual desire disorder in women and described it as "the major female psychosexual dysfunction (132)." However, little evidence suggests that the disorder can be traced to hormonal inadequacies in women. Hypogonadal women (with androgen deficiency due to pathophysiologic problems that affect androgen production in the ovaries and/or adrenal glands) do demonstrate an increase in sexual interest after androgen replacement (133).

Androgen substitution should be administered as an adjuvant treatment to counseling in women with low libido only when low androgen levels are due to inadequate ovarian and/or adrenal function in the presence of normal estrogen levels. Administration of androgens to women without low androgen levels who complain of decreased sexual interest or desire is not recommended (134). The "normal" ranges for androgens and estrogens, especially as related to female sexual dysfunction, remain a subject of controversy (135). The possible adverse effects from testosterone therapy in women include breast cancer, fluid retention, masculinization (hisutism, acne, temporal balding, voice deepening, clitoromegaly), and hepatocellular damage (with high doses).

For women, intramuscular or subcutaneous injections, transdermal patches, or topical agents are available. But, again, the only clinical indications for testosterone replacement in women are symptomatic testosterone deficiency following natural menopause, or due to surgical menopause, chemotherapy or irradiation, premature ovarian failure, or pre-menopausal loss of libido with diminished serum free testosterone. Aging is associated with a decline in testosterone in normal premenopausal women (136).

Increasing age may result in a gradual hypogonadal state in men, referred to as andropause. The age of presentation for erectile dysfunction and andropause, or "partial androgen deficiency in aging men," typically occurs in the fifties and beyond, and these health issues may be harbingers for other related diseases such as cardiovascular disease and depression (137). Treatment with hormone replacement is controversial, and a recent statement from Committee on Assessing the Need for Clinical Trials of Testosterone Replacement Therapy of The Institute of Medicine argues for caution. Testosterone can cause gynecomastia, testicular atrophy, congestive heart failure, and stroke, and can accelerate the growth of prostate cancer (138).

For men, testosterone delivery systems include depo-testosterone, scrotal patches (scrotal or nonscrotal), or a drying gel. Oral administration is associated with hepatic injury. Intramuscular injections, favored by bodybuilders and competitive athletes, produce a fast rise and fall in levels. Testosterone injections biweekly for 6 weeks increased the frequency of sexual thoughts in a group of eugonadal men with low libido compared with placebo. However, no effect was observed in men with inhibited erectile dysfunction (139). Apparently testosterone increases sexual interest in men with pretreatment levels in the normal range. This study also suggests that men with hyposexual sexual desire disorder may benefit from testosterone injections even if serum levels are within the normal range. Additional research is needed, however, because the study included only 20 men.

Human chorionic gonadotropin was used as a treatment in 45 men with erectile failure and 6 men with lack of sexual desire (140). The treatment period was 1 month with twice weekly injections of 5,000 IU or placebo in a double-blind design. The investigators reported that 47% of treated patients had a "good result" compared with 12% of the placebo group; however, they did not separate the cases of erectile failure from the cases of low sexual interest or fully define "good result."

Antidepressants

Although many antidepressants (tricyclic antidepressants and monamine oxidase inhibitors) have been noted to cause a variety of sexual side effects, others have been noted to improve sexual functioning in patients without brain injuries, including both serotonin agents and buproprion, which inhibits reuptake of dopamine. Fluoxetine has been associated with orgasm dysfunction (141). Researchers postulate an excitatory mechanism for adrenergic systems and an inhibitory role for serotonergic systems but in view of reports of both increased and decreased sexual functioning, the neurochemical effects are unclear. Trazodone and fenfluramine have been associated with improvement in libido in a number of case reports (142–144), although both also have been reported to cause sexual dysfunction. Buproprion has also been shown to improve libido in individuals with hypoactive sexual desire disorders. In a study of 60 female and male outpatients with psychosexual dysfunction (sexual aversion, inhibited sexual desire, inhibited sexual excitement, and/or inhibited orgasm), 12 weeks of double blind treatment with bupropion resulted in significantly greater improvements in sexual functioning among treated patients than in the placebo group. Only 3% of placebo-treated patients reported improvement compared with 63% of the medicated group (145).

Opiate Antagonists

Opioids have also been implicated in sexual function. (159) In a small study involving 7 men, 25–50 mg/day led to full return of erectile function as well as nocturnal penile tumescence in 6 patients (32). In a study of 30 men (age 25–50 years) with idiopathic impotence, naltrexone, an opiate antagonist, increased "sexual performance" (defined as intercourse) in 11 of 15 treated patients (31).

Natural Compounds

A number of compounds from nature have been identified as treatments for erectile dysfunction. These include yohimbine, Citrulline, pyrano-isoflavones, bererine, forskolin, and Korean red ginseng (146, 147). Yohimbine, an alpha-adrenoceptor blocker, has been investigated in multiple studies of sexual dysfunction (148–153). Identifying the cause of impotence (arterial insufficiency) may also identify potential responders to yohimbine (153). Tobacco may negatively influence its effectiveness (149). Yohimbine administered with L-arginine glutamate (a nitric oxide-precursor) resulted in substantially increased physiologic (vaginal pulse amplitude) responses in a group of women with female sexual arousal disorder (154). Similarly, this combination treatment was effective in improving erectile function in male patients with mild to moderate erectile dysfunction (155).

Other Treatments for Erectile Dysfunction

Intracavernosal injection (papaverine, phentolamine, prostaglandin E1, vasoactive intestinal peptide), transurethral vasoactive agents (prostaglandin E1), vacuum erection devices, vascular surgery and penile prostheses are other therapeutic strategies for erectile dysfunction (156).

Self-injection of papaverine (a smooth muscle relaxant) or papaverine with phentolamine (an alpha-adrenergic blocker) is a treatment modality for impotence due to neurological or vasculogenic causes. Nearly all patients with neurogenic impotence and 60–70% of patients with vasculogenic impotence respond to intracavernous injections (157). Priapism, fibrosis of erectile tissues, hematomas, vasovagal reflex, and chemical hepatitis have been reported (158). Intracavernous injection of prostaglandin E1 is another approach, although painful erection occurs in up to 20% of patients, perhaps related to concentration and/or neuropathy (159, 160). Papaverine (with or without phentolamine) and prostaglandin E1 acts by increasing arterial inflow through vasodilatation and decreasing venous outflow by occluding draining venules, probably through relaxation of smooth muscle in the corpus cavernosum. Unilateral injection results in bilateral effects through cross-circulation.

Prosthetic surgery is less frequently chosen because other alternatives are available for men with erectile disorders. The two major categories of penile prostheses are the semi-rigid and the inflatable prosthesis. Complications include mechanical failure, infection, pain, and perforation, but the rate of complications is now lower because of technologic advances. Other alternatives include vacuum constriction devices, vascular reconstruction, and arterial and venous surgery. Nerve grafts, nerve growth factors, neuroprotection and nerve regeneration, explored at a basic science level, and may offer promise for the management of erectile dysfunction (161).

Other Alternatives for Women

Lubrication can be effective to promote sexual arousal in women with inadequate secretion and to treat dyspareunia and vaginismus. Some components of the sexual response continuum, including engorgement, elevation, and elongation of the vagina and clitoral erection, are not influenced by lubricants alone. Oral-genital stimulation and the use of vibrators may be helpful for some women.

Zestra for Women is a botanical feminine massage oil (containing borage seed oil, evening primrose oil, special extracts of angelica, coleus forskolin, antioxidants, and vitamin E) formulated to enhance female sexual pleasure and arousal. The formulation has been show to improve level of arousal, level of desire, satisfaction with arousal, genital sensation, ability to have orgasms, and sexual pleasure in a group of women with and without sexual arousal disorder in a randomized, placebo-controlled, double blind, crossover design trial (162).

INTERVENTIONS FOR SEXUAL BEHAVIOR DISORDERS

As pointed out by Simpson (163) the literature on sexually aberrant behavior is fraught because of a lack of consensus in defining and delineating the boundaries of such behavior among researchers and clinicians. Documentation of sexual behavior disorders after traumatic brain injury is recorded in surveys and case reports (42, 164–167). Research documents such types of behaviors in animals.

Sexual offending disorders are defined as sexual acts against another person that cause affront or distress (163). These behaviors include touching (frotteurism, toucherism), exhibitionism, voyeurism, and sexual aggression. In one study of 445 patients with TBI, 6.5% were identified as individuals who had committed some form of sexual offense. Alcohol was a factor in only three. The most common offenses were inappropriate touching, followed by exhibitionism and overt sexual aggression (162).

The individual with brain injury may have reduced social skills and this can be demonstrated in disinhibited interpersonal behaviors. These behaviors may cause responses from care providers based on individual sexual attitudes. Unwanted sexual advances may occur and require redirection. Sexual acting out is a result of disinhibition, which creates a variety of inappropriate behaviors and social interactions with sexual implications (84).

The term disinhibition, associated with orbitofrontal injury, presents the underlying force leading to hypersexual, or inappropriate behaviors. Such behaviors are usually described in the context of interpersonal contact but also may manifest as perseverative self-directed behaviors, such as excessive masturbation. Such behaviors may represent response to injury, loss of self-esteem, or need to act out psychological conflict. Changes in sexual preference may represent release of inhibitions from frontal damage (42). Behavior modification may also be helpful in reducing the frequency of some of these behaviors (168).

Sexual offenders have been treated with hormonal therapy such as medroxyprogesterone and other antiandrogens (e.g., cyproterone) that are progesterone derivatives and these agents have been used successfully in treatment of aggressive hypersexual behavior in patients with brain injury to decrease levels of serum testosterone (168, 169). Such interventions have not been thoroughly studied in brain-injured patients, and violent sexual behaviors are rare in this population. Brain-injured persons are more likely to be victims of sexual abuse by others than perpetrators of violent crimes (170).

SEX THERAPY

Sex therapy focuses on various strategies to improve sexual functioning in both individuals and couples in which one or both partners may have some type of sexual dysfunction. Although sex therapy is more commonly conducted within the context of relationships, individuals without current partners may benefit from some of the techniques used. As previously mentioned, a thorough assessment of the problem(s) is essential to the development of a problem-oriented treatment plan. In this way, sex therapy focuses on the specific area of dysfunction. In addition, sex therapy often involves collaboration between the sex therapist and physicians (171). Therefore, treatment may include medication or change of medications and behavioral and cognitive psychotherapeutic techniques.

LoPiccolo (172) presented the concept of direct treatment of sexual dysfunction which included some basic therapeutic principles such as viewing sexual dysfunction within the context of the relationship, provision of basic sexual education and information, examination about sexual attitudes, addressing performance anxiety, improving sexual communication, improving the partners' ability to use sexual techniques, prioritizing sexual activity, and providing specific techniques to change behavior. Therefore, in addition to common couples therapy, techniques such as exploration of feelings and direct communication strategies, cognitive therapy techniques such as reframing and coping skills development are also utilized (173).

Behavioral strategies may include increasing affectionate behaviors, relaxation, behavioral rehearsal and/or more sex specific strategies such as desensitization, nondemand pleasuring, directed masturbation, Kegel exercises, non-demand stimulation, start-stop techniques, the squeeze technique, and the quiet vagina exercise (18, 174). Such techniques vary in effectiveness and require intervention by therapists with specific training in both sex therapy and experience in treating individuals with TBI. In this way, standard approaches to sex therapy can be appropriately modified to accommodate any physical, emotional, behavioral, or cognitive impairments that may be present. These techniques of sex therapy may be useful for persons with brain injury and their partners as they explore new ways of relating intimately and sexually to each other.

Treatment of premature ejaculation (PE) is an example of the usefulness of sex therapy techniques. PE is defined as, "Persistent or recurrent ejaculation with minimal sexual stimulation before, on, or shortly after penetration and before the person wishes it . . . the disturbance causes marked distress or interpersonal difficulty(8)." Estimates of incidence vary from 30% to 75% in men and suggest that it is a common problem (175). Given the demographics, cognitive, and behavioral characteristics of males with TBI, PE may be a common but unidentified problem. Treatment of PE can involve several components including an exploration of early sexual or masturbatory experiences in adolescence or young adulthood that may have reinforced rapid arousal and ejaculation as well as interactions within a sexual relationship that may be reinforcing or influencing decreased ejaculatory control. Specific information about the frequency of PE, sexual expectations and their negative effects, and the usefulness of improving communication during sex are also helpful. Treatment may also include masturbation exercises coupled with techniques such as the squeeze technique, visualization or relaxation exercises, the start-stop technique, and graduated steps to increased stimulation. Using these approaches within the broader context of sex therapy can lead to good outcomes for these individuals and their partners (175).

PROFESSIONAL AND PATIENT EDUCATION

For many individuals and couples, the essential aspects of programs addressing sexuality are education and counseling. In both disabled and non-disabled populations,

lack of education may result in problems establishing and maintaining healthy intimate, sexual relationships. Loss of sexual capacity may be related to failure of the rehabilitation program to address sexuality needs of clients (40). The goal of rehabilitation is to look holistically at the person with a disability and this perspective includes sexuality (176). Quality of life is a goal of rehabilitation and a commitment to including sexuality education as a component of information provided is essential. Education is an integral component of inpatient, outpatient, and residential programs.

Educational program development and implementation requires that healthcare professionals are knowledgeable and comfortable discussing the topic, and value the importance of addressing sexuality. The healthcare professional must have an awareness of the perceptions and feelings that may influence communication of information to patients, partners and families. Barriers identified that result in sexual education not being addressed in healthcare settings include inadequate knowledge, a perceived lack of time, an assumption that someone else is providing the education, and poor patient/family readiness to learn (177).

Staff education can be a method of exploring staff attitudes, awareness, and values. Key goals of education are to increase both the staff's comfort level and knowledge and to gain skills in communicating about sexuality with their peers, patients and families. Discussions can explore the normal development of sexuality throughout the life cycle, human sexual response, cultural differences, and the impact of traumatic brain injury on sexual function (178, 179). In a recent study, results indicated that persons with traumatic brain injury had more negative feelings about their sexuality and relationships than did participants without brain injury. Education in sexuality and ego adaptability for persons working with them is identified as a need (180).

Determining the best time for presenting information and education related to sexuality for the person with brain injury and partners and families is subject to debate, but is probably best provided in the early phase after injury. Sexual dysfunction can develop later in recovery, and follow up with patients regarding sexual function, and integration of prevention programs is essential program components (181). Lack of awareness of deficit can be prolonged, and education is helpful before and after return to the community (182). Nevertheless, learning readiness needs to be determined on an individual basis. The timing, topic areas, amount and method of education should be individualized.

In some settings, sexuality is not addressed until socially inappropriate behavior occurs. Common behaviors seen in persons emerging from coma may be touching genitalia, and self-stimulation, including masturbation. As the individual regains speech, verbal expression that includes sexual references may occur. Patients may be disinhibited and express sexual feelings to staff or family members. Privacy, safety for patients, and education and support are critical. It is important for partners and families to be prepared for such behaviors. Staff are the most common targets for inappropriate social behaviors. Education is important for all members of the treatment team in inpatient and outpatient settings (163, 183, 184).

Health promotion and prevention is essential. Key topics to include in education of patients and family are potential changes after TBI that may impact sexuality. Of crucial importance is the provision of information about sexually transmitted diseases, including gonorrhea, chylamydial infections, herpes simplex viral infections, syphilis, parasitic infections, hepatitis, genital warts, urethritis, prostatitis, and acquired immunodeficiency syndrome. Safer sex practices include a careful selection of partners, mutual screening as necessary, and use of condoms and spermicides. Information on contraception should be provided, as well as strategies to address memory and compliance challenges due to cognitive impairments (84). Individuals with brain injury are at Increased vulnerability to sexual abuse (170).

Education to prepare the person with brain injury for optimal independent living, making informed choices, and socially appropriate behavior will facilitate a successful sexual adjustment (178). Addressing issues of self-esteem directly may be helpful (184). Social and communication skills, integral to initiating and sustaining relationships, should be included in education. Clinical practice guidelines for interventions may be helpful. Three psychosocial components of the guidelines are one-to-one verbal interpersonal skills, one-to-one nonverbal interpersonal skills and strategies to deal with rejection. The guidelines provide specific interventions to foster the development of necessary social skills in long-term traumatic brain injury clients (185).

Education on psychosocial and sexual issues can be accomplished through group education meetings, social skills groups, family/patient meetings, community skills training, and individual or group counseling (182). Role-playing and more concrete and structured, repetitive styles are better choices for presenting education (38). The group setting for patient education also provides experience with improving social skills. Treatment is adapted to the level of awareness of the individual (182). Identifying the person's preferred learning style is important, as well as combining various teaching methods to improve retention of the information. Providing written materials, at an appropriate reading level and font size, are particularly important when there are cognitive impairments.

An interdisciplinary team approach, with all professional staff prepared to discuss sexuality issues in an atmosphere of permission is ideal. Leadership that fosters a team approach with the expectation that sexuality education is consistently delivered as part of the program will result in the best outcomes (178).

The PLISSIT model is a structure to guide interventions for sexual counseling and education. Permission (P) can be achieved by simply asking patients an open-ended question to identify concerns. This can be accomplished during the initial assessment and validates for the patient that you are open to discussing sexuality and lead to further questions and dialogue. Limited Information (LI) may include factual information related to concerns such as how the disability can affect sexual functioning. Specific Suggestion (SS) may include information on problem solving or when to seek medical attention/intervention. Intensive Therapy (IT) is individualized treatment provided by sex therapists and counselors. This model recognizes that there may be individual comfort levels and abilities among staff members (88, 176, 177).

A sexuality education program should include both professional and patient/family educational components and be integrated into the interdisciplinary rehabilitation programs in both inpatient and outpatient settings. A comprehensive sexuality education program, implemented in the Statewide Head Injury Program in Massachusetts, outlines both staff and patient education programs, implemented in residential and day treatment programs for adults with traumatic brain injury. Components of the program include patient and staff needs assessments and evaluation measures, and policies and procedures. Sexuality education for staff occurs at the orientation level with advanced level workshops and professional readings programs. Patient education classes are presented in a style adapted to enhance learning, with various strategies in written, question and answer format with prompt feedback and reinforcement, role-playing, and pre-post testing (186).

REPRODUCTIVE ISSUES FOR WOMEN WITH BRAIN INJURY

A full discussion of reproductive issues for women with brain injury is beyond the scope of this chapter. However, a number of articles and books, written by women with disabilities, are useful for persons with brain injury as well as the professionals who care for and advise them. Although the specific effects of the brain injury on pregnancy, labor, and delivery have not been investigated, other sources offer practical recommendations (86, 187, 188).

Several issues with particular relevance to women with traumatic brain injury are addressed below, including (1) amenorrhea, (2) seizure disorders and anticonvulsant medications, (3) other drugs with teratogenic potential, (4) management of pregnant women in coma or vegetative state, (5) contraception, and (6) infertility.

Amenorrhea

Although female reproductive dysfunction after brain injury is largely unstudied, amenorrhea is frequently observed. Hypopituitarism after head trauma results in amenorrhea, among other clinical signs, but many cases of amenorrhea after brain injury are not associated with hypopituitarism. A pregnancy test should be performed initially when indicated. A low or normal serum prolactin level indicates anovulation, and medroxyprogesterone for 5–10 days will produce withdrawal bleeding, indicating stress and trauma as a likely cause. If there is no response, then a serum LH and FSH level should be obtained. A low or normal level may indicate hypopituitarism or hypothalamic disorder. Consultation with an endocrinologist or gynecologist is recommended.

Seizures and Pregnancy

The risk of malformations associated with use of anticonvulsant drugs during pregnancy in women with epilepsy is clear (189). The absolute risk of major malformations in neonates exposed to anti-epileptic drugs in utero is 7–10%, which is 3–5% higher than for the general population. Barbiturates and phenytoin are associated with congenital heart malformations and craniofacial anomalies. The fetal hydantoin syndrome is further characterized by prenatal and postnatal growth deficiencies, mental retardation, and limb defects; less often microcephaly, ocular defects, hypospadias, and hernias may be caused by other epileptic agents (190). Valproate and carbamazepine are associated with spinal bifida and hypospadias (191). High daily dosage, high serum concentration, low folate levels, and poly-therapy are additional risk factors (189). Infants of epileptic mothers may develop hemorrhagic disorders, apparently due to a deficiency of vitamin K-dependent factors (192). Despite such risks, 90% of women with seizure disorders deliver normal infants.

Because teratogenicity of anticonvulsant medications is associated with elevated levels of oxidative metabolites, an enzymatic marker may be useful in determination of risk. Low enzymatic activity was found in 4 of 19 fetuses, and the predicted high risk for fetal hydantoin syndrome was confirmed postnatally (190).

The risk of seizures during pregnancy, labor, and delivery is increased in 40% of women with epilepsy, although 50% have no change and 10% have a decrease in seizures (193).

In one study, however, 68% of pregnancies in which seizure frequency increased were associated with non-compliance with treatment recommendations (194). Pregnancy can affect anticonvulsant levels, which decline over time, because of emesis, decreased absorption, and due to increases in plasma volume, liver metabolism, and renal clearance. In addition, hormone changes may lead to increased seizures, and protein binding may be altered.

The International League Against Epilepsy (ILAE) published guidelines for the care of women with epilepsy who may become pregnant (195). The recommendations include: counseling about the risk of seizures, bleeding, and toxemia in pregnant women; counseling about malformations, prematurity, seizures, and developmental disorders in fetus and infant; ultrasound evaluation for neural tube defects, heart malformations, and craniofacial anomalies, and amniotic fluid analysis of alpha-fetoprotein for neural tube defects; counseling about options for termination of pregnancy; careful choice of anticonvulsant and monitoring of anticonvulsant levels, both during pregnancy (when they may decrease) and after delivery (when they may increase); adequate amounts of folate (192, 196).

Anticonvulsant drugs have different rates of transmission in breast milk: 5–10% for valproate, 30% for phenytoin, 40% for phenobarbital, 45% for carbamazepine, 60% for primidone, and 90% for ethosuximide (195). Other medications, including antidepressants, antipsychotic agents, and antimigraine medications, prescribed to persons with traumatic brain injury with relative frequency, may have adverse effects on the fetus. These include antidepressants, antipsychotic agents, and antimigraine medications (197).

Coma and Vegetative State

Pregnant women with moderate to severe brain injury who are hospitalized in trauma centers may be in coma, vegetative state, or be classified as in a state of "maternal brain death" during pregnancy. Some may emerge from coma during pregnancy, but a small percentage, evolve into and remain in a vegetative state. Both maternal survival and emergence from the vegetative state are possible. Medical as well as ethical and legal questions are raised.

Dillon and associates (198) recommend maternal life-support measures at 24–27 weeks of gestation, followed by cesarean section at 28 weeks, but no extraordinary measures at less than 4 weeks for mother or fetus. Others (199) recommend continued maternal support until 32–34 weeks to increase survival rates. Obviously, for the fetus that does not survive the trauma suffered by the mother, the pregnancy must be terminated to save the mother's life. Experimental evidence suggests that the fetus may be less vulnerable to acute asphyxia than the mother. Redistribution of blood flow to vital organs, anaerobic metabolism, and decreased oxygen consumption may be the essential mechanisms (200).

Contraception

Options for contraception are not usually limited by medical considerations in patients with brain injury. Poor patient compliance because of memory difficulties may dictate choice; oral contraception may be ill advised for this reason. Long-acting injectable techniques may be preferable; permanent solutions, if desired, include vasectomy and tubal ligation. Subdermal delivery of the synthetic progesin levonorgestrel has a failure rate of 4 or 5/1,000 users/year compared with 20–50/1,000 users for oral contraceptives; for persons taking phenytoin or carbamazepine, pregnancy rates are higher (201). Oral hormonal contraception may increase the risk of venous thrombosis, and this must be considered in women historically or potentially at risk (84, 86).

Infertility

In patients with traumatic brain injury, initial evaluations should include hormonal assays, including LH, FSH, prolactin, thyroid function studies, and total testosterone. Low concentrations of LH, FSH, and testosterone suggest hypopituitary or hypothalamic injury, and a releasing hormone stimulation test should be conducted. Hypothalamic ovulatory dysfunction may be treated with clompheneitrate, menotropins (human menopausal gonadotropins or LH and FSH), or gonadotropin-releasing hormone. In men, hypothalamic-pituitary failure may be treated with menotropins, human chorionic gonadotropin, or gonadotropin-releasing hormone. Testosterone promotes virilization and may enhance sexual function but has no effect on spermatogenesis.

CONCLUSION

This chapter has focused on the pathophysiology of sexual dysfunction and the contributions of medical, psychological, social and cultural factors that influence sexual functioning in disabled populations. Whenever possible, we have attempted to focus on the specific needs of the TBI population. Updates for the evaluation and treatment of sexual dysfunction, depending on etiology, are provided to practitioners in the field of rehabilitation. Other areas of focus have included neuroendocrine disorders and women's health care in regard to both sexuality and reproduction in this population. Further research is needed to further clarify the incidence and prevalence of these disorders, and effective treatment approaches for optimal outcomes for this population of men and women with disabling injury. In addition, additional attention to the needs of sexual minorities, including gay, lesbian, and transgendered individuals is required to further advance our understanding of sexuality across the entire disabled and non-disabled population. Despite gaps in our basic science and clinical knowledge base, major advances over the last decade have been made in the evaluation and treatment of sexual, reproductive, and neuroendocrine dysfunction that will be of benefit to our patients with traumatic brain injury. Rapid development in these areas of research will no doubt lead to many new interventions in the not too distant future.

References

1. Bell KR, Pepping M. Women and traumatic brain injury. *Phys Med Rehabil Clin N Am.* 2001;12 (1):169–82.
2. Masters WH, Johnson VE. *Human Sexual Response.* Boston: Little, Brown 1966.
3. Kaplan HS. Hypoactive sexual desire. *J Sex Marital Ther.* 1977;3(1):3–9.
4. Fourcroy JL. Female sexual dysfunction: potential for pharmacotherapy. *Drugs.* 2003;63(14):1445–57.
5. Levine SB. Erectile dysfunction: why drug therapy isn't always enough. *Cleve Clin J Med.* 2003;70(3):241–6.
6. Basson R. The female sexual response: a different model. *J Sex Marital Ther.* 2000;26(1):51–65.
7. World Health Organization. *International Classification of Disease – 10, 10th Revision.* Geneva: WHO 1992.
8. American Psychiatric Association. *Diagnostic and Statistical Manual of Mental Disorders, DSM IV.* Washington, DC: American Psychiatric Association 1994.
9. Sipski ML. A physiatrist's views regarding the report of the International Consensus Conference on Female Sexual Dysfunction: potential concerns regarding women with disabilities. *J Sex Marital Ther.* 2001;27(2):215–6.
10. Basson R, Berman J, Burnett A, et al. Report of the international consensus development conference on female sexual dysfunction: definitions and classifications. *J Urol.* 2000b;163(3):888–93.
11. Avis NE, Stellato R, Crawford S, et al. Is there an association between menopause status and sexual functioning? *Menopause.* 2000a;7(5):297–309.
12. Avis NE. Sexual function and aging in men and women: community and population-based studies. *J Gend Specif Med.* 2000b; 3(2):37–41.
13. Laumann EO, Paik A, Rosen RC. Sexual dysfunction in United States: prevalence and predictors. *JAMA.* 1999;281(6):537–44.
14. Baumeister RF, Catanese KR, Vohs KD. Is there a gender difference in the strength of sex drive? Theoretical views, conceptual distinctions, and a review of relevant evidence. *Personality and Soc Psychol Rev.* 2001;5(3):242–73.
15. Angier N. *Woman: An Intimate Geography.* New York: Houghton Mifflin 1999.
16. Leiblum SR. Sexual problems and dysfunction: epidemiology, classification, and risk factors. *J Gend Specif Med.* 1999;2(5):41–5.
17. McKenna K. The brain is the master organ in sexual function: Central nervous system control of male and female sexual function. *Int J of Impot Res.* 1999;11(Suppl 1):S48-S55.
18. Allgeier WE, Allgeier AR. *Sexual Interactions, 4th edition.* Lexington, MA: DC Heath 1995.
19. Guiliano FA, Rampin O, Benoit G, et al. Neural control of penile erection. *Urol Clin North Am.* 1995;22(4):747–66.
20. Berard EJ. The sexuality of spinal cord injured women: physiology and pathophysiology. *Paraplegia.* 1989;27(2):99–112.
21. MacLean PD. Brain mechanisms of primal sexual functions and related behavior. In SandIer M, Gessa G (eds.). *Sexual Behavior: Pharmacology and Biochemistry.* New York: Raven Press 1975.
22. Marson L, Platt KB, McKenna KE. Central nervous system innervation of the penis as revealed by the transneuronal transport of pseudorabies virus. *Neuroscience.* 1993;55(1):263–80.
23. Hulter B, Lundberg PO. Sexual function in women with hypothalamo-pituitary disorders. *Arch Sex Behav.* 1994;23(2):171–83.
24. Lilly R, Cummings JL, Benson DF, et al. The human Kluver-Bucy syndrome. *Neurology.* 1983 33(9):1141–5.
25. Goscinski I, Kwaitkowski S, Polak J, et al. The Kluver-Bucy syndrome. *J Neurosurg Sci.* 1997;41(3):269–72.
26. Herzog AG, Russell V, Vaitukaitis JL, et al. Neuroendocrine dysfunction in temporal lobe epilepsy. *Arch Neurol.* 1982; 39(3):133–135.

27. Herzog AG, Seibel MM, Schomer DL, et al. Reproductive endocrine disorders in men with partial seizures of temporal lobe origin. *Arch Neuro*. 1986a;43(4):347–50.

28. Herzog AG, Seibel MM, Schomer DL, et al. Reproductive endocrine disorders in women with partial seizures of temporal lobe origin. *Arch Neurol*. 1986b;43(4):341–46.

29. Walker AE. The neurological basis of sex. *Neurol India*. 1976;24(1):1–13.

30. Horn LJ, Zasler ND: Neuroanatomy and neurophysiology of sexual dysfunction. *J Head Trauma Rehabil*. 1990;5(2):1–13.

31. Fabbri A, Jannini EA, Gnessi L, et al. Endorphins in male impotence: evidence for naltrexone stimulation of erectile activity in patient therapy. *Psychoneuroendocrinology*. 1989;14(1–2):103–11.

32. Goldstein JA. Erectile failure and naltrexone. *Ann Intern Med*. 1986;105:799.

33. Thomsen IV. Late outcome of very severe blunt head trauma: a 10–15 year second follow-up. *J Neurol Neurosurg Psychiatry*. 1984;47(3):260–8.

34. Rosenbaum M, Najenson T. Changes in life patterns and symptoms of low mood as reported by wives of severely brain-injured soldiers. *J Consul Clin Psychol*. 1976;44(6):881–8.

35. Lezak MD. Living with the characterologically altered brain injured patient. *J Clin Psychiatry*. 1978;39(7):592–8.

36. Bond MR. Assessment of the psychological outcome of severe head injury. *Acta Neurochir (Wien)*. 1976;34(1–4):57–70.

37. Garden FH, Bonke CF, Hoffman M. Sexual functioning and marital adjustment after traumatic brain injury. *J Head Trauma Rehabil*. 1990;5(2):52–9.

38. Kreuter, M. Sullivan, M., Dahllof, AG, et al. Partner relationships, functioning, mood, and global quality of life in persons with spinal cord injury and traumatic brain injury. *Spinal Cord*. 1998; 36(4):252–61.

39. Hibbard MR, Gordon WA, Flanagan S, et al. Sexual dysfunction after traumatic brain injury. *NeuroRehabilitation*. 2000;15(2): 107–20.

40. Kreuter M, Dahllof AG, Gudjonsson G, et al. Sexual adjustment and its predictors after traumatic brain injury. *Brain Inj*. 1998; 12(5):349–68.

41. Kosteljanetz M, Jensen TS, Norgard B, et al. Sexual and hypothalamic dysfunction in the postconcussional syndrome. *Acta Neurol Scand*. 1981;63(3):169–80.

42. Miller BL, Cummings JL, McIntyre H, et al. Hypersexuality or altered sexual preference following brain injury. *J Neurol Neurosurg Psychiatry*. 1986;49(8):867–73.

43. Kreutzer JS, Zasler ND. Psychosexual consequences of traumatic brain injury: methodology and preliminary findings. *Brain Inj*. 1989;3(2):177–86.

44. Zasler ND, Horn LJ. Rehabilitative management of sexual dysfunction. *J Head Trauma Rehabil*. 1990;5(2):14–24.

45. O'Carroll RE, Woodrow J, Maroun F. Psychosexual and psychosocial sequelae of closed head injury. *Brain Inj*. 1991; 5:303–13.

46. Corrigan JD. Substance abuse as a mediating factor in outcome from traumatic brain injury. *Arch Phys Med Rehabil*. 1995; 76(4):302–9.

47. Kelly MP, Johnson CT, Knoller N, et al. Substance abuse, traumatic brain injury, and neuropsychological outcome. *Brain Inj*. 1997;11(6):391–402.

48. Sparadeo FR, Barth JT, Stout CE. Addiction and traumatic brain injury. In Stout CE, Levitt JL, Ruben DH (eds). *Handbook for Assessing and Treating Addictive Disorders*. New York: Greenwood Press 1992.

49. Delmonico RL. Sexuality and substance abuse in traumatic brain injury independence. *Brain Inj Source*. 2001;5:24–6.

50. Aloni, R, Katz S. A review of the effect of traumatic brain injury on the human sexual response. *Brain Inj*. 1999;13(4):269–80.

51. Sandel ME, William KS, Dellapietra L, et al. Sexual functioning following traumatic brain injury. *Brain Inj*. 1996;10(10):719–28.

52. Derogatis LR. *Derogatis Interview For Sexual Function (DISF)*. Baltimore: Clinical Psychometric Research 1987.

53. Center for Research on Women with Disabilities. National Study of Women with Physical Disabilities. Internet: www.bcm.tmc.edu/crowd/national_study/MAJORFIN.htm, retrieved 7/28/02.

54. Olkin R. *What Psychotherapists Should Know About Disability*. New York: Guilford Press 1999, pp. 226–237.

55. Aloni R, Katz S. *Sexual Difficulties After Traumatic Brain Injury And Ways To Deal With It*. Springfield, IL: Charles C. Thomas 2003, pp. 9–19.

56. Glass C, Soni B. ABC of sexual health: sexual problems of disabled patients. *BMJ*. 1999;318(7182):518–21.

57. Kaiser Permanente National Diversity Council and the Kaiser Permanente National Diversity Department. *A Provider's Handbook on Culturally Competent Care: Lesbian, Gay, Bisexual and Transgendered Population*. Oakland, CA: Kaiser Permanente 2000.

58. Garnets, LD. Sexual orientations in perspective. *Cultur Divers Ethnic Minor Psychol*. 2002;8(2):115–29.

59. O'Dell MW, Riggs RV. Traumatic brain injury in gay and lesbian persons:Practical and theoretical considerations. *Brain Inj Source*. 2001;5(3):22–3.

60. Mapou RL. Traumatic brain injury rehabilitation with gay and lesbian individuals. *J Head Trauma Rehabil*. 1990;5(2):67–72.

61. Horn, LJ, Glenn M. Update on pharmacology. *J Head Trauma Rehabil*. 1988;3(2):87–90.

62. Horn, LJ, Glenn M. Update on pharmacology, part 2. *J Head Trauma Rehabil*. 1988;3(3):86–90.

63. Labi ML. Neuroendocrine disorders after traumatic brain injury, In Horn LJ, Zasler ND. *Medical Rehabilitation of Traumatic Brain Injury*. Philadelphia: Hanley and Belfus 1996, pp.539–555.

64. Barreca T, Perria C, Sannia A, et al. Evaluation of anterior pituitary function in patients with posttraumatic diabetes insipidus. *J Clin Endocrinol Metab*. 1980;51(6):1279–82.

65. Edwards OM, Clark JD. Post-traumatic hypopituitarism. Six cases and a review of the literature. *Medicine*. 1986;65:281–90.

66. Clark JD, Raggatt PR, Edwards 0M. Hypothalamic hypogonadism following major head injury. *Clin Endocrinol*. 1988;29(2):153–65.

67. Benvenga S, Campenni A, Ruggeri RM, et al. Clinical review 113: Hypopituitarism secondary to head trauma. *J Clin Endocrinol Metab*. 2000;85(4):1353–61.

68. Kelly DF, Gonzalo IT, Cohan P, et al. Hypopituitarism following traumatic brain injury and aneurysmal subarachnoid hemorrhage: a preliminary report. *J Neurosurg*. 2000;93(5):743–52.

69. Lieberman SA, Oberoi AL, Gilkison CR, et al. Prevalence of neuroendocrine dysfunction in patients recovering from traumatic brain injury. *J of Clin Endocrinol Metab*. 2001;86(6):2752–6.

70. Ghigo E, Masel B, Aimaretti G, et al. Consensus guidelines on screening for hypopituitarism following traumatic brain injury. *Brain Injury*, August 2005;19(9):711–724.

71. Ishikawa SE, Saito T, Kaneko K, et al. Hyponatremia responsive to fludrocortisone acetate in elderly patients after head injury. *Ann Intern Med*. 1987;106(2):187–91.

72. Stewart, DG, Cifu, DX. Management of Neuroendocrine Disorders after Brain Injury. *Phys Med Rehabil Clin N Am*. 1997;8(4): 827–42.

73. Kern KB, Meislin HW. Diabetes insipidus: occurrence after minor head trauma. *J Trauma*. 1984;24(1):69–72.

74. Notman DD, Mortek MA, Moses AM. Permanent diabetes insipidus following head trauma:observations on ten patients and an approach to diagnosis. *J Trauma*. 1980;20(7):599–602.

75. Barton RN, Stoner HB, Watson SM. Relationships among plasma cortisol, adrenocorticotropin, and severity of injury in recently injured patients. *J Trauma*. 1987;27(4):384–92.

76. Klachko DM, Winer N, Burns TW, et al. Traumatic hypopituitarism occurring before puberty: Survival 35 years untreated. *J Clin Endocrinol Metab*. 1968;28(12):1768–72.

77. Shaul PW, Towbin RB, Chernausek SD. Precocious puberty following severe head trauma. *Am J Dis Child*. 1985;139(5):467–9.

78. Blendonohy P, Philip PA. Precocious puberty in children after traumatic brain injury. *Brain Inj*. 1991;5(1):63–8.

79. Attella MJ, Nattinville A, Stein DG. Hormonal state affects recovery from frontal cortex lesions in adult female rats. *Behav Neural Biol*. 1987;48 (3):352–267.

80. Roof RL, Hall ED. Estrogen-related gender difference in survival rate and cortical blood flow after impact-acceleration head injury in rats. *J Neurotrauma*. 2000;17(12):1155–69.

81. Groswasser Z. Cohen M., Keren O. Female TBI patients recover better than males. *Brain Inj*. 1998;12(9):805–8.

82. Jennett B, Teasdale G. *Management of Head Injuries*. Philadelphia: F.A. Davis 1981.

83. Sipski ML, Alexander CJ. *Sexual Function in People With Disability and Chronic Illness: A Health Professionals Guide*. Gaithersberg: Aspen 1997.

84. Griffith ER, Lemberg S. *Sexuality and the Person with Traumatic Brain Injury: A Guide for Families*. Philadelphia: F.A. Davis 1993.

85. Kroll K, Levy Klein E. *Enabling Romance: A Guide to Love, Sex, and Relationships for the Disabled*. New York: Harmony Books 1992.

86. Haseltine F, Cole SS, Gray DB. *Reproductive Issues for Persons with Physical Disabilities*. Baltimore: PH Brookes 1993.

87. Ducharme S, Gill KM. Sexual values, training and professional roles. *J Head Trauma Rehabil*. 1990;5:38–45.

88. Annon J. The PLISSIT model: a proposed conceptual scheme for the behavioral treatment of sexual problems. *J Sex Ed Therapists* 1976;5:1–15.

89. Schover LR. Sexual problems in chronic illness. In Leiblum SR, Rosen RC (eds.). *Principles and practice of sex therapy, 3rd Ed*. New York: Guilford 2000, pp. 398–422.

90. Schover LR, Friedman JM, Weiler SJ, et al. Multiaxial problem-oriented system for sexual dysfunctions: an alternative to DSM-III. *Arch Gen Psychiatry*. 1982;39:614–9.

91. LoPiccolo L, Heiman JR. Sexual assessment and history interview. In LoPiccolo J, LoPiccolo L (eds.). *Handbook of sex therapy*. New York: Plenum Press 1978, pp. 103–113.

92. Beck AT, Steer RA, Brown GK. *BDI-II: Beck Depression Inventory Manual*. San Antonio: The Psychological Corporation 1996.

93. Butcher JN, Graham JR, Ben-Porath YS, et al. *MMPI-2 (Minnesota Multiphasic Personality Inventory – 2): Manual for administration, scoring, and interpretation, Revised Edition*. Minneapolis: University of Minnesota Press 2001.

94. Millon T, Davis R, Millon C. *MCMI-III: Millon clinical multiaxial inventory – III manual second edition*. Minneapolis: National Computer Systems Inc. 1997.

95. Rust J, Golombok S. The Glomobok-Rusk Inventory of Sexual Satisfaction (GRISS). *Br J Clin Psychol*. 1985;24(Pt 1):63–4.

96. Siosteen A, Lundqvist C, Blomstrand C, et al. Sexual ability, activity, attitudes, and satisfaction as part of adjustment in spinal cord-injured subjects. *Paraplegia*. 1990;28:285–95.

97. Rosen R, Brown C, Heiman J, et al. The Female Sexual Function Index (FSDI): a multidimensional self-report instrument for the assessment of female sexual function. *J Sex Marital Ther*. 2000;26(2):191–208.

98. Derogatis LR, Rosen R, Leiblum S, et al. The Female Sexual Distress Scale (FSDS): initial validation of a standardized scale for assessment of sexually related personal distress in women. *J Sex Marital Ther*. 2002;28(4):317–30.

99. Quirk FH, Heiman JR, Rosen RC, et al. Development of a sexual function questionnaire for clinical trials of female sexual dysfunction. *J Womens Health Gend Based Med*. 2002;11(3):277–89.

100. Rosen RC, Lane RM, Menza M. Effects of SSRIs on sexual function: a critical review. *J Clin Psychopharmacol*. 1999;19(1):67–85.

101. Seidman SN, Pesce VC, Roose SP. High-dose sildenafil citrate for selective serotonin reuptake inhibitor-associated ejaculatory delay: open clinical trial. *J Clin Psychiatry*. 2003;64(6):721–5.

102. Sitsen JMA. Prescription drugs and sexual function. In Money J, Musaph H (eds.). *Handbook of Sexology. Vol VI*. Amsterdam/New York/London: Elsevier 1988, pp. 425–61.

103. Drugs that cause sexual dysfunction. *Med Lett Drugs Ther*. 1983;25(641):73–6.

104. Abboud CF. Laboratory diagnosis of hypopituitarism. *Mayo Clin Proc*. 1986;61:35–48.

105. Kaneko S, Bradley WE. Evaluation of erectile dysfunction with continuous monitoring of penile rigidity. *J Urol*. 1986;136(5):1026–9.

106. Morales A, Condra M, Reid K. The role of nocturnal penile tumescence monitoring in the diagnosis of impotence: a review. *J Urol*. 1990;143(3):441–6.

107. Thase ME, Reynolds CF 3rd, Jennings JR, et al. Nocturnal penile tumescence is diminished in depressed men. *Biol Psychiatry*. 1988;24(1):33–46.

108. Assessment: Neurological evaluation of male sexual dysfunction. Report of the Therapeutics and Technology Assessment Subcommittee of the American Academy of Neurology. *Neurology*. 1995;45(12):2287–92.

109. Lundberg PO, Ertekin C, Ghezzi A, et al. Neurosexology. *European J Neurology*. 2001;8(Supp 3):2–24.

110. Deliganis AV, Maravilla KR, Heiman JR, et al. Female genitalia: dynamic MR imaging with use of MS-325 initial experiences evaluating female sexual response. *Radiology*. 2002;225(3):791–9.

111. Sipski ML, Behnegar A. Neurogenic female sexual dysfunction: a review. *Clin Auton Res*. 2001;11(5):279–83.

112. Fink HA, MacDonald R, Rutks IR, et al. Sildenafil for male erectile dysfunction: a systematic review and meta-analysis. *Arch Intern Med* 2002;162(12):1349–60.

113. Gans WH, Zaslau S, Wheeler S, et al. Efficacy and safety of oral sildenafil in men with erectile dysfunction and spinal cord injury. *J Spinal Cord Med*. 2001;24(1):35–40.

114. Padma-Nathan H, Steidle C, Salem S, et al. The efficacy and safety of a topical alprostadil cream, Alprox-TD, for the treatment of erectile dysfunction: two phase 2 studies in mild-to-moderate and severe ED. *Int J Impot Res*. 2003;15(1):10–7.

115. Porst H, Young JM, Schmidt AC, et al. Efficacy and tolerability of vardenafil for treatment of erectile dysunction in patient subgroups. *Urology*. 2003;62(3):519–23; discussion 523–4.

116. Sanchez Ramos A, Vidal J, Jauregui ML, et al. Efficacy, safety and predictive factors of therapeutic success with sildenafil for erectile dysfunction in patients with different spinal cord injuries. *Spinal Cord*. 2001;39(12):637–43.

117. Carrier S. Pharmacology of phosphodiesterase 5 inhibitors. *Can J Urol*. 2003;10 Suppl 1:12–6.

118. Herschorn S. Cardiovascular safety of PDE5 inhibitors. *Can J Urol*. 2003;10 (Suppl 1):23–8.

119. Gonzalo ML, Brotzman M, Trock BJ et al. Clinical efficacy of sildenafil citrate and predictors of long-term response. *J Urol*. 2003;170(2Pt1):503–6.

120. Atmaca M, Kuloglu M, Tezcan E. Sildenafil use in patients with olanzapine-induced erectile dysfunction. *Int J Impot Res*. 2002; 14(6):547–9.

121. Nurnberg HG, Hensley PL, Gelenberg AJ, et al. Treatment of antidepressant-associated sexual dysfunction with sildenafil: a randomized controlled trail. *JAMA*. 2003;289(1):56–64.

122. Yap RL, McVary KT. Topical agents and erectile dysfunction: is there a place? *Curr Urol Rep*. 2002;3(6):471–6.

123. Steidle C, Padma-Nathan H, Salem S, et al. Topical alprostadil cream for the treatment of erectile dysfunction: a combined analysis of the phase II program. *Urology*. 2002;60(6):1077–82.

124. Bechara A, Bertolino MV, Casabe A, et al. Duplex Doppler Ultrasound assessment of clitoral hemodynmaics after topical administration of alprostadil in women with arousal and orgasmis disorders. *J Sex Marital Ther*. 2003;29(Suppl 1):1–10.

125. Benkert O, Crombach G, Kockott G. Effect of L- dopa on sexually impotent patients. *Psychopharmacologia*. 1972;23(1):91–5.

126. Montorsi F, Perani D, Anchisi D, et al. Apomorphine-induced brain modulation during sexual stimulation: a new look at central phenomena related to erectile dysfunction. *Int J Impot Res*. 2003;15(3):203–9.

127. Montorsi F, Perani D, Anchisi D, et al. Brain activation patterns during video sexual stimulation following the administration of apomorphine: results of a placebo-controlled study. *Eur Urol*. 2003;43(4):405–11.

128. Hagemann JH, Berding G, Bergh S et al. Effects of visual sexual stimuli and apomorphine SL on cerebral activity in men with erectile dysfunction. *Eur Urol*. 2003;43(4):412–20.

129. Lal S, Ackman D, Thavundayil JX, et al. Effect of apomorphine, a dopamine receptor agonist, on penile tumescence in normal subjects. *Prog Neuropsychopharmacol Biol Psychiatry*. 1984; 8(4–6):695–9.

130. Lal S. Apomorphine in the evaluation of dopaminergic function in man. *Prog Neuropsychopharmacol Biol Psychiatry*. 1988; 12(2–3):117–64.

131. Lammers, PI, Rubio-Aurioles E, Castell R, et al. Combination therapy for erectile dysfunction: a randomized, double blind,

unblinded active-controlled, cross-over study of the pharmaco-dynamics and safety of combined oral formulations of apomorphine hydrochloride, phentolamine mesylate and papverine hydrochloride in men with moderate to severe erectile dysfunction. *Int J Impot Res.* 2002;14(1):54–9.

132. O'Carroll RE. Sexual desire disorders: a review of controlled treatment studies. *J Sex Res.* 1991;28(4):607–24.

133. Sherwin BB, Gelfand MM. The role of androgen in the maintenance of sexual functioning in oopherectomized women. *Psychosom Med.* 1987;49(4):397–409.

134. Apperloo MJ, Van Der Stege JG, Hoek A, Weijmar Schultz WC. In the mood for sex: the value of androgens. *J Sex Marital Ther.* 2003;29(2):87–102.

135. Anastasiadis AG, Davis AR, Salomon L, et al. Hormonal factors in female sexual dysfunction. *Curr Opin Urol.* 2002;12(6):503–7.

136. Zumoff B, Strain GW, Miller LK, et al. Twenty-four-hour mean plasma testosterone concentration declines with age in normal premenopausal women. *J Clin Endocrinol Metab.* 1995;80(4):1429–30.

137. Tan RS. Novel treatment options for overlapping yet distinct erectile dysfunction and andropause syndromes. *Curr Opin Investig Drugs.* 2003;4(4):435–8.

138. Liverman CT, Blazer DG, editors. *Testosterone and aging – clinical research directions. Committee on Assessing the Need for Clinical Trials of Testosterone Replacement Therapy, Board of Health Sciences Policy, Institute of Medicine.* Washington DC: The National Academies Press 2003.

139. O'Carroll RE, Bancroft J. Testosterone therapy for low sexual interest and erectile dysfunction in men: A controlled study. *Br J Psychiatry.* 1984;145:146–51.

140. Buvat J, Lemaire A, Buvat-Herbaut M. Human chorionic gonadotropin treatment of nonorganic erectile failure and lack of sexual desire: a double-blind study. *Urology.* 1987;30(3):216–9.

141. Zajecka J, Fawcett J, Schaff M, et al. The role of serotonin in sexual dysfunction: fluoxetine-associated orgasm dysfunction. *J Clin Psychiatry.* 1991;52(2):66–8.

142. Gartrell N. Increased libido in women receiving trazodone. *Am J Psychiatry.* 1986;143(6):781–2.

143. Mathews A, Whitehead A, Kellet J. Psychological and hormonal factors in the treatment of female sexual dysfunction. *Psychol Med.* 1983;13(1):83–92.

144. Stevensen RW, Solyom L. The aphrodisiac effect of fenfluramine: two case reports of a possible side effect to the use of fenfluramine in the treatment of bulimia. *J Clin Psychopharmacol.* 1990;10(1):69–71.

145. Crenshaw TL, Goldberg JP, Stern WC. Pharmacologic modification of psychosexual dysfunction. *J Sex Marital Ther.* 1987;13(4):239–52.

146. Drewes SE, George J, Khan F. Recent findings on natural products with erectile-dysfunction activity. *Phytochemistry.* 2003;62(7):1019–25.

147. Hong B, Ji YH, Hong JH, et al. A double-blind crossover study evaluating the efficacy of Korean red ginseng in patients with erectile dysfunction: a preliminary report. *J Urol.* 2002;168(5):2070–3.

148. Danjou P, Alexandre L, Warot D, et al. Assessment of erectongenic properties of apomorphine and yohimbine in man. *Br J Clin Pharmacol.* 1988;26(6):733–9.

149. Guay AT, Spark RF, Jacobson J, et al. Yohimbine treatment of organic erectile dysfunction in a dose-escalation trial. *In J Impot Res.* 2002;14(1):25–31.

150. Morales A, Condra M, Owen JA, et al. Is yohimbine effective in the treatment of organic impotence? Results of a controlled trial. *J Urol.* 1987;137(6):1168–72.

151. Reid K, Surridge DH, Morales A, et al. Double-blind trial of yohimbine in treatment of psychogenic impotence. *Lancet.* 1987;2(8556):421–3.

152. Sondra LP, Mazo R, Chancellor MB. The role of yohimbine for the treatment of erectile impotence. *J Sex Marital Ther.* 1990;16(1):15–21.

153. Susset JG, Tessier CD, Wincze J, et al. Effect of yohimbine hydrochloride on erectile impotence: a double-blind study. *J Urol.* 1989;141(6):1360–3.

154. Meston CM, Worcel M. The effects of yohimbine plus L-arginine glutamate on sexual arousal in postmenopausal women with sexual arousal disorder. *Arch Sex Behav.* 2002;31(4):323–32.

155. Lebret T, Herve JM, Gorny P, et al. Efficacy and safety of a novel combination of L-arginine glutamate and yohimbine hydrochloride: a new oral therapy for erectile dysfunction. *Eur Urol.* 2002;41(6):608–13.

156. Kalsi JS, Minhas S, Kell PD, et al. Oral agents for erectile dysfunction. *Hosp Med.* 2003;64(5):292–5.

157. Sidi AA. Vasoactive intercavernous pharmacotherapy. *Urol Clin North Am.* 1988;15(1):95–101.

158. Levine SB, Althof SE, Turner LA, et al. Side effects of self-administration of intracavernous papaverine and phentolamine for the treatment of impotence. *J Urol.* 1989;141(1):54–7.

159. Ishii N, Watanabe H, Irisawa C, et al. Intracavernous injection of prostaglandin E1 for the treatment of erectile impotence. *J Urol.* 1989;141(2):323–5.

160. Stakl W, Hasun R, Marberger M. Intracavernous injection of prostaglandin E1 in impotent men. *J Urol.* 1988;140(1):66–8.

161. Burnett AL. Neuroprotection and nerve grafts in the treatment of neurogenic erectile dysfunction. *J Urol.* 2003;170(2 Pt2):S31–4;discussion S34.

162. Ferguson DM, Steidle CP, Singh GS, et al. Randomized, placebo-controlled, double blind, crossover design trial of the efficacy and safety of Zestra for Women in women with and without female sexual arousal disorder. *J Sex Marital Ther.* 2003;29 Suppl 1:33–44.

163. Simpson G, Blaszczynski A, Hodgkinson A. Sex offending as a psychosocial sequela of traumatic brain injury. *J Head Trauma Rehabil.* 1999;14(6):567–80.

164. Lusk MD, Kott JA. Effects of head injury on libido. *Med Aspects Hum Sex.* 1982;16(10):22–30.

165. Weinstein EA, Kahn RL. Patterns of sexual behavior following brain injury. *Psychiatry.* 1961;24:69–78.

166. Weinstein EA. Sexual disturbances after brain injury. *Med Aspects Hum Sex.* 1974;8(10):10–16,18 passim.

167. Weinstein EA. Effects of brain damage on sexual behavior. *Med Aspects Hum Sex.* 1981;15(11):158, 163–4.

168. Britton KR. Medoxyprogesterone in the treatment of aggressive hypersexual behaviour in traumatic brain injury. *Brain Inj.* 1998;12(8):703–7.

169. Emory LE, Cole CM, Meyer WJ. Use of Depo-Provera to control sexual aggression in persons with traumatic brain injury. *J Head Trauma Rehabil.* 1995;10(3):47–58.

170. Cole S. Facing the challenges of sexual abuse in persons with disabilities. *J Sex Disabil.* 1986;7(3–4):71–8.

171. Leiblum SR, Rosen RC. Introduction: sex therapy in the age of Viagra. In Leiblum SR, Rosen RC (eds.). *Principles and practice of sex therapy, 3rd Ed.* New York: Guilford 2000, pp. 1–13.

172. LoPiccolo J. Direct treatment of sexual dysfunction. In LoPiccolo J, LoPiccolo L (eds.). *Handbook of sex therapy.* New York: Plenum Press 1978, pp. 1–17.

173. Pridal CG, LoPiccolo J. Multielement treatment of desire disorders: Integration of cognitive, behavioral, and systemic therapy. In Leiblum SR, Rosen RC (eds.). *Principles and practice of sex therapy, 3rd Ed.* New York: Guilford 2000, pp. 57–81.

174. Althof SE. Erectile dysfunction: psychotherapy with men and couples. In Leiblum SR Rosen RC (eds.). *Principles and Practice of Sex Therapy, 3rd edition.* New York, Guilford 2000, pp. 242–275.

175. Polonsky, DC. Premature ejaculation. In Leiblum SR, Rosen RC (eds.). *Principles and practice of sex therapy, 3rd Ed.* New York: Guilford 2000, pp. 305–32.

176. Duldt BW, Pokorny ME. Teaching communication about human sexuality to nurses and other healthcare providers. *Nurse Educ.* 1999;24(5):27–32.

177. Herson L, Hart KA, Gordon MJ, et al. Identifying and overcoming barriers to providing sexuality information in the clinical setting. *Rehabil Nurs.* 1999;24(4):148–51.

178. Hough S. Sexuality within the head-injury rehabilitation setting: A staff's perspective. *Psychol Rep.* 1989;65(3 Pt 1):745–6.

179. Medlar TM, MedlarJ. Nursing management of sexuality issues. *J Head Trauma Rehabil.* 1990;5(2):46–51.

180. Gaudet L, Crethar HC, Burger S, et al. Self reported consequences of traumatic brain injury: A study of contrasting TBI and non TBI participants. *Sexuality and Disability*. 2001;19(2)111–19.

181. Aloni A, Keren O, Cohen M, et al. Incidence of sexual dysfuncion in TBI patients during the early post-traumatic in-patient rehabilitation phase. *Brain Inj*. 1999;13(2):89–97.

182. Dombrowski LK, Petrick JD, Strauss D. Rehabilitation treatment of sexuality issues due to acquired brain injury. *Rehabil Psychol*. 2000;45(3):299–309.

183. Kotch MJ. Agitation:understanding and managing challenges on the nursing unit. *Brain Inj Source*. 2001;5(3):8–11.

184. Zencius A, Wesolowski MD, Burke WH, et al. Managing hypersexual disorders in brain-injured clients. *Brain Inj*. 1990;4(2):175–81.

185. Gutman S, Deger D. Enhancement of one-on-one interpersonal skills necessary to initiate and maintain intimate relationships: a frame of reference for adults having sustained a traumatic brain injury. *Occup Ther Ment Health*. 1997;13(2):51–67.

186. Medlar T. The sexuality education program of the Massachusetts statewide head injury program. *Sex Disabil*. 1998;16(1):11–19.

187. Patel M, Bonke C. Impact of traumatic brain injury on pregnancy. *J Head Trauma Rehabil*. 1990;5(2):60–6.

188. Rogers JG, Matsumura M. *Mother-To Be: A Guide to Pregnancy and Birth for Women with Disabilities*. New York: Demos 1991.

189. Lindhout D, Omtzigt JG. Pregnancy and risk of teratogenicity. *Epilepsia*. 1992;33(Suppl 4):S41–8.

190. Buehler BA, Delimont D, van Waes M, et al. Prenatal prediction of risk of the fetal hydantoin syndrome. *N Engl J Med*. 1990;322(22):1567–72.

191. Rosa FW. Spina bifida in infants of women treated with carbamazepine in pregnancy. *N Engl J Med*. 1991;324(10):674–7.

192. Werler MM, Shapiro S, Mitchell AA. Periconceptional folic acid exposure and risk of occurrent neural tube defects. *JAMA*. 1993;269(10):1257–61.

193. Dalessio DJ. Current concepts. Seizure disorders and pregnancy. *N Engl J Med*. 1985;312(9):559–63.

194. Schmidt D, Canger R, Avanzini G, et al. Change of seizure frequency in pregnant epileptic women. *J Neurol Neurosurg Psychiatry*. 1983;46:751–5.

195. Guidelines for the care of women of childbearing age with epilepsy. Commission on Genetics, Pregnancy, and the Child, International League against Epilepsy. *Epilepsia*. 1993;34(4): 588–9.

196. Czeizel AE, Dudas I. Prevention of the first occurrence of neural-tube defects by periconceptual vitamin supplementation. *N Engl J Med*. 1992;327(26):1832–5.

197. Briggs, GG, Freeman RK, Yaffe SJ. *Drugs in Pregnancy and Lactation: A Reference Guide to Fetal and Neonatal Risk, 4th ed*. Baltimore: Williams & Wilkins 1994.

198. Dillon WP, Lee RV, Tronolone MJ, et al. Life support and maternal death during pregnancy. *JAMA*. 1982;248(9):1089–91.

199. Hill LM, Parker D, O'Neill BP. Management of maternal vegetative state during pregnancy. *Mayo Clin Proc*. 1985;60(7):469–72.

200. Cohn HE, Sacks EJ, Heymann MA, et al. Cardiovascular responses to hypoxemia and acidemia in fetal lambs. *Am J Obstet Gynecol*. 1974;120(6):817–24.

201. A subdermal progestin implant for long-term contraception. *Med Lett Drugs Ther*. 1991;33(839):17–8.

medical findings, but also physiological, behavioral, and cognitive-affective functioning, including vulnerabilities and strengths. Martelli, Nicholson and Zasler, in chapter 39 of this text, provide a thorough review of the most useful pain assessment instruments, along with a model and method of pain assessment.

Importantly, a comprehensive, multimodal, biopsychosocial assessment becomes critical when pain is chronic, and should address beliefs about the individual's pain condition, pain coping strategies, psychological adjustment, activity level and quality of life (34, 35). The impact of various cognitive processes on the subjective perception of the patient's pain must be considered in the context of a comprehensive pain assessment. Turk has emphasized the importance of understanding and addressing the important role of patient pain appraisals, beliefs and expectancies (36). Furthermore, Dr. Turk has noted that patients who have chronic pain resulting from traumatic events tend to view any physical sensation as harmful and noxious, thereby increasing anxiety, as well as, subjective pain perceptions ultimately leading to further avoidance of activities and greater functional limitations which only serves to facilitate further deconditioning perpetuating this cycle.

Components of emotion that are relevant to the pain experience include: the subjective experience of how the pain feels, autonomic arousal associated with bodily reactions to pain, cognitive appraisal(s) of the painful experience as related to the personal meaning of the pain or the learned responses to pain and injury, non-verbal behaviors including facial expressions and body language associated with pain, and lastly, affective reactions to pain including anxiety (more typical acutely) and depression (more typical chronically) (37). People who have chronic pain have a much higher predilection and incidence of depression, anxiety, as well as, anger. Diathesis-stress models have been proposed to explain the higher rate of depression in this patient population, however, the implications are likely applicable to other psychoemotional responses to chronic pain as well.

Finally, psychological assessment is now a required element of pain treatment programs accredited by the Commission on Accreditation of Rehabilitation Facilities (38) as well as several managed care companies. Again, readers are referred to Chapter 39 in this text for a more thorough review of pain assessment methodology. This chapter includes a survey of general classes and useful pain assessment instruments including a model of assessment based on previous work (39).

PAIN MANAGEMENT STRATEGIES

The management of pain represents a significant public health issue in the United States. It is both costly to our health care system and devastating to the patient's quality of life. The need to improve pain outcomes is reflected by the congressional declaration of the present decade as the "Decade of Pain Control and Research," and the acknowledgment in January 2001 of pain as the "fifth vital sign" by the Joint Commission of Healthcare Organizations.

The goal of pain management is to modulate and ideally negate the associated physical and psychological symptoms of pain, prevent chronicity and reduce functional disability. Realistic endpoints of pain relief consistent with the clinical situation should be established. Pain management methods include both non-pharmacologic and/or pharmacologic methods and are optimized when provided in a coordinated interdisciplinary and multidisciplinary fashion (see Chapter 39). Clinicians should strive to identify pain generators and treat them as directly as possible versus simply treating the symptom of pain. The simplest, least invasive, lowest risk and most cost effective management approaches that allow for optimization of patient compliance and maximal functional restoration should be used whenever possible. When pharmacologic agents are used, analgesia should be delivered with minimal adverse effects and inconvenience to the patient, with clearly defined treatment expectancies, all of which will optimize compliance.

Medical Management: General Considerations

In the acute care setting, already compromised neurological status may limit the array of pharmacotherapeutic agents that might be appropriate to use in a patient where the neurosurgical and neurological status is either stabilized and/or static. Medications that potentially alter any aspect of the neurological assessment should be used with caution in the acute care setting if there is a more significant brain injury and/or neurologic instability. Additionally, consideration should be given to medications with reversible effects (e.g. opiate reversal with naltrexone) whenever there is question of medication effect versus ongoing deterioration of neurological status.

During the acute care phase, the primary pain generators in trauma patients will be fractures, intra-abdominal injuries, soft tissue injuries and pain associated with invasive procedures. Pain treatment should be tailored to the degree of pain assessed and reported via metric (e.g. Visual Analog Scale) or qualitative (e.g. mild, moderate, severe and excruciating) descriptors. For neurologically compromised patients with response limitations, prophylactic pain management should be practiced based upon injuries sustained and clinical presentation. Pharmacologic prophylaxis of pain should be considered in low level patients with TBI (e.g. vegetative and/or minimally conscious) given: a) difficulty in assessment of pain in this patient sub-group, as well as, controversies regarding pain appreciation and suffering in patient's whose awareness of pain may be difficult if not impossible to confirm and b) the negative impact of pain (even in patients in a vegetative state) related to sub-cortical physiologic responses to nociceptive stimuli including increased tone/posturing, tachycardia, tachypnea, diaphoresis in addition to other adverse effects.

In the sub-acute setting, many of the same issues present in the acute care setting will continue to serve as pain generators. As patients are weaned from pain medication, pain severity can increase and acute pain generators can evolve into sub-acute pain generators. Ongoing attention to pain management must be continued as patients are moved to neurosurgical step-down units and/or inpatient rehabilitation units. Changes in patient status in the sub-acute setting may reflect underlying neural changes that are adaptive or maladaptive. Maladaptive changes can result in additional pain generators (e.g., progression and/or increase of tonal abnormalities resulting in hypertonicity and rigidity) as well as central pain phenomena. Pain often affects functional assessment in lower level neurologic patients and must be adequately assessed and treated. This includes pain associated with spasticity, posturing, fractures, pressure sores, peripheral nerve changes, complex regional pain syndrome (CRPS) and post-surgical incisional pain.

Chronic pain has many elements of acute and sub-acute pain but is generally promulgated by additional factors including psychological ones. Current evidence strongly supports mechanisms of central sensitization in chronic pain phenomena which are not present in the acute and sub-acute periods. The patient suffering from chronic pain should be treated just as aggressively as a patient with acute or sub-acute pain, but because peripheral pain triggers are frequently less obvious, with different modalities. With chronic pain, biopsychosocial models for assessment and management are indicated and inclusion and integration of behavioral and psychological interventions usually optimizes treatment outcome.

It is critical in the context of assessment to take an adequate pain history in order for the clinician to provide an adequate foundation for identifying possible or probable pain generators. Clinicians are cautioned against assumptions that commonly reported pain symptoms are due to the brain injury itself (e.g. post-traumatic headache) when pain is more commonly produced by extra-cerebral injury. Evaluating clinicians should be familiar with both the broad array of pain symptoms that may be reported by post trauma patients, as well as assessment methodologies for the various types of pain seen in this population. Clinicians are referred to various other sources for a more detailed description of patient assessment methodologies for persons with pain disorders including dual diagnoses of TBI and pain for more in-depth discussions of this topic (40, 41).

Pharmacological Management

Mild pain medicines that should be considered typically include aspirin, acetaminophen and non-steroidal anti-inflammatory drugs. For moderate pain the following may be considered: high dose aspirin or acetaminophen, oral NSAIDs, newer generation NSAIDs such as Cox II inhibitors (now limited to the single agent, celecoxib), injectable NSAIDs, mixed narcotic analgesics with aspirin or acetaminophen (with or without caffeine) and tramadol. For severe pain, medications to consider would include: parenteral narcotics (Morphine Sulfate = standard), mixed agonists/antagonists (pentazocine, nalbuphine), partial agonist narcotics (buprenorphine), antidepressants, anticonvulsants, and/or atypical agents. Stimulants such as methylphenidate are used with opioid analgesics as an adjuvant analgesic and to help manage opioid-induced sedation and cognitive impairment. Common medications used in pain management are included in Table 38-1.

Nerve damage with both peripheral and central pain generators is not uncommon in post-trauma patients. Some post-trauma patients may present with both opioid sensitive and opioid insensitive pain at different sites and due to different etiologies. Medications that have been used for opioid insensitive pain include non-steroidal anti-inflammatory drugs (42), tricyclic anti-depressants, newer generation antidepressant agents such as venlafaxine or duloxetine, tizanidine, anti-epileptic medications, and various topical medications (some of which may need to be produced through compounding pharmacies), among other pharmacotherapeutic options.

Adjuvant analgesics are drugs that are analgesic in specific circumstances but have primary indications other than for pain management. Adjuvant analgesics are usually combined with analgesics. Corticosteroids, such as prednisone, are commonly used as short-term therapy to decrease pain and nausea and improve mood, appetite, and general sense of well being. Adverse effects of short-term corticosteroid use include edema, dyspepsia, and neuropsychiatric changes. Diabetic patients should be counseled about careful blood glucose monitoring while taking corticosteroids due to their hyperglycemic effect.

Antidepressants and anticonvulsants are used to manage a variety of neuropathic pain states that have not been responsive to opioid analgesics (see Table 38-4). Tricyclic antidepressants (TCAs), particularly amitriptyline, have shown efficacy in the management of diabetic neuropathy, and are used for other neuropathic states. TCAs can also manage underlying depression in pain states. Other TCAs such as nortriptyline, imipramine, and desipramine are also used. Agents that are SNRIs such as venlafaxine (Effexor) and duloxetine (Cymbalta) have also been found effective in certain pain conditions due to apparent antinociceptive properties. TCA adverse

TABLE 38-2
Medications for Pain

ANTIDEPRESSANTS		ANTICONVULSANTS	
Bedtime dose helps sleep and pain		*Especially for lancinating/neuropathic pain*	
DRUG	TYPICAL DOSE	DRUG	TYPICAL DOSE
Amitriptyline	75 mg qhs	Carbamazepine	200 mg q 8 h
Desipramine	75 mg qhs	Valproic acid	250 mg q 8 h
Nortriptyline	75 mg qhs	Phenytoin	100 mg q 8 h
Fluoxetine	20 mg qd	Clonazepam	0.5 mg q 8 h
Paroxetine	20 to 40 mg qd	Gabapentin	600 mg q 8 h
		Lamotrigine	100–400 mg/d
Venlafaxine	75–300 mg./d	Pregabalin	50–100 mg/tid
Duloxetine	40 to 60 mg/d	Levetiracetam	500–1500 mg/bid
Analgesics		*Local Anesthetics*	
Acetaminophen	650 mg q 4–6 h	Lidocaine	1.5 mg/kg IV
Tramadol	100 mg q 4–12 h	Mexiletine	225 mg q 8 h
		Flecainide	150 mg q 12 h
Steroids			
Prednisone	20–80 mg qd	*Topical*	
Dexamethasone	4–16 mg qd	Capsaicin	Topical qid
		"Speed Gel"	Topical tid – qid

TABLE 38-3
Opioid Analgesics

SHORT-ACTING OPIOIDS[1]			LONG-ACTING OPIOIDS[1]		
DRUG	EQUIVALENT DOSES		DRUG	EQUIVALENT DOSES	
	ORAL	PARENTERAL		ORAL	PARENTERAL
Morphine	30 mg q 3–4 h	10 mg q 3–4 h	MS-Contin	90 - 120 mg q 12 h	–
Hydromorphone	7.5 mg q 3–4 h	1.5 mg q 3–4 h	Levorphanol	4 mg q 6–8 h	2 mg q 6–8 h
Codeine	200 mg q 3–4 h	–	Methadone	20 mg q 6–8 h	10 mg q 3–6 h
Hydrocodone	30 mg q 3–4 h	–	Oramorph SR	90 - 120 mg q 12 h	–
Oxycodone	30 mg q 3–4 h	–	Oxymorphone	–	1 mg q 3–4 h
Meperidine	300 mg q 2–3 h	100 mg q 3 h			
Fentanyl	IM or IV		Fentanyl	Transdermal: 25 g patch 45–135 mg Morphine p.o. over 24 h	
Opioid-naive adults and children ≥50 kg body weight					

Note: The above mentioned drugs are only a partial listing of available opioids.

effects include anti-cholinergic effects (dry mouth, sedation); weight gain; orthostatic hypotension; and cardiac arrhythmias. Secondary amines such as nortriptyline and desipramine have fewer adverse effects and should be used in patients, such as the elderly, when there is concern for anticholinergic effects, sedation, and orthostatic hypotension. Antidepressants generally should be initiated at a low dosage and titrated up slowly based on pain relief and patient tolerance.

Anticonvulsants, such as carbamazepine and gabapentin, can be effective for the management of neuropathic pain, particularly lancinating or paroxysmal pain. Because carbamazepine can decrease platelets, neutrophils, and red blood cells, patients on carbamazepine should have complete blood counts performed routinely. Gabapentin has shown efficacy in diabetic neuropathy and post—herpetic neuralgia, and generally has a milder adverse effect profile consisting of sedation, ataxia, and does not require routine lab work. A recent Cochrane review examining the role of AEDs (anti-epileptic drugs) for acute and chronic pain noted that although they are widely used in chronic pain surprisingly few trials show analgesic effectiveness. They noted that there was no evidence for anticonvulsant effectiveness in acute pain, however, in chronic pain syndromes it was suggested that aside from treatment of trigeminal neuralgia, that AEDs be relegated to basically third line treatment. Lastly, it was noted that there was no evidence to support the contention that gabapentin was superior to other AEDs in neuropathic pain management (43). As with the antidepressants, one should institute treatment at a low dosage and titrate the dose up slowly to improve tolerance and optimize compliance. Valproate, oxcarbazepine, lamotrigine, topamax, levetiracetam, phenytoin and clonazepam are other anticonvulsants that also have been used for neuropathic pain. Newer AEDs, such as pregabalin, an alpha2-delta ligand, recently approved for certain types of neuropathic pain may also prove useful in the management of post-traumatic pain conditions (44, 45).

Newer agents such ziconotide (Prialt), a synthetic neuronal N-type calcium channel blocker, which has received recent FDA approval, may also offer promise for treatment of intractable severe chronic pain in patients intolerant of or refractory to other forms of treatment (46). This agent, like other intraspinal (intrathecal or epidural) analgesics should only be tried when other standard treatments have failed and must be administered via a programmable implanted microinfusion device for long term users. Morphine is the only other agent that is FDA approved for intrathecal use for chronic pain, although other agents including ketamine, midazolam, clonidine and various local anesthetics (i.e. lidocaine and bupivacaine) have been used, alone or in combination, in this application on an off-label basis (47).

Other agents that have more recently been recognized as adjuvants in the pharmacologic management of pain include tizanidine (Zanaflex) and sodium amobarbital (Amytal). Tizanidine has been shown to be effective in a variety of pain conditions including fibromyalgia, as well as, tension type headache, possibly on the basis of modulation of substance P and/or owing to its alpha-adrenergic effects (48). Mailis and Nicholson (49) have provided an excellent review of the use of sodium amytal infusion in the assessment and treatment of chronic pain (and functional disorders).

Capsaicin can be used topically to help decrease pain associated with peripheral neuropathies. Capsaicin depletes peptides such as substance P that mediate nociceptive transmission. Application of capsaicin is associated usually with a burning sensation, which may be severe enough to require pre-medication with either an oral analgesic or a topical lidocaine cream or ointment. Patients should be counseled not to touch mucous membranes after applying capsaicin.

Compounded agents, typically formulated through "compounding pharmacies" may also play a role in pain management of the patient after TBI. Agents that have been used in topical formulations for pain include: local anesthetics, antidepressants, alpha-2 agonists, opioids, glutamate antagonists such as Gabapentin, calcium channel blockers, skeletal muscle relaxants, capsaicin, Ketamine, menthol, and NSAIDs. Standard topical formulas such as "speed gel", which contains amitriptyline, lidocaine, guaifenesin and ketoprofen, can work quite well for neuropathic/neuralgic scalp pain, scar pain, and post-traumatic myalgias. Similar compounded topicals with varying ingredients such as gabapentin, ketamine and clonidine may be more helpful as adjuvants for CRPS related pain (50).

Surgery produces pain by releasing pain and inflammatory mediators via damaged tissue. This pain is acute pain and will improve as the wound heals and the patient convalesces. The goal of postoperative pain management is to provide continuous and effective analgesia with minimal adverse effects. NSAIDs such as parenteral ketorolac are used both intra-operatively and post-operatively to decrease the production of inflammatory prostaglandins released at the site of injury. The ketorolac dose is dependent on route, patient age, and weight, and should only be continued at the appropriate dosage for five days due to the development of renal dysfunction and GI toxicity. Opioid analgesics are the most commonly used medications for acute and sub—acute post-operative pain, usually administered intramuscularly or intravenously on an as needed basis. This approach can lead to delays in the patient receiving adequate analgesia due to medication administration delays and intramuscular route absorption.

Patients should be switched to oral opioid analgesics when oral administration is tolerated. Patient-controlled analgesia (PCA) is a process where the patient is allowed to self-administer low doses of intravenous opioid analgesics to maintain analgesia. To use PCA, a patient should be sufficiently cognizant to understand the goals of PCA and understand the use of the equipment. Patients who are confused or cognitively impaired are not good candidates for PCA. The number of injections and attempted injections can be monitored for efficacy and adverse effects, in addition to the patient's report of pain. Opioid analgesics can also be administered into the epidural or intrathecal space, combined with local anesthetics such as bupivacaine or ropivacaine for postoperative pain management. Patient-controlled epidural analgesia may be considered in specific circumstances.

Opioid analgesics stimulate the opioid receptors (mu, Kappa, and delta subtypes) that are widely distributed throughout the brain, spinal cord and peripheral nervous system. The opiate receptors appear to function at presynaptic potassium channels and indirectly affect voltage gated sodium channels to reduce the release of excitatory amino acids and substance P. Analgesia occurs primarily via action at the mu receptors, and less so at the kappa and delta receptors. Mu receptor stimulation is also responsible for some other opiate effects such as miosis, depressed gastric motility, and respiratory depression. Kappa stimulation does influence spinal analgesia, and also causes miosis and respiratory depression. Stimulation of delta receptors seems to account for hallucinations, confusion and stimulation of respiratory and vasomotor centers (51).

Desirable clinical effects of opioid analgesics include analgesia and reduced anxiety. Undesirable effects include sedation, urinary retention, respiratory depression, tolerance and dependence. Circumstantial side effects include euphoria, depressed bowel motility, and depressed cough. Tolerance to side effects develops fairly rapidly as compared to analgesic effects. Tolerance is simply a shift in the dose-response curve to achieve a desired therapeutic effect – one needs to either increase the dose or shorten the dosing interval. This phenomenon is not unique to opiates and occurs with a variety of medications. Physical dependence refers to the phenomena of the body becoming accustomed to the presence of the medication and that an abstinence syndrome may be precipitated by abrupt withdrawal of the medication, again a phenomenon not unique to narcotics (e.g. also seen with SSRI's). In the case of narcotics, abstinence syndrome symptoms may include lacrimation, diaphoresis, nausea and vomiting and typically does not persist for more than 72 hours; however, associated sleep disturbances and depression can last several weeks. Tolerance and physical dependence are simply physiologic responses to opioid exposure and do not imply aberrant drug use. Addiction is a complex set of maladaptive behaviors resulting in physical, psychological or social harm. There is an alteration in central nervous system function which the affected individual finds desirable resulting in a craving for the drug in question, often associated with tolerance for the non-analgesic, desired effect, resulting in unsanctioned dose escalation and preoccupation with acquisition of the drug and resultant adverse psychosocial consequences. The term pseudo-addiction refers to behaviors similar to those in addiction, but more specific to desired analgesic affects. The behaviors cease when appropriate analgesic management leads to adequate pain control (in other words, the physician has failed to provide sufficient medication or alter dosing in response to expected physiologic tolerance) (51, 52).

"Cognitive" and affective side-effects do occur with opiate medications. Euphoria, or dysphoria, sedation, hypnagogic or hypnopompic hallucinations appear typically within 3–7 days of dose initiation or escalation, but abate within the same time frame (52). Any worsening of cognitive performance occurs within the first few days of use, or first few hours after a dose, but tolerance develops to this phenomenon. There are relatively few differences found in cognitive performance in patients taking opioids compared to their performance before opioids or with the performance of a comparable pain population not taking opioids (53). Overall, there is no evidence that there are any long term cognitive side effects from narcotics, and adequate pain control may enhance cognitive performance (54, 51). In a study of 144 patients with low back pain, Jamison administered Digit Symbol and Trail-Making Test B prior to taking opiates and then at 90 and 180 day intervals. Test scores significantly improved while patients were taking opioids for pain (55). Finally, a TBI clinician must consider the fact that the opiate system is intimately involved in learning and reward. In the rodent model, genetic absence of the mu receptor, but not the kappa receptor, results in severe impairments in spatial learning (56). Therefore, the possibility exists that narcotic use in TBI may not simply be humane (analgesic properties) and without any significant long term negative cognitive consequences, but may also promote certain cognitive or affective improvements. However, practitioners must be aware that there may be adverse cognitive effects in those persons taking undue/excessive amounts of opioid medications, either due to inappropriate physician prescribing practices or patient noncompliance. Other potential reasons for occurrence of opioid related cognitive impairment include drug sensitivity, concurrently use of other substances (e.g. alcohol), or temporary impairment associated with increasing of opioid dose.

There are a variety of derived and synthetic narcotics available, each with different potencies and properties. Meperidine, and to a lesser extent, propoxyphene have mixed opioid agonist and antagonist properties and may cause severe cognitive problems in the elderly, including hallucinations. Neither drug, nor should most narcotics, be used with MAO inhibitors secondary to a risk of hypertensive crisis or autonomic dysregulation. Moderate potency narcotics (hydrocodone and oxycodone) are metabolized by liver P450 enzymes into morphine and if given with other drugs that inhibit metabolism via this enzyme (SSRI's for example) a given dose of these narcotics may produce less than optimal pain relief. Similarly, the low potency synthetic narcotic tramadol should be used with caution with SSRI's and other anti-depressants secondary to increased seizure risk (more likely a function of its agonistic properties on NE and 5HT receptors, that may also be desirable in dampening central sensitization)(57).

The use of narcotics in chronic non-malignant pain management remains controversial. Poppy derivatives and opioid medications have demonstrated proven pain relieving properties for hundreds of years. It has only been in the last century that a significant social stigma has been attached to the use or prescription of narcotics for chronic pain treatment. Now, the pressures from agencies like JCAHO to provide appropriate and thorough pain management appear to be at odds with legislative and legal considerations imposed by State Boards of Medicine. Physicians and patients are concerned about addiction, tolerance, and side effects from narcotics, all of which may generally be more hyperbole than fact although such concerns may sometimes be very real such as in the case where a patient becomes addicted to medication due to inappropriate prescribing or monitoring practices of their treating physician.

Furlan et al. (submitted) (58) have recently completed a systematic review of opioids for CNCP (chronic non-cancer pain) that will serve as the CPSO's (College of Physicians and Surgeons of Ontario) updated guidelines to be released this year (2005). This systematic review of 38 Randomized Controlled Trials (RCTs) concluded that: (1) Opioids are effective in the treatment of CNCP by reducing pain and improving functional outcomes when compared to placebo (2). Opioids are equally effective for both nociceptive and neuropathic pain syndromes when compared to placebo (3). Opioids are effective in fibromyalgia by reducing pain, but did not improve functional outcomes when compared to placebo (4). Opioids were superior to other drugs (e.g., NSAIDS, tricyclic antidepressants), in reducing pain, but failed to improve functional outcomes (5). Constipation and nausea were noticeable side effects more commonly associated with opioids (6). While recent studies indicate development of significant endocrinological abnormalities and erectile dysfunction on chronic opioids, the majority of the studies did not inquire about sexual dysfunction. The only two studies that provided a sexual activity score showed that patients on opioids actually reported they were better in terms of sexual behaviour compared to controls. Improvement of mood or adjustment secondary to better pain control may account for this result (7). However, addiction/abuse in patients with chronic pain can not be assumed not to exist (despite popular statements), because the existing literature a) excluded high risk populations (therefore it is not representative of chronic pain patients seen particularly in pain clinics); b) is methodologically not designed to look for "addiction", and c) the duration of the trials is too short to allow for development of the disorder (even if appropriate definitions and screening tools for addiction had been used).

Most patients taking long acting opioids should be supplied with a fast acting rescue opioid to treat breakthrough pain. Oral rescue medicine may be needed every 2–4 hours. The usual dose is the analgesic equivalent of 5–15% of the 24 hour baseline dose of the scheduled long acting opioid analgesic. As with any pain medication and/or intervention, the prescribed agent should be titrated to achieve optimal pain relief with minimal side-effects. Clinicians should discuss treatment expectancies prior to issuing prescriptions for any pain medication.

Clinicians treating patients with TBI may be especially concerned about cognitive side effects and slowing of cognitive recovery; again, a concern that may be overemphasized. Indeed, for non-brain injured patients with multiple fractures or other injuries, physicians would have no qualms about administering narcotics, especially in the acute care setting. Yet in the acute and sub-acute phases of brain injury, when the patient may be unable to communicate or have severely altered consciousness, physicians are reticent to provide adequate analgesia with narcotics. From a practical perspective, it would be appropriate to use narcotics for analgesia if the physician can reasonably assume that a patient with brain injury has opiate responsive sources of pain, even if they have limited ability to communicate. In fact, a common contributor to "agitation" in the acute care or rehabilitation setting may be inadequate analgesia. On the other hand, there is evidence that patients in a vegetative state do not have conscious awareness of nociceptive stimuli; specifically, there is activation of brainstem, thalamic and primary somatosensory cortices, but not of secondary association cortex (59). The implication is that patients who are truly in a vegetative state (i.e. arousal without awareness) and not MCS may in fact be incapable of "suffering" (in line with historical neurologic community dogma that persons in VS do not feel pain). Opioid analgesic treatment could, however, be considered even in patients in VS if they were experiencing dysautonomic type symptoms from a suspected nociceptive stimulus and/or were manifesting significant physiologic reactivity associated with noxious stimuli including tachycardia, tachypnea, diaphoresis and rigidity. Good clinical care would dictate that every attempt to modulate and/or minimize nociceptive stimuli should be made before using opiate analgesics.

Clinicians should be familiar with important documents concerning the use of controlled substances such as opiate medications. In 2004, the Federation of State Medical Boards of the United States published a *Model Policy for the Use of Controlled Substances for the Treatment of Pain* which was developed in collaboration with pain experts around the country to provide guidance to state medical boards in developing state pain policies and regulations. Written in the form of a model policy document, the guidelines provide model language that may be used to by states to clarify their positions regarding the use of controlled substances to treat pain, alleviate physician uncertainty about such practice and encourage better pain management. In 2004, the Federation's House of Delegates adopted recommendations and revised the pain policy to reflect new medical insights in pain treatment, particularly with regard to the undertreatment of pain (60). As prescribers, professionals should also be aware of the myriad issues that may confront both the clinician and the patient when opiate medications are utilized for chronic pain management (61). One must also remain aware of the current evidence based medicine regarding the utility of chronic opioid therapies in specific types of pain conditions, such as chronic, non-malignant, neuropathic pain (62, 63).

Current consensus among pain specialists dictates that concerns regarding addiction are generally not a contraindication to opioid treatment for otherwise intractable pain although the possible problems associated with inappropriate opioid treatment should be kept in mind. In particular, the need and efficacy of opioids with chronic pain patients having prior drug abuse histories or addiction prone personalities should be carefully assessed and monitored when being considered for or treated with opiates. The effectiveness of opioids with respect to both reduction in pain severity ratings as well as effect on functional capacity should be considered. Clinicians should always use a "controlled substance agreement" when using such agents for pain management to protect not only the patient's safety but also their own given the litigious nature of our society (64). Ultimately, clinicians must have insight into the fact that chronic pain should be managed in a rational manner via integration of pharmacological approaches with behavioral and traditional rehabilitation interventions (65).

General Guidelines for Pain Pharmacotherapy

The physician should aim for drug prescriptions that optimize compliance and minimize potential side-effects. Particularly in cognitively impaired patients, physicians should aim for once to twice a day drug dosing. Patients should be counseled on the goals of treatment and what to expect regarding adverse effects, especially constipation with opioid analgesics or GI side-effects with NSAIDs. As possible, significant others should also be informed of treatment regimen and possible complications.

Depending on the severity of the pain and the patient's pain tolerance, consider a trial of acetaminophen as an initial management strategy. If prescribing a nonselective NSAID for more that 10–14 days then consider co-administration of a mucoprotectant agent such as a proton pump inhibitor and/or misoprostol. For elderly patients, a gastroprotectant should be used regardless of the duration of NSAID therapy. Only proceed to opiate-like and/or opiate medications when the pain level and functional disability associated with the pain are moderate to severe (42).

When using opioid analgesics, fears regarding dependence should be openly discussed as should any sexual function side-effects. Ideally, the clinician should aim for decreasing polypharmacy, however, when appropriate, combination drug regimens should be considered. It is critical to ascertain whether patients are taking their medicine correctly (e.g. taking scheduled medicine on a prn basis) and /or supplanting their prescribed medications with over the counter (OTC) products.

Non-pharmacologic Medical Management

A wide variety of medical rehabilitative interventions focusing on physical modalies (e.g., physiotherapy, exercise, chiropractic, massage, etc.), as well as, other non-pharmacological medical interventions for chronic pain may be helpful in ameliorating pain complaints and suffering following TBI (66, 67). However, more recent evidence suggests that many such treatments may be of questionable value relative to placebo or no treatment. Depending upon the etiology of the pain generator in question, numerous non-pharmacologic medical and psychological approaches may be considered in the management of pain conditions including use of physical agents and modalities, injection therapies, exercise, biofeedback, adaptive equipment and/or psychological interventions. These treatment modalities should all be given adequate consideration in conjunction with possible pharmacologic alternatives if physicians are to develop adequate functionally oriented treatment regimens for addressing chronic pain issues in persons with TBI. Readers are referred to chapter 39 for details regarding the behavioral and psychological management of pain following TBI.

Physical Modalities

Physical agents utilized to modulate pain may include superficial heat and cold. The most common modalities used are hot/cold packs, heat lamps (incandescent or infrared), paraffin baths and cryotherapy. Hydrotherapy interventions for pain management may involve prescription of whirlpool or contrast baths. Various diathermy techniques may also be utilized to facilitate pain control including ultrasound, phonophoresis, as well as, short-wave and microwave diathermy. There are also a number of electrical stimulation techniques utilized in pain management such as transcutaneous electrical stimulation (TENS) and iontophoresis that are commonly employed as adjuvants for pain control. Although historically used for chronic pain modulation, a recent Cochrane (68) review examining the efficacy of TENS in the aforementioned application found inconclusive results with published trials not providing information on the stimulation parameters most likely to provide optimum pain relief, nor the effectiveness of long term treatment. A more recent study (69) found that evidence was lacking, limited or conflicting for efficacy in mechanical neck disorder management for electrotherapy interventions including PEMF (pulsed electromagnetic field) therapy, galvanic current, iontophoresis, TENS, diadynamic current, and electrical muscle stimulation. Cranial Electrical Stimulation (CES) is a treatment for pain reduction that, unlike TENS, targets central nervous system function. The technique involves attachment of electrodes carrying microcurrent across the scalp and induces an approximate 15Hz cortical rhythm. Many controlled studies support that it is a safe and useful treatment for pain, especially chronic pain and its associated symptomatology of anxiety, depression and insomnia (70).

Physical modalities tend to play a more predominant role in the treatment of pain complaints of musculoskeletal origin and may include traction, manual medicine techniques (e.g. joint manipulation, myofascial release techniques and strain counter-strain), as well as, massage (71). Body-work techniques and bioenergetics, although not well studied aside from acupuncture, are two additional classes of intervention that may also be used as adjutants in chronic pain management (e.g. Reiki, Alexander, Trager and meridian, acupuncture, polarity, respectively). Injection techniques including intra-articular, peri-articular, peritendinous, ligamentous/fibrous tissue (i.e. prolotherapy) and trigger point can all be used in various types of musculoskeletal pain disorders (72). Axial injections such as epidurals, zygapophyseal joint, and sympathetic blocks may all be relevant considerations for pain treatment in this population, depending on the presumptive pain generators.

Exercise, is an underappreciated and therefore under-prescribed treatment intervention in persons post-TBI or for that matter many other patients with pain complaints. Exercise can play a significant role in controlling pain both on a central and peripheral basis improving deconditioning that may be resulting in nocicption and concurrently improving weight control, affect, and general state of health and well-being (73, 74). Exercise has also been shown to elevate beta endorphin levels as much as five times that of resting levels (75). Additionally, recent information strongly supports the argument that exercise results in up-regulation of brain-derived neurotrophic factor (BDNF) and therefore may play a role in promoting neural repair and enhance learning and memory by increasing neurotrophic support (76). Of course, the benefits of exercise are dependent upon the patient taking an active invovlvement in rehabilitation.

Adaptive equipment such as reachers, sock aides, long handled scrubbers and/or brushes, as well as, ergonomically modified task analyses for ADLs, mobility and work environments are a few of the many different interventions that may also facilitate greater pain modulation and

tolerance. Appropriate education regarding pacing and energy conservation techniques may also add to further improvement in functional status depending upon the type of chronic pain condition being treated.

SPECIAL TOPICS IN PAIN MANAGEMENT IN PERSONS WITH TBI

Post-Traumatic Headache

Background Information

Headache (e.g. cephalalgia) is the most common physical complaint reported after mild brain injury/concussion and cranial (i.e. head) trauma. Headache is also very frequently associated with cervical injuries and post-traumatic cervicalgia. Historically, head pain or headache was believed to be reported far less commonly in more severe injuries (77). More recent research suggests that even persons status post moderate to severe traumatic brain injury suffer from acute headache symptoms, most often on a daily basis and in a frontal location and tended to improve with time with recovery generally leveling off by 6 months post-injury (78). The general experience, however, continues to indicate a trend towards greater levels of subjective complaints of headache among those individuals with milder brain injuries as opposed to more severe ones. Zasler (79) has speculated that the primary cause for such headaches is in fact related to cervical injury and that early treatment rendered to persons with more severe TBI, such as chemical paralysis and protracted bedrest, may actually be therapeutically, albeit inadvertently, prophylaxing against the development of PTHA.

Post-traumatic headache and in particular post-concussive headaches seldom connote serious underlying neurological problems. Clinicians should be aware, however, of various significant clinical conditions that may be responsible for PTHA and therefore should always appropriately consider the differential diagnosis of this condition including late intracranial, extra-axial hematomas, tension pneumocephalus due to dural leaks, communicating hydrocephalus, ventriculoperitoneal shunt malfunction resulting in low or high pressure headaches, post-traumatic epilepsy (whether convulsive or non-convulsive) and carotid-cavernous fistulas (80).

There continue to be significant disparities in classification and nomenclature regarding post-traumatic headache (PTH), often because these are arbitrary and not predicated on physiology or established time courses for symptom manifestation (79). The etiology, course, pathophysiology and treatment remain poorly understood (81). The International Headache Society published their revised classification system in 2004 (82). As per the revised classification, there are two broad categories of headache including acute PTHA and chronic PTHA. Acute PTHA is further divided into headache associated with moderate to severe (5.1.1) and that associated with mild head injury (5.1.2). Chronic PTHA is divided into the following sub-classifications: chronic headache due to moderate to severe head injury (5.2.1) and chronic headache due to mild head injury (5.2.2). There are many consternations regarding this classification and more importantly the specifics of the criteria including onset time, duration of headache, misuse of the modifier "chronic" (which typically is used to modify pain when pain duration is six months or greater), causation criteria, use of "head injury" as opposed to "brain injury", among other problems. It should be noted that there are further classifications for: acute, as well as, chronic headache attributed to whiplash injury, headache due to traumatic intracranial hematoma, headache associated with other head and/or neck injury, as well as, post-craniotomy headache. Interestingly, there are no specific headache classifications for post-trauma migraine, tension headache or neuritic/neuralgic headache (82).

Potential sources of head pain that may be relevant in the assessment of a patient presenting with post-traumatic headache include the dura, venous sinuses, cranial cavities including sinuses, eye socket, ear, nasal and oral pharynx. The skin, nerves, muscles and periosteum of the cranium are all pain sensitive. Cervical/cranial joint capsules (including the temporomandibular joint), cervical facets/zygapophyseal joints and the cervical sympathetic plexus may all be primary nociceptive pain generators that produce local or referred head pain (83, 84). One of the most common, yet often overlooked, sources of head pain is referred cervical myofascial pain emanating from any of the four layers of posterior cervical musculature secondary to cervical acceleration deceleration injuries generally associated with the traumatic events that caused the brain injury in the first place (85, 86) (see Figures 38-6–9).

Clinical Evaluation of Post-traumatic headache

The distinction between various types of post-traumatic headache has become somewhat blurred in the majority of the scientific literature. Defining variables used in various studies may actually overlap headache subtypes. Furthermore, as discussed above, the presence of primary and

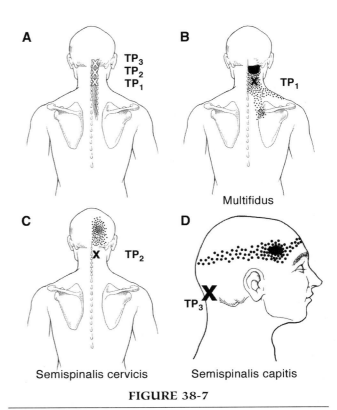

FIGURE 38-7

Posterior cervical muscles prone to development of trigger points producing referred pain perceived as cervicalgia and/or cephalalgia

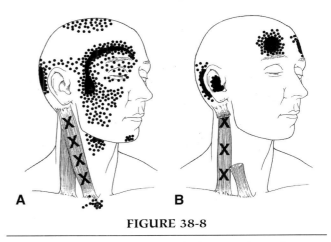

FIGURE 38-8

Referred pain patterns for sternocleidomastoid muscle trigger points, sternal division (A) and clavicular division (B)

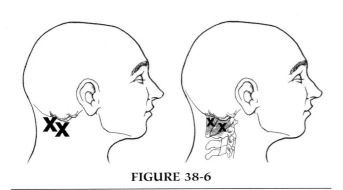

FIGURE 38-6

Sub-occipital muscle trigger points

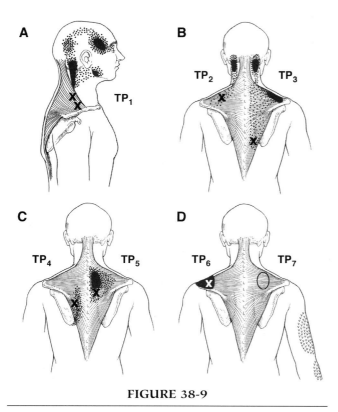

FIGURE 38-9

Trapezius muscle trigger point referral patterns

secondary peripheral sensitization, along with windup and central sensitization, along with the concepts of resulting expanded receptive fields and "convergence-projection" may make the identification of the original nociceptive generator quite difficult. This may indeed be moot, since it may be beneficial to treat both the primary pain generator and the secondary/concurrent pain generators in order to reduce the disabling consequences of post-traumatic headache. It remains important, however, to identify likely sources of pain (primary and secondary) in order to treat them. Readers interested in PTHA should consult more comprehensive treatises for a more complete overview (79, 81).

Historical information regarding mechanism of injury can help distinguish types of headache. The physical forces involved in post-traumatic headache include impact and/or acceleration/deceleration (inertial) loading; the latter typically involves "whiplash" type injury to the neck. In more generalized post-traumatic headache, surgical intervention provides yet another "external physical force" that may produce head pain.

On review of systems, it is useful to use the acronym "*COLDER*"; Character: dull, throbbing, lancinating, sharp, etc.; Onset: any precipitants, relationship to menses, time of day, temporal relationship to injury; Location: Unilateral, bilateral, occipital, radiating, frontal, bitemporal, etc.; Duration: length of headache

episodes; Exacerbation: stooping, valsalva, bending, touch, stress, poor sleep, menses, weather changes, etc.; Relief: Medications that work, modalities that help, sleep, etc. Other questions that should be asked include the severity of the headache (where 0 is none and 10 is the worst imaginable), frequency of the headache, associated symptoms (nausea, vomiting, photophobia, and/or phonophobia), presence of an aura, as well as the degree of functional disability associated with headache episodes including their vocational impact (e.g. how many days of work missed per month) (84, 80).

The physical examination should include observation (for traumatic changes, asymmetries and general posture), neurological examination, cervical ROM, palpation of cervical and cranial musculature, palpation of GON and LON egress points, provocative movements, ocular examination and auscultation for carotid, mastoid, temporal and ocular bruits. Although an in-depth discussion of myofascial pain is beyond the scope of this chapter, the reader is referred to other more extensive resources (84, 85, 87). Myofascial pain is very common in the sternocleidomastoids and trapezius after whiplash or inertial injury. It is interesting to note that the zone of referred pain for the sternocleidomastoid extends to retro-orbital and periorbital areas; associated "autonomic" symptoms include vertigo, tinnitus, and a sense of fullness in the ear, as well as, ear pain (commonly confused for otitis externa). These symptoms may be explained by convergence projection theory in that there is overlap in the sensory dermatomes for the SCM and the trigeminal tract as discussed above. The cervical musculature is also a major source of afferents to the vestibular systems integrating eye, head and neck movement, thereby making dizziness a common complaint in this patient population (so called cervical vertigo). The zone of referred pain to the ear overlaps the sensory area for the vagus; theoretically, peripheral sensitization in the SCM could lead to central sensitization within the vestibular and possibly vagal systems (80) (See Figures 38-6–9).

Common Clinical Subtypes and Features of Post-Traumatic Headache

Musculoskeletal Headache

Musculoskeletal headache is classically characterized as a cap-like discomfort, but varies with the offending musculature. The sternocleidomastoid is notorious for referring pain retro or peri-orbitally. The pain may be constant or intermittent, relieved by application of heat, cold, massage and many over the counter medications including NSAIDs. There may be autonomic components to specific muscles. TMJ or craniomandibular syndrome may be considered a variant of musculoskeletal or tension headache and is almost always seen in conjunction with direct trauma to the craniomandibular complex when traumatic in origin. This type of headache is also frequently overlooked as a primary or contributory cause for PTH (88). In TMJ, clicking, popping or malocclusion of the jaw may be noticed (89). Other etiologies of TMJD must be assessed for that may have little to nothing to do with the traumatic injury in question, whether in relation to stress or tension, dental malocclusion, and/or prior psychosexual abuse.

Many of the patients with musculoskeletal headache have as a primary or secondary component, myofascial pain. The therapeutic targets are pain relief, stretch to normal length (establish normal range of motion), and then strengthening of the involved musculature. Efforts to correct postural or skeletal problems, as well as, disordered sleep cycles, should be undertaken as well. Pharmacological interventions for myofascial pain include NSAIDs, TCAs and possibly muscle relaxants. TCA's, particularly amitryptiline, may help with disordered sleep. "Muscle relaxants" have no proven efficacy, although some resemble TCA's in their chemical structure and clinical effect. Anti-spasticity drugs are seldom used, although tizanidine may have some theoretical benefit over other traditional anti-spasticity agents due both to selectivity and anti-nociceptive properties. The hallmark of treatment of myofascial pain has been the treatment of trigger points, as well as, promulgating factors (90). These may be approached with acupressure or dry needling, but most practitioners use injections of local anaesthetic, followed by stretch of the involved muscle group and/or physical interventions directed at "myofascial release" techniques (91). Recently, the use of botulinum toxin (off label) has been advocated for modulation of chronic myofascial pain (92). Theoretically, this should allow for increased ability to stretch the muscle, but may impede later phases of treatment related to strengthening. Non-pharmacologic treatment of myofascial pain involves the use of modalities and therapy. Various heating modalities are well tolerated by most patients, and allow for muscle relaxation for therapeutic stretch. Some patients respond well to cooling with fluorimethane spray for the same purposes. Patients should be taught a home program of stretching, and then a gradual strengthening program. Current literature does not strongly support the use of physical treatments per se in the management of headache disorders (93).

Within the broad category of musculoskeletal headache, other etiologies beyond the almost omnipresent myofascial pain include cranio-mandibular syndrome, cervical zygapophyseal joint disorders (see section below on cervicogenic headache), and "cranial and somatic dysfunction." In craniomandibular disorder, there may be internal derangement of the temporomandibular joint and almost always a myofascial component related to muscles of mastication (temporalis, pterygoids, or masseter). These muscular problems should be treated as described above. Often intervention is supplemented by the use of intra-oral appliances such as occlusal splints (bite blocks), dietary changes relative to softer food consistency and jaw exercises. Non-surgical treatment is effective in managing more than 80% of patients with craniomandibular disorders (94). In the case of joint pathology, which may be identified with MRI, arthroscopic intervention is indicated. Open arthrotomy or arthroplasty is rarely needed, and often associated with suboptimal outcomes.

Cervicogenic Headache

Cervicogenic headaches may be related to dysfunction of the facet joints. Others have hypothesized that chronic pain following cervical acceleration-deceleration type injuries may be due to central sensitization (95).

Preliminary diagnostic criteria were developed in 1987 and were consolidated into a formal statement in 1990. Obligatory for the diagnosis were unilateral head pain without side-shift and symptoms or signs of cervical involvement, the latter which could include provocation of pain by neck movement or by external pressure to the upper posterior neck, concurrent cervicalgia or reduced cervical range of motion. Subsequent, Sjaastad et al. (96) further amended the criteria by moving the cervical involvement to the first major criteria and relaxing the criterion for unilaterality to the point of even accepting bilateral occurrence. Emphasis to date has been on the nosologic validity of the criteria and no studies have established that patients who meet the diagnostic criteria actually have a cervical source for their pain (97). The IHS criteria of 2004 further refined the diagnostic criteria for cervicogenic headache and included a parameter noting that pain would resolve within three months after successful treatment of the causative disorder or lesion. Most patients present with unilateral (albeit sometimes bilateral) sub-occipital pain as well as secondary oculo-frontotemporal discomfort/pain.

Dysfunction of the cervical zygapophyseal joints, particulary at C2 and C3 may refer pain to the head (see Figure 38-10). Treatment considerations include injection of local anaesthetic intra-articularly, or block of the medial branches of the dorsal rami supplying the joint. At a more subtle level is the concept, which remains somewhat controversial from an allopathic perspective, of cranial and cervical somatic dysfunction. These disorders are typically treated with osteopathic techniques designed to re-align dysfunctional units. Cervical mobilization and manipulation may be effective in the treatment of chronic headaches (98). Various techniques may be used, but caution should be exercised with high velocity procedures due to risk of cervical fracture and/or vertebral artery damage, the latter which is generally avoided by avoiding mobilization in extension.

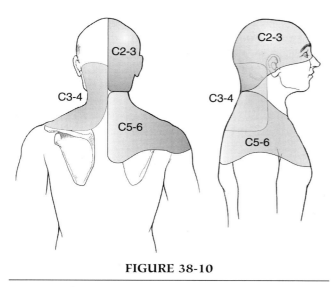

FIGURE 38-10

Cervical sensory dermatomes for sensory roots C2-6

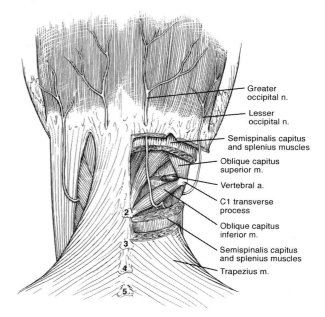

FIGURE 38-11

Anatomy of upper posterior cervical region with specific reference to C2 terminal branches of the lesser and greater occipital nerves

Cervicogenic headache is quite common following trauma (99). Some have argued that it is likely the most common etiology of post-traumatic headache (100, 101). Numerous treatments have been assessed, most with suboptimal study methodologies (102). The studies suggest that in appropriate cases manual therapy (103), exercise and blocks (diagnostic as well as therapeutic) may play important roles in modulating cervicogenic headache pain (97).

Neuritic and Neuralgic Head Pain

Neuritic scalp pain may occur from local blunt trauma, surgical scalp incision or penetrating scalp injuries. Occasionally, neuromatous lesions may form after scalp nerve injury and serve as a pain nidus. Pain complaints may vary from only report dysesthetic "numbness" discomfort on touching to lacinating type pain that spontaneously occurs without provocative measures. Neuralgic pain may occur secondary to occipital neuralgia (greater and/or lesser), supra-orbital and/or infra-orbital as the most common clinical post-traumatic cephalic and/or facial neuralgias seen in clinical practice although certainly other post-traumatic neuralgias/neuropathies may be observed (104).

Occipital neuralgia (ON) may occur following cervical acceleration deceleration type injuries, as well as, direct trauma to the craniocervical junction. ON may be perpetuated by contraction or myodystonia of the splenius muscle, which it penetrates. Pain is typically felt at the craniocervical junction and the sensory distribution of the nerve (e.g. C2). The affected nerve is tender to palpation and palpation generally replicates the pain associated with the headache (e.g. stabbing quality). There is frequently referral of pain into the ipsilateral frontotemporal scalp

and less frequently retro-orbitally (also ipsilaterally) secondary to ephaptic transmission between the proximal part of the C2 origin of the nerve and the ophthalmic branch of the fifth cranial nerve (86).

Whether the etiology is local neuroma formation in scar tissue in the scalp, or greater or lesser occipital neuralgia, the systemic pharmacological interventions are essentially the same and include NSAID's, TCA, and anticonvulsants, particularly, gabapentin. Injection of local anaesthetic with or without steroid may also be indicated for both diagnostic and therapeutic purposes for neuritic and neuralgic pain disorders. For greater and lesser occipital neuralgia, in particular, clinicians should be familiar with the anatomy of the region given risks of aberrantly placed injections (see Figure 38-11). In either situation, myofascial pain may be a secondary or perpetuating pain generator and must be treated as well on a concurrent basis. Rarely, surgical decompression or nerve lysis (surgical, cryotherapy) is necessary for these types of neuropathic cephalalgias.

Post-Traumatic Migraine

Post-traumatic migraine (PTM) or neurovascular headache is more common than originally thought although its true incidence is poorly defined in the available scientific literature. Patients with PTM may have a genetic predisposition to development of migraine following trauma to either the head/brain and/or neck (105).

There is inadequate information to stipulate how acute PTM may differ mechanistically and otherwise from chronic PTM.

PTM is most likely to be described as throbbing. Vascular headache is usually unilateral and is exacerbated by coughing, bending over; cold may help, but heat usually makes the pain worse. There may be associated nausea, vomiting, or anorexia. Hemicranial allodynia may occur after central sensitization takes place.

The aim of treatment of migraine or neurovascular headache is to prevent or reduce the frequency of the onset of headache (prophylactic treatment) and/or to abort a headache rapidly should it occur (as well as sustain the headache relief once aborted). The precise trigger for migraine or vascular headache remains obscure and controversial; this is especially true in relation to post-traumatic vascular headache. What is clear is that the trigeminal afferent system becomes sensitized by a sterile inflammatory "soup" that includes excitatory neurotransmitters, nitric oxide, histamine, prostaglandin E2; this sensitization then produces vasodilatation of extra-cerebral vessels, including those in the meninges, and accentuates the inflammatory response. The pounding headache of migraine appears to originate from dilatation of large cranial vessels innervated by the trigeminovascular system and the associated release of CGRP, substance P and neurokinin A from trigeminal neurons; sensitized trigeminal afferents may provide nociceptive input from simple mechanical stimulation of the dilated vessels, akin to a vascular allodynia. Triptans block the release of CGRP at 5HT1B and D receptors. However, stimulation of 5HT2B receptors promote migraine; TCA's may block these receptors (106). Second order neurons in the brainstem are sensitized; the periaqueductal gray seems particularly vulnerable in migraine (13).

Prophylactic migraine medications include some NSAIDs, beta-blockers, calcium channel blockers, TCA's and depakote as more traditional treatments. Naturopathic agents such as butterbar and feverfew can also be considered as can nutritional therapies such as B complex vitamins and magnesium supplementation. Abortive medications may include ergot derivatives, dihydroergotamine derivatives, triptans, parenteral atypical antipsychotics (107) and/or narcotics, among other drugs. However, triptans, as a class, may be ineffective if their use is delayed and allodynia develops (10). Many of the drugs were used for their vasoconstrictive properties (ergot derivatives) even though extra-cerebral vasodilation is a secondary phenomenon in migraine; they have significant systemic or cardiac side effects; If patients experience chronic daily headache and use abortive analgesics, they are at risk for developing rebound or medication overuse headache. Stimulation of various analgesic receptors in the brainstem affects 5HT. Short term use (including acetaminophen) increases 5HT release from raphe spinal

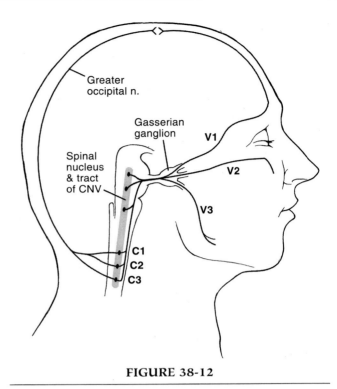

FIGURE 38-12

Schematic representation of interconnectivity between the spinal nucleus and tract of cranial nerve V, upper three cervical roots and the ophthalmic branch of the fifth cranial nerve through the gasserian ganglion

pathways, and has a therapeutic effect. However, long term use may lead to 5HT depletion and up-regulation of 5HT2A receptors particularly. Whereas stimulation of 5HT1b and 1D receptors aborts acute migraine (e.g. triptans), 5HT2A stimulation increases neuronal excitability and potentiates nociceptive transmission. The increased density of 5HT2 A receptors could lead to an "excitable brain," a hyperalgesic state, with increased headache frequency and severity. It also undercuts the antagonism of 5HT2 which is a common mechanism underlying preventative medications in migraine management (22). Caffeine over-use may also contribute to patients becoming refractory to abortive medications containing this substance.

Again, due to central overlap of primary nociceptive afferents involved in true vascular headache and those related to cervical sensory nerves, the patient may present with a combination of vascular, neuralgic, and/or musculoskeletal headache, all of which may require treatment. Cervical nociceptive input may also promulgate migraine through the trigeminocervical complex (108) and therefore must be addressed as part and parcel of comprehensive migraine assessment and treatment (23) (see Figure 38-12).

Botulinum toxin has also been used (off label) to treat migraine headache (109). Botulinum toxin may exert this effect not only through muscle relaxation but through inhibiting release of sensitizing neurotransmitters such as glutamate and substance P. Current research with botulinum toxin seems to be focusing on specific headache sub-types, specifically, chronic daily headache (110) and not trigeminovascular type headache disorders.

Post-Traumatic Tension Headache

Tension-type headache (TTHA) is one of the most common primary headache disorders and like many other headache conditions can be considered a spectrum disorder. Per ICDH-2 criteria 2.1 to 2.4 diagnostic categories for TTHA include: infrequent episodic TTHA, frequent episodic TTHA, chronic TTHA and probable TTHA (111).

Advances in basic pain and clinical research have improved the understanding of the pathophysiologic mechanisms of tension-type headache. Increased excitability of the central nervous system generated by repetitive and sustained pericranial myofascial input may be responsible for the transformation of episodic tension-type headache into the chronic form. Studies of nitric oxide (NO) mechanisms suggest that NO may play a key role in the pathophysiology of tension-type headache and that the anti-nociceptive effect of nitric oxide synthase inhibitors may become a novel principle in the future treatment of chronic headache (112). It should be noted, however, that other neurochemicals including calcitonin gene-related peptide (CGRP), serotonin, substance P, neuropeptide Y and vascoactive intestinal peptide (VIP) have all been in either episodic and/or chronic TTHA (111).

The mechanisms by which trauma, either to the neck, cranium or cranial adnexal structures or the brain itself may trigger tension type headaches are poorly understood. TTHA may result from an interaction between changes in the descending control of second order trigeminal brain stem nociceptors and interrelated peripheral changes, such as myofasical mediated pain and/or pericranial muscles nociceptive afferent input. Clearly, stress and negative emotional states (mediated through limbic circuitry) may trigger such headaches through central mechanisms; what role TBI itself has in potentially triggering such headaches in susceptible individuals is less clear. With more frequent episodes of headache, central changes have been theorized to become increasingly more important. With greater duration, long term sensitization of nociceptive neurons and decreased activity in the anti-nociceptive system gradually leads to chronic TTHA. Current consensus is that peripheral mechanisms are most likely involved in episodic TTHA and central mechanisms play a more important role in chronic TTHA. There is still debate as to whether the pain in TTHA originates from peripheral (e.g. myofascial) versus central origins.

Treatment of TTHA should include pharmacotherapy, both acute and prophylactic, as well as, non-pharmacologic approaches (111). The mainstay of acute pharmacotherapy are NSAIDs sometimes in conjunction with caffeine, sedatives and/or tranquilizers. Adequate doses of NSAIDs must be utilized prior to labeling a trial as a failure. There is no scientific evidence to support the use of traditional muscle relaxants in TTHA. Prophylactic pharmacotherapy for TTHA is much more diversified with various drug classes being utilized including tricyclic antidepressants, tizanidine, botulinum toxin and certain SNRIs such as venlafaxine (113). Nitric oxide synthase inhibitors may also hold therapeutic promise (114). Non-pharmacological treatments may include relaxation therapy as well as EMG biofeedback, cognitive behavioral therapies including stress management, limited contact treatment, physical therapy when apropos, and lastly, oromandibular treatment in selected patients.

Rare Post-Traumatic Headache Subtypes: Dysautonomic Headache, Cluster and Paroxysmal Hemicrania

Various dysautonomic headaches have been reported and although rare should be considered in the differential diagnostic work-up of a patient with PTHA. Clues to a dysautonomic source of headache pain include a unilateral episodic throbbing pain and hyperactive sympathetics involving the ipsilateral face during the attack (miosis, sweating) but between attacks, a mild Horner's syndrome (115). Trigeminal autonomic headaches have also been reported (116). Post-traumatic cluster headache and paroxysmal hemicrania are relatively rare types of post-traumatic headache (117, 118). It should be noted, however, that with less common headache variants there is always a question about the causal relationship of the injury to the headache onset and promulgation. The literature is scant in proving a causal link between trauma and these headache sub-types.

Analgesic Rebound Headache

Analgesic rebound headache may be seen from overuse of a variety of analgesic and/or abortive headache agents including ergotamines, opiates, caffeine, triptans and/or barbiturates (119). Overuse of these medications may lead to development of chronic daily headache (CDH). Patients may become dependent on these symptomatic headache medications. Drug withdrawal normally results in worsening of headache this is particularly noted when medication is stopped suddenly as opposed to being slowly weaned with concurrent alternative headache management options prescribed. Headache medication overuse may also make headaches refractory to prophylactic headache medication (120).

Post-Traumatic Sinus Headache

Sinus headaches, which may be post-traumatic or unrelated (or both), may be steady or have a throbbing quality. They may be seasonal or associated with allergic symptoms. A history of sinus or facial fractures is relevant. The daily pattern of sinus headaches relates to drainage angles: frontal and ethmoid are often worse with recumbency at night and better during the day when upright, whereas, maxillary and sphenoid sinus headache improves with recumbency at night.

Neuropathic Pain

Neuropathic pain is defined as a chronic pain condition that occurs or persists after a primary lesion or dysfunction of the peripheral or central nervous system. Traumatic injury of peripheral nerves also increases the excitability of nociceptors in and around nerve trunks and involves components released from nerve terminals (neurogenic inflammation) and immunological and vascular components from cells resident within or recruited into the affected area. Action potentials generated in nociceptors and injured nerve fibers release excitatory neurotransmitters at their synaptic terminals such as L-glutamate and substance P and trigger cellular events in the central nervous system that extend over different time frames.

Neuropathic pain has been shown to be mediated by both peripheral and central nervous system phenomena. In the peripheral nervous system mechanisms that have been posited to be involved with neuropathic pain include, but are not necessarily limited to, spontaneous ectopic discharges, neuroimmune factors such as inflammatory cytokines and sympathetic sensory coupling. Central nervous system mechanisms that are theorized to be involved with neuropathic pain include central sensitization, disinhibition, as well as, astrocyte and microglia activation (121).

Short-term alterations of neuronal excitability, reflected for example in rapid changes of neuronal discharge activity, are sensitive to conventional analgesics, and do not commonly involve alterations in activity-dependent gene expression. Novel compounds and new regimens for drug treatment to influence activity-dependent long-term changes in pain transducing and suppressive systems (pain matrix) are emerging. At present, therapeutic options are largely limited to drugs approved for other conditions, including anticonvulsants (carbamazepine, gabapentin, pregabalin), antidepressants (TCAs, venlafaxine, duloxetine), antiarrhythmics (e.g. mexiletine), tramadol and opioid analgesics. However, treatment based on the underlying disease state may be less than optimal, in that two patients with the same neuropathic pain syndrome may have different symptomatologies and thus respond differently to the same treatment. Increases

in our understanding of the function of the neurologic system over the last few years have led to new insights into the mechanisms underlying pain symptoms, especially chronic neuropathic pain.

Neurosurgical options may need to be considered when enteral pharmacotherapeutic options fail or produce sub-optimal pain control. Surgical options include modulative techniques, such as neurostimulation or implanted drug delivery systems, and ablative procedures such as DREZotomies (122).

Central Pain Syndromes

Central pain is defined as "pain associated with lesions of the central nervous system." People with TBI may experience central pain akin to that recognized as post-stroke pain, but may also have associated spinal cord injury with spinal pain. Sixty to seventy percent of patients with SCI have pain that is often chronic in nature (123). Diffuse pain below the level of the lesion may be due to involvement of the posterior spinal tracts, there may be a band-like pain at the transitional zone, or in pain developing late after injury, the source may be a syrinx (124).

Evident from the discussion of the anatomy and neurochemistry of nociceptive transmission, multiple systems contribute to the development of central pain. It is prudent to be cautious in medication and other treatment choices, given the overlap in plasticity mechanisms subserving central sensitization and more positive dynamic neurological functions such as learning, memory and motor recovery. However, it would also be clinically appropriate to consider combinations of medications with different mechanisms of action (whether in the same or different "class" of drug) in an effort to effectively treat the pain syndromes after TBI.

Brain-related central pain develops in about 8% of stroke patients, although its incidence and prevalence following TBI are unclear. It is classically seen with lesions of the thalamus, particularly the ventrocaudal nuclei. Changes in thalamocortical processing may include loss of inhibition or sensitization. Allodynia and dysesthesias, sometimes involving the entire hemicorpora are hallmarks of brain-related pain. Central pain syndromes have often been very challenging for both the treating physician and the suffering patient.

Intravenous morphine and intravenous lidocaine may be effective for treatment. Enteral opioid pain medications may be effective but are sometimes poorly tolerated on a chronic treatment basis. Similarly, oral mexilitine does not seem to be as effective as its IV counterpart, lidocaine (125, 126). Tricyclic antidepressants have been used for decades, but caution must be observed in those over 65 because of anticholinergic side effects (127). Anticonvulsants have also been used; there appears to be some effectiveness with lamotrigine in doses of

200–400 mg/day for both brain and spinal cord pain (128). Gabapentin may also be effective (129), but topiramate does not seem to have clinical benefit (130).

Non-pharmacological interventions have also demonstrated benefit in some patients who are refractory to pharmacologic management. Such interventions have included transection of spinal nerves or cordotomy (although 60–80% of patients may have recurrence of pain after 2 years), spinal cord or deep brain stimulation, which appears to enhance GABA transmission (124).

Complex Regional Pain Syndrome (CRPS)

CRPS remains a much debated clinical condition with perhaps as much misinformation as information (131). The latest research developments suggest that this condition is multidimensional with neuropathic, nociceptive and inflammatory components with associated sympathetic system dysfunction. Current consensus opinion also indicates that CRPS is likely associated with central sensitization phenomena as well as motor abnormalities. Treatments that have been shown to be efficacious include a gamut of physical interventions, pharmacotherapeutic measures, and interventional treatments. Research has suggested that interdisciplinary programs emphasizing functional restoration may offer the optimal treatment paradigm. As noted by Harden (132), "Functional restoration should provide different interventional and non-interventional modalities in a timely manner to facilitate reanimation and normalization of use and movement of the affected limb". Pharmacotherapeutic interventions for pain can be considered as either "maintenance" or "rescue/abortive" and include such diverse drug classes as tricyclic antidepressants, opioids, anticonvulsants, NSAIDs, clonidine, nifedipine, alpha-adrenergic antagonists (e.g. phenoxybenzamine and phentolamine), biphosphonates, calcitonin, among the most well studied (132). Interventional treatments that have shown benefit include both sympathetic and epidural blocks.

Conclusion

Pain clearly is a complex clinical phenomena (133, 134). Treatment of post-traumatic pain conditions is even more multidimensional, whether in the acute or chronic phase post-injury. Judicious use of medical interventions must rely not only on sound medical knowledge that remains up to date with current accepted practice but also on keen observational, interview and examination skills. A sound familiarity with the post-traumatic pain literature, as well as, the myriad conditions that can be seen following multi-trauma and/or traumatic brain injury (135) is paramount to recognizing these clinical conditions when they present themselves. As was once said by Goethe, "We see what we look for, we look for what we know".

References

1. Lahz, S., Bryant, R.A. Incidence of Chronic Pain Following Traumatic Brain Injury, *Archives of Physical Medicine and Rehabilitation* 1996;77:889–891.
2. Beetar JT, Guillmette TJ, Sparadeo FR. Sleep and pain complaints in symptomatic traumatic brain injury and neurologic population. *Arch Phys Med Rehabil* 1996;77:1298–1302.
3. Apkarian AV, Bushnell MC, Treede RD, Zubieta JK: Human brain mechanisms of pain perception and regulation in health and disease. *European Journal of Pain* 2005;9:463–484.
4. Walker W: Pain pathoetiology after TBI: neural and non-neural mechanisms. *JHTR* 2004;19(1):72–81.
5. McMahon S.B., David L.H., Bevan S.: Inflammatory mediators and modulators of pain. In: SB McMahon & M. Koltzenburg (Eds.): *Wall and Melzack's Textbook of Pain*. 5th Edition. Elsevier/Churchill Livingstone. Philadelphia. Pgs. 49–72, 2006.
6. Rao S: .The neuropharmacology of centrally-acting analgesic medications in fibromyalgia. *Rheum Dis Clinics of North America*, 28(2), 2002.
7. Pollock DS, Bainbridge JL: Rational pharmacotherapy of neuropathic pain. *The Pain Practitioner* 2004;14(2):24–31.
8. Li J, Simone D, Larson A: Windup leads to characteristics of central sensitization. *Pain* 1999;79:75–82.
9. Tetzlaff J. Treatment of acute pain in the orthopedic patient. *Pain Management* 2004;July/August: 12–24.
10. Burstein R, Goor-Aryeh I, Jakubowski M: Migraine, sensitization of trigeminovascular neurons and triptan therapy. *Headache Currents* 2004;1(2):25–32.
11. Bolay H, Moskowitz M: Mechanisms of pain modulation in chronic syndromes. *Neurology* 2002;59(5).
12. Rao S: The neuropharmacology of centrally-acting analgesic medications in fibromyalgia. *Rheum Dis Clinics of North America*, 2002;28(2).
13. Welch KM: Contemporary concepts of migraine pathogenesis. *Neurology*, 2003;61(Suppl 4):S2–S8.
14. Eisenberger NI, Lieberman MD, Williams KD: Does rejection hurt? An FMRI study of social exclusion. *Science*. 2003;302(5643): 237–239.
15. Peyron R, Laurent B, Garcia-Larrea L: Functional imaging of brain responses to pain. A review and meta-analysis. *Neurophysiol Clin* 2000;30(5):263–288.
16. Firestone, L. Gyulai F, Mintun M, et al. Human brain activity response to fentanyl imaged by positron emission tomography. *Anesthesia and analgesia* 1996;82:1247–61.
17. Young RF, Tronnier V, Rinaldi PC. Chronic stimulation of the Kölliker-Fuse nucleus region for relief of intractable pain in humans. *J Neurosurg* 1992;76(6):979–85.
18. Bartsch T, Goadsby P: Increased responses in trigeminocervical nociceptive neurons to cervical input after stimulation of the dura mater. *Brain* 2003;126:1801–1813.
19. Goadsby P, Knight Y, Hoskin K: Stimulation of the greater occipital nerve increases metabolic activity in the trigeminal nucleus caudalis and cercial dorsal horn of the cat. *Pain*, 23–28, 1997.
20. Shevel E, Speirings E: Cervical muscles in the pathogenesis of migraine headache. *J. Headache Pain* 2004;5:12–14.
21. Arendt-Nielsen L, Laursen R, Drewes A: Referred pain as an indicator for neural plasticity. *Prog Brain Res* 2000;129:343–356.
22. Lake A, Saper J: Chronic headache: new advances in treatment strategies. *Neurology*, 2002;59(Suppl 2):S8–13.
23. Knight Y: Brainstem modulation of caudal trigeminal nucleus: a model for understanding migraine biology and future drug targets. *Headache Currents*. 2(5):108–118.
24. Weiller C, May A, Limmroth V, et al. Brain Stem activation in spontaneous human migraine attacks. *Nature Med*, 1995;1: 658–660.
25. Terhors G, Meijler W, Korf J, Kemper R: Trigeminal nociception-induced cerebral Fos expression in the conscious rat. *Cephalalgia*, 2001;21:963–975.
26. Bromm B, Desmedt JE (eds).: *Pain and the brain: From nociception to cognition*. Raven Press: New York, 1995.
27. Vogt, BA, Sikes, RW and Vogt, LJ: Anterior cingulate cortex and the medial pain system. In: BA. Vogt and M Gabriel, eds.,

Neurobiology of cingulate cortex and limbic thalamus: A comprehensive handbook, 1993;pp. 313–344.

28. Willis WD, Westlund, KN: Neuroanatomy of the pain system and of the pathways that modulate pain. *Journal of Clinical Neurophysiology.* 1997;14:2–31.

29. Albe-Fessard D, Berkley KJ, Kruger L, et al.: Diencephalic mechanism of pain sensation. *Brain Res.* 356(3):217–296, 1985.

30. Chapman, CR: Limbic processes and the affective dimension of pain. In G. Carli & M. Zimmerman (eds) *Progress in brain research*, Vol 10, Elsevier. 1996.

31. Gabriel, M. The role of pain in cingulate cortical and limbic thalamic mediation or dance learning, in: J.M. Besson, G. Guilbaud and H. Ollat, eds. *Forebrain areas involved in pain processing*, pp. 197–211. John Libbey Eurotext: Paris, 1995.

32. Melzack R. Pain and the neuromatrix in the brain. *J Dent Educ.* 2001;65:1378–1382.

33. Galer, B.S. and Jensen, M.F. The development and preliminary validation of a pain measure specific to neuropathic pain: The Neuropathic Pain Scale, *Neurology*, 1997;48:332–338.

34. Gatchel, RJ and Turk, DC (Eds.): *Psychosocial Factors in Pain.* The Guilford Press: New York, 1999.

35. Gatchel RJ, Lou L, and Kishino N: Concepts of Multidisciplinary Pain Management. In Boswell MV, Cole BE (Eds.) Weiner's Pain Management: *A Practical Guide for Clinicians (Am. Acad. of Pain Management)* . New York: Taylor & Francis Group, 2006; 1501–1508.

36. Turk DC: Understanding pain sufferers: the role of cognitive processes. *The Spine Journal.* 2004;4:1–7.

37. Ong KS, Seymour RA: Maximizing the safety of non-steroidal anti- inflammatory drug use for post-operative dental pain: an evidence based approach. *Anesth Prog.* 2003;50(3):62–74.

38. Gonzales, VA., Martelli, MF. and Baker, JM.: Psychological assessment of persons with chronic pain. *NeuroRehabilitation*, 2000; 14(2):69–83.

39. Martelli, MF and Zasler, ND: Useful psychological instruments for assessing persons with functional medical disorders. In ND Zasler and MF Martelli (Eds): *Functional Medical Disorders, State of the Art Reviews in Physical Medicine and Rehabilitation*, pp. 147–162. Phila.: Hanley and Belfus, 2002.

40. Turk, DC and Melzack, R: The measurement of pain and the assessment of people experiencing pain, in: DC Turk and R Melzack, eds. *Handbook of Pain Assessment* (pp 3–14), The Guilford Press: New York, 1992.

41. Zasler, ND & Martelli, MF (eds): Pain Management. *The Journal of Head Trauma Rehab.* 19(1), 2004.

42. Kaplan RJ: Current status of non-steroidal anti-inflammatory drugs in physiatry. *Am J Phys Med Rehabil.* 2005;84:885–894.

43. Wiffen P, Collins S, McQuay H, Carroll D, Jadad A, Moore A: Anticonvulsant drugs for acute and chronic pain. *Cochrane Review.* 4:2003.

44. Dworkin RH, Corbin AE, Young MS, et al.: Pregabalin for the treatment of post-herpetic neuralgia. A randomized, placebo-controlled trial. *Neurology.* 2003;60:1274–1283.

45. Shneker BF, McAuley JW: Pregabalin: a new neuromodulator with broad therapeutic indications. *Ann Pharmacother.* 2005;39(12): 2029–2037.

46. *The Medical Letter.* Ziconotide (Piralt) for Chronic Pain. 2005; 47(1223/1224):103–104.

47. Hassenbusch SJ, Portenoy RK, Cousins M, et al.: Polyanalgesic Consensus Conference 2003: an update on the management of pain by intraspinal drug delivery – report of an expert panel. *J Pain Symptom Manage.* 2004;27(6):540–563.

48. Chou R, Peterson K, Helfand M: Comparative efficacy and safety of skeletal muscle relaxants for spasticity and musculoskeletal conditions: a systematic review. *J Pain Symptom Manage* 2004;28(2): 140–175.

49. Mailis, A, Nicholson, K: The use of sodium amytal in the assessment and treatment of functional or other disorders. In: ND Zasler and MF Martelli (Eds): *Functional Medical Disorders, State of the Art Reviews in Physical Medicine and Rehabilitation*, pp. 131–146. Phila.: Hanley and Belfus, 2002.

50. Argoff CE: Topical treatments for pain. *Current Pain & Headache Reports*, 2004;8:261–7.

51. Leong M, Royal M: Opioid therapy in chronic non-cancer pain management. *Practical Pain Management*, Sept/Oct, 43–47, 2004.

52. Hewitt DJ, Chapman SL: Chronic Pain. In: M. Rizzo & PJ Eslinger (Eds.): *Principles and Practice of Behavioral Neurology and Neuropsycyhology.* W.B. Saunders. Philadephia. 2004;Pgs. 737–76.

53. Chapman S: Effects of intermediate and long-term use of opioids on cognition in patients with chronic pain. *Clin J Pain*, 2002;18: S83–90.

54. Tassain V Attal N, Fletcher D, et al: Long term effects of oral sustained release morphine on neuropsychological performance in patients with chronic non-cancer pain. *Pain*, 104: 389–400, 2003.

55. Jamison R: Neuropsychological effects of long-term opioid use in chronic pain patients. *J Pain Symptom Manage*, 2003;26(4): 913–921.

56. Jamot L, Matthes H, Simmonin F, et al: Differential involvement of the mu and kappa opioid receptors in spatial learning. *Genes Brain Behav*, 2003;2(2): 80–92.

57. Sammons M:. Pharmacological Management of Chronic Pain: Fibromyalgia and Neuropathic pain. *Prof Psychol Res Pr*, 2004;35:206–210.

58. Furlan AD, Sandoval JA, Mailis-Gagnon A, Tunks E: Opioids for chronic non-cancer pain: a meta-analysis of effectiveness and side-effects. Submitted for publication. *Canadian Medical Association Journal.*

59. Laureys S, Faymonville, M, Peigneux P et al: Cortical processing of noxious somatosensory stimuli in the persistent vegetative state. *Neuroimage*, 2002;17:732–41.

60. Federation of State Medical Boards of the United States, Inc. *Model Policy for the use of controlled substances for the treatment of pain.* 2004.

61. Bloodworth D: Issues in opioid management. *Arch of Phys Med Rehabil.* 2005;84(S3):42–55.

62. Chou R: Drug class review on long acting opioid analgesics. Oregon evidence based practice center. *OHSU.* April 2004.

63. Eisenberg E, McNicol ED, Carr DB: Efficacy and safety of opioid agonists in the treatment of neuropathic pain of non-malignant origin. Systematic review and meta-analysis of randomized controlled trials. *JAMA.* 2005;293:3043–3052.

64. Hansen H, Jordan A, Bolen J: Controlled substances and risk management. In Boswell MV, Cole BE (Eds.) Weiner's Pain Management: *A Practical Guide for Clinicians (Am. Acad. of Pain Management)* . New York: Taylor & Francis Group, 2006;1417–1455.

65. Gallagher RM: Rational integration of pharmacologic, behavioral, and rehabilitation strategies in the treatment of chronic pain. *Arch Phys Med Rehabil.* 2005;84(S3):64–76.

66. McQuay H. & Moore, A.: *An evidence based resource for pain relief.* Oxford: Oxford University Press, 1998.

67. College of Physicians and Surgeons of Ontario: Evidence-based recommendations for medical management of chronic non-malignant pain, November, 2000.

68. Carroll D, Moore RA, McQuay HJ, Fairman F, Tramer M, Leijon G: Transcutaneous electrical nerve stimulation (TENS) for chronic pain. *Cochrane Review.* 4:2003.

69. Kroeling P, Gross AR, Goldsmith CH (Cervical Overview Group): A Cochrane review of electrotherapy for mechanical neck disorders. *Spine.* 2005;30(21):E641–648.

70. Kirsch, DL and Smith, RB: The use of cranial electrotherapy in the management of chronic pain: A review. *NeuroRehabilitation*, 2000;14(2):85–94.

71. Craig E, Kaelin D: Physical Modalities. In: *Physical Medicine and Rehabilitation.* The Complete Approach. M. Grabois, S.J. Garrison, K.A. Hart, L.D Lehmkuhl (Eds). Pages: 440–457. Blackwell Science. London. 2000.

72. Slipman CW, Palmitier RA, DeDianous DK: *Injection Techniques. The Complete Approach.* M. Grabois, S.J. Garrison, K.A. Hart, L.D. Lehmkuhl (Eds). Pages: 458–486. Blackwell Science. London. 2005.

73. Frontera W: Exercise in Physical Medicine and Rehabilitation. In: *Physical Medicine and Rehabilitation. The Complete Approach.* M. Grabois, S.J. Garrison, K.A. Hart, L.D. Lehmkuhl (Eds). Pages: 487–503. Blackwell Science. London. 2000.

74. Hoffman MD, Shepanski MA, Mackenzie SP: Experimentally induced pain perception is acutely reduced by aerobic exercise in

people with chronic low back pain. *J Rehabil Res Dev* 2005;42(2):183–90.

75. Angelopoulos, TJ: Beta-endorphin immunoreactivity during high-intensity exercise with and without opiate blockade. *Eur J Appl Physiol* 86(1):92–6. 2001.

76. Vaynman S, Gomez-Pinilla, F: License to run: exercise impacts functional plasticity in the intact and injury central nervous system by using neurotrophins. *Neurorehabil Neural Repair* 2005;19:283–295.

77. Yamaguchi M. Incidence of headache and severity of head injury. *Headache*, 1992;32(9):427–431.

78. Walker WC, Seel RT, Curtiss G, Warden DL: Headache after moderate and severe traumatic brain injury: a longitudinal analysis. *Arch Phys Med Rehabil*. 2005;86(9):1793–1800.

79. Zasler ND (Ed.): Post-traumatic headache. *J Head Trauma Rehabil*. 1999;14(1).

80. Zasler, ND & Martelli, MF. Post-traumatic headache: Practical approaches to diagnosis and treatment. In: R.B. Weiner (Ed.): *Pain Management: A Practical Guide for Clinicians*, 6th edition. Boca Ratan, FL: St. Lucie Press, 2002;313–344, 125–138.

81. Evans RW: Post-traumatic headaches. In Evans RW (Ed.) *Neurologic Clinics*, 22(1), 237–249. Philadelphia: Saunders, 2004.

82. International Headache Society. The International Classification of Headache Disorders. 2nd Edition. *Cephalalgia*. 24(Suppl 1), 2004.

83. Packard RC: Epidemiology and pathogenesis of post-traumatic headache. *J Head Trauma Rehabil*. 1999;14(1):9–21.

84. Zafonte R, Horn L: Clinical assessment of post-traumatic headache. *J Head Trauma Rehabil*. 1999;14:22–33.

85. Travell JG, Simons DG: *Myofascial pain and dysfunction. The trigger point manual*. Vol. 1. Baltimore, MD. Williams & Wilkins, 1992.

86. Hecht JS: Occipital nerve blocks in post-concussive headaches: a retrospective review and report of ten patients. *J Head Trauma Rehab*. 2004;19(1):58–71.

87. Russell IJ, Bieber CS: Myofascial pain and fibromyalgia syndrome. In: SB McMahon & M. Koltzenburg (Eds.): *Wall and Melzack's Textbook of Pain*. 5th Edition. Elsevier/Churchill Livingstone. Philadelphia. 2006;669–682.

88. Duckro P, Chibnall J, Greenberg M. Prevalence of temporomandibular dysfunction in chronic post-traumatic headache patients. *Headache Q*, 1997;8:228–233.

89. Dionee RA, Kim H, Gordon SM: Acute and chronic dental and orofacial pain. In: SB McMahon & M. Koltzenburg (Eds.): *Wall and Melzack's Textbook of Pain*. 5th Edition. Elsevier/Churchill Livingstone. Philadelphia. 2006;819–832.

90. Gerwin RD: A review of myofascial pain and fibromyalgia – factors that promote their persistence. *Acupunct Med*. 2005;23(3): 121–134.

91. Hou CR, Tsai LC, Cheng KF, et al: Immediate effects of various physical therapeutic modalities on cervical myofascial pain and trigger-point sensitivity. *Arch Phys Med Rehabil* 2002;83(10): 1406–1414.

92. Mense S: Neurobiological basis for the use of botulinum toxin in pain therapy. *J Neurol*. 2004;251 (Suppl 1):11–7.

93. Biondi DM: Physical treatments for headache: a structured review. *Headache*. 2005;45:738–746.

94. Dimitroulis G, Gremillion H, Dolwick M, Walter J. Temporomandibular disorder. 2.Non-surgical treatment. *Aust Dent J.*, 1995;40(6):372–376.

95. Curatolo M, Arendt-Nielsen L, Petersen-Felix S: Evidence, mechanisms and clinical implications of central hypersensitivity in chronic pain after whiplash injury. *Clin J Pain*. 2004;20(6):469–477.

96. Sjaastad O, Fredriksen TA, Pfaffenrath V: Cervicogenic headache: diagnostic criteria. *Headache*. 1998;38:442–445.

97. Bogduk N: Distinguishing primary headache disorders from cervicogenic headache: clinical and therapeutic implications. *Headache Currents*. 2005;2(2):27–36.

98. Jensen O, Nielsen F, Vosmar L: An open study comparing manual therapy with the use of cold packs in the treatment of post-traumatic headache. *Cephalalgia*. 1990;10:241–250.

99. Bogduk N: The neck and headaches. *Neurol Clin N Am*. 2004; 22:151–171.

100. Zasler ND (Ed.): Post-traumatic headache. *J Head Trauma Rehabil* 199;14(1).

101. Packard RC: The relationship of neck injury and post-traumatic headache. *Current Pain and Headache Reports* 2002;6:301–307.

102. Ribeiro S, Palmer SN, Antonaci F: Cervicogenic headache. *American Journal of Pain Management*. 2005;15:48–58.

103. Gross AR, Hoving JL, haines TA, et al: A Cochrane review of manipulation and mobilization for mechanical neck disorders. *Cochrane Database Syst Rev*. 2004;(1):CD004249.

104. Aguggia M: Typical facial neuralgias. *Neurol Sci* 2005;2:s68–70.

105. Weiss HD, Stern BJ, Goldberg J: Post-traumatic migraine: chronic migraine precipitated by minor head or neck trauma. *Headache*. 1991;31:451–456.

106. Weber C, Moskowitz M: Therapeutic implications of central and peripheral neurologic mechanisms in migraine. *Neurology*. 2003;61(Suppl 4):S9–20.

107. Siow HC, Young WB, Silberstein SD: Neuroleptics in headache. *Headache*. 2005;45:358–371.

108. Goadsby PJ: Primary neurovascular headache. In: SB McMahon & M. Koltzenburg (Eds.): *Wall and Melzack's Textbook of Pain*. 5th Edition. Elsevier/Churchill Livingstone. Philadelphia. 2006; 851–874.

109. Aoki K: Evidence for anti-nociceptive activity of botulinum toxin type A in pain management. *Headache* 2003;43(Suppl 1):S9–S15.

110. Silberstein SD, Stark Lucas, et al: Botulinum toxin type A for the prophylactic treatment of chronic daily headache: a randomized, double- blind, placebo-controlled trial. *Mayo Clin Proc*. 2005; 80(9):1119–1121.

111. Schoenen J: Tension-type headache. . In: SB McMahon & M. Koltzenburg (Eds.): *Wall and Melzack's Textbook of Pain*. 5th Edition. Elsevier/Churchill Livingstone. Philadelphia. 2006; 875–886.

112. Ashina S, Bendtsen L, Ashina M: Pathophysiology of tension-type headache. *Curr Pain Headache Rep*. 2005;9(6):415–422.

113. Lenaerts ME: Pharmacoprophylaxis of tension-type headache. *Curr Pain Headache Rep*. 2005;9(6):442–447.

114. Stillman MJ: Pharmacotherapy of tension type headaches. *Curr Pain Headache Rep*. 2002;6:408–413.

115. Vijayan N. A new post-traumatic headache syndrome;clinical and therapeutic observations. *Headache*. 1977;17:19–22.

116. Putzki N, Nirkko A, diener HC: Trigeminal autonomic cephalalgias: a case of post-truamtic SUNCT syndrome? *Cephalalgia*. 2005;25(5):395–397.

117. Formisano R, Angelini A, DeVuojno G, Calisse P, Fiacco F, Catarci T, Bozzao L, Cerbo R: Cluster-like headache and head injury: case report. *Ital J Neurol Sci*. 1990;11(3):303–5.

118. Matharu MJ, Goadsby PJ: Post-traumatic chronic paroxysmal hemicrania (CPH) with auta. *Neurology*. 2001;56(2):273–5.

119. Couch JR: Rebound-withdrawal headache (medication overuse headache). *Curr Treat Options Neurol*. 2006;8(1):11–19.

120. Warner J, Fenichel G. Chronic post-traumatic headache - often a myth? *Neurology* 1996;46:915–916.

121. Bennett GJ: Pain mechanisms in peripheral neuropathies. Progress in Neuropathic Pain. *American Academy of Pain Management*. April 2005.

122. Sindou M, Mertens P: Neurosurgical management of neuropathic pain. *Stereotact Funct Neurosurg*. 2000;75(2–3)76–80.

123. Nicholson K: Pain assocaited with lesion, disorder or dysfunction of the central nervous sytem, *NeuroRehabilion* 2000;14(1): 3–14.

124. Nicholson BD: Evaluation and treatment of cental pain syndromes. *Neurology*. 2004;62(5 Suppl S):S30–6.

125. Attal N, Gaude V, Brasseur L, et al: Intravenous lidocaine in central pain: a double blind placebo controlled, psychophysical study. *Neurology*. 2000;54:564–574.

126. Attal N, Guirimand F, Brasseur L, et al: effects of IV morphine in central pain: a randomized placebo-controlled study. *Neurology*. 2002;58:554–563.

127. Leijon G, Boivie J: Central post-stroke pain – a controlled trial of amitryptiline and carbamazepine. *Pain*. 1989;36:27–26.

128. Vestergaard K, Andersen G, Gottrup H et al: Lamotrigine for central post- stroke pain: a randomized controlled trial. *Neurology*. 2001;5:184–190.

129. Tai QQ, Kirshblum S, Chen B, et al.: Gabapentin in the treatment of neuropathic pain after spinal cord injury: a prospective randomized double-blind cross-over trial. *J Spinal Cord Med.* 2002;25:100–105.

130. Canavero S, Bonicalzi V, Paolotti R: Lack of effect of topiramate for central pain. *Neurology.* 2002;58,831–832.

131. Pearce JMS: Chronic regional pain and chronic pain syndromes. *Spinal Cord.* 2005;43:263–268.

132. Harden N: Pharmacotherapy of complex regioinal pain syndrome. *Arch Phys Med Rehabil.* 2005;84(S3):17–28.

133. Miller L: Neurosensitization: a model for persistent disability in chronic pain, depression and post-traumatic stress disorder following injury. *Neurorehabilitation.* 2000;14(1):25–32.

134. Nicholson, K, Martelli, MF & Zasler, ND: Myths and misconceptions about chronic pain: The problem of mind body dualism. In R.B. Weiner (Ed.): *Pain Management: A Practical Guide for Clinicians,* 6th edition, pp. 465- 474. Boca Raton, FL: St. Lucie Press, 2002.

135. Zasler, N.D. Martelli, M.F., Nicholson, K.: Chronic pain. In: J.M. Silver, T.W. McAllister, S.C. Yudofsky (Eds.): *"Textbook of Traumatic Brain Injury",* 2nd Edition. American Psychiatric Publishing, Inc. 2004;419–436.

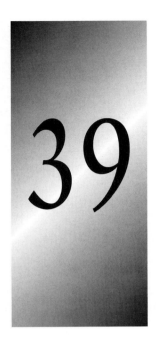

39

Psychological Approaches to Comprehensive Pain Assessment and Management Following TBI

Michael F. Martelli
Keith Nicholson
Nathan D. Zasler

INTRODUCTION

The purpose of this chapter is to help illustrate the important components and increase awareness and understanding of psychological approaches to assessment and management of pain in persons with TBI. This illustration is intended to assist with the making of appropriate referrals, and promoting effective carryover and integration of pain management principles into care of persons with concomitant TBI. It is not intended as a substitute for the necessary training and experience that is prerequisite to providing effective assessment and treatment of pain in persons with TBI.

A Brief Overview of Pain: An Informed Conceptualization

Pain is defined by the International Association for the Study of Pain (1) as a "psychological state" characterized by "an unpleasant sensory and emotional experience associated with actual or potential tissue damage, or described in terms of such damage." An important distinction, with associated differences in definition, pathophysiology, phenomenological experience, plus assessment and treatment focus, relates to chronicity. Acute pain, usually occurring in response to identifiable tissue damage or a noxious event, has more clearly identifiable triggers and neuroanatomical pathways, and

communicates useful information that provokes adaptive responses. It has a time-limited course during which treatment is aimed at providing relief as well as promoting resolution or correction of underlying pathophysiological processes.

As time passes without resolution of an acute pain problem, subjective components may become more pronounced, identifiable triggers and neuroanatomic pathways can become obscure, and behavioral responses can become more disproportionate to underlying pathophysiology and even obstructive to resolution and adaptation. Chronic pain, simply defined as pain persisting beyond six months, may or may not be associated with any obvious tissue damage or pathological process, but can disrupt virtually all life areas and produce marked emotional and behavioral changes. Frequent concomitants of chronic pain include: maladaptive protective responses or pain behaviors; protracted courses of medication use and minimally effective or even iatrogenic medical services; and marked behavioral or emotional changes, including restrictions in daily activities. Pain related avoidance behaviors and reduced activity are likely to result in a cyclic disability-enhancing pattern. The longer pain persists, the more recalcitrant it becomes and the more treatment goals focus on improved coping with pain and its concomitants (2, 3). Finally, there is acceptance that persistent pain is often associated with peripheral or central sensitization effects in which hyper-responsiveness or spontaneous discharge of components of the pain system develops (4, 5). Numerous functional imaging studies have begun to document the interaction of psychologic and neurobiologic processes in chronic pain patients (6–13).

Pain is best conceptualized as a multidimensional subjective experience mediated by emotion, attitudes and other perceptual influences. Variability in pain responses is the rule rather than the exception and appears to reflect complex biopsychosocial interactions between genetic, developmental, cultural, environmental, and psychological and injury/illness related factors (14, 15). Important distinctions between pain and suffering(16), sensory and affective experience, and impairment and disability (17) (WHO) reflect the variability in response to pain problems. While some pain patients appear to present with unusual and possibly exaggerated suffering or disability, others present with a kind of "la belle indifference" in which extremely high reported pain severity may be associated with no apparent affective distress, pain behavior or interference in many life activities. In some cases, the onset, maintenance, severity or exacerbation of pain is primarily associated with psychological factors and may warrant a DSM-IV (18) diagnosis of Pain Disorder Associated with Psychological Factors. In this regard, it has been noted that there is an association between post-traumatic stress reactions and development of chronic pain (19–22), with uncontrollable pain following physical injury potentially representing the core-trauma resulting in post-traumatic symptomatology (23). However, it is cautioned that one should avoid the pitfalls of mind-body dualism and always consider both psychological and organic factors in the presentation of any chronic pain patient (24).

It should be emphasized that pain may arise from a combination of numerous physical and psychological factors. Complexities in pain presentation warrant referral to pain management specialists and/or specialty interdisciplinary pain programs (25). This is particularly true in cases of "intractable" and functionally disabling pain. It is always best to intervene when "pre-chronic", where competent, specialized, early intervention offers the greatest hope of facilitating adaptation.

The importance of assessing and managing pain has been incorporated into the prevailing standards of healthcare practice in the United States. The Joint Commission on Accreditation of Healthcare Organizations (JCAHO), in its recent accreditation manuals, acknowledges that while pain coexists with a number of diseases and injuries, it requires explicit attention (JCAHO, 2000). Overall, the standards require organizations to: 1) recognize individual's rights to appropriate pain assessment and management; 2) identify persons with pain in initial and ongoing assessments; and 3) educate patients, residents, clients and families about pain management.

Traumatic Brain Injury and Pain

There is a very high comorbidity of chronic pain problems with cranial trauma whether or not there is traumatic brain injury (TBI). Indeed, headache is the primary complaint in virtually all surveys of the post-concussive syndrome (26). The frequency of post traumatic headache (PTH) in the immediate post-accident period has been estimated to be as high as 90%, with problems continuing beyond six months in as many as 44% (3), although there is generally poor understanding of the incidence, etiology or many other aspects of PTH (27).

In addition to headache, many other pain problems may follow trauma, including neck and back pain, complex regional pain syndrome, and fibromyalgia, among others. Curiously, most studies report that pain problems are much more common in less severe as compared with more severe TBI (3, 26, 28) although pain problems may also be common in the latter (29). Importantly, more severe brain injuries may result in reduced sensitivity to pain due to lesions of the CNS structures involved in processing pain, as observed in some dementias (4, 30). Those with more severe TBI may also enjoy optimal post traumatic healing due to reduced activity and extended rest periods (31). In contrast, it has also been suggested that there is increased likelihood for developing a central sensitization or neurosensitization effect (20, 26) after milder injuries, where there is not only no damage to CNS pain processing structures, but less time for healing and rest before return to usual activities with greater opportunity for psychophysiologic arousal .

Traumatic Brain Injury, Pain, and Neuropsychological Function

There is increasing awareness of the role that pain may play in symptom presentation following traumatic brain injury, especially with regard to cognitive complaints. Several recent reviews (3, 24, 26, 31–36) have examined literature objectively assessing these complaints. The available evidence strongly supports the conclusion that chronic pain, especially head pain and neck pain, and pain related symptomatology, independent of TBI or neurologic disorder, can and often do produce impairment of cognitive functioning. Multiple lines of evidence, including studies of acute and chronic pain, animal and human studies, experimental and clinical studies and neurophysiologic studies support this conclusion. A brief summary of the converging evidence that supports this conclusion, based on a review by (37) Dr. Martelli, is presented in Table 39-1. Notably, attentional capacity, processing speed, memory, and executive functions, as assessed on neuropsychological tests, are the cognitive domains most likely to be affected.

TABLE 39-1
Evidence of Negative Effects of Pain on Cognition in Animals and Humans

1. Experimental animal and human information processing / attentional capacity literature indicates that distracters less aversive than pain disrupt attention, as does pain;

2. Experimental rodent and other mammalian studies showing pain related disrupted maze and other learning for both appetitive (e.g, food reward) and avoidant (eg, shock) stimuli;

3. Experimental rodent studies showing improved performance with cessation of pain;

4. Experimental rodent and other mammalian studies showing improved performance after administration of pain relieving medications known to disrupt cognition;

5. Experimental human studies showing improved cognitive performance after discontinuation of pain stimulus and/ or administration of psychoactive opioid pain relievers;

6. Animal studies showing that stress (including chronic pain) is associated with damage to the hippocampus, inhibition of neurogenesis, and deficits in hippocampal-based memory function;

7. PTSD findings of deficits in hippocampal-based declarative verbal memory associated with smaller hippocampal volume;

8. Recent preclinical evidence showing that selective serotonin reuptake inhibitor (SSRI) antidepressants promote neurogenesis, reverse effects of stress on hippocampal atrophy, improve cognitive deficits observed in OCD, depression, etc;

9. A majority of studies indicating pain cognitive interference effects, at least attention dysregulation, in chronic and acute pain patients. Study designs including experimental pain, neuropathic pain, neurophysiologic measures, combination neuropsychologic and neurophysiologic measures, and reward designs helped to bolster conclusions about interference effects despite failure of most studies to utilize explicit response bias detection measures for pain and cognition.

10. Consistent neurophysiologic studies showing very specific neurophysiologic (e.g. anterior cingulated cortex (ACC)) effects associated with chronic pain and attentional disruption, often co-existing with other patterns, consistent with other disorders also having reasonable evidence of cognitive impairments and neurophysiologic expressions (e.g., hypofrontality and depression);

11. Neural plasticity / cerebral reorganization associated with chronic pain showing functional cerebral changes (e.g. studies showing expansion of sensory cortex (e.g., Flor (11));

12. Neuroendocrine and HPA perturbation in chronic pain and evidence that pain and chronic stress (and depression) are linked via chronic stress-induced HPA dysfunction (along with evidence of combined muscle energy depletion and serotonin deficiency (peripherally, but also centrally), along with depressed levels of somatomedin C, caused by deficit of stage 4 sleep dependent release of GH, and elevated NE response levels in fibromyalgia;

13. Amassing neurophysiologic evidence of central sensitization (38)and disrupted pain inhibitory mechanisms associated with dysfunctional ACC functioning of both anterior / ventral and posterior/ dorsal quadrants (associated with cognitive and affective regulation, respectively), plus evidence that less severe and less disruptive chronic pain is associated with a greater habituation response to painful stimuli (vs. sensitization) and not associated with cognitive disruption. The newest integration of these findings link a biopsychosocial model where genetics, learning history and psychological variables interact, with a clear role played by anxiety and avoidance conditioning to produce a pattern of pain arousal that mimics OCD, chronic or severe depression, PTSD or high trait anxiety, with hypoaroused inhibition (ACG hypofunction) of pain, obsessional thoughts, anxiety, somatic concerns, intrusive associations/ memories) and disrupted allocation of attentional resources;

14. Evidence that the concomitants of chronic pain alone may account for cognitive disruption; sleep disturbance / deprivation (e.g., metaanalytic studies showing impaired attention and psychomotor function, including greater impairment compared to alcohol intoxication; studies indicating significant trait-like interindividual variability in sleep deprivation effects that are stable within individuals); pain medications; depression and anxiety; and suggestion that combinations are additive;

15. Consistent findings showing both normalization of neuropathophysiology and cognitive function (for performance and self reported improvements in cognition) after effective pain reduction interventions.

16. Indications that chronic pain, as well as depression, are associated with structural cerebral changes. For example, chronic pain has been associated with decreased prefrontal and thalamic gray matter density compared with matched controls, suggesting that the pathophysiology of chronic pain includes thalamocortical processes.

Adapted from Martelli (37).

These reviews indicate that the concomitants of chronic pain may be as important or more important than pain itself in producing cognitive impairment. Specifically, cognitive impairment in chronic pain patients has been associated with mood change/emotional distress, somatic preoccupation and pain catastrophization, sleep disturbance, fatigue, and perceived interference with daily activities that are potential sources of chronic stress. For example, major depression is frequently found following mild TBI, is associated with higher postconcussion symptom endorsement, poor functional outcome, high distress levels, disability and cognitive impairment which typically remit after effective treatment for depression (39). In a metaanalytic review, (40) Pilcher and Huffcutt found that partial sleep deprivation impairs cognitive and motor performance. More interestingly, in a review of experimental human and animal studies, (41) Kundermann, Krieg, Schreiber and Lautenbacher found that sleep deprivation produces hyperalgesic changes and can counteract analgesic medication effects via disruption of both serotonergic and opioidergic processes.

Mahmood et al. (30) examined the previously observed association between sleep disturbance, cognitive and pain complaints and TBI (e.g., Beetar, Guilmette, Sparadeo, (42)). They noted that, while severe TBI is more likely to produce subcortical damage and reduce pain experience, mild TBI is associated with increased pain and sleep disturbance, and that sleep disturbance is associated with frontal hypoactivation that, especially when associated with depression, may render post TBI individual especially vulnerable to cognitive dysfunction. They observed that measures sensitive to executive functioning and information processing speed were associated with sleep quality scores. Consistent with these findings, Mooney et al.'s (39) review of poor recovery following mild TBI found that most of the variance in recovery of mild TBI compensation seekers seems to be explained by depression, pain and response bias versus brain injury variables.

Importantly, these associated factors have consistently been found to be more strongly associated with both cognitive complaints and impairments than is pain severity, although problems with the assessment of pain severity (e.g., response biases to report pain and the restricted range of measurements) may account for the relatively weak predictive power of pain severity ratings. Further, metaanalytic studies and increasing recent evidence have associated these individual factors with decrements in cognitive functioning, independent of chronic pain or combination effects (24, 26, 32–34, 36).

Hart, Wade & Martelli (34) reviewed studies of cognitive functioning in patients with chronic pain with an emphasis on the role of emotional distress and the mechanisms of stress-related effects. The association between psychological distress and cognitive impairment was found to be especially significant for pain-related negative emotions and variables that mediate suffering, such as interference with activities and increased somatic vigilance. This relationship was independent of the effects of pain intensity. It was noted that the anterior cingulate cortex (ACC) plays an important role in pain processing, attention and affective-motivational experience, and that the ACC appears to mediate the impact of pain-related emotional distress on cognitive functioning through allocation of attentional resources. Further, maladaptive physiologic stress responses and dysregulation of the hypothalamic-pituitary-adrenocortical (HPA) axis can produce negative effects on hippocampal function and memory. The underlying mechanism for cognitive impairment that Hart et al. (34) postulated is the anticipation of unpredictable pain symptoms, especially in individuals high in trait neuroticism. This presents a significant stressor that repeatedly activates both the HPA axis and ACC areas and results in disruption of cognitive efficiency. Hart et al. (34) did not address what remains a potentially important research area, i.e., how these putative mechanisms might interact in cases of persons with brain injury where neurologic impairments and additional sources of stress are operative.

Clearly, chronic pain and associated problems can complicate the symptom picture in TBI. Especially in cases of persistent sequelae following mild TBI, increasing evidence suggests that chronic head and other pain and associated problems can present a differential diagnostic challenge, and contribute to or maintain symptoms. This evidence provides strong support for the argument that resolution of the post concussive syndrome and successful adaptation to residual sequelae frequently relies on successful coping with post traumatic pain and/or other pain and associated symptomatology. In addition, careful consideration of pain in the differential diagnosis of brain injury is required. Some recommended procedures for conducting neuropsychological assessment of persons when pain is a significant complaint have been included in Table 39-2.

PAIN ASSESSMENT

Pain is a complex and subjective perceptual process comprised of behavioral, affective, cognitive, and sensory components. Especially when chronic, it often has no clear cut objective pathophysiological correlates. The complexity of this subjective and multidimensional experience is highlighted by independent replicated functional imaging studies showing that anticipation of pain produces similar activation of cortical networks as does pain itself (7, 12, 43). Dualistic (i.e., organic/biologic versus functional/ psychologic) models that explain disease and health primarily in terms of measurable biomedical variables have generally not proven useful for measuring or

TABLE 39-2

Recommendations for Assessing and Minimizing the Confounding Effects of Pain During Neurocognitive Examination

1. Always assess pain when present, when post traumatic adaptation seems compromised by pain and related symptomatology, or limitations in daily functioning, and decrements in test performance seem atypical. Clarify the frequency, intensity and character of pain during the examination and more generally, the characteristics of the chronic pain experience and related problems.
2. Assess problems that are commonly associated with chronic pain (e.g., sleep disturbance, fatigue, somatic preoccupation, anxiety, depression) as these all have the potential to markedly disrupt aspects of cognitive functioning.
3. Repeat administration of measures sensitive to the effects of fatigue (e.g., sustained, attention-demanding, timed tests) during examinations to help identify or corroborate fatigue-related deficits.
4. Always assess effort, motivation and response bias during examination, especially with regard to symptom complaints.
5. Consider postponing cognitive assessment in cases where pain and related symptomatology have not been appropriately or aggressively treated.
6. Use accommodating? procedures during examinations where possible (e.g., optimizing comfort, providing frequent breaks, allowing frequent position changes and use of personal orthotics [cushions, heating or ice pads, etc.], modifying lighting and sound, etc.).

treating pain. Biopsychosocial models better explain variability in health care outcomes and direct more effective interventions for challenging chronic health care situations, including chronic pain rehabilitation (44).

A biopsychosocial stress and coping formulation conceptualizes adaptation to injury as a series of stressful demands which require interactions between existing coping resources and injury related stresses and demands. Hence, identification of coping liabilities is an integral prerequisite to bolstering coping resources and improving long term adaptation. A biopsychosocial assessment perspective affords the optimal understanding of the patient with pain and the myriad of factors that might contribute to this subjective experience and complicate, or otherwise affect symptom presentation (45). Such factors include not only the patient's medical findings, but also physiological, behavioral, and cognitive-affective functioning, including vulnerabilities and strengths.

A comprehensive, biopsychosocial assessment should be considered the standard of care when pain is chronic (46, 47). Initial assessment should address self report, via interview of patient and relevant others, and use of appropriate assessment instruments, in the following areas:

1. Pain intensity
2. Affective response
3. Quality / characteristics, and
4. Location.

History from the patient regarding the presentation of the pain problem is as important as examination results, and should include inquiry about such questions as: onset and course (e.g.,when, where, how; sudden or progressive, fluctuating or steady, etc.), intensity level, duration, activities preceeding an exacerbation, stress related effects, variability across the day and night, effect of movement and posture change, irritating and relieving factors, medications employed and effects, current activities and pain related activity changes, specific effect of pain on mood, activity, cognition, affect, sleep, appetite, and more general effects of pain in the persons life. Importantly, special assessment procedures are indicated in cases of persons with response limitations or significant cognitive impairments. These include special versions of instruments and reliance on observation and structured interview of relevant others and observers, and integration of this information with physical examination procedures (see Hadjistavropoulos, von Baeyer, and Craig (48), for an extensive review of self-report, observational and physiological measures used in pain assessment of adults with impaired communication abilities).

A comprehensive assessment should also address the following areas:

5. Pain behaviors and environmental effects / responses
6. Beliefs about the pain condition
7. Coping strategies and effectiveness
8. Psychosocial context and social responses to pain,
9. Personality and psychoemotional status and adjustment, including how this affects or is affected by pain, and
10. Activity, level of function / disability and quality of life.

A brief survey of general classes and useful instruments for inclusion in a comprehensive pain assessment, updated from previous work (49) is included in Table 39-3. Also included in this table are special instruments designed for persons with significant response limitations and/or cognitive impairment, including the very young and elderly.

TABLE 39-3

General Classes and Instruments Commonly Included in an Assessment of Pain and Psychological Variables Relevant to Adjustment and Coping

---

Specific Pain Domain Instruments: Self Reported Pain Intensity and Location

- *Visual Analogue Pain Scale* (VAS (1)): is a brief graphical, nonpsychometric measure of subjective pain intensity represented by a straight line with typical endpoints of no pain and worst possible pain. It is widely used to quickly assess pain report, track changes during treatment, and assess outcome (50).
- *Verbal Rating Scale* (VRS) is a similar measure where pain intensity is indicated on a linear scale with verbal anchors ranging from no pain to worst possible pain and including mild, moderate, severe and very severe (50, 51).
- *Numeric Rating Scale* (NRS) is another similar measure where pain intensity is indicated verbally or by pointing at a number from 0 or 1 to 10 (50, 52).
- *Pain Drawing* ((53, 54)) is a measure of the location aspect of pain. It is the most common instrument used for this type of self-report (50).
- *McGill Pain Questionnaire*, short form (SF-MPQ: (55)) was designed to measure descriptive aspects of pain via selection of adjectival pain descriptors. It provides three classes of pain descriptors: Sensory (burning, sharp, sore), Affective (e.g., exhausting, punishing), and Intensity (e.g., intense, excruciating). Different combination of descriptors may be associated with different nociceptive or psychological factors.
- *Pain Diaries* are temporal measures of frequency, duration and intensity of pain episodes (56, 57). They typically ask subjects to self-report, in a journal for several days or weeks, when and in what situations pain increases or decreases. More complete versions typically assess such areas as: location, intensity, onset (e.g., sudden or progressive; fluctuating or steady, etc.), characteristics (e.g., throbbing, dull aching), duration, preceding activities, stress, effects of pain on activities, cognition, affect, sleep, appetite, and factors affecting pain mitigation or exacerbation (e.g., weather, activity, stress, medications, distraction).

Instruments Designed for Children and Adults with Significant Cognitive Impairment

- *FACES Scale* (51) was designed for young children and consists of six cartoon faces ranging from a smiling face for "no pain" to a tearful face for "worst pain". Versions have been adapted for cognitively impaired adults.
- *Oucher Scale* (58) consists of sequenced pictures of a child's face, ranging from "no hurt" to "the biggest hurt you could ever have", which are shown and explained to a child who selects which exemplifies current pain level. It is designed for children and can be used with adults with significant cognitive problems (59). Versions are available for most ethnicities.
- *FLACC* (FACE, LEGS, ACTIVITY, CRY, CONSOLABILITY) Scale is a standardized rating composite measure of observed physical indicators of pain in infants and preverbal children who are unable to provide verbal report. It can also be used in children and adults with severe cognitive impairments (see McGrath and Gillespie (60)).
- *Observational Pain Scale* (61) is a standardized rating measure for estimating pain level in cognitively impaired patients who can't respond to VAS, Numeric or Oucher Scales. It produces a composite pain score based on observation of: facial expressions, verbalizations/ vocalizations and body movements; changes in interpersonal interactions; changes in activity patterns or routines; changes in mental status; and/or physiologic changes.

Pain Specific Measures of Functioning: Pain Quality, Affect and Behavioral, Cognitive/ Attitudinal and Emotional Coping

- *Multidimensional Pain Inventory* (62) employs a biopsychosocial conceptualization to assess relevant psychosocial, cognitive, and behavioral aspects of responses to pain. This well researched instrument has 61 items, includes 13 scales and measures pain severity, patient-perceived pain interference, affective distress, life control, social support, response from others, and disability. It includes specific norms for different statistically derived chronic pain subtypes (63): interpersonally distressed with inadequate social support; globally dysfunctional coping; and adaptive coping. An inexpensive software scoring program is available (64). This multiaxial classification system is a psychometrically sound and objective method of evaluating chronic pain patients, may be integrated with useful psychological information from multiple other sources, and offers benefit for matching patients to types of pain management interventions. In a recent study (65) the MPI successfully classified chronic whiplash associated disorders into homogenous subgroups
- *Pain Affect Visual Analogue Scale* (VAS) can also be used to quickly assess affective pain distress (52) versus sensory intensity, and similarly offers utility for assessing treatment changes and outcome.
- *Pain Patient Profile* (P3) (66) is a screening measure for depression, anxiety, & excessive somatization in pain patients. It is a double normed (both healthy controls and chronic pain patients) screening test developed to measure psychological factors related to chronic pain conditions in order to help identify those who would likely benefit from mental health treatment as part of their treatment plan.
- *Battery for Health Improvement* (BHI) assessment (68) is a dual normed (community samples and pain patients) instrument designed for multidimensional assessment and computerized progress tracking to identify affective,

TABLE 39-3 (*continued*)

characterological, psychophysiological and social factors that affect pain, recovery and rehabilitation progress, vocational training or job placement readiness, and impairment and disability. It can contribute useful information regarding psychosocial factors underlying pain reports, perceived disability, somatic preoccupation, design for interventions and outcome. A recent revision, the BHI-2, offers expanded national norms and multiple reference groups, along with expanded and updated scales.

- *Profile of Chronic Pain: Screen* (PCP:S:) (68) is a brief 15-item measure designed to identify individuals who merit more detailed psychosocial evaluation. It assesses the psychological impact of chronic pain in terms of: pain severity, functional interference, and pain-related emotional burden. Random national sample data were employed to demonstrate good validity and minimal social desirability response. National norms are available by gender for three age groups.

- *Profile of Chronic Pain: Extended Assessment Battery* (PCP:EA) (69) is a very new, 86-item instrument with: (a) 33 items assessing pain location and severity, pain characteristics (e.g. worst daily pain), medication use, health care status, the identity of the most important person in the patient's life, and functional limitations in 10 areas of daily living; (b) 13 multi-item subscales addressing aspects of coping (guarding, ignoring, task persistence, and positive self-talk), catastrophizing, pain attitudes and beliefs (including disability beliefs, belief in a medical cure for pain, belief in pain control, and pain-induced fear), and positive (tangible and emotional) and negative (insensitivity and impatience) social responses. National stratified samples across three age groups, two survey studies providing strong evidence for the hypothesized factor structure, internal consistency, independence from response bias, and validity, and the presence of normative data suggest good diagnostic and prescriptive utility.

- *Pain Stages of Change Questionaire* (PSOCQ) (70, 71) has good demonstrated reliability and validity in predicting patient readiness to adopt new beliefs and coping responses to pain. More recent research (72, 73) suggests some utility in identifying patient cluster types that differentially respond to specific multidisciplinary or cognitive-behavioral pain treatments consistent with a self-management approach to chronic pain problems.

- *Survey of Pain Attitudes* (SOPA-R-35:(74)) is a well-researched instrument that assesses patient feelings about pain control, solicitude (solicitous responses from others in response to one's pain), medication (as appropriate treatment for pain), pain-related disability, pain and emotions (the interaction between emotions and pain), medical cures for pain, and pain-related harm (pain as an indicator of physical damage or harm)

- *Pain Catastrophizing Scale* (PCS;(75)) is a brief, well-researched measure of the negative mental set in the presence, or anticipation of pain marked by magnification, rumination and helplessness. Pain catastrophizing is a robust predictor of analgesic use, distress, psychosocial dysfunction, & disability, and superior in comparisons to disease severity, pain levels, age, sex, depression, or anxiety. It also demonstrates benefit as a therapeutic measure of cognitive restructuring as a therapeutic tool (76). A child version is also available (77).

- *Pain Anxiety Symptoms Scale* (PASS) (78) is a measure of fear of pain across cognitive, overt behavioral and physiological domains. It has good correlations with related measures of anxiety and disability and has been found to predict disability and interference due to pain when controlling for emotional distress and pain.

- *Kinesiophobia Scale* (K-Scale:(79)) is a quick screening measure of unreasonable or irrational fear of pain and painful reinjury upon physical movement. It assesses pain-phobias or avoidance conditioned pain related disability (i.e., unhealthy pain maintaining habits that are a major contributor to pain related disability) and correlates highly with similar measures. High scores, once malingering factors are ruled out, signal the need for combination therapies with emphasis on reeducation, countering maladaptive phobic responses and promoting adaptive attitudes and treatment participation/ cooperation (e.g., graduated exposure, cognitive reinterpretation and systematic desensitization). Recently, a version has been adapted for use in the general population (80).

- *Cogniphobia Scale* (C-Scale) (81), adapted from the K-Scale, quickly screens unreasonable or irrational fear of headache or painful reinjury upon cognitive effort / exertion. The C-Scale is designed to assess anxiety based avoidant behavior with regard to cognitive exertion. Like the Kinesiophobia scale, this instrument measures anxiety based avoidant behavior and offers information about need for combination therapies that include such anxiety reduction procedures.

- *Chronic Pain Coping Inventory* (CPCI:(82)) is a 65-item measure of strategies used by patients to cope with chronic pain across 11 pain coping dimensions. In cross validational studies, four scales (Guarding, Resting, Asking for Assistance, and Task Persistence) reliably predicted patient- and significant other-reported patient adjustment. Eight scales (Guarding, Opioid Medication Use, NSAID Use, Sedative-Hypnotic Medication Use, Resting, Asking for Assistance, and Exercise/ Stretch) demonstrated moderate-to-strong consistency between patient and significant-other versions.

- *Chronic Pain Acceptance Questionnaire* (CPAQ) (83) and a revised version (84) is a measure of acceptance of pain. The 20-item revised form has 2 empirically derived subscales: Activity Engagement (i.e., degree to which respondents are living a normal life despite pain) and Pain Willingness (i.e., degree to which respondents have pain experiences without avoidance or control efforts). In a very recent large sample (85) the CPAQ scales were reliably stronger predictors of distress and disability compared with coping variables, suggesting that a pain management efforts can benefit from shaping a more accommodating view of pain experience for certain individuals or circumstances.

TABLE 39-3 (continued)

- *Psychosocial Pain Inventory* (PPI:) (86) is a 25-item, eight-page structured interview designed to assess the influence of psychosocial factors in chronic pain syndromes in 10 areas: 1) pain behavior (e.g., up time, time in bed), 2) social reinforcement, 3) life changes, 4) litigation, 5) financial status, 6) use of alcohol, 7) medication use. 8) coping strategies, 9) social environment, and 10) environmental stress. In also includes questions concerning personal and family histories, past and current medical histories, and reactions and adjustments to the pain and medical treatments.
- *Hendler Chronic Pain Screening Test* (87) assesses contribution of physical versus psychological variables to pain behavior. Higher scores reflect strong psychologically influenced or motivated pain behavior, and suggest recommendations for conservative treatments with multimodality treatment programs. Very high scores typically require further psychological or psychiatric intervention.
- *Headache Disability Rating* procedure of Packard and Ham (88) is a scale that estimates impairment from headache rated on frequency, severity and duration of attacks and how activities impact on functional skills and activities of daily living. Importantly, it includes a modifier variable for rating motivation (i.e., treatment motivation, exaggeration/ over concern, and legal interest) that are used to adjust the total impairment rating.
- *Pain Assessment Battery – Research Edition* (PAB) (89): four measures that provide information regarding patient stress, pain reports with qualitative pain analysis and pain coping strategies, including nonorganic pain complaints. Format allows serial computerized administrations and tracking.
- *Oswestry Low Back Pain Disability Questionnaire* (90) assesses the amount of restriction pain imposes on functional levels. Assessment areas include intensity, personal care, lifting, walking, sitting, standing, sleeping, sex life, social life, and traveling. The percentage of endorsed items gives an indication of the amount of disability. It has been proposed that up to 20% indicates minimal disability, 20 to 40% indicated moderate disability, 40 to 60% indicates severe disability, and greater than 60% indicates severe disability.
- *Vanderbilt Pain Management Inventory* (91) measures chronic pain coping strategies (e.g., active, passive) and provides useful information for treatment planning and recommendations
- *Cognitive Coping Strategies Inventory* (92) assesses the degree to which patients engage in adaptive and maladaptive cognitive coping strategies.
- *Coping Strategies Questionnaire* (64) is a 48-item scale that rates the frequency of engagement in 8 different behavioral and cognitive coping strategies in response to pain or physical symptom experience.

Measures of General Health Functioning and Behavior

- *Millon Behavioral Health Inventory* (MBHI) and its recent upgrade, the *Millon Behavioral Medicine Diagnostic test* (MBMD) (93) is one of the most frequently used health inventories for medical populations in the US. The MBHI provides information across four broad categories: basic coping styles, psychogenic attitudes, specific disease syndromes, and prognostic indices. It has good psychometric properties, a large normative database of representative medical patients, with specific disease scales developed for specific patient groups. The MBMD has updated and expanded the research base and clinical scales (165-items, 38 scales, 3 validity scales). The MBMD assists with: identification of significant psychiatric problems, making specific recommendations; pinpointing personal and social assets to facilitate adjustment; identifying medical regimen compliance problems; structuring post-treatment plans and self-care responsibilities in the patient's social network. Computerized scoring and an interpretive report facilitate use.
- *The SF-36 Health Survey* (SF-36) (94) surveys general health status in terms of physical and mental health and functional status. Widely used in research, and as an outcome measure (95), it assesses 8 areas, including limitations in physical functioning and social functioning and roles and activities, pain, mental health, vitality and health perceptions.
- *The Neurobehavioral Functioning Inventory* (NFI) (96). The NFI is a multipurpose inventory designed to measure current cognitive, physical, and emotional functioning in persons with traumatic brain injury or other neurobehavioral disorders. It is comprised of six independent scales reflecting problems frequently experienced by persons with neurobehavioral disorders: depression, somatic, memory/attention, communication, aggression and motor functioning. This well researched instrument includes separate forms for patient and family, demonstrates concurrent validity with neuropsychological test data and objective personality inventory profiles, can assist with treatment planning and allows measurement of change over time.
- *The Sickness Impact Profile* (SIP) (97) is a behaviorally based measure of health status designed to assess both psychosocial and physical dysfunction. It has sound psychometric properties, is used widely with chronic pain patients and can provide relevant information regarding degree of functional limitation in daily activity.
- *The Illness Behavior Questionnaire* (IBQ:(98, 99))provides useful information about attitudes, perceived reactions of others and psychosocial variables. It delineates 7 factors that include general hypochondriasis, disease conviction, psychological vs. somatic focusing, affective disturbance, affective inhibition, denial, and irritability. In addition, it has value in identifying patients who rely on illness behaviors as a coping style for need procurement.

TABLE 39-3 (*continued*)

General Psychological Measures: Mood, Anger and Anxiety

- *The Beck Depression Inventory – 2* (BDI-2) (100) is a common self-report measure that assesses depressive symptomatology. It has been reported to differentiate chronic pain patients with and without major depression utilizing an optimal cutoff score of 21 (101) and has well documented predictive validity.
- *The Zung Self-rating Depression Scale* (SDS) (102), seems especially well suited for medical settings, and has several advantages over other measures. It is shorter, simpler to administer and score, requires a lower reading level, fits well with medical and injury situations and can be easily administered in an interview format (62). Items are self ratings on a scale ranging from 1 to 4 ("Not at all" to "Most or all of the time") and are scored in the direction of increased depressive symptomatology, with a raw score cutoff for mild depression of approximately 40 points.
- *The State-Trait Anger Expression Inventory-2* (STAXI-2) (103)and its recent update is a reliable, well-normed instrument for assessing the experience, expression and control of both current state and trait anger. Anger Expression and Anger Control scales assess four relatively independent anger-related traits: (a) expression of anger outward; (b) holding anger in; (c) controlling outward expression; and (d) controlling internal angry feelings. This instrument provides information regarding how experience, expression and control of anger may contribute to psychophysiologic arousal and symptoms and increase risk for developing somatic symptoms and medical problems. Indirectly, it offers suggestions for the direction of appropriate interventions. Importantly, anger is a frequent concomitant of chronic pain that has been unfortunately underappreciated (57).
- *The Beck Anxiety Inventory* (BAI) (104) is a screening measure of severity of patient anxiety. Specifically designed to reduce overlap with symptoms of depression, it assesses both physiological and cognitive components of anxiety in 21 items describing subjective, somatic, or panic-related symptoms. The BAI differentiates well between anxious and non-anxious groups in a variety of clinical settings.
- *The Perceived Stress Scale* (PSS) (105) is a widely used instrument for measuring the degree to which situations in one's life are appraised as stressful. Items measure how unpredictable, uncontrollable, and overloaded respondents find their lives and directly queries current levels of experienced stress. Higher PSS scores have been associated with greater vulnerability physical and psychological symptoms following stressful life events.

Comprehensive Personality Assessment Instruments

- *The Minnesota Multiphasic Personality Inventory* (MMPI:(106) MMPI-2 (107)) is the most widely used psychological assessment instrument in the US. The MMPI is a 567 item (true/false) objective measure of personality function and emotional status with 10 clinical and 3 (7 in revised version) validity scales that were derived through empirical discrimination). Its predictive abilities are based on more than fifty years of actuarial data collection and analysis. It is a very sensitive measure of psychological states, traits and styles (e.g., excessive anxiety, tension, depression, hostility and problematic anger, somatization tendencies, sociopathy, substance abuse, deviant thinking and experience, social withdrawal, etc.). Through configural interpretation of the relative scale elevations, tentative hypothesis regarding personality and coping style and relative degree of particular types of psychological disturbance can be gleaned. Importantly, although the MMPI can and is frequently misused and misinterpreted (e.g., application of psychiatric norms to medical patients tends to beg psychiatric interpretations), it represents one of the most useful adjuncts to personality assessment and treatment planning. A cursory summary of potential utility of MMPI profile interpretation for assessing psychological reactions and contributions to physical conditions was offered by Fordyce (101), and roughly includes configural guidelines for interpreting: 1) Willingness to display physical symptom behaviors; 2) Distress/discomfort about illness ("How comfortably sick?"); 3) Poor general coping skills; 4) Depression complicating physical symptoms; 5) Tension (and sympathetic arousal) contributing to physical symptoms (High back, head, neck, shoulder, etc.); 6) Treatment outcome issues. A number of subtypes of chronic have been identified by other researchers although, as with other measures, it remains unclear to what extent results may inform the degree to which complaints are associated with organic (especially peripheral pathology) versus psychologic contributions to patient presentation (108, 109).
- *The Personality Assessment Inventory* (PAI) (110) a good measure of general psychopathology that can help with identification of a wide variety of risk factors that could adversely affect adjustment. It has good psychometric properties and contains 340 items, with 22 scales, including 4 validity scales. As with most other general psychological assessment measures, it has no norms for chronic pain and tends to overpathologize this group.
- *Millon Clinical Multiaxial Inventory*, 3rd edition (MCMI-III:) (111): includes scales assessing DSM-IV based psychiatric disorders, including affective, personality and psychotic disorders, somatization and others. It is useful for the differential diagnosis of personality disorders and psychological vulnerabilities for adaptation to pain. Like other psychiatric measures, it has limited pain group norms and may be prone to overpathologizing patients.

TABLE 39-3 (continued)

Pain Assessment Measures with Built In Response Bias Indicators

Pain Assessment Battery (PAB) (89): – Research Edition: *Proposed* clinical hypothesis procedure evaluating:	• Symptom Magnification Frequency (SMF) > 40% • Extreme Beliefs Frequency (EBF) > 35% • Four other "validity" indicators (i.e., alienation, rating percent of max, % extreme ratings (2 scales)
Millon Behavioral Health Inventory (MBHI) (93)	Elevation on three built-in validity scales
Hendler Chronic Pain Screening Test (87)	• Scores of 21–31 (Exaggerating) • Scores >31 (Primary psychological influence)

Factors Suggestive of Significant Exaggeration, Illness Behavior or Malingering
Main & Spanswick Indicators (112)
• Failure to comply with reasonable treatment
• Report of severe pain with no associated psychological effects
• Marked inconsistencies in effects of pain on general activities
• Poor work record and history of persistent appeals against awards
• Previous litigation

These instruments are intended to be integrated with a thorough history taking, interview of patient and relevant others as available, and examination of relevant medical and allied health records.

The understanding derived from a comprehensive biopsychosocial pain assessment provides the framework for designing individually tailored treatment interventions and recommendations. Examining the impact of various cognitive processes on the subjective perception of the patient's pain is a critical component of this comprehensive assessment. Turk (113) has emphasized the importance of understanding and addressing the important role of patient pain appraisals, beliefs and expectancies. He, and others (e.g., Asmundson, Nicholas & Carleton (114)), note that patients with chronic pain resulting from traumatic events are predisposed to experiencing physical sensations as harmful and noxious which increases both anxiety and subjective pain perceptions. This, in turn, leads to further activity avoidance and functional limitations that block recovery and facilitate increased deconditioning, creating increased risk for developing chronic and disabling pain.

Important psychoemotional components relevant to the assessment of chronic pain (115) include: the subjective experience of pain; autonomic arousal associated with bodily reactions to pain; cognitive appraisal(s) of the painful experience as related to the personal meaning of the pain or the historically learned responses to pain and injury; nonverbal behaviors including facial expressions and body language associated with pain; and affective reactions to pain, including anxiety and depression. Persons with chronic pain have a much higher predilection and incidence of depression and anxiety as well as anger. A diathesis-stress model has been proposed to explain the higher rate of depression in this patient population, and likely applies to other psychoemotional responses to chronic pain (116).

Finally, pain assessment and treatment strategies are best conceptualized in terms of suitability to a multidimensional process that evolves significantly as it persists over time. The stages of pain processing model (117–119) is an illustrative model that distinguishes the sensory, affective, cognitive-evaluative, and behavioral dimensions of pain as it changes with increasing chronicity. The first two stages involve sensory discrimination and associated affective responses. The former is commonly assessed by ratings of pain intensity and location, while the latter is assessed by ratings of pain unpleasantness. The third stage involves the meaning and implications of pain for the patient and associated emotional suffering, and is commonly assessed by measuring pain-related emotional states (e.g., depression, anxiety, frustration) and beliefs (e.g., perceived ability to control or endure pain). The fourth stage refers to illness behavior (e.g., lifestyle and role disruption, avoidance) and can be assessed through self and collaborated ratings and observation (e.g., pain behaviors manifested at home, work, clinical interview). As pain persists, there is a transition of the focus of assessment from the first two stages to the latter two.

Response Bias Assessment

Diagnosis and treatment is the usual reason for assessment of chronic pain, along with impairment and disability evaluation in compensation situations. Importantly, assessments can involve contexts with strong financial, personal, social and/or other incentives. Hence, chronic pain patients may present with response bias, or the tendency to report or present pain or related disability in a less than fully truthful, accurate or valid fashion. For example, many assessments occur in such forensic contexts as health care insurance policy coverage, disability insurance policy application, social security disability application, personal injury litigation, worker's compensation claims, functional capacity evaluations and determination of capacity for work. These contexts often present strong financial (120) and numerous other and often more powerful vocational, social, personal and other incentives (see Martelli, Nicholson et al., Chapter 64, in this text).

Response bias in pain presentation can range from symptom minimization to symptom exaggeration and malingering. Hence, assessment of examinee veracity in report and attribution of symptoms, and motivation during presentation and assessment, becomes critical with regard to increasing diagnostic accuracy. This is prerequisite to provision of appropriate and timely treatment, prevention of iatrogenic impairment and disability reinforcement, and appropriate legal compensation decisions (Martelli, Nicholson, Zasler & Bender, Chapter 64 in this text).

A thorough analysis of response bias in chronic pain is beyond the scope of this chapter. Chapters that more fully explore the topic of response bias assessment in chronic pain can be found in Martelli, Zasler, Nicholson et al. (121) and Nicholson and Martelli (36). Chapter 64 in this text is specifically devoted to the general assessment of response bias and provides background, relevant measures and a general model for assessment. Measures specific to response bias regarding pain report are included, and readers are referred to that chapter for a detailed review. Additional pain response bias measures with potential utility are included in Table 39-3.

Importantly, because Chapter 64 emphasizes assessment of neurocognitive response bias, additional clarification of the unique nature of pain and the challenges in pain assessment is indicated. Pain, unlike cognitive impairment from brain injury, is a subjective complaint that is more viscerally, directly and universally noxious. It is much more difficult to assess than neurocognitive impairment due to limitations of existing measures and is, in fact, extremely difficult to verify or refute. (122–128). Assessment of pain presents a significant diagnostic challenge for all but the most conspicuous cases of severe, functionally disabling physical pathology. The advances that are being made in assessment, treatment and outcomes in chronic pain owe to new biopsychosocial models and psychophysiological advancements. These are based on discarding simple dichotomous models in favor of evidence of central processing factors and psychophysiologic etiologies, as a preponderance of data are accumulating to indicate that chronic pain is often represented in dysfunctional cerebral processing and not only the same peripheral mechanisms as acute pain on which medical assessments are more usually conducted (24, 35).

Unfortunately, there remains predominant overrepresentation of simplistic and uninformed dichotomous pain conceptualizations. These persist despite failed attempts to make dichotomous discriminations between "organic" and "nonorganic" pain using either medical or psychological measures. For example, in Fishbain et al's (126, 127) metaanalytic review, it was concluded that the Waddell signs, the most relied upon measure of "nonorganicity" in medicine and physical therapy, are invalid. That is, even when properly used, they do not discriminate organic from nonorganic problems, are associated with higher pain levels, may represent an organic phenomenon and are neither correlated with psychological distress or secondary gain. It shouldn't be surprising that many psychological measures have proven inadequate, given that they were derived from prediction of physical measures of nonorganicity that were invalid.

The lack of any reliable or valid measures of presence or degree of pain and pain exaggeration or malingering necessarily weakens the utility of psychological measures designed to make such predictions. Nonetheless, attempts to develop methods and guidelines for the detection of response bias and malingered pain are continuing. Malingering, or the act of willful, deliberate, and fraudulent feigning, or significant exaggeration of pain is only one variant of response bias, and an extreme one. The presence of response bias, which may not be an uncommon response to aversive stimuli, is much more easily documented than malingering. However, the two are often confounded and used synonymously in professional neuropsychological publications and practice, where response bias measures are frequently referred to, explicitly or implicitly, as "malingering tests". Inferences about malingering, especially in a restrictive health care environment with strong gate keeping pressures, are inherently problematic. In the absence of dependent measures or clinical methods with demonstrated validity for assessment of possible malingering of pain, inferences about pain malingering using current measures and procedures necessarily produce fallible judgments with unknown false positive rates.

Despite the absence of reliable or valid measures and methodologies for detecting degree of pain exaggeration or malingering (35, 124, 128–130), estimates, unreliable as they must be, have been proffered. Fishbain (124) in his systematic review of available samples and methodologies estimated that malingering may occur in 1.25 – 10.4% of chronic pain patients, while Mendelson and Mendelson (129) concluded that notable exaggeration or malingering of chronic pain across settings is less than 20%.

However, it must be emphasized that, in the case of chronic pain, malingering and exaggeration are usually distinct entities that are not simply differentiated by degree. Exaggeration, which appears much more commonly, can be distinguished from malingering in several important ways. While deliberate exaggeration and malingering are typically driven by external monetary or other incentives, chronic pain mechanisms frequently involve dysregulation of central pain processing mechanisms and derive from exaggerated neurophysiologic pain responses (see Zasler, et al., Chapter 41 in this text), including allodynia (pain from stimuli that are not usually painful), hyperalgesia (increased response to painful stimuli) and hyperesthesia (abnormal acuteness of sensitivity to sensory stimuli). In addition, suboptimal psychological adaptation to chronic pain frequently involves catastrophization and related processes rather than exaggeration for purposes of monetary or other secondary gain. Finally, pain is, by nature, highly aversive and associated with physiologic and behavioral avoidance reflexes that are genetically programmed and present at birth, and accompanied by anxieties and aversive emotions that are both highly conditionable and strongly and inherently disruptive of adaptive behavior. This not only makes differentiating exaggerated from non-exaggerated pain responses difficult and necessarily reliant on value judgments, but represents a clearly distinct phenomenon in contrast with exaggeration for the purposes of secondary gain.

The task of making determinations regarding genuine pain severity and impact and related functional impairment and disability is complicated by numerous factors. These factors are not necessarily fully appreciated except by the most informed chronic pain management specialists, and usually misunderstood by nonspecialists. These factors should be considered as reasons for considerable caution in making inferences about response bias and malingering during chronic pain assessments. In brief summary, they include:

- The subjective and complex nature of pain, as previously noted;
- The lack of valid measures of presence, severity, exaggeration or malingering of pain;
- The lack of formal, scientifically validated conceptual models and "rating systems" of pain associated impairment and disability;
- Numerous methodological problems with response bias assessment measures generally, including those designed for domains that are much easier to assess than chronic pain (e.g., problems with reliability, validity; sensitivity, specificity, misclassification, generalizability, lack of mutual exclusion, etc.; see Chapter 64 in this text for a review of generally problems with available response bias measures)
- The challenge of disentangling not only the multiple contributors to subjective pain experience, but also to associated functional disability;
- The context of assessment, where referral may be for treatment or compensation (e.g., where the latter is typically associated with higher rates of response bias and malingering; see Chapter 64 in this text) and numerous factors may be exerting motivational influence

- The nature of aversive events and anxiety, which are known to produce strong classical and operant conditioning, especially relating to avoidance behavior, and to decompensate efficient behavior and adaptation in animals and humans. That is, pain, by its aversive nature, predisposes organisms to avoidance as a typically adaptive, biological survival mechanism. However, the presence of anxiety, distress and avoidance behavior is often misinterpreted as a sign of "nonorganicity", exaggeration and/or malingering in physical examinations, or as a psychogenic etiologic factor, when evidence indicates it is most often a reaction to pain or an indicator of severity (14, 59, 126, 127). The failure of the highly relied upon Waddell signs as a purported indicator of nonorganicity, and the evidence that they are in fact not associated with secondary gain and appear more associated with organic phenomenon and severity of pain, is a good illustration of how this misconception has contributed to misdiagnosis and associated misunderstanding and mistreatment of persons with chronic pain.
- Western cultural tendencies to interpret distress responses and avoidance to aversive pain experience as inherently pathological. Evidence of this comes from the misrepresentation and misinterpretation of the "fight-flight" response. The overwhelming majority of ethological and human evidence indicates that flight attempts almost invariably precede fight attempts in coping with aversive events, in the following sequence: freeze, flee, fight, fright (131). In fact, adaptation to chronic pain requires learning to overcome the avoidance responses that are innate to all organisms.
- The distinct nature of exaggeration versus malingering of pain. Mechanisms underlying development of central and peripheral sensitization that lead to allodynia and hyperesthesia are becoming better understood. These, by definition and appearance, represent an exaggerated response. However, they are neurophysiologically based and not driven by external incentives like secondary gain. Similarly, pain catastrophization and related processes represents an exaggerated pain response, but are explained by suboptimal psychological coping and must be differentiated from deliberate exaggeration for purposes of secondary gain.
- The critically important distinction between acute and chronic pain. Chronic pain is distinct from acute pain not only with regard to the absence of clearly identifiable peripheral tissue damage or neuroanatomical pathways, but, as recent neuroscience evidence shows, also in terms of how it is processed in the central nervous system. In addition to previously noted differences, recent reviews of functional

neuroimaging studies clearly demonstrate that chronic pain is processed differently than acute pain both in terms of the lateral versus medial pain systems and the activation of affective-evaluative mechanisms (see Zasler, et al, chapter 39 in this text, or Apakarian (6) for a review). When these distinctions are blurred, and chronic pain is assessed in terms of standards for acute pain, as is generally practiced in medicine and psychology, the absence of clearly identifiable pain triggers and greater emotional activation leads to conclusions that erroneously infer deliberate exaggeration and malingering. Given strong external incentives in a restrictive health care environment (Martelli et al, in Chapter 64 of this text) with increasing preponderance of insurance and adversarial medicolegal referrals, an inflation of false positive diagnoses of malingering might be expected.

The unique nature of chronic pain and limitations with regard to its assessment require caution with regard to over-interpretation of response bias procedures and emphasize the importance of integrating multiple data sources and making thoughtful inferences only after integration of thorough historical information, interview, assessment, behavioral observations, collaborative interview and data sources, and so on. Importantly, Martelli (132) and Nicholson (133) have argued that assessments conducted by persons without specialty chronic pain training and experience likely violate professional ethical standards.

PAIN MANAGEMENT

Early after the emergence of pain, and when pain is in the acute stage, treatment nterventions invariably address amelioration of distress, correction of underlying pathophysiology and promotion of healing. Inherent in all pain management interventions is the prevention of chronicity, which is undoubtedly the most important purpose and most effective accomplishment in pain management. Zasler et al. (Chapter 39 in this text) address the medical approaches involving assessment and treatment of acute pain. They emphasize the importance of effective assessment and treatment by using the compliment of medical and pharmacologic agents and other strategies designed to minimize distress while correcting underlying pathophysiology and restoring function. Although acute pain management interventions are primarily medical in nature, behavioral and psychological pain management interventions still play an important role in cases where associated psychological distress is significant, medical interventions do not produce expected pain relief, and/or where correction of pathology is complicated or where

traditional analgesic medications or other medical interventions cannot be employed.

Unfortunately, acute pain is not always resolved. As it persists, it becomes chronic and more intractable. The goal of preventing chronicity gradually transforms to include reducing the severity and persistence of pain related distress, associated psychological and physical symptoms, functional disability and life interference, and improving adaptation and coping with pain. Although the goals of comprehensive chronic pain management interventions can vary with individuals and settings, they can generally be summarized as addressing the following areas:

- Modulation and reduction of intensity, frequency and duration of sensory, as well as cognitive-evaluative and affective distress responses related to pain experience
- Modulation and reduction of associated physical and psychological symptoms and concomitants of pain, especially as they relate to mood and emotions, cognition, energy, sleep, eating, physiological arousal and general physical and emotional health
- Reduction of functional disability, maladaptive avoidance and illness behavior, and interference with regular and preferred activities, including regular daily activities and preferred family, social, avocational, vocational and recreational function and activities
- Increasing self management to actively utilize available strategies to minimize pain related distress, functional disability and life interference

Because persistent pain may be associated with a combination of physical and psychological factors, combination treatments and a multidisciplinary approach to chronic pain management, consisting of pain specialists in medicine, psychology, physical therapy, occupational and/or vocational and/or other allied health professions, are indicated. This approach is widely accepted as the most clinically successful and cost effective process in treating chronic pain (25, 134–137). This is best conducted, and can usually only be effectively accomplished, within the context of a specialty pain clinic. Specialty pain clinics are the treatment of choice for chronic pain conditions, with clinical efficacy supported by several recent reviews (134, 138–141). Referral to pain management specialists and specialty pain clinics should be considered the standard of care for the treatment of persons with chronic pain.

When the person with pain has also sustained a TBI, additional recommendations are warranted. In persons with TBI and pain, there is evidence that pain is harder to manage (29), that it takes longer to complete a pain management program (142), and that special attention is required because of cognitive difficulties (26).

Hence, referral to pain specialty pain programs with experience in treating persons with TBI, and/or consultation with such providers to allow expectation of extended treatment periods and incorporation of cognitive compensatory strategies, is indicated

Model for Conceptualizing Chronic Pain Treatments

There is considerable evidence and growing acceptance that many or most forms of chronic pain involve central and/or peripheral sensitization (143). Evidence for a neuromuscular conceptualization of many chronic pain problems has grown very fast and represents a convergence of findings across multiple specialties (38). Most forms of chronic pain are now considered (4, 5, 26, 38, 144) to possibly include a hyper-responsiveness of the pain system involving "wind up" or sensitization in the CNS / brain. Conceptually, the thrust of current efforts in chronic pain management seem to be toward "desensitization" of the CNS through combination treatments. In addition, multidisciplinary and multicomponent or combination treatment packages represent the most effective treatments in chronic pain, especially when comorbid with brain injury (3, 20, 31).

The authors have proposed a preliminary classification model for planning and conceptualizing chronic pain management interventions (143, 31). This model, summarized in Table 39-4, can include combination of any of the included treatments. It facilitates the classification of currently available and potentially useful chronic pain treatment approaches according to specific area and manner of desensitization targeted, which can include any of the treatments included. This model offers

a potentially useful classification system for conceptually organizing the wide variety of available treatment interventions and in planning combination treatments.

It should be noted that Tyrer and Lievesley (145), among others, recommend the development of pain management facilities specifically designed for persons with brain injuries. The emotional disturbances associated with pain are also frequently comorbid with TBI, highlighting the importance of a biopsychosocial perspective. Such a perspective allows for a holistic conceptualization of the patient, incorporating multimethod, multimodal assessments that facilitate individualized treatment planning. Treatment goals include not only the reduction/relief from pain, but also increased self-control, increased adaptation to life changes secondary to pain and brain injury, and improved functioning and quality of life.

Behavioral–Psychological Management

Behavioral and psychological services are an important component of comprehensive pain management services. A review by McCracken and Turk (146) identified more than 200 studies confirming that behavioral medicine interventions such as cognitive-behavioral therapy, biofeedback, and relaxation, are effective in reducing pain and pain related distress. Table 39-5 includes a summary of some of the most frequently used and empirically supported strategies. This table borrows from the review by Martelli et al. (3), but readers are referred to additional reading for more comprehensive summaries in the work of McQuay and Moore (147), reviews of evidence-based recommendations for management of chronic non-malignant pain (e.g., College of Physicians and Surgeons (148)), or the

---

TABLE 39-4
A Desensitization Model for Chronic Pain Treatment Interventions

Desensitizing Peripheral CNS Procedures
- EMG and Temperature Biofeedback; Various Relaxation and Imagery Procedures; Transcutaneous Electrical Nerve Stimulation (TENS)

Desensitizing CNS Medications
- Anti-epileptic drugs, tizanidine HCL, Amytal, neuroimmunomodulators, SSRI's etc.

Desensitizing Behavioral Activity Procedures
- Operant behavioral activity programs; graduated exposure / graduated activity programs; relaxation, imagery, refocusing; cognitive behavioral reinterpretive strategies

Desensitizing Psychotherapeutic Procedures
- Emotional desensitization of catastrophic reaction to injury and pain and other fears and trauma; splinting of emotional reactions and calming of catastrophic reactions and hypervigilance to pain; specific formal pain and fear desensitization procedures; pain exposure / desensitization procedures; cognitive behavioral reinterpretive strategies

Desensitizing Neurophysiologic Procedures
- Cranioelectrotherapy Stimulation (CES). Consider EEG Biofeedback or other potentially helpful adjunctive relaxation procedures such as sound and light (AudioVisualStimulation, AVS) and Transcranial Magnetic Stimulation and Brain Electrical Stimulation.

TABLE 39-5
Summary of Useful Behavioral Treatments for Chronic Pain

Patient Education: The most conspicuous and malleable factor that contributes to psychophysiologic arousal and stress responding is patient expectancy and knowledge about symptom management. For example, Ham and Packard (154) found that headache patients that desired an explanation of their headache at least as much as pain relief. In the case of mild TBI, education about expected symptoms and course has been shown to reduce the anxiety and selective attention and misattribution that can unnecessarily prolong symptoms (155). The best education treatment packages generally contain elements targeting numerous factors. Accurate information and expectancies help with this and also assist with coping with pain more adaptively. Stress management information and strategies can assist with reducing sympathetic arousal / discharge that exacerbates pain, while specific postural training and sleep hygiene can assist with postural rehabilitation and normalizing sleep patterns.

Cognitive-Behavioral Treatments: Cognitive approaches incorporate the physical, psychological and behavioral aspects of the pain experience in promoting patient self management of pain. They typically emphasize learning of self regulation and self control skills and taking greater personal responsibility for lifestyle habit change, especially with regard to identifying and replacing maladaptive beliefs about pain. Specific training is provided in cognitive strategies and skills to replace such inappropriate negative expectations and beliefs as catastrophization and associated magnification, rumination and helplessness that maintain physiologic arousal and maladaptive avoidance and illness behaviors that complicate symptom resolution (113). A comprehensive multimodal approach should include education, skills acquisition, cognitive and behavioral rehearsal, homework and generalization and maintenance (156).

Relaxation Training: Progressive muscle relaxation (PMR) is the most studied relaxation procedure (157). PMR involves the systematic tensing and relaxing of various muscle groups to elicit a deepening relaxation response, usually with combination of muscle groups and addition of diaphragmatic breathing to shorten the protocol. Meta-analytic reviews generally conclude that relaxation training and biofeedback training are equally effective. Relaxation training presumable serves to (1) reduce proprioceptive input to the hypothalamus, thereby decreasing sympathetic nervous system activity (150) and (2) directly reduce muscle tension or pre-headache vasoconstriction (158).

Operant Treatment: Operant based treatment strategies require altering environmental contingencies to eliminate reinforcement of pain and illness behaviors (e.g., verbal complaints, inactivity, avoidance) while rewarding "well" behaviors (e.g., incrementally increased exercise, activity level, involvement and participation).

Biofeedback: Extensive research supports the utility of EMG or thermal biofeedback for headache pain, and chronic musculoskeletal pain disorders more generally. The forehead, trapezii, frontal-posterior neck, and neck areas are frequent EMG feedback sites. Patterns of pathophysiologic neuromuscular activity that underlie pain complaint and functional limitations, which can be remediated through feeding back physiologic information to allow self-correction, include: a) Stress-related hyperarousal in musculoskeletal or other physiologic systemts; b) Postural dysfunction; c) Hyper- or hypo- tonicity induced by reflex systems activated by inflammation, active trigger points and cumulative strain or recurrent trauma; d) Learned guarding or bracing to mitigate anticipated pain or injury; e) Learned inhibition or avoidance of muscle activation / activity; e) Chronic compensation for joint hypermobility/hypomobility (e.g., muscles taking over the role of damaged joint tissue); f) Faulty motor schema and muscle imbalance reflecting development of one or more of the preceding syndromes, and resulting in the lack of coordination and stability between typically coordinated muscle groups. Recently, data are emerging which indicates that EEG biofeedback, and associated EEG driven stimulation offers efficacy in treatment of some persistent pain and persistent post-concussive symptoms (159, 160). Finally, evidence has been reported that individuals can gain specific voluntary control over rostral anterior cingulate activation to directly control pain perception in severe, chronic clinical pain (161).

Social and Assertiveness Skills Training: Skills training may help some patients with more effective communication of needs. Increased need fulfillment decreases distressful emotions which reduces physiological arousal that contributes to pain experience (162).

Imagery and Hypnosis: Using some combination of autohypnosis, suggestions of relaxation and visual imagery, patients are generally instructed to visualize the pain (i.e., give it form) and focus on altering the image to reduce the pain. Imagery based treatment is most effective following establishment of a good therapeutic alliance in order to facilitate compliance (163).

Habit Reversal: These treatment packages teach pain patients to detect, interrupt, and reverse maladaptive habits (e.g., maladaptive head/jaw posture, jaw tension, negative cognitions). Specific skills are taught to both reverse poor functional habits and stressful thoughts as well as feelings that precipitate/perpetuate them (164).

many systematic reviews prepared for the Cochrane Collaboration (149). Although there is a paucity of studies examining pain management in persons with TBI, the interventions used are the same, qualified by understanding that treatment may take somewhat longer and require cognitive compensatory strategies, commensurate with cognitive impairments, to assist with learning.

When persons with TBI initially present to psychologists for pain management services, the initial assessment process is always benefited by establishment of a therapeutic rapport. This includes countering any patient resistances or misconceptions (e.g., that pain must be in "their head" because they are seeing a psychologist) and engendering accurately informed and hopeful expectancies. Psychological management of persons with pain and TBI begins with an assessment that identifies all variables relevant for treatment. In addition to areas such as personality and emotional status, coping style and strategies, social support, and pain specific factors (see Table 39-3 and preceding pain assessment section), evaluation must also include specific sequelae associated with brain injury. An integration of this information is necessary to ensure that the full constellation of residual sequelae and strengths are considered to optimize an individually designed treatment plan that anticipates and implements compensatory strategies for all potential obstacles to benefit from behavioral interventions. For example, deficits in memory, attention, or executive functioning might be addressed through task-analytic instruction and compensatory memory notebooks with provision of external reminders for completion of at-home assignments. The patients specifically tailored treatment plan should provide a framework and outline for treatment, define goals and patient / therapist expectations and sequences, and provide psychoeducational information about the particular type of chronic pain and rationale for treatment.

Despite the previously noted dearth of outcome studies examining the behavioral treatment of pain after traumatic brain injury, the available literature suggests general similarities in clinical presentations, pathophysiologies and treatment responses, with somewhat greater similarities for traumatic versus not traumatic chronic pain, and some evidence suggesting greater treatment resistance for the latter type (150).

In cases of post traumatic pain, the severity and frequency of pain attacks or exacerbations and chronic pain-related sequelae such as coping abilities, depression, and anxiety are significantly improved by combined psychological treatment protocols (64, 151–153). Supportive counseling that begins early after trauma and is continuous results in better patient response (64).

Table 39-5 includes a summary of some of the most frequently used and empirically supported strategies (3), but readers are again referred to additional reading for more comprehensive summaries (McQuay & Moore (147);

College of Physicians and Surgeons (148); The Cochrane Library (149)).

Conclusion

Chronic pain is a frequent concomitant of TBI. However, the assessment and treatment of persons with pain is a complicated and challenging process. Pain, by itself, can have a more disabling effect across a wider range of functions than brain or many other types of injuries. In addition to the absence of clear and objective measures for assessment and monitoring of pain, pervasive misconceptions dominate modern medical and psychological practice. Fortunately, recent advances in chronic pain assessment and treatment can be attributed to adoption of a biopsychosocial perspective. The most promising current treatment interventions are combination treatments that are holistic in nature and target the patient's reaction to pain within his/her daily life and ability to exercise self-control. Multicomponent treatment packages are currently the preferred treatment choice for chronic pain (3, 20, 162), especially when it accompanies TBI. The current chapter is intended to promote familiarity with many important issues and current knowledge required to increase awareness and understanding of psychological approaches to assessment and management of pain in persons with TBI. This will hopefully assist with the making of appropriate referrals, and promoting effective carryover and integration of pain management principles into care of persons with concomitant TBI.

*R*eferences

1. Merskey H, Bogduk N (eds.):*Classification of Chronic Pain*. 2nd Ed., IASP Press: Seattle, 1994.
2. Kulich RJ, Baker WB: A guide for psychological testing and evaluation for chronic pain. In Aranoff GM (ed.) *Evaluation and Treatment of Chronic Pain*, pp. 301–312. Baltimore, MD: Williams and Wilkins, 1999
3. Martelli MF, Grayson R, Zasler ND: Post-traumatic headache: Psychological and neuropsychological issues in assessment and treatment. *J Head Trauma Rehabil* 1999;1:49–69.
4. Nicholson K: Pain associated with lesion, disorder or dysfunction of the central nervous sytem. *NeuroRehabilitation* 2000b;14(1): 3–14.
5. Nicholson K: At the crossroads: Pain in the 21st century. *NeuroRehabilitation* 2000c;14(2):57–68.
6. Apkarian AV, Bushnell MC, Treede RD, Zubieta JK: Human brain mechanisms of pain perception and regulation in health and disease. *Eur J Pain.* 2005;9(4):463–484.
7. Wager, T. D., Rilling, J. K., Smith, E. E., Sokolik, A., Casey, K. L., Davidson, R.J., Kosslyn, S. M., Rose, R. M. & Cohen, J. D. (2004). Placebo-induced changes in FMRI in the anticipation and experience of pain. *Science*, 303, 1162–1167.
8. Apkarian AV, Sosa Y, Sonty S, Levy RM, Harden RN, Parrish TB, Gitelman DR. Chronic back pain is associated with decreased prefrontal and thalamic gray matter density *J Neurosci.* 2004; 24(46):10410–5.
9. Salomons TV, Johnstone T, Backonja MM, Davidson RJ: Perceived Controllability Modulates the Neural Response to Pain. *J of Neurosci* 2004;24(32):7199–7203.
10. Giesecke T, Gracely RH, Grant MA, Nachemson A, Petzke F, Williams DA, Clauw DJ: Evidence of augmented central pain

processing in idiopathic chronic low back pain. *Arthritis Rheum.* 2004;50(2):613–23.

11. Flor H: Cortical Reorganization and Chronic Pain: Implications for Rehabilitation. *J Rehabil Med* 2003;41:66–72.

12. Porro CA: Functional Imaging and Pain: Behavior, Perception, and Modulation. *Neuroscientist* 2003;9(5):354–369.

13. Zasler, N.D., Martelli, M.F. Nicholson K: Post-traumatic pain disorders: Medical Assessment and Management. In:*Brain Injury Medicine: Principles and Practice.* N. Zasler, D. Katz, R. Zafonte (Eds.). New York. Demos Publishers. In preparation.

14. Hinnant DW: Psychological evaluation and testing. In Tollison DC, Satterwhite JR, Tollison JW (eds.) *Handbook of Chronic Pain Management*, pp. 18–35. Baltimore, MD: Williams & Wilkins, 1994.

15. Turk DC, Holzman AD: Chronic pain: Interfaces among physical, psychological and social parameters. In Holzman AD, Turk DC (eds.) *Pain Management: A Handbook of Psychological Treatment Approaches*, pp. 1–9). New York, Pergammon Press, 1986.

16. Fordyce WE: Pain and suffering: A reappraisal, *Am Psychol* 1988; 43:276–283.

17. World Health Organization: International Classification of Impairments, Disabilities and Handicaps. Geneva: WHO, 1980.

18. American Psychiatric Association, *Diagnostic and Statistical Manual of Mental Disorders*, 4th Edition. American Psychiatric Association: Washington, 1994.

19. Bryant RA, Marosszeky JE, Crooks J, Baguley IJ, Gurka JA: Interaction of posttraumatic stress disorder and chronic pain following traumatic brain injury. *J Head Trauma Rehabil* 1999;14: 588–594.

20. Miller L: Neurosensitization: A model for persistent disability in chronic pain, depression, and posttraumatic stress disorder following injury. *Neurorehabilitation*, 2000;14:1,25–32.

21. Sharp TJ & Harvey AG: Chronic pain and posttraumtic stress disorder: Mutual maintenance? *Clin Psychol Rev* 2001;21:857–877.

22. Williams WH, Evans JE: Brain injury and emotion: An overview to a special issue on biopsychosocial approaches in neurorehabilitation. *Neuropsychol Rehabil* 2003;13(1/2):1–11.

23. Schreiber S, Galai-Gati T: Uncontrolled pain following physical injury as the core-trauma in post-traumatic stress disorder. *Pain* 1993;54(1):107–110.

24. Nicholson K, Martelli MF, Zasler ND: Myths and misconceptions about chronic pain: The problem of mind body dualism. In Weiner RB (ed.) *Pain Management: A Practical Guide for Clinicians*, 6th edition, pp. 465–474. Boca Ratan, FL: St. Lucie Press, 2002.

25. Branca B, Lake AE: Psychological and Neuropsychological Integration in Multidisciplinary Pain Management After TBI. *J Head Trauma Rehabil* 2004;19(1):40-57.

26. Nicholson K: Pain, Cognition and Traumatic Brain Injury. *NeuroRehabilitation* 2000a;14:95–104.

27. Evans RW: Post-traumatic headaches. In Evans RW (Ed.) *Neurologic Clinics*, 22(1), 237–249. Philadelphia: Saunders, 2004.

28. Zasler ND, Martelli MF: Post-traumatic headache: Practical approaches to diagnosis and treatment. In Weiner RB (ed.) *Pain Management: A Practical Guide for Clinicians*, 6th edition. Boca Ratan, FL: St. Lucie Press, 2002.

29. Lahz S. Bryant RA: Incidence of Chronic Pain Following Traumatic Brain Injury, *Arch Phys Med Rehabil.* 1996;77:889–891.

30. Mahmood O, Rapport LJ, Hanks RA, Fichtenberg NL: Neuropsychological performance and sleep disturbance following traumatic brain injury. *J Head Trauma Rehabil* 2004;19(5): 378–90.

31. Zasler ND, Martelli MF, Nicholson K: Chronic Pain (and Traumatic Brain Injury). In Silver JM, McAllister TW, Yudofsky SC (eds) *Textbook of Traumatic Brain Injury.* Arlington, VA: American Psychiatric Publishing, 2005.

32. Hart RP, Martelli MF, Zasler ND: Chronic pain and neuropsychological functioning. *Neuropsychol Rev* 2000;10(3):131–149.

33. Martelli MF, Zasler ND, Nicholson K and Hart RP: Masquerades of Brain Injury. Part I: Chronic pain and traumatic brain injury. *The Journal of Controversial Medical Claims* 2001;8(2):1–8.

34. Hart RP, Wade JB, Martelli MF: Cognitive Impairment in Patients with Chronic Pain: The Significance of Stress. *Current Pain and Headache Reports.* 7:116–226. 2003.

35. Nicholson K, Martelli MF: The problem of Pain. *J Head Trauma Rehabil* 2004;19(1):2–9.

36. Nicholson K, Martelli MF: Malingering Motivation and Compensation. In Young G, Kane A, Nicholson K (Eds) *Causality: Psychological Evidence for Court.* Springer, New York, in press.

37. Martelli MF: Pain, the Brain and Neuropsychological Effects. Workshop presented at the 33rd annual meeting of the International Neuropsychological Society (INS), St. Louis, 2005a. Downloadable at: http://villamartelli.com/#TLK Direct Link: http://villamartelli.com/INS_2005PainBrainFinal2.pdf

38. Jay GW, Krusz JC, Longmire DR, McLain, DA:*Current Trend in the Diagnosis and Treatment of Chronic Neuromuscular Pain Syndromes: Myofascial Pain Syndrome, Chronic Tension-Type Headache, and Fibromyalgia.* Sonora. CA: American Academy of Pain Management, 2001.

39. Mooney G, Speed J, Sheppard S: Factors related to recovery after mild traumatic brain injury. *Brain Injury* 2005;19(12):975–87.

40. Pilcher JJ, Huffcutt AL: Effects of sleep deprivation on performance: A meta analysis. *Sleep* 1996;19:318-326.

41. Kundermann B, Krieg JC, Schreiber W, Lautenbacher S: The effect of sleep deprivation on pain. *Pain Res Manag.* 2004;9(1): 25–32.

42. Beetar JT, Guilmette TJ, Sparadeo FR: Sleep and pain complaints in symptomatic traumatic brain injury and neurologic populations. *Arch Phys Med Rehabil* 1996;77(12):1298–302.

43. Porro CA, Baraldi P, Pagnoni G, Serafini M, Facchin P, Maieron M, Nichelli P: Does anticipation of pain affect cortical nociceptive systems? *J Neurosci.* 2002;15;22(8):3206–14.

44. Martelli MF, Zasler ND, MacMillan P: Mediating the relationship between injury, impairment and disability: A vulnerability, stress & coping model of adaptation following brain injury. *NeuroRehabilitation:An interdisciplinary journal* 1998;11(1):51–66.

45. Martelli MF, Zasler ND, Mancini AM, MacMillan P: Psychological assessment and applications in impairment and disability evaluations. In May RV, Martelli MF (eds.) *Guide to Functional Capacity Evaluation with Impairment Rating Applications*, pp.3-1–3-84. Midlothian, VA: NADEP Publications, 1999.

46. Gatchel RJ. Turk DC (eds.):*Psychosocial Factors in Pain.* New York: The Guilford Press, 1999.

47. Schnall E: Pain assessment and the mental health practitioner: A mind-body approach. *Einstein Journal of Biological Medicine* 2003;20:10–13.

48. Hadjistavropoulos T, von Baeyer C, Craig KD: Pain assessment in persons with limited ability to communicate. In Turk DC, Melzack R (eds) *Handbook of pain assessment*, 2nd edition. New York: The Guilford Press, pp. 134–149, 2001.

49. Martelli, MF and Zasler, ND: Useful psychological instruments for assessing persons with functional medical disorders. In Zasler ND, Martelli MF (eds):*Functional Medical Disorders, State of the Art Reviews in Physical Medicine and Rehabilitation*, pp. 147–162. Phila.:Hanley and Belfus, 2002.

50. Jensen MP, Karoly, P: Self-report scales and procedures for assessing pain in adults. In Turk DC, Melzack R (eds.) *Handbook of pain assessment*, 2nd edition. New York: The Guilford Press, pp. 15–34, 2001.

51. Whaley LF, Wong DL:*Nursing Care of Infants and Children*, 3rd ed. St Louis: Mosby, 1987.

52. Gracely RH, McGrath P, and Dubner R. Ratio scales of sensory and affective verbal pain descriptors. *Pain* 1978;5:5–18.

53. Rainsford AO, Cairns D, Mooney V: The pain drawing as an aid to the psychologic evaluation of patients with lower back pain. *Spine* 1974;1:127–134

54. Margolis RB, Tait RC, Krause SJ: A rating system for use with patient pain drawings. *Pain* 1986;24:57–65.

55. Melzack R: The Short-Form McGill Pain Questionnaire. *Pain* 1987;30:191–197.

56. Jensen M.P: The validity and reliability of pain measures in adults with cancer. *J Pain* 2003;4(1):2-21.

57. Turk DC, Burwinkle TM: Assessment of chronic pain in rehabilitation: Outcomes measures in clinical trials and clinical practice. *Rehabil Psychol.* 2005;50(1):56–64.

58. Knott C, Beyer J, Villarruel A, Denyes M, Erickson, V, Willard G: Application of the Oucher in Practice: A developmental approach

to pain assessment in children. *Journal of Maternal-Child Nursing* 1994;19(6):314–320.

59. Hadjistavropoulos T, LaChapelle DL: Extent and nature of anxiety experience during physical examination of chronic low back pain. *Behavior Research and Therapy* 2000;38(1)13–18.

60. McGrath PA, Gillespie J: Pain assessment in children and adolescents. In: Turk DC, Melzack R (eds.) *Handbook of pain assessment*, 2nd edition, pp. 97–118. New York: The Guilford Press, 2001.

61. Gagliese L: Assessement of Pain in Elderly People. In Turk DC, Melzack R (eds.) *Handbook of pain assessment*, 2nd edition. New York: The Guilford Press, pp. 119–133, 2001.

62. Rudy TE, Turk DC:*Multiaxial assessment of pain: Multidimensional pain inventory computer program user manual version 2.1.* Pittsburgh, PA, University of Pittsburgh, 1989.

63. Turk DC: Cognitive behavioral techniques in the management of pain. In Foreyt JP, Rathjen RP (eds.) *Cognitive Behavior Therapy: Research and Application.* New York: Plenum Publishing Company, 1978.

64. Rosensteil AK, Keefe FJ: The use of coping strategies in chronic low back pain patients: Realtionship to patient characteristics and current adjustment. *Pain* 1983;17:33–44.

65. Söderlund A, Denison E: Classification of patients with whiplash associated disorders (WAD):Reliable and valid subgroups based on the Multidimensional Pain Inventory (MPI-S). *Eur J Pain* in press.

66. Tollison CD, Langley JC:*Pain Patient Profile (P3).* Minneapolis, MN: National Computer Systems; 1992.

67. Bruns D, Disorbio JM, Copeland-Disorbio J:*Battery for Health Improvement (BHI).* Minneapolis, MN: National Computer Systems; 1996.

68. Ruehlman LS, Karoly P, Newton C, Aiken LS: The development and preliminary validation of a brief measure of chronic pain impact for use in the general population. *Pain* 2005;113:82-90.

69. Ruehlman LS, Karoly P, Newton C, Aiken LS: The development and preliminary validation of the Profile of Chronic Pain: Extended Assessment Battery. *Pain* in press.

70. Kerns RD, Rosenberg R, Jamison RN, Caudille MA, Haythornthwait J: Readiness to adopt a self-management approach to chronic pain: the Pain Stages of Change Questionnaire (PSOCQ). *Pain* 1997;72(1–2):227–234.

71. Jensen MP, Nielson WR, Romano JM, Hill ML, Turner JA: Further evaluation of the pain stages of change questionnaire: is the transtheoretical model of change useful for patients with chronic pain? *Pain* 2000;86:255–264.

72. Burns JW, Glenn B, Lofland K, Bruehl S, Harden RN: Stages of change in readiness to adopt a self-management approach to chronic pain: the moderating role of early-treatment stage progression in predicting outcome. *Pain* 2005;115(3):322–31.

73. Kerns RD, Wagner J, Rosenberg R, Haythornthwaite J, Caudill-Slosberg M: Identification of subgroups of persons with chronic pain based on profiles on the pain stages of change questionnaire. *Pain* 2005;116(3):302–10.

74. Jensen MP, Turner JA, Romano JM, Lawler BK: Relationship of pain-specific beliefs to chronic pain adjustment. *Pain* 1994;57: 301–309.

75. Sullivan, MJL, Bishop S, Pivik J: The Pain Catastrophizing scale: development and validation. *Psychological Assessment* 1995; 7:524–532.

76. Thorn BE, Boothby JL, Sullivan MJL. Targeted treatment of catastrophizing for the management of chronic pain. *Cognitive and Behavioral Practice* 2002;9:127–138.

77. Crombez G, Bijttebier P, Eccleston C, Mascagni T, Mertens G, Goubert L, Verstraeten K: The child version of the pain catastrophizing scale (PCS-C):a preliminary validation. Pain. 2003 Aug;104(3):639–46.

78. McCracken LM, Zayfert C, Gross RT: The Pain Anxiety Symptoms Scale: development and validation of a scale to measure fear of pain. *Pain* 1992 Jul;50(1):67–73.

79. Todd DD: Kinesiophobia: The relationship between chronic pain and fear-induced disability. *The Forensic Examiner* 1998;7(5/6): 14–20.

80. Houben RM, Leeuw M, Vlaeyen JW, Goubert L, Picavet HS: Fear of Movement/Injury in the General Population: Factor Structure and Psychometric Properties of an Adapted Version of the Tampa Scale for Kinesiophobia. *J Behav Med.* 2005;27:1–10.

81. Todd DD, Martelli MF, Grayson, RL. *The Cogniphobia Scale (C-Scale):A measure of headache impact.* Glen Allen, VA: Concussion Care Centre of Virginia (Test in the public domain), 1998.

82. Jensen MP, Turner JA, Romano JM, Strom SE: The Chronic Pain Coping Inventory: development and preliminary validation. *Pain* 1995;60:203-216.

83. Geiser DS: A comparison of acceptance-focused and control-focused psychological treatments in a chronic pain treatment center, Unpublished doctoral dissertation, University of Nevada, Reno, 1992.

84. McCracken LM, Vowles KE, Eccleston C: Acceptance of chronic pain: component analysis and a revised assessment method. *Pain* 2004;107:159–166.

85. McCracken LM, Eccleston C. A comparison of the relative utility of coping and acceptance-based measures in a sample of chronic pain sufferers. *Eur J Pain* 2006;10(1):23–29.

86. Heaton RK, Lehman RAW, Getto CJ: Psychosocial Pain Inventory. Odessa, FL: Psychological Assessment Resources, 1985

87. Hendler N, Vienstein P, Gucer P, Long D: A preoperative screening test for chronic back pain patients. *Psychosomatics* 1979; 20:801–808.

88. Packard RC Ham LP: Impairment rating for posttraumatic headache. *Headache.* 1993;33(7):359–364.

89. Eimer BN, Allen LM: Psychological Assessment and Treatment of Chronic Pain and Related Disability. *User's Guide to the Pain Assessment Battery-Research Edition.* Durham, NC: CogniSyst, Inc. 1995.

90. Fairbank JC, Mbaot JC, Davies JB, O'Brien JP: The Oswestry low back pain and disability questionnaire. *Physiotherapy* 1980;66: 271–273.

91. Brown GK, Nicassio PM: The development of a questionnaire for the assessment of active and passive coping strategies in chronic pain patients. *Pain* 1987;31:53–65.

92. Butler R, Damarin F, Beaulieu C, Schwebel A, Doleys D: Assessing cognitive coping strategies for acute post-surgical pain. Psychological assessment. J Consult Clin Psychol 1989;1:41–45.

93. Millon T: The MBHI and the MBMD. In S. Strack (ed.) *Interpretive Strategies for the Millon Inventories.* New York: Wiley, 1999.

94. Ware JE, Kosinski M, Gandek B: SF-36 *Health Survey: Manual and interpretation guide.* Lincoln, RI: QualityMetric, Inc., 2000.

95. Callahan CD, Young PL, Barisa MT: Using the SF-36 for longitudinal outcomes in rehabilitation. *Rehabil Psychol* 2005;50(1): 65–70.

96. Kreutzer JS, Marwitz JH, Seel R, Serio CD: Validation of a neurobehavioral functioning inventory for adults with traumatic brain injury. *Arch Phys Med Rehabil.* 1996;77:116–124.

97. Bergner M, Bobbitt RA, Carter WB, Gilson BS: The Sickness Impact Profile, Development and final revision of a health status measure. *Medical Care* 1981;19:787–805.

98. Pilowsky I, Spence ND: Patterns of illness behavior in patients with intractable pain. *J Psychosom Res* 1975;19:279–287.

99. Pilowsky I, Spence ND: Illness behavior syndromes associated with intractable pain. *Pain* 1976;2:61–71.

100. Beck AT, Ward CH, Mendelson M, Mock J, Erbaugh, J: An inventory for measuring depression. *Arch Gen Psychiatry* 1961;4: 561–571.

101. Fordyce WE: Use of the MMPI in the Assessment of Chronic Pain. In Butcher J, Dahlstrom G, Schofield W (eds.) *Clinical Notes on the MMPI.* Number three in the series. University of Washington Press, 1983.

102. Zeigler DK, Paolo AM: Headache symptoms and psychological profile of headache-prone individuals: A comparison of clinic patients and controls. *Arch Neurol* 1995;52(6):602–606.

103. Skevington SM: A standardized scale to measure beliefs about controlling pain (BPCQ):A preliminary study. *Psychology and Health* 1990;4:221–232.

104. Beck AT:*Beck Anxiety Inventory*(r) (BAI(r)) San Antonio: Harcourt Assessment, Inc., 1990, 1993.

105. Cocchiarella L, Andersson GBJ (eds.):*Guides to the evaluation of permanent impairment, 5th edition.* Chicago, AMA Press, 2001

106. Dahlstrom WG, Welsh GS & Dahlstrom LE:*An MMPI handbook: Research applications (Vol. 2)*, Minneapolis: University of Minnesota Press, 1975.

107. Butcher JN, Dahlstrom WG, Graham JR, Tellegren, A, Kaemmer B:*MMPI-2:Manual for Administration and Scoring*. Minneapolis, MN: University of Minnesota, 1989.

108. Keller LS, Butcher JN:*Assessment of chronic pain patients with the MMPI-2. MMPI-2 Monographs*. Minneapolis, MN. University of Minnesota Press, 1991.

109. Vendrig AA: The Minnesota Multiphasic Personality Inventory and chronic pain: a conceptual analysis of a long-standing but complicated relationship. *Clin Psychol Rev* 2000;20:533–559.

110. Morey, L.C. *Personality Assessment Inventory - Professional Manual*. Florida, USA: Psychological Assessment Resources, Inc, 1991.

111. Millon, T. *MCMI-II Manual*. Minneapolis, MN: National Computer Systems;1977.

112. Main CJ, Spanswick CC: Functional overlay and illness behaviour in chronic pain: distress or malingering? Conceptual difficulties in medico-legal assessment of personal injury claims. *J Psychosom Res* 1995;39:737–754.

113. Turk DC: Understanding pain sufferers: the role of cognitive processes. *Spine J*. 2004;4:1–7.

114. Asmundson GJ, Nicholas Carleton R: Fear of Pain is Elevated in Adults with Co-Occurring Trauma-Related Stress and Social Anxiety Symptoms. *Cognitive Behavior Therapist* 2005;34(4): 248–55.

115. Ong KS, Seymour RA: Evidence-based medicine approach to preemptive analgesia. *American Journal of Pain management* 2003; 13:158–172.

116. Banks SM, Kerns, RD: Explaining high rates of depression in chronic pain: A diathesis-stress framework. *Psychological Bulletin*. 119(1):95–110. 1996.

117. Price DD:*Psychological and Neural Mechanisms of Pain*. New York: Raven, 1988.

118. Price DD, Riley JL, Wade JB: Psychosocial approaches to measurement of the dimensions and stages of pain. In Turk DC, Melzack R (eds) *Handbook of Pain Assessment*, pp 53-75. New York: Guilford Press, 2001.

119. Wade JB, Dougherty L, Hart RP, *et al*. A canonical correlation analysis of the influence of neuroticism and extraversion on chronic pain, suffering, and pain behavior. *Pain*. 1992;51:67–73.

120. Rohling ML, Binder LM: Money matters: A meta-analytic review of the association between financial compensation and the experience and treatment of chronic pain. *Health Psychology* 1995; 14(6):537.

121. Martelli MF, Zasler ND, Nicholson K, Hart RP, Heilbronner RL: Masquerades of Brain Injury. Part II: Response Bias in Medicolegal Examinees and Examiners. *The Journal of Controversial Medical Claims* 2001;8(3):13–23.

122. Merskey H: Classification of chronic pain, descriptions of chronic pain syndromes and definitions of pain terms. *Pain*, 3, S10–S11, S13–S24, 1986.

123. Hall HV, Pritchard DA:*Detecting Malingering and Deception: Forensic Distortion Analysis*. Delray Beach, FL: St. Lucie Press, 1996.

124. Fishbain DA, Cutler RB, Rosomoff HL, Rosomoff RS: Chronic pain, disability exaggeration/malingering research and the application of submaximal effort research (1961–1999). *Clin J Pain* 1999;15(4):244–274.

125. Martelli MF, Zasler ND, Nicholson K, Pickett TC, May VR: Assessing the veracity of pain complaints and associated disability. In Weiner RB (ed.):*Pain Management: A Practical Guide for Clinicians*, 6th edition. Boca Ratan, FL: St. Lucie Press, 2001.

126. Fishbain DA, Cole B, Cutler RB, Lewis J, Rosomoff HL, Rosomoff RS: A structured evidence-based review on the meaning of nonorganic physical signs: Waddell signs. *Pain Med*. 2003 Jun;4(2):141–81.

127. Fishbain DA, Cutler RB, Rosomoff HL, Rosomoff RS: Is There a Relationship Between Nonorganic Physical Findings (Waddell Signs) and Secondary Gain/Malingering? *Clin J Pain* 2004;20(6): 399–408.

128. Sullivan M: Exaggerated Pain Behavior: By What Standard? *Clin J Pain* 2004;20(6):433–439.

129. Mendelson G, Mendelson D: Malingering Pain in the Medicolegal Context. (review). *Clin J Pain* 2004;20(6):423–432.

130. Robinson, ME, Dannecker, EA: Critical Issues in the Use of Muscle Testing for the Determination of Sincerity of Effort. *Clin J Pain* 2004;20(6):392–398.

131. Bracha HS, Ralston TC, Matsukawa JM, Matsunaga SM, Williams AI, Bracha AS: Does "Fight or Flight" Need Updating? *Psychosomatics* 2004;45:448–449.

132. Martelli MF: Ethical Challenges in the Neuropsychology of Pain, Part 1. In S.S. Bush (Ed.) *A Casebook of Ethical Challenges in Neuropsychology*. New York: Swets & Zeitlinger, 2005b.

133. Nicholson K: Ethical Challenges in the Neuropsychology of Pain, Part 2. In S.S.Bush (Ed.) *A Casebook of Ethical Challenges in Neuropsychology*. New York: Swets & Zeitlinger, 2005.

134. Gatchel RJ, Lou L, and Kishino N: Concepts of Multidisciplinary Pain Management. In Boswell MV, Cole BE (Eds) Weiner's *Pain Management: A Practical Guide for Clinicians* (Am. Acad. of Pain Management) . New York: Taylor & Francis Group, 2006.

135. Lemstra M, Stewart B, Olszynski WP. Effectiveness of multidisciplinary intervention in the treatment of migraine: a randomized clinical trial. *Headache*. 2002;42(9):845–854.

136. Loeser JD: Multidisciplinary pain programs. In Loeser JD (Ed.) *Bonica's management of pain*. Philadelphia: Lippincott, Williams & Wilkins, 2001.

137. Ashburn MA, Staats PS: Management of chronic pain. *Lancet* 1999;353:1865–1869.

138. Campbell A, Cole BE: Interdisciplinary Pain Management Programs: The American Academy of Pain Managmement Model. In Boswell MV, Cole BE (Eds) Weiner's *Pain Management: A Practical Guide for Clinicians* (Am. Acad. of Pain Management) . New York: Taylor & Francis Group, 2006.

139. Gustafsson M, Ekholm J, Broman L. Effects of a multiprofessional rehabilitation programme for patients with fibromyalgia syndrome. *J Rehabil Med*. 2002;34(3):119–127.

140. Okifuji A, Turk DC, Kalauokalani D: Clinical outcome and economic evaluation of multidisciplinary pain centers, in, *Handbook of pain syndromes: Biopsychosocial perspectives*. In Block AR, Kremer EF, Fernandez E (eds) *Handbook of Pain Syndome*, pp. 77–97. Mahwah, New Jersey: Lawrence Erlbaum Associates, 1999.

141. Flor H, Fydrick T, Turk DC. Efficacy of multidisciplinary pain treatment centers: a meta-analytic review. *Pain*.1992;49:221–230.

142. Andary MT, Crewe N, Ganzel SK, Haines PC, Kulkarni MR, Stanton DF, Thompson A, & Yosef M: Traumatic brain injury/chronic pain syndrome: A case comparison study. The *Clin J Pain* 1997;13:244–250.

143. Martelli M.F, Zasler ND, Nicholson K, Bender MC: Psychological, neuropsychological and medical considerations in the assessment and management of pain. *J Head Trauma Rehabil* 2004; 19(1):10–28.

144. Katz WA, Rothenberg R: Section 3:The nature of pain: pathophysiology. *J Clin Rheumatol*. 2005 Apr; 11(Suppl 2): S11–5.

145. Tyrer S, Lievesley A. Pain following traumatic brain injury: Assessment and management. *Neuropsychol Rehabil* 2003; 13(1/2):189–210.

146. McCracken LM, Turk DC. Behavioral and cognitive behavioral treatment for chronic pain: outcome, predictors of outcome, and treatment process. *Spine*. 2002;27(22):2564–2573.

147. McQuay H, Moore A:*An evidence based resource for pain relief*. Oxford: Oxford University Press, 1998.

148. College of Physicians and Surgeons of Ontario:*Evidence-based recommendations for medical management of chronic non-malignant pain*, November, 2000.

149. *The Cochrane Library*:Issue 2 (2002). Oxford, UK: Update Software Ltd, 2002 (www.Cochrane.org).

150. Andrasik F: Relaxation and Biofeedback Self Management for Pain. In Boswell MV, Cole BE (Eds) Weiner's *Pain Management: A Practical Guide for Clinicians* (Am. Acad. of Pain Management). New York: Taylor & Francis Group, 2006.

151. Jensen MP, Turner JA, Romano JM: Self-efficacy and outcome expectancies: Relationship to chronic pain coping strategies and adjustment. *Pain* 1987;44:263–269.

152. Lazarus RS. Folkman S:*Stress, appraisal, and coping*. New York: Springer, 1984.

153. Grayson RL: *EMG biofeedback as a therapeutic tool in the process of cognitive behavioral therapy: preliminary single case results*. Poster presented at the Association for Advancement of Behavior Therapy (AABT), 31st annual convention, Miami, Florida, November, 1997.

154. Ham LP, Packard RC: A retrospective, follow-up study of biofeedback-assisted relaxation therapy in patients with post-traumatic headache. *Biofeedback Self Regul* 1996;21(2):93–104.

155. Mittenberg W, Trement G, Zielinski RE, et al. Cognitive-behavioral prevention of postconcussion syndrome. *Arch Clin Neuropsychol* 1996;11:139–145.

156. Brown KS, DeCarvalho, LT: Psychotherapeutic Approaches in Pain Management. In Boswell MV, Cole BE (Eds) Weiner's *Pain Management: A Practical Guide for Clinicians* (Am. Acad. of Pain Management) . New York: Taylor & Francis Group, 2006.

157. Blanchard EB: Behavioral medicine and health psychology. In: Bergin, Garfield (eds) *Handbook of Psychotherapy and Behavior Change*. New York: John Wiley & Sons, 1994.

158. Auerbach SM and Gramling SE:*Stress Management: Psychological Foundations*. New York: Prentice-Hall, Inc, 1998.

159. DeVore JR: Applied Psychophysiology: State of the Art. In Zasler ND, Martelli MF (eds): *Functional Medical Disorders, State of the Art Reviews in Physical Medicine and Rehabilitation*. Philadelphia: Hanley and Belfus, 2002.

160. Othmer S and Other S: Efficacy of Neurofeedback for Pain Management. In Boswell MV, Cole BE (Eds.) Weiner's *Pain Management: A Practical Guide for Clinicians* (Am. Acad. of Pain Management) . New York: Taylor & Francis Group, 2006.

161. Decharms RC, Maeda F, Glover GH, Ludlow D, Pauly JM, Soneji D, Gabrieli JD, Mackey SC. Control over brain activation and pain learned by using real-time functional MRI. *Proc Natl Acad Sci* 2005;102(51):18626–631.

162. Miller L:*Psychotherapy of the Brain Injured Patient*. New York: WW Norton & Comany, Inc, 1993.

163. Martin PR:*Psychological Management of Chronic Headaches*. New York: The Guilford Press, Guilford Publications, Inc, 1993.

164. Gramling SE, Neblett J, Grayson RL, Townsend D: Temporomandibular Disorder: efficacy of an oral habit reversal treatment program. *J Behav Ther Exp Psychiatry* 1996;27:212–218.

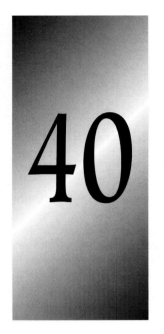

40

Neurorehabilitation Nursing of Persons with TBI: From Injury to Recovery

Terri Antoinette

INTRODUCTION

It is critical for nurses who will provide neurorehabilitation nursing care to persons who have sustained a traumatic brain injury (TBI) to possess highly specialized knowledge and acute clinical assessment skills. This must be based on an understanding of the pathophysiologic effects of the TBI, the potential medical complications which can affect all body systems, and the physical, cognitive, neurobehavioral, psychosocial, and functional impact of the TBI on the person and the significant others in his/her life.

The delivery of rehabilitation nursing care extends far beyond the delivery of care at the bedside. The licensed, registered, professional nurse: (1) collaboratively practices with the physician and the interdisciplinary team to implement rehabilitation interventions based on evidenced-based practice, (2) provides ongoing support and supervision to licensed practical nurses and direct care givers (i.e. certified nursing assistants) in the delivery of quality care, and (3) conducts patient/family teaching to promote the achievement of individualized quality outcomes.

This chapter presents an overview of neurorehabilitation nursing care issues throughout the continuum of care from prehospital management through acute/ subacute, neurobehavioral, and post-acute rehabilitation.

PRIMARY AND SECONDARY BRAIN INJURY

Primary brain injuries occur at the time of impact and result from an immediate biomechanical disruption of brain tissue and vasculature. Primary injuries may include: (1) concussions, contusions, lacerations, and skull fractures, (2) epidural, subdural and intracerebral hematomas, (3)penetrating injuries,(4) subarachnoid and intraventricular, hemorrhages,and (5) diffuse axonal injuries (DAI) (1, 2).

Secondary brain injuries may begin within minutes after the initial injury and throughout the early posttraumatic hours, days, and weeks. The pathophysiology of secondary injury has numerous etiologies. This include neurochemical changes and physiological events which precipitate a metabolic cascade effect followed by cerebral edema, increased intracranial pressure (ICP) and increased metabolic demand with resultant hypoxia, cerebral ischemia, impaired cerebral autoregulation, altered ion homeostasis, additional neuronal destruction, and cell death (2–7).

In a study by Jones et al. (8), involving 124 severely injured patients, 91% were found to have secondary injuries and mortality was associated with the duration of hypotension, hypoxia, and hyperthermia (9). The role of the nurse is paramount in the assessment, intervention and ultimate prevention and minimization of these injuries.

PREHOSPITAL NURSING CARE

The Guidelines for the Management of Severe Head Injury (10–12) provide evidence-based recommendations for practice which guide the delivery of critical care nursing interventions and clinical pathways from pre-hospital resuscitation through intensive care treatment to adults who have sustained a severe TBI with Glasgow Coma Scores (GCS) of 3 to 8 (13–18).

Critical care nurses may be involved in the care of the patient both at the scene as well as in route to the emergency department. Prompt intervention at the scene has been associated with improved outcome. An advanced trauma life support (ATLS) evaluation is conducted and the person's airway, breathing and circulation assessed. Fluid resuscitation is initiated with isotonic solutions, a patent airway established, ventilation and rapid physiologic resuscitation performed and emergency intervention for mulitsystem injuries instituted (10–12, 16–18).

Although the incidence of concomitant cervical spinal cord injuries has been cited as 2%–6% (19–21), iatrogenic post-traumatic spinal cord injuries after arrival to the hospital have been estimated to range from 10% to 25% (22). Emergency nursing and paramedic personnel should implement spinal cord injury precautions specific to modification of resuscitative techniques, airway stabilization, neck immobilization and spinal stabilization (16, 19).

During the brief pre-hospital assessment phase, the nurse should continuously assess vital signs (pulse, respiration, blood pressure and pain), perform the Glasgow Coma Scale, and observe pupillary responses for size, shape, symmetry and reactivity to light, eye position, and extraoccular movement. Observation should also occur for fluid/bleeding from the ears or nares and a determination made as to whether or not the fluid is cerebral spinal fluid (CSF). Additional assessments to be performed include muscle strength grading and observation for weakness, asymmetry of facial movements, paralysis, pain, decerebrate and decorticate posturing (4, 5, 17, 18, 23).

The skill of the nurse in astutely assessing the patient is of paramount importance. These assessment findings serve as a baseline of comparison for subsequent serial neurological exams, for interventional decision making, and for evaluating treatment effectiveness to minimize secondary brain injury (6, 15).

Valuable information to obtain from the patient, or if not possible, from witnesses at the scene include: (1) mechanism of injury (e.g. blow to the head, fall, ejection from the vehicle), (2) time of injury and extrication time, (3) presence of protective devices (e.g. seat belt, airbags, helmet), (4) loss of consciousness or change in cognitive status, (5) progressively worsening headache, repeated vomiting, (6) periods of apnea or cyanosis, (7) the presence of hypotension (8), amount of blood loss, (9) signs of substance abuse, (10) the position in which the person was found (i.e. lying face down) and (11) medication history (5, 16, 19, 23).

If the person is conscious and able to converse, a history should be taken and an assessment of level of consciousness (LOC) should include orientation to person, time, place, and situation, assessment of confusion, attention, level of arousal and the ability to follow commands (5, 16, 23).

Key determinants of survival are the adequacy of resuscitation efforts (restoration of circulating blood volume, blood pressure, oxygenation and ventilation), the identification of injury severity and the expeditious transfer to a facility with neurosurgical capabilities (10–12, 15).

CRITICAL CARE NURSING MANAGEMENT

This section will focus on the rationale and the general principles which guide the nursing care of the TBI patient in the ICU. The reader is referred to other chapters in this text for more detailed, clinically specific information regarding acute management.

The priority of nursing care in the ICU is protecting the brain from secondary injury and includes: (1) maintaining the ICP and cerebral perfusion pressure (CPP) within normal limits, (2) avoiding systemic hypotension, hypoxia, and hypercapnia, (3) controlling cerebral metabolic rate (e.g seizure control, normothermia, sedation) (4) assuring adequate fluid volume status, (5) maintaining serum glucose level at 80-120mg/dL, and (6) providing nutritional support. The use of mannitol, barbiturates and hyperventilation will vary depending on the course and severity of neurological deterioration (3, 6, 10–12, 18).

Because of the extreme sensitivity of the traumatized brain, the nurse must conscientiously interpret the benefits and risks of each potential intervention. Implementing clinically appropriate treatment is paramount because even a brief delay can result in further neurological insult (3).

Hypoxia

Immediate correction is imperative for episodes of hypoxia (partial pressure of arterial oxygen (PaO_2) less than 60mmHg or arterial oxygen saturation (SaO_2) less than 90% if pulse oximetry is used). Studies from the Traumatic Coma Data bank reported a mortality rate of 50% for patients with hypoxia versus 27% for those without (8, 18, 24).

Acute respiratory failure has been reported in 20% of patients with neurological trauma (6, 25). Ongoing assessment of respirations includes airway clearance, rate, pattern and characteristics of breath sounds, and monitoring of arterial blood gas (ABG), and oxygen saturation levels. In ventilated patients, the nurse must detect airway obstruction complications by monitoring the position of tubes, cuff pressures and problems with mucous plugs. An ambu bag and mask must be available for emergency use (26).

Early detection of respiratory complications is paramount. A study from the Traumatic Coma Data Bank revealed that 41% of patients in the study developed pneumonia and pulmonary insufficiency was reported in 28% (8, 27). Other complications include adult respiratory distress syndrome, pulmonary contusion, neurogenic pulmonary edema, pulmonary empyema, atelectasis, pulmonary embolus, hemothorax or pneumothorax (6, 18).

Hypotension

The nurse must immediately intervene to correct hypotension (systolic blood pressure less than 90 mm Hg). Hypotension that is tolerated in healthy individuals is not well tolerated in the injured brain and can lead to disruption of cerebrovascular autoregulation, a drop in CPP, elevated ICP and ischemic injury (3, 8).

Chestnut et al. (24) reported that a single episode of hypotension from the time of injury through resuscitation increased mortality 150% and also increased morbidity. Fearnside, (28) in a prospective study, reported that hypotension occurring anytime during a patient's prehospital and in-hospital course independently predicted increased mortality and morbidity.

Increased ICP

Increased ICP significantly influences morbidity and mortality. Saul et al. (29) reported a mortality rate of 15% for patients whose ICP remained below 25 mm Hg as opposed to 69% for those persons with ICP values in excess of 25 mm Hg. ICP values greater than 40 mm Hg is considered to be intracranial hypertension that is life threatening (8, 29, 30).

Cushing's triad (hypertension/widening pulse pressure, bradycardia and irregular respiratory pattern) is an ominous sign associated with rising ICP, pressure on the medullary center of the brainstem and irreversible damage (6, 16).

Suctioning

Since ICP can increase with endotracheal suctioning, it is important that the nurse adhere to patient specific protocols regarding the timing and appropriateness of the procedure, administration of medication prior to the procedure, hyperoxygenation of the lungs before suctioning, and instructions specific to the number and time limits for each of the suctioning attempts. Suctioning of the nasal passage should not occur until the possibility of basal skull fracture and dural tear have been ruled out (6, 14, 26).

Positioning

One of the most frequently performed activities that ICU nurses perform is that of therapeutically positioning the patient. Prior to any positioning it is imperative that spinal cord injury is ruled out. It is important to maintain neutral alignment of the head and neck and avoid disruption of cerebral venous outflow due to tight cervical collars or taped endotracheal tubes. Rotation of the head and flexion of the neck can increase ICP, decrease jugular venous outflow, and affect changes in cerebral blood flow (3, 14, 31–34).

Positioning recommendations based on neurological criteria, while at times conflicting, generally cite that elevating the head of the bed up to 30 degrees may decrease ICP, enhance venous return and decrease cerebral vasoconstriction. Caution must be taken, however, because cardiovascular, pulmonary and other body system responses to positioning may influence hemodynamic stability, cerebral perfusion pressure and systemic oxygenation. For example, in patients who are hypovolemic, hypotension may worsen if the head of the bed is elevated (3, 14, 31–35).

Turning and repositioning for contracture and spasticity management and to prevent skin breakdown must also be considered. Hip flexion of greater than 90 degrees may also elevate ICP. It is important for the nurse to obtain individualized patient specific instructions from the physician regarding positioning (3, 14, 18, 31–34, 36).

Nutrition

The body's initial response to severe TBI is that of a hypermetabolic/ hypercatabolic state. The Guidelines for the Management of Severe Head Injury recommend enteral or parenteral nutrition (particularly jejunal feeding) to replace 140% of resting metabolism expenditure in nonparalyzed patients and 100% in paralyzed patients (10–12, 16).

Options for feeding include parenteral, enteral-gastric and enteral-jejunal. Advantages of jejunal feeding include: (1) improved absorption of nutrients and gastric tolerance, (2) improved nitrogen retention (3) greater increases in serum prealbumin, (4) increased caloric intake, and (5) lower rate of pneumonia. When compared with parenteral feeding, the advantage of jejunal feeding includes: (1) lower theoretical risk of infection and sepsis, (2) decreased risk of hyperglycemia, and (3) lower cost. Once gastric tolerance is attained, enteral gastric feedings have practical advantages specific to the resumption of the normal digestive process and the capability for the delivery of bolus feedings (10–12, 18, 37–39).

Neurological Complications

In order to recognize subtle neurological improvement or deterioration, nurses must perform a systematic, organized neurological assessment which includes the Glascow Coma Scale, level of consciousness (arousal, awareness, higher cognitive functioning, speech and language), pupillary reflexes, cranial nerve function, sensory and motor function, and deep tendon reflexes. A Mini-Mental Status Examination should be done when clinically appropriate (4, 40).

The nurse should be able to accurately describe and recognize all classifications of seizures. Familiarity with the patient's history in regard to the time and onset of seizures, side effects of anticonvulsants, and familiarity with the recommendations for anticonvulsants from the Severe Head Injury Guidelines is paramount (10–12). Detailed information regarding neurological complications will be discussed elsewhere in this text.

Pain

Pain can adversely effect ICP and CPP and interfere with the accuracy of some parameters of vital signs and neurological assessment (e.g. pupillary response, sedation). If the patient is unable to consciously respond to questions regarding pain intensity, it is important for the nurse to observe for facial grimacing, body movement, crying, restlessness, elevated blood pressure and heart rate and agitation (6).

Multisystem Complications

Stabilization of systemic injuries is paramount to minimize blood loss and to prevent complications. The patient is also at risk for the development of multisystem complications such as coagulation disorders, deep venous thrombosis (DVT), cardiac arrhythmias, syndrome of inappropriate anti-diuretic hormone, electrolyte abnormalities, and glucose fluctuations. Nosocomial infections (i.e. pulmonary, urinary tract, vascular catheter, and wound) can be life threatening and require prompt assessment and appropriate treatment. Serious gastric complications include the development of stress ulcers, gastrointestinal bleeding, malabsorption syndromes and increased potential of aspiration. Hyperthermia must be closely monitored and rapidly treated (antipyretics, cooling blankets and antibiotics when indicated) since it increases cerebral metabolic demands (4, 5, 18, 41).

Noxious Stimuli

Environmental noise, lights, loud conversations and nursing activities have been reported to increase ICP in some patients, particularly those with minimal reserves of intracranial compliance. It is important that the nurse monitor if ICP and CPP increases during nursing care activities and be prepared to stop and place the patient in a neutral position if the ICP increases above a level predetermined by the physician (26).

The nurse must monitor the environment to protect the patient from excessive stimulation and plan and organize patient care to assure that nursing procedures (i.e. turning positioning, bathing, oral care, suctioning) are done in a manner that minimizes noxious stimulation to the degree possible. It is also important for the nurse to educate the family regarding the effects of noxious stimuli (6, 14, 26).

Clinical Pathways

Protocols and clinical pathways are valuable clinical tools which describe observable and measurable outcomes with specified time frames and provide an organized, systematic model for analysis of trends which require intervention by various members of the interdisciplinary team (6, 13, 26). Mcilvoy (41), in a study of the effect of implementing a TBI clinical pathway at a level one trauma center, noted decreases in hospital length of stay and reduction in costs.

Family Dynamics/Supportive Interventions in the ICU

The concept of family focused nursing in the ICU is based on the premise that the family is the primary unit of health care and the patient is best understood within the context of the family system rather than in isolation. It is essential that communication occur with the family/significant others as early as possible. Loved ones can provide pertinent information about the patient's preinjury medical history and, if present, details surrounding the events preceding the TBI. Also, the patient emerging from coma may demonstrate less confusion/agitation in the presence of a loved one (42–44).

The need for medical information was identified as a priority in several studies which investigated the needs of family members whose loved ones sustained a brain injury (44–46). Ideally, the nurse should be present when the physician discusses the patient's medical condition and prognosis with the family (44, 47). The nurse can then reinforce this information in a caring manner with kind, clear, realistic explanations of the patient's medical condition.

Because of the severe nature of TBI, the family of the injured person often demonstrates symptoms of shock, disbelief, denial, anxiety, and anger. This anger can be displaced onto the nursing staff, since it is the nursing staff who provide care around the clock and have more contact with the families than other health care professionals (45).

Hainesworth (48), in a study of acute care nurses caring for neurologically devastated patients, reported that nurses expressed feelings of severe stress and anxiety when they had to endure verbal and occasional physical outbursts from family members. Villaneuva (49) and Bell (50) reported that the experience level of the nurse and the responsivity of the patient accounted for many of the variations of how nurses interact with patients and families. For some nurses, particularly novice ones, the technical care in of itself can be overwhelming and the nurse, if not provided with support, may have a tendency to focus more on the technological aspects of care and less on the patient as a person.

Educational instruction specific to family dynamics, the recovery process, and strategies for intervention should be an integral part of the training that nurses receive. Villanueva (49) stressed the importance of experienced nurses serving as role models in the sharing and teaching of the knowledge they have acquired to help ease the transition of the new nurse. The nurse's inclusion as part of the interdisciplinary team also serves to allay a sense of isolation and provides a consistent, consensual approach to dealing with family members who are demonstrating challenging interpersonal interactions.

Rehabilitation Services in the ICU

The initiation of interdisciplinary rehabilitative services in the ICU should begin once it is determined that sufficient medical stabilization has occurred (51, 52). A 1992 study by MacKay et al. (53) assessed the occupational and long-term benefits of a formal early intervention program which provided physical, occupational and speech-language therapy services to a group of patients two days after admission compared with a nonformalized group who received rehabilitation services after an average of twenty three days into their hospital stay. The study demonstrated a dramatic reduction in inpatient (acute care and rehabilitation facility) length of stay in the formalized intervention group from 10 months to 5 months. Ninety-four percent of the patients from the formalized group were able to be discharged home as compared with fifty seven percent from the nonformalized group.

ACUTE/SUBACUTE REHABILITATION

Due to increasingly shortened lengths of stay in the acute care hospital, patients are being discharged sooner to acute/sub-acute settings with multiple medical complications and neuropsychological sequela. The intent of this section is to provide a concise multi-system overview that briefly outlines the nursing care issues most commonly encountered. The reader is referred to the other chapters in this text for in-depth discussions.

Care of Persons in Low-Level Neurologic States

The goals of nursing management for patients functioning at the Rancho Los Amigos Levels I, II and III who are admitted to an acute/subacute rehab facility are the same as in the acute care hospital. The Rancho Los Amigos Levels of Cognitive Function scale, while less valid and reliable than the Disability Rating Scale and other outcome measurement tools, is useful as a descriptive tool to categorize behavioral criteria that describe the patient's level of awareness and capacity to appropriately interact with the environment (54, 55).

Nursing staff are in an ideal position to observe spontaneous eye opening, purposeful versus nonpurposeful movement, the person's cognitive/behavioral level of responsiveness to stimulation and commands and the return of sleep-wake cycles. It is important that nurses understand the definitions and diagnostic criteria for the various disorders of consciousness (e.g. coma, vegetative state, minimally conscious state) (56).

After a diagnosis has been established, and consideration given to the etiology and location of injury, length of time since injury, comorbidity of medical complications, age, and knowledge of the patient's wishes, the physician may choose to discuss treatment alternatives (i.e. do not resuscitate (DNR) orders, mechanical ventilation, dialysis, administration of blood/ blood products, the administration of antibiotics and other medications, artificial hydration/nutrition) with the family/decision maker (57–59).

The nurse will be directly involved in supporting the family/decision maker throughout this process. It is, therefore, helpful to have the nurse present whenever the physician discusses these treatment alternatives. In addition to the medical rationale underlying treatment alternatives, the nurse must be cognizant of the legal and ethical policies of the health care facility and the need for compliance with state laws (statutory or court recognized) regarding advance directives (60).

Factors to consider include the emotional readiness of the family, the prognosis for functional recovery (56, 57, 59), (See other chapters for detailed prognostic information) and, most importantly, respect for the patient's wishes. Religious and cultural beliefs and the family's feeling of needing to deal with "unfinished business" all impact on this process.

Sensory/Environmental Stimulation of Persons in Low-Level Neurological States

Persons may present to the rehab setting from the ICU with orders for multiple medications (e.g., anticonvulsants, benzodiazepines, narcotics, antihistamines, neuroleptics, antispasticity agents, gastrointestinal agents, anticholinergics, antiemetics, hypnotics) that may potentially impair recovery. As medications that can potentially impair arousal are discontinued and cognitive enhancing medications initiated, the nurse must objectively observe the patient's level of neurobehavioral responsiveness, recognize potential side effects and promptly report objective assessment findings to the physician and the interdisciplinary team (59).

While caring for the patient, the nurse should be respectful of the possibility that the patient may be able to hear and possibly understand what is being said. The nurse should always address the patient by name, provide simple reality orientation to person, time and place and always talk calmly in a clear and concise manner to prepare the patient for what procedure or treatment is going to next occur (6, 61, 62).

The nurse can encourage the family to interact with their loved one through therapeutic touch, hand-holding and passive range of motion exercises, if clinically appropriate. Bringing in familiar objects from home and playing music and television programs that the patient enjoyed may provide meaningful visual and auditory stimulation. If the person begins to follow even one step verbal or written commands, a simple communication system can be established with head nods, eye blinks, up and down eye movements, or finger raising yes-no signals (6, 61, 62).

The nurse should educate the family regarding the importance of preventing over stimulation and alert the family that possible causes of restlessness may include pain, irritation from tubes/positioning devices, full bladder/bowel, constipation and other noxious stimuli (6, 61).

Respiratory Abnormalities

Clinical conditions which can increase the propensity toward respiratory complications include chest trauma, weakened or absent gag reflex, dysfunction of the lower esophageal sphincter, dysphagia, ineffective airway clearance, aspiration, recurrent regurgitation, and decreased mobility (61, 63–65). Bontke et al. (63) in a study of rehabilitation patients in the TBI Model System Programs identified respiratory failure (defined as requiring artificial ventilation for more than one week) in 39% of cases followed by pneumonitis (26%) as the most common extracerebral complications seen after brain injury.

Monitoring for a patent airway, rate, depth and pattern of respirations, auscultation for breath sounds, assessment of cough reflex, turning and positioning every one to two hours to mobilize secretions, humidification and suctioning are critical nursing interventions. Secretions should be observed for viscosity, color and odor (6, 61). Decannulation protocols may be initiated when deemed clinically appropriate, but in the low level patient, an individual risk versus benefit decision must be made regarding the suppressed ability to cough and clear secretions versus complications from long-term tracheostomies (59, 63, 64).

Aspiration is a major cause of pneumonia. Unless clinically contraindicated, the head of the bed should be maintained at 30–45 degrees. To prevent aspiration associated with enteral feedings, an initial swallowing study should be performed with high-risk patients, correct placement of feeding tubes monitored, gastric residuals routinely checked, stomach contents aspirated to determine gastric pH, and ongoing assessment performed of the benefit/risk of continuous versus intermittent feedings (65).

Cardiovascular Abnormalities

Life-threatening arrythmias, changes in cardiac rate and conduction, and alterations in blood pressure may be neurogenic in origin and can occur during the acute/subacute rehab stay. The nurse should ongoingly perform a comprehensive cardiovascular assessment which includes the monitoring of vital signs and the rate, rhythm and quality of apical pulses. An admission ECG can serve as baseline to determine changes in cardiac status (6, 16, 68, 69).

Post traumatic hypertension can resolve spontaneously. Labi and Horn (68) reported that only 45% of persons who had been receiving antihypertensive medications during their rehabilitation stay, required them at the time of discharge. It is important that the nurse keep the physician apprised of blood pressure readings so that a determination can be made by the physician regarding the appropriateness of weaning and/or discontinuing these medications, particularly those with sedating and central nervous system side effects, which could impair recovery (69).

After major brain trauma, the incidence of deep venous thrombosis (DVT) has been reported to be as high as 54% (69, 70). The nurse should monitor vital signs, assess peripheral pulses and Homans'sign, perform bilateral circumferential leg measurements, and examine extremities for redness, pain, tenderness, edema, and dilated superficial veins. DVT and pulmonary embolism may occur, however, without warning thereby making prophylaxis essential (71).

Compression stockings are mechanical methods of prophylaxis and should be fitted in accordance with the manufacturer's sizing chart. Stockings which are too large will not provide adequate support to the extremities and stockings too small may cause circulatory impairment. The patient's legs should be elevated prior to application, wrinkles in the stockings avoided and the patient observed for allergic reactions, skin irritation and thrombophlebitis (72).

Pneumatic compression boots are also used as a mechanical prophylaxis to DVT; however, the boots must be applied in accordance with manufacturer's instructions. Camerota et al. (73) reported that only 48% of patients in an acute care facility and 33% in a nursing home had the boots correctly applied.

Several studies (66, 74, 75) have reported a greater reduction in the incidence of thromboembolic events when pneumatic compression boots were used in combination with anticoagulant therapy. The use of anticoagulant therapy; however, requires a case specific risk versus benefit determination by the physician (66, 69).

Genitourinary Abnormalities

Urinary elimination patterns are frequently altered after brain injury. Patients typically present with uninhibited detrusor hyperreflexia (e.g. spastic bladder), and demonstrate symptoms of urge incontinence which include urgency, frequency, decreased bladder capacity, normal bladder sensation and normal to low post void residuals (61, 76).

Other types of incontinence (i.e. stress, reflex, functional, overflow, mixed) may also occur secondary to urinary retention, pudendal nerve damage, trauma to the urinary tract, benign prostatic hypertrophy, spinal cord injury, or cognitive impairment (62, 69, 76–78).

Transient causes of incontinence which need to be ruled out may include delirium, UTI's, atrophic urethritis or vaginitis, impaction, restricted mobility and even depression. Excess urine output can also be related to endocrine problems, hyperglycemia, hypercalcemia, congestive heart failure and peripheral edema (77, 79). Cognitive and behavioral disturbances, lack of initiation, decreased awareness, agitation, confusion, disorientation, communication and mobility issues also may contribute to incontinence (78, 79).

Medications such as benzodiazepines may cause confusion and secondary incontinence. Diuretics may lead to incontinence due to polyuria, frequency and urgency. Anticholinergic agents (including antihistamines, antidepressants, antipsychotics, opiates, antispasmodics, antiparkinsonian agents), alpha-adrenergic agonists (such as those found in over the counter decongestants and diet pills), beta-adrenergic agonists and calcium-channel blockers may also cause urinary retention and overflow incontinence (77).

Persons often enter the acute/subacute rehab setting with indwelling urethral catheters. A study by Yost (80) reported the development of urinary tract infections (UTI's) within 72 hours of first use in 70% of the patients studied. Additional complications from indwelling catheters may include hematuria, obstruction, pain, bladder spasms, urethral erosion, stones, epididymitis, periurethral abscess, fistula formation, chronic renal inflammation, bacteremia and pyelonephritis (77–79).

In June of 2005, the Centers for Medicare and Medicaid Services (CMS) released a revision to the State Operations Manual (SOM) specific to Surveyor Guidance for Incontinence and Catheters. This memorandum specifies that an assessment for the appropriateness of an indwelling catheter should be performed on admission and ongoingly and catheter use restricted to: (1) urinary retention that cannot be treated or medically/surgically corrected (i.e. post void residual volumes over 200 milliliters, unsuccessful management of retention/incontinence with intermittent catheterization and persistent overflow incontinence, symptomatic infections and/or renal dysfunction), (2) the need to prevent further contamination of Stage III or Stage IV pressure ulcers or (3) use as a comfort measure in terminally ill patients where changing is painful and disruptive (78).

The first step in assuring that the patient with bladder incontinence receives appropriate treatment to prevent UTI's and restore bladder function, is the performance of a thorough assessment. Discussion with the patient/family should occur prior to starting a bladder management program and information obtained specific to previous elimination patterns and premorbid urinary tract complications. A pelvic and rectal examination should be done to rule out factors which may affect incontinence (i.e. prolapsed uterus or bladder, prostate enlargement, fecal impaction). Several post-void residuals, preferrably thru ultrasonographic assessment, should also be obtained to ensure adequate emptying and a cough stress test performed to determine if urine leakage is provoked (77, 78).

The two essential components of a bladder program are a schedule of fluid management and a pre-established voiding schedule. Unless clinically contraindicated, overhydrating in the morning and early afternoon serves to cue the patient to a sensation of a full bladder. To promote rest, fluids are restricted after 7p.m. (especially caffeinated drinks). The fluid needs for an average person is 2500cc per 24 hour period but may vary depending on clinical variables (77–79).

Programs range from care-giver dependent (scheduled check and change) to those requiring active patient involvement. "Habit training/scheduled voiding," a behavioral technique whereby toileting is scheduled to coincide with a predetermined analysis of the patient's voiding patterns and times of fluid intake, can begin when the person is cognitively functioning at Rancho Level V (77–79).

"Prompted voiding" may be appropriate with patients who can recognize some degree of bladder fullness, ask for assistance or are able to respond to the staff when prompted to toilet. The patient receives positive feedback if they void successfully when prompted or remain dry after declining toileting. As the program progresses, the patient may learn to recognize the need to void, to ask for help or respond when prompted (77, 78).

In a study involving nursing home residents, a 40% reduction in incontinent episodes occurred in response to prompted voiding techniques regardless of the type of urinary incontinence or cognitive deficit (residents were able to say their name or reliably point to one of two objects) (81).

"Bladder rehabilitation/bladder retraining" is appropriate for cognitively intact patients and requires the capability to delay voiding and to urinate according to a timetable. Based on the baseline assessment of voiding times, the person is encouraged to lengthen the time between voids by consciously suppressing the urge. Bladder training can also be combined with pelvic muscle (Kegel) exercises and pelvic floor electrical stimulation therapy (77, 78). A cystometrogram EMG is sometimes done to determine the patient's degree of sensation and voluntary control (54).

Most importantly, the success of bladder programs requires the commitment and compliance of the direct care staff to implement the program and the support of administrative staff to provide adequate numbers of staff.

Anticholinergic medications are sometimes used to relax smooth muscle in the urinary tract, increase bladder capacity and increase the threshold volume for overactive bladder contractions. Caution is advised, however, due to side effects such as urinary retention, sedation and memory impairment (54, 66). Anticholinergics are contraindicated in patients with narrow-angle glaucoma (77).

Male external collection devices (i.e. condom catheters) are available, but also are associated with increased risk of UTI's (82). Patients must be carefully evaluated prior to use for symptomatic UTI, urinary retention and upper tract damage. These devices should not be used in patients with chronic obstruction. Proper application is critical and the patient must be routinely monitored for contact dermatitis, maceration and irritation of the penis, ischemia, penile obstruction and UTI (61, 77, 78).

External collection devices for females are not widely used. Reported adverse reactions include periurethral erythema, perineal itching, skin abrasions, and adherence problems (77, 78, 83). Incontinence briefs are typically used in females. After each episode of incontinence, the skin should be checked for breakdown, a moisture barrier applied and the skin kept clean and dry.

Gastrointestinal Abnormalities

After TBI, the patient is at risk for the development of gastritis, duodenitis, gastroparesis, lower esophageal sphincter dysfunction, gastric atony, and stress ulcers (74). Gastrointestinal bleeding is a serious complication which has been reported in up to 80% of patients who have sustained TBI's (84). Medications such as steroids, nonsteroidal anti-inflammatory agents, aspirin and anticoagulants may also exacerbate the problem due to their propensity to increase GI bleeding (66).

Antacids, H_2 blockers, or sucralfate may be used prophylactically in the acute phase after TBI; (74, 85) however, the patient must be closely monitored due to the increased risk of pneumonia which has been reported with the use of antacids or H_2 blockers (86, 87).

Metoclopramide, a central dopamine receptor antagonist, has been historically used to treat gastroparesis and gastroesophageal reflux but observation must occur for deleterious effects such as sedation and extrapyramidal symptoms (54, 87, 88).

A gastrointestinal assessment should include auscultation of the abdomen in all four quadrants for bowel sounds, palpation for signs of pain or distention, testing of stool for occult blood and monitoring vital signs and serial Hgb and Hct for changes indicative of hemorrhage. Checking stool for frequency, color and consistency is important due to the predisposition for constipation secondary to immobility, opiates and fluid restrictions. Conversely, diarrhea may occur due to intolerance to tube feeding or antibiotics (61). Other serious bowel complications include, impaction, intestinal obstruction, paralytic ileus and clostridium difficile colitis (16, 26, 76).

After brain injury, bowel incontinence typically occurs secondary to upper motor neuron damage which results in uninhibited neurogenic bowel; however, co-existing spinal cord and traumatic injuries and preexisting gastrointestinal diseases can also effect bowel continence. Prior to implementation of a bowel program, it is important to determine the type/s of neurogenic bowel dysfunction. A rectal exam should be performed to assess the condition of external and internal hemorrhoids and a physical assessment done to determine if saddle sensation, the bulbocavernosus and anal reflexes are intact (76, 89).

Discussion should occur with the family to determine preexisting elimination patterns and a baseline assessment conducted to determine the time of day and frequency of stools. Based on identified patterns, a toileting schedule can be developed preferably 15–30 minutes after meals, to facilitate the effect of the gastrocolic reflex. Unless clinically contraindicated, left side-lying or sitting will also facilitate evacuation. Adequate fluid intake and close monitoring of tube feeding to assure adequate amounts of fiber, roughage and fluid is also important (61, 76, 89).

Stool softeners and bulk formers should be utilized and dosages and times of administration adjusted as needed. Digital stimulation is not appropriate in bowel programs to manage uninhibited neurogenic bowel, but suppositories or products such as Theravac SB™, a 4cm³ mini-enema/stool softener laxative may be used to trigger the defecation reflex. A daily bowel movement is not necessary but a patient should not go for more than 3 days without a bowel movement. Continuity of the program is maintained even if the patient has a bowel movement between training times (61, 76, 89, 90).

Nutrition and Feeding

In a study of patients admitted to a rehabilitation unit, Brooke and Barbour (91) reported an average weight loss of 29 pounds. The need for increased nutritional support

X

COGNITIVE AND
BEHAVIORAL PROBLEMS

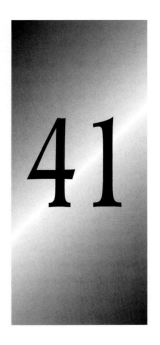

41

Cognitive Rehabilitation

Keith D. Cicerone

Cognitive impairments are often the most persistent and prominent sequelae of brain injury in patients with moderate or good neurologic recovery. Interventions designed to promote the recovery of cognitive functioning and reduce cognitive disability are an integral aspect of brain injury rehabilitation programs after traumatic brain injury (TBI) (1). Despite this, as many as 80% of persons who have sustained a TBI believe that their need to improve their cognition had not been met at one year post-injury (2). The growth in clinical services directed at the rehabilitation of cognitive impairments has recently been matched by efforts to establish the empirical basis for cognitive rehabilitation (3). This chapter is intended to integrate some of the clinical issues involved in the remediation of cognitive impairments after TBI, with a discussion of the empirical literature. The discussion of the literature relies primarily on studies that provide evidence for the "best available practices" in cognitive rehabilitation, but includes some discussion of clinically important or innovative therapies.

RECOVERY OF NEUROCOGNITIVE FUNCTIONS

In a seminal text on the *Restoration of Function after Brain Injury*, Luria (4) described a number of different

mechanisms to support the re-organization of higher cortical functions after brain injuries. This description rests on the distinction between the two meanings of "function." The concept of function may be used to refer to the specific activity performed by a tissue or organ; however, in relation to the physiology of higher nervous activity and the psychology of higher cognitive processes, "function" refers to a complex adaptive activity consisting of a group of multistage representations, which are organized in a dynamic relationship, and directed toward performance of a particular task. This conceptualization of function might be better described as a "functional system," similar to the current concept of distributed cortical networks (5). A fundamental characteristic of a functional system is that different processes may be utilized to carry out a given task under different conditions, a property which increases the adaptability of higher cognitive functions. The mechanisms for recovery of function follow a similar evolution from simple to complex. In cases of damage to the primary cerebral areas serving sensory and motor functioning, re-organization after injury may take place through (a) the ability of intra-systemic processes to take over role of damaged tissue, and (b) the intact influence of higher cortical centers on lower levels of function. At the highest levels of cerebral functional systems, recovery takes place through a process of inter-systemic re-organization, which may include completely different components that formerly served widely different functions.

Luria (4) was eloquent in relating these principles of recovery to specific methods of rehabilitation. He also identified several factors considered to moderate recovery, such as the extent of neurologic damage and the developmental level and premorbid integrity of the disturbed function. One of the principle factors determining the success of restoration of higher cognitive functioning is the patient's level of motivation (or "capacity for mental tension") since recovery at this level requires active, effortful, and conscious compensation.

The neurological mechanisms underlying recovery have continued to receive attention, with several attempts to apply these principles to neurorehabilitation (6, 7). However, few interventions for cognitive impairment after TBI have been derived explicitly from such principles. Current approaches to cognitive rehabilitation do at least implicitly incorporate some of the proposed principles of recovery. Therapies may focus on modification of inherent cognitive processes and abilities, or on the external environmental conditions that affect performance. Therapies may also emphasize retraining of multiple, basic neurocognitive components or the retraining of more integrative abilities and functional skills. Finally, the therapeutic approach can be "bottom-up," based on the sequential building from elementary to complex skills, or "top-down" via the application of superordinate controls over subordinate processes.

Process-Specific Remediation

Skill-specific or process-specific models of cognitive remediation assume that specific interventions can impact differentially on component neurocognitive deficits. Sohlberg and Mateer (8) developed an influential, process-specific approach to cognitive rehabilitation in which treatments are directed, in highly targeted manner, at specific cognitive areas. The process-specific approach is based on the assumption that direct retraining of specific cognitive processes, through multiple repeated trials of stimulation and activation of the targeted cognitive process, can lead to the reorganization of higher level neurologic and cognitive processes. Treatments are provided in accordance with a hierarchical model of cognitive functioning from lower to higher components of cognitive functioning, in order to provide continuous stimulation and activation of the cognitive process. It is assumed that improvements in functioning at the process-specific level will generalize to tasks that contain similar cognitive requirements, and eventually to improvements in everyday functioning. Gordon and colleagues (9) also combined specific, well-controlled training procedures in basic scanning, somatosensory stimulation and size estimation, and visual-spatial organization into a comprehensive perceptual remediation program. The training program was effective in promoting improvement on psychometric

measures closely related to the training areas. Limited generalization of improvements to measures not specifically related to the training tasks occurred, although the investigators noted more time spent in recreational reading after treatment

Functional Skills Training

Functional skills training concentrates on the patient's ability in domain-specific, context-specific areas of functioning and the retraining of "competencies of daily life" (10) rather than the putative underlying deficits. Mayer et al. (10) suggested several approaches to training, such as (1) repetition of a whole skill in a natural context (e.g., drinking from a cup during breakfast), (2) training of component parts (e.g., looking for the cup, reaching, grasping, etc) followed by whole-skill training, and (3) various attempts to substitute new procedures to perform the desired activity. Although conceptualizing behavior and presumable interventions according to a hierarchy of pre-skills, individual skills, and routine and activity patterns, this approach did not consider the cognitive task attributes distinct from the functional skills being trained. Following Tsvetkova's (11) notion of retraining within the context of a broader function, they suggest that the remediation of cognitive impairments should not address specific components through training exercises in memory, attention, reasoning, and so on, but to address these impairments only in so far as they are embedded within functional activities. Though the work of Glisky and Schacter (12) is derived from neurocognitive-oriented work on spared memory abilities after brain injury, their training approach is very functionally oriented in its emphasis on the acquisition of domain-specific knowledge by memory-impaired patients. They utilized a method of "vanishing cues" to teach four brain-injured amnesic patients computer-related vocabulary words. Consistent with a functional approach, the training was intended to provide the patients with specific knowledge in an area important to the patient's everyday lives (computer terms) rather than produce general improvements in memory function. Glisky and Schacter (12) suggested that the same procedure might be applied toward the acquisition of complex forms of knowledge by brain-injured patients, as well as the possibility of training patients to become expert in specific, defined content areas. In each of these functional approaches the patient is trained on the same task that he or she is expected to perform in the context of daily activities, and training is specific to that situation. Generalization to other related situations is not expected as a consequence of the initial training. Thus the necessity of training a wide range and number of specialized, context-specific skills and routines is characteristic of the functional model.

Metacognitive Remediation

Metacognition refers to the subjective knowledge and experience of one's own cognitive processes, which can be used to guide cognitive activity (13). Metacognitive training therefore places its major emphasis on increasing awareness of deficits, self-monitoring of errors, and self-regulation in order to improve the ability to independently recognize or anticipate the need for compensatory strategies and utilize those strategies in the appropriate situations. Shallice's (14) neuropsychological model distinguishes between the cognitive levels of *processing structures* and two levels of *cognitive control*. Processing structures consist of special-purpose cognitive subsystems such as object recognition, semantic comprehension, spatial orientation, and so on, that can be analyzed by fractionation of the subsystems into the involved components. These cognitive sub-systems can also be organized into relatively invariant functional routines, or schema, such as eating breakfast or driving home from work. *Routine* control of activity is accomplished through relatively automatic and rapid selection of habitual schemata and the inhibition of weaker competing schemata. However, an additional level of voluntary, strategic, and *nonroutine* control is required when planning is required, when the correction of unexpected errors is required, when the required response is novel or not well learned, or when habitual responses need to be inhibited.

Reliance on the underlying assumption that patients will be able to develop sufficient awareness and insight to apply strategies in a variety of situations is a distinctive aspect of the metacognitive approach. Crosson et al. (15) has distinguished between intellectual, emergent, and anticipatory levels of awareness after brain injury. Different degrees of compensation may be available to patients, depending on their degree of awareness deficit. For example, patients with marked deficits of intellectual awareness may require external, task-specific compensation whereas patients with minimal awareness deficits may compensate by recognition or anticipation of problems while moving from one environment to another several times in the course of their daily functioning.

REMEDIATION OF ATTENTION DEFICITS

Remediation of Attention Deficits

Various components of attention have been identified and related to different cerebral networks. Posner and Rothbart (16) identified three different attention networks. The posterior attention network involves the parietal cortex, pulvinar and reticular thalamic nuclei and superior colliculus and is involved in orienting to and locating sensory stimuli in space. The anterior attention network involves the anterior cingulate gyrus and supplementary motor

area and appears active in the detection and selection of target stimuli and inhibition of responses to irrelevant stimuli. Although selectivity may occur on an automatic or unconscious level, situations which are novel or complex will require conscious and strategic control over attention. The vigilance network involves the locus coeruleus and brainstem reticular connections with cerebral cortex, especially lateral frontal cortex. This system may be responsible for maintaining alertness and vigilance. Whyte (17) also reviewed evidence suggesting that attention was not a single cognitive process controlled by a focal brain region and indicated that the neural control of attention was mediated by various structures including the brain stem, subcortical structures, and cerebral cortex, which interact in a richly interconnected network. Whyte (17) suggested that the distribution of attention across this dense neural network had two important clinical implications. First, he suggested that different brain lesions could produce qualitatively different attention deficits due to disruption of distinct aspects of the attentional network. Second, lesions to different brain regions could produce similar attentional impairments due to the distributed and integrative nature of the attentional system. The effectiveness of remedial interventions would, in principle, depend upon providing treatment directed at the precise nature of the attentional deficit.

Impairments of attention are common after TBI, and include reductions of processing speed, difficulty sustaining the focus of attention (e.g., maintaining concentration or a train of thought), and limitations in the ability to regulate the allocation of attention in complex situations (e.g., shifting attention to multiple speakers, or between several ongoing tasks). Therefore it is not surprising that some of the earliest formal attempts at cognitive remediation after TBI were directed at deficits of attention. In an early study of attention process training (APT), Sohlberg and Mateer (18) provided the training to four patients and compared it with training for visual perceptual abilities, using a multiple baseline across subjects design. The patients were all at least one year, and up to 6 years, after injury, so it is likely that their deficits were stable. All four subjects demonstrated gains on a single attentional-outcome measure following APT, but not after the visual-perceptual treatment. The measure used to assess improvements in attention was similar in several respects to the training tasks, so it is likely that the improvements reflected some degree of familiarity and practice with the task demands and near transfer to the outcome measure.

A more recent study of APT (19) used a randomized crossover design to compare APT with a "placebo" condition that consisted of education and support. The 14 patients with acquired brain injury were again all at least one year post-injury, ranging as far as 22 years post-injury. Most of the patients had sustained severe TBI, including positive neuroimaging, and they all exhibited impairments of attention on neuropsychological evaluation and subjective report by the participant and/or a significant other. The APT tasks were again administered in accordance with a hierarchical approach, although the training exercises were selected for each of the patients based on their specific profiles of attention deficits. Treatment effects in this study were evaluated on a range of outcome measures, including neuropsychological measures intended to reflect specific components of attention, standardized questionnaires, and structured interviews. Significant benefits of APT, compared with therapeutic support, were most apparent in patients' self-reported changes in attention and memory functioning. Improvements in cognitive functioning on neuropsychological measures intended to assess the anterior attentional network for the regulation of attention (but not measures of spatial orienting or vigilance) were also greater following APT, and paralleled the patients' self-reports of improved functioning. The specificity of improvements on an aspect of attention related to the regulation of attention, and relationship of these improvements to patients' subjective improvements in their daily functioning, argues against the interpretation that the benefits of treatment were due either to generalized stimulation or task-specific practice effects. These findings also suggest that the benefits of training are due to patients' improved ability to control their attention, rather than restoration of more basic attentional processes.

Several additional prospective, randomized, controlled studies are consistent with the view that treatment for attention deficits are effective during the postacute phase of recovery from TBI, and related primarily to patients' ability to understand the nature of their deficits and use appropriate compensations in functional situations. One study (20) treated 26 people who had sustained a TBI between one and six years earlier and were living in the community. The attention treatment consisted of computer-based tasks directed at improving participants, ability to focus their attention or allocate their attention between tasks; in addition to practice on the computer-based tasks a significant portion of each treatment session was devoted to providing participants with feedback about their performance and implementing strategies to compensate for their attention difficulties. The group receiving the attention treatment improved significantly over the course of treatment, although these effects were relatively weak and did not transfer to additional measures. In another study (21) attention remediation was compared with a "placebo" condition of recreational computing. The patients varied widely in their time post injury and severity of deficits, and included etiologies of both TBI and stroke, although neither of the latter two factors was related to the effects of treatment. Training was intended to address attention control processes such as manipulating information in working memory or dividing attention between two tasks, and was compared with the effects of recreational computing. Some benefit of the attention treatment were apparent immediately after treatment, but were more evident six months after treatment, at which time the patients who received the attention treatment showed continued improvement while the patients who used recreational computing did not improve, and in some cases their performance deteriorated. The treatment group's pattern of modest initial improvement followed by increased benefits over time may have represented their increased proficiency in the use of strategies in their daily functioning. This pattern of prolonged benefits of treatment being related to the active use of strategies, and lack of benefits when strategies are no longer used, is evident in a number of studies and consistent with the view that improvements in functioning are related to patients' ability to learn and implement compensatory strategies in their everyday functioning.

This approach also served as the basis for an intervention that was intended specifically to teach patients with TBI to compensate for the experience of "information overload" due to their slowed information processing during the performance of daily tasks (22). Twenty-two patients with TBI, most of whom were more than six months post-injury, received either "Time Pressure Management" training or generic instructions to improve their concentration. The Time Pressure Management (TPM) was intended to increase patients' awareness of errors and use of strategies to manage demands under distracting conditions that were likely to be encountered in their everyday lives. Participants receiving TPM showed significantly greater use of self-management strategies during task performance, particularly on more complex tasks that allowed them to adjust their approach to the task, but not on basic reaction time tasks in which such a strategy could not be applied.

Patients with mild TBI often complain of difficulties with the more complex aspects of attention, and are likely to exhibit selective impairments of attention functioning in the context of generally intact cognitive functioning. One small, observational study (23) has evaluated the effectiveness of an intervention intended to improve "working attention" in four patients with mild TBI, compared with four patients who did not receive treatment. The intervention emphasized the use of strategies to allocate attention resources and manage the rate of information during task performance. The patients receiving attention treatment demonstrated "clinically significant gains" on objective measures of attention and significant reductions of self-reported attentional difficulties in their daily functioning.

Overall, these studies suggest that significant benefits can be obtained by patients with attentional difficulties during the postacute period of recovery from TBI.

Gains on objective measures of attention are related to subjective improvements in patients' everyday functioning. Finally, these benefits appear to be related to patients' abilities to apply compensatory strategies in their daily functioning, even for relatively basic deficits such as reduced processing speed, rather than by restoration of the underlying attention processes. The evidence for generalized, functional improvements in attention functioning after treatment in the above cited studies rests primarily on patients' subjective report. However, one single-subject study has reported beneficial effects of an intervention intended to facilitate control over attention during functional activities, such as decreasing the frequency of lapses in attention while the patient was reading novels and texts (24).

The benefits of remediation for attention deficits during the acute period of rehabilitation for TBI are not readily apparent, and it does not appear possible to distinguish the effects of specific attentional training (such as APT) from the more general effects of acute brain injury rehabilitation (25) or spontaneous recovery (26).

REMEDIATION OF MEMORY DEFICITS

Memory complaints are ubiquitous after brain injury. However, the memory difficulties seen after TBI typically do not reflect a classic amnesic disorder. Instead, memory difficulties are likely to be due to a number of different factors, and are unlikely to represent a unitary deficit. For example, attention deficits such as distractibility or slowed processing are commonly believed to cause impairments in the acquisition of information, and executive impairments may cause memory failures due to the failure to adequately organize material or initiate efficient memory retrieval processes (27).

One of the first descriptions of remediation for memory deficits after brain injury (28) presented two case studies on the use of semantic elaboration and visual imagery techniques to improve the encoding of information. After the effectiveness of these techniques was demonstrated in the laboratory, they were applied to the patient's presenting problem of reduced academic performance. The success of treatment was assessed by the patient's improved subjective ratings of her memory functioning and reduction of negative self-statements, and her ability to remain in her academic classes with less subjective difficulty. Review of her academic performance suggested that she was able to apply the procedure in her everyday life, although the effects were not as great as were seen in the laboratory situation.

Ryan and Ruff (29) examined the general effectiveness of compensatory memory remediation by combining a number of strategies for improving verbal and non-verbal memory capacities in a comprehensive remediation program. Treatment was provided to ten patients with TBI who exhibited persistent mild to moderate memory deficits. Interventions included instruction and practice in the use of rehearsal, elaborative semantic encoding and associative strategies, imagery construction, "personalized emotional techniques", external memory strategies, and group education and practice with the various memory compensations. Individualized cuing procedures were developed for each patient and practiced on a daily basis. Control patients participated in recreational activities and psychosocial support. At the completion of the treatment both groups demonstrated significant improvement on memory measures, without any apparent specific benefits from the specialized memory remediation program. Subsequent analysis did suggest that the patients with relatively milder cognitive deficits showed greater benefit from the memory remediation strategies, while those with moderate residual impairments did not benefit from treatment. This study is important for several reasons. First, the treatment more closely resembled a multidimensional, clinical protocol than in many experimental studies. Second, the study evaluated the differential effectiveness of treatment in relation to the severity of cognitive impairment. Finally, the study provided an explicit comparison between active, specialized memory remediation and a nonspecific intervention.

Kaschel and colleagues (30) conducted a prospective, controlled study of a visual imagery technique for the rehabilitation of participants with mild memory impairment after acquired brain injury. The intervention consisted of a standardized imagery-acquisition procedure to promote imagery-generation, overlearning and automatization, and included an individually-tailored training period directed at the transfer of the strategy to everyday relevant materials. Visual imagery was compared with "pragmatic memory training" that included practical guidelines to improve memory and the use of notebooks and calendars. Twenty-four patients with TBI had initially been referred for memory rehabilitation, and memory problems were considered to be of primary importance, although patients with severe memory impairment were excluded. Significant improvement was apparent only for the imagery condition on the recall of verbal material, consistent with the expected effects of treatment. The improvements associated with visual imagery training were paralleled by positive changes in relatives' ratings of patients' memory functioning and were maintained at three month follow-up.

Another randomized controlled trial (31) has specifically compared "repetitive drill and practice" on memory tasks with training in cognitive strategies to improve memory functioning after TBI. Cognitive strategies to improve memory functioning were explained, demonstrated, and practiced three times a week for six weeks, and patients received daily homework stressing the importance of application of memory strategies in everyday life. Intervention was highly individualized, with the specific memory problems selected for training based on the subjects' report of difficulties experienced in their daily functioning. Patients in both the strategy training and "drill and practice" groups reported subjective improvements in memory functioning, but significant effects on objective memory performance could only be demonstrated in the strategy training group, and this difference was maintained at 4 month follow-up.

In a follow-up study four years after the initial training (32), subjective memory and objective memory performance were the same for both patient groups and equivalent to a no-treatment brain injury control group (and still well below the level of normal control subjects). Of note, several subjects in the strategy training group showed a decline in their performance, while the "pseudotreatment" group showed continued, significant improvements despite the fact that patients were between five and 25 years post injury at the time of follow-up. In contrast with this study, Wilson (33) evaluated 26 patients with traumatic head injury who had been referred for memory therapy five to 10 years earlier. On standardized memory testing, most patients remained stable and 8 patients showed improved performance. It was noted that many subjects were using more memory aids and strategies at the time of follow-up assessment than they were at the completion of their initial memory rehabilitation, which may have accounted for the positive findings (34).

Prospective Memory The ability to remember to do something at some future time, referred to as prospective memory, appears to be one of the most common memory problems for patients with acquired brain injury (35). Prospective memory interventions may be based on modifications of other memory interventions, such as space-retrieval and distributed practice techniques or use of elaborative encoding strategies. A series of case studies (36, 37) described a specific prospective memory training procedure in five patients with severe traumatic brain injury. Training consisted of giving the patients simple, repetitive, one-step prospective memory tasks to be carried out at increasingly longer time intervals following instructions, ranging from two to ten minutes. The patients all improved with practice on the prospective memory tasks, with some evidence of improvement on neuropsychological measures and observations of daily memory functioning. However, the limited time between the assignment of tasks and their execution, lack of intervening or complex tasks, and degree of therapist control all limit the relevance of the training to real life demands.

External Memory Compensations Patients with memory impairments after TBI are commonly taught to use a memory notebook or diary to compensate for their difficulties in spontaneous, or unassisted, recall of information. One randomized controlled trial (38) has compared notebook training with supportive therapy for eight patients with TBI, all more than two years post injury. The treatment consisted of teaching a specific protocol for use of a memory notebook, and individualized modifications to address the subjects' personal needs and application to novel settings. Patients who received the notebook training reported fewer observed, everyday memory failures than the supportive therapy subjects. Three of the subjects who received the memory remediation were still actively using the memory notebook to assist with their daily activities at six month follow-up.

In this study, and in the studies described above using some form of strategy training, the patients who benefited from treatment all exhibited relatively mild memory difficulties. In contrast, patients with severe memory deficits after TBI appear more likely to require training in the use of specific compensations that can be applied to specific tasks, rather than attempts to remediate their underlying memory deficits through the use of strategies. For example, the use of a memory notebook has been shown to be superior to verbal rehearsal strategies when patients are required to remember specific information, particularly for patients with more severe memory impairments (39). While external memory compensations such as memory notebooks are commonly employed in cognitive rehabilitation, patients with severe memory difficulties are likely to require an extended period of training to ensure the practical application of a memory notebook (40, 41).

External Cuing and Environmental Compensations In the last several years there has been increased development of external cuing and assistive technologies as a compensation for memory impairments after TBI. For example, three studies have described the use and effectiveness of a portable voice organizer to help patients to recall their therapy goals (42) or to prospectively remember to perform relevant everyday tasks (43, 44). The use of existing technologies to assist people with memory deficits will typically require additional training, and consideration of multiple factors that influence the selection of an external cuing system (e.g., the patient's cognitive strengths and weaknesses, knowledge and familiarity with specific technologies, and the necessary resources and "user friendliness" to support programming and maintenance of the assistive device (45, 46).

Several assistive devices have been developed specifically with the intent of improving the cognitive functioning of people with acquired neurocognitive impairments, such as the Essential Steps cognitive orthotic system (47), the ISAAC cognitive prosthetic system (48) and the NeuroPage paging service (49–51). Initial evidence for the effectiveness of these systems is limited to descriptive case studies (47–49). More recently, Wilson and her colleagues (50) have evaluated the effectiveness of the NeuroPage portable paging system to reduce everyday memory failures during the performance of functional activities, such as remembering to take one's medication or shut off appliances. A randomized controlled trial of the paging system was conductive for patients with persisting memory difficulties, many of whom had been referred only after previous interventions had failed. For each patient, the use of the pager was adapted to address specific problems in their typical daily functioning (e.g., keeping appointments) identified by the patient or a relative. Significant improvements in the ability of participants to carry out everyday tasks with the use of the pager were apparent, compared with no-treatment and baseline conditions. The paging system was noted to be most useful for those people who needed to carry out certain tasks on a regular basis and had some insight into their memory deficits. Based on this research, a commercial service offering NeuroPage was subsequently established through the National Health Service in the United Kingdom (51). Among the first 40 patients, with diverse etiologies of memory dysfunction, who were recruited into this study, 31 were reportedly able to use the pager successfully. The most frequent types of reminders were related to taking medication, daily orientation (e.g., getting up in the morning) and daily household activities (e.g., making lunch, taking a shower, doing the laundry) and these accounted for about 75% of messages provided by the pager. Among the patients who used the paging system consistently for some time, the authors noted several patterns of use. One group of patients continued to use the pager on a consistent basis for many months with no appreciable change in the messages required each week. Another group of patients continued to use the pager, but adjusted the number of messages they required. Some clients found that they were able to discontinue use of the pager after some time, suggesting that the pager served to establish their routine and they could then manage alone or use a different type of self-directed reminder. It is unclear whether these different patterns of use correspond to different patient characteristics (e.g, severity of memory impairment, presence of neurocognitive co-morbidites, level of motivation) although this might provide important clinical information in the future. It is clear that different forms of memory compensations are best selected only after careful consideration of these, and other, patient characteristics.

REMEDIATION FOR DEFICITS IN EXECUTIVE FUNCTIONING

Disturbances in executive functioning are prevalent after acquired brain injury, and represent significant obstacles to social functioning, work and rehabilitation. Disorders of executive functioning may affect the ability to anticipate the effects of our actions, appreciate alternative perspectives, and to recognize other people's reactions to our behavior and modify our actions accordingly. Disturbances of executive functioning may be apparent after various types of cortical or subcortical damage, but are often associated with damage to the frontal lobes. The dorsolateral frontal cortex has extensive connections with polysensory posterior association areas (52) and appears to be related to deficits in complex discrimination and association (53). The medial prefrontal cortex has been implicated in the processes of motor initiation and motor regulation and also appears to play a role in tasks requiring complex attention and planning (52). The orbitofrontal cortex is part of paralimbic cortex (5) has been related to disturbances of complex social and emotional behavior in humans (54, 55).

Patients with frontal-lobe damage may exhibit dissociation between the relative preservation of verbal knowledge, and the failure of this knowledge to guide behavior in pursuit of the appropriate goals and actions. This tendency to disregard the requirements of a given task, even when these are verbally appreciated, represented a fundamental aspect of executive dysfunction, referred to as *goal neglect* (56). Levine and his colleagues (57) developed a formalized intervention for executive dysfunction, referred to as goal management training (GMT), based on the theory of goal neglect. The process of GMT involves five discrete stages of what is essentially a general purpose, problem-solving algorithm starting with an evaluation of the relevant goals in a situation, through the selection of sub-goals, and then monitoring the results of one's attempts at a solution; in the event of a mismatch the entire process is repeated. Thirty patients with mild to severe TBI were randomly assigned to receive either GMT or an alternative treatment of motor skills training. GMT consisted of a single session in which participants were instructed to apply the problem solving algorithm to two functional tasks. Patients in the motor skills training condition practiced reading and tracing mirror-reversed text and designs. Treatment effectiveness was assessed on several paper and pencil tasks which resembled the training tasks, and were intended to simulate the kind of unstructured everyday situations which might elicit goal management deficits. Participants who received GMT demonstrated significant reduction in errors and prolonged time to task completion (presumably reflecting increased care and attention to the tasks) on two of the three outcome measures following the intervention. The entire treatment in this study consisted of one hour of intervention, which may be adequate to suggest the potential efficacy of GMT but provides little evidence of its clinical effectiveness.

Another prospective randomized controlled study (58) utilized a problem solving intervention intended to facilitate patients' ability to reduce the complexity of a multistage problem by breaking it down into manageable subgoals. Training was provided 37 patients who were identified as poor problem solvers on formal tests of planning and response regulation. Twenty participants received an intervention directed at remediation of executive function deficits, while 17 participants received an alternative intervention consisting of memory retraining. Patients who received the problem solving training demonstrated significant gains on neuropsychological measures of planning ability as well as improvement on behavioral ratings of executive dysfunction, such as awareness of cognitive deficits, goal-directed ideas, and problem-solving ability.

Rath and his colleagues (59) evaluated the effectiveness of an "innovative" treatment for problems-solving deficits, compared with a "conventional" neuropsychological group treatment for patients with TBI. The patients were described as being "higher functioning" but with documented, persistent impairments in social and vocational functioning (e.g., job loss, marital difficulties), an average of 4 years post-injury. The conventional treatment consisted of group exercises intended to improve cognitive skills and provide support for coping with emotional reactions and changes after injury. The innovative problem-solving intervention focused on the development of emotional self-regulation strategies as the basis for maintaining an effective problem-orientation, along with a "clear thinking" component that included training in problem solving skills using role-plays of real-life examples of problem situations. Both groups showed significant improvement of their memory functioning after treatment. Only the problem solving group treatment resulted in significant beneficial effects on measures of executive functioning, self-appraisal of "clear thinking", self-appraisal of emotional self-regulation, and objective observer-ratings of interpersonal problem solving behaviors in naturalistic simulations.

These three randomized controlled studies demonstrate that training patients with TBI to use formal problem-solving methods can be an effective intervention. The study by Rath et al. (59) suggests that the development of strategies to improve emotional self-regulation may be particularly relevant to the clinical treatment of patients with executive functioning deficits after TBI, and provides the clearest evidence that this intervention may improve patients' performance in everyday situations.

Several studies have attempted to remediate executive function impairments through the development and internalization of strategies for effective self-regulation. According to Luria (60), self-regulation is achieved through the covert, verbal mediation ("inner speech") of purposeful activity. However, simply having the patient repeat the task instruction is insufficient to re-establish self-regulation (61). Cicerone and Wood (62) used a self-instructional training procedure to encourage planning and self-monitoring, while inhibiting inappropriate behaviors. The training procedure included three stages of self-verbalization, progressing from overt verbalization, through faded verbal self-instruction, to covert verbal mediation of appropriate responses. Over the course of training, there was a dramatic reduction in task-related errors as well as more gradual reduction and eventual cessation of off-task behaviors. Generalization to his functional, real-life behaviors were observed only with additional instruction and practice in the application and self-monitoring of the verbal mediation strategy to his everyday behaviors. A subsequent study (63) replicated this finding with six patients who exhibited impaired planning and self-monitoring after frontal lobe injury. Five of the six patients showed marked reduction of task-related errors and perseverative responses, suggesting that the effectiveness of training was related to the patients' improved ability to inhibit inappropriate responses. Self-instructional training has also been shown to be an effective component of interventions directed at attention (22, 64) or memory (65).

There is a potential paradox in attempts to remediate disorders of executive functioning, in that these disorders effect the processes of self-monitoring and self regulation that are an inherent aspect of remedial compensations. Successful compensation appears to require some residual capacity to deliberately and consciously apply strategies. A recent, uncontrolled group study (66) of patients with documented frontal lobe damage, severe cognitive impairments and poor self-awareness has demonstrated improvements after four months of treatment in patients' knowledge and use of self-regulatory strategies, and the self-rated effectiveness of strategies in their daily functioning. Several case studies have also described interventions that improved the patients' ability to self-monitor their behavior (67, 68). In each of these studies, the goal of cognitive remediation was not the training of task-specific performance, but the training and internalization of regulatory cognitive processes. In contrast, limited success was observed in two descriptive case studies of patients with orbitofrontal damage that resulted in social cognition and affective regulation. In both cases, the patients were able to improve specific behaviors in the situations in which they had been trained, but could not effectively modify their problematic social and emotional responses in novel, real-life situations, despite extensive treatment (69, 70).

Remediation of Pragmatic Communication Deficits

Deficits in executive functioning may be expressed as a disturbance of the social and affective and pragmatic aspects of communication, as noted by Eslinger in this volume. Thus, while classic neurologic syndromes of language impairment are not commonly seen after TBI, patients with TBI frequently exhibit impairments of pragmatic communication. These may include the loss of coherence and cohesiveness during narrative discourse, difficulty interpreting subtle, contextual aspects of communication (e.g., humor, sarcasm, irony), and failure to interpret or respond to non-verbal cues in the context of social communications. Helffenstein and Wechsler (71) evaluated the effectiveness of a group intervention designed to improve interpersonal communication skills, in which the central aspect of treatment was to provide patients with systematic review and feedback concerning their interpersonal, communication interactions. Beneficial effects were noted following this procedure, compared with a sample of subjects with TBI who received equivalent treatment contact without the systematic feedback. Specific improvements were noted on self-report measures of self-concept, ratings of interpersonal and communications skills, and the effectiveness of interpersonal communication in non-therapy, social settings. Several uncontrolled group studies (72, 73) and single-case studies (74, 75) have reported improved pragmatics and conversational skills following treatment that included systematic feedback and self-monitoring of interpersonal communications. The focus of the group-based treatment was to improve patients' communication competence in social contexts, including initiation, topic maintenance, turn taking, and active listening. Within each of these skill areas, treatment addressed the subjects' awareness of obstacles to effective communication, practice of effective communication, and generalization to natural contexts. The goal of the generalization phase was to apply the trained skills to relevant activities and settings in each individual's particular community, incorporating practice with parents and peers (72). One case study (76) has indicated that improvements in narrative discourse that were seen in treatment did not transfer to the patients' functional conversations. This lack of generalization was attributed to the "acontextual" nature of the treatment, and can be contrasted with the treatments that included specific interventions to promote the generalization of communications skills to the patients' real-life contexts and activities.

INTENSIVE-HOLISTIC COGNITIVE REHABILITATION

Cognitive rehabilitation of TBI may best be achieved through a comprehensive, *holistic* approach to the treatment of cognitive, emotional, and functional impairments and disability. Comprehensive-holistic neuropsychological rehabilitation is centered around the goals of fostering patients' awareness of their functional potential and adapting to the chronic limitations imposed by their injury, in order to alleviate disability in everyday, social functioning. Ben-Yishay was perhaps the first clinician to delineate and advocate the need for a holistic approach to the neuropsychological rehabilitation of individuals with brain injury (77). In discussing the rationale for the holistic, or therapeutic milieu, approach to neuropsychological rehabilitation, Ben-Yishay and Gold (78) emphasized that the neurobehavioral manifestations after traumatic brain injury are dynamic and multidetermined. They suggest that "it is meaningless to make rigid distinctions between higher and lower level cognitive functions or between physiogenic and psychogenic factors in emotional disturbances" after brain injury (p. 194). Thus, neither isolated cognitive remedial exercises to improve attention, memory, and or other "fragmentary" deficits, nor a focus exclusively on traditional psychotherapeutic interventions, are likely to be effective. Instead, an effective rehabilitation program must systematically integrate interventions directed at the remediation of cognitive deficits, functional skills, and interpersonal functions. Improvements in functioning are typically accomplished by an improvement in the effective functional application of residual cognitive abilities, rather than restoration of the underlying cognitive deficits, per se.

An early study of the relationship between holistic cognitive rehabilitation and employability (79) evaluated the effectiveness of a clinical program consisting of three phases. The first phase consisted of individual modules of cognitive remediation and group treatments to improve interpersonal communication, social competence, and awareness and acceptance of the consequences of brain injury. Treatment was provided within the model of a "therapeutic community" which included the engagement of family members and significant others in the treatment process. The second phase of treatment was devoted to structured work trials, and the third stage involved actual work placements. Employability ratings suggested that 84% of the previously unemployed patients were able to engage in some form of productive activity following the neuropsychological rehabilitation program. A subsequent study (80) suggested that patient characteristics related to motivation, affective regulation, and accurate self-appraisal were more closely related to effective functioning after treatment than neurologic or neuropsychological characteristics.

The relative contributions of individualized cognitive remedial interventions and small-group based exercises in interpersonal communication within the context of a holistic neuropsychological rehabilitation program have been explicitly evaluated (81). One group of patients received a mixture of cognitive and interpersonal interventions. A second group of patients received the individualized cognitive remedial interventions but did not receive interpersonal communication training. The third group received the initial, basic attentional training followed by the interpersonal remediation, while the individualized cognitive interventions were withheld. Only the two groups receiving the individualized cognitive remediation showed improvement on near transfer measures of cognitive functioning, which may have reflected practice effects as these measures were similar to the tasks used in treatment. There was a tendency for patients receiving the interpersonal training to show improvement on measures of affect regulation, self appraisal and self esteem. These findings are consistent with the holistic approach to treatment, indicating that the greatest gains in functioning may be achieved through the integrated treatment of both cognitive and interpersonal functioning.

There have been two prospective, randomized controlled studies of comprehensive rehabilitation for patients with TBI. Both studies are best considered as efficacy studies, in that treatment was provided to selected patients in a highly constrained environment. The first of these studies (82) compared the effects of structured cognitive rehabilitation with treatment providing professional attention and psychosocial support. Participants with moderate-to-severe TBI, one to seven years post-injury, were recruited from the community and "quasi-randomly" assigned to treatment conditions. Potential participants with expressive or receptive language disturbance, significant visual deficits, prior neuropsychiatric disturbance, or poor motivation were excluded from treatment. Subjects in the neuropsychological treatment condition received specific treatments directed at improving attention, memory, visuospatial ability, and problem solving. Subjects in the alternative, psychosocial treatment condition received an equivalent amount of treatment directed at coping skills, interpersonal functioning, and personal development. Both groups improved, but there was little overall difference between the two groups on measures of neuropsychological functioning or emotional adjustment. The findings suggest that non-specific factors (e.g., establishment of a therapeutic alliance and expectations for improvement) contributed to the effects of treatment in both conditions.

Salazar and colleagues (83) evaluated the efficacy of cognitive rehabilitation for 120 people with moderate to severe TBI (an average of 38 days post injury) within a single, military medical referral center. The program was based on the principles of a "therapeutic milieu" modified to meet the needs of patients returning to active military duty. Patients were randomly assigned to receive either a multidisciplinary, in-hospital cognitive rehabilitation program or home-based education and encouragement from a psychiatric nurse. There was no difference between groups on either return to work or fitness for military duty one year after treatment. The groups also did not differ on measures of neuropsychological functioning, although participants with more severe injuries demonstrated greater improvement after the cognitive rehabilitation program.

In both of these studies, the ability to generalize the results to the typical clinical situation is limited. Length of treatment was relatively brief (eight weeks) in both studies, and significant subject selection biases were apparent. Salazar (83) noted the "extraordinarily high return-to-work rates" and suggested that participants' high pre-injury education and level of functioning, significant degree of spontaneous recovery, and ready availability of (military) employment after injury might have limited the ability to detect any differential benefits from the cognitive rehabilitation program.

Clinical studies of comprehensive-holistic cognitive rehabilitation have generally reported more positive results. One prospective, non-randomized study evaluated the benefits of either a "standard" program of postacute neurorehabilitation or a more structured and intensive milieu-based rehabilitation program (84). Treatment was provided to 56 patients with primarily moderate-to-severe TBI who had been referred for cognitive rehabilitation, either from acute rehabilitation or from the community. All patients were screened and assigned to one of the treatment programs based on clinician's judgments regarding the most appropriate treatment. As a result of this selection process, patients who received the more intensive-holistic cognitive rehabilitation program were further post-injury, more likely to exhibit impaired self-awareness, and exhibited lower initial levels of community functioning on admission to rehabilitation. Overall, patients in both treatment conditions showed significant improvements in community integration; the patients who received the intensive-holistic treatment program showed greater improvement despite the fact that they were less functional and further post-injury at the time of admission. Improvements in overall neuropsychological functioning were associated with clinically significant improvement in community integration. Patients' satisfaction with their cognitive functioning after treatment was also a strong indication of successful community integration, again suggesting the contribution of psychological factors in patients' ability to benefit from cognitive rehabilitation.

A number of retrospective studies have also reported positive benefits from comprehensive neuropsychological rehabilitation programs, compared with patients who did not receive rehabilitation (85–87). Observational studies in this area have also demonstrated significant improvements in community functioning after treatment (88–90) that persist for many years (91, 92). These clinical studies support the effectiveness of a programmatic approach to cognitive rehabilitation for people with TBI, including those who have been unable to resume effective functioning several years after injury.

CONCLUSIONS

Cognitive rehabilitation is an integral part of the neurorehabilitation of TBI. The first published case studies on remediating memory deficits in brain damaged individuals appeared in 1977 (28). The clinical practice of cognitive rehabilitation has matured substantially in the ensuing 25 years. Empirical evidence for the effectiveness of cognitive rehabilitation is beginning to catch up with clinical practice. Recent systematic reviews of the literature (3, 93) have identified 20 randomized, controlled trials addressing the remediation of higher cognitive deficits in patients with TBI, with 35% of these published within the last 5 years. In clinical practice, there is general consensus that cognitive rehabilitation (regardless of the specific approach taken) should be directed at improving patients' everyday functioning and quality of life. Most studies of interventions for specific cognitive functions have been limited to assessing the effectiveness of treatment at the impairment level, although several recent studies have demonstrated clinically meaningful improvements in community integration following comprehensive-holistic cognitive rehabilitation.

Efforts to provide patients with the best available treatment, and to evaluate the effectiveness of cognitive rehabilitation, need to consider the complex nature of the interventions, the heterogeneity of patients with TBI, and the need to individualize treatment according to the unique and varied demands of patients' lives. For these reasons, the practice of cognitive rehabilitation will continue to rely upon clinical judgment and experience. Cognitive rehabilitation is not a distinct form of service, or the purview of any single discipline, but a specialized form of rehabilitation that requires adequate professional training in the nature of brain-behavior relationships, the neurologic basis of intact and impaired cognitive function, and the rehabilitation of cognitive disorders (94). It is also essential for clinicians who practice cognitive rehabilitation to maintain their knowledge of the literature and the empirical basis for the effectiveness of interventions as a means of guiding treatment selection and implementation. The increasing emphasis on evidence-based (cognitive) rehabilitation is not intended to supplant clinical judgment, but to inform it through the best available scientific evidence.

The ability to secure adequate reimbursement for cognitive rehabilitation remains a challenge in many cases, sometimes due to the position taken by referral sources and payers that cognitive rehabilitation remains an "investigational" procedure. The increasing evidence for the effectiveness of cognitive rehabilitation, and familiarity with evidence-based recommendations for cognitive rehabilitation by practicing clinicians, should help to facilitate this process. There is already evidence that some major insurance providers are incorporating the current evidence for effectiveness of cognitive rehabilitation in their clinical policy bulletins. In other cases, clinicians who are providing treatment in accordance with evidence-based recommendations may be able to obtain approval for cognitive rehabilitation through the external claim review process that is available in many states.

From a scientific perspective, the evaluation of the effectiveness of cognitive rehabilitation is, of course, a continuous and ongoing process. There continues to be some debate regarding the most appropriate methodology for conducting research on cognitive rehabilitation. Well-designed single-case studies can provide important information, especially regarding novel or innovative interventions. Highly controlled, clinical trials remain the most sure way to subject an intervention to rigorous confirmation of its efficacy. The selection of an appropriate research methodology will depend on multiple considerations, including the state of the already existing evidence, the ability to standardize the intervention across subjects or settings, and the availability of resources required to conduct the study. Perhaps the most compelling need in this area is the establishment of sustained programs of research that develop and evaluate the effectiveness and utility of an intervention through increasingly rigorous and practical methods, including the replication of findings across settings. This has generally not been achieved in the field of cognitive rehabilitation, with some exceptions (18, 19, 49–51). There is also a need to assess the external validity of cognitive rehabilitation, particularly through the use of outcome measures that are congruent with the research intentions. For example, the use of functional imaging may provide information about the degree of functional plasticity and nature of cerebral reorganization (if any) associated with a specific intervention. However, it can not be assumed that changes in the pattern of cerebral activation, even when present, are related to improvements in the individual's neuropsychological performance or everyday functioning. This will require that these interventions be assessed with an appropriate range of relevant health-outcome measures (e.g., functional limitations, community integration, subjective well-being). It is only through a sustained program of research that cognitive rehabilitation will fulfill its clinical and scientific promise, to improve the quality of lives for people with neurocognitive disability.

*R*eferences

1. Mazmanian PE, Kreutzer JS, Devany CW, Martin KO. A survey of accredited and other rehabilitation facilities: education, training and cognitive rehabilitation in brain-injury programmes. *Brain Injury* 1993;7:319–331.
2. Corrigan JD, Whiteneck G, Mellick MA: Perceived needs following traumatic brain injury. *J Head Trauma Rehabil* 2004;19: 205–16.
3. Cicerone KD, Dahlberg C, Kalmar K, Langenbahn DM, Malec JF, Bergquist TF et al. Evidence-based cognitive rehabilitation: recommendations for clinical practice. *Arch Phys Med Rehab* 2000;81;1596–1615.

4. Lura AR. Restoration of Function after Brain Injury. Oxford: Pergamon Press. 1963.

5. Mesulam M-M. *Principles of Behavioral and Cognitive Neurology* (2nd. Edition) New York: Oxford University Press. 2000.

6. Roberson IH, Murre JM. Rehabilitation of brain damage: brain plasticity and principles of guided recovery. *Psych Bull* 1999; 125:544–575.

7. Bach-y-Rita P. Theoretical basis for brain plasticity after a TBI. *Brain Injury* 2003;17:643–651.

8. Sohlberg MM, Mateer CA. *Introduction to Cognitive Rehabilitation: Theory and Practice.* New York: Guilford Press, 1989

9. Gordon WA, Hibbard MR, Egelko S, Diller L, Shaver MS, Lieberman A, Ragnarsson K. Perceptual remediation in patients with right brain damage: a comprehensive program. *Arch Phys Med Rehabil* 1985;66:353–9.

10. Mayer NH, Keating DJ, Rapp D. Skills, routines and activity patterns of daily living: A functional nested approach. In B Uzzell, Y Gross (eds.) *Clinical neuropsychology of intervention.* 1986, Boston:Martinus Nijhoff.

11. Tsvetkova LS. Basic principles of a theory of reeducation of brain-injured patients. *Journal of Special Education,* 1972;6:135–144.

12. Glisky EL, Schacter DL. Acquisition of domain-specific knowledge in organic amnesia: Training for computer-related work. *Neuropsychologica* 1987;25:893–906.

13. Flavell JH. Metacognition and cognitive monitoring: A new area of psychological inquiry. *American Psychologist,* 1979;34: 906–911.

14. Shallice T. Neurologic impairment of cognitive processes. *British Medical Bulletin,* 1981;37:187–192.

15. Crosson B, Barco PP, Velozo CA, Bolesta MM, Cooper PV, Werts D, Brobeck TC. Awareness and compensation in post-acute head injury rehabilitation. *Journal of Head Trauma Rehabilitation,* 1989;4(3), 46–54.

16. Posner MI, Rothbart MK. Attentional mechanisms and conscious experience. In AD Milner, MD Rugg (eds), *The Neuropsychology of Consciousness.* 1992 (pp. 91–111). New York: Academic Press.

17. Whyte J. Neurologic disorders of attention and arousal: Assessment and treatment. *Archives of Physical Medicine and Rehabilitation,* 1992;73:1094–1103.

18. Sohlberg MM, Mateer CA. Effectiveness of an attentional training program. *J Clin Exp Neuropsychol* 1987;9:117–130.

19. Sohlberg MM, McLaughlin KA, Pavese A, Heidrich A, Posner MI. Evaluation of attention process training and brain injury education in persons with acquired brain injury. *J Clin Exp Neuropsychol* 2000;22:656–676.

20. Niemann H, Ruff RM, Baser CA. Computer assisted attention retraining in head injured individuals: A controlled efficacy study of an out-patient program. *J Consult Clin Psychol* 1990;58; 811–817.

21. Gray JM, Robertson I, Pentland B, Anderson S. Microcomputer-based attentional retraining after brain damage: A randomized group controlled trial. *Neuropsychol Rehabil* 1992;2:97–115.

22. Fasotti, L, Kovacs, F., Eling PATM, Brouwer WH. Time pressure management as a compensatory strategy training after closed head injury. *Neuropsychological Rehabilitation,* 2000;10:47–65.

23. Cicerone KD. Remediation of 'working attention' in mild traumatic brain injury. *Brain Injury,* 2002;16:185–195.

24. Wilson B, Robertson IH. A home based intervention for attentional slips during reading following head injury: A single case study. *Neuropsychol Rehabil* 1992;2:193–205

25. Novack TA, Caldwell SG, Duke LW, Berquist T. Focused versus unstructured intervention for attention deficits after traumatic brain injury. *J Head Trauma Rehabilil* 1996;11(3):52–60.

26. Ponsford JL, Kinsella G. Evaluation of a remedial programme for attentional deficits following closed head injury. *J Clin Exp Neuropsychol* 1988;10:693–708.

27. DeLuca J, Schultheis MT, Madigan NK, Christodoulou C, Averill A. Acquisition versus retrieval deficits in traumatic brain injury: Implications for memory rehabilitation. *Arch Phys Med Rehabil* 2000;81:1327–1333.

28. Glasgow RE, Zeiss RA, Barrera M, Lewinsohn PM. Case studies on remediating memory deficits in brain damaged individuals. *J Clin Psychol* 1977;33:1049–1054.

29. Ryan TV, Ruff RM. The efficacy of structured memory retraining in a group comparison of head trauma patients. *Arch Clin Neuropsychol* 1988;3:165–179.

30. Kaschel R, Della Sala S, Cantagallo A, Fahlbock A, Laaksonen R, Kazen M. Imagery mnemonics for the rehabilitation of memory: A randomised group controlled trial. *Neuropsych Rehab,* 2002;12:127–153.

31. Berg I, Konning-Haanstra M, Deelman B. Long term effects of memory rehabilitation. A controlled study. *Neuropsychol Rehabil* 1991;1:97–111.

32. Milders MV, Berg IJ, Deelman BG. Four-year follow-up of a controlled memory training study in closed head injured patients. *Neuropsychological Rehabilitation,* 1995;5:223–238.

33. Wilson B. Recovery and compensatory strategies in head injured memory impaired people several years after insult. *Journal of Neurology, Neurosurgery and Psychiatry,* 1992;55:177–80.

34. Evans JJ, Wilson B, Needhan P, Brentnall S. Who makes good use of memory aids? Results of a survey of people with acquired brain injury. *J Int Neuropsych Soc,* 2003;9:925–935.

35. Mateer CA, Sohlberg MM, Crinean J. Perceptions of memory function in individuals with closed head injury. *J Head Trauma Rehabil* 1987;2(3): 74–84.

36. Sohlberg MM, White W, Evans E, Mateer C. An investigation of the effects of prospective memory training. *Brain Injury,* 1992a; 6:139–154.

37. Raskin SA, Sohlberg MM. The efficacy of prospective memory training in two adults with brain injury. *Journal of Head Trauma Rehabilitation,* 1996;11(3):32–51.

38. Schmitter-Edgecombe M, Fahy J, Whelan J, Long, C. Memory remediation after severe closed head injury. Notebook training versus supportive therapy. *J Consult Clin Psychol* 1995;63:484–489.

39. Zencius A, Wesolowski MD, Burke WH. A comparison of four memory strategies with traumatically brain-injured clients. *Brain Injury* 1990;4:33–38.

40. Burke J, Danick J, Bemis B, Durgin C. A process approach to memory book training for neurological patients. *Brain Injury* 1994;8:71–81.

41. Sohlberg MM, Mateer CA. Training use of compensatory memory books: A three stage behavioral approach. *J Clin Exp Neuropsychol* 1989;11:871–891.

42. Hart T, Hawkey K, Whyte J. Use of a portable voice organizer to remember therapy goals in traumatic brain injury rehabilitation: A within-subjects trial. *J Head Trauma Rehabil* 2002;17:556–570.

43. van den Broek MD, Downes J, Johnson Z, Dayus B, Hilton N. Evaluation of an electronic memory aid in the neuropsychological rehabilitation of prospective memory deficits. *Brain Injury,* 2000;14:455–452.

44. Yasuda K, Misu T, Beckman B, Watanabe O, Ozawa Y, Nakamura T. Use of an IC Recorder as a voice output memory aid for patients with prospective memory impairment. *Neuropsych Rehab,* 2002;12:1155–166.

45. O'Connel ME, Mateer CA, Kerns KA. Prosthetic systems for addressing problems with initiation: Guidelines for selection, training and measuring efficacy. *NeuroRehab,* 2003;18:9–20.

46. LoPresti EL, Mihailidis A, Kirsch N. Assistive technology for cognitive rehabilitation: State of the art. *Neuropsychol Rehabil* 2004;14:5–39.

47. Bergman MM. The Essential Steps cognitive orthotic. *NeuroRehab,* 2003;18:31–46.

48. Gorman P, Dayle R, Hood CA, Rumrell L. Effectiveness of the ISAAC cognitive prosthetic system for improving rehabilitation outcomes with neurofunctional impairment. *NeuroRehab,* 2003;18:57–67.

49. Wilson BA, Emslie H, Quirk K, Evans J. George: Learning to live independently with NeuroPage. *Rehabilitation Psychology,* 1999;44:284–296.

50. Wilson BA, Emslie HC, Quirk K, Evans JJ. Reducing everyday memory and planning problems by means of a paging system. a randomised control crossover study. *J Neurol Neurosurg Psychiat,* 2001;70:477–482.

51. Wilson BA, Scott H, Evans J, Emslie H. Preliminary report of a NeuroPage service within a health care system. *NeuroRehab,* 2003;18:3–8.

52. Barbas H, Pandya DN. Patterns of connections of the prefrontal cortex in the rhesus monkey associated with cortical architecture. In Levin HS, Eisenberg, HM & Benton, AL (editors) *Frontal lobe function and dysfunction*. 1991, New York: Oxford University Press, 35–58.

53. Rezai K, Andreasan NC, Alliger R, Cohen G, Swayze V, O'Leary DS. The neuropsychology of the prefrontal cortex. *Archives of Neurology* 1993;50:636–642.

54. Lhermitte F. Human autonomy and the frontal lobes. Part II: Patient behavior in complex and social situations: The "environmental dependency syndrome". *Annals of Neurology*, 1986;19: 335–343.

55. Eslinger PJ, Damasio AR: Severe disturbance of higher cognition after bilateral frontal ablation: Patient EVR. *Neurology* 1985;35:1731–1741.

56. Duncan, J, Emslie H, Williams P, Johnson R, Freer C. Intelligence and the frontal lobe: The organisation of goal-directed behaviour. *Cognitive Psychology*, 1996;30:2257–303.

57. Levine B, Robertson IH, Clare L, Carter G, et al. Rehabilitation of executive functioning: an experimental-clinical validation of goal management training. *J Int Neuropsychol Soc* 2000;299–312.

58. von Cramen DY, Mathes-von Cramen, Mai N. Problem solving deficits in brain injured patients. A therapeutic approach. *Neuropsychol Rehabil* 1991;1:45–64

59. Rath JF, Simon D, Langenbahn DM, Sherr RL, Diller L. Group treatment of problem-solving deficits in outpatients with traumatic brain injury: a randomized outcome study. *Neuropsychol Rehabil* 2003;13:461–488.

60. Luria AR. *Higher Cortical Functions in Man*. 1980, New York: Basic Books.

61. Luria AR, Pribram KH, Homskaya ED. An experimental analysis of the behavioral disturbance produced by a left frontal arachnoidal endothelioma. *Neuropsychologia* 1964;2:257–280.

62. Cicerone KD, Wood JC: Planning disorder after closed head injury: A case study. *Arch Phys Med Rehabil* 1987;68:111–115.

63. Cicerone KD, Giacino JT. Remediation of executive function deficits after traumatic brain injury. *NeuroRehabilitation* 1992;2(3):12–22.

64. Webster JS, Scott RR. The effects of self-instructional training of attentional deficits following head injury. *Clin Neuropsychol* 1983;5:69–74.

65. Ownsworth TL, McFarland K. Memory remediation in long-term acquired brain injury: two approaches in diary training. *Brain Injury*, 1999;13:605–626.

66. Ownsworth TL, McFarland K, Young RmcD. Self-awareness and psychosocial functioning following acquired brain injury: an evaluation of a group support programme. *Neuropsychol Rehabil* 2000;10:465–484.

67. Sohlberg MM, Sprunk H, Metzelaar K. Efficacy of an external cuing system in an individual with severe frontal lobe damage. *Cog Rehabil* 1988;6:36–41.

68. Alderman N, Fry RK, Youngson HA. Improvement of self monitoring skills, reduction of behaviour disturbance and the dysexecutive syndrome. *Neuropsychological Rehabilitation* 1995;5:193–222.

69. von Cramen DY, Matthes-von Cramen G. Back to work with a chronic dysexecutive syndrome? (a case report). *Neuropsycholl Rehabil* 1994;4:399–417.

70. Cicerone KD, Tanenbaum LN. Disturbance of social cognition after traumatic orbitofrontal brain injury. *Arch Clin Neuropsychol* 1997;12:173–188.

71. Helffenstein D, Wechsler R. The use of interpersonal process recall (IPR) in the remediation of interpersonal and communication skill deficits in the newly brain injured. *Clin Neuropsychol* 1982; 4:139–143.

72. Wiseman-Hakes C, Stewart ML, Wasserman R, Schuller R. Peer group training of pragmatic skills in adolescents with acquired brain injury. *J Head Trauma Rehabil* 1998;13(6):23–38.

73. Ehrlich J, Sipes A. Group treatment of communication skills for head trauma patients. *Cognitive Rehabilitation* 1985;3: 32–37.

74. Gajar A, Schloss PJ, Schloss CN, Thompson CK. Effects of feedback and self-monitoring on head trauma youths' conversational skills, *J App Beh Anal* 1984;17:353–358.

75. Giles GM, Fussey I, Burgess P. The behavioral treatment of verbal interaction skills following severe head injury: A single case study. *Brain Injury* 1988;2:75–79.

76. Cannizzaro MS, Coelho CA. Treatment of story grammar following traumatic brain injury: a pilot study. *Brain Injury* 2002;16:1065–1073

77. Ben-Yishay Y, Rattok J, Lakin P, Piasetsky E, Ross B, Silver S, Zide E, Ezrachi O. Neuropsychologic rehabilitation: Quest for a holistic approach. *Seminars in Neurology* 1985;5:252–259.

78. Ben-Yishay Y, Gold J. Therapeutic milieu approach to neuropsychological rehabilitation. In RLl Woods (ed.) *Neurobehavioral Sequelae of Traumatic Brain Injury*. 1990 Taylor & Francis: New York.

79. Ben-Yishay Y, Silver SM, Piasetsky E, Rattok J. Relationship between employability and vocational outcome after intensive holistic cognitive rehabilitation. *Journal of Head Trauma Rehabilitation,* 1987;2(1):35–48.

80. Ezrachi O, Ben-Yishay Y, Kay T, Diller L, Rattok J. Predicting employment in traumatic brain injury following neuropsychological rehabilitation. *Journal of Head Trauma Rehabilitation,* 1991;6(3), 71–84.

81. Rattok J, Ben-Yishay Y, Ezrachi O, Lakin P, Piasetsky E, Ross B, Silver S, Vakil E, Zide E, Diller L. Outcome of different treatment mixes in a multidimensional neuropsychological rehabilitation program. *Neuropsychology* 1992;6(4):395–415.

82. Ruff RM, Baser CA, Johnston JW, Marshall LF. Neuropsychological rehabilitation: An experimental study with head-injured patients. *J. Head Trauma Rehabil* 1989;4(3):20–36.

83. Salazar AM, Warden DL, Schwab K, Spector J, et al. Cognitive rehabilitation for traumatic brain injury: a randomized trial. *JAMA* 2000;283:3075–3081.

84. Cicerone KD, Mott T, Azulay JA, Friel J. Community integration and satisfaction with functioning after intensive cognitive rehabilitation for traumatic brain injury. *Archives of Physical Medicine and Rehabilitation* 2004;85:1643–1650.

85. Goranson TE, Graves RE, Allison D, La Freniere R. Community integration following multidisciplinary rehabilitation for traumatic brain injury. *Brain Injury* 2003;17:759–774.

86. Prigatano GP, Fordyce DJ, Zeiner HK, Roueche JR, Pepping M, Wood BC. Neuropsychological rehabilitation after closed head injury in young adults. *J Neurol Neurosurg Psychiat* 1984;47: 505–13.

87. Prigatano GP, Klonoff PS, O'Brien KP, Altman IM, Amin K, Chiapello D, Shepherd J, Cunningham M, Mora M. Productivity after neuropsychologically oriented milieu rehabilitation. *J Head Trauma Rehabil* 1994;9(1):91–102.

88. Malec J. Impact of comprehensive day treatment on societal participation for persons with acquired brain injury. *Arch Phys Med Rehab* 2001;82:885–895.

89. Seale GS, Caroselli JS, High WM, Becker CL, Neese LE, Scheibel R. Use of the Community Integration Questionnaire (CIQ) to characterize changes in functioning for individuals with traumatic brain injury who participated in a post-acute rehabilitation programme. *Brain Injury* 2002;16:955–967

90. Klonoff PS, Lamb DG, Henderson SW, Shepherd J. Outcome assessment after milieu-based neurorehabilitation: new considerations. *Arch Phys Med Rehabil,* 1998;79:684–690.

91. Sander AM, Roebuck TM, Struchen MA, Sherer M, High WM. Long-term maintenance of gains obtained in post-acute rehabilitation by persons with traumatic brain injury. *J Head Trauma Rehab* 2001;16:356–373

92. Klonoff PS, Lamb DG, Henderson SW. Milieu-based neurorehabilitation in patients with traumatic brain injury: outcome at up to 11 years postdischarge. *Arch Phys Med Rehab* 2000;81:1535–1537.

93. Cicerone KD, Dahlberg C, Malec JF, Harley JP, Langenbahn DM. *Update on evidence-based cognitive rehabilitation*. Presented at ACRM-ASNR Joint Conference on Evidence-Based Rehabilitation, Ponte Verde, FL; September 9, 2004.

94. Harley JP, Allen C, Braciszeski TL, Cicerone KD, Dahlberg C, Evans S, Foto M, Gordon WA, Harrington D, Levin W, Malec JF, Millis S, Morris J, Muir C, Richert J, Salazar E, Schiavone DA, Smigielski JS. Guidelines for Cognitive Rehabilitation. *NeuroRehab* 1992;2(3):62–67.

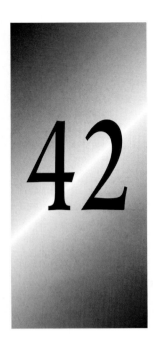

42 Cognitive Impairments After TBI

Paul J. Eslinger
Giuseppe Zappalà
Freeman Chakara
Anna M. Barrett

INTRODUCTION

Traumatic brain injury (TBI) is associated with several types of pathophysiology that damage cerebral cortex and subcortical nuclear structures as well as white matter connections (see chapter by Povlishock and Bullock for more details). The resulting changes in brain anatomy and physiology disrupt the typical functioning of specific structures and the larger neural networks they comprise, leading to subsequent neurological and neurobehavioral impairments. In addition to these direct brain-behavior effects of TBI, there can be many complicating medical and psychological problems that contribute to post-traumatic cognitive, behavioral and emotional impairments. These are detailed in several chapters throughout the text and underscore the complex nature of TBI. Despite their prevalence, cognitive impairments must be carefully evaluated on an individual basis, as they may be influenced by pre-existing conditions (e.g., learning disabilities, attention deficit hyperactivity disorder, substance abuse, prior head trauma), co-morbid conditions (e.g., seizures, major depression, pain, and medication side-effects) and differences in TBI effects and recovery. As an example, recent study identified a significant effect of major depression in lowering cognitive test scores after TBI (1). Hence, a multidisciplinary and comprehensive approach to TBI is necessary for best treatment outcomes.

Attentional and memory problems after TBI are among the most common cognitive impairments reported by patients, their family members and clinicians (2, 3). Recent study has also emphasized that prominent working memory impairments occur after TBI (4). Such cognitive deficits are frequently accompanied by a spectrum of other cognitive, social, emotional and behavioral changes as well. This chapter provides an overview of cognitive impairments that are commonly associated with TBI in adults. Accompanying chapters by Kreutzer (*Neuropsychological Assessment and Treatment*), Cicerone (*Cognitive Rehabilitation*), Murdoch (*Speech Disorders*), Wehamn (*Vocational Rehabilitation*), Coelho (Language and Communication), Arciniegas and Silver (*Cognitive Psychopharmacology*) and Johnston (*Functional Assessment and Outcome Evaluation*) address important interrelated aspects of cognition and TBI. The importance of these topics stem from the fact that the long-term effects of TBI on personal, social and occupational ability and disability can often be related to cognitive, behavioral and emotional functioning. Indeed, cognitive measures are among the most important predictors of patients' return to work and independent living, even among those with good medical recoveries (4–7).

NEUROPSYCHOLOGICAL EVALUATION

Neuropsychological assessment encompasses clinical and psychometric testing procedures that survey and objectively measure the effects of cerebral damage on cognitive, behavioral, social and emotional functioning (8, 9). These procedures typically employ a wide range of standardized cognitive tests and survey instruments, together with comprehensive interview and clinical assessment. Neuropsychological test scores can change in different ways depending upon TBI pathophysiology. To this end, a variety of specific assessment techniques have been developed to evaluate a patient's relative strengths and weaknesses in multiple neurobehavioral domains such as memory, language, attention, spatial cognition, executive functions, and social cognition. Scores are then interpreted in reference to available normative data that provide the typical range and variation in test performance. Interpretation of neuropsychological test scores is meant to identify the type and severity of cognitive impairments that in turn reflect general location and severity of brain injury. While some clinicians employ fixed neuropsychological batteries that administer the same compilation of tests to all patients, most clinicians use a flexible battery approach that focuses on specific problem areas identified through clinical exam and observation. The flexible battery approach also places a very strong emphasis on evaluating the patient's *pattern* of performance; that is, the possible causes for their impaired test score. For example, an impaired memory test score may be reflect attentional and encoding deficiencies, memory consolidation deficits, or poor retrieval of information. Delineating specific processing impairments may provide a more direct and efficient approach to remediation services that target impaired processes. Therefore, neuropsychological assessment, along with assessments provided through medical and diverse therapy services (i.e., physical, occupational, speech and recreational specialists) is geared toward identifying how best to intervene in the remediation of cognitive, behavioral, social and emotional impairments that are caused by TBI (see chapters by Cicerone and by Wehman for further discussion of this interface). The following sections cover specific cognitive processing domains that are particularly important in TBI.

INFORMATION PROCESSING AND ATTENTION

Information processing measures are typically designed to determine the speed and accuracy of sensory-perception and perceptual-motor responses. These processes are mediated by diverse brain structures that include multiple cortical regions, subcortical nuclei and many white matter connections. The pathophysiology of head trauma may affect information processing in several ways. Sarno et al. (10) recently demonstrated that head trauma was associated with prolonged simple and choice reaction times to visual, auditory and tactile stimuli. Tactile stimuli

presented particular difficulty in comparison to vision and audition (i.e., sensory-specific deficit) as well as in combination with those modalities (i.e., cross-modal deficits). Mathias et al. (11) confirmed that reaction time speed was compromised after mild TBI, particularly as visual task difficulty increased and when inter-hemispheric transfer of information was required. The level of difficulty and transfer deficits were more evident for visual than tactile tasks in their study. Tinius (12) reported that similar to adults with attention deficit disorder, those with mild TBI were impaired on reaction time measures, underscoring the frequent finding of slowed reaction time after head trauma (13). However, reaction time changes interact with the particular type of tasks presented. For example, simple reaction time tasks are often completed in normal fashion after head trauma, but choice or complex reaction time tasks are frequently more difficult and lead to detectable impairments (14–16).

Zoccolotti and colleagues (17) sought to compare multiple information processing and attentional measures in a group of 106 patients with generally more severe TBI drawn from multiple European sites. The sample was tested at least 5 months after injury and 80% of participants suffered coma of 8 days or longer. Patients were presented with 4 computerized tasks with responses limited to button presses to measure accuracy and latency. The first 2 tasks were designed to require *intensive attention* and included measures of: (1) alertness (reaction time with and without a tonal warning) and (2) sustained attention (15 minutes of vigilant observation of horizontal bar movements). The final 2 tasks were considered measures of *selective attention* and hypothesized to be problematic for patients. These included: (3) selective attention (go no-go and design detection tasks) and (4) divided attention (simultaneous visual and auditory tasks, each to detect a specific pattern during continuous stimulus presentations). Patients showed considerably more difficulty in the selective attention tasks requiring go- no go responding (combining working memory with inhibitory control) or divided attention (increasing the working memory load), with up to one-half demonstrating deficits. Some difficulties were also evident in the more straightforward intensive attention conditions, varying between 9–33% of patients. However, coma severity had no statistically significant effects on the intensive attention measures of alertness and vigilance. Analyses also indicated considerable variability in performance amongst patients. This is not unexpected given the diverse trauma and personal characteristics of the sample. At least three subgroups were identified:

- A severely impaired subgroup, with a similar attention deficit profile as the overall sample (greater impairment in selective and divided attention tasks). This subgroup, comprising nearly 50% of the sample, also had more severe trauma and longer length of coma. While all patients with mild and moderate levels of coma completed the divided attention task, 5% of severe and 26% of very severe coma patients were unable to complete the task.

- A less impaired subgroup with a large dissociation between normal alertness scores and poor divided attention scores. Nearly 44% of the sample showed this pattern of performance that argues against a nonspecific or generalized slowing of performance and supports the possibility of a specific divided attention deficit. We have encountered such deficits commonly in clinical practice, where they can be described as disorganized behavior, losing track of objects, paperwork and activities, and being able to undertake only one activity or task at a time.

- A third possible subgroup (comprising only 7% of the sample) included those with very long reaction times in both alertness and divided attention tasks, suggesting very slowed psychomotor speed.

The prolonged reaction times of TBI patients appear to be influenced by both the type of task and the working memory load that it requires, usually represented by the number of competing stimuli and choices. These cognitive deficits may be a behavioral index of diffuse cerebral damage that subsequently limits speed of information processing particularly as environmental demands increase, becoming either more concentrated or sustained over time. Hence, TBI patients must exert greater mental effort in cognitive and occupational tasks that may have been readily managed prior to injury. This can lead to increased physical and mental fatigue, even headaches, that may be mistaken for stress effects. In these cases, a reduced work load and schedule is usually recommended. In some TBI cases, the degree of attentional change is sufficient to warrant evaluation of attention deficit-type symptoms. This is typically undertaken with a combination of standardized tests of attention (such as the Working Memory Index from the Wechsler Adult Intelligence Scale and continuous performance tasks) and behavioral survey of attentional behaviors (such as the Brown Adult ADD Scale). Treatment of adult TBI patients with low dose stimulants can be of significant benefit to their occupational and daily functioning, particularly when combined with cognitive compensatory strategies.

UNAWARENESS OF DEFICITS (ANOSOGNOSIA)

Anosognosia (meaning, literally, "without knowledge of disease," a term introduced by Babinski (18)) is a common behavioral disorder occurring in neurological conditions, characterized by limited acknowledgement or denial of neurological dysfunction. The symptoms of which the patient is unaware may vary, and include memory and cognitive deficits, hemiparesis, visual and other sensory disturbances, gait disorder and deficits of naturalistic action/limb apraxia (19, 20)

Patients' inability to recognize functionally-relevant problems is known to be a major barrier to rehabilitation after closed-head injury (21). Disavowal of neurological impairment can take several forms, including lack of emotional concern for acknowledged deficits (anosodiaphoria), verbal denial of deficits that are implicitly acknowledged (e.g. patients claim that they can walk but never actually attempt to get out of bed), combined explicit and implicit denial of deficits, denial of ownership of an impaired body part (asomatagnosia or somatoparaphrenia), and, at the far end of the continuum, dislike or hatred of a dysfunctional body part (misoplegia) (19, 22). Patients with this disorder can evidence dramatic abnormalities in behavior, such as throwing themselves from their beds "in order to get rid of that awful leg." Although occurring in conjunction with other clinical syndromes such as spatial neglect, amnesia, and even thought disorders, dissociations of awareness of deficit from each of the associated clinical syndromes are reported, and thus anosognosia may be best characterized as an independent syndrome, at this time without a single neuroanatomic basis.

Impact of Anosognosia

Although there are no formal studies of the possible contribution of anosognosia to a delay in seeking medical attention after closed head injury, numerous anecdotal reports suggest that unawareness of deficit (sometimes theorized to be partly due to a functional adaptation, e.g. "shock") may keep patients from presenting promptly to a medical care provider or emergency room after head injury, especially if patients lack other bodily injuries. Currently, no treatments for closed head injury are available that depend critically upon initiation within a short period after an injury occurs, but in the administration of acute thrombolytic therapies after stroke it has been suggested that anosognosia is a barrier to treatment delivery (19).

The most relevant impact of anosognosia on rehabilitation after closed head injury is in patients' acceptance of the rationale for participation in treatment (engagement in the rehabilitative program), and in their ability to participate in the program once having agreed to do so (19, 22, 23). It is reasoned that patients may put forward inadequate or inconsistent effort, preventing gains in strength and endurance. However, anosognosia and decreased motivation has not in formal studies been universally associated with a poorer rehabilitation outcome (24). The scope of rehabilitation for anosognosic patients may be more limited because of safety and supervision needs, and fewer challenging tasks may be attempted in order to ensure that patients will not expose themselves to further harm or attempt to perform tasks of which they are incapable. Lastly, anosognosia presents a barrier to studying outcomes in head trauma rehabilitation. After traumatic brain injury, patients consistently report better cognitive, physical and emotional outcomes than do their loved ones and clinicians (25–29). This creates problems in interpretation of patient self-report data, which might under other circumstances be considered to be of greater validity than that of external observers (30).

Mechanisms of Anosognosia

Proposals to account for unawareness of neurological deficits include: *psychological denial*, *modular dysfunction* at the level of an isolated cognitive or neurological subsystem or in a single semantic domain, *monitoring dysfunction* at a level of superordinate cognitive processing, and *multifactorial* theories postulating dysfunction in several cognitive domains (19, 22).

A detailed discussion of the putative mechanisms underlying anosognosia after brain injury is beyond the scope of this chapter. However, because of the importance of this theory, we will briefly discuss evidence regarding the mechanism of psychological denial. Weinstein and Kahn (31) first proposed that psychological denial may produce inability to acknowledge neurological deficits after stroke such as hemiparesis. Important clinical observations, however, are inconsistent with the psychological defense mechanism hypothesis. A coping strategy should be more utilized as recovery progresses, cognition improves, and chronic losses become apparent. Anosognosia is most apparent immediately post-injury, and gradually improves (19, 21, 22, 27, 30). A denial syndrome should be most severe for deficits posing the greatest potential ego threat, and less marked for deficits not likely to produce disability. However, modular dissociations in anosognosia not clearly based on subjective deficit severity (e.g. unawareness of visual problems but awareness of gait problems) are reported after head injury (22, 32). In subjects without brain injury, anosognosia can be induced by selective hemispheric anesthesia (19), but in the same individuals, this occurs more commonly after right- than left-sided injection. This asymmetry is difficult to explain on a psychological basis. Most critically, in brain-injured patients, it is unclear that anosognosia confers even temporary functional advantage, either in reducing subjective distress (33) or in improving function (34), which is central to the concept of a psychological defense. Schacter and Prigatano (35) wrote an excellent summary of the controversy about this issue:

> Although most observers agree that defensive denial of a kind that can be observed in non-brain-damaged patients plays *some* role in the unawareness phenomena exhibited by *some* brain-damaged patients, the nature

and extent of the contribution is still the subject of debate . . . The critical problem . . . is to develop adequate criteria for distinguishing between defensive and nondefensive forms of unawareness and to delineate the underlying bases for them.

Management and Treatment of Anosognosia

Unfortunately, large controlled trials of specific management and treatment methods for subjects with anosognosia after closed head injury are not yet available. A number of approaches are reported to be symptomatically useful (36–41). These include *explicit* techniques in which therapists have subjects self-assess and then perform straightforward, quantifiable tasks and help them to measure assessment-performance discrepancies, *implicit* techniques in which subjects are asked to perform in both preserved and deficient areas in order to experience the contrast between these abilities, and techniques involving *external and off-line feedback*, such as videotaping and later viewing task performance, and reviewing it in a group setting with performance assessment from other group members. Related to the external/off-line method is *intervention based on third person assessments*, in which patients make judgments about pictured scenaria in which others fail to perform tasks, preselected to resemble their impairments (42). Although reinforcement with these methods has traditionally been behavioral, positive results have been reported when increased accuracy of self-assessment is reinforced with monetary rewards (43).

A general difficulty with these clinical reports, however, is that although patients' awareness of deficit may have improved, the effect on daily living activities has not been well-studied. In at least one instance, there was a failure of the improved self-awareness to generalize to untrained tasks (38). Therefore, further studies are needed to identify the most effective interventions for anosognosia after TBI. In typical practice, such interventions are team-based and often require continued efforts by educated caregivers after hospital discharge.

INTELLECTUAL FUNCTIONING

Measures of intellectual functioning are frequently employed in the neuropsychological assessment of brain-injured patients to ascertain a broad range of cognitive capacities (44, 45). Although several instruments have been designed for the purpose of evaluating intelligence, the Wechsler scales are currently favored by most clinicians. The Wechsler Adult Intelligence Scale has several important features:

1. It surveys a broad range of verbal and nonverbal cognitive abilities with standardized instructions and materials

2. Test items are presented in ascending difficulty and usually discontinued after a certain number of incorrect responses, allowing for assessment of many different abilities without undue frustration for patients

3. The scale provides multiple scores for comparison such as verbal, performance and full scale IQ, and index scores for verbal comprehension, perceptual organization, working memory and processing speed

4. Interpretation of multiple subtest and composite scores is possible through extensive normative data that provide statistical comparisons, enhancing the strong reliability and validity indicators of the scale.

Interpretation of IQ tests requires highly trained clinical expertise particularly because there is no single or specific profile of intellectual impairment that results from brain damage (46). From available studies, however, it is possible to identify several common patterns of findings related to TBI effects, as follows:

1. A generalized pattern of intellectual decline is most likely to be observed in patients whose TBI is at least moderate to severe (47, 48).

2. The Wechsler Processing Speed Index is particularly sensitive to brain dysfunction, due mainly to the sensitivity of the digit-symbol coding and symbol search subtests. In contrast, other subtests (e.g., Matrix Reasoning, Vocabulary) appear resistant to the incremental effects of TBI (47, 49).

3. A large discrepancy between Verbal and Performance IQ scores is not always synonomous with brain damage; nor does it necessarily imply damage to one hemisphere versus the other. For example, a lower Performance IQ may be related to slowed visuomotor processing rather than right hemisphere damage per se, and a lower Verbal IQ may be related to impaired attention and concentration rather than left hemisphere damage per se. However, discrepancies of 15 points or more deserve close scrutiny for cognitive dysfunction (50, 51) as these differences are reaching statistically improbable levels for typical cognitive functioning. This entails ruling out other premorbid or concurrent causes of test impairment and supporting any inferences about localized brain damage (e.g., left or right hemisphere, frontal or temporal cortical) with additional specific indicators.

4. In reasoning about and explaining any left vs. right hemisphere disparities in intellectual processing, investigators have emphasized that the left hemisphere tends to fundamentally process information sequentially whereas the right hemisphere engages in more simultaneous information processing (51). Thus, left vs. right hemisphere deficits, at least as expressed through verbal vs. performance IQ score differences, should not be interpreted as simply verbal vs. visuospatial differences; rather, they may reflect different levels and approaches to information processing.

5. In studies of localized cerebral damage, left hemisphere injuries often result in lower digit span and arithmetic subtest scores, whereas picture arrangement deficiencies have been associated with right hemisphere lesions (52).

6. Impairment on the block design subtest has been associated with damage to the parietal lobes regardless of the side of cerebral dysfunction (46).

7. Vocabulary and picture completion subtests have been employed in estimating premorbid intellectual functioning because of their robust resistance to brain injury (49, 52).

8. Deficits on the similarities subtest has been associated predominantly with left frontal injury because of its reliance on verbal concept formation and abstraction (51, 53).

9. In interpreting intellectual test scores and patterns, the important contributions of unique personal attributes must be assessed including educational level, premorbid functioning, learning disability, cultural/linguistic factors and others that are likely to affect IQ test scores.

The foregoing summary should not be considered immutable; rather, clinicians engaged in assessing intellectual functioning among TBI patients utilize these principles to guide interpretation and hypotheses about related functional deficits, their causes and their remediation. Similarly, the cognitive strengths observed in IQ testing may point clinicians in the direction of harnessing intact patient abilities to compensate for possible limitations. In our clinical experience, we do not rely on one sign of TBI as being sufficient for rendering diagnosis. Similarly, the presence of atypical IQ scores by itself should not be taken to suggest cerebral impairment without further investigation. For individuals with unusual IQ profile scores, review of their school testing records can disclose significant pre-existing discrepancies in verbal and mathematical/spatial abilities. Competent neuropsychological evaluations take many factors into account as part of understanding TBI effects. IQ scores, therefore, should not be considered in isolation from measures of attention, memory, language, etc; similarly, test data should not be emphasized in the absence of a clear patient history, neurological evaluation and related data from other service providers.

MEMORY

Learning and memory are among the most fundamental and important capacities that underlie human development and adaptation. The neurobiological bases of how we acquire and subsequently retain vast amounts of information and experiences remain enigmatic though there is increasing understanding of the neural structures and processes that mediate functional memory systems. In scientific and clinical studies of TBI there is viable evidence for both alterations to memory-related structures and disruption of memory processing. The effects of post-traumatic memory impairments can be disabling and significantly limit an individual's ability to live independently, handle a job, and interact productively with others (54). Subjective complaints of memory impairment after TBI are quite common, even among those with mild TBI and good medical recovery (55). Although not always substantiated by objective memory testing, physiological brain changes underlying such complaints have been verified in some scientific studies but not others. The controversy arises in part from the wide individual variability in the effects of TBI on learning and memory abilities. Differences in patient sampling (e.g., consecutive series vs. patients referred for assessment) and in how learning and memory are assessed may lead to dissimilar results and conclusions. Differences in the length of time post-injury, age, and severity of TBI can also contribute to contrasting outcomes. Complicating effects of chronic pain, sleep disturbance, depression, stress due to loss of income etc. are known to contribute to learning and memory problems, and must be considered in both etiology and treatment plans. Despite these many cautions, reliable correlation has been found between memory performance and brain volumetric measures in the temporal lobe of adults with mild TBI (56). Specifically, decreased hippocampal and temporal white matter volumes were significantly related to memory impairment. Despite normal MRI or CT imaging in 15 of 20 patients with mild TBI, Umile et al. (57) reported that dynamic brain imaging (including SPECT and PET) detected abnormalities in 18 of the 20 patients, with 15 of 20 having abnormalities in the temporal lobe, primarily the hippocampal region. There are also functional imaging data suggesting that the brain activity patterns of TBI patients become altered during tasks of memory retrieval. Specifically, patients engaged increased levels of frontal, anterior cingulate and occipital activity while showing reduced right dorsomedial thalamic activation and attenuated hemispheric asymmetry that was characteristic of controls (58).

Post-Traumatic Amnesia

Post-traumatic amnesia (PTA) refers to the immediate and dramatic amnesic effects of TBI. Patients can be described as *confused*, *agitated*, *repeating questions*, and *disoriented* in this acute/post-acute phase. PTA is defined as the period during which patients are neither encoding nor retaining any new information and experiences, and can last from a few moments to several weeks and even months after TBI. Although patients are awake and alert during this period, they subsequently recall little to no information regarding the accident and such post-traumatic events as transportation to the hospital, medical evaluation, and even visits of family members. Patients with PTA are disoriented to time, place and reason for hospitalization, and may even think that they are at school or in their hometown. As described previously, they may show anosognosia during this period as well as a range of behavioral difficulties and agitation.

PTA is variable in both extent of amnesia and pattern of recovery. It is considered a general marker of neurological impairment and in most cases gradually improves. Sometimes the term 'shrinking post-traumatic amnesia' is used to refer to the gradual reduction in severity and temporal extent of amnesia (in both retrograde and anterograde spheres). PTA can be assessed with standardized instruments such as the Galveston Orientation and Amnesia Test (59). Recovery of orientation and short-term memory can be reliably predicted from early daily screening and is generally predictive of functional independence upon discharge (60, 61). It is important during this period to rule out contributing effects of sleep disturbance, pain medications, and other complicating factors on post-traumatic attention and memory deficits.

An interesting implication of PTA concerns its relationship to post-traumatic stress disorder (PTSD). That is, does loss of consciousness and memory after TBI necessarily preclude the development of PTSD symptoms that typically involve the re-experiencing of the traumatic events as well as heightened emotion with anxiety and avoidance behaviors. If the event cannot be remembered, can PTSD symptoms still be possible? Turnbull, Campbell and Swann (62) examined the inter-relationship in 53/371 TBI cases. Results indicated that those with traumatic memories of the TBI event (n = 26) reported the highest psychological distress followed by those with no traumatic memories (n = 14) who reported less severe and non-intrusive symptoms. Reviews by Bryant (63) and Harvey et al. (64) have generally favored the view that PTA and PTSD can co-exist though in ways that may be different than in non-TBI PTSD cases. The latter review underscored a number of caveats, related either to imprecise criteria for TBI and/or limited assessment of stress-related symptoms (PTSD and acute stress disorder). Further research is needed to clarify the causes and management of these co-morbid conditions.

Information Processing Aspects of Memory

Memory is neither a unitary nor an automatic process. Although there is individual variation in learning styles, cognition and interests that affects subsequent retention, there are several well-standardized tests of learning and memory that permit identification of specific memory impairments. Information processing approaches to memory and the brain have identified 3 principal aspects: *encoding, consolidation* and *retrieval*. Encoding typically refers to the acquisition of new information and experiences through sensory-perceptual and attentional mechanisms. Encoding is believed to be mediated by several cortical/cortical sensory-perceptual systems together with attentional/executive resources that are allocated according to information load, difficulty, prior knowledge etc. Consolidation pertains to biological mechanisms that are necessary to maintaining a memory trace, thought to involve interactive processing between cortical sensory association areas and limbic system structures, particularly the hippocampus and related medial temporal lobe areas. Retrieval refers to the recovery of stored information either through recall or recognition processes. The neural basis of retrieval remains unclear but may involve executive processes mediated by the prefrontal cortex for search and comparison of familiarity. Given this model of memory and the diversity of neural structures and connections that subserve memory, it becomes easier to understand how memory complaints may be so common after TBI, since large scale coordination of attentional, sensory-perceptual, limbic and executive processing systens is usually required.

Studies investigating TBI and memory continue to show diverse results. While some studies have identified principally encoding deficits, others have identified consolidation and retrieval deficits (65, 66). Curtis et al. (67) suggested that subgroups of memory impaired TBI patients can present with mainly consolidation or retrieval deficits. Particularly in patients with mild TBI, memory impairments may not be apparent on some standardized testing and become evident only under certain conditions such as when patients must divide attention during the encoding phase (68). The latter investigators reported that patients with severe TBI can also present with variable memory results, depending upon whether they attended to the target stimuli or distracting stimuli during encoding. There are a number of other cognitive and learning parameters that can affect memory retention in patients. For example, strategies of clustering similar semantic information (e.g., chunking) can improve verbal retention, while spaced repetition of words can also contribute to more effective learning (69). An important clinical guideline that is emerging from extant literature is the realization that interactive effects of processing speed, working memory and episodic memory impairments may combine to influence learning and memory capacities in naturalistic settings (70). In addition to the importance of cognitive remediation strategies for these deficits, some researchers have suggested that that pro-cholinergic medications may be helpful in recovery (71, 72).

CONFABULATIONS AND DELUSIONS

TBI can cause both confabulations and delusions. These disorders lie at the interface of memory, self-awareness/self-monitoring, visual perceptual and executive function abilities after TBI and occur as direct effects of brain injury and as associated features of organic psychoses. Some patients show confabulations within the context of significant amnesia, attempting to fill in gaps of memory loss with overlearned knowledge about themselves and others. This kind of confabulation is thought to involve a combination of amnesia and disinhibited responding, usually associated with temporal and frontal dysfunction. Several delusional misidentification syndromes have been described, centering around altered ability to recognize people and the belief that people are disguising themselves in some way. These have been associated with combined damage to frontal (usually bilateral) and right posterior hemisphere regions. Examples include Capgras syndrome, defined as the impaired belief that someone well known to the patient has been replaced with a look-alike imposter (also described as reduplicative paramnesia) (73), and Fregoli syndrome in which the patient believes that a stranger (e.g., another patient or a staff member) is actually a familiar person (such as their mother) (74). Confabulations and delusions generally resolve over time, but are also know to persist chronically. Challenging patients's false beliefs is often not helpful in recovery and family members as well as providers often must accommodate these fixed beliefs. A single delusion can occur or there may be several co-occurring delusions, not necessarily inter-related. Misidentification and delusional syndromes can occur after TBI without other features of pyschosis.

SPATIAL COGNITION

Spatial cognition subserves a variety of adaptive behaviors, from navigation within diverse environments to spatial-related attention, memory and reasoning. Spatial cognition is obviously critical to daily activities such as driving, ambulation, dressing, self-care and keeping track of items maintained in home and work settings. TBI infrequently causes the striking hemispatial neglect syndrome often associated with right parietal lobe damage, but can lead to changes in attention to spatial cues, visuomotor scanning that underlies spatial search, constructional praxis, and learning/memory of places as well as various spatial patterns and complex scenes (66, 75, 76). Exploratory deficits and other motor-intentional spatial disorders commonly occur after TBI, associated with medial frontal cortical dysfunction and hypokinesia (77). Most often, spatial cognitive deficits associated with TBI have not been singled out per se, but rather discussed within the context of attention, intelligence, memory and executive functions. Spatial representational and spatial-motor dysfunction after TBI have been less fully investigated.

CHEMICAL SENSES

TBI can dramatically affect both olfaction and taste. Olfactory deficits have been associated with multiple types of trauma to the head as well as trauma to the nasal cavity, olfactory epithelium, and the olfactory nerve as it travels through the cribiform plate to the olfactory bulb. Brain pathophysiology from inflammation, white matter shearing, hemorrhage, contusion and other effects can cause particular damage to the main olfactory structures of the brain including the olfactory bulb, tract, and interconnected subcortical and piriform cortical regions in the basal and medial aspects of the frontal and temporal lobes (78). In a comprehensive study of 268 patients with TBI, studied at a specialty smell and taste center, Doty and colleagues (77) reported that 66.8% showed anosmia (complete loss of smell) and 20.5% demonstrated microsmia (partial loss of smell). The incidence of these deficits was higher than other reports probably because of specialty center referral patterns. Performance was based on scores from the University of Pennsylvania Smell Identification Test, a 40-odorant scratch and sniff, multiple choice recognition test. About one-half of the cases suffered head trauma from motor vehicle accident, with head trauma from falls the second most likely cause. Follow-up testing of 66 patients, varying from 1 month to 13 years later (mean follow-up period was 5.5 years, with mean age 41.25 years, and the sample 55% male), showed that 36% improved slightly while 45% experienced no change and 18% worsened in their olfactory deficit. Three patients actually regained normal olfaction although none had anosmia to begin with. The incidence of parosmia (olfactory distortions) decreased from 41% to 15.5% over an 8-year follow-up period. Parosmias varied from transient to intermittent to persistent in severity. There were no significant effects of age, sex or time since injury on olfactory deficits. Other changes in olfaction include decreased threshold, hallucination (usually associated with post-traumatic epilepsy), and decreased recognition memory.

Taste can be affected by TBI in a variety of ways, although usually not as severe as olfaction. Quantitative changes in gustation include altered threshold levels and decreased intensity of taste that are often described as ageusia or hypogeusia (80). Occasional increased sensitivity or hypergeusia can occur as well. Changes in taste are typically measured in relationship to detection and recognition of the four basic taste stimuli: salty, sweet, sour, and bitter. Qualitative changes in gustation are often described as onset of unpleasant tastes such as bitterness, metallic and even rancid, and as a loss of typical taste

preferences. Deems et al. (81) reported that 18% of all taste problems evaluated at a specialty smell and taste clinic were related to trauma. These disorders are generally not amenable to treatment once other modifiable causes have been ruled out (e.g., oral hygiene, sinus, oral secretions, toxic exposures, smoking). Subcortical-cortical gustatory regions and pathways are less vulnerable to damage from head trauma than olfaction. Complaints of decreased taste can be related in many cases to olfactory loss, leading to decreased flavor detection and perception rather than gustatory deficit per se.

EXECUTIVE FUNCTIONS

Executive functions encompass cognitive and emotional processes that underlie many aspects of human adaptation, adjustment, and achievement. These processes have often been defined in terms of complex cognitive activities such as planning, judgment, decision-making and anticipation that require the coordination of multiple subprocesses to organize behaviour and achieve particular goals. Associated cognitive operations include working memory, prospective memory, strategic planning, cognitive flexibility, abstract reasoning and self-monitoring. Executive functions have also been implicated in the goal-directed *regulation* of attentional resources, sensory-perception, and actions in order to manage transitions from one activity to another throughout the day and across diverse settings (8, 82–85).

The neural systems involved in executive functions include the prefrontal cortex most prominently, together with interconnected neural circuitry forming prefrontal-cortical and subcortical networks. Some of these networks have been described under the terms *dorsolateral*, *orbital* and *medial* (86, 87). The dorsolateral prefrontal circuit is thought to mediate many higher cognitive aspects of behaviour such as abstract reasoning, planning and working memory. The orbital prefrontal circuit has been implicated mainly in social and emotional aspects of behavior including certain kinds of decision-making, theory of mind, emotional-based learning and social judgment. The medial prefrontal circuit has been related to motivational and attentional processes including initiation, inhibition and maintainance of behavior. In studies of TBI-related pathology, orbital and medial regions of the prefrontal cortex have been found to be especially vulnerable to damage by mechanisms of shearing and stretching of fibers as well as direct injury from impact against the irregular base of the skull. The orbital-medial prefrontal region is especially affected by strong blunt impact as well as physical acceleration/deceleration forces. Applied force vectors and tissue compliance influence the intensity of the coup, countercoup, angular and rotational forces that stretch and lacerate brain tissue centrifugally, from midline sagittal aspects (i.e., medial and orbital pre-frontal cortex impacting against the lamina cribrosa and the roof of the orbit as well as against the wing of the sphenoid bone) toward the surface of the cortex (lateral prefrontal cortex) and the deep connections with the striatum, thalamus and other subcortical nuclei such as the amygdala.

TBI-related damage to prefrontal neural circuits has been linked to the variety of executive function deficits. Impairments on measures of working memory (e.g., Paced Auditory Serial Addition Test), divided attention and sequencing (e.g., Trail Making), verbal associative fluency, learning and memory as well as planning and set shifting have been reported, even in cases after mild TBI (88, 89). Some clinical disorders such as distractability and impulsivity have been found to be related to measured attentional and executive function deficits (90, 91). Significant correlations between measures of executive functions and regional cerebral glucose metabolism have been found in the mesial and lateral prefrontal regions and the cingulate gyrus. Interesting, the correlations were evident despite the absence of detectable structural lesions on brain MRI. These findings confirmed those reported previously by Goldenberg et al. (92) who also noted correlation of executive measures with reduced blood flow in the thalamic region. Hence, impairments of executive functions may be related not only to focal traumatic lesions of the prefrontal cortex but also to white matter disconnection (i.e., diffuse axonal injury) of prefrontal-related networks that link to the thalamus and other important cortical and subcortical regions.

Some behavioral disorders after TBI have not been linked to cognitive deficits per se and may be due to alterations in emotion-related processing. For example, Rolls et al. (93) reported that patients with ventral frontal damage after TBI had particular difficulty in reward-based contingency learning. That is, after successfully learning an initial stimulus-reward association, they were impaired in both reversal learning (when the stimulus signalling reward was reversed) and in extinction learning (when the stimulus no longer signalled reward). The impairments were correlated to surveyed behavioral deficits that included disihibition, social difficulties, lack of initiative and perseveration. Interestingly, the behavioral deficits were not correlated with verbal IQ, paired associate learning or Tower of London performance. Emotion processing may also be an integral part of decision-making capacities when one must rely on judgment of chance and probability of consequences such as gambling. This has been operationalized into a standardized task (The Iowa Gambling Task) in which subjects must learn to choose cards from stacks that are rigged to have different levels of risk and pay-off, varying from high risk-high win to low risk-low win (94). Patients with ventral frontal damage performed poorly on this task, choosing high risk

options that led to huge losses. Furthermore, many did not generate the anticipatory skin conductance responses that might typically signal risk-taking effects. Another facet of emotion-related processing involves recognition of common forms of emotional expressions. Hornak et al. (95) showed that ventral frontal damage from head trauma (and other etiologies as well) was associated with deficient recognition of emotional facial expressions and correlated with subjective emotional change and social behavior of patients.

Both focal and diffuse frontal lesions disrupt activities of daily living (ADL) and executive impairment may represent a main component of ADL failure (96, 97). In particular, executive abilities of planning, self-monitoring and self-correction, decision-making and judgement are considered critical for independent, adaptive functioning within real world settings (98). Deficits of inattentiveness, mental slowing, impulsivity, and lack of prospective memory can all contribute to functional impairments after TBI. The impact of such impairments can be viewed as damaging a complex cognitive-emotional *macrostructure* or *managerial knowledge unit* (including strategic planning, procedural memory, working memory) that underlies most multi-step requirements of real life, such as meal preparation or a recreational activity (97, 99). Meal preparation or going to a movie may well be more difficult than many cognitive tasks presented during a formal cognitive testing session in the laboratory because of the need to impose structure and invest executive resources in planning, implementing and accomplishing the many aspects of the task (82, 83, 99, 100). In cognitive testing the patient typically is administered a single problem with instructions, learning trials may be short, initiation is prompted and feedback is often given at the end of the task. Certainly it is not the same in real world settings, where situational constraints, priorities and requirements are not always clear, and success depends on timely, internally-generated and self-monitored processing without the benefit of feedback. Most neuropsychological tests do not specifically explore strategic planning, competitive skills, or prospective memory. A notable exception to this is the experimental Strategic Management Simulation technology that has shown promise in detecting executive impairments in TBI patients with good medical recovery and few neuropsychological test deficits (101). An important priority in both assessment and linkage to cognitive remediation is the development of further paradigms that tap multiple problem solving variables in real time and with varying degrees of structure and feedback.

Social Cognition and Behavior

Humans are naturally social creatures, born to live and thrive within social settings with many complex forms of interaction that have emotional coloring and context. Hence, an important facet of human cognition and executive functioning extends beyond the strictly intellectual endeavors of planning, concept formation, and problem-solving to domains such as metacognitive thinking, social skills, moral beliefs, personality traits, and "theory of mind", a special faculty of the human brain that mediates interpretation and appreciation of other people's feelings and mental states (8, 102, 103). Fronto-temporal damage from TBI can lead to dramatic alterations of conduct, personality, and psychosocial integration, at times leaving most cognitive and sensory-motor functions relatively intact. From a clinical standpoint, there is often a spectrum of social-behavioral symptoms associated with TBI rather than definite syndromes. Some patients become puerile, profane, facetious, irresponsible, irascible, and aggressive as forms of social disinhibition. Others lose spontaneity, initiative, curiosity, and develop mental and behavioral inertia as forms of abulia and apathy (104). Still others develop lack of awareness and insight, loss of creativity and emotional vitality. Some of these deficits are expressed as loss of pragmatic aspects of communication, loss of empathy and inability to understand and appreciate sarcasm, jokes, irony, and other vital social communication tools (105, 106). Although many of these social-emotional deficits are difficult to objectively evaluate and measure, they are important and problematic sequelae of TBI that must be evaluated and managed. The combined use of clinical interview with patient and family members and behavioral inventories can uncover many of these deficits. Experimental measures of social judgment, theory of mind abilities, social knowledge and emotion-related processing are beginning to shed light on deficits underlying these real-life problems and are increasingly targeted in experimental intervention programs.

SUMMARY

Cognitive impairments after TBI often present significant challenges for recovery and return to premorbid levels of occupational and social functioning. In early stages, patients' lack of awareness of their deficits (anosognosia), impaired self-regulation, and post-traumatic amnesia constitute major limitations to participation in rehabilitation services and safety. Often there is a combination of attentional, memory, perceptual, processing speed, executive function and social-emotional deficits that require multimodal therapy services and a gradual return to independent daily activities. Cognitive and social-emotional deficits are frequently slower to recover than physical injuries and require outpatient therapy services with medical follow-up care. Education of caregivers is particularly important for monitoring and continued remediation of such impairments within home and community settings. When cognitive deficits remain persistent, individualized therapy is usually required combining aspects of skill retraining, compensatory strategies, and environmental supports to optimize functional cognitive capacities.

References

1. Rapoport MJ, McCullagh S, Shammi P, Feinstein A. Cognitive impairment associated with major depression following mild and moderate traumatic brain injury. *J Neuropsychiat Clin Neurosci* 2005;17:61–65.
2. van Zomeren AH, van den Burg W. Residual complaints of patients two years after severe head injury. *J Neurol Neurosurg Psychiat* 1985;48:21–28.
3. Ponsford J, Kinsella G. Attentional deficits following closed head injury. *J Clin Exp Neuropsychol* 1992;14:822–838.
4. Park NW, Moscovitch M, Robertson IH. Divided attention impairments after traumatic brain injury. *Neuropsychologia* 1999;37:1119–1133.
5. Brooks DN. Measuring neuropsychological and functional recovery. In Levin HS, Grafman J, & Eisenberg HM (Eds.) *Neurobehavioral Recovery from Head Injury* (pp. 57–72). New York: Oxford University Press 1987.
6. Dikmen SS, Ross BL, Machamer JE et al. One year psychosocial outcome in head injury. *J Intl Neuropsychol Soc* 1995; 1:67–77.
7. Drake AI, Gray N, Yoder S. Pramuka M, Llewellyn M. Factors predicting return to work following mild traumatic brain injury: A discriminant analysis. *J Head Trauma Rehabil* 2000;15: 1103–1112.
8. Eslinger P, Grattan L, Geder L. Neurologic and neuropsychologic aspects of frontal lobe impairments in postconcussive syndrome. In Rizzo M, Tranel D (Eds.) *Head Injury and Postconcussive Syndrome* (pp. 415–440) New York: Churchill Livingstone, 1996.
9. Jones RD, Anderson SW, Cole T, Hathaway-Nepple J. Neuropsychological sequelae of traumatic brain injury. In Rizzo M, Tranel D (Eds.) *Head Injury and Postconcussive Syndrome* (pp. 395–414) New York: Churchill Livingstone, 1996.
10. Sarno S, Erasmus L-P, Lipp B, Schlaaegel W. Multisensory integration after traumatic brain injury: A reaction time study between pairings of vision, touch, and audition. *Brain Injury* 2003;17: 413–426.
11. Mathias JL, Beall JA, Bigler ED. Neuropsychological and information processing deficits following mild traumatic brain injury. *J intl Neuropsychol Soc* 2004;1:286–297.
12. Tinius T. The Integrated Visual and Auditory Continuous Performance Test as a neuropsychological measure. *Arch Clin Neuropsychol* 2003;18:439–454.
13. Miller E. Simple and choice reaction time following severe closed head injury. *Cortex* 1970;6:121–127.
14. Ponsford J, Kinsella G. Attentional deficits following closed head injury. *J Clin Exp Neuropsychol* 1992;14:822–838.
15. Stuss DT, Stethern LL, Hugenholtz H, Picto T, Pivik J, Richard MJ. Reaction time after head injury: Fatigue, divided and focussed attention and consistency of performance. *J Neurol Neurosurg Psychiat* 1989;52:742–748.
16. von Zomeren AH, Brouwer P. *Clinical Neuropsychology of Attention.* Oxford: Oxford University Press, 1994.
17. Zollolotti P, Matano A, DeLoche G et al. Patterns of attentional impairment following closed head injury: A collaborative European study. *Cortex* 2000;36:93–107.
18. Babinski J. Contribution a l'etude dies troubles mentaux dans l'hemiplegie organique cerebrale (anosognosia). *Revue Neurologique* (Paris) 1914;27:845–847.
19. Adair JC, Schwartz RL, Barrett AM. Anosognosia. In Heilman KM and Valenstein E (Eds). *Clinical Neuropsychology, fourth edition* (pp. 185–214). New York: Oxford University Press, 2003.
20. Hart T, Giovannetti T, Montgomery MW, Schwartz MF. Awareness of errors in naturalistic action after traumatic brain injury. *J Head Trauma Rehabil* 1998;13:16–28.

21. Prigatano GP, Schacter DL. *Awareness of Deficit After Brain Injury: Clinical and Theoretical Issues.* New York: Oxford University Press, 1991.

22. Giacino JT, Cicerone K. Varieties of deficit unawareness after brain injury. *J Head Trauma Rehabil* 1998; 13:1–15.

23. Prigatano GP, Wong JL. Cognitive and affective improvement in brain dysfunctional patients who achieve inpatient rehabilitation goals. *Arch Phys Med Rehabil* 1999;80:77–84.

24. Fleming JM, Strong J, Ashton R. Cluster analysis of self-awareness levels in adults with traumatic brain injury and relationship to outcome. *J Head Trauma Rehabil* 1998;13:39–51.

25. McKinlay WW, Brooks DN. Methodological problems in assessing psychosocial recovery following severe head injury. *J Clin Neuropsychl* 1984;6:87–99.

26. Abreu BC, Seale G, Scheibel RS, Huddleston N, Zhang L, Ottenbacher KJ. Levels of self-awareness after acute brain injury: How patients' and rehabiitation specialists' perceptions compare. *Arch Phys Med Rehabil* 2001;82:49–56.

27. Powell JM, Machamer JE, Temkin NR, Dikmen SS. Self-report of extent of recovery and barriers to recovery after traumatic brain injury: A longitudinal study. *Arch Phys Med Rehabil* 2001;82: 1025–1030.

28. Wallace CA, Bogner J. Awareness of deficits: Emotional implications for persons with brain injury and their significant others. *Brain Injury* 2000;14:549–562.

29. Prigatano GP, Bruna O, Mataro M, MuÒoz JM, Fernandez S, Junque C. Initial disturbances of consciousness and resultant impaired awareness in Spanish patients with traumatic brain injury. *J Head Trauma Rehabil* 1998;13:29–38.

30. Lanham RA, Weissenburger JE, Schwab KA, Rosner MM. A longitudinal investigation of the concordance between individuals with traumatic brain injury and family or friend ratings on the Katz Adjustment Scale. *J Head Trauma Rehabil* 2000;15: 1123–1138.

31. Weinstein EA, Kahn RL. *Denial of Illness: Symbolic and Physiological Aspects.* Springfield, IL: Charles C. Thomas, 1955.

32. Dalla Barba G, Bartolomeo P, Erigs AM, Boisse MF, Bachoud-Levi AC. Awareness of anosognosia following head trauma. *Neurocase* 1999;5:59–

33. Starkstein SE, Federoff JP, Price TR, Leiguarda R, Robinson RG. Anosognosia in patients with cerebrovascular lesions: a study of causative factors. *Stroke* 1992;23:1446–1453.

34. Scherer M, Bergloff P, Levin E, High WM, Oden KE, Nick TG. Impaired awareness and employment outcome after traumatic brain injury. *J Head Trauma Rehabil* 1998;13:52–61.

35. Schacter DL and Prigatano GP, 1991. Forms of unawareness. In Prigatano GP, Schacter DL (Eds). *Awareness of Deficit after Brain Injury: Clinical and Theoretical Issues.* New York: Oxford University Press, 1991.

36. Sohlberg MM, Mateer CA, Penkman L, Glang A, Todis B. Awareness intervention: who needs it? *J Head Trauma Rehabil* 1998; 13:62–78.

37. Langer KG, Padrone FJ. Psychotherapeutic treatment of awareness in acute rehabilitation of traumatic brain injury. *Neuropsychol Rehabil* 1992;2:59–70.

38. McGlynn SM, Schacter DL. Unawareness of deficits in neuropsychological syndromes. *J Clin Exp Neuropsychol* 1989;11: 143–205.

39. Schlund MW. Self awareness: Effects of feedback and review on verbal self reports and remembering following brain injury. *Brain Injury* 1999;13:375–380.

40. Sohlberg MM, Johansen A, Geyer S, Hoornbeck S. *Training in the Use of Compensatory Systems after Head Injury.* Puyallup, Washington: Association for Neruropsychological Research and Development, 1999.

41. Daniels-Zide E, Ben-Yishay Y. Therapeutic milieu day program. In Christensen A-L, Uzell BP (Eds.) *International Handbook of Neuropsychological Rehabilitation. Critical issues in Neuropsychology* (pp. 183–193. New York: Kluwer Academic/Plenum, 2000.

42. Sohlberg MM and Rawlings-Boyd J. *Picture this! Strategies for Assessing and Increasing Awareness of Memory Deficits.* San Antonio, TX: The Psychological Corporation. 1996.

43. Rebmann MJ, Hannon R. Treatment of unawareness of memory deficits in adults with brain injury: Three case studies. *Rehabil Psychol* 1995;40:279–287.

44. Fisher DC, Ledbetter MF, Cohen NJ, Marmor D, Tulsky DS. (2000). WAIS-III and WMS-III profiles of mildly to severely brain-injured patients. *Appl Neuropsychol* 2000;7:126–132.

45. Yeates KO, Taylor HG, Wade SL, Drotar D, Stancin T, Minich N. A prospective study of short and long-term neuropsychological outcomes after traumatic brain injury in children. *Neuropsychol* 2002;16:514–523.

46. Lezak MD. *Neuropsychological Assessment (3rd ed.).* New York: Oxford University Press, 1995.

47. Martin TA, Donders J, Thompson E. Potential of and problems with measures of psychometric intelligence after traumatic brain injury. *Rehabil Psychol* 2000;45:402–408.

48. O'Connell MJ. Prediction of ceturn to work following traumatic brain injury: Intellectual, memory, and demographic variables. *Rehabil Psychol* 2000;45:212–217.

49. Axelrod BN, Fichtenberg NL, Liethen PC, Czarnota MA, Stucky K. Performance characteristics of postacute traumatic brain injury patients on the WAIS-III and WMS-III. *Clin Neurosychol* 2001; 15:516–520.

50. Groth-Marnat, G. *Handbook of Psychological Assessment (4th ed.).* Hubuken, NJ: John Wiley & Sons, 2003.

51. Kaufman AS, Lichtenberger EO. *Assessing Adolescent and Adult Intelligence.* Boston: Allyn & Bacon, 2002.

52. Reitan RM, Wolfson D. *The Halstead-Reitan neuropsychological test Battery: Theory and Clinical Interpretation (2nd ed.).* Tucson, AZ: Neuropsychological Press, 1993.

53. Dobbins, C. & Russell, EW. Left temporal lobe brain damage pattern on the Wechsler Adult Intelligence Scale. *J Clin Psychol* 1990;46:863–868.

54. Drake AI, Gray N, Yoder S, Pramuke M., Llewellyn M. Factors predicting return to work following mild traumatic brain injury: A discriminant analysis. *J Head Trauma Rehabil* 2000;15: 1103–12.

55. Rimel RW, Giordani B, Barth JT, Boll TJ, Jane JA. Disability caused by minor head injury. *Neurosurg* 1981;9:221–8.

56. Bigler ED, Anderson CV, Blatter DD, Anderson CV. Temporal lobe morphology in normal aging andtraumatic brain injury. *Am J Neuroradiol* 2002;23:255–66.

57. Umile EM, Sandel ME, Alavi A, Terry CM, Plotkin RC. Dynamic imaging in mild traumatic brain injury: Support for the theory of medial temporal vulnerability. *Arch Phys Med Rehabil* 2002; 83:1506–13.

58. Levine B, Carbeza R, McIntosh AR, Black SE, Grady CL, Stuss DT. Functional reorganisation of memory after traumatic brain injury: A study with H(2)(15)O positron emission tomography. *J Neurol Neurosurg Psychiat* 2002;73:173–81.

59. Levin HS, Benton AL, Grossman RG. Neurobehavioral Consequences of Closed Head Injury. Oxford University Press: New York, 1982.

60. Tate RL, Perdices M, Pfaff A, Jurjevic L. Predicting duration of post-traumatic amnesia (PTA) from early PTA measurements. *J Head Trauma Rehabil* 2001;16:525–42.

61. Alderso AL, Novack TA. Measuring recovery of orientation during acute rehabilitation for traumatic brain injury: Value and expectations of recovery. *J Head Trauma Rehabil* 2002; 17:210–9.

62. Turnbull SJ, Campbell EA, Swann IJ. Post-traumatic stress disorder symptoms following a head injury: Does amnesia for the event influence the development of symptoms? *Brain Injury* 2001;15: 775–85.

63. Bryant RA. Post-traumatic stress disorder and traumatic brain injury: Can they co-exist. *Clin Psychol Rev* 2001;21:931–48.

64. Harvey AG, Brewin CR, Jones C, Kopelman MD. Co-existence of post-traumatic stress disorder and traumatioc brain injury: Towards a resolution of the paradox. *J Intl Neuropsychol Soc* 2003;9:663–676.

65. DeLuca J, Schultheis MT, Madigan NK, Christodoulou C, Averill A. Acquisition versus retrieval deficits in traumatic brain injury: Implications for memory rehabilitation. *Arch Phys Med Rehabil* 2000;81:1327–33.

66. Vanderploeg RD, Curtiss G, Schinka JA, Lanham RA. Material-specific memory in traumatic brain injury: Differential effects during acquisition, recall, and retention. *Neuropsychol* 2001;15: 174–84.

67. Curtiss G, Vanderploeg RD, Spencer J, Salazar AM. Patterns of verbal learning and memory in traumatic brain injury. *J Intl Neuropsychol Soc* 2001;7:574–85.

68. Mangels JA, Craig FI, Levine B, Schwartz ML, Stuss DT. Effects of divided attention on episodic memory in chronic traumatic brain injury: A function of severity and strategy. *Neuropsychologia* 2002;40:2369–85.

69. Hillary FG, Schultheis MT, Challis BH, Millis SR, Carnevale GJ, Galashi T, DeLuca J. Spacing of repetitions improves learning and memory after moderate and severe TBI. *J Clin Exp Neuropsychol* 2003;25:49–58.

70. Perbal S, Couillet J, Azouvi P, Pouthas V. Relationships between time estimation, memory, attention, and processing speed in patients with severe traumatic brain injury. *Neuropsychologia* 2003;41:1599–1610.

71. Griffin SL, vanReekum R, Masanic C. A review of cholinergic agents in the treatment of neurobehavioral deficits following traumatic brain injury. *J Neuropsychiat Clin Neurosci* 2003;15:17–26.

72. Morey CE, Cilo M, Berry J, Cusick C. The effect of Aricept in persons with persistent memory disorder following traumatic brain injury: A pilot study. *Brain Injury* 2003;17:809–15.

73. Alexander MP, Stuss DT, Benson DF. Capgras syndrome: A reduplicative phenomenon. *Neurology* 1979;29:334–339.

74. Box O, Laing H, Kopelman M. The evolution of spontaneous confabulation, delusional misidentification and a related delusion in a case of severe head injury. *Neurocase* 1999;5:251–262.

75. Vecera S, Rizzo M. Spatial attention: Normal processes and their breakdown. *Neurol Clin* 2003;21:575–607.

76. Skelton RW, Bukach CM, laurance HE, Thomas KG, Jacobs JW. Humans with traumatic brain injuries show place-learning deficits in computer-generated space. *J Clin Exp Neuropsychol* 2000;22:157–75.

77. Heilman KM. Intentional neglect. *Frontiers in Bioscience* 2004.

78. Eslinger PJ, Damasio AR, Van Hoesen GW: Olfactory dysfunction in man: Anatomical and behavior aspects. *Brain and Cognition* 1982;1:259–85.

79. Doty RL, Yousem DM, Pham LT, Kreshak AA, Geckle R, Lee WW. Olfactory dysfunction in patients with head trauma. *Arch Neurol* 1997;54:1131–1140.

80. Pritchard TC, Eslinger PJ, Wang J, Yang Q. Smell and taste disorders. In Rizzo M & Eslinger PJ (Eds.) *Principles and Practice of Behavioral Neurology and Neuropsychology* (pp. 335–360). Saunders: Philadelphia, 2004.

81. Deems DA, Doty RL, Settle RG et al. Smell and taste disorders: A study of 750 patients from the University of Pennsylvania Smell and Taste Center. *Arch Otolaryngol Head Neck Surg* 1991;117: 508–528.

82. Shallice T, Burgess PW. Deficits in strategy application following frontal lobe damage in man. *Brain* 1991;114:727–741.

83. Levine B, Dawson D, Schwartz ML, Boutet I, Stuss DT. Assessment of strategic self-regulation in traumatic brain injury: Its relationship to injury severity and psychosocial outcome. *Neuropsychol* 2000;14:491–500.

84. Eslinger PJ. Conceptualizing, describing, and measuring components of executive function. In Lyon GR, Krasnegor (Eds.) *Attention, Memory, and Executive Function* (pp. 367–396). Baltimore: Paul H. Brookes, 1996.

85. Andres P, Van der Linden M. Are central executive functions working in patients with focal frontal lesions? *Neuropsychologia* 2002;40:835–845.

86. Eslinger PJ, Geder L. Behavioural and emotional changes after focal frontal lobe damage. In Bogousslavsky J, Cummings JL (Eds). *Behavior and Mood Disorders in Focal Brain Lesions* (pp. 217–260).Cambridge: Cambridge University Press, 2000.

87. Barbas H. Connections underlying the synthesis of cognition, memory and emotion in primate prefrontal cortices. *Brain Res Bull* 2000;15:319–330.

88. Grafman J, Jones B, Salazar A. Wisconsin Card Sorting performance based on location and size of neuroanatomic lesion in Vietnam veterans with penetrating head injury. *Percept Mot Skill* 1990;74:1120–22.

89. Allegri RF, Harris P. Prefrontal cortex in memory and attention processes. *Rev Neurol* 2001;32:449–453.

90. Baddeley A, Della Sala S, Papagano C, Spinnler H. Dual task performance in dysexecutive and nondysexecutive patients with a frontal lesion. *Neuropsychol* 1997;11:187–94.

91. Burgess PW, Alderman N, Evans J, Emslie H, Wilson BA. The ecological validity of tests of executive function. *J Intl Neuropsychol Soc* 1998;4:547–558.

92. Goldenberg G, Oder W, Spatt J, Podreka I. Cerebral correlates of disturbed executive function and memory in survivors of severe closed head injury: A SPECT study. *J Neurol Neurosurg Psychiat* 1992;55:362–8.

93. Rolls E.T, Hornak J, Wade D, McGrath J. Emotion-related learning in patients with social and emotional changes associated with frontal lobe damage. *J Neurol Neurosurg Psychiat* 1994;57: 1518–24.

94. Bechara A, Tranel D, Damasio H, Damasio AR. Failure to respond autonomically to anticipated future outcomes following damage to prefrontal cortex. *Cereb Cortex* 1996;6: 215–225.

95. Hornak J, Rolls ET, Wade D. Face and voice expression identification in patients with emotional and behavioral changes following ventral frontal lobe damage. *Neuropsychologia* 1996; 34:247–61.

96. Eslinger PJ, Damasio AR. Severe disturbances of higher cognition after bilateral frontal lobe ablation: Patient EVR. *Neurol* 1985;35:1731–41.

97. Fortin S, Godbout L, Braun CMJ. Cognitive structure of exeutive deficits in frontally lesioned head trauma patients performing activities of daily living. *Cortex* 2003;39:273–291.

98. Acker MBA. Review of ecological validity of neuropsychological tests. In D E Tupper and K D Cicerone (Eds). *The Neuropsychology of Everyday Life: Assessment and Basic Competncies* (pp. 19–55). Boston: Klucer Ac. Publ., 1990.

99. Grafman J. Similarities and distinctions among current models of prefrontal cortical functions. *Ann NY Acad Sci* 1995;769: 337–368.

100. Channon S, Crawford S. Problem-solving in real-life type situations: the effects of anterior and posterior lesions on performance. *Neuropsychologia* 1999;37:757–70.

101. Satish U, Streufert S, Eslinger PJ. Complex decision-making after orbitofrontal danage: Neuropsychological and strategic management simulation assessment. *Neurocase* 1999;5:355–364.

102. Stuss DT, Gallup GG, Alexander MP. The frontal lobes are necessary for "theory of mind". *Brain* 2001;124:279–86.

103. Fine C, Lumsden J, Blair RJR. Dissociation between "theory of mind" and executive functions in a patient with early left amygdala damage. *Brain* 2001;124:287–298.

104. Trexler LT, Zappalà G. Neuropathological determinants of acquired attention disorders in traumatic brain injury. *Brain Cogn* 1988;8:291–302.

105. Eslinger PJ. Neurological and neuropsychological bases of empathy. *Eur Neurol* 1998;39:193–9.

106. McDonald S, Flanagan S. Social perception deficits after traumatic brain injury: Interaction between emotion recognition, mentalizing ability, and social communication. *Neuropsychol* 2004; 18:572–9.

43 Neuropsychological Assessment and Treatment of TBI

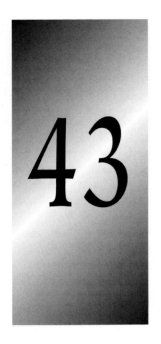

Laura A. Taylor
Lee A. Livingston
Jeffrey S. Kreutzer

C linical neuropsychologists are professionals within the field of clinical psychology who have special expertise in the area of brain-behavior relationships. According to the National Academy of Neuropsychology (NAN) definition (1), clinical neuropsychologists use "psychological, neurological, cognitive, behavioral, and physiological principles, techniques, and tests to evaluate patients' neurocognitive, behavioral, and emotional strengths and weaknesses and their relationship to normal and abnormal central nervous system functioning." Results from comprehensive evaluations are utilized for identification and diagnosis of neurobehavioral disorders, prognostication, development of treatment plans, and rehabilitation of individuals with neurologic conditions, health problems, neurodevelopmental disorders, cognitive problems, learning disorders, and psychiatric conditions. Many neuropsychologists are also responsible for the development and implementation of individual, group, and family therapy and education programs. This chapter will review guiding principles for neuropsychologists, the process of neuropsychological assessment and report writing, the contribution of neuropsychological assessment to the development of treatment recommendations, and neuropsychologist's role in rehabilitation and treatment. This chapter further strives to explore the role of neuropsychology in rehabilitation and a holistic approach to patient care.

PRINCIPLES GUIDING THE PRACTICE OF CLINICAL NEUROPSYCHOLOGY

Neuropsychologists play a key role in the evaluation and treatment of individuals with traumatic brain injury (TBI). Some view neuropsychology as a purely technical field with practitioners focusing on cognitive testing and functional neuroanatomy. More recently, neuropsychologists have taken a holistic perspective on practice focusing on issues of emotional adjustment, family functioning, and treatments to help patients return to normal life.

A set of guiding principles has been developed to help neuropsychologists develop a more holistic practice. Consideration of the following principles can help clinicians more efficiently achieve positive outcomes and effect greater levels of client satisfaction:

- empower patients and their families to take an active role in the evaluation and treatment process
- believe that people with neurological disabilities are more like people without neurological disabilities
- convey honesty and caring in personal interactions to form an adequate foundation for a strong therapeutic relationship
- develop practical plans for rehabilitation and explain rehabilitation techniques in language that patients, families, and interdisciplinary professionals are likely to understand

- help patients and their families understand the common neurobehavioral sequelae of brain injury and the typical recovery course
- recognize that change is inevitable and help the patient and family develop plans to deal with changes as they arise over time
- remember that every patient is important and deserves to be treated with respect
- remember that patients and families often have different perspectives; consider their individuality when formulating treatment approaches
- be willing to refer to other professionals if a case extends beyond personal areas of expertise and clarifies roles of various treatment providers.

TABLE 43-1

The Caring, Understanding, Respecting, and Trust-Building Checklist

---

- Review the patient's chart before seeing them; try to remember important details, and bring the details into your conversations.
- Go beyond your job description, at least sometimes.
- Ask the patient if they have questions or want to mention something that has not come up in conversation; answer their questions in language they can understand.
- When you can't help, refer to others who can.
- Discuss your ideas about helping the patient and your plans to do so.
- When asked by the patient, communicate to significant others about the patient's needs and care.
- Listen carefully.
- Give the patient time to finish what they are saying.
- Paraphrase what the patient says to convey your understanding.
- Maintain eye contact and face the patient when talking to them.
- Be on time for appointments and apologized on the rare occasions when you are not.
- Address patients by their proper surname (Mr., Mrs., or Ms.) unless instructed by them to do otherwise.
- Frequently inquire about the patient's needs, priorities, and perceptions of progress.
- Ask the patient for ideas about how to make things better and try to use their ideas.
- Carefully explain and discuss the limits of your expertise.
- Do what you say you will when you say you will.
- Respect the patient's right to confidentiality.
- Acknowledge when circumstances prevent you from doing what you agreed to and discuss acceptable alternatives.

Adapted from *The Brain Injury Handbook: A Guide for Rehabilitation Providers for Improving Therapeutic Relationships* (Kreutzer, Kolakowsky-Hayner, & West, 1999) (2).

To facilitate a positive and effective practice, many rehabilitation professionals employ a variety of trust-building behaviors with their patients. Table 43-1 displays a checklist of behaviors, which neuropsychologists and other rehabilitation professionals are encouraged to incorporate into their standard practice.

COMPREHENSIVE NEUROPSYCHOLOGICAL ASSESSMENT

Comprehensive neuropsychological evaluation typically involves clarification of the referral question, review of records, clinical interviews, behavioral observation, and administration of standardized measures. Standardized measures are used to assess cognitive, academic, neurobehavioral, and emotional functioning. In addition, the impact of the acquired brain injury on the family, pain, substance abuse, vocational potential, motivation, effort, judgment, and safety are also areas of emphasis in neuropsychological assessment. The following sections will describe these evaluation techniques in more detail.

Referral Question

The first step in neuropsychological assessment is identifying issues of concern and clarifying referral questions. Doing so allows selection of relevant assessment methods. Directly answering the referral source's questions and addressing their concerns is a hallmark of a beneficial neuropsychological report.

Referral sources often request information in three areas: (1) information pertaining to diagnosis, prognosis, and neuropsychological, neurobehavioral, and emotional functioning; (2) information about functional abilities, including level of independence and academic and vocational functioning; and (3) information about treatment and rehabilitation needs. Tables 43-2, 43-3, and 43-4 depict common referral questions encountered by neuropsychologists in each of these three areas. The variety of referral questions highlight the variety of complex issues and questions which neuropsychologists are often asked to address in their assessments. Answering these questions appropriately necessitates comprehensive, holistic assessment. They also provide insight into potential recommendations and treatment needs.

Records Review

Thorough review of the records is the foundation of the evaluation process, providing guidance for the interview, test selection, and treatment planning. In addition, familiarity with records allows the examiner to ask the patient relevant questions during the initial interview and communicates to the patient that the examiner is well-prepared

---

TABLE 43-2

Referral Questions Regarding Cognitive, Emotional, and Neurobehavioral Functioning

- Is there any evidence of preexisting cognitive, emotional, or neurobehavioral difficulties? Describe levels of functioning in each area relative to preinjury.
- How has the neurological injury impacted their cognitive, emotional, or neurobehavioral functioning?
- Are current symptoms consistent with preexisting difficulties, psychological disorder, brain injury, or a combination of factors?
- Is there evidence that emotional/psychological difficulties contribute to cognitive deficits?
- To what extent does pain or unresolved physical problems contribute to emotional or cognitive impairments?
- Is the patient at risk of harming him/herself or others?
- Is there evidence of posttraumatic stress disorder, depression, anxiety, or other psychological disorders?
- Within each area of cognitive, intellectual, and psychomotor functioning, compare the patient's performance to the normal population. Which areas would you consider to be relative strengths and which areas would you consider to be weaknesses?
- Compare the patient's level of functioning in each area to the patient's last evaluation. Which skills have improved, declined, and remained stable? Identify potential factors which may have contributed to improvements or limited change.
- What is the prognosis for future improvements or declines?
- When will it be helpful to evaluate the patient again? for what purposes?
- Is the patient eligible for special services, programs, or benefits?

TABLE 43-3

Referral Questions Pertaining to Adaptive, Educational, and Vocational Functioning

- Is the patient safe to drive? If not, what are the patient's needs with respect to driving evaluation, driver's training, and instruction in use of public transportation? Is the patient eligible for transportation services for persons with disabilities?
- Is the patient safe to live independently? If not, what supervision level or alternative living arrangements are recommended?
- Is the patient competent to manage their finances?
- Can the patient manage their medication independently?
- Please provide information about the patient's judgment and safety.
- How will the patient's neurobehavioral status impact parenting?
- What is the patient's potential for academic and vocational success?
- How has the injury impacted the patient's academic and vocational potential?
- Is the patient able to manage part-time or full-time work schedule?
- What kinds of training, accommodations, and interventions are most likely to increase their potential for academic or vocational success in the current school/work environment?
- Can the patient succeed in the present academic/work environment? Should an alternative academic placement or employment opportunity be considered?
- How will the patient's neurobehavioral status impact their ability to interact with coworkers, customers, family, friends, etc.?
- Identify which neuropsychological factors are primarily contributors to functional impairments.
- Is there evidence that emotional/psychological difficulties contribute to functional impairments?

---

and interested in the patient's well being. Review of medical, psychological, criminal, academic, and vocational records is strongly recommended. Review of medical and rehabilitation records provides information about pre- and post-injury history of health problems and treatment. Information pertaining to mechanism of injury, injury severity, injury-related cognitive and physical sequelae, and rehabilitation services may also be obtained. Pre- and post-injury mental health records provide an invaluable source of information about long-standing emotional issues and substance misuse and post-injury emotional, neurobehavioral, and personality changes. Mental health records also provide information about treatments and medications which have been effective. Criminal records may elucidate difficulties with authority, antisocial behavior, mental health issues, substance abuse problems, and litigation history.

In reviewing school records, the neuropsychologist gains information about history of learning difficulties, academic potential, and information about the patient's strengths and weaknesses. Vocational records review includes examination of performance reviews, job descriptions, and information about wage history, attendance records, grievances, and disciplinary actions. Based upon review of vocational records, the neuropsychologist has the opportunity to ascertain pre- and post-injury work experience, habits, attitudes, and accomplishments. In addition, records review provides information about the patient's ability to function within structured environments, response to authority figures, and interpersonal skills. Academic and vocational history provides the basis for making recommendations about vocational and academic potential, optimal work/school settings, and appropriate accommodations. In addition, review of academic and vocational records provides an opportunity for estimating patients' premorbid or expected level of functioning.

TABLE 43-4
Referral Questions Pertaining to Treatment Issues

- What types interventions have the potential to benefit the patient (e.g., medication, rehabilitation services, psychotherapy, support group, vocational rehabilitation, etc.)?
- Provide information about reasonable treatment goals, priorities for intervention, optimal frequency of services, potential service providers, and associated costs.
- Which factors will affect the patient's ability to benefit from rehabilitation interventions and treatment? Are there interventions that would minimize limiting factors (e.g., pharmacologic, compensatory)?
- Is the patient a good candidate for individual, group, marital, or family therapy?
- What is the patient's prognosis for improvement with and without intervention?
- Is the family a good support system? How are family members helping the patient or contributing to present difficulties?
- What are the family's expectations regarding recovery and the patient's ability to return to previous activities? What are the family's needs with respect to education about the recovery process?
- What support and education programs would benefit family members? Describe potential service providers, optimal frequency of services, and associated costs.

Establishing the premorbid level of functioning provides the basis for judging current levels of impairment.

Behavioral Observations

Behavioral observation during the course of interview and testing affords the examiner with the opportunity to assess behaviors, which are not readily tapped by quantitative assessment devices. Table 43-5 depicts information that is typically gathered through behavioral observation. Observation across different settings, by different observers, and at different times is optimal. Interviewing patients in their home or current living situations is an excellent means of obtaining information about how patients react in their home environments. If home-based observation is not possible, family members and caregivers may be able to provide additional information about behavior observed in the home. Neuropsychologists also gather information about behaviors from members of the interdisciplinary team members who may have the opportunity to observe the patient in other settings.

Clinical Interview

The clinical interview provides a valuable sample of behavior. The examiner has the opportunity to observe how the patient interacts and responds to questions. In addition, the clinical interview affords an opportunity for clarifying information from the records, gathering historical information, and ascertaining primary presenting concerns. During the clinical interview, special care is taken to collect the following information: presenting complaints; family/caregiver concerns; injury information; postconcussive symptoms; academic and vocational history; family and social functioning; medical and psychological history; history of prior TBI's; and current daily living situation and functional capabilities. Every effort is made to interview the patient and one or more family members/caregivers. If in-person interview with family members is not possible, telephone interview may be a viable option. Interviewing employers, teachers, and treating providers is also valuable.

Quantitative Assessment

Quantitative neuropsychological assessment findings provide a useful complement to data gathered through behavioral observation and clinical interview. Quantitative assessment provides the opportunity to gather data about neuropsychological functioning in a standardized way, allowing the examiner to make comparisons to normative data and to make comparisons over time with repeated testing (3). In determining which assessment instruments to use, neuropsychologists consider several factors. First, comprehensive assessment is multidimensional and multimethod, covering a range of functioning areas using a variety of measures to assess each area. Second, tests are selected with emphasis placed upon problem areas endorsed by the patient, his or her family, and the referral source. Third, measures are chosen based upon ease of completion and administration time whenever possible. Finally, in determining which tests to use, neuropsychologists consider the test reliability and validity, normative samples, and research findings specific to brain injury.

This section does not provide encyclopedic knowledge about the function and process of quantitative neuropsychological assessment. On the contrary, we purport to offer a broad overview of the topic emphasizing the importance of evaluating patients as multi-faceted beings with significant pre-injury histories, interpersonal relationships, emotional reactions to injury and so forth. Those interested in comprehensive reviews of this subject are encouraged to peruse Lezak's text, *Neuropsychological Assessment* (3) and the chapter entitled, "Neuropsychological Evaluation of the Patient with Traumatic Brain Injury" in *Rehabilitation of the Adult and Child with Traumatic Brain Injury* (4).

Evaluation of Cognitive and Academic Functioning

Following TBI, individuals commonly experience cognitive difficulties. Comprehensive assessment of cognitive

TABLE 43-5
Behavioral Observations Relevant to Neuropsychological Assessment

GENERAL OBSERVATION AREA	SPECIFIC AREAS TO ASSESS
Appearance	• Dress • Physical condition • Hygiene • Eye contact
Motor abilities and stamina	• Gait/ambulation • Reaction time • Quality of movements • Signs of restlessness/agitation • Fatigue and stamina
Affect	• Range • Appropriateness to situation and content • Consistency with reported mood • Level of frustration tolerance • Signs of anxiety, grief, depression, euphoria, or emotional withdrawal • Emotional lability
Communication	• Speech quality (e.g., rate, volume, tone) • Fluency, articulation, intelligibility, and spontaneity of speech • Word-finding problems/anomia • Grammar and vocabulary • Auditory comprehension abilities • Ability to understand and carry out task instructions
Thought patterns	• Organization of thoughts • Evidence of hallucinations, delusions, or paranoia • Ability to remain on topic and other unusual thinking patterns (e.g., tangentiality, circumstantiality, derailment, paraphasia, clanging, neologisms, blocking, perseveration) • Flexibility or rigidity in thinking • Appropriateness of responses
Attitude toward examiner and testing	• Cooperation and interest level • Consistency of effort • Persistence • Openness to questions • Level of comfort
Attitude toward self/level of self-awareness	• Level of self-confidence • Awareness of errors and error correction • Reaction to successes and failures • Accuracy of performance rating • Insight and level of awareness • Attainability of goals
Reactions to test items	• Level of frustration tolerance • Expressed concern about task difficulty • Increase or decrease in effort with increasing task difficulty • Persistence
Work habits and approach to testing	• Response rate, response latency, and processing speed • Deliberate versus impulsive responding • Planning and organization abilities • Problem-solving approach to tasks • Flexibility in shifting between tasks • Handwriting accuracy • Reaction to praise

TABLE 43-6
Tests and Their Corresponding Area of Functioning

FUNCTIONING AREA	TEST(S)
Academic Skills	
Arithmetic Calculation	Arithmetic (Wide Range Achievement Test - Third Edition: WRAT3); Numerical Operations (Wechsler Individual Achievement Test – 2nd edition: WIAT-II)
Arithmetic Reasoning	Arithmetic (Wechsler Adult Intelligence Scale–Revised & 3rd edition: WAIS-R & WAIS-III); Mathematics Reasoning (WIAT-II)
Reading Comprehension	Gray Oral Reading Test-Revised (GORT-R); Reading Comprehension (WIAT-II); Test of Reading Comprehension – Third Edition (TORC-3)
Word Reading	GORT-R; Pseudoword Decoding and Word Reading (WIAT-II); Reading (WRAT3); TORC-3
Spelling	Spelling (WRAT3); Spelling (WIAT-II)
Writing	Spelling (WRAT3); Spelling and Written Expression (WIAT-II)
Attention and Concentration	Continuous Performance Test; Dementia Rating Scale (Attention scale); Digit Span and Digit Symbol (WAIS-R & WAIS-III); Letter-Number Sequencing (WAIS-III & WMS-III); Mental Control (Wechsler Memory Scale-Revised & 3rd edition: WMS-R & WMS-III); Paced Auditory Serial Addition Test (PASAT); Spatial Span Forward and Backward (WMS-III); Speech Sounds Perception Test, Rhythm Test, and Trail Making Test: Parts A and B (Halstead-Reitan Battery: HRB); Stroop Color Word Test; Symbol Digit Modalities Test (SDMT)
Motor and Sensory Functions	
Speed and Dexterity	Finger Tapping Test (HRB); Grooved Pegboard
Grip Strength	Hand Dynamometer (HRB)
Coordinated Bilateral Movement	Luria Motor Tests
Hand-Eye Coordination	Digit Symbol (WAIS-R & WAIS-III); Grooved Pegboard; Luria Motor Tests; SDMT (written); Trail Making Test: Parts A & B (HRB)
Sensory & Sensorimotor	Tactile Perception, Tactile Form Recognition, Tactile Localization, and Fingertip Writing (HRB); Tactual Performance Test (TPT; HRB)
Nonverbal Memory	
Immediate	Benton Visual Retention Test; Corsi Block Test; Dementia Rating Scale (Memory scale); Family Pictures and Faces (WMS-III); Motor Free Visual Perception Test; Visual Reproduction (WMS-R & WMS-III)
Delayed	Dementia Rating Scale (Memory scale); Family Pictures and Faces delay (WMS-III); Recognition Memory Test; Rey Osterrieth Complex Figure Test (ROCF); Visual Reproduction (WMS-R & WMS-III)
Learning	Digit Symbol (WAIS-R & WAIS-III); Spatial Span (WMS-III); SDMT
Incidental Learning	Coding (WISC-III); SDMT; TPT (Memory and Location)
Verbal Memory	
Immediate	California Verbal Learning Test: CVLT (Trial I); Logical Memory and Verbal Paired Associates (WMS-R & WMS-III); Rey Auditory Verbal Learning Test: RAVLT (Trial I); Word Lists (WMS-III)
Delayed	CVLT (delay and recognition); Logical Memory and Verbal Paired Associates delay (WMS-R & WMS-III); RAVLT (delay and recognition); Word Lists delay (WMS-III)
Remote Memory and Fund of Information	Information (WAIS-R & WAIS-III)
Learning	CVLT; RAVLT
Visual Based Skills	
Visuoperception and Visual Reasoning	Digit Symbol, Object Assembly, Picture Completion, and Picture Arrangement (WAIS-R & WAIS-III); Hooper Visual Organization Test; Judgment of Line Orientation Test; Line Bisection Test; Motor Free Visual Perception Test; SDMT (oral & written); Visual Form Discrimination Test

TABLE 43-6 (continued)

FUNCTIONING AREA	TEST(S)
Visuomotor & Visuoconstruction	Digit Symbol, Block Design and Object Assembly (WAIS-R & WAIS-III); ROCF; SDMT; Trail Making Test A and B
Language Skills	
Vocabulary	Clinical Interview; Vocabulary (WAIS-R & WAIS-III)
Oral Fluency	Controlled Oral Word Association Test
Naming	Boston Naming Test
Expressive Language	Aphasia Screening Test (HRB); Boston Diagnostic Aphasia Examination; Clinical Interview; Oral Expression (WIAT-II)
Receptive Language	Behavioral observation of instruction following; Clinical Interview; Listening Comprehension (WIAT-II); Token Test
Reasoning and Judgment	
Verbal Reasoning	Comprehension and Similarities (WAIS-R & WAIS-III)
Nonverbal Reasoning	Category Test (HRB); Picture Arrangement (WAIS-R & WAIS-III); Ravens Progressive Matrices; Trail Making Test B (HRB); Wisconsin Card Sorting Test
Judgment of Safety	Comprehension (WAIS-R & WAIS-III); Independent Living Scales; Judgment and Safety Screening Inventory (JASSI) – Patient and Informant Versions
Self-Awareness	Clinical Interview; Judgment and Safety Screening Inventory (JASSI), comparison of patient and family responses; Neurobehavioral Functioning Inventory (NFI), comparison of patient and family responses

and academic functioning can help elucidate deficits. Areas which are typically assessed in comprehensive evaluation of cognitive and academic functioning include: academic skills, attention and concentration, motor abilities, sensation, learning and memory, visuoperception, visuoconstructional abilities, language, and reasoning. Table 43-6 depicts specific tests and the corresponding areas of functioning assessed. The reader is referred to Lezak's (3) seminal text on neuropsychological assessment for further information about tests which are commonly used to assess cognitive and academic functioning.

Assessment of Emotional, Personality, and Neurobehavioral Functioning

Neurobehavioral and personality changes are common following TBI. In addition, survivors typically have difficulty adjusting to injury-related changes, increasing the risk of emotional difficulties. As such, comprehensive neuropsychological evaluation involves assessment of neurobehavioral, emotional, and personality functioning. Table 43-7 describes several measures which are commonly administered to assess these areas of functioning.

Concern has been expressed that measures of emotional and personality functioning have limited utility for patients with TBI. First, many instruments were developed specifically for people with psychiatric difficulties, not for those with neurological disorders. Many individuals with TBI may be diagnosed with psychiatric disorders secondary to the overlap between sequelae of TBI and psychiatric symptoms. Witol and colleagues (6) caution clinicians to consider the contributions of TBI when interpreting the results of measures of emotional and personality functioning. The Neurobehavioral Functioning Inventory (NFI; 10) and the Neurobehavioral Rating Scale (NBRS; 11) were developed for use with TBI populations, and may be good alternatives. Second, reliance on self-report is difficult following TBI secondary to difficulties with self-awareness. As such, clinicians seek out corroborating information from family members and records review. Finally, many measures are long and require at least a sixth grade reading level. Many individuals experience reading comprehension problems, visual disturbances, pain, and attention and concentration problems. Each of these injury-related sequelae can negatively impact patients' abilities to respond to the questionnaires. If concerns about a patient's ability to respond to the questionnaire emerge, clinicians may wish to consider clinician-rated measures such as the NBRS and the Hamilton Depression Rating Scale (HDRS; 8).

Evaluation of Judgment and Safety

Safety is a common area of concern for families and referral sources following TBI. Questions often arise surrounding safety in the following situations: driving, living alone, working, and managing finances and medications. In assessing safety issues, evaluating patient's

TABLE 43-7
Measures Used to Assess Emotional, Personality, and Neurobehavioral Functioning

MEASURE	BRIEF DESCRIPTION
Beck Depression Inventory (BDI)	The BDI is a 21-item, self-report measure designed to detect the presence and severity of depression symptoms (5). The multiple-choice format requires a sixth grade reading level. Repeated administrations permit monitoring of treatment effects. Notably, the BDI emphasizes the vegetative symptoms of depression which may be consistent with TBI and medical illness (6).
Brief Symptom Inventory (BSI)	The BSI, a shortened version of the Symptom Checklist-90-R, is a 53-item self-report measure, which is designed to evaluate the severity of psychiatric symptoms (7). A sixth grade reading level is required. Few studies have been conducted with TBI populations. Witol and colleagues (6) expressed concern about the possibility neurobehavioral symptoms would be labeled as psychiatric.
Hamilton Depression Rating Scale (HDRS)	The HDRS is a 17-item screening instrument, which was designed to assess the cognitive, emotional, and physical symptoms of depression (8). The measure is completed by the clinician during the clinical interview with the patient and family and records review. As such, the measure is useful for screening depression in individuals who have limited reading abilities or vision problems which preclude reading. There is limited research examining the validity of using the HDRS with TBI populations. Witol and colleagues (6) expressed concern that many of the items are consistent with neurobehavioral sequelae of TBI.
Minnesota Multiphasic Personality Inventory – 2nd Edition (MMPI-2)	The MMPI-2 is a 567-item, self-report measure of personality and emotional functioning in adults (9). A 6th grade reading level is required, but audiotaped versions are available. Concern has been expressed about overpathologizing of individuals with TBI on the MMPI-2. Witol and colleagues (6) urge clinicians to consider the contributions of TBI when interpreting the results of the MMPI-2.
Neurobehavioral Functioning Inventory (NFI)	Developed for use with a TBI population, the NFI is an 83-item measure which was designed to examine the frequency of neurobehavioral difficulties post-injury (10). The measure can be administered in a self-report format or orally. Patient and family versions are available, allowing for comparison of responses. Normative data, based upon age and injury severity, is available. Information is gathered about functioning in six domains: depression, somatic symptoms, memory/attention, communication, aggression, and motor abilities.
Neurobehavioral Rating Scale (NBRS)	Adapted from the Brief Psychiatric Rating Scale, the NBRS was designed to assess behavioral and emotional symptoms, which are commonly exhibited post-TBI (11). The 27-item scale is completed by a clinician based upon observations during an interview. Items are rated on a scale from 1 (not present) to 7 (extremely severe). Witol and colleagues (6) assert that the NBRS is an extremely useful tool for assessing neurobehavioral functioning acutely.

judgment is critical. To assess judgment and safety, the examiner may ask patients and their family members about daily functioning. For example, with regard to driving, information may be gathered about recent accidents or traffic violations and about patient and family members' concerns. Medication issues include forgetting medications and not taking medications as prescribed. With respect to financial management, the examiner may ask about bounced checks, late or missed bills, and utilities being turned off.

The Judgment and Safety Screening Inventory (12) was designed to assess judgment and safety concerns in

TABLE 43-8
Methods Used to Assess Substance Use

MEASURE	BRIEF DESCRIPTION
Addiction Severity Index (ASI)	The ASI assesses recent and lifetime alcohol and illicit drug use difficulties and gathers information regarding legal issues, medical and vocational history, and family/social functioning (21). The ASI has been found to have good reliability and validity (22); however, research on the ASI and acquired brain injury populations is very limited.
Brief Michigan Alcoholism Screening Test (B-MAST)	The B-MAST, a shortened version of the MAST, contains 10 of the original 25 MAST items and is highly correlated with the MAST (23). The B-MAST has been found to be useful in the detection of alcohol abuse among individuals with TBI (20).
CAGE	The CAGE is a four-question screening tool, which is easily administered and scored. Each question follows a yes/no format. Two or more positive responses are suggestive of alcohol problems. The CAGE has been shown to be highly effective in detecting alcohol abuse in the general population (24) and in individuals with TBI (20).
Michigan Alcoholism Screening Test (MAST)	The MAST is a 25-item screening questionnaire that focuses on lifetime problems and consequences of drinking in the areas of social, vocational, and family functioning (25).
Quantity-Frequency-Variability Index (QFVI)	The QFVI is a self-report measure, with patient and informant versions. The QFVI classifies drinking behavior in one of five categories: abstinent, infrequent, light, moderate, or heavy (26, 27). The QFVI has been shown to be effective in assessing pre- and post-injury alcohol use among survivors of TBI (28). Concordance rates between family members' and patients' reports on the QFVI have been found to exceed 90% (29).
Substance Abuse Subtle Screening Inventory (SASSI)	The SASSI is a 78-item, self-report alcohol and drug abuse assessment instrument, which has been found to have high sensitivity and specificity when used with the general population. However, the SASSI appears to be less effective in detecting substance abuse problems among individuals with TBI (30).

the following areas: travel; financial management; interpersonal functioning; food and kitchen; use of appliances, tools, and utensils; household issues; medications and alcohol; fire safety; and firearm safety. Respondents are asked to identify their concern level (none, little, much, or very) about different aspects of each functioning area. Space is provided for open-ended responses from patients and other informants. Patient and informant versions allow for comparisons between respondents.

Substance Abuse Assessment

Substance abuse is a significant problem for individuals with TBI and occurs more frequently among survivors of TBI than in the general population (13–16). In a comprehensive review study, Corrigan (17) indicated that approximately two thirds of individuals with TBI have a history of substance abuse pre-injury, and one third to one half of individuals hospitalized are intoxicated at the time of injury. In a study by Hall and colleagues (18), approximately 30% of participants with a brain injury were alcohol dependent whereas 20% were drug dependent at two years post-injury.

Given the significance of this problem among survivors of TBI, substance abuse screening is an important part of comprehensive neuropsychological evaluation. Substance abuse assessment involves administration of standardized assessment measures and thorough review of records. Measures designed to assess substance abuse in the general population are often used to assess pre- and post-injury substance use in persons with acquired brain injury. Research reveals that composite measures are helpful in diagnosing and treating substance abuse problems among persons with brain injury (19). Assessment measures frequently used include the Michigan Alcoholism Screening Test (MAST), Brief Michigan Alcoholism Screening Test (B-MAST), CAGE, Quantity-Frequency-Variability Index (QFVI), Addiction Severity Index (ASI), and Substance Abuse Subtle Screening Inventory (SASSI). Table 43-8 provides descriptions of each measure. Overall, research suggests that the CAGE or B-MAST are more effective screening instruments for TBI populations and less time-consuming than the SASSI and ASI (20).

Self-report measures are easily administered and relatively inexpensive, and as such, they are often the cornerstones of substance abuse assessment. However, self-report measures are limited due to their reliance upon individuals' willingness and ability to disclose information accurately. Patients may be reluctant to admit the extent of alcohol or drug use. Patients with memory problems or limited self-awareness may also be unreliable historians (29). Family members' reports may also be inaccurate secondary to minimization or denial of problems, personal substance abuse history, perceptions about substance use, or lack of information regarding the patient's use (30). Given the aforementioned limitations, accurate assessment of substance use may be compromised if one relies predominantly on information provided by one source. To address these limitations, neuropsychologists solicit information from a variety of informants, including family members, caregivers, and employers. Records review also allows for corroboration of informant and patient reports.

Pain Assessment

Pain, a common complaint of individuals who have sustained TBI, often contributes to cognitive deficits and negatively impacts quality of life secondary to activity restrictions. Individuals' response to pain varies significantly based upon the meaning of pain to the individual and the impact of pain on their life. Thorough pain assessment may include administration of standardized measures, such as the McGill Pain Inventory (31) and visual analog scales (32). Information is gathered about pain intensity, frequency, duration, quality, location, date of onset, history of pain problems, family history, and treatments and their effectiveness. In addition, behaviors which exacerbate and improve pain are important to assess. Patients are often asked to rate their pain on a 1 (no pain) to 10 (extreme pain) scale throughout the assessment in order to establish if poor performances are related to pain. During the evaluation, examiners are alert to pain behaviors (e.g., shifting in seat, rubbing areas of pain focus) and to medication side effects (e.g., fatigue). The reader is referred to the chapter in this book entitled, "Pain Assessment and Management," by Drs. Zasler, Nicholson, Martelli, and Bender for detailed information about the assessment and treatment of pain among individuals with TBI.

Assessment of Motivation and Effort

Comprehensive neuropsychological assessment typically incorporates evaluation of patients' motivation and effort during the evaluation. As a general practice, patients are often encouraged to exert maximum effort during the testing process to reduce concerns about malingering (33). When there is a question of malingered neuropsychological impairment, practitioners have several techniques to discourage and identify such activity. Neuropsychologists look for consistency in performance across tests, consistency of

test performance and presenting complaints with those expected given injury severity, and consistency between observed behaviors and presenting complaints.

Neuropsychological and psychological tests may be used to assess legitimate versus malingered memory impairments or exaggerated symptoms. Mittenberg, Azrin, Millsaps, and Heilbronner (34) found a pattern of scores on the Wechsler Memory Scale-Revised (35) that differentiated individuals instructed to malinger head trauma symptoms from patients with head injury. Discrepancy between predicted and obtained scores on the Wechsler Adult Intelligence Scale-Revised (36) may be used to discriminate between patients with TBI and those producing insufficient effort (37).

Specialized tests developed specifically for detection of malingering are available for inclusion in neuropsychological test batteries, including the following: Portland Digit Recognition Test (38), Recognition Memory Test (39), Rey 15-Item Test (40), Test of Memory Malingering (41), and the Word Memory Test (42). Normative data on the F(p) Scale of the MMPI also aids in the identification of unusual response patterns suggestive of insufficient effort or symptoms exaggeration (43).

Secondary gain issues are important to consider, including revenge, attention seeking, escape from responsibility, and pending lawsuits, Worker's compensation hearings, or disability benefit hearings. History of litigation and benefit seeking should be ascertained during interview and records review. The reader is referred to the chapter in this book entitled, "Assessment of Response Bias," by Drs. Martelli, Zasler, and Bender for a thorough review of assessment techniques for evaluating motivation and effort.

Vocational Assessment

Research suggests that a majority of persons with moderate or severe TBI are unable to sustain employment (44–47). Vocational issues are a primary concern for patients and their families, and referral sources frequently list return to work among their primary concerns for patients. Referral questions often focus on individuals' readiness to return to work, potential work capacity, and needed accommodations and rehabilitation services. Prognostication about vocational potential should be based upon thorough return to work assessment and comprehensive neuropsychological evaluation revealing strengths and limitations. Comprehensive assessment reveals potential obstacles to successful return to work, including cognitive deficits, emotional issues, interpersonal difficulties, transportation issues, anger management problems, and pain and other physical symptoms.

Areas which are commonly assessed in comprehensive assessment include the following: (1) job responsibilities, including special training required, equipment used, and interpersonal interaction with co-workers and customers; (2) conditions set by employer regarding return to work; (3) the patient's perceptions about obstacles to working and about their ability to return to work on a part-time or full-time basis; (4) transportation requirements for the job; (5) work schedule issues (e.g., hours required, over time, swing shift work, possibility of working part-time, flexibility of position, openness to accommodations); (6) safety issues on the job, including history of prior injuries on the job; (7) work-place response to others with injuries and disabilities; (8) relationship with supervisor; (9) supervisor's knowledge of the injury and extent of injury-related sequelae; (10) pre-injury work history; (11) patient perceptions about job security; and (12) the patient's career goals, desire to return to work, and willingness to consider other job options. In addition, consideration of the nature of the job in question is valuable. Individuals tend to be most successful returning to work in family-owned or small businesses, which are supportive and allow for accommodations.

Family and Caregiver Assessment

As the length of hospital and rehabilitation stays decrease (48, 49), family members have had to take on the principal caretaking role soon after injury. Caregiving places significant burden on the family. Research reveals that caregiving family members are at risk for emotional difficulties (50–58). Given the importance of the family's role in caring for the survivor, assessment of the impact of injury on the family is critical to ensure they have the support needed to continue performing their vital role. Family and caregiver assessment should center around gaining an understanding of the impact of injury on emotional functioning, relationship quality, financial situation, life plans, quality of life, and daily responsibilities (e.g., work, child care, household responsibilities). In addition, clinical neuropsychologists often explore existing supports and consider additional support needs. Written recommendations that include options for increasing family supports are extremely beneficial. Special care should be taken to help the caregiving family member(s) understand that they will be unable to support the survivor if they do not take care of themselves and seek assistance in managing their increasing responsibilities. The reader is referred to James Malec, Ph.D.'s chapter in this text entitled, "Family and Caregiver Issues and Interventions," for information about issues related to assessment and treatment of family members and caregivers.

Comparison to Premorbid Functioning

Neuropsychologists are often asked to determine whether or not the injury resulted in cognitive, academic, neurobehavioral, or emotional impairments. Determining deficits requires comparison of current functioning to premorbid functioning. Three methods may be employed to estimate premorbid functioning. First, several indicators are highly correlated with intelligence, and as such, provide an estimate of premorbid functioning. These indicators include grades, scores on standardized testing, and educational and vocational attainment. Review of records and clinical interview are avenues of gathering this information. Second, some measures of cognitive functioning (e.g., single-word reading) are highly correlated with intelligence and are typically not affected by TBI (59). Scores on these standardized measures will likely be comparable to premorbid levels of functioning. Finally, within the "best performance method," the highest test scores obtained during comprehensive neuropsychological evaluation are considered in the estimation of pre-injury abilities (3).

PROGNOSTICATION AND TREATMENT PLANNING

Prognostication

Questions about future prognosis are typically among the primary questions posed by referral sources. As such, clinical neuropsychologists are often called upon to provide information about long-term academic, vocational, and independent living potential. In addition, questions are often posed about an individual's likelihood of benefiting from rehabilitation services and potential treatment benefits. Thorough review of the research literature on outcomes following TBI provides the foundation for prognostic estimation. Several factors need to be considered when making predictions about an individual's outcome, including age, premorbid level of functioning, injury type and severity, additional injuries (e.g., orthopedic), pre-existing medical and psychological issues, extent and chronicity of deficits, daily functioning, and availability of support services and interventions (3).

Recommendations and Treatment Planning

Comprehensive neuropsychological assessment culminates in the development of practical, feasible recommendations and the development of treatment plans. The goal is to develop recommendations and identify interventions, which will enhance patients' and families' well being and optimize functioning. Referral for medical follow-up, psychological services, psychiatric intervention, support, vocational/academic assistance, and other rehabilitation services in the community are commonly included. Compensatory strategies to address impairments are typically provided. Repeated neuropsychological testing is often suggested to monitor progress or deterioration. Based upon findings from re-evaluation, amendments may be made to the existing treatment plan. Table 43-9 depicts recommendations that may be provided to address problems in a variety of functional areas.

TABLE 43-9
Post-Injury Problem Areas and Aample Recommendations

FUNCTIONAL AREA	RECOMMENDATIONS
Academic skills	
Arithmetic	• use a calculator for all but the most basic mathematical operations; check work carefully; rely on family for assistance with financial management
Reading comprehension	• use chapter headings to outline material; take notes and highlight or underline key words while you are reading; use self-sticking notepaper to create indexes in the reading material to facilitate reviewing information; use the PQRST method (preview, question, read, study, test)
Spelling	• use an electronic spelling aid or word processing spell checker; purchase a portable electronic spell checker for home use; spell the word out loud, or mouth each letter as you spell the word to help focus your attention as you write; keep a small speller's dictionary near where you write; use index cards to make flash cards of words you find yourself missing often and test yourself; play Scrabble; work cross-word and other puzzles
Writing	• focus on quality versus quantity; allow ample time for task completion; dictation; remedial training
Attention and concentration	• reduce distractions (e.g., ear plugs, sit facing wall, clear desk before beginning work); avoid interruptions (e.g., use 'do not disturb' sign); use self-coaching to stay on task; schedule breaks throughout the day; avoid multi-tasking; before changing tasks, record information about stopping point
Motor/sensory functioning	
Coordination and motor slowing	• occupational and physical therapy; fitness training; sports and recreational activities; pace tasks; allow adequate time for task completion and transition between tasks; organize environment for efficiency (e.g., gather all needed materials prior to initiating project); set realistic timelines for task completion
Vision	• neuro-ophthalmologic evaluation; corrective lenses; vision therapy; use large print reading materials and thick pen when writing notes to be read by client; audiotape instructions/reading material; make sure there is appropriate light; avoid glare
Hearing	• audiology examination; ask others to speak loudly and enunciate clearly; hearing aids
Smell	• smoke detectors; label and date perishable foods
Learning and memory	• present information in many forms (e.g., auditory, visual, kinetic); use to-do lists, calendars, memory notebook, and other assistive devices; repeat information; use mnemonics and imagery; demonstrate tasks; record and replay information; break tasks down into small steps and introduce new steps as earlier steps are accomplished
Visually based skills	• use a blank piece of paper or fold the sheet to mask extraneous details on a page; use a straight edge, ruler, or finger to follow a line of text; always check work in the same order; describe a design or task in words rather than rely on a mental image; take part in activities which require hand-eye coordination
Language	
Instruction following	• improve instructional format (e.g., short, simple sentences); simplify or reduce variety of tasks; reduce distractions; provide instructions in multiple formats; shaping
Judgment and safety	
Judgment and safety issues	• consider supervised living situations; 24-hour supervision; respite for family; seek feedback from others before beginning a task
Problem solving	• teach structured problem solving; develop and maintain mentor relationship; ask client how they plan to approach task prior to beginning

TABLE 43-9 (*continued*)

FUNCTIONAL AREA	RECOMMENDATIONS
Driving	• take precautions to maximize safety (e.g., avoid driving in inclement weather or traffic, drive with licensed driver, take breaks on long trips, drive familiar routes, drive only when well rested, reduce distractions); driving evaluation; driver's training; training in use of public transportation; exploration of other transportation options (family, friends, neighbors, and area resources);
Financial management	• rely on family to assist with financial management; use an organizer with dated slots and place bills in slots one week before they are due; record due dates for bills in a calendar or planner; use a calculator; check work carefully; take care of challenging tasks only when well rested and distractions are minimized
Medication management	• use a compartmentalized medication box, distributing medication in appropriate compartments at the beginning of the week; set an alarm to cue when to take medication
Fatigue/sleep problems	• promote sleep hygiene (e.g., regular sleep schedule, limit caffeine/exercise before bed); medication consultation (stimulants and sleep medication); consider sleep study; adjust work schedule; schedule breaks; schedule most challenging tasks at times of peak energy level
Emotional issues	
Depression	• supportive psychotherapy; medication management; enhance support network; increase activity level and participation in pleasant activities; encourage focus on progress; avoid comparisons to the past; monitor sources of stress
Frustration, irritability, and anger problems	• stress management and relaxation training; anger management; assertiveness, conflict resolution, and social skills training; medication management
Feeling misunderstood by others	• communication and social skills training; educate client about how to discuss injury with others; education of coworkers, employers, and family; supportive psychotherapy; support group; enhance social support

DIFFERENTIAL DIAGNOSIS

Patients with TBI present for assessment and treatment with myriad cognitive, behavioral, emotional, and somatic symptoms. Differential diagnosis is often the culmination of a comprehensive neuropsychological assessment. Differential diagnosis requires a breadth of knowledge about the spectrum of the *Diagnostic and Statistical Manual of Mental Disorders, 4th edition* (60) conditions and proficient interviewing skills. Information about the onset, nature, intensity, and duration of symptoms provides valuable insights into conditions, which should be considered as possible diagnoses. Oftentimes, the confirmation of a diagnosis follows long-term evaluation and treatment of the patient. Exacerbation or abatement of symptoms, as well as the emergence of additional problems, are monitored to facilitate differential diagnosis.

Neuropsychological evaluators and rehabilitation treatment providers incorporate a multitude of data collection strategies to glean pertinent information for differential diagnosis. Clinicians may enlist assistance from family members, friends, or significant others in order to procure thorough medical, social, and psychiatric patient

and family history. Unstructured, semi-structured, or structured interviews are often utilized to this end. The *Structured Clinical Interview for DSM-IV Axis I Disorders—Clinical Version* (61) is an assessment tool available to practitioners for determining pre and post-injury psychological difficulties. Glenn (62) advised conducting a structured search in order to best discover etiology and recommended the following information be ascertained: pre-injury diagnosis, neuropsychological disorders, sensorimotor disorder, medical disorders, adverse effects of medication, reactive mood and anxiety disorders, and sleep disorders.

There is often considerable overlap between symptoms of medical and psychological disorders. For example, cognitive impairments are typical consequences of most neurological conditions, including frontotemporal dementia and TBI (63). However, impairments in cognition are often evident in individuals with psychiatric disorders, including major depressive disorder and anxiety disorders. As such, differentiation between the etiologies of cognitive impairments may be challenging.

Differentiation between pre-existing conditions and post-injury complications is often critical to forming an accurate diagnosis and to planning effective treatment. Premorbid psychological or personality disorders, learning disabilities, drug or alcohol problems, and medical conditions (e.g., cerebrovascular disease, hypertension, diabetes, epilepsy, prior TBI) are potential mediating variables that commonly influence the course of a TBI. In conducting a comprehensive evaluation, neuropsychologists attempt to tease out premorbid problems from current injury-related complications and sequelae. In order to assist clinicians in differentiating between premorbid problems and post-injury complications, Table 43-10 provides referral questions to consider during comprehensive neuropsychological assessment.

Identification of comorbid conditions is one of the principal aims of comprehensive neuropsychological assessment. Psychological comorbidities are quite common after a TBI. Hibbard and her colleagues (64) found two or more Axis I diagnoses post-TBI, representing 44% of their sample. Depression and anxiety disorders (e.g., PTSD, OCD, panic disorder, GAD) were the most frequently cited post-injury affective problems of this sample. Researchers have found that approximately 60% of individuals with a TBI meet criteria for major depression at some point after a brain injury (64). Research indicates the frequency of reported emotional difficulties is directly proportional to injury severity, except in the most severe cases of TBI (65). Table 43-11 depicts common co-morbidities encountered in the clinical practice of patients with TBI.

Neuropsychological evaluators consider the impact of comorbidities such as mood disorders or psychosis on patients' assessment findings. For example, conditions that alter mental status (e.g., delirium, vegetative states, or active hallucinations) may invalidate results of assessment. Screening with measures such as the Mini-Mental Status Examination (66) or the Minnesota Multiphasic Personality Inventory-II (67) is recommended. These instruments help to rule-out potentially confounding factors of diminished consortium or significant affective disturbance, respectively. Table 43-12 provides a list of test measures least and most susceptible to the affect slowed mental processing and/or psychomotor performance often observed with certain mood disorders.

Mild head injury offers unique challenges to evaluators in terms of differential diagnosis than moderate and severe neurological damage. Clear physiological

---

TABLE 43-11
Common Comorbidities

- Adjustment Disorder with Anxiety or Depressed Mood
- Adjustment Disorder with Mixed Emotional Features and Disturbed Conduct
- Major Depressive Disorder
- Mood Disorder due to General Medical Condition
- Personality Change Secondary to General Medical Condition
- Polysubstance Abuse
- Post-traumatic Stress Disorder
- Substance Abuse or Dependence

TABLE 43-10
Questions to Facilitate Differentiation Between Premorbid Problems and Injury-Related Sequelae

- Did patient have problems with substance misuse prior to the TBI?
- Did the individual have a pre-injury personality disorder?
- Was the patient receiving mental health treatment for a mood disorder or other psychological problem before the injury?
- Did the patient have pre-existing learning difficulties?
- Were pain or sleep problems apparent prior to the patient having a TBI?
- How was the patient's daily functioning prior to the injury? Explore areas such as relationships, occupational or educational pursuits, and recreational activities.
- Have others noticed a change in the patient's functioning since the injury?
- When did emotional difficulties or substance use issues arise?

TABLE 43-12
Tests Least and Most Susceptible to Affect of Mood Disorders

Least Susceptible	Most Susceptible
Category Test	Symbol Digit Modalities Test
WAIS Verbal Subtests Vocabulary Comprehension Similarities	WAIS Performance Subtests Block Design Digit Symbol-Coding
Rey-Osterrieth Complex Figure Test	Trail Making Test: Parts A & B
Wide Range-Achievement Test Reading Spelling	Grooved Pegboard Test
Token Test	Controlled Oral Word Association Test

consequences of serious brain injury are unquestionable, such as positive CT or MRI findings. For mild brain damage, however, hard neurological signs of injury may not be present. Comorbid problems with somatic functioning may complicate differential diagnosis after mild head injury. Practitioners are encouraged to be familiar with difficulties associated with somatic problems. According to the DSM-IV (60), there are a number of distinct disorders with a physical presentation, including Pain Disorder, Hypochondriasis, Somatization Disorder, and Conversion Disorder. Table 43-13 depicts highlights of the DSM-IV criteria for each of these diagnoses.

TABLE 43-13
DSM-IV Diagnoses and Associated Criteria for Selected Disorders

DSM-IV DIAGNOSIS	**CRITERIA**
Pain Disorder	<ul><li>pain reported at one or more anatomical sites</li><li>pain is sufficient in severity to warrant clinical attention</li><li>pain causes significant distress or impairment in functioning</li><li>psychological factors have an important role in onset, severity, exacerbation, or maintenance of pain</li><li>symptoms or deficits are not better accounted for by another mental condition (i.e., mood, anxiety, or psychotic disorder) and does not meet criteria for Dyspareunia</li><li>symptoms or deficits are not intentionally feigned</li></ul>
Hypochondriasis	<ul><li>preoccupation with fears of having a serious disease</li><li>fear is often based on the person's misinterpretation of bodily symptoms</li><li>preoccupation persists despite appropriate medical evaluation and reassurance</li><li>belief is not of delusional intensity and is not restricted to a circumscribed concern about appearance</li><li>preoccupation causes clinically significant distress or impairment in functioning</li><li>duration of the disturbance is at least 6 months</li><li>preoccupation is not better accounted for by Generalized Anxiety Disorder, Obsessive-Compulsive Disorder, Panic Disorder, a Major Depressive Episode, Separation Anxiety, or another Somatoform Disorder</li></ul>
Somatization Disorder	<ul><li>history of many physical complaints beginning before age 30 years</li><li>complaints must continue for several years and result in treatment being sought</li><li>after appropriate investigation, each of the physical symptoms cannot be fully explained by a known medical condition or the direct effects of a substance (e.g., a drug of abuse, a medication)</li><li>when there is a related general medical condition, the physical complaints or resulting impairment are in excess of what would be expected from the history, physical examination, or laboratory findings</li><li>patient reports or displays symptoms at any time during the course of the disturbance as described below:<ul><li>four pain symptoms</li><li>two gastrointestinal symptoms</li><li>one sexual symptom</li><li>one pseudoneurological symptom</li></ul></li></ul>
Conversion Disorder	<ul><li>one or more symptoms or deficits affecting voluntary motor or sensory function</li><li>symptoms are suggestive of a neurological or other medical condition and may not be intentionally produced or feigned<ul><li>symptom cannot, after appropriate investigation, be fully explained by a general medical condition, or by the direct effects of a substance, or as a culturally sanctioned behavior or experience</li><li>symptom causes clinically significant distress or impairment in social, occupational, or other important areas of functioning or warrants medical evaluation</li><li>symptom is not limited to pain or sexual dysfunction, does not occur exclusively during the course of Somatization Disorder, and is not better accounted for by another mental disorder</li></ul></li></ul>

NEUROPSYCHOLOGICAL REPORT WRITING

Communicating results from the neuropsychological assessment to referral sources, treating providers, patients, and their families is a critical task for neuropsychologists. If test results are not communicated effectively, the utility of the entire assessment process comes into question. When writing a helpful report, neuropsychologists consider the following:

1. Review records thoroughly to ensure that historical information, pre-existing conditions, and injury severity are understood and considered in formulating impressions and recommendations.
2. In formulating diagnostic impressions, consider the impact of pre-existing conditions, psychological and emotional issues, motivation, effort, self-awareness, and pain.
3. Write reports in a language that patients and lay people can understand, avoiding use of jargon.
4. Tailor reports to each specific patient rather than being generic.
5. Write and disseminate reports in a timely fashion. Review test results with the patient and discuss findings in a meaningful way. Encourage the patient and his or her family to ask questions.

6. Take special care to ensure reports address and answer the referral source's questions and concerns.
7. Consider the patient's and family's concerns and the meaning of the injury to the patient during report development.
8. Consider the patient's reactions to test findings and impressions, and take special care to ensure the presentation of the findings and conclusions will be palatable to the patient.
9. Highlight strengths as well as deficits.
10. Translate test results into recommendations which will make patients' lives better.

Although practitioners are encouraged to develop unique reports which are specific to each patient, structure is an important way to provide a familiar framework for referral sources. Placing information in similar sections with distinct headings allows readers to locate information quickly. Structured report formats also provide a way to organize large amounts of information and to increase efficiency. Table 43-14 depicts important sections that may be included in comprehensive neuropsychological reports and content which may be included in each section.

TABLE 43-14
Report Structure and Content

REPORT SECTION	CONTENT OF SECTION
Confidentiality Statement	• Include statement indicating that report contents are "strictly confidential" and should not be disseminated or reproduced without the patient's explicit permission
Agency Contact Information	• Include agency name, complete mailing address, telephone number, fax number
Demographic Information and Referral Source	• Include patient's name, address, race, marital status, handedness, date of birth, age, current medications, date of injury, and referral source
Presenting Problem and Reason for Referral	• Highlight presenting problems, including injury date, etiology, and injury specifics • Identify specific referral questions
Basis of Evaluation	• Provide sources of interview information • Identify records which were reviewed • Provide checklist of tests administered in the appendices
Behavioral Observations	• Describe behavioral observations during the testing process, including information presented in Table 43-4 (general behavioral observations included in "Behavioral Observations" section and specific test related behaviors included in "Test Results" section)
Current Symptoms	• Identify current problems reported by the patient and his or her family members • Include current neurobehavioral symptoms endorsed on the Neurobehavioral Functioning Inventory, listing specific items endorsed in a table • Highlight changes in functioning compared to pre-injury

TABLE 43-14 (continued)

REPORT SECTION	CONTENT OF SECTION

Historical Information	• Include information about the following:
	  • Academic/vocational history
	  • Family/social history
	  • Medical/mental health history; current treatment
	  • Pre- and post-injury substance use
	  • Criminal history

Summary of Medical Records	• Provide summary of principal medical and mental health records reviewed
Daily Living Abilities	• Identify current living situation, daily activities, and ability to perform activities independently and safely (e.g., hygiene, driving, medication compliance, financial management) • Note any post-injury change in living situation, daily activities, and independence • Highlight judgment and safety issues, with table depicting responses on the Judgment and safety Screening Inventory
Test Results	• Provide behavioral observations pertaining to approach to testing and reaction to testing • Note level of motivation and effort • Estimate pre-injury abilities (Impaired to High Average) • Describe of test performance in each functional area • Provide table comparing test data to pre-injury estimates, prior tests, and normative data • Provide graphical depictions of selected test results in appendices (e.g., performance across trials on verbal learning tasks, figure depicting MMPI-2 results)
Impressions	• Integrate information from various report sections • Note and discuss consistencies between various information sources • Provide diagnostic formulation and support for each diagnosis • Provide table depicting DSM-IV and ICD diagnoses • Respond to referral questions clearly • Highlight interactions between cognitive, emotional, neurobehavioral, pain, and medical factors • Provide conclusions about prognosis for improvement and future academic and vocational functioning
Recommendations	• Provide practical, feasible recommendations that address cognitive, neurobehavioral, and emotional issues • Provide recommendations regarding judgment, safety, and daily living activities • Provide referrals for services which may improve functioning (e.g., medical follow-up, evaluation, therapy, support group) (see Table 43-9 for sample recommendations)

NEUROPSYCHOLOGICAL TREATMENT

Neuropsychologists specialize in the assessment and treatment of neurobehavioral disorders encountered across the lifespan. As treatment providers, neuropsychologists offer invaluable expertise in developing compensatory strategies and identifying resources to help patients cope with disruptions in their daily functioning. Neuropsychological treatments and interventions are ideally created with appreciation of individuals' unique characteristics and needs. Treatment plans aim to accentuate patients' strengths, to help them overcome neurocognitive and behavioral challenges identified by assessment, and to maximize coping. Staples of neuropsychological rehabilitation include education and referral, individual and family psychotherapy, support groups, behavior management, cognitive remediation, and job advocacy and planning.

Education and Referral

Research has found that family members of people with TBI most frequently cited health information as an important need (68). Rehabilitation professionals strive to provide reliable and accurate information about TBI to patients, family members, friends, teachers, employers, and other treatment providers. Bibliotherapy is chosen by many professionals to facilitate communication of vital medical knowledge. Patients may be provided with written material for review and discussion. For example, *Getting Better and Better after Brain Injury: A Guide for Families, Friends, and Caregivers* by Kreutzer and Kolakowsky-Hayner (69) offers pertinent information about consequences of TBI and the recovery process. Rehabilitation specialists may also be called upon to provide referral sources with information about the common manifestations of TBI. Providers of adjunctive therapies are likely to profit from understanding an individual patient's neurobehavioral or cognitive post-injury difficulties.

Patients often demonstrate needs outside the realm of a neuropsychologist's expertise. Treatment providers are encouraged to be mindful of adjunctive treatments which may prove beneficial to patients. Appropriate and timely referrals to alternative treatment professionals are encouraged. The identification of services likely to be helpful to patients is the first step. Rehabilitation professionals may consider patients' abilities and willingness to fully participate and make use of additional treatments. Examples of adjunctive services include substance abuse treatment, psychotropic medication, vocational rehabilitation, clubhouse programs, support groups, or comprehensive driver's evaluation.

Individual Psychotherapy

Psychotherapy is considered an essential component of holistic treatment for patients with TBI by many rehabilitation professionals (70–73). Qualified neuropsychologists play a vital role in providing psychotherapy for individuals with TBI (71). Individual therapy with patients and family members is a useful and commonly practiced mode of inpatient and outpatient rehabilitation. Patients may benefit from attending sessions without their family members present for private discussions of personal issues. Conversely, family members may be invited to sessions in order to obtain psychoeducation about the patient's injury or to provide input about the patient's functioning outside of session.

Psychotherapy further offers people with TBI the opportunity to learn skills to better deal with dramatic life changes encountered after a TBI. Practitioners and patients with TBI determine mutually acceptable therapy goals to address areas of deficiency. Improving emotional adjustment, communication skills, and symptom management are examples of typical therapy goals. Training in anger or stress management, social skills, and strategies to manage depression or anxiety are therapeutic strategies often employed with patients following a TBI.

Family and Marital Intervention

Research supports the need for interventions following TBI for families. (68, 74–76). Researchers have found that nine out of 10 patients are discharged to home after inpatient rehabilitation (48). Family members of patients have an understandably difficult time coping with role changes, increased responsibilities, and stress associated with TBI (e.g., insurance issues, financial strain, and medical appointments). Despite the efforts of rehabilitation staff to prepare families for patients' discharge, many family members report feeling overwhelmed and ill-equipped to manage the long-term needs of survivors (18, 77).

Most families do not receive professional emotional support following the TBI of a family member (68). Research on caregiver burden revealed that over one-third of caregivers endorsed clinically significant levels of depression and anxiety (55). Emotional reactions of families following the brain injury of a loved one may also include intense feelings of anger, blame, and guilt. Reassuring family members that these reactions are normal responses to a tragic event can enhance long-term functioning.

Family interventions not only provide a valuable means for improving emotional support, but also may help with symptom reduction and coping skills enhancement. Some family members receive individual therapy as an adjunct to or as a substitution for family therapy. Neuropsychologists are often pro-active in recommending and implementing treatments tailored for the needs of a family or an individual family member.

Psychotherapy provides patients and their families the opportunity to share their feelings of grief, loss, and helplessness in a supportive and understanding environment. Treatment providers also impart information regarding the patients' neurological condition through patient-family education. Information commonly shared with family members includes the effects of brain injury, the process of recovery from TBI, and compensatory strategies. Dysfunction in sexuality may also be addressed as a component of therapy. Psychosocial treatment approaches are associated with helping survivors and their families cope with post-injury issues of such as impaired sexual performance or disinhibition (78). Readers interested in additional information about families of patients with TBI are referred to the chapter in this text by James Malec, Ph.D., "Family and Caregiver Issues and Interventions."

Support Groups

Support groups for survivors of TBI and their family members or friends provide a number of benefits to participants. Community based support programs offer survivors of brain injury and their family members or friends help in managing a wide range of disability-related stressors. For example, support groups are a source of emotional support, education, and social networking. Participants in a peer oriented group for survivors reported having increased knowledge about TBI, enhanced quality of life, improved general outlook, and better emotional coping (79). Patients and their families often benefit emotionally from the shared experiences of others. Support group members commonly disclose information regarding resources or coping strategies they have found useful in recovering from TBI. People are given the opportunity to extend their social connections within the community through their participation in support groups. An organization such as the Brain Injury Association of America, Inc. provides referral services and information about local support groups for interested parties. Common objectives of a group for persons with TBI may include discussing needs of survivors and families, sharing information, identifying local resources, and networking. Rehabilitation specialists are encouraged to be familiar with such organizations and groups in their area.

Behavior Management

Behavior management is another tool available to treatment professionals for patients demonstrating disruptive or dangerous behavior. Behavior management may incorporate aspects of cognitive remediation in applying interventions. Behavioral approaches providing emotional support and maintaining sensitivity to the contextual environment of the patient are recommended (80). Yody and colleagues (81) advocate for behavior management training that reduces unwanted behaviors by reinforcing alternative behaviors serving similar functions or purpose. Families and other service providers (e.g., teachers, nursing staff, and employers) may benefit from learning behavior management techniques. Problems such as impulsivity and aggressiveness can greatly interrupt patients' social functioning at work, home, or in treatment facilities. For example, behavior modification techniques to enhance the inhibitory control of patients have demonstrated effectiveness (82).

COGNITIVE REMEDIATION

Ben-Yishay and Diller (83) argued for an integrative, holistic approach to cognitive remediation that considered issues of awareness, self-concept, and self-efficacy. Mateer and colleagues (84) further recommended integrating cognitive and emotional interventions given the interaction between the two domains of functioning. The authors indicated that successful integration maximizes treatment potential.

Direct intervention to address cognitive deficits incurred as a result of a TBI may be obtained through cognitive retraining (85). Neurocognitive domains (e.g., attention/concentration, memory, learning, and planning) and

academic skills may be amenable to remediation efforts. The preponderance of evidence indicates there is some benefit of cognitive rehabilitation programs across a continuum of services (86). Cicerone and colleagues (87) reported that therapies for skill acquisition and domain-specific knowledge could be beneficial for individuals with moderate to severe memory impairments. Research suggests that enhancement of specific skills areas may account for the majority of noted benefits observed from cognitive retraining in such domains as attention (88).

Cognitive rehabilitation typically includes training patients in compensatory strategies to enhance functioning compromised by neurological damage. Patients' strengths and skills are often exploited in attempts to overcome areas of relative neurocognitive weakness. For example, rehabilitation specialists train patients in the effective use of memory logs, checklists, mnemonic devices, and self-monitoring to help them compensate for cognitive deficits. Keith Cicerone, Ph.D., addresses this topic more thoroughly in the chapter entitled "Cognitive Rehabilitation." Table 43-15 depicts programs and strategies developed to ameliorate cognitive dysfunction.

Job Advocacy and Planning

As TBI frequently occurs to young people in arguably the most productive years of their working lives, employment is an especially important issue (111). A common goal for adults who have experienced a TBI is employment or return-to-work (112). Following comprehensive evaluation, neuropsychologists often advocate for services their patients need to successfully return to work. Specific cognitive skills (i.e., concept formation, cognitive flexibility, and problem solving) are cornerstones of functional recovery and successful rehabilitation that may be disrupted by a TBI and identified during the assessment process (111).

Persons recovering from brain injury often require additional programs and supports to supplement traditional models of vocational rehabilitation. Wehman, West, Kregel, Sherron, and Kreutzer (113) conducted a study about the efficacy of a supportive employment program for survivors of severe brain injury. Program participants were matched with a job opening based on preliminary assessments. Interventions such as work and social skills training, job modifications, and counseling were completed. Patients also received assistance with addressing common obstacles to employment (e.g., interpersonal conflicts, or lack of transportation or housing) by an employment specialist. Helping survivors find financially and socially rewarding jobs and appropriate vocational supports enhances the probability patients will experience a successful return to work after a TBI. Wehman and colleagues (114) investigated the long-term follow-up of persons with TBI after being involved in supported employment. Findings suggested that

TABLE 43-15
Remediation Strategies or Programs Applicable to Various Functional Skill Areas

FUNCTIONAL SKILLS AREAS	COGNITIVE REMEDIATION	REFERENCES
Academic Skills		
Reading	Phonological & strategy-based	Lovett et al., 2000 (89)
Spelling	Lexical treatment program	Brunsdon et al., 2002 (90)
Arithmetic	Arithmetic problem solving	Delazer, Bodner, & Benke, 1998 (91)
Attention		
	Computer-assisted attention retraining	Gray, Robertson, Pentland, & Anderson, 1992 (92); Wood & Fussey, 1987 (93)
	Attention Process Training	Sohlberg & Mateer, 1987a (94); Park, Proulx, & Towers, 1999 (95)
	Cognitive remediation programme (CRP)	Stevenson et al., 2002 (96)
	Remediation of "working attention"	Cicerone, 2002 (97)
	Virtual reality cognitive training	Cho et al., 2002 (98)
Memory / Learning	Prospective memory training	Sohlberg et al., 1992 (99)
	Explicit memory & errorless learning	Wilson et al., 1994 (100)
	Memory strategy training	Yerys et al., 2003 (101)
	Memory book training	Burke, et al., 1994 (102); Sohlberg & Mateer, 1987b (103)
	Electronic memory aids	Van den Broek et al., 2000 (104)
	Structural memory retraining	Ryan & Ruff, 1988 (105)
Planning / Organization	Self-instructional training	Cicerone & Wood, 1987 (106)
	Cognitive & metacognitive approaches	Ellis & Lenz, 1990 (107)
	Goal setting, task analysis, and monitoring outcome	Ellis & Friend, 1991 (108)
Problem Solving	Problem-solving training	Von Cramon et al., 1991 (109)
	Cognitive-behavioral training	Suzman et al., 1997 (110)

supported employment was cost-effective for individuals with TBI.

The 2005 article by Wehman, Targett, West, and Kregel (115) reviews the research literature with respect to TBI and employment, and provides a series of recommendations for future research and public policy. The reader is referred to the chapter in this book entitled, "Vocational Rehabilitation Issues," by Dr. Paul Wehman for detailed information about employment services for individuals following a TBI.

SUMMARY

Early on, neuropsychologists were primarily involved in quantifying cognitive abilities and endeavoring to localize brain dysfunction. Over the past several decades many neuropsychologists working in rehabilitation settings have expanded their practice to address the diverse and long-term needs of persons with brain injury and their families. Neuropsychologists have had important roles on rehabilitation teams addressing issues relating to behavioral management, emotional adjustment, substance abuse, family functioning, and return to work. With larger numbers of people surviving traumatic brain injury, neuropsychologists have had an opportunity to play an increasingly important role in rehabilitation. Undoubtedly, many persons with brain injury face long-term difficulties adjusting and returning to productive lives. Neuropsychologists are often well qualified to help patients and their families, and many have chosen to expand their roles far beyond that of cognitive evaluator.

References

1. Barth, J. T., Pliskin, N., Axelrod, B., Faust, D., Fisher, J., Harley, J. P., Heilbronner, R., Larrabee, G., Puente, A., Ricker, J., & Silver, C. Introduction to the NAN 2001 definition of a clinical neuropsychologist. *Archives of Clinical Neuropsychology* 2003;18:551–555.

2. Kreutzer, J., Kolakowsky-Hayner, S., West, D. *The Brain Injury Handbook: A Guide for Rehabilitation Providers for Improving Therapeutic Relationships and Outcomes.* Richmond, VA: The National Resource Center for Traumatic Brain Injury 1999.

3. Lezak, M. D., Howieson, D. B., Loring, D. W., Hannay, H. J., & Fischer, J. S. *Neuropsychological Assessment* (4th Edition). New York: Oxford University Press 2004.

4. Putnam, S., Fichtenberg, N. Neuropsychological examination of the patient with traumatic brain injury. In M. Rosenthal, J. Kreutzer, E. Griffith, B. Pentland (Eds). *Rehabilitation of the Adult and Child with Traumatic Brain Injury* (pp. 147–166). Philadelphia, PA: F. A. Davis Co 1999.

5. Beck, A. T., Rush, A. J., Shaw, B. F., Emery, G. *Cognitive therapy of depression.* New York: Guilford 1979.

6. Witol, A. D., Kreutzer, J. S., Sander, A. M. Emotional, behavioral, and personality assessment after traumatic brain injury. In M. Rosenthal, E. R. Griffith, J. S. Kreutzer, & B. Pentland (Eds.), *Rehabilitation of the adult and child with traumatic brain injury.* Philadelphia: F. A. Davis Company 1990.

7. Derogatis, L. R. *Brief symptom inventory.* Baltimore: Clinical Psychometric Research 1975.

8. Hamilton, M. Development of a rating scale for primary depressive illness. *British Journal of Social and Clinical Psychology* 1967;6:278–296.

9. Butcher, JN, et al. *Minnesota Multiphasic Personality Inventory-2 (MMPI-2):Manual for administration and scoring.* Maryland: University of Minnesota Press 1989.

10. Kreutzer J., Seel, R. T., Marwitz, J. H. *The Neurobehavioral Functioning Inventory.* San Antonio (TX):Psychological Corporation 1999.

11. Levin, H., High, W., Goethe, K., Sisson, R., Overall, J., Rhoades, H., Eisenberg, H., Kalisky, Z., Gary, H. The Neurobehavioral Rating Scale: assessment of the behavioral sequelae of head injury by the clinician. *Journal of Neurology, Neurosurgery, & Psychiatry* 1987;48:556–563.

12. Kreutzer, J. S., West, D. D., Marwitz, J. H. *Judgment and Safety Screening Inventory: Administration manual.* Richmond, VA: National Resource Center for Traumatic Brain Injury 2001.

13. Bogner, J. A., Corrigan, J. D., Mysiw, W. J., Clinchot, D., Fugate, L. A comparison of substance abuse and violence in the prediction of long-term rehabilitation outcomes after traumatic brain injury. *Archives of Physical Medicine & Rehabilitation* 2001; 82(5):571–577.

14. Kolakowsky-Hayner, S. A., Gourley, E. V., Kreutzer, J. S., Marwitz, J. H., Cifu, D. X., McKinley, W. O. Pre-injury substance abuse among persons with brain injury and persons with spinal cord injury. *Brain Injury* 1999;13(8):571–581.

15. Kolakowsky-Hayner, S. A., Kreutzer, J. S. Pre-injury crime, substance abuse, and neurobehavioral functioning after traumatic brain injury. *Brain Injury* 2001;15(1):53–63.

16. Kreutzer, J. S., Marwitz, J. H., Witol, A. D. Interrelationships between crime, substance abuse, and aggressive behaviours among persons with traumatic brain injury. *Brain Injury* 1995; 9(8):757–768.

17. Corrigan, J. D. Substance abuse as a mediating factor in outcome from traumatic brain injury. Archives of Physical Medicine & Rehabilitation 1995;76(4):302–309.

18. Hall, K., Karzmark, P., Stevens, M., Englander, J., O'Hare, P., Wright, J. Family stressors in traumatic brain injury: A two-year follow-up. *Archives of Physical Medicine and Rehabilitation* 1994;75 (8):876–884.

19. Cherner, M., Temkin, N. R., Machamer, J. E., Dikmen, S. S. Utility of a composite measure to detect problematic alcohol use in persons with traumatic brain injury. *Archives of Physical Medicine & Rehabilitation* 2001;82(6):780–786.

20. Fuller, M. G., Fishman, E., Taylor, C. A., Wood, R. B. Screening patients with traumatic brain injuries for substance abuse. *Journal of Neuropsychiatry & Clinical Neurosciences* 1994;6(2): 143–146.

21. McLellan, A. T., Luborsky, L., Woody, G. E., O'Brien, C. P. An improved diagnostic evaluation instrument for substance abuse patients. The Addiction Severity Index. *Journal of Nervous & Mental Disease* 1980;168(1):26–33.

22. McLellan, A. T., Luborsky, L., Cacciola, J., Griffith, J., Evans, F., Barr, H. L., O'Brien, C. P. New data from the Addiction Severity Index. Reliability and validity in three centers. *Journal of Nervous & Mental Disease* 1985;173(7):412–423.

23. Pokorny, A. D., Miller, B. A., Kaplan, H. B. The brief MAST: a shortened version of the Michigan Alcoholism Screening Test. *American Journal of Psychiatry* 1972;129 (3):342–345.

24. Ewing, J. A. Detecting alcoholism. The CAGE questionnaire. *JAMA* 1984;252(14):1905–1907.

25. Selzer, M. L. The Michigan alcoholism screening test: the quest for a new diagnostic instrument. *American Journal of Psychiatry* 1971;127(12):1653–1658.

26. Cahalan, D., Cisin, I. H. American drinking practices: summary of findings from a national probability sample. II. Measurement of massed versus spaced drinking. *Quarterly Journal of Studies on Alcohol* 1968a;29(3):642–656.

27. Cahalan, D., Cisin, I. H. American drinking practices: Summary of findings from a national probability sample: I. Extent of drinking by population subgroups. *Quarterly Journal of Studies on Alcohol* 1968b;29:130–151.

28. Kreutzer, J. S., Doherty, K. R., Harris, J. A., Zasler, N. D. Alcohol use among persons with traumatic brain injury. *Journal of Head Trauma Rehabilitation* 1990;5(3):9–20.

29. Sander, A. M., Witol, A. D., Kreutzer, J. S. Alcohol use after traumatic brain injury: concordance of patients' and relatives' reports. *Archives of Physical Medicine & Rehabilitation* 1997;78(2):138–142.

30. Arenth, P. M., Bogner, J. A., Corrigan, J. D., Schmidt, L. The utility of the Substance Abuse Subtle Screening Inventory-3 for use with individuals with brain injury. *Brain Injury* 2001;15(6):499–510.

31. Melzack, R. The McGill Pain Questionnaire: Major properties and scoring methods. *Pain* 1975; 16:277–299.

32. Huskisson, E. C. Visual analogue scales. In Melzack, R. (Ed.) *Pain measurement and assessment* (pp. 33–37.). New York: Raven Press 1985.

33. Kreutzer, J., Harris-Marwitz, J., & Myers, S. (1990). Neuropsychological issues in litigation following traumatic brain injury. *Neuropsychology* 1990;4(4):249–260.

34. Mittenberg, W., Azrin, R., Millsaps, C., & Heilbronner, R. Identification of malingered head injury on the Wechsler Memory Scale-Revised. *Psychological Assessment* 1993;5:34–40.

35. Wechsler, D. *Wechsler Memory Scale-Revised* 1987; New York: Psychological Corporation.

36. Wechsler, D. Wechsler Adult Intelligence Scale-Revised 1981;San Antonio, TX: Psychological Corporation.

37. Demakis, G., Sweet, J., Sawyer, T., Moulthrop, M., Nies, K., Clingerman, S. Discrepancy between predicted and obtained WAIS-R IQ scores discriminates between traumatic brain injury and insufficient effort. *Psychological Assessment* 2001;13 (2):240–248.

38. Binder, L. M. *Portland Digit Recognition Test Manual (2nd ed.)* 1993 Portland, OR: Author: Binder, L. M.

39. Warrington, E. K. (1984). *Recognition Memory Test Manual* 1984; UK: NFER-Nelson.

40. Rey, A. *L'examen clinique en psychologie.* Paris: Presses Universitaires de France 1964.

41. Tombaugh, T. N. *Test of Memory Malingering.* Canada: Muli-Health Systems, Inc. 1996.

42. Green, P., Allen, L. M., Astner, K.. *The Word Memory Test: A user's guide to the oral and computer-administered forms, US Version 1.1* 1996;Durham, NC: CogniSyst.

43. Rothke, S., Friedman, A., Jaffe, A., Greene, R., Wetter, M., Cole, P., Baker, K. Normative data for the F(p) Scale of the MMPI-2:Implications for clinical and forensic assessment of malingering. *Psychological Assessment* 2000;12(3):335–340.

44. Brooks, N., McKinlay, W., Symington, C, Beattie, A., & Campsie, L. Return to work within the first seven years of severe head injury. *Brain Injury* 1987;1:5–19.

45. Gollaher, K., High, W., Sherer, M., Bergloff, P., Boake, C., Young, M. E., Ivanhoe, C. Prediction of employment outcome one to three years following traumatic brain injury. *Brain Injury* 1998; 12:255–263.

46. Jacobs, H. E. The Los Angeles head injury survey: Procedures and findings. *Archives of Physical Medicine and Rehabilitation* 1988; 69:425–431.

47. Kreutzer, J. S., Marwitz, J. H., Walker, W., Sander, A., Sherer, M., Bogner, J., Fraser, R., Bushnik, T. Moderating factors in return to work and job stability after traumatic brain injury. *Journal of Head Trauma Rehabilitation* 2003;18(2):128–138.

48. Harrison-Felix, C., Newton, C. N., Hall, K., Kreutzer, J. Descriptive findings from the Traumatic Brain Injury Model Systems national database. *Journal of Head Trauma and Rehabilitation* 1996;11(5):1–14.

49. Kreutzer, J. S., Kolakowsky-Hayner, S. A., Ripley, D., Cifu, D. X., Rosenthal, M., Bushnik, T., Zafonte, R., Englander, J., High, W. Charges and lengths of stay for acute and inpatient rehabilitation treatment of traumatic brain injury 1990–1996. *Brain Injury* 2001;15(9):763–774.

50. Gervasio, A., Kreutzer, J. Kinship and family member's psychological distress after traumatic brain injury: a large sample study. *Journal of Head Trauma Rehabilitation* 1997;12(3):14–26.

51. Harris, J., Godfrey, H., Partridge, F., Knight, R. Caregiver depression following traumatic brain injury (TBI):a consequence of adverse effects on family members? *Brain Injury* 2001;15(3):223–238.

52. Kreutzer J., Gervasio A., Camplair, P. Primary caregiver's psychological status and family functioning after traumatic brain injury. *Brain Injury* 1994a;8(3):197–210.

53. Kreutzer J., Gervasio, A., Camplair, P. Patient correlates of caregiver's distress and family functioning after traumatic brain injury. *Brain Injury* 1994b;8(3):211–230.

54. Livingston, M. G., Brooks, D. N., Bond, M. R. Three months after severe head injury: psychiatric and social impact on relatives. *Journal of Neurology, Neurosurgery, & Psychiatry* 1985;48:870–875.

55. Marsh, N. V., Kersel, D. A., Havill, J. H., Sleigh, J. W. Caregiver burden at 1 year following severe traumatic brain injury. *Brain Injury* 1988;12(12):1045–1059.

56. Oddy, M., Humphrey, M., Uttley, D. Subjective impairment and social recovery after closed head injury. *Journal of Neurology, Neurosurgery, & Psychiatry* 1978;41:611–6.

57. Panting, A., Merry, P. H. The long term rehabilitation of severe head injuries with particular reference to the need for social and medical support for the patient's family. *Rehabilitation* 1972;38:33–37.

58. Perlesz, A., Kinsella, G., Crowe, S. Psychological distress and family satisfaction following traumatic brain injury: injured individuals and their primary, secondary, and tertiary carers. *Journal of Head Trauma Rehabilitation* 2000;15(3):909–929.

59. Stebbins, G. T., Wilson, R. S. Estimation of premorbid intelligence in neurologically impaired individuals. In P. J. Snyder & P. D. Nussbaum (Eds), *Clinical neuropsychology: A pocket handbook for assessment*. Washington, D. C.:American Psychological Association 1988.

60. American Psychiatric Association (APA). *Diagnostic and statistical manual of mental disorders (4th ed.)* 2000. Washington, DC: American Psychiatric Press.

61. First, M. B., Spitzer, R., Gibbon, M., Williams, J. (1997). *Structured Clinical Interview for DSM-IV Axis I Disorders—Clinical Version (SCID-CV)* 1997;Washington, DC: American Psychiatric Press.

62. Glenn, M. B. A differential diagnostic approach to the pharmacological treatment of cognitive, behavioral, and affective disorders after traumatic brain injury. *Journal of Head Trauma Rehabilitation* 2002;17(4):273–283.

63. Zakzanis, K., Leach, L., Kaplan, E. *Neuropsychological Differential Diagnosis*. Lisse, the Netherlands: Swets & Zeitlinger 1999.

64. Hibbard, M. R., Uysal, S., Kepler, K., Bogdany, J., Silver, J. Axis I pathology in individuals with traumatic brain injury. *Journal of Head Trauma and Rehabilitation* 1998;13(4):24–39.

65. Golden, Z., & Golden, C. Impact of brain injury severity on personality dysfunction. *International Journal of Neuroscience* (2003);113 (5):733–745.

66. Folstein M. F., Folstein, S. E., & McHugh, P. R. Mini-Mental State: A practical method for grading the state of patients for the clinician. *Journal of Psychiatric Research* 1975;12:189–198.

67. Ben-Porath, Y., Butcher, J., Dahlstrom, W. G., Graham, J., & Tellgan, A. *Minnesota Multiphasic Personality Inventory-II* (2nd ed) 2001;Minneapolis, MN: University of Minnesota Press.

68. Kolakowsky-Hayner, S., Miner, K., Kreutzer, J. Long-term Life Quality and Family Needs after Traumatic Brain Injury. *Journal of Head Trauma Rehabilitation* 2001;16(4):374–385.

69. Kreutzer, J., Kolakowsky-Hayner, S. *Getting Better (and Better) after Brain Injury: A Guide for Family, Friends, and Caregivers*. Richmond, VA: The National Resource Center for Traumatic Brain Injury 1999.

70. Butler, R., Satz, P. Individual psychotherapy with head injured adults: Clinical notes for the practitioner. *Professional Psychology: Research & Practice* 1988;19(5):536–541.

71. Prigatano, G. Psychotherapy after brain injury. In *Neuropsychological Rehabilitation after Brain Injury*. Baltimore, MD: The John Hopkins University Press 1986.

72. Prigatano, G. Disordered mind, wounded soul: The emerging role of psychotherapy in rehabilitation after brain injury. *Journal of Head Trauma Rehabilitation* 1991;6(4):1–10.

73. Prigatano, G., Ben-Yishay, Y. Psychotherapy and psychotherapeutic interventions in brain injury rehabilitation. In M. Rosenthal, J. Kreutzer, E. Griffith, B. Pentland (Eds). *Rehabilitation of the Adult and Child with Traumatic Brain Injury* (pp. 271–282). Philadelphia, PA: F. A. Davis Co 1999.

74. Moules, S., Chandler, B. A study of the health and social needs of carers of traumatically brain injured individuals served by one community rehabilitation team. *Brain Injury* 1999;13(12):983–993.

75. Serio, C., Kreutzer, J., Gervasio, A. Predicting family needs after brain injury: implications for intervention. *Journal of Head Trauma and Rehabilitation* 1998;10(2):32–45.

76. Rotondi, A. J., Sinkule, J., Spring, M. An interactive web-based intervention for persons with TBI and their families: Use and evaluation by female significant others. *Journal of Head Trauma Rehabilitation* 2005; 20(2):173–185.

77. Gillen, R., Tennen, H., Affleck, G., Steinpreis, R. Distress, depressive symptoms, and depressive disorder among caregivers of patients with brain injury. *Journal of Head Trauma Rehabilitation* 1998;13(3):31–43.

78. Dombrowski, L. K., Petrick, J. D., Strauss, D. Rehabilitation treatment of sexuality issues due to acquired brain injury. *Rehabilitation Psychology* 2000;45(3):299–309.

79. Hibbard, M., Cantor, J., Charatz, H., Rosenthal, R., Ashman, T., Gundersen, N., Ireland-Knight, L., Gordon, W., Avner, J., Gartner, A. Peer support in the community: initial findings of mentoring program for individuals with traumatic brain injury and their families. *Journal of Head Trauma and Rehabilitation* 2002;17(2):112–131.

80. Ylvisaker, M., Jacobs, H., Feeney, T. Positive supports for people who experience behavioral and cognitive disability after brain injury: A review. *Journal of Head Trauma Rehabilitation* 2003;18(1): 7–32.

81. Yody, B., Schaub, C., Conway, J., Peters, S., Strauss, D., Helsinger, S. Applied behavior management and acquired brain injury: Approaches and assessment. *Journal of Head Trauma Rehabilitation* 2000;15(4):1041–1060.

82. Alderman, N., Burgess, P. Integrating cognition and behaviour: A pragmatic approach to brain injury rehabilitation. In R. Wood and I. Fussey (Eds.), *Cognitive Rehabilitation in Perspective.* (pp. 204–228). Basingstoke: Taylor Francis 1990.

83. Ben-Yishay, Y., Diller, L. Cognitive remediation in traumatic brain injury: Update and issues. *Archives of Physical Medicine and Rehabilitation* 1993;74 (2):204–213.

84. Mateer, C. A., Sira, C. S., O'Connell, M. E. Putting Humpty Dumpty together again: The importance of integrating cognitive and emotional interventions. *Journal of Head Trauma Rehabilitation* 2005;20(1):62–75.

85. Sohlberg, M., Mateer, C. *Introduction to Cognitive Rehabilitation.* New York: Guilford Press 1989.

86. Katz, D. I., Mills, V. Traumatic brain injury: Natural history and efficacy of cognitive rehabilitation. In D. Stuss, G. Winocur, & I. H. Robertson (Eds), *Cognitive Rehabilitation* (pp. 279–301). United Kingdom: University Press: Cambridge 1999.

87. Cicerone, K., Dahlberg, C., Kalmar, K., Langenbahn, D., Malec, J., et al. Evidence based cognitive rehabilitation: Recommendations for clinical practice. *Archives of Physical Medicine and Rehabilitation* 2000;81:1596–1615.

88. Park, N., Ingles, J. L. Effectiveness of attention rehabilitation after acquired brain injury: A meta-analysis. *Neuropsychology* 2001; 15(2):199–210.

89. Lovett, M., Lacerenza, L., Borden, S., Frijters, J., Steinbach, K., DePalma, M. Components of effective remediation of developmental reading disabilities: Combining phonological and strategy-based instruction to improve outcomes. *Journal of Educational Psychology* 2000;92:263–283.

90. Brunsdon, R., Hannan, T., Coltheart, M., & Nickels, L. Treatment of lexical processing in mixed dyslexia: A case study. *Neuropsychological Rehabilitation* 2002;12:385–418.

91. Delazer, M., Bodner, T., Benke, T. Rehabilitation of arithmetical text problem solving. *Neuropsychological Rehabilitation* 1998; 8:401–412.

92. Gray, J., Robertson, I., Pentland, B., Anderson, S. Microcomputer-based attentional retraining after brain damage: A randomized group controlled trial. *Neuropsychological Rehabilitation* 1992;2:97–115.

93. Wood, R., Fussey, I. Computer-based cognitive retraining: A controlled study. *International Disability Studies* 1987;9:149–153.

94. Sohlberg, M., Mateer, C. Effectiveness of an attention training program. *Journal of Clinical and Experimental Neuropsychology* 1987;19:117–130.

95. Park, N., Proulx, G., Towers, W. Evaluation of the Attention Process Training program. *Neuropsychological Rehabilitation* 1999;9(2):135–154.

96. Stevenson, C., Whitmont, S., Bornholt, L., Livesey, D., Stevenson, R. A cognitive remediation programme for adults with Attention Deficit Hyperactivity Disorder. *Australian & New Zealand Journal of Psychiatry* 2002;36:610–616.

97. Cicerone, K. D. Remediation of 'working attention' in mild traumatic brain injury. *Brain Injury* 2002;16:185–195.

98. Cho, B., Ku, J., Pyojang, D., Kim, S., Lee Y., Kim, I., Lee, J., Kim, S. The effect of virtual reality cognitive training for attention enhancement. *Cyberpsychology & Behavior* 2002;5:129–137.

99. Sohlberg, M., White, O., Evans, E., Mateer, C. Background and an initial investigation of the effects of prospective memory training. *Brain Injury* 1992;5:139–154.

100. Wilson, B., Baddeley, A., Evans, J., Shiel, A. Errorless learning in the rehabilitation of memory impaired people. *Neuropsychological Rehabilitation* 1994;4:307–326.

101. Yerys, B., White, D., Salorio, C., McKinstry, R., Moinuddin, A., Debaun, M. Memory Strategy Training in children with cerebral infarcts related to sickle cell disease. *Journal of Pediatric Hematology/Oncology* 2003;25:495–498.

102. Burke, J., Danick, J., Bemis, B., Durgin, C. A process approach to memory book training for neurological patients. *Brain Injury* 1994;8:71–81.

103. Sohlberg, M., Mateer, C. Training use of compensatory memory books: a three stage behavioral approach. *Journal of Clinical and Experimental Neuropsychology* 1987b;11:871–891.

104. Van den Broek, M. D., Downes, J., Johnson, Z., Dayus, B., Hilton, N. Evaluation of an electronic memory aid in the neuropsychological rehabilitation of prospective memory deficits. *Brain Injury* 2000;14(5):455–462.

105. Ryan, T., Ruff, R. The efficacy of structural memory retraining in a group comparison of head trauma patients. *Archives of Clinical Neuropsychology* 1988;3:165–179.

106. Cicerone, K. D., Wood, J. C. Planning disorder after closed head injury: A case study. Archives of Physical Medicine and Rehabilitation 1987;68:111–115.

107. Ellis, E., Lenz, K. Techniques for mediation content-area learning: Issues and research. *Focus on Exceptional Children* 1990; 22:1–16.

108. Ellis, E., Friend, P. Adolescents with learning disabilities. In B. Y. L. Wong (Ed.), *Learning about learning disabilities* (pp. 506–563). Orlando, FL: Academic Press 1991.

109. Von Cramon, Matthes-von Cramon, G., Mai, N. Problem solving deficits in brain injured patients: A therapeutic approach. *Neuropsychological Rehabilitation* 1991;1:45–64.

110. Suzman, K., Morris, R., Morris, M., Milan, M. Cognitive-Behavioral remediation of problem solving deficits in children with acquired brain injury. *Journal of Behavior Therapy & Experimental Psychiatry* 1997;28:203–212.

111. Doninger, N., Heinemann, A., Bode, R., Sokol, K., Corrigan, J., & Moore, D. Predicting community integration following traumatic brain injury with health and cognitive status measures. *Rehabilitation Psychology* 2003;48(2):67–76.

112. Vandiver, V., Johnson, J., Christofero-Snider, C. Supporting employment for adults with acquired brain injury: a conceptual model. *Journal of Head Trauma Rehabilitation* 2003;18(5): 457–463.

113. Wehman, P., West, M., Kregel, J., Sherron, P, Kreutzer, J. Return to work for persons with severe traumatic brain injury: A database approach to program development. *Journal of Head Trauma Rehabilitation* 1995;10(1):27–39.

114. Wehman, P., Kregel, J., Keyser-Marcus, L., Sherron-Targett, P, Campbell, L., West, M., Cifu, D. X. Supported employment for persons with traumatic brain injury: A preliminary investigation of long-term follow-up costs and program efficiency. *Archives of Physical Medicine and Rehabilitation* 2003;84:192–196.

115. Wehman, P., Targett, P., West, M., Kregel, J. Productive employment for persons with traumatic brain injury: What have we learned after 20 years? *Journal of Head Trauma Rehabilitation* 2005;20(2):115–127.

44 Principles of Behavioral Analysis and Modification

Robert L. Karol

INTRODUCTION

Psychological considerations are integral to the treatment of persons with brain injury. Most of the elements people use to define their self-worth, such as intelligence, physical prowess, financial status, etc., are vulnerable after brain injury. Moreover, coping skills may decline and behavioral dyscontrol may increase due to alterations in cognition. Treatment protocols that de-emphasize psychological status are less likely to be successful than therapy programs that incorporate psychological deliberations.

Often treatment programs focus on medical, physical, and cognitive factors: (1) walking, balance, transfers between a bed and a chair, or transferring into a car; receptive and expressive language deficits; upper extremity use and activities of daily living; and medical stability. It is natural to give weight to these functions. It is apparent to all professionals when persons with brain injury are unable to walk, talk, or care for themselves. Physicians are trained to intervene when there is medical instability. Moreover, persons with brain injury and their families are exquisitely aware of these problems and they want professionals to fix them. They assume that recovery of personality will accompany physical recovery (2).

Hence, persons with brain injury become a set of symptoms. The term "medicalization" describes this process (3). In part, the power of this process is based upon our society's expectation for health care. People in our society expect our health care professionals to act in a certain way – to use medications and high technology to focus on symptom cure – stemming from people's familiarity with acute medical care, sometimes from media entertainment (4) or from media reporting of advances in research. Professionals accommodate people's expectations. After all, expectations are an important element in care (5). However, fulfilling this expectation can leave persons with brain injury and their families dissatisfied. Psychological variables determine their comfort level with care, but frequently persons with brain injury and their families articulate poorly their psychological needs. The challenge is that psychological variables seem nebulous and indistinct. Yet, in the long term, factors associated with psychological variables and quality of life can have a greater impact on persons with brain injury and their families than other variables, (6) and cognitive and behavioral concerns tend to be most burdensome (7). To be more helpful, rehabilitation ought to address higher needs related to satisfaction with life (8).

Unfortunately, third party reimbursement sources compound the potential inattention to psychological considerations. Insurance system changes are leading to shorter hospital stays, and there is more pressure on families to provide care at home (9). Nevertheless, insurance often fails to cover community support services (10).

When persons with brain injury are able to walk, talk, perform activities of daily living, and are medically stable, insurers press for program discharge, regardless of whether persons with brain injury or their families are psychologically ready for return to the natural environment, or even for transfer to another program or care setting. Furthermore, there is little attention paid to the willingness to perform skills that professionals have taught persons with brain injury and their families.

It is a mistake when professionals, persons with brain injury, families, and insurers downplay psychological variables. Psychosocial sequelae may be a better predictor of outcome than physical symptoms (11). Also, outcome itself can be a function of psychological care. The intensity of psychological care correlates with cognitive gains (12). Hopefully, this is familiar knowledge among rehabilitation professionals. Behavioral or emotional dysfunction can be hard to treat and untreated can disrupt the care of cognitive and physical functioning (13). The satisfaction persons with brain injury and their families express regarding their rehabilitation is likely to be influenced by their perceptions of their treatment. Awareness of the importance of psychological variables is important. Sadly, families report being inadequately informed about brain injury and rate professionals as unhelpful (14).

Hence, this chapter will address behavioral and psychological care. The intent of the chapter is to provide an overview of assessment and intervention methods and issues, identify important behavioral and psychological process variables in rehabilitation, and highlight selected applications.

PRINCIPLES OF ASSESSMENT AND INTERVENTION

Assessment

Introduction to Assessment   Professionals ought to predicate treatment on thorough assessment. Psychological assessment dovetails with evaluations by all other disciplines because psychological variables affect the outcome of all disciplines' evaluations and their treatment efforts. For example, low effort due to depression can contaminate the findings of physical therapists. Hopelessness can interfere with the educational efforts of nurses leading to poor reliability in the self-administration of medications. The beliefs of persons with brain injury influence compliance with physicians' recommendations. Therefore, psychological assessment is essential for the provision of services to persons with brain injury, not just for psychological care, but also for success by all disciplines.

Psychological assessment primarily covers three domains: emotional, behavioral, and cognitive functioning. Emotional status includes factors such as depression,

anger, anxiety, etc. The examples in the preceding paragraph derive from emotional variables that have behavioral implications. Behavioral considerations range from noncompliance to aggression. Cognitive functioning includes executive processes, memory and learning, intellectual abilities, etc. and are evaluated using clinical observation and neuropsychological testing.

Assessment of Emotional Status   Emotional disturbance is a significant component of brain injury. The National Institute of Health Consensus Statement (15) states, "Mood disorders, personality changes, altered emotional control, depression, and anxiety are also prevalent after TBI" (p. 12). Because the brain regulates emotional functioning, (16–18) organic damage can cause direct emotional changes. In addition, the recognition and expression of emotions can be altered by brain lesions (19). There is also the emotional adjustment to having and living with a disability. There have been numerous reports of the emotional sequelae of brain injury (11, 20–22). Recently, researchers have also paid particular attention to grief as distinct from depression (23).

Professionals can use clinical acumen and psychometric assessment to determine emotional functioning. They should decide how to balance these two approaches based upon the setting and the level of functioning of the persons with brain injury with whom they are working. For instance, in a community-based setting with higher-functioning individuals, psychometric evaluation may be feasible, but at Rancho Los Amigos Level V (24) it is untenable with people newly arrived from an intensive care unit fresh out of coma.

Clinical assessment of emotional functioning occurs through a combination of diagnostic interview and observation. Interview can provide clues as to what persons with brain injury are experiencing. How persons with brain injury express emotions can provide insight into their coping abilities. Of course, professionals need to be aware of deficits in the expression of emotion, such as aprosdia (the loss of speech tone that conveys affective data), that might mislead professionals in their judgment regarding emotional status. Observation when persons with brain injury demonstrate emotional dyscontrol provides clues as to what they are feeling. Fluctuations in emotional intensity throughout the day, from day to day, or across events offer professionals the opportunity to study emotional patterns. Professionals must observe the antecedents and the consequences of emotions as well as the qualitative and quantitative aspects of the emotions to fully understand the expression of emotions. Experienced professionals, for example, might determine upon close observation that a diagnosis in the chart of depression is, in fact, anxiety. Trained observation of emotional events is often worth much more than only obtaining professionals' reports or reading the record. A combination of interview, providing leads in regard to emotional status, and observation of emotions in practice during behavioral events can assist professionals in the exact delineation of emotional functioning.

In the case of psychometric assessment, there is an unending array of published psychological test instruments for the determination of emotional functioning. These range from measures of particular emotional variables (e.g., Beck Depression Inventory) (25, 26) to broad personality inventories (e.g., MMPI). There are also rating scales, questionnaires, and interview formats that include emotional or adjustment variables (e.g., Neurobehavioral Rating Scale-Revised, (27, 28) Functional Assessment Measure, (29–31) Mayo-Portland Adaptability Inventory (32–34)). Interview, observation, or both ought to accompany any psychometric assessment of emotional variables. Qualitative variables can be crucial in emotional assessment: how persons with brain injury experience or express emotions provides insight into their functioning beyond psychometric tools.

Professionals must consider the appropriateness of any instrument for the evaluation of emotional status for persons with brain injury. First, it is helpful when there are norms for persons with brain injury for the particular instrument. While it is important to be able to determine if persons with brain injury deviate from the general population, it is also useful for rehabilitation to know if they diverge from the normal experiences of other persons with brain injury. Publishers of standardized, mass-marketed tests of emotional adjustment generally fail to include a subgroup of persons with brain injury during test development. Furthermore, when they include persons with brain injury in a sample, the subject characteristics in any particular study of the brain injury population may differ in some significant fashion from the persons with brain injury being seen by a given professional. Important distinctions may exist on variables including the nature of onset, location of damage, time post onset, pre-morbid personality dimensions, etc.

Second, cultural variables can play a critical role in the psychometric assessment of adjustment after brain injury. Professionals may be aware of the impact of cultural factors on personality assessment in mental health populations, but they are potentially less in tune to the intersection of culture and coping with disturbances in physical health, particularly various cultures' differing views on appropriate approaches to brain injury. Behaviors that may appear pathological in one culture may represent normative beliefs in another culture (35). In light of the alterations in personality and cognitive functioning that can occur after brain injury, people have a complex emotional response to brain injury symptoms based on their social and cultural views of the symptoms.

Third, the neurological experiences of persons with brain injury are unique contaminants to the assessment of emotional status. Many markers of emotional states in mental health populations include neurological or physiological functioning (e.g., impaired concentration or memory, sleep disturbances, alterations in initiation or energy level). However, for many persons with brain injuries these are normal reflections of organic impairment and may be unrelated to emotional disturbance. There have been investigations of the impact of such factors on emotional assessment, for example for depression, and the effect of these variables varies (36–38).

Yet, many persons with brain injury have had experiences that would indicate clear emotional pathology in mental health populations. When persons with brain injury report histories of periods of "blacking out" or "out of body episodes," they could be due to coma or seizures; reports of hallucinations may be recollections of emergence from coma; acknowledgment of "delusional thoughts" could be confabulations during rehabilitation. While it is certainly possible that persons with brain injury have had blackouts, out of body episodes, delusions, hallucinations, etc. as a function of emotional pathology, the attribution of these symptoms ought to include the differential diagnosis of normal brain injury sequelae. Professionals must adjust their interpretations of psychometric instruments that utilize symptoms commonly occurring after organic brain injury.

Self report by persons with brain injury can also be a concern due to the injury. Memory deficits, in particular, can be a barrier to psychometric assessment of coping. When a test requires recall of personality based preferences, coping styles, past emotional experiences, or previous behavioral episodes, persons with brain injury may not be able to remember what they have done or what type of people they were in the past. It is common for persons with brain injury to relate that they are unable to remember how they were feeling at a particular point in time. Sometimes denial or lack of awareness can have a global effect on self report measures. A person with brain injury might self report an emotional picture that substantially conflicts with the one that professionals would obtain from significant others about their loved one with the injury (e.g., a person with brain injury might fail to report depression that is clearly present to other observers). Since many tests rely on self-reported recall of preferences, emotions, and behaviors, professionals must be cautious in the interpretation of psychometric test results of adjustment and coping styles for some persons with brain injury.

Finally, professionals must take care in the actual administration of psychometric tests of adjustment to persons with brain injury. Cognitive deficits can impair the ability of persons with brain injury to complete the tests or they can lead professionals to misinterpret the results because the findings are affected by cognitive deficits during test administration. Reading ability is one obvious determinant for the suitability of a test. Other factors range from concentration (partial attention paid to test items as well as variable effort in completing the test) to comprehension and aphasia (understanding the directions and the test items) to even visual-perceptual ability (for visual analog or Likert scale measures). Even difficulty with decision making can interfere with responding to test items.

Assessment of Behavior   It is essential that professionals formulate any intervention program for behavioral problems on sound behavioral assessment. The principles of behavioral analysis and assessment are well-established (39–41). Furthermore, their application to brain injury care has been detailed for some time (42, 43). Behavioral assessment routinely begins with decisions about which behaviors to assess. This is crucial. If professionals fail to appreciate the nature of their raw observations before measurement, they will operationalize and measure the wrong events or the unimportant aspects of events. Good clinical judgment must precede behavioral measurement. Next, behavioral assessment entails professionals defining in operational terms the behaviors they select. They then can observe behaviors and record frequency, severity, duration, etc.

Standardized rating of behavior is an alternative to individualized assessment of operationally defined target behaviors unique for each person. In this approach, behaviors such as aggression, noncompliance, or irritability are rated using predefined definitions of behaviors. Ratings can be completed by professionals, families, persons with brain injury, or someone else. The Agitated Behavior Scale (44) is an example of a rating scale with items covering impulsivity, violence, wandering, etc., as is the Neurobehavioral Rating Scale (45) with items including disinhibition, agitation, hostility/uncooperativeness, etc.

Regardless of the approach, two hurdles loom large related to the nature of behavioral dyscontrol after brain injury. First, the behaviors that most concern professionals, families, and others after brain injury are exceedingly complex. The process of defining behaviors in operational terms takes considerably more time and effort than many professionals anticipate. Second, overly simple behavioral assessment that involves just recording easily correctable aspects of behavior will miss important antecedents and qualitative variables that provide clues to treatment. This is especially so in light of cognitive and emotional impairments after brain injury that complicate behavioral etiology. Unfortunately, professionals in rehabilitation settings often approach record keeping for behavioral problems with ambivalence (46). The combination of needing excellent assessment, with the difficulty of knowing what to assess, and professionals' challenges in implementing assessment procedures can defeat efforts at treatment.

Assessment of Cognition   A keystone for successful behavioral treatment of persons with brain injury is evaluation of their cognitive functioning. Cognitive disturbance has far reaching implications. It affects emotional coping, behavioral dyscontrol, participation in physical and medical care, and return to independence and productivity. The foundation of cognitive assessment is neuropsychological evaluation. Neuropsychological evaluations are addressed in the chapter by Drs. Taylor, Livingston, and Kreutzer; however, there are two aspects of cognitive evaluations that are particularly pertinent to the current discussion.

The first aspect is the utilization of neuropsychological information to help formulate the treatment of emotional issues and behavioral dysfunction (47). Neuropsychological data greatly facilitates the treatment of emotional and behavioral problems, (48) though care must be taken to not rely solely on neuropsychological data (49). Still, many emotional and behavioral problems are partially based upon cognitive difficulties. For example, paranoia can be a reflection, in part, of attentional and memory deficits when persons with brain injury have perceptions of other people that are inaccurate because of a failure to attend to and recall all of the elements of an interaction. Similarly, speed of processing deficits can cause anger outbursts when persons with brain injury are unable to keep up in conversations, leading to frustration with getting their needs heard. Any study of behavioral dyscontrol or emotional distress ought to include cognitive processing assessment.

Second, professionals need to realize the importance of clinical observation for the determination of cognitive deficits. Sometimes issues of injury severity or noncooperation render formal neuropsychological testing impractical, forcing professionals to rely solely on observation of cognition, while at other times observation of cognitive deficits is a crucial adjunct to testing. Experienced professionals should watch an emotional or behavioral event with an eye towards noticing how cognitive deficits influence the timing, severity, and nature of the event, as well as the effect of cognitive deficits on coping strategies. Also, observation of the impact cognition has on emotion and behavior provides excellent hypotheses for neuropsychological testing. The converse is also true: neuropsychological data can help refine professionals' observations, making the time spent on observation more productive.

Intervention

Contingency Management   The rubric contingency management, in brief, refers to the application of reinforcement and punishment to alter and control behavior. The principles of contingency management are well delineated, (40, 50) and professionals traditionally use these procedures for the treatment of behavioral dyscontrol after brain injury. It behooves professionals, however, to be certain that they correctly apply these procedures.

Many professionals across disciplines who attempt to utilize contingencies assume that they are simply to apply, whereas, in fact, they are quite complicated.

Technically, a reward is something that increases a behavior and a punishment is something that decreases a behavior. Professionals can explore a wide range of rewards and punishments (e.g., social, tangible, tokens/points) (51). Unfortunately, sometimes professionals independently believe something is a reward or a punishment and then apply it to change the behaviors of a particular person. This is problematic because the consequence may not be a reward or a punishment for that individual. Professionals should observe behaviors and discuss rewards or punishments with the person before plan implementation. It can be helpful to use access to naturally occurring behavior as a reward for the performance of lower probability behaviors that professionals want to encourage (52).

A positive reinforcer, when *presented*, increases a behavior; a negative reinforcer, when *removed*, increases a behavior. Many professionals often misunderstand the latter: negative reinforcement is not punishment! Both positive and negative reinforcement are rewarding. Punishment also can occur in two ways: the *application* of something unpleasant (positive punishment) or the *removal* of something pleasant (negative punishment) (52). Both forms of punishment decrease behavior. Table 44-1 summarizes the relationship between reinforcement and punishment, with examples.

Punishment is frequently misapplied. Punishment will not increase a desired behavior. Professionals cannot teach correct behavior with punishment. Moreover, punishment typically suppresses a behavior, but can be impermanent: when the punishment stops, the behavior may return (40). Also, as punishment begins behavior may worsen. There may be significant emotional responses and punishment may lead to aggression (39, 52). If professionals endure the period of worse behavior, persistent application of punishment may eventually suppress behavior. However, the severity of aggression or other behaviors that adults with brain injury can produce in response to punishment is usually beyond what most professionals or programs are willing to tolerate.

Punishment can be detrimental to the process of treatment. It can impair rapport. Professionals may find that those persons to whom they are administering punishment avoid them (39). At the same time, however, persons with brain injury receiving punishment may learn from professionals to use punishment to change the behavior of other people. Professionals who provide punishment may be seen as models for how to act (52).

Punishment carries with it numerous significant ethical and moral concerns, beyond its ineffectiveness in teaching adaptive compensation strategies. In addition, there are regulatory standards regarding the use of aversive or psychologically risky procedures (53). Skilled professionals generally advise against the use of punishment (54). It is unnecessary, and it is fraught with risk for misuse. Still, punishment requires discussion because professionals working with persons with brain injury can slip into punitive paradigms. Punishment can even be reinforcing for professionals because it may rapidly decrease unwanted behaviors (52). Punitive acts may include discharge from rehabilitation by overwhelmed professionals who label persons with brain injury as dishonest or unmotivated (55).

In contrast, professionals can utilize reinforcement to teach appropriate behavior because it works to increase behaviors. However, the pattern of reinforcement influences how subsequent behavior occurs. There are four primary schedules of reinforcement. The first one is "fixed ratio:" the frequency of responses required to achieve reinforcement is set, and reinforcement occurs based on that frequency (e.g., every fourth time). This schedule encourages fast bursts of responding because the faster people perform, the more reinforcement they receive. However, there tend to be behavioral pauses after reinforcement. Typically, reinforcement is given every time (continual reinforcement) at the start of treatment and faded over time to a less frequent rate (intermittent reinforcement).

The second schedule of intermittent reinforcement is called "variable ratio." Professionals provide reinforcement on a schedule with an average frequency of required responses (e.g., on average every fourth time), but with random variation around the average. This produces a higher rate of responding with more uniformity than fixed ratio schedules.

The third intermittent schedule is "fixed interval." In this schedule, reinforcement happens after a set interval

---

TABLE 44-1
Positive and Negative Reinforcement and Punishment

TYPE	ACTION	
	PROVIDE	**REMOVE**
Desirable	*Positive Reinforcement* Increases behavior (Salary at work)	*Negative Punishment* Decreases behavior (Revoking driver's license)
Undesirable	*Positive Punishment* Decreases behavior (Spanking)	*Negative Reinforcement* Increases behavior (Potential early prison parole)

of time. This schedule can cause a "scallop" effect in which appropriate behavior increases as the time for reinforcement approaches and then declines after reinforcement.

The fourth intermittent schedule is known as "variable interval." Variable interval schedules eliminate the scallop effect because reinforcement happens after the passage of an average amount of time, not a consistent, set amount of time. Learning with variable intervals of reinforcement is fairly resistant to extinction (the cessation of a desired behavior during periods of a lack of reinforcement). Variable interval schedules produce a more uniform response than fixed interval schedules.

It can be difficult for professionals who are unfamiliar with reinforcement schedules to keep in mind the various options. Table 44-2 provides familiar examples of the four basic schedules of reinforcement to help identify them. Of course, there are other schedules of reinforcement and professionals may even form schedules including conjunctive schedules that require adherence to two or more performance requirements to receive reinforcement or they may chain different schedules together (52). The variations are countless.

Professionals must carefully examine how they deliver reinforcement compared to how they intend to provide it. There must be consistency in reinforcement across all professionals. Problems surface when a single professional is inconsistent or there is variability among many professionals. When one professional is inconsistent, treatment effectiveness will decline and may induce confusion or anger from persons with brain injury. If some professionals provide reinforcement, but other professionals do not, staff-splitting by persons with brain injury will likely ensue. Similarly, professionals may be pitted against family members, for example, when one group reinforces or extinguishes behaviors and the other set does not. Reinforcement will fail when there is inconsistency across professionals or between professionals and families.

Professionals must also be certain that the way a team of professionals reinforces behavior matches the treatment plans. For example, suppose a person with brain injury is to be encouraged whenever the person attempts a particular desirable behavior or coping strategy

(fixed ratio/continual reinforcement). Instead, busy or unaware professionals provide encouragement at the end of their workday in the late afternoon for efforts during that shift (fixed interval). Chart entries note better behavior in the afternoon with gradual improvement as time passes (scallop effect). This is occurring because of the inadvertent change in the schedule of reinforcement.

Consistency with plans is essential when using reinforcement. Furthermore, social attention (positive reinforcement) in response to maladaptive behavior (e.g., aggression) or escape from unwanted activities (negative reinforcement) such as difficult rehabilitation treatment due to behavioral dyscontrol (e.g., noncompliance) can unintentionally maintain undesirable behaviors (56).

The use of reinforcement is more complicated than just deciding on reinforcement schedules. A behavior must first occur for professionals to reinforce it. Professionals can prompt behaviors using cues and instruction so as to initiate behaviors; once behaviors have begun, professionals can reinforce them. Thereafter, professionals can gradually discontinue the prompts. Also, desirable behaviors may begin in rudimentary forms. Professionals must shape the behavior by reinforcing successive approximations of the behavior, progressively requiring more sophisticated approximations of the final behavior before reinforcement occurs. Professionals can also chain behaviors together.

Generalization occurs when behaviors that one learns in a particular setting occur in other settings, even without reinforcement of the behaviors in the new setting. Of course, professionals can encourage generalization with prompting and initial reinforcement. Professionals may also observe response generalization of the behavior to similar behaviors: learning a behavior influences the frequency of similar behaviors. This can be quite beneficial. For example, increased willingness to take showers may generalize to increased room cleaning.

Extinction is an additional tool. When professionals fail to provide reinforcement following behaviors they are using an extinction paradigm. When professionals ignore an emotional outburst on the part of a person with brain injury, they are extinguishing the behavior. As powerful as extinction can be, professionals must appreciate crucial factors in its use. Often, after extinction begins, there is a surge in the behavior. If the behavior is dangerous (e.g., aggression or self-injurious behaviors), the burst of behavior carries increased risk. There may also be periods of spontaneous recovery: after the behavior declines or stops, it may temporarily reappear. Professionals must take care to avoid unintentionally reinforcing either a burst or spontaneous recovery of the behavior. It is important to note that the schedules of reinforcement under which behaviors were acquired influences their resistance to extinction. Finally, extinction is best paired with reinforcement of alternative behaviors.

TABLE 44-2
Examples of Reinforcement Schedules

Schedule	Example
Fixed Interval	Weekly paycheck
Variable Interval	Good performance on pop quizzes
Fixed Ratio	Factory piecework
Variable Ratio	Slot machine payouts

Behaviors often must be situation specific. As well as learning what to do, persons with brain injury must learn where and when to act. Professionals must reinforce behaviors in certain settings and not in others, teaching when and where behaviors ought to occur. Persons with brain injury often need instruction in reading social cues and context. Otherwise, they may do behaviors appropriate for home, for example, in other settings or they may attempt conversations acceptable with intimate friends when they are with strangers.

Professionals can use contingencies selectively. There are at least four useful procedures: differential reinforcement of other behavior (DRO), differential reinforcement of incompatible behavior (DRI), differential reinforcement of alternative behavior (DRA), and differential reinforcement of low-rate behavior (DRL) (57). In DRO, professionals provide reinforcement when an identified undesirable behavior does not occur. Using DRI, professionals reinforce a behavior that interferes with or prohibits an undesirable behavior. For DRA, reinforcement happens for a desirable behavior while ignoring an unwanted behavior. Lastly, in DRL, reinforcement occurs in response to the reduction of an unwanted behavior.

Token economies are a special format for the implementation of contingency management treatment. In token economies, professionals establish explicit rules for the delivery, withholding, or debiting of tokens (or some other accounting system, such as points) based upon the performance or absence of behaviors that professionals delineate. These tokens can be exchanged by persons with brain injury for reinforcing items, activities, etc. that professionals specify. In essence, the tokens substitute for money in a real economy (41). Tokens serve as conditioned (or secondary) generalized reinforcers (41, 52). They are conditioned or secondary in that people learn to associate them with things that are reinforcing (i.e., tokens by themselves have little inherent value without a relationship to what one can exchange for them). They are generalized because one can exchange them for several sources of reinforcement. Of course, unlike money, tokens can only be redeemed within the closed token economy of defined rewards.

Token economies have a number of advantages over simpler contingency management efforts (40). There may be less satiation than would occur with a set reward because a variety of reinforcers may be purchased with the tokens. For persons with brain injury this can also provide a sense of choice. They may choose diverse rewards or settle on particularly desirable ones. The flexibility may help persons with brain injury feel engagement with the process of behavioral change, though professionals should similarly involve persons with brain injury in the selection of reinforcers in even simpler contingency management plans.

Since persons with brain injury can accumulate tokens toward a valuable or large reinforcer, professionals can use them to permit a measured acquisition of a valuable reinforcer. A corollary of this is the specification that a person can choose to save tokens, as permitted by the economy rules, or to spend the tokens shortly after they earn them. Still, tokens can prove to be strong reinforcers because of their power to translate into significant rewards. Also, tokens can decrease the delay between behavior and reinforcement because professionals can provide them expeditiously. Rather than disrupting the flow of behavior by immediately giving a reinforcing item or event, professionals can easily provide tokens. Professionals must take care, however, in that tokens can become a stimulus for when to perform well and behavior may be different when they are not available (40).

Professionals must recognize that in many ways they are administering an *actual* economy. In the real economy people sometimes under perform and expect to be paid, use legalistic arguments regarding precise procedural concerns to reduce debits for improper behavior (e.g., financial penalties for crime), seek ambiguities in the specification of permissible behavior (e.g., analysis of tax code loopholes) to retain more money, commit theft to increase funds, hide inappropriate behavior, blame other people for their own acts, etc. In a token economy, persons with brain injury may also attempt to outfox the rules through procedural challenges, loopholes, theft, hiding behavior, blaming others, etc. For example, they may seek tokens for behaviors close to those behaviors that professionals specify as due reinforcement or they may claim that certain behaviors do not warrant a debit because the behaviors are not exactly the behaviors listed in the token economy behavioral descriptions (e.g., touching someone's hair does not count as touching the *person* or standing three inches away from someone does not count as *touching* them).

Professionals must consider devoting extra time to the design and implementation of token economies. Token economies can be intrusive in care environments and they can be cumbersome (39). Professionals must delineate each behavior. They must carefully codify in detail what they will use as tokens, how much each behavior earns or costs, how many earned tokens can accumulate, what reinforcers tokens can purchase, how tokens will be exchanged for reinforcers, how the token economy will terminate, etc (39). Obsessiveness helps. However, once in place token economies can provide professionals with a structure to address behavioral dyscontrol (58) and can be used across disciplines (59).

Token economies can be helpful for behavioral issues arising from brain injury. Professionals can implement a token economy with a single person with a brain injury (60) or in a programmatic fashion (61). However, as with any treatment, professionals must individualize treatment.

The use of any contingency management procedure is complex. There is no practical cookbook to guide professionals about which procedure to utilize with which symptom or person. Since treatment must be founded on individual, multifaceted symptom patterns and causes, any pre-determined treatment algorithms will fail to capture the extraordinary diversity of clinical presentations and etiological variables upon which professionals should base treatment. Moreover, as has been reviewed in the preceding discussion, contingency management encompasses a breadth of actual procedures that are highly intricate. Still, contingency management is likely to work best when three conditions are met.

First, they are more effective when persons with brain injury accept the idea of explicitly receiving reinforcement from another adult to alter their behavior. Not surprisingly, many persons with brain injury reject the idea that professionals are intentionally reinforcing their behavior. They dislike the manipulative feeling that apparent contingency procedures engender. While adults may use consequences to alter the behavior of children, adults in our society resist the idea that other people may attempt to apply contingencies to their own behavior. Persons with brain injury feel similar in this regard to any other adult and may resist contingency paradigms that remind them of being treated by professionals as if they are children whose behavior is to be controlled by others. Certainly, using contingencies with persons with brain injury who are suspicious or paranoid is contraindicated (62).

Second, when persons with brain injury act in their own best interests contingency management is more effective. Some persons with brain injury fail to do so because of their cognitive impairments, even when they understand and recall the likely consequences. Despite their awareness, factors such as lability, rigidity, nonverbal processing deficits, impulsivity, and executive dysfunctions lead to the failure of consequences to change behavior. Persons with brain injury may strike someone and later acknowledge having had awareness of the consequences, but they still proceeded. These persons may report either they could not stop themselves or could not think about the consequences quick enough to change their behavior. Sometimes they will state that the need for emotional release overrode their reflections about consequences.

Third, contingency management is likely to be more useful when memory difficulties do not interfere. Professionals must consider the impact of memory deficits on the effectiveness of contingency procedures. Many persons with brain injury forget their own behavior before professionals have an opportunity to respond with consequences. This defeats the purpose of linking behavior with consequences. Some persons with brain injury, when they are in a situation where they might choose a behavior that professionals have previously reinforced, forget the previous event. Because they forget that there were consequences last time, the previous consequences have no influence. Both of these scenarios can defeat the use of consequences. However, there is evidence that in younger persons with brain injury consequences can work even when there exists impairment in explicit memory (memory of consciously recalled information) (63). Still, consequence-oriented behavior management outside of controlled environments can be relatively ineffective (64).

Errorless Learning in Intervention   The errors people make at the start of learning are an additional concern in the use of contingency techniques. There are potential cognitive (e.g., interference with acquisition) and emotional (e.g., frustration, self-esteem) issues that arise with persistent errors. In contrast, errorless learning provides structure and cues, with initial performance demands set at an achievable level, so that as task complexity increases persons with brain injury perform correctly at each step. Correct responses can be provided to insure avoidance of errors. When applied to cognitive learning tasks, there is evidence of the benefit of errorless learning procedures (65–67). Professionals can apply errorless learning procedures to behavioral concerns (68). In doing so professionals insure that the situations persons with brain injury confront are of a type and level of complexity they can handle, with adequate prompts and training, before proceeding to more difficult emotional and behavioral challenges. Comprehensive programs can be built around errorless learning that adopt a holistic approach (69). Of course, contingency techniques, including reinforcement, stimulus fading, and cueing, can be incorporated into errorless protocols.

The Impact of Modeling on Intervention   People receive vicarious reinforcement from observing other people receiving contingencies (70). Therefore, persons with brain injury may benefit from their observations of other people receiving reinforcement. If they see other people obtaining desirable consequences for certain actions, they may imitate the same behavior in anticipation of obtaining the same results. Moreover, they may determine that certain behaviors are socially acceptable upon observing the results of those behaviors. Professionals must take care, therefore, that they publicly encourage only behaviors that they wish to have emulated.

There are two issues, in particular, that professionals have to attend to regarding modeling. First, in some instances, professionals will reward one person with a brain injury for a particular behavior when doing so is part of the treatment plan, but not the same behavior from another person. Suppose professionals award a particular reward to someone who achieves a relatively low behavioral milestone, but one that is difficult for that person to reach. A much higher level functioning person with brain injury, who has loftier goals, observes this.

The second person, who is capable of much better behavior, demands rewards for behaviors similar to those of the first person, despite that behavior being well below the second person's capabilities. Individualized treatment plans based upon ability and goals are essential, but professionals must be astute in their application of the plans so that they avoid cross contamination.

Second, professionals must be cognizant of the modeling effect of their own behavior (46). Professionals are being watched: persons with brain injury notice professionals' behavior. For example, professionals may have difficulty teaching physical boundaries when persons with brain injury observe them patting each other on the back; professionals who are heard telling each other off-color jokes may struggle to teach sound sexually appropriate behavior; professionals who make an offhand comment about another professional contribute to staff-splitting and noncompliance by persons with brain injury. There are no off-the-record statements, attitudes, or behaviors on the part of professionals if they can be observed, detected, or implied by the persons with brain injury whom they serve. Professionals must constantly be attentive to the powerful impact of modeling.

Of course, modeling can also be a very powerful positive influence. Professionals can model appropriate behavior, emotions, and skills. Modeling can range from specific skills to more pervasive attitudes. Appropriate modeling can accelerate learning (71).

Environmental Intervention Environmental change strives to influence behavior by alteration of antecedent conditions. In general, how other people act toward persons with brain injury and physical elements in the environment comprise the antecedent conditions. Of the two, how other people act is probably the more crucial. In one estimate, 95% of maladaptive behaviors were felt to be a function of how professionals acted (72).

Environmental control emphasizes the establishment of environments conducive to appropriate behavior. The correct environment will vary for persons with brain injury depending upon their cognitive and emotional functioning. Ideally, professionals' attention to neuropsychological and psychosocial factors will permit the creation of a "Neuropsychosocial Environment," (48) one based on the etiological "phenomenology of dyscontrol" of each person. In "Neuropsychosocial Intervention" all of the elements that contribute to the occurrence of behaviors constitute the phenomenology of dyscontrol, including the obvious — cognition and emotions; the discoverable — self image, values, family influences, expectations, pre-morbid personality; and the subtle — noise tolerance, privacy needs, responses to others' appearance, sleep cycle effects, professionals' attitudes, etc. Once professionals comprehensively consider all of the factors that determine the occurrence of each behavior, they can formulate the neuropsychosocial environment, a psychological and physical world, for each person that obviates the need for undesirable behaviors or interferes with their occurrence. The goal is to create a world consisting of the behaviors of others and physical plant elements that matches the capabilities of each person (48). In essence, persons with brain injury encounter only situations they can handle.

An environmental approach can address severe behaviors. However, there are two challenges: the need for careful observation and generalization (73). Systematic observational assessment is necessary to precisely determine the antecedent conditions leading to behavioral dyscontrol. Professionals must decipher the exact behavioral triggers in a complex social world for persons with impairment in cognitive and emotional functioning. Second, since the approach is not skill building, but environmental engineering, generalization can be a concern. Professionals must therefore strive for changes that are effective, transferable to additional settings, and doable by core people constituting the natural environment.

Environmental change is useful on its own or as an adjunct to other treatment. For example, it can be beneficial until skill building can take place (68). Positive behavioral supports (64, 74) designed to organize antecedent conditions combine skill building with environmental structuring. Moreover, professionals can arrange specific environments that match the abilities of persons with brain injury and then modify them as they can tolerate changes (75). Finally, professionals can use environmental control early in recovery as persons with brain injury emerge from coma (76).

In general, an environmental approach is proactive (before an episode of behavioral dyscontrol happens) in contrast to contingency management, which is reactive (after behavior occurs). Persons with brain injury encounter a positive world, one they can handle, individualized for each person. This creates a framework for success. One notable effect of an environmental approach is that treatment plans describe how professionals should act before behavioral dyscontrol occurs, not merely how they should act afterwards (74).

Counseling and Intervention Psychotherapy is an information exchange. Professionals convey ideas or, at least, encourage certain ideas. With new information, or enhanced awareness of previously known information, persons with brain injury, or anyone else in counseling for that matter, gain insight and skills. The usual intent is to influence emotion and behavior, although sometimes experiences during counseling sessions can be beneficial emotional events.

For many persons with brain injury the insights and skills they learn through counseling are invaluable. After all, most persons with brain injury arrive at their injury with little or no knowledge of what to expect. They are often afraid and worried. It is very difficult to cope and adjust without knowledge, and they must do so with a brain that is impaired in its information processing skills.

There are a myriad of issues that persons with brain injury must face. These concerns begin in the acute rehabilitation center. Professionals need to be aware of how persons with brain injury perceive rehabilitation. From the professionals' perspective, rehabilitation professionals are the "good guys," there to help people who are critically injured become healthy enough to leave the hospital with the skills and knowledge to thrive. In fact, excellent rehabilitation centers seek to help persons with brain injury achieve goals that they have set for themselves to reintegrate into society.

From the perspective of persons with brain injury, there may be a very different reality. The rehabilitation center can be an unfamiliar, busy place with procedures and rules that are implicit, not explicit, or confusing. Persons with brain injury can feel uncertain in the rehabilitation center, not just because of their lack of experience with the physical space, but because of inexperience with the operational characteristics of rehabilitation: roles, schedules, regulations, procedures, and culture. Treatment environments following brain injury are alien places to most people (77). Also, professionals are strangers and therefore, at least initially, are untested sources of reassurance.

Persons with brain injury can struggle early with their sense of loss of control. Professionals must appreciate how hard it is for persons with brain injury to cope with the imposition of rules and schedules for sleep, nursing care, meals, therapies, and visits from family or friends. Even when professionals provide choices, the professionals set the parameters for the decision-making. Professionals assign the label "non-compliant" to persons with brain injury who fail to adhere to the choices that professionals permit.

Counseling can assist persons with brain injury to adapt to the rehabilitation experience. Early reassurance regarding how the rehabilitation team functions is essential. Counseling can provide rationales for professionals' decisions and place them within the context of recovery. It can also address issues of self-esteem that arise when formerly independent adults find themselves dependent on other people who make decisions about them.

Alternatively, counseling can assist persons with brain injury to learn to assert their desires in an effective manner. Professionals traditionally conduct rehabilitation with assumptions about processes, values, and goals that persons with brain injury might not share. Counseling can help bridge paradigm mismatches that would otherwise lead to conflicts between persons with brain injury and professionals. It can help persons with brain injury to delineate their perspectives with the intent of influencing how rehabilitation professionals provide services to them and what services they want.

Counseling should continue after discontinuation of acute rehabilitation. Major life issues that professionals ought to have broached during rehabilitation typically come to the forefront of attention after hospitalization. Being confronted by the reality of a situation is emotionally different than preparatory, theoretical discussions. Issues that loom large usually include interpersonal relationships, work, driving, finances, sexuality, chemical use, supervision, and living arrangements. Some of the most important counseling happens after acute rehabilitation.

Professionals who provide counseling can face a difficult situation when persons with brain injury confront these issues. Many persons with brain injury want to assert themselves by returning to previous activities. In part, the role of professionals should be to help fulfill this desire when possible, but when persons with brain injury have limitations that require them to adapt to alterations in lifestyle or when society will not adjust to their strengths and weaknesses, it can fall upon professionals to facilitate awareness and coping. This is a complex challenge. Poor awareness is a highly complex symptom often with multiple aspects and determinants; (78–83) its treatment can be exceedingly difficult. Professionals must learn to be the voice of insight and, simultaneously, the source of support.

It is crucial that professionals build rapport with persons with brain injury before helping them confront reality. An empathetic treatment ambiance is essential when counseling persons with brain injury (84). Trust is essential to help persons with brain injury through the rapids of life. However, professionals should prepare for persons with brain injury to reach the point in time when they no longer want guidance. Many persons with brain injury want to strike out on their own, trying out their own ideas and abilities. Professionals must know when to prohibit plans and when to permit trial and error learning. Dangerous plans require professionals' prohibitions. For example, professionals should intervene when someone lacking the required skills intends to drive or return to a dangerous job, such as welding. On the other hand, even if neuropsychological and other data suggest a person may struggle with a particular endeavor, it can be a learning experience for the person to try it. If the person is resolved to make an attempt, professional resistance may lower rapport just when the person needs the most guidance. Professionals can help the person succeed to the degree possible. Still, the real world imposes consequences (e.g., being fired) with a stronger impact than the consequences that professionals can manipulate. The role of professionals in such circumstances is to be available for emotional support and to renew realistic planning. A nonjudgmental approach is essential to accomplish this.

Professionals must modify counseling for the cognitive abilities of persons with brain injury (4). Professionals have to consider the neuropsychological status of each person and adjust accordingly. There are numerous variables to weigh, including length of session (attention span), speed of speech (processing speed), sophistication of concepts or use of analogies (verbal reasoning), use of gestures (nonverbal processing), diagrams on a white board (visual-spatial ability), etc. One size does not fit all. Too often in health care for persons with brain injury, professionals pay insufficient attention to how well they are truly communicating; inadequate reflection on the actual impact of communication can destroy counseling effectiveness. Finally, it is important that there be consideration of professionals' characteristics and approach to counseling to insure a good match between professionals and persons with brain injury (55).

There are innumerable counseling approaches. It is impossible to discuss the application of all of them to brain injury. Still, many fall into one of three schools of thought: (85) cognitive-behavioral (e.g., Ellis' Rational Emotive Therapy and Beck's Cognitive Therapy), humanistic (e.g., Roger's Person Centered Therapy and Perl's Gestalt Therapy), and psychodynamic (e.g., Freud's Classical Psychoanalysis and Jung's Analytic Therapy). Very briefly, approaches from the cognitive-behavioral school focus on the facilitation of suitable, observable behavior and the alteration of thoughts that directly influence behavior; humanistic approaches emphasize self actualization, the growth of human potential, and the enhancement of the ability to experience one's feelings; professionals using psychodynamic approaches seek for people to increase control over unconsciousness influences and to understand the relationship between mental structures (85). Parenthetically, many rehabilitation professionals may be surprised at the inclusion of psychodynamic approaches. Yet, psychodynamically oriented therapists are increasingly addressing persons with brain injury (86). There are efforts to link research in brain function with psychoanalysis (87). Of course, psychoanalytical case conceptualization of emotional and behavioral functioning must recognize those issues that derive organically and not just attend to psychoanalytic formulation (88), but this is true of any psychological approach.

Professionals may choose to use approaches from any of these schools to assist persons with brain injury or they may decide to combine elements from more than one school. In the case of the more insight-oriented approaches (i.e., humanistic and psychodynamic) the premise is that insights garnered in treatment will change the perspectives of persons with brain injury. Such alterations should subsequently lead to emotional and behavioral improvement. This works best when persons with brain injury have sufficient cognitive processing ability to accomplish two aspects of this treatment. First, they should be able to formulate and express their thoughts and feelings. Second, they should be able to utilize changes in perspectives to effect change in emotional responses and behavioral repertoire.

Threats to the former include aphasia, impaired vocabulary, verbal reasoning deficits, memory impairment, etc. Obstacles to the latter include deficits in divided attention, set shifting, memory, impulsivity, rigidity, etc. Sometimes, in fact, persons with brain injury can articulate, and believe, insightful perspectives, but organic impairment interferes with real world performance.

In contrast, cognitive-behavioral approaches seek to more directly correct actions and those thoughts that immediately attend upon behaviors. The principle is that efficacious behavioral improvement happens by a straight forward focus on requisite behavioral changes. This occurs most successfully when existential issues are less prominent, though professionals can use cognitive interventions to address existential issues. Furthermore, professionals vary in their emphasis on the cognitive versus behavioral end of the spectrum, either philosophically or on a case by case basis. In the more cognitive range, persons with brain injury often need abilities similar to those necessary to participate in insight oriented therapy. At the more behavioral tail, deficits in memory and learning can be impediments. In addition, recognition of the need to change is important, particularly for sophisticated behaviors that require complex social skills.

Skill building can be a corollary of counseling. This can entail skills that persons with brain injury develop implicitly from new insights gained in counseling or skills taught to them explicitly in counseling. Skill sets may range from cognitive compensation techniques to anger management skills to social skills (the latter will be discussed later in this chapter). In regard to cognitive rehabilitation, it behooves professionals to avoid artificial barriers between counseling and training in cognitive compensation methods. An integrated approach, using counseling combined with cognitive rehabilitation, should be part of professionals' armamentarium (89). For anger management skills, professionals should adapt the skills for the abilities of persons with brain injury (90).

REHABILITATION PROCESS CHALLENGES

The Importance of Early Attention to Psychological Variables

Rehabilitation is a formative time for persons with brain injury. Professionals can set the tone for the future experience of living with brain injury (91). Often, later in life, persons with brain injury still reflect on their early experiences (92–94). Sometimes there is gratitude; sometimes there is anger; sometimes there is disappointment.

Early assessment and intervention for emotional and behavioral concerns can help influence the direction of care and the perspectives of persons with brain injury.

In some settings, consultation on emotional or behavioral variables occurs only after there is a problem. In such places, prophylactic evaluation and case involvement by professionals with expertise on these issues is deemed secondary to initiation of physical, occupational, speech, and recreational therapies. This is unfortunate.

The gold standard for rehabilitation ought to be the automatic inclusion of evaluation and treatment of emotional and behavioral variables. Treatment teams should act proactively and avoid waiting for these problems to develop (46, 47). It is an error to assume that rehabilitation and accompanying adjustment on the part of persons with brain injury will proceed smoothly. Rather, professionals should function with the premise that brain injury is likely to be devastating, entailing cognitive, behavioral, and emotional traps, until the course of a case proves otherwise.

There are numerous benefits that accrue from this perspective. To begin with, professionals can detect behavioral and emotional issues as they start to initiate early intervention. For example, professionals can address depression before it becomes overwhelming or noncompliance before it is entrenched. It is easier to gently help re-conceptualize concerns as they emerge than to have to terraform the emotional and behavioral landscape.

Furthermore, guidance in how persons with brain injury conceive rehabilitation and their interactions with professionals can enhance the impact of other therapies. Professionals can facilitate motivation and effort in treatment. Willingness to perform necessary skills may otherwise be given less attention in rehabilitation than is acquisition of those skills. Knowing *how* to do something does not automatically imply *wanting* to do something, even if it is beneficial and necessary.

Finally, it is advantageous to include emotional and behavioral assessment and intervention at the start of rehabilitation so that persons with brain injury view attention to those variables as a natural part of everyone's rehabilitation. This removes the stigma of being singled out for help with emotional and behavioral responses to rehabilitation and brain injury. It also allows time to build rapport before any difficulty starts so that a relationship is in place on which to build further treatment, if necessary. In essence, evaluation and treatment of behavioral and emotional issues ought to be a standard, automatic component of rehabilitation, initiated upon admission to rehabilitation.

Goal Setting

Rehabilitation is a collaborative effort requiring input from professionals, families, and persons with brain injury, among others. In intensive care units, the relationship of professionals to persons with brain injury is one of parent to infant, with professionals keeping the person alive.

In acute care settings, the relationship is one of parent to child, with professionals providing care and nurturance. However, in rehabilitation the relationship ought to be adult to adult, with professionals bringing knowledge and experience to a shared endeavor that includes recognition of the contribution of persons with brain injury. Fortunately, there is an increasing awareness of the importance of viewing treatment as a joint venture. For example, in the realm of behavioral treatment, the model of utilizing positive supports (74) to achieve successful behavioral functioning is based on an alliance with the person with brain injury. It takes a conceptual shift to view persons with brain injury as partners (95). Professionals' attitude toward persons with brain injury can have a large impact on treatment (46). In addition, it is essential that professionals be cognizant of cultural variables (96).

Professionals have a responsibility to avoid interpreting system problems, including societal attitudes or funding challenges, as organically imposed limits, while still facilitating awareness of organically determined limits. On one hand, it is unfair for professionals to be overly restrictive because of system issues or biases while, on the other hand, it is a failure of treatment to ignore anasognosia or unawareness, allowing pursuit of goals that really are unobtainable. Accurate feedback is good care, but being accurate (not over- or under- inclusive of limits) and compassionate (not too harsh in one's presentation) can be a challenge for professionals.

Family Issues

Families are ordinarily unprepared to cope with brain injury. In part, there is a mismatch between their expectations for treatment outcome and the reality of recovery after brain injury. In our society, families expect the health care system to cure people after injury or at least leave them with minimal residual problems. Mass media, such as television, promulgate this expectation. Television portrays miraculous recoveries after all sorts of injuries, including brain injury. Rarely do shows demonstrate the true aftermath of brain injury. In addition, families' own experience with health care after acute illnesses fosters this expectation. When families take a child with an earache to their physician, they anticipate that the physician will cure the child, not that the child will be permanently deaf. When people break bones, they expect their physician to fix them, and they anticipate they will have little residual difficulty. However, when families experience the onset of a chronic condition in a loved one (e.g., spinal cord injury, kidney failure requiring recurrent dialysis, diabetes, AIDS, brain injury), there is no eventual cure and families do not know what to do. Persons with brain injury are not cured even when families, employees, friends, insurers, physicians, professionals, etc. all fulfill their roles and provide excellent help.

Families are unequipped for a health condition that violates all of their expectations and that requires them to adopt roles for which they had no previous training. They can feel resentment at the failure of the societal compact regarding health care. They perform their *acute* care roles (visits to the hospital, time off work, support of compliance with the treatment and medications, etc.), and yet the health care system fails them (i.e., there is no cure). Dr. Sanders' chapter on family intervention addresses family issues more thoroughly, but the impact of families' functioning is pertinent here in so far as it affects the psychological and behavioral status of persons with brain injury.

It is incumbent upon professionals to provide assistance to families if they wish to achieve successful rehabilitation. They should address the families' anger and frustration with the health care system. In addition, families may need help with their own guilt over their failure to protect their loved one from harm before onset and their powerlessness to obtain a cure afterwards (97). Professionals can help by exploring reasonable expectations for families and encouraging appropriate roles.

For example, many families attempt to be ever-present during rehabilitation, similar to their behavior during acute illnesses. This is detrimental to families because they are unable to maintain such vigilance indefinitely, despite feeling that they should be able to do so, and they burn out. Professionals can assist families to accept that involvement at a reduced level that can be maintained for years is better than total involvement early, with burn out shortly past acute rehabilitation.

Families may ignore their own needs (98). Yet, all aspects of caregivers' lives may be altered after brain injury (9). Moreover, there can be stressful changes not just for the primary caregiver, but for other relatives as well (99). While some family members may do relatively well, (100) the greatest stressors relate to behavioral, personality, and emotional changes in their loved ones after brain injury (101). Families may go through a crisis in how they relate and interact (102).

Professionals should also be alert for another scenario. Sometimes families have unresolved issues regarding the nature of behavioral care of their loved one, either during hospitalization or in the years following rehabilitation. When family members struggle with the necessity of implementing behavior plans, their needs merit attention. Their untoward reactions to behavior plans can range from disagreement accompanied by withdrawal to efforts that directly undermine behavior plans. This problem is similar to the challenge that professionals encounter with family agendas, sometimes hidden, that are at odds with professionals' other treatment efforts. For example, families may render assistance with return to work ineffective because of their own emotional needs (55) or there may be enabling issues interfering with chemical dependency treatment. Of course, usually family members are strong allies in the implementation of behavioral treatment, and they are frequently quite insightful about how to proceed, but occasionally families need help to engage appropriately.

Despite the overwhelming nature of brain injury for families, professionals can greatly impact family perspectives after injury onset. For instance, a structured program that focuses on helping families can positively address the need families have for health information and emotional, community, and professional support (103). Obviously, families' need for help continues after acute rehabilitation. Families can benefit from ongoing support and guidance, even when professionals provide it by phone (104). Still, it can be very difficult to relieve family stress when behavioral dyscontrol persists (105).

SELECTED APPLICATIONS

For a variety of issues in rehabilitation, emotional, behavioral, and neuropsychological assessment underlie the application of contingency, environmental, and counseling techniques, in conjunction with family intervention. The need to assess and treat some issues seems to arise repeatedly. A comprehensive review of all psychological difficulties is unfeasible here, but selected topics are worthy of mention.

Aggression

Physical aggression may be the most distressing of all brain injury symptoms to other people. People will tolerate memory problems, depression, or the need for a wheelchair, but they will not permit physical assaults. When physical aggression occurs it commands attention.

As the severity of aggression increases, it requires an increasingly comprehensive approach. Environmental change can address the antecedents of aggression. The main variable to manipulate in a stimulus control paradigm is the behavior of professionals and other people. As already noted, their behavior often proves to be the primary antecedent for physical aggression.

Contingency techniques can be used after physical aggression, though they may prove more useful as an adjunct to antecedent control. Recall, however, the challenges in applying contingency procedures after brain injury. Moreover, when persons with brain injury direct aggression at professionals, it is particularly tempting for some professionals to be punitive. In this sense, contingency techniques can be notably difficult for professionals to positively and correctly implement.

Counseling with persons with brain injury can be essential to facilitate interpretation of antecedent and contingency changes, the utilization of skill based techniques for anger management, cognitive restructuring of frustrating events, and preparation for future stressful events. Counseling can decrease errors and enhance errorless learning.

It is essential that professionals attend to variables that influence the expression of aggression. Treatment is less likely to be successful if two different people who apparently exhibit the same behavior receive the same treatment without an understanding of the behavioral etiology. Professionals must attend to the contribution of emotional variables leading to aggression and not just focus on the superficial behavioral symptom of aggression. Similarly, cognitive processing often plays a crucial role in the expression of aggression.

Families need particularly attentive support when there is physical aggression. Aggression may embarrass or frighten family members, especially when it is directed at the family. Professionals may need to encourage family members to consider their own safety. Alternatively, professionals may need to work with them regarding their own stimulus value and behavior as an environmental antecedent.

Noncompliance

Noncompliance is a difficult problem for professionals. The obstacle to avoid is the automatic assumption that noncompliance is an intentional challenge to authority. Noncompliance can be due to a variety of factors. These include true dyscontrol (in which refusal is based on post-onset organic difficulty with acquiescence), manipulation for secondary gain, communication or memory deficits, pre-morbid oppositional personality, or attempts to reassert self-determination. It is also easy to miss the contribution to noncompliance of fatigue and poor sleep, depression, and initiation or impulsivity problems. As with all behaviors, determination of behavioral etiology is paramount for intervention.

Intervention may be multifaceted. Avoidance of power struggles is important. Education about the implications of noncompliance can be useful, particularly when unawareness is present. Sometimes negotiation can determine alternatives to achieve creative solutions. Alterations in schedules or the use of reminders, as well as other environmental changes can be successful.

Unfortunately, noncompliance can lead to paradoxical outcomes for persons with brain injury. Other people may view noncompliance as evidence for the need to restrict independence, despite its occurrence as an effort by persons with brain injury to expand their choices. They want the freedom to choose, and other people want to control poor choices. Treatment of noncompliance requires a careful balance of necessary rules and maximization of personal choice.

Impulsivity

Impulsivity can be a particularly frustrating behavior for professionals and families, and, for that matter, for persons with brain injury. For professionals and families, impulsivity is difficult to address because it crosses other behaviors (e.g., social inappropriateness, risk to elope, suicidal ideation, noncompliance, hoarding, physical and verbal aggression) causing a worsening of whatever symptoms would occur anyway. For persons with brain injury, impulsivity can be embarrassing if there is sufficient self-awareness, because they act contrary to how they might otherwise behave. Oftentimes, upon post hoc guided reflection, persons with brain injury will express regret regarding impulsive behavior.

Two scenarios exist regarding impulsivity. First, persons with brain injury may act too intensely or prematurely. The resulting behavior appears as "too much, too soon." The behavior is too much of a good thing. Professionals find themselves trying to modulate behavior that would be acceptable if performed in a different setting, more slowly, or less intensely. Second, persons with brain injury may fail to stop inappropriate behavior, acts that ought not to occur at all. Professionals tend to describe these behaviors as risky or dangerous to persons with brain injury or to other people. There is a failure to inhibit impulses toward aggression, elopement, suicide, etc. Behavior in the first scenario appears as overly activated responses, and behavior in the second situation presents as uncontrolled behavior. Persons with brain injury find themselves being told to slow down in the first instance and stop in the second case. Impulsivity, therefore, may represent over activation or under control (48).

Impulsivity would appear to be a prominent component of the complaint of personality change after brain injury (106). It is likely to contribute to some of the more troublesome behaviors of aggression, sexual acting out, verbal abuse, etc. Moreover, the negative consequences associated with such behaviors tend not to alter their occurrence when impulsivity is a factor (74). As such, environmental changes, decreasing stimuli associated with impulsive responding, and skill building, when appropriate, may be more effective.

Depression, Grief, Catastrophic Reaction, and Post-Traumatic Stress Disorder

Many persons with brain injury experience depression, (107) and the risk of suicide increases after brain injury (108). Depression can worsen as time passes post onset (109) and may correlate with increases in awareness or setbacks in the real world. Depression may be related to loss of self-esteem, uncertainty about the future, disruption of social supports, or particular events (e.g., loss of job). There are neuroanatomical and neurochemical factors as well, (11) and it is unclear as to whether depression after brain injury is the same phenomena as depression without brain injury (107). Moreover, grief ought to be considered separate from depression *per se* (23). In light of experimental findings of brain activation during grief, (110) persons with brain injury may experience or demonstrate grief differently than others.

Furthermore, the typical stages of grief seen when people contemplate death may not apply well to the experience of brain injury (111). Rather, the emotional responses to brain injury may be better conceived as an identity crisis (112). However, the crisis may persist as the injury requires continual adaptation. There is an ongoing dynamic between brain injury and changing life circumstances, and it requires recurrent adjustment. This is characterized by uncertainty and has been described as a "mobile-mourning" process (113). Even after acute recovery, brain injuries do not appear static for many persons with brain injury. As they counter new life situations, unsuspected aspects of their injuries emerge to challenge them.

In addition, the people in the support system available to persons with brain injury are usually unprepared for survival of the person with alterations in cognitive, emotional, and behavioral functioning. They are unprepared to help. There is no known societal role for them to follow (114). As with persons with brain injury, family grief does not follow an orderly progression to resolution (97).

Persons with brain injury may also experience a catastrophic condition (115). They face lack of self actualization. This arises when impairment in abstract conceptual ability interferes with their accounting for performance failure on various tasks or activities. The resulting discord between impaired ability and an acceptable self-formulation of their shortcomings leads to the catastrophic condition and anxiety.

Deft handling of the catastrophic condition, or reaction, is important for successful rehabilitation. Pushing activities that highlight deficits and enhances struggles, or failures, can be contraindicated. In fact, two of the foundations of "Holistic Habit Retraining," (69) a neurorehabilitation methodology, are errorless learning and a supportive approach, to help avoid the anxiety, frustration, despair, and resignation of the catastrophic condition that would otherwise interfere with learning.

Professionals must remain cognizant of the potential of catastrophic reactions as person with brain injury become more aware of deficits. There is the potential for catastrophic reactions as they advance from impaired self awareness to some awareness or to denial of deficit (116). Professionals may encounter accusations that they are making persons with brain injury worse during rehabilitation as awareness increases. This may be accompanied by a range of responses including withdrawal, noncompliance, resistance, anger, hostility, and aggression as persons with brain injury struggle with a mixture of perplexity and increasing despair.

Catastrophic reactions may vary in their presentation (117). In one scenario persons with brain injury may feel overwhelmed while experiencing shame, anxiety, and hopelessness. The loss of sense of self can drive frustration. Alternatively, in a second situation professionals may primarily observe passivity and withdrawal. Affect can appear flat. In a third variation persons with brain injury may respond with aggression and acting out behaviors (e.g., chemical abuse). There is likely to be hostility and resentment. In a fourth presentation there may be efforts to mask anxieties through superficial acquiescence and attempts to hide difficulties. This may prove difficult to maintain, however, since it requires persistent concealment of problems. In all instances persons with brain injury are attempting to cope with the underlying loss of integrity of the self. Finally, it should be apparent that any given person may have a combined clinical picture.

The development of post traumatic stress disorder (PTSD) is an additional factor that can complicate the care of persons with brain injury (118). There is documentation of PTSD after brain injury; (119) yet, there is debate regarding the co-occurrence of PTSD and brain injury (120) since traumatic brain injury can result in loss of consciousness and amnesia. Researchers have proposed avenues for the evolution of PTSD, however (121, 122). PTSD could arise from implicit memories occurring without conscious recall. Conditioned fear could cause PTSD in some cases. There may be later cognitive representations that lead to PTSD symptoms. Also, stressful events subsequent to immediate onset may be the basis for PTSD. Finally, neurobiological changes may contribute to PTSD.

Social Skills

Social skills are a broad set of human interaction variables. They range from relatively narrow elements, such as eye contact or gestures, to broader factors including sensitivity to context and language-communication skills. Professionals need to address social self regulation (e.g., disinhibition, inertia), social self awareness (i.e., knowledge of one's impact on other people), social insensitivity (i.e., understanding another person's perspective or emotions) and social problem solving (i.e., interpersonal issue resolution) (123). Without social skill competency, brief, seemingly simple, everyday exchanges become episodes of miscommunication and sources of frustration. Worse, the lack of proficiency in social skills impairs the establishment or maintenance of ongoing supportive relationships.

It is important to recognize that social skill enhancement is challenging for a number of reasons. First, underlying cognitive deficits can impair learning new skills or remembering to apply them. Second, emotional factors, such as anger or frustration, or social pressure, such as the desire to perform in a certain fashion to impress some-one else, can distort how persons with brain injury perform skills. Third, persons with brain injury may relapse back to older, more over learned, dysfunctional skills.

Fortunately, research shows that persons with brain injury can learn skills for the social setting (124). This may involve specific skills, though there may be an increased difficulty in acquiring complex skills (125). When behavioral dyscontrol has resulted in the attainment of desirable goals in the past, then training in socially acceptable alternative methods to reach the same goal can mitigate behavioral problems (68). In the broader context of the utilization of social ability, social participation is also a function of perceived self-efficacy and determination, as well as energy level (126). Training can focus on general social competency that involves learning underlying principles for communication and social skills (127).

Substance Abuse

Psychological considerations play a role in the treatment of substance abuse following brain injury. Professionals are likely to encounter three common patterns: social users whose use remains unchanged, but whose brain can no longer tolerate even a social level of consumption; social users whose use increases after onset, becoming abusive; and pre-onset abusers whose use remains abusive (and whose use may have contributed to their injury onset). Regardless of the amount and pattern of use, the best advice is abstinence: "zero, forever."

Still, it can be a considerable challenge for professionals to help persons with brain injury achieve abstinence. There are tremendously strong factors encouraging the use of alcohol and illicit drugs, including poor insight, denial, lack of information, peer pressure, depression, addiction, etc. Some persons with brain injury even report that the place they feel most normal is a bar, where their brain injury symptoms, including slurred speech, balance problems, memory difficulties, and social-sexual forwardness are commonplace among patrons without brain injuries. Hence, early discussion of chemical use and integration with other rehabilitation efforts helps set the stage for any future more comprehensive intervention.

Elsewhere in this book, Dr. Corrigan devotes a complete chapter to substance abuse. However, from a behavioral standpoint two concerns bear comment. The message of abstinence should be consistent across all professionals and family members. To be successful, professionals have to be attentive to issues of co-dependency (128). Moreover, professionals should be aware of any family members who may also have substance abuse problems and who will be unreliable participants in providing a united front on this issue.

Second, at times persons with brain injury may reject treatment advice. There are three typical objections: past adverse treatment experiences, claims of familiarity with chemical dependency treatment messages, or resistance to time away from community integration. Professionals must prepare to answer these concerns. Specialized programs for persons with brain injury who have substance abuse problems should differ from past treatment programs sufficiently enough so as to address the first two objections.

Persons with brain injury often experience frustration in traditional programs because of cognitive processing variables. They struggle in group treatment that fails to accommodate comprehension, language, memory, and processing speed variables. Furthermore, many persons with brain injury require help with abstinence because of their injury, not because of pre-morbid life devastation due to drugs or alcohol (e.g., alcohol use may have been at acceptable social levels prior to onset). It is important to remember that many persons with brain injury incur their injuries unrelated to any chemical use on their part (e.g., falls, sports, motor vehicle crash victims). Hence, traditional program messages regarding the need to redesign a dysfunctional life seem inappropriate to many persons with brain injury.

The integrated inclusion of a spiritual aspect in some programs can also be a difficulty. Some persons with brain injury, while accepting the need for treatment to achieve abstinence, reject faith-based messages in their brain injury recovery. This may be a function of their religious beliefs or the course of their emotional or psychological healing.

Finally, traditional follow-up support groups do not always readily welcome persons with brain injury and other participants may relate poorly to the experiences of persons with brain injury. Persons with brain injury may find that their social skill difficulties are at times misunderstood. Their cognitive problems can frustrate other group members.

Therefore, specialized programs can help after brain injury by structuring care around the cognitive needs of persons with brain injury and by tailoring their message to fit the circumstances of persons with brain injury. Also, professionals should have available materials that cover chemical use and brain injury. For example, it can be helpful to use workbooks specifically designed for chemical use after brain injury (129–131) or, if using a 12-step program, to use the 12-steps modified for persons with brain injury (132).

Professionals will find it easier to respond to the third objection (time away form community reintegration) when they link chemical health treatment to rehabilitation for brain injury. If professionals present it as a component of the overall plan of brain injury recovery, persons with brain injury may view it as more acceptable.

SUMMARY

Issues of emotional and behavioral functioning require significant attention on the part of professionals. These concerns can influence the outcome of rehabilitation and can have a significant impact on persons with brain injuries and their families. Yet, there are forces ranging from insurers' perspectives to the inherent complexities in addressing psychological variables that impede treatment. Professionals will most benefit the people they serve when they are diligent about providing care for psychological needs.

Professionals should base intervention on solid assessment. This ought to include clinical observation, interview, and psychometric assessment of cognitive, behavioral, and emotional functioning. There is an array of possible intervention strategies. Treatment techniques include contingencies, environmental manipulation, counseling and skill building. Professionals should be aware of the advantages of starting care early after onset, the needs of families, and the nature of goal setting after brain injury. In fact, throughout behavioral care, during every type of evaluation and treatment for all emotional and behavioral problems, professionals must keep in the forefront of their decision making the unique nature of brain injury and its interaction with psychological functioning.

ACKNOWLEDGMENT

Grateful acknowledgment is due Marti Beltz, Ann Reese, and Lindsey Schafer for their assistance with library research and manuscript preparation.

References

1. Delmonico RL, Hanley-Peterson P, Englander J. Group psychotherapy for persons with traumatic brain injury: Management of frustration and substance abuse. *J Head Trauma Rehabil* 1998;13(6):10–22.
2. Stansfield K. Adaptation of family members of brain-injured patients: Perceptions of the hospitalization event. *Axon* 1990; Dec:71–75.
3. Gainer R. *The resumption of social role activities following severe brain injury: A decade later*. Best Practices in Brain Injury Service Delivery XIII, Brain Injury Association of Iowa Conference 2005, Des Moines, IA.
4. Folzer SM. Psychotherapy with "mild" brain-injured patients. *Am J Orthopsychiatry* 2001;71(2):245–251.
5. Torrey EF. *The Mind Game – Witchdoctors and Psychiatrists*. New York: Emerson Hall Publishers, Inc, 1972.
6. Tennant A, MacDermott N, Neary D. The long-term outcome of head injury: Implications for service planning. *Brain Inj* 1995; 9(6):595–605.
7. Man DW. Family caregivers' reactions and coping for persons with brain injury. *Brain Inj* 2002;16(12):1025–1037.
8. Fugl-Meyer AR, Fugl-Meyer KS. The coping process after traumatic brain injury. *Scand J Rehabil Med Suppl* 1988;17:51–53.
9. Dring R. The informal caregiver responsible for home care of the individual with cognitive dysfunction following brain injury. *J Neurosci Nurs* 1989;21(1):42–45.
10. Bellenir K. *Head Trauma Sourcebook*. Detroit: Omnigraphics, Inc, 1997, Vol 23.
11. Rosenthal M, Christensen BK, Ross TP. Depression following traumatic brain injury. *Arch Phys Med Rehabil* 1998;79(1):90–103.
12. Heinemann AW, Hamilton B, Linacre JM, Wright BD, Granger C. Functional status and therapeutic intensity during inpatient rehabilitation. *Am J Phys Med Rehabil* 1995;74(4):315–326.
13. Burke WH, Lewis FD. Management of maladaptive social behavior of a brain injured adult. *Int J Rehabil Res* 1986;9(4):335–342.
14. McMordie WR, Rogers KF, Barker SL. Consumer satisfaction with services provided to head-injured patients and their families. *Brain Inj* 1991;5(1):43–51.
15. *Rehabilitation of Persons with Traumatic Brain Injury.NIH Consensus Statement* 1998;16 (1):1–41.
16. Bear MF, Connors BW, Paradiso MA. *Neuroscience – Exploring the Brain*. Baltimore: Williams & Wilkins, 1996.
17. Beatty J. *The Human Brain – Essentials of Behavioral Neuroscience*. Thousand Oaks: Sage Publications, Inc, 2001.
18. McGee JM. Insight – Neuroanatomy of behavior after brain injury or you don't like my behavior? You'll have to discuss that with my brain directly. *Premier Outlook* 2004;4(2):24–32.
19. Stringer AY. *A Guide to Adult Neuropsychological Diagnosis*. Philadelphia: F.A. Davis Company, 1996.
20. Jorge RE, Robinson RG, Starkstein SE, Arndt SV. Depression and anxiety following traumatic brain injury. *J Neuropsyc Cl Neurosciences* 1993;5:369–374.
21. Levin HS, Goldstein FC, MacKenzie EJ. Depression as a secondary condition following mild and moderate traumatic brain injury. *Semin Clin Neuropsychiatry* 1997;2(3):207–215.
22. Rapoport MJ, McCullagh S, Streiner D, Feinstein A. The clinical significance of major depression following mild traumatic brain injury. *Psychosomatics* 2003;44(1):31–37.
23. Niemeier JP, Kennedy RE, McKinley WO, Cifu DX. The Loss Inventory: A measure of emotional and cognitive responses to disability. *Disabil Rehabil* 2004;26(10):614–623.
24. Hagen C, Malkmus D, Durham P. *Levels of Cognitive Functioning*. Downey: Rancho Los Amigos Hospital, 1972.
25. Beck AT. *Depression – Causes and Treatment*. Philadelphia: University of Pennsylvania Press, 1967.
26. Beck AT, Rush AJ, Shaw BF, Emery G. *Cognitive Therapy of Depression*. New York: The Guilford Press, 1979.
27. Levin GS, Grossman MD. Behavioral sequelae of closed head injury. *Arch Neurol* 1978;35:720–726.
28. Vanier M, Mazaux JM, Lambert J, Dassa C, Levin HS. Assessment of neuropsychologic impairments after head injury: Interrater reliability and factorial and criterion validity of the Neurobehavioral Rating Scale-Revised. *Arch Phys Med Rehabil* 2000;81(6):796–806.
29. Hall KM, Hamilton BB, Gordon WA, Zasler ND. Characteristics and comparisons of functional assessment indices: Disability Rating Scale, Functional Independence Measure, and Functional Assessment Measure. *J Head Trauma Rehabil* 1993;8(2):60–74.
30. Turner-Stokes L. Standardized outcome assessment in brain injury rehabilitation for younger adults. *Disabil Rehabil* 2002;24(7): 383–389.
31. Tesio L, Cantagallo A. The Functional Assessment Measure (FAM) in closed traumatic brain injury outpatients: A Rasch-based psychometric study. *J Outcome Meas* 1998;2(2):79–96.
32. Bohac DL, Malec JF, Moessner AM. Factor analysis of the Mayo-Portland Adaptability Inventory: Structure and validity. *Brain Inj* 1997;11(7):469–482.
33. Malec JF, Moessner AM, Kragness M, Lezak MD. Refining a measure of brain injury sequelae to predict postacute rehabilitation outcome: Rating scale analysis of the Mayo-Portland Adaptability Inventory. *J Head Trauma Rehabil* 2000;15(1):670–682.
34. Malec JF, Thompson JM. Relationship of the Mayo-Portland Adaptability Inventory to functional outcome and cognitive performance measures. *J Head Trauma Rehabil* 1994;9(4):1–15.
35. Niemeier JP, Burnett DM, Whitaker D. Cultural competence in the rehabilitation setting: Are we falling short of meeting needs? *Arc Phys Med Rehabil*, 2003;84:1240–1245.
36. Green A, Felmingham K, Baguley IJ, Slewa-Younan S, Simpson S. The clinical utility of the Beck Depression Inventory after traumatic brain injury. *Brain Inj* 2001;15(12):1021–1028.

37. Rowland SM, Lam CS, Leahy B. Use of the Beck Depression Inventory-II (BDI-II) with persons with traumatic brain injury: Analysis of factorial structure. *Brain Inj* 2005;19(2):77–83.

38. Sliwinski M, Gordon WA, Bogdany J. The Beck Depression Inventory: Is it a suitable measure of depression for individuals with traumatic brain injury? *J Head Trauma Rehabil* 1998;13(4):40–46.

39. Cooper JO, Heron TE, Heward WL. *Applied Behavior Analysis.* Upper Saddle River, NJ: Prentice Hall, 1987.

40. Kazdin AE. *Behavior Modification in Applied Settings, 6th Edition.* Belmont, CA: Wadsworth/ Thomson Learning, 2001.

41. Pierce WD, Cheney CD. *Behavior Analysis and Learning, 3rd Edition.* London: Lawrence Erlbaum Associates, 2004.

42. Ashley MJ, Krych DK, Persel CS, Persel CH. *Working with Behavior Disorders – Strategies for Traumatic Brain Injury Rehabilitation.* San Antonio: Communication Skill Builders, The Psychological Corporation, 1995.

43. Wesolowski MD, Zencius AH. *A Practical Guide to Head Injury Rehabilitation – A Focus on Postacute Residential Treatment.* New York: Plenum Press, 1994.

44. Corrigan JD. Development of a scale for assessment of agitation following traumatic brain injury. *J Clin Exp Neuropsychol* 1989;11(2):261–277.

45. Levin HS, High WM, Goethe KE, Sisson RA, Overall JE, Rhoades HM, Eisenberg HM, Kalisky Z, Gary HE. The neurobehavioural rating scale: Assessment of the behavioural sequelae of head injury by the clinician. *J Neurol, Neurosurg, and Psychiatry* 1987;50:183–193.

46. Mattheis BK, Kreutzer JS, West DD. *The Behavior Management Handbook – A Practical Approach to Patients with Neurological Disorders.* San Antonio: Therapy Skill Builders, The Psychological Corporation, 1997.

47. Franzen MD. Neuropsychological assessment in traumatic brain injury. *Crit Care Nurs Q* 2000;23(3):58–64.

48. Karol RL. *Neuropsychosocial Intervention – The Practical Treatment of Severe Behavioral Dyscontrol After Acquired Brain Injury.* Boca Raton: CRC Press LLC, 2003.

49. Sbordone RJ. Limitations of neuropsychological testing to predict the cognitive and behavioral functioning of persons with brain injury in real-world settings. *NeuroRehabil* 2001;16:199–201.

50. Bower GH, Hilgard ER. *Theories of Learning, 5th Edition.* Upper Saddle River, NJ: Prentice Hall, 1998.

51. Fasotti L, Spikman J. Cognitive rehabilitation of central executive disorders. In Brouwer W, van Zomeren E, Berg I, Bouma A, Haan E (eds.), *Cognitive Rehabilitation – A Clinical Neuropsychological Approach.* Amsterdam: Boom Publishers, 2002, 107–123.

52. Powell RA, Symbaluk DG, MacDonald SE. *Introduction to Learning and Behavior, 2nd Edition.* Belmont, CA: Wadsworth/Thomson Learning, 2005.

53. Joint Commission on Accreditation of Healthcare Organizations. *Comprehensive Accreditation Manual for Hospitals: The Official Handbook.* Oakbrook Terrace: Joint Commission Resources, 2004.

54. Franzen MD, Lovell MR. Behavioral treatments of aggressive sequelae of brain injury. *Psychiatric Annals* 1987;17(6):389–396.

55. Pepping M, Prigatano GP. Psychotherapy after brain injury: Costs and benefits. In Prigatano GP, Pliskin NH (eds.), *Clinical Neuropsychology and Cost Outcome Research: A Beginning.* New York: Psychology Press, 2003, 313–328.

56. Treadwell K, Page TJ. Functional analysis: Identifying the environmental determinants of severe behavior disorders. *J Head Trauma Rehabil* 1996;11(1):62–74.

57. Beatty C. Perception & reality – Interventions for behavioral problems after brain injury. *Premier Outlook* 2004;4(2):4–12.

58. Gloag D. Rehabilitation after head injury:2-Behavior and emotional problems, long term needs, and the requirements for services. *Brit Med J* 1985;290:913–916.

59. Giles GM, Clark-Wilson J. The use of behavioral techniques in functional skills training after severe brain injury. *Am J Occupational Ther* 1988;42 (10):658–665.

60. Hegel MT. Application of a token economy with a non-compliant closed head-injured male. *Brain Inj* 1988;2(4):333–338.

61. Eames P, Wood R. Rehabilitation after severe brain injury: A follow-up study of a behaviour modification approach. *J Neurol Neurosurg Psychiatry* 1985;48:613–619.

62. Prigatano GP, O'Brien KP, Klonoff PS. The clinical management of paranoid delusions in postacute traumatic brain-injured patients. *J Head Trauma Rehabil* 1988;3(3):23–32.

63. Slifer KJ, Tucker CL, Gerson AC, Cataldo MD, Sevier RC, Suter AH, Kane AC. Operant conditioning for behavior management during posttraumatic amnesia in children and adolescents with brain injury. *J Head Trauma Rehabil* 1996;11(1):39–50.

64. Feeney TJ, Ylvisaker M, Rosen BH, Greene P. Community supports for individuals with challenging behavior after brain injury: An analysis of the New York state behavioral resource project. *J Head Trauma Rehabil* 2001;16(1):61–75.

65. Kessles, RPC, de Haan EHF. Implicit learning in memory rehabilitation: A meta-analysis on errorless learning and vanishing cues methods. *J Cl Exp Neuropsych* 2003;25(6):805–814.

66. Squires EJ, Humkin NM, Parkin, AJ. Errorless learning of novel associations in amnesia. *Neuropsychologia* 1997;35(8):1103–1111.

67. Tailby R, Haslam C. An investigation of errorless learning in memory-impaired patients: Improving the technique and clarifying theory. *Neuropsychologia* 2003;41:1230–1240.

68. Ducharme JM. Treatment of maladaptive behavior in acquired brain injury: Remedial approaches in postacute settings. *Clin Psychol Rev* 2000;20(3):405–426.

69. Martelli MF, Zasler ND, Tiernan PR. Skill acquisition and automatic process development after brain injury: A holistic habit retraining (HHR) model for community reentry. *Brain Inj Professional* 2005;2(1):10–16.

70. Bandura A. *Principles of Behavior Modification.* New York: Holt, Rinehart and Winston, Inc, 1969.

71. Wood R. Management of behavior disorders in a day treatment setting. *J Head Trauma Rehabil* 1988;3(3):53–61.

72. Yody BB, Schaub C, Conway J, Peters S, Strauss D, Helsinger S. Applied behavior management and acquired brain injury approaches and assessment. *J Head Trauma Rehabil* 2000;15(4):1041–1060.

73. Ducharme JM. A conceptual model for treatment of externalizing behaviour in acquired brain injury. *Brain Inj* 1999;13(9):645–668.

74. Ylvisaker M, Jacobs HE, Feeney TJ. Positive supports for people who experience behavioral and cognitive disability after brain injury: A review. *J Head Trauma Rehabil* 2003;18(1):7–32.

75. Hayden ME, Moreault AM, LeBlanc J, Plenger PM. Reducing level of handicap in traumatic brain injury: An environmentally based model of treatment. *J Head Trauma Rehabil* 2000;15(4):1000–1021.

76. Nielsen L, Beaver C, Hovedy W. *A Systematic Approach to Maximizing Recovery via the Environment.* Boise: Idaho Elks Rehabilitation Hospital, 1998.

77. Eames P. Behavior disorders after severe head injury: Their nature and causes and strategies for management. *J Head Trauma Rehabil* 1988;3(3):1–6.

78. Hart T, Sherer M, Whyte J, Polansky M, Novack TA. Awareness of behavioral, cognitive, and physical deficits in acute traumatic brain injury. *Arch Phys Med Rehabil* 2004;85(9):1450–1456.

79. Martin C, Viguier D, Deloche G, Dellatolas G. Subjective experience after traumatic brain injury. *Brain Inj* 2001;15(11):947–959.

80. Newman AC, Garmoe W, Beatty P, Ziccardi M. Self-awareness of traumatically brain injured patients in the acute inpatient rehabilitation setting. *Brain Inj* 2000;14(4):333–344.

81. Prigatano GP, Schacter DL. *Awareness of Deficit After Brain Injury – Clinical and Theoretical Issues.* New York: Oxford University Press, 1991.

82. Sherer M, Hart T, Nick TG. Measurement of impaired self-awareness after traumatic brain injury: A comparison of the patient competency rating scale and the awareness questionnaire. *Brain Inj* 2003;17(1):25–37.

83. Sherer M, Hart T, Nick TG, Whyte J, Thompson RN, Yablon SA. Early impaired self-awareness after traumatic brain injury. *Arch Phys Med Rehabil* 2003;84(2):168–176.

84. Klonoff PS. The art and science of milieu-oriented neurorehabilitation. *Barrow Quarterly* 2005;21(2):14–21.

85. Nelson-Jones R. *Six Key Approaches to Counseling & Therapy.* New York: Continuum, 2000.

86. Harvey M. *Neuropsychoanalytic Perspectives in Rehabilitation for Individuals with Brain Injury.* American Psychological Association Conference 2005, Washington, DC.

87. Milton J, Polmear C, Fabricius J. *A Short Introduction to Psychoanalysis.* London: Sage Publications, 2004.

88. McWilliams N. *Psychoanalytic Case Formulation.* New York: Guilford Press, 1999.

89. Prigatano GP, Borgaro S, Caples H. Non-pharmacological management of psychiatric disturbances after traumatic brain injury. *Int Rev Psych* 2003;15:371–379.

90. O'Neill H. *Managing Anger.* London: Whurr Publishers Ltd, 1999.

91. Howard ME. Behavior management in the acute care rehabilitation setting. *J Head Trauma Rehabil* 1988;3(3):14–22.

92. Pflug JN. *Miles to Go Before I Sleep – My Grateful Journey Back from the Hijacking of EgyptAir Flight 648.* Center City: Hazelden, 1996.

93. Stoler DR, Hill BA. *Coping with Mild Traumatic Brain Injury.* Garden City Park: Avery Publishing Group, 1998.

94. Swanson KL. *I'll Carry the Fork! Recovering a Life After Brain Injury.* Los Altos: Rising Star Press, 1999.

95. Conduleci A. *Interdependence: The Route to Community, 2nd Edition.* Winter Park: GR Press, Inc, 1995.

96. Lipson JG, Dibble SL. *Culture & Clinical Care.* San Francisco: UCSF Nursing Press, 2005.

97. Testani-Dufour L, Chappel-Aiken L, Gueldner S. Traumatic brain injury: A family experience. *J Neurosci Nurs* 1992;24(6):317–323.

98. Man DWK, Lam CS, Bard CC. Development and application of the Family Empowerment Questionnaire in brain injury. *Brain Inj* 2003;17(5):437–450.

99. Perlesz A, Kinsella G, Crowe S. Psychological distress and family satisfaction following traumatic brain injury: Injured individuals and their primary, secondary, and tertiary carers. *J Head Trauma Rehabil* 2000;15(3):909–929.

100. Ponsford J, Olver J, Ponsford M, Nelms R. Long-term adjustment of families following traumatic brain injury where comprehensive rehabilitation has been provided. *Brain Inj* 2003; 17(6):453–468.

101. Kreutzer JS, Marwitz JH, Kepler K. Traumatic brain injury: Family response and outcome. *Arch Phys Med Rehabil* 1992;73(8): 771–778.

102. Soderstrom S, Fogelsjoo A, Fugl-Meyer KS, Stenson S. Traumatic brain injury crisis intervention and family therapy—Management and outcome. *Scand J Rehabil Med Suppl* 1992;26:132–141.

103. Kreutzer J, Taylor LA. *Innovative tools for effective family intervention following neurotrauma.* American Psychological Association Conference 2005, Washington, DC.

104. Albert SM, Im A, Brenner L, Smith M, Waxman R. Effect of a social work liaison program on family caregivers to people with brain injury. *J Head Trauma Rehabil* 2002;17(2):175–189.

105. Carnevale GJ, Anselmi V, Busichio K, Millis SR. Changes in ratings of caregiver burden following a community-based behavior management program for persons with traumatic brain injury. *J Head Trauma Rehabil* 2002;17(2):83–95.

106. McAllister TW. Neuropsychiatric sequelae of head injuries. *Psychiatr Clin North Am* 1992;15(2):395–413.

107. Busch CR, Alpern HP. Depression after mild traumatic brain injury: A review of current research. *Neuropsychol Rev* 1998; 8(2):95–108.

108. Teasdale TW, Engberg AW. Suicide after traumatic brain injury: A population study. *J Neurol Neurosurg Psychiatry* 2001;71(4): 436–440.

109. Fordyce DJ, Roueche JR, Prigatano GP. Enhanced emotional reactions in chronic head trauma patients. *J Neurol Neurosurg Psychiatry* 1983;46:620–624.

110. Gundel H, O'Connor M, Littrell L, Fort C, Lane RD. Functional neuroanatomy of grief: An fMRI study. *Am J Psychiatry* 2003; 160(11):1946–1953.

111. Tadir M, Stern JM. The mourning process with brain injured patients. *Scand J Rehabil Med Suppl* 1985;12:50–52.

112. Persinger MA. Personality changes following brain injury as a grief response to the loss of sense of self: Phenomenological themes as indices of local lability and neurocognitive structuring as psychotherapy. *Psychol Rep* 1993;72:1059–1068.

113. Muir CA, Haffey WJ. Psychological and neuropsychological interventions in the mobile mourning process. In Edelstein BA, Couture ET (eds.), *Behavioral Assessment and Rehabilitation of the Traumatically Brain-Damaged.* New York: Plenum Press, 1984;247–271.

114. Guerriere D, McKeever P. Mothering children who survive brain injuries: Playing the hand you're dealt. *J Soc Pediatr Nurs* 1997;2(3):105–115.

115. Goldstein K. The effect of brain damage on the personality. *Psychiatry* 1952;15:245–260.

116. Prigatano GP, Klonoff PS. A clinician's rating scale for evaluating impaired self-awareness and denial of disability after brain injury. *Clin Neuropsychologist* 1998;12(1):56–67.

117. Klonoff PS, Lage GA, Chiapello DA. Varieties of the catastrophic reaction to brain injury: A self psychology perspective. *Bull Menninger Clin* 1993;57(2):227–241.

118. Bryant RA, Marosszeky JE, Crooks J, Baguley IJ, Gurka JA. Post-traumatic stress disorder and psychosocial functioning after severe traumatic brain injury. *J Nerv Ment Dis* 2001;189(2): 109–113.

119. Turnbull SJ, Campbell EA, Swann IJ. Post-traumatic stress disorder symptoms following a head injury: Does amnesia for the event influence the development of symptoms? *Brain Inj* 2001; 15(9):775–785.

120. Sbordone RJ, Liter JC. Mild traumatic brain injury does not produce post-traumatic stress disorder. *Brain Inj* 1995;9(4): 405–412.

121. Bryant RA. Posttraumatic stress disorder and traumatic brain injury: Can they co-exist? *Clin Psychol Rev* 2001;21(6):931–948.

122. Joseph S, Masterson J. Posttraumatic stress disorder and traumatic brain injury: Are they mutually exclusive? *J Trauma Stress* 1999;12(3):437–453.

123. Grattan LM, Ghahramanlou M. The rehabilitation of neurologically based social disturbance. In Eslinger PJ (ed.), *Neuropsychological Interventions – Clinical Research and Practice.* New York: The Guilford Press, 2002;266–293.

124. Coelho CA, DeRuyter F, Stein M. Treatment efficacy: Cognitive-communicative disorders resulting from traumatic brain injury in adults. *J Speech Hear Res* 1996;39(5):S5–17.

125. Brotherton FA, Thomas LL, Wisotzek IE, Milan MA. Social skills training in the rehabilitation of patients with traumatic closed head injury. *Arch Phys Med Rehabil* 1988;69(10):827–832.

126. Dumont C, Gervais M, Fougeyrollas P, Bertrand R. Toward an explanatory model of social participation for adults with traumatic brain injury. *J Head Trauma Rehabil* 2004;19(6):431–444.

127. McGann W, Werven G, Douglas MM. Social competence and head injury: A practical approach. *Brain Inj* 1997;11(9): 621–628.

128. Seaton JD, David CO. Family role in substance abuse and traumatic brain injury rehabilitation. *J Head Trauma Rehabil* 1990; 5(3):41–46.

129. Ohio Valley Center for Head Injury Prevention and Rehabilitation. *Substance Use and Abuse After Brain Injury: A Programmer's Guide.* Columbus: The Ohio State University, 2003.

130. Ohio Valley Center for Brain Injury Prevention and Rehabilitation. *User's Manual for Faster More Reliable Operation of a Brain After Injury.* Columbus: The Ohio State University, (n.d.).

131. Karol R, Sparadeo F. *Alcohol, Drugs, and Brain Injury.* Loretto, MN: Vinland Center, 1993.

132. Accessible Space, Inc. *The Twelve Steps for Head Injury.* St. Paul, MN: Accessible Space, Inc, 1988.

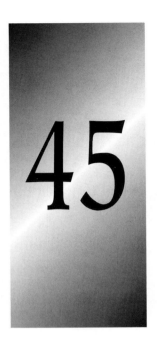

45 Neuropsychiatric Aspects of TBI

Thomas W. McAllister

INTRODUCTION

To the casual observer deficits in speech and language function or ambulation may be the most readily apparent changes after a traumatic brain injury (TBI). However it is often changes in personality and behavior that cause the most distress to survivors and their family/caregivers. Such alterations in the core sense of who the individual is, or who their loved ones believe them to be, can be devastating. Frequently these issues are the rate-limiting step in various rehabilitation settings, interfere with return to work and the ability to achieve the maximum quality of life within the least restrictive environment (1–6). The cost to the nation in care expenditures, lost productivity and family disruption is staggering (7).

Some individuals with mild traumatic brain injury and virtually all individuals who survive moderate and severe TBI are left with significant long-term neurobehavioral sequelae (8–10). The reduction in TBI-associated mortality rates over the last several decades (11) has led to a significant increase in the number of individuals with long-term neurobehavioral disorders related to TBI (5, 12). In addition to the agitation, aggression, and confusion often seen in the acute recovery period, TBI is associated with an increase in the relative risk of developing many psychiatric disorders including mood disorders, psychotic disorders, anxiety disorders, obsessive-compulsive disorder and others (13–16). TBI may well be a critical risk factor in the development of schizophrenia in those with a genetic vulnerability to this illness (17).

Even apart from formal psychiatric disorders, behavioral challenges abound. Syndromes such as apathy, disorders of impulse control and affect, though perhaps not meeting formal criteria for specific psychiatric disorders are a source of excess disability. Environmental and psychosocial factors play key roles in the genesis and maintenance of these neurobehavioral problems, but so does the profile of regional brain injury.

The overarching theme of this chapter is that the assessment and treatment of the neurobehavioral sequelae of TBI follow logically from an understanding of the typical profile of traumatic injury. Thus the relationship of the neuropathophysiology of TBI to the neurobehavioral sequelae commonly encountered by individuals with TBI is outlined. An approach to the evaluation and treatment of these sequelae is suggested.

RELATIONSHIP OF PROFILE OF INJURY TO NEUROBEHAVIORAL SEQUELAE

Our knowledge of the neuropathophysiology of TBI has increased dramatically over the last decade (18). Advances in molecular biology, molecular genetics, neuroimaging, neuropsychology, and other neurodiagnostic techniques make possible a much finer resolution of brain injury profile associated with specific neuropsychiatric sequelae. The neuropathophysiology of TBI is more thoroughly discussed in chapters 6–8 (18). It is important to highlight some features of the neuropathology of TBI in that they help to explain the special vulnerability to neurobehavioral challenges seen in TBI survivors.

In brief, most injuries result from the brain coming into contact with an object (which might include the skull, or some external object) or from rapid acceleration or deceleration of the brain. Contact mechanisms often result in damage to scalp, skull, and brain surface (e.g., contusions, lacerations, intracerebral hematomas) (18). Acceleration/deceleration mechanisms are associated with shear, tensile, and compression forces that have maximum impact on axons and blood vessels resulting in axonal injury, tissue tears, and intracerebral hematomas. Injury from both mechanisms occurs immediately (referred to as primary injury) and may also evolve over time due to a variety of factors including massive release of neurotransmitters with subsequent triggering of excitotoxic injury cascades, and other injury-related factors such as hypoxia, edema, and elevated intracranial pressure (referred to as secondary injury).

With respect to brain tissue, contact mechanisms tend to produce focal injuries such as surface contusions and lacerations. In addition, rapid acceleration or deceleration results in differential motion of the partially tethered brain within the skull. Surface contusions can thus be seen where the swirling motion of the brain comes into contact with bony protuberances on the interior of the skull. Frequent sites of such injury are the anterior temporal poles, the lateral and inferior temporal cortices, the frontal poles, and the orbital frontal cortices. Acceleration and deceleration mechanisms also produce more widespread or diffuse injury ("diffuse axonal injury") to white matter. Particular areas of vulnerability include the corpus callosum, the rostral brainstem, and sub-frontal white matter (18).

Secondary injury appears to occur at least in part from mechanical distortion of the neurons resulting in massive release of neurotransmitters. Although this probably occurs throughout the brain, the excitotoxic cascades and other forms of secondary injury such as hypoxia/ischemia have a disproportionate effect on certain brain regions such as the hippocampus, even in the context of an otherwise fairly mild injury (19).

Thus the typical profile of injury involves a combination of primary injury (occurs at time of application of force) and secondary injury (evolves over time subsequent to the primary injury) as well as a combination of focal and diffuse injury. Furthermore, although the damage may be diffuse or multi-focal, there are certain

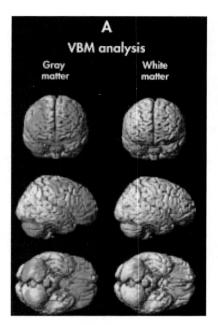

FIGURE 45-1

Results of voxel-bashed morphometry demonstrating areas of reduced gray and white matter density in individuals with TBI compared to controls. Red areas show frontal and temporal abnormalities. From Bigler E. "Structural Imaging." In Silver JM, McAllister TW, Yudofsky SC (eds). *Textbook of Traumatic Brain Injury.* American Psychiatric Press, Washington D.C. 2005, p. 87. Used with permission

brain regions which are highly vulnerable to injury and account for the high rate of challenging behaviors and the increased rates of psychiatric illness that are associated with TBI. These include the frontal cortex and sub-frontal white matter, the deeper midline structures including the basal ganglia, the rostral brainstem, and the temporal lobes including the hippocampi (see figure 45-1).

RELATIONSHIP OF TBI INDUCED NEUROTRANSMITTER CHANGE TO NEUROBEHAVIORAL SEQUELAE

In addition to the profile of regional brain injury described above there is evidence that neurotransmitters with important roles in modulating common neurobehavioral sequelae of TBI (such as regulation of mood, anxiety, motivation, impulse control, and aggression) are altered in TBI. This evidence is briefly summarized to set the stage for rational psychopharmacological interventions for these sequelae.

Catecholaminergic System Changes   There is significant evidence for dysfunction of catecholaminergic systems associated with TBI (20–22). This is important because the catecholamines (epinephrine, norepinephrine, dopamine) play critical roles in a variety of domains important in behavioral homeostasis. Animal studies and observations from the use of catecholamine agonists in clinical practice suggest that epinephrine and norepinephrine play important roles in arousal, cognition, reward behavior, and mood regulation (23–25). Deficits in central adrenergic tone and thus associated with deficits in arousal, attention, memory, motivated behavior (apathy), and mood regulation. Dopaminergic tone and proper dopamine signaling are particularly important in the modulation of motivated behavior, attention, and working memory (see (22, 26, 27) for reviews).

As noted there is evidence of disruption of catecholaminergic homeostasis after injury. TBI results in activation of the sympathoadrenomedullary axis with subsequent alterations in hemodynamic parameters and cardiopulmonary function. Plasma norepinephrine (NE) levels are elevated after TBI and this elevation correlates with injury severity indicators (28). Circulating levels of dopamine, norepinephrine, and epinephrine may be markers of injury severity and likelihood of recovery (20, 21). Animal models of TBI have also shown a relationship between injury severity, increasing circulating levels of epinephrine and norepinephrine, and secondary complications such as cardiac arrhythmias (29). Transient hypoxia, common in more severe injuries, can result in dramatic releases of hippocampal norepinephrine (30).

Animal studies suggest that alterations in dopamine, norepinephrine, and epinephrine levels can be prolonged after TBI, associated with alterations in catecholaminergic receptors in damaged cortical areas, and can impair catecholaminergic function after trauma (29, 31). Administration of certain catecholaminergic agents may enhance recovery from brain injury (32–34), even after one-time doses (32, 35–37). Conversely, catecholaminergic *antagonists* can slow rate of recovery from certain types of brain injury (38). Some agents that augment catecholaminergic tone reduce the cognitive effects of TBI in animal models. For example Zhu et al. (39) administered L-deprenyl, a selective and irreversible MAO-B inhibitor to rats subjected to combined fluid percussion TBI and entorhinal cortical lesions and found significantly reduced cognitive impairment (Morris water maze performance) compared to the rats treated with vehicle only. There is good evidence that in individuals with TBI, methylphenidate, which augments both the dopaminergic and adrenergic systems, is effective in ameliorating certain cognitive deficits (40). Another study (41) showed significant improvement in executive function tasks with bromocriptine, a dopamine agonist.

Cholinergic System Changes Central cholinergic tone is critical to the modulation of most cognitive and behavioral domains, appearing to facilitate signal to noise ratios. It is of particular importance however with respect to attention and memory (Perry and Perry 2004).

Alterations in central cholinergic tone may also play a role in the genesis of mood disorders, particularly depression (see (42)). Cerebral cholinergic neurons and their ascending projections are vulnerable to trauma (43). Acutely, cholinergic neurons release large amounts of acetylcholine. Subsequently there is evidence for long-term reductions in cerebral acetylcholine levels (44). Sudden release of acetylcholine at the time of injury may contribute to the extent of injury through facilitation of excitotoxic cascades. Cholinergic antagonists can be neuroprotective in models of TBI (see (43) for review). Several studies have shown damage to the nucleus basalis of Meynert, as well as reduced levels of choline acetyl transferase (a marker of cholinergic afferents) in brain regions vulnerable to trauma including temporal cortex, cingulate and posterior parietal regions in humans who died within several weeks of injury (43, 45–47). Post-synaptic muscarinic and nicotinic receptors remained intact (45–47), suggesting cholinergic agonists as a potential point of intervention for cognitive deficits (43).

Serotonergic System Changes Central serotonergic tone is important in the modulation of normal mood states and aggression. Medications that increase serotonergic function are effective antidepressants and anxiolytics, and can reduce the frequency and intensity of aggressive behavior. As with the catecholaminergic and cholinergic systems, the serotones system is activated in TBI with increased levels of serotonin evident in areas of significant tissue damage, and in association with lowered regional cerebral glucose utilization (18, 48–50).

Summary Several cortical regions including frontal cortex, temporal cortex, and hippocampus are particularly vulnerable to TBI. Furthermore sub-cortical white matter, particularly in frontal regions and the corpus callosum, are often damaged. In addition catecholaminergic, cholinergic, and serotonergic systems are vulnerable to disruption acutely and chronically in TBI. This profile of structural and neurochemical injury plays a direct role in the common neurobehavioral sequelae associated with TBI.

CHANGES IN PERSONALITY

Survivors and family/caregivers frequently describe the effects of the injury as "changes in personality". Lifelong patterns of responding to external cues, situations in the environment, and internal drives or motivations, can be significantly altered. This takes two different forms: exaggeration of pre-injury traits, or fundamental changes in response patterns. Within the latter category, careful inspection usually reveals that this can be further parsed into alterations in the frequency or intensity of predictable responses to environmental cues or stimuli, or unpredictable response patterns. Several common clusters of symptoms that characterize the "personality changes" are recognizable.

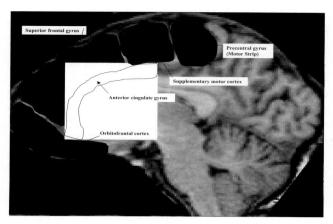

FIGURE 45-2

Mid-saggital view of the brain showing prominent regions associated with executive functions. From McDonald et al. Executive dysfunction following traumatic brain injury: Neural substrates and treatment strategies NeuroRehabilitation 17 (2002) 333–344. Used with permission

Dysexecutive Syndromes   Motivated behavior can be thought of as sets of behavioral responses that are more likely to occur than can be accounted for by chance alone. There are generally three components to motivated behaviors including initiation, procurement, and self-monitoring. These components, along with decision making, and mental flexibility are often referred to as executive functions. In fact much of the altered and distressing changes in behavior or personality after TBI can be subsumed under the rubric of impaired executive function (or "dysexecutive syndromes") (see (51) for review).

Three broad (and somewhat overlapping) domains comprise executive functions:

(i)   *higher order cognitive function* (including mental flexibility, problem solving, set-shifting),

(ii) *social comportment* (including context specific awareness of one's behavior relative to past individual and societal norms, self-monitoring and self-correction), and

(iii) *motivated/ reward-related behavior* (including initiation, sequencing, achieving/consuming).

As noted, these are not fully distinct domains but rather are more interactive and overlapping. This complex relationship is mirrored clinically in the observation that one can see individuals with prominent deficits in one, two, or all three domains to varying degrees. From the clinical standpoint, the prominent challenging behaviors brought to the clinician's attention flow from these domains and can be usefully grouped into the following categories:

(i) Cognitive Syndromes
Cognitive deficits after TBI are covered in greater detail in Chapter 44. It is worth highlighting that initial and

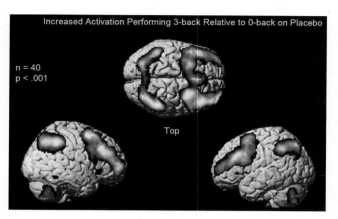

FIGURE 45-3

Activation of working memory regions as shown with functional MRI. The above image shows the mean group image of 40 participants performing a WM task (3-back). Note extensive yet selective bifrontal, biparietal, and cerebellar activation associated with the task

persistent cognitive deficits are the most common complaints after traumatic brain injury (TBI) (52, 53) and the major hindrance to normalization in the areas of independent living, social re-adaptation, family life, and vocational endeavors (54, 55). There are several predictable areas of impairment including short-term memory, speed of information processing, and attention (56–66). Obviously these are not completely independent domains, and in fact the typical profile of attention and memory deficits could be reasonably subsumed under the construct of working memory (WM), the ability to hold information in mind and manipulate that information in light of incoming information. Much progress has been made defining the circuitry and neurochemistry of WM (see McAllister et al. 2004 for review; (26, 67–69) and suggests that (1) the parietal cortices (70–73), (2) the frontal speech areas such as Broca's area (inferior frontal gyrus) and the supplemental motor areas, and (3) the prefrontal area (74, 75) play major roles in WM function. The conceptualization of WM as a core deficit in TBI may have particular significance in that the brain regions implicated in WM circuitry are the same regions that are vulnerable to injury in the typical TBI.

(ii) Social Comportment
Impulsivity   One of the more common concerns of patients and family/caregivers alike is that survivors have difficulty with impulse control. This can be manifested in verbal utterances, physical actions, snap decisions, and poor judgment flowing from the failure to fully consider the implications of a given action. This is closely related to the concept of stimulus boundedness in which the individual responds to the most salient cue in the environment or attaches exaggerated salience to a particular cue

without regard to previously determined foci of attention or priorities.

Irritability Another very common concern of patients and family/caregivers pertains to the modulation of anger. Survivors describe themselves as more irritable or more easily angered. Although a particular cue might be perceived as a legitimate aggravation of some sort, the response is characteristically out of proportion to the precipitating stimulus. Responses can range from verbal outbursts to dangerous aggressive and assaultive behavior. This modulatory deficit differs in intensity, onset, and duration from the pre-injury pattern for any given individual.

Affective Instability Survivors and family/caregivers frequently describe a change in affective stability characterized by exaggerated displays of emotional expression which seem out of proportion to both the precipitating stimulus and the injured individual's previous range of response to similar stimuli. Cues or events that previously might have elicited momentary sadness may now precipitate weeping or crying. Events which in the past might have provoked a frown or reply laced with irritation now result in loud angry verbal outbursts associated with marked sympathetic arousal. The hallmarks of this instability typically include a paroxysmal onset, brief duration, and an exaggerated intensity of response out of proportion to the precipitating stimulus. This phenomenon is common to a variety of disorders affecting the CNS and has been given a variety of terms including pathological affect, affective lability, pseudobulbar affect, and affective incontinence (see (76) for review).

Awareness Deficits The burden of the above changes in personality and behavior is often complicated by a surprising and at times devastating lack of awareness of these changes (see (77, 78) for reviews). The injured individual may be unable to appreciate that their behavior is different since the injury, in stark contrast to family/caregivers and providers who may be painfully aware that the injured individual has changed in fundamental ways and can often provide detailed lists of these changes.

Alternatively an individual with TBI may have a vague sense that he or she is different or "not who I used to be" and yet struggle to define the specific ways in which their behavior or personality differs from prior to the injury. Awareness is not a unitary concept (79) and thus it is important to characterize the nature and extent to which an individual suffers from this problem. Of particular interest to this discussion is that individuals with TBI are less likely to be aware of changes in behavior and executive function than changes in more concrete domains such as motor function (e.g., (80)). Furthermore the degree of awareness has been found to correlate with functional and vocational outcome in many (81–84) though not all studies (85).

As is the case with disorders of affective stability, problems with awareness of deficits are not unique to individuals with TBI but rather occur in a broad range of disorders of the CNS including severe and persistent mental disorders such as schizophrenia (78). The literature suggests that lack of awareness of illness is not simply a function of global cognitive deficits but perhaps is more related to frontal-executive dysfunction (86–88, 89–92). Studies of the neuranotomical correlates of illness awareness deficits in these disorders, and in overlapping syndromes such as anosagnosia suggest that injury to certain brain regions carries a heightened vulnerability to awareness deficits (78). Stuss (93, 94) suggests that frontal systems generate self-awareness, self-reflectiveness, and self-monitoring. Other work has suggested that lack of awareness in schizophrenia is associated with selective structural brain changes, including smaller brain size and selective atrophy of certain subregions of the frontal lobes (77, 95). Furthermore, using a self-reflective task while undergoing functional MRI, Flashman et al. have been able to show very high correlations of degree of unawareness with frontal activation in individuals with schizophrenia (78). Because frontal systems also play a critical role in the modulation of key social skills and behaviors (e.g., initiation, motivation, problem solving, and affective modulation), frontal lobe damage can affect the ability to understand the impact that deficits have on day-to-day function and how to apply that knowledge to a current situation. In individuals with TBI, this dimension is frequently the focus of family/caregiver concern yet is often not recognized by individuals with TBI (5, 96–100). Even when the individual admits to some difficulties, he or she is often unable to predict the implications of these deficits in current or future social situations.

(iii) Disorders of Motivation

Apathy The underlying deficit associated with apathy is in the realm of motivated behavior (101). Although not as overtly disturbing or alarming as some of the other changes in personality described above, it can be disturbing to family/caregivers, and is frequently the reason that injured individuals fail to progress in rehabilitation programs. Furthermore it is often misinterpreted as either laziness or depression and may be somewhat paradoxically linked to aggression when for example attempts to engage the individual in activities in which they have little interest can precipitate assaultive behavior (25).

Apathy is quite common after TBI. Kant et al. (102) found that apathy (mixed with depression) occurred in 60% of their sample of individuals with TBI. Andersson et al. (103) found that almost half of their sample of individuals with TBI had significant degrees of apathy. Deficits in motivated behavior can occur in association with injury to the circuitry of "reward" which includes behavior specific (thirst, sex, hunger) hypothalamic centers (25, 104), and a more general reward system linking the forebrain to the midbrain. Key nodal points in this circuitry include the amygdala, hippocampus, caudate, entorhinal and cingulate cortices, the ventral tegmental area and the medial forebrain bundle. Catecholaminergic systems, particularly the mesolimbic dopaminergic system appear to play critical roles in the modulation of the reward system (see (25, 104) for reviews).

RELATIONSHIP OF PROFILE OF INJURY TO PERSONALITY CHANGES

A full discussion of the neuroanatomical substrates of the above behaviors is beyond the scope of this chapter. However the link between the injury profile in a typical TBI and some of these behaviors is fairly simply understood.

Five major frontal-subcortical circuits have been identified, one orchestrating primarily motor function, one primarily oculomotor function, and three that have significant roles in non-motor forms of behavior (see (105, 106) for reviews). Each of the latter three circuits can affect motivated behavior, though in somewhat different ways. Each circuit is named for its site of origin in the frontal cortex (e.g. the dorsolateral frontal-subcortical circuit, the orbitofrontal-subcortical circuit, and the anterior cingulate-subcortical circuit) (see Figure 45-4). Each circuit follows a similar path starting from the site of origin in the frontal cortex projecting to the striatum, from there to the globus pallidus, then to the thalamus and back to the frontal cortex. Each circuit is thought to be a more or less closed loop with some additional input

from other functionally related brain regions. The circuits differ from each other with respect to exact pathways through the key nodal points. Thus for example the dorsolateral frontal circuit projects to the dorsal caudate, the orbitofrontal circuit to the ventral caudate, and the anterior cingulate to the medial striatum/nucleus accumbens respectively. Similar topographic differences can be traced through the global pallidus and the thalamus as well.

Examination of the brain regions vulnerable to injury in the typical TBI and the neuroanatomical substrate of core cognitive and behavioral domains (executive functions, social comportment, motivation) suggests why these areas are so often a source of distress to survivors and their family/caregivers after TBI. The frontal-subcortical circuits responsible for these critical domains of higher intellectual function and empathic, motivated, nuanced human behavior are highly vulnerable to injury in the typical TBI. Damage to the dorsolateral prefrontal cortex and its circuitry impairs executive functions such as working memory, decision making, problem solving and mental flexibility.

Damage to the orbitofrontal cortex and related nodal points impairs intuitive, reflexive, social behaviors and the capacity to self-monitor and self-correct in real time within a social context.

Damage to anterior cingulate and related circuitry impairs motivated and reward-related behaviors. Injury to medial temporal regions further impairs other aspects of memory and the smooth integration of emotional memory with current experience and real-time assessment of stimulus salience. In short the profile of injury vulnerability predicts the neuropsychiatric sequelae of injury (see Figure 45-5).

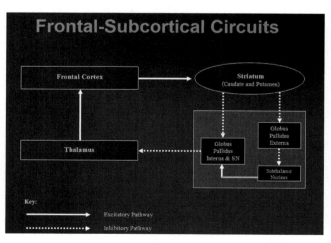

FIGURE 45-4

Outline of key nodal points in the five major frontal-subcortical circuits. Adapted from Arciniegas D, Beresford T. *Principles of Neuropsychiatry: An Introductory Approach,* Cambridge University, 2001. Cambridge, UK. p. 62. Used with permission

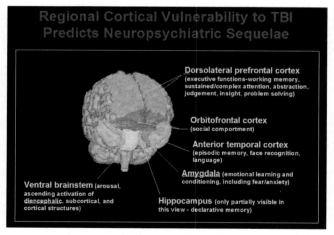

FIGURE 45-5

Relationship of brain regions vulnerable in typical TBI to predictable neurobehavioral sequelae. Adapted from Arciniegas D, Beresford T. *Principles of Neuropsychiatry: An Introductory Approach,* Cambridge University, 2001. Cambridge, UK. p. 370. Used with permission

This principle then should be the foundation on which a good neuropsychiatric evaluation is based. The process of elucidating the profile of injury, the profile of current signs and symptoms, and mapping the latter onto the former to assess goodness of fit is the work of the neuropsychiatric evaluation. Signs and symptoms which are not accounted for by the profile of injury must be explained on another basis or the profile of injury should be re-assessed. The clinical picture should make sense in the context of the brain damage.

RELATIONSHIP OF TBI TO PSYCHIATRIC DISORDERS

In addition to the changes in cognition, behavior, and personality described above, a significant body of evidence suggests that TBI results in an increased relative risk of developing psychiatric disorders including mood and anxiety disorders, and psychotic syndromes (13, 15, 16, 107) (see Table 45-1). For example Koponen et al. (16) studied 60 individuals 30 years after their TBI and found that almost half (48%) developed a new Axis I psychiatric disorder after their injury. The most common diagnoses were depression, substance abuse, and anxiety disorders. Rates of lifetime and current depression (26%, 10%), panic disorder (8%, 6%), and psychotic disorders (8%, 8%), were significantly higher than base rates found in the Epidemiologic Catchment Area (ECA) study (108).

Hibbard et al. (15) studied 100 adults on average, 8 years after TBI. A significant number of individuals had Axis 1 disorders prior to injury. After TBI, the most frequent Axis I diagnoses were major depression and anxiety disorders (ie, PTSD, OCD, and panic disorder).

Almost half (44%) of individuals had two or more disorders. More recently (109) this group reported a longitudinal study of 188 individuals enrolled within four years of injury and assessed at yearly intervals on at least two occasions. Once again they found elevated rates of psychiatric disorders prior to injury. Subsequent to TBI, there were increased rates of depression, PTSD, and other anxiety disorders. This was particularly true of those with pre-injury psychiatric disorders. Furthermore, the rates were greatest at the initial assessment point after injury and stabilized or decreased over time (see Table 45-2). Van Reekum et al. (13) carefully reviewed the literature on the relationship of TBI to a variety of psychiatric disorders and using the ECA data for baseline rates concluded that TBI was associated with an increase in the relative risk for several psychiatric disorders (see Table 45-1).

Fann et al. (110) recently published findings on a cohort study of the medical records of about 1,000 HMO members who sustained a TBI classified as either mild (LOC <1hr) or moderate to severe, and followed for three years. Compared to non-injured controls, the individuals with TBI had increased indicators of psychiatric illness, especially in the first year after injury, and there was some evidence of a biologic grandient (49% in the moderate-severe group, 34% in the mild group, 18% in the non-injured comparison group). In injured individuals without history of psychiatric illness the Odds Ratio of developing psychiatric illness in the first 6 months was 4.0 in the moderate-severe group. Wei et al. (111) in a study of Medicaid beneficiaries in four states found that 18% of ~3,600 individuals diagnosed with TBI suffered severe mental illness, and another 16.5% had other mental disorders. Those with mental illness had significantly higher expenditures.

TABLE 45-1
TBI and Psychiatric Disorders

DISORDER	TOTAL N (# STUDIES)	MAX DURATION OF FOLLOW-UP (YRS)	# WITH DISORDER	% WITH DISORDER	RELATIVE RISK
Depression	653(8)	7.5	289	44	7.5
Bipolar Affective Disorder	354(5)	7.5	15	4.2	5.3
Gen. Anxiety Dis	398(5)	7.5	36	9.1	2.3
OCD	282(3)	7.5	18	6.4	2.6
Panic Dis	282(3)	7.5	26	9.2	5.8
PTSD	441(6)	7.5	62	14.1	1.8

From van Reekum et al. Can traumatic brain injury cause psychiatric disorders? *J Neuropsychiatry* 12:316–327, 2000. Used with permission.

TABLE 45-2
Prevalence (%) of Axis I Disorders at All Time Points (109)

DIAGNOSIS	COMMUNITY BASE RATES*	PRE-TBI (N=188)	T1 (N=188)	T2 (N=188)	T3 (N=188)
Depression†	6	20	35	24	21
Substance abuse‡	17	32	14	10	17
PTSD	8	10	30	18	21
Other anxiety‖	2–13	16	27	19	9
Any other Axis I¶	–	5	9	5	0

From Ashman et al. Psychiatric challenges in the First 6 Years after Traumatic Brain Injury: Cross-Sequential Analyses of Axis I Disorders. *Arch Physical Medicine and Rehabilitation* 85:S36–42, 2004.
*Bourdon et al.
†Includes major depression, depression not otherwise specified, and dysthymia.
‡Includes alcohol abuse, alcohol dependence, drug abuse, and drug dependence.
‖Includes obsessive-compulsive disorders (OCD), panic, phobias, and generalized anxiety disorder (GAD).
¶Excludes depression disorders, substance abuse and dependency, PTSD, OCD, panic, phobias, and GAD.

Diagnostic and Labeling Issues

It is important to address several issues with respect to the above studies and the question of psychiatric disorders in general after TBI.

Symptoms vs. Disorder   As with any potentially disabling condition, individuals with TBI report a variety of symptoms in a variety of domains (discouragement, frustration, fatigue, anxiety etc). Not all of these symptoms will rise to the level of a disorder. However symptoms that are consistent and sustained over time (usually weeks), and that are of sufficient severity to interfere with social or occupational function or quality of life, are legitimately considered disorders. In the studies cited above, standardized criteria encompassing those principles were used and thus argue strongly that TBI acts as a gateway to the development of many psychiatric disorders. The consistent observation that individuals who sustain a TBI have higher base rates of psychopathology prior to injury suggests that there is a reciprocal interaction: psychopathology predisposes to TBI, and TBI in turn predisposes the individual to develop psychiatric disorders.

Labeling Issues   Many individuals resist the idea that they have an illness. This is not unique to individuals with TBI, but rather reflects a general dislike of being labeled as having a disease. There is an even greater resistance to seeing oneself as having a psychiatric illness. Again this is equally true of injured and non-injured populations. However effective treatment can follow appropriate diagnosis. To avoid a diagnosis because of a societal or individual resistance to it is not in the interest of the individual suffering with the symptoms.

Use of Diagnostic and Statistical Manual of Mental Disorders (DSM) Nomenclature   As with most diagnostic schemes the DSM approach has strengths and weaknesses. Its reliance on standardized phenomenological criteria has been helpful, particularly when sorting out idiopathic psychiatric disorders. It is less helpful when approaching diagnosis in neuropsychiatric populations, including those with TBI. There are several reasons for this. In the DSM, psychiatric disorders in the context of neurological illness can be coded as "diagnosis" x "secondary to a general medical condition". The use of the modifier "secondary to a general medical condition" implies that it is possible to accurately assess causality when for example a depressive syndrome follows a TBI by some time interval. Although this may be true, (and probably often is the case), proof is lacking and thus such a label reflects the impression or bias of the clinician.

The terms used to describe the changes in behavior and personality flowing out of damage to the various frontal-subcortical circuits described above are "personality change secondary to . . .". Although this represents a significant improvement over "organic personality disorder" (DSM III), it does not do justice to the subtle and nuanced alterations present after a brain injury.

Perhaps most importantly the current schema does not recognize or allow for the alteration of syndromic presentations by brain injury. The question of how to diagnose depression in a non-verbal individual for example is not addressed in the DSM. The idea that depression can be expressed in other ways is not reflected directly in the menu of symptom options. For example so called "depressive equivalents" must be inferred by creative clinicians. Thus the diagnostic schema requires further refinement that hopefully will be reflected in future editions of the DSM. Despite these limitations it is helpful to review what is known about the association of TBI and certain psychiatric disorders.

MOOD DISORDERS

Depression   Depression after brain injury is common, with estimates that 25–60% of individuals with TBI experience a depressive episode (DSM-IV criteria) within 8 years of injury (15, 112). These rates do not take into account individuals who have depressive symptoms but who fail to meet DSM-IV diagnostic criteria. It is also important to note that depression is associated with poorer cognitive, social, and functional outcome (112, 113) and can act as an amplifier of other neurobehavioral challenges including anxiety and aggression (7, 15, 112). The increased rate of depression and associated symptoms in TBI compared to other injuries suggests that CNS trauma and/or factors in plasticity/repair may play a role in the genesis of mood disorders.

Neural Circuitry of Depression Over the last decade substantial progress has been made in outlining the brain regions and related circuitry of mood regulation (see (114–116)), and not surprisingly they overlap with the areas vulnerable to the typical TBI. A thorough review of this topic is well beyond the scope of this chapter but several points are worth noting. Much of the insights come from functional imaging studies (see Refs. 114, 117 for thorough discussion) that have indicated metabolic abnormalities in dorsolateral prefrontal cortex (DLPFC) and anterior cingulate (reduced activity), and ventrolateral prefrontal cortex (increased activity) associated with depression. Although there is some variability of findings, other regions including temporal lobe and basal ganglia have also been found to have reduced activity (114).

A second group of studies has explored induced changes in mood state in depressed patients before and after manipulations such as sleep deprivation and tryptophan depletion, or before and after induced sadness in healthy individuals. The weight of evidence from these studies suggests that interventions leading to a less depressed state are associated with increased activity in DLPFC and anterior cingulate, and decreased activity in ventrolateral prefrontal cortex – largely consistent with the resting baseline studies (see (114)). Taken together this evidence suggests that the two frontal-striatal-thalamo-cortical circuits originating in orbitofrontal and dorsolateral prefrontal cortex function abnormally in depression. It may be that the orbitofrontal circuit with its limbic connections is the substrate of disordered emotional processing and vegetative symptoms common in depression, whereas dysfunction in the dorsolateral circuit may result in the cognitive deficits associated with depression (114, 116, 117).

Neurochemistry of Depression Several neurotransmitter systems play key roles in normal mood regulation and depression. Evidence of monoamine dysfunction in depression comes from the putative mechanisms of action of antidepressant compounds, most of which increase release, block re-uptake, or interfere with metabolism of norepinephrine, serotonin, or dopamine (see (118) for recent review). Interventions that reduce central monoaminergic tone (for example the

medication reserpine) are associated with an increased rate of depression. However, it is clear that a simple "imbalance of monoamines" explanation is inadequate. Several drugs (e.g., CNS stimulants) increase release of monoamines but are poor antidepressants. The effects of antidepressant compounds on monoamine transmitters can be demonstrated within hours, yet the mood altering effects take several weeks and not all depressed individuals respond equally to the same antidepressant. Thus, much remains to be learned.

An alternative theory of the genesis of depression posits that there is an imbalance of cholinergic and adrenergic tone with a relative cholinergic hyperactivity (see (42)). There are several reasons to postulate a role for cholinergic systems in mood regulation. Relative to healthy controls, depressed patients have a variety of exaggerated physiological responses to cholinergic agonists. The cholinergic agonists arecoline and physostigmine induce dysphoria in normals and can worsen depressive symptoms in individuals with mood disorders (42). The majority of antidepressants, including the tricyclics and SSRIs, have anticholinergic properties. Recent magnetic resonance spectroscopy (MRS) studies suggest that there may be elevated levels of the acetylcholine precursor choline in orbitofrontal cortex and other brain regions of individuals with depression (119, 120). The nicotinic receptor blocker mecamylamine has also recently been shown to have some antidepressant properties (42, 121).

It is important to note that antidepressants can effect neural response to injury and repair. For example several recent reports have suggested that antidepressants may have neurotrophic effects including facilitating regeneration of catecholamine terminals in cortical and hippocampal regions (42, 122, 123).

Treatment With respect to treatment of depression after TBI, there is a lack of good data. A brief selective review of this literature is provided (see Silver and Arciniegas, Chapter 55 for detailed review). Several papers address the use of tricyclic antidepressants although this is a relatively old literature and the results are somewhat conflicting. Wroblewski and colleagues (124) reported a small randomized, placebo-controlled prospective study, in which 10 individuals with severe TBI and depression were given placebo and desipramine in a crossover fashion. Desipramine was found to be more effective than placebo. Dinan and Mobayed (125) in a cohort study of 13 patients with mild TBI matched with 13 depressed patients without brain injury found amitriptyline to be less effective in the TBI group. Saran (126) using amitriptyline in an open label design found less reduction in depression scores in a mild TBI group than a non-injured group. Significant methodological issues limit the strength of the evidence from all three of the above studies.

A large number of case series and case reports address the treatment of depression after TBI with a variety of other agents. However methodological problems such as the use of mixed populations (e.g. stroke, penetrating brain injury, TBI, epilepsy) (127, 128), absence of clear diagnostic criteria (127, 129–131), absence of validated outcome measures (129, 130, 131–133), or the use of more than one intervention at a time, limit the conclusions that can be drawn from many of these reports.

Several similar reports have addressed the use of selective serotonin re-uptake inhibitors in this population, but again basic methodological flaws, and small numbers make it difficult to draw conclusions from these papers.

Overall several important points can be made with respect to depression after TBI. The brain regions and circuitry implicated in the genesis of depression overlap to a great extent with those regions at greatest risk for damage in the typical TBI. Furthermore, the major neurotransmitter systems felt to play key modulatory roles in the regulation of mood and affect are the same as those known to be altered by TBI (ie adrenergic, dopaminergic, cholinergic, and serotonergic systems). When one considers the additional roles of stress, loss, social isolation, and other common psychosocial insults common in TBI, it is surprising that the frequency of depression following TBI is not higher.

MANIC SYNDROMES

Mania is characterized by episodes of sustained (longer than one week) changes in mood (euphoria or irritability) and increased psychomotor activity. It may be associated with increased energy, decreased need for sleep, and a penchant for dangerous behavior (reckless activities, increased spending, increased sexual activity). Some manic episodes can be accompanied by psychotic symptoms such as grandiose delusions or thought process disturbances such as loosened associations or flight of ideas. Mania is a well-described complication of many disorders of the CNS including TBI (134, 135). Robinson et al. (134) found 6 of 66 (9%) carefully characterized TBI patients developed manic episodes. In these patients mania was not associated with severity of injury, post-traumatic epilepsy, family or past personal history of mania. It was associated with lesions in the temporal and orbitofrontal cortices. Shukla et al. (136) reported on 20 individuals with TBI and mania and found that nine of their patients had epileptogenic activity on EEG. Irritable mood not euphoria was more commonly observed. Van Reekum et al. (13) reviewed the literature and suggested that TBI was associated with a five-fold increase in relative risk of developing bipolar disorder relative to base rates in the population. The role of genetic loading in the etiology of mania after TBI is not clear. For example Malaspina et al. (17) did not find an increase in exposure to TBI in her large bipolar pedigree study.

A variety of other small series and case reports suggest that mania can be seen in association with all injury severities including some cases with brief or no documented loss of consciousness (133, 137–139). The full array of phenomenologic variants of mania can be seen including a bipolar course, rapid cycling, and triggering of manic episodes by antidepressant medications (132, 136, 138, 140, 141).

It is difficult to determine the exact role that profile of injury plays in mania as the underlying circuitry of this disorder is less well established than that for depression. In mania occurring after CNS disorders (not solely TBI) there is a marked preponderance of right fronto-temporal and basal ganglia injury (5, 134, 142).

Treatment   Although there are many case reports and small series of TBI-related manic syndromes in the literature there are no systematic studies of this issue that one can use to inform treatment. Even the case series and case reports available do not give sufficient data to allow firm conclusions about treatment response. However the impression from this literature and clinical experience suggests that the same agents used in idiopathic bipolar disorder can be effective in TBI-related manic episodes. Thus the usual approach is to control acute manic episodes with an antipsychotic agent such as risperidone, olanzapine, or haloperidol while starting an anticycling agent such as valproic acid or lithium for longer-term prophylaxis of the illness.

PSYCHOTIC SYNDROMES

The term psychosis refers to a cluster of symptoms, which includes problems in both thought content and thought process. Delusions and hallucinations typically characterize disorders of thought content. Alterations in the structure and flow of speech and language such as loosening of associations, flight of ideas, thought blocking, and production of nonsense words or neologisms, are characteristic of disordered thought process. Psychosis is often equated with schizophrenia, but is more accurately viewed as a syndromic manifestation of many neuropsychiatric conditions, including depression, bipolar affective disorder, delirium, and dementia, to name a few.

Although psychosis is a relatively rare complication of TBI, it does occur more frequently than in the general population. It is a good example of a low frequency, high impact complication of TBI, causing enormous distress to individuals and their caregivers. There are several contexts in which psychotic syndromes following TBI can occur including during the period of post-traumatic amnesia, as a complication of post-traumatic epilepsy, in the context of TBI-related mood disorders, or associated with a chronic, schizophrenia-like syndrome. It is necessary to distinguish these different contexts, in so far as it is possible, to guide appropriate interventions (143, 144).

Relatively few studies directly address the association and causal connections between TBI and psychosis. Davison and Bagley (145) summarized the results of eight long-term (15 to 20 years) follow-up studies of individuals with brain injuries published between 1917 and 1960. Across these studies, the percentage of TBI patients developing a schizophrenia-like psychosis varies from 0.7% to 9.8%, suggesting an observed incidence of schizophrenia-like psychosis that is 2 to 3 times greater than that expected by chance in the TBI population. Van Reekum et al. (13) reviewed the literature and found a more modest relative risk associated with TBI. The role of genetic vulnerability is also not clear. Davison and Bagley found no evidence of increased genetic loading for schizophrenia in TBI patients who developed psychotic symptoms. Malaspina and colleagues (17) however studied 1830 individuals who were first-degree relatives of people with schizophrenia or bipolar disorder, looking for a relationship between these illnesses and TBI. Compared to other first-degree relatives with similar genetic vulnerabilities, those with a history of TBI were at significantly greater risk to develop schizophrenia. The authors propose a synergistic effect between TBI and genetic risk in families with two or more members with schizophrenia.

Based on the studies to date, it seems reasonable to conclude that psychotic disorders do occur in individuals with a TBI at rates greater than in the non-injured population. The more severe the injury, the greater is the likelihood of psychosis. Psychotic syndromes may occur soon after the TBI, or after a delay of months to many years (see Table 45-3). In cases with delayed onset, the injury is almost certainly not the only etiologic factor, although it is interesting to note the high rate of previous TBI in patients with schizophrenia. Furthermore, it appears that TBI can interact with genetic vulnerability

to greatly increase the risk of developing illnesses such as schizophrenia.

As noted, psychotic symptoms can occur in the context of a seizure disorder, a relatively common complication of TBI. A relationship between seizures and mental disorders, particularly psychotic syndromes, has been commented on for centuries (146) and is the subject of a somewhat confusing literature. In a comprehensive review of studies looking at the prevalence of psychosis in epileptic populations, McKenna and colleagues (147) found prevalence rates ranging from 0% to 27% in small clinic-based studies and rates of 2.8% and 3.2% in larger surveys of patients attending epilepsy clinics. Two large-scale Scandinavian community surveys of individuals with epilepsy found prevalence rates for psychosis of 2% (148) and 7.1% (149), both of which are higher than prevalence rates in individuals without epilepsy.

Epileptic psychosis is overwhelmingly associated with complex partial seizures, occurring four to 12 times more frequently in temporal lobe epilepsy than in other types of epilepsy. Psychotic syndromes are most likely to occur in conjunction with left-sided temporal lobe lesions (150–153). This is particularly the case for schizophrenia-like syndromes and paranoid syndrome.

Psychotic syndromes associated with posttraumatic epilepsy can occur predominantly in the peri-ictal period (either during seizures or in the immediate post-ictal period), or inter-ictally, in which case the psychotic symptoms are more commonly chronic rather than episodic (154). Most commonly seen is a post-ictal acute confusional state characterized by generalized confusion, fluctuating sensorium, agitation, hallucinations, and delusions, which is similar to the posttraumatic delirium described above. This condition generally resolves within a few hours of the seizure, although rarely it may persist for several days.

Less commonly psychotic symptoms occur as part of the seizure ictus. The clinical picture is one of paroxysmal onset of psychotic symptoms which can include auditory, visual or somatosensory hallucinations, delusions

TABLE 45-3
Interval of Injury to Development of Psychosis in Selected Studies

STUDY	SAMPLE	LATENCY
Achte et al. 1969, 1991. (Psychopath 24:309–315)	WWII veterans, mainly penetrating TBI	2 days to 48 yrs, 42% occurring 10 yrs after
Fujii and Ahmed, 1996 (Neuropsychiatry, Neurospych, Beh Neurol. 9:133–138)	State hospital sample	3 mos – 19 yrs, mean of 5.9 yrs
Feinstein and Ron 1998 (J Neuropsychiatry 10:448–452)	44 subjects with psychosis after neurological disorders	0–54 yrs, mean of 11.7 yrs

(often paranoid, grandiose or religious), as well as alterations in thought process (loosened associations, flight of ideas, cognitive disorganization). As with other seizure phenomena, these symptoms usually recede quickly (over several minutes) unless they are associated with repetitive seizures of a more prolonged inter-ictal psychotic syndrome. The most useful clue clinically is the time course of the psychotic symptoms, characterized by the paroxysmal onset, rapid resolution (most commonly), and relative absence of such symptoms in between events (155).

Relationship of Profile of Injury to Psychosis A full discussion of the neuroanatomical substrate of schizophrenia and psychotic symptoms is not possible. However a brief overview is instructive. No single brain region has been identified as the site or cause of schizophrenia, rather several brain regions appear to play important roles in the genesis and phenomenology of this disorder. These regions overlap with those vulnerable to injury in the typical TBI. Computed axial tomography (CT) scan and magnetic resonance imaging (MRI) studies of patients with schizophrenia have identified enlarged lateral and third ventricles (156, 157), reduced frontal and temporal lobe volumes (158), reduced thalamic volumes (159), and enlargement of basal ganglia, particularly the caudate and globus pallidus (160–162). Functional imaging studies have also focused on frontal, temporolimbic, and basal ganglia areas. Positron-emission tomography (PET) studies of drug-free schizophrenics have suggested reduced metabolism in the cingulate gyrus and hippocampus, (163, 164) and reduced metabolism in the basal ganglia (165, 166). Some schizophrenic patients have abnormal patterns of frontal activation when engaged in cognitive tasks that require frontal function (163, 166).

Recent neuropathological studies of patients with schizophrenia have suggested abnormalities in regions of the dorsolateral pre-frontal cortex and the hippocampus. Selemon and colleagues (167) reported prefrontal (Brodmann's area 9), as well as more widespread increased neuronal density in association with reduced cortical thickness. They thought this finding might be related to reduction of neuropil. Akbarian and colleagues (168, 169) reported abnormal distribution of nicotinamide adenine dinucleotide phosphate diaphorase-expressing neurons in both dorsolateral prefrontal cortex and temporal cortex. They postulated that these findings were consistent with altered (incomplete) migration of this population of neurons. Furthermore, these cells participate in subsequent guidance of other migrating neurons, pruning, programmed cell death, and overall modulation of proper "connectivity."

The temporal lobes, particularly the left temporal lobe and the hippocampal formation appear to play a role in auditory hallucinations and in delusions of passivity and control. Dysfunction of the prefrontal cortex is also implicated in delusion formation. It is not surprising then

that psychotic syndromes occur with increased frequency in patients after a TBI. There is significant overlap between the regions implicated in the etiology of schizophrenia and its prominent symptoms, and those regions which are commonly affected in TBI, including the frontal lobes (both dorsolateral cortex and orbitofrontal cortex), temporal lobes, basal ganglia, and thalamus. In some respects, it is surprising that psychotic syndromes are not seen more commonly after TBI.

Treatment Issues A critical first step in the evaluation and treatment of psychotic symptoms is making an accurate diagnosis and determining the etiology of the psychotic symptoms. This necessitates distinguishing psychotic symptoms from other brain injury-related symptoms such as confabulation, misidentification syndromes, and delusions (170). Once the presence of psychotic symptoms has been clearly established, a diligent search for underlying causes is necessary. A history of any earlier psychiatric illness must be aggressively sought. A positive family history of psychiatric illness can give valuable clues about the patient's diagnosis. It is important to determine whether the psychotic symptoms are related to a posttraumatic seizure disorder, a mood disorder (either depression or mania with psychotic features), concurrent or past substance abuse, or a manifestation of a schizophrenialike disorder.

Treatment approaches follow logically from this differential diagnosis. Seizure-related symptoms are best managed with adjustment of the anticonvulsant regimen or consideration of surgical approaches in refractory cases. Mood disorders are best treated with antidepressants or anti-cycling agents (12, 171–173). Single agents should be tried initially, but a combination of drugs may be necessary. Antipsychotic agents may be needed in the initial phases of treatment of a mood disorder with psychotic features, but these should be tapered and discontinued once the mood disturbance has been successfully treated. Treatment of associated substance abuse can be very difficult, but must be attempted (174).

Should these initial treatments efforts fail, or when a psychotic syndrome is the primary psychopathology (i.e., the patient appears to have a schizophrenia-like disorder), then antipsychotic agents must be used. There are several potential problems with the use of these agents. It is therefore critical that they be used sparingly and for the treatment of true psychotic symptoms, not for the management of nonspecific agitation. Problems with motor function, gait, arousal, and speed of information processing are common in brain-injured patients and can be exacerbated by the sedation, psychomotor slowing, parkinsonism, and anticholinergic side effects associated with the common antipsychotic agents. TBI may also increase the likelihood of tardive dyskinesia (175). Clinicians often report this increased sensitivity to side effects of psychotropics, although there is little systematic evidence to confirm these observations (5, 12, 171, 173, 176). It is prudent to start with one third to one half of the usual starting doses and to lengthen the interval between dosage increases. Newburn (177) reviewed the pharmacotherapy of psychiatric disorders associated with TBI, advising caution with drugs having prominent anticholinergic, antihistaminic, or antidopaminergic effects because of risk of adverse effects on cognition. Also, traditional antipsychotic drugs should be cautiously used because they might decrease synaptic plasticity.

Atypical Antipsychotics Atypical antipsychotic drugs have emerged as first line drugs for treatment of psychotic disorders. They are also being used with increasing frequency to treat ill-defined anxiety syndromes and mood disorders. Unless there is evidence that psychotic signs and symptoms are a direct result of some other treatable condition, such as cerebral dysrhythmia, one of these drugs should be employed. Six such drugs are currently available: clozapine, risperidone, olanzapine, quetiapine, aripiprazole, and ziprasidone. These drugs offer two main advantages over conventional neuroleptic drugs. They have greater efficacy, especially in decreasing negative as well as positive symptoms of schizophrenia, and in decreasing agitation and aggression. The latter effect can be of particular benefit in some individuals with TBI. Most importantly, the atypical antipsychotics carry significantly less risk of causing extrapyramidal symptoms (EPS) and tardive dyskinesia. Like all drugs with antipsychotic activity, the atypicals have some blocking effect on dopamine-2 (D_2) receptors, but proportionally less so than conventional drugs. The atypical class also shows a preference for limbic D_2 receptors with minimal nigrostriatal effects, and thus less risk of EPS. Affinity for $5\text{-}HT_{2A}$ receptors is thought to also contribute to decreased EPS risk (178).

Clozapine is considered the most potent and effective of the atypical antipsychotic agents. However, it is also associated with the most side effects, including a heightened risk of agranulocytosis. Clozapine also has the most prominent anticholinergic effects and can cause orthostatic hypotension (178, 179). Drooling and sedation can be distressing problems with clozapine. Weight gain can occur with all of the atypicals but is probably more likely with clozapine and olanzapine. Clozapine carries greater risk of causing seizures, which is a consideration in treating patients with a history of brain injury. Due to this side effect profile, clozapine will not usually be the first of the atypicals to try. It is rational to try at least two of the other atypical antipsychotic drugs before beginning a clozapine trial. Among the other four, none shows clearly superior efficacy. A particular patient's history of previous response, minimizing certain side effects, and the clinician's familiarity with one drug or another all affect choice of drug. In some instances, one might wish to use a side effect, such as sedation or tendency to cause weight gain to advantage.

A variety of case reports and small case series that suggest most of the atypical antipsychotics can be used to effectively treat psychosis resulting from TBI (131, 180–183), though there are no randomized controlled trials to date. For example Butler (180) reported persecutory and nihilistic delusions, Capgras delusions, and depersonalization in a 17-year-old man after TBI. The delusions completely resolved within 2 weeks of beginning treatment with olanzapine, 5 mg daily. Feinberg and colleagues (181) reported a 61-year-old man who developed misidentification delusions of the Fregoli type after suffering right frontal and left temporoparietal contusions. Umansky and Geller (182) reported successful treatment with olanzapine of psychosis and affective disturbance after severe TBI with frontal lobe injury in a 42-year-old man. Laddomada and colleagues (183) reported successful treatment of psychosis after TBI with clozapine in a 25-year-old man. Previous treatment with clonazepam and carbamazepine had not helped.

Thus, psychosis in a brain-injured patient can be successfully treated, but requires a thorough diagnostic assessment to discern the underlying cause, and the rational pharmacotherapeutic approach that follows logically from this diagnostic process. Medication approaches must be adjusted for the particular characteristics and vulnerabilities of the patient with a TBI.

ANXIETY DISORDERS

Anxiety is a common complaint in injured and noninjured populations alike. There are several different patterns of anxiety including generalized anxiety, panic disorder, phobic disorders, obsessive-compulsive disorder, and post-traumatic stress disorder. There are relatively few studies however addressing the incidence of these disorders after TBI and even fewer studies addressing treatment options (see (184) for review).

Generalized Anxiety Disorder (GAD) Van Reekum et al. (13) reported a 2.3 fold increase in relative risk for GAD based on five studies that met their inclusion criteria. For example in a study by Fann et al. (7), 24% of their sample (the majority of whom had mild TBI) evaluated 2–3 years after injury met criteria for generalized anxiety disorder. Many had co-morbid depression and many had symptoms that pre-dated their TBI. Robinson and Jorge (185) also found high rates of co-morbid anxiety and depression. 76% of their sample of depressed TBI patients also met criteria for generalized anxiety disorder (GAD). 22% of the non-depressed group also met GAD criteria.

Hibbard et al. (15) also found high rates of several different anxiety disorders (PTSD, 19%; obsessive-compulsive disorder, 15%; panic disorder, 14%; GAD, 9%) in their sample of 100 individuals with mixed injury severity studied an average of 8 years after injury. Deb et al. (107) found a high rate of panic disorder (7%) but no change in rates for GAD or obsessive compulsive disorder relative to the general population.

The question of anxiety symptoms and their link to post-concussive symptoms is an important one. There is a significant overlap between many postconcussive symptoms and core symptoms in generalized anxiety disorder. Thus, many patients endorse complaints of headache, dizziness, blurred vision, irritability, and sensitivity to noise or light after mild brain injury (56, 186, 187). It is less clear how many patients actually experience anxiety and how many have diagnosable anxiety disorders. Although 55% of Dikmen's group (186) of 20 patients with mild brain injury complained of subjective anxiety, 45% of the matched control subjects had similar complaints (a statistically nonsignificant difference). Schoenhuber and Gentilini (188) were unable to find a significant difference in mean anxiety scores in their study of 35 patients with mild brain injury and matched control subjects.

Obsessive-Compulsive Disorder   Three studies (13, 15, 189) assessed their TBI populations for obsessive – compulsive disorder. As pointed out by Van Reekum et al. (13) these studies represent a combined sample of 282 subjects followed for a maximum of 7.5 years. 6.4% had obsessive compulsive disorder which represents about a 2-fold increase in relative risk compared to the general population.

Post-Traumatic Stress Disorder (PTSD)   There is an increasing awareness of the relationship between PTSD and brain injury. Initially it was assumed that the presence of post-traumatic amnesia prevented the development of PTSD by preventing the formation of what was felt to be a core component of the syndrome – the exquisitely vivid memories and re-experiencing of the traumatic life-threatening event. In fact there is evidence that individuals with loss of consciousness, particularly 15 minutes or more do have reduced rates of PTSD (184, 190, 191). However this is by no means an absolute rule. McMillan (192) reported on 10 individuals who met criteria for PTSD despite amnesia for the traumatic event and several others have reported similar findings (193–195). However it is more common to see PTSD and PTSD-like syndromes in individuals with at least partial recall of the events. Patients with a history of mild brain injury seem to manifest signs and symptoms suggestive of PTSD fairly commonly. Symptoms may include sleep disturbance, recurrent nightmares, exaggerated startle responses, daytime flashbacks, and avoidant behaviors such as refusing to drive or leave home. Driving phobias may become prominent. Lishman (1), in his review of the psychiatric sequelae of brain injury, refers to PTSD-like symptoms, concluding that "the circumstances of the accident may recur vividly in dreams, maintain states of

anxiety, or become the focus for obsessional rumination or conversion hysteria" (p. 306). McMillan (196) described PTSD symptoms in a woman with a severe brain injury despite amnesia for the event itself and a PTA of approximately 6 weeks.

Bryant and Harvey have reported a series of studies of individuals hospitalized after motor vehicle accidents, some with and some without TBI (usually mild TBI). They have shown that rates of acute stress disorder 1 month after an accident are comparable in the two groups, and that acute stress disorder is a good predictor of those who go on to develop PTSD 6 months after injury (197–199). For example, they studied 46 individuals admitted to a hospital after an MTBI (LOC with PTA <24 hours) and 59 survivors of motor vehicle accidents without evidence of TBI 6 months after their accidents (194, 200). Twenty percent of the TBI group and 25% of the non-TBI group had PTSD. The TBI group had more postconcussive symptoms than did the non-TBI group. Furthermore, the TBI group with PTSD was significantly more symptomatic than the TBI without PTSD group. This suggests that, like other psychiatric disorders such as depression, PTSD can amplify postconcussive symptoms after an MTBI and complicate recovery. In a sample of individuals with mild TBI (LOC <15 minutes), Mayou et al. (2000) found that almost half (48%) of those with definite loss of consciousness had PTSD 3 months after injury, and one-third of their subjects with MTBI had PTSD 1 year after injury. Although it might at first seem strange that those with LOC could develop PTSD with intrusive memories, it has been suggested that the intrusive memories are of events immediately before or after the accident, or there may be patchy amnesia with some islands of preserved memory.

Warden et al. suggest that a PTSD-like syndrome does occur after TBI but that the phenomenology may be different from that seen in individuals without TBI. They studied 47 members of the Armed Forces who sustained moderate to severe TBI. Using the strict definition of PTSD defined in DSM-III-R, none of the individuals met full criteria for PTSD. However when the re-experiencing criteria was dropped under the assumption that the traumatic amnesia would make this symptoms less likely, 13% met these revised criteria. This study is particularly instructive in that it raises the issue of subsyndromal levels of PTSD. As Warden et al. described, patients who do not meet formal criteria for PTSD yet manifest many of the core symptoms (apart from the re-experiencing) are commonly seen. This highlights the fact that clinicians must be aware of the profile of injury through which psychiatric symptoms will be expressed following a TBI. In this case the injury associated memory loss alters one of the key components of PTSD seen in the non-injured population, and yet the rest of the core symptoms are present, can cause enormous disability, and need aggressive treatment. Failure to appreciate this altered clinical phenomenology on the one hand, or excessively rigid reliance on DSM criteria developed without the TBI population in mind can lead the clinician astray.

Thus it seems that GAD, panic disorder, obsessive-compulsive disorder, and PTSD do occur at increased rates in individuals with TBI compared to the general population. As with the other psychiatric disorders discussed, the phenomenology of the disorders may be altered by the "filter" through which the symptoms are expressed.

Treatment Very little information is available with respect to treatment of these disorders in individuals with TBI (see Chapter 55). Warden and Labbate (184) suggest that education and cognitive-behavioral therapy have an important role in treatment. There are no systematic medication trials. Thus the usual approach is to follow the same treatment algorithm for anxiety disorders in the non-injured population. Selective serotonin re-uptake inhibitors such as sertraline or citalopram are useful first-line agents for both GAD and obsessive-compulsive disorder, and arguably for panic disorder and PTSD. Benzodiazepines can be useful but are often second line agents due to their effects on cognition and the high rate of substance abuse disorders in the TBI population. Atypical antipsychotics such as risperidone, quetiapine, and olanzapine are increasingly being used to treat anxiety. However these should be third line agents due to the potential for weight gain or full metabolic syndrome and the less likely but real concern for the development of tardive dyskinesia. Aripiprazole and ziprazidone may be better choices in individuals who are already overweight or at risk for metabolic syndrome. Buspirone can also be of benefit to some individuals. It is important to give this agent a several week trial before assessing efficacy as it takes this long to have an effect.

SUBSTANCE ABUSE

Use of alcohol and other substances can play an important role in TBI including etiology, neuropathophysiology, recovery, and functional outcome (see Chapter 40). For example about half of all traumatic brain injuries involve the use of alcohol, and about one half of these individuals are intoxicated at the time of injury (174). The majority of these individuals have pre-injury patterns suggestive of addictive drinking (alcohol dependence)(201). In fact alcohol use is the single greatest risk factor for TBI, and TBI is often an irreversible consequence of alcohol and drug abuse (201). The presence of alcohol at the time of injury predicts longer durations of unconsciousness (202), increased challenging behaviors during the acute hospitalization (203), cognitive outcome (204) and overall outcome including mortality(205).

Individuals with pre-injury substance abuse problems often continue to struggle with these issues after their injury. Ashman et al. (109) found that their TBI population had an almost 2-fold increased rate of substance use disorders (drug/alcohol abuse/dependency) relative to the general population (32% vs. 17%) *prior* to injury. Subsequent to injury the rates went down initially probably reflecting enforced abstinence related to hospitalization and rehabilitation stays. However by the third assessment point the rate was identical to that seen in the general population (17%). In an earlier study of 100 individuals studied at least one year (mean 7.6 years) after injury, 28% of the sample struggled with substance use disorders (15).

Treatment A full discussion of this topic can be found in Chapter 40. In the acute hospitalization period it is important to be alert to the potential for substance withdrawal syndromes. Treatment of withdrawal from alcohol and drugs in addicted patients with TBI are similar to those employed in patients without TBI, with some important exceptions. The identification of alcohol and drug intoxication and withdrawal follows the general principles of pharmacological dependence. The use of blood and urine toxicology is important to identify the presence and levels of alcohol and drugs for assessment of intoxication and anticipation of withdrawal. The use of vital signs, particularly blood pressure, pulse, and temperature, are critical in determining the presence and severity of the withdrawal state (206).

After the acute and sub-acute rehabilitation phase, it is often desirable to prescribe aggressive treatment for substance abuse problems that appear likely to persist. However there are a variety of issues that complicate this process in individuals with TBI. Although counseling and the use of group therapy and 12-step recovery models remain the mainstay of treatment (see (201) for review) the cognitive deficits of many with TBI makes these interventions more difficult in that there is often relatively little or no carry-over of issues discussed from one session to the next.

There is often a significant problem with denial. Disorders of substance use are frequently associated with a resistance or psychological denial with respect to the impact that the substance use has on an individual's life. This can be greatly compounded by the deficits of awareness that were described earlier (see (78)). Thus there is a double denial (denial of substance abuse and TBI-related deficits) that can hamper establishment of a therapeutic alliance around the need for treatment.

There are also difficulties related to the usual treatment settings. Individuals with TBI can find group meetings (e.g. AA or NA meetings) over stimulating. This can result in further difficulties processing the informational content of the meetings. Furthermore the difficulties in social comportment described earlier can become quite apparent in group settings and when individuals are over stimulated. This can result in the individual being asked to leave or not being welcome at future meetings. There can be a culture within groups that discourages or down-plays the need for psychotropic medications and this can be detrimental to individuals who are already wavering in their commitment to medication compliance especially if they are not convinced that they have a problem in need of treatment.

Despite the above difficulties, the tried and true interventions remain the cornerstone of treatment. Thus additional supports are needed to enhance their efficacy in individuals with TBI. Basic principles used in working with individuals with TBI work in addiction treatment as well. Individuals will do better with concrete and structured settings. Whenever possible programs should be geared to the cognitive level of the individual. When this is not possible the use of a buddy system to help to translate or operationalize the information from individual or group sessions to real life can be effective. It is important for the treatment team to have a thorough understanding of both addiction and TBI to provide a consistent, cogent, and effective treatment plan (201).

Techniques such as keeping treatment interventions simple, focused, and concrete are critical in both patient populations(201). Clinicians may find a need to be more directive and supportive than they are accustomed to with other patient populations (174). Redirection using appropriate cues and reinforcers is often needed more than in other populations. It is important to teach substance use prevention skills that can be used in more than one life setting to maximize generalizability. As noted it is important to never assume understanding or memory of content from previous session. This requires the therapist to be redundant both within and between sessions. It can be helpful to summarize previous progress and then restate where the previous meeting left off (i.e. be redundant) (174, 201).

Dementia

Dementia is defined in the DSM as a syndrome characterized by impairment in memory and at least one other domain of higher cognitive function ("memory plus") that is of sufficient severity to interfere with social and or occupational function. Although progression is often inferred this need not be the case. Thus many individuals with TBI who have significant impairments in memory and executive function meet this definition of dementia. However the larger issue is whether exposure to a TBI increases the risk of a progressive dementing disorder such as Alzheimer's dementia (SDAT) later in life (see Chapter 32 for discussion of the full scope of late complications of TBI). At this time it is not possible to say definitively whether TBI, particularly mild TBI is a risk factor for Alzheimer's disease. This topic has been recently reviewed

by Jellinger (207) who concluded that both SDAT and TBI are associated with abnormalities in amyloid and tau protein deposition and that several epidemiological studies have suggested either that SDAT occurs with increased frequency in individuals with TBI or that the age of onset of SDAT is reduced after TBI relative to non-injured controls. Furthermore the possibility exists that the two conditions share common genetic vulnerabilities with respect to polymorphisms in the apolipoprotein E (ApoE) gene.

ApoE is a complex glycolipoprotein that facilitates the uptake, transport, and distribution of lipids. It appears to play an important role in neuronal repair and plasticity after injury (208). A four exon gene codes for ApoE on chromosome 19 in humans. There are three major alleles: e2, e3, and e4. These alleles differ in amino acids at positions 112 and 158: e2 (cysteine/cysteine), e3 (cysteine/arginine), and e4 (arginine/arginine). Animal models suggest a link between the e4 allele and increased mortality, extent of damage, and poor repair following trauma (208, 209). The human e4 allele has been associated with a variety of disorders with prominent cognitive dysfunction including normals with memory complaints (210), AD, and poor outcomes in stroke and TBI (208, 211). Several studies have reported that the e4 allele is associated with poor outcomes following TBI, using a variety of measures (212, 213). Crawford et al. (214), for example, found poorer memory performance in their sample of 30 individuals with TBI with at least one e4 allele compared to 80 TBI patients without an e4 allele. Lichtman et al. (215) found lower total functional independence measure scores in seven e4(+) patients with TBI compared to the 24 individuals with TBI but without an e4 allele. Friedman et al. (216) found a significantly higher percentage of poor outcome indicators both acutely (prolonged loss of consciousness), and at 6–8 months after injury (significant dysarthria, global functional outcome rating) in 27 individuals with TBI and the e4 allele compared to 42 individuals with TBI but without an e4 allele. Liberman et al. (217) found lower cognitive performance on several cognitive measures at 3 weeks but not 6 weeks after injury in the e4(+) patients. In a recent 30 year follow up study of individuals with TBI Koponen et al. (218) found that 6 of 19 e4 (+) individuals had definite or probable SDAT, whereas none of the 41 e4 (−) individuals had developed SDAT.

The mechanism by which the e4 allele exerts its negative effect is unclear. ApoE4 shows an increased affinity for beta amyloid and thus an increased propensity to promote aggregation of beta amyloid (216). Rather than an active detrimental effect, it may be that the ApoE4 is less effective than ApoE3 in promoting neuronal repair, and neuritic growth and branching. There may be a cholinergic link between the ApoE and cognitive impairment (see (219)). In AD, the degree of reduction of choline acetyl transferase, one of the markers for the disease, is correlated with the "dose" of e4 (208). Parasuraman et al. (220) have argued based on accumulated neuropsychological, electrophysiological, and neuroimaging evidence that the cognitive effects of the e4 allele are mediated through reduced cholinergic input to posterior parietal systems regulating selective attention.

Thus similarities in neuropathological findings and response to neurotrauma, genetic vulnerabilities with respect to apolipoprotein E, and some (though not all) epidemiological studies suggest that there is a link between TBI and subsequent development of SDAT. However further clarification is needed. From a clinical standpoint the important issue is the stability of cognitive deficits over time. Any individual who has had stable cognitive function after the period of spontaneous recovery that begins to show evidence of cognitive decline must have an aggressive evaluation for the underlying cause as this is not the typical course following TBI.

NEUROPSYCHIATRIC ASSESSMENT

It is clear from the above that a careful assessment of neurobehavioral concerns should be an important component of the evaluation and rehabilitation of individuals with TBI. A full discussion of all the dimensions of a neuropsychiatric assessment will not be attempted (see (221) for review). However it is worth highlighting several points.

Need for Multiple Sources of Information The cognitive deficits that frequently accompany a TBI alter the neuropsychiatric assessment, particularly the history taking. The presence of short-term memory deficits, problems with sequencing events in time, and difficulties with self-monitoring and self-awareness can make it very challenging for an individual to give a clear and consistent history. This puts the onus on the clinician to identify other sources of information (family members, friends, employers, primary medical/school/vocational records) that can help clarify the history and current clinical picture. The clinician must also obtain permission from the injured individual and work hard to explain the need for others to be involved in the treatment as observers and sources of critical information.

Assessment of Pre-Injury Baseline Assessment of the effects of an injury must start with a thorough understanding of what the individual was like prior to the injury. Absent such information there is a significant risk of mis-attributing life-long traits, characteristics, and behaviors to the brain injury. The following domains should be carefully explored and efforts made to gain primary records and reliable history with respect to:

- *Medical history*
- *Neurobehavioral traits and characteristics* (e.g. history of psychiatric illness)
- *Intellectual capacity* (indicators include educational history, vocational history, parental education)
- *Functional performance* (profile of personal, professional, and vocational accomplishments)
- *Personality style* (indicators include patterns of coping with stress, stability of key relationships)

Proper information on the above domains helps to paint a picture of life before the injury. Ideally such information is obtained shortly after the injury. The more time that passes from the point of injury, the greater the tendency to (mis) attribute more issues and life events to the injury. It is important to not simply take the word of injured individuals and their family/caregivers that "he was always perfectly normal" but make efforts to get primary documentation, not just "hearsay".

Assessment of Post-Injury Changes Once the baseline picture is complete, the clinician is positioned to accurately assess the changes that have occurred since the time of the injury. It is important to carefully review the functional domains that are frequently affected by injury including cognition, personality, mood regulation, speech/language, mobility, and higher order domains such as vocational performance, major role performance within the family or equivalent context. It can be helpful to use standardized assessment scales and tools that serve to sample the full array of common problems such as the Neurobehavioral Rating Scale-revised (222) or the Neuropsychiatric Inventory (223). Alternatively one can use scales and instruments that offer a more detailed approach to a given problem area specific to the individual being assessed such as the Overt Aggression Scale (224) or Apathy Evaluation Scale (225). For bedside assessment of cognition it is helpful to supplement a standardized instrument such as the Mini Mental Status Exam (226) with something that helps to assess frontal executive functions such as the Frontal Assessment Battery or the Behavior Rating Inventory of Executive Function (BRIEF, (227, 228)), (see Table 45-4).

Attribution of Etiology It is important to emphasize that temporal association does not guarantee causality. There are several ways that neurobehavioral change can be associated with brain injury. Change may be a direct effect of the insult to neural tissue with subsequent disruption of the functions sub-served by the damaged tissue. For this to be properly assessed requires accurate, sometimes fine-grained knowledge of the profile of regional brain injury and the relationship of the related circuitry to the functional change in question (the "neural component").

Alternatively the change may reflect the development of a new illness or disorder that is the driving force behind the behavioral change. For example an individual may develop various endocrine complications of their brain injury related to pituitary damage, chronic pain

TABLE 45-4
NeuroBehavioral Rating Instruments Useful in TBI

NAME OF INSTRUMENT	COMMENTS	FORMAT	NUMBER OF ITEMS	APPROXIMATE TIME TO ADMINISTER	OUTPUT
BEDSIDE MEASURES OF COGNITION					
Mini-Mental Status Exam (226)	Not a good measure of frontal executive functions	Rater administered	30	5 minutes	Score range to 30
Frontal Assessment Battery (230)	Good measure of executive function	Rater Administered	6	5–10 minutes	Score range to 18
BRIEF-A (228)	Good measure of executive function	Self-report or Family/caregiver report	75	10–15 minutes	Total and subscales
MEASURES OF SPECIFIC BEHAVIORS					
Beck Depression Inventory (231)	Requires self-awareness, ability to read, some memory skills	Self-report	21	5 minutes	Normal score less than 10
Spielberger State Trait Anxiety Inventory (232)	Measures both current (state) and trait anxiety. Requires self-awareness, ability to read, some memory skills	Self-report	40	5 minutes	Scores range from 20 to 80
Overt Aggression Scale (224)	Good coverage of common aggressive behaviors	Rater administered	16	5 minutes	Total and domain scores
Apathy Evaluation Scale (225)	Good coverage of common symptoms suggestive of apathy	Self-report and informant	18	10 minutes	Total score
Scale to Assess Unawareness of Mental Disorders (233)	Assesses patient view of whether an individual is aware of problems in personality and behavior	Rater administered	20	10 minutes	Assess awareness and attribution of specific psychotic symptoms
PCL-S (234)	Assesses symptoms commonly associated with PTSD	Self-report	17	5–10 minutes	Total scores
SURVEYS OF BEHAVIOR					
Neuropsychiatric Inventory (223)	Excellent coverage of common symptoms. Somewhat lengthy	Rater administered	91	10–20 minutes	Total score and 12 domain scores
Neurobehavioral Rating Scale – Revised (222)	Excellent coverage of common symptoms	Rater administered	57	15 minutes	Total score, domain scores

from orthopedic injuries, or depression that more reasonably explains the behaviors in question (the "biological component"). It is equally plausible that behavioral change could be caused by the meaning of the accident or injury, a reaction to a loss of self-esteem due to disfiguring injury, loss of mobility, or unemployment (the "psychological component"). Finally, changes in environment such as living situation, change in caregivers, or change in routine or flow of daily life can have an enormous impact on the behavior and adaptation of an individual with brain injury (the "social component").

Formulation and Interpretation All of the above factors can reasonably be attributed to the event of the injury. For example the individual would not have endocrine abnormalities save for the injury-related pituitary damage, or may well have not developed depression absent the injury. However the degree of linkage to neural tissue damage varies across these factors. An individual showing new, aggressive outbursts associated with a change in residential care providers may be better served by working to further train the residential provider rather than by the aggressive use of medications. On the other hand if this patient has clear evidence of orbitofrontal damage, it may be that their threshold for tolerating frustration is so lowered that treatment will require both medication approaches and environmental manipulation.

The proper assessment and formulation of the relative weighting or contribution of each of these factors to the genesis of the challenging behaviors frames what can be termed a neurobiopsychosocial paradigm. It differs from more traditional psychiatric assessments with respect to the critical importance placed on understanding the profile of regional brain injury, and the array of complex behavioral circuitry that this profile would reasonably disrupt. Thus the work of the neuropsychiatric assessment can be summarized as the process of matching the profile of brain injury with the changes that have occurred in cognition, behavior, and overall function, and gauging the "goodness of fit" between predicted and actual outcomes. This is followed by an interpretative process whereby the clinician assigns relative weights to the various contributions made by the neural, biological, psychological, and social components. Treatment interventions should flow logically from this formulation. It is important to point out that even experienced clinicians can make mistakes in this process due to the complexity of clinical presentations and the incomplete data available. Thus the final critical component to this process is the regular re-evaluation of intervention efficacy. Essentially each formulation should be hypothesis driven and each intervention flow logically and in an empirically testable fashion (e.g. "I believe the increase in aggression is due to depression, thus I will prescribe antidepressants"). Poor or incomplete response to the intervention should prompt a re-evaluation and formulation of a new and testable hypothesis. It is acceptable to be wrong, it is not acceptable to engage in sloppy thinking.

PRINCIPLES IN TREATMENT

A detailed approach to specific syndromes and disorders can be found in Chapter 55 (Silver and Arciniegas), and Chapter 56 (Arciniegas and Silver). However several general treatment principles are worth emphasizing.

Variability in Presentation It is important to be aware that the presentation of psychiatric syndromes in individuals with TBI may differ from the presentation in the non-injured population. In general, the more mild the TBI, the more similar the presentation is. However special challenges arise in more severely injured individuals with cognitive, motor, and speech/language deficits. There are three broad factors that contribute to variability in clinical presentation.

Mood Instability and Affective Lability Due to the instability in mood and affect accompanying disruption of the aforementioned frontal-subcortical circuits, it is necessary to pay attention to an extended baseline of behavior. Individuals with TBI are subject to more rapid fluctuation in mood and affect and this overall instability should not be equated with the more sustained alteration in mood that is the hallmark of depression. Attributing internal feelings to external behavior is more difficult due to the frequent presence of pathological or "pseudobulbar" affect (76).

Alterations in Speech and Language Function Varying degrees of speech/language impairment are commonly seen following TBI, particularly in individuals with more severe injuries. These changes can range from subtle problems with naming and word finding to global aphasia. Dysarthria and articulation problems can be seen. The ability to modulate the prosody of speech can also be altered (229). This is manifested by difficulties in modulating speech tone, pitch, and amplitude (expressive aprosody), or in decoding and interpreting these components in the speech of others (receptive aprosody). The result of these deficits is an uncoupling of the content or propositional component of speech from the emotional valence and related non-verbal components of language. Patients with receptive dysprosody may have difficulty reading social cues and this may contribute to problems in social comportment. Those with expressive dysprosody may express distressing thought content without seeming to have appropriate accompanying affect (e.g. "I am depressed and suicidal" expressed in a flat monotone without depth of feeling) leading the clinician to be somewhat confused about the clinical significance of what is being expressed.

Effects of Associated Neurological Impairments
One must also consider the effect that injury-related neurological deficits may have on clinical symptoms of psychiatric disorders. For example how will depression be expressed or manifested in non-verbal patients? How will delusions and hallucinations be evident in these same patients? In an individual with quadriplegia, what does manic hyperactivity look like? How will PTSD present in someone with amnesia for the event? Thus the clinician must become adept at envisioning what the psychiatric illness would look like if expressed through the filter of the individual's neurological and functional deficits.

Effects of Cognitive Impairment   Individuals with poor self-monitoring, impaired memory, distorted sense of time, or time-sequencing deficits will have significant problems presenting an accurate history. The clinician must rely not only on what the individual reports but must strive to get additional information from family/caregivers.

Heightened Vulnerability to Medication Side Effects
Individuals with TBI as well as other neuropsychiatric disorders often manifest an increased sensitivity to medication side effects. This may take several forms. The first is a tendency to develop typical side effects associated with the given medication at a lower than usual dose. The second is a lowered threshold at which the individual develops a delirium or toxic encephalopathy. The third is a worsening of the neurological deficits associated with the TBI. For example it is not uncommon to observe worsening of tremor or gait problems, increased emotional lability, or increased slowing of speed of information processing associated with psychotropic drug use. In other words the very symptoms the clinician is treating may be made worse by the medications prescribed. This highlights the need to take a careful medication history encompassing not only the current medications but medications used in the past as well as the response to those agents. Furthermore it is important to clarify whether a history of "that medicine didn't help" reflects a true lack of response or more a manifestation of the heightened vulnerability to side effects just described.

The above issues contribute to diagnostic and treatment challenges that can be outlined as follows:

(1) *Atypical Clinical Presentations* – As noted earlier, clinical presentations of common psychiatric disorders may not meet standard diagnostic criteria as outlined in the DSM. Thus it is reasonable to have a "relaxed fit" criteria when approaching diagnoses in individuals with TBI.

(2) *Trait vs. State Presentations* – It is important to point out that there are two broad factors that contribute to the neurobehavioral sequelae of TBI; the injury induced changes in personality, and the increased rate of psychiatric disorders. A problem arises when the latter presents as a heightening or worsening of the former. For example it is quite common for an individual with TBI to have a baseline of increased irritability or lowered frustration tolerance. It is also quite common for these traits to be exaggerated in the presence of a superimposed episode of depression or mania (or some other psychiatric disorder). If the clinician does not carefully tease out the post-injury baseline and clearly ascertain whether there is a change in the frequency and/or intensity of the challenging behaviors, it is easy to misattribute challenging behavior to a dysexecutive syndrome only, as opposed to a dysexecutive syndrome exacerbated worse by the presence of an Axis I psychiatric disorder.

(3) *Treat syndromes or disorders not symptoms (diagnosis before treatment)* – It goes without saying that it is best to have a clear sense of what is causing the challenging behavior before designing a treatment plan. Yet many clinicians are inclined to prescribe antipsychotics or SRI's without formulating a hypothesis for what they are treating. This is a symptomatic approach – similar to treating a fever associated with a bacterial infection with acetaminophen but not antibiotics. In the neuropsychiatric arena, the symptomatic approach should be a last resort after having carefully ruled in or out the presence of an Axis I disorder (e.g. depression, mania, psychosis), neuromedical conditions that would account for the behavior (e.g. complex partial seizures, pain, iatrogenic complications, medication side effects), or factors in the environment that are causing the change in behavioral symptoms. Again it is important to restate that being wrong sometimes is unavoidable, but sloppy diagnostic thinking is avoidable.

(4) *Role of behavioral metaphors* – There are times, especially when data is difficult to obtain or when the neurological deficits through which challenging behaviors are being expressed are severe, that one is at a loss to account for the etiology of a given behavior or behaviors, and thus not clear about a treatment strategy. A fallback position is to attempt to conceptualize the cluster of behaviors as if they were a particular syndrome or as if they represented what Tariot et al. (235, 236) have termed a "behavioral metaphor". For example an individual expressing increased negativism, loss of interest in activities, and/or self-destructive or self-injurious behavior might be conceptualized as having a depressive syndrome (see Table 45-5) and thus could reasonably be prescribed an antidepressant regimen. An individual with increased irritability, increased arousal and activation, and a significant reduction in sleep might be conceptualized as having an irritable manic-like syndrome and thus be started on an anti-cycling

TABLE 45-5
Examples of Behavioral Metaphors

TYPE	BEHAVIOR	INITIAL TREATMENT
Depressive	Negativistic, lack of interest in activities, Weepy, aggressive or self-injurious behavior	SSRI's or other antidepressants
Manic	Increased level of arousal and activity, irritability, decreased need for sleep, increased sexual activity	Mood stabilizers or anti-cycling agents (e.g. anticonvulsants, lithium)
Psychotic	Consistent misinterpretation of environment in a paranoid fashion, apparent response to internal stimuli, aggression th at "comes out of nowhere" but may flow out of paranoid misinterpretation of events	Antipsychotics (e.g. low dose risperidone)
Anxiety	Challenging behaviors most apparent in setting of anticipation of events, change in routine, consistently difficult *or* novel situations	Anxiolytics

Adapted from: Ryan JM. Kidder SW. Daiello LA. Tariot PN. (2002) Psychopharmacologic interventions in nursing homes: what do we know and where should we go? *Psychiatric Services.* 53(11):1407–13.

regimen or mood stabilizers. The critical issue is that these are testable hypotheses and should be treated as such. Target behaviors and baseline frequencies should be identified prior to treatment and an adequate but time-limited trial prescribed. It should be clearly decided what the endpoint is and if the desired goal is not attained, the medication should be discontinued and an alternative conceptual scheme considered.

Role of Behavioral and Environmental Interventions

It is important to point out that individuals with cognitive impairment of all kinds, including individuals with TBI have a heightened sensitivity not only to medications, but to the environment in which they live. This is related to several factors.

Stimulus Boundedness As mentioned earlier one of the characteristics of damage to frontal-subcortical circuits with attendant problems in executive function and social comportment is that individuals have great difficulty with components of attention including complex, selective, and sustained attention. This results in difficulty with prioritization of incoming stimuli and the gating out of stimuli that would ordinarily be deemed of secondary importance. At its essence this may be a problem assigning or decoding proper salience to the constant influx of environmental cues and stimuli. In any event the result is that the individual becomes hostage for at least very sensitive to, events in their immediate environment.

Fondness for Routine Individuals with cognitive deficits are often quite sensitive to changes in routine or schedule. This may relate to the afore-mentioned deficits in executive function in which problems with problem solving and mental flexibility can be quite apparent. Over time individuals (injured or non-injured) develop routines that tend to maximize predictability and efficient function, and minimize stress. Changes in these routines call for mental flexibility and problem solving skills to maintain environmental homeostasis. Individuals challenged in these domains will often respond with anxiety, irritability, or even catastrophic reactions to these changes in routine. This tendency can be apparent in response to both changes in people in their environment or changes in time or schedule. The latter may relate to basic impairments in both sense of time and memory, resulting in ongoing anxiety and perseverative requests for information or re-assurance with respect to upcoming events or activities. Family/caregivers and staff often function as cognitive prosthetic devices that the individual relies upon to supply ongoing memory for events, maintenance of schedule, and overall sense of time. Being deprived of these human prosthetic devices is a frightening experience and can result in appearance of some very challenging behaviors.

Predictability of Response Injured and non-injured individuals alike base much of minute to minute and long-term decisions and actions on predictions of the response a given action will produce. Increasing the probability of favorable responses and decreasing the likelihood of undesirable responses are powerful forces in shaping behavior. However certain executive deficits such as inferential reasoning, self-monitoring, self-correction, and episodic memory are critical to the successful application of these experiences to shaping behavior. In this context predictability of response becomes even more critical to maximize contextual learning and generalize these lessons to other novel settings. Individuals existing in an environment in which the same behaviors elicit different responses from different people at different times can become confused, anxious, and agitated.

Thus it is critical to carefully consider these factors when performing a neuropsychiatric assessment. To ignore the environment and factors that may be provoking challenging behaviors will greatly reduce the efficacy of any prescribed medication even if it is the proper medication. On the other hand, without the properly prescribed medication, even massive efforts at applied behavioral analysis and environmental manipulation may be in vain. The therapeutic issue should not be: "Do we prescribe a drug, or write a behavioral plan?" Rather the question is better framed as "Which medicine prescribed in the context of what changes in environment and strategies for shaping behavior has the best potential for success?".

CONCLUSIONS

Attention to the diagnosis and management of the neurobehavioral sequelae of TBI can serve a critical role in advancing the rehabilitative process. It requires a knowledge and understanding of the profile of regional structural and neurochemical injury associated with the typical TBI and how that profile predicts the common neurobehavioral sequelae. Careful assessment requires an accurate description of the individual's functional and neurobehavioral status prior to the injury, and how that has changed subsequent to the injury. It is helpful to be aware of the problems in diagnosis in individuals who have a fluctuating behavioral baseline, who may have significant cognitive deficits, or in whom the usual connection between internal feeling state and external behaviors may be uncoupled. Treatment should follow from a clearly articulated diagnostic scheme and should be time-limited and re-evaluated in the presence of poor or incomplete response.

References

1. Lishman WA: The Psychiatric Sequelae of Head Injury: A Review. *Psychol Med* 1973;3:304–318.
2. McKinlay WW, Brooks DN, Bond MR, et al.: The Short Term Outcomes of Severe Blunt Head Injury as Reported by Relatives of the Injured Persons. *J Neurol Neurosurg Psychiatry* 1981;44: 527–533.
3. Oddy M, Humphrey M, Uttley D: Subjective Impairment and Social Recovery after Closed Head Injury. *Journal of Neurology, Neurosurgery & Psychiatry* 1978;41:611–616.
4. Goethe KE, Levin HS: Behavioral Manifestation During the Early and Long-Term Stages of Recovery after Closed Head Injury. *Psychiatric Annals* 1984;14:540–546.
5. McAllister TW: Neuropsychiatric Sequelae of Head Injuries. *Psychiatric Clinics of North America* 1992;15:395–413.

6. Arciniegas D, Topkoff J: The Neuropsychiatry of Pathological Affect:An Approach to Evaluation and Treatment. *Seminars in Clinical Neuropsychiatry* 2000;5:290–306.
7. Fann JR, Katon WJ, Uomoto JM, Esselman PC: Psychiatric Disorders and Functional Disability in Outpatients with Traumatic Brain Injuries. *American Journal of Psychiatry* 1995;152: 1493–1499.
8. DHHS: *Department of Health and Human Services: Interagency Head Injury Task Force Report.* In Washington DC, US Department of Health and Human Services, 1989.
9. Levin HS, Gary HE, Eisenberg HM, et al.: Neurobehavioral Outcome 1 Year after Severe Head Trauma: Experience of the Traumatic Coma Data Bank. *Journal of Neurosurgery* 1990;73: 699–709.
10. Sorenson SB, Kraus JF: Occurrence, Severity, and Outcome of Brain Injury. *Journal of Head Trauma Rehabilitation* 1991; 5:1–10.
11. Sosin DM, Sniezek J, Thurman D: Incidence of Mild and Moderate Brain Injury in the United States. *Brain Injury* 1991;10:47–54.
12. Arciniegas DB, Topkoff J, Silver JM: Neuropsychiatric Aspects of Traumatic Brain Injury. *Current Treatment Options in Neurology* 2000;2:169–186.
13. van Reekum R, Cohen T, Wong J: Can Traumatic Brain Injury Cause Psychiatric Disorders? *Journal of Neuropsychiatry and Clinical Neuroscience* 2000;12:316–327.
14. Silver J, Weissman M, Kramer R, Greenwald S: Association between Severe Head Injuries and Psychiatric Disorders: Findings from the New Haven Nimh Epdemiologic Catchment Area Study. *Journal of Neuropsychiatry and Clinical Neuroscience* 1997; 9:640.
15. Hibbard MR, Uysal S, Kepler K, Bogdany J, Silver J: Axis I Psychopathology in Individuals with Traumatic Brain Injury. *Journal of Head Trauma Rehabilitation* 1998;13:24–39.
16. Koponen S, Taiminen T, Portin R, Himanen L, Isoniemi H, Heinonen H, Hinkka S, Tenovuo O: Axis I and Ii Psychiatric Disorders after Traumatic Brain Injury: A 30-Year Follow-up Study. *American Journal of Psychiatry.* 2002;159:1315–1321.
17. Malaspina D, Goetz R, Friedman J, et al.: Traumatic Brain Injury and Schizophrenia in Members of Schizophrenia and Bipolar Disorder Pedigrees. *American Journal of Psychiatry* 2001;158: 440–446.
18. Gennarelli T, Graham D: *Neuropathology.* in Silver J, McAllister T, Yudofsky S (eds): Textbook of Traumatic Brain Injury. Washington, DC: American Psychiatric Press, 2005, 27–50.
19. Umile EM, Sandel ME, Alavi A, Terry CM, Plotkin RC: Dynamic Imaging in Mild Traumatic Brain Injury: Support for the Theory of Medial Temporal Vulnerability. *Archives of Physical Medicine & Rehabilitation* 2002;83:1506–1513.
20. McIntosh TK: Neurochemical Sequelae of Traumatic Brain Injury: Therapeutic Implications. *Cerebrovascular and Brain Metabolism Reviews* 1994;6:109–162.
21. McIntosh TK, Juhler M, Wieloch T: Novel Pharmacologic Strategies in the Treatment of Experimental Traumatic Brain Injury: 1998. *Journal of Neurotrauma* 1998;15:731–769.
22. McAllister TW, Flashman LA, Sparling MB, Saykin AJ: Working Memory Deficits after Mild Traumatic Brain Injury: Catecholaminergic Mechanisms and Prospects for Catecholaminergic Treatment–a Review. *Brain Injury* 2004;18:331–350.
23. Smeets WJ, Gonzalez A: Catecholamine Systems in the Brain of Vertebrates: New Perspectives through a Comparative Approach. *Brain Research – Brain Research Reviews* 2000;33:308–379.
24. Charney DS: Monoamine Dysfunction and the Pathophysiology and Treatment of Depression. *Journal of Clinical Psychiatry* 1998; 59 Suppl 14:11–14.
25. McAllister TW: Apathy. *Seminars in Clinical Neuropsychiatry.* 2000;5:275–282.
26. Arnsten AFT: Catecholamine Modulation of Prefrontal Cortical Cognitive Function. *Trends in Cognitive Sciences* 1998;2: 436–447.
27. McAllister TW: Evaluation and Treatment of Neurobehavioral Complications of Traumatic Brain Injury – Have We Made Any Progress? *Neurorehabilitation* 2002;17:263–264.
28. Jennett B, Teasdale G: *Management of Head Injuries.* in Contemporary Neurology Series. Philadelphia: Davis, 1981, vol 20, 114–140.

29. Prasad MR, Tzigaret C, Smith DH, Soares H, McIntosh TK: Decreased Alpha-Adrenergic Receptors after Experimental Brain Injury. *Journal of NeuroTrauma* 1993;9:269–279.

30. Globus M, Busto R, Dietrich W, Martinez E, Valdes I, Ginsberg M: Direct Evidence for Acute and Massive Norepinephrine Release in the Hippocampus During Transient Ischemia. *Journal of Cerebral Blood Flow and Metabolism* 1989;9:892–896.

31. McIntosh TK: Neurochemical Sequelae of Traumatic Brain Injury: Therapeutic Implications. *Cerebrovascular and Brain Metabolism Reviews* 1994;6:109–162.

32. Feeney DM, Boyeson MG, Linn RT, Murray HM, Dail WG: Responses to Cortical Injury. 1. Methodology and Local Effects of Contusions in the Rat. *Brain Research* 1981;211:67–77.

33. Feeney DM, Hovda DA: Amphetamine and Apomorphine Restore Tactile Placing after Motor Cortex Injury in the Cat. *Psychopharmacology* 1983;79:67–71.

34. Feeney DM, Sutton RL: Pharmacotherapy for Recovery of Function after Brain Injury. *Critical Review of Neurobiology* 1987; 1987:135–197.

35. Boyeson MG, Feeney DM: The Role of Norepinephrine in Recovery from Brain Injury. *Society of Neuroscience Abstracts* 1984; 10:68.

36. Romhanyi R, Tandian D, Hovda DA, Kawamata T, Yoshiro A, Cristescu SV, Becker DP: Catecholaminergic Stimulation Enhances Recovery of Function Following Concussive Brain Injury. *Journal of Neurotrauma* 1990;9:164.

37. Tandian D, Romhanyi R, Hovda DA, Yoshino A, Kawamata T, Badaday NF, Becker DP: Amphetamine Enhances Both Behavior and Metabolic Recovery Following Fluid Percussion Brain Injury. *Journal of Neurotrauma* 1990;9:174.

38. Sutton RL, Feeney DM: Alpha-Noradrenergic Agonists and Antagonists Affect Recovery and Maintenance of Beam-Walking Ability after Sensorimotor Cortex Ablation in the Rat. *Restorative Neurology and Neuroscience* 1992;4:1–11.

39. Zhu J, Hamm RJ, Reeves TM, Povlishock JT, Phillips LL: Postinjury Administration of L-Deprenyl Improves Cognitive Function and Enhances Neuroplasticity after Traumatic Brain Injury. *Experimental Neurology* 2000;166:136–152.

40. Whyte J, Vaccaro M, Grieg-Neff P, Hart T: Psychostimulant Use in the Rehabilitation of Individuals with Traumatic Brain Injury. *Journal of Head Trauma Rehabiliation* 2002;17:284–299.

41. McDowell S, Whyte J, D'Esposito M: Differential Effect of a Dopaminergic Agonist on Prefrontal Function in Traumatic Brain Injury Patients. *Brain* 1998;121:1155–1164.

42. Shytle RD, Silver AA, Sheehan KH, Sheehan DV, Sanberg PR: Neuronal Nicotinic Receptor Inhibition for Treating Mood Disorders: Preliminary Controlled Evidence with Mecamylamine. *Depression & Anxiety* 2002;16:89–92.

43. Arciniegas DB: The Cholinergic Hypothesis of Cognitive Impairment Caused by Traumatic Brain Injury. *Curr Psychiatry Rep* 2003;5:391–399.

44. Dixon CE, Liu SJ, Jenkins LW, et al.: Time Course of Increased Vulnerability of Cholinergic Neurotransmission Following Traumatic Brain Injury in the Rat. *Behavioural Brain Research* 1995;70: 125–131.

45. Dewar D, Graham DI: Depletion of Choline Acetyltransferase but Preservation of M1 and M2 Muscarinic Receptor Binding Sites Temporal Cortex Following Head Injury: A Preliminary Human Postmorten Study. *Journal of Neurotrauma* 1996;13:181–187.

46. Murdoch I, Perry EK, Court JA, Graham DI, Dewar D: Cortical Cholinergic Dysfunction after Human Head Injury. *Journal of Neurotrauma* 1998;15:295–305.

47. Murdoch I, Nicoll JA, Graham DI, Dewar D: Nucleus Basalis of Meynert Pathology in the Human Brain after Fatal Head Injury. *J Neurotrauma* 2002;19:279–284.

48. Pappius HM: Local Cerebral Glucose Utilization in Thermally Traumatized Rat Brain. *Annals of Neurology* 1981;9:484–491.

49. Prasad MR, Tzigaret CM, Smith D, Soares H, McIntosh TK: Decreased Alpha 1-Adrenergic Receptors after Experimental Brain Injury. *Journal of Neurotrauma* 1992;9:269–279.

50. Tsuiki K, Takada A, Nagahiro S, Grdisa M, Diksic M, Pappius HM: Synthesis of Serotonin in Traumatized Rat Brain. *Journal of Neurochemistry* 1995;64:1319–1325.

51. McDonald BC, Flashman LA, Saykin AJ: Executive Dysfunction Following Traumatic Brain Injury: Neural Substrates and Treatment Strategies. *NeuroRehabilitation* 2002;17:333–344.

52. Lovell M, Franzen M: *Neuropsychological Assessment.* in Silver JM YS, Hales RE, eds. (ed.): Neuropsychiatry of Traumatic Brain Injury. Washington, D.C.: American Psychiatric Press, Inc., 1994, 133–160.

53. Whyte J, Polansky M, Cavallucci C, Fleming M, Lhulier J, Coslett H: Inattentive Behavior after Traumatic Brain Injury. *J of the International Neuropsychological Society* 1996;2:274–281.

54. Ben-Yishay Y, Diller L: Cognitive Remediation in Traumatic Brain Injury: Update and Issues. *Archives of Physical Medicine & Rehabilitation* 1993;74:204–213.

55. Cicerone K, Dahlberg C, Kalmar K, Langenbahn DM, Malec J, Bergquist TF, Felicetti T, Giacino JT, Harley JP, Harrington DE, Herzog J, Kneipp S, Laatsch L, Morse PA: Evidence-Based Cognitive Rehabilitation: Recommendations for Clinical Practice. *Archives of Physical Medicine and Rehabilitation* 2000;81: 1596–1615.

56. Binder LM: Persisting Symptoms after Mild Head Injury: A Review of the Post-Concussive Syndrome. *J Clin Exp Neuropsychol* 1986;8:323–346.

57. Binder LM: A Review of Mild Head Trauma 2: Clinical Implications [Review]. *Journal of Clinical & Experimental Neuropsychology* 1997;19:432–457.

58. Binder LM, Rohling ML, Larrabee J: A Review of Mild Head Trauma. Part I: Meta-Analytic Review of Neuropsychological Studies. *Journal of Clinical and Experimental Neuropsychology* 1997;19:421–431.

59. Cripe LI: The Neuropsychological Assessment and Management of Closed Head Injury: General Guidelines. *Cognitive Rehabilitation* 1987;5:18–22.

60. Gentilini M, Nichelli P, Schoenhuber R: *Assessment of Attention in Mild Head Injury.* in Levin H, Eisenberg H, Benton A (eds): Mild Head Injury. New York: Oxford University Press, 1989, 163–175.

61. Gronwall D: *Cumulative and Persisting Effects of Concussion on Attention and Cognition.* in Levin H, Eisenberg H, Benton A (eds): Mild Head Injury. New York: Oxford University Press, 1989, 153–162.

62. Gronwall D: Minor Head Injury. *Neuropsychology* 1991; Vol. 5:253–265.

63. Leininger BE, Gramling SE, Farrell AD, et al.: Neuropsychological Deficits in Symptomatic Minor Head Injury Patients after Concussion and Mild Concussion. *J Neurol Neurosurg Psychiatry* 1990;53:293–296.

64. Levin HS, Grossman RG: Behavioral Sequelae of Closed Head Injury. *Archives of Neurology* 1978;35:720–727.

65. Levin HS, Amparo EG, Eisenberg HM, et al.: Magnetic Resonance Imaging and Computerized Tomography in Relation to the Neurobehavioral Sequelae of Mild and Moderate Head Injuries. *J Neurosurg* 1987;66:706–713.

66. Levin HS, Goldstein FC, High WM, Eisenberg HM: Disproportionately Severe Memory Deficit in Relation to Normal Intellectual Functioning after Closed Head Injury. *Journal of Neurology, Neurosurgery, and Psychiatry* 1988;51:1294–1301.

67. Smith EE, Jonides J: Neuroimaging Analyses of Human Working Memory. *Proceedings of the National Academy of Sciences of the United States of America* 1998;95:12061–12068.

68. Smith ES, Jonides J, Marshuetz C, Koeppe RA: Components of Verbal Working Memory: Evidence from Neuroimaging. *Proceedings of the National Academy of Sciences of the United States of America* 1998;95:876–882.

69. Baddeley AD, Hitch GJ: Developments in the Concept of Working Memory. *Neuropsychology* 1994;8:485–493.

70. Paulesu E, Frith CD, Frackowiak RS: The Neural Correlates of the Verbal Component of Working Memory. *Nature* 1993;362: 342–345.

71. Awh E, Jonides J, Smith EE, Schumacher EH, Koeppe RA, Katz S: Dissociation of Storage and Rehearsal in Verbal Working Memory. *Psychol. Sci.* 1996;7:25–31.

72. Jonides J, Smith EE, Marshuetz C, Koeppe RA, Reuter-Lorenz PA: Inhibition in Verbal Working Memory Revealed by Brain Activation. *Proceedings of the National Academy of Sciences of the United States of America* 1998;95:8410–8413.

73. Smith EE, Jonides J, Koeppe RA: Dissociating Verbal and Spatial Working Memory Using Pet. *Cerebral Cortex* 1996;6:11–20.

74. Smith EE, Jonides J, Marshuetz C, Koeppe RA: Components of Verbal Working Memory: Evidence from Neuroimaging. *Proc Natl Acad Sci* 1998;95:876–882.

75. Smith EE, Jonides J: Storage and Executive Processes in the Frontal Lobes. *Science* 1999;283:1657–1661.

76. Arciniegas DB, Lauterbach EC, Anderson K, Chow T, Flashman L, Hurley R, Kaufer D, McAllister T, Reeve A, Schiffer R, Silver J: The Differential Diagnosis of Pseudobulbar Affect (Pba): Distinguishing Pba from Disorders of Mood and Affect. *CNS Spectrums* 2005, in press.

77. Flashman LA, McAllister TW, Johnson SC, Rick JH, Green RL, Saykin AJ: Specific Frontal Lobe Subregions Correlated with Unawareness of Illness in Schizophrenia: A Preliminary Study. *Journal of Neuropsychiatry & Clinical Neurosciences* 2001;13: 255–257.

78. Flashman LA, Roth RM, McAllister TW, Vidaver RM, Koven N, Saykin AJ: Self-Reflection Impairment in Patients with Schizophrenia and Relationship to Awareness of Illness. (submitted).

79. Flashman LA, McAllister TW: Lack of Awareness and Its Impact in Traumatic Brain Injury. *NeuroRehabilitation* 2002;17: 285–296.

80. Fahy TJ, Irving MH, Millac P: Severe Head Injuries. *The Lancet* 1967;2:475–479.

81. Trudel TM, Tryon WW, Purdum CM: *Closed Head Injury, Awareness of Disability and Long Term Outcome.* In New Hampshire Brain Injury Association Annual Meeting. Center of New Hampshire Convention Center, Manchester, NH, 1996.

82. Ezrachi O, Ben-Yishay Y, Kay T, et al.: Predicting Employment in Traumatic Brain Injury Following Neuropsychological Rehabilitation. *Journal of Head Trauma Rehabilitation* 1991;6:71–84.

83. Sherer M, Bergloff P, Levin E, High WM, Oden KE, Nick TG: Impaired Awareness and Employment Outcome after Traumatic Brain Injury. *Journal of Head Trauma Rehabilitation* 1998;13: 52–61.

84. Sherer M, Boake C, Levin E, Silver BV, Ringholz G, High WMJ: Characteristics of Impaired Awareness after Traumatic Brain Injury. *Journal of the International Neuropsychological Society* 1998;4:380–387.

85. Cavallo MM, Kay T, Ezrachi O: Problems and Changes after Traumatic Brain Injury: Differing Perceptions within and between Families. *Brain Injury* 1992;6:327–335.

86. Cuesta MJ, Peralta V: Lack of Insight in Schizophrenia. *Schizophrenia Bulletin* 1994;20:359–366.

87. Cuesta MJ, Peralta V, Caro F, de Leon J: Is Poor Insight in Psychotic Disorders Associated with Poor Performance on the Wisconsin Card Sorting Test? [Erratum Appears in Am J Psychiatry 1996; Feb;153(2):270.]. *American Journal of Psychiatry.* 1995; 152:1380–1382.

88. David A, Van Os J, et al.: Insight and Psychotic Illness: Cross-Sectional and Longitudinal Associations. *British Journal of Psychiatry* 1995;167:621–628.

89. Lysaker P, Bell M: Insight and Cognitive Impairment in Schizophrenia: Performance on Repeated Administrations of the Wisconsin Card Sorting Test. *Journal of Nervous and Mental Disease* 1994;182:656–660.

90. McEvoy JP, Apperson LJ, Applebaum PS, et al.: Insight into Schizophrenia: Its Relationship to Acute Psychopathology. *Journal of Nervous and Mental Disease* 1989;177.

91. Mohamed S, Fleming S, Penn DL, Spaulding W: Insight in Schizophrenia: Its Relationship to Measures of Executive Functions. *Journal of Nervous and Mental Disorders* 1999;187:525–531.

92. Young DA, Davila R, Scher H: Unawareness of Illness and Neuropsychological Performance in Chronic Schizophrenia. *Schizophrenia Research* 1993;10:117–124.

93. Stuss DT: *Disturbance of Self-Awareness after Frontal System Damage.* in Prigatano GP, Schacter DL (eds): Awareness of Deficit after Brain Injury. New York: Oxford University Press, 1991.

94. Stuss DT (ed.): *Self, Awareness, and the Frontal Lobes: A Neuropsychological Perspective.* Berlin, Springer, 1991.

95. Flashman LA, McAllister TW, Andreasen NC, Saykin AJ: Smaller Brain Size Associated with Lack of Awareness in Patients with Schizophrenia. *American Journal of Psychiatry* 2000;157: 1167–1169.

96. Ford B: Head Injuries - What Happens to Survivors. *The Medical Journal of Australia* 1976;1:603–605.

97. Miller H, Stern G: The Long-Term Prognosis of Severe Head Injury. *The Lancet* 1965;1:225–229.

98. Oddy M, Coughlan T, Tyerman A, et al.: Social Adjustment after Closed Head Injury: A Further Follow-up Seven Years after Injury. *Journal of Neurology, Neurosurgery and Psychiatry* 1985; 48:564–568.

99. Ota Y: *Psychiatric Studies on Civilian Head Injuries.* in Walker AE, Caveness WF, Critchley M (eds): The Late Effects of Head Injury. Springfield, IL: Charles L. Thomas, 1969, 110–119.

100. Prigatano GP: *Disturbances of Self-Awareness of Deficit after Traumatic Brain Injury.* in Prigatano GL, Schacter DL (eds): Awareness of Deficit after Brain Injury. New York: Oxford University Press, 1991, 111–126.

101. Marin RS: Apathy: A Neuropsychiatric Syndrome. *Journal of Neuropsychiatry & Clinical Neurosciences.* 1991;3:243–254.

102. Kant R, Duffy JD, Pivovarnik A: Prevalence of Apathy Following Head Injury. *Brain Injury* 1998;12:87–92.

103. Andersson S, Krogstad JM, Finset A: Apathy and Depressed Mood in Acquired Brain Damage: Relationship to Lesion Localization and Psychophysiological Reactivity. *Psychological Medicine* 1999;29:447–456.

104. Chau DT, Roth RM, Green AI: The Neural Circuitry of Reward and Its Relevance to Psychiatric Disorders. *Current Psychiatry Reports* 2004;6:391–399.

105. Cummings JL: Frontal-Subcortical Circuits and Human Behavior. *Archives of Neurology* 1993;50:873–880.

106. Mega MS, Cummings JL: *Frontal Subcortical Circuits.* in S.P. Salloway PFM, and J.D. Djuffy (ed.): The Frontal Lobes and Neuropsychiatric Illness. 2001.

107. Deb S, Lyons I, Koutzoukis C: Neuropsychiatric Sequelae One Year after a Minor Head Injury. *Journal of Neurology, Neurosurgery & Psychiatry* 1998;65:899–902.

108. Bourdon KH, Rae DS, Locke BZ, Narrow WE, Regier DA: Estimating the Prevalence of Mental Disorders in U.S. Adults from the Epidemiologic Catchment Area Survey. *Public Health Reports* 1992;107:663–668.

109. Ashman TA, Spielman LA, Hibbard MR, Silver JM, Chandna T, Gordon WA: Psychiatric Challenges in the First 6 Years after Traumatic Brain Injury: Cross-Sequential Analyses of Axis I Disorders. *Archives of Physical Medicine & Rehabilitation* 2004;85: S36–42.

110. Fann JR, Burington B, Leonetti A, Jaffe K, Katon WJ, Thompson RS: Psychiatric Illness Following Traumatic Brain Injury in an Adult Health Maintenance Organization Population.[See Comment]. *Archives of General Psychiatry* 2004;61:53–61.

111. Wei W, Sambamoorthi U, Crystal S, Findley PA: Mental Illness, Traumatic Brain Injury, and Medicaid Expenditures. *Archives of Physical Medicine & Rehabilitation* 2005;86:905–911.

112. Jorge RE, Robinson RG, Moser D, Tateno A, Crespo-Facorro B, Arndt S: Major Depression Following Traumatic Brain Injury. *Archives of General Psychiatry* 2004;61:42–50.

113. Jorge RE, Robinson RG, Arndt S, Forrester AW, Geisler FH, Starkstein SE: Depression Following Traumatic Brain Injury: A 1 Year Longitudinal Study. *Journal of Affective Disorders* 1993;27.

114. Brody AL, Barsom MW, Bota RG, Saxena S: Prefrontal-Subcortical and Limbic Circuit Mediation of Major Depressive Disorder. *Seminars in Clinical Neuropsychiatry.* 2001;6:102–112.

115. Drevets WC, Raichle ME: Neuroanatomical Circuits in Depression: Implications for Treatment Mechanisms. *Psychopharmacology Bulletin* 1992;28:261–274.

116. Liotti M, Mayberg HS: The Role of Functional Neuroimaging in the Neuropsychology of Depression. *Journal of Clinical & Experimental Neuropsychology* 2001;23:121–136.

117. Drevets WC: Functional Anatomical Abnormalities in Limbic and Prefrontal Cortical Structures in Major Depression. *Progress in Brain Research* 2000;126:413–431.

118. Elhwuegi AS: Central Monoamines and Their Role in Major Depression. *Progress in Neuro-Psychopharmacology & Biological Psychiatry* 2004;28:435–451.

119. Charles HC, Lazeyras F, Krishnan KR, Boyko OB, Payne M, Moore D: Brain Choline in Depression: In Vivo Detection of Potential Pharmacodynamic Effects of Antidepressant Therapy Using Hydrogen Localized Spectroscopy. *Progress in Neuro-Psychopharmacology & Biological Psychiatry* 1994;18:1121–1127.

120. Steingard RJ, Yurgelun-Todd DA, Hennen J, Moore JC, Moore CM, Vakili K, Young AD, Katic A, Beardslee WR, Renshaw PF: Increased Orbitofrontal Cortex Levels of Choline in Depressed Adolescents as Detected by in Vivo Proton Magnetic Resonance Spectroscopy. *Biological Psychiatry* 2000;48:1053–1061.

121. Shytle RD, Silver AA, Sanberg PR: Comorbid Bipolar Disorder in Tourette's Syndrome Responds to the Nicotinic Receptor Antagonist Mecamylamine (Inversine). *Biological Psychiatry* 2000;48:1028–1031.

122. Duman RS, Heninger GR, Nestler EJ: A Molecular and Cellular Theory of Depression. *Archives of General Psychiatry* 1997;54:597–606.

123. Duman RS, Malberg J, Nakagawa S, D'Sa C: Neuronal Plasticity and Survival in Mood Disorders. *Biological Psychiatry* 2000;48:732–739.

124. Wroblewski BA, Joseph AB, Cornblatt RR: Antidepressant Pharmacotherapy and the Treatment of Depression in Patients with Severe Traumatic Brain Injury: A Controlled, Prospective Study. *J Clin Psychiatry* 1996;57:582–587.

125. Dinan TG, Mobayed M: Treatment Resistance of Depression after Head Injury: A Preliminary Study of Amitriptyline Response. *Acta Psychiatrica Scandinavica* 1992;85:292–294.

126. Saran AS: Depression after Mild Closed Head Injury: Role of Dexametharone Suppression Test and Antidepressants. *J Clin Psychiatry* 1985;1985:335–338.

127. Smith MC, DeFrates-Densch N, Schrader TO, Crone SF, Davis D, Pumo DJ, Runne JT, Van Loon PC: Age and Skill Differences in Adaptive Competence. *Int J Aging Hum Dev* 1994;39: 121–136.

128. Ruedrich SL, Chu CC, Moore SL: Ect for Major Depression in a Patient with Acute Brain Trauma. *American Journal of Psychiatry* 1983;140:928–929.

129. Wroblewski BA, Leary JM, Phelan AM, et al.: Methylphenidate and Seizure Frequency in Brain Injured Patients with Seizure Disorders. *J Clin Psychiatry* 1992;53:86–89.

130. Mas F, Prichep LS, Alper K: Treatment Resistant Depression in a Case of Minor Head Injury: An Electrophysiological Hypothesis. *Clinical Electroencephalography* 1993;24:118–122.

131. Schreiber S, Klag E, Gross Y, Segman RH, Pick CG: Beneficial Effect of Risperidone on Sleep Disturbance and Psychosis Following Traumatic Brain Injury. *International Clinical Psychopharmacology* 1998;13:273–275.

132. Stewart JT, Hemsath RN: Bipolar Illness Following Traumatic Braininjury: Treatment with Lithium and Carbamazepine. *J Clin Psychiatry* 1988;49:74–75.

133. Bracken P: Mania Following Head Injury. *Br J Psychiatry* 1987;150:690–692.

134. Robinson RG, Boston JD, Starkstein SE, et al.: Comparison of Mania and Depression after Brain Injury: Causal Factors. *Am J Psychiatry* 1988;145:172–178.

135. Starkstein SE, Boston JD, Robinson RG: Mechanisms of Mania after Brain Injury:12 Case Reports and Review of the Literature. *J Nerv Ment Dis* 1988;176:87–100.

136. Shukla S, Cook BL, Mukherjee S, et al.: Mania Following Head Trauma. *Am J Psychiatry* 1987;144:93–96.

137. Riess H, Schwartz CE, Klerman GL: Manic Syndrome Following Head Injury: Another Form of Secondary Mania. *J Clin Psychiatry* 1987;48:29–30.

138. Pope HG, McElroy SL, Satlin A, et al.: Head Injury, Bipolar Disorder, and Response to Valproate. *Compr Psychiatry* 1988;29:34–38.

139. Nizamie SH, Nizamie A, Borde M, et al.: Mania Following Head Injury: Case Reports and Neuropsychological Findings. *Acta Psychiatr Scand* 1988;77:637–639.

140. Cohn CK, Wright JR, Vaul RAD: Post Head Trauma Syndrome in an Adolescent Treated with Lithium Carbonate - Case Report. *Diseases of the Nervous System* 1977;38:630–631.

141. Hale MS: Lithium Carbonate in the Treatment of Organic Brain Syndrome. *J Nerv Ment Dis* 1982;170:362–365.

142. Starkstein SE, Mayberg HS, Berthier ML, et al.: Mania after Brain Injury: Neuro-Radiological and Metabolic Findings. *Ann Neurol* 1990;27:652–659.

143. McAllister TW: Traumatic Brain Injury and Psychosis: What Is the Connection? *Semin Clin Neuropsychiatry* 1998;3:211–223.

144. McAllister TW, Ferrell RB: Evaluation and Treatment of Psychosis after Traumatic Brain Injury. *NeuroRehabilitation* 2002;17:357–368.

145. Davison K, Bagley CR: Schizophrenia-Like Psychosis Associated with Organic Disorders of the Central Nervous System. *Br J Psychiatry* 1969;114:113–184.

146. Trimble MR: The Psychoses of Epilepsy. *Clin Neuropharmacol* 1985;8:211–220.

147. McKenna P, Kane J, K P: Psychotic Syndromes in Epilepsy. *American Journal of Psychiatry* 1985;142:895–904.

148. Krohn W: A Study of Epilepsy in Northern Norway, Its Frequency and Character. *Acta Psychiatry Neurol Scan* 1961 (suppl); 150:215–225.

149. Gudmundsson G: Epilepsy in Iceland - a Clinical and Epidemiological Investigation. *Acta Neurol Scand* 1966 (suppl);25:1–25.

150. Toone B, Dawson J, Driver M: Psychoses of Epi-Lepsy: A Radiological Evaluation. *Br J Psychiatry* 1982;140:244–248.

151. Trimble MR, Perez M: *The Phenomenology of the Chronic Psychosis of Epilepsy.* in Koella W, Trimble MR (eds): Temporal Lobe Epilepsy, Mania, and Schizophrenia. Basel: Karger, 1982, 98–105.

152. Flor-Henry P: Psychosis and Temporal Lobe Epilepsy: A Controlled Investigation. *Epilepsia* 1969;10:363–395.

153. Sherwin I, Peron-Magnan P, Bancaud J, Bonis A, Talairach J: Prevalence of Psychosis in Epilepsy as a Function of the Laterality of the Epileptogenic Lesion. *Archives of Neurology* 1982;39:621–625.

154. Trimble MR: Interictal Psychoses of Epilepsy. *Adv Neurol* 1991;55:143–152.

155. Tucker G, Price T, Johnson V, McAllister T: Phenomenology of Temporal Lobe Dysfunction: A Link to Atypical Psychosis—a Series of Cases. *J of Nervous and Mental Disease* 1986;174:348–356.

156. Waldman A: Neuroanatomic/Neuropathoogy Corre-Lates in Schizophrenia. South Med J 85:907–916, 1992 54. Stevens Jr: Anatomy of Schizophrenia Revisited. *Southern Medical Journal* 1997;85:907–916.

157. Waldman AJ: Neuroanatomic/Neuropathologic Correlates in Schizophrenia. *South Med J* 1992;85:907–916.

158. Stevens JR: Anatomy of Schizophrenia Revisited. *Schizophrenia Bulletin* 1997;23:373–383.

159. Turetsky B, Cowell P, Gur R, et al.: Frontal and Temporal Lobe Brain Volumes in Schizophrenia: Relationship to Symptoms and Clinical Subtype. *Arch Gen Psychiatry* 1995;52:1061–1070.

160. Andreasen NC, Arndt S, Swayze V, Cizadlo T, Flaum M, O'Leary D, Ehrhardt JC, Yuh WT: Thalamic Abnormalities in Schizophrenia Visualized through Magnetic Resonance Image Averaging. *Science* 1994;266:294–298.

161. Buchanan RW, Breier A, Kirkpatrick B, Elkashef A, Munson RC, Gellad F, Carpenter WT, Jr.: Structural Abnormalities in Deficit and Nondeficit Schizophrenia. *Am J Psychiatry* 1993;150:59–65.

162. Jernigan TL, Zisook S, Heaton RK, Moranville JT, Hesselink JR, Braff DL: Magnetic Resonance Imaging Abnormalities in Lenticular Nuclei and Cerebral Cortex in Schizophrenia. *Archives of General Psychiatry* 1991;48:881–890.

163. Swayze VW, 2nd, Andreasen NC, Alliger RJ, Yuh WT, Ehrhardt JC: Subcortical and Temporal Structures in Affective Disorder and Schizophrenia: A Magnetic Resonance Imaging Study. *Biological Psychiatry* 1992;31:221–240.

164. Tamminga CA: *Neuropsychiatric Aspects of Schizophrenia.* in Yudofsky SC, Hales RE (eds): The American Psychiatric Press Textbook of Neuropsychiatry. Washington, DC: American Psychiatric Press, 1997, 855–882.

165. Tamminga CA, Thaker GK, Buchanan R, Kirkpatrick B, Alphs LD, Chase TN, Carpenter WT: Limbic System Abnormalities Identified in Schizophrenia Using Positron Emission Tomography with Fluorodeoxyglucose and Neocortical Alterations with Deficit Syndrome. *Archives of General Psychiatry* 1992;49:522–530.

166. Buchsbaum MS, Haier RJ, Potkin SG, Nuechterlein K, Bracha HS, Katz M, Lohr J, Wu J, Lottenberg S, Jerabek PA: Frontostriatal Disorder of Cerebral Metabolism in Never-Medicated Schizophrenics. *Archives of General Psychiatry* 1992;49:935–942.

167. Selemon LD, Rajkowska G, Goldman-Rakic PS: Abnormally High Neuronal Density in Two Widespread Areas of the Schizophrenic Cortex: A Morphometric Analysis of Prefrontal Area 9 and Occipital Area 17. *Archives of General Psychiatry* 1995; 52:805–818.

168. Akbarian S, Kim JJ, Potkin SG, Hagman JO, Tafazzoli A, Bunney WE, Jr., Jones EG: Gene Expression for Glutamic Acid Decarboxylase Is Reduced without Loss of Neurons in Prefrontal Cortex of Schizophrenics. *Archives of General Psychiatry* 1995; 52:258–266.

169. Akbarian S, Kim JJ, Potkin SG, Hetrick WP, Bunney WE, Jr., Jones EG: Maldistribution of Interstitial Neurons in Prefrontal White Matter of the Brains of Schizophrenic Patients. *Archives of General Psychiatry* 1996;53:425–436.

170. McAllister TW: Neuropsychiatric Aspects of Delusions. *Psychiatric Annals* 1992;22:269–277.

171. McAllister TW: Mixed Neurologic and Psychiatric Disorders: Pharmacological Issues. *Compr Psychiatry* 1992;33:296–304.

172. McAllister TW, Price TRP: *Depression in the Brain Injured: Phenomenology and Treatment.* in Endler NS, McCann CD (eds): Depression: New Directions in Theory, Research, and Practice. Toronto, Canada: Wall and Emerson, 1990, 361–387.

173. Gualtieri CT: Pharmacotherapy and the Neurobehavioral Sequelae of Traumatic Brain Injury. *Brain Inj* 1988;2:101–129.

174. Sparadeo FR, Strauss D, Bartels JT: The Incidence, Impact, and Treatment of Substance Abuse in Head Trauma Rehabilitation. *J Head Traum Rehabil* 1990;5:108.

175. Kane J, Honigfeld G, Singer J, Meltzer H: Clozapine for the Treatment-Resistant Schizophrenic. A Double-Blind Comparison with Chlorpromazine. *Archives of General Psychiatry* 1988;45: 789–796.

176. Silver JM, Hales RE, Yudofsky SC: *Neuropsychiatric Aspects of Traumatic Brain Injury.* in Yudofsky SC, Hales RE (eds): The American Psychiatric Press Textbook of Neuropsychiatry. Washington, D.C.: American Psychiatric Press, Inc., 1992, 179–190.

177. Newburn G: Psychiatric Disorders Associated with Traumatic Brain Injury, Optimal Treatment. *CNS Drugs* 1998;9:441–456.

178. Tandon R, Milner K, Jibson M: Antipsychotics from Theory to Practice: Integrating Clinical and Basic Data. *Journal of Clinical Psychiatry* 1999;60:21–28.

179. Maixner S, Mellow A, Tandon R: The Efficacy, Safety, and Tolerability of Antipsychotics in the Elderly. *Journal of Clinical Psychiatry* 1999;60:29–41.

180. Butler P: Diurnal Variation in Cotard's Syndrome Copresent with Capgras Delusion Following Traumatic Brain Injury. *Australian & New Zealand Journal of Psychiatry* 2000;34:684–687.

181. Feinberg T, eaton L, Roane D, Giacino J: Multiple Fregoli Delusions after Traumatic Brain Injury. *Cortex* 1999;35:373–387.

182. Umansky R, Geler V: Olanzapine Treatment in an Organic Hallucinosis Patient. *International Journal of Neuropsychopharmacology* 2000;3:81–82.

183. Laddomada A, LaCroce M, Paluello M, Serri L, Altamura A: Clozapine Treatment and Post-Traumatic Psychotic Disorders, a Case Report. *Eur. Neuropsychopharmacology* 1999;9:257–258.

184. Warden D, Labatte L: Posttraumatic Stress Disorder and Other Anxiety Disorders. in Silver J, McAllister T, Yudofsky S (eds): Textbook of Traumatic Brain Injury. Arlington, VA: American Psychiatric Publishing, Inc., 2005, 231–244.

185. Robinson RG, Jorge RE: *Mood Disorders.* in Silver J, Yudofsky SC, Hales RE (eds): Neuropsychiatry of Traumatic Brain Injury. Washington, D.C.: American Psychiatric Press, 1994, 219–250.

186. Dikmen S, McLean A, Temkin N: Neuropsychological and Psychosocial Consequences of Minor Head Injury. *Journal of Neurology, Neurosurgery, and Psychiatry* 1986;49:1227–1232.

187. Levin HS, Mattis S, Ruff RM, Eisenberg HM, Marshall LF, Tabaddor K, High WM, Jr., Frankowski RF: Neurobehavioral Outcome Following Minor Head Injury: A Three-Center Study. *Journal of Neurosurgery* 1987;66:234–243.

188. Schoenhuber R, Gentilini M: Anxiety and Depression after Mild Head Injury: A Case Control Study. *J Neurol Neurosurg Psychiatry* 1988;51:722–724.

189. Deb S, Lyons I, Koutzoukis C: Neurobehavioural Symptoms One Year after a Head Injury. *British Journal of Psychiatry* 1999; 174:360–365.

190. Sbordone RJ, Liter JC: Mild Traumatic Brain Injury Does Not Produce Post-Traumatic Stress Disorder. *Brain Injury* 1995;9: 405–412.

191. Mayou RA, Black J, Bryant B: Unconsciousness, Amnesia and Psychiatric Symptoms Following Road Traffic Accident Injury. *British Journal of Psychiatry* 2000;177:540–545.

192. McMillan TM: Post-Traumatic Stress Disorder Following Minor and Severe Closed Head Injury:10 Single Cases. *Brain Injury* 1996;10:749–758.

193. McMillan TM: Post-Traumatic Stress Disorder and Severe Head Injury. *Br J Psychiatry* 1991;159:431–433.

194. Bryant RA, Harvey AG: The Influence of Traumatic Brain Injury on Acute Stress Disorder and Post-Traumatic Stress Disorder Following Motor Vehicle Accidents. *Brain Injury* 1999;13: 15–22.

195. King N: Mild Head Injury: Neuropathology, Sequelae, Measurement and Recovery. *British Journal of Clinical Psychology* 1997;36:161–184.

196. McMillan: Post-Traumatic Stress Disorder and Severe Head Injury. *British Journal of Psychiatry* 1991;159:431–433.

197. Bryant RA, Harvey AG: Relationship between Acute Stress Disorder and Posttraumatic Stress Disorder Following Mild Traumatic Brain Injury. *American Journal of Psychiatry* 1998;155: 625–629.

198. Harvey AG, Bryant RA: Acute Stress Disorder after Mild Traumatic Brain Injury. *Journal of Nervous & Mental Disease* 1998; 186:333–337.

199. Harvey AG, Bryant RA: Predictors of Acute Stress Following Mild Traumatic Brain Injury. *Brain Injury* 1998;12:147–154.

200. Bryant RA, Harvey AG: Postconcussive Symptoms and Posttraumatic Stress Disorder after Mild Traumatic Brain Injury. *Journal of Nervous & Mental Disease* 1999;187:302–305.

201. Miller N, Adams J: *Alcohol and Drug Disorders.* in Silver J, McAllister T, Yudofsky SC (eds): Text Book of Traumatic Brain Injury. Arlington, VA: American Psychiatric Publishing, Inc., 2005, 509–532.

202. Edna TH: Alcohol Influence and Head Injury. *Acta Chirurgica Scandinavica* 1982;148:209–212.

203. Sparedeo F, Gill D: Effects of Prior Alcohol Use on Head Injury Recovery. *Journal of Head Trauma Rehabilitation* 1989;4:75–82.

204. Brooks N, Symington C, Beattie A, Campsie L, Bryden J, McKinlay W: Alcohol and Other Predictors of Cognitive Recovery after Severe Head Injury. *Brain Injury* 1989;3:235–246.

205. Ruff RM, Niemann H: Cognitive Rehabilitation Versus Day Treatment in Head-Injured Adults: Is There an Impact on Emotional and Psychosocial Adjustment? *Brain Injury* 1990;4: 339–347.

206. Miller JD: Pathophysiology and Management of Head Injury. *Neuropsychology* 1991;5:235–261.

207. Jellinger KA: Head Injury and Dementia. *Current Opinion in Neurology* 2004;17:719–723.

208. Chen Y, Lomnitski L, Michaelson DM, Shohami E: Motor and Cognitive Deficits in Apolipoprotein E-Deficient Mice after Closed Head Injury. *Neuroscience* 1997;80:1255–1262.

209. Hartman RE, Laurer H, Longhi L, Bales KR, Paul SM, McIntosh TK, Holtzman DM: Apolipoprotein E4 Influences Amyloid Deposition but Not Cell Loss after Traumatic Brain Injury in a Mouse Model of Alzheimer's Disease. *Journal of Neuroscience* 2002;22:10083–10087.

210. Laws SM, Clarnette RM, Taddei K, Martins G, Paton A, Hallmayer J, Almeida OP, Groth DM, Gandy SE, Forstl H, Martins RN: Apoe-Epsilon4 and Apoe -491a Polymorphisms in Individuals with Subjective Memory Loss. *Molecular Psychiatry* 2002; 7:768–775.

211. Nathoo N, Chetty R, van Dellen JR, Barnett GH: Genetic Vulnerability Following Traumatic Brain Injury: The Role of Apolipoprotein E. *Molecular Pathology* 2003;56:132–136.

212. Nathoo N, Chetry R, van Dellen JR, Connolly C, Naidoo R: Apolipoprotein E Polymorphism and Outcome after Closed Traumatic Brain Injury: Influence of Ethnic and Regional Differences. *Journal of Neurosurgery* 2003;98:302–306.

213. Chiang MF, Chang JG, Hu CJ: Association between Apolipoprotein E Genotype and Outcome of Traumatic Brain Injury. *Acta Neurochirurgica* 2003;145:649–653; discussion 653–644.

214. Crawford FC, Vanderploeg RD, Freeman MJ, Singh S, Waisman M, Michaels L, Abdullah L, Warden D, Lipsky R, Salazar A, Mullan MJ: Apoe Genotype Influences Acquisition and Recall Following Traumatic Brain Injury. *Neurology* 2002;58:1115–1118.

215. Lichtman SW, Seliger G, Tycko B, Marder K: Apolipoprotein E and Functional Recovery from Brain Injury Following Postacute Rehabilitation. *Neurology* 2000;55:1536–1539.

216. Friedman G, Froom P, Sazbon L, Grinblatt I, Shochina M, Tsenter J, Babaey S, Yehuda B, Groswasser Z: Apolipoprotein E-Epsilon4 Genotype Predicts a Poor Outcome in Survivors of Traumatic Brain Injury. *Neurology* 1999;52:244–248.

217. Liberman JN, Stewart WF, Wesnes K, Troncoso J: Apolipoprotein E Epsilon 4 and Short-Term Recovery from Predominantly Mild Brain Injury. *Neurology* 2002;58:1038–1044.

218. Koponen S, Taiminen T, Kairisto V, Portin R, Isoniemi H, Hinkka S, Tenovuo O: Apoe-Epsilon4 Predicts Dementia but Not Other Psychiatric Disorders after Traumatic Brain Injury. *Neurology* 2004;63:749–750.

219. Parasuraman R, Greenwood PM: The Apolipoprotein E Gene, Attention, and Brain Function. *Neuropsychology* 2002;16:254–274.

220. Parasuraman R, Greenwood P, Sunderland T: The Apolipoprotein E Gene, Attention, and Brain Function. *Neuropsychology* 2002:254–274.

221. Ovsiew F, Bylsma FW: The Three Cognitive Examinations. *Seminars in Clinical Neuropsychiatry* 2002;7:54–64.

222. McCauley S, Levin H, Vanier M, Mazaux J, Boake C, Goldfader P, Rockers D, Butters M, Kareken D, Lambert J, Clifton G: The Neurobehavioural Rating Scale-Revised: Sensitivity and Validity in Closed Head Injury Assessment. *J Neurol Neurosurg Psychiatry* 2001;71:643–651.

223. Cummings JL, Mega M, Gray K, Rosenberg-Thompson S, Carusi DA, Gornbein J: The Neuropsychiatric Inventory: Comprehensive Assessment of Psychopathology in Dementia. *Neurology* 1994;44:2308–2314.

224. Yudofsky S, Silver J, Jackson W, Endicott J, Williams D: The Overt Aggression Scale for the Objective Rating of Verbal and Physical Aggression. *Am J. Psychiatry* 1986;143:35–39.

225. Marin RS, Biedrzycki RC, Firinciogullari S: Reliability and Validity of the Apathy Evaluation Scale. *Psychiatry Research*. 1991;38:143–162.

226. Folstein MF, Folstein SE, McHugh PR: "Mini Mental State": A Practical Method for Grading the Cognitive State of Patients for the Clinician. *Journal of Psychiatry Research* 1975;12:189–198.

227. Gioia GA, Isquith PK, Guy SC, Kenworthy L: *Brief: Behavior Rating Inventory of Executive Function*. Odessa, Florida, Psychological Assessment Resources, Inc., 2000.

228. Roth RM, Isquith PK, Gioia GA: *Behavioral Rating Inventory of Executive Function – Adult Version*. Lutz, Fl., Psychological Assessment Resources, Inc., 2005.

229. Ross DA, Olsen WL, Ross AM, Andrews BT, Pitts LH: Brain Shift, Level of Consciousness, and Restoration of Consciousness in Patients with Acute Intracranial Hematoma. *Journal of Neurosurgery* 1989;71:498–502.

230. Dubois B, Slachevsky A, Litvan I, Pillon B: The Fab: A Frontal Assessment Battery at Bedside. *Neurology* 2000;55:1621–1626.

231. Beck AT, Steer RA, Brown GK: *Beck Depression Inventory-Ii (Bdi-Ii)*. San Antonio, TX, The Psychological Corporation, 1996.

232. Spielberger CD: *State-Trait Anxiety Inventory*. Palo Alto, California, Consulting Psychologists Press, Inc., 1983.

233. Amador XF, Strauss DH, Yale SA, et al.: Awareness of Illness in Schizophrenia. *Schizophrenia Bulletin* 1991;17:113–132.

234. Weathers F, Litz BT, Herman DS, Huska JA, Keane TM: *The Ptsd Checklist: Reliability, Validity, & Diagnostic Utility*. In Annual Meeting of the International Society for Traumatic Stress Studies. San Antonio, TX, 1993.

235. Tariot PN, Loy R, Ryan JM, Porsteinsson A, Ismail S: Mood Stabilizers in Alzheimer's Disease: Symptomatic and Neuroprotective Rationales. *Advanced Drug Delivery Reviews* 2002;54:1567–1577.

236. Tariot PN: The Older Patient: The Ongoing Challenge of Efficacy and Tolerability. *Journal of Clinical Psychiatry* 1999;60 (Suppl 23):29–33.

XI

SPEECH, LANGUAGE, AND SWALLOWING PROBLEMS

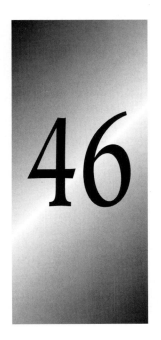

46 Assessment and Treatment of Speech and Language Disorders in TBI

Bruce E. Murdoch
Brooke-Mai Whelan

COMMUNICATION DISORDERS FOLLOWING TBI: AN INTRODUCTION

Traumatic brain injury (TBI) is the result of impact-induced biomechanical forces upon neural tissue, including compression, acceleration–deceleration and rotational acceleration (1, 2). Associated neurological injuries may be focal, multifocal, or diffuse, involving direct trauma, as well as tension-related tearing of tissue and/or shearing as a consequence of rotational force (1). In relation to communication skills, the potentially wide-ranging and heterogeneous nature of TBI accommodates an infinite range of prospective motor speech and language disturbances, through effects on the cortical, subcortical, bulbar and/or cerebellar systems.

Of particular note, the integrity of an individual's communication skills subsequent to TBI is often a critical factor in determining post-injury quality of life (3). Indeed, it has been recognized that speech and language deficits resulting from TBI may impose substantial social (4, 5) and vocational (6) ramifications. In the case of adults, the speech and language corollary of TBI is accountable for social segregation, academic failure, and/or vocational demotion following injury (2). In the case of children, TBI has been documented to cause immediate communication deficits, as well as a potential predisposition to speech and/or language impediments evident during the formative years, whereby infants fail to meet milestones as they proceed along an anticipated motor-cognitive developmental continuum (2). Until recently, the remediation of communication problems associated with TBI has been considered subordinate to the management of related medical conditions (7). In light of the potentially adverse psychosocial impact that a loss of an ability to communicate may impose upon individuals with TBI, however, it must be emphasized that effective speech-language rehabilitation can no longer be viewed as an ancillary treatment objective.

Dysarthria represents a frequently documented symptom of TBI. It reportedly constitutes more than one-third of the communication deficits within this population (8). Furthermore, a diverse range of dysarthric subtypes has been observed in individuals subsequent to TBI (8). Within these subtypes, reported levels of motor speech dysfunction have been documented to vary from mild articulatory imprecision to nonfunctional speech (9). In contrast, apraxia of speech constitutes a rarely documented motor speech anomaly associated with TBI (10–12); however, it has been reported to manifest in tandem with dysarthria and aphasic symptoms in some cases (11). We are precluded in this chapter from discussing this further due to the limited amount of research available pertaining to apraxia in TBI, and the frequently encountered diagnostic conundrum faced by clinicians with respect to delineating between the symptoms of simultaneous motor programming and muscular control deficits.

Current knowledge about the impact of TBI upon linguistic function is somewhat secondary to that about influences upon motor speech control. This discrepancy may be attributed to the fact that individuals with TBI have been historically reported to perform within normal limits on assessments of general language function (13), largely resulting in the exclusion of this population from supplemental linguistic analysis. Utilizing appropriately sensitive measures of higher-order, in addition to primary language function, deficits at the cognitive–linguistic interface, have been recently identified in TBI subjects (14). Similarly to motor speech sequelae, the nature of linguistic impairments resulting from head injury have been reported as variable (13). Incidence rates with respect to language dysfunction, however, have been documented to be as high as 100% in some research (15), highlighting TBI patients as a clinically viable population for language screening and intervention.

Mild TBI (mTBI) has received attention in the popular media as a public health concern (16, 17). Despite the fact that the majority of neurobehavioral alterations that result from mTBI have been documented to resolve within months of the related trauma, recent evidence suggests that premorbid levels of functioning may never be returned to after an injury (16). Of note, speech and language constitute neurobehavioral domains implicated within this population (18). Clearly, TBI encompassing the full spectrum of severity levels has the capacity to have an impact upon communication proficiency. It is the aim of this chapter, therefore, to describe the speech and language deficits that may manifest in individuals with TBI, as well as to provide a summary of applied assessment and treatment techniques that may be readily integrated within contemporary rehabilitation programs.

ASSESSMENT AND TREATMENT OF MOTOR SPEECH DISORDERS IN TBI

The variable nature of the neuropathology resulting from TBI predicts the potential involvement of isolated or manifold motor speech subsystems. Consequently, emergent motor speech profiles in TBI subjects may include articulatory, velopharyngeal, laryngeal and/or respiratory deficiencies. A characteristic common to the dysarthria associated with TBI, however, is its intractable nature (8). Of note, it has been documented that although frequently presenting in tandem with language impairments at onset, the dysarthria of TBI endures long after initial linguistic deficits have resolved (3, 19, 20). Recent outcome studies, however, have indicated that the dysarthria of TBI

may respond effectively to a range of treatment techniques, documented to facilitate improvements in clinical speech features, functional communication skills, and physiological substrates (21–28). The following section outlines the nature of motor speech impairments associated with TBI, suitable assessment techniques and relevant treatment approaches.

The Dysarthria of TBI: Neuroanatomical Classification and Clinical Features

As mentioned previously, the precise nature of the dysarthria that manifests as a consequence of TBI is governed by the location and scope of neural damage endured (8). The inherently diffuse nature of TBI, however, typically accommodates potential disruption at exponential loci along the neural axis, implicating upper as well as lower motor neuron systems. Indeed, classifications of spastic (29), hyperkinetic/hypokinetic (30, 31), flaccid (32, 33), ataxic (27, 34, 35) and mixed (29, 36) dysarthria have been reported within the TBI literature (37); however, spastic (37) and more recently mixed (i.e., spastic-ataxic) (36) subtypes have been highlighted as the most prevalent motor speech disturbances in this population. This motor speech profile is consistent with diffuse bilateral hemispheric damage following head injury (37), potentially implicating terminal loci of the neural fulcrum, such as the frontal lobes (38–40) and cerebellum, as the neuropathological substrates of the dysarthria of TBI.

Spastic Dysarthria

Spastic dysarthria, resulting from upper motor neuron damage implicating cortical motor areas and/ or associated descending motor tracts (41), reportedly manifests as a result of wide-ranging disturbance across the motor speech subsystems, characterized by hypertonicity of the muscles and reduced range, speed and strength of muscle excursion (42). Perceptually, this physiological symptom complex is typically characterized by strained-strangled vocal quality, as well as reduced alternate motion and speech rates (42).

Hyperkinetic and Hypokinetic Dysarthria

Although less common than spastic dysarthria, upper motor neuron damage as a consequence of TBI has also been reported to result in hypokinetic or hyperkinetic dysarthric subtypes (37). Neuropathologically defined within extrapyramidal nuclei such as the basal ganglia and divisions of the brain stem, hyperkinetic motor behavior denotes aberrantly excessive movement and hypokinesia, diminished and decelerated movement (1). Clinically, hyperkinetic dysarthria is characterized by disturbances in the rhythm and rate of oromotor movements as a consequence of involuntary motor actions, and variability in muscle tone (43, 44). Perceptually, this profile is most often distinguished by prosodic deviations including impairments in pitch and volume control, stress, rate, phrase as well as inter-word and phoneme duration, but may also include additional aberrant speech features such as sudden respiratory inhalations and exhalations, vocal arrest, strained-strangled vocalization, articulatory imprecision and hypernasality (43–46).

In contrast, the clinical characteristics of hypokinetic dysarthria embody oromotor deviations associated with rigidity, diminished range as well as force of movement, and variations in movement velocity (47, 48). Perceptually, these neuromuscular disturbances commonly manifest as monopitch, monoloudness, reduced stress, festinatory speech (i.e., short rushes), hoarse and/ or breathy vocal quality, articulatory imprecision, phoneme repetition, low pitch, overall increased but variable speech rate and diminished volume control (47–49).

Flaccid Dysarthria

In keeping with the inherently heterogeneous nature of neurological damage associated with TBI, motor speech disturbances consistent with lower motor neuron lesions have also been observed within this population. Resulting from damage to the motor cranial and/ or spinal nerves, flaccid dysarthria is characterized by muscular weakness, absent or reduced reflexes, muscle atrophy and fasciculations (1). Clinically, the motor speech deficits associated with this neurological profile may vary, dependent upon the specific cranial nerves implicated (50, 51). A common assemblage of deviant speech features, however, has been observed in flaccid dysarthric populations including breathiness, audible inspiration, hypernasality, nasal emission, reduced phrase length, consonant imprecision, vocal harshness, monopitch and monoloudness (45). Of particular note, the resonatory and phonatory deficiencies frequently seen in flaccid dysarthria have been described as largely unique to this dysarthric subtype (50).

Ataxic Dysarthria

Extending further along the neural axis, cerebellar damage has also been reported as a possible outcome of TBI (8). Ataxic dysarthria constitutes the resultant motor speech deficit and is typically characterized by articulatory and prosodic insufficiencies (52). Perceptually, these insufficiencies translate as articulatory imprecision (encompassing both consonants and vowels), articulatory breakdowns, excess and equal stress, prolongation of phonemes and inter-word intervals, diminished speech rate, monopitch, monoloudness and harsh vocal quality (53). This motor speech profile has been reported to specifically represent the neuromuscular effects of reduced tone and co-ordination, effecting slow and inaccurate motor behaviors

relevant to the force, range, timing and direction of speech musculature movement (52, 54).

Mixed Dysarthria

The heterogeneous and often pervasive nature of TBI, respecting lesion location, has also been associated with the clinical presentation of mixed dysarthria, concomitantly encompassing the motor speech deviations of several dysarthric subtypes (1, 37, 55). Notably, a recent body of research identified mixed dysarthria as the most prevalent from of motor speech impairment in cohort of TBI subjects, including spastic-ataxic, spastic-hypokinetic, spastic-flaccid, flaccid-ataxic and spastic-flaccid-ataxic subtypes (8, 36). Of further interest, within this group individuals classified with mixed dysarthric subtypes demonstrated the most qualitatively severe motor speech disturbances, suggesting that more diffuse brain damage may correlate with more severe speech disturbances.

Dysarthria Acquired During Childhood

The aforementioned neuroanatomical classification of dysarthric subtypes and associated clinical features largely relate to motor speech anomalies acquired in adulthood or at neurodevelopmentally stable life stages. Historically, this taxonomy has been adopted as a frame of reference to classify dysarthria resulting from TBI in childhood, however, not without recognised limitations (56). It has been eloquently acknowledged that the pathophysiological mechanisms underlying childhood TBI may be disparate to those which take hold within the adult brain, particularly when considered within the context of developmental hierarchies and neuroplasticity capabilities (56). Indeed, TBI in childhood has been documented to recover more rapidly than that endured in adulthood, as a consequence of distinctive neuroplasticity mechanisms (57). Furthermore, children have been reported to predominantly endure brain injuries as a result of low speed motor vehicle accidents or falls, in opposition to adolescents and adults, commonly involved in high-speed collisions (57). These factors suggest that the mechanisms of child versus adult TBI may be incongruent, with greater rotational acceleration effects and consequently more diffuse brain damage expected in adult populations (56, 57).

Until recently, the perceptual and physiological features of dysarthria resulting from TBI in childhood have been relatively unexplored (58). Contemporary research, however, has revealed similar dysarthric profiles in children as compared to adults following TBI, with respect to the presentation of a variable array of disturbances in prosodic, resonatory, phonatory and articulatory aspects of speech production (56). Despite these clinical parallels, future research investigating the nature of interactions between developmental and acquired factors is considered critical to the better elucidation of mechanisms underpinning dysarthrias contracted in childhood (59). In particular, resultant motor speech impairments may represent a maturation-sensitive consequence of head injury, within the context of developmental neurological systems. As such, longitudinal monitoring of motor speech abilities in children with TBI is considered pivotal to the prompt identification and remediation of speech deficits that may potentially manifest at any point during the course of motor development.

The Dysarthria of TBI: Perceptual, Acoustic and Physiological Evaluation

Conventionally, perceptual speech analysis has provided the main stay of dysarthria assessment (56). Despite offering qualitative insights into the audible deviations apparent in dysarthric speech, these methods proffer little with respect to empirically identifying the neuromuscular locus or neurophysiological basis of the presenting deficits. Recently, advancements in technology have catalysed the development of more objective motor speech assessment tools, affording the compilation of quantitative acoustic and physiological profiles by way of state of the art instrumentation. Notwithstanding the value of the data generated via instrumental assessments, speech is by its very nature an audible entity, its "normalcy" considered by some to be most efficiently judged by the human ear. To this end, perceptual and instrumental techniques combined have been recommended as the most effective means of evaluating motor speech dysfunction (56), taking into consideration relevant pathophysiological substrates as well as deviant perceptual features impacting upon functional communication proficiency. The proceeding summary of assessment methods utilized in the evaluation of dysarthria is largely applicable to both adult and paediatric populations. Recommendations have been made, however, with respect to the screening of developmental articulatory/ phonological processes, and/ or accommodating literacy related limitations in children.

Perceptual Assessment

Comprehensive perceptual evaluations of motor speech function have been described as those which evaluate the 5 major elements of speech production, including: respiration, phonation, resonance, articulation and prosody (56). The perceptual motor speech assessment battery utilized in our research laboratory adheres to this recommendation, providing qualitative judgements pertaining to deviant speech dimensions (i.e., speech feature analysis (60); Fisher–Logemann Test of Articulation Competence (61)), speech intelligibility (i.e., Assessment of Intelligibility of Dysarthric Speech (ASSIDS) (55)) and subsystem dysfunction (i.e., Frenchay Dysarthria Assessment (FDA)(62)). For a more detailed summary of specific assessments applicable to TBI, refer to Table 46-1.

TABLE 46-1
Comprehensive Perceptual Motor Speech Assessment Battery Applicable to TBI

- Assessment of Intelligibility of Dysarthric Speech (55)
  - standardized assessment of severity of dysarthric speech
  - incorporates measure of speech intelligibility at both single word and sentential levels, overall speech rate, rate of intelligible speech and a ratio of communication efficiency
- Frenchay Dysarthria Assessment (62)
  - standardized assessment of neuromuscular systems associated with motor speech production, including: reflexive, respiratory, articulatory, resonatory and phonatory mechanisms
  - provides composite profile relative to status of motor speech subsystem functioning
- Speech feature analysis (60)
  - following reading aloud of a standard citation such as "The Grandfather Passage" (45) or in the case of children who may not be able to read, an oral picture description task, speech samples are analysed and rated according to the presence and severity of 33 possible deviant speech dimensions
  - relevant dimensions encompass five domains of speech production, namely: prosody (i.e., pitch, loudness, phrasing, rate, stress); respiration (i.e., breath support for speech); resonance (i.e., nasality); phonation (i.e, vocal quality); and articulation (i.e., consonant precision, length of phonemes, precision of vowels)
  - also provides an overall rating of speech intelligibility
- Fisher-Logemann Test of Articulation Competence (61)
  - *relevant to childhood TBI*, this assessment generates an articulatory profile which may be further analysed relating to the nature of deviant speech productions within the context of developmental articulatory and phonological errors

Instrumental Assessment

The instrumental evaluation of dysarthria encompasses both acoustic and physiological assessment techniques. Acoustic assessment is specifically dedicated to the evaluation of voice, providing measures of frequency, amplitude, perturbation and signal noise, as well as temporally constrained aspects of phonation (e.g., maximum phonation time and voice onset time) (63) and is certainly applicable to TBI populations. A number of acoustic analysis systems are available commercially, including the Computerised Speech Lab® (CSL) (Kay Elemetrics Corp.), VisiPitch® (Kay Elemetrics Corp.), CSpeech®, the Canadian Speech Research Environment® (CSRE), MacSpeech Lab II®, and Dr. Speech Science for Windows® (Tiger Electronics) (64, 65). The CSL and VisiPitch, however, represent the most commonly employed acoustic analysis programs, rated as user friendly via the provision of real-time visual displays of acoustic parameters and the facility to store and analyse data (63).

Physiological assessments represent a corpus of instrumentation dedicated to the evaluation of the neuromuscular control mechanisms underlying speech. Available physiological apparatus not only evaluate phonatory aspects of speech production, but also extend to the assessment of articulation, resonance and respiration, including devices such as the Laryngograph, Electromagnetic articulograph, Nasometer and Respitrace. Refer to Table 46-2 for summary of physiological instrumentation that may be utilized in the assessment of individuals with TBI.

TABLE 46-2
Physiological Instrumentation Utilized in the Assessment of Dysarthria Following TBI

Laryngeal function	❏ electroglottographic assessment (Laryngograph®) ❏ aerodynamic assessment (Aerophone II®)
Respiratory function	❏ spirometric assessment ❏ kinematic assessment (Respitrace®) ❏ aerodynamic assessment (AerophoneII ®)
Articulatory function	❏ lip and tongue pressure transduction systems ❏ electropalatography (EPG) ❏ electromagnetic articulography (EMA)
Velopharyngeal function	❏ Nasometer® (Kay Elemetrics) ❏ accelerometric assessment

Physiological Measures of Laryngeal Function

In relation to the physiological assessment of laryngeal function, electroglottography (EGG) and measures of laryngeal aerodynamics represent two of the most commonly applied physiological tools in the clinical assessment of voice (63). EGG provides a means of representing vocal fold vibratory patterns (66, 67) and aerodynamic measures generate information pertaining to the interaction of various phonatory parameters. Waveforms generated via electroglottographic methods (e.g., Fourcin® Laryngograph) correspond to the opening and closing phases of the glottal cycle, and the velocity at which the vocal folds adduct (65). Measures of laryngeal aerodynamics such as the Aerophone II®, provide indices relating to the interplay of various laryngeal mechanisms in the production of voice, such as subglottal pressure, phonatory air flow, sound pressure level and laryngeal airway resistance (63). In addition to the parameters mentioned above, the Aerophone II® is also capable of measuring vocal fold adduction-abduction rates (68). Of note, high variability rates in performance have been reported in studies of aerodynamic laryngeal function (63). In order to counteract these variability effects, it has been recommended that the average of at least 5 repetitive samples, should be established as a representative illustration of laryngeal function on such measures (69). Within the context of TBI, however, fatigue effects as a result of effortful or repetitive physiological assessment tasks must also be considered in the interpretation of such data (63).

Physiological Measures of Respiratory Function

Assessments of laryngeal function routinely co-occur with an evaluation of respiratory mechanisms underlying speech production (63). Physiological measures of speech breathing may be divided into 2 broad categories: 1) spirometric (i.e., direct measures of lung volume and capacity) and 2) kinematic (i.e., indirect measures of lung function by way of monitoring chest wall activity during breathing cycles and speech production tasks). Dry spirometers provide a means of measuring a range of respiratory parameters, including: vital capacity, inspiratory capacity, expiratory and inspiratory reserve volumes, forced expiratory volume, respiration rate, tidal volume and volume/ flow relationships. Furthermore, each of the parameters obtained may be compared to predicted age, height and sex-based values by way of formulae weighted for age and/ or height (70, 71).

Kinematic measures of speech breathing provide independent yet simultaneous recordings of alterations in rib cage and abdomen volumes during speech and non-speech tasks. A range of kinematic instrumentation has been applied to the study of speech breathing in neurologically impaired populations (68), including magnetometers, strain-gauge belt pneumographs and inductance plethysomography (72–74). Respitrace®, an inductance plethysomographic measure of respiratory function, is the instrument of choice in our research laboratory. This instrument monitors changes in chest wall circumference via electrical inductance. Wires contained within elasticised straps placed around the chest and abdomen register dimensional alterations during specified tasks. A visual display signal is generated for analysis purposes and may also function as a biofeedback tool during therapy.

Physiological Measures of Articulatory Function

In relation to the evaluation of articulatory function, pressure transduction systems are commonly employed to measure lip and tongue strength, endurance, velocity of movement, and fine force control. Within our research laboratory a miniaturised pressure transducer (Entran Flatline®, Entran Devices Inc., Model EPL 20001–10) with factory calibration, mounted upon an aluminium strip, is used to measure interlabial pressures during speech and nonspeech tasks, resembling that initially described by (75). Similarly a rubber-bulb pressure transduction system is utilized to evaluate tongue function, in line with that described by (76–78).

Electropalatography (EPG) and electromagnetic articulography (EMA) represent measures of dynamic articulatory function. More specifically, EPG provides a means of evaluating the positioning and timing of tongue to hard palate contacts during speech, via a thin acrylic palate studded with miniature sensory electrodes, fitted within a subject's oral cavity. Contact patterns during speech are subsequently acquired and stored in an external processing unit for analysis. By way of transmitter and receiver coil systems generating electromagnetic fields, the Electromagnetic Articulograph® (EMA) AG-100 (Carstens Medizinelektronic, Germany) provides a two-dimensional representation of articulatory movements (79). More specifically, the EMA has the capacity to generate kinematic articulatory parameters, including trajectory, velocity, duration and acceleration, via the tracking of displacement relative to receiver coils positioned on the midline of the tongue, upper and lower lips, velum and mandible.

Physiological Measures of Velopharyngeal Function

Measures of nasal airflow, air pressure, vibration and oro-nasal acoustic output offer non-invasive, clinically viable methods of assessing velopharyngeal competence (80). Nasal accelerometry and measures of oro-nasal acoustic output ratios represent the assessments of velopharyngeal function utilized routinely within our research laboratory. Nasal accelerometry involves the placement of miniature, vibration sensitive accelerometers upon the lateral nasal cartilage and thyroid lamina, which detect nasal and laryngeal vibrations during speech. The magnitudes of vibration detected are then used to calculate a ratio of nasal to laryngeal vibration, providing an index of nasality, the Horri Oral Nasal Coupling (HONC) index (81, 82). High HONC indices are considered representative of velopharyngeal incompetence.

The Nasometer® (Kay Elemetrics) offers a measure of nasality via the generation of oro-nasal acoustic output ratios (83–85). Two directional microphones separated by a sound-separating plate are positioned anterior to the nose and mouth which record acoustic output signals. Accompanying software calculates nasalance scores which effectively represent nasal to oral acoustic output ratios during various speech tasks. High scores are considered representative of velopharyngeal dysfunction.

The Dysarthria of TBI: Treatment Approaches

The treatment of the dysarthria of TBI in both child and adult populations has been described as a convoluted and protracted process, necessitating consideration of individual deficits within the context of functional communication requirements (86). The International Classification of Functioning, Disability, and Health (ICF) offers a widely-accepted framework for intervention relative to domains of health (87), which encompass communication skills. Within this model, the treatment of dysarthria is viewed from a three-tiered perspective, including: (1) integrity of body function and structure; (2) associated activity limitations and participation restrictions; (3) contextual factors facilitating functional improvements/ reduction in disability.

The inherently heterogeneous nature of the dysarthria associated with TBI respecting lesion site and severity, has largely precluded the reporting of group outcome studies relative to individual treatment techniques (88). By and large, research pertaining to treatment effects has been conducted via single case study designs, reporting the impact of a range of behavioral, instrumental and prosthetic approaches (22–26, 89–97).

Behavioral Approach

The behavioral approach to the rehabilitation of dysarthric speech involves the teaching of compensatory strategies via traditional methods, which encompass the presentation of therapeutic stimuli and the establishment of response contingencies (98). The principle goal of this approach is to facilitate functional gains in speech intelligibility (99) via neuromuscular therapeutic techniques (100). These therapies include active exercises (e.g., strength training), stretching (e.g., to increase or decrease tone), passive exercises (e.g., massage to relax musculature), and the use of physical modalities such as heat (to reduce pain), cold (to reduce spasticity) and electrical stimulation (to elicit voluntary contractions) (100). Historically, traditional/ behavioral techniques have provided the mainstay of dysarthria therapy, given their economic viability and wide-ranging environmental utility (101). Although failing to constitute an unabridged stockpile of behavioral dysarthria therapy techniques, Table 46-3 represents a number of commonly utilized traditional approaches in the remediation of phonatory, respiratory, resonatory, articulatory and prosodic deficits.

Instrumental Approach

The instrumental therapeutic approach incorporates techniques which offer direct physiological or biofeedback pertaining to motor speech subsystem function during therapy tasks. Biofeedback tools provide a means of re-establishing motor control patterns by way of unconventional or adjunct sensory channels (113). Sensory channels may incorporate auditory, visual or tactile modalities, however, visual feedback signals have been documented as the most effective in the remediation of dysarthria (114–116). Table 46-4 highlights a range of biofeedback techniques currently utilized in the treatment of

respiratory, phonatory, resonatory, articulatory and prosodic disorders.

Prosthetic/ Surgical Approach

Prosthetic and/ or surgical interventions, which effectively modify the physical configuration of specific motor speech subsystems (98), are commonly employed in the remediation of severe dysarthria (101). Table 46-5 summarises a range of prosthetic/ surgical techniques utilized the treatment of motor speech impairments, usually employed subsequent to an ineffective trial of more traditional therapeutic approaches.

CASE REPORTS: CLINICAL MANAGEMENT OF DYSARTHRIA FOLLOWING TBI

The ability to apply the previously highlighted principles of dysarthria assessment and treatment to the management of a clinical caseload represents a requisite skill for any clinician. Within the context of the framework for intervention outlined in the ICF (87), the following vignettes constitute proposed clinical management plans relevant to the treatment of dysarthria following TBI, in a 26 year old adult and a 14 year old child.

TABLE 46-3

Behavioral Therapeutic Approaches in the Treatment of Dysarthria Following TBI

TARGETED MOTOR SPEECH SUBSYSTEM	METHOD
• Phonation	❏ *Hyperadduction reduction techniques*: aim to alleviate excessive vocal fold adduction by way of tension reduction techniques such as *chewing* (102), *yawn-sigh* and *gentle voice onset* methods (103)
	❏ *Hypoadduction reduction techniques*: aim to achieve effective vocal fold adduction and effective phonation in dysphonic patients via the application of *push/pull* (104), *hard glottal attack* (105), and *increased phonatory effort* (106) methods
• Respiration	❏ *Manipulating posture* to maximize respiratory control (107) via the provision of visual, tactile and/ or auditory cues
	❏ *Inspiratory checking* (108) technique aims to increase breath support and enhance respiratory control during exhalation via drills which encourage the regulation of air flow and volume during vocalization
• Resonance	❏ Exercises aimed at increasing range of movement and strength of velum including *blowing, gagging and sucking* (101), as well as palatal awareness via *visual feedback* (101), *palatal massage* (109) and *icing/ brushing* (110) techniques
• Articulation	❏ Aim to normalise function of the articulators (i.e., lips, tongue and jaw) via the *modification of muscle tone* (e.g., hypertonia versus hypotonia), *maximising muscle strength* (i.e., isotonic and isometric oromotor exercises (109, 111)) and *articulation/ speech drills* of increasing complexity (98)
• Prosody	❏ Methods aimed at remediating stress patterning (e.g., *contrastive stress drills* (109)), intonation (e.g., *altering respiratory capacity and patterning* (112)) and rate (e.g., *intersystemic reorganization* (109) involving therapist directed pacing of speech)

TABLE 46-4

Instrumental Therapeutic Approaches in the Treatment of Dysarthria Following TBI

TARGETED MOTOR SPEECH SUBSYSTEM	METHOD
• Phonation	❏ Use of apparatus with the facility to display vocal parameters such as pitch, intensity and duration during speech output (e.g., Vocalite (117), Visipitch (112), Visispeech (118), Speech Viewer (91), storage oscilloscope (119))
• Respiration	❏ *U-tube manometer:* requires patient to maintain specific water level over designated period of time via controlled exhalation (109)
	❏ *Kinematic instrumentation (e.g., Respitrace®):* provides visual representation of chest wall movements during speech tasks. Feedback shown to be effective in increasing lung volumes, increasing abdominal contributions to breathing as well as enhancing co-ordination of speech breathing (95, 120)
• Resonance	❏ *Endoscopy* and *flexible fibre nasopharyngoscopy* provides direct visual feedback pertaining to velar and posterior pharyngeal wall excursion during speech (121, 122)
	❏ *Velograph* provides real time representation of velar movement via an oscilloscope (123)
	❏ *Nasometer®* provides bar graphs and/or real time visual displays of nasalance during speech (101)
• Articulation	❏ *Electromyography (EMG)* represents a biofeedback tool with applications for altering labial and lingual muscle tone and strength (26, 92, 124–126)
	❏ *Electropalatography (EPG)* may be utilized as a biofeedback device to alter lingual postures during speech (127, 128)
• Prosody	❏ *Speech Viewer* (129) provides both visual and auditory feedback pertaining to fundamental frequency and vocal intensity. Documented as successful device in improving pitch, intonation and rate of speech (130)
	❏ Modification of speech rate during reading via *PACER computerised rhythmic cueing* (131)
	❏ *Delayed Auditory Feedback (DAF)* documented as useful biofeedback device in reducing rate, increasing vocal intensity and enhancing overall speech intelligibility (132–134)

TABLE 46-5

Prosthetic and/or Surgical Approaches in the Treatment of Dysarthria Following TBI

TARGETED MOTOR SPEECH SUBSYSTEM	METHOD
• Phonation	❏ *Voice amplifiers:* electronic device aimed at increasing voice volume (112, 135)
	❏ *Botox injections* (136), *laryngeal nerve resections* (137) in the treatment of hyperadduction
	❏ *Reinnervation of paralysed vocal folds* (138), *collagen/ Teflon implants* (139, 140) and *arytenoid adduction* (141) in the treatment of hypoadduction
• Respiration	❏ *Abdominal muscle girdling* by way of elasticised bandages (109). Enhances expiratory control during speech by facilitating recoil of the abdominal musculature.
	❏ Postural enhancement by use of *overhead slings* (109). Provides surface upon which individuals may bear down to establish expiratory force for speech.
• Resonance	❏ *Palatal lift prosthesis* aims to achieve palatopharyngeal closure (142, 143)
• Articulation	❏ *Bite block* to increase jaw stability and maximize function of other articulators and/ or *palatal augmentation prosthesis* which aims to facilitate tongue/ palatal contacts required for articulation otherwise compromised by reduced range of movement or elevation of tongue (143, 144)
• Prosody	❏ *Pacing* (145)/ *alphabet board* (146) encourages speech rate reduction

Case 1 (Adult): Moderate Spastic-Ataxic Dysarthria (86).

Case History: Jacob is a 26-year-old male who sustained a TBI as the result of a motor vehicle accident. On admission to hospital a Glasgow Coma of score of 5 was reported, indicative of severe head injury. MRI investigations revealed bilateral subcortical hemorrhages and multiple contusions. At the time of his accident, Jacob was married and working as a practicing accountant. His family and employer were reportedly committed to his rehabilitation and return to the work force.

Motor Speech Profile: Moderate Spastic-ataxic Dysarthria: Perceptual assessment results revealed: reduced speech intelligibility, consonant imprecision, reduced breath support for speech, hypernasality, strained-strangled vocal quality, reduced pitch and loudness control, reduced speech rate and impaired stress patterning. Physiological assessment revealed wide-ranging motor speech subsystem dysfunction, incorporating: reduced respiratory support for speech, hyperfunctional laryngeal activity, velopharyngeal insufficiency and reduced range and speed of labial and lingual movement.

Clinical Management Plan: A multisystem approach was adopted in the rehabilitation of Jacob's speech, involving a combination of behavioral and instrumental treatment techniques. Consistent with the ICF, his presenting motor speech deficit was considered in relation to structural and functional impairments, imposed activity limitations and participation restrictions as well as manipulable contextual factors. Refer to Table 46-6 for the proposed rehabilitation schedule.

Case 2 (Child): Moderate Spastic Dysarthria (147)

Case History: Max is a 14-year-old male who sustained a TBI following a pedestrian/ motor vehicle accident. On admission to hospital a Glasgow Coma of score of 5 was reported, indicative of severe head injury. Computed tomographic (CT) scan revealed soft tissue hematoma over right temporal and left zygomatic regions as well as an area of high attenuation in left lentiform nucleus and additional foci scattered over peripheral grey/ white region anteriorly and superiorly. No significant mass effect was observed. At the time of his accident, Max was a high-achieving year 9 high-school student with a range of extracurricular interests, including: debating, football and tennis.

Motor Speech Profile: Moderate Spastic Dysarthria: Subsequent to TBI, Max endured a 5-month period of mutism. Perceptual assessment of speech function following this period revealed: severely reduced range and speed of lingual movement; moderately reduced range and speed of labial movement, consonant imprecision, strained-strangled vocal quality, hypernasality, reduced breath support for speech, slow speech rate, monopitch and moderately reduced speech intelligibility. Physiological assessment also revealed wide-ranging motor speech subsystem dysfunction, incorporating: reduced lung volumes and capacities as well as reduced abdominal excursion during speech, laryngeal hyperfunction, velopharyngeal insufficiency and reduced labial and lingual strength and endurance.

Clinical Management Plan: A multisystem approach was again adopted in the rehabilitation of Max's speech, involving a combination of behavioral and instrumental treatment techniques. Consistent with the ICF, his presenting motor speech deficit was considered in relation to structural and functional impairments, imposed activity limitations and participation restrictions as well as manipulable contextual factors. Refer to Table 46-7 for the proposed rehabilitation schedule. Furthermore, longitudinal monitoring of Max's speech and language abilities was considered pivotal in maximising educational and subsequently vocational potential, as he continued to mature from adolescence into adulthood.

ASSESSMENT AND TREATMENT OF LANGUAGE DISORDERS IN TBI

Detailed investigations of linguistic integrity subsequent to TBI have been afforded limited consideration within the scientific literature thus far (13). The forerunning explanation for this lack of inquiry may rest with the observation that TBI subjects tend to perform within normal limits on tests of general language function, routinely incorporated within linguistic screening batteries. Despite this admission, however, recent evidence indicates that TBI proffers distinct ramifications for cognitive-linguistic substrates underpinning complex language processes, the rudiments of which fail to be adequately evaluated via standard aphasia tests.

Consequently, the proceeding sections of this Chapter highlight the nature of language impairments following TBI, appropriately sensitive assessments of linguistic function for use within adult and pediatric populations, as well as relevant treatment strategies.

Linguistic Deficits and TBI: Taxonomy and Neural Substrates

Despite being reported to largely perform within the range of normal on assessments of general language function, individuals with TBI frequently demonstrate deficiencies in relation to functional communication

TABLE 46-6

Multisystem Approach to the Rehabilitation of Moderate Spastic Dysarthria Following TBI in an Adult: Jacob

TREATMENT GOAL	METHOD

• Reducing impairment in body structure and function. Remediate physiological dysfunction within motor speech subsystems.
  ○ Enhance cooordination of chest wall movements during speech
  ○ Remediate hyperadduction of vocal folds
  ○ Increase velopharyngeal competence
 	
  ○ Increase strength and range of labial and lingual movements
	➤ Kinematic instrumentation to offer visual feedback of chest wall movement
	➤ Chewing/ yawn-sigh, gentle voice onset techniques
	➤ Use of Nasometer® to provide visual feedback of nasalance during speech
	➤ Isometric and isotonic lip and tongue exercises

• Reducing activity limitations and participation restrictions. Enhance speech intelligibility.
  ○ Modify stress and intonation patterns
  ○ Increase speech rate
  ○ Enhance articulatory precision
	➤ Contrastive stress and intonation drills
	➤ PACER technique
	➤ Articulation drills

• Maximising communicative success across a range of communication environments
  ○ Increasing communication partner awareness of conversational topics and contextual cues
  ○ Repairing communication breakdowns
 	
  ○ Capitalizing upon situational and environmental recompense to maximize effectiveness of communication
	➤ Practice routinely identification of contextual cues and establishment of topic of conversation
	➤ Clarify if communication partner has comprehended intended message and provide strategies for communication partners to request clarification
	➤ Limit communicative interactions when fatigued and maximize interaction when energy levels are at their peak; avoid noisy environments

• Manipulating contextual factors. Enhancing opportunities for participation across social and vocational contexts	
• Providing information to family/ friends/ workmates pertaining to nature of communicative disability and strategies to enhance communicative effectiveness within social and vocational environments	➤ Provide resources outlining: the cause and nature of presenting communication deficit; strategies to maximize communicative success with unfamiliar communication partners (e.g., sitting in front partner, requesting clarification in the event of misunderstood message) ➤ Provide assistance in communicatively taxing situations (e.g., board meetings; face to face client contact)

*Note: References pertaining to individual treatment techniques may be located in Tables 46-3, 46-4, and 46-5.

skills (148–153). Furthermore, where TBI individuals do present deficits in primary language function such as naming, verbal association, reading and/ or auditory comprehension (150, 154, 155), error profiles generally fail to meet the criteria for classification within traditional Bostonian taxonomies (149). On the basis of these characteristics, a coherent conceptualisation of the nature of linguistic deficits associated with TBI has been hindered thus far.

Most recently, however, measures of high-level linguistic functioning including probes of metalinguistic ability, lexical-semantic manipulation and language integration, have been recognised as sensitive indices of cognitive-linguistic breakdown in TBI populations (14). Tasks involving: the interpretation of ambiguous sentences, making inferential judgements, semantically constrained sentence generation, interpretation of metaphorical expressions and humour, formation of semantic associations, identification of semantic absurdities, synonym and antonym generation, definition and multiple definition formulation have been specifically implicated. These tasks are considered to be complex in nature, potentially necessitating the interplay of cognitive (e.g., attention, memory, executive

TABLE 46-7

Multisystem Approach to the Rehabilitation of Moderate Spastic Dysarthria Following TBI in a Child: Max

TREATMENT GOAL	METHOD
• Reducing impairment in body structure and function. Remediate physiological dysfunction within motor speech subsystems	
○ Increase strength, range and speed of labial and lingual movements	➤ Isometric and isotonic lip and tongue exercises; timed alternate motion exercises
○ Increase breath support for speech	➤ Inspiratory checking technique
○ Remediate hyperadduction of vocal folds	➤ Chewing/ yawn-sigh, gentle voice onset techniques
○ Enhance velopharyngeal closure	➤ Use of accelerometer to provide visual biofeedback during nasal/ non-nasal contrasts
• Reducing activity limitations and participation restrictions. Enhance speech intelligibility.	
○ Enhance articulatory precision	➤ Articulation drills
○ Increase speech rate and enhance pitch variation	➤ Speech Viewer® to provide auditory and visual feedback re: rate and pitch parameters during speech tasks
• Maximising communicative success across a range of communication environments	
○ Increasing communication partner awareness of conversational topics	➤ Max to consistently orient communication partner to topic of conversation and to maximize use of contextual cues (e.g., environmental props)
○ Repairing communication breakdowns	➤ Clarify if communication partner has comprehended intended message and offer revisions when needed
	➤ Write message if not understood
○ Capitalizing upon situational and environmental recompense to maximize effectiveness of communication	➤ Avoid noisy environments; utilize friends and family to assist in communicative interactions with unfamiliar partners or in unfamiliar environments
• Manipulating contextual factors. Enhancing opportunities for participation across social and educational contexts	
➤ Providing information to family/ friends/ teachers pertaining to nature of communicative disability and strategies to enhance communicative effectiveness within social and educational environments	➤ Provide resources outlining: the cause and nature of presenting communication deficit; strategies to maximize communicative success with unfamiliar communication partners (e.g., ask for clarification if Max's speech is unable to be understood; ask him to write messages in the event of communication breakdown; move to a quiet environment; affirm comprehension of conversational topic with close friends
	➤ Oral assessment items/ debating (e.g., english orations may be written by Max and tape recorded by family member/ friend for class presentation)
	➤ Utilization of flash cards for scoring when umpiring game of tennis

*Note: references pertaining to individual treatment techniques may be located in Tables 46-3, 46-4, and 46-5.

function) and linguistic processes (156). It is this interface that appears to be most susceptible to the effects of TBI, as opposed to more general language processes.

Overall communicative competence has also been postulated to necessitate the interplay of cognitive-linguistic processes which facilitate access to and manipulation of the semantic system within contextually defined environments (13), extending well beyond the domain of operational or primary level language (157). Indeed, some research has highlighted frontal lobe dysfunction as the primary substrate underlying the language impairments associated with TBI, on the basis of diminished neuropsychological test results pertaining to frontal lobe integrity in tandem with reduced language performance (158). In support of this postulate, closed head injury has been hypothesised to yield its greatest impact upon the prefrontal cortex, by virtue of skull configuration (159). It is plausible, therefore, that the interplay of frontal lobe-dependent cognitive domains such as attention, memory, executive function etc. with linguistic processes may be subsequently impaired as a result of TBI.

Linguistic deviations interwoven within a tapestry of cognitive deficits represents a commonly accepted view of the language symptom complex associated with TBI (13, 149, 155, 160). The precise nature of cognitive-linguistic interactions within this population, respecting a hierarchy of domain-specific influences upon language function, however, remains largely unknown (13). Recently, TBI performance profiles on tasks of lexical-semantic manipulation (e.g., TWT-R) have been strongly correlated with the cognitive variables of memory and attention (14), potentially earmarking these variables as integral to the mediation of certain linguistic operations.

In a similar manner to motor speech correlates, the linguistic sequelae of TBI have been documented as extremely variable from case to case (14), perhaps best attributed to variations in neuropathology across subjects. Despite this heterogeneity, however, several studies have identified subgroups within TBI populations respecting language performance (161–163). Global cognitive-linguistic impairment to near normal levels of functioning have been reported, with and without concomitant combinations of attentional, memory and/ or visuospatial deficits (162, 163). These profiles suggest that certain aspects of language are indeed influenced and perhaps directed by cognition, evidenced by distinct yet variable levels of discernable association subsequent to brain injury.

Thus far, the focus of the discussion pertaining to linguistic impairments associated with TBI has been directed at adult populations. Brain injury within childhood, or developmentally formative life stages with respect to cognitive skill acquisition, however, must be afforded special consideration. In a similar manner to adult language disturbances as a result of TBI, children with head injuries have been documented to present a form of "subclinical aphasia"(164), or rather, symptom complexes which fail to comply with the primary characteristics of traditional aphasic syndromes. For example, previous studies have specifically reported impairments on task of verbal fluency (165–168), confrontation naming (167, 169–171), verbal repetition (170, 171) and written expression (164, 172). Although not representative of frank aphasic deficits, it has been hypothesized that these atypical profiles may reflect the impact of TBI upon language processes in developmental ascendency at the time of insult (164).

In line with adult research, post-TBI language profiles in children suggest impairment of a high-level linguistic nature, particularly when the aforementioned deficits are considered within the context of well-documented neuropsychological deviations, including: disturbances of memory, attention, visuospatial ability and executive function (173–175). Indeed, following this line of investigation, reduced scores on sentence generation, as well as ambiguity and figurative language interpretation tasks have been identified in children with TBI (176).

Despite the many clinical parallels that may be drawn between language syndromes associated with adult and pediatric TBI, children potentially present deficits against a developmental backdrop, providing distinctive implications for assessment and treatment. Of most note, TBI in children has been documented to disproportionately disturb the acquisition of new language skills as compared to the recovery of already established abilities (177), and the younger a child is at the time of injury, the more profound the effect on language function (172, 178). Furthermore, latent behavioral deficits have also been reported to manifest in children with TBI (179, 180), posing definite ramifications for educational and vocational potential. These caveats indicate that assessment and treatment plans must be carefully mapped out in the treatment of paediatric head injury, as much as to enhance communicative competence as to maximize the quality of present and future life opportunities.

Linguistic Deficits and TBI: Assessment

In general, individuals with TBI have been reported to demonstrate distinctive deficits on high-level language tasks which entail: (i) the application of metalinguistic competence; (ii) linguistic integration/ reasoning; (iii) divergent language production; (iv) lexical-semantic manipulation (i.e., judgement, organization, retrieval) (13). Subsequently, assessment batteries utilized in the evaluation of TBI individuals should incorporate such measures. Relevant assessments as they relate to adult and pediatric populations have been listed in Tables 46-8 and 46-9, respectively. Acknowledging the potential for varying levels of deficit severity in TBI populations, assessments of primary language function may also be required to delineate impairments in some individuals. As per high-level language evaluation, refer to Tables 46-8 and 46-9 for recommended assessments of general language function as they apply to adult and pediatric cases.

It has also been acknowledged that the conversational speech of TBI subjects is frequently characterized by verbosity, tangentiality and idiosyncratic phraseology (152). Parameters such as these are inadequately assessed via standard aphasia batteries. Consequently, contemporary research has begun to focus upon the assessment of more dynamic versus static linguistic functions in TBI, including discourse, or language in its most naturalistic form (181). A comprehensive summary of discourse and its analysis as it relates to TBI is beyond the scope of this Chapter. Suffice

---

TABLE 46-8

Recommended Linguistic Assessment Battery:
Adult TBI (14, 181)

General Language Function
- ☐ Western Aphasia Battery (WAB) (182)
- ☐ Boston Diagnostic Aphasia Examination (BDAE) (183)
- ☐ Boston Naming Test (BNT) (184)
- ☐ Neurosensory Centre Comprehensive Examination for Aphasia (NCCEA) (185)
- ☐ The Revised Token Test (186)

High-level Linguistic Function
- ☐ Test of Language Competence-Expanded (TLC-E) (187)
- ☐ The Word Test-Revised (TWT-R) (188)
- ☐ The Test of Word Knowledge (TOWK) (189)
- ☐ Wiig-Semel Test of Linguistic Concepts (WSTLC) (190)
- ☐ The Right Hemisphere Language Battery (RHLB) (191)

Discourse
- ☐ Story Retell: The Businessman and the Tramp (181)

TABLE 46-9

Recommended Linguistic Assessment Battery:
Childhood TBI (192)

General Language Function
- ☐ Receptive-Expressive Emergent Language Test, Second Edition (REEL 2) (INFANTS) (193)
- ☐ Preschool Language Scale–3 (PLS–3) (Birth–6 years) (194)
- ☐ Clinical Evaluation of Language Fundamentals, Preschool (CELF-P) (3–6 years) (195)
- ☐ Clinical Evaluation of Language Fundamentals, Third Edition (CELF 3) (6–16 years) (196)
- ☐ Peabody Picture Vocabulary Test, Third Edition (PPVT-III) (197)
- ☐ Hundred Pictures Naming Test (HPNT) (198)
- ☐ Boston Naming Test (BNT) (184)

High-level Linguistic Function
- ☐ Test of Language Competence, Expanded (TLC-E)
- ☐ Test of Word Knowledge (TOWK) (189)
- ☐ Test of Problem Solving. Elementary (TOPS-Elementary) (199)
- ☐ Test of Problem Solving, Adolescent (TOPS-Adolescent) (200)

Phonological Awareness
- ☐ Queensland University Inventory of Literacy (QUIL) (201)
- ☐ Test of Phonological Awareness (TOPA) (202)

Discourse
- ☐ School Age Oral Language Assessment (SAOLA) (203)

---

to report that discourse analysis of non-interactional (e.g., narrative, procedural, expository) and interactional language samples has provided valuable insights into the nature of the functional linguistic impairments associated with TBI (181). Discourse analysis may involve the evaluation of syntactic, thematic and/or information variables (181) as well as the more pragmatic aspects of communication, or the application of social rules (204), including turn-taking, maintenance of topic, comprehension of verbal and nonverbal cues etc. (205–207). Possible methods of language sample acquisition for discourse analysis have been listed in Tables 46-8 and 46-9, however, for a detailed discussion of analysis techniques, the reader is referred to (181, 208, 209).

Linguistic Deficits and TBI: Treatment Approaches

The rehabilitation of cognitive disorders resulting from TBI, including language deficits, essentially involves three general approaches, including: restorative, compensatory and/or behavioral techniques (210–213). Restorative techniques involve the undertaking of repetitive tasks targeting specific neural processes, with the aim of restoring function. Compensatory techniques involve the development of strategies and/or competencies which overcome prevailing deficits via the acquisition of functional skills (213). Behavioral techniques engage behavior modification strategies in the development of targeted skills (210). In most cases, these strategies are used in combination, the restoration of behaviors and behavioral compensations representing the products of intervention.

Behavioral/ Restorative Approach

Specifically targeting impairments, traditional/ restorative approaches to language rehabilitation involve the repetitive undertaking of structured linguistic tasks, the nature of which are determined following a psycholinguistic evaluation of cognitive–linguistic integrity (214, 215). Refer to Table 46-10 for some examples of restorative therapy tasks.

Compensatory Approach

The compensatory approach to linguistic rehabilitation entails the development of self-initiated strategies to overcome particular communicative deficits, by way of physical props (e.g., written notes), external cues (e.g., requests for repetition of information) or internalized or self-cueing (208, 216). The success of compensatory approaches has been reported to rely upon the user's ability to apply them automatically (208). Consequently, compensatory strategies utilized naturally by a particular individual will be automatized more quickly than those strategies that are foreign or unfamiliar. For examples of compensatory strategies, please refer to Table 46-11.

TABLE 46-10

Restorative Therapeutic Strategies in the Treatment of Linguistic Deficits Following TBI (208)

Deficit	Therapy Task
• Lexical–semantic Processing	➤ Generating synonyms and antonyms ➤ Word-definition matching ➤ Convergent and divergent naming
• Comprehension of complex linguistic information	➤ Interpreting abstract expressions ➤ Proverb/metaphor explanation ➤ Discriminating between fact and opinion ➤ Following instructions of increasing length and complexity
• Organization of verbal expression	➤ Sequencing tasks ➤ Story retelling ➤ Narrative production using specified schemas

TABLE 46-11

Compensatory Therapeutic Strategies in the Treatment of Linguistic Deficits Following TBI (208)

DEFICIT	STRATEGY
• Verbosity with good insight into maladaptive behavior	➤ Frequent clarification with communication partner that they are following conversation
• Verbosity with poor insight into maladaptive behavior	➤ Obtain assistance of external communication partner regarding relevance of verbal output
• Word retrieval problems with natural tendency to circumlocute	➤ Utilize circumlocution as a means of facilitating word retrieval
• Ineffective functional communication	➤ Identify where communication breakdowns occur (i.e., in what environments), formulate communication strategies for use in those environments and develop skills by way of functional therapy tasks (e.g., role playing)

TREATMENT APPROACHES: PEDIATRIC CONSIDERATIONS

By and large, the same treatment approaches may be applied to the rehabilitation of linguistic deficits as a consequence of TBI endured in childhood. In the case of pediatric populations, however, therapeutic hierarchies must not only focus on the remediation of skills already established at the time of injury, but must also take into account the future acquisition of developmental language processes. Of particular note, the impact of TBI on cognitive-linguistic functioning may not always manifest immediately following insult in children (208). Associated language deficits may only become apparent when the child fails to successfully acquire specific language processes relevant to a developmental continuum. As a result, children with acquired brain injuries should be monitored longitudinally in order to permit the prompt identification and remediation of potential cognitive-linguistic anomalies, with a view to promoting a sound educational and vocational platform.

CASE REPORTS: CLINICAL MANAGEMENT OF LINGUISTIC IMPAIRMENTS FOLLOWING TBI

The following vignettes present clinical management plans relative to the rehabilitation of linguistic deficits following TBI in a 23-year-old adult and a 9-year-old child.

Case 1: Linguistic Impairment Following TBI in Adulthood

Case History: Kylie was a 23-year-old kindergarten teacher and part-time student at the time she sustained a TBI as the result of a motor vehicle accident. She was unconscious at the accident scene. However, no Glasgow Coma Score was recorded. Neuroimaging investigations failed to identify any focal neurological damage. At the commencement of her rehabilitation program, returning to work as a kindergarten teacher was her consummate goal.

Language Profile:

- Primary-level language largely intact with evidence of word retrieval deficits
- Natural inclination to utilize circumlocution as a means of facilitating word retrieval
- High-level linguistic deficits evident. Reduced performance on tasks of lexical semantic manipulation (e.g., forming semantic associations, defining words with multiple meanings, constructing semantically constrained sentences).
- Narrative discourse analysis revealed a proliferation of verbal disruptions, general verbosity

- Conversational discourse presented a similar profile, marked by intricate details in the presentation of information whereby the original theme of the message was often times forgotten. Kylie was insightful pertaining to her verbose communication style, frequently acknowledging her tendency to ramble.
- Often demonstrated overfamiliarity and inappropriate communicative behaviors with unfamiliar communication partners, with little insight pertaining to these character traits.

Based on the above information and within the context of the framework for intervention promoted by the ICF, a functional cognitive-linguistic communication plan for Kylie's rehabilitation was devised (208), 3 months subsequent to injury. This plan specifically targeted levels of impairment, activity limitation and participation restriction, and has been illustrated in Table 46-12.

Case 2: Linguistic Impairment Following TBI in Childhood

Case History: Sally was a 9-year-old primary school student who sustained a TBI as the result of a fall from a horse. No loss of consciousness was observed at the time of injury but she was not responsive to commands. A Glasgow Coma Score of 7 was recorded at hospital admission. CT scan failed to reveal any focal neurological damage, however, a left occipital skull fracture was indicated.

Two days after hospital admission, Sally's condition deteriorated to a state of deep coma, requiring ventilation for a period of 1 week. Subsequent CT scan revealed right cerebral oedema, compressed ventricles and midline shift. Limited verbal output was observed post-injury with the gradual return of simplified yet socially appropriate language, 4 weeks following insult. Speech/ language evaluation at this time revealed:

Language Profile:

- Primary-level language largely intact with evidence of deficiencies in aspects of spoken language production, such as confrontation naming
- Conversational discourse was marked by circumlocutory behaviors, frequent repetition of utterances, difficulty interpreting humour and comprehending complex instructions
- Delayed responses to test items evident
- Overall, high-level linguistic impairment impacting upon communicative competence was diagnosed. General profile was characterized by reduced verbal fluency and word retrieval skills in the presence of impaired performance on tasks requiring comprehension of complex concepts and instructions.

TABLE 46-12
Cognitive-Linguistic Rehabilitation Plan Following Adult TBI: Kylie

GOAL	METHOD
Providing effective instructions to children the preschool setting	Maximize verbal retrieval and planning by way of: (i) utilising circumlocution as a means of facilitating word retrieval; (ii) plan one sentence explanations increasing hierarchically to more complex structures; (iii) structured lexical-semantic tasks (e.g., naming to definition; convergent naming; divergent naming etc) Provide opportunities for role playing and rehearsal
Reduce verbosity in conversation	Discuss content categories such as relevant, irrelevant and embellishment Discuss narrative structure Identify presence and absence of content within conversations Establish self-initiated cues to reduce verbosity Provide opportunities for role playing, video feedback, group therapy
Develop appropriate conversational style with unfamiliar communication partners	Discuss various communication contexts, appropriate and inappropriate communication styles Provide opportunities for role-playing and video feedback to enhance self-monitoring skills

Based on the above information and within the context of the framework for intervention promoted by the ICF, a functional cognitive-linguistic communication plan for Sally's rehabilitation was devised (217). Refer to Table 46-13 for specific treatment schedule. Sally received 6 months of intensive speech pathology intervention with regular monitoring of progress including a formal language review at 12 months post-injury. At this point, the majority of linguistic deficits had resolved with the exception of subtle word finding difficulties in conversation. Ongoing speech pathology intervention involved monitoring of language recovery, as well as the implementation of compensatory strategies, tailored to changeable educational and social needs over the course of Sally's academic life.

TABLE 46-13
Cognitive–Linguistic Rehabilitation Plan
Following Childhood TBI: Sally (217)

GOAL	METHOD
• Reduce word finding difficulty	➤ Convergent naming
	➤ Identify salient features relative to specified items
	➤ Utilize salient features strategy to facilitate word retrieval in conjunction with communication partner
	➤ Story retell/ story construction
• Enhance comprehension of complex material	➤ Following instructions of increasing length and linguistic complexity
	➤ Interpreting ambiguous sentences and figurative language; explaining jokes
	➤ Provide opportunities to request repetition of information when information not understood (e.g., role play in classroom environment)
	➤ Provide classroom strategies: request teachers to write complex instructions down when not understood; provide written summary of each class; engage in tutorials at end of lesson to ensure Sally has understood main concepts; regular contact with parents and monitoring of academic progress

MILD TBI: MORE THAN MEETS THE EYE?

To date, TBI research has largely focused upon the effects of moderate to severe level trauma, typically incorporating cases that have demonstrated extended periods of lost consciousness (18). It has been long acknowledged, however, that an absence of frank neurological disturbance subsequent to head injury does not guarantee an unmarred recovery (218). Indeed, physical, cognitive and affective disturbances constitute frequently documented sequelae associated with concussion or mTBI (219).

The majority of mTBI behavioral research to date has been neuropsychologically-based, lacking in-depth linguistic analyses (220). Reduced processing speed, concentration, attention and memory (219) have been identified as common cognitive deficits in mTBI patients.

Respecting language, deficits in verbal fluency, story recall/ verbal memory and anomaly detection (221–224) have also been reported, suggesting that higher-level linguistic processes may be implicated following mTBI. Indeed, a comprehensive language evaluation recently conducted within our laboratory was in support of this hypothesis. Deficits in lexical access, complex lexical-semantic manipulation at single word and sentential levels, as well as the organization and monitoring of responses were highlighted in a single mTBI case, nearly 2 years post-injury (225).

Potential high-level language implications in mTBI are supported by a neuroanatomical rationale. In an absence of frank neurological disturbance, dynamic imaging studies relating to cerebral perfusion and metabolism, have revealed frontal and temporal lobe abnormalities in mTBI cases (226–229). In terms of localisation theory, these findings have evident implications for language function. The mTBI language profile identified within our laboratory closely paralleled that of frontal lobe disconnection populations previously studied (230–235). This finding supports the notion that mTBI mechanisms may also preferentially implicate frontal lobe systems involved in the recruitment and directed interplay of the frontal lobes with other language areas, perhaps via neuronal fall out processes (236).

With respect to speech, it has been generally accepted that motor speech disturbances commonly accompany severe TBI (237). Within the domain of mTBI, however, speech deficits have also been documented (172, 238–240). The precise nature of these disturbances remains unexplored, with detailed perceptual and physiological investigations of motor speech function sorely lacking.

Acceleration-deceleration trauma without explicit neurological deficit has been recognized in simian research to evoke diffuse degenerative changes in axonal functioning (241). Shear strain (238) induced axonal injury has been hypothesised to result in the degeneration of synaptic terminals as well as disturbed neuronal input (242–244). Evidently, the extent of axonal damage subsequent to mTBI may involve the complete neural axis, extending from the cortical regions mentioned previously, to terminal aborizations within the brain stem (241). These neurophysiological alterations resulting as a consequence of mTBI, provide a platform for explaining the physical, cognitive and affective sequelae frequently associated with this syndrome. The potentially wide-ranging neuropathological profile of mTBI also offers possible ramifications for speech and language function, including manifestations of subclinical oromuscular and cognitive-linguistic alterations that may be undetected by standard assessments of fine motor control and cognitive abilities.

If we consider that the demands placed upon mTBI patients are greater at any given time after injury than that of patients with severe brain trauma (245), the challenge lies ahead for researchers and clinicians to evaluate and apply appropriately sensitive methods of assessment to this population, in an effort to better delineate the nature of associated communication deficits. Special attention must be afforded to mTBI endured in childhood, considering that subtle symptoms may be easily camouflaged by inherent variabilities in maturational rates, particularly in regard to neuropsychological factors (18). Furthermore, ascertaining whether or not the communicative sequelae of mTBI demonstrate responsivity to traditional treatment techniques is yet to be determined.

The neuropsychological literature currently provides the mainstay of data pertaining to the assessment and treatment of mTBI cohorts (220). Contemporary studies have recently reported efficacious outcomes subsequent to a process-specific approach to the remediation of working attention/ memory deficits (246), and the implementation of compensatory strategies for functional impairments of memory, attention, reasoning and additional components of executive function (247). The development and application of cognitive communication rehabilitation techniques relative to this population, however, is much needed. To this end, it is anticipated that Speech-Language Pathologists may have a potentially valuable role to play in the future educational and/ or vocational rehabilitation of individuals with mTBI, as the precise nature of the motor/ cognitive sequelae associated with this syndrome continue to be unraveled.

References

1. Murdoch BE. *Acquired Speech And Language Disorders: A Neuroanatomical And Functional Neurological Approach*. London: Chapman and Hall; 1990.
2. Murdoch BE, Theodoros DG. Introduction: Epidemiology, neuropathophysiology, and medical aspects of traumatic brain injury. In: Murdoch BE, Theodoros DG, editors. *Traumatic Brain Injury: Associated Speech, Language And Swallowing Disorders*. San Diego: Singular Thomson Learning; 2001. pp. 1–23.
3. Najenson T, Sazbon L, Fiselzon J, Becker E, Schecter I. Recovery of communicative functions after prolonged traumatic coma. *Scand J Rehabil Med* 1978;10:15–21.
4. Oddy M. Head injury and social adjustment. In: Brooks N, ed. *Closed Head Injury: Psychological, Social And Family Consequences*. New York: Oxford University Press; 1984. pp. 108–122.
5. Malkmus DD. Community re-entry: Cognitive-communication intervention within a social skill context. *Topics Lang Disord* 1989;9:50–66.
6. Brooks N, McKinlay W, Symington C, Beattie A, Campsie L. Return to work witihn the first seven years of severe head injury. *Brain Inj* 1987;1:5–19.
7. Murdoch BE, Theodoros DG, editors. *Traumatic Brain Injury: Associated Speech, Language And Swallowing Disorders*. San Diego: Singular Thomson Learning; 2001.
8. Theodoros DG, Murdoch BE, Goozee JV. Dysarthria following traumatic brain injury: Incidence, recovery and perceptual features. In: Murdoch BE, Theodoros DG, editors. *Traumatic Brain Injury: Associated Speech, Language and Swallowing Disorders*. San Diego: Singular Thomson Learning; 2001. p. 27–52.
9. Taylor Sarno M, Buonaguro A, Levita E. Characteristics of verbal impairment in closed head injury patients. *Arch Phys Med Rehabil* 1986;67:400–405.
10. Ewing-Cobbs L, Fletcher JM, Levin HS. Neurobehavioral sequelae following head injury in children: Educational implications. *J Head Trauma Rehabil* 1986;1:57–65.
11. Yorkston KM, Beukelman DR. Motor speech disorders. In: Beukelman DR, Yorkston KM, eds. *Communication Disorders Following Traumatic Brain Injury*. Texas: Pro-Ed; 1991. pp. 251–315.
12. Dworkin JP, Abkarian GG. Treatment of phonation in a patient with apraxia and dysarthria secondary to severe closed head injury. *J Med Speech Lang Pathol* 1997;4:105–115.
13. Hinchliffe FJ, Murdoch BE, Theodoros DG. Linguistic deficits in adults subsequent to traumatic brain injury. In: Murdoch BE, Theodoros DG, editors. *Traumatic Brain Injury: Associated Speech, Language and Swallowing Disorders*. San Diego: Singular Thomson Learning; 2001. p. 199–222.
14. Hinchliffe FJ, Murdoch BE, Chenery HJ. Towards a conceptualisation of language and cognitive impairment in closed head injury: Use of clinical measures. *Brain Inj* 1998;12:109–132.
15. Sarno M. The nature of the verbal impairment after closed head injury. *J Nerv Ment Dis* 1980;168(11):685–692.
16. Lustig AP, Tompkins CA. An examination of severity classification measures and subject criteria used for studies on mild pediatric traumatic brain injury. *J Med Speech Lang Pathol* 1998; 6(1):13–25.
17. Ferguson RJ, Mittenberg WM, Barone DF, Schneider B. Postconcussion syndrome following sports-related head injury: Expectation as etiology. *Neuropsychology* 1999;13(4):582–589.
18. Segalowitz SJ, Lawson S. Subtle symptoms associated with self-reported mild head injury. *J Learn Disabil* 1995;28(5):309–319.
19. Levin HS. Aphasia in closed head injury. In: Sarno M, editor. *Acquired Aphasia*. New York: Academic Press; 1981. pp. 427–463.
20. Sarno M, Levin HS. Speech and language disorders after closed head injury. In: Darby JK, editor. *Speech Evaluation In Neurology: Adult Disorders*. New York: Grune and Stratton; 1985. p. 323–339.
21. Aten JL. Spastic dysarthria: Revising understanding of the disorder and speech treatment procedures. *J Head Trauma Rehabil* 1988;3:63–73.
22. Brand HA, Matsko TA, Avart HN. Speech prosthesis retention problems in dysarthria: Case report. *Arch Phys Med Rehabil* 1988;69:213–214.
23. Enderby P, Crowe E. Long-term recovery patterns of severe dysarthria following head injury. *Br J Disord Commun* 1990;25:341–354.
24. Kuehn DP, Wachtel JM. CPAP therapy for treating hypernasality following closed head injury. In: Till JA, Yorkston KM, Beukelman DR, eds. *Motor Speech Disorders: Advances In Assessment And Treatment*. Baltimore: Paul H. Brookes Publishing; 1994. p. 207–212.
25. Light J, Beesley M, Collier B. Transition through multiple augmentative communication systems: A three-year case study of a head injured adolescent. *Aug Alternat Commun* 1988;4:2–14.
26. Nemec RE, Cohen K. EMG biofeedback in the modification of hypertonia in spastic dysarthria: Case report. *Arch Phys Med Rehabil* 1984;65:103–104.
27. Simmons N. Acoustic analysis of ataxia dysarthria: An approach to monitoring treatment. In: Berry W, editor. *Clinical Dysarthria*. San Diego: College-Hill Press; 1983. p. 283–294.
28. Workinger M, Netsell R. Restroation of intelligible speech 13 years post-head injury. *Brain Inj* 1992;6:183–187.
29. Groher M. Language and memory disorders following closed head trauma. *J Speech Hear Res* 1977;20:212–223.
30. Kent RD, Netsell R, Bauer L. Cineradiographic assessment of articulatory mobility in the dysarthrias. *J Speech Hear Disord* 1975;40:467–480.
31. Lehiste I. Some acoustic charcteristics of dysarthric speech. *Bibl Phonet* 1965;2:1–124.
32. Netsell R, Daniel B. Dysarthria in adults: Physiologic approach in rehabilitation. *Arch Phys Med Rehabil* 1979;60:502–508.
33. von Cramon D. Traumatic mutism and the subsequent reorganization of speech functions. *Neuropsycholgia* 1981;19:801–805.
34. Yorkston KM, Beukelman DR. Ataxic dysarthria: Treatment sequence based on intelligibility and prosodic considerations. *J Speech Hear Disord* 1981;46:398–404.

35. Yorkston KM, Beukelman DR, Minifie FD, Sapir S. Assessment of stress patterning in dysarthric speakers. In: McNeil MR, Aronson AE, Rosenbeck JC, eds. *The Dysarthrias: Physiology, Acoustics, Perception, Management.* San Diego: College-Hill Press; 1984. pp. 131–162.

36. Theodoros DG, Murdoch BE, Chenery HJ. Perceptual speech characteristics of dysarthric speakers following severe closed head injury. *Brain Inj* 1994;8:101–124.

37. Marquardt TP, Stoll J, Sussman H. Disorders of communication in traumatic brain injury. In: Bigler ED, editor. *Traumatic Brain Injury: Mechanisms Damage, Assessment, Intervention, And Outcome.* Ausitn: Pro-Ed; 1990. pp. 181–205.

38. Langfitt TW, Obrist WD, Alavi A, Grossman RI, Zimmerman R, Jaggi J, et al. Computerised tomography, magnetic resonance imaging, and positron emission tomography in the study of head trauma. *J Neurosurg* 1986;64:760–767.

39. Netsell R, Lefkowitz D. Speech production following traumatic brain injury: Clinical and research implications. *American Speech-Language-Hearing Association Special Interests Division: Neurophysiology and Neurogenic Speech and Language Disorders* 1992;2:1–8.

40. Wilson JTL, Hadley DM, Weidmann KD, Teasdale GM. Intercorrelations of lesions detected by magnetic resonance imaging after closed head injury. *Brain Inj* 1992;6:391–399.

41. Thompson-Ward EC. Spastic dysarthria. In: Murdoch BE, ed. *Dysarthria: A Physiological Approach to Assessment and Treatment.* Cheltenham: Stanley Thornes Ltd; 1998. p. 205–241.

42. Duffy JR. Spastic dysarthria. In: Duffy JR, editor. *Motor Speech Disorders: Substrates, Differential Diagnosis, and Management.* St. Louis: Mosby; 1995. pp. 128–144.

43. Duffy JR. Hyperkinetic dysarthria. In: Duffy JR, editor. *Motor Speech Disorders: Substrates, Differential Diagnosis, and Management.* St. Louis: Mosby; 1995. pp. 189–221.

44. Theodoros DG, Murdoch BE. Hyperkinetic dysarthria. In: Murdoch BE, editor. *Dysarthria: A Physiological Approach to Assessment and Treatment.* Cheltenham: Stanley Thornes Ltd; 1998. pp. 314–336.

45. Darley FL, Aronson AE, Brown JR. *Motor Speech Disorders.* Philadelphia: W.B. Saunders Company; 1975.

46. Zraick RI, LaPointe LL. Hyperkinetic dysarthria. In: McNeil MR, editor. *Clinical Management of Sensorimotor Speech Disorders.* New York: Theime; 1997. pp. 249–260.

47. Duffy JR. Hypokinetic dysarthria. In: Duffy JR, ed. *Motor Speech Disorders: Substrates, Differential Diagnosis and Management.* St. Louis: Mosby; 1995. pp. 166–188.

48. Theodoros DG, Murdoch BE. Hypokinetic dysarthria. In: Murdoch BE, ed. *Dysarthria: A Physiological Approach to Assessment and Treatment.* Cheltenham: Stanley Thornes Ltd; 1998. pp. 266–313.

49. Darley FL, Aronson AE, Brown JR. Clusters of deviant speech dimensions in the dysarthrias. *J Speech Hear Res* 1969;12:462–496.

50. Duffy JR. Flaccid dysarthria. In: Duffy JR, editor. *Motor Speech Disorders: Substrates, Differential Diagnosis, and Management.* St. Louis: Mosby; 1995. pp. 99–127.

51. Murdoch BE, Thompson-Ward EC. Flaccid dysarthria. In: Murdoch BE, editor. *Dysarthria: A Physiological Approach to Assessment and Treatment.* Cheltenham: Stanley Thornes Ltd; 1998. pp. 176–204.

52. Duffy JR. Ataxic dysarthria. In: Duffy JR, editor. *Motor speech disorders: Substrates, differential diagnosis, and management.* St. Louis: Mosby; 1995. pp. 145–165.

53. Brown JR, Darley FL, Aronson AE. Ataxic dysarthria. *Int J Neurol* 1970;7:302–318.

54. Murdoch BE, Theodoros DG. Ataxic dysarthria. In: Murdoch BE, ed. *Dysarthria: A Physiological Approach to Assessment and Treatment.* Cheltenham: Stanley Thornes Ltd; 1998. pp. 241–265.

55. Yorkston KM, Beukelman DR. *Assessment of Intelligibility of Dysarthric Speech.* Austin: Pro-Ed; 1981.

56. Cahill LM, Murdoch BE, Theodoros DG. Dysarthria following traumatic brain injury in childhood. In: Murdoch BE, Theodoros DG, eds. *Traumatic brain injury: Associated speech, language, and swallowing disorders.* San Diego: Singular Thomson Learning; 2001. pp. 121–153.

57. Levin HS, Benton AL, Grossman RG. *Neurobehavioral Consequences of Closed Head Injury.* New York: Oxford University Press; 1982.

58. van Mourik M, Catsman-Berrevoets CE, Paquier PF, Yosef-Bak E, van Dongen HR. Acquired childhood dysarthria: Review of its clinical presentation. *Pediatr Neurol* 1997;17(4):299–307.

59. Murdoch BE, Hudson-Tennet LJ. Speech disorders in children treated for posterior fossa tumors: Ataxic and developmental features. *Eur J Disord Commun* 1994;29:379–397.

60. FitzGerald FJ, Murdoch BE, Chenery HJ. Multiple Sclerosis: Associated speech and language disorders. *Aust J Hum Commun Disord* 1987;15:15–33.

61. Fisher HB, Logemann JA. *The Fisher-Logemann Test of Articulation Competence.* Boston: Houghton Mifflin Co.; 1971.

62. Enderby P. *Frenchay Dysarthria Assessment.* San Diego: College-Hill Press; 1983.

63. Theodoros DG, Murdoch BE. Laryngeal dysfunction following traumatic brain injury. In: Murdoch BE, Theodoros DG, eds. *Traumatic Brain Injury: Associated Speech, Language and Swallowing Disorders.* San Diego: Singular Thomson Learning; 2001. pp. 89–109.

64. Thompson-Ward EC, Theodoros DG. Acoustic analysis of dysarthric speech. In: Murdoch BE, ed. *Dysarthria: A Physiological Approach to Assessment and Treatment.* Cheltenham: Stanley Thornes Ltd; 1998. pp. 102–129.

65. Colton R, Casper JK. The voice history, examination and testing. In: Colton R, Casper JK, editors. *Understanding Voice Problems: A Physiological Perspective for Diagnosis and Treatment.* 2nd ed. Baltimore: Williams & Williams; 1996. pp. 186–240.

66. Colton R, Conture EG. Problems and pitfalls of electroglottography. *J Voice* 1990;4:10–24.

67. Hanson DG, Gerratt BR, Karin RR, Berke GS. Glottographic measures of vocal fold vibration: An examination of laryngeal paralysis. *Laryngoscope* 1988;98:541–548.

68. Theodoros DG, Murdoch BE. Laryngeal dysfunction in dysarthric speakers following severe closed head injury. *Brain Inj* 1994;8:667–684.

69. Hammen V, Yorkston KM. Effect of instruction on selected aerodynamic parametres in subjects with dysarthria and control subjects. In: Till JA, Yorkston KM, Beukelman DR, eds. *Motor speech disorders: Advances in assessment and treatment.* Baltimore: Paul H, Brookes Publishing Co; 1994. pp. 161–173.

70. Boren HG, Kory RC, Synder JC. The Veterans Administration–Army cooperative study of pulmonary function II. The lung volume and its subdivisions in normal men. *Am J Med* 1966;41:96–114.

71. Kory RC, Callahan R, Boren HG. The Veterans Administration–Army cooperative study of pulmonary function I. Clinical spirometry in normal men. *Am J Med* 1961;30:243–258.

72. Hoit JD, Hixon TJ. Body type and speech breathing. *J Speech Hear Res* 1986;29:313–324.

73. Solomon N, Hixon TJ. Speech beathing in Parkinson's disease. *Journal Speech Hear Res* 1993;36:294–310.

74. Stathopoulos ET, Sapienza C. Respiratory and laryngeal function of women and men during vocal intensity variation. *J Speech Hear Res* 1993;36:64–75.

75. Hinton VA, Luschei ES. Validation of modern miniature transducer for measurement of interlabial contact pressure during speech. *J Speech Hear Res* 1992;35:245–251.

76. Murdoch BE, Attard MD, Ozanne AE, Stokes PD. Impaired tongue strength and endurance in developmental verbal dyspraxia: A physiological analysis. *Eur J Disord Commun* 1995;30:51–64.

77. Robin DA, Somodi CB, Luschei ES. Measurement of tongue strength and endurance in normal and articulation disordered subjects. In: Moore CA, Yorkston KM, Beukelman DR, editors. *Dysarthria and apraxia of speech: Perspectives on management.* Baltimore: Paul H. Brooks; 1991. pp. 173–184.

78. Goozee JV, Murdoch BE, Theodoros DG. Physiological assessment of tongue function in dysarthria following traumatic brain injury. *Logopedics Phoniatrics Vocology* 2001;26:51–65.

79. Goozee JV, Murdoch BE, Theodoros DG, Stokes PD. Kinematic analysis of tongue movements in dysarthria following traumatic brain injury using electromagnetic articulography. *Brain Inj* 2000;14:153–174.

80. Theodoros DG, Murdoch BE. Velopharyngeal dysfunction following traumatic brain injury. In: Murdoch BE, Theodoros DG, editors. *Traumatic Brain Injury: Associated Speech, Language, and Swallowing Disorders*. San Diego: Singular Thomson Learning; 2001. pp. 75–88.

81. Horri Y. An accelerometric approach to nasality measurement: A preliminary report. *Cleft Pal J* 1980;17:254–261.

82. Horri Y. An accelerometric measure as a physical correlate of perceived hypernasality in speech. *J Speech Hear Res* 1983;26: 476–480.

83. Dalston RM, Seaver EJ. Relative values of various standardized passages in the nasometric assessment of patients with velopharyngeal impairment. *Cleft Pal Craniofac J* 1992;29:17–21.

84. Dalston RM, Warren DW, Dalston ET. A preliminary investigation concerning the use of nasometry in identifying patients with hyponasality and/ or nasal airway impairment. *J Speech Hear Res* 1991;34:11–18.

85. Nellis JL, Neiman GS, Lehman JA. Comparison of nasometer and listener judgements of nasality in the assessment of velopharyngeal function after pharyngeal flap surgery. *Cleft Pal Craniofac J* 1992;29:157–163.

86. Theodoros DG, Murdoch BE. Treatment of dysarthria following traumatic brain injury. In: Murdoch BE, Theodoros DG, editors. *Traumatic Brain Injury: Associated Speech, Language and Swallowing Disorders*. San Diego: Singular Thomson Learning; 2001. pp. 155–196.

87. Organization, World Health. *ICF: International Classification of Functioning, Disability and Health*. Geneva: World Health Organization; 2001.

88. Yorkston KM. Treatment efficacy: Dysarthria. *J Speech Hear Res* 1996;39:S46-S57.

89. Bellaire K, Yorkston KM, Beukleman DR. Modification of breath patterning to increase naturalness of a mildly dysarthric speaker. *J Commun Disord* 1986;19:271–280.

90. Beukleman DR, Yorkston KM. A communication system for the severely dysarthric speaker with an intact language system. *J Speech Hear Disord* 1977;42:265–270.

91. Bougle F, Ryalls J, Le Dorze G. Improving fundamental frequency modulation in head trauma patients: A preliminary comparison of speech-language therapy conducted with and without IBM's Speech Viewer. *Folia Phoniatr Logop* 1995;47:24–32.

92. Draizar D. Clinical EMG feedback in motor speech disorders. *Arch Phys Med Rehabil* 1984;65:481–484.

93. Goldstein P, Ziegler W, Vogel M, Hoole P. Combined palatal-lift and EPG-feedback therapy in dysarthria: A case study. *Clin Linguist Phonet* 1994;8:210–218.

94. Murdoch BE, Pitt G, Theodoros DG, Ward EC. Real-time continuous feedback in the treatment of speech breathing disorders following childhood traumatic brain injury: Report of one case. *Pediatr Rehabil* 1999;3:5–20.

95. Murdoch BE, Sterling D, Theodoros DG. Physiological rehabilitation of disordered speech breathing in dysarthric speakers following severe closed head injury. In: Conference proceedings of the *Australian Society for the Study of Brain Impairment*; 1995; Hobart, Tasmania; 1995.

96. Stewart DS, Rieger WJ. A device for the management of velopharyngeal incompetence. *J Med Speech Lang Pathol* 1994;2: 149–155.

97. Stringer AY. Treatment of motor aprosodia with pitch biofeedback and expression modelling. *Brain Inj* 1996;10:583–590.

98. Kearns KP, Simmons NN. The efficacy of speech-language pathology intervention: Motor speech disorders. *Semin Speech Lang* 1990;11:273–295.

99. Ray J. Orofacial myofunctional therapy in dysarthria: A study on speech intelligibility. *Int J Orofac Myology* 2002;28:39–48.

100. Clark HM. Neuromuscular treatments for speech and swallowing: A tutorial. *Am J Speech Lang Pathol* 2003;12(4):400–415.

101. Theodoros DG, Thompson-Ward EC. Treatment of dysarthria. In: Murdoch BE, editor. *Dysarthria: A Physiological Approach to Assessment and Treatment*. Cheltenham: Stanley Thornes Ltd; 1998. p. 130–175.

102. Froeschels E. Chewing method as therapy. *Arch Otolaryngol* 1952;56:427–434.

103. Boone DR. *The Voice and Voice Therapy*. 2nd ed. Englewood Cliffs, NJ: Prentice-Hall 1977.

104. Froeschels E, Kastein S, Weiss D. A method of therapy for paralytic conditions of the medchanisms of phonation, respiration and glutination. *J Speech Hear Disord* 1955;20:365–370.

105. Boone DR, McFarlane SC. *The voice and voice therapy*. 4th ed. Englewood Cliffs, NJ: Prentice-Hall; 1988.

106. Ramig LO, Bonitati CM, Lemke JH, Horri Y. Voice treatment for patients with Parkinson's disease: Development of an approach and preliminary efficacy data. *J Med Speech Lang Pathol* 1994;2:191–209.

107. Netsell R, Rosenbeck JC. Treating the dysarthrias. In: Darby JK, editor. *Speech and language evaluation in neurology: Adult Disorders*. Orlando: Grune & Stratton; 1995. pp. 363–392.

108. Netsell R, Hixon TJ. Inspiratory checking in therapy for individuals with speech breathing dysfunction. *J Am Speech Hear Assoc* 1992;34:152.

109. Rosenbeck JC, LaPointe LL. The dysarthrias: Description, diagnosis and treatment. In: Johns D, editor. *Clinical Management of Neurogenic Communication Disorders*. Boston: Little, Brown & Co.; 1991. pp. 97–152.

110. Dworkin JP, Johns DF. Management of velopharyngeal incompetence in dysarthria: A historical review. *Clin Otolaryngol* 1980;5:61–74.

111. Robertson S. The efficiay if oro-facial and articulation exercises in dysarthria following stroke. *Int J Lang Commun Disord* 2001;36 Suppl:292–297.

112. Yorkston KM, Beukelman DR, Bell KR. *Clinical Management of Dysarthric Speakers*. Boston: Little, Brown & Co.; 1988.

113. Volin RA. Clinical applications of biofeedback. *Am Speech Hear Assoc* 1993;September:43–51.

114. Garber SR, Burzynski CM, Vale C, Nelson R. The use of visual feedback to control vocal intensity and nasalisation. *J Commun Disord* 1979;12:399–410.

115. Prosek RA, Montgomery AA, Walden BE, Schwartz DM. EMG biofeedback in the treatment of hyperfunctional voice disorders. *J Speech Hear Disord* 1978;43:282–294.

116. Rubow R. Role of feedback, reinforcement, and compliance on training and transfer in biofeedback-based rehabilitation of motor speech disorders. In: McNeil MR, Rosenbeck JC, Aronson AE, editors. *The Dysarthrias: Physiology, Acoustics, Perception, Management*. San Diego: College-Hill Press; 1984. pp. 207–230.

117. Scott S, Caird FI. Speech therapy for Parkinson's disease. *J Neurol Neurosurg Psychiatry* 1983;46:140–144.

118. Johnson JA, Pring TR. Speech therapy and Parkinson's disease: A review and further data. *Br J Disord Commun* 1990;25: 183–194.

119. Berry WR, Goshorn EL. Immediate visual feedback in the treatment of ataxia dysarthria: A case study. In: Berry WR, editor. *Clinical Dysarthria*. San Diego: College-Hill Press; 1983. pp. 253–265.

120. Thompson EC, Murdoch BE. Treatment of speech breathing disorders in dysarthria: A biofeedback approach. In: Conference Proceedings of the *Australian Association of Speech and Hearing*; 1995; Queensland, Australia; 1995.

121. Siegel-Sadewitz VL, Shprintzen RJ. Nasopharyngoscopy of the normal verlopharyngeal sphincter: An experiment of biofeedback. *Cleft Pal J* 1982;19:194–200.

122. Witzel M, Tobe J, Salyer K. The use of nasopharyngoscopy biofeedback therapy in the correction of inconsistent velopharyngeal closure. *Int J Pediatr Otorhinolatyngol* 1988;15: 137–142.

123. Kunzel H. First applications of a biofeedback device for the therapy of velopharyngeal incompetence. *Folia Phoniatr* 1982;34: 92–100.

124. Hand CR, Burns MO, Ireland E. Treatment of hypertonicity in muscles of lip retraction. *Biofeedback and Self-Regulation* 1979; 4:171–181.

125. Booker HE, Rubow RT, Coleman PJ. Simplified feedback in neuromuscular retraining: An automated approach using electromyographic signals. *Arch Phys Med Rehabil* 1969;50: 621–625.

126. Gallegos K, Medina R, Espinoza E, Bustamante A. Electromyographic feedback in the treatment of bilateral facial paralysis: A case study. *J Behav Med* 1992;15:533–539.

127. Gibbon F, Dent H, Hardcastle W. Diagnosis and therapy of abnormal alveolar stops in speech-disordered child using electropalatography. *Clin Linguist Phonet* 1993;7:247–267.

128. Hardcastle WJ, Morgan Barry RA, Clark CJ. Articulatory and voicing characteristics of adult dysarthric and verbal dyspraxic speakers: An instrumental study. *Br J Disord Commun* 1985;20:249–269.

129. Machines) IIB. *Speech Viewer: Guide de l'Utilisateur.* Paris: IBM; 1989.

130. Le Dorze G, Dionne L, Ryalls J. The effects of speech and language therapy for a case of dysarthria associated with Parkinson's disease. *Eur J Disord Commun* 1992;27:313–324.

131. Beukelman DR, Yorkston KM, Tice B. *Pacer/Tally.* Arizona: Communication Skill Builders; 1988.

132. Downie WW, Low JM, Lindsay DD. Speech disorder in Parkinsonism-Usefulness of delayed auditory feedback in selected cases. *Br J Disord Commun* 1981;16:135–139.

133. Hanson W, Metter E, J. DAF as instrumental treatment for dysarthria in progressive supranuclear palsy: A case report. *J Speech Hear Disord* 1980;45:268–275.

134. Hanson W, Metter E. DAF speech rate modification in Parkinson's disease: A report of two cases. In: Berry WR, editor. *Clinical Dysarthria.* San Diego: College-Hill Press; 1983. pp. 231–251.

135. Allen CM. Treatment of nonfluent speech resulting from neurological disease-Treatment of dysarthria. *Br J Disord Commun* 1970;5:3–5.

136. Blitzer A, Brin M, Fahn S, Lovelace R. Localisaed injections of botulinum toxin for the treatment of focal laryngeal dystonia (spastic dysphonia). *Laryngoscope* 1988;98:193–197.

137. Dedo HH. Recurrent laryngeal nerve section for spastic dysphonia. *Ann Otol Rhinol Laryngol* 1979;85:451–459.

138. Facs MM, Beery Q. Muscle-nerve pedicle laryngeal reinnervation. *Laryngoscope* 1986;96:1196–1200.

139. Ford CN, Martin DW, Warner TF. Injectable collagen in laryngeal rehabilitation. *Laryngoscope* 1984;94:513–518.

140. Hammarberg B, Fritzell B, Schiratzki H. Teflon injection of 16 patients with paralytic dysphonia: Perceptual and acoustic elevations. *J Speech Hear Disord* 1984;49:72–82.

141. Isshiki N, Tanada M, Sawada M. Arytenoid adduction for unilateral vocal cord paralysis. *Arch Otolaryngol* 1978;104:555–558.

142. Gonzalez JB, Aronson AE. Palatal lift prosthesis for treatment of anatomic and neurologic palatopharyngeal insufficiency. *Cleft Pal J* 1970;7:91–104.

143. Light J, Beer Edelman S, Alba A. The dental prosthesis used for intraoral muscle therapy in the rehabilitation of the stroke patient. *New York State Dental Journal* 2001;67(5):22–27.

144. Netsell R. Construction and use of bite-block for use in evaluation and treatment of speech disorders. *J Speech Hear Disord* 1985;50:103–106.

145. Helm NA. Management of palilalia with a pacing board. *J Speech Hear Disord* 1979;44:350–353.

146. Beukelman DR, Yorkston KM. Communication options for patients with brain stem lesions. *Arch Phys Med Rehabil* 1978;59:337–340.

147. Murdoch BE, Horton SK, Theodoros DG, Thompson EC. Clinical application of speech science instrumentation in the determination of treatment priorities in acquired and congenital childhood dysarthria. In: Hulstijn W, Peters HFM, Van Lieshout PHH, eds. *Speech Production: Motor Control, Brain Research and Fluency Disorders.* Amsterdam: Elsevier Science B.V.; 1997.

148. Hagen C. Language disorders in head trauma. In: Holland A, ed. *Language disorders in adults: Recent advances.* San Diego: Colleg-Hill Press; 1984. pp. 245–281.

149. Holland A. When is aphasia aphasia? The problem of closed head injury. In: *Clinical Aphasiology.* Minneapolis: BRK Publishers; 1982. pp. 345–349.

150. Levin HS, Grossman RG, Rose SE. Long term neuropsychological outcome of closed head injury. *J Neurosurg* 1979;50:412–422.

151. Milton S, Prutting C, Binder G. Appraisal of communication competence in head injured adults. In: Brookshire R, editor. *Clinical Aphasiology.* Minneapolis: BRK Publishers; 1984. pp. 114–123.

152. Prigatano G, Rousche J, Fordyce D. Nonaphasic language disturbances after brain injury. In: Prigatano G, editor. *Neuropsychological Rehabilitation After Brain Injury.* Baltimore: John Hopkins University Press; 1986. pp. 18–28.

153. Thompsen IV. Evaluation and outcome of aphasia in patients with severe closed head trauma. *J Neurol Neurosurg Psychiatry* 1975;38:713–178.

154. Sarno M, Buonaguro A, Levita E. Characteristics of verbal impairment in closed head injured patients. *Arch Phys Med Rehabil* 1986;67:400–405.

155. Levin HS, Grossman RG, Kelly PJ. Aphasia disorder in patients with closed head injury. *J Neurol Neurosurg Psychiatry* 1976;39:1062–1070.

156. Association AS-L-H. Guidelines for speech-language pathologists serving persons with language, socio-communicative and/or cognitive-communication impairments. *ASHA* 1991;33(Suppl. 5):21–28.

157. Bloom L, Lahey M. *Language Development and Language Disorders.* New York: Wiley; 1978.

158. McDonald. Pragmatic language skills after closed head injury: Ability to meet the information needs of the listener. *Brain Lang* 1993;44:28–46.

159. Mayer NH, Schwartz MF. Executive function disorders. *J Head Trauma Rehabil* 1993;8(1):1–119.

160. Chapman S, Levin S, Culhane KA. *Language impairment in closed head injury.* New York: Marcel Decker; 1995.

161. Hartley L, Jensen PJ. Three discourse profiles of closed head injured speakers: Theoretical and clinical implications. *Brain Inj* 1992;5:267–285.

162. Hinchliffe FJ, Murdoch BE, Chenery HJ, Baglioni AJ, Harding-Clark J. Cognitive-linguistic subgroups in closed head injury. *Brain Inj* 1998;12:109–132.

163. Coppens P. Subpopulations in closed head injury: Preliminary results. *Brain Inj* 1995;9:195–208.

164. Ewing-Cobbs L, Fletcher JM, Levin HS, Landry SH. Language disorders after pediatric head injury. In: Darby JK, ed. *Speech and Language Evaluation in Neurology: Childhood Disorders.* Florida: Grune & Stratton; 1985. pp. 97–112.

165. Chadwick O, Rutter M, Brown G, Schaffer D, Traub M. A prospective study of children with head injuries: II Cognitive sequelae. *Psychol Med* 1981;11:49–61.

166. Chadwick O, Rutter M, Shaffer D, Shrout PE. A prospective study of children with head injuries: IV. Specific cognitive deficits. *J Clin Neuropsychol* 1981;3:101–120.

167. Jordan FM, Ozanne AE, Murdoch BE. Performance of closed head-injured children on a naming task. *Brain Inj* 1990;4:27–32.

168. Slater EJ, Bassett SS. Adolescents with closed head injuries. *Am J Dis Child* 1988;142:1048–1051.

169. Jordan FM, Ozanne AE, Murdoch BE. Long-term speech and language disorders subsequent to closed head injury in children. *Brain Inj* 1988;2:179–185.

170. Levin HS, Eisenberg HM. Neuropsychological impairment after closed head injury in children and adolescents. *J Pediatr Psychol* 1979;4:389–402.

171. Levin HS, Eisenberg HM. Neuropsychological outcome of closed head injury in children and adolescents. *Child Brain* 1979;5:281–292.

172. Ewing-Cobbs L, Levin HS, Eisenberg HM, Fletcher JM. Language functions following closed head injury in children and adolescents. *J Clin Exp Neuropsychol* 1987;9:575–592.

173. Fletcher JM, Ewing-Cobbs L, Miner ME, Levin HS, Eisenberg HM. Behavioral changes after closed head injury. *J Consult Clin Psychol* 1990;58:93–98.

174. Levin HS, Culhane KA, Medelsohn D, Lilly MA, Bruce D, Fletcher JM, et al. Cognition in relation to magnetic resonance imaging in head injured children and adolescents. *Arch Neurol* 1993;50:897–905.

175. Perrott SB, Taylor HG, Montes JF. Neuropsychological sequelae, familial stress, and environmental adaptation following pediatric head injury. *Dev Neuropsychol* 1991;7:69–86.

176. Jordan FM, Cremona-Meteyard S, King A. High-level Lingusitic disturbances subsequent to childhood closed head injury. *Brain Inj* 1996;10:729–738.

177. Hebb DO. The effect of early and late brain injury upon test scores and the nature of abnormal adult intelligence. Proceedings of *the American Philosophical Society* 1942;1:265–292.

178. Ewing-Cobbs L, Miner ME, Fletcher JM, Levin HS. Intellectual motor and language sequelae following closed head injury in children. *J Pediatr Psychol* 1989;9:575–592.

179. Bates E, Reilly J, Marchman E. Discourse and grammar after early focal brain injury. In: Conference Proceedings of the *Academy of Aphasia*; 1992; Toronto, Canada; 1992.

180. Chapman S, Levin HS. Discourse abilities and executive function in head-injured children. In: Conference Proceedings of the *American Speech-Language and Hearing Association*; 1994; New Orleans; 1994.

181. Hinchliffe FJ, Murdoch BE, Theodoros DG. Discourse production in traumatic brain injury. In: Murdoch BE, Theodoros DG, editors. *Traumatic Brain Injury: Associated Speech, Language and Swallowing Disorders*. San Diego: Singular Thomson Learning; 2001. pp. 223–242.

182. Kertesz A. *The Western Aphasia Battery*. New York: Grune & Stratton; 1982.

183. Goodglass H. *Boston Diagnostic Aphasia Examination*. 3rd ed. Philadelphia: Lippincott Williams & Wilkins; 2001.

184. Kaplan E, Goodglass H, Weintraub S. *Boston Naming Test*. Philadelphia: Lippincott Williams & Wilkins; 1983.

185. Spreen O, Benton AL. *Neurosensory Centre Comprehensive Examination for Aphasia*. Victoria: University of Victoria; 1969.

186. McNeil MR, Prescott TE. *Revised Token Test*. Baltimore: University Park Press; 1978.

187. Wiig EH, Secord W. *Test of Language Competence-Expanded Edition*. New York: Psychological Corporation; 1989.

188. Huisingh R, Barrett M, Zachman L, Blagden C, Orman J. *The Word Test-Revised: A Test of Expressive Vocabulary and Semantics*. Illinois: Linguisystems; 1990.

189. Wiig EH, Secord W. *Test of Word Knowledge*. New York: Psychological Corporation; 1992.

190. Wiig EH, Semel E. Development of comprehension of logical grammatical sentences by grade school children. *Percept Mot Skills* 1974;38:171–176.

191. Bryan K. *The Right Hemisphere Language Battery*. Southhampton: Far Communications; 1989.

192. Murdoch BE, Theodoros DG. Language disorders following traumatic brain injury in childhood. In: Murdoch BE, Theodoros DG, eds. *Traumatic Brain Injury: Associated Speech, Language and Swallowing Disorders*. San Diego: Singular Thomson Learning; 2001. pp. 247–271.

193. Bzoch KR, League R. *Receptive-Expressive Emergent Language Test*, 2nd edition. Austin: Pro-Ed; 1991.

194. Zimmerman IL, Steiner VG, Pond RE. *Preschool Language Scale-3*. San Antonio: Psychological Corporation; 1992.

195. Wiig EH, Secord W, Semel E. *Clinical Evaluation of Language Fundamentals–Preschool*. San Antonio: Psychological Corporation; 1992.

196. Semel E, Wiig EH, Secord W. *Clinical Evaluation of Language Fundamentals*, 3rd edition. San Antonio: Psychological Corporation; 1995.

197. Dunn LM, Dunn LM, Williams KT. *Peabody Picture Vocabulary Test*, 3rd Edition. Minnesota: American Guidance Service; 1997.

198. Fisher JP, Glenister JM. *The Hundred Pictures Naming Test*. Victoria: ACER; 1992.

199. Bowers L, Huisingh R, Barrett M, Orman J, LoGuidice C. *Test of Problem Solving–Elementary*. Queensland: Pro-Ed; 1994.

200. Bowers L, Huisingh R, Barrett M, Orman J, LoGuidice C. *Test of Problem Solving–Adolescent*. Queensland: Pro-Ed; 1991.

201. Dodd B, Holm A, Oerlemans M, McCormack M. *Queensland University Inventory of Literacy*. Queensland: The University of Queensland; 1996.

202. Torgenson JK, Bryant BR. *Test of Phonological Awareness*. Queensland: Pro-Ed; 1994.

203. Allen L, Leitao S, Donovan M. *School Age Oral Language Assessment*. Fremantle: Language-Learning Materials, Research and Development; 1993.

204. Marsh N. Social skill deficits following traumatic brain injury: Assessment and treatment. In: McDonald S, Togher L, Code C, editors. *Communication Disorders Following Traumatic Brain Injury*. East Sussex: Psychology Press Ltd.; 1999. pp. 175–210.

205. Brown P, Levinson S. *Politeness: Some Universals in Language Use*. Cambridge: Cambridge University Press; 1987.

206. Clark HH. Responding to indirect speech acts. *Cog Psychol*1979; 11:430–477.

207. Grice HP. Logic and conversation. In: Cole F, Morgan JL, editors. *Syntax and Semantics 3: Speech Acts*. New York: Academic Press; 1975. pp. 41–58.

208. Hinchliffe FJ, Murdoch BE, Theodoros DG. Treatment of cognitive-linguistic communication disorders following traumatic brain injury. In: Murdoch BE, Theodoros DG, eds. *Traumatic Brain Injury: Associated Speech, Language, and Swallowing Disorders*. San Diego: Singular Thomson Learning; 2001. pp. 273–309.

209. Body R, Perkins MR. Validation of linguistic analyses in narrative discourse after traumatic brain injury. *Brain Inj* 2004; 18(7):707–724.

210. Uzzell B, Gross Y, editors. *Clinical Neuropsychology of Intervention*. New York: Guilford; 1986.

211. Diller L. Neuropsychological rehabilitation. In: Meier MJ, Benton AL, Diller L, editors. *Neuropscyhological Rehabilitation*. London: Churchill-Livingston; 1987. pp. 1–17.

212. Coelho CA, DeRuyter F, Stein M. Treatment efficacy: Cognitive-communicative disorders resulting from traumatic brain injury in adults. *J Speech Hear Res* 1996;39:S5–S17.

213. Mazaux JM, Richer E. Rehabilitation after traumatic brain injury in adults. *Disabil Rehabil* 1998;20:435–447.

214. Mateer CA, Sohlberg MM, Youngman PK. The management of acquired attention and memory deficits. In: Wood RL, Fussey I, eds. *Cognitive Rehabilitation in Perspective*. London: Taylor & Francis; 1990. pp. 68–95.

215. Sohlberg MM, Mateer CA, editors. *Introduction to Cognitive Rehabilitation: Theory and Practice*. New York: Guilford; 1989.

216. Johns D, ed. *Clinical Management of Neurogenic Communicative Disorders*. Boston: Little Brown and Company; 1985.

217. Jordan FM. Speech and language disorders following childhood closed head injury. In: Murdoch BE, ed. *Acquired Neurological Speech/Language Disorders in Childhood*. London: Taylor & Francis; 1980. pp. 124–147.

218. Klove H, Cleeland CS. The relationship of neuropsychological impairment to other indices of severity of head injury. *Scand J Rehabil Med* 1972;4:55–60.

219. Borgaro S, Prigatano G, Kwasnica C, Rexer JL. Cogntive and affective sequelae in complicated and uncomplicated mild traumatic brain injury. *Brain Inj* 2003;17(3):189–198.

220. Duff MC, Proctor A, Haley K. Mild traumatic brain injury (MTBI): Assessment and treatment procedures used by speech-langauge pathologists (SLPs). *Brain Inj* 2002;16(9):773–787.

221. Anderson V, Catroppa C, Morse S, Haritou F, Rosenfeld J. Outcome from mild head injury in young children: A prospective study. *J Clin Exp Neuropsychol* 2001;23(6):705–717.

222. Goldstein FC, Levin HS, Goldman WP, Clark AN, Altonen TK. Cognitive and neurobehavioral functioning after mild versus moderate traumatic brain injury in older adults. *J Int Neuropsychol Soc* 2001;7:373–383.

223. Hanten G, Dennis M, Zhang L, Barnes M, Roberson G. Childhood head injury and metacognitive processes in language and memory. *Dev Neuropsychol* 2004;25(1&2):85–106.

224. Williams DH, Levin HS, Eisenberg HM. Mild head injury classification. *Neurosurg* 1990;27(3):422–428.

225. Whelan B-M, Murdoch BE. Delineating communication deficits associated with mild traumatic brain injury (mBI): A case report. In: *Conference Proceedings of the 7th International Neurotrauma Symposium*; 2004; Adelaide, South Australia; 2004.

226. Umile EM, Sandel E, Alavi A, Terry CM, Plotkin RC. Dynamic imaging in mild traumatic brain injury: Support for the theory of medial temporal vulnerability. *Arch Phys Med Rehabil* 2002; 83:1506–1513.

227. Humayun MS, Presty SK, LaFrance ND. Local cerebral glucose abnormalities in mild closed head injured patients with cognitive impairments. *Nuclear Medicine Communications* 1989;10: 335–44.

228. Varney NR, Bushnell DL, Nathan M. NeuroSPECT correlates of disabling mild head injury: Preliminary findings. *J Head Trauma Rehabil* 1995;10(3):18–28.

229. Gross H, Kling A, Henry G, Herndon C, Lavretsky H. Local cerebral glucose metabolism in patients with long-term behavioral and cognitive deficits following traumatic brain injury. *J Neuropsychiatry* 1996;8:324–334.

230. Whelan B-M, Murdoch BE, Theodoros DG, Hall B, Silburn PA. Defining a role for the subthalamic nucleus within operative theoretical models of subcortical participation in language. *J Neurol Neurosurg Psychiatry* 2003;74:1543–1550.

231. Whelan B-M, Murdoch BE, Theodoros DG, Silburn PA, Hall B. A role for the dominant thalamus in language? A linguistic comparison of two cases subsequent to unilateral thalamotomy procedures in the dominant and nondominant hemispheres. *Aphasiology* 2002;16(12):1213–1226.

232. Whelan B-M, Murdoch BE, Theodoros DG, Silburn PA, Hall B. Re-appraising contemporary theories of subcortical participation in language: Proposing an interhemispheric regulatory function for the subthalamic nucleus (STN) in the mediation of high-level linguistic processes. *Neurocase* 2004;10(5): 345–352.

233. Whelan B-M, Murdoch BE, Theodoros DG, Silburn PA, Hall B. Redefining functional models of basal ganglia organization: Role for the post-eroventral pallidum in linguistic processing. *Mov Disord* 2004;19(11):1267–1278.

234. Whelan B-M, Murdoch BE, Theodoros DG, Silburn PA, Hall B. Borrowing from models of motor control to translate cognitive processes: Evidence for hypokinetic-hyperkinetic linguistic homologues. *J Neurolinguistics*. [AU: Please supply full reference.]

235. Whelan B-M, Murdoch BE, Theodoros DG, Silburn PA, Harding-Clark J. Towards a better understanding of the role of subcortical nuclei participation in language: The study of a case

following bilateral pallidotomy. *Asia Pacific Journal of Speech Language and Hearing* 1000;5:93–112.

236. Gronwall D. Cumulative and persisting effects of concussion on attention and cognition. In: Levin HS, Eisenberg HM, Benton AL, eds. *Mild Head Injury*. New York: Oxford University Press; 1989.

237. Chadwick O. Psychological sequelae of head injury in children. *Dev Med* 1985;27:69–79.

238. Boll T, Barth J. Mild head injury. *Psych Dev* 1983;3:263–275.

239. Levin H, Amparo E, Eisenberg J, Williams D, High W, McArdle C, et al. Magnetic resonance imaging and computerized tomography in relation to the neurobehavioral sequelae of mild and moderate head injuries. *J Neurosurg* 1987;66:706–713.

240. Levin H, Mattis S, Ruff R, Eisenberg HM, Marshall LF, Tabaddor K. Neurobehavioral outcome following minor head injury: A 3-centre study. *J Neurosurg* 1987;66:234–243.

241. Gennarelli T. Mechanisms of brain injury. *J Emergency Med* 1993;11:5–11.

242. Hayes R, Povlishock J, Singha B. Pathophysiology of mild head injury. *Phys Med Rehabil* 1992;6:9–20.

243. Miller L. Neuropsychology and pathophysiology of mild head injury and the post-concussion syndrome: Clinical and forensic consideration. *J Cog Rehabil* 1996;15:8–23.

244. Povlishock J. Traumatically-induced axonal injury: Pathogenesis and pathobiological implications. *Brain Pathol* 1992;2:1–12.

245. Ponsford J. Psychological sequelae of closed head injury: Time to redress the imbalance. *Brain Inj* 1990;4(2):111–114.

246. Cicerone KD. Remediation of "working attention" in mild traumatic brain injury. *Brain Inj* 2002;16(3):185–195.

247. Walker JP. Functional outcome: A case for mild traumatic brain injury. *Brain Inj* 2002;16(7):611–625.

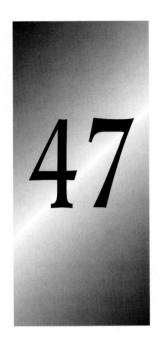

47

Evaluation and Treatment of Swallowing Problems After TBI

Jeri A. Logemann

Traumatic brain injury in children or adults can affect swallowing in a variety of ways (1–4). It is important for the clinician to investigate the history of the patient's original injury and acute care for that injury in order to understand the type(s) of swallowing disorders that may be present. The neural damage resulting from traumatic brain injury and the incident causing the injury can vary tremendously from patient to patient. There is the direct neural damage at the site of trauma, the contrecoup injury or the opposite side of the brain trauma as the brain bounces in the brain case, and there is the twisting or torquing of the brainstem during the injury. Thus, there is rarely a direct relationship between the location of the trauma and the nature of the swallow disorders. However, the clinician should learn the locus of the direct injury and results of any other testing of neural function to identify other areas of damage (5).

In addition to the neural damage, there is potential structural damage during the injury that could affect swallowing. For example, if the patient's neck is broken as their head is injured, they may exhibit problems in swallow related to cervical spine injury (6). If the patient flies from a motor vehicle and lands on a foreign body such as a stick or piece of metal, there may be penetrating wounds into the neck that affect swallowing. Thus, the exact nature of the patient's damage at the scene of the accident is quite important. Another factor in identifying swallowing disorders in the patient who has suffered a traumatic brain injury, is to define any emergency medical care that could affect swallowing (7). This would include an emergency tracheostomy, which might be placed higher in the neck than normal and damage laryngeal function. If intubation to establish an airway is done traumatically, it can cause dislocation of one or both arytenoid cartilages or other damage to the larynx, particularly the true vocal folds. Understanding the nature of the patient's injuries and the medical care they received is important in accurately assessing dysphagia in the head-injured patient. The key to successful recovery/rehabilitation of dysphagia after brain injury is to define the exact structural or physiologic abnormalities in the swallow and to design the therapy program to address these disorders.

Swallowing Disorders Seen in Brain Injury A broad range of swallowing disorders is seen in patients after brain injury, probably because of the wide range of damage that can cause dysphagia in these patients. If the patient exhibits upper motor neuron damage with high muscle tone, there may be difficulty in opening the mouth, controlling the oral tongue and the soft palate. Most commonly, there is a delay in triggering the pharyngeal swallow or even an absent pharyngeal swallow. There may be reduced motor control of the pharyngeal stage of swallow when it triggers, involving reduced movement of the tongue base to generate pressure to move the food into the pharynx, reduced laryngeal elevation because of scar tissue, tracheostomy, etc., or there may be reduced pharyngeal wall contraction resulting in reduced pressure generation. Dysfunction in the airway protection provided by the larynx does not occur frequently in head-injured individuals nor does a dysfunction at the upper esophageal sphincter at the entrance of the esophagus. However, patients with structural damage can have scar tissue in place that affects either airway closure or opening of the upper esophageal sphincter. Myoclonus may occur in any oral or pharyngeal structure including the oral tongue, tongue base, soft palate, pharyngeal walls, larynx, and completely discoordinate the swallow. It is critical that the speech language pathologist define the exact nature of the patient's swallowing disorder(s) in order to define appropriate therapy/management for the patient's swallowing problem(s).

Counseling the Patient's Family   In a patient who has suffered a severe brain injury, swallowing is often one of the last things to be evaluated. Sometimes, patients are allowed to eat because they exhibit no symptoms of a swallow disorder such as coughing or choking. Then, later, as recovery progresses, the patient begins to exhibit some signs of dysphagia while swallowing particular types of food. It is important that clinicians talk with the patient's physician and family as soon as possible regarding the possibility of swallowing disorders and the potential need to evaluate swallowing. Families often think that if the patient is not visibly struggling to eat, coughing and choking, their swallowing is fine. If the patient is allowed to eat and then later has an assessment which identifies a significant swallow impairment, families and patients can become very angry, complaining that they were allowed to eat at an earlier stage in recovery sometimes at another institution, but now the clinician is "making them go backwards" and delaying their recovery. Because of this reaction, it's important that clinicians introduce the possibility of a swallow impairment early, even if evaluation isn't possible immediately because of the patient's medical status.

Evaluation of Dysphagia in Brain Injured Patients: When and How   The evaluation of dysphagia in brain injured patients should begin as they are admitted to the acute care hospital. However, in some situations, the patient receives a severe enough injury that swallowing evaluation is not even considered until the patient has been stabilized and life is no longer threatened. **For some patients this may be days or weeks.** The initial screening assessment may simply indicate that the patient is not ready for a full swallowing assessment. Many patients are

in a coma initially. A small amount of data point to the fact that the longer the coma, the more severe the swallow problems are likely to be (3). When the patient is consistently awake and exhibits some level of alertness, dysphagia assessment should begin at the bedside. Formal swallowing evaluation and therapy have been found to improve dysphagia outcomes in brain injured patients (8)

Bedside assessment usually includes an oral motor assessment, a review of receptive and expressive language and ability to understand direction, history of medications used since the injury, and oral sensory testing to identify any abnormal oral reflexes or postural abnormalities (9). The major purpose of the bedside clinical assessment is to identify oral motor difficulties in the face, lips, tongue, palate, pharynx, and larynx, and to determine whether there is significant risk of a pharyngeal stage swallowing impairment. Pharyngeal stage swallowing impairments cannot be diagnosed at the bedside and require an instrumental assessment in order to define the exact nature of the swallowing problem and its sequelae such as inefficient swallow or aspiration. A review of the patient's medications may identify medications that could negatively affect swallow including tranquilizers, psychotropics, and medications that cause xerostomia (10). Oral sensory assessment examining two point discrimination and light touch sensitivity is important in determining the patient's ability to recognize where food is located in the mouth and whether or not all of the food has been cleared in any swallow attempt. Some brain injured individuals exhibit severely slowed oromotor control such that opening the mouth can take 3 to 5 minutes. In this situation, there is generally significant hypertonicity in facial musculature which requires rotary massage on one cheek while digital pressure downward is applied firmly to the chin and the patient is given repeated directions to try to open their mouth. Even with this assist to heighten sensory awareness, the patient may take 3 to 5 minutes to open their mouth. In such a patient who is also nonverbal, an instrumental swallow assessment must be delayed until they are able to open their mouth in under 30 seconds. The rotary massage and continuous digital pressure to the chin will facilitate faster oral opening as well as an understanding of the patient's neural and structural damage causing the swallowing problem. Family members should be counseled regarding the fact that the patient is not yet ready to have an instrumental swallow assessment but rather needs to build control over their oral mechanism instead. The patient's ability to manage their own saliva and awareness of their saliva is also an important component of the bedside assessment. At the end of a bedside assessment, the clinician should be able to describe the patient's level of alertness, their ability to follow direction, behavior control, their oral motor function and their saliva control as well as understand the patient's neural and structural damage causing the swallowing problem. Patients should also be assessed for their ability to vocalize and to coordinate respiratory and laryngeal function. If the patient has been given food or is eating, the clinician should observe the patient swallowing to identify any dysphagic symptoms. Unfortunately, the bedside clinical examination cannot define pharyngeal physiology or pharyngeal symptoms of swallow disorders such as aspiration (11).

Instrumental Assessments Instrumental assessments may include a radiographic evaluation, fiberoptic endoscopic examination of swallow (FEES) or manometric assessment. Radiographic assessment is the simplest for the patient who has sustained a brain injury since no tube or other instrumentation must be placed into their nose or mouth. During the radiographic assessment, the patient must be able to be positioned into the fluoroscopy equipment so that the head and neck can be viewed in the lateral plane (Figures 47-1 and 47-2). Even this can be difficult for some low level patients. However, in many instances the patient can be moved into the equipment and positioned between the fluoroscopy tube and the table on a cart or gurney, thus requiring no voluntary motor control on their part.

The radiographic study is designed to define the anatomy and the physiology of the oral preparatory, oral and pharyngeal phases of swallow and to identify therapy procedures to improve the swallow if needed. The goal of the test is to find ways for the patient to swallow successfully, not to keep them from eating (12). The patient is given measured volumes of thin liquids, pudding and,

if the patient is capable of chewing, a material requiring mastication, generally a Lorna Doone cookie. Other foods can be given as needed. The patient is presented with measured volumes of thin liquid beginning with a small amount (1 ml) and asked to swallow it. The material is a flavored barium. The patient is given 2 swallows of each bolus volume or food type and the swallow is observed fluoroscopically. In total, the patient should receive 2 swallows each of 1, 3, 5, 10 ml of thin liquids, cup drinking of thin liquids, pudding and masticated material. The bolus volumes of thin liquid are increased sequentially as long as the patient swallows the smaller volume successfully, that is, without aspiration or large amounts of residual food left in the mouth or pharynx. If the patient exhibits a significant swallow impairment which results in aspiration or large amounts of oral or pharyngeal residue, the patient should be given treatment strategies during the x-ray study to improve the swallow and eliminate these sequelae of swallow disorders. Generally, when selected treatment techniques are introduced during the radiographic study, three types of techniques are attempted in the following order: 1) postural change; 2) heightening sensory awareness; and 3) voluntary swallow maneuvers. The specific postural techniques, sensory enhancements and voluntary swallow maneuvers to be introduced with a particular patient will depend upon the nature of their swallowing disorders revealed by the diagnostic portion of the test and the level of their ability to follow direction. The purpose of introducing therapy strategies into the radiographic diagnostic study is to determine which procedures are the most efficacious for the patient and to do so in a way that

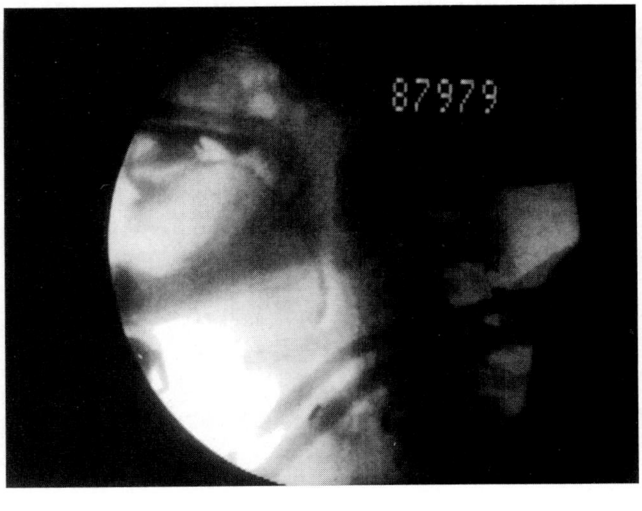

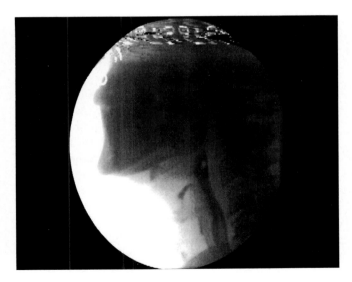

FIGURE 47-1

Lateral radiographic view of the oral cavity and pharynx after a swallow in a brain injured patient who is also spinal cord injured and is wearing a neck brace. There is significant residue in the mouth and the tongue base is also coated with material

FIGURE 47-2

Lateral radiographic view of the oral cavity and pharynx at mid swallow in a patient post brain injury. The airway should be completely closed at this time but there is penetration and aspiration present

documents their effectiveness. If none of these strategies improve the safety or efficiency of the swallow, the clinician can introduce other food consistencies such as nectar- or honey-thickened liquids to determine whether or not the patient can gain a safe and fairly efficient swallow with a diet change. At the end of the radiographic study, the clinician should be able to define the patient's swallow physiology and safety, the best treatment procedures for the patient's swallow disorder(s) and the optimal diet as well as safety of the swallow. The report provided after the study should provide this information in a concise and accurate format.

Another instrumental assessment is the fiberoptic endoscopic evaluation of swallowing or FEES which involves the nasal insertion of a fiberoptic tube in order to view the pharynx from above. This procedure does not enable observation of the oral preparatory or oral phases of swallow, nor does it permit assessment of the pharyngeal stage of swallow during the moment of laryngeal elevation, tongue base retraction and upper esophageal sphincter opening (6, 13–14). It does enable observation of the bolus entering the pharynx over the base of tongue, the initial movements of the pharyngeal stage of swallow and any aspiration that may occur as the bolus appears in the pharynx. It also enables viewing of the pharynx after the swallow when any bolus residual may be aspirated. In summary, endoscopy provides a superior view of the pharynx and enables the clinician to observe selected aspects of the oral pharyngeal swallow (see Figure 47-3). Endoscopy has the advantage of involving no radiographic exposure and enabling the clinician to bring the equipment to the patient's bedside (15). The question the clinician must answer is whether or not the endoscopic examination will provide the information needed for management of the patient's swallowing disorder(s).

If the question the clinician needs answered in the swallow assessment is whether or not the pressure generated during swallow is adequate, then manometry may be the appropriate procedure to be used. Many swallowing disorders, including difficulties with the oral tongue, tongue base or pharyngeal wall, lead to reduced pressure generation in the pharynx including reduced movement of the base of tongue, reduced movement of the pharyngeal walls and reduced laryngeal elevation and forward movement. While the radiographic study or the fiberoptic endoscopic study can give a perception of reduced pressure to clear food through the pharynx, actual measurements of pressure can only be made with manometry. Manometry, too, involves placement of a tube transnasally into the pharynx and the top of the cervical esophagus. Generally, this is done under fluoroscopy in order to assure where the pressure sensors in the manometric tube are located (see Figure 47-4) and to determine what structures are touching the manometric tube that may create pressure changes (16).

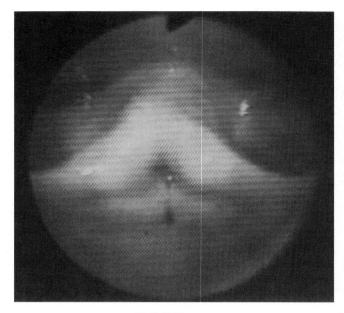

FIGURE 47-3

A superior endoscopic view of the larynx and the pharynx with the false vocal folds closely approximated prior to swallow. The arytenoids and pyriform sinuses are also in view. The upper esophageal sphincter (UES) is located at the top of the image behind the arytenoids and is closed. Opening of the UES is not usually visible during endoscopy as the endoscopic image disappears as the larynx elevates during the first third of the pharyngeal swallow (24, 25)

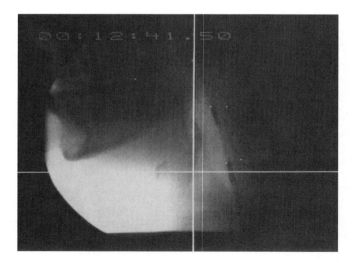

FIGURE 47-4

Lateral radiographic view of the oral cavity and pharynx prior to a swallow with a solid state manometric catheter in place prior to swallow. The manometric catheter is a 3 mm diameter flexible tube containing the solid state pressure sensors represented by the dark elongated rectangles resting on the pharyngeal wall first at the level of the tongue base, and second at the level of the laryngeal entrance

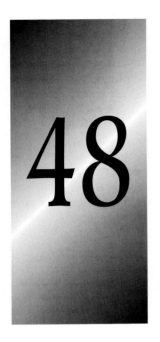

48 Cognitive-Communication Deficits Following TBI

Carl A. Coelho

anguage is best defined within the context of communication. Human communication involves the sharing and exchange of information between people. Language refers to communication through the use of words or other symbols and entails the use of multiple modalities such as: speaking, auditory comprehension, reading, writing, and gesture (1). Language use is frequently displayed through speech. Speech has developed into a highly efficient system for the exchange of even the most complex ideas. However, speech is the end product of a multifaceted cognitive process. For example in a situation in which two people are interacting; the speaker has to organize his thoughts, or communicative intent, decide what he wants to say and put what he wants to say into an appropriate linguistic form. This occurs by selecting the right words and phrases to express the intended meaning, and then placing these words in the correct order specified by the grammatical rules of the language. The next stage involves the formulation of motor commands necessary for programming the speech mechanism (i.e., the neural and muscular activities for activating respiration, phonation, resonance, articulation, and prosody) to produce an acoustic signal that accurately represents the words selected to communicate the speaker's intent. The final step in this process is the execution of the commands resulting in the production of speech (2).

Brain injuries may disrupt the process of communication at a variety of levels. Speech disorders (e.g., apraxia of speech or the dysarthrias) will not be discussed in the present chapter. The reader is referred to chapter 46 for a thorough discussion of that topic. Rather this chapter will focus on language disorders following traumatic brain injury (TBI).

LANGUAGE DISORDERS FROM A SITE OF LESION PERSPECTIVE

The nature of a brain injury will in large measure determine the characteristics of the subsequent language disorder. For example, strokes are typically associated with focal lesions to either hemisphere or subcortical structures, resulting in fairly predictable deficit patterns. By contrast, TBI may result in focal injury to specific regions of the brain (e.g., coup and contrecoup sites of impact), diffuse axonal injury (i.e., stretching, tearing, shearing of nerve fibers), or a combination of both. This mechanism of injury yields a far less homogenous array of deficits. Language disorders resulting from lesions to the left hemisphere, right hemisphere, subcortical regions, and diffuse damage are reviewed separately below.

Focal Left Hemisphere Damage—Aphasia

McKinley and colleagues (3) have noted that language is disturbed in 75% or more of individuals with TBI. However, the nature of this language disturbance, that is, whether it is aphasic or nonaphasic, is not clear-cut. Aphasia is defined as an acquired impairment of language processes underlying receptive and expressive modalities caused by damage to areas of the brain that are primarily responsible for language function (4). Aphasia is characterized by grammatical disturbances, deficits of word retrieval, auditory comprehension, reading, and writing, in the presence of relatively intact cognitive abilities (e.g., orientation, attention, memory). Lesions associated with aphasia are usually located in the left hemisphere in the region of the posterior frontal lobe, anterior temporal lobe, and/or inferior parietal lobe (i.e., anywhere along the distribution of the left middle cerebral artery). The incidence of aphasia secondary to TBI reported in the literature varies greatly. Reports range from approximately 2% of 750 (5) and 614 (6) consecutive admissions to two city hospitals, to nearly 50% (7, 8). Sarno, Buonaguro, and Levita (9) reported on a group of 125 individuals with closed head injuries admitted to a rehabilitation center. The individuals studied fell into three groups: those with classic aphasia (30%), those with dysarthria accompanied by subclinical aphasia (34%), and those with subclinical aphasia (36%). The authors classified individuals as aphasic if their use of speech for expression and/or reception was impaired. Subclinical aphasia referred to evidence of linguistic processing deficits on formal testing in the absence of clinical manifestations of linguistic impairment. The apparent discrepancies regarding the incidence of aphasia following TBI are difficult to resolve because of the lack of consistency in the descriptions of the individuals with TBI studied, the different aphasia assessment tools employed, as well as the varied definitions of aphasia applied. An examination of specific linguistic deficits following TBI reported in the literature indicates that anomia, difficulty retrieving words, (5, 7, 9–13) and impaired auditory comprehension (7, 9) are the most commonly observed symptoms. Holland (14) noted that there is overlap in these deficit areas between individuals with aphasia and those with TBI, as well as in the associated reading and writing deficits both groups often demonstrate. However, it is the qualitative differences in the naming errors between the two groups which may be most useful in distinguishing between aphasic and nonaphasic responses. Both individuals with aphasia and those with TBI (particularly those in the acute stages) produce circumlocutions and various paraphasias and have reduced fluency in the generation of category-specific words; individuals with TBI, however, demonstrate additional naming errors. For example, they may also produce naming errors related to their personal situations or make errors of confabulation (i.e., sometimes bizarre responses related to the individual's disorientation). Milton and colleagues (15) have described a system for qualitatively evaluating naming behavior for individuals with TBI. The system permits descriptions of correct responses, and, when responses are incorrect, descriptions of their semantic, phonemic, and other relationships to the target. For example, for the target stimulus "apple" semantically-related responses might include such utterances as: "fruit", "Granny Smith", or "pear". Phonemically-related responses might include such utterances as: "able" or "ubel". Other responses might include such things as "saw" or "We grew them in our backyard".

Focal Right Hemisphere Damage

As noted by Myers (16) it has only been in the last 25 years that the cognitive and communcative deficits associated with the right hemisphere have been considered. As was the case for left hemisphere damage most instances of focal lesions to the right hemisphere are the result of cerebrovascular accidents (CVA). Localization of specific functions related to language processing in the right hemisphere has been a confusing endeavor. Some investigators have observed that the difficulty localizing the component processes involved in maintaining semantic information may be attributable to the involvement of both anterior and posterior cerebral regions and their interconnections (17). Although it is beyond the scope of the present chapter to discuss in any detail the nature of deficits that result from right hemisphere damage (RHD), this section will summarize some of the characteristic features. Generally speaking the range of deficits linked to RHD may be placed into five broad categories (16). The first is attentional deficits which includes problems with: arousal, orientating, vigilance, sustained and selective attention. The next category is neglect which involves a reduction of: attention to left-sided input, use of left limbs, awareness and recognition of left-sided body parts, and awareness of illness. The third category involves visuoperceptual deficits including: visual attention, integration, and memory, and spatial and topographical orientation. A fourth category is affective and emotional deficits including reductions in: the use of facial expression to convey emotion, sensitivity to facial expressions of others, use of prosody to convey emotion, and comprehension of emotional prosody. The final category is cognitive and communicative deficits, included here are reduced: discourse comprehension and production, communicative efficiency and specificity, processing of complex inferences as well as alternative and ambiguous meanings, sensitivity to contextual information, and appreciation of shared knowledge.

With regard to specific linguistic impairments, individuals with RHD typically perform adequately on language tasks that involve convergent processing (i.e., those requiring a limited number of responses and familiar word meanings) such as confrontation naming, yes/no questions, and providing definitions. Divergent language tasks (i.e., those involving a wide range of meanings which diverge from a single semantic concept such as verbal fluency, open-ended questions, or resolving ambiguities) present more difficulty for this group. They often have trouble understanding intended meanings because of a decreased ability to generate, maintain, or inhibit additional, alternate, and related meanings when the dominant meaning is inappropriate to the context (16).

Focal Subcortical Damage

There is a growing body of literature which documents that right-handed individuals who sustain damage to the left basal ganglia or left thalamus can also develop aphasia (18–20). Three subcortical aphasia syndromes have been described by Naeser and associates. The first, anterior syndrome, results from damage in the internal capsule, lenticular nucleus, and anterior white matter. This syndrome is characterized by hemiplegia; slow, dysarthric speech with near normal phrase length and prosody; poor confrontation naming; good repetition; good comprehension; and poor oral reading and writing. The second is posterior syndrome, which is associated with damage in the putamen and internal capsule, and the posterior white matter. Features of this syndrome are hemiplegia, fluent speech without dysarthria, good single word repetition but poor sentence repetition, impaired confrontation naming, poor comprehension, reading and writing. The third pattern described, anterior-posterior syndrome, results from capsular-putamenal damage with anterior and posterior white matter involvement. Characteristics include a combination of symptoms seen in both Broca's and Wernicke's aphasias. Robin and Scheinberg (21) have cautioned that aphasia caused by lesions in the basal ganglia result in a variety of speech and language impairments that are not all accounted for by the three syndromes described by Naeser and associates.

Aphasia resulting from damage to the left thalamus is typically characterized by hemiplegia and difficulty initiating spontaneous speech. In addition, speech may be echolalic and contain neologistic errors. Fairly good auditory comprehension and reading are usually noted, while writing and word retrieval are impaired. These individuals have also been observed to be perseverative with fluctuating performance moment to moment (22).

Diffuse Axonal Damage

Although individuals with TBI may incur focal lesions, a far more common type of brain pathology following TBI, and specifically closed head injury, is diffuse axonal injury. This pattern of injury is typically associated with what has been termed confused language (10, 23–25). Confused language is described as receptive/expressive language that may be phonologically, syntactically, and semantically intact, yet lacking in meaning because responses are irrelevant, confabulatory, circumlocutory, or tangential in relation to a specific topic, and lacking a logical sequential relationship between thoughts (26). Such language dysfunction may be mistaken for a fluent aphasia but is more appropriately considered cognitive in nature as opposed to linguistically-based, that is, as a symptom of cognitive rather than linguistic deficits. Traumatic brain injuries frequently result in significant disruption of cognitive processes such as (attention, memory and executive functions). More recent considerations of language disruption following TBI have suggested use of the term cognitive-communicative disorders as being a more accurate description of these impairments. Cognitive-communicative disorders involve difficulty with any aspect of communication secondary to cognitive dysfunction (27). Some individuals with TBI exhibit language disorders most consistent with aphasia, some with communicative deficits comparable to those seen in RHD, and some, particularly in the acute stages of recovery from TBI, demonstrate language behavior consistent with confused language. Regardless, a primary component of language dysfunction in the majority of TBI survivors pertains to disordered language use (i.e., pragmatics). Pragmatics refers to the set of rules which govern the use of language in context (28). Sohlberg and Mateer (29) observed that whereas individuals with aphasia may communicate better than they talk, individuals with TBI appear to talk better than they communicate. Pragmatic deficits are probably most prevalent in those individuals with frontal lobe injuries. Although the frontal lobes are not thought to be responsible for primary cognitive functions, it appears they are involved in coordinating and actualizing many functions involved in cognitive processing such as attention, motivation, regulation, and self-monitoring (30). Individuals with prefrontal injury frequently demonstrate problems, among other things, with: disorganized discourse; inappropriate social interactions (e.g., difficulty interpreting social cues); and abstract forms of language (e.g., irony or sarcasm) (31).

DISCOURSE ANALYSIS

Just as predominant impairments of language caused by focal lesions may mask subtle cognitive disturbances, primarily cognitive disturbances resulting from diffuse brain injury, may mask subtle language deficits (32). Such deficits typically go undetected, or are incompletely delineated by the traditionally used language assessment tools, such as aphasia batteries. In an effort to document such pragmatic deficits many investigators of verbal communicative ability following TBI have chosen to analyze *discourse* (33–43). Discourse is a series of related linguistic units that convey a message. The length of a given discourse is determined by the communicative function of the message. There are various types of discourse and each type has different cognitive and linguistic demands (44). It has been suggested that discourse is the most natural and basic unit of normal verbal communication (45). Furthermore, accurate production or comprehension of a narrative requires a complex interaction of linguistic, cognitive, and social abilities (i.e., language use) that are sensitive to the particular disruption following TBI.

Discourse analyses begin with the elicitation of a spoken *narrative*, minimally five sentences in length. A variety of types of discourse may be studied including *procedural* (e.g., describing how to change a tire), *descriptive* (e.g., describing a favorite activity), *story narratives*, and *conversational*. The discourse samples are audiotaped and transcribed verbatim. Once transcribed, the narratives are divided into basic units for analysis, such as T-units (i.e., an independent clause plus any dependent clauses associated with it). A T-unit is similar to a sentence but is more reliably identified. Segmenting narratives into sentences is often problematic because of the tendency of some speakers to link sentences of a narrative with conjunctions such as *and*, *or*, and *then*, making it difficult to delineate sentence boundaries (46). Depending on the type of discourse and the focus of the analysis, the actual discourse analysis may be done at a variety of levels (see Table 48-1). For example, in a narrative story, at the sentence level the number of T-units may be tallied as a measure of narrative length, or the number of subordinate clauses may be

counted as a measure of grammatical complexity. Across-sentence analyses may involve examining how speakers link meaning units across several sentences (e.g., counting complete or incomplete ties), referred to as intersentential cohesion. In story narrative analysis, episodes may also be examined. Episode components are defined as information units pertaining to stated goals, attempts at solutions, and consequences of these attempts. Additional analyses include productivity measures such as total words produced or total speaking time, content measures such as accurate or irrelevant content units, and measures of conversational speech, for example, appropriateness of an utterance or topic maintenance.

DISCOURSE DEFICITS FOLLOWING TBI

Functional communication requires language competence in a variety of settings ranging from informal social interactions to formal educational or work-related tasks (42). Findings of recent investigations have demonstrated that individuals with TBI experience difficulty with communicative effectiveness across a number of discourse genres (see 47–49 for reviews). What follows is a summary of several studies of discourse in individuals with TBI. Prior to beginning, a clarification on the use of the term TBI is offered. Although both closed and penetrating head injuries are classified as TBI, there are distinct differences between the two types, both in terms of array of deficits and recovery, the discussion of which is beyond the scope of this chapter. Throughout the review, which follows, the generic term TBI will be used because in many instances authors have not specified whether the individuals with brain injuries studied, had a penetrating or closed head injury. This review is organized by the level analysis. Prior to beginning this summary a brief overview of the levels of analysis for discourse production is provided. The most basic distinction in the analysis of discourse is whether the discourse genre of interest involves a monologue (narratives such as telling a story) or is interactive in nature (such as participating in a conversation). At the most general level, analyses of narrative discourse are focused on within-sentence processes, termed microlinguistic, or between-sentence processes, referred to as macrolinguistic . Under each of these broad categories are sublevels such as, lexical, syntactic, and lexical-semantic for the within-sentence analyses, and under the between-sentence analyses are the sublevels of local (microstructure) and global (macrostructure). Each of the sublevels has corresponding measures or analyses (see Table 48-1). Conversational analyses can be broken down in terms of the role of the participant during an interaction, that is, whether the individual functions as an initiator or as a responder. In each role there sublevels again with corresponding measures in the analysis.

TABLE 48-1
Various Levels in the Analysis of Narrative Discourse Production

GENERAL LEVELS	SUBLEVELS	EXAMPLES OF MEASURES
Within-Sentence microlinguistic	Lexical	Lexical errors
	Syntactic	Completeness Complexity
	Lexical-semantic	Propositional analysis
Between-Sentence macrolinguistic	Local (microstructure)	Cohesion
		Local coherence
	Global (macrostructure)	Global coherence Story grammar

TABLE 48-2
Examples of Narrative Story Analyses (Coelho, 2002)

DISCOURSE MEASURES	DESCRIPTION	EXAMPLE
Sentence Production Words per T-unit	Total words in story divided by number of T-units	118 words/6 T-units = 19.7
Subordinate clauses per T-unit	Number subordinate clauses in story divided by number of T-units	3 subord. clauses/6 T-units = .5
Cohesion Cohesive adequacy– Percent complete ties of total ties	Each occurrence of a cohesive tie judged as to its adequacy. Number of complete ties in story divided by total number of cohesive ties.	**Complete tie** – The girl was hungry. *She* ate her lunch. **Incomplete tie** – The boys walked home from the mall. *They* stopped at his house for a snack. **Erroneous tie** – Dave and Joe drove to the game. *He* forgot the tickets.
Story Grammar Number of total episodes	Total number of complete and incomplete episodes in a story.	**Complete episode –** *[Initiating event]* and this fly comes in. and the Father's bothered by this. *[Attempt]* so he decides to swat or hit the fly. and he hits his wife. *[Direct consequence]* and she goes down. **Incomplete episode –** *[Attempt]* and he hits his daughter *[Direct consequence]* and the daughter goes down to the floor.
Proportion of T-units within episode structure	Number of T-units in episode structure divided by total number of T-units in story.	10 T-units in episodes/ 16 total T-units = .62

Narrative Discourse

For each of the levels of analysis for narrative discourse a brief description is provided of each analysis followed by a summary of the findings from the TBI discourse literature. Examples of some of the more commonly used narrative analyses appear in Table 48-2. This will be followed by a comparable discussion of the analyses of conversational discourse.

Microlinguistic Analyses

Lexical Production Examinations of lexical production typically involve measures such as lexical diversity (i.e., number of different words produced) and the occurrence of paraphasic errors. The literature on lexical problems in discourse following TBI has been somewhat equivocal. For example some authors have reported a reduction in the number of different words produced (50) or a greater frequency of verbal paraphasias (51) following TBI, while others have noted that lexical production was not a problem for the individuals with TBI they studied (52, 53). Difficulties with verbal fluency and word retrieval following TBI reported in the discourse literature must be interpreted cautiously. Some of these studies have included, within their participant groups, individuals with TBI who were aphasic (e.g., 37, 51).

Syntax Syntactic aspects of discourse have been examined in several studies with mixed findings. Syntactic complexity, as measured by percentage of T-units containing dependent clauses (33), embeddedness of subordinate clauses (51), subordinate clauses per T-unit (54), and words per T-unit (55), was comparable to that of normal controls. Further, syntactic complexity was not judged as being a primary deficit when rated on various pragmatic rating scales (52, 53, 56). By contrast, other investigators have reported syntactic impairments in the discourse of individuals with TBI. For example Campbell and Dollaghan (50) noted that syntactic complexity, as measured by percentage of utterances containing two or more lexical verbs, was decreased in six of nine participants they studied. In addition an increased incidence of grammatical errors (e.g., omissions of the subject, main verb and other required grammatical morphemes, word order transpositions, verb tense and agreement errors) have also been noted for participants with TBI versus normal controls (51, 57). Once again these findings may have been partially contaminated by the presence of aphasia for some of the brain-injured participants.

Lexical-Semantic The contradictory findings, noted for lexical production and syntax, have prompted other investigators to examine the microlinguistic dysfunction in the discourse of individuals with TBI through semantic analyses, specifically propositional analysis. The advantage of propositional analysis is that it permits the examination of semantic complexity of an utterance apart from sentence structure and grammaticality (58). Propositions are meaning units identified with respect to a predicate (i.e., verb, modifier) and its arguments (i.e., agent, instrument). Any sentence may contain several propositions (59). Using a measure of words per proposition, Chapman and colleagues (33) did not find deficiencies in information flow for a group of adolescents with TBI. However, McDonald (39) tallied unspecified propositions in explanations of a board game by two individuals with TBI and found that one participant provided less detail than the non-brain-injured controls. Another study that applied propositional analyses, noted that individuals with TBI appeared to have difficulty with the planning and organization of language (60). Similarly, individuals with TBI were noted to produce significantly fewer propositions per T-unit than normal controls. In other words, they demonstrated a decreased ability to insert multiple ideas into single sentences (61). By contrast, the non-brain-injured (NBI) participants' appeared to chunk information, and that appeared to be a mechanism for linking propositions together, which increased the likelihood that the listener might understand multiple ideas as a connected semantic unit. The participants with TBI appeared less adept at applying this strategy to facilitate discourse organization.

Macrolinguistic Analyses

Continuing with the review of narrative discourse analyses, the focus now shifts to the macrolinguistic analyses which examine discourse performance between or across sentences.

Cohesion Sentences are connected by various kinds of meaning relations described as cohesive markers or ties. A word is considered a cohesive marker if its meaning cannot be adequately interpreted without the listener searching the text, beyond that sentence, for the completed meaning. Cohesional analyses, as described by Halliday and Hasan (45), have been undertaken in several studies of discourse and TBI. Discourse samples of individuals with TBI have been described as lacking continuity as evidenced by their production of fewer cohesive ties than normal controls in both narrative and procedural discourse tasks (37, 40). However, other investigators have reported that individuals with TBI produced a comparable number of cohesive ties as NBI participants in narrative discourse (39, 51, 54, 62). Differences in the proportional use of ties across discourse tasks have been reported for individuals with TBI (40, 54). Mentis and Prutting observed that their TBI participants used different cohesional patterns which appeared to be related to their reduced linguistic processing abilities, their reduced pragmatic abilities, as well as their attempts to compensate for the linguistic deficits. Liles and colleagues noted that, in a story retelling task, similar proportions of referential (e.g., *Tom is an engineer. **He** works in Ohio.*), lexical (e.g., *I gave Frank our tickets. The **idiot** lost them all.*), and conjunctive (e.g., *Bill worked all night. **And his hammering kept the rest of us awake.***) markers occurred for both the TBI and NBI groups. In the story generation task however, a distinction between the groups appeared in which the individuals with TBI showed a reversal of the pattern used in the story retelling task. In story generation all of the TBI participants decreased the proportional use of reference and increased the proportion of lexical ties. This shift in the proportional use of types of cohesive ties across the story tasks was attributed to the TBI groups' apparent direct reference to the stimulus picture. These direct references were characterized as interjected descriptors of the picture that were unrelated to the rest of the text. The individuals with TBI rarely integrated these lexical items into the text structure and consequently they were often judged to be incomplete ties. The TBI participants' tendency to refer outside their texts suggested that they were unable to detach themselves from the perceptual salience of the stimulus picture in order to organize their language for story development. In a final study, Coelho and colleagues (35) examined cohesion in discourse samples from a story generation task gathered longitudinally from two individuals with TBI. One individual demonstrated poor cohesive adequacy with meaningful content, as measured by story structure, and the second, fair to good cohesion with poor content. These findings emphasize the clinical utility of monitoring discourse abilities longitudinally and of employing a multilevel analysis procedure.

Coherence Coherence refers to the conceptual organization of discourse. The coherence of a text depends on the speaker's ability to maintain thematic unity (63). Coherence is typically considered from two perspectives, global and local. Global coherence pertains to how discourse is organized with respect to a general goal, plan, or topic. Local coherence refers to the maintenance of meaningful conceptual links between individual sentences within a text. Coherence has been specifically examined in the narrative discourse of individuals with TBI (39, 51, 62) and the findings have been mixed. With the exception that the participants with TBI produced more unexplained references, McDonald (39) noted that their texts were as coherent as those of the normal controls. Similarly, Van Leer and Turkstra (62) found no differences in the coherence ratings for their groups of TBI and NBI participants. However, Glosser and Deser (51) reported that the individuals with TBI they studied were significantly impaired relative to the normal controls in measures of local and global coherence, with global coherence most impaired. These authors suggested that coherence depends on intact access to semantic memory representations of real-world knowledge, as well as perceptual and conceptual integration necessary to maintain the plan and overall organization of discourse. In addition, the ability to produce discourse perceived as coherent requires simultaneous attention and mental manipulation of several bits of information including integration of the speaker's plan and the listener's perspective. The TBI participants' greater impairment with the maintenance of global versus local coherence, suggested that their discourse impairment was more related to a disruption of macro-organizational abilities as opposed to problems with meaning relationships between contiguous concepts (51).

Story Grammar Story grammar pertains to the purported regularities in the internal structure of stories that direct an individual's comprehension and production of the logical relationships between people and events. Story grammar knowledge is typically measured by complete episodes. An episode consists of (a) an initiating event that prompts a character to formulate a goal-directed behavior, (b) an action, and (c) a direct consequence marking attainment or nonattainment of the goal. An episode is considered complete only if it contains all three components (64). A variety of difficulties with story grammar has been reported for individuals with TBI. For example, Chapman and colleagues (33) noted that their severely impaired group of individuals with TBI demonstrated a reduction in the number of essential story components, failed to signal new episodes with setting information, and often omitted essential action information. These authors commented that it was unclear whether this difficulty was a reflection of an underlying impairment of the internal story schema or difficulty implementing story schema during discourse production. In another study NBI participants and those with TBI produced comparable numbers of complete episodes in a story-retelling task, but three of the four individuals with TBI produced no episodes in story generation (54). The TBI participants' apparent inability to use episode structure in the story generation task, in spite of having been able to produce complete episodes in the story retelling task, suggested that the story generation task required an interaction of cognition and language use in which the

TBI participants could not consistently engage. A reduction in the number of total episodes produced was also noted in a later study by the same authors (35). Finally, Coelho (65) noted that a group of 55 TBI participants produced fewer T-units within episode structure (i.e., the proportion of total T-units that contributed to episodic structure) than did a group of 47 NBI individuals. Although the TBI and NBI participants were not different in terms of the number of total episodes produced, which had been reported in previous studies (35,54), the NBI participants produced more T-units within the structure of episodes. In other words, the NBI group produced fewer extraneous T-units—that is, T-units that did not contribute to episodic structure. This measure was considered to be an indication of participants' ability to use story grammar as an organizational plan for language.

Miscellaneous Measures

Informativeness. The measurement of informativeness in discourse production has focused on three aspects primary aspects: amount of information communicated, quality of information (incompassing such descriptors as irrelevant, redundant, off topic, over personalized, etc.), and efficiency of information (66). The discourse output of TBI participants has been described as reduced in a number of studies as measured by number of words (and/or meaningful words), utterances or sentences; mean length of utterance in morphemes or communication units (comparable to T-units); or some combination of these measures such as number of words per T-unit or syllables per story grammar element, and percentage of syllables or utterances in mazes (33, 37, 42, 50, 55, 65, 67). Individuals with TBI have also been described as comparable to normal controls in terms of the amount of pertinent content expressed and in narrative length, but significantly slower in the rate of information produced (36, 55). These individuals appeared to "talk past the point of diminishing returns", their oral narratives were lengthier and slower relative to the amount of content provided (36, p. 6). Other investigators have reported normal productivity for individuals with TBI in terms of the number of T-units or sentences in narrative tasks (40, 54).

Other indices of informativeness have included such measures as: number of essential steps included in a description of a procedure (42), amount of pertinent content (36), content units (37), amount of essential information, accuracy of story, and implied meanings (68) and number of concepts introduced (55). In general mixed findings have been noted with essential steps and pertinent content the TBI participants being comparable to the normal controls (36, 42), but in other studies the individuals with TBI produced fewer content units and concepts and demonstrated some difficulty with implied meanings (37, 55, 68).

Summary of Findings on Narrative Discourse

Numerous investigations have illustrated the clinical utility of narrative discourse analyses with the TBI population (33–37, 39, 40–42, 50, 51, 54, 55, 60, 62, 65, 67, 68). In terms of microlinguistic processes, findings on lexical production and syntactic aspects of discourse have been noted to be somewhat ambiguous. Some investigators have reported difficulties in these areas for individuals with TBI, and others have observed that these abilities remain intact following injury. Results from some of these studies have been confounded by the inclusion of individuals who were also aphasic as a result of their TBI. Although some individuals with TBI in the acute stages of rehabilitation may demonstrate impairments with word retrieval and syntax, such discourse deficits are not characteristic of this population in the chronic stages (65). When microlinguistic processes are examined by means of semantic analyses the findings are more straightforward. Individuals with TBI demonstrate consistent problems with the planning and organization of language as reflected in their difficulties inserting multiple ideas into single sentences (60, 61).

Narrative discourse performance has also been evaluated extensively in terms of of macrolinguistic processes, namely cohesion, coherence, and story grammar. Cohesion has been noted to be an area of inconsistent impairment and performance may vary considerably depending on the discourse elicitation task presented (40, 54). For example, the cohesive adequacy of individuals with TBI has been reported to be comparable to that of normal speakers in story retelling, but impaired for story generation (54). Similarly, the proportion of types of cohesive ties used by participants with TBI changed from story retelling to story generation, which was not the case for the normal speakers (40, 54). Similar to cohesion, TBI participants' ability to generate complete episodes was frequently effected by the nature of the task, with story retelling being easier than story generation. Story generation required a complex interaction of language and various cognitive abilities that were difficult for even mildly impaired individuals with TBI (54, 65). It has also been noted that TBI participants produced more T-units that did not contribute to episodic structure. It appears that these individuals have difficulty using story grammar to organize language (65). Along similar lines, conceptual organization of discourse (i.e., coherence) has also been noted to be problematic for individuals with TBI. Specifically, their greater difficulty with the maintenance of global (i.e., general plan or goal) versus local (i.e., conceptual links between sentences) coherence suggests a disruption of macro-organizational processes for discourse (51). Analyses of story grammar (i.e., the generation of episodes) and cohesion enable discourse samples to be examined at multiple levels allowing for the delineation of distinct discourse patterns (35).

Finally, the applicability of findings on narrative discourse productivity and content analysis of individuals with TBI have also been limited by the inclusion of individuals with aphasia and dysarthria in the groups studied. However, in general terms, the TBI participants studied demonstrated decreased discourse efficiency, generating information at a slower rate in lengthier utterances than controls (36, 55).

Conversational Discourse

The analysis of conversational discourse is of particular interest for the study of the TBI population because of its importance in the process of socialization. The development and maintenance of social relationships has been noted to be challenging for survivors of TBI. The consequences of this difficulty are social isolation, increased reliance on family for social support, and significant problems returning to work, school, and premorbid avocations. It has been suggested that these interactional problems are the result of social skills deficits, and that these deficits in social skills are felt to be a reflection of subtle impairments in pragmatic language use during conversation (69, 70). There have been numerous reports pertaining to the analysis of conversational discourse following TBI. These reports are summarized below by type of analysis.

Response Appropriateness

The appropriateness of TBI participants' utterances within conversations utilizing procedures described by Blank and Franklin (71) has been described (72, 73). A greater number of turns per conversation were noted for the participants with TBI than for the normal controls. This increased number of turns resulted from their shorter length of utterance per turn and their conversational partner's higher percentage of oblige production (i.e., utterances for which a response is expected, as in a question) (72). In a follow-up to the original study, which involved 5 individuals with TBI, Coelho and colleagues (73) studied 32 individuals with TBI, all of whom had recovered a high level of functional language, and were all rated as Rancho Los Amigos Level of Cognitive Functioning (74) VII (automatic-appropriate) or above. As a group the individuals with TBI did not initiate a great deal and appeared dependent on the examiner to maintain the momentum of the interaction. They produced fewer spontaneous obliges and comments (i.e., utterances for which a response is not required) than did the NBI controls and functioned primarily as "responders". Further, when they did respond, they provided more information than was requested. Although this extra information was not inappropriate or bizarre, it did not facilitate disclosure on the part of the conversational partner. The function of disclosure in social interaction is to allow the opportunity to talk about oneself or subjects of interest to oneself, in order to establish, sustain and enjoy social interaction (69).

Analysis of Topic

The proficiency by which participants manage conversational topics is critical to the success of an interaction. Topic management pertains to how participants in a conversation extend or maintain a given topic, as well as how discussion of a topic is discontinued, and how and when participants change topics (75). The specific contribution of speakers and their conversational partners to topic maintenance and development through analysis of ideational intonation units has been examined (76). Ideational describes a concept borrowed from Halliday (77) and pertains to the idea that discourse is about something or contributes some content. Therefore, ideational units can be assumed to represent what speakers contribute to topic maintenance and development, and to exist as a function of cognitive processes. For example, there are categories of ideational units for new information appropriate to the topic contributed by a speaker and categories representing no new information but still maintaining a topic. Thus it is reasonable to assume that production of ideational intonation units is likely to be disrupted in persons with brain injuries and cognitive impairments. Mentis and Prutting (76) found differing patterns of production between an adult with TBI and a NBI control in their intonation unit analysis across unspecified, concrete, and abstract conversational contexts. The individual with TBI produced fewer units containing novel information not specifically requested, fewer clarification and confirmation requests, and more agreement and acknowledgement units. In a follow-up study this analysis procedure was applied to conversational samples of a group of ten individuals with TBI and ten NBI controls (78). The intonation unit analysis did not distinguish high functioning individuals with TBI from controls matched for age, gender, and socioeconomic status. The method of eliciting conversation, with the examiner directing the conversation, may have constrained the context and, thereby, masked deficits commonly attributed to this population's difficulty in social interchanges.

Other approaches to the analysis of topic management have involved the examination of how topics are introduced and changed during a conversation (73, 79). Any participant in a conversation may introduce topics. Topics are changed in one of three ways: (a) at the beginning of the conversation, or by ending discussion of one topic and initiating another, referred to as a novel introduction; (b) by means of a smooth shift, in which discussion of one topic is subtly switched to another; or (c) by means of a disruptive shift, in which discussion of one topic is abruptly or illogically switched to another

topic. Findings on this measure have been mixed. Coelho et al. (79) observed that five individuals with TBI demonstrated difficulty initiating and sustaining topics compared to five matched controls. However, when a group of 32 individuals with TBI were compared to an NBI group of 43 individuals, the group with TBI produced comparable numbers of Novel Introductions and Smooth Shifts as the NBI group during their conversations with an examiner. Neither group produced many Disruptive Shifts (73).

Systemic Functional Linguistics

Systemic Functional Linguistics (SFL) describes language use as a series of choices (77, 80). When a speaker produces an utterance, choices are made pertaining to what will be said and how it will be said. The listener and the situation in turn, influence the what and the how of the utterance. The impact of context on language use is an important consideration of SFL. Context has been described as a combination of three components: field, mode, and tenor. Field pertains to the nature of the social interaction taking place (e.g., a speech or a conversation with friends). Mode refers to the modality by which the discourse is produced (e.g., written or oral). Tenor describes who is involved in the interaction, their relationship to each other, and their roles or status (e.g., teacher and student, two strangers, clerk and customer) (43). Two additional components of SFL are genre, which pertains to the influence of culture on language (i.e., the step-by-step structure that are followed to achieve goals) and ideology, which involves the participants' biases and personal perspectives. Three types of SFL analyses have been used to study the nature of language structures, which are used to establish and maintain interpersonal interactions of individuals with TBI. These have included: exchange structure analysis, generic structure potential, and mood and modality analysis. Each of these is described briefly below.

Exchange structure analysis. Exchange structure analysis (ESA) involves the examination of who has the knowledge (i.e., the primary knower) in an interaction and how that information is transferred (to the secondary knower). This approach has been applied to interactions of individuals with TBI during a variety of service encounters (e.g., calling about: bus schedules, getting a driver's license, therapy schedules, and therapy goals) (43, 81, 82). Investigators studied whether TBI participants and NBI controls altered their communicative behavior with different conversational partners who varied in terms of familiarity (e.g., an information operator, a policeman, their mother, or a therapist). In reviewing the findings from this analysis the authors examined the communication partners' responses to the TBI versus control participants. Results indicated that the therapists gave more information to the normal controls than to the TBI participants. The mothers tended to provide more information to their NBI sons than to their sons with TBI, but this difference was not significant. In terms of requesting information therapists asked more questions of the normal controls than of the individuals with TBI, while the police asked more questions of the TBI participants than of the NBI individuals. Finally, therapists generated more clarifications and checking utterances with the individuals with TBI than with the NBI group. There were no other significant differences for the communication partners. In comparing the individuals with TBI to the NBI controls across the four conditions a number of significant differences were reported. First of all the TBI group produced more information in the police encounter than did the control group. Some of the information offered was inappropriate (i.e., more information than was requested, which was similar to the findings of Coelho and colleagues (72, 73)). The individuals with TBI provided more information in their interactions with the police than in those with the therapists and the operators at the bus station. This was felt to be due in part to the greater number of questions produced by the police. Because the mothers did not request much information from their sons with TBI, that group provided less information to their mothers as compared to the NBI group. In addition, the TBI group requested more information from the therapists than did the controls. The individuals with TBI generated more requests for clarifications than the NBI groups when conversing with the therapists. Finally, the TBI group asked for clarifications more with the police than with their mothers or the operators at the bus station (81, 82). Overall, results indicated that the discourse performance of the participants with TBI varied according to their conversational partner.

Generic structure potential analysis. This analysis addresses the issue of which aspects of language use appear to be influenced by particular dimensions of the context. Togher and colleagues (82) examined the core structural elements (e.g., greeting, address, service initiation, service request, service compliance, close, goodbye, etc.) that would be expected in two types of interactions (i.e., the bus information operator, and the police) for TBI and NBI participants. Results indicated that the generic structural elements in the TBI service encounters were different in terms of length and content than those of the controls. The TBI group had difficulties opening sequences and with the main service requests. This group also produced repetitious and at times inappropriate elements not seen with the NBI group. There were several significant differences noted between the police and bus information encounters as well. When the control participants interacted with the police the greeting sequences were shorter and promptly followed by succinct service requests. In addition the closing/goodbye sequences were

longer when they spoke to the police than when they interacted with the bus information operator. By contrast, when the participants with TBI interacted with the police they had longer greeting sequences and shorter goodbyes (82). The authors comment that opening and closing sequences facilitate the development of interpersonal relationships by establishing credibility, confirming the success of the encounter, and encouraging future contact. During the longer closing sequences of the NBI participants, the police encouraged them to call again, however this was not observed during the shorter closing sequences of the TBI group. This analysis of the overall structure of an interaction facilitates the identification of specific structural elements that may be problematic. These can then be further analyzed in terms of mood and modality.

Mood and Modality Analysis   The analysis of mood may be used to study the lexical and grammatical choices made at the clause level to establish the degree of directness being expressed (e.g., statements such as "I will be home on Tuesday" are direct, whereas a declarative statement with rising intonation such as "You'll be home Tuesday?" are less direct and considered to be more polite). A direct statement may be either positive or negative (e.g., "I will be home" or "I won't be home"). Between these two poles a speaker may indicate uncertainty or directness through expressions of modality such as *might, must, possibly, probably*, or comments such as *I think*. Definiteness decreases as the speaker's expression of modality increases. Mood and modality has been examined in the interactions of TBI and NBI speakers in four interactions (with: a bus information operator, police, mother, therapist). Results indicated that the TBI participants were able to access a variety of politeness strategies, however they appeared less adept at applying these strategies across the four different interactions when compared to the NBI group (83).

Conversation Analysis

Other highly structured analyses have also been applied to conversational samples. One such system is conversation analysis (CA) which was developed to delineate the structural organization and sequential ordering of talk. Friedland and Miller (84) have applied CA to conversational samples of an individual with TBI. The authors commented that CA was sensitive for identifying pragmatic deficits in this individual. Specifically it identified the precise locale of conversational breakdowns and hoe these were repaired or not. Further, it demonstrated how one conversational partner adapted to these breakdowns and was successful during interactions with the TBI participant and another was not.

Pragmatic Rating Scales

In contrast to the very structured analysis procedures of SFL and CA a number of investigators have utilized pragmatic rating scales to investigate conversational abilities (56, 85–90). Although some of the pragmatic dimensions rated within these scales are redundant, each scale has a rather novel approach to looking at conversation. For example, some scales rate both nonverbal (e.g., intonation, facial expression, eye contact, gesture) and verbal (conversation initiation, turn taking, topic maintenance, response length, presupposition and referencing) communication (87). While others focus on specific aspects of the verbal message such as intelligibility, sentence formation, and coherence of narrative (56). Some theoretically-based scales focus on aspects of pragmatics such as utterance acts (e.g., vocal intensity, voice quality, prosody), propositional acts (e.g., lexical selection, word order, stylistic variations), and illocutionary and perlocutionary acts (e.g., speech acts, topic, turn taking) (88). Other scales are questionnaires completed during an observation or from personal knowledge which deal with such issues as "Does client: make rapid and inappropriate changes in conversational topic without clues to the listener? or fail to attend to cues for conventional turns, interrupting frequently or failing to hold up his or her end of the conversation?" (85, 91). Observations on the use of such pragmatic rating scales for assessing individuals with TBI have been generally positive. The scales are not labor intensive, which is the case for most of the other formal analysis procedures, and they are useful for assessing selected communicative behaviors unobtrusively, in real-world settings.

Social Information Processing

A final category of analysis views communication as an integral aspect of social pragmatic skills. A universally accepted definition of social skills is absent from the enormous literature on this topic. Similarly, numerous conceptual models of social skills have been described (92). The ability to communicate effectively is the basis of socially skilled behavior, and in humans, language is the primary method of communication. Ylvisaker, Urbanczyk, and Feeney (93) suggested a conceptualization of social skills following TBI that specifically incorporated the dimension of communication. Five components are included: (a) the individual's knowledge of self; (b) the extent to which an individual attends to their personal appearance; (c) social cognition (i.e., social perception, social knowledge, and social decision making); (d) communication, and (e) the social environment (i.e., significant people in the individual's natural environment). Analysis procedures pertaining to social cognition have examined such skills as cooperation, turn-taking, politeness, negotiation, topic management, and sensitivity to role and status of all participants. For example, McDonald (39) studied two individuals with TBI and 12 NBI participants explaining a novel procedure to a blind-folded third person. The productions of the TBI participants were rated as disorganized, confusing, and ineffective as compared to the controls. The disorganization was attributed to errors in sequencing and inclusion of irrelevant propositions. In a second study individuals with TBI and NBI controls participated in a barrier task, which required that the participants explain a board game to a listener not present in the room (94). The authors noted that the TBI participants appeared to be bound to the physical properties of the stimulus before them, and omitted important details from their explanations that the listener needed to understand the game. Similar findings were noted for adolescents using the same task (95). The investigators concluded that overall performance was limited by the TBI participants' decreased ability at role taking which in turn was associated with frontal lobe damage. In a final study, Turkstra and colleagues (96) studied social cognition of 10 adolescents with TBI and 60 NBI peers. Two tasks were presented: emotion recognition and conversation judgment. In the emotion recognition task, the participants were asked to identify the emotion depicted by an actor (happy, sad, peeved, angry, disgusted). For the conversation judgment task, six conversation skills were depicted: (a) attentive listening; (b) perception of nonverbal cues; (c) detection of sarcasm; (d) sharing the conversational burden; (e) humility; and (f) speaking at the listener's level. Each participant was asked to make judgments about the actor during videotaped vignettes (e.g., "Is the person a good listener?", "What makes you think so?"). Results indicated that the TBI group differed significantly from the NBI group for both recognition of emotion and the conversational judgments. Most of the errors on the conversation skills task were related to the detection of sarcasm and the feelings it might evoke in a listener. This finding was consistent with those of McDonald (97) which demonstrated impaired understanding of sarcasm and other forms of social inference in adults with TBI.

Summary of Findings on Conversational Discourse

The analysis of conversational discourse has been conducted from a variety of perspectives and the procedures applied have ranged from rating scales or check lists to highly structured analysis protocols. Although not entirely consistent, results from various pragmatic rating scales, and analyses of response appropriateness and topic management suggest that individuals with TBI experience difficulty when called upon to function as a partner in communicative dyads, whether in conversation or referential communication. These individuals demonstrate problems initiating and sustaining topics in conversation and frequently rely on their discourse partner to assume a greater proportion of the communicative burden to ensure a successful interchange of information (39, 56, 72, 73, 76, 91).

The role of individuals with TBI as participants in conversational dyads will vary according to the tenor relationships. In addition, the factors of familiarity and status appear to influence the language choices made by conversational partners during these interactions. These language choices are the result of the different roles the conversational participants assume and how conversational partners respond to the disability of the participant with TBI (43).

Finally when conversation is considered as a component of social skills or social cognition, a decreased ability for role taking has been identified as a primary deficit for individuals with TBI. Problems with the recognition of emotion and interpretation of sarcasm and inference also compromise their social functioning (96, 97).

INTERPRETATIONS OF DISCOURSE DEFICITS FOLLOWING TBI

The present review has indicated that individuals with TBI frequently demonstrate discourse impairments. These difficulties cross discourse genres and are revealed by a variety of discourse analyses. This chapter has focused primarily on descriptions of narrative and conversational discourse deficits. If it is assumed that these types of discourse are different in terms of underlying requisite processes, then the reasons for difficulty with narrative and conversational discourse should also be different. What follows are interpretations of narrative and conversational discourse impairments following TBI.

Narrative Discourse Impairments

Kintsch and van Dijk (98) have proposed that semantic information may be represented at multiple levels. These levels include: the surface structure, the text base; consisting of the microstructure (i.e., meaning contained in words and phrases) and macrostructure (i.e., topic- or gist-level information), and the mental model where the listener constructs a representation of the situation described (i.e., comprehends the text). The notion that a text's representations occur at a number of levels implies that discourse analysis must be performed at multiple levels as well. The primary division in such structural analyses occurs between the analysis of linguistic (e.g., lexical, syntactic, and cohesion analyses) and of conceptual or semantic representations (e.g., propositional and frame [i.e., higher level of semantic structure specifying constituents and relations among constituents]) levels (99). Two broad types of cognitive functions, assumed to be involved in discourse processing, further characterize these levels of analysis, that is whether an analysis is micro- or macrolinguistic in nature. Microlinguistic functions are language-specific procedures for processing

phonological and syntactic aspects of single words and sentences in the absence of context. Macrolinguistic functions involve cognitive procedures for integrating linguistic and nonlinguistic knowledge for the purposes of maintaining the conceptual, semantic, and pragmatic organization of discourse. The critical distinction between these two categories is that the macrolinguistic processes involve analyses of language units as contextual events (63).

With regard to microlinguistic analyses, the TBI participants have been noted to have comparable scores to normal controls on measures of lexical diversity (100) and syntactic complexity (65). For measures of macrolinguistic processes, no consistent differences between the groups have been noted for cohesive adequacy, however TBI participants typically have lower scores on measures of story grammar performance than normal controls (65). In addition, individuals with TBI demonstrate lower propositional density scores (61). As a group TBI participants demonstrate relatively preserved microlinguistic discourse functioning. The impairments noted in their narrative discourse production are associated with problems in macrolinguistic functions, that is, with the interaction of linguistic and conceptual structures. The finding that the TBI participants present with predominantly macrolinguistic discourse deficits is consistent with the diffuse pathology associated with TBI and closed head injury in particular. Glosser and Deser (51) have specified that microlinguistic, language-specific, functions are dependent on the integrity of a specialized neural system within the left hemisphere. Conversely macrolinguistic functions depend on different neural systems that are nonfocal and bilaterally distributed.

To better understand how macrolinguistic discourse functions are disrupted in TBI, Huber's (101) description of text processing may be considered. Two distinct modes are involved: macroprocessing in which the speaker focuses primarily on the critical ideas in a text, and microprocessing in which the speaker deals with individual meaning units and their relationships as conveyed by various syntactic devices. Microprocessing requires linguistic knowledge and an algorithmic processing mode that is rule governed facilitating the analysis of linguistic elements. Macroprocessing involves general world knowledge and pragmatic reasoning and the mode of processing is heuristic. Lexical information, such as key words and idioms, is picked from the text and matched with experiential knowledge and expectations about persons, events, and situations. As soon as a plausible match is obtained, the interpretation process ends (101). This macroprocessing mode is the likely source of narrative discourse breakdown among the group of TBI participants reported on above (61, 65, 100).

There are a variety of cognitively-based explanations for this breakdown that are also reasonable avenues to pursue in future studies of narrative discourse following

TBI. First, optimal discourse processing involves simultaneous micro- and macroprocessing. However, such processing will be hindered by limitations of working memory, potentially resulting in incomplete integration or understanding of all propositional elements within a text. Previous findings of significant correlations between working memory and linguistic cohesion in discourse of individuals with TBI support this notion (37). Other investigators have also emphasized the critical role working memory plays in discourse (102–105). Secondly, individuals who are proficient at discourse processing are able to integrate prior real-world knowledge to facilitate interpretation of the ongoing discourse. This integration of prior experiences is facilitated through the use of story schemas and script knowledge. Schemas and scripts are cognitive structures that generate expectations about the way a story might progress and organize the understanding of real-world events and their consequences. Both scripts and story schemas are attempts to characterize prerequisite memory representations of contextual information. Inclusion of irrelevant information during the production of discourse may reflect attentional or memory problems (106). Finally, the formation of story macrostructure requires knowledge about goals and actions, difficulty with story grammar may reflect problems with executive functions or goal-directed behavior in general. The relationship between executive functioning and discourse would appear to be quite logical. It has been suggested that discourse proficiency involves an interaction of cognitive and linguistic organizational processes, which requires executive control (107). Recent findings have demonstrated several significant, but modest, correlations between scores from the Wisconsin Card Sorting Test (WCST) (108, 109), a purported test of executive functioning, and measures of story narratives (65). This relationship between executive functioning and narrative discourse production in adults with TBI corroborates findings of previous investigations (68, 110).

Conversational Discourse Impairments

The complexities of conversational discourse have been well described in a number of studies (43, 49, 111–113). Effective participation in a conversation is dependent on a variety of factors such as: topic maintenance, turn taking, appropriate referencing, sensitivity to the conversational partner, and general cognitive abilities such as attention, vigilance, and memory. Social cognition (i.e., social: perception, knowledge, and decision making) will also have important influences on conversational skill. Galski and colleagues (114) have commented that the success of an individual's social, vocational, familial, and academic integration rests on the recovery of effective communication.

Although individuals with TBI demonstrate difficulty with many narrative discourse tasks, conversational discourse appears to be more difficult for this population. This may be attributed to the interactive nature of conversation. Consistent with this explanation, is the report that individuals with TBI produced more discourse errors in conversation than in a structured referential communication task. The authors suggested that conversations are more complex because due to social aspects, such as the relationship between conversational partners that is, familiarity, status, and role, as well as the face-saving strategies used for politeness when communication breakdowns occur (115). Such factors typically are not at issue in non-interactive types of discourse. Additional support for the contention that conversation may be more challenging than narrative discourse for individuals with TBI comes from a study which entered measures of both narrative and conversational discourse into a discriminant factor analysis (DFA). The goal was to determine which type of discourse analysis would best discriminate TBI from NBI participants. Results of the DFAs run with both sets of discourse data indicated that the conversational measures were most accurate in discriminating the groups (116). It appears that because the conversational measures were pragmatic in nature and more sensitive to the communicative dysfunction displayed by individuals with TBI than the more structurally focused narrative measures.

An additional explanation pertains to the potential cognitive factors that have been suggested to be important for meaningful participation in conversation. For example, topic maintenance and appropriate referencing requires both selective and sustained attention. Further, functional memory is required to recall what the speaker has said as well as the listener (112). Social competence requires the ability to apply social skills flexibly in accordance with the rules of an interaction. It has been argued that the inability to flexibly apply behavior according to rules, which entails executive functioning, may account for conversational difficulty following TBI (70). Support for the notion that executive functioning may be an important factor in conversational proficiency comes from findings of significant correlations between measures of conversational performance and scores from the WCST (117). Finally, comprehension of sarcasm and implicit language may also influence the effectiveness of a conversational participant (97).

CONCLUSIONS

This chapter has reviewed the nature of language dysfunction following TBI. Although some individuals with TBI will demonstrate aphasia, most will present with language deficits that are cognitively-based versus linguistic, referred to as cognitive-communicative impairments. The majority of these individuals will present with pronounced difficulties with pragmatics, that is with the use of language in context. These pragmatic deficits are not readily apparent when the assessment of language is focused on single words or isolated sentences. Rather, language should be evaluated in terms of discourse. Discourse permits the analysis of language at multiple levels (i.e., micro- and macrolinguistic, micro- and macroprocessing) which may be differentially impaired after TBI. Further, the analysis of interactive discourse (i.e., conversation) will reveal difficulties with social cognition that cannot be observed in the typical acontextual assessment settings.

Most survivors of TBI will demonstrate a variety of narrative and conversational discourse deficits. The underlying bases for these impairments are probably different but in many ways similar as well. Problems with narrative discourse are attributed to disruption of macrolinguistic processes involved in the organization of semantic information. This organizational process more than likely involves executive control. Meaningful interactions involve the flexible application of social rules which is also associated with executive functions. Delineation of the processes which subserve discourse will provide important treatment implications for cognitive-communicative impairments.

References

1. Tanner, D.C. *Exploring communication disorders*. Boston: Allyn & Bacon, 2003.

2. Denes, P.B., Pinson, E.N. *The speech chain*. Baltimore: Williams & Wilkins, 1964.

3. McKinlay, W.W., Brooks, D.N., Bond, M.R., Martinage, D.P., Marshall, M.M. The short-term outcome of severe blunt head injury as reported by the relatives of the injured person. *Journal of Neurology, Neurosurgery, and Psychiatry*, 1981;44,527–533.

4. Davis, A. *A survey of adult aphasia and related language disorders*. Englewood Cliffs, NJ: Prentice Hall, Inc., 1993.

5. Heilman, K.M., Safran, A., Geschwind, N. Closed head trauma and aphasia. *Journal of Neurology, Neurosurgery, and Psychiatry*, 1971;34:265–269.

6. Schwartz-Cowley, R., Stepanik, M.J. Communication disorders and treatment in the acute trauma center setting. *Topics in Language Disorders*, 1989;9:1–9.

7. Levin, H.S., Grossman, R.G., Kelly, P.J. Aphasic disorders in patients with closed head injury. *Journal of Neurology, Neurosurgery, and Psychiatry*, 1976;39:119–130.

8. Thomsen, I.V. Evaluation and outcome of aphasia in patients with severe closed head trauma. *Journal of neurology, neurosurgery, and psychiatry*, 1975;38:713–718.

9. Sarno, M.T., Buonaguro, A., Levita, E. Characteristics of verbal impairment in closed head injury. *Archives of Physical Medicine and Rehabiliation*, 1986;67:400–404.

10. Levin, H.S., Grossman, R.G., Rose, J.E., Teasdale, G. Long-term neuropsychological outcome of closed head injury. *Journal of Neurosurgery*, 1979;50:412–422.

11. Levin, H.S., Benton, A.L., Grossman, R.G. *Neurobehavioral consequences of closed head injury*. (pp. 140–161). New York: Oxford University Press, 1982.

12. Sarno, M.T. The nature of verbal impairment after closed head injury. *Journal of Nervous and Mental Disease*, 1980;168: 685–692.

13. Thomsen, I.V. Evaluation and outcome of traumatic aphasia in patients with severe verified lesions. *Folia Phoniatrica*, 1976;28: 362–377.

14. Holland, A.L. When is aphasia aphasia? The problem of closed head injury. In R.H. Brookshire (Ed.) *Clinical Aphasiology Conference Proceedings*, 1982;12:345–349.

15. Milton, S.B., Turnstall, C., Wertz, R.T. Dysnomia: A rose by any other name may require elaborate description. In R.H. Brookshire (Ed.) *Clinical Aphasiology Conference Proceedings*, 1983;14: 114–123.

16. Myers, P.S. *Right hemisphere damage*. San Diego: Singular Pub., 1999.

17. Molloy, R., Brownell, H.H., Gardner, H. (1990). Discourse comprehension by right-hemisphere stroke patients: Deficits of prediction and revision. In Y. Joanette, H.H. Brownell (Eds.) *Discourse ability and brain damage: Theoretical and empirical perspectives*. New York: Springer-Verlag. (pp. 113–130).

18. Crosson, B., Nadeau, S.E. (1998). The role of subcortical structures in linguistic processes: Recent developments. In B. Stemmer, H.A. Whitaker (Eds. *Handbook of neurolinguistics*. San Diego: Academic Press. (pp. 431–445).

19. Nadeau, S.E., Rothi, L.G. (2001). Rehabilitation of subcortical aphasia. In R. Chapey (Ed.) *Language intervention strategies in aphasia and related neurogenic communication disorders*, 4th edition. Philadelphia: Lippincott Williams & Wilkins. (pp.457–470).

20. Naeser, M.A., Alexander, M.P., Helm-Estabrooks, N., & associates Aphasia with predominantly subcortical lesion sites: Description of three capsular putamenal aphasia syndromes. *Archives of Neurology*, 1982;39:2–14.

21. Robin, D.A., Scheinberg, S. Subcortical lesions and aphasia. *Journal of Speech and Hearing Disorders*, 1990;55:90–100.

22. Brookshire, R.H. *Introduction to neurogenic communication disorders*, 6th edition. St. Louis, MO: Mosby., 2003.

23. Groher, M. Language and memory disorders following closed head trauma. *Journal of Speech and Hearing Research*, 1977;20:212–223.

24. Halpern, H., Darley, F., Brown, J.R. Differential language and neurologic characteristics in cerebral involvement. *Journal of Speech and Hearing Disorders*, 1973;38:162–173.

25. Prigatano, G. *Neuropsychological rehabilitation after brain injury*. Baltimore:Johns Hopkins Press, 1986.

26. Hagan, C. Language disorders in head trauma. In A. Holland (Ed.), *Language disorders in adults: Recent advances*. (pp. 245–282). San Diego: College-Hill Press, 1984.

27. American Speech-Language-Hearing Association Roles of speech-language pathologists in the identification, diagnosis, and treatment of individuals with cognitive-communication disorders. Position statement. *ASHA Supplemen* 24: in press, 2004.

28. Newhoff, M., Apel, K. Impairments in pragmatics. In L.L. LaPointe (Ed.) *Aphasia and related neurogenic language disorders*, 2nd ed. New York: Thieme, 1997.

29. Sohlberg, M.M. & Mateer, C.A. *Introduction to cognitive rehabilitation theory and practice*. New York: Guilford Press, 1989.

30. Stuss, D.T., Benson, D.F. *The frontal lobes*. New York: Raven Press, 1986.

31. Alexander, M.P., Benson, D.F., Stuss, D.T. Frontal lobes and language. *Brain and Language*, 1989;37:656–691.

32. Adamovich, B.L.B. Cognition, language, attention, and information processing following closed head injury. In J.S. Kreutzer, P.H. Wehman (Eds.) *Cognitive rehabilitation for persons with traumatic brain injury*. Baltimore: Brookes, 1991.

33. Chapman, S.B., Culhane, K.A., Levin, H.S., Harward, H., Mendelsohn, D., Ewing-Cobbs, L., Fletcher, J.M., Bruce, D. Narrative discourse after closed head injury in children and adolescents. *Brain and Language*, 1992;43:42–65.

34. Coelho, C.A., Liles, B.Z., Duffy, R.J. The use of discourse analyses for the evaluation of higher level traumatically brain-injured adults. *Brain Injury*, 1991a;5:381–392.

35. Coelho, C.A., Liles, B.Z., Duffy, R.J. Discourse analyses in closed head injured adults: Evidence for differing patterns of deficits. *Archives of Physical Medicine and Rehabilitation*, 1991b;72: 465–468.

36. Ehrlich, J.S. Selective characteristics of narrative discourse in head injured and normal adults. *Journal of Communication Disorders*, 1988;21:1–9.

37. Hartley, L., Jensen, T. Narrative and procedural discourse after closed head injury. *Brain Injury*, 1991;5:267–285.

38. Hartley, L., Jensen, T. Three discourse profiles of closed head injured speakers: Theoretical and clinical implications. *Brain Injury*, 1992;6:271–282.

39. McDonald, S. Pragmatic language skills after closed head injury: Ability to meet the informational needs of the listener. *Brain and Language*, 1993;44:28–46.

40. Mentis, M., Prutting, C.A. Cohesion in the discourse of normal and head-injured adults. *Journal of Speech and Hearing Research*, 1987;30:583–595.

41. Snow, P., Douglas, J., Ponsford, J. Discourse assessment following traumatic brain injury: A pilot study examining some demographic and methodological issues. *Aphasiology*, 1995;9:365–380.

42. Snow, P., Douglas, J., Ponsford, J. Procedural discourse following traumatic brain injury. *Aphasiology*, 1997;11:947–967.

43. Togher, L., Hand, L., Code, C. Exchanges of information in the talk of people with traumatic brain injury. In S. McDonald, L. Togher, C. Code (Eds.), *Communication skills following traumatic brain injury* (pp. 113–145). Hove, UK: Psychology Press, 1999.

44. Cherney, L.R. Pragmatics and discourse: An introduction. In L.R. Cherney, B.B. Shadden, C.A. Coelho (Eds.) *Analyzing discourse in communicatively impaired adults.* (pp. 1–8). Gaithersburg, MD: Aspen, 1998.

45. Halliday, M.A.K., Hasan, R. *Cohesion in English.* London:Longman Group Limited, 1976.

46. Hughes, D., McGillivray, L., Schmidek, M.A. *Guide to narrative language:Procedures for assessment.* Eau Claire, WI: thinking Publications, 1997.

47. Coelho, C.A. Discourse production deficits following traumatic brain injury: A critical review of the recent literature. *Aphasiology*, 1995;9:409–429.

48. Snow, P., Douglas, J. Conceptual and methodological challenges in discourse assessment with TBI speakers: Towards an understanding. *Brain Injury*, 2000;10:397–415.

49. Togher, L. Discourse sampling in the 21st century. *Journal of Communication Disorders*, 2001;34:131–150.

50. Campbell, T.F., Dollaghan, C.A. Expressive language recovery in severely brain-injured children and adolescents. *Journal of Speech and Hearing Disorders*, 1990;55:567–581.

51. Glosser, G., Deser, T. Patterns of discourse production among neurological patients with fluent language disorders. *Brain and Language*, 1990;40:67–88.

52. Milton, S.B., Prutting, C.A., Binder, G.M. Appraisal of communicative competence in head injured adults. In R.H. Brookshire (Ed.) *Clinical Aphasiology Conference Proceedings*, 1984;14:114–123.

53. Penn, C., Cleary, J. Compensatory strategies in the language of closed head injured patients. *Brain Injury*, 1988;2:3–17.

54. Liles, B.Z., Coelho, C.A., Duffy, R.J., Zalagens, M.H. Effects of elicitation procedures on the narratives of normal and closed head injured adults. *Journal of Speech and Hearing Disorders*, 1989;54:356–366.

55. Stout, C.E., Yorkston, K.M., Pimentel, J.I. Discourse production following mild, moderate, and severe traumatic brain injury: A comparison of two tasks. *Journal of Medical Speech-Language Pathology*, 2000;8:15–25.

56. Ehrlich, J., Barry, P. Rating communication behaviors in the head-injured adult. *Brain Injury*, 1989;3:193–198.

57. Peach, R.K., Schaude, B.A. *Reformulating the notion of "preserved" syntax following closed head injury.* Paper presented at the annual convention of the American Speech-Language-Hearing Association, November, 1986.

58. Kamhi, A.G., Johnston, J.R. Semantic assessment: Determining prepositional complexity. In W.E. Secord, J.S. Damico (Eds.), *Best practices in school speech-language pathology: Descriptive/nonstandardized language assessment.* (pp. 99–105). New York: The Psychological Corp. Harcourt Brace Jovanovich, 1992.

59. Kintsch, W. The psychology of discourse processing. In M.A. Gernsbacher (Ed.), *Handbook of psycholinguistics* (pp. 721–740). San Diego: Academic Press, 1994.

60. Biddle, K.R., McCabe, A., Bliss, L.S. Narrative skills following traumatic brain injury in children and adults. *Journal of Communication Disorders*, 1996;29:447–469.

61. Coelho, C.A., Grela, B., Corso, M., Gamble, A., Feinn, R. Microlinguistic deficits in the narrative discourse of adults with traumatic brain injury. *Brain Injury*, 2005;19:1139–1145.

62. Van Leer, E., Turkstra, L. The effect of elicitation task on discourse coherence and cohesion in adolescents with brain injury. *Journal of Communication Disorders*, 1999;32:327–349.

63. Glosser, G. (1993). Discourse production patterns in neurologically impaired and aged populations. In H.H. Brownell, Y. Joanette (Eds.) *Narrative discourse in neurologically impaired and normal aging adults.* San Diego, CA: Singular. (pp. 191–212).

64. Stein, N.L., Glenn, C.G. An analysis of story comprehension in elementary school children. In R.O. Freedle (Ed.) *New directions in discourse processing.* (pp. 53–120). Norwood, NJ: Ablex, 1979.

65. Coelho, C.A. Story narratives of adults with closed head injury and non-brain-injured adults: Influence of socioeconomic status, elicitation task, and executive functioning. *Journal of Speech, Language, and Hearing Research*, 2002;45:1232–1248.

66. Shadden, B.B. Information analyses. In L.R. Cherney, B.B. Shadden, C.A. Coelho (Eds.) *Analyzing discourse in communicatively impaired adults.* (pp. 85- 114). Gaithersburg, MD: Aspen, 1998.

67. Snow, P., Douglas, J., Ponsford, J. Narrative discourse following severe traumatic brain injury: A longitudinal follow-up. *Aphasiology*, 1999;13:529–552.

68. Tucker, F.M. & Hanlon, R.E. Effects of mild traumatic brain injury on narrative discourse production. *Brain Injury*, 1998;12:783–792.

69. Bond, F. & Godfrey, H.P.D. Conversation with traumatically brain-injured individuals: A controlled study of behavioural changes and their impact. *Brain Injury*, 1997;11:319–329.

70. Godfrey, H.P.D. & Shum, D. Executive functioning and the application of social skills following traumatic brain injury. *Aphasiology*, 2000;14:433–444.

71. Blank, M., Franklin, E. Dialogue with pre-schoolers: A cognitively-based system of assessment. *Applied Psycholinguistics*, 1980;1:127–150.

72. Coelho, C.A., Liles, B.Z., Duffy, R.J. Analysis of conversational discourse in head injured adults. *Journal of Head Trauma Rehabilitation*, 1991c;6:92–99

73. Coelho, C.A., Youse, K.M., Le, K.N. Conversational discourse in closed- head-injured and non-brain-injured adults. *Aphasiology*, 2002;16:659–672.

74. Hagan, C., Malkmus, D., Durham, P. Levels of cognitive functioning. In *Rehabilitation of the head injured adult: Comprehensive physical management.* Downey, CA: Professional Staff Association of Rancho Los Amigos Hospital, 1980.

75. Brinton, B., Fujiki, M. *Conversational management with language-impaired children.* Rockville, MD: Aspen, 1989.

76. Mentis, M., Prutting, C.A. Analysis of topic as illustrated in a head-injured and normal adult. *Journal of Speech and Hearing Research*, 1991;34:88–98.

77. Halliday, M.A.K. *An introduction to functional grammar.* London: Edward Arnold, 1985.

78. Wozniak, R.J., Coelho, C.A., Duffy, R.J., Liles, B.Z. Intonation unit analysis of conversational discourse in closed head injury. *Brain Injury*, 1999;13:191–203.

79. Coelho, C.A., Liles, B.Z., Duffy, R.J., Clarkson, J.V., Elia, D. Conversational patterns of aphasic, closed head injured, and normal speakers. *Clinical Aphasiology*, 1993;12:145–155.

80. Halliday, M.A.K. *An introduction to functional grammar* (2nd Ed.). London: Edward Arnold, 1994.

81. Togher, L, Hand, L, Code, C. Measuring service encounters in the traumatic brain injury population. *Aphasiology*, 1997a;11:491–505.

82. Togher, L., Hand, L., Code, C. Analyzing discourse in the traumatic brain injury population: Telephone interactions with different communication partners. *Brain Injury*, 1997b;11:169–189.

83. Togher, L., Hand, L. Use of politeness markers with different communication partners: An investigation of five subjects with traumatic brain injury. *Aphasiology*, 1998;12:755–770.

84. Friedland, D., Miller, N. Conversation analysis of communication breakdown after closed head injury. *Brain Injury*, 1998;12:1–14.

85. Damico, J. Clinical discourse analysis: A functional language assessment technique. In C.S. Simon (Ed.) *Communication skills and classroom success:* Assessment of language-learning disabled students (pp.165–206). San Diego: College-Hill, 1985.

86. Gerber, S., Gurland, G. *Interactive analysis of pragmatic-linguistic abilities in acquired aphasia.* Paper presented at the annual convention of the American Speech-Language-Hearing Assoc., Seattle, WA, November, 1990.

87. Halper, A.S., Cherney, L.R., Burns, M.S., Mogil, S.I. *Clinical management of right hemisphere dysfunction* (2nd Ed.). Gaithersberg, MD: Aspen, 1996.

88. Prutting, C., Kirchner, D. Applied pragmatics. In T.M. Gallagher, C.A. Prutting (Eds.) *Pragmatic assessment and intervention issues in language* (pp. 29–64). San Diego: College-Hill, 1983.

89. Roth, F., Spekman, N. Assessing the pragmatic abilities of children: Part I. Organizational framework and assessment parameters. *Journal of Speech and Hearing Disorders,* 1984a;49: 2–11.

90. Roth, F., Spekman, N. Assessing the pragmatic abilities of children: Part II. Guidelines, considerations, and specific evaluation procedures. *Journal of Speech and Hearing Disorders,* 1984b; 49:12–17.

91. Snow, P., Douglas, J., Ponsford, J. Conversational discourse abilities following severe traumatic brain injury: A follow-up study. *Brain Injury,* 1998;12:911–935.

92. Marsh, N.V. Social skill deficits following traumatic brain injury: Assessment and treatment. In S. McDonald, L. Togher, C. Code (Eds.) *Communication disorders following traumatic brain injury.* New York: Psychology Press, 1999.

93. Ylvisaker, M., Urbanczyk, B., Feeney, S.F. Social skills following traumatic brain injury. *Seminars in Speech and Language,* 1992;13:308–322.

94. McDonald, S., Pearce, S. The 'dice' game: A new test of pragmatic language skills after close-head injury. *Brain Injury,* 1995; 9:255–271.

95. Turkstra, L.S., McDonald, S., Kaufman, P. Assessment of pragmatic communication skills in adolescents after traumatic brain injury. *Brain Injury,* 1996;10:329–345.

96. Turkstra, L.S., McDonald, S., DePompei, R. Social information processing in adolescents: Data from normally-developing adolescents and preliminary data from their peers with traumatic brain injury. *Journal of Head Trauma Rehabilitation,* 2001;16:469–483.

97. McDonald, S. Differential pragmatic loss after closed head injury: Ability to comprehend conversational implicature. *Applied Psycholinguistics,* 1992;13:295–312.

98. Kintsch, W., van Dijk, T.A. Towards a model of text comprehension and production. *Psychological Review,* 1978; 85:363–394.

99. Frederiksen, C.H., Bracewell, R.J., Breuleux, A., Renaud, A. (1990). The cognitive representation and processing of discourse: Function and dysfunction. In Y. Joanette, H.H. Brownell (Eds.) *Discourse ability and brain damage: Theoretical and empirical perspectives.* New York: Springer-Verlag. (pp. 69–112).

100. Coelho, C.A., Grela, B. *Indices of lexical diversity in narratives of adults with closed head injuries.* Unpublished manuscript, 2003.

101. Huber, W. (1990). Text comprehension and production in aphasia: Analysis in terms of micro- and macrostructure. In Y. Joanette, H.H. Brownell (Eds.) *Discourse ability and brain damage:*

Theoretical and empirical perspectives. New York: Springer-Verlag. (pp. 154—179).

102. Baddeley, A. *Working memory.* Oxford, U.K.: Clarendon Press, 1987.

103. Connor, L.T., MacKay, A.J., White, D.A. Working memory: A foundation for executive abilities and higher-order cognitive skills. In G. Ramsberger (Ed.) Executive functions: Description, disorders, assessment, management. *Seminars in Speech and Language* 2000;21:109–120.

104. Tompkins, C.A. *Right hemisphere communication disorders, theory and management.* San Diego: Singular, 1995.

105. van Dijk, T.A., Kintsch, W. *Strategies of discourse comprehension.* New York: Academic Press, 1983.

106. Ulatowska, H.K., Allard, L., Chapman, S.B. (1990). Narrative and procedural discourse in aphasia. In Y. Joanette, H.H. Brownell (Eds.) *Discourse ability and brain damage: Theoretical and empirical perspectives.* New York: Springer-Verlag. (pp. 180–198).

107. Ylvisaker, M., Szekeres, S.F., Feeney, T. Communication disorders associated with traumatic brain injury. In: R. Chapey (Ed.) *Language intervention strategies in aphasia and related neurogenic communication disorders* (pp. 745–800). Philadelphia: Lippincott , Williams & Wilkins, 2001.

108. Grant, D.A., Berg, E.A. A behavioral analysis of degree of reinforcement and ease of shifting to new response in a Weigl type card sorting problem. *Journal of Experimental Psychology,* 1948;38:404–411.

109. Heaton, R.K., Chelune, G.J., Talley, J.L., Kay, G.G., Curtiss, G. *Wisconsin Card Sorting Test manual: Revised and expanded.* Odessa, FL: Psychological Assessment Resources, 1993.

110. Coelho CA, Liles BZ & Duffy RJ Impairments of discourse abilities and executive functions in traumatically brain injured adults. *Brain Injury,* 1994;9:471–477.

111. Doyle, P.J., Goda, A.J., Spencer, K.A. The communicative informativeness and efficiency of connected discourse by adults with aphasia under structured and conversational sampling conditions. *American Journal of Speech-Language Pathology,* 1995;4:130–134.

112. Mackenzie, C. Adult spoken discourse: The influences of age and education. *International Journal of Language and Communication Disorders,* 2000;35:269–285.

113. Wilkinson, R. Sequentiality as a problem and resource for intersubjectivity in aphasic conversation: Analysis and implications for therapy. *Aphasiology,* 1999;13:327–343.

114. Galski, T., Tompkins, C., Johnston, M.V. Competence in discourse as a measure of social integration and quality of life in persons with traumatic brain injury. *Brain Injury,* 1998;12: 769–782.

115. Prince, S., Haynes, W.O., Haak, N.J. Occurrence of contingent queries and discourse errors in referential communication and conversational tasks: A study of college students with closed head injury. *Journal of Medical Speech-Language Pathology,* 2002;10:19–39.

116. Coelho, C.A., Youse, K.M., Le, K.N., Feinn, R. Narrative and conversational discourse of adults with closed head injuries and non-brain-injured adults: A discriminant analysis. *Aphasiology,* 2003;17:499–510.

117. Coelho, C.A., Youse, K.M. *Conversational abilities and executive functions following closed head injury.* International Neuropsychological Society Conference, Baltimore, MD, February, 2004.

XII

MOTOR RECOVERY, FUNCTIONAL MOBILITY, AND ACTIVITIES OF DAILY LIVING

49 Neuroscientific Basis for Occupational and Physical Therapy Interventions

Randolph J. Nudo
Numa Dancause

INTRODUCTION

The field of neurorehabilitation is currently undergoing a fundamental change in approach to therapy after central nervous system injury. In the past, occupational and physical therapy after stroke or traumatic brain injury (TBI) was based almost exclusively on empirical data and without a full understanding of the neural processes or correlates of recovery mechanisms. Since the early 1980's, experimental data has been accumulating to provide compelling evidence that the adult brain is capable of significant anatomical and physiological plasticity. These data have contributed to a renewal of the long-debated theory of vicariation, or the taking over of function of damaged brain regions by spared, healthy regions. It has become clear that in both humans and in experimental animal models, the injured brain compensates in a variety of ways that contribute to the spontaneous return of function, and that behavioral interventions are perhaps the most powerful modulators of post-injury plasticity.

Based on this growing evidence for behaviorally-driven neural plasticity after brain injury, and the increasing number of scientists and clinicians that have begun to design therapeutic approaches grounded in the latest neuroplasticity principles, some have suggested that we are fast approaching an impending paradigm shift in neurorehabilitation therapy (1). In the coming years, advances in behavioral principles, robotics, pharmacotherapeutics, brain imaging, genetics, genomics, nanoelectronics, and neural prosthetics are likely to change the landscape of functional restoration after brain injury. The purpose of this chapter is to introduce the reader to the underlying principles of functional brain plasticity and how they may be applied to restoration of function after brain injury. What circumstances gave rise to the fundamental changes in emerging therapeutic principles? What factors modulate brain structure and function in the healthy and injured brain? How can contemporary therapeutic interventions be improved based on principles of neural plasticity? What does the future hold for further development of therapeutic approaches? While the answers to these questions are still fragmentary, it is hoped that this chapter will help to prepare students and practitioners of neurorehabilitation for the paradigm shift that is already in progress.

It is important to note that most of the clinical examples and animal models of plasticity are based on recovery after ischemic infarct, rather than on TBI *per se*. This is primarily because the vast majority of the literature on post-injury plasticity associated with recovery focuses on stroke or ischemia. In many ways, post-stroke plasticity is an easier phenomenon to investigate and understand. The injury is typically focal and well-circumscribed. The surviving cortical and subcortical tissue is essentially undamaged. In TBI, injuries may be diffuse or multi-focal. Whether these same plasticity principles based on post-stroke recovery generalize to TBI is still an unanswered question. However, the description of the various modulators of post-stroke plasticity and their neuroanatomical and neurophysiological bases provides a fundamental understanding of the potential for the role of neuroplasticity in post-TBI recovery.

MATURATION OF OUR UNDERSTANDING OF BRAIN PLASTICITY AND RECOVERY PRINCIPLES

The modern era of the application of brain plasticity principles to recovery after injury began in the mid-1980s with a series of experiments demonstrating use-dependent modulation of the functional organization of somatosensory cortex (2–6). These studies demonstrated that after amputation of a digit or transection of a peripheral nerve in experimental animals, the deafferented cortex quickly became responsive to inputs from adjacent skin surfaces. While later studies eventually showed that these functional alterations could be attributed, in part, to modulation of pre-existing divergent connections in the lemniscal pathway (such as diverging thalamocortical arbors), other changes, such as alterations in local cortical circuits and long-term anatomical changes have also been reported within the cortex, thus making it clear that the functional organization of the cerebral cortex is modifiable (Figure 49-1).

Results demonstrating use-dependent (and skill-dependent) modulation of auditory cortex, visual cortex,

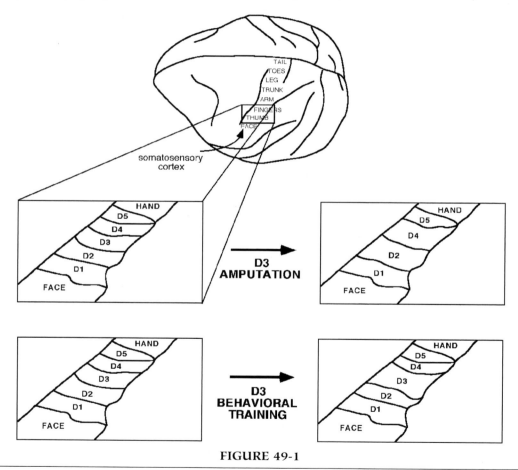

FIGURE 49-1

Classic neurophysiological studies in primary somatosensory cortex (area 3b) of non-human primates demonstrating that the functional topography of cerebral cortex is modifiable after peripheral injury and after repetitive use. Top experiment shows the area 3b hand map before and a few months after amputation of a single digit. Prior to the amputation, area 3b displays the normal topographic pattern, with neurons responding to light touch on individual digits progressing from ulnar to radial aspects of the hand as a microelectrode is introduced from more medial to more lateral locations. Each digit's representational territory in cortex is demarcated by a sharp border. After a digit 3 amputation, neurons in the former digit 3 cortical territory become response to stimulation of skin surfaces adjacent to the missing digit, i.e., to stimulation of digits 2 and 4. Adapted from (2, 6). Bottom experiment depicts changes in the digit 3 representation in area 3b following several weeks training on a sensorimotor task in which digit 3 is repetitively stimulated. The representation of the stimulated digit expands and receptive field sizes become smaller (132)

and motor cortex eventually erased any lingering doubts that topographic plasticity may be a methodological epiphenomenon, or specific to only certain portions of the cerebral cortex. Behavioral improvement appeared to correlate with neurophysiologic map plasticity, suggesting that these changes were an adaptive response of the cerebral cortex to novel behavioral requirements.

However, even in the early 19th century, clinicians and scientists began to ask specific questions regarding brain plasticity, though their knowledge of underlying neuronal mechanisms was rudimentary. While better known for his study of phrenology (with Gall), Johann Spurzheim wrote that brain and muscles can increase with exercise "because the blood is carried in greater abundance to the parts which are excited and nutrition is performed by the blood". In the mid-19th century, Jean-Pierre Flourens, one of the first experimental brain researchers, asserted that after restricted lesions of the cerebellum, recovery could occur as the result of compensation by other brain areas. This view was later to be incorporated in Lashley's principle of equipotentiality that states that all parts of the neocortex (or at least, all parts within a localized functional area, such as visual cortex or somatosensory cortex) play an equal role in memory storage, or in a particular physiological function (7).

Several other investigators took up the question of brain recovery mechanisms throughout the first half of the 20th century, including Sherrington, Franz, Glees, Denny-Brown, Kuypers and others using behavioral and neurophysiological techniques (8–13). But it was in the final two decades of the century when solid evidence from experimental animal models accumulated to give adequate credence to the notion that cortical functions are not static in adulthood (14). Parallel human neuroimaging studies confirmed that these same processes could probably be generalized to humans (15).

Thus, the recent intensive interest in recovery after brain injury has come about as a result of two nearly simultaneous events: 1) the maturation of our understanding of brain plasticity principles, and 2) the rapid development of sophisticated neuroimaging techniques. In addition, specifically with regard to stroke recovery, interest has been spurred by the initial effectiveness of pharmacologic and physiotherapeutic interventions introduced during the acute or chronic stages after stroke (i.e., thrombolytic agents, amphetamine, constraint-induced movement therapy) (16–18). These recently developed interventions were largely based on neuroscientific and behavioral principles developed from animal models of post-injury recovery.

While results demonstrating neuroplasticity in healthy brains as a result of experience, and in injured brains as a result of trauma or stroke were largely phenomenological in the initial stage of discovery, the molecular and cellular mechanisms regulating these events are now being investigated intensively. The coming decade will be important in defining which of the many potential features of neuroplasticity represent adaptive mechanisms, which represent maladaptive mechanisms and which are epiphenomenal.

NEURAL CORRELATES OF SKILLED MOTOR CONTROL

Because many of the same underlying adaptive neurological processes are thought to occur in both normal and injured brains, to appreciate the events that shape anatomical and physiological plasticity and promote functional motor recovery after brain injury, it is first necessary to understand how repetitive use and motor skill acquisition modulate the structure and function of the normal, uninjured brain. In this section, the organization of the motor cortex will be reviewed briefly. Then, the modulatory role of sensorimotor behavior will be discussed.

Organization of Motor Cortex

The motor cortex is composed of a number of interconnected cortical regions that are distinguishable from surrounding areas primarily on the basis of cytoarchitecture, thalamocortical and intracortical connectivity (hodology), and electrophysiological properties. In addition to the extensively studied primary motor cortex (M1) located in the precentral gyrus, there are several other motor areas that play important roles in motor control. These include the premotor cortex (dorsal and ventral premotor cortex, or PMd and PMv, respectively), the supplementary motor area (SMA), and the cingulate motor cortex (CM). Each of these motor regions can be further subdivided based on histochemical, hodological and neurophysiological properties (Figure 49-2).

The primary pathway through which the motor cortex directs motor commands to the spinal cord motor neurons is the corticospinal tract. Corticospinal neurons originate from each of the cortical motor regions in the frontal cortex, i.e., from CM, PMv, PMd, SMA and from M1. Additional corticospinal neurons originate from parietal cortex, though their precise function in motor control is still unclear. Monosynaptic corticomotoneuronal neurons (i.e., neurons with somata located in cerebral cortex with fibers terminating directly onto motor neurons in the spinal cord) are thought to originate primarily from M1.

Each of the cortical motor areas is reciprocally interconnected with the others, though to varying degrees. Thus, M1 receives input from premotor, supplementary motor and cingulate motor areas, and emanates corticocortical axons to terminate in these same regions. In addition, cortical motor areas receive substantial input from

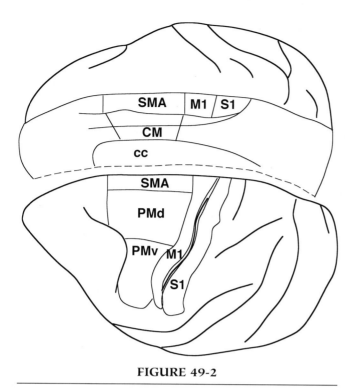

FIGURE 49-2

Location of motor areas in the cerebral cortex of a macaque monkey. At least five subdivisions can be recognized on the basis of structural and functional properties. These include the primary motor cortex located in the precentral gyrus (M1), the dorsal and ventral premotor cortex located anterior to M1 (PMd and PMv, respectively), the supplementary motor area located medial to PMd on the medial aspect of the cortex (SMA) and the cingulate motor areas located in the cingulate gyrus on the medial wall (CM). Each of these main motor areas can be subdivided further based on cytoarchitectonic, neurophysiologic, and chemoarchitectonic criteria. Note that much of the M1 representation is buried in the central sulcus (i.e., on the anterior bank of the precentral gyrus) in most primates (including humans). Thus, access for detailed neurophysiological mapping studies is limited. Certain non-human primate species (e.g., squirrel monkeys, marmoset monkeys) possess a relatively shallow central sulcus allowing more access to the posterior aspect of M1

parietal cortex, specifically from somatosensory regions. Thus, the motor cortex cannot be considered strictly as a motor structure, but instead, is a site of somatosensory-motor integration, with a primarily motor output function based on its corticospinal connections, primarily its monosynaptic connections with motor neurons. In fact, when focal ischemic lesions are made in either the primary somatosensory cortex (S1) or M1 of non-human primates, deficits are quite similar when performance on sensorimotor tasks is assessed (17, 18). For example, in addition to a decrement in manual skill, monkeys with lesions in either S1 or M1 display a type of sensory agnosia. The sensory agnosia eventually subsides, possibly due to the

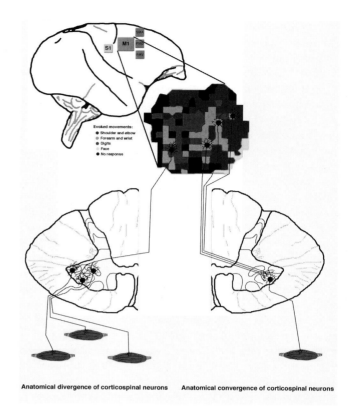

FIGURE 49-3

Anatomical divergence and convergence of corticospinal neurons. Upper: Example of a motor map of evoked movements in the primary motor cortex (M1) derived from intracortical microstimulation techniques. The map shows the intermingling of evoked digits (red), wrist and forearm (green) movements clustered in the middle of more proximal (elbow and shoulder; blue) movements. Lower left: Corticospinal divergence. One cell located in the digit representation of M1 projects to several motoneuronal pools in the spinal cord that, in turn, project to different arm muscles. This result has been demonstrated using both axonal tracing and spike-triggered averaging techniques (133, 134). Functionally, this illustrates that one very small area of the motor map can have a very widely distributed influence on the musculature of the arm. Lower right: Corticospinal convergence. Several cells located at various locations within the wrist and forearm representations in M1 all project to the same motoneuronal pool in the spinal cord, which then projects to a single muscle of the arm. This has been demonstrated using both intracortical microstimulation and stimulus-triggered averaging techniques (135, 136). Functionally, this illustrates that a wide surface area of the motor map can have a very focal influence on the musculature of the arm

use of visual guidance to compensate for deficits in somatosensory-motor integration (19).

The functional representation of the skeletal motor apparatus is represented in cortical motor areas in a topographic fashion, with the contralateral leg represented more medially and the hand and face represented more laterally in M1. However, due to anatomical divergence of corticospinal neurons, a strict topography is not apparent when the spatial organization is examined on a more refined scale. It has been estimated that each corticomotoneuronal cell innervates about four or five separate motor neuron pools (20). Further, neurons originating corticomotoneuronal fibers innervating a single motor neuron pool are located in multiple sites within a topographic region in M1 (Figure 49-3). This anatomical divergence and convergence of corticospinal fibers, along with a dense network of local intracortical connections within M1 results in a substrate that provides a great deal of flexibility in its functional arrangement. In other words, it appears that motor cortex is expressly designed to allow for plastic reorganization of its local circuitry and ultimately, of its functional outputs.

Use-Dependent and Skill-Dependent Modification of Motor Cortex Topography

A common technique for demonstrating the detailed topography of cortical motor areas in experimental animals is known as intracortical microstimulation (ICMS) (21). Based on ICMS results in non-human primates, the general topographic representation of specific body parts is quite consistent in M1, but substantial individual variability exists in the detailed topography on a more refined level, e.g., within the hand representation (Figure 49-4). The size of the hand representation can vary by over 100% in different monkeys, a difference that cannot be accounted for on the basis of the animal's size alone. It has been hypothesized that individual variation in motor maps is a result of each individual's sensorimotor experiences leading up to the motor mapping procedure (22).

The modifiability of the motor map has now been studied extensively in M1 of humans, non-human primates and rodents (caudal forelimb area) (23, 24). Soon after the learning of a new fine motor skill, the representations of the movements involved in the skilled task are enlarged. At least in experimental animals, specific combinations of movements used in the task emerge in ICMS maps (25). Presumably, local functional networks are established within the reorganized cortex, potentially reflecting the emergence of muscle and movement synergies within M1. Long-term potentiation of intracortical connections is likely to play a role in the emergent properties of reorganized cortex (26, 27). Plasticity in motor maps resulting from the acquisition of motor skills is both progressive and reversible.

Plasticity in motor cortex organization as a result of motor skill learning has also been shown in humans using fMRI techniques. While neuroimaging results represent a very different form of data, skill-dependent changes can be demonstrated during the acquisition of skilled motor

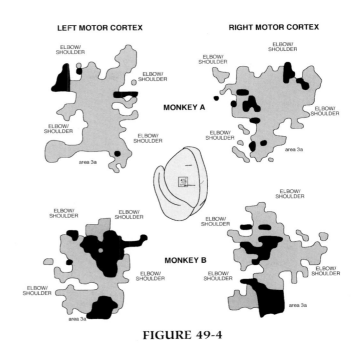

FIGURE 49-4

Individual variability in M1 maps in non-human primates. When the M1 maps of the hand representation are compared between hemispheres of the same animal, the mosaical patterns are similar on the two sides. For example, in both Monkeys A and B, the pattern of digit flexion representations (black) in the left motor cortex is roughly a mirror image of the pattern in the right motor cortex. However, when the digit flexion representation is compared between Monkeys A and B, the patterns are strikingly different, if not complementary. This high degree of individual variability in motor maps may result from the differential motor experiences of the animals prior to the mapping experiment. Graig denotes non-digit distal forelimb areas. Adapted from Ref. 22

tasks. However, the timing of the learning events may be critical to the particular changes that are observed (28). While the relationship between acquired skills and the size of motor representations holds for M1, the story may be more complex for other motor areas or for other motor tasks. For example, during the sequential learning of foot movements, cerebral blood flow was increased bilaterally in the dorsal premotor cortex and cerebellum during the execution of the movement. After a one-hour training session, blood flow in these regions was no longer increased during foot movement (29). As the authors suggest, these areas may be involved in cognitive strategies and motor routines to execute the foot movements, but are no longer involved once the sequence of movements is learned.

Structural changes in motor cortex also occur during the acquisition of motor skills. In rodents assigned to a skilled reaching task, reaching accuracy increased significantly at 3, 7 and 10 days of training. However, synaptogenesis (synapses per neuron) increased after 7 or 10 days of training, but not after 3 days of training. Motor map plasticity occurred at 10 days of training only. Motor learning-dependent synaptogenesis is localized only to those motor regions undergoing the motor map changes (30) (Figure 49-5). Thus, structural and functional changes in motor cortex are co-localized, and are evident only in late stages of training, possibly related to the consolidation of motor skills rather than their initial acquisition (31). This late change in motor maps and motor cortex synaptogenesis is important in interpreting differences between fMRI results in human motor learning studies with electrophysiological and anatomical results in animal studies. The typical human studies are conducted over relatively short time intervals (minutes to hours), and thus, may be reflecting very different aspects of motor learning-dependent neuroplasticity.

From the standpoint of developing new rehabilitative interventions based on neuroplasticity principles, it is important to contrast the effects of skill learning with repetitive, but non-skilled motor activity (Figure 49-5). In experimental animals, repetitive motor activity that does not induce improvements in motor skill or motor learning fail to alter motor map topography or synapse number (30, 32, 33) albeit induces angiogenesis (34, 35). This phenomenon has not yet been extensively studied, but may play a very important role in recovery at particular stages after brain injury.

ACUTE AND CHRONIC CHANGES IN PERI-LESIONAL AND REMOTE REGIONS AFTER BRAIN INJURY

Following injury to the brain via trauma or stroke, a cascade of molecular and cellular events is set into motion in the surrounding tissue that results in both temporary and permanent changes in the anatomy and physiology of the affected structures (36). Many of these changes are pathological consequences of the injury (e.g., edema) and

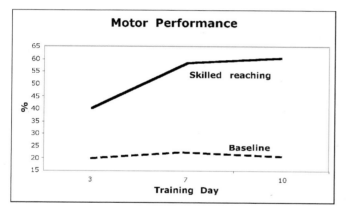

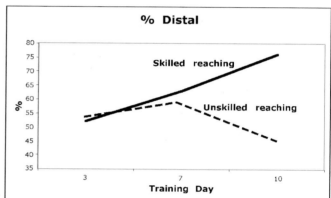

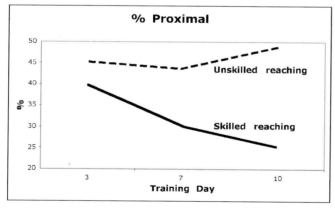

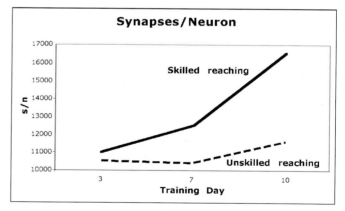

FIGURE 49-5

Functional and structural changes in motor cortex related to improvements in motor skill. As rats develop skill at a reach and retrieval task (upper left), distal representations occupy a progressively greater portion of the forelimb area (upper right), while proximal representations occupy a progressively smaller portion (lower left). In addition, synaptogenesis occurs during motor skill acquisition, especially during the later phases of motor learning (i.e., mostly at 10 days, but not substantially at 3 or 7 days; lower right). Simple repetitive tasks that do not require acquisition of new motor skills result in no neurophysiological map changes or synapse changes. Adapted from Ref. 31

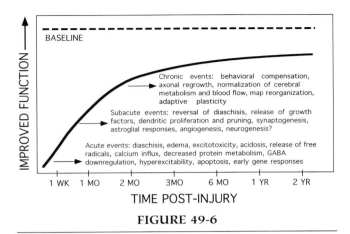

FIGURE 49-6

Cascade of acute, sub-acute and chronic events that are triggered by cortical injury. As acute pathogenesis subsides, improved sensorimotor function occurs. During the subacute phase, presumed restorative mechanisms are set in motion, such as dendritic arborization, release of growth factors and angiogenesis. Finally, functional and structural changes are consolidated in chronic phases as evidenced by alterations in axonal pathways and functional map configuration

have potentially damaging results. However, many adaptive processes may begin early in the post-injury stage and result in reduction of pathophysiological events or in neuroplastic changes leading to at least some restoration of function (37, 38) (Figure 49-6). While a thorough understanding of these processes at the molecular, cellular and network levels is just beginning, sufficient knowledge is now available to begin testing hypotheses about the effects of specific post-injury interventions on functional recovery and its underlying neuroanatomical and neurophysiological bases.

Theories of Recovery

At least three general theories have been proposed to explain the substantial recovery that often follows brain injury, referred to here as reversal of diaschisis, compensation and adaptive plasticity (or vicariation of function) (Figure 49-6). As early as 1914, von Monokow discussed the role of diaschisis, or the temporary reduction in function of structures interconnected with an injured brain region, in the acute stages after injury (39). It is well known that both cerebral blood flow and metabolism are decreased in the region immediately adjacent to the injured tissue. Further, structures anatomically connected with the injured region undergo similar reductions in blood flow and metabolism. Gradually, blood flow and metabolism returns to the connected regions. Since this disruption is temporary, functional recovery is likely to be related, in part, to a gradual reduction in diaschisis.

Compensation in motor behavior is a common consequence of brain injury as the individual attempts to

supplant lost functions with alternative strategies. As an extreme example of compensatory behavior, a stroke survivor may begin to use the less-impaired limb for completing common tasks. However, more subtle changes in movement patterns occur even during use of the impaired limb. Stroke survivors with impaired function of the arm and hand may use proximal musculature in compensatory strategies to propel the limb forward (40). Depending upon the specificity of the motor endpoint that is assessed, such compensatory behavior could be missed, leading to the suggestion that motor performance has normalized. Even with the smallest experimental ischemic infarcts that can be made reliably in experimental monkeys, subtle changes in the kinematics of motor strategies take place, leading to the question of whether "true recovery", i.e., return to normal, pre-lesion behavior, ever occurs (41). This is an extremely important, but often overlooked aspect of recovery that is critical for interpreting studies of neuroplasticity mechanisms after injury. Since use-dependent and learning-dependent changes are observable in the anatomy and physiology of normal, intact brains, it must be presumed that the development of compensatory motor patterns post-injury also alter brain structure and function.

A third general theory posits that functional recovery is largely dependent upon adaptive plasticity of intact, remaining brain structures. Various alternative terms have also been used to describe this theory, including "vicariation of function" and "neural compensation". While this theory is also at least a century old, it has received considerable support in the past two decades from correlative studies in both experimental animals and in humans after brain injury. Underlying mechanisms thought to be involved in adaptive plasticity include unmasking of existing connections, long-term potentiation, long-term depression, axonal sprouting, dendritic sprouting, synaptogenesis and angiogenesis. Also, while the role of neurogenesis after brain injury is still controversial, some studies now suggest that brain injury can induce this process at least in some regions, and that neurogenesis may contribute to functional recovery (42).

Neurophysiologic Alterations in Intact Structures After Brain Injury

Focal injury to the cerebral cortex does not simply result in a "hole" in the affected structure. Adjacent, intact cortical regions, as well as more remote cortical regions interconnected with the damaged area, undergo substantial physiological and anatomical changes. As early as 1950, Glees and Cole, using cortical surface stimulation techniques, demonstrated that if the motor representation of the thumb in primary motor cortex (M1) was destroyed in experimental monkeys, it reappeared in the adjacent, intact motor cortex (10). Later, it was demonstrated that a focal ischemic infarct in the primary somatosensory cortex that eliminated the sensory representation of a single digit resulted in the eventual re-emergence of the digit representation in the adjacent tissue (43). These results would seem to support the adaptive plasticity or vicariation hypothesis. However, when newer intracortical microstimulation (ICMS) techniques were applied to M1, the vicariation phenomenon could not be replicated (25). Instead, when small, focal infarcts were made in the digit representation of M1, a further loss in digit representation occurred in the adjacent M1. While it may be tempting to dismiss the earlier results of Glees and Cole based on the spatially crude surface mapping techniques that were used, another important factor was found to contribute to the findings. This factor – the post-injury motor experience of the animal – has great impact on the ultimate, chronic condition of the motor map, and, very likely on the ultimate motor performance that can be achieved.

To determine the effects of post-injury experience on reorganization of motor maps, Nudo and colleagues encouraged the use of the impaired limb by placing a restrictive jacket on experimental monkeys. The jacket contained a long sleeve that extended the length of the less-impaired forelimb, and ended in a soft mesh mitt on the hand. The restricted hand could still be used for climbing, but was ineffective for grasping small objects, a task that was difficult to perform with the affected hand. Beginning about five days post-injury, two half-hour sessions of reach/grasp training were conducted each day. Several days to weeks were required to retrain skilled use of the affected hand, but eventually motor performance on the experimental task was similar to pre-lesion levels. Following this recovery period, the ICMS-derived motor maps revealed that the digit representations in the intact areas were maintained. In some cases, they expanded into regions where prior mapping revealed proximal representations (44). Thus, motor experience after injury can drastically alter the ultimate functional organization of motor cortex (Figure 49-7).

This phenomenon is not limited to the adjacent cortex. In other non-human primate experiments employing slightly larger lesions encompassing the entire M1 hand area, hand representations in the premotor cortex were enlarged several months later, even in the absence of post-injury training. Further, the magnitude of the premotor enlargement was directly related to the size of the injury in M1 (45) (Figure 49-7). Since premotor cortex has reciprocal connections with M1, it is not surprising that this region is altered. But the enlarged representation related to the size of the M1 injury suggests that it may play a significant vicarious role in recovery.

Anatomical Alterations in Intact Cortical Structures After Brain Injury

In concert with behavioral recovery and neurophysiological remodeling, injured brains undergo significant

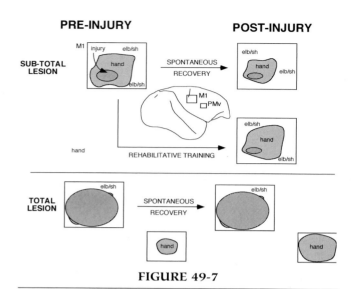

FIGURE 49-7

Functional alteration of local and distant cortical organization following focal injury. Sub-total lesion: If the injury is small enough, reorganization is primarily confined to the local adjacent tissue. For example, a subtotal injury to the M1 hand area results in changes in representational maps in the spared hand area adjacent to the injury. Post-injury rehabilitative training can have a profound influence on the inevitable map configuration. Total lesion: After a total lesion of the M1 hand area, other motor regions interconnected with M1 are stimulated to reorganize. For example, the hand representation in the ventral premotor cortex (PMv) enlarges. This premotor area normally has reciprocal connections with the injured M1. Adapted from (45)

anatomical plasticity in neuronal and non-neuronal structures. In rat motor cortex, intracortical fibers in the bordering intact tissue display orientations different from those seem in normal animals, suggesting that injury induces local axonal sprouting (46). Arteriolar collateral growth and new capillaries also form in the ischemic border (47). Significant neuroanatomical changes also occur in the contralesional (intact) motor cortex, but the role of this cortex in functional recovery of the affected limb is still a subject of debate. Recent results from animal studies suggest that the neuroanatomical changes in the intact cortex occur as a use-dependent or skill-dependent change due to increased use of the less-affected limb (48).

The latent potential for enhancing neuroanatomical plasticity mechanisms after stroke has been demonstrated by the use of mutant mouse strains that lack the Nogo receptor. Nogo is a protein involved in the inhibition of axonal growth. Mice lacking the Nogo receptor recover motor function after stroke better than controls. Further, rats subjected to anti-Nogo antibody treatment initiated one week after stroke resulted in better behavioral recovery compared with controls. Further, sprouting of contralateral corticorubral and ipsilateral corticospinal fibers was observed (49). Pharmacologic treatment with D-amphetamine after stroke has also been shown to enhance neocortical sprouting, synaptogenesis and behavioral recovery after stroke (50).

PHYSIOTHERAPEUTIC TREATMENT FOR MOTOR DISABILITY AFTER BRAIN INJURY: CURRENT PRACTICE

Since it is now clear that certain types of behavioral and pharmacologic interventions have the potential to alter neurophysiological activity and neuroanatomical structure, it may be helpful to examine the various therapeutic approaches used in post-injury rehabilitation, and consider their potential for maximization of recovery based on neuroplasticity principles. This discussion may lead to a better understanding of the underlying mechanisms of rehabilitative therapy by pointing out the current gaps in our basic knowledge. It also may help us to refine therapeutic interventions to take advantage of the modulatory role that specific behavioral and pharmacological therapies play.

The Maximization of Motor Recovery Through Diverse Approaches

Treatment of upper limb impairments following brain injury (such as that occurring after stroke) follows either: 1) principles of neurofacilitation or 2) principles of functional retraining. Traditionally, the choice between these rehabilitation strategies has been based on the phase of stroke recovery. Whereas in the acute/subacute phase, therapy typically focuses on the prevention of maladaptive compensatory strategies while promoting the recovery of normal function, in the chronic phase, the emphasis is placed on maximizing function, often through the teaching of compensatory strategies (51).

Principles of Neurofacilitative Approaches Neurofacilitative approaches, such as Rood, Brunnstrom, Bobath, Proprioceptive Neuromuscular Facilitation (PNF) and Sensory Integration (SI) therapy, are usually used in early post-injury stages to favor motor recovery following a stroke, when most of the recovery seems to occur (52). These approaches focus on the recovery of normal movement. Unwanted movements and spasticity are inhibited and normal patterns are facilitated under the assumption that regaining of voluntary control over key movements will transfer to functional improvement. These approaches are based on empirical assumptions that motor impairments are a consequence of a disruption of central nervous system (CNS) hierarchical and reflex motor control

(53–57). In the traditional view of these approaches, recovery of motor function follows the same chronology that is observed in neurodevelopmental stages, supposedly reflecting the CNS efforts to reestablish its internal hierarchical order that was disrupted by the neuronal loss consequent to the injury. Therefore, these approaches utilize neurophysiological phenomena (e.g. reflex pathways) to favor 'normal' motor behaviors and are largely based on neurodevelopmental knowledge (58). Whereas largely used and trusted by therapists (59, 60), in general they have not resulted in substantial impact on patients' recovery when examined in controlled trials (61–64) and seem to result in similar behavioral outcomes when compared to each other (65–67).

Currently, to our knowledge no studies have explored physiological or morphological effects of neurofacilitative approaches on the CNS. This contrasts with the large number of mechanistic studies that are related to approaches based on movement repetition and retraining. However, it should be noted that the current absence of basic research investigating the effects of these approaches may be due to technical challenges rather than a weaker scientific rationale. Among the technical difficulties, because the NDT approach is specifically adapted for the individual's particular needs and because it involves a high level of therapist manual expertise, inter-subject and inter-therapist variability is very high, making it quite difficult to standardize protocols. Hopefully, in the near future, the mechanisms of action of these approaches will be investigated. Currently, the urge for experimental support for the widely used clinical practice is felt and underlined by the NDT community (68). The desire to provide an evidence-based practice is supported by the Neuro-Developmental Treatment Association, which is currently providing financial support for research and favoring the development of a consistent knowledge base among therapists.

Principles of Functional Retraining Recently, studies evaluating the mechanisms underlying motor acquisition and motor control have resulted in the elaboration of behavioral treatment approaches based on practice (51, 69, 70). In these approaches, it is believed that the hemiparetic subject has distorted central motor programs resulting from CNS cell death. Based on the assumption that repetition of movements has the same effects as the ones reported for normal individuals (71), it is believed that practice establishes novel motor plans for the resolution of encountered motor problems (72). Additionally, it is taught that movement repetition improves behavior by affecting muscle weakness, an important problem affecting upper limb function (73–75).

Initial evaluations of the efficacy of repetition of movement, in order to improve motor outcomes following stroke, have provided encouraging results. Several studies have shown that repetitive, concentrated practice improves motor outcomes (14, 76–80). Additionally, diverse practice approaches have been explored in order to maximize retention and transferability (81–88). At this point, whereas it is well established that practice improves motor outcomes and function following stroke, currently a consensus on a precise and consistent protocol to use to maximize the recovery is far from established. The elaboration of standardized training protocols based on principles of motor learning, retention and transferability specific to the hemiparetic population, is one of the most urgent needs for patient management.

While animal models have frequently been used to optimize basic therapeutic strategies in preclinical drug trials, their utility has been under-appreciated. Surely, animal research allows investigation of mechanisms through which practice favors recovery and the identification of morphological and physiological processes that accompany improved motor performances. Whereas physiological changes at the level of the motor cortex induced by practice following stroke has been shown (44), the impact of diverse types of practice, intensity or even the time at which practice is most beneficial for the modulation of adaptive physiological and or morphological changes has yet to be investigated. For example, it was recently shown that rats undergoing training consisting of repetitive movements demonstrated functional and structural plasticity within the same cortical regions (30). This study provides strong evidence that synapse formation and physiological expansion of cortical representation of movement are concomitant and probably inter-dependent adaptive processes playing important roles in learning. Knowing that learning and practice are so influential in the recovery from stroke, the investigation of the parallel changes of dendritic arbors and physiological reorganization of motor maps in M1 or in premotor cortex will be of great interest. In the near future, the choice of treatment, intensity and schedule of therapy at different stages of stroke (e.g. acute, chronic) could be directed to take advantage of the most prolific stages of morphological and physiological reorganization.

Although it is a long held belief that most of the rehabilitation of stroke patients occurs in the first few weeks to months following stroke (Duncan and Lai, 1997), there is little evidence available indicating that physical rehabilitation is effective for patients with chronic CVA, and the literature is even equivocal on the value of physical rehabilitation for sub-acute patients (89, 90). However, the fact that some patients with a given extent and locus of lesion recover more movement than others suggests that additional factors may be involved. Taub and colleagues suggested that some motor abilities were possible, but were not reinforced. In the vernacular of classical conditioning, these behaviors were extinguished or actively inhibited (89). From this assumption, it was stipulated that function could be improved in chronic stroke patients. In particular, this group has developed an innovative approach known as constraint-induced movement therapy (CIT) that has received a great deal of attention in the last decade. The idea behind the application of CIT originates from fundamental experiments conducted in non-human primates following peripheral deafferentation (91). In these experiments, disuse of the affected upper limb of non-human primates was observed following the injury. This maladaptive behavior persisted if no manipulation was introduced, even after a three to six month spontaneous recovery period. At that point, the function of the deafferented limb could be greatly enhanced by forcing its use by restraining the non-affected limb (92). This led to the 'learned non-use' hypothesis which stipulates that non-use, or less than maximal use, of the deafferented limb results from negatively reinforced attempts to use the affected limb. This negative feedback would consist of unsuccessful behavioral consequences of attempts to use the affected upper limb (e.g., absence of reward for goal-directed activity, or painful execution). After the initial recovery period, when the ability to use the affected limb is stable, behavioral sequelae caused by the learned non-use remain. Therefore, because of the phenomenon, the actual use of the affected limb is much less than its true potential (89, 93, 94). Strong support for the learned non-use formulation came from a study where restraint was applied directly following the deafferentation of the upper limb of an animal for a 3-month duration, therefore preventing the learned non-use phenomenon to occur (95). When the restraint was removed, the animals used their deafferented limb. Also, when deafferented prenatally, animals exhibited purposive use of the deafferented limb from the first day of extrauterine life (96, 97). In that experimental paradigm, the use of the upper limb following the lesion was also restricted because of the limited intrauterine space, thus preventing the negative feedback from unsuccessful usage of the limb and supposedly the learned non-use phenomenon from developing.

Physiologically, it can be assumed that deafferentation is a lesion which, like potentially many others, such as traumatic brain injury or stroke, creates a disruption of sensorimotor integration loops (98–100). By this logic, disruption would result in initial poor motor behavior. The progressive reestablishment of sensorimotor integration loops through motor behavior favoring CNS adaptive mechanisms may underlie a substantial amount of spontaneous recovery from these lesions. However, during the adaptive period, the learned non-use phenomenon would negatively intervene, making the subjects subconsciously or consciously learn that the use of the affected limb results in poor behavioral outcomes. The negative feedback from these outcomes would reinforce preferential usage of the non-affected limb. In that view, the learned non-use phenomenon would not only be present following deafferentation, but also following any injury disrupting sensorimotor integration loops. Therefore, the application of a restraint on the unaffected limb, to force the use of the affected limb, should result in improvement of motor outcomes in numerous neurologic, and even orthopedic, conditions (101).

In the original application of the learned non-use hypothesis to the hemiparetic population, a simple arm-restraint was employed (102). In that study, stroke and head-injured patients were required to keep their uninvolved upper extremities within a hand-enclosed sling during waking hours over a two-week interval. Functional improvements in diverse tasks and in force were reported, and most of them were maintained when examined in a one-year follow-up assessment. The results supported the hypothesis that learned non-use occurs in select neurological patients and that this maladaptive behavior can be reversed through application of a forced-use paradigm. In a second experiment (103), use of the sling for 14 days was combined with six hours of practice of functional movements with the impaired limb for 10 of those days. The behavioral training paradigm consisted of operant conditioning (104). Patients demonstrated improvements beyond what had been reported with the sole use of the sling, and improvements in motor performance were maintained during a two-year period of follow-up. The increase of motor improvements obtained from the combination of behavioral training with the wearing of the sling is a strong indication that, in addition to reversal of learned non-use, additional factors may be involved in the recovery in chronic stroke patients[1].

Positive results using the CIT paradigm have been reported in several experiments (94, 105, 106) and by unrelated research groups (107, 108), repeatedly demonstrating large effect sizes for the Motor Activity Log (MAL) and for the Wolf Motor Function Test (WMFT). In addition, more recent studies using a modified CIT demonstrate that upper extremity function can be improved after TBI. Most importantly, improvement in motor skill made by the patients has been shown to be transferable to other activities in their daily lives. It should be pointed out that the constraint increases the time of treatment to up to 90% of waking hours of the subject. Thus, it imposes a discipline that might otherwise be difficult to achieve in practice. It can be argued that it probably is the simplest and most reliable way to reach such a high level of intensity for a clinical intervention. In the absence of constraint, if a task introduces too many obstacles to execute with the affected limb, the subject will naturally have the tendency perform it with the other limb, therefore limiting the learning

experience with the impaired limb. The constraint forces the patient to immediately apply the motor skills he is learning during daily treatment in a natural and very significant location: at home. Learning is context-dependent, meaning that an important factor in the retention of motor skills is the relationship between the context of practice and the context of application (109). Therefore, the level of intensity of intervention and direct context-dependent application of the learned motor patterns during the day might explain why the therapy has such a high impact on the performance level on tests evaluating functional motor state of the patient (e.g. MAL; WMFT).

The paradigm used in non-human primate experiments is strikingly similar to CIT. Monkeys wore a jacket with a long sleeve restricting fine control by the less affected limb. Thus, these animal experiments may be very useful for evaluating various aspects of the CIT protocol (e.g., timing, intensity, specific behavioral factors, etc.). From the monkey studies, it would appear that the repetitive behavior is the more important factor in CIT, rather than the presence of the constraint device. Recovery of hand representations in primary motor cortex is very rapid when the use of the restraint jacket is combined with repetitive training. However, when the restraint device is the sole source of motivation to use the impaired limb, normalization of motor maps occurs extremely slowly, if at all. Monkeys that wore a restraint jacket for up to one year did not display as much map recovery as monkeys engaged in repetitive training for only two weeks (110).

A series of experiments to evaluate the presence of cortical representation changes, paralleling the behavioral changes resulting from CIT, has also been performed (91, 111, 112). These studies reported increased cortical representation areas of the affected arm following treatment, an upper limb representational map size that was similar in both affected and less-affected hemispheres at a 6 months follow up, and shifts of the center of the output map, suggesting recruitment of adjacent brain areas examination. This last result has been related by the authors to the phenomenon that has been reported in monkeys undergoing repetition of movement therapy following a cortical ischemic lesion (44). Therefore, human studies now support the hypothesis that CIT modulates recovery through processes that are similar to the ones that are known to occur following motor learning through practice and repetition.

As previously mentioned, one of the interesting results that came from these studies was that, in addition to the reversal of the learned non-use phenomena, other factors appeared to be involved in the motor recovery of chronic stroke subjects. In fact, it was even shown that subjects that were undergoing intensive physical therapy, consisting of aquatic therapy, neurophysiological facilitation,

---

[1]Discussion of this particular topic can be found below.

and task practice showed a level of improvement similar to that of sling restraint of the less-affected arm, combined with intensive task practice or shaping (94, 105). However, in these experiments, the intensive therapy control groups showed higher levels of decrement of arm use at the two year follow up in comparison to the CIT group. Therefore, it appears that one of the advantages of the usage of a sling is the higher retention of use of the affected limb at the two-year follow-up, and that the common factor in all techniques producing an equivalently large treatment effect is repeated use of the more-affected upper extremity (89). It thus can be suggested that chronic hemiparetic patients have the capacity for functional motor learning and that they have not maximized their motor potential after traditional acute care.

In conclusion, we would tend to consolidate the preceding literature into one treatment hypothesis: Intensive treatment based on repetition creates plastic changes that are associated with learning (which might include reversal of learned nonuse). This probably acts through positive behavioral conditioning of the use of the impaired limb resulting in learning and amelioration of the general motor schema of the upper limb.

Too Much, Too Early?

After injury to the sensorimotor cortex in rats, extreme use of the affected limb can result in an enlargement of the lesion and further motor impairment (113). If the unimpaired limb is placed in a restrictive cast after cortical injury, rats must rely heavily on the impaired limb for posture and locomotion. Forced overuse of the impaired limb during the first week after injury results in expansion of the injury and poorer motor performance (114). Forced overuse during the next seven days does not result in injury expansion, but nonetheless resulted in poorer motor performance. More recently, it has been shown that after TBI in rats, neuroplasticity-related intracellular signaling proteins are disrupted if voluntary exercise is provided within the first week post-injury (115). These studies strongly suggest that there are specific vulnerable periods for maladaptive effects of use after injury. Timing of these maladaptive effects must be considered along with timing of adaptive effects in any rational therapeutic design for treatment of motor deficits after injury.

Assessment of Efficacy

The assessment of efficacy of clinical approaches is an important issue, not only for stroke and brain injury recovery, but for the entire field of neurorehabilitation in general. Particularly in the cases of stroke recovery, one important question surrounding this topic is: Should we focus on the return of "normal" movement (true recovery) or just on return of function at any cost (i.e., compensatory

strategies)? This question extends beyond the clinical field and is also debated in the literature discussing animal models of stroke (40, 41, 116). It also raises the question of evaluative tools. Obviously, very different tools are needed to evaluate the divergence from 'normality' of movement and functional capacities of a patient. Whereas evaluation tools focusing on the 'abnormalities' of movements are much more useful and appropriate to the practice of neurodevelopmental approaches, newer, strictly functional scales are used in several research protocols to measure the impact of movement repetition based treatments. Particularly, in the cases of CIT, the validity of the clinical tests they traditionally use to assess motor recovery has been questioned (106, 117, 118). These tests only evaluate function and use, and do not evaluate the use of compensatory strategies. In fact, the treatment effects become much more uncertain when using evaluation tools monitored by trained therapists, such as the Fugl-Meyer (119) or the Barthel index (118). It can be argued that the WMFT and MAL are self-reports that could circumvent the blinding process (118); familiarizing patients with the MAL questions on a daily basis may permit recollection of previous responses, thereby narrowing the choice points on the MAL. This effectively reduces the variability, and enhances the effect size (119). On the other hand, it can also be argued that the ultimate goal of therapy, specifically at a chronic stage, is to improve function and use of the affected limb and that the WMFT and MAL are specifically designed and were shown to do this well (117). Alternatively, for the validation and evaluation of learning processes, movement kinematics could be assessed. A recent study showed that in chronic patients, when immobilizing the trunk, the subjects use their shoulder and elbow joints in a more normal way (120). The use of the trunk helps patients to create end-point trajectories that are more similar to healthy subjects. This study underlines that compensatory behavior can potentially be detrimental to maximization of function, in this case, limiting the range of reaching. Whereas maximization of function is the goal of rehabilitative approaches, the identification of these detrimental compensatory strategies is necessary to achieve this goal. Novel evaluation scales are being developed (121) and will hopefully help clinicians in that task.

Treatment Groups and Valid Controls

It now seems obvious that the evaluation of treatment outcomes must take into consideration the type of treatment and the initial level of function of the targeted population (52, 122). Intrinsic, non-treatment-related elements are key determinants in the level of potential benefits a patient derives from a particular treatment. Whereas the initial level of function (as reflected by clinical assessments such as the Fugl-Meyer) has traditionally been used as the main predictor for recovery, other factors are now identified as better predictors. The initial grade of paresis appears to be the most important clinical predictor for motor recovery (123). Additionally, motor evoked potentials (MEP) seem to be highly predictive for the occurrence of motor recovery (124–126). It was shown to be a much better predictor than clinical examination, infarct size and location, age, gender, and stroke type (infarction versus hemorrhage). Also, preservation of the corticospinal tract with MRI imaging was also found to correlate with good recovery, confirming the TMS studies (127). This confirms that studies evaluating the efficacy of different clinical approaches need to have stringent selection criteria for their subjects. Recovery from strokes can vary largely between individuals. For example, purely cortical stroke survivors recover better than purely subcortical or mixed cortical-subcortical strokes. Decreases in the level of recovery can be observed from cortex, corona radiata, and posterior limb of internal capsule (128). This suggests that recovery of upper limb movement is heavily dependent on the preservation of corticofugal fibers (128, 129). Also, the recovery period is approximately twice as long for patients with severe paresis (15wk), compared to patients with mild paresis (6.5wk) (130). Therefore, to truly evaluate the impact of a treatment on stroke survivors, studies should be designed to include patients with similar predicted outcomes in each experimental group. Additionally, if some subjects have intrinsic conditions rendering them unable to benefit from a certain approach, they should be studied separately to identify the substrate of this failure and the potential alternative approaches from which they could benefit more. For example, a preliminary study to investigate the integrity of short-term motor memory in stroke subjects indicated that patients with low Fugl-Meyer and executive function scores had problems modifying their motor commands based on previous experience (131). Such results raise important questions concerning the use of movement repetition in this particular population of hemiparetic patients.

SUMMARY

Our understanding of recovery from damage to the central nervous system has evolved tremendously in the last few decades. Fundamental research on the diverse physiological, morphological, molecular and genetic changes resulting from ischemic damage and the association of certain phenomena to behavioral recovery has drastically impacted stroke management. Evolving knowledge of plastic changes accompanying functional recovery coming from both animal studies and technological advancements in humans (e.g., fMRI) might create a entire new set of outcome predictors and or surrogate markers of recovery states useful for both study design and patient treatment choices. These novel indicators might also direct the type, intensity and duration of treatments. For example, cortical representation of body segments evaluated with TMS could become a means to identify the endpoint for treatment. When patients demonstrate a plateau in physiological reorganization, this could imply that most of the adaptive changes have already taken place. Whereas much work has been done, obviously, many questions are still unanswered. Most of the experiments that have been performed so far have included only subjects showing high functional scores. Unfortunately, a large proportion of hemiparetic stroke patients show mild improvements with currently available treatments. Surely, significant work in both animals and humans needs to be accomplished to better understand and provide more efficient treatments to individuals with brain injury.

References

1. Taub, E., Uswatte, G., Elbert, T., New treatments in neurorehabilitation founded on basic research, *Nat Rev Neurosci* 2002;3(3):228–36.
2. Kaas, J. H., Merzenich, M. M., Killackey, H. P., The reorganization of somatosensory cortex following peripheral nerve damage in adult and developing mammals, *Annual Review of Neuroscience* 1983;6:325–356.
3. Killackey, H. P., Gould, H. J.,3rd, Cusick, C. G., Pons, T. P., Kaas, J. H., The relation of corpus callosum connections to architectonic fields and body surface maps in sensorimotor cortex of new and old world monkeys, *J Comp Neurol* 1983;219(4): 384–419.
4. Merzenich, M. M., Kaas, J. H., Wall, J., Nelson, R. J., Sur, M., Felleman, D., Topographic reorganization of somatosensory areas 3b and 1 in adult monkeys following restricted deafferentation, *Neuroscience* 1983;8:33–55.
5. Merzenich, M. M., Kaas, J. H., Wall, J. T., Sur, M., Nelson, R. J., Felleman, D. J., Progression of change following median nerve section in the cortical representation of the hand in areas 3b and 1 in adult owl and squirrel monkeys., *Neuroscience* 1983;10(3): 639–665.
6. Merzenich, M. M., Nelson, R. J., Stryker, M. P., Cynader, M. S., Schoppmann, A., Zook, J. M., Somatosensory cortical map changes following digit amputation in adult monkeys, *Journal of Comparative Neurology* 1984;224:591–605.
7. Finger, S., *Origins of Neuroscience* Oxford University Press, New York, 1994.
8. Sherrington, C. S., *The Integrative Action of the Nervous System* C. Scribner and Sons, New York,1906.
9. Franz, S. I., Variations in distribution of the motor centers, *Psychological Monographs* 1915;19:80–162.
10. Glees, P. and Cole, J., Recovery of skilled motor functions after small repeated lesions in motor cortex in macaque, *Journal of Neurophysiology* 1950;13:137–148.
11. Denny-Brown, D., Motor mechanisms-introduction: the general principles of motor integration, in *Handbook of Physiology. Neurophysiology*, sect. I, vol. 2, ch. 32 ed. Am. Physiol. Soc., Washington, DC,1960, pp. 781–796.
12. Lashley, K. S., Temporal variation in the function of the gyrus precentralis in primates, *Am. J. Physiol.* 1923;65:585–602.
13. Lawrence, D. G. and Kuypers, H. G. J. M., The functional organization of the motor system in the monkey. I. The effects of bilateral pyramidal lesions, *Brain* 1968;91:1–14.
14. Bach-y-Rita, P., Wood, S., Leder, R., Paredes, O., Bahr, D., Wicab Bach-y-Rita, E., Murillo, N., Computer-assisted motivating

rehabilitation (CAMR) for institutional, home, educational late stroke programs, *Top Stroke Rehabil* 8 (4),1–10,2002.

15. Chollet, F., DiPiero, V., Wise, R. J., Brooks, D. J., Dolan, R. J., Frackowiak, R. S., The functional anatomy of motor recovery after stroke in humans: a study with positron emission tomography, *Annals of Neurology* 29 (1),63–71,1991.

16. Walker-Batson, D., Smith, P., Curtis, S., Unwin, H., Greenlee, R., Amphetamine paired with physical therapy accelerates motor recovery after stroke. Further studies, *Stroke* 26(12), 2254–9,1995.

17. Papadopoulos, S. M., Chandler, W. F., Salamat, M. S., Topol, E. J., Sackellares, J. C., Recombinant human tissue-type plasminogen activator therapy in acute thromboembolic stroke, *J Neurosurg* 1987;67(3):394–8.

18. Feeney, D. M., Gonzalez, A., Law, W. A., Amphetamine, haloperidol, and experience interact to affect rate of recovery after motor cortex injury, *Science* 1982;217(4562):855–7.

19. Nudo, R. J., Friel, K. M., Delia, S. W., Role of sensory deficits in motor impairments after injury to primary motor cortex, *Neuropharmacology* 2000;39(5):733–42.

20. Cheney, P. D., Fetz, E. E., Palmer, S. S., Patterns of facilitation and suppression of antagonist forelimb muscles from motor cortex sites in the awake monkey, *J Neurophysiology* 1985;53: 805–820.

21. Asanuma, H. and Rosèn, I., Topographical organization of cortical efferent zones projecting to distal forelimb muscles in the monkey, *Experimental Brain Research* 1972;14:243–256.

22. Nudo, R. J., Jenkins, W. M., Merzenich, M. M., Prejean, T., Gedela, R., Neurophysiological correlates of hand preference in primary motor cortex of squirrel monkeys, *Journal of Neuroscience* 1992;12(8):2918–2947.

23. Donoghue, J. P., Plasticity of adult sensorimotor representations, *Current Opinion in Neurobiology* 1995;5(6):749–754.

24. Nudo, R. J., Adaptive plasticity in motor cortex: implications for rehabilitation after brain injury, *J Rehabil Med* (41 Suppl), 7–10, 2003.

25. Nudo, R. J. and Milliken, G. W., Reorganization of movement representations in primary motor cortex following focal ischemic infarcts in adult squirrel monkeys, *Journal of Neurophysiology* 1996;75:2144–2149.

26. Hess, G. and Donoghue, J. P., Long-term potentiation of horizontal connections provides a mechanism to reorganize cortical motor maps, *J Neurophysiol* 1994;71(6):2543–2547.

27. Flynn, C., Monfils, M. H., Kleim, J. A., Kolb, B., McIntyre, D. C., Teskey, G. C., Differential neuroplastic changes in neocortical movement representations and dendritic morphology in epilepsy-prone and epilepsy-resistant rat strains following high-frequency stimulation, *Eur J Neurosci* 2004;19(8):2319–28.

28. Karni, A., Meyer, G., Rey-Hipolito, C., Jezzard, P., Adams, M., Turner, R., Ungerleider, L., The acquisition of skilled motor performance: fast and slow experience-driven changes in primary motor cortex, *Proceedings of the National Academy of Sciences, USA* 1998;95:861–868.

29. Lafleur, M. F., Jackson, P. L., Malouin, F., Richards, C. L., Evans, A. C., Doyon, J., Motor learning produces parallel dynamic functional changes during the execution and imagination of sequential foot movements, *Neuroimage* 2002;16(1):142–57.

30. Kleim, J. A., Barbay, S., Cooper, N. R., Hogg, T. M., Reidel, C. N., Remple, M. S., Nudo, R. J., Motor learning-dependent synaptogenesis is localized to functionally reorganized motor cortex, *Neurobiol Learn Mem* 2002;77(1):63–77.

31. Kleim, J. A., Hogg, T. M., VandenBerg, P. M., Cooper, N. R., Bruneau, R., Remple, M., Cortical synaptogenesis and motor map reorganization occur during late, but not early, phase of motor skill learning, *J Neurosci* 2004;24(3):628–33.

32. Plautz, E. J., Milliken, G. W., Nudo, R. J., Effects of repetitive motor training on movement representations in adult squirrel monkeys: role of use versus learning, *Neurobiol Learn Mem* 2000;74(1):27–55.

33. Remple, M. S., Bruneau, R. M., VandenBerg, P. M., Goertzen, C., Kleim, J. A., Sensitivity of cortical movement representations to motor experience: evidence that skill learning but not strength training induces cortical reorganization, *Behav Brain Res* 2001;123(2):133–41.

34. Kleim, J. A., Cooper, N. R., VandenBerg, P. M., Exercise induces angiogenesis but does not alter movement representations within rat motor cortex, *Brain Res* 2002;934(1):1–6.

35. Black, J., Isaacs, K., Anderson, B., Alcantara, A., Greenough, W., Learning causes synaptogenesis whereas motor activity causes angiogenesis in cerebellar cortex of adult rats, *Proceedings of the National Academy of Sciences, USA* 1990;87:5568–5572.

36. Farooqui, A. A., Haun, S. E., Horrocks, L. A., Ischemia and Hypoxia, in *Basic Neurochemistry*, Siegel, G. J., Agranoff, B. W., Albers, R. W.,Molinoff, P. B. Raven Press, New York,1994, pp. 867–883.

37. Cramer, S. C. and Bastings, E. P., Mapping clinically relevant plasticity after stroke, *Neuropharmacology* 2000;39(5):842–851.

38. Witte, O. W., Buchkremer-Ratzmann, I., Schiene, K., Neumann-Haefelin, T., Hagemann, G., Kraemer, M., Zilles, K., Freund, H. J., Lesion-induced network plasticity in remote brain areas, *Trends Neurosci* 20(8),348–9.,1997.

39. Finger, S., Koehler, P. J., Jagella, C., The Monakow concept of diaschisis: origins and perspectives, *Arch Neurol* 2004;61(2): 283–8.

40. Cirstea, M. C. and Levin, M. F., Compensatory strategies for reaching in stroke, *Brain* 123(Pt 5),940–53,2000.

41. Friel, K. M. and Nudo, R. J., Recovery of motor function after focal cortical injury in primates: compensatory movement patterns used during rehabilitative training, *Somatosens Mot Res* 1998; 15(3):173–89.

42. Zhang, R., Zhang, Z., Wang, L., Wang, Y., Gousev, A., Zhang, L., Ho, K. L., Morshead, C., Chopp, M., Activated neural stem cells contribute to stroke-induced neurogenesis and neuroblast migration toward the infarct boundary in adult rats, *J Cereb Blood Flow Metab* 2004;24(4):441–8.

43. Jenkins, W. M. and Merzenich, M. M., Reorganization of neocortical representations after brain injury: a neurophysiological model of the bases of recovery from stroke, *Progress in Brain Research* 1987;71:249–266.

44. Nudo, R. J., Wise, B. M., SiFuentes, F., Milliken, G. W., Neural substrates for the effects of rehabilitative training on motor recovery after ischemic infarct, *Science* 1996;272:1791–1794.

45. Frost, S. B., Barbay, S., Friel, K. M., Plautz, E. J., Nudo, R. J., Reorganization of remote cortical regions after ischemic brain injury: a potential substrate for stroke recovery, *J Neurophysiol* 2003; 89(6):3205–14.

46. Carmichael, S. T., Wei, L., Rovainen, C. M., Woolsey, T. A., New patterns of intracortical projections after focal cortical stroke, *Neurobiol Dis* 2001;8(5):910–22.

47. Wei, L., Erinjeri, J. P., Rovainen, C. M., Woolsey, T. A., Collateral growth and angiogenesis around cortical stroke, *Stroke* 2001; 32(9):2179–84.

48. Bury, S. D. and Jones, T. A., Facilitation of motor skill learning by callosal denervation or forced forelimb use in adult rats, *Behav Brain Res* 2004;150(1–2):43–53.

49. Lee, J. K., Kim, J. E., Sivula, M., Strittmatter, S. M., Nogo receptor antagonism promotes stroke recovery by enhancing axonal plasticity, *J Neurosci* 2004;24(27):6209–17.

50. Stroemer, R. P., Kent, T. A., Hulsebosch, C. E., Enhanced neocortical neural sprouting, synaptogenesis, behavioral recovery with D-amphetamine therapy after neocortical infarction in rats, *Stroke* 1998;29(11):2381–93.

51. Shumway-Cook, A. and Woollacoot, M., *Motor Contro: Theory and Practical Applications* Williams & Wilkins, Baltimore, MD, 1995.

52. Duncan, P. W. and Lai, S. M., Stroke recovery, *Topics in Stroke Rehabilitation* 1997;4(3):51–58.

53. Brunnstrom, S., *Movement therapy in hemiplegia: a neurophysiological approach* Harper & Row, New York,1970.

54. Bobath, K. and Bobath, B., The neurodevelopmental treatment., in *Man Palsy. Clin Dev Med No 90.*, Scrutton, D. Heinemann, London, 1984, pp. 16–18.

55. Bobath, B., *Adult Hemiplegia: Evaluation and Treatment.*, 3rd ed. ed. Heinemann Medical Books, Oxford,1990.

56. Montgomery, P., Neurodevelopmental treatment and sensory integrative theory, in *II Step Conference*, problems, C. m. o. m. c. APTA, Alexandria, VA,1991.

57. Voss, D., Ionata, M., Myers, B., *Proprioceptive Neuromuscular Facilitation: Patterns and Techniques*, 3rd. ed. Harper & Row, Philadelphia,1985.

58. Gordon, J., Assumptions underlying physical therapy intervention: theoritical and historical perspectives., in *Movement sciences: foundations for physical therapy in rehabilitation*, Carr, J. H., Shepherd, R. B., Gordon, J., Andal, E. MD: Aspen, Rockville, 1987, pp. 1–30.

59. Lennon, S., Physiotherapy practice in stroke rehabilitation: a survey, *Disabil Rehabil* 2003;25(9):455–61.

60. Lennon, S., Baxter, D., Ashburn, A., Physiotherapy based on the Bobath concept in stroke rehabilitation: a survey within the UK, *Disabil Rehabil* 2001;23(6):254–62.

61. Dickstein, R., Hocherman, S., Pillar, T., Shaham, R., Stroke rehabilitation. Three exercise therapy approaches, *Phys Ther* 1986; 66(8):1233–8.

62. Logigian, M. K., Samuels, M. A., Falconer, J., Zagar, R., Clinical exercise trial for stroke patients, *Arch Phys Med Rehabil* 1983;64(8):364–7.

63. Wagenaar, R. C., Meijer, O. G., van Wieringen, P. C., Kuik, D. J., Hazenberg, G. J., Lindeboom, J., Wichers, F., Rijswijk, H., The functional recovery of stroke: a comparison between neurodevelopmental treatment and the Brunnstrom method, *Scand J Rehabil Med* 1990;22(1):1–8.

64. Basmajian, J. V., Gowland, C. A., Finlayson, M. A., Hall, A. L., Swanson, L. R., Stratford, P. W., Trotter, J. E., Brandstater, M. E., Stroke treatment: comparison of integrated behavioral-physical therapy vs traditional physical therapy programs, *Arch Phys Med Rehabil* 68(5 Pt 1),267–72,1987.

65. Crow, J. L., Lincoln, N. B., Nouri, F. M., De Weerdt, W., The effectiveness of EMG biofeedback in the treatment of arm function after stroke, *Int Disabil Stud* 1989;11(4):155–60.

66. Paci, M., Physiotherapy based on the Bobath concept for adults with post-stroke hemiplegia: a review of effectiveness studies, *J Rehabil Med* 2003;35(1):2–7.

67. Woldag, H. and Hummelsheim, H., Evidence-based physiotherapeutic concepts for improving arm and hand function in stroke patients: a review, *J Neurol* 2002;249(5):518–28.

68. Howle, J. M., *Neuro-Developmental Treatment Approach: Theoretical Foundations and Principles of Clinical Practice* Neuro-Developmental Treatment Association, Laguna Beach, California, 2004.

69. Shumway-Cook, A. and Horak, F. B., *Balance rehabilitation in the neurological patient* NERA, Seattle,1992.

70. Horak, F. and Shumway-Cook, A., Clinical implications of postural control in research., in *Balance.*, Duncan, P. W. APTA, Alexandria, VA,1990.

71. Gottlieb, G. L., Corcos, D. M., Jaric, S., Agarwal, G. C., Practice improves even the simplest movements, *Exp Brain Res* 1988;73(2):436–40.

72. Whiting, H. T. A., Dimensions of control in motor learning., in *Tutorials in motor behavior.*, Stelmach, G. E. andRequin, J. North Holland, New York,1980, pp. 537–550.

73. Gillen, G. and Burkhard, A., *Stroke rehabilitation: a function-based approach* Mosby,1998.

74. Bogousslavsky, J., Van Melle, G., Regli, F., The Lausanne Stroke Registry: analysis of 1,000 consecutive patients with first stroke, *Stroke* 1988;19(9):1083–92.

75. Bourbonnais, D. and Vanden Noven, S., Weakness in patients with hemiparesis, *Am J Occup Ther* 1989;43(5):313–9.

76. Basmajian, J. V., Gowland, C., Brandstater, M. E., Swanson, L., Trotter, J., EMG feedback treatment of upper limb in hemiplegic stroke patients: a pilot study, *Arch Phys Med Rehabil* 1982;63: 613–616.

77. Balliet, R., Blood, K. M., Bach-y-Rita, P., Visual field rehabilitation in the cortically blind?, *J Neurol Neurosurg Psychiatry* 1985; 48(11):1113–24.

78. Butefisch, C., Hummelsheim, H., Denzler, P., Mauritz, K. H., Repetitive training of isolated movements improves the outcome of motor rehabilitation of the centrally paretic hand, *J Neurol Sci* 1995;130(1):59–68.

79. Sunderland, A., Tinson, D. J., Bradley, E. L., Fletcher, D., Langton Hewer, R., Wade, D. T., Enhanced physical therapy improves recovery of arm function after stroke. A randomised controlled trial, *J Neurol Neurosurg Psychiatry* 1992;55(7): 530–5.

80. Langhammer, B. and Stanghelle, J. K., Bobath or motor relearning programme? A comparison of two different approaches of physiotherapy in stroke rehabilitation: a randomized controlled study, *Clin Rehabil* 2000;14(4):361–9.

81. Adams, J. A., A closed-loop thoery of motor learning, *J Mot Behav* 1971;3(1):111–49.

82. Shea, C. H., Shebilske, W., Worchel, S., *Motor learning and control* Prentice Hall, Englewood Cliffs, NJ,1993.

83. Kottke, F. J., From reflex to skill: the training of coordination, *Arch Phys Med Rehabil* 1980;61(12):551–61.

84. Stallings, L. M., Retention and transfer, in *Motor learning. From theory to practice*, Stallings, L. M. Mosby, St. Louis,1982, pp. 197–218.

85. Smyth, M. M., Memory for movements, in *The psychology of movement*, Smyth, M. M. andWing, A. M. Academic Press, San Diego,1984, pp. 83–117.

86. Gentile, A. M., Skill acquisition: Action, movement, and neuromotor processes, in *Movement science: Foundations for physical therapy in rehabilitation*, Carr, J. H., Shepherd, R. B., Gordon, J., Gentile, A. M.,Held, J. M. Aspen, Rockville, MD,1987, pp. 93–154.

87. Winstein, C. J., Motor learning considerations in stroke rehabilitation, in *Stroke Rehabilitation: The Recovery of Motor Control*, Duncan, P. andBadke, M. Year Book Medical Publishers, Inc., Chicago,1987, pp. 109–134.

88. Schmidt, R. A., *Motor control and learning.*, 2nd ed. Human Kinetics, Champaign, IL,1988.

89. Taub, E., Uswatte, G., Pidikiti, R., Constraint-Induced Movement Therapy: a new family of techniques with broad application to physical rehabilitation – a clinical review, *J Rehabil Res Dev* 1999;36(3):237–51.

90. Taub, E. and Morris, D. M., Constraint-induced movement therapy to enhance recovery after stroke, *Curr Atheroscler Rep* 2001;3(4):279–86.

91. Taub, E., Uswatte, G., Morris, D. M., Improved motor recovery after stroke and massive cortical reorganization following Constraint-Induced Movement therapy, *Phys Med Rehabil Clin N Am* 14(1 Suppl), S77–91, ix, 2003.

92. Knapp, H. D., Taub, E., Berman, A. J., Movements in monkeys with deafferented limbs., *Exp Neurol* 1963;7:305–315.

93. Andrews, K. and Stewart, J., Stroke recovery: he can but does he?, *Rheumatol Rehabil* 1979;18(1):43–8.

94. Taub, E. and Wolf, S. L., Constraint induced movement techniques to facilitate upper extremity use in stroke patients, *Topics in Stroke Rehabilitation* 1997;3(4):38–61.

95. Taub, E., Movement in nonhuman primates deprived of somatosensory feedback, *Exercise and Sports Sciences Reviews* 1977;4:335–374.

96. Taub, E., Perrella, P., Barro, G., Behavioral development after forelimb deafferentation on day of birth in monkeys with and without blinding, *Science* 1973;181(103):959–60.

97. Taub, E., Goldberg, I. A., Taub, P., Deafferentation in monkeys: pointing at a target without visual feedback, *Exp Neurol* 1975; 46(1):178–86.

98. Asanuma, H. and Pavlides, C., Neurobiological basis of motor learning in mammals, *Neuroreport* 8(4), i–vi,1997.

99. Keller, A., Arissian, K., Asanuma, H., Formation of new synapses in the cat motor cortex following lesions of the deep cerebellar nuclei, *Exp Brain Res* 1990;80(1):23–33.

100. Keller, A., Arissian, K., Asanuma, H., Synaptic proliferation in the motor cortex of adult cats after long-term thalamic stimulation, *Journal of Neurophysiology* 1992;68:295–308.

101. Catania, A. C., *Learning.*,4th ed. ed. Prentice Hall, Upper Saddle river, NJ,1998.

102. Wolf, S. L., Lecraw, D. E., Barton, L. A., Jann, B. B., Forced use of hemiplegic upper extremities to reverse the effect of learned nonuse among chronic stroke and head-injured patients, *Exp Neurol* 1989;104(2):125–32.

103. Taub, E., Miller, N. E., Novack, T. A., Cook, E. W., 3rd, Fleming, W. C., Nepomuceno, C. S., Connell, J. S., Crago, J. E.,

Technique to improve chronic motor deficit after stroke, *Arch Phys Med Rehabil* 1993;74(4):347–54.

104. Taub, E., Overcoming learned nonuse: a new approach to treatment in physical medicine, in *Clinical Applied Psychophysiology*, Carlson, J. G., Seifert, A. R., Birbaumer, N. Plenum, New York, 1994.

105. Taub, E., Crago, J. E., Uswatte, G., Constraint-Induced (CI) Therapy: a new approach to treatment in physical rehabilitation., *Rehabil Psychol* 1998;43:152–170.

106. Kunkel, A., Kopp, B., Muller, G., Villringer, K., Villringer, A., Taub, E., Flor, H., Constraint-induced movement therapy for motor recovery in chronic stroke patients, *Arch Phys Med Rehabil* 1999;80(6):624–8.

107. Levy, C. E., Nichols, D. S., Schmalbrock, P. M., Keller, P., Chakeres, D. W., Functional MRI evidence of cortical reorganization in upper-limb stroke hemiplegia treated with constraint-induced movement therapy, *Am J Phys Med Rehabil* 2001;80(1):4–12.

108. Miltner, W. H., Bauder, H., Sommer, M., Dettmers, C., Taub, E., Effects of constraint-induced movement therapy on patients with chronic motor deficits after stroke: a replication, *Stroke* 1999;30(3):586–92.

109. Hochstenbach, J. and Mulder, T., Neuropsychology and the relearning of motor skills following stroke, *Int J Rehabil Res* 1999;22(1):11–9.

110. Friel, K. M., Heddings, A. A., Nudo, R. J., Effects of postlesion experience on behavioral recovery and neurophysiologic reorganization after cortical injury in primates, *Neurorehabil Neural Repair* 2000;14(3):187–98.

111. Liepert, J., Bauder, H., Wolfgang, H. R., Miltner, W. H., Taub, E., Weiller, C., Treatment-induced cortical reorganization after stroke in humans, *Stroke* 2000;31(6):1210–6.

112. Liepert, J., Miltner, W. H., Bauder, H., Sommer, M., Dettmers, C., Taub, E., Weiller, C., Motor cortex plasticity during constraint-induced movement therapy in stroke patients, *Neurosci Lett* 1998;250(1):5–8.

113. Kozlowski, D. A., James, D. C., Schallert, T., Use-dependent exaggeration of neuronal injury after unilateral sensorimotor cortex lesions, *J Neurosci* 1996;16(15):4776–4786.

114. Humm, J. L., Kozlowski, D. A., James, D. C., Gotts, J. E., Schallert, T., Use-dependent exacerbation of brain damage occurs during an early post-lesion vulnerable period, *Brain Res* 1998;783(2):286–292.

115. Griesbach, G. S., Gomez-Pinilla, F., Hovda, D. A., The upregulation of plasticity-related proteins following TBI is disrupted with acute voluntary exercise, *Brain Res* 2004;1016(2):154–62.

116. Roby-Brami, A., Feydy, A., Combeaud, M., Biryukova, E. V., Bussel, B., Levin, M. F., Motor compensation and recovery for reaching in stroke patients, *Acta Neurol Scand* 2003;107(5):369–81.

117. Morris, D. M. and Taub, E., Constraint-induced therapy approach to restoring function after neurological injury, *Top Stroke Rehabil* 2001;8(3):16–30.

118. Dromerick, A. W., Edwards, D. F., Hahn, M., Does the application of constraint-induced movement therapy during acute rehabilitation reduce arm impairment after ischemic stroke?, *Stroke* 2000;31(12):2984–8.

119. van der Lee, J. H., Wagenaar, R. C., Lankhorst, G. J., Vogelaar, T. W., Deville, W. L., Bouter, L. M., Forced use of the upper extremity in chronic stroke patients: results from a single-blind randomized clinical trial, *Stroke* 1999;30(11):2369–75.

120. Michaelsen, S. M., Luta, A., Roby-Brami, A., Levin, M. F., Effect of trunk restraint on the recovery of reaching movements in hemiparetic patients, *Stroke* 2001;32(8):1875–83.

121. Levin, M. F., Desrosiers, J., Beauchemin, D., Bergeron, N., Rochette, A., Development and validation of a scale for rating motor compensations used for reaching in patients with hemiparesis: the reaching performance scale, *Phys Ther* 2004;84(1):8–22.

122. Lincoln, N., Parry, R., Vass, C., Randomized, controlled trial to evaluate increased intensity of physiotherapy treatment of arm function after stroke, *Stroke* 1999;30:573–579.

123. Hendricks, H. T., van Limbeek, J., Geurts, A. C., Zwarts, M. J., Motor recovery after stroke: a systematic review of the literature, *Arch Phys Med Rehabil* 83(11),1629–37.,2002.

124. Heald, A., Bates, D., Cartlidge, N. E., French, J. M., Miller, S., Longitudinal study of central motor conduction time following stroke. 2. Central motor conduction measured within 72 h after stroke as a predictor of functional outcome at 12 months, *Brain* 116(Pt 6),1371–85,1993.

125. Escudero, J. V., Sancho, J., Bautista, D., Escudero, M., Lopez-Trigo, J., Prognostic value of motor evoked potential obtained by transcranial magnetic brain stimulation in motor function recovery in patients with acute ischemic stroke, *Stroke* 1998;29(9):1854–9.

126. Pennisi, G., Rapisarda, G., Bella, R., Calabrese, V., Maertens De Noordhout, A., Delwaide, P. J., Absence of response to early transcranial magnetic stimulation in ischemic stroke patients: prognostic value for hand motor recovery, *Stroke* 1999;30(12):2666–70.

127. Binkofski, F., Seitz, R. J., Hacklander, T., Pawelec, D., Mau, J., Freund, H. J., Recovery of motor functions following hemiparetic stroke: a clinical and magnetic resonance-morphometric study, *Cerebrovasc Dis* 2001;11(3):273–81.

128. Shelton, F. N. and Reding, M. J., Effect of lesion location on upper limb motor recovery after stroke, *Stroke* 2001;32(1):107–12.

129. Werring, D. J., Clark, C. A., Barker, G. J., Miller, D. H., Parker, G. J., Brammer, M. J., Bullmore, E. T., Giampietro, V. P., and Thompson, A. J., The structural and functional mechanisms of motor recovery: complementary use of diffusion tensor and functional magnetic resonance imaging in a traumatic injury of the internal capsule, *J Neurol Neurosurg Psychiatry* 1998;65(6):863–9.

130. Jorgensen, H. S., Nakayama, H., Raaschou, H. O., Olsen, T. S., Recovery of walking function in stroke patients: the Copenhagen Stroke Study, *Arch Phys Med Rehabil* 1995;76(1):27–32.

131. Dancause, N., Barbay, H. S., Frost, S. B., Plautz, E. J., Friel, K. M., Stowe, A. M., Zoubina, E. V., Nudo, R. J., Redistribution of premotor cortical connections after an ischemic lesion in primary motor cortex, *Society for Neuroscience Abstracts* Program No. 262.9, 2002.

132. Jenkins, W. M., Merzenich, M. M., Ochs, M. T., Allard, T., Guic-Robles, E., Functional reorganization of primary somatosensory cortex in adult owl monkeys after behaviorally controlled tactile stimulation, *Journal of Neurophysiology* 1990;63:82–104.

133. Shinoda, Y., Yokota, J. I., Futami, T., Divergent projection of individual corticospinal axons to motoneurons of multiple muscles in the monkey, *Neuroscience Letters* 1981;23:7–12.

134. Cheney, P. D. and Fetz, E. E., Comparable patterns of muscle facilitation evoked by individual corticomotoneuronal (CM) cells and by single intracortical microstimuli in primates: evidence for functional groups of CM cells, *Journal of Neurophysiology* 1985;53:786–804.

135. Park, M. C., Belhaj-Saif, A., Gordon, M., Cheney, P. D., Consistent features in the forelimb representation of primary motor cortex in rhesus macaques, *J Neurosci* 2001;21(8):2784–92.

136. Donoghue, J. P., Leibovic, S., Sanes, J. N., Organization of the forelimb area in squirrel monkey motor cortex: representation of digit, wrist, and elbow muscles, *Exp Brain Res* 1992;89(1):1–19.

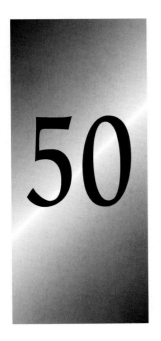

50

Therapy Interventions for Mobility Impairments and Motor Skill Acquisition After TBI

Katherine J. Sullivan

Innovations in mobility rehabilitation after brain injury derive from recent advances in neuroplasticity and neurorecovery. In particular, our understanding of motor recovery after brain injury is being influenced by basic science work that demonstrates that the process of motor skill acquisition is essential to promote both behavioral changes in motor performance and morphologic changes in neural structures within the motor cortex. (Please refer to Chapter by Nudo & Dancause for discussion of neuroplasticity and effects on brain injury recovery). The complexities of rehabilitation after brain injury comes from the usual situation that both neural structures that interfere with normal movement (i.e., corticospinal neurons and their connections) as well as those that impact the cognitive processes associated with motor learning are affected. Therefore, physical neurorehabilitation needs to include intervention strategies that address impairment level motor deficits that result after brain injury such as weakness, abnormal movement synergies, and abnormal tone as well as the intrinsic and extrinsic factors that promote motor learning and the acquisition of motor skills needed to increase function.

The field of neurorehabilitation needs to experience a paradigm shift. Advances in basic science research provide important understanding of the physiologic events that occur after brain injury and the neural processes that modify and impact recovery. The challenge for neurorehabilitation specialists who work with individuals with brain damage is to incorporate the strategies that are elucidated by the animal studies and ultimately design the clinical trial studies that will systematically examine these treatment paradigms within the clinical setting. Unfortunately, clinical trials that specifically examine treatment efficacy in human populations with traumatic brain injury (TBI) are sparse. However, evidence from the work done in individuals with stroke-related brain damage may provide a basis for the design of future TBI trials.

The intent of this chapter is to focus on rehabilitation approaches that address motor recovery; specifically, primary and secondary impairments that affect mobility and the process of motor skill acquisition after brain damage. This chapter will discuss factors that affect motor skill acquisition after brain injury, review traditional treatment approaches that address physical impairments that affect mobility, and present some examples of innovations in therapeutic interventions that address the acquisition of skills and promotion of meaningful functional recovery.

DISABLEMENT MODEL

Recovery from brain damage is multi-factorial and involves more than just the recovery and reorganization of neural structures. Contextual factors such as environmental influences like physical barriers, social support system and access to funds and services or personal factors such as age, gender, health status and personal lifestyle behaviors are all powerful predictors of outcome after TBI. For this reason, it is helpful to use an organizing framework such as the International Classification of Functioning, Disabilities, and Health (ICF) disablement model when approaching problem identification, goal formulation, and treatment planning. Additionally, the multiple dimensions of this model reflects the need for an interdisciplinary team to adequately address all of the contributing factors to disability after TBI.

The ICF disablement model is a classification system developed and disseminated by the World Health Organization (WHO) (1). The ICF characterizes the impact of a condition such as TBI according to the following dimensions: body function and structures, activities, and participation.

- *Loss of body functions and structures* include the impairments that result as a primary or secondary consequence of the brain injury. The neuromuscular motor impairments that will be discussed in this chapter include such things as impairments in voluntary movement, balance and postural control, and abnormal tone that result from direct insult to brain structures. Secondary impairments are the musculoskeletal conditions that result from immobility or excessive muscle tone such as muscle contractures, restricted joint mobility, and disuse weakness and deconditioning.
- *Activities* are the tasks that the individual performs such as walking, feeding, dressing, and other self-care related functions. Activity limitations reflect the difficulty that the person has in functional task performance.
- *Participation* reflects the individual's involvement in life and societal activity. There are 9 participation domains that include: personal maintenance, mobility, exchange of information, social relationships, home life and assistance to others, education, work and employment, economic life, and community, social, and civic life. The focus of this chapter will be therapeutic approaches associated with improving participation in mobility related tasks and activities.

Disablement models are a meaningful way to determine and evaluate the consequences of disease or injury. The original intent of the ICF classification (and its predecessor the ICIDH-2) was to evaluate the process of health care delivery, which required the need to develop and measure outcomes at each level of the disablement process (2). Because of this, recent trends in rehabilitation literature (particularly in randomized clinical trials that examine the efficacy and effectiveness of rehabilitation interventions)

include levels of measurement that reflect outcomes at the impairment, activity, and participation levels.

Another application of the disablement schema is to provide an organizing framework for rehabilitation intervention such that rehabilitation approaches could be developed and standardized in order to identify goals that are aimed to address problems at the levels of impairment, activity, or participation. Designed to assess the consequences of disease or injury, the disablement classification system has an implicit assumption that interventions that improve impairments will lead to improvements in functional limitations, and hence, reduce disability. Quinn and Gordon (3) propose that one of the limitations of using the disablement model as a framework for intervention is that it takes a reductionist approach to rehabilitation. A reductionist approach would emphasize that disease or injury leads to disablement; therefore, reduction of disease or injury-related impairments would be the focus of rehabilitation. In contrast, they suggest that the process of rehabilitation is the reverse, such that, rehabilitation interventions are designed to lead to recovery (Figure 50-1). A physical rehabilitation approach that emphasizes recovery would 1) identify the roles related to self-care, social and recreational pursuits, and occupation that an individual desires to assume or reassume after injury, 2) identify the skills required to successfully achieve these pursuits, 3) determine the physical limitations and cognitive processes that are impaired and contribute to the functional deficits, and 4) design interventions that address physiologic mechanisms of recovery at both the impairment and skill levels.

Recent advances in neuroplasticity provide mechanistic validation to a rehabilitation approach that emphasizes

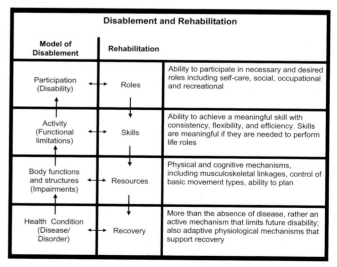

Disablement and Rehabilitation

Model of Disablement	Rehabilitation	
Participation (Disability)	Roles	Ability to participate in necessary and desired roles including self-care, social, occupational and recreational
Activity (Functional limitations)	Skills	Ability to achieve a meaningful skill with consistency, flexibility, and efficiency. Skills are meaningful if they are needed to perform life roles
Body functions and structures (Impairments)	Resources	Physical and cognitive mechanisms, including musculoskeletal linkages, control of basic movement types, ability to plan
Health Condition (Disease/ Disorder)	Recovery	More than the absence of disease, rather an active mechanism that limits future disability; also adaptive physiological mechanisms that support recovery

FIGURE 50-1

Conceptual framework of functioning and health in rehabilitation. Adapted from Quinn and Gordon (79)

recovery and skill acquisition. Consistently, animal models of recovery after brain damage demonstrate that the process of motor skill acquisition is a critical component that subserves both functional and neurological recovery (4–11). One of the major premises of a paradigm shift in physical rehabilitation of individual's with brain injury is the need to design therapeutic interventions that promote the acquisition of motor skill as well as address the direct and indirect impairments that occur to the neuromuscular system.

PRINCIPLES OF FUNCTIONAL TRAINING AND MOTOR SKILL ACQUISITION

The recent advances in neuroplasticity discussed by Nudo and Dancause in Chapter 49 of this book provide substantial evidence for the neurophysiologic and neuroanatomic mechanisms that underlie the process of motor skill acquisition and the importance of skill acquisition in recovery after brain damage. Clinicians in the neurorehabilitation field need to develop strategies to integrate the concepts

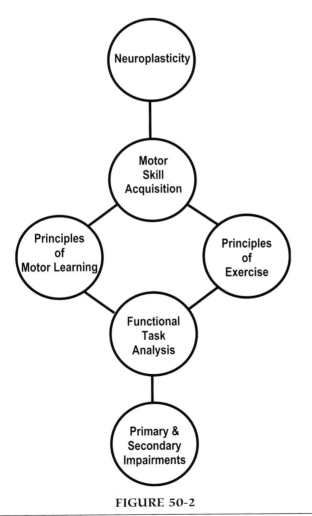

FIGURE 50-2

Theoretical model for neurologic therapeutic intervention

of neuroplasticity and motor recovery with the clinical environment where the learning of motor skills occurs. Figure 50-2 proposes a Theoretical Model for Neurologic Therapeutic Intervention that incorporates our current understanding of neuroplasticity and neurorecovery. This model is based on the assumption that neuroplasticity is driven by the acquisition of motor skills. What are the therapeutic principles that should be incorporated into therapy sessions in order to optimize the learning experience and maximize the level of skill acquisition for our patients? Recent research in neurorehabilitation suggests that key principles of motor skill acquisition and learning and principles of exercise can be applied to increase neurorehabilitation effectiveness and include the importance of practice and feedback, task-specificity, and training intensity. These principles provide important guidelines for the design and delivery of therapeutic interventions. Another important aspect of the neurotherapeutic model is at the level of assessment, whereby, the therapist analyzes functional task performance and determines the primary and secondary impairments that contribute to functional deficits. The organization of this chapter is to elucidate each of the critical factors that guide the clinician in the design of therapeutic programs that drive neuroplasticity through the process of skill acquisition. In addition, this chapter discusses the mechanisms and intervention strategies of the primary and secondary impairments of the neuromuscular and musculoskeletal systems that most commonly affect mobility after TBI.

Process of Motor Skill Acquisition After Brain Injury

Motor skill acquisition is the process by which an individual learns a motor skill. As with other cognitive processes such as language, verbal learning or declarative memory, motor learning occurs within various regions of the cortical and subcortical structures that are involved in the formation of a motor program that is parameterized in time and space to accurately meet a task goal. For example, a child learning to hit a baseball has to develop the strength and coordination to swing a bat with the speed and accuracy to meet the ball as it passes over the plate. The development of the sensorimotor representation of an action plan occurs in cortical sensorimotor structures such as the primary and secondary motor and sensory cortices. However, the initiation and retention of an action plan occurs in prefrontal, basal ganglia, and cerebellar structures. Therefore, motor skill acquisition and retention occurs throughout a neural network that involves all of these movement-related cortical and subcortical areas (12–14). Obviously, the impact of TBI on motor skill acquisition is profound since individual's post-TBI can have involvement with structures that directly impact force production (i.e., motor cortex and direct connections to corticospinal tract of spinal cord) and coordination (i.e., cerebellum and basal ganglia effects on motor control) as well as with other cortical and subcortical areas associated with action plan development, initiation, and retention.

When working on motor skill learning with individuals with TBI, it is particularly important to appreciate the distinction between declarative (explicit) and non-declarative memory (implicit) systems since it is common that patients will present with cognitive deficits which interfere with their ability to have declarative recall but may not interfere with their ability to learn motor skills. The explicit and implicit learning systems are functionally and neuroanatomically distinct (15, 16). Declarative memory is memory for facts and events and is mediated by the medial temporal areas that include the hippocampus and diencephalic nuclei. Patients' post-TBI who are in the period of post-traumatic amnesia have declarative memory deficits as a result of damage in this neural system. In contrast, implicit or non-declarative memory is a collection of abilities that includes the formation of skills and habits, priming and perceptual learning, classical conditioning, and nonassociative learning. The implicit learning systems are not dependent upon the medial temporal areas that support declarative learning. Motor skill learning is a form of implicit learning in which changes in motor performance with practice can occur without conscious awareness of all of the movement-related abilities that are being learned. The areas associated with implicit learning are those that participated in the original learning; therefore, the sensorimotor, prefrontal, basal ganglia, and cerebellar areas, which comprise the neural network for movement, are the areas that are most likely to subserve the implicit motor skill learning system.

The dissociation between declarative awareness and skill learning has been demonstrated in healthy individuals(17) as well as those with brain damage due to Alzheimer's disease (18, 19), Parkinson's disease (20, 21), encephalitis and anoxia (22), and TBI (23, 24). Clinically, this dissociation is significant since it reveals that there is not a direct relationship between the ability to learn new declarative information and the ability to learn motor skills. This dissociation between learning systems confirms that the ability to learn motor skills is retained even in the presence of profound declarative memory loss. Clinical strategies that can be effective when working on motor skill acquisition with individuals who have profound short term declarative memory loss include task-specific training that focuses on the direct acquisition of skills, adaptation of daily routines or the environment such that cues for functional skills can be provided that do not require declarative recall (e.g., memory boards, prearranged functional setups, pictures), and monitoring responsiveness to therapeutic interventions by more sensitive measures of motor performance such as measurement of the time to complete tasks (25).

Motor skill acquisition occurs as a result of practice. The process of motor learning occurs in stages. Fitts and Posner (26) described three stages of motor skill acquisition. The *cognitive* phase is the initial phase of learning where the learner develops the execution requirements of the skill to be learned. During the *cognitive* phase, the learner has frequent errors and variable performance as he/she develops an understanding of what to do. The learner is dependent on visual and verbal environmental cues to organize the movement. As errors decrease, other forms of feedback such as kinesthetic information will be used for error detection and correction. In this early stage of learning, therapists serve as important sources of augmented verbal, visual or tactile feedback. Feedback that provides information of movement outcome is knowledge of results (KR) and information of movement errors is knowledge of performance (KP) (27). When a therapist reports the time it took to complete a 10-meter walk they are providing KR; a description of the gait deficits during that walk is an example of KP. Due to the high cognitive and attentional demands during this initial phase of skill acquisition, practice in an environment with few distractions is recommended. This is particular relevant when working with individuals with brain damage who have impairments such as slowed information processing, attention deficits, and high distractibility.

With additional practice, the learner shifts to the *associative* phase of learning. In this phase, the learner shifts from what to do to how to best complete the action. The learner begins to rely less on visual and verbal cues and attends to kinesthetic cues in order to develop an internal reference of correctness. As kinesthetic awareness develops, the learner has a greater ability to detect movement errors and their consequences. After extended practice, the learner shifts to the *autonomous* phase in which motor tasks are performed more automatically and with less error. During this phase, cognitive effort is less and attentional demands directed to the task are reduced. Patients with brain injury can be introduced to more environmental complexity and distraction as they advance to these later phases of skill acquisition.

In summary, motor skill learning is a purposeful, problem-solving thought process in which the learner develops the coordination of perception and action in order to perform motor skills efficiently and effectively (28). Physical practice of a motor skill is the most important requirement in order to promote skill acquisition and motor learning. Therapists are instrumental in setting up the therapeutic learning environment in such a way as to promote the process of skill acquisition. Understanding that motor learning occurs in stages that have varying cognitive demands is especially important when planning a therapeutic session for someone with brain injury. In addition, it is important to be aware that the level of performance proficiency (i.e., cognitive, associative, autonomous) will vary with the task and environmental demands (29). In other words, a functional task such as a wheelchair transfer may be performed at an autonomous level in the structured and quiet atmosphere of an individual treatment room. However, on the nursing unit where environmental demands are high or during a car transfer where task demands are more difficult performance proficiency may regress to a lower level until sufficient practice with these additional challenges has occurred.

Principles of Motor Learning

Motor learning is a process associated with practice or experience that leads to a relatively permanent change in the ability to produce skilled movements (27). However, in the clinic, learning processes are not directly observed since learning is a reflection of internal neural processes such as enhanced synaptic efficacy within motor-related neural networks. Motor performance is the level of skill execution or how a person completes a movement or functional task. Motor performance is the directly observable action. Motor learning is inferred when an individual reliably and accurately performs a motor skill in various settings and across various points of time. We can infer that an individual has truly learned a motor skill when motor performance can be retained or transferred to a novel situation. The motor performance versus motor learning distinction is very important since conditions of practice and feedback, which can positively impact motor performance, can interfere with the cognitive processes that are required to promote motor learning.

Practice and feedback are two of the most important training variables that can affect motor performance and learning. Motor learning research of both healthy controls and individuals with brain damage demonstrates that practice and feedback can be manipulated in such a way that performance gains during training can be very high; yet, measures of learning such as performance during a retention or transfer test can be detrimentally affected. Clinically, we observe motor performance as a patient practices a task during a therapy session. How would a therapist determine if the patient learned the motor task? In the clinical setting, a retention test would be the observed performance on the following therapy session with no feedback or cueing provided. Performance at this moment would reveal the task-related learning that occurred from the previous therapy session. In contrast, a transfer test reveals the generalizability of what was learned in one condition to another similar but different condition. For example, it has been demonstrated in individuals with stroke that practice in a static balance activity did not transfer to the balance requirements needed during walking (30). In contrast, practice of treadmill walking at speeds closer to normal walking speeds

results in very good transfer in that walking speed increases are observed overground (31).

Practice conditions can be manipulated to vary the presentation of tasks (i.e., practice schedule) across a training session or the presentation of feedback within a training session of a particular task. Conditions of practice or feedback that invoke greater cognitive effort appear to be more effective for motor learning. Cognitive effort involves the perceptual and motor as well as decision-making processes that occur during skill acquisition (32). When cognitive effort is high during task practice, performance may be degraded; however, retention performance is better compared to task practice with less cognitive effort. Cognitive effort as a construct that underlies motor learning processes has profound implications for the generalizability of motor learning principles derived from young, healthy adults to motor skill learning in individuals with impaired cognitive processing. What is the interaction between practice or feedback conditions that require greater cognitive effort in individuals who have impaired cognitive ability? It is not yet clear what the impact of cognitive processing deficits post-brain injury will have on mental processes associated with motor learning. The following section will review the limited literature that investigates the manipulation of practice and feedback on motor learning in individuals with brain damage.

Effects of Practice Conditions   Structuring the practice session includes the determination of the tasks to be practiced and the order of this task practice during the therapy session (33). Part-task vs. whole-task practice is one example of a practice schedule where either a task is practiced in its separate components or is practiced in its entirety. Consistently, it has been demonstrated in young, able-bodied individuals that the effectiveness of whole- vs. part-practice relies upon the nature of the task being learned (34). If a task is serial in nature, a part-task practice schedule can be effective. A serial task is a task that can be broken into discrete tasks that when ordered appropriately result in a meaningful functional outcome. For example, a patient learning to brush his teeth in the morning must learn to unscrew the toothpaste and apply it to the brush, move the brush to clean his teeth, and reach for a glass in order to rinse his mouth. Each discrete component of this functional task sequence can be practiced individually then practiced as a whole. In contrast, continuous tasks such as walking, pushing a wheelchair, or steering a car cannot be parsed into discrete components since successful task performance requires interaction and responsiveness to environmental conditions.

Variable and random-order practice are two practice conditions that have been demonstrated to be more effective for motor learning in young, able-bodied populations. Variable practice reflects the variety of conditions in which a task is practiced such as walking on a treadmill at different speeds or practicing a transfer to different surfaces. This is in contrast to constant practice where the same task and conditions are repeatedly practice. Theoretically, variable practice is a more effective method of invoking the cognitive processes to establish a motor program and the flexibility of processing needed to parameterize this program to meet environmental goals (35). Unfortunately, there are very few motor learning studies in populations with brain-damage that have tested these hypotheses. In fact, there is some evidence that variable practice effects in healthy, able-bodied populations may not be as applicable to individuals with profound declarative memory impairments (18) or motor deficits (31).

Random order practice is a practice schedule in which the order of, for example, 3 different tasks are scheduled throughout a therapy session. This is in contrast to a blocked schedule where the 3 tasks would be ordered and practiced in a block such that practice of task 1, is followed by task 2 and so forth. The effectiveness of random-order practice in comparison to blocked practice has been attributed to the *contextual interference effect* (36, 37). Contextual interference is the cognitive interference introduced when several tasks are practiced together. Random practice induces a form of forgetting that requires the learner to reconstruct the motor memory from a previous, but not immediately preceded, practice trial. The evidence for random-order practice in individuals with brain injury is limited and not consistent. Random practice has been demonstrated to be effective in individuals with stroke learning a series of functional grasps (38) but has not been investigated in individuals with more profound declarative memory and cognitive processing deficits. It is not clear how brain injury that affects various higher-level cognitive processes such as memory and attention may influence practice condition effectiveness. Further work is needed to determine if practice conditions that promote deeper levels of information processing will be as effective in individuals with brain injury that have information processing deficits.

Effects of Feedback   Feedback has a powerful influence on motor performance. A patient learning a motor skill receives intrinsic feedback from visual, auditory, and proprioceptive systems that may or may not be impaired due to brain injury. In addition, a patient receives augmented feedback from the therapist in the form of KR or KP as the therapist provides verbal, visual, or tactile information during a therapeutic procedure or functional training session. Augmented feedback can interfere with the more permanent learning effect that one hopes to achieve with practice. If given too frequently or continuously, feedback can interfere with the problem solving thought process that should occur during practice and instead "guide" the patient to the optimal response (39). Studies

that have examined the effects of feedback in healthy subjects (40), older individuals (41, 42), individuals with stroke (43), and TBI (44) demonstrate that post-response feedback (feedback provided after the skill is performed) given with less frequency can result in motor performance during a retention or transfer test that is more accurate or consistent then feedback provided more frequently or concurrently. In these types of studies, feedback is provided after every trial (100%), with reduced relative feedback (i.e., 50% of trials), or concurrently in which feedback is provided at the same time as the task is performed.

Concurrent feedback consistently degrades learning compared to post-response feedback with less frequency (45). Yet, therapeutic interventions that use biofeedback, computer-generated feedback, or continuous physical guidance by a therapist are examples of concurrent feedback that is typically observed in the clinical environment. One method that appears to be particularly effective in clinical settings to promote motor learning is the use of a faded feedback schedule in which the relative frequency of feedback is decreased within or between practice sessions. With a faded feedback schedule, feedback presentation is high during early learning and then decreased in frequency in the later phases. In this way, feedback is provided in the early stages when the learner needs much information to learn what to do and how to perform the task but feedback is faded as the learner is encouraged to develop the problem solving and self-discovery needed to actually learn a motor skill.

Summary   The importance of practice, the effective scheduling of practice and the frequency of feedback are important principles of motor learning that can be applied to the treatment of individuals with brain injury. However, evidence guiding clinical application is limited and at times inconsistent. In particular, there is a need for motor learning studies that examine the interaction between the cognitive processes invoked during the motor learning process with the cognitive impairments that result from brain injury. Sherwood and Lee (32) propose that the depth of cognitive processing and the degree of cognitive effort have a profound effect on motor learning processes. This has implications for the application of motor learning principles in the rehabilitation of individuals with brain damage. Individuals with profound cognitive impairments in attention and memory may respond differently to conditions of practice or feedback frequency that require greater depths of information processing or cognitive effort. Further work is needed to understand these relationships; however, therapist can take concepts presented here and apply it to the clinical setting. Blocked practice and frequent feedback, which have lower information processing demands, may be more appropriate for individuals with severe cognitive processing deficits. However, over the course of recovery, conditions of practice and feedback that require greater cognitive effort would be appropriate.

Principles of Exercise

Therapeutic exercise is the method most commonly used to address mobility problems after brain injury. Therapeutic exercise incorporates exercise principles into the design of therapeutic interventions in which the goal is to increase functional performance and decrease specific movement-related dysfunction. Traditionally, therapeutic exercise programs have been designed to remediate impairment specific mobility problems. For example, if range of motion is limited due to muscle shortening, exercise techniques can be used that will effectively lengthen the shortened muscle. While impairment-focused interventions may be effective in the rehabilitation of specific impairments (evidence for impairment-focused interventions will be discussed later in the chapter), there is building evidence from meta-analysis that impairment-focused interventions have no effect on functional performance (46).

A recent trend in therapeutic exercise is to incorporate sport physiologic training principles in the design of exercise programs that increase aerobic capacity and strength in individuals with brain damage (47, 48). This is an important consideration since the dosing of exercise can influence treatment outcome. Task-specificity (what is the nature of the task or skill to be learned?) and training intensity (what is the frequency, duration, time, and demand of the activity?) appear to be 2 important factors that affect therapeutic exercise effectiveness after brain injury.

Task-Specific Training   Since the writings of Bernstein in the early 1900's (49), the importance of movement and task-specific learning has been well recognized in the psychological sciences. It has only been in the past 10–15 years that the emphasis on task-specific training has been incorporated into the rehabilitation setting.[1] The effectiveness of task-specific training derives from the specificity of learning hypothesis proposed by Henry in the 1950's who suggested that the most effective conditions for motor learning occur when performance during practice is well-matched to the performance requirements needed during retention or transfer conditions (50). Motor learning reflects a neural specificity of practice since motor skill acquisition involves the integration of

the sensory and motor information that occurs during practice, and ultimately, leads to the sensorimotor solution that results in accurate, consistent, and skillful movements (27).

The importance of repetitive, task-oriented practice in the recovery of upper limb function (51–53) and walking (31, 54–57) has been consistently demonstrated in clinical trials of stroke-related brain damage and is beginning to emerge in TBI populations as well (58–61). In these studies, interventions are designed that involve specific task practice that incorporates the upper limb in various functional activities or in repetitive activity such as walking on a treadmill.

A recent and comprehensive systematic review compiled by Van Peppen et al. (46) of physical therapy interventions post-stroke demonstrated strong evidence for greater patient benefit due to functional task practice than impairment-focused interventions. Functional improvement was associated with interventions such as aerobic training, constraint-induced movement therapy, transfer training, and treadmill training with or without body weight support. In contrast, exercise programs that focused on muscle strengthening, muscular re-education with biofeedback or neuromuscular stimulation showed improved impairment level outcomes such as strength and range of motion but failed to result in significant functional outcomes. In addition, Van Peppen et al. (46) demonstrated no evidence for improved functional outcomes to support the use of neurophysiologic treatment approaches such as neurodevelopmental treatment (NDT), proprioceptive neuromuscular facilitation (PNF) or Brunnstrom (62–64).

Our understanding of the mechanisms that subserve functional recovery and responsiveness to task-specific training is elucidated by eloquent animal work that demonstrate that repetitive task practice that involves the acquisition of a motor skill results in neuroplasticity in both synaptic and neuronal morphology and in cortical reorganization (6, 65, 66) These findings of experience-dependent neuroplasticity are corroborated in humans with brain damage through recent neuroimaging studies that use transcranial magnetic stimulation (TMS) and functional magnetic resonance imaging (fMRI) to demonstrate the potential for cortical reorganization as a result of task-specific therapeutic interventions for both upper limb and lower limb recovery (67–70).

Training Intensity   Time spent in exercise training and increasing the difficulty or physiologic demands of the exercise session are examples of methods to increase training intensity. Exercise dosing can have differential effects that vary as a function of the time in the activity (min/day), frequency of sessions (times/wk) and the duration of training (weeks of training). Kwakkel et al. (71) demonstrated that specific skills training post-stroke for

---

[1]Note that task-specific training is distinguished from ADL training. Task-specific training implies that the training event is designed to improve motor skill acquisition in a specific task. ADL training implies that the training event is designed to decrease the level of physical assistance to complete a functional task; therefore, ADL training may allow the use of compensatory strategies or assistive devices in order to enhance task completion.

30 min/day, 5 days/wk for 20 wks in addition to a standard rehabilitation program was most effective if the specialized training was specifically focused on active arm or leg focused training. Winstein et al. (53) have also demonstrated the preferential effect of additional therapy time in functional task training. The added significance of this study is that functional training in the early rehabilitation period post-stroke resulted in significant differences in both strength and function at 9 months post-injury compared to strength training or usual care groups. This study illustrates the impact that early functional training in the period immediately post-injury may have on future limb use and function later in the recovery process.

A recent systematic review specifically investigated the effects of exercise intensity as measured by time in therapy on ADL, walking, and dexterity in patients with stroke (72). The results of this meta-analysis suggests that more intensive therapy that includes approximately 16 hrs of additional task-specific training in the first 6 months post-brain injury particularly dedicated to lower limb and ADL activities is more effective than standard therapy programs. Limitations of this meta-analysis include the inability to determine the precise treatment contrast that separates the longer time in therapy from the control comparison. At this time there is insufficient literature in TBI populations to conduct a meta-analysis; however, there is some evidence that the findings from stroke may be somewhat generalizable to individuals with TBI. Eng et al. (73) in a prospective study in the inpatient rehabilitation setting compared mobility outcomes between patients with stroke and TBI. Overall, patients with TBI had higher mobility status at admission and discharge; however, the improvement in mobility status per day was not different between the diagnostic groups. Cifu et al. (74) specifically examined the effect of therapy intensity (time in therapy/ length of stay) and found that therapy intensity predicted the amount of motor function improvement a discharge. While the level of evidence may not be as high as the evidence from stroke, there is clearly a trend that shows similar responsiveness in patients with TBI. Collectively, this literature reflects the need for studies that investigate the optimal dosing of exercise programs designed to improve mobility especially in populations with brain beyond stroke.

Incremental increases in task difficulty and increasing the physiologic demand of the exercise are additional methods to manipulate training intensity. Adaptive task practice is a method whereby the therapist adjusts the difficulty of the task as they observe performance and provide feedback during practice. Task difficulty is adjusted such that the patient experiences progressive challenge across training. Adaptive task practice is one of the practice strategies used in CI therapy as the optimal movements develop or a "shaped" during therapy. Strong evidence exists for CI therapy as a treatment to increase dexterity

of the hemiparetic arm and appears to be related to the high intensity dosing of task-specific upper limb training (46). Case study series in individuals with TBI using a modified CI therapy approach are beginning to demonstrate a similar responsiveness to this type of training (60).

Increasing physiologic demand is another effective strategy to increase training intensity. In studies of treadmill training with and without body weight support, it has been demonstrated that treadmill training at higher speeds is more effective then training at constant or variable speeds that are within the range of the patient's typical overground walking speed (75, 76). In addition, fast walking results in improvements in body and limb kinematics and muscle activation patterns in individuals that have impaired walking due to hemiparesis (77). Training within a task at maximum capability is one of the tenets of training specificity and appears to be applicable to individuals with brain injury relearning a functional task. The equivocal evidence found in the recent Cochrane review of treadmill training with or without body weight support may be due to the high degree of variability between studies in the frequency, duration, and timing of the intervention as well as the level of physiologic intensity used across studies (78).

Summary   Task-specificity and intensity are important principles of exercise that can be applied to the treatment of individuals with brain injury. There is strong evidence that intensive, functional task training is effective in individuals with stroke-related brain damage; however, there is limited (yet developing) evidence in populations with TBI. Most likely, principles of exercise incorporated into therapeutic interventions will extend to other populations with brain damage such as those with TBI. It is unknown if cognitive and behavioral problems, common post-TBI, will interfere with the compliance needed to achieve the desired training effect.

THE LINK BETWEEN ACQUISITION OF SKILLS AND AVAILABLE RESOURCES

At this point, we return to the rehabilitation model proposed by Quinn and Gordon (79) (Figure 50-1). This chapter has focused on the acquisition of skill including the evidence that neuroplasticity and neurorecovery are promoted through the skill acquisition process, conditions of practice and feedback frequency affect the retention and generalizability of motor skill learning, and training intensity and specificity appear to be important parameters that drive functional training effectiveness. Skills are required in order for our patients with brain damage to participate in desired roles related to self-care, social and recreational pursuits, and occupation. However, post-TBI there is a myriad of physical, behavioral, and cognitive limitations that contribute to the functional deficits. Typically, rehabilitation specialists classify these limitations as impairments that have to be remediated. The perspective developed by Quinn and Gordon suggests that the goal of therapy is to determine what resources the patient needs to successfully accomplish the functional task. In essence, the diagnostic challenge for the therapist is to identify the impairments that prevent functional task performance and develop an intervention program that develops the necessary resources to successfully complete the task. This section of the chapter will address the therapeutic interventions and strategies used to develop patient resources and address impairment level problems.

Behavioral Treatment Strategies

In the days, weeks, and months after TBI, patients present with a variety of potential behavioral disorders that may impact their ability to participate in therapy. This can be compounded by organic deficits in cognition (e.g., confusion and disorientation, decreased short term memory, decreased problem-solving and reasoning ability, delayed processing, motor and verbal disinhibition, lack of initiation and concrete reasoning), perception (e.g., visual, auditory or tactile hyper- or hypo-sensitivity, neglect, visual-field deficits, right-left discrimination problems), and communication (e.g., expressive or comprehension aphasia, decreased understanding, delayed responsiveness) as well

TABLE 50-1
Behavioral Treatment Strategies

LOCF	RECOVERY PHASE	APPROACH
I, II, III	Minimal response	Sensory stimulation Preventative maintenance Monitoring response to early mobilization
IV	Confused, agitated	Structured environment Directed activity Monitor response to stimulation Brief, frequent activity changes
V, VI	Confused	Structured environment Directed activity Consistent approach Complexity to tasks varied gradually Environmental distractions varied gradually
VII, VIII	Automatic	Reduce structure Greater self-monitoring Progressively challenging tasks

LOCF – Levels of Cognitive Function from Rancho Los Amigos Rehabilitation Hospital (Hagen, 1079).

as their personal reactions to injury and disability such as loss of control, frustration and anger, lack of insight, and depression. The challenge for the therapist working on mobility issues is to adjust performance expectations and to adapt the therapeutic learning environment. The Table 50-1 summarizes common therapeutic strategies that can be applied as the patient progresses through the various behavioral and cognitive phases associated with TBI recovery.

The overall therapeutic goal is to progress the patient through the various stages of cognitive function recovery through systematic and gradated stimulation and activity (29). The following descriptions provide an overall behavioral strategy that would be appropriate as specific mobility training or preventive maintenance of musculoskeletal deformity is being applied. It is important to note that the stages of motor learning discussed earlier have applicability within each of these stages particularly at the mid- and high-level management phases. Motor performance proficiency increases as the learner moves from the cognitive, associative, and autonomous phases of skill acquisition. Similar strategies such as monitoring environmental distraction and task complexity apply as well when an individual with brain injury is progressing through the levels of cognitive function (80, 81).

It is important to note the level of evidence for most recommendations on cognitive management used for physical rehabilitation are primarily at the level of clinical expertise. A recent Cochrane review of sensory stimulation for individuals with TBI in a coma or vegetative state revealed that most of the literature in this particular area of cognitive-physical rehabilitation is primarily at the level of case study or case series (82). Three studies met inclusion criteria for an RCT; however, there were serious methodological limitations that led the authors to conclude that there was no reliable evidence to rule in or out the use of sensory stimulation in patients in coma. Given the need for additional RCT's that address the issue of cognitive and physical management post-TBI, the following summarize what is regarded as best available practice in this area using the Rancho Los Amigos Levels of Cognitive Function (LOCF) Scale to delineate low-, mid-, and high-level cognitive groups (80).

Low-Level Cognitive Management Patients who are considered within the LOCF levels of I, II, and III have low-levels of responsiveness that range from unresponsive to any stimulation (LOCF I), generalized response that is limited and non-purposeful (LOCF II), to localized responsiveness in which the patient may follow simple commands (LOCF III). This decrease level of responsiveness is often accompanied by severe postural tone and paralysis that can lead to secondary musculoskeletal impairments. Specific strategies to address these secondary impairments will be discussed later. In addition, to preventing complications due to immobility and impaired motor control therapists, in collaboration with other team members, usually begin some form of sensory stimulation program to encourage arousal and responsiveness. Once the patient is medically stable, upright mobility activities are initiated progressing from bed mobility to upright postures in a wheelchair or tilt table. Observationally, changes in posture and upright positions appear to be effective in evoking increased levels of responsiveness in patients in these lower levels.

Mid-Level Cognitive Management   The transition from unresponsiveness to LOCF IV is often accompanied by confusion and agitation. A patient at this level is easily confused and disoriented and may present with aggressive and inappropriate behavior. His responses during this phase appear to be due to internal confusion. During this phase, the patient cannot readily engage in self-care activity and episodes of incontinence are frequent due to lack of internal and external awareness. The therapeutic strategy at this phase is to provide a structured and safe environment with minimal distraction that can allow the patient to move about. Within this structured environment, brief, directed activity can be introduced. Frequent, short treatments that are interspersed across the day would be the ideal therapy schedule for a patient in this phase.

Patients' post-TBI at LOCF V and VI are non-agitated but continue to present with confusion and profound declarative memory deficits. At LOCF V, the patient responds to commands and is more alert but is easily distractible with difficulty concentrating on tasks. Agitated outbursts and inappropriate verbal responses still occur when the patient is frustrated. At LOCF VI, that patient has more consistent goal-directed behavior but needs cuing. Greater participation in ADLs is evident as the individual is developing greater awareness of self and others. This level is associated with the period of post-traumatic amnesia in which the ability to develop new declarative memories is seriously impaired. The Rancho Cognitive levels state that during these phases individuals cannot learn new information. However, the distinction between the explicit (declarative) and implicit (non-declarative) memory systems would suggest that patients during post-traumatic amnesia do have the capability to learn new motor skills, and in fact, has been demonstrated in individuals' post-TBI during post-traumatic amnesia (23, 24).

The most effective therapeutic strategies during this phase would include task-specific training in structured environments. Treatment approach at this level would encourage successful performance through adaptive task practice in which task practice is challenging, yet, successful. The expectation is that repetitive task practice during this phase of recovery would lead to a gradual improvement in motor performance as the patient acquires motor skills that may be independent of any verbal recollection of the task training. For patients with confusion, a consistent approach to the daily schedule, treatment setting, activities, instruction, and team members is most effective. Task complexity and changes in the structure of practice (i.e., increased variability) and feedback (i.e., decreased frequency) can be progressed as the patient's cognitive status improves.

High-Level Cognitive Management   The progression from the previous levels to LOCF VII and VIII is marked by improvements in short term memory with more appropriate and purposeful behavior. During this phase, there is less confusion, better recall, and increased self-awareness and interaction with others and the environment. However, limitation in insight, abstract reasoning and problem solving can still exist, particularly for those in LOCF VII. At this level, it is realistic to expect completion of ADLs with relative independence. Therapy focuses on the tasks and skills needed to facilitate community integration. This phase is primarily focused on skill acquisition in the tasks that will assist the individual to participate in their desired self-care, social, occupational, and recreational goals.

Physical Impairment-Focused Interventions

Mobility impairments after brain injury are either directly related to the damage of neural structures such as impairments in voluntary movement, abnormal tone, and balance or are secondary impairments that result from these neural system impairments. Secondary mobility impairments result in limitation of the musculoskeletal system such as muscle contractures, joint mobility restrictions, and disuse weakness. Both neural and musculoskeletal impairments can be major contributors to functional deficits after brain injury. The following section provides a brief overview of current therapeutic strategies to address these problems.

Neural System Impairments

Voluntary and Purposeful Movement   Impairments in voluntary movement associated with TBI can be due to an upper motor neuron weakness syndrome that includes inability to do selective joint movements out of synergy, decreased force production, and impaired initiation of purposeful voluntary movement. The primary mechanisms for these movement deficits post-TBI can be attributed to diffuse axonal injury due to scatted white matter infarctions in the descending motor pathways, focal cortical contusions or deep cerebral hemorrhage that results in direct damage to the corticospinal tract as it passes through the striatocapsular region, and transtentorial herniation where compression of motor pathways in the upper brain stem can occur (83). Diffuse axonal injury and/or major brainstem contusion can result in low levels of consciousness in which reflexive movement patterns within decorticate and decerebrate postures can result from motor output of subcortical motor brainstem systems that include the rubrospinal, reticulospinal, and vestibulospinal systems (84).

In contrast to stroke where 70% of all stroke survivors will present with a motor hemiparesis (85), only 17% of patients post-TBI will have arm/hand paresis with synergistic movement and of these individuals motor recovery is good such that only 3% will have synergistic hemiparesis at 4 months post-injury (83). The predominate motor deficit in patients post-TBI is impaired force production leading to decreased power generation and strength and impaired integration of voluntary movement with the other cortical, subcortical, and cerebellar motor systems involved in the planning, initiation, completion and retention of accurate and consistent goal-directed movement. Weakness and impaired power generation can be a major factor along with sensory integration and cognitive deficits that interfere with performance of mobility tasks. The differential diagnosis and treatment of movement dysfunction after brain injury requires the therapist to determine what are primary contributors to impaired task completion (i.e., force generation, synergistic movement), how can these primary contributors be addressed (i.e., strength training, muscle re-education), and how can the learning environment be structured to result in the acquisition of skill when considering both the cognitive and motor deficits of the patient (i.e., task-specific training).

There are numerous therapeutic strategies employed by therapist to address issues of neural motor control that can vary in emphasis across the recovery continuum from the acute care phase (86) where lower level management strategies are needed to later in the recovery process where the focus is to incorporate motor control strategies with task training (81, 87–89). Current approaches to muscle re-education and therapeutic exercise use an interactive systems model that emphasizes that task accomplishment emerges from a complex interaction of biomechanical, motor, and sensory effects that are modified by environmental constraints (90). Typically, therapists interact with the patient as they manipulate the mechanical demand of the task within the sensorimotor conditions that optimize task performance.

Traditionally, neurophysiologic therapeutic approaches such as neurodevelopmental treatment (NDT) (91), proprioceptive neuromuscular stimulation (PNF) (92), and the Brunnstrom approach (93) were commonly used to facilitate motor and postural control. These approaches were derived from the neurophysiologic understanding of the time such as the hierarchical organization of the nervous system, that proprioceptive afferent sensory stimulation can be used to modify abnormal tone and

facilitate a patient's movement pattern, and that recovery from brain damage occurs in a predictable sequence that corresponds to development (94). With current advances in neuroscience (5) and greater understanding of motor control (95) as well as the trend for evidence-based practice, there is building consensus that the traditional neurophysiologic treatment approaches are not effective compared with usual care that emphasizes functional training (46). It would be remiss to treat patients with a traditional neurophysiologic treatment approach alone since it appears that these approaches emphasize impairment-focused intervention and have not been shown to be effective in improving functional gains. However, important therapeutic principles have emerged from these traditional neurophysiologic approaches that continue to influence practice today. The importance of proximal control and midline alignment, the use of resistance and developmental postures as ways to increase demand needed for functional tasks, and the quantification of recovery as patients develop more isolated joint movement and control all derive from these approaches. Current best practice would incorporate these important therapeutic principles with our understanding of motor learning and exercise physiology to promote skill acquisition in our patients with brain injury.

Abnormal Muscle Tone   Clinically, therapists are confronted with two major problems related to the impaired regulation of muscle tone. Abnormal muscle tone includes problems with velocity-dependent increases in phasic stretch reflexes associated with the upper motor neuron syndrome (i.e. spasticity) (96) and abnormal postural control interfering with the ability to maintain upright head, neck, and trunk postures against gravity (86). Pierson (97) describes a wide range of clinical assessment tools that can be used to assess treatment effectiveness and functional outcomes as it relates to abnormal tone particularly spasticity. These tools include goniometry to assess range of motion limitations that can result from muscle imbalance, the modified Ashworth Scale that is an ordinal scale to quantify tone intensity, and functional tests such as the Jebsen Taylor Hand Function test, gait speed, and the Berg Balance scale to determine the effects of abnormal tone on function. These outcome measures are commonly used; however, a recent review of the reliability and validity of spasticity assessments suggest that further work is needed to develop more objective measures as well as measures that capture the real-world impact of spasticity on function (98).

The approach to abnormal tone management is twofold. One is to address the primary issues related to spasticity and postural control by providing therapeutic interventions that attempt to decrease tone or increase upright control in functional postures such as sitting and standing. The second approach is to address the secondary musculoskeletal impairments that can occur when severe and unrelenting increases in abnormal muscle tone result in muscle contracture and joint deformity. Specific approaches to address these secondary tone-related impairments will be discussed in the next section.

Therapeutic interventions that use weight bearing through the extremities and trunk are often used in various functional positions to decrease tone as the patient develops appropriate motor control to maintain upright postures and to complete functional tasks (86, 88). The goal of the therapy is to facilitate more effective motor unit recruitment, and due to the task-oriented nature of the training, appears to be more effective then interventions that focus on the reduction of spasticity alone. For example, in a recent double-blind, placebo-controlled multi-site RCT, botulinum toxin intramuscular injections reduced muscle tone in patients with upper limb spasticity after stroke but there was no change in disability or quality of life (99). In a similarly controlled RCT, botulinum toxin injections to the gastrocs were effective at reducing muscle tone and limb pain but were no more effective than placebo in improving gait function (100). In both studies, no specific splinting or physical therapies were incorporated into the treatment. One explanation for the lack of functional improvement is that treatment only focused at the impairment level (i.e., the reduction of muscle tone) and did not potentiate the benefit of tone reduction with the process of skill acquisition. More effective approaches to tone management may include the integration of pharmacologic interventions with the task-specific training required to make significant functional improvements.

Balance and Vestibular Disorders   Balance and vestibular disorders after TBI can be due to damage of the peripheral vestibular sensory apparatus or central structures that respond to the vestibular sensory inputs such as the vestibular nuclear complex, central pathways of the vestibulo-ocular and vestibulospinal reflexes, the brainstem, and cerebellum (101). Peripheral vestibular dysfunction after TBI can be reduced (hypofunction) which results in vertigo, dysequilibrium, and impaired gaze stability if the damage is unilateral. If bilateral, patients may have less severe complaints of vertigo but present with severe dysequilibrium and gait ataxia. Trauma to the head can also result in benign paroxysmal positional vertigo (BPPV) caused when otoconia either are displaced into the semicircular canals or is floating in the endolymph. BPPV results in distorted vestibular function that is gravity-sensitive; therefore, episodes of severe vertigo and positional nystagmus occur with head position changes. Central vestibular disorders can commonly occur as a result of diffuse damage to white matter tracts that interact with vestibular areas of the brainstem and the cerebellum. Severe episodes of vertigo and dizziness are not

as common with central vestibular disorders. Patients will usually have a wide range of symptoms, which include constant feelings of vertigo that are also accompanied by nausea, nystagmus, ataxia, or dysequilibrium. Whether from central or peripheral causes, balance deficits and dizziness have been identified as major factors affecting functional prognosis and return to work after TBI (102, 103).

Patients post-TBI commonly present with gait instability and are at high risk for falls. Balance deficits can be a result of the combined effects of visual, somatosensory, and vestibular impairments as well as motor control deficits that result in weakness and incoordination. The Dynamic Gait Index (DGI) is a clinical tool that can be used to assess fall risk in individuals with balance disorders (90). Whitney et al. (104) demonstrated that gait instability as measured by the DGI was related to falls history. Individuals with vestibular disorders that were either from peripheral (e.g., BPPV, labyrinthine concussion, labryinthitis), central (e.g., stroke, head trauma, cerebellar dysfunction) or combined peripheral and central vestibular dysfunction were 2.58 times more likely to fall if they scored =19/24 on the DGI.

Vestibular rehabilitation post-TBI can include vestibular adaptation exercises such as gaze stabilization exercises, balance retraining, sensory organization exercises with progressively more difficult static and dynamic activity, and canalith repositioning maneuvers (101). There is good evidence that vestibular rehabilitation that incorporates various balance retraining strategies that are designed to address specific patient problems can be effective (105, 106). The two exercise approaches used for the treatment of vestibular hypofunction include vestibular adaptation exercises to improve gaze stability and balance exercises that foster the use of visual and somatosensory information to improve postural stability (see Herdman (105) for detailed description of vestibular, balance, and gait exercises used for balance rehabilitation). Canalith repositioning maneuvers are specific techniques used to treat patients with BPPV (107). It is beyond the scope of this chapter to discuss the appropriate application of all these various balance interventions since they are designed to address specific vestibular deficits based upon the patient's history, age, and diagnosis. Excellent sources are available to provide greater background in this rehabilitation specialty area (105, 108).

Musculoskeletal Impairments

Muscle Conctracture and Joint Mobility   Impaired voluntary motor control and spasticity are the primary cause of muscle contracture and joint deformity after TBI. Hypertonia in combination with immobility due to paralysis and altered mechanical properties of muscle and connective tissues due to disuse can result in severe deformity of the upper and lower extremities. In addition, heterotopic ossification can further complicate joint mobility management. Common patterns of deformity that result from spastic motor patterns includes shoulder adductor/internal rotation, elbow flexion, forearm pronation, wrist and finger flexion contractures of the upper limb and equinovarus foot with clawed toes, valgus foot, stiff or flexed knee, and hip adductor and flexor contractures of the lower limb (109). Spastic deformities interfere with bed positioning, sitting and standing, transfers and walking as well as self-care activities such as hygiene and dressing. In addition to interfering with function, spastic deformities can be a major source of pain (97). The cumulative effect of these secondary musculoskeletal impairments can seriously impact quality of life or the potential for recovery especially for individuals who have been in coma for extended periods of time.

The primary therapeutic goal is to prevent or correct muscle contractures. Various preventative methods are employed in the acute care setting immediately post-injury such as performing passive range of motion and stretching or using preventive bed position including the use of wedges, splints, and pillows to improve limb alignment (86, 110). Various therapeutic interventions are effective to increase passive range of motion or to prevent its loss and include stretching (111, 112), serial casting (113, 114), dynamic splinting (110, 115), orthotic management (116), and, in combination with these types of physical approaches, pharmacologic management such as motor point blocks (116), and intrathecal baclofen (117). In severe cases, when more conservative management has not been effective, surgical management for tendon lengthening or releases may be indicated (110).

Weakness and Deconditoning One area that is beginning to receive more study it the effect of immobility on work capacity in individuals with brain injury. Peak exercise capacity and cardiorespiratory fitness of individuals with moderate to severe brain injury is reported to be 60–70% of the capacity of normal healthy adults of similar age (118). It is common in the acute phase that patients with TBI are confined to bedrest for days, weeks, or months depending upon the initial brain injury severity. The adverse effects of prolonged bedrest are well documented in humans but little attention has been given to the additive effects of immobility to chronic disease or injury (119). Immobility due to bedrest as well as a reduction in physical activity results in decreased muscular strength and aerobic capacity that leads to reduced work capacity. Additionally, prolonged immobility can result in osteopenia, which can interfere with fracture healing for patients who may also present with multiple fractures in addition to the brain injury (120).

Thirty days of bedrest can result in 18–20% reduction in knee extensor peak torque; however, strength can recover within 92% of pre-bedrest levels within 30 days after bedrest (120). Findings such as these highlight the importance of active muscle contraction during bedrest and the introduction of early intermittent ambulation and physical activity to attenuate the effects of immobility in patients with TBI. Responsiveness and tolerance of individuals with moderate to severe TBI to aerobic or circuit training has been demonstrated in both the acute and sub-acute phases post-TBI (47, 48). Peak work rate improved in patients with TBI recruited within 24 ± 14 wks of injury that completed resisted cycling for a goal of 30 min (actual cycling time achieved 23 ± 5 min) at 60–80% age-predicted maximum heart rate for 24 sessions over 8 wks (47). Forty-five minutes of circuit training (combination of aerobic exercise, muscular strength, and endurance training) at 60% age-predicted maximum heart rate for 3 sessions per week for 12 wks increased peak power output and VO_2 peak in 14 individuals approximately 17 wks post-injury (48). Clearly, exercise and early mobility training are indicated to lessen the impact of secondary causes of weakness and decreased endurance. With proper supervision and monitoring of cardiovascular responses to exercise, individuals with TBI can engage in intensive strength and conditioning training.

INNOVATIONS IN PHYSICAL REHABILITATION

Constraint induced (CI) movement therapy and the use of treadmill training with body weight support (BWS) are examples of innovations in rehabilitation that are derived from basic science work in neuroplasticity and neurorecovery and incorporate principles of motor learning and exercise into the therapeutic intervention. The therapeutic goal of each of these interventions is to increase skill in functional tasks.

The scientific rationale for CI therapy is derived from studies in non-human primates in which 2 important findings impact the clinical application of this paradigm. First, Taub (121) observed that deafferented monkeys who wore a restraining jacket that constrained the non-affected limb had greater use of the limb then monkeys that were not constrained. However, Nudo (122) demonstrated that greatest amount of motor cortical reorganization and functional recovery occurred in primates who wore the restraining jacket *and* engaged in repetitive skills training. As a result, CI therapy has developed as a therapeutic intervention where use of a constraint device and intensive task practice is used to promote upper limb recovery in individuals who have hemiparesis due to stroke (Fig. 50-3).

The effectiveness of this approach in individuals post-stroke who meet a minimum motor criteria was first described by Wolf (123) and Taub (124) and is currently being investigated in a multi-site, RCT funded by the NIH

(125). The paradigm under investigation includes individuals post-stroke in either the subacute period (4–9 months post-stroke) or chronic period (>1 yr post-stroke) who at a minimum must be able to actively extend the wrist, thumb, and at least 2 other digits 10°. The intervention occurs 5 days/wk for two weeks for 6 hr/day in training with therapist supervision that combines the use of a constraint device (mitt on unaffected hand) with task practice and adapted task practice (shaping). The patient signs a behavioral contract and agrees to wear the mitt 90% of waking hours and to maintain a daily diary of activities. The results of the trial have not been published; however, smaller experimental trials have demonstrated the effectiveness of this intervention and the specific effectiveness of this practice schedule (126–128). Several recent studies have found that a modified CI therapy (Figure 50-3) can be effective after stroke (129, 130) and TBI (60). These researchers found that a modified practice schedule of CI therapy for 3 times/wk for 10 wks for 30 min/day of supervised therapist training in combination with the restraint use 5dy/wk for 5 hrs/day during patient-identified times

of high frequency upper limb use results in improved motor function and self-perceived use of the limb. One of the advantages of a modified practice schedule is that it is more compatible with the delivery of services reimbursed for rehabilitation at this time.

Step training on a treadmill with body weight-support (BWS) is a neurotherapeutic intervention used to promote locomotor recovery in individuals with spinal cord or brain injury that is derived from basic science animal research. Adult cats with low thoracic spinal transaction recovered the ability to step on a treadmill after training with trunk support and assistance with paw placement (131–133). These findings precipitated a movement in rehabilitation to use body weight support systems in locomotor rehabilitation of humans with spinal cord injury (134–136) and stroke (31, 56) (Figure 50-4). The effectiveness of this type of training is attributed to the intense and

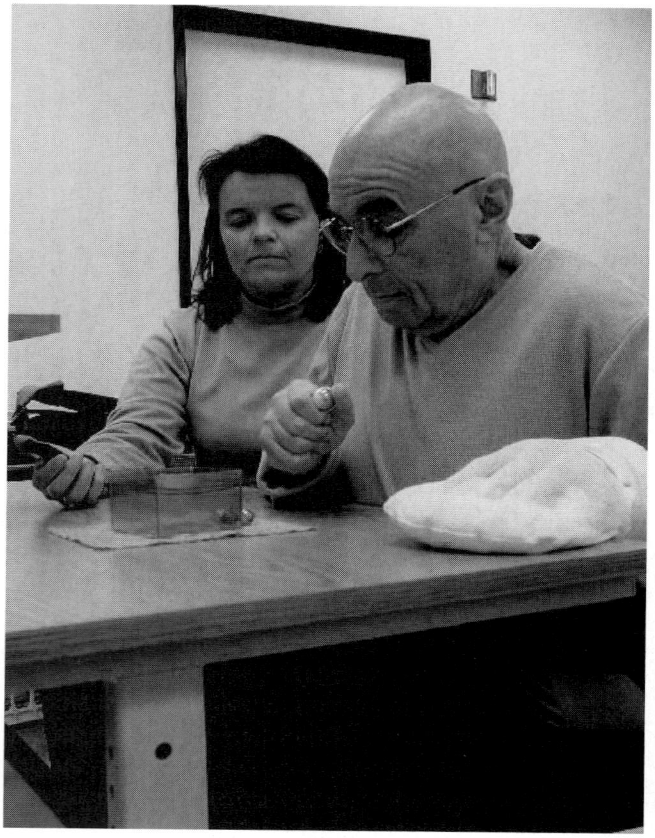

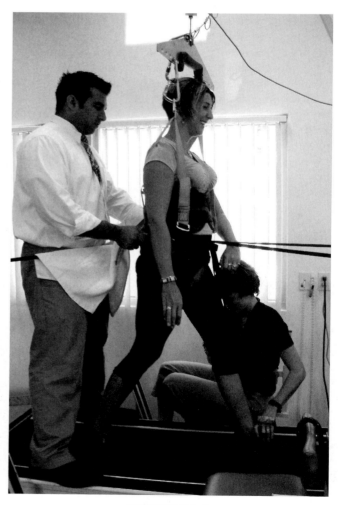

FIGURE 50-4

Step training on a treadmill with body weight support is an example of intense, task-specific training that incorporates the repetitive practice of walking

FIGURE 50-3

Constraint induced (CI) movement therapy is a therapeutic intervention where use of a constraint device and intensive task practice is used to promote upper limb recovery in individuals with hemiparesis

task-specific nature of walking on a treadmill in which the appropriate afferent inputs associated with walking provide the input needed to induce experience-dependent changes in neuroplasticity at spinal and supraspinal levels (137–139).

Despite several investigations of treadmill training with or without BWS in individuals with stroke-related brain injury, a recent Cochrane review found weak evidence supporting the effectiveness of this approach (78). However, what this Cochrane report did reveal is that there is tremendous variability in the time post-injury that the intervention occurred and the frequency, duration, and intensity of the protocols being studied. In fact, subsequent studies that specifically addressed training parameters have demonstrated that training intensity as determined by treadmill speed is an important parameter of training effectiveness (31, 76), yet, none of the studies in the Cochrane review used speeds or other training parameters known to affect exercise effectiveness.

At this time, preliminary work in individuals with stroke-related brain damage does suggest that functional changes in overground walking velocity can occur with a training program that includes a minimum of 12 sessions for at least 3x/wk for 4 wks that results in at least 20 minutes of treadmill walking time at speeds within 1.5 – 2.0 mph (31). Clearly, more systematic work is needed to determine the most effective training parameters for this intervention. There is one study that has demonstrated both the effectiveness and challenge of applying this intervention in individuals with severe brain injury (61). The authors have developed the Missouri Assisted Gait (MAG) Scale to identify the small but significant changes in motor ability during gait recovery of patients with TBI.

What is it about these two rehabilitation innovations that make them distinctly different from usual therapeutic approaches? What is the active ingredient that appears to result in functional changes that appear to be more substantial than in other treatment paradigms? Both interventions incorporate the principles of motor learning and exercise that have been described in this chapter. First, the interventions focus on task practice with appropriate feedback monitored and gradated by the therapist. In both CI therapy and treadmill training with BWS, the patient actively engages in task practice for periods of time that are substantially greater than what is typically provided in therapy. Second, the therapies focus on intense, task-specific training. It is more than just the time in task therapy that appears to be effective. The training must be a challenge or engage the patient in higher levels of performance than is normally experienced. Third, task-specificity is incorporated into training protocols that have defined training parameters for frequency, intensity, and duration. In order to achieve a training effect, the patient must engage in enough exercise or task practice, which is systematically progressed in order to induce a physiologic or neural response. Finally, these interventions address the impairments and deficit in functional skills that are unique to the needs and capabilities of the individual patient.

The Theoretical Model for Neurologic Therapeutic Intervention presented in Figure 50-2 proposes that the theoretical foundation for physical rehabilitation after brain injury is based on the premise that 1) skill acquisition promotes neuroplasticity, 2) motor learning and exercise principles are used to enhance the acquisition and retention of motor skills, 3) skills to be learned are identified through functional task analysis and patient perspective (i.e., the individual's self-perceived goals and expectations), and 4) the differential diagnosis process for therapists involves the identification of the primary and secondary impairments that interfere with functional performance.

Implication for Future Directions

This is a very exciting time for physical rehabilitation specialist since it is evident that physical activity, particularly the acquisition of motor skills, provides the stimulus that the nervous system needs to recover. The challenge for researchers in this area is to conduct the clinical trials that will define the tasks and training parameters that result in effective therapeutic interventions. In addition, these trials must be expanded to include other populations with brain damage in order to provide greater generalizability for clinicians. The challenge for clinicians is to incorporate an evidence-based treatment approach, which integrates their individual clinical expertise with advances in neuroscience and incorporates the perspective from patients and family members. The ability to learn the necessary skills our patients need to return to meaningful and productive roles are the changes that will truly improve the quality of life for our patients with brain injury.

References

1. *International Classification of Functioning, Disability and Health: ICF.* Geneva, World Health Organization 2001.
2. Gray D. B., Hendershot G. E. The ICIDH-2: developments for a new era of outcomes research. *Arch Phys Med Rehab* 2000;81 (12 Suppl 2): S10–4.
3. Quinn L., Gordon J. *Functional Outcomes: Documentation for Rehabilitation* St. Louis: Saunders; 2003.
4. Nudo, R. J., Plautz, E. J., and Milliken, G. W. Adaptive plasticity in primate motor cortex as a consequence of behavioral experience and neuronal injury. *Seminars in Neurosci* 1997;9:13–23.
5. Nudo R. J., Barbay S., Kleim J. A. Role of neuroplasticity in functional recovery after stroke. In: Levin H. S., Grafman J., eds. *Cerebral reorganization of function after brain damage.* New York: Oxford University Press; 2000;168–97.
6. Kleim J. A., Barbay S., Nudo R. J. Functional reorganization of the rat motor cortex following motor skill learning. *J Neurophysiol.* 1998;80:3321–25.

7. Nudo R. J., Milliken G. W., Jenkins W. M., Merzenich M. M. Use-dependent alterations of movement representations in primary motor cortex of adult squirrel monkeys. *J Neurosci* 1996;16:785–807.

8. Kleim J. A., Hogg T. M., VandenBerg P. M., Cooper N. R., Bruneau R., Remple M. Cortical synaptogenesis and motor map reorganization occur during late, but not early, phase of motor skill learning. *J Neurosci* 2004;24(3):628–33.

9. Jones, T. A., Hawrylak, N., Klintsova, A. Y., and Greenough, W. T. Brain damage, behavior, rehabilitation, recovery, and brain plasticity. *Mental Retardation and Developmental Disabilities* 1998;4:231–237.

10. Bury S. D., Jones T. A. Unilateral Sensorimotor Cortex Lesions in Adult Rats Facilitate Motor Skill Learning with the "Unaffected" Forelimb and Training-Induced Dendritic Structural Plasticity in the Motor Cortex. *J Neurosci* 2002;22:8597–606.

11. Jones T. A., Chu C. J., Grande L. A., Gregory A. D. Motor skills training enhances lesion-induced structural plasticity in the motor cortex of adult rats. *J Neurosci* 1999;19:10153–10163.

12. Karni A. The acquisition of perceptual and motor skills: a memory system in the adult human cortex. *Brain Res Cogn* 1996;5:39–48.

13. Shadmehr R., Holcomb H. H. Neural correlates of motor memory consolidation. *Science* 1997;277:821–25.

14. Grafton S. T., Hazeltine E., Ivry R. B. Abstract and effector-specific representations of motor sequences identified with PET *J Neurosci* 1998;18:9420–9428.

15. Squire L. R. Declarative and nondeclarative memory: Multiple brain systems supporting learning and memory. *J Cogn Neurosci* 1992;4:232–43.

16. Squire L. R., Zola S. M. Structure and function of declarative and nondeclarative memory systems. *Proc Natl Acad Sci U S A* 1996;93:13515–22.

17. Willingham D. B., Nissen M. J., Bullemer P. On the development of procedural knowledge. *J Exp Psych: Learn Mem Cog* 1989;15(6):1047–60.

18. Dick M. B., Shankle R. W., Beth R. E., Dick-Muehlke C., Cotman C. W., Kean M. L. Acquisition and long-term retention of a gross motor skill in Alzheimer's disease patients under constant and varied practice conditions. *J Gerontol B Psychol Sci Soc Sci* 1996;51:103–11.

19. Jacobs D. H., Adair J. C., Williamson D. J., Na D. L., Gold M., Foundas A. L. et al. Apraxia and motor-skill acquisition in Alzheimer's disease are dissociable. *Neuropsychologia* 1999;37(7):875–80.

20. Guadagnoli M. A., Leis B., Van Gemmert A. W., Stelmach G. E. The relationship between knowledge of results and motor learning in Parkinsonian patients. *Parkinsonism & Related Disorders* 2002;9(2):89–95.

21. Mochizuki-Kawai H., Kawamura M., Hasegawa Y., Mochizuki S., Oeda R., Yamanaka K. et al. Deficits in long-term retention of learned motor skills in patients with cortical or subcortical degeneration. *Neuropsychologia* 2004;42(13):1858–63.

22. Cavaco S., Anderson S. W., Allen J. S., Castro-Caldas A., Damasio H. The scope of preserved procedural memory in amnesia. *Brain* 2004;127(Pt 8):1853–67.

23. Ewert J., Levin H. S., Watson M. G., Kalisky Z. Procedural memory during posttraumatic amnesia in survivors of severe closed head injury. Implications for rehabilitation. *Arch of Neuro* 1989;46(8):911–6.

24. Mutter S. A., Howard J. H., Jr., Howard D. V. Serial pattern learning after head injury. *J Clin Expl Neuropsych* 1994;16(2):271–88.

25. Sullivan K. J. Functionally distinct learning systems of the brain: Implications for brain injury rehabilitation. *Neurology Report* 1998;22:126–31.

26. Fitts P. M., Posner M. I. *Human Performance.* Belmont, CA: Brooks/Cole, 1967.

27. Schmidt R. A., Lee T. D. *Motor Control and Learning: A Behavioral Emphasis* 3rd ed. Champaign, IL: Human Kinetics Publishers, Inc 1998.

28. Wishart L. R., Lee T. D., Ezekiel H. J., Marley T. L., and Lehto N. K. Applications of motor learning principles: The physiotherapy client as a problem solver I. Concepts. *Physiotherapy Canada* 2000 (Summer), 229–232.

29. Sullivan K. J. Cognitive Rehabilitation. In: Montgomery J., ed. *Physical Therapy for Traumatic Brain Injury.* New York: Churchill Livingstone, Inc 1995;33–54.

30. Winstein C. J., Gardner E. R., McNeal D. R., Barto P. S., Nicholson D. E. Standing balance training: effect on balance and locomotion in hemiparetic adults. *Arch Phys Med Rehabil* 1989;70:755–62.

31. Sullivan K., Knowlton B., Dobkin B. Step training with body weight support: Effect of treadmill speed and practice paradigms on post-stroke locomotor recovery. *Arch Phys Med Rehabil* 2002; 83:683–91.

32. Sherwood D. E., Lee T. D. Schema theory: critical review and implications for the role of cognition in a new theory of motor learning. *Res Q Exerc Sport* 2003;74(4):376–82.

33. Marley T. L., Ezekiel H. J., Lehto N. K., Wishart L. R., and Lee T. D. Application of motor learning principles: The physiotherapy client a problem-solver II. Scheduling practice. *Physiotherapy Canada* 2000 (Fall), 315–319.

34. Chamberlin C., Lee T. D. Arranging Practice Conditions and Designing Instruction. In: Singer R. N., Murphey M., Tennant L. K., eds. *Handbook of Research on Sport Psychology.* New York: Macmillan; 1993;213–41.

35. Shea C. H., Kohl R. M. Specificity and variability of practice. *Res Q Exerc Sport.* 1990;61:169–77.

36. Shea J. B., Morgan R. L. Contextual interference effects on the acquisition, retention, and transfer of a motor skill. *J Exp Psych: Human Learn Mem* 2005;5:179–87.

37. Hall K. G., Magill R. A. Variability of practice and contextual interference in motor skill learning. *J Motor Beh* 1995;27:299–309.

38. Hanlon R. E. Motor learning following unilateral stroke. *Arch Phys Med Rehabil.* 1996;77:811–15.

39. Winstein C. J., Schmidt R. A. Reduced frequency of knowledge of results enhances motor skill learning. *J Exp Psych: Learn Mem Cog* 1990;16:677–91.

40. Ezekiel H. J., Lehto N. K., Marley T. L., Wishart L. R., and Lee T. D. Application of motor learning principles: The physiotherapy client as a problem-solver III. Augmented feedback. *Physiotherapy Canada* (Winter) 2001;33–39.

41. Swanson L. R., Lee T. D. Effects of aging and schedules of knowledge of results on motor learning. *J Ger: Psych Sci* 1992;47:406–11.

42. Behrman A. L., Vander Linden D. W., Cauraugh J. H. Relative frequency of knowledge of results: Older adults learning a force-time modulation task. *J Hum Movement Sci* 2005;37:975–87.

43. Winstein C. J., Merians A. S., Sullivan K. J. Motor learning after unilateral brain damage. *Neuropsychologia* 1999;37:975–87.

44. Thomas D. M., Harro C. C. Effects of relative frequency of knowledge of results on brain injured and control subjects learning a linear positioning task. *Neurology Report* 2005;20:60–62.

45. Winstein C. J., Pohl P. S., Cardinale C., Green A., Scholtz L., Waters C. S. Learning a partial-weight-bearing skill: effectiveness of two forms of feedback *Phys Ther* 1996;76:985–93.

46. Van Peppen R. P. S., Kwakkel, G., Wood-Dauphinee, S., Hendricks H. J. M., Van der Wees P. J., and Dekker J. The impact of physical therapy on functional outcomes after stroke: What's the evidence? *Clin Rehabil* 2004;18:833–862.

47. Bateman A., Culpan F. J., Pickering A. D., Powell J. H., Scott O. M., Greenwood R. J. The effect of aerobic training on rehabilitation outcomes after recent severe brain injury: a randomized controlled evaluation. *Arch Phys Med Rehabil* 2001;82(2):174–82.

48. Bhambhani Y., Rowland G., Farag M. Effects of circuit training on body composition and peak cardiorespiratory responses in patients with moderate to severe traumatic brain injury. *Arch Phys Med Rehabil* 2005;86(2):268–76.

49. Bernstein N. A. The co-ordination and regulation of movements. Oxford: Pergamon Press; 1967.

50. Henry F. M. Specificity vs. generality in learning motor skill. In: Brown R. C., Kenyon G. S., eds. *Classical Studies on Physical Activity.* Englewood Cliffs, NJ: Prentice-Hall; 1968;341–40.

51. Wolf S. L., Lecraw D. E., Barton L. A., Jann B. B. Forced use of hemiplegic upper extremities to reverse the effect of learned nonuse among chronic stroke and head-injured patients. *Exp Neurol.* 1989;104:125–32.

52. Taub E., Wolf S. Constraint induced movement techniques to facilitate upper extremity use in stroke patients. *Topics in Stroke Rehab.* 1997;3:38–61.

53. Winstein C. J., Rose D. K., Tan S. M., Lewthwaite R., Chui H. C., Azen S. P. A randomized controlled comparison of upper-extremity rehabilitation strategies in acute stroke: A pilot study of immediate and long-term outcomes. *Arch Phys Med Rehabil* 2004; 85(4):620–8.

54. Richards C. L., Malouin F., Wood-Dauphinee S., Williams J. I., Bouchard J. P., Brunet D. Task-specific physical therapy for optimization of gait recovery in acute stroke patients. *Arch Phys Med Rehabil.* 1993;74:612–20.

55. Malouin F., Potvin M., Prevost J., Richards C. L., Wood-Dauphinee S. Use of an intensive task-oriented gait training program in a series of patients with acute cerebrovascular accidents. *Phys Ther.* 1992;72:781–89.

56. Visintin M., Barbeau H., Korner-Bitensky N., Mayo N. E. A new approach to retrain gait in stroke patients through body weight support and treadmill stimulation. *Stroke* 1998;29:1122–8.

57. Salbach N. M., Mayo N. E., Wood-Dauphinee S., Hanley J. A., Richards C. L., Cote R. A task-orientated intervention enhances walking distance and speed in the first year post stroke: a randomized controlled trial. *Clin Rehab* 2004;18(5):509–19.

58. Neistadt M. E. The effects of different treatment activities on functional fine motor coordination in adults with brain injury. *Am J Occupational Ther* 1994;48(10):877–82.

59. Giles G. M., Ridley J. E., Dill A., Frye S. A consecutive series of adults with brain injury treated with a washing and dressing retraining program. *Am J Occupational Ther* 1997;51(4):256–66.

60. Page S., Levine P. Forced use after TBI: promoting plasticity and function through practice. *Brain Injury* 2003;17(8):675–84.

61. Wilson D. J., Swaboda J. L. Partial weight-bearing gait retraining for persons following traumatic brain injury: preliminary report and proposed assessment scale. *Brain Injury* 2002;16(3):259–68.

62. Lord J. P., Hall K. Neuromuscular reeducation versus traditional programs for stroke rehabilitation. *Arch Phys Med Rehabil* 1986; 67(2):88–91.

63. Hesse S., Bertelt C., Jahnke M. T., Schaffrin A., Baake P., Malezic M. et al. Treadmill training with partial body weight support compared with physiotherapy in nonambulatory hemiparetic patients. *Stroke* 1995;26:976–81.

64. Langhammer B., Stanghelle J. K. Bobath or motor relearning programme? A comparison of two different approaches of physiotherapy in stroke rehabilitation: a randomized controlled study. *Clin Rehab* 2004;14(4):361–9.

65. Nudo, R. J., Plautz, E. J., and Milliken, G. W. Adaptive plasticity in primate motor cortex as a consequence of behavioral experience and neuronal injury. *Seminars in Neruosci* 1997;9:13–23.

66. Jones T. A., Chu C. J., Grande L. A., Gregory A. D. Motor skills training enhances lesion-induced structural plasticity in the motor cortex of adult rats. *J Neurosci* 1999;19:10153–63.

67. Liepert J., Bauder H., Wolfgang H. R., Miltner W. H., Taub E., Weiller C. Treatment-induced cortical reorganization after stroke in humans. *Stroke* 2000;31:1210–1216.

68. Koski L., Mernar T. J., Dobkin B. H. Immediate and long-term changes in corticomotor output in response to rehabilitation: correlation with functional improvements in chronic stroke. *Neurorehab Neural Repair* 2004;18(4):230–49.

69. Sullivan K. J., Dobkin B. H., Tavakol M., Davis B., Knowlton B. J., Harkema S. J. Post-stroke cortical plasticity induced by step training. *Society for Neuroscience Proceedings* 2001.

70. Dobkin B. H., Firestine A., West M., Saremi K., Woods R. Ankle dorsiflexion as an fMRI paradigm to assay motor control for walking during rehabilitation. *Neuroimage* 2004;23:370–381.

71. Kwakkel G., Wagenaar R. C., Twisk J. W., Lankhorst G. J., Koetsier J. C. Intensity of leg and arm training after primary middle-cerebral-artery stroke: a randomised trial. *Lancet* 1999;354: 191–96.

72. Kwakkel G. P., van Peppen R. M. P., Wagenaar R. C. P., Dauphinee S. W. P. P., Richards C. P., Ashburn A. P. et al. Effects of Augmented Exercise Therapy Time After Stroke: A Meta-Analysis. *Stroke* 2004;35:2529–36.

73. Eng J. J., Rowe S. J., McLaren L. M. Mobility status during inpatient rehabilitation: a comparison of patients with stroke and traumatic brain injury. *Arch Phys Med Rehabil* 2002;83(4):483–90.

74. Cifu D. X., Kreutzer J. S., Kolakowsky-Hayner S. A., Marwitz J. H., Englander J. The relationship between therapy intensity and rehabilitative outcomes after traumatic brain injury : a multicenter analysis. *Arch Phys Med Rehabil* 2003;84(10):1441–8.

75. Sullivan K., Knowlton B., Dobkin B. Step training with body weight support: Effect of treadmill speed and practice paradigms on poststroke locomotor recovery. *Arch Phys Med Rehabil* 2002; 83:683–91.

76. Pohl M. M. Speed-dependent treadmill training in ambulatory hemiparetic stroke patients: a randomized controlled trial. *Stroke* 2002;33(2):553–8.

77. Lamontagne A., Fung J. Faster is better: implications for speed-intensive gait training after stroke. *Stroke* 2004;35(11):2543–8.

78. Moseley A. M., Stark A., Cameron I. D., Pollock A. *Cochrane Database of Systematic Reviews* 2005.

79. Quinn L., Gordon J. *Functional Outcomes: Documentation for Rehabilitation.* St. Louis: Saunders;2003.

80. Hagen C., Malkmus D., Durham P. *Levels of cognitive functioning. Rehabilitation of the Head Injured Adult: Comprehensive Management.* Downey, C. A. : Rancho Los Amigos Hospital; 1979.

81. Blanton S., Porter L., Smith D., Wolf S. L. Strategies to Enhance Mobility in Traumatic Brain Injured Patients. In: Rosenthal M., Griggith E. R., Kreutzer J. S., Pentland B., eds. *Rehabilitation of the Adult and Child with Brain Injury* 3rd ed. Philadelphia: F.A. Davis Company; 1999;219–41.

82. Lombardi F., Taricco M., De Tanti A., Telaro E., Liberati A. *Cochrane Database of Systematic Reviews.* 2005.

83. Katz D. I., Alexander M. P., Klein R. B. Recovery of arm function in patients with paresis after traumatic brain injury. *Arch Phys Med Rehabil* 1998;79(5):488–93.

84. Saper C. B. Brain Stem Modulation of Sensation, Movement, and Conciousness. In: Kandel E. R., Schwartz J. H., Jessell T. M., eds. *Principles of Neural Science* 4th ed. New York: McGraw-Hill; 2000;889–909.

85. Jorgensen H. S., Nakayama H., Raaschou H. O., Vive-Larsen J., Stoier M., Olsen T. S. Outcome and time course of recovery in stroke. Part II: Time course of recovery. The Copenhagen Stroke Study. Arch Phys Med Rehabil. *Arch Phys Med Rehabil* 1995;76:406–12.

86. Gill-Body K. M., Giorgetti M. M. Acute Care and Prognostic Outcome. In: Montgomery J, ed. *Physical Therapy for Traumatic Brain Injury.* New York: Churchill-Livingstone, Inc; 1995;1–31.

87. Gowland C., Gambarotto C. A. Assessment and Treatment of Physical Impairments Leading to Disability after Brain Injury. In: Finlayson M. A. J., Garner S. H., eds. *Brain injury rehabilitation: Clinical considerations.* Baltimore: Williams & Wilkins;1994;102–23.

88. Fisher B. E., Woll S. Consideration in the Restoration of Motor Control. In: Montgomery J, ed. *Physical Therapy for Traumatic Brain Injury.* New York: Churchill-Livingston, Inc 1995;55–78.

89. Winkler P. Head Injury. In: Umphred D. A., ed. *Neurological Rehabilitation* 3rd ed. Philadelphia: Mosby 1995;421–767.

90. Shumway-Cook A., Woolcott M. H. Motor Control: Theory and Practical Application. 2nd ed. Baltimore: Williams & Wilkins;2001.

91. Bobath B. *Adult Hemiplegia: Evaluation and Treatment* 3rd ed. London: William Hinneman Medical Books; 1990.

92. Knott M., Voss D. E. *Proprioceptive neuromuscular facilitation* 2nd ed. New York: Harper and Row; 1968.

93. Brunnstrom S. *Movement therapy in hemiplegia.* New York: Harper & Row; 1970.

94. Gordon J. Assumptions Underlying Physical Therapy Intervention: Theoretical and Historical Perspectives. In: Carr J. H., Shepherd R. B., Gordon J., Gentile A. M., Held J. M., eds. *Movement Science: Foundations for Physical Therapy in Rehabilitation.* Rockville, M. D. : Aspen Publishers, Inc 1987;1–30.

95. Latash M. L., Anson J. G. What are "normal movements" in atypical populations? *Behavior Brain Sci* 1996;19:55–106.

96. Mayer N. H. Clinicophysiologic concepts of spasticity and motor dysfunction in adults with an upper motoneuron lesion. *Muscle & Nerve* 1997; Supplement 6:S1–13.

97. Pierson S. H. Outcome measures in spasticity management. *Muscle & Nerve* 1997; Supplement 6:S36–60.

98. Elovic E. P., Simone L. K., Zafonte R. Outcome assessment for spasticity management in the patient with traumatic brain injury: the state of the art. *J Head Trauma Rehabil* 2004;155–77.

99. Childers M. K., Brashear A., Jozefczyk P., Reding M., Alexander D., Good D. et al. Dose-dependent response to intramuscular botulinum toxin type A for upper-limb spasticity in patients after a stroke. *Arch Phys Med Rehabil* 2004;85(7):1063–9.

100. Pittock S. J., Moore A. P., Hardiman O., Ehler E., Kovac M., Bojakowski J. et al. A double-blind randomised placebo-controlled evaluation of three doses of botulinum toxin type A (Dysport) in the treatment of spastic equinovarus deformity after stroke. *Cerebrovascular Diseases* 2003;15(4):289–300.

101. Gill-Body K. M. Current concepts in the management of patients with vestibular dysfunction. *PT Magazine* 2001;39–58.

102. Greenwald B. D., Cifu D. X., Marwitz J. H., Enders L. J., Brown A. W., Englander J. S. et al. Factors associated with balance deficits on admission to rehabilitation after traumatic brain injury: a multicenter analysis. *J Head Trauma Rehabil* 2001;16(3):238–52.

103. Chamelian L., Feinstein A. Outcome after mild to moderate traumatic brain injury: the role of dizziness. *Arch Phys Med Rehabil* 2004;85(10):1662–6.

104. Whitney S. L., Hudak M. T., Marchetti G. F. The dynamic gait index relates to self-reported fall history in individuals with vestibular dysfunction. *J Vest Research* 2000;10(2):99–105.

105. Herdman S. J., Schubert M. C., Tusa R. J. Strategies for balance rehabilitation: fall risk and treatment. *Annals of the New York Academy of Sciences* 2001;942:394–412.

106. Hall C. D., Schubert M. C., Herdman S. J. Prediction of fall risk reduction as measured by dynamic gait index in individuals with unilateral vestibular hypofunction. *Otology & Neurology* 2004;25(5):746–51.

107. Herdman S. J., Blatt P. J., Schubert M. C. Vestibular rehabilitation of patients with vestibular hypofunction or with benign paroxysmal positional vertigo. *Current Opinion in Neurology* 2000;13(1):39–43.

108. Herdman S. J. *Vestibular Rehabilitation*. 2nd ed. Philadelphia: FA Davis, Co. 2000.

109. Mayer N. H., Esquenazi A., Childers M. K. Common patterns of clinical motor dysfunction. *Muscle & Nerve* 1997; Supplement 6:S21–35.

110. Anderson D. Management of Decreased ROM from Overactive Musculature and Hetertopic Ossification. In: Montgomery J, ed. *Physical Therapy for Traumatic Brain Injury.* New York: Churchill-Livingstone, Inc 1995;79–99.

111. Zhang L. Q., Chung S. G., Bai Z., Xu D., van Rey E. M., Rogers M. W. et al. Intelligent stretching of ankle joints with contracture/spasticity. *IEEE Transactions on Neural Systems & Rehabilitation Engineering* 2002;10(3):149–57.

112. Singer B. J., Dunne J. W., Singer K. P., Jegasothy G. M., Allison G. T. Non-surgical management of ankle contracture following acquired brain injury. *Disability Rehabil* 2004;26(6):335–45.

113. Singer B. J., Jegasothy G. M., Singer K. P., Allison G. T. Evaluation of serial casting to correct equinovarus deformity of the ankle after acquired brain injury in adults. *Arch Phys Med Rehabil* 2003;84(4):483–91.

114. Mortenson P. A., Eng J. J. The use of casts in the management of joint mobility and hypertonia following brain injury in adults: a systematic review. *Phys Ther* 2003;83(7):648–58.

115. Lannin N. A., Horsley S. A., Herbert R., McCluskey A., Cusick A. Splinting the hand in the functional position after brain impairment: a randomized, controlled trial. *Arch Phys Med Rehabil* 2003;84(2):297–302.

116. Blanton S., Grissom S. P., Riolo L. Use of a static adjustable ankle-foot orthosis following tibial nerve block to reduce plantar-flexion contracture in an individual with brain injury. *Phys Ther* 2002;82(11):1087–97.

117. Meythaler J. M., Guin-Renfroe S., Grabb P., Hadley M. N. Long-term continuously infused intrathecal baclofen for spastic-dystonic hypertonia in traumatic brain injury: 1-year experience *Arch Phys Med Rehabil* 1999;80(1):13–9.

118. Bhambhani Y., Rowland G., Farag M. Reliability of peak cardiorespiratory responses in patients with moderate to severe traumatic brain injury. *Arch Phys Med Rehabil* 2003;84(11):1629–36.

119. Convertino V. A., Bloomfield S. A., Greenleaf J. E. An overview of the issues: physiological effects of bed rest and restricted physical activity. *Med Sci Sports Exerc* 1997;29(2):187–90.

120. Bloomfield S. A. Changes in musculoskeletal structure and function with prolonged bed rest. *Med Sci Sports Exerc* 1997;29(2):197–206.

121. Taub E. Movement in nonhuman primates deprived of somatosensory feedback. *Exerc & Sport Sci Reviews* 1976;4:335–74.

122. Nudo R. J., Wise B. M., SiFuentes F., Milliken G. W. Neural substrates for the effects of rehabilitative training on motor recovery after ischemic infarct *Science* 1996;272:1791–94.

123. Wolf S. L., Lecraw D. E., Barton L. A., Jann B. B. Forced use of hemiplegic upper extremities to reverse the effect of learned nonuse among chronic stroke and head-injured patients. *Exp Neurol* 1989;104:125–32.

124. Taub E., Miller N. E., Novack T. A., Cook E. W. d., Fleming W. C., Nepomuceno C. S. et al. Technique to improve chronic motor deficit after stroke. *Arch Phys Med Rehabil* 1993;74:347–54.

125. Winstein C. J., Miller J. P., Blanton S., Taub E., Uswatte G., Morris D. et al. Methods for a multisite randomized trial to investigate the effect of constraint-induced movement therapy in improving upper extremity function among adults recovering from a cerebrovascular stroke. *Neurorehabilitation & Neural Repair* 2003;17(3):137–52.

126. Wolf S. L., Lecraw D. E., Barton L. A., Jann B. B. Forced used of hemiplegic upper extremities to reverse the effect of learned nonuse among chronic stroke and healthy injured patients. *Exp Neurology* 1989;104:125–32.

127. Taub E., Miller N. E., Novack T. A., Cook E. W., III, Fleming W. C., Nepomuceno C. S. et al. Technique to improve chronic motor deficit after stroke. *Arch Phys Med Rehabil* 1993;74:347–54.

128. Blanton S., Wolf S. L. An application of upper-extremity constraint-induced movement therapy in a patient with subacute stroke. *Phys Ther* 1999;79(9):847–53.

129. Page S. J., Sisto S. A., Levine P. Modified constraint-induced therapy in chronic stroke. *Am J Phys Med Rehabil* 2002;81(11):870–5.

130. Page S. J., Sisto S. A., Levine P., Johnston M. V., Hughes M. Modified constraint induced therapy: a randomized feasibility and efficacy study. *J Rehabil Res Dev* 2001;38(5):583–90.

131. Barbeau H., Rossignol S. Recovery of locomotion after chronic spinalization in the adult cat. *Brain Res* 1987;412:84–95.

132. de Leon R. D., Hodgson J. A., Roy R. R., Edgerton V. R. Locomotor capacity attributable to step training versus spontaneous recovery after spinalization in adult cats. *J Neurophysiol* 1998;79:1329–40.

133. Lovely R. G., Gregor R. J., Roy R. R., Edgerton V. R. Effects of training on the recovery of full-weight-bearing stepping in the adult spinal cat. *Exp Neurol* 1986;92:421–35.

134. Finch L., Barbeau H., Arsenault B. Influence of body weight support on normal human gait: development of a gait retraining strategy. *Phys Ther* 1991;71:842–55.

135. Behrman A. L., Harkema S. J. Locomotor training after human spinal cord injury: a series of case studies. *Phys Ther* 2000;80:688–700.

136. Harkema S. J., Hurley S. L., Patel U. K., Requejo P. S., Dobkin B. H., Edgerton V. R. Human lumbosacral spinal cord interprets loading during stepping. *J Neurophysiol* 1997;77:797–811.

137. Barbeau H. Locomotor training in neurorehabilitation: emerging rehabilitation concepts. *Neurorehabilitation & Neural Repair* 2003;17(1):3–11.

138. Barbeau H., Fung J. The role of rehabilitation in the recovery of walking in the neurological population. *Current Opinion in Neurology* 2001;14(6):735–40.

139. Dobkin B. H. Overview of treadmill locomotor training with partial body weight support: A neurophysiologically sound approach whose time has come for randomized clinical trials. *Neurorehabilitation and Repair* 1999;13:157–65.

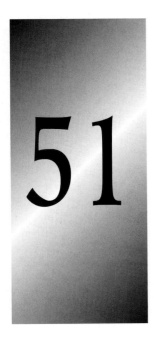

51 Therapy for Activities of Daily Living: Theoretical and Practical Perspectives

Robin McNeny

THERORETICAL PERSPECTIVES: FOCUS ON ADL ASSESSMENT AND INTERVENTION

Activities of Daily Living as Human Occupations

The term "activities of daily living" was first introduced by a physical therapist in 1949 as part of a published checklist she designed to assess her patient's performance of daily living tasks (1). Humans engage in activities of daily living in order to maintain themselves, create an outlet for self-expression, fulfill roles, and to bring meaning into their lives. Occupational therapists regard these activities as "human occupations". As Fisher says *occupation* is the "action of seizing, taking possession of, or occupying space or time" (2). Therefore occupation is about doing and therapy directed toward resumption of occupational tasks is significant as it enables "people to perform the actions they need and want to perform so that they can engage in and 'do' the familiar, ordinary, goal-directed activities of every day in a manner that brings meaning and personal satisfaction" (3).

Engagement in occupation is vital to the human spirit and to health (4). Through engagement in occupation, we become competent. Engagement in occupation begins at birth and continues throughout the life span. Occupations are ordered around routines and patterns for living. Humans learn about and make adaptive responses to their world through the pursuit of occupation. Humans bring rhythm to life as they engage in ordinary tasks through the course of days and weeks. This rhythm set within the appropriate context brings healthy balance to life. Healthy rhythm and balance includes involvement in what Adolph Meyer refers to as the "big four": work, play, rest and sleep (5). These four areas of occupation form the core of human activity.

Assessment of and intervention for impairments in occupational performance are based on a view that clients are occupational beings. Because each person possesses an "occupational identity", each person has a life centered on personal values, interests and roles. While values, interests and roles are abstract, occupational identity is concretely expressed through doing (6). Participation in everyday occupations develops skills, promotes competence, establishes connections with others, expands one's sense of belonging and community while giving meaning and purpose to life (7).

Capturing the depth and meaning of ordinary daily tasks within the culture and context of an individual's life is a central concept of occupation as a scientific guide to practice. Insight into the client's culture and context for living are fundamental to an understanding of the client's occupations. Because American clinicians are often entrenched in westernized middle-class culture, we have a tendency to view clients through that cultural bias (8). Modern rehabilitationists are challenged to analyze more deeply the "whys" and "hows" behind the readily observed actions of our clients as they perform activities of daily living. Such an analysis helps the clinician understand the meaning the individual client assigns to the tasks the client chooses to do.

Areas of Occupation

Clinicians practicing in acute rehabilitation settings usually focus on two areas of occupation: self care skills, often called personal activities of daily living (PADL's) and independent living skills, referred to as instrumental ADL's (IADL's). Occupations focused on work and play, while important, are usually addressed later in the continuum of care. PADL's include tasks commonly performed as part of a daily routine: feeding, dressing, grooming, toileting, bathing and transfers. More individual characterization and variation are found in IADL's. However, we do a disservice to our clients when we narrow the focus of the therapy program to a mere set of ADL's. Such a restricted focus minimizes the complexity and richness of occupational performance.

Brain injury interrupts life. Abruptly an individual loses his or her place in the world. Roles are disrupted. Rhythm and balance are lost. The capacity to engage in meaningful tasks is restricted. Occupational identity is shaken if not totally lost. The capacity to "do" is flawed or perhaps totally absent. Where once there was routine, now there is chaos. Where once there was satisfaction and meaning, now there is confusion. Suddenly participation in life becomes toil. In occupational therapy, the client engages in the process of "relocation of self" where skills required to resume essential life roles are taught (4).

To set the proper stage for this relocation process, the occupational therapist conducts a client-centered assessment of occupational performance. Law (7) states that each person "has unique interests and occupations through which they find satisfaction". A client-centered assessment defines the client's occupations while simultaneously determining how the brain injury has affected participation in valued activities. A well-conducted client-centered assessment provides the foundation for a client-centered treatment plan designed to promote occupational performance and in turn, health.

ASSESSING OCCUPATIONAL PERFORMANCE

Focusing the Assessment

Fisher (9) defines assessment as "a process of collecting, organizing and interpreting the relevant information that is necessary to plan and implement a meaningful, effective program of treatment". Trombly recommends a "top-down" evaluative approach (10) where the first stage of assessment is exploration of the client's occupational performance issues.

Clinicians have access to a plethora of ADL assessment tools that "score" an individual's performance on PADL's and in some cases, IADL's: the Klein-Bell Scale (11), the Barthel Index (12), the Kenny Self-Care Evaluation (13), the Assessment of Motor and Process Skills (14), the A-One Evaluation (15), the Canadian Occupational Performance Measure (16), the Allen Cognitive Test (17), Rabideau Kitchen Evaluation (18) and the Kohlman Evaluation of Living Skills (19). Table 51-1 explores some of these ADL assessment tools in greater depth.

Many clinicians employ "homemade" ADL checklists in their practices rather than using published checklists and assessments. These facility-developed evaluations are compatible with the program's focus and mission. Many are derived from the Functional Independence Measure (20) commonly used by rehabilitation teams as a comprehensive tool for functional assessment of PADL's and IADL's.

The advantage of using a standardized and reliable tool for assessment of ADL's is the ability to retest the client's performance over time, regardless of the testing environment. Communication between clinicians along the continuum of care is clearer when the same evaluative tool is used to assess performance. Improvements in ADL performance are apparent and reliable. However, standardized assessments often take longer to administer and to score. Though clinically important information is gained from assessments such as the AMPS and A-One, clinicians feel they lack the time to devote to such thorough, occupationally oriented evaluations.

With so many assessments available for use, clinicians must identify the goal of the ADL evaluation before selecting an assessment tool. The evaluation might have a descriptive purpose. That is, the therapist chooses to assess the client's ADL performance at a given moment in time to describe the degree of impairment and need for therapy intervention. The evaluation could have a predictive purpose where the clinician ascertains through ADL performance the patient's capacity to live alone, function in the community or support primary life roles. The ADL evaluation also might serve an evaluative purpose where the clinician documents progress in performance over the course of time (1, 21). Clearly some ADL assessments are better for descriptive assessment and others more appropriate for predictive assessment. Law and Letts provide a thoughtful, comprehensive comparison of 13 ADL assessments in their paper which may serve as a guide for assessment tool selection (21).

Undoubtedly, there is more to the assessment of activities of daily living than simply scoring patient's performance using an ordinal scale. Though the scales and measures available for the rehabilitation clinician and

TABLE 51-1

ASSESSMENT	POPULATION	STANDARDIZATION	COMMENTS
Klein-Bell ADL Scale	Adults in a rehabilitation program	Good	Test-retest reliability is good; content validity is very good; lengthy evaluation to administer
Barthel Index	Adults in a rehabilitation program	Good	Test-retest reliability and content validity are excellent; lengthy to administer
Kenny Self-Care Evaluation	General adult rehabilitation	Good	Test-retest reliability poor; content validity is good; lengthy to administer
Assessment of Motor and Process Skills	A variety of populations; a school version is available and studies continue assessing the use of AMPS with different cultures	Good	Reliable and valid; can be individualized to the patient's occupations; new test items are being evaluated to expand utility of assessment
The A-One Evaluation	Adults with neurobehavioral impairment	Good	Reliable and valid however certification in the interpretation of the evaluation is recommended; can be administered during the course of routine ADL's
Canadian Occupational Performance Measure	Variety of ages and populations	Good	Reliable and valid; intended for use as an outcome measure; allows clinician to focus on client's goals
The Allen Cognitive Test	Adults with psychiatric diagnoses; some work has been done with adults with brain injury	Good	Based on Allen's Cognitive Theory, the instrument is reliable and valid but training in testing procedure and interpretation is recommended
Rabideau Kitchen Evaluation	Adults with rehabilitation diagnoses	Non-standardized	Face validity; good inter-rated reliability; provides standard way to evaluate patient performance on kitchen tasks
Kohlman Evaluation of Living Skills	Adults and adolescents, including adults with brain injury	Good	Reliable and valid; useful in determining client safety in the home/ community

*more in-depth analysis is available in *A Critical Review of Scales of Activities of Daily Living* by Law and Letts (21).

team quantify and objectify the client's performance, a thorough assessment of ADL's requires clinicians to analyze the full spectrum of the patient's performance. The best assessment begins with an understanding of the client as an occupational being, therefore the occupational profile interview is a proper starting point.

The Occupational Profile

The occupational profile is a semi-structured interview conducted with the client to determine the client's roles, habits, interests, values and to confirm the client's goals for the rehabilitative process. Frequently, after a brain injury, the client is unable to reliably provide information for the occupational profile due to disorientation, cognitive deficits, language impairments or behavioral issues. In such situations, the clinician should interview family or close friends to gather this vital information.

The occupational profile promotes an understanding of the client (6). Following the interview, the clinician is able to answer the following important questions about the client:

- How does my client describe himself?
- How do my client's occupations define and maintain her identity?
- In what ways does my client's engagement in occupations allow for self-expression?
- What are my client's goals given her present disability and how do they relate to her occupations?

The occupational profile consolidates information on the client's environment, daily routine, educational achievement, social support system as well as primary areas of interest. This data defines the patient's and/ or significant other's goals for rehabilitation. These stated goals become primary drivers for the treatment planning process yet to come.

Assessing Performance in Areas of Occupation

The assessment of occupational performance involves analytically watching clients "do", utilizing what Padilla, Barrett and Walker have identified as "mindful observation" (8). In the intensive care setting where persons with brain injury usually are dependent in ADL's, the therapist assesses the client's PADL's while managing potential complications to minimize or eliminate the impact on later occupational performance. The OT working in the ICU monitors range of motion, muscle tone and provides splints and positioners as needed to prevent deformity and contracture. Often the occupational and physical therapists conduct co-evaluations in the ICU. As the patient improves and begins in-patient rehabilitation, the OT assesses the client's performance of relevant PADL's. Information from the occupational profile provided by the client or family guide the performance evaluation process. Assessment begins with PADL's of greatest value and priority to the client and family. As therapy continues in day rehabilitation and outpatient therapy, the OT assessment of ADL performance is refined to focus on higher level skills to promote maximal independence in the home and community. Through the continuum of rehabilitation, occupational therapists, as "experts in occupation", analyze the methods used by their clients to complete ADL tasks (1). The therapists discern whether observed errors are attributable to problems in range of motion, strength, coordination, balance, visual-perceptual function or executive skills and use this information to design treatment programs.

As clients transition from the hospital setting into the community, the therapist broadens the assessment of occupational performance. The home health occupational therapist has the benefit of assessing the client in his natural environment, which allows the therapist to ascertain the effects of the natural environment, culture, and support network on performance (1). Some studies suggest that assessment performed in a client's natural environment provides the most accurate picture of ADL performance (22). Because assessment in the out-patient setting occurs in a clinical environment, the clinician must listen carefully to the client and family's descriptions of specific ADL performance carried out at home in order to identify areas of performance breakdown or client/family concern.

Several of the evaluation tools previously mentioned comprehensively assess occupational performance, rather than just ADL skills. Use of these assessments enhances the clinician's insight into the meaning, function and form of occupational performance for the individual client while elucidating performance components that influence performance (6). The Canadian Occupational Performance Measure (16) assesses self-maintenance, productivity and leisure roles with an eye to those areas that the client regards as valuable and meaningful. The Assessment of Motor and Process Skills (14) guides the clinician's observation of the client as he engages in tasks of his choice selected from an extensive list of varied occupations. During the course of task performance, the clinician identifies the motor or process skills that facilitate or impede task performance. The Arnadottir OT-ADL Neurobehavioral Evaluation (15), clinically known as the A-One, aids the clinician's detection of potential neurobehavioral deficits that are impacting the quality of or completion of occupational task performance. Use of any of these occupationally-based assessment tools gives the clinician a fuller appreciation of the client's occupational performance assets and impairments while promoting a more holistic and hearty assessment than that which is available through a simple ADL checklist.

Best Practice Methods for Assessing Occupational Performance

The use of real versus simulated tasks during the assessment process is an important consideration. Simulated assessments lack the influence of context, which may shape, either positively or negatively, a client's performance. Occupational performance is influenced by the context surrounding the occupation itself. Context includes physical elements such as the physical environment, the area's topography or even the level of lighting or noise. Spiritual context involves the client's sense of a higher being and purpose to life, both of which contribute to motivation and the inspiration to "do". Temporal context, such as the time of year or a stage in life, have bearing on task selection and performance. A homemaker doing a cooking evaluation three days before Thanksgiving may engage with greater motivation in the preparation of apple pies for her family dinner than she would in the preparation of a soup-and-sandwich lunch for herself using a menu planned by her therapist (23). Context is an inescapable part of the assessment process.

Simulated activities as a form of assessment, while not ideal, are necessary in many clinical settings. Clinicians working in hospitals may employ several strategies to improve the quality of simulated assessments. Through interviews, clinicians may obtain detailed information about the client's home environment and insert as many of these features as possible into the assessment. For example, the therapist might learn that the client's bedroom contains a low chair routinely used for dressing. During the dressing assessment, the clinician utilizes a chair of the same height to determine the effect of sitting on a lower surface during dressing. Some OT kitchens have moveable islands that allow therapists to configure the kitchen as similarly as possible to the client's home. If the patient plans to use a regular bed at home, the therapist should perform all bed-related assessments with the hospital bed flat and the rails down. Real coins and bills improve the quality of money management skills assessment. Provision of the client's own grooming tools and supplies in the bag or container used at home enhances the physical context of the task.

Assessing Client Factors that Affect Performance

At times, therapists find it necessary to assess specific components of functional performance further to identify the nature of or severity of an underlying problem. Known as client factors, these components are peculiar to the individual client and play a role in the client's ability to perform functional tasks. Client factors include mental functions, sensory functions, neuromusculoskeletal and movement-related functions, visual and speech functions. Table 51-2 provides some examples of client factors (23). Perhaps the therapist notices while assessing bathing that the client cannot reach her lower back. A specific evaluation of the client's upper extremity range of motion and strength reveals that though her shoulder range of motion is within normal limits, her antigravity strength is insufficient to support washing her lower back. In another case, during an assessment of a client's self-feeding skills, the clinician notices that the client over-reaches for her milk carton, closes one eye when scooping food with her fork and sometimes closes both eyes when chewing. A quick assessment of ocular alignment reveals a diplopia that is interfering with the client's comfort and precision during PADL's.

TABLE 51-2
Examples of Client Factors

Mental functions	Level of arousal, orientation, personality, motivation, attention, visual-perceptual function, judgment, mathematical calculations, motor planning
Sensory functions	visual acuity, hearing, balance, taste, smell, tactile discrimination, pain
Neuromusculoskeletal and movement-related functions	range of motion, mobility, strength, muscle tone, reflexive responses, eye-hand coordination, tics and tremors, ability to ambulate
Skin and related structure functions	skin integrity including the presence of wounds

---

Formal testing of client factors, such as visual-perceptual or memory assessments, is based upon an assumption that there is a relationship between the factor being tested and the client's ability to perform the daily living task (9). Tests such as the Toglia Cognitive Assessment (TCA) (24), the Lowenstein Occupational Therapy Cognitive Assessment (25) and the Contextual Memory Test (26) are used to assess client factors. Researchers continue to seek evidence of a correlation between tests such as these and occupational performance (27).

The complete occupational performance assessment provides a picture of the client's occupations within context, an understanding of the client's and/or significant other's goals for the therapy process as well as information on impairments in client factors that limit overall performance. Armed with a good assessment, the clinician proceeds to plan treatment to promote the client's relocation of self, all the while keeping the client's priorities and goals for the treatment process in mind.

GOAL SETTING STRATEGIES

In times past, health care providers paternalistically offered advice and treatment to clients to remediate their conditions or symptoms. This advice and the prescribed intervention was offered with the client's best interests in mind. In most cases, clients accepted the health care provider's advice and treatment without question, believing that the health care provider knew best. Whatever priorities the health care provider set were "fine"– even if they didn't match the client's own priorities.

Times have changed. Now individuals receiving medical services are more informed, more involved in decision-making and more vocal about their preferences. Client-centered goal setting is now routine in many health care settings. Major health care accrediting agencies, such as JCAHO and CARF, require evidence of the client's and significant others' input into the goal-setting process. Current research demonstrates that client-identified goals yield the best therapy outcomes. Therefore, goal setting with the client and caregiver is an integral part of the rehabilitative process. Often goals identified by clients and especially by caregivers focus on areas which, if improved, make return to home and care in the home easier. Those clients who initially are unable to state their rehabilitation goals must be given the chance to provide input once able (28). At times, clients set lofty long-term goals, such as driving, returning to school or work or staying home alone. In such situations, the clinician works with the client to outline realistic and attainable short-term goals, never losing sight of the client's long-term goals.

Once ADL-related treatment goals are set, intervention focuses on the client's ability "to do" (29). A well-defined treatment goal integrates the client's expressed

---

TABLE 51-3
Examples of Goal with Qualifiers

Patient will place arms in sleeves of shirt with moderate assist while sitting in wheelchair.

Patient will calculate money up to $2.00 in coins with 40% accuracy.

Patient will bring washcloth to face with maximal assistance.

Patient will prepare shopping list for a simple breakfast using a planned menu, with minimal assist.

Patient will complete entire morning grooming routine in 30 minutes with supervision.

Each of these areas of consideration are important and should be kept in mind during the treatment process.

---

skills and desires with the environmental context in which the client functions. The treatment program includes tasks, activities, and instruction to meet these goals. As Baum et al. says so well: "The unique contribution of occupational therapy is to maximize the fit between what the person wants and needs to do and his or her capability to do it" (1).

Well-formulated treatment goals are functional, measurable, specific, clear to the reader and reflective of the client's priorities. Achievement of treatment objectives is easily determined when goals are written well. Goal qualifiers enhance both the specificity and the achievability of treatment goals. Goal qualifiers may include quantifiable measures such as the frequency with which a task is performed, the rate of accuracy achieved during performance, the setting in which a task is performed, or the number of rest breaks required during task performance. Table 51-3 lists several different types of goal qualifiers.

As treatment goals are achieved, the clinician in collaboration with the client sets new functional goals. New areas of occupational performance are introduced into the treatment program as the client demonstrates readiness for engagement in advanced tasks. Good communication between clinicians about goal achievement and the client's goal priorities as the client progresses through the continuum of care facilitates progression of the treatment plan.

The clinician may employ one of several strategies to solicit client involvement in the goal setting and goal progression process. Team conferences that include clients and families provide a forum for the entire team to review progress and establish treatment priorities. A review of treatment goals by clinicians at the beginning of each treatment session gives the treatment session focus. Memory notebooks may include a section devoted to mapping treatment goals. One recent study recommended the use of a "goal notebook" to improve clinician-client discussions and to remind both the client and the clinician about active treatment goals (30).

ADL INTERVENTION: BRINGING MEANING BACK TO LIFE

Improving Personal Activities of Daily Living

Personal activities of daily living (PADL) include bathing, bowel and bladder management, dressing, eating, hygiene and grooming and functional mobility (23). Each person performs PADL's in personally unique and individually customized sequences. Clients with severe brain injury frequently experience limits on their ability to perform these most basic and familiar tasks (31). Many factors contribute to deficits in self-care performance, including impaired function of the upper and lower extremities, cognitive deficits, visual-perceptual impairments, communication impairments and behavioral problems.

The comprehensive PADL treatment program provides retraining opportunities that incorporate multiple considerations associated with PADL performance. These parameters include:

1. the *context* in which the tasks are performed
2. the client's *habits and routines* related to task performance
3. *safety* during performance of tasks
4. the efficacy of *adaptive devices and compensatory techniques*
5. *interdisciplinary team involvement*, including the caregivers
6. the client's ability to *self-monitor and correct errors*

Knowledge of *context* related to PADL's performance is critical. Cultural context influences the client's choice of attire, food choices and grooming preferences. Knowledge of the physical context in which PADL's are performed helps the clinician design strategies to overcome architectural barriers, such as inaccessible bathrooms or out-of-reach clothes closets. An awareness of context helps eliminate the imposition of the therapist's values on the client. For example, the therapist might insist during treatment that the client place the dinner napkin in his lap during meals only to discover that the client and his family always keep napkins, as well as their elbows, on the table during meals. Treatment programs must be contextually relevant or they are ultimately of little value to the client.

PADL's are habit-driven. *Habits* are "automatic behavior that is integrated into more complex patterns" which facilitate daily performance of self-care (23). PADL's are so habitual that most people proceed through morning and evening self-care tasks without much conscious thought. It is helpful to the retraining program to know the client's pre-injury habits (32). Knowledge of pre-injury habits helps the clinician formulate a treatment program that draws upon familiar patterns of behavior that may hasten skill competence. Did the client put socks on before or after trousers? Did the client shower in the morning or evening? Was moisturizer used under makeup? Sometimes clients serve as the source of this information. However, if the client cannot provide information regarding pre-injury habits, the clinician needs to obtain this information from families. Unfortunately, because many PADL's are performed privately, families may have limited insight into the client's pre-injury habits.

The motor, cognitive, behavior and visual-perceptual sequelae common after brain injury often make performance of some PADL's risky. *Safety* is a primary concern for the clinician. Clients with dysphagia require assistance or supervision for self-feeding. Clients with balance problems may not be able to safely stand during self-dressing. Problems with incoordination, muscle weakness or visual-perceptual function can make shaving or the application of eye make-up hazardous. In addition, the unpredictability associated with impulsivity creates an environment wrought with potential safety risks. A portion of the treatment regimen must be devoted to training in the integration of safety-enhancing strategies. The therapist might advise that dressing be performed in supine in bed or that the client use an electric razor instead of a straight razor. Caregiver instruction should include training in safety concerns as well as the admonition to expect the unexpected, especially if the client has impaired self-awareness, demonstrates impulsivity, has apraxia or is confused.

Adaptive devices may prove helpful when motor impairments interfere with task performance. However, when memory impairments are marked, clients often forget that they have adaptive devices and thus, fail to use them. Clients who utilize elastic shoelaces may proceed to untie their shoes when undressing. Apraxia may impede the client's ability to learn to operate an adaptive device, provoking the client to abandon its use in frustration. Clients experiencing disorganization and poor sequencing may lose track of adaptive devices or fail to have them handy at the critical moment. Clinicians should consider carefully the real benefit of adaptive aids to clients with brain injury. Likewise care should be taken when devoting precious treatment time to training in the use of adaptive devices.

Clients with brain injury frequently must learn to do familiar tasks in a new ways. The use of *compensatory strategies* during PADL performance is often successful. Compensatory strategies address areas of performance breakdown. The clinician performs task analysis to identify elements critical to task performance. Task analysis involves in-depth study of the physical, cognitive and behavioral requirements of a given activity. Task analysis is applicable to any occupation, from the simplest of self-care tasks to work-related tasks. A comparison of the task requirements with the client's abilities and limitations reveals the points in task performance where compensation or adaptation must occur to facilitate successful performance.

When teaching compensatory strategies, the clinician first structures the task, adding new elements to address the areas of breakdown. Clients unable to maintain standing need to learn to dress and bathe in a sitting or supine position. Clients with homonymous hemianopsia must learn to purposefully look to their "blind side" during feeding, grooming and dressing. Clients with severe sequencing deficits may require a written checklist to complete their morning PADL routine. A client with tonal dysfunction that worsens during strenuous activity may need a tone-reducing orthosis during ADL's. With the therapist close at hand, the client proceeds through the PADL's incorporating compensatory strategies while receiving either verbal and/or physical assistance as needed.

Once the PADL's are structured, the client practices task performance to facilitate learning. Chunking instruction in compensatory techniques may reduce the chance of overwhelming the client (32). The chunking strategy may be used, for example when addressing impairments in self-dressing with a client with hemiplegia. The therapist first teaches a compensatory technique for upper extremity dressing. The upper extremity dressing technique is practiced daily with the therapist providing assistance with lower extremity dressing. Once the client masters the upper extremity dressing technique, treatment progresses to lower extremity dressing. A compensatory strategy to facilitate independence with lower extremity dressing is taught by the therapist. Therapy focuses on practice of lower extremity dressing strategies with the therapist providing physical and verbal assistance. Once the client demonstrates competence with the two parts of dressing separately, the dressing sequence is put together and practiced until mastered.

Chaining and prompting techniques are used to facilitate learning of compensatory strategies. Because functional tasks are comprised of sequences of steps, retraining of task performance may be accomplished by forward, backward or whole-task chaining. Forward chaining involves teaching the first task step first, adding subsequent steps as the client is ready. Backward chaining entails teaching the final step task first, such as teaching a client to put on and tie his shoes first before other garments are taught. Once the last task step is mastered, the clinician works backward toward the first step of the task as the client demonstrates readiness to learn. Whole-task chaining, which proved most successful in a study by Giles, presents all task steps in their proper sequence coupled with repeated practice until competence is demonstrated (33).

Chaining allows the client to use completed steps as cues to initiate subsequent steps. Therapists either verbally assist the client through the chain of steps or provide written cue cards that outline the task sequence.

When the client is unable to move on to the next step, the therapist may query the client. Questions such as "You've put sugar in your coffee. What do you do next?" or "You've finished washing your face. What comes next?" often triggers the client's recall of the next step or his need to reference his cue card. As the client's competence with the task improves, fewer cueing queries from the clinician are required.

Though the area of PADL is typically the domain of the occupational therapist, the entire *interdisciplinary team* including the caregiver must be involved in the PADL treatment process. Performance of PADL's occurs throughout the 24-hour day necessitating the participation of nurses, other therapy staff, residential staff, caregivers and family to ensure carryover of newly learned techniques, to provide consistency in cueing, to ensure safety and to promote learning thus increasing proficiency. Communication among the interdisciplinary team members regarding PADL performance must occur routinely. In-patient programs often rely on boards posted at clients' bedsides upon which clinicians record self care performance information. Memory diaries that document PADL performance and strategies are used in in-patient programs, outpatient programs and in the community. Videos of clients performing self-care help clarify levels of performance and provide instruction for distant caregivers. Team meetings provide an opportunity to discuss self-care performance. Communication is fundamental to providing the consistency that is essential in all areas of brain injury rehabilitation.

Throughout the retraining process, the client must be taught to *monitor performance for errors* and to initiate self-correction. Feedback is one method for teaching error recognition. Feedback may involve the clinician showing a client mistakes made during task performance. While this approach works, the clinician or another individual is essential to such a feedback process.

A better technique involves guiding the client through a sequence of activity prediction, self-critique and problem solving. In activity prediction, the client estimates how he will do on a given task before the task commences. Using information from prior performances, the client identifies areas where breakdown might occur. Once the client completes the task, the client engages in self-critique, comparing actual performance with predicted performance. Activity prediction followed by self-critique improves the client's self-awareness and improves performance (34).

Some clients repeatedly commit the same errors, at times due to an inability to approach a task in a novel, potentially more successful manner. One approach to reduce repeated errors is to help the client generate alternative approaches to a task. When a therapist notes that an error is occurring repeatedly, the therapist should work with the client to identify areas of performance breakdown noticed during task performance. Some clients are able to identify errors spontaneously but others require the assistance of the therapist to review each step of the task. Once the pattern of error is identified, the clinician guides the client through an analysis of possible alternatives to task performance that could eliminate the repeated errors. The alternatives are then employed during task performance and analyzed by the client and therapist. Those that prove beneficial to the quality of performance are incorporated into the task routine.

Interventions for Deficits in Instrumental Activities of Daily Living

Instrumental activities of daily living (IADL's) are those activities "oriented toward interacting with the environment" and are often multifaceted in nature (23). Completion of IADL's is usually essential to an individual's capacity to live independently in the community. In some cases, family members may rely upon the individual to complete specific IADL's to keep the family unit running. IADL's include activities such as caring for other humans or pets, use of communication equipment, community-based mobility, home management, providing food for self and perhaps others and managing finances.

Because IADL's are so complex, they are very susceptible to significant disruption after brain injury. Physical limitations such as hemiplegia, impaired balance and incoordination impact IADL's that require bilateral extremity use to complete, such as folding laundry as well as activities that entail precision, such as dialing a cell phone or chopping vegetables for a salad. The complexity of IADL's places a high demand on cognitive function, including memory function, executive skills, reasoning, judgment and problem-solving. Visual-perceptual-motor dysfunction such as impaired spatial skills, apraxia and hemi-inattention make accurate, independent performance of many IADL's very difficult, if not impossible. Functional communication, money management and home management depend to some degree on language function.

Each person possesses a unique repertoire of IADL's. Valued IADL's are related to a person's life roles such as parent, home maintainer, worker, student, or volunteer. Competency requirements for specific roles vary from person to person.

There is no "cook book" of interventions for treatment of dysfunction in IADL's though treatment-oriented resources are available to the clinician (8, 22, 31, 35–39). Limited research into the effectiveness of some therapeutic approaches has been done (19, 22, 28, 36, 37, 40–44). The optimal intervention for disruption in IADL performance is personalized for each client based on the client's preferences, willingness to adapt task performance, the nature of the task itself and the impact of the sequelae of brain injury on task performance.

During treatment planning, the clinician should be mindful of several important points. Though the approach, strategies and techniques employed to provide intervention for IADL's vary with each patient, these considerations supply a guide for the treatment planning and implementation process.

1. the *client and family's goals* relative to previously performed IADL
2. the *setting* in which treatment for IADL's is occurring
3. facilitation of *generalization of skills* learned
4. selection of *treatment tasks*
5. utility of *technology* during task performance
6. *educational needs* of the client and family

The over-riding goal of rehabilitation is to enable the person receiving care to attain a satisfying quality of life. Disturbing data exists regarding quality of life after brain injury. In one study, at follow-up, a small proportion of patients was competitively employed. Of those studied, 12% rarely left their home because of continuing functional limitations (41). While each person defines "quality of life" differently, it is imperative that the *clients and their significant others' goals for rehabilitation and perception of quality within their own lives* form the foundation for treatment. Some families tolerate role changes within the family system better than others. While one husband is perfectly comfortable assuming all the responsibilities of home management given his wife's disability, another husband may regard his wife's ability to manage laundry, prepare meals and do housework to the extent she is able as a vital necessity to the family. Many family units need the client to be able to stay alone for a period of time during the day in order for family members to work or attend school. In such cases, the therapist must address the numerous activities essential to that client's safety and independence while home alone. In addition, clients often state a desire to resume tasks that bring special meaning to life, such as participation in religious worship or participation in the weekly bridge club. Therapists who listen carefully to their clients are able to determine the client's treatment priorities.

Once treatment priorities are identified, the therapist begins the intervention process. Clinicians must not underestimate the power of client investment on the outcome of treatment. As Pierce articulately states: "The appeal of a therapeutic activity, and thus, its treatment power, always depends on the degree to which the patient perceives it as offering desirable levels of pleasure, productivity and restoration" (45).

The *setting* in which IADL treatment naturally occurs influences the types of activities used in remediation and the nature of the treatment itself. Without question, a familiar environment enhances performance because well-known task elements serve as prompts for the client. In fact, some researchers have concluded that treatment in an unfamiliar environment is fraught with distraction and thus is a hindrance to the client (22).

Despite shortening lengths of stay, in-patient treatment programs often begin the IADL treatment program. The in-patient therapist is challenged to provide the most realistic treatment environment possible within the hospital setting. Some in-patient rehabilitation programs feature Easy Street[1], a mock naturalistic environment that includes a retail shopping area. Though not equivalent to working with the client in the "real world", mock environments like Easy Street or even the hospital gift shop and eateries enhance context. Functional tasks such as ordering from a menu, handling money, following directional signs, use of public restrooms and managing architectural barriers may be practiced in such environments. At least one paper reports a longer length of stay and less favorable FIM scores for patients who received treatment only in a clinic setting as compared to patients who had at least one session in the Easy Street environment (46). In-patient settings without benefit of the Easy Street environment may enhance contextual relevance by using the client's own recipes during cooking tasks or working on financial management using copies of the client's bills. A collection of phone directories from surrounding regions for use during phone skills retraining improves familiarity. Community outings to grocery stores, shopping centers, and restaurants formerly frequented by the client provide excellent environments for therapy. Use of more natural and contextually relevant therapeutic media within the clinical setting is recommended. The standard collection of pegs and cones can be replaced with functional task modules such as car maintenance kits, pet care supplies, a set of greeting cards to practice writing skills and coupons for sorting (36, 37). In an age where provider productivity and efficiency are mandated within the clinical setting, greater creativity is required of the clinician who desires to provide maximally relevant treatment to clients. The extra effort though is worth it when contextual relevance is improved.

Much IADL treatment occurs in outpatient, day rehabilitation and home settings as clinicians work with clients who are actively re-integrating into their naturalistic environment. Outpatient and day rehabilitation efforts may be augmented by "homework" assigned by the clinician and performed between clinical appointments. The home health therapist has the real benefit of engaging the patient in IADL retraining in the most familiar environment.

---

[1]*Product Information* Easy Street – Exclusively manufactured, sold and installed by Chamberlain West, Inc, 7300 E. Acoma Drive, Scottsdale, Arizona 85260

As the treatment program progresses, the clinician must be concerned about the client's ability to *generalize into the natural environment the skills being mastered* in the treatment session. Generalization involves the client's ability to do as well in the home setting as in the clinical setting. Cases have been reported where clients do less well when the clinician or the clinical setting are withdrawn from the context of the activity (22, 42). Neistadt emphasizes that clients with brain injury often depend on a "data-driven mode of information processing" during pursuit of IADL's. Such behavior causes inflexibility in thinking, demonstration of stimulus-bound behavior and failure to generalize (42). Techniques developed by Toglia (34, 38) and Ben-Yishay (22) create a therapeutic environment where cues and assistance are provided but gradually faded as performance progresses. Neistadt describes application of these strategies to food preparation tasks (42). Maximization of generalization is achieved by providing opportunities for practice in as many contexts as possible. Inclusion of family in the treatment session provides one alteration to task context. Practice of tasks either in a transitional apartment, while on pass or in the home between outpatient sessions provides variation in contexts. In some situations, generalization simply doesn't occur. In those situations, therapists should shift the treatment program to the practice of specific tasks in specific contexts to gain the highest level of performance competence.

When planning treatment for IADL's, the clinician should weigh the client's *choices of treatment tasks* carefully as well as the appropriate approach to treatment. All IADL's may be therapeutically graded to provide a suitable level of challenge. Grading techniques involve changing specific task parameters such as tools needed for task completion, the amount of environmental distraction, the complexity of the task and the amount of cueing offered by another person. Treatment always begins at a level where clients are challenged but not frustrated. The selection of treatment activity is guided by the client's stated goal and should be an activity in which the client has expressed interest. As performance improves, the elements of the treatment task are advanced to more greatly challenge the patient.

An occupational therapist treating a client with topographical disorientation, right-left confusion and hemi-inattention focuses the treatment plan on the client's expressed interest in meal planning. The client clips coupons to help reduce her food costs. One treatment modality employed to address the hemi-inattention and right-left confusion could be sorting coupons for food products to the left and cleaning products to the right. The OT might introduce map reading as a therapy activity. The therapist orients the patient to the map, incorporating directional terms. The complexity of the maps used increases as the client shows improved map reading skills. Once improvements in right-left sorting and map reading tasks are noted, therapy progresses past the confines of the OT clinic into the medical facility. The OT provides written directions for a route from the OT clinic to the facility's front door. As part of the treatment session, the client uses the written directions to travel to the prescribed route. The written directions contain landmarks on the right and left that the client must note along the way. In addition to in-clinic therapy, the OT provides a homework assignment requiring the client to use written directions to find the OT clinic on the next visit, asking for assistance as needed. As treatment progresses and improvements are noted, the clinical treatment program and homework assignments are made more difficult. Advanced treatment could include having the client read directions to the person who provides transportation to OT appointments, training with the OT in the use of public transportation or the use of a state map to plan a vacation. Clinicians must make deliberate treatment modality selections based on the client's occupations and then progress the task complexity as the patient demonstrates readiness.

Ever-evolving *technology* has great potential for many clients with brain injury. Staying current with technological advances is a challenge for busy therapists and funding assistive technology is often difficult, if not impossible, for many individuals with brain injury. However, technology does provide some tremendous possibilities. Low-tech devices available at modest cost allow clients with severe motoric impairments to control their environment, such as turning on lights and using the telephone. Computers provide voice-activated options as well as adaptive peripherals which facilitate word processing for individuals without hand function (47). Electronic aids to daily living (EADL's) dial telephones, unlock doors and provide many options for environmental control.

Cognitive orthotics, sometimes called assistive technology devices (ATD's), provide "support for weakened or ineffective brain functions" (43). Such orthoses provide cues, assist with task completion, maximize self-management, allow a higher level of self-sufficiency and often promote self-esteem and self-confidence (43, 44, 48). Individuals without brain injury employ cognitive orthoses such as portable digital assistants (PDA's), portable tape recorders, watch alarms and computer-based schedulers routinely. The ISAAC cognitive prosthetic system has shown great promise in assisting clients with brain injury. A recent report (49) demonstrates the utility of this small device. Its advantages over other cognitive prosthetics include its compact size, portability, its adaptability to the individual client's needs, and its immense programming possibilities. Cognitive prosthetics have shown utility with clients with brain injury (48) and have the added advantage of being a tool used by people without disability, unlike traditional memory notebooks.

As clinicians seek technological solutions for their clients, several factors must be kept in mind. First, the client's desire to employ a technological solution must be explored. The therapist needs to determine the client's overall awareness of his deficits and how technology, when properly employed, may help. The therapist must conduct a task analysis of the client's remaining abilities and strengths that could support use of technology while also considering the intactness of client factors often essential to technological use, such as vision, language skills, ability to keep up with the device and the ability to manipulate the device (48). The cost of technology also needs to be considered. Care must be taken when introducing potentially life-changing technology to a client who lacks the financial means to purchase the device. Alternative funding sources, such as vocational rehabilitation services or even charitable organizations, are sometimes available. The motivated client can partner with a clinician to look for alternate funding. Finally, the clinician should consider the client's overall familiarity with technological devices. A client with an information technology or engineering background may more quickly learn how to use an EADL than a client who has never used a computer and who has no mechanical background. Technology has awesome potential to assist individuals with brain injury manage IADL's despite their physical or cognitive sequelae.

Throughout the IADL treatment process, clinicians must remain alert to the *educational needs of the client and family*. It is difficult for clinicians to imagine or anticipate the many issues and concerns of the caregiver, especially if the clinician has never provided personal support for a person with a brain injury. Understanding the complexity of brain injury is not easy for clients or for families. During the treatment process, families may wonder why their loved one doesn't do the things that he is perfectly capable of performing. For example, a wife may say to the therapist: "I saw my husband fix his own lunch with you. Why is it when I come home from work I discover that he hasn't gotten off the couch all day. Why doesn't he fix his own lunch at home?" Clients may wonder why they never seem to be able to finish any task they start. Education about the significant impact of impaired executive function is usually helpful for families and clients who may have received considerable instruction on performance of transfers, the administration of medications and home exercises but who have not learned sufficiently about perseveration, impaired initiation and decreased planning. As stated by McDonald et al. (50): "Impairment in executive abilities has significant implications for the day-to-day life of those who have sustained traumatic brain injury" – implications that families and clients don't always understand.

Clients and families also benefit from intense instruction in safety related to performance of IADL's. Clear advice regarding supervision needs, use of dangerous implements such as power tools and the operation of motor vehicles must be given. Families need guidance on activities the client may safely and capably do alone, whether in the home or in the community. Discussions regarding the client's degree of self-awareness may be relevant. Lack of awareness is a common sequelae of brain injury and can lead to all manner of difficulties including resistance to rehabilitative efforts, deliberate involvement in unsafe activities and interpersonal conflict (51). As intervention is employed to improve the client's self-awareness, support and education for the caregivers may foster their ability to carry on and cope.

Families will often ask whether the client can do particular IADL's that the therapist has not yet addressed clinically. Clinicians must take care when basing judgments about a client's ability to perform tasks at home and in the community on testing of component skills or on simulated activities. For example, a therapist might state that a client is unable to stay home alone because the client performed poorly on a visual-perceptual test. While some component testing has shown encouraging relationships to IADL performance, there clearly is a disconnection between performance on a paper-pencil task related to an IADL and performance of IADL itself (22, 27). Likewise, asserting that a client is incapable of certain IADL's based on a simulated task is a stretch. Clinicians may offer predictions based on an analysis of performance components and results of simulated activities, but with caution. The best approach is to engage the client in the task in question to determine the client's actual skill level. Otherwise clinicians find themselves stating their best guess based on previous experience and the data at hand.

Clinicians do well to maintain an open door for clients and families to ask questions and receive education, not only during active treatment but also after formal treatment has ended. Improvements in as well as deterioration of IADL performance occur long after the therapy program ends. The desire and need for therapy also changes over time. One study reports that some survivors of brain injury sense a greater readiness for therapy long after the course of therapy is completed (41). Clients and families need to understand what is "expected" and "normal" after a brain injury and what constitutes a situation of concern. Referring clients and caregivers to brain injury support groups may provide a valuable resource over time.

OCCUPATIONAL THERAPY IN BRAIN INJURY REHABILITATION

The occupational therapist functions as a part of the interdisciplinary brain injury team. Occupational therapists are trained to view clients holistically as occupational beings for whom participation in daily life is a vital part of existence. Occupational therapists seek to improve the health of those receiving occupational therapy services while engaging clients in meaningful activity. The best occupational therapy utilizes treatment modalities that inspire and motivate the client while providing relevant experience.

Occupational therapy educational coursework includes basic sciences, anatomy, physiology, neuroanatomy, kinesiology as well as instruction in disease and disability. In addition, occupational therapy students study psychology, sociology and human development. The language of occupational therapy theory and practice is found in the *Occupational Therapy Practice Framework* that describes the domain and process of occupational therapy (23).

Occupational therapists who practice in brain injury rehabilitation programs benefit from continuing education focused on cognitive function, behavior management and intervention techniques. While the occupational therapy educational curriculum provides a basic foundation in these areas, further education sharpens the clinician's skills. The ever-evolving field of assistive technology demands that the occupational therapist continually review the literature for developments applicable to persons with brain injury.

The most significant contribution of the occupational therapist to the brain injury rehabilitation team is the therapist's understanding of and insight into the individual client's ability to participate in activities of daily living of interest and importance to the client and the family. The occupational therapist's ability to analyze task performance is critical to the team's understanding of the client's need for assistance and supervision in the community. Occupational therapists are not "ADL retrainers". Rather occupational therapists alter context during treatment in order to clarify important issues in functional task performance for the client, family and treatment team while facilitating maximal participation in activities of importance to the client.

Utilizing a collaborative approach, the physician and occupational therapist do well to mesh their understanding of the client's participation in daily life prior to the brain injury with the client's and family's stated rehabilitation goals. While a full restoration to pre-injury participation isn't always possible, the physician and OT must work with the client and family to establish reasonable, achievable expectations for improvement and performance. The physician should encourage the occupational therapy staff to be creative and innovative in treating patients. The occupational therapist and physician should work together in setting parameters on client activity, especially in the areas of driving, return to work and living situation based on the therapist's evaluation and intervention with the client in a variety of tasks and

contexts and the physician's knowledge of the client's medical condition.

CONCLUSION

Law states (7) that "participation in the everyday occupations of life is a vital part of human development and lived experience". Brain injury can radically affect an individual's level of participation in everyday activities. Reduced participation in important life tasks affects the client's sense of competency within the environment as well as overall satisfaction with life. Therapeutic efforts directed toward improved participation in occupations must be uniquely designed to capture the client's interest as together the client and clinician work toward the client's return to quality of life and relocation of self.

References

1. Law M. Evaluating activities of daily living: Directions for the future. *AJOT* 1993;47:233–237.
2. Fisher A. G. Uniting practice and theory in an occupational framework. *AJOT* 1998;52:509–521.
3. American Occupational Therapy Association. Position paper: Occupation. *AJOT* 1995;49:1015–1018.
4. Yerxa E. Health and the human spirit for occupation. *AJOT* 1998;52:412–422.
5. Meyer A. The philosophy of occupational therapy. *Archives of Occupational Therapy* 1922;1:1–10.
6. Hocking C. Implementing occupation-based assessment. *AJOT* 2001;55:464–469.
7. Law M. Participation in the occupations of everyday life – 2002 Distinguished scholar lecture. *AJOT* 2002;56:640–649.
8. Padilla R., Barrett K., Walker L. Culture and the occupational therapy practitioner. *OT Practice* April 21,2003:33–40.
9. Fisher A. G., Liu Y., Velozo C. A., Pan A. W. Cross-cultural assessment of process skills. *AJOT* 1992;46:876–885.
10. Trombly C (ed.). *Occupational Therapy for Physical Dysfunction – 4th edition*. Baltimore: Williams and Wilkins 1995.
11. Klein R. M., Bell B. Self care skills: Behavioral measurement with the Klein-Bell ADL Scale. *Archives of Physical Medicine and Rehabilitation* 1982;63:335–338.
12. Mahoney F. I., Barthel D. W. Functional evaluation: The Barthel Index. *Maryland State Medical Journal* 1965;14:61–65.
13. Schoening H. A., Anderegg L., Bergstrom D., Fonda M., Steinke N., Ulrich P. Numerical scoring of self care status of patients. *Archives of Physical Medicine and Rehabilitation* 1965;47:689–697.
14. Fisher A. The assessment of motor and process skills (AMPS) in N. Katz (ed) *Cognitive Rehabilitation: Models for interventions in occupational therapy*. Boston: Andover 1991.
15. Arnadottir G. *The Brain and Behavior: Assessing Cortical Dysfunction through Activities of Daily Living*. St.Louis: CV Mosby 1990.
16. Law M., Baptiste S., Carswell A., McColl M. A., Polatajko H., Pollock N. *Canadian Occupational Performance Measure*.Ottawa: Canadian Association of Occupational Therapists 1998.
17. Allen C. K. *Allen Cognitive Test Manual*. Colchester, CT: S&S Worldwide 1990.
18. Neistadt M. : The relationship between constructional and meal preparation skills. *Archives of Physical Medicine and Rehabilitation* 1993;74:144–148.
19. McGourty L. K. Kohlman Evaluation of Living Skills in B J Hemphill (ed) *Mental Health Assessement in Occupational Therapy*. Thorofare NJ: Slack 1988.

20. Granger C. V., Divan N., Fieldler R. C. Functional assessment scales: a study of persons with traumatic brain injury. *Archives of Physical Medicine and Rehabilitation* 1995;74:107–113.

21. Law M., Letts L. A critical review of scales of activities of daily living. *AJOT* 1989;43:522–528.

22. Arilotta C. Performance in areas of occupation. *Physical Disabilities Special Interest Section Quarterly* 2003;26:1–3.

23. Occupational therapy practice framework: Domain and process. *AJOT* 2002;56:609–639.

24. Toglia J. P. *Toglia Categorization Assessment Manual*. Pequannock NJ: Maddak 1994.

25. Katz N., Itsovich M., Auerbach S., Elazar B. LOTCA Battery for brain-injured patients: Reliability and validity. *AJOT* 1989; 43:184–192.

26. Toglia J. P. *The Contextual Memory Test Manual*. Tucson: Therapy Skill Builders 1993.

27. Goverover Y., Hinojosa J. Categorization and deductive reasoning: Predictors of Instrumental Activities of Daily Living. *AJOT* 2002;56:509–516.

28. Trombly C. A., Radomski M. V., Trexel C., Burnett-Smith S. E. Occupational therapy and achievement of self identified goals by adults with acquired brain injury. *AJOT* 2002;56:489–498.

29. Baum C., Law M. : Occupational therapy practice: Focusing on occupational performance. *AJOT* 1997;51:277–288.

30. Gagne D. E., Hoppes S. : The effects of goal-focused occupational therapy on self care skills: A pilot study. *AJOT* 2003;57:215–219.

31. McNeny R. Activities of daily living in M. Rosenthal, E. R. Griffith, J. S. Kreutzer, B. Pentland (eds) *Rehabilitation of the Adult and Child with Traumatic Brain Injury*. Philadelphia: FA Davis 1999.

32. Giles G. M., Shore M. Clinical notes: A rapid method for teaching severely brain-injured adults how to wash and dress. *Archives of Physical Medicine and Rehabilitation* 1989;70:156–158.

33. Giles G. M., Ridley J. E., Dill A., Frye S. A consecutive series of adults with brain injury treated with a washing and dressing retraining program. *AJOT* 1997;51:256–266.

34. Abreu B. C., Toglia J. P. Cognitive rehabilitation: A model for occupational therapy. *AJOT* 1987;14:439–448.

35. Christiansen C. H., Little B. R., Bockman C. Personal projects: A useful approach to the study of occupation. *AJOT* 1998;52: 439–446.

36. Asher D., Newman S. Replacing cones and pegs with functional tasks. *OT Practice* February 28,2000:16–18.

37. Deshaies L. D., Bauer E. R., Berro M. Occupation based treatment in physical disabilities rehabilitation. *OT Practice* July 2,2001: 13–17.

38. Toglia J. P. Attention and memory in CB Royeen (ed) *AOTA Self-Study Series: Cognitive Rehabilitation*. Rockville MD: AOTA 1993.

39. Zemke R. Task skills, problem solving and social interaction in CB Royeen (ed) *AOTA Self-Study Series: Cognitive Rehabilitation*. Rockville MD: AOTA 1993.

40. Gardarsdotti S., Kaplan S. Validity of the Arnadottir OT-ADL Neurobehavioral Evaluation (A-ONE): Performance in activities of daily living and neurobehavioral impairments of persons with left and right hemisphere damage. *AJOT* 2002;56:499–508.

41. Huebner R. A., Johnson K., Bennett C. M., Schneck C. Community participation and quality of life. *AJOT* 2003;57:177–185.

42. Neistadt M. A meal preparation treatment protocol for adults with brain injury. *AJOT* 1994;48:431–438.

43. Bergman M. M. The Essential Steps (r) cognitive orthotic. *Neurorehab* 2003;18:31–46.

44. Wilson B. A., Scott H., Evans J., Emslie H. Preliminary report of a NeuroPage service within a health care system. *Neurorehab* 2003;18:3–8.

45. Pierce D. The issue is: What is the source of occupation's treatment power? *AJOT* 1998;52:490–491.

46. Hecox R., roach K. E., Das Varna J. M., Giraud J. E., Davis C. M., Neulen K. Functional independence measurement of patients receiving Easy Street: A retrospective study. *Phys and Occup Therapy in Geriatrics* 1994;12:1731.

47. Bergman M. The benefits of a cognitive orthotic in brain injury rehab. *JHTR* 2002;17:431–445.

48. O'Connel M. E., Mateer C., Kerns K. Prosthetics systems for addressing problems with initiation: Guidelines for selection, training and measuring efficacy. *Neurorehab* 2003;18:9–20.

49. Gorman P., Dayle R., Hood C. A., Rumrell L. Effectiveness of the ISAAC cognitive prosthetic system for improving rehabilitation outcomes with neurofunctional impairment. *Neurorehab* 2003; 18:57–67.

50. McDonald B. C., Flashman L. A., Saykin A. J. Executive dysfunction following traumatic brain injury: Neural substrates. *Neurorehab* 2002;17:333–344.

51. Flashman L. A., McAllister T. W. Lack of awareness and its impact in traumatic brain injury. *Neurorehab* 2002;17:285–296.

XIII

NEUROPSYCHO-PHARMACOLOGY AND ALTERNATIVE TREATMENTS

AGGRESSION AND AGITATION

Aggressive and/or agitated behavior is a major source of disability to individuals with brain injury and a major source of stress to families of persons with this problem. Additionally, these behaviors can endanger the safety of not only patients and their families but also the professionals providing care to them. A multimodal, multidisciplinary, collaborative approach to treatment is necessary in most cases. The concurrent use of family treatments, psychopharmacologic interventions, and psychotherapeutic approaches is often required. In establishing a treatment plan for patients with agitation or aggression, the overarching principle is that diagnosis comes before treatment. It is essential to determine the mental status of the patient before the agitated or aggressive event, the nature of the precipitant, the physical and social environment in which the behavior occurs, the ways in which the event is mitigated, and the primary and secondary gains related to agitation and aggression (149, 150).

Although there is no medication that is approved by the FDA specifically for the treatment of aggression, medications are widely used (and commonly misused) in the management of patients with acute or chronic aggression. Unfortunately, there is a paucity of rigorous double-blind, placebo controlled studies (i.e. "Level I" studies) or even prospective cohort studies (i.e. "Level II") to guide clinicians in the use of pharmacologic interventions. The International Brain Injury Association has assembled a task force on reviewing the literature on this literature pertaining to the neurobehavioral consequences of TBI (in progress). At this time, we suggest utilizing the Consensus Guidelines for the Treatment of Agitation in the Elderly with Dementia as a framework for the assessment and management of agitation and aggression after TBI (151), with the caveat that the effectiveness of these medications is highly variable in persons with TBI.

Medications for posttraumatic aggression and/or agitation are generally selected with one or another hypothesis in mind regarding the neurochemistry of these problems. For example, hypothesized strategies for treatment of aggression and agitation include inhibition of excessive activity in temporolimbic areas with anticonvulsants, reduction of "hyperactive" limbic monoaminergic neurotransmission with β-adrenergic receptor antagonists (i.e., propranolol) or dopamine receptor antagonists (i.e., haloperidol), augmentation of orbitofrontal and/or dorsolateral prefrontal cortical activity with monoaminergic agonists (i.e., amantadine, methylphenidate, and perhaps buspirone), or modulation of limbic and frontal activity through augmentation of serotonergic activity (e.g., SSRIs). However, the neurochemistry of posttraumatic aggression is not well understood and may differ between individuals. Consequently, the pharmacologic treatment

of this problem often entails a trial-and-error approach to find a medication that is both effective and tolerable.

After appropriate assessment of possible etiologies of these behaviors, treatment is focused on the occurrence of comorbid neuropsychiatric conditions (depression, psychosis, insomnia, anxiety, delirium). When present, aggression or agitation may be a manifestation of these problems rather than an independent diagnosis. Therefore, comorbid neuropsychiatric conditions should be treated prior to developing an independent treatment approach to the patient's agitation or aggression. Additionally, it is important to consider whether there the behavior is occurring in the acute (hours to days) or chronic (weeks to months) phase after TBI, and also the severity of the behavior (mild to severe). The differential diagnosis of posttraumatic aggression varies as a function of time since injury, with confusional states being more common in the early post-injury period and other neuropsychiatric problems such as psychosis being more common in the late post-injury period. The effects of these treatments may vary depending on the presence of other neuropsychiatric conditions and the time since injury. Finally, clinicians should bear in mind that patients may not respond to just one medication, but may require combination treatment, similar to the pharmacotherapeutic treatment for refractory posttraumatic depression.

Acute Aggression

Antipsychotics

Antipsychotics are the most commonly used medications in the treatment of aggression. Although these agents are appropriate and effective when aggression arises as a result of psychosis, the use of typical antipsychotic agents to treat chronic aggression in the absence of psychosis is often ineffective and may result in serious treatment-related complications such as tardive dyskinesia. Usually, it is the sedative side effects rather than the antipsychotic properties of antipsychotics that are used (i.e., misused) to "treat" (i.e., mask) the aggression. Often, patients develop tolerance to the sedative effects of the neuroleptics and, therefore, require increasing doses. As a result, extrapyramidal and anticholinergic-related side effects occur. Paradoxically (and frequently), akathisia may result from the use of these agents and thereby worsen agitation and restlessness. As the dose of neuroleptic is increased, especially when a high-potency antipsychotic such as haloperidol is administered, these symptoms predictably worsen. Akathisia is often mistaken for increased irritability and agitation, setting in motion a cycle of increasing neuroleptics and worsening akathisia.

There is some evidence from studies of injury to motor neurons in animals that have found that haloperidol decreases recovery. This effect was only seen when animals actively participated in a behavioral task and not when the animals were restrained after drug administration (135). It is possible that the effect on decreasing dopamine and inhibiting neuronal function, which may be the mechanism of action to treat aggression, may have other detrimental effects on recovery. As noted earlier, Rao et al. (1985) (136) found that patients treated with haloperidol in the acute period following TBI experienced significantly longer periods of posttraumatic amnesia. This finding raises important potential risk/benefit issues that must be considered before antipsychotic drugs are used to treat aggressive behavior in patients with neuronal damage.

In patients with brain injury, psychosis, and aggression, we recommend atypical antipsychotics as first-line treatments for acute agitation following TBI. Starting does of these medications should be low (i.e., risperidone 0.5 mg) and repeated at short intervals (sometimes as frequent as every hour) until control of aggression is achieved. If after several administrations of risperidone the patient's aggressive behavior does not improve, the hourly dose may be increased until the patient is so sedated that he or she no longer exhibits agitation or violence. Once the patient is not aggressive for 48 hours, the daily dosage should be decreased gradually (i.e., by 25%/day) to ascertain whether aggressive behavior reemerges. In this case, consideration should then be made about whether it is best to increase the dose of risperidone and/or to initiate treatment with a more specific anti-aggressive medication or nonpharmacologic intervention. Other atypical antipsychotic medications such as olanzapine, quetiapine (which produces little in the way of extrapyramidal symptoms), or ziprasidone may be used, although there is no published experience with these medications in persons with TBI.

Benzodiazepines

The literature regarding the effects of the benzodiazepines in the treatment of aggression is inconsistent, at best. The sedative properties of benzodiazepines are helpful in the management of acute agitation and aggression in many cases. Paradoxically, increased hostility, aggression, and the induction of rage may occur in patients treated with benzodiazepines, and particularly persons with neurological problems, although this phenomenon is rare (152). Benzodiazepines can produce amnesia, and preexisting memory dysfunction can be exacerbated by the use of benzodiazepines. Brain-injured patients may also experience increased problems with coordination and balance with benzodiazepine use. For this reason, we do not recommend the use of benzodiazepines for the treatment of acute aggression in patients with TBI.

Chronic Aggression

If a patient continues to exhibit periods of agitation or aggression over weeks to months, prophylactic use of medications may be required to decrease or prevent these behaviors. Consideration of such medications should be undertaken only after evaluation of the antecedents and consequences of these behaviors and attempts to address these issues in the service of decreasing aggression and agitation nonpharmacacologically.

Antipsychotics

If, after thorough clinical evaluation, it is determined that the aggressive episodes result from psychosis, such as paranoid delusions or command hallucinations, then antipsychotic medications will be the treatment of choice. There have been double-blind placebo controlled studies of risperidone showing efficacy in the treatment of agitation in elderly patients with dementia (153, 154), as well as children with autism and serious behavioral problems (155). Olanzapine appears to be more sedating, and quetiapine produces more limited extrapyramidal symptoms than does risperidone. Quetiapine appears to be the antipsychotic medication (except for clozapine) least likely to produce extrapyramidal effects in vulnerable populations, such as those with Parkinson's disease (156). Clozapine may have greater antiaggressive effects than other atypical antipsychotic medications (142), but its propensity to impair cognition and increase seizure risk, and as well as the arduous hematologic monitoring required during its use, may offset its potential benefits in this population. Based on the available evidence and our own clinical experience, we suggest that when atypical antipsychotics are used for posttraumatic aggression or agitation, risperidone, olanzapine, and quetiapine should be considered first-line before the other even newer atypical antipsychotic agents.

Buspirone

Serotonin appears to be a key neurotransmitter in the modulation of aggressive behavior. In preliminary open case studies, buspirone, a 5-HT$_{1A}$ agonist, has been reported to be effective in the management of aggression and agitation for patients with head injury (105, 106, 157), as well as dementia, and developmental disabilities and autism (150). In rare instances, we have found that some patients become more aggressive when treated with buspirone. We recommend that buspirone be initiated at low dosages (i.e., 5 mg BID) and increased to 10 mg BID after one week. Dosages of 45–60 mg/day may be required before there is improvement in aggressive behavior, although we have sometimes observed dramatic improvement within one week of treatment initiation.

Benzodiazepines

Clonazepam may be effective in the long-term management of aggression, although evidence is restricted to case reports. Freinhar and Alvarez (1986) (159) found that clonazepam decreased agitation in three elderly patients with organic brain syndromes. Keats and Mukherjee (1988) (160) reported anti-aggressive effects of clonazepam in a patient with schizophrenia and seizures. We use clonazepam when pronounced aggression and anxiety occur together, or when aggression occurs in association with neurologically-induced tics and similarly disinhibited motor behaviors. Doses should be initiated at 0.5 mg BID and may be increased to as high as 2–4 mg BID, as tolerated. Unfortunately, sedation and ataxia are frequent side effects during treatment with this agent among persons with TBI. As noted earlier, the risk:benefit ratio of benzodiazepine use in this population should be given serious consideration prior to initiating treatment with these agents.

Anticonvulsants

Carbamazepine has been shown to be effective for the treatment of idiopathic bipolar disorder and has also been advocated for the control of aggression in both epileptic and nonepileptic populations. Open-label studies have indicated that carbamazepine may be effective in decreasing aggressive behavior associated with developmental disabilities, schizophrenia, and patients with a variety of other organic brain disorders (150). Several of these studies included individuals with TBI. Chatham-Showalter (1996) (161) observed improvement in seven TBI patients treated in an open-label fashion with carbamazepine, and observed these improvements after only four days of treatment. In an open-label study of carbamazepine on assaultive behavior in eight patients with "organic brain diseases" (only two had brain injury from gunshot wounds), Patterson (1987) (162) reported that the number of episodes decreased by over 50% as documented by nursing staff. In a study by Azouvi and coworkers (1999) (163), ten patients presenting with agitation and anger outbursts after severe TBI experienced significant reduction in such behaviors as assessed using six relevant items on the Neurobehavioral Rating Scale-Revised (164) during 8 weeks of treatment with carbamazepine (mean dose of 9.47 ± 2.9 mg/kg/day). However, four of the ten patients experienced significant drowsiness during the course of the study, necessitating use of lower doses than had been initially planned and that may thereby have reduced the effectiveness of this treatment. An additional patient developed a significant allergic cutaneous reaction necessitating discontinuation of carbamazepine. While the authors of this study report no significant changes in cognition during the course of this trial, their primary measure of cognition was the Mini-Mental State Examination – a measure which is widely regarded as a poor instrument for the assessment of cognition following traumatic brain injury due to its insensitivity to executive

dysfunction and to impairments of the speed and efficiency of information processing. Hence, a failure to find no change in cognition in this study must be regarded with some caution since the measure used is unlikely to be sensitive to such changes in persons with TBI.

In our experience and that of others, the anticonvulsant valproic acid may also be helpful to some patients with organically induced aggression (165–167), although there are only a few open-label case reports regarding the use of this agent among persons with aggression following TBI. Horne and Lindley (1995) (168) report a case of a 70 year-old woman whose posttraumatic emotional lability and irritability improved during treatment with valproate. Wroblewski et al. (1997) (169) observed significantly reduced posttraumatic aggression among five individuals, and report that those improvements occurred within 1–2 weeks of treatment initiation.

Gabapentin may be beneficial for the treatment of agitation in patients with dementia (170, 171). Doses have ranged from 200–2400 mg/day. However, Childers and Holland (1997) (172) report an increase in anxiety and restlessness (i.e, agitation) in two cognitively impaired TBI patients for whom gabapentin was used primarily to reduce chronic pain. Although this report is not consistent with our use of this agent among persons with TBI, it is unclear whether or to what extent gabapentin is of benefit for the treatment of posttraumatic agitation and/or aggression.

For patients with aggression and epilepsy whose seizures are being treated with anticonvulsant drugs such as phenytoin and phenobarbital, switching to carbamazepine or to valproic acid may treat both conditions and reduce adverse side effects (i.e., sedation, confusion, disinhibition) that is sometimes seen in persons treated with the older anticonvulsants such as phenobarbital. Oxcarbazepine may be an alternative to carbmazepine in light of its relative lack of hepatic autoinduction, more favorable drug-drug interaction profile, and more limited cognitive and motor effects, but there are no published reports of its use among persons with aggression following TBI at the time of this writing.

Lithium

Although lithium is known to be effective in controlling aggression related to manic excitement, many studies suggest that it may also have a role in the treatment of aggression in selected, nonbipolar patient populations. These include patients with mental retardation who exhibit self-injurious or aggressive behavior, children and adolescents with behavioral disorders, prison inmates, and those with other organic brain syndromes (150). Two individuals in state psychiatric facilities with brain-injury related aggression (one patient with TBI and one with post-anoxic encephalopathy) responded to an open-label trial of lithium (173). Glenn and colleagues (1989) (98) reported their experience using lithium in the treatment of ten "brain-injured patients with severe, unremitting, aggressive, combative, or self destructive behavior or severe affective instability." Five patients had a "dramatic response."

As noted earlier, individuals with brain injury have increased sensitivity to the neurotoxic effects of lithium (174, 175). Because of lithium's potential for neurotoxicity, we limit the use of lithium in those patients whose aggression is related to manic effects or recurrent irritability related to cyclic mood disorders.

Antidepressants

The antidepressants that have been reported to control aggressive behavior include those that act preferentially (amitriptyline) or specifically (trazodone, sertraline, and fluoxetine) on serotonin. In open studies, Mysiw et al. (1988) (176) and Jackson et al. (1985) (177) reported that amitriptyline (maximum dose 150 mg/day) was effective in the treatment of twenty patients with recent severe brain injury whose agitation had not responded to behavioral techniques. Improvement was documented in 12/17 patients within the first week of treatment. Szlabowicz and Stewart (1990) (178) successfully treated a 43-year-old man with aggressive behavior subsequent to anoxic encephalopathy with amitriptyline 75 mg Qhs. Trazodone has also been reported to be effective in the treatment of aggression that occurs with organic mental disorders (150). As noted earlier in this chapter, Kant et al. (1998) (18) conducted an open-label 8-week open trial of sertraline in 13 patients with irritability and aggression after TBI. Behaviors were monitored using the Overt Aggression Scale-Modified for outpatients, and sertraline was administered up to 200 mg/day. This treatment produced a significant reduction in irritability and aggression.

Fluoxetine, a potent serotonergic antidepressant, has been reported to be effective in the treatment of aggressive behavior in a patient who suffered brain injury as well as in patients with personality disorders and depression, and adolescents with mental retardation and self-injurious behavior (150). We have used selective serotonin reuptake inhibitors with considerable success in aggressive patients with brain lesions. The dosages used are similar to those for the treatment of mood lability and depression, and should be guided by the ease-of-use considerations discussed in the preceding sections of this chapter.

Stimulants

There have been several studies that have examined the role of dopaminergic medications and stimulants in the treatment of agitation and aggression. Nickels et al. (1994) (118) report improvement during treatment with amantadine in two of three subjects with post-coma agitation, and Chandler et al. (1988) (117) report improvement during treatment with amantadine in two patients with agitation and aggression in the post-acute injury period. Mooney and Haas (1993) (179) conducted a randomized, pretest, posttest, placebo-controlled, single-blind study of the effect of methylphenidate 30 mg/day for six weeks on brain injury related anger in 38 individuals with "serious" TBI occurring six or more months prior to treatment. Patients treated with methylphenidate had a lower level of anger. Although we do not recommend these agents as first-line treatments for agitation or aggression following TBI, they should be considered in patients in who there is evidence from neuroimaging of sufficient remaining frontal cortex to permit these agents to augment function in that area and restore its ability to inhibit or modulate limbically-mediated behaviors. In the absence of remaining frontal cortex, these agents pose the risk of further increasing limbic drive and worsening agitated or aggressive behavior.

β-Adrenergic Receptor Antagonists

Since the first report of the use of β-adrenergic receptor antagonists ("β-blockers") in the treatment of acute aggression in 1977, over 25 articles describing the use of β-blockers with over 200 patients with aggression have appeared in the neurologic and psychiatric literature (150). Most of these patients had been unsuccessfully treated with antipsychotics, minor tranquilizers, lithium, and/or anticonvulsants before treatment with β-blockers. The agents in this medication class that have been investigated in controlled prospective studies include propranolol (a lipid-soluble, nonselective β-adrenergic receptor antagonist), nadolol (a water-soluble, nonselective β-adrenergic receptor antagonist), and pindolol (a lipid-soluble, nonselective β-adrenergic receptor antagonist with partial sympathomimetic activity).

The effectiveness of propranolol in reducing agitation has been demonstrated during the initial hospitalization after TBI in a double-blind placebo-controlled study in 21 subjects with severe TBI (180). The maximum intensity of episodes and the numbers of episodes were less after propranolol than they were after placebo as assessed using the Overt Aggression Scale. Unfortunately, the authors of this study do not list the number of patients who dropped out at each time point during the study, thus diminishing the reliability of the conclusions. Greendyke and colleagues (1986) (181) performed a double-blind randomized placebo-controlled crossover study of propranolol in ten patients with aggression (mean dose 520 mg/day). Only 5 patients had TBI, and the response of these patients varied. These authors later performed a double-blind randomized placebo-controlled crossover study of pindolol (doses up to 60 mg/day) in 11 patients with behavioral problems, including aggression (182). It appears that most of these patients also participated in their earlier propranolol study, and again only five of these were patients with TBI. Although the patients as a group demonstrated improvement in assaultiveness, hostility, and uncooperativeness, we are unable to assess whether the TBI patients responded differentially. Alpert and colleagues (1990) (183) used nadolol in chronically hospitalized patients with aggression, and observed improvements in this symptom during treatment with this agent. Unfortunately, these patients did not have TBI.

Collectively, the literature suggests that β-adrenergic receptor antagonists are effective agents for the treatment of aggressive and violent behaviors, particularly those related to "organic brain syndromes" such as TBI. Patients with reactive airway disease (asthma), chronic obstructive pulmonary disease, insulin-dependent diabetes mellitus, congestive heart failure, persistent angina, significant peripheral vascular disease, and hyperthyroidism are not good candidates for treatment with β-blockers. Among patients without cardiovascular or cardiopulmonary problems, propranolol may be initated at doses of 60 mg/day and increased by this amount every 3 days. Among patients with hypotension or bradycardia, treatment is usually initiated with a single test-dose of 20 mg/day and treatment should not proceed if patients develop symptoms related to these problems, if severe dizziness, ataxia, or wheezing occurs, and/or if the pulse rate is reduced below 50 beats per minute or systolic blood pressure is less than 90 mmHg. When this initial test dose is tolerated, doses of propranolol are gradually increased to 12 mg/kg body weight or until aggressive behavior is under control. Doses of 800 mg or less of propranolol are usually sufficient to control aggressive behavior. Patients should be maintained on the highest tolerable dose of propranolol for at least 8 weeks before concluding that the patient is not responding to this medication.

Given the potential for drug-drug interactions with propranolol, plasma levels of all antipsychotic and anticonvulsive medications should be monitored during treatment. In particular, propranolol is associated with significant increases in plasma levels of thioridazine, and the combination of these two medications should be avoided. When a patient requires the use of a once-a-day medication because of compliance difficulties, long-acting propranolol or nadolol may be of use. When patients develop bradycardia that prevents prescribing therapeutic dosages of propranolol, pindolol can be substituted, using one-tenth the dosage of propranolol. Pindolol's intrinsic sympathomimetic activity stimulates the β-adrenergic receptor and may limit the development of symptomatic bradycardia.

As suggested above, the major side effects of β-blockers when used to treat aggression are a lowering of blood pressure and pulse rate. Because peripheral β-adrenergic receptors are fully blocked in doses of 300–400 mg/day, further changes in these vital signs usually do not occur even when doses are increased beyond those levels. Despite reports of depression with the use of β-blockers, controlled trials and our experience indicate that it is a rare occurrence.

SLEEP

Evaluation of sleep disturbances following TBI should first include assessment of other neuropsychiatric problems (e.g., depression, mania, anxiety, delirium) that may better account for the sleep disturbance. Independent of these problems, TBI may result in significant sleep disturbances including impaired rapid-eye-movement (REM) recovery and multiple nocturnal awakenings (184). Hypersomnia that occurs after severe penetrating head injury most often resolves within the first year after injury, whereas insomnia that occurs in patients with long periods of coma and diffuse injury has a more chronic course (185). Barbiturates and long-acting benzodiazepines should probably be avoided in this population, and if they are prescribed at all then they such should be used with great caution. These drugs interfere with REM and stage 4 sleep patterns, and may contribute to persistent insomnia (186). Clinicians should warn patients of the dangers of using over-the-counter preparations for sleeping and for colds because of the prominent anticholinergic side effects of these agents.

Trazodone, a sedating antidepressant medication that is devoid of anticholinergic side effects, is the preferred agent for the treatment of insomnia following TBI. A dose of 50 mg should be administered initially. If this dose is ineffective, doses up to 150 mg may be prescribed. Nonpharmacological approaches should be used regardless of whether or not medications are used, and should include minimizing daytime naps, maintaining regular sleep onset times, and engaging in regular physical activity during the day.

FATIGUE

Fatigue is a common symptom among persons with traumatic brain injury, and may occur independent of other posttraumatic neuropsychiatric disturbances. When treatment of other posttraumatic neuropsychiatric problems does not adequately improve fatigue, specific treatment of this problem may be required. Psychostimulants and amantadine are the most commonly used agents for the treatment of fatigue in persons with TBI, and may be of some benefit toward that end. In our experience, dosing of these agents similar that employed for the treatment of diminished arousal and attention is usually sufficient to treat posttraumatic fatigue. These medications may be of particular benefit in patients with posttraumatic depression in whom fatigue persists despite improvement in mood during treatment with antidepressants.

Modafinil, a medication recently approved for the treatment of excessive daytime somnolence in patients with narcolepsy, also may have a role in treatment of post-TBI fatigue. Although the exact mechanism of action of modafinil is not clear, animal studies suggest that its promotion of wakefulness may result from an indirect, dose-dependent reduction of the release of GABA in the cerebral cortex, medial preoptic area, and posterior hypothalamus (187, 188), activation of hypocretin (orexin) neurons in the lateral hypothalamus (189), and dose-dependent increases in glutamate release in the ventrolateral and the ventromedial thalamus (190). Some combination of these mechanisms in humans may increase arousal via activation in regions critical to this purpose, either directly via glutamatergic thalamic activation, indirectly via reduction of GABA function, or through the secondary effects of lateral hyopothalamic projections to regions involved in control of arousal and sleep-wake cycle (tubero-mammilary nucleus and the locus coeruleus) (191).

Studies of the effect of modafinil on fatigue and excessive sleepiness in patients with multiple sclerosis (192, 193) and Parkinson's disease (194) suggest benefit. Elovic (2000) (195) has suggested that modafinil may be of similar benefit in patients with TBI. Teitelman (2001) (196) described his use of modafinil among 10 outpatients with nonpenetrating traumatic brain injury and functionally significant excessive daytime sleepiness and in two patients with somnolence due to sedating psychiatric medications. The patients included in his report were between the ages of 42 to 72 years, all were outpatients, and were treated in an open-label fashion. Doses of modafinil ranged between 100 mg to 400 mg taken once each morning. Nine of these patients reported improvements in excessive daytime sleepiness, and some patients also reported subjective improvements in attention as well as other cognitive benefits. Although this medication was generally well tolerated, this report also describes treatment intolerance due to increased "emotional instability" in two women with brain injury complicated by multiple other medical conditions and receiving multiple additional medications. At the time of this writing there are no published clinical studies with which to evaluate the effectiveness or tolerability of modafinil for post-traumatic hypersomnolence or fatigue. If used in this population, dosages should start with 100 mg in the morning, and can be increased to up to 400 mg/day administered in either a single daily dose or two divided doses (i.e., 200 mg in the morning, and 200 mg in the afternoon). Higher doses (up to 600 mg/day) are sometimes used, but there is no evidence in any patient population that such doses offer benefit beyond that achieved with 400 mg/day.

COLDNESS

Complaints of feeling cold, without actual alteration in body temperature, are occasionally seen in patients who have suffered brain injury. This feeling can be distressing to those who experience it. Patients may wear excessive amounts of clothing, and may adjust the thermostat in their homes to the point that other members of the family are made uncomfortable. While this is not a commonly reported symptom of traumatic brain injury (TBI), Hibbard et al. (1998) (197) report that in a sample of 331 individuals with traumatic brain injury, 27.9% complained of changes in body temperature, and 13% persistently felt cold. Eames (1997) (198), while conducting a study of the cognitive effects of vasopressin nasal spray in patients with TBI, reported that thirteen patients had the persistent feeling of coldness, despite normal sublingual temperature. All were treated with nasal vasopressin spray for one month. Eleven of these patients stopped complaining of feeling cold after one month of treatment, and one other patient had incomplete improvement in this symptom.

Silver and Anderson (1999) (199) performed a pilot study of the effects of intranasal vasopressin (DDAVP) twice daily for one month among six patients who complained of persisting coldness after brain injury. Five of the six patients had a dramatic response to DDAVP – some as soon as one week after initiating treatment – and no longer complained of feeling cold. This response persisted even after discontinuation of treatment. Patients denied any side effects from treatment with this agent. The authors of this study suggest that DDAVP may reverse physiologic effects of a relative deficit in vasopressin in the hypothalamus caused by injury to the vasopressin precursor producing cells in the anterior hypothalamus, and may thereby correct an internal temperature setpoint disrupted by the brain injury.

OTHER ISSUES IN THE PHARMACOTHERAPY OF NEUROPSYCHIATRIC DISTURBANCES FOLLOWING TBI

There has been a bias held by patients, families, and some treatment centers against the use of medications for the treatment of neuropsychiatric disorders in patients with brain injury. The bias against the use of psychiatric medications may have several bases, including the stigma associated with mental illness and psychiatric treatment, and in some cases the patient's previous and often suboptimal experience with psychotropic medications. Stigma may relate to the view that psychiatric symptoms are signs of weakness, indolence, or even moral decline. We have suggested that the neuropsychiatric paradigm – one that rejects the misleading demarcation between "brain" and "mind" and emphasizes the neurobiological bases of all cognitive, emotional, and behavioral problems regardless of the relationship of such problems to brain injury – is the most useful response to such biases. Patients struggling to accept treatment in the face of old stigmas may benefit from an explanation of symptoms as the products of alterations in neurotransmitters, brain structures, brain networks, or some combination of these, and from the presentation of treatments as designed to allieviate or compensate for such brain dysfunctions.

Unfortunately, particularly for patients with TBI, the experience of treatment with psychotropic medications has often been a negative one and their biases against treatment with some of these medications are not entirely without merit. Antipsychotic medications, and particularly typical antipsychotics, are widely misused as a general "tranquilizer" to sedate patients agitated after TBI, with resulting impairment in alertness, cognition, and (in some cases) the production of severe extrapyramidal symptoms. For example, we evaluated in consultation one patient who had been treated with low-dose fluphenazine to control agitated behavior. One month later, the staff and family complained that she was "underaroused." On our examination, the patient had severe cogwheel rigidity that had not been diagnosed previously. One hour after administration of benztropine 1 mg, she was "active" again.

Another fear about medication is that it will interfere with a "natural healing process" that occurs after TBI. Evidence obtained from animal models suggests that certain drugs, particularly agents that potently antagonize dopamine type-2 receptors, may interfere with recovery following neuronal injury. Feeney et al. (1982) (135) studied the effect of D-amphetamine on recovery from hemiplegia after ablation of the sensorimotor cortex in rats. They found that D-amphetamine accelerated the rate of recovery, and that this effect was blocked by haloperidol. In addition, haloperidol, when administered alone, resulted in delayed recovery. Importantly, recovery was affected only when the animal was allowed to move during drug administration. This implies that haloperidol delays the recovery process during active rehabilitation, rather than interfering with spontaneous recovery per se. In another model, Hovda et al. (1985) (200) found that haloperidol blocked the positive effect of D-amphetamine on recovery of depth perception after visual cortex injury.

It has been suggested that the mechanism of action of haloperidol in delaying recovery also operates through its effects as an α-adrenergic antagonist (201). Clonidine, an α2-adrenergic agonist, and prazosin, an α1-adrenergic antagonist, reinstate deficits after sensorimotor cortex ablation (202), an effect not seen with propranolol (203). Other studies have demonstrated that clonidine has deleterious effects on recovery (204, 205). It should be noted that these experimental methods in animals do not produce the same neuropathological findings as contusions or diffuse axonal injury in humans, and, therefore, may not apply fully to our understanding of the effects α-adrenergic antagonism following TBI in humans.

In animal studies involving the neurotransmitter γ-aminobutyric acid (GABA), increased GABA function has been associated with greater neuromotor deficits and poorer recovery (206). Increased production of GABA associated with benzodiazepine administration may result in greater glutamate neurotoxicity (207). Diazepam has been found to block recovery of sensory deficits after rat neocortex ablation (208).

The studies cited above relating psychotropic use to impaired neuronal recovery after laboratory-induced brain injury have all used animal models. The study by Rao et al. (1985) (136) appears to offer support for the notion of delayed recovery following administration of haloperidol by virtue of its demonstration of increased duration of posttraumatic amnesia among patients receiving this medication. However, there have been no carefully controlled clinical trials of this important relationship in humans. Interestingly, when the medical records of recovering stroke patients were reviewed, the use of antihypertensive medications or haloperidol was associated with poorer recovery (209). Goldstein and Davis (1990) (205) found that when patients who had had ischemic strokes were administered phenytoin, benzodiazepines, dopamine receptor antagonists, clonidine, or prazosin, they showed poorer sensorimotor function and lower activities of daily living than stroke patients who did not receive those drugs.

Many patients are prescribed anticonvulsant drugs (ACDs) after TBI, and may still be receiving them at the time of neuropsychiatric consultation in the period following acute rehabilitation. As noted previously, it is important to ascertain whether such agents were prescribed for the treatment of active seizures, for seizure prophylaxis, or for the treatment of another neuropsychiatric problem. Treatment with anticonvulsant drugs can produce de novo cognitive and emotional symptoms (210–212). Phenytoin appears to adversely affect cognition more than carbamazepine (213). Dikmen et al. (1991) (214) described greater cognitive impairment during treatment with phenytoin for prophylaxis of posttraumatic seizures when compared to placebo in a study with 244 patients with TBI. Intellectual deterioration in children on chronic treatment with phenytoin or phenobarbital also has been documented (215). Dikmen et al. (2000) (216) found no adverse cognitive effects of valproate when administered for 12 months after TBI. In a double-blind placebo-controlled study of the cognitive and emotional effects of phenytoin (40 patients) and carbamazepine (42 patients) in TBI patients being treated with these medications for seizure prophylaxis, Smith et al. (1994) (217) noted that both of these medications (but particularly carbamazepine) produced significantly more cognitive and motor slowing than did placebo. They found that both phenytoin and carbamazepine had negative effects on cognitive performance, especially those that involved motor and speed performance. Although, in the patient group as a whole, the effects were of questionable clinical significance, some patients experienced clinically significant negative cognitive effects during treatment with either of these agents. This is concordant with other observations of carbamazepine's potential to significantly impair cognition in persons with neurological conditions that confer a vulnerability to such effects (218).

However, some patients do tolerate the cognitive effects of valproate and/or carbamazepine relatively well. Minimal impairment in cognition was found with both valproate and carbamazepine in a group of patients with epilepsy (219). Although those included in this study were not TBI patients, this observation suggests that at least some neurologically vulnerable patients may not experience significant cognitive impairment during treatment with these agents. Similarly, Persinger (2000) (220) reported that 12 of 14 patients treated with carbamazepine in the late period following TBI retrospectively reported improvements in episodes of confusion and depression, increases in attention and focus, and reduction or elimination of subtle psychotic-like experiences ("aversive sensed presence"). The author of this study suggests that this finding suggests an electrical (although not epileptic) nature for such symptoms that may be amenable to treatment with carbamazepine or other anticonvulsants.

Among the newer anticonvulsant medications, topiramate, but not gabapentin or lamotrigine, has been demonstrated to adversely affect cognition in healthy young adults (221). Treatment with more than one anticonvulsant (polytherapy) has been associated with increased adverse neuropsychiatric reactions (211). Hoare (1984) (222) found that the use of multiple anticonvulsant drugs to control seizures resulted in an increase in disturbed behavior in children.

Patients who have a seizure immediately after brain injury often are placed on an anticonvulsant drug for seizure prophylaxis. Temkin et al. (1990) (223) showed that the administration of phenytoin acutely after traumatic injury had no prophylactic effect on seizures that occurred subsequent to the first week after injury. Similarly, valproate did not demonstrate any efficacy in preventing late posttraumatic seizures (223). It should be noted that there was a non-significant trend towards a higher mortality during treatment with valproate in this context. Anticonvulsant medications are not recommended after one week of injury for prevention (prophylaxis) of posttraumatic seizures (225). Any patient with TBI who is treated with anticonvulsant medication requires regular reevaluations to substantiate continued clinical necessity for such treatment.

These studies suggest that careful monitoring of cognition, motor function, and other neurobehavioral functions during treatment with any psychotropic compound in persons with TBI is warranted. In general, treatment with these medications should be reserved for patients with neuropsychiatric disturbances that are not fully amenable to treatment through nonpharmacologic means.

CONCLUSIONS

In this chapter, we have reviewed the role of medication in the treatment of the most frequently occurring neuropsychiatric disturbances that are associated with TBI. Ideally, it would be desirable if the neuropsychiatric problems resulting from TBI could be controlled by nonpharmacologic means alone. However, posttraumatic neuropsychiatric disturbances are associated with significant distress and considerable functional disability, and some of these problems may also endanger the patient and others. In many cases, behavioral treatment and cognitive rehabilitation are of less than optimal benefit in the absence of effective psychopharmacologic treatments of neuropsychiatric disturbances. In other psychiatric conditions such as major depression, there is evidence that delay of effective treatment may result in refractoriness of the condition. For example, Post (1992) (226) reported that recurrent affective disorder becomes more difficult to treat the longer the condition persists. Thus there are theoretical reasons for prompt initiation of pharmacological treatment of neuropsychiatric disturbances in patients with TBI. When appropriately administered, medications may significantly alleviate these problems, improve rehabilitation efforts, and contribute to improved quality of life among persons with TBI.

*R*eferences

1. Levin et al. 1987 Levin HS, High WM, Goethe KE, Sisson RA, Overall JE, Rhoades HM, Eisenberg HM, Kalisky Z, Gary HE. The neurobehavioural rating scale: assessment of the behavioural sequelae of head injury by the clinician. *J Neurol Neurosurg Psychiatry* 1987;50:183–193.
2. McCauley SR, Levin HS, Vanier M, Mazaux JM, Boake C, Goldfader PR, Rockers D, Butters M, Kareken DA, Lambert J, Clifton GL. The neurobehavioural rating scale-revised: sensitivity and validity in closed head injury assessment. *J Neurol Neurosurg Psychiatry* 2001;71:643–651.
3. Cummings JL, Mega M, Gray K, Rosenberg-Thompson S, Carusi DA, Gornbein J. The Neuropsychiatric Inventory: comprehensive assessment of psychopathology in dementia. *Neurology* 1994; 44(12):2308–14.
4. Silver JM, Yudofsky SC. The Overt Aggression Scale: Overview and clinical guidelines. *J Neuropsychiatry Clin Neurosci* 1991, 3 (suppl):S22–S29.
5. Marin RS, Biedrzycki RC, Firinciogullari S. Reliability and validity of the Apathy Evaluation Scale. *Psychiatry Res* 1991;38(2):143–162.
6. American Psychiatric Association. *Practice Guideline for the Treatment of Patients With Major Depressive Disorder, Second Edition*. Washington DC: American Psychiatric Press, Inc. 2000.

7. Arciniegas DB, Topkoff J, Silver JM. Neuropsychiatric aspects of traumatic brain injury. *Current Treatment Options in Neurology* 2000;2(2):169–186.

8. Silver JM, Hales RE, Yudofsky SC. Psychopharmacology of depression in neurologic disorders. *J Clin Psychiatry* 1990; 51 (suppl 1):33–39.

9. Silver JM, Yudofsky SC, Hales RE. Depression in traumatic brain injury. *Neuropsychiatry, Neuropsychology, and Behavioral Neurology* 1991;4:12–23.

10. McAllister TW, Arciniegas DB. Evaluation and Treatment of Postconcussive Syndrome. *NeuroRehabilitation* 2002;17(4):265–83.

11. Arciniegas DB, Topkoff J. The neuropsychiatry of pathological affect: an approach to evaluation and treatment. *Seminars in Clinical Neuropsychiatry* 2000;5(4):290–306.

12. Hurley RA, Taber KH. Emotional disturbances following traumatic brain injury. *Current Treatment Options in Neurology* 2002;4(1):59–76.

13. Fann JR, Uomoto JM, Katon WJ. Sertraline in the treatment of major depression following mild traumatic brain injury. *J Neuropsychiatry Clin Neurosci* 2000;12:226–232.

14. Turner-Stokes L, Hassan N, Pierce K, Clegg F. Managing depression in brain injury rehabilitation: the use of an integrated care pathway and preliminary report of response to sertraline. *Clinical Rehabilitation* 2002;16(3):261–281.

15. Fann JR, Uomoto JM, Katon WJ. Cognitive improvement with treatment of depression following mild traumatic brain injury. *Psychosomatics* 2001;42:48–54.

16. Schmitt JA, Kruizinga MJ, Reidel WJ. Non-serotonergic pharmacological profiles and associated cognitive effects of serotonin reuptake inhibitors. *J Psychopharmacol* 2001;15(3):173–179.

17. Meythaler JM, Depalma l, Devivo MJ, Guin_renfoe S, Novack TA. Sertraline to improve arousal and alertness in severe traumatic brain injury secondary to motor vehicle crashes. *Brain Inj* 2001; 15(4):321–331.

18. Kant R, Smith-Seemiller L, Zeiler D. Treatment of aggression and irritability after head injury. *Brain Inj* 1998;12(8):661–666.

19. Cassidy JW. Fluoxetine: a new serotonergically active antidepressant. *J Head Trauma Rehabil* 1989;4:67–69.

20. Wroblewski BA, Guidos A, Leary J, Joseph AB. Control of depression with fluoxetine and antiseizure medication in a brain-injured patient. *Am J Psychiatry* 1992;149:273.

21. Bessette RF, Peterson LG. Fluoxetine and organic mood syndrome. *Psychosomatics* 1992;33:224–226.

22. Horsfield SA, Rosse RB, Tomasino V, Schwartz BL, Mastropaolo J, Deutsch SI. Fluoxetine's effects on cognitive performance in patients with traumatic brain injury. *International Journal of Psychiatry in Medicine* 2002;32(4):337–344.

23. Rickels K, Schweizer E. Clinical overview of serotonin reuptake inhibitors. *J Clin Psychiatry* 1990;51:10.

24. Patterson DE, Braverman SE, Belandres PV. Speech dysfunction due to trazodone-fluoxetine combination in traumatic brain injury. *Brain Inj* 1997;11(4):287–291.

25. Spinella and Eaton 2002 Spinella M, Eaton LA. Hypomania induced by herbal and pharmaceutical psychotropic medicines following mild traumatic brain injury. *Brain Inj* 2002;16(4):359–367.

26. Breen R, Goldman CR. Response to "Evaluation of brain injury related behavioral disturbances in community mental health centers". *Comm Mental Health J* 1997;33:359–364.

27. Fujishiro J, Imanishi T, Onozawa K, Tsushima M. Comparison of the anticholinergic effects of the serotonergic antidepressants, paroxetine, fluvoxamine and clomipramine. *Eur J Pharmacol* 2002;454(2–3):183–188.

28. Perino C, Rago R, Cicolini A, Torta R, Monaco F. Mood and behavioural disorders following traumatic brain injury: clinical evaluation and pharmacological management. *Brain Inj* 2001; 15(2):139–148.

29. Saran AS. Depression after minor closed head injury: role of dexamethasone suppression test and antidepressants. *J Clin Psychiatry* 1985;46:335–338.

30. Dinan TG, Mobayed M. Treatment resistance of depression after head injury: a preliminary study of amitriptyline response. *Acta Psychiatr Scand* 1992;85:292–294.

31. Varney NR, Martzke JS, Roberts RJ. Major depression in patients with closed head injury. *Neuropsychology* 1987;1:7–9.

32. Wroblewski BA, Joseph AB, Cornblatt RR. Antidepressant pharmacotherapy and the treatment of depression in patients with severe traumatic brain injury: a controlled, prospective study. *J Clin Psychiatry* 1996;57 :582–587.

33. Robinson RG, Schultz SK, Castillo C, Kopel T, Kosier JT, Newman RM, Curdue K, Petracca G, Starkstein SE. Nortriptyline versus fluoxetine in the treatment of depression and in short-term recovery after stroke: a placebo-controlled, double-blind study. *Am J Psychiatry* 2000;157(3):351–359.

34. De Smet Y, Ruberg M, Serdaru M, Dubois B, Lhermitte F, Agid Y. Confusion, dementia, and anticholinergics in Parkinson's disease. *J Neurol Neurosurg Psychiatry* 1982;45:1161–1164.

35. Dubois B, Pillon B, Lhermitte F, Agid Y. Cholinergic deficiency and frontal dysfunction in Parkinson's disease. *Ann Neurol* 1990; 28:117–121.

36. Dixon CE, Hamm RJ, Taft WC, Hayes RL. Increased anticholinergic sensitivity following closed skull impact and controlled cortical impact traumatic brain injury in the rat. *J Neurotrauma* 1984;11:275–287.

37. Dixon CE, Liu SJ, Jenkins LW, Bhattachargee M, Whitson JS, Yang K, Hayes RL. Time course of increased vulnerability of cholinergic neurotransmission following traumatic brain injury in the rat. *Behav Brain Res* 1995;70:125–131.

38. Wroblewski BA, McColgan K, Smith K, Whyte J, Singer WD: The incidence of seizures during tricyclic antidepressant drug treatment in a brain-injured population. *J Clin Psychopharmacol* 1990;10: 124–128.

39. Khouzam HR, Donnelly NJ. Remission of traumatic brain injury-induced compulsions during venlafaxine treatment. *General Hospital Psychiatry* 1998;20(1):62–63.

40. Teng et al. 2001 Teng CJ, Bhalerae S, Lee Z, Farber J, Morris H, Foran T, Tucker W. The use of bupropion in the treatment of restlessness after a traumatic brain injury. *Brain Inj* 2001;15(5): 463–467.

41. Davidson J. Seizures and bupropion: a review. *J Clin Psychiatry* 1989;50:256–261.

42. Pinder RM, Brogden RN, Speight TM, Avery GS. Maprotiline: a review of its pharmacological properties and therapeutic efficacy in mental states. *Drugs* 1977;13:321–352.

43. Johnston JA, Lineberry CG, Ascher JA, Davidson J, Khayarallah MA, Feighner JP, Stark P. A 102-center prospective study of seizure in association with bupropion. *J Clin Psychiatry* 1991;52(11): 450–456.

44. Newburn G, Edwards R, Thomas H, Collier J, Fox K, Collins C. Moclobemide in the treatment of major depressive disorder (DSM–3) following traumatic brain injury. *Brain Inj* 1999;13: 637–642.

45. Gualtieri CT, Evans RW. Stimulant treatment for the neurobehavioural sequelae of traumatic brain injury. *Brain Inj* 1988; 2:273–290.

46. Ruedrich I, Chu CC, Moore SI. ECT for major depression in a patient with acute brain trauma. *Am J Psychiatry* 1983;140: 928–929.

47. Zwil AS, McAllister TW, Price TRP. Safety and efficacy of ECT in depressed patients with organic brain disease: review of a clinical experience. *Convulsive Therapy* 1992;8:103–109.

48. Crow S, Meller W, Christenson G, Mackenzie T. Use of ECT after brain injury. *Convulsive Therapy* 1996;12(2):113–116.

49. Kant R, Coffey CE, Bogyi AM. Safety and efficacy of ECT in patients with head injury: a case series. *J Neuropsychiatry Clin Neurosci* 1999;11:32–37.

50. Ojemann LM, Baugh-Bookman C, Dudley DL. Effect of psychotropic medications on seizure control in patients with epilepsy. *Neurology* 1987;37:1525–1527.

51. Dubovsky SL. Psychopharmacological treatment in neuropsychiatry. In Yudofsky SC, Hales RE (eds). *The American Psychiatric Press Textbook of Neuropsychiatry, 2nd Edition*. Washington DC: American Psychiatric Press, Inc. 1992, 663–701.

52. Jalil P. Toxic reaction following the combined administration of fluoxetine and phenytoin: two case reports. *J Neurol Neurosurg Psychiatry* 1992;55:414–415.

53. Sovner R, Davis JM. A potential drug interaction between fluoxetine and valproic acid. *J Clin Psychopharmacol* 1991; 11:389.

54. Grimsley SR, Jann MW, Carter JG, D'Mello AP, D'Souza MJ. Increased carbamazepine plasma concentration after fluoxetine coadministration. *Clin Pharmacol Ther* 1991;50:10–15.

55. Parmelee DX, O'Shanick GJ. Carbamazepine-lithium toxicity in brain-damaged adolescents. *Brain Inj* 2:305–308.

56. Stewart JT, Hemsath RH. Bipolar illness following traumatic brain injury: treatment with lithium and carbamazepine. *J Clin Psychiatry* 1988;49:74–75.

57. Starkstein SE, Boston JD, Robinson RG. Mechanisms of mania after brain injury: 12 case reports and review of the literature. *J Nerv Ment Dis* 1988;176:87–100.

58. Starkstein SE, Mayberg HS, Berthier ML, Fedoroff P, Price TR, Dannals RF, Wagner HN, Leiguarda R, Robinson RG. Mania after brain injury: neuroradiological and metabolic findings. *Ann Neurol* 1990;27:652–659.

59. Bamrah JS, Johnson J. Bipolar affective disorder following head injury. *Br J Psychiatry* 1991;158:117–119.

60. Zwil AS, McAllister TW, Cohen I, Halpern LR. Ultra-rapid cycling bipolar affective disorder following a closed–head injury. *Brain Inj* 1993;7:147–152.

61. Massey EW, Folger WN. Seizures activated by therapeutic levels of lithium carbonate. *South Med J* 1984;77:1173–1175.

62. Schiff HB, Sabin TD, Geller A, Alexander L, Mark V. Lithium in aggressive behavior. *Am J Psychiatry* 1982;139:1346–1348.

63. Hornstein A, Seliger G. Cognitive side effects of lithium in closed head injury. *J Neuropsychiatry Clin Neurosci* 1989;1:446–447.

64. Nizamie SH, Nizamie A, Borde M, Sharma S. Mania following head injury: case reports and neuropsychological findings. *Acta Psychiatr Scand* 1988;77:637–639.

65. Stewart JT, Hemsath RH. Bipolar illness following traumatic brain injury: treatment with lithium and carbamazepine. *J Clin Psychiatry* 1988;49:74–75.

66. Sayal K, Ford T, Pipe R. Case study: bipolar disorder after head injury. *J Am Acad Child Adolesc Psychiatry* 2000;39:525–528.

67. Massagli TL: Neurobehavioral effects of phenytoin, carbamazepine, and valproic acid: implications for use in traumatic brain injury. *Arch Phys Med Rehabil* 1991;72:219–226.

68. Marangell LB, Silver JM, Yudofsky SC. Psychopharmacology and Electroconvulsive Therapy. In Hales RE, Yudofsky SC, Talbott JA (eds): *Essentials of Clinical Psychiatry*. Washington DC: American Psychiatric Press, Inc. 1999, 705–800.

69. Pleak RR, Birmaher B, Gavrilescu A, Abichandri C, Williams DT. Mania and neuropsychiatric excitation following carbamazepine. *J Am Acad Child Adolesc Psychiatry* 1988;27:500–503.

70. Pope HG Jr, McElroy SL, Satlin A, Hudson JL, Keck PE Jr, Kalish R. Head injury, bipolar disorder, and response to valproate. *Compr Psychiatry* 1988;29:34–38.

71. Monji A, Yoshida A, Koga H, Tashiro K, Tashiro N. Brain injury-induced rapid-cycling affective disorder successfully treated with valproate. *Psychosomatics* 1999;40:448–449.

72. Dreifuss FE, Santilli N, Langer DH, Sweeney KP, Moline KA, Menander KB. Valproic acid hepatic fatalities: a retrospective review. *Neurology* 1987;37:379–385.

73. Bakchine S, Lacomblez L, Benoit N, Parisot D, Chain F, Lhermitte F. Manic-like state after bilateral orbitofrontal and right temporoparietal injury: efficacy of clonidine. *Neurology* 1989; 39:777–781.

74. Dubovsky SL, Franks RD, Allen S. Verapamil: a new antimanic drug with potential interactions with lithium. *J Clin Psychiatry* 1987;48(9):371–372.

75. Levy NA, Janicak PG. Calcium channel antagonists for the treatment of bipolar disorder. *Bipolar Disorders* 2000;2(2):108–119.

76. Clark AF, Davison K. Mania following head injury: a report of two cases and a review of the literature. *Br J Psychiatry* 1987; 150:841–844.

77. Poeck K. Pathological laughter and crying. In Fredericks JAM (ed): *Handbook of Clinical Neurology* 1985;45(1):219–225.

78. Zeilig G, Drubach DA, Katz-Zeilig M, Karatinos J. Pathological laughter and crying in patients with closed traumatic brain injury. *Brain Inj* 1996;10:591–597.

79. Jorge R, Robinson RG. Mood disorders following traumatic brain injury. *Int Rev Psychiatry* 2003;15(4):317–327.

80. Lauterbach EC, Schweri MM. Amelioration of pseudobulbar affect by fluoxetine: possible alteration of dopamine-related pathophysiology by a selective serotonin reuptake inhibitor. *J Clin Psychopharmacol* 1991;11:392–393.

81. Panzer MJ, Mellow AM. Antidepressant treatment of pathologic laughing or crying in elderly stroke patients. *J Geriatr Psychiatry Neurol* 1992;4:195–199.

82. Schiffer RB, Herndon RM, Rudick RA. Treatment of pathological laughing and weeping with amitriptyline. *N Engl J Med* 1985; 312:1480–1482.

83. Seliger GM, Hornstein A, Flax J, Herbert J, Schroeder K. Fluoxetine improves emotional incontinence. *Brain Inj* 1992;6: 267–270.

84. Sloan RL, Brown KW, Pentland B. Fluoxetine as a treatment for emotional lability after brain injury. *Brain Inj* 1992;6:315–319.

85. Lawson IR, MacLeod DM. The use of imipramine ("Tofranil") and other psychotropic drugs in organic emotionalism. *Br J Psychiatry* 1969;115:281–285.

86. Robinson RG, Parikh RM, Lipsey JR, Starkstein SE, Price TR. Pathological laughing and crying following stroke: validation of a measurement scale and a double-blind treatment study. *Am J Psychiatry* 1993;150:286–293.

87. Andersen G, Vestergaard K, Riis JO. Citalopram for post-stroke pathological crying. *Lancet* 1993;342:837–839.

88. Udaka F, Yamao S, Nagata H, Nakamura S, Kameyama M. Pathologic laughing and crying treated with Levodopa. *Neurology* 1984;41:1095–1096.

89. Sandyk R, Gillman MA. Nomifensine for emotional incontinence in the elderly. *Clin Neuropharmacol* 1985;8:377–378.

90. Evans RW, Gualtieri CT, Patterson D. Treatment of chronic closed head injury with psychostimulant drugs: a controlled case study and an appropriate evaluation procedure. *J Nerv Ment Dis* 1987;175:106–110.

91. Nahas Z, Arlinghaus KA, Kotrla KJ, Clearman RR, George MS. Rapid response of emotional incontinence to selective serotonin reuptake inhibitors. *J Neuropsychiatry Clin Neurosci* 1998;10: 453–455.

92. Brown KW, Sloan RL, Pentland B. Fluoxetine as a treatment for post-stroke emotionalism. *Acta Psychiatrica Scandinavica* 1998; 98(6):455–458.

93. Breen R, Goldman CR. Response to "Evaluation of brain injury related behavioral disturbances in community mental health centers". *Comm Mental Health J* 1997;33:359–364.

94. Muller U, Murai T, Bauer-Wittmund T, von Cramon DY. Paroxetine versus citalopram treatment of pathological crying after brain injury. *Brain Inj* 1999;13:805–811.

95. Andersen G, Stylsvig M, Sunde N. Citalopram treatment of traumatic brain damage in a 6-year-old boy. *J Neurotrauma* 1999; 16:341–344.

96. Allman P. Drug treatment of emotionalism following brain damage. *J Royal Soc Med* 1992;85:423–424.

97. Gualtieri T, Chandler M, Coons TB, Brown LT. Amantadine: a new clinical profile for traumatic brain injury. *Clin Neuropharmacol* 1989;12:258–270.

98. Glenn MB, Wroblewski B, Parziale J, Levine L, Whyte J, Rosenthal M. Lithium carbonate for aggressive behavior or affective instability in ten brain-injured patients. *Am J Phys Med Rehabil* 1989;68:221–226.

99. Lewin J, Sumners D. Successful treatment of episodic dyscontrol with carbamazepine. *Br J Psychiatry* 1992;161:262.

100. American Psychiatric Association. *Diagnostic and Statistical Manual of Mental Disorders, 4th Edition*. Washington, DC: American Psychiatric Press Inc. 1994.

101. Angus WR, Romney DM: The effect of diazepam on patients' memory. *J Clin Psychopharmacol* 1984;4:203–206.

102. Lucki I, Rickels K, Geller AM. Chronic use of benzodiazepines and psychomotor and cognitive test performance. *Psychopharmacol* 1986;88:426–433

103. Roth T, Hartse KM, Saab PG, Piccione PM, Kramer M. The effects of flurazepam, lorazepam, and triazolam on sleep and memory. *Psychopharmacol* 1980;70:231–237.

104. Walburga van Laar M, Volkeerts ER, van Willigenburg APP. Therapeutic effects and effects on actual driving performance of chronically administered buspirone and diazepam in anxious outpatients. *J Clin Psychopharmacol* 1992;12:86–95.

105. Gualtieri CT. Buspirone for the behavior problems of patients with organic brain disorders. *J Clin Psychopharmacol* 1991;11:280–281.

106. Gualtieri CT. Buspirone: neuropsychiatric effects. *J Head Trauma Rehabil* 1991;6:90–92.

107. Marin RS, Fogel BS, Hawkins J, Duffy J, Krupp B. Apathy: a treatable syndrome. *J Neuropsychiatry Clin Neurosci* 1995;7:23–30.

108. Andersson S, Gundersen PM, Finset A. Emotional activation during therapeutic interaction in traumatic brain injury: effect of apathy, self-awareness and implications for rehabilitation. *Brain Inj* 1999;13(6):393–404.

109. Krupp BH, Fogel BS. Motivational impairment in primary psychiatric and medical illness. *Psychiatric Ann* 1997;27:34–38.

110. Marin RS: Differential diagnosis of apathy and related disorders of diminished motivation. *Psychiatric Ann* 1997;27:30–33.

111. Kant R, Duffy JD, Pivovarnik A: Prevalence of apathy following head injury. *Brain Inj* 1998;12(1):87–92.

112. Andersson S, Bergedalen AM. Cognitive correlates of apathy in traumatic brain injury. *Neuropsychiatry Neuropsychol Behav Neurol* 2002;15(3):184–191.

113. Hoehn-Saric R, Lipsey JR, McLeod DR. Apathy and indifference in patients on fluvoxamine and fluoxetine. *J Clin Psychopharmacol* 1990;10:343–345.

114. McAllister TW. Apathy. *Semin Clin Neuropsychiatry* 2000;5:275–282.

115. Kraus MF, Maki PM. Effect of amantadine hydrochloride on symptoms of frontal lobe dysfunction in brain injury: case studies and review. *J Neuropsychiatry Clin Neurosci* 1997;9(2):222–230.

116. Van Reekum R, Bayley M, Garner S, Burke IM, Fawcett S, Hart A, Thompson W. N of 1 study: amantadine for the amotivational syndrome in a patient with traumatic brain injury. *Brain Inj* 1995;9:49–53.

117. Chandler MC, Barnhill JL, Gualtieri CT. Amantadine for the agitated head-injury patient. *Brain Inj* 1988;2:309–311.

118. Nickels JL, Schneider WN, Dombovy ML, Wong TM. Clinical use of amantadine in brain injury rehabilitation. *Brain Inj* 1994;8:709–718.

119. Drake ME, Pakalnis A, Denio LS, Phillips B. Amantadine hydrochloride for refractory generalized epilepsy in adults. *Acta Neurol Belg* 1991;91(3):159–164.

120. Shields WD, Lake JL, Chugani HT. Amantadine in the treatment of refractory epilepsy in childhood: an open trial in 10 patients. *Neurology* 1985;35(4):579–581.

121. Powell JH, al-Adawi S, Morgan J, Greenwood RJ: Motivational deficits after brain injury: effects of bromocriptine in 11 patients. *J Neurol Neurosurg Psychiatry* 1996;60(4):416–421.

122. Eames P. The use of Sinemet and bromocriptine. *Brain Inj* 1989;3:319–320.

123. Catsman-Berrevoets CE, Harskamp FV. Compulsive pre-sleep behavior and apathy due to bilateral thalamic stroke: response to bromocriptine. *Neurology* 1988;38:647–649.

124. Rothman KJ, Funch DP, Dreyr NA. Bromocriptine and puerperal seizures. *Epidemiology* 1990;1:232–238.

125. Lal S, Merbitz CP, Grip JC. Modification of function in head-injured patients with Sinemet. *Brain Inj* 1988;2:225–233.

126. Debette S, Kozlowski O, Steinling M, Rousseaux M: Levodopa and bromocriptine in hypoxic brain injury. *J Neurol* 2002;249(12):1678–82.

127. Lipper S, Tuchman MM. Treatment of chronic post-traumatic organic brain syndrome with dextroamphetamine: first reported case. *J Nerv Ment Dis* 1976;162:266–371.

128. Glenn MB. Methylphenidate for cognitive and behavioral dysfunction after traumatic brain injury. *J Head Trauma Rehabil* 1998;13:87–90.

129. Cummings JL. Cholinesterase inhibitors: A new class of psychotropic compounds. *Am J Psychiatry* 2000;157:4–15.

130. Levy ML, Cummings JL, Kahn-Rose R. Neuropsychiatric symptoms and cholinergic therapy for Alzheimer's disease. *Gerontology* 1999;45 Suppl 1:15–22.

131. Wroblewski B, Glenn MB, Cornblatt R, Joseph AB, Suduikis S. Protriptyline as an alternative stimulant medication in patients with brain injury: a series of case reports. *Brain Inj* 1993;7:353–362.

132. Reinhard DL, Whyte J, Sandel ME. Improved arousal and initiation following tricyclic antidepressant use in severe brain injury. *Arch Phys Med Rehabil* 1996;77(1):80–83.

133. Stanislav SW. Cognitive effects of antipsychotic agents in persons with traumatic brain injury. *Brain Inj* 1997;11(5):335–341.

134. Sandel ME, Olive DA, Rader MA. Chlorpromazine-induced psychosis after brain injury. *Brain Inj* 1993;7(1):77–83.

135. Feeney DM, Gonzalez A, Law WA. Amphetamine, haloperidol, and experience interact to affect rate of recovery after motor cortex injury. *Science* 1982;217:855–857.

136. Rao N, Jellinek HM, Woolston DC. Agitation and closed head injury: haloperidol effects on rehabilitation outcome. *Arch Phys Med Rehabil* 1985;66:30–34.

137. Wolf B, Grohmann R, Schmidt LG, Ruther E. Psychiatric admissions due to adverse drug reactions. *Compr Psychiatry* 1989;30:534–545.

138. Rosebush P, Stewart T. A prospective analysis of 23 episodes of neuroleptic malignant syndrome. *Am J Psychiatry* 1989;146:717–725.

139. Vincent FM, Zimmerman JE, Van Haren J. Neuroleptic malignant syndrome complicating closed head injury. *Neurosurg* 1986;18:190–193.

140. Yassa R, Nair V, Schwartz G. Tardive dyskinesia and the primary psychiatric diagnosis. *Psychosomatics* 1984;25:135–138.

141. Yassa R, Nair V, Schwartz G. Tardive dyskinesia: a two-year follow-up study. *Psychosomatics* 1984;25:852–855.

142. Michals ML, Crismon ML, Roberts S, Childs A. Clozapine response and adverse effects in nine brain-injured patients. *J Clin Psychopharmacol* 1993;13(3):198–203.

143. Burke JG, Dursun SM, Reveley MA. Refractory symptomatic schizophrenia resulting from frontal lobe lesion: response to clozapine. *J Psychiatry Neurosci* 1999;24(5):456–461.

144. Schreiber S, Klag E, Gross Y, Segman RH, Pick CG. Beneficial effect of risperidone on sleep disturbance and psychosis following traumatic brain injury. *Int Clin Psychopharmacol* 1998;13:273–275.

145. Wilkinson R, Meythaler JM, Guin-Renfroe S. Neuroleptic malignant syndrome induced by haloperidol following traumatic brain injury. *Brain Inj* 1991;13(12):1025–1031.

146. Rosebush PI, Stewart T, Mazurek MF. The treatment of neuroleptic malignant syndrome: are dantrolene and bromocriptine useful adjuncts to supportive care? *Br J Psychiatry* 1991;159:709–712.

147. Oliver AP, Luchins DJ, Wyatt RJ. Neuroleptic-induced seizures: an in vitro technique for assessing relative risk. *Arch Gen Psychiatry* 1982;39:206–209.

148. Lieberman JA, Kane JM, Johns CA. Clozapine: guidelines for clinical management. *J Clin Psychiatry* 1989;50:329–338.

149. Corrigan PW, Yudofsky SC, Silver JM. Pharmacological and behavioral treatments for aggressive psychiatric inpatients. *Hosp Comm Psychiatry* 1993;44:125–133.

150. Yudofsky SC, Silver JM, Hales RE. Treatment of Agitation and Aggression. In Schatzberg AF, Nemeroff CB (eds). *American Psychiatric Press Textbook of Psychopharmacolgy, 2nd Edition*. Washington DC: American Psychiatric Press, Inc. 1998, 881–900.

151. Alexopoulos GS, Silver JM, Kahn DA. Treatment of agitation in older persons with dementia. The Expert Consensus Panel for agitation in dementia. *Postgrad Med* 1998;1–88.

152. Dietch JT, Jennings RK. Aggressive dyscontrol in patients treated with benzodiazepines. *J Clin Psychiatry* 1988;49:184–189.

153. De Deyne PP, Rabheru K, Rasmussen A, Bocksberger JP, Dautzenberg PL, Eriksson S, Lawlor BA. A randomized trail of risperidone, placebo, and haloperidol for behavioral symptoms of dementia. *Neurology* 1999;53:946–955.

154. Katz IR, Jeste DV, Mintzer JE, Clyde C, Napolitano J, Brecher M. Comparison of risperdone and placebo for psychosis and behavioral disturbances associated with dementia: a randomized, double-blind trial. Risperidone Study Group. *J Clin Psychiatry* 1999;60:107–115.

155. McCracken JT, McGough J, Shah B, Cronin P, Hong D, Aman MG, Arnold LE, Lindsay R, Nash P, Hollway J, McDougle CJ, Posey D, Swiezy N, Kohn A, Scahill L, Martin A, Koenig K, Volkmar F, Carroll D, Lancor A, Tierney E, Ghuman J, Gonzalez NM, Grados M, Vitiello B, Ritz L, Davies M, Robinson J, McMahon D; Research Units on Pediatric Psychopharmacology Autism Network. Risperidone in children with autism and serious behavioral problems. *N Engl J Med* 2002;347:314–321.

156. Fernandez HH, Trieschmann ME, Burke MA, Friedman JH. Quetiapine for psychosis in Parkinson's disease versus dementia with Lewy bodies. *J Clin Psychiatry* 2002;63:513–515.

157. Ratey JJ, Leveroni CL, Miller AC, Komry V, Gaffar K. Low-dose buspirone to treat agitation and maladaptive behavior in brain-injured patients: two case reports. *J Clin Psychopharmacol* 1992; 12:362–364.

158. Levine AM. Buspirone and agitation in head injury. *Brain Inj* 1988;2:165–167.

159. Freinhar JP, Alvarez WA. Clonazepam treatment of organic brain syndromes in three elderly patients. *J Clin Psychiatry* 1986; 47(10):525–526.

160. Keats MM, Mukherjee S. Antiaggressive effect of adjunctive clonazepam in schizophrenia associated with seizure disorder. *J Clin Psychiatry* 1988;49:117–118.

161. Chatham-Showalter PE: Carbamazepine for combativeness in acute traumatic brain injury. *J Neuropsychiatry Clin Neurosci* 1996;8:96–99.

162. Patterson JF. Carbamazepine for assaultive patients with organic brain disease. *Psychosomatics* 1987;28(11):579–581.

163. Azouvi P, Jokic C, Attal N, Denys P, Markabi S, Bussel B. Carbamazepine in agitaton and aggressive behaviour following severe closed-head injury: results of an open trial. *Brain Inj* 1999;13:797–804.

164. Vanier M, Mazaux J-M, Lambert J, Dassa C, Levin HS. Assessment of neuropsychologic impairment after head injury: interrater reliability and factorial and criterion validity of the neurobehavioral rating scale-revised. *Arch Phys Med Rehabil* 2000;81:796–806.

165. Geracioti TD Jr. Valproic acid treatment of episodic explosiveness related to brain injury. *J Clin Psychiatry* 1994;55(9): 416–417.

166. Giakas WJ, Seibyl JP, Mazure CM. Valproate in the treatment of temper outbursts (letter). *J Clin Psychiatry* 1990;51:525.

167. Mattes JA. Valproic acid for nonaffective aggression in the mentally retarded. *J Nerv Ment Dis* 1992;180:601–602.

168. Horne M, Lindley SE. Divalproex sodium in the treatment of aggressive behavior and dysphoria in patients with organic brain syndromes. *J Clin Psychiatry* 1995;56(9):430–431.

169. Wroblewski BA, Joseph AB, Kupfer J, Kalliel K. Effectiveness of valproic acid on destructive and aggressive behaviours in patients with acquired brain injury. *Brain Inj* 1997;11(1):37–47.

170. Herrmann N, Lanctot K, Myszak M. Effectiveness of gabapentin for the treatment of behavioral disorders in dementia. *J Clin Psychopharmacol* 2000;20:90–93.

171. Roane DM, Feinberg TE, Meckler L, Miner CR, Scicutella A, Rosenthal RN. Treatment of dementia-associated agitation with gabapentin. *J Neuropsychiatry Clin Neurosci* 2000;12:40–43.

172. Childers MK, Holland D. Psychomotor agitation following gabapentin use in brain injury. *Brain Inj* 1997;11(7):537–540.

173. Bellus SB, Stewart D, Vergo JG, Kost PP, Grace J, Barkstrom SR. The use of lithium in the treatment of aggressive behaviours with two brain-injured individuals in a state psychiatric hospital. *Brain Inj* 1996;10(11):849–860.

174. Hornstein A, Seliger G. Cognitive side effects of lithium in closed head injury. *J Neuropsychiatry Clin Neurosci* 1989;1:446–447.

175. Moskowitz AS, Altshuler L. Increased sensitivity to lithium-induced neurotoxicity after stroke: a case report. *J Clin Psychopharmacol* 1991;11:272–273.

176. Mysiw WJ, Jackson RD, Corrigan JD. Amitriptyline for post-traumatic agitation. *Am J Phys Med Rehabil* 1988;67:29–33.

177. Jackson RD, Corrigan JD, Arnett JA. Amitriptyline for agitation in head injury. *Arch Phys Med Rehabil* 1985;66:180–181.

178. Szlabowicz JW, Stewart JT. Amitriptyline treatment of agitation associated with anoxic encephalopathy. *Arch Phys Med Rehabil* 1990;71:612–613.

179. Mooney GF, Haas LJ. Effect of methylphenidate on brain injury-related anger. *Arch Phys Med Rehabil* 1993;74:153–160.

180. Brooke MM, Questad KA, Patterson DR, Bashak KJ. Agitation and restlessness after closed head injury: a prospective study of 100 consecutive admissions. *Arch Phys Med Rehabil* 1992;73: 320–323.

181. Greendyke RM, Kanter DR, Schuster DB, Verstreate S, Wootton J. Propranolol treatment of assaultive patients with organic brain disease: a double-blind crossover, placebo-controlled study. *J Nerv Ment Dis* 1986;174:290–294.

182. Greendyke RM, Kanter DR. Therapeutic effects of pindolol on behavioral disturbances associated with organic brain disease: a double-blind study. *J Clin Psychiatry* 1986;47:423–426.

183. Alpert M, Allan ER, Citrome L, Laury G, Sison C, Sudilovsky A. A double-blind, placebo-controlled study of adjunctive nadolol in the management of violent psychiatric patients. *Psychopharmacol Bull* 1990;28:367–371.

184. Prigatano GP, Stahl ML, Orr WC, Zeiner HK. Sleep and dreaming disturbances in closed head injury patients. *J Neurol Neurosurg Psychiatry* 1982;45:78–80.

185. Askenasy JJM, Winkler I, Grushkiewicz J. The natural history of sleep disturbances in severe missile head injury. *Journal of Neurological Rehabilitation* 1989;3:93–96.

186. Buysse DJ, Reynolds III CF. Insomnia., In Thorpy MJ (ed). *Handbook of Sleep Disorders*. New York: Marcel Dekker, 1990, 373–434.

187. Ferraro L, Tanganelli S, O'Connor WT, Antonelli T, Rambert F, Fuxe K. The vigilance promoting drug modafinil decreases GABA release in the medial preoptic area and in the posterior hypothalamus of the awake rat: possible involvement of the serotonergic 5-HT3 receptor. *Neurosci Lett* 1996;220:5–8.

188. Ferraro L, Antonelli T, O'Connor WT, Tanganelli S, Rambert FA, Fuxe K. Modafinil: an antinarcoleptic drug with a different neurochemical profile to d-amphetamine and dopamine uptake blockers. *Biol Psychiatry* 1997;42:1181–1183.

189. Chemelli RM, Willie JT, Sinton CM, Elmquist JK, Sammell T, Lee C, Richardson JA, Williams SC, Xiong Y, Kisanuki Y, Fitch TE. Narcolepsy in orexin knockout mice: molecular genetics of sleep regulation. *Cell* 1999;98:437–451.

190. Ferraro L, Antonelli T, O'Connor WT, Tanganelli S, Rambert F, Fuxe K. The antinarcoleptic drug modafinil increases glutamate release in thalamic areas and hippocampus. *Neuroreport* 1997;8: 2883–887.

191. Lin L, Faraco J, Li R, Kadotani H, Rogers W, Lin X, Qiu X, de Jong PJ, Nishino S, Mignot E. The sleep disorder canine narcolepsy is caused by a mutation in the hypocretin (orexin) receptor 2 gene. *Cell* 1999;98:365–376.

192. Rammohan KW, Rosenberg JH, Lynn DJ, Blumenfeld AM, Pollak CP, Nagaraja HN. Efficacy and safety of modafinil (Provigil) for treatment of fatigue in multiple sclerosis: a two centre phase 2 study. *J Neurol Neurosurg Psychiatry* 2002;72:179–183.

193. Zifko UA, Rupp M, Schwarz S, Zipko HT, Maida EM. Modafinil in treatment of fatigue in multiple sclerosis Results of an open-label study. *J Neurology* 2002;249(8):983–987.

194. Nieves AV, Lang AE. Treatment of excessive daytime sleepiness in patients with Parkinson's disease with modafinil. *Clin Neuropharmacol* 2002;25(2):111–114.

195. Elovic E. Use of provigil for underarousal following TBI. *J Head Trauma Rehabil* 2000;15(4):1068–1071.

196. Teitelman E. Off-label uses of modafinil. *Am J Psychiatry* 2001;158:1341.

197. Hibbard MR, Uysal S, Sliwinski M, Gordon WA. Undiagnosed health issues in individuals with traumatic brain injury living in the community. *J Head Trauma Rehabil* 1998;13(4):47–57.

198. Eames P. Feeling cold: an unusual brain injury symptom and its treatment with vasopressin. *J Neurology Neurosurg Psychiatry* 1997;62(2):198–199.

199. Silver JM, Anderson K. Vasopressin treats the persistent feeling of coldness after brain injury. *J Neuropsychiatry Clin Neurosci* 1999;11(2):248–252.

200. Hovda DA, Sutton RL, Feeney DM. Haloperidol blocks amphetamine-induced recovery of binocular depth perception after bilateral visual cortex ablation in cat. *Proc West Phramacol Soc* 1985;28:209–211.

201. Sutton RL, Weaver MS, Feeney DM. Drug-induced modifications of behavioral recovery following cortical trauma. *J Head Trauma Rehabil* 1987;2:50–58.
202. Sutton RL, Feeney DM. Yohimbine accelerates recovery and clonidine and prazosin reinstate deficits after recovery in rats with sensorimotor cortex ablation (abstract). *Soc Neurosci Abstr* 1987;13:913.
203. Boyeson MG, Feeney DM: The role of norepinephrine in recovery from brain injury. *Soc Neurosci Abstr* 1984;10:68.
204. Feeney DM, Westerberg VS. Norepinephrine and brain damage: alpha noradrenergic pharmacology alters functional recovery after cortical trauma. *Can J Psychol* 1990;44:233–252.
205. Goldstein LB, Davis JN. Clonidine impairs recovery of beam-walking after a sensorimotor cortex lesion in the rat. *Brain Res* 1990;508:305–309.
206. Boyeson MG. Neurochemical alterations after brain injury: clinical implications for pharmacologic rehabilitation. *Neurorehabilitation* 1991;2:33–43.
207. Simantov R. Gamma-aminobutyric acid (GABA) enhances glutamate cytotoxicity in a cerebellar cell line. *Brain Res Bull* 1990; 24:711–715.
208. Schallert T, Hernandez TD, Barth TM. Recovery of function after brain damage: severe and chronic disruption by diazepam. *Brain Res* 1986;379:104–111.
209. Porch B, Wyckes J, Feeney DM. Haloperidol, thiazides and some antihypertensives slow recovery from aphasia (abstract). *Soc Neurosci Abstr* 1985;11:52.
210. Rivinus TM. Psychiatric effects of the anticonvulsant regimens. *J Clin Psychopharmacol* 1982;2(3):165–192.
211. Reynolds EH, Trimble MR. Adverse neuropsychiatric effects of anticonvulsant drugs. *Drugs* 1985;29:570–581.
212. Smith DB. Cognitive effects of antiepileptic drugs. *Adv Neurol* 1991;55:197–212.
213. Gallassi R, Morreale A, Lorusso S, Procaccianti G, Lugaresi E, Baruzzi A. Carbamazepine and phenytoin: comparison of cognitive effects in epileptic patients during monotherapy and withdrawal. *Arch Neurol* 1988;45:892–894.
214. Dikmen SS, Temkin NR, Miller B, Machamer J, Winn HR. Neurobehavioral effects of phenytoin prophylaxis of posttraumatic seizures. *JAMA* 1991;265:1271–1277.
215. Corbett JA, Trimble MR, Nichol TC. Behavioral and cognitive impairments in children with epilepsy: the long-term effects of anticonvulsant therapy. *J Am Acad Child Psychiatry* 1985;24: 17–23.
216. Dikmen SS, Machamer JE, Winn HR Anderson GD, Temkin NR. Neuropsychological effects of valproate in traumatic brain injury: a randomized trial. *Neurology* 2000;54(4):895–902.
217. Smith KR Jr, Goulding PM, Wilderman D, Goldfader PR, Holterman-Hommes P, Wei F. Neurobehavioral effects of phenytoin and carbamazepine in patients recovering from brain trauma: a comparative study. *Archives of Neurology* 1994;51:653–660.
218. Meador KJ, Loring DW, Ray PG, Murro AM, King DW, Nichols ME, Deer EM, Goff WT. Differential cognitive effects of carbamazepine and gabapentin. *Epilepsia* 1999;40:1279–1285.
219. Prevey ML, Delaney RC, Cramer JA, Cattanach L, Collins JF, Mattson RH. Effect of valproate on cognitive functioning. Comparison with carbamazepine. The Department of Veterans Affairs Epilepsy Cooperative Study 264 Group. *Arch Neurol* 1996; 53(10):1008–1016.
220. Persinger MA. Subjective improvement following treatment with carbamazepine (Tegretol) for a subpopulation of patients with traumatic brain injuries. *Perceptual & Motor Skills* 2000;90: 37–40.
221. Martin R, Kuzniecky R, Ho S, Hetherington H, Pan J, Sinclair K, Gilliam F, Faught E. Cognitive effects of topiramate, gabapentin, and lamotrigine in healthy young adults. *Neurology* 1999; 52(2):321–327.
222. Hoare P. The development of psychiatric disorder among schoolchildren with epilepsy. *Dev Med Child Neurol* 1984;26(1):3–13.
223. Temkin NR, Dikmen SS, Wilensky AJ, Keihm J, Chabal S, Winn HR. A randomized, double-blind study of phenytoin for the prevention of post-traumatic seizures. *N Engl J Med* 1990;323: 497–502.
224. Temkin NR, Dikmen SS, Anderson GD, Wilensky AH, Holmes MD, Cohen W, Newell DW, Nelson P, Awan A, Winn HR. Valproate therapy for prevention of posttraumatic seizures: a randomized trial. *J Neurosurg* 1999;91(4):593–600.
225. Brain Injury Special Interest Group of the American Academy of Physical Medicine and Rehabilitation. Practice parameter: antiepileptic drug treatment of posttraumatic seizures. *Arch Phys Med Rehabil* 1998;79(5):594–597.
226. Post RM. Transduction of psychosocial stress into the neurobiology of recurrent affective disorder. *Am J Psychiatry* 1992; 149(8):999–1010.

53 Pharmacotherapy of Cognitive Impairment

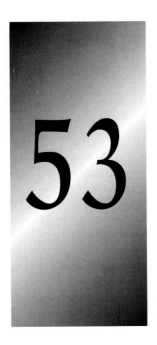

David B. Arciniegas
Jonathan M. Silver

INTRODUCTION

Cognitive impairments are among the most common neuropsychiatric sequelae of traumatic brain injury (TBI) at all levels of severity, and typically include impairments of arousal, speed of information processing, attention, memory, language and social communication, and executive functioning (1–5). Although each of these domains of cognitive function may be disrupted by direct injury to cortical, subcortical, or brainstem elements of the distributed cerebral networks that support them, injury to the axons connecting these elements or providing them with the neurochemical input required for their function also contributes to posttraumatic cognitive impairments (6–8). Understanding the neurochemical bases of cognition and the neurochemical consequences of TBI facilitates the development of rational approaches to the pharmacotherapy of posttraumatic cognitive impairments. Although the state of knowledge regarding these issues is at present incomplete, clinicians working with persons with cognitive impairments are well served to stay apprised of this rapidly growing body of information in order to make informed decisions regarding the use of medications in this population.

Toward that end, this chapter provides a review of the pharmacotherapy of cognitive impairment following TBI. To frame that review, definitions of the major domains of cognition most commonly affected by TBI, their basic neuroanatomy and, where known, their neurochemistry is offered. Next, the neurochemical consequences of TBI particularly relevant to understanding the pharmacotherapy of cognitive and other neuropsychiatric consequences of TBI are reviewed. Thereafter, studies of pharmacotherapies for cognitive impairment following TBI are reviewed and recommendations for the application of those pharmacotherapies are presented.

COGNITION: DEFINITIONS, NEUROANATOMY, AND NEUROCHEMISTRY

Arousal

Arousal is the most fundamental cognitive function, and is supported by a set of selective distributed reticulothalamic, thalamocortical, and reticulocortical networks (9, 10). The principal component of the reticulothalamic portion of the arousal system consists of cholinergic projections arising from the penduculopontine and laterodorsal tegmental nuclei. These projections terminate in the body of the thalamus as well as the reticular nucleus of the thalamus, the balance of activity between which appears to modulate the degree of thalamic activity. Thalamocortical projections, which are predominantly glutamatergic, activate cortex and prepare it for information processing. The level of cortical arousal, or the readiness of cortex to engage in information processing, is modulated by the reticulocortical portion of the arousal system. This portion of the arousal system consists of dopaminergic projections arising from the ventral tegmental area of the midbrain, noradrenergic projections arising from the locus ceruleus, serotonergic projections arising from the median and dorsal raphe nuclei, and cholinergic projections arising from the medial septal nucleus and vertical limb of the diagonal band of Broca (to medial temporal structures) and also the nucleus basalis of Meynert (to neocortical, and especially frontal, areas). These projections appear to modulate the activity of widespread areas of neocortex. Collectively, the relative balance between and reciprocal influences of the reticulothalamic and reticulocortical systems determine the individual's clinical level of arousal.

Mechanical injury to any of these elements of the arousal system may impair this most basic cognitive function (6, 8). In more severe injuries, and particularly those in which rotational forces produce shearing or frank hemorrhage in the upper brainstem (i.e., Duret's hemorrhage), arousal may be severely compromised as a result of damage to reticular structures and their reticulothalamic and reticulocortical projections (11). Mechanical injuries of the thalamus, particularly when bilateral, may also compromise cortical arousal and produce persistent vegetative or minimally conscious states (12). Unfortunately, this type of injury is frequently associated with post-TBI fatality (13). Mechanical injury to white matter fibers connecting the several portions of the arousal system (i.e., diffuse axonal injury) produces varying degrees of impaired arousal, decreased speed and efficiency of information processing, and contributes to disturbances in other aspects of cognition (14, 15). Neurochemical perturbations resulting from mechanical injury to these systems, including acute excesses of glutamate, acetylcholine, dopamine, norepinephrine, and serotonin, also contribute to acute disturbances in arousal (16–23). Chronic disturbances in arousal may be due in part to injury-induced deficits in one or more of these neurotransmitters. The role of acute and chronic neurotransmitter dysfunction in disturbances of posttraumatic arousal and other cognitive impairments is discussed in more detail in the next section of this chapter.

Attention

Sensory gating, selective attention, and sustained attention (vigilance or concentration) are relatively basic cognitive functions. Sensory gating is a pre-attentive process that permits filtering of incoming stimuli in order to admit only a limited amount of information into attentional processing networks (7, 24–26). Selective attention refers to the direction of attentional resources to a stimulus, sustained attention refers to the maintenance of attentional processing on a stimulus, and working memory denotes the ability to maintain attention to that stimulus in the period immediately following its absence (27).

The boundaries of attentional processes overlap with those of many other cognitive processes, including arousal, perception, recognition, memory, and executive function. Accordingly, attentional disturbances may exacerbate impairments in these other domains of cognition. For example, impairments of attention may interfere with encoding of information (new learning), and thereby produce or exacerbate memory impairments. Similarly, higher-level attentional processes may overlap substantially with executive function, both conceptually and as well as practically given the methods by which executive functions are assessed clinically.

Attentional processes are predicated on several large-scale, selective, distributed neural networks (28; see Mesulam 2000 (9) for a detailed review). These networks include those involved in arousal described above, since arousal is a prerequisite for even the most basic aspects of attention. Additionally, primary and secondary sensory cortices, heteromodal parietal cortical areas, medial temporal (i.e., hippocampal and entorhinal) areas, the striatum and pallidum, several prefrontal (i.e., cingulate, inferolateral, and dorsolateral) cortices, and the axonal connections between them are components of these distributed attentional networks (29–31).

Electrophysiological studies suggest that the neurobiological bases of sensory gating, selective attention, and sustained attention are different (26, 32). Sensory gating appears most strongly related to the function of a cholinergically-dependent hippocampal inhibitory circuit, and is a pre-requisite for the development of selective attention within sensory cortical-hippocampal-frontal networks. Sustained attention is most strongly related to the function of inferior frontal-subcortical and dorsolateral prefrontal-subcortical circuits. The function of these circuits is dependent on a complex set of interactions between the major neurotransmitter systems, including those regulating the availability and function of cortical dopamine, norepinephrine, serotonin, acetylcholine, glutamate, and gamma-aminobutyric acid.

Spatial attention and visuospatial function appear to be served by a network that includes elements of the reticular system, thalamus, superior colliculus, striatum, posterior parietal cortex, frontal eye fields, and parietal cortex (9). As with other attentional processes, most of the major neurotransmitter systems are involved in spatial attention and visuospatial function. Unlike other attentional processes, spatial attention and visuospatial function display a pattern of marked right hemispheric specialization (33, 34). Disruptions in the structure and/or functioning of these networks produce a range of clinical symptoms, although the classic attentional disturbances arising from these right hemisphere attentional networks include acute confusional states (delirium) and left hemi-inattention (neglect).

As with arousal, acute and chronic neurochemical dysfunction within the networks serving these attentional functions most likely contributes to posttraumatic attentional impairments (24, 35, 36). Impairments in attention may also contribute to problems with the speed of information processing, although the latter is a complex cognitive process predicated not only on attention but also the efficiency and connectivity of the various networks involved in attentional processing and the executive control of attention.

Memory

Memory is a multifaceted cognitive function that includes both new learning (encoding) and recall (retrieval) of both declarative and non-declarative (implicit and/or procedural) information (37–39). Declarative memory refers to encoding and retrieval of both semantic (or fact) and episodic (or event) information; in other words, declarative memory serves learning and recall of information regarding "who," "what," "when," and "where." The process of declarative learning, whether verbal or nonverbal, is a hippocampally-dependent process (40, 41). Highly processed multimodal sensory information is transmitted from the inferior parietal (heteromodal) association cortices to the entorhinal-hippocampal complex. When that information produces a sufficiently robust signal in the hippocampus (a process that is, at least in part, predicated on assignment of motivational, emotional, or other "survival-related" significance by amygdala-hippocampal interactions), the process of long-term potentiation is initiated and that information is encoded for later recall. After declarative information is consolidated by this hippocampally-dependent process, retrieving declarative information requires frontal structures to activate the selective distributed networks in which that information was originally encoded. Declarative memory is also therefore highly associative, meaning that memories may be retrieved by reactivation of nearly any part of the network involved in the original encoding of that information or by activation of other networks whose constituent elements are shared by the network involved in the original encoding of that information.

Declarative memory disturbances are relatively frequent consequences of TBI, and may result from injury to the cortical, subcortical, and white matter elements of the networks that serve the various aspects of memory. From a neurochemical perspective, acute excesses of glutamate produce a series of excitotoxic events (i.e., increases in intracellular calcium and activation of second messenger systems) that damage entorhinal and hippocampal areas involved in the development of memory. Damage to these areas results in chronic impairments declarative

memory (42–46). Persistent neurochemical dysfunction in these and other structures required for declarative memory, including alterations in glutamatergic function (43–46) and cholinergic function (7, 24, 47–50), may contribute to posttraumatic impairments in new learning. Injury to the frontal-subcortical elements of this system appears to result in difficulties with efficient retrieval of previously learned information. Information retrieval may be affected by structural and/or neurochemical damage to the frontal-subcortical circuits that subserve this function. In particular, deficits in the availability of dopamine, norepinephrine, and acetylcholine to these circuits appear to contribute to impairments in memory retrieval (51–54).

Procedural memory involves the learning of information of non-declarative nature, and for our purposes is best understood as memory for "how" to perform certain tasks. Procedural memory is predicated on the development and fine-tuning of the sensorimotor-subcortical-cerebellar networks that required for learning and efficiently retrieving complex sensorimotor programs. As such, procedural memory is not hippocampally-dependent and its function and dysfunction are dissociable from declarative memory. Additionally, procedural memory is not associative, but is instead dedicated: it is inflexibly limited to the context (i.e., the specific sensorimotor processes) involved in procedural learning.

Ward et al. (2002) (55) note that procedural memory appears to be less affected by traumatic brain injury than is declarative memory. Recognition of the dissociation between posttraumatic procedural and declarative memory deficits may be relevant to the design of rehabilitation strategies to improve functional memory performance in this population (56). Although procedural memory may be distinguished from declarative memory on anatomical grounds, normal performance in this cognitive domain is dependent on many of the same neurotransmitters required by the frontal-subcortical circuits involved in retrieval of declarative information (57).

Language

Language refers to the symbolic (both verbal and written) means of communicating thought, and is generally a function of the dominant cerebral hemisphere. The principal domains of language include fluency, comprehension, repetition, and naming, each of which is associated with a selective distributed network specialized to serving its respective language domains (see Damasio and Damasio (2000) (58) for review). Fluency is predicated on a network of frontal structures involving at least dorsolateral, prefrontal motor association, and anterior insular cortices, white matter and subcortical structures through which these areas are connected, and the frontal opercular (Broca's) area. Output from this network of structures requires that primary motor cortex and the physical structures needed to communicate verbally or by writing are intact, although communication impairments related to disturbances in elementary motor function are generally distinguishable from true language disturbances (aphasias).

Comprehension of language is predicated on a network of temporoparietal structures, including at least the superior temporal language association cortex (Wernicke's area), inferior parietal heteromodal association cortex, and the white matter structures connecting them. Input to these areas requires that the sensory structures, their connections to primary sensory cortices, and the connection of these areas to sensory association systems are intact. Communication disturbances due to impairments in sensory structures and primary sensory cortices are also generally distinguishable from true language impairments.

The neural networks serving fluency and comprehension are distinct and dissociable, resulting in the production of aphasias referable to dysfunction in their respective networks. Disturbances in the networks subserving fluency produce the "anterior" aphasias, including Broca's and transcortical motor aphasias. The hallmark feature of these aphasias is impaired language syntax (i.e., agrammatisms), reduced phrase length, and undue word finding pauses. Disturbances in the networks subserving comprehension produce the "posterior" aphasias, including Wernicke's and transcortical sensory aphasias. The hallmark feature of these aphasias is impaired language semantics, including impaired understanding of word or phrase meaning and ineffective monitoring of language output (e.g., substitutions, phonemic paraphasias, neologisms, etc.).

Repetition is served by a distinct network comprised of Wernicke's area, a phonological output area at the anterior border of Wernicke's area, Broca's area, and the arcuate fasciculus which connects the posterior and anterior language areas. Disruption of any of these areas produces deficits in repetition. Disruption of the phonological output area or arcuate fasciculus may produce an isolated disruption of repetition, a problem referred to clinically as conduction aphasia. The neural networks subserving naming are widely distributed, and overlap substantially with those upon which fluency, comprehension, and repetition are predicated. Consequently, impairments of naming are commonly associated with any disruption sufficient to produce impairments in these other areas of language.

Disturbances of language and functional communication are not uncommon among persons with TBI (59–64), and may negatively affect functional outcome after TBI (65). Frank aphasias are generally associated with direct injury to cortical language areas or their subcortical white matter connections, and are relatively less common after TBI than are more subtle functional communication impairments. These subtle language disturbances, such as mild word-finding and naming problems, are common consequences of TBI across the spectrum of injury severity, and tend to be more strongly associated with anterior (i.e., frontal and temporopolar) rather than posterior (temporoparietal) lesions (63).

The neurochemistry of posttraumatic language impairments is less clearly understood than is the neurochemistry of posttraumatic impairments of arousal, attention, and memory. Several reports of the pharmacotherapy of aphasia suggest a role for augmentation of dopamine (66–72) and acetylcholine (73) in the treatment of language disturbances in persons with stroke and TBI, although findings from such studies are not universally positive (74). While inferential reasoning of the neurochemistry of language from pharmacotherapeutic interventions should be undertaken with caution, these reports suggest that dopaminergic and/or cholinergic systems may be reasonable targets for the treatment of posttraumatic language disturbances.

Prosody

Prosody refers to the affective import and kinesics of language (75, 76). Disturbances of prosody, or the aprosodias, demonstrate a pattern of non-dominant hemispheric specialization. The nondominant hemisphere structures and networks serving prosody are simplistically understood as homologous with those in the dominant hemisphere serving the syntax and semantics of language. Impaired function of the nondominant frontal structures involved in language may produce disturbances in the affective and kinesic aspects of language production, resulting in flat or monotonous expression that fails to communicate effectively the emotional relevance and subtlety of the information expressed. Impaired function of the non-dominant temporoparietal structures involved in language may produce disturbances in the appreciation of the affective and kinesic aspects of the communications of others.

At present, little is known about the frequency of either the posttraumatic aprosodias or their neurochemistry. It has been suggested that dopaminergic dysfunction may influence prosody (77). However, Raymer et al. (2001) (66) observed no improvements in prosody despite improvements in fluent language in a patient with a poststroke aphasia treated with bromocriptine. Although the neurochemistry and pharmacotherapy of the aprosodias is poorly understood, clinicians should be mindful of such language disturbances as they may mask affective or mood disturbances experienced by persons with TBI and may impair the ability of these individuals to engage in effective social communication despite otherwise intact language.

Praxis

Praxis refers to the on-demand integration of task understanding and execution, and impairments of this ability are referred to as apraxias (78, 79). Ideomotor apraxia denotes a condition in which an individual is unable to perform on demand a relatively simple (ostensibly "single-step") task such as brushing one's hair or teeth, pointing to objects, or pantomiming simple actions. Ideational apraxia denotes a condition in which the sequential linking of several ideomotor tasks is impaired.

Praxis displays a pattern of dominant hemisphere specialization, and the neural networks subserving this domain of cognition appear to overlap substantially with those serving language (10, 80). Consequently, the apraxias tend to be associated with the aphasias, and particularly with the nonfluent aphasias. The neurochemistry of praxis is not well understood, although it has been suggested that striatal dopamine deficits may contribute to the development of apraxia (81). As such, interventions targeting the aphasias, when effective, may be expected to improve concurrent disturbances of praxis. However, Raymer et al. (2001) (66) observed no improvement in limb apraxia despite improvement in nonfluent aphasia in a patient with post-stroke aphasia treated with bromocriptine. The specific neurochemistry of apraxia therefore remains uncertain, as does the neurochemical basis for pharmacotherapy of posttraumatic impairments in praxis.

Complex Cognition

Complex cognitive functions, including comportment ("social intelligence"), motivation, and executive function are also frequently impaired after TBI (82–86). Comportment describes the manner in which one interacts with others, and involves the integration of emotional (i.e., limbic and paralimbic) information with an understanding of the rules of social interaction. As such, we have described this function as the foundation of "social intelligence" (87). This term refers to the ability to understand and integrate self-assessment with social cueing, and deficits in social intelligence may result in socially inappropriate and maladaptive behavior. This cognitive function is most often ascribed to the lateral orbitofrontal-subcortical circuit (88), given the role of this cortical area in the integration of limbic-paralimbic information with other socially or environmentally relevant information.

Motivation refers to the process of generating, directing, and sustaining goal-directed cognition, emotion, and behavior. Dysfunction of this process results in apathy: a reduction in goal-directed motor, emotional, and cognitive activity (89). Motivation is most often ascribed to the anterior cingulate-subcortical circuit (88–90).

Although the occurrence and treatment of both comportmental and motivational impairments overlap substantially with those of impaired cognition, these impairments typically are more commonly regarded as behavioral rather than cognitive disturbances *per se*. As such, treatment of these problems is discussed in the chapter describing pharmacotherapies of neuropsychiatric disturbances elsewhere in this volume.

Executive function refers to a collection of abilities including: categorization and abstraction; systematic memory searching and information retrieval; problem solving; self-direction; planning and organization of cognition and behavior; independence from external environmental contingencies; maintenance of and fluent shifting between information or behavior sets; and use of language to guide behavior. These are the functions that are most immediately regarded as "intelligence" by patients, their families, and their care providers.

Executive function is most often ascribed to the dorsolateral prefrontal-subcortical circuit, and in particular its ability to integrate the processing and interaction of more "basic" cognitive processes carried on elsewhere in the brain. Executive dysfunction is a relatively common consequence of TBI, and may arise as a direct effect of injury to the dorsolateral prefrontal cortex, the subcortical elements connect to this cortical area, or the axonal connections between them (82). The function of the dorsolateral prefrontal-subcortical circuit serving executive function is dependent on a host of neurotransmitters including glutamate (serving as the primary excitatory neurotransmitter), acetylcholine, dopamine, norepinephrine, serotonin, (serving various modulatory functions), and gamma-aminobutyric acid (GABA, serving as the primary inhibitory neurotransmitter), among others (87, 88, 91). Consequently, posttraumatic disturbances in the function of any of these neurotransmitters may contribute to executive function impairments. By extension, pharmacotherapies that improve the function of posttraumatic impairments in these neurotransmitter systems would be expected to produce improvements in executive function.

Summary of the Neuroanatomic and Neurochemical Bases of Cognition

In this section we reviewed the basic neuroanatomy and neurochemistry of several cognitive domains in which posttraumatic impairments are common. Although normal cognition ultimately depends on a complex set of neurotransmitter, neuroactive peptides, neurohormones, second messenger system, and genetically-regulated neurochemical processes and interactions, several simple themes relevant to currently available pharmacotherapies are apparent. Glutamate-mediated neuronal damage and/or long-term glutamatergic dysfunction (either excess or deficit) may adversely affect a host of cognitive functions, including arousal, attention, memory, and executive function. Catecholamine (i.e., dopamine and norepinephrine) dysfunction appears particularly important to cortical aspects of arousal attention, speed of processing, language, executive function, and perhaps also memory retrieval. The role of serotonin in cognition is uncertain; augmentation of serotonin via nonselective serotonin reuptake inhibitors does not appear to be of direct benefit to cognition, but may indirectly affect cognition via improvement of comorbid disorders such as depression (92). Whether more limited alteration of serotonergic activity (e.g., alteration of action at 5HT-3 receptors) improves cognition directly or indirectly through modulation of other neurotransmitter systems is a matter of present investigation (see Buhot et al. 2000 (93) for review). Cholinergic function appears important to both subcortical and cortical aspects of arousal, attention, and memory, and may also play an important role in language and executive function. In the next section of this chapter, we will review the evidence for neurotransmitter dysfunction following TBI in order to frame the neurochemical basis of pharmacotherapies for posttraumatic cognitive impairments.

THE NEUROBIOLOGICAL BASES OF COGNITIVE IMPAIRMENT FOLLOWING TBI

Cognitive deficits arising from penetrating and/or focal trauma are often understandable given the functions known to be subserved by the site of injury; for example, executive impairments following severe bifrontal contusion and/or white matter injury, impaired anterograde memory following bilateral entorhinal-hippocampal injury, and so on (94). However, the etiology of cognitive impairments following non-penetrating (or "non-focal") injuries is relatively less well understood. Cytotoxic processes such as calcium and magnesium dysregulation, free radical injury, neurotransmitter (especially glutamate and cholinergic) excitotoxicity, and diffuse axonal injury due to straining and shearing biomechanical forces result from non-penetrating, non-contusional injuries (see McIntosh et al. (1999) (95) and Halliday (1999) (96) for review). These processes functionally and structurally disrupt the neural networks subserving neuropsychiatric function (i.e., cognition, emotion, and behavior). Studies of neurochemical changes subsequent to TBI suggest that alterations in neurotransmitter production and/or delivery occur within these networks both acutely and chronically, and therefore play a role in the development of cognitive impairments following TBI. As discussed in the following sections of this chapter, all of the major neurotransmitter systems, including glutamate, dopamine, norepinephrine, serotonin, and acetylcholine, are elevated in the acute period following TBI, a process that we

suggest may be simplistically understood as an acute traumatically-induced "neurotransmitter storm." However, the timing and/or eventual recolution of these neurotransmitter elevations influences the relevance of each of these systems to acute and/or chronic posttraumatic cognitive impairments.

Glutamate

TBI-induced glutamatergic disturbances are almost certainly important in the genesis of injury to areas critical to neuropsychiatric function (see Obrenovitch and Urenjak (1997) (19) for a detailed review). Excessive release of the amino acid neurotransmitters glutamate and aspartate appears to be at least in part responsible for traumatically-induced neuronal injury, particularly to areas in which these neurotransmitters play key roles (i.e., hippocampus and frontal cortices) (97–99). The degree of elevation of these excitatory amino acid neurotransmitters appears to be associated with the severity of injury and post-injury survival (100–102). The principal neurotoxic effects of glutamate are generally attributed to its action at N-methyl-D-aspartate (NMDA) receptors. When glutamate activates an NMDA receptor, it opens a channel in the cell membrane that permits influx of calcium. When excessive amounts of calcium enter the cell, oxidative processes and activation of proteolytic enzymes ensue, and the axonal terminus of the neuron is injured or destroyed. Even where such excesses are not directly excitotoxic, they tend to "drive" glucose utilization, which may exceed the capacity of the brain for oxidative metabolism, thereby producing toxic accumulations of lactate (103).

Cerebral glutamate levels are elevated within hours following TBI and appear to remain elevated for at least the first week following TBI in humans (104–107). The rate of return to normal levels of glutamate may be adversely affected by concurrent hypoxia (108). With or without such complicating factors, the rate at which glutamate levels return to pre-injury baseline – if they do indeed completely normalize after TBI – is uncertain. The rate of decline of glutamate levels observed in studies performed to-date suggests a trend towards normalization of cerebral glutamate in the weeks following TBI. However, early elevations of glutamate may permanently damage cortical areas (109) and thereby contribute to persistent posttraumatic cognitive impairments.

Animal models suggest that antagonism of glutamate receptors may attenuate the severity of neuronal injury following either focal ischemia (110) or trauma (98, 99). Additionally, glutamate-mediated excitotoxicity may be attenuated by therapeutically induced, but not spontaneous, cerebral hypothermia delivered in the acute post-injury period (111). Unfortunately, there are at present no widely available pharmacotherapies that effectively limit the destructive effects of acute excesses of glutamate or that ameliorate cognitive or other neuropsychiatric problems predicated on glutamate-induced neuronal damage (112).

Memantine and amantadine, two moderate-affinity uncompetitive NMDA receptor antagonists, are of theoretical interest to both the prevention of glutamate-mediated neurotoxicity in TBI and also the remediation of posttraumatic cognitive impairments predicated on glutamatergic dysfunction. Although there is evidence that memantine confers neuroprotection from glutamate-mediated excitotoxicity when administered shortly after experimental TBI in animals (113), there are at present no studies demonstrating neuroprotection from either amantadine or memantine in human TBI. Memantine and amantadine appear to indirectly increase striatal, prefrontal cortical, and nucleus accumbens dopamine function through their actions at glutamate receptors on midbrain dopaminergic neurons (114–117) or other yet undetermined mechanisms (118). The effects of these medications on both glutamate function and dopaminergic function may account for the purported benefit of memantine among persons with cognitive impairments due to Alzheimer's disease (119–122), cerebrovascular disease (120–123), and Wernicke-Korsakoff syndrome (124). As discussed in the next section, amantadine has been observed to improve arousal, attention, motivation, and other frontally-mediated functions in persons with TBI (125–129). Although encouraging of the potential application of this medication and other uncompetitive NMDA receptor antagonists to the treatment of posttraumatic cognitive impairments, the role of the glutamatergic properties of these agents towards that end is at present uncertain.

Catecholamines

Discrete lesions to ascending monoaminergic projections may interfere with the cognitive function served by the networks dependent upon them (130). Monoaminergic afferents course from the brain stem anteriorly, curving around the hypothalamus, the basal ganglia, and the frontal cortex, placing them in anatomical areas that are especially vulnerable to strain and shear forces that occur during TBI. Catecholamines alter the signal-to-noise ratio in the circuits that process information (131–133). In the setting of optimal catecholamine levels, the processing of contextually relevant cognitive, emotional, or behavioral information (signal) is enhanced and processing of background information (noise) is inhibited. As such, catecholamines serve as key modulators of information processing circuits in the brain. Because dopamine and norepinephrine exhibit an inverted U-shaped dose-response curve with respect to their effects on cortical information processing (9), either deficient or excessive dopamine may interfere with this process.

Two studies found markedly elevated plasma catecholamine levels after acute head injury in humans (22, 134). Acute elevations of these neurotransmitters are predictive of poor recovery from TBI (17, 22, 23). Whether such elevations are themselves sufficiently injurious to contribute to poor recovery after TBI or are instead simply a proxy for injury severity is not clear.

Also unclear is the role of catecholaminergic dysfunction in the development of persistent posttraumatic cognitive impairments. Tang et al. (1997) (18) suggested that striatal hyperdopaminergia contributes to post-TBI memory deficits in recently injured animals, antagonism of which improved visual memory performance. This finding appears to contradict the inference of reduced dopamine function drawn from observations of cognitive benefits following augmentation of dopaminergic function (using methylphenidate, for example) among persons with TBI in the days to weeks following injury (135, 136) and the observation that robust dopamine antagonism delays recovery from posttraumatic amnesia (137). However, it is consistent with the suggestion that either hyper- or hypodopaminergia may interfere with cognition following TBI. Very few other experimental-injury studies (20, 138) offer support for the hypothesis that cerebral catecholamine levels are chronically altered by TBI, and only one human study offers indirect evidence of relationship markers of dopaminergic or noradrenergic function and long-term cognitive deficits in traumatically brain-injured humans. Konrad et al. (2003) (35) studied 26 children with TBI, 31 children with attention deficit hyperactivity disorder (ADHD), and 26 healthy comparison children. Subjects with TBI and ADHD excreted significantly more urinary normetanephrine in resting situations and less urinary epinephrine after cognitive stress, and showed a decreased blink rate (an indirect measure of dopamine function) compared to normal controls. Children with TBI also demonstrated a higher excretion of metanephrine in the resting situation in comparison to children with ADHD and controls. Children with ADHD showed a higher tonic activity of the noradrenergic system and a less adaptive epinephrine excretion in response to cognitive stress, and children with TBI were impaired in their tonic epinephrine excretion. These observations suggest the possibility of long-term alterations in systemic monaminergic function following TBI, but they offer only indirect evidence of posttraumatic dysfunction in cerebral monaminergic systems.

Although evidence of direct, persistent, and statistically significant injury to catecholaminergic afferents following TBI is at present lacking (139), genetically-determined individual differences in the metabolism of these neurotransmitters by catechol-O-methyltransferase (COMT) may contribute to posttraumatic cognitive impairments. Substitutions in the gene sequence for COMT at codon 158 (Val/Met) result in expression of an enzyme with either high activity (COMT-val) or low activity (COMT-met) (140). Persons homozygous for the COMT-val isoform appear to metabolize catecholamines more efficiently than persons homozygous for the COMT-met isoform, and heterozygotes (i.e., COMT-val/met) metabolize catecholamines with an intermediate level of efficiency. In a study of 123 persons with TBI and posttraumatic executive dysfunction, Lipsky et al. (2002) (141) observed the highest levels of executive dysfunction on the Wisconsin Card Sorting Task (generally regarded as a measure of executive function) among subjects homozygous for the fast-acting COMT enzyme, intermediate levels of impairment among heterozygotes, and the lowest levels of impairment among subjects homozygous for the slow-acting COMT enzyme. This finding suggests that even if TBI produces only modest injury to reticulocortical catecholaminergic projections, individual differences in the metabolism of these neurotransmitters might in some persons (i.e., those with the fast-acting COMT enzyme) transform modest structural injury into substantial functional impairments in catecholamine-dependent cognitive functions.

In summary, while the extent of dopaminergic and noradrenergic dysfunction in the late period following TBI remains uncertain, pre-injury genetic differences in the metabolism of these neurotransmitters may contribute to posttraumatic cognitive impairments. The implications of such finding with respect to long-term neuropsychiatric disturbances require further study.

Serotonin

Serotonergic projections to frontal cortical areas are susceptible to biomechanical injury, and both diffuse axonal injury and contusions may produce dysfunction in this neurotransmitter system. Secondary neurotoxicity that is caused by excitotoxins and lipid peroxidation may also damage serotoninergic projections (142). Pappius (1989) (21) demonstrated widespread increases in hemispheric serotonin levels following experimentally induced brain injury in rats, and noted that increases in serotonin appeared to produce decreases in cerebral glucose utilization. Busto et al. (1997) (143) observed a prompt increase in the extracellular levels of serotonin in cortical regions adjacent to the impact site in an experimental injury study in rats. Tsuiki et al. (1995) (144) demonstrated in an experimental injury paradigm that serotonin synthesis was significantly increased in cortical areas throughout the injured hemisphere, particularly in the dorsal hippocampus and hippocampal area CA3, in the medial geniculate nucleus, and in the dorsal raphe nucleus. These authors observed depression in cortical glucose use in areas with increased serotonin synthesis. Eghwrudjakpor et al. (1997) (20) demonstrated a rapid increase in hemispheric concentrations of serotonin,

dopamine, and norepinephrine shortly after trauma experimentally induced traumatic brain injury in rats, with continued increases to three to four times control levels by 24 to 48 hours postinjury. These authors also report significant regional differences in serotonin levels after experimental TBI, with increases in the cerebral hemispheres but decreases in the spinal cord.

Findings regarding posttraumatic cerebral serotonin levels are discrepant, but such discrepancies may be attributable to between-study differences in the sites from which CSF samples are obtained. For example, Vecht et al. (1975) (145) and Bareggi et al. (1975) (146) found that lumbar cerebrospinal fluid (CSF) 5-hydroxyindoleacetic acid (5-HIAA) was below normal in conscious patients and normal in patients who were unconscious. Decreased CSF levels of serotonin are reported by Karakucuk et al. (1997) (142) in 45 adults undergoing minor surgery with spinal anesthesia within 24 hours of TBI. However, Porta et al. (1975) (147) demonstrated elevated ventricular CSF 5-HIAA levels in patients within days of severe TBI. These findings suggest that ventricular sampling in humans may more accurately reflect alterations in cerebral serotonin levels after TBI than lumbar cerebrospinal fluid sampling. Additionally, focal and diffuse lesions may result in differences with respect to monoaminergic alterations after TBI. For example, Van Woerkom et al. (1977) (148) investigated patients with frontotemporal contusions and those with diffuse contusions. They documented decreased levels of 5-HIAA in patients with frontotemporal contusions, but increased 5-HIAA levels in those with more diffuse contusions.

The evidence in both animal and human studies suggests that TBI results in acute increases in hemispheric serotonin levels and also that such increases are associated with decreased cerebral glucose utilization. As a result of decreasing cortical metabolism, acute elevations of serotonin may in part contribute to posttraumatic cognitive impairments during the acute injury period. It stands to reason that augmentation of serotonergic function in the acute injury period would be of little benefit cognitively. Consistent with that reasoning, Meythaler et al. (2001) (149), in a placebo-controlled trial of sertraline for arousal and attentional impairments in 11 subjects with severe TBI in the acute rehabilitation setting, failed to find a statistically significant treatment effect on these cognitive functions. Although their small sample size precludes generalization of their findings, they suggest that augmentation of serotonergic function alone is insufficient to produce marked improvements in cognition among persons with recent severe TBI. Similarly, Wilson and Hamm (2002) (150) observed no improvement in memory function in experimentally-injured rats treated with fluoxetine. These findings suggest that selective serotonin reuptake inhibitors (SSRIs) such as these should not at the present time be regarded as agents with direct cognitive-enhancing properties in the setting of acute severe TBI.

Whether the SSRIs are without such effects in the late period follow TBI is uncertain. Schmitt et al. (2001) (151) investigated the cognitive effects of several SSRIs and demonstrated significant improvements in verbal fluency among healthy middle-aged adults treated with sertraline 50–100 mg when compared to treatment with placebo. The authors of this study attributed that effect to sertraline's modest ability to inhibit dopamine reuptake. Fann et al. (2001) (92) describe improvements in psychomotor speed, recent verbal memory, recent visual memory, general cognitive efficiency, and patient-reported perception of cognitive symptoms during treatment of post-TBI depression with sertraline. It is possible that treatment with sertraline may confer cognitive benefits on the basis of resolving depression alone, as a function of augmenting either frontal serotonergic or dopaminergic function, or by both these and other mechanisms.

Similarly, Horsfield et al. (2002) (152) performed an eight-month open-label study of the effects of fluoxetine 20–60 mg/day in five patients with TBI and varying levels of depression in order to determine whether this medication conferred mood and/or cognitive benefits. They observed improvements in mood among persons with such symptoms, and demonstrated improvement on several measures of attention, processing speed, and working memory in this small group of patients. Their findings are consistent with the observations of Fann et al. (2001) (92) with respect to improved cognition in association with reduced depressive symptoms, but extend that finding to suggest a possible benefit of this serotonergic augmentation on cognition more generally. The authors of this study also note fluoxetine's ability to stimulate expression of brain-derived neurotrophic factor and its specific tyrosine kinase receptor. Such effects have been demonstrated to produce neuritic elongation and increased dendritic branching density of some hippocampal neurons in rodents. Although it is possible that similar mechanisms may be operative in humans, the sample size and findings of the Horsfield et al. (2002) (152) study do not support this interpretation at present. Instead, interpreting their findings as reflecting the activating effects of fluoxetine (which may operate through a variety of neurochemical mechanisms) is both simpler and more likely to be correct.

At present, it appears that serotonergic augmentation using SSRIs may be of benefit in the treatment of depression following TBI, and that alleviation of depression is associated with improvement in cognition. It is not clear that these agents, which are non-selective with respect to their effects at a receptor level, confer any direct benefit on cognition alone. Receptor-specific modulation of serotonergic function (i.e., agonism of 5-HT$_{2A}$, 5-HT$_{2C}$ or 5-HT$_4$ receptor, or antagonism of 5-HT$_{1A}$ or 5-HT$_3$

and 5-HT$_{1B}$ receptors) may afford cognitive benefits (93). Consistent with that suggestion, Kline et al. (2001) (153) demonstrated improvement in spatial memory in experimentally-injured rats treated with the 5HT$_{1A}$ receptor antagonist repinotan. Additional studies are needed to clarify the cognitive effects of agents that modify receptor specific serontonergic activity among persons with TBI.

Acetylcholine

Findings from both basic and clinical studies suggest that TBI produces acute elevations and long-term deficits in cortical cholinergic function. Multiple studies (48, 154–160) demonstrate this pattern of cholinergic dysfunction following experimentally-induced TBI in rodents, as well as a robust relationship between chronic posttraumatic cholinergic deficits and spatial memory impairments. One of the most compelling demonstrations of relatively selective cholinergic injury following TBI is the report of Schmidt and Grady (1995) (139). They induced a fluid-percussion head injury sufficient to cause a 13- to 14-minute loss of righting reflex in rats anesthetized with halothane. Rats with experimentally induced midline injury suffered significant bilateral reductions in cholinergic neurons, including reductions in area Ch1 (medial septal nucleus; 36%), Ch2 (nucleus of the diagonal band of Broca; 44%), and Ch4 (nucleus basalis of Meynert; 41%). Among animals with lateralized injuries, similarly severe losses of cholinergic neurons were observed ipsilateral to the injury site and lesser but nontrivial (11–28%) losses were observed contralaterally. The authors note that these losses did not extend to brainstem cholinergic nuclei (Ch5 and Ch6), and there were no observable effects on forebrain dopaminergic or noradrenergic innervation. These findings suggest that cholinergic deficits may be the most prominent type of chronic posttraumatic neurotransmitter disturbance.

TBI in humans produces the same pattern of cholinergic dysfunction as is reported in the experimental injury literature, with acute elevations of cerebral acetylcholine followed by chronic cholinergic deficits. Grossman et al. (1975) (161) demonstrated that patients with TBI had elevated acetylcholine levels in fluid obtained from either intraventricular catheters or lumbar puncture in the acute period following TBI. Dewar and Graham (1996) (162), Murdoch et al. (16, 163) demonstrated loss of cortical cholinergic afferents with concurrent preservation of post-synaptic muscarinic and nicotinic receptors several weeks after severe and fatal TBI. Arciniegas et al. (7, 25, 26), using the hippocampally-mediated cholinergically-dependent P50 evoked waveform response to paired auditory stimuli as a marker of cholinergic function, demonstrated electrophysiologic abnormalities in patients with chronic symptoms of impaired auditory gating, attention, and memory in the late (>1 year) period following TBI. In a subsequent study, Arciniegas et al. (2003) (24) demonstrated that this electrophysiologic abnormality is present in the majority of persons with persistent attention and memory complaints in the late period following TBI. Collectively, these findings support the hypothesis that cholinergic function is chronically deficient among many persons with TBI and that cholinergic deficit may be a significant contributor to posttraumatic cognitive impairments.

Given the role of acetylcholine in arousal and attention (9, 10), memory (164, 165), and executive function (166), and the evidence suggesting that cholinergic deficits contribute to posttraumatic cognitive impairments, pharmacotherapies that augment cholinergic function may improve posttraumatic cognitive impairments. These therapies are discussed in more detail in the next section of this chapter.

Summary of Post-Traumatic Neurochemical Disturbances

Animal and human studies suggest that most of the major neurotransmitter systems are acutely activated by mechanical brain injury. These excesses appear to result in a complex set of cerebral, and hence cognitive, dysfunctions. Neurotransmitter disturbances appear to be not only consequences of TBI but also contributors to brain injury. Excesses of glutamate are excitotoxic and may permanently damage areas with dense glutamatergic innervation, including frontal, striatal, and medial temporal (i.e., hippocampal) areas. There is, at present, no evidence to support chronic reductions in glutamatergic function after TBI. However, it is conceivable that improving the efficiency of glutamatergic neurotransmission with agents like memantine, amantadine, or neramexaane (another uncompetitive NMDA receptor antagonist presently under study in humans) may improve cognitive and other neurobehavioral functions in persons with TBI.

Acute catecholaminergic excesses after TBI appear predict poor outcome following TBI; when present, such increases may simply be a marker of injury severity in the studies in which they were assessed. Although evidence of chronic reductions in catecholaminergic function after TBI and/or a relationship of such to posttraumatic cognitive impairments in humans is lacking, more modest reductions in these neurotransmitters may in some genetically vulnerable persons (i.e., those with a fast-acting COMT enzyme) contribute to posttraumatic impairments in catecholamine-dependent cognitive functions. Alternatively, persons with traumatic lesions to catecholamine projections would be expected to develop cognitive impairments in the areas to which the lesioned fibers project. The cognitive functions served by the cerebral (i.e., frontal) areas to which these catecholaminergic fibers project are at greatest risk for disruption, including arousal, attention, speed and efficiency of information processing, executive function, and perhaps also language.

At present, there is also a dearth of evidence to support a relationship between posttraumatic dysfunction in serotonergic systems and cognitive impairment. Acute serotonergic excesses are associated with decreased cortical metabolism in the areas in which such excesses occur. In the acute post-injury period, sertononin-induced cerebral hypometabolism may contribute to cognitive dysfunction. It is not clear whether such excesses normalize, persist, or transition to posttraumatic deficits in serotonergic function. There is some evidence that treatment with the sertraline (92) or fluoxetine (152) may facilitate cognitive improvements in persons with depression following TBI. However, it does not appear that these agents facilitate cognitive improvements alone, at least not among persons with severe TBI (149). Consequently, the contribution of serotonergic dysfunction to posttraumatic cognitive impairments in the absence of comorbid posttraumatic depression is uncertain.

There is considerable animal and human evidence of acute posttraumatic excesses of acetylcholine and chronic posttraumatic reductions in cholinergic function. Because acetylcholine is a major contributor to the function of brain systems involved in arousal, attention, memory, language, and executive function, cholinergic deficits would be expected to contribute posttraumatic cognitive impairments.

The pharmacotherapy of TBI should be considered in the context of these findings. As will become clear in the next section of this chapter, the pharmacotherapeutic studies performed to-date appear to support most strongly the suggestion that augmentation of catecholaminergic and cholinergic function, and perhaps also glutamatergic function, are useful neurochemical targets for pharmacologic intervention among persons with posttraumatic cognitive impairments.

PHARMACOTHERAPY OF POST-TRAUMATIC COGNITIVE IMPAIRMENTS

As with any pharmacotherapy for the neuropsychiatric (i.e., cognitive, emotional, or behavioral) sequelae of TBI, the basic principles of pharmacotherapy (see Chapter 52, "Pharmacotherapy of Neuropsychiatric Disturbances") in this population should be followed. For purposes of this discussion, we will assume that prior to initiating any pharmacologic treatment for posttraumatic cognitive impairments the treating clinician has first completed a thorough psychiatric, developmental, and neurological evaluation. When subsequently considering pharmacotherapy of cognition, two issues require additional attention. First, the presenting cognitive complaints must be carefully assessed, defined, and operationalized, preferably though the use of objective measures of cognition. These measures may include "bedside" tests such as the Mini-Mental State Examination (167), any of several versions of the Clock Drawing Test, the Frontal Assessment Battery (168) or other similar measures of frontally-mediated cognition, but are better assessed through formal neuropsychological testing. Measures that are sensitive to both global cognitive impairment as well as impairments of speed of information processing, attention, memory, language, and executive function should be included in any pre-treatment cognitive assessment.

Second, the use and effectiveness of all ongoing treatments must be reevaluated, including both pharmacologic and non-pharmacologic therapies (whether prescribed and/or self-administered). Several classes of medications are of particular concern. Anticonvulsants such as phenytoin and carbamazepine may exacerbate cognitive impairments among persons with TBI. In a double-blind placebo-controlled study of phenytoin (40 patients) and carbamazepine (42 patients) in TBI patients being treated with these medications for seizure prophylaxis, Smith et al. (1994) (169) report that both of these medications (but particularly carbamazepine) produced significantly more cognitive and motor slowing than did placebo. Dikmen et al. (1991) (170) also observed greater cognitive impairment during treatment with phenytoin for prophylaxis of posttraumatic seizures when compared to placebo in a study with 244 patients with TBI. Additionally, phenytoin conferred no benefit against the development of post-traumatic seizures when used after the first week post-TBI. Both studies suggest that careful monitoring of cognition during treatment with anticonvulsants in brain-injured patients is warranted, and that such treatment should be reserved for patients with clearly established posttraumatic seizure disorders. Typical antipsychotic medications (e.g., haloperidol, fluphenazine, thioridazine, chlorpromazine) may exacerbate cognitive impairments among persons with TBI (171) and may prolong the period of posttraumatic amnesia (137). Benzodiazepines are known to impair memory and other aspects of cognition even among individuals without brain injuries (172), and there is some evidence supporting the common clinical belief that these agents impair cognitive performance among persons with TBI (173). It is concerning that prescription of anticonvulsants, typical antipsychotics, and benzodiazepines remains common in this population. It is sometimes the case that such treatments have not been properly applied, are predicated on misdiagnosis of the problem, or are the result of poor communication among treating professionals regarding the problem in question. When treating posttraumatic cognitive impairments, the most appropriate first pharmacological recommendation is to eliminate

these medications. If after eliminating these medications there remain cognitive, emotional, or behavioral problems that require treatment, nonpharmacologic therapies should be offered. When these interventions fail to afford improvement in posttraumatic cognitive performance, then medications may be required.

As noted in the previous sections of this chapter, advances in our understanding of the neurochemistry of TBI have been used to develop *a priori* hypotheses to guide the selection of pharmacotherapeutic agents in some treatment studies. While these studies are few in number, continued development of the pharmacotherapeutic literature in this area should be predicated on such *a priori* hypothesis rather than on the basis of extrapolation from the treatment of other neuropsychiatric disorders. At present, our understanding of the neurochemical consequences of TBI yields three principal themes in the pharmacotherapy of posttraumatic cognitive impairments: modulation of glutamatergic function, augmentation of catecholaminergic function, and enhancement of cholinergic function.

There are at present no proven therapies with which to limit the effects of glutamate-mediated excitotoxic injury among traumatically brain-injured persons. It is also not clear whether or to what extent acute alterations or long-term dysfunction of glutamate function contribute to posttraumatic cognitive impairments. This is likely to be an area of increasing research in the field of TBI, and clinicians should be aware of the possibility that agents affecting glutamatergic function may find applications in the pharmacotherapy of posttraumatic cognitive impairments. However, given the lack of data regarding this approach we will not consider further this issue.

The majority the pharmacotherapeutic literature in this field focuses on augmentation of catecholaminergic function, cholinergic function, or both. As discussed above, chronic cholinergic and/or catecholaminergic dysfunction contribute to cognitive impairments following TBI. While the experimental and human literature offers stronger evidence of chronic posttraumatic cholinergic dysfunction, clinical evidence suggests a potentially useful role for augmentation of either or both of these neurotransmitter systems in persons with posttraumatic cognitive impairments. However, the interindividual response to such agents is not uniform (136). Some patients respond to psychostimulants, some to cholinesterase inhibitors, some require medications from both classes, and some respond to neither class of medication. Selecting an appropriate treatment for a given patient might be made easier if clinical markers of dysfunction in these systems were available. However, simple, inexpensive, and widely available markers of *in vivo* neurotransmitter function are at present lacking.

In the absence of widely available markers of neurotransmitter dysfunction, pharmacotherapeutic studies performed to-date generally employ agents observed to be effective for the treatment of cognitive impairments among persons with phenotypically similar but etiologically distinct neuropsychiatric disorders. For example, the attention deficits of persistently impaired TBI survivors sometimes superficially resemble those of patients with attention-deficit hyperactivity disorder (ADHD). Given this similarity, psychostimulants (e.g., methylphenidate, dextroamphetamine) and dopaminergically active medications (amantadine, bromocriptine, L-dopa/carbidopa, etc.) have been used with some success for the treatment of posttraumatic impairments of arousal, processing speed, attention, and executive function. Because posttraumatic memory disturbances may in some respects resemble those observed among persons with Alzheimer's disease, agents used for the treatment of cognitive impairments in Alzheimer's disease have been studied in persons with similar problems following TBI. Although there are some differences in the relative predominance of encoding and retrieval deficits between these conditions, the cholinesterase inhibitors have been used with some success among patients with posttraumatic memory impairments.

Complicating the matter of selecting the agent most likely to improve posttraumatic cognitive impairment in an individual patient is the relative paucity of rigorously conducted clinical studies upon which to base treatment decisions. Although the pharmacotherapy of posttraumatic cognitive impairments is the most extensively studied area of neuropsychiatric treatment in this population to-date, the limited number and methodological problems of these studies limit their generalizability to everyday clinical practice.

In this section, studies of pharmacotherapies for posttraumatic cognitive impairments are organized according to medication class. Included in the discussion of the agents are the types of cognitive impairments they appear to improve. These studies include some double-blind placebo-controlled studies, uncontrolled open-label studies, and also case series or single-case reports. The strength of the evidence they provide for the use of these agents in clinical practice is a matter of considerable debate, and most offer evidence sufficient to support the use of these agents only as treatment options for posttraumatic cognitive impairments. Guided by the published literature and our own clinical experience, we offer preliminary recommendations regarding the pharmacotherapy of posttraumatic cognitive impairments. However, we encourage clinicians to consider the application of these agents to the treatment of in an individual patient a matter of empiric trial, and we suggest that clinicians consider reviewing the articles referenced herein prior to using these agents in their clinical practice.

Psychostimulants

The effects of psychostimulants such as methylphenidate and dextroamphetamine on central monoaminergic systems are complex. Methylphenidate and dextroamphetamine increase the release of dopamine and norepinephrine and, at higher doses, block the reuptake of these monoamines. These agents also appear to inhibit monoamine oxidase, which in combination with their other effects increases the effectiveness of monoaminergic neurotransmission. The effect of increased catecholaminergic activity in the ascending reticular activating system, the striatum, and the several cortical-subcortical circuits appears to be an increase in arousal, speed of processing, and attention. Such agents may afford such benefits in both the acute inpatient rehabilitation and post-acute outpatient settings, and there are theoretical reasons to suggest that stimulants may also facilitate neuronal recovery after brain injury by a variety of dopaminergically-mediated mechanisms (174).

Methylphenidate

Evans et al. (1987) (175) performed a single-case controlled study of methylphenidate (.15 mg/kg BID and .3 mg/kg BID) in a 21-year old male with a remote severe TBI. They observed improvements on measures of sustained attention, processing speed, motor speed, memory, and also mood. Subsequently, Gualtieri and Evans (1988) (176) performed a double-blind placebo-controlled crossover design study of methylphenidate among 15 adult patients with severe TBI. Subjects were 5–12 months post-injury, and were treated with methylphenidate .15 mg/kg BID and .3 mg/kg BID. They report treatment-related mood and behavioral, but not cognitive, improvements. In a similarly designed study, Speech et al. (1993) (177) treated 12 adult subjects with moderate to severe TBI with methylphenidate .3 mg/kg BID one year or more after their injuries. They observed a nonsignificant trend towards improvement in mood and performance on measures of vigilance and distractibility. They observed no improvements in memory, processing speed, or social interaction.

Plenger et al. (1996) (178) demonstrated a significant effect of methylphenidate on attention, Disability Rating Scale scores, and motor performance during subacute recovery from TBI in a randomized, double-blind, placebo-controlled study during which 23 subjects were treated for 30 days. They found that attention and functional performance were significantly improved by treatment with methylphenidate at day 30, but were not different from placebo treatment at day 90. In this study, methylphenidate treatment did not affect the ultimate level of recovery on these measures but appeared to improve the rate of recovery. However, analysis of data from this study is complicated by subject dropouts: only 12 subjects remained in the study at 30 days and only 9 subjects remained at 90 days. Consequently, it is difficult to fully evaluate the effects of methylphenidate in this cohort. Whyte et al. (2002) (136) suggest that random variations in initial injury severity of these subjects might either account for or potentially mask true drug effects. In a similar study, Kaelin et al. (1996) (179) describe the effect of methylphenidate 15 mg twice daily on the course of recovery in 11 patients with TBI during acute inpatient rehabilitation setting. Using an A-A-B-A design, they demonstrated that methylphenidate significantly improved attention as measured by performance on digit span and symbol search tasks and was associated with improved Disability Rating Scale scores. Although one subject was withdrawn from the study due to tachycardia, methylphenidate was generally well tolerated. Although these studies are not without methodological problems and their findings are modest, they suggest that methylphenidate may improve cognitive function and the rate of recovery following TBI.

More recently, Whyte et al. (1997) (135) performed a randomized, double-blind, placebo-controlled, repeated crossover design to assess the effect of methylphenidate on attention in 19 subjects with nonpenetrating TBI recruited from either inpatient or outpatient settings. Referral for study participation was based on attending physician's recommendation of this treatment for clinically apparent problems with attention. Subjects were excluded if they had a history of prior TBI or other neurological disease, major mental illness, learning disability, attention deficit disorder, or if they were taking any psychoactive medication other than carbamazepine (which two subjects were taking at the time of study). Eleven of these patients participated in a task assessing distractibility and phasic arousal and 19 participated in an assessment of behavioral inattention. Patients were on average 31 years old (median age 27), had an average of 12 years of education, and were in general in the post-acute period following TBI (mean interval since injury = 514 days, median interval since injury = 145 days). Subjects underwent six serial assessments, typically separated by 1–3 days. Task administration was randomly assigned to methylphenidate or placebo in pairs over the course of the study in order to facilitate interpretation of individual subject performance patterns and to distinguish practice from treatment effects. Methylphenidate was administered at a dose of 0.25 mg/kg (rounded to the nearest 2.5 mg) BID, and assessments were performed approximately 90 minutes after administration of methylphenidate or placebo. The study tasks created 22 performance variables for analysis. Methylphenidate significantly improved arousal and speed of processing, but did not improve most aspects of vigilance (sustained attention), distraction, or motor speed.

Placed in the context of other studies of methylphenidate in adults with posttraumatic cognitive impairments, the findings of Whyte et al. (135) suggest that principal benefit of this agent is on processing speed and to a lesser extent on subjective ratings of behavior and mood. This finding stands in contrast to the more common clinical use of methylphenidate for impairments of vigilance and distractibility. They note that there is, at present, little data to support the use of methylphenidate for posttraumatic memory impairments. It stands to reason that improvements in attention might secondarily benefit memory, although the studies performed to-date offer little support for this suggestion. Whether methylphenidate has benefits on aspects of attention other than processing speed remains uncertain, but common clinical experience suggests that at least some persons with attentional impairments benefit from treatment with this agent.

Two studies (180, 181) describe the use of methylphenidate in the treatment of children and adolescents with posttraumatic cognitive impairments. In the study by Mahalick et al. (1998) (180), methylphenidate .3 mg/kg BID was administered in a crossover design study of 14 subjects (age 5–14 years) approximately 1.2 years after mild-to-moderate TBI. They observed statistically significant improvements in vigilance, processing speed, and distractibility. In a similarly designed study, Williams et al. (1998) (181) examined the effects of methylphenidate 5–10 mg BID (adjusted for subject weight) in 10 subjects (age 5–16 years) who were on average 2 years post-injury (of unspecified severity). They observed no significant effects of this treatment on cognition, although there was suggestion in their data of improved accuracy on a continuous performance task. They report a trend towards behavioral improvements as assessed by teachers using the Conners Rating Scale (a scale commonly used in the assessment of children with attention deficit disorder), but parents ratings on this scale did not support teacher ratings. Considered together, these studies leave uncertain the possible benefits of methylphenidate in children and adolescents with posttraumatic cognitive impairments.

Dextroamphetamine

Dextroamphetamine is frequently used in the treatment of attention and memory impairment following TBI, and is thought to have additional beneficial effects on depression, anergia, and impaired motivation. However, there are only three reports to support its use in this population. Evans and Gualtieri (1987) (176) assessed cognition, mood, and behavior during treatment with dextroamphetamine .1 mg/kg BID and .2 mg/kg BID. They describe treatment-related improvement in measures of vigilance (sustained attention), processing speed, motor speed, memory, and mood during treatment with dextroamphetamine. Bleiberg et al. (1993) (173) conducted a double-blind, crossover study of the effects of dextroamphetamine, lorazepam, and placebo on measures of processing efficiency and speed in a 55-year old male who suffered a complicated mild TBI (5 minutes loss of consciousness and left subdural hematoma) approximately

5 years prior to study. They observed improvements in cognitive speed and stability of performance (correct responses per unit of time) during treatment with dextroamphetamine but not placebo, and also observed decrements in cognitive function during treatment with lorazepam. Hornstein et al. (1996) (182) reviewed the use of dextroamphetamine in the treatment of individuals during acute rehabilitation after TBI in the context of a larger review of this subject. Of the 27 patients so treated, 15 appeared to benefit from treatment with dextroamphetamine as measured by Glascow Outcome Scale.

Methylphenidate and Dextramphetamine in Clinical Practice

Although psychostimulants would be predicted to improve catecholaminergically-dependent cognitive functions among persons with TBI, the literature is variable with respect to their beneficial effects. In light of the relative lack of *in vivo* evidence of long-term dopaminergic or noradrenergic dysfunction following TBI presented earlier in this chapter, the variability of benefit in the published reports is not surprising. Additionally, methodological issues (e.g., small sample sizes, study design, assessment measures, study period, interval since injury, etc.) in the studies performed to-date make interpretation of the cognitive and neurobehavioral benefits of psychostimulants in persons with TBI difficult, at best. Nonetheless, common clinical experience suggests that some patients do experience cognitive improvements during treatment with psychostimulants. To the extent that an individual's posttraumatic cognitive impairments are related to catecholaminergic dysfunction, whether from injury to afferent projections, synaptic catecholamine metabolism (i.e., COMT enzymatic activity) that exceeds catecholamine availability, or some combination of these factors, methylphenidate and related psychostimulants may afford some degree of cognitive improvement among persons with TBI, and may in particular be useful for the treatment of posttraumatic impairments in arousal, speed of processing, and possibly attention.

In clinical practice, careful assessment of arousal, speed of processing, and attention should be undertaken before and during treatment with these agents. Although such assessments may be difficult to undertake in some clinical practices (183), they are important to perform in order to determine whether these medications impart sufficient benefit to merit their continued use in a given patient. Assessment with appropriate neuropsychological tests (for example, continuous performance tests or other standardized tests of reaction time or processing speed) may be particularly helpful in this regard. In the absence of improvement on such measures during treatment with these agents, reports of subjective improvement in cognition or daily function during treatment with these agents are frequently used as a measure of treatment response. While such reports may be used to justify continued use of these agents, the observation of subjective improvement but lack of improvement on objective measures should prompt reconsideration of the etiology of the impairments reported. Since psychostimulants may improve mood, increase motivation, or lessen fatigue, subjective improvements without evidence of demonstrable cognitive improvements may suggest that the primary problem lies in posttraumatic depression, apathy, fatigue, or some combination of these non-cognitive problems.

Unlike many other medications used to treat neuropsychiatric conditions, stimulants generally take effect quickly (within 0.5–1 hour following administration) and also lose effect after only a few hours. Therefore, the first issue in the administration of these agents is determining the optimally effective dosage and dosing frequency required to sustain that effect. Methylphenidate and dextroamphetamine are generally administered twice daily, typically at breakfast and again at midday. Initial dosing with either agent generally begins at 5 mg BID and is gradually increased in increments of 5 mg BID until either beneficial effect or medication intolerance is achieved. Most studies suggest that optimal doses of either methylphenidate or dextroamphetamine are in the range of 10–20 mg BID, although some clinicians use of considerably higher doses (i.e., 40 mg or more BID). Some individuals may require relatively frequent dosing (i.e., readministration every 3–4 hours) of methylphenidate or dextroamphetamine in order to sustain cognitive benefits from them throughout the course of the day. Multiple longer-acting methylphenidate or dextroamphetamine preparations are available. Individuals requiring relatively high and frequent doses of methylphenidate or dextroamphetamine may benefit from use of longer-acting preparations of these medications.

Adverse reactions to these medications are most often related to increases in cerebral dopamine, and to a lesser extent cerebral norepinephrine, activity. Dextroamphetamine and methylphenidate have the potential to produce paranoia, dysphoria, anxiety, agitation, and irritability, although these adverse effects are in practice very uncommon at doses typically used to treat posttraumatic cognitive impairments. Psychosis is a relatively rare consequence of adminstration of these medications. Even among persons with posttraumatic psychosis, these agents may be of benefit for cognitive impairments and without untoward effects on psychotic symptoms when used in combination with an atypical antipsychotic medication. However, combined therapy with psychostimulants and antipsychotics is not recommended unless the patient is under the care of a neuropsychiatrist with expertise in the use of this medication combination. Mild increases in heart rate and/or blood pressure may occur during treatment with psychostimulants, although these tend to occur relatively infrequently in patients without other cardiac or vascular problems and are only rarely of sufficient magnitude to merit discontinuation of these agents. Use of these agents during pregnancy is discouraged, and their use is contraindicated among patients receiving monoamine oxidase inhibitors (MAOIs) and women who are breastfeeding. Clinicians are advised to avoid use of these agents among persons with comorbid Tourette's syndrome and other tics, glaucoma, untreated hypertension or cardiovascular problems, and symptomatic hyperthryoidism. These agents may potentiate the effects of phenobarbital and phenytoin by delaying gastrointestinal absorption, increase the noradrenergic effects of tricyclic antidepressants, increase the dopaminergic effects of antiparkinsonian agents, and potentiate the analgesic properties of meperidine. Because depressed mood and increased fatigue may develop following abrupt discontinuation of psychostimulants, these medications should be discontinued gradually among patients receiving them chronically.

Clinicians are sometimes reluctant to make use of psychostimulants out of concern that they might lower seizure threshold in patients with TBI. Wroblewski et al. (1992) (184) examined changes in seizure frequency after initiation of methylphenidate among 30 patients with both severe brain injury and posttraumatic seizures. The frequency of seizures was monitored for 3 months before treatment with methylphenidate, 3 months during treatment, and 3 months after treatment was discontinued. They found that only 4 patients experienced more seizures during methylphenidate treatment, and 26 had either fewer or the same number of seizures during treatment. Although many patients in this study were treated concurrently with anticonvulsant medications, 13 of these experienced fewer seizures when treated with methylphenidate. While this finding should not be misunderstood as suggesting an anticonvulsant effect of methylphenidate, it does suggest that methylphenidate does not substantially increase seizure risk among persons with TBI, including those with posttraumatic epilepsy.

Similarly, in a double-blind placebo-controlled study of the effects of methylphenidate (0.3 mg/kg body weight bid) in 10 children with well-controlled seizures and attention-deficit disorder, no seizures occurred during the 4 weeks of treatment with either active drug or placebo (185). Although this observation was not made among persons with TBI, it supports the thesis that methylphenidate itself does not appear to increase the risk of seizure even among patients with established epilepsy. Interestingly, dextroamphetamine has been used adjunctively in the treatment of refractory seizures (186). While most clinicians would not regard this agent as an adjunctive therapy for seizures, this report echoes other observations of a relative lack of adverse effect of stimulants

on seizure frequency. It appears that this class of medications is generally well tolerated with respect to its effects on seizure frequency, and that even established epilepsy should not preclude treatment with this agent when a clinician deems it to be of potential benefit to an individual patient.

Bromocriptine

Bromocriptine appears to act directly on postsynaptic dopamine receptors – particularly dopamine type 2 (D2) receptors – and serves as an agonist in dopaminergically-mediated cerebral systems. At low doses, bromocriptine acts as a pre-synaptic D2 agonist, and thereby reduces dopaminergic release and function in dopaminergically-mediated systems. Its net effect at mid-range doses appears to be augmentation of cerebral dopaminergic systems (187). Accordingly, Eames (1989) (188) suggest that bromocriptine may be useful in treating "cognitive initiation" problems of brain injury patients who are at least 1 year post-injury. McDowell et al. (1998) (189) studied 24 subjects using a counterbalanced, double-blind, placebo-controlled crossover design. Bromocriptine improved performance on some frontally-mediated tasks, such as executive function and dual-task performance, but did not improve working memory. No other effects of bromocriptine on posttraumatic cognitive dysfunction were observed.

Others report benefits on nonfluent aphasia (71), akinetic mutism (190), and apathy (191) during treatment with this bromocriptine among patients with such problems following stroke. These effects have been attributed to dopaminergic augmentation of frontal function (192). Unlike the psychostimulants, bromocriptine has not been demonstrated to have a consistent effect on affective lability or mood disorders due to TBI, stroke, or other neurological conditions.

Treatment with this agent generally begins with 2.5 mg/day and is gradually titrated to the highest dose tolerated. Common side effects during treatment with bromocriptine include dizziness, drowsiness, faintness, syncope, nausea, vomiting, abdominal cramps, constipation, and diarrhea, although these are generally of mild severity. Uncontrolled hypertension and hypersensitivity to ergot alkaloids are strict contraindications to the use of bromocriptine. Although use of this agent among women who are breastfeeding their infants is contraindicated, use during pregnancy does not appear to be associated with significant increased adverse events among pregnant patients or on fetal development. It has been suggested that bromocriptine may possess some anticonvulsant properties (193). Although this suggestion should not be misunderstood as an endorsement of bromocriptine for the adjunctive treatment of posttraumatic epilepsy, it may offer some reassurance of its safety for use among cognitively impaired TBI survivors with this problem.

Amantadine

The effects of amantadine on dopaminergic function are not entirely clear, but include increasing dopamine release, decreasing presynaptic dopamine reuptake, stimulation of dopamine receptors, and/or enhancement of postsynaptic dopamine receptor sensitivity. As such, amantadine is generally regarded as an agent whose principal effects on posttraumatic cognitive and neurobehavioral disturbances are mediated through indirect augmentation of dopaminergic function. As noted previously, amantadine is an uncompetitive antagonist at NMDA receptors (194). The clinical effects of amantadine's NMDA receptor antagonist properties are uncertain, although it is possible that it may contribute to stabilization and/or augmentation of glutamatergic function. Additionally, amantadine also appears to stimulate striatal acetylcholine release indirectly via its effects on NMDA receptors in this brain region. To the extent that improved striatal cholinergic function contributes to improvements in cognition dependent on frontostriatal circuits, amantadine might also be of benefit via this mechanism of action. However, the relative contributions of NMDA receptor antagonism and/or indirect striatal pro-cholinergic effects to the clinical effects produced by amantadine are at present a matter of speculation.

Kraus and Maki (1997) (125) administered amantadine 400 mg/day to six patients with TBI and observed improvements in motivation, attention and alertness, and executive function. They also observed treatment-related improvements in impulsivity and emotional (affective) lability. It has also been suggested that amantadine improve posttraumatic anergia, abulia, mutism, anhedonia, perseveration, and/or agitation (126–129).

Amantadine is often started at a dose of 50 mg BID, and is usually increased every week by 100 mg/day to either symptomatic improvement or medication intolerance. In the experience of the authors, amantadine may be of use in the treatment of hypoarousal and/or fatigue following TBI. Amantadine 100 mg BID is often sufficient to impart improvement in these symptoms without undue side effects. When higher doses are necessary, the maximum dosage of amantadine should not exceed a total daily dose of 400 mg. When used at higher doses, treatment-emergent adverse effects may be more common.

Headache, nausea, diarrhea, constipation, anorexia, dizziness, lightheadedness, orthostatic hypotension may occur during treatment with amantadine. Anxiety, irritability, depression, and hallucinations may also develop during treatment with this agent, but are relatively uncommon. At higher doses, psychosis and confusion may occur. These treatment-emergent symptoms may be

the result of excessively strong NMDA receptor antagonism, dopaminergic excess, or some combination of these effects. Abrupt withdrawal has been associated (rarely) with neuroleptic malignant syndrome. Adverse reactions to amantadine appear to occur more often in elderly patients than in younger patients. Additionally, coadminstration of triamterene/hydrochlorothiazide may decrease renal excretion of amantadine, resulting in medication intolerance at doses that would ordinarily be regarded as within the usual therapeutic range.

Although amantadine does not possess direct anticholinergic activity *per se* at conventional therapeutic doses, it is not uncommon for patients treated with this agent to develop anticholinergic-like symptoms. Additionally, amantadine may potentiate the effects of anticholinergic agents and other psychostimulants. These observations leave open the question of amantadine on cholinergic function *in vivo*, as the basic science studies of the neurotransmitter effects of this agent would not predict these effects.

It has been reported that amantadine may lower seizure threshold (128). However, this suggestion is contentious. Two studies (195, 196) investigated amanatdine as an adjunctive anticonvulsant therapy among persons with refractory epilepsy. These studies report improved seizure control in about 30%, no change in seizure frequency in 30–40%, and worsened seizures in 20–30% among patients treated with amantadine. These findings suggest that amantadine does not invariably precipitate or worsens seizure frequency, even among persons with refractory epilepsy. Nonetheless, it is prudent to be vigilant for the development or worsening of seizures when amantadine is used among persons with TBI.

Carbidopa/L-Dopa

L-dopa (levodopa) is a dopamine precursor. When coupled with carbidopa to decrease the extent of its metabolism in the periphery, L-dopa increases dopamine levels in the central nervous system. Although this medication is uncommonly used in clinical practice for these purposes, it may be an alternative to the traditional psychostimulants for the treatment of cognitive impairments and other neurobehavioral disturbances following TBI.

Lal et al. (1988) (197) describe the use of carbidopa/ L-dopa among 12 patients with brain injury (including several patients with hypoxic-ischemic brain injuries). During treatment with L-dopa/carbidopa 10/100 to 25/250 QID, patients demonstrated improvements in alertness and concentration, decreased fatigue, hypomania, and sialorrhea, as well as improved memory, mobility, posture, and speech.

Treatment with carbidopa/L-dopa should begin with low doses (10/100 BID) and may be gradually increased to doses of 25/250 QID. Consultation with a neurologist or neuropsychiatrist experienced in the use of this agent in this population is suggested when clinicians unfamiliar with carbidopa/L-dopa elect to use this agent in this population. Common side effects are predominantly related to its central dopaminergic effects, and may include dykinesias, anxiety, hallucinations (especially visual), paranoia or overt psychosis. Nausea may be a treatment-limiting side effect in some patients, and is more common during treatment with preparations with relatively lower doses of carbidopa (i.e., 10/100 vs. 25/100). Other less frequent side effects include palpitations, orthostatic hypotension, anorexia, vomiting, and dizziness. Rare but serious adverse effects include gastrointestinal hemorrhaging, duodenal ulcer, hypertension, phlebitis, leukopenia, agranulcytosis, thrombocytopenia, and hemolytic or nonhemolytic anemia. Carbidopa/ L-dopa does not appear to reduce seizure threshold clinically, but there is insufficient data with which to assess the risk of seizures during treatment with this agent among persons with TBI.

Modafinil

Modafinil, a medication recently approved for the treatment of excessive daytime somnolence in patients with narcolepsy, may have a role in treatment of post-TBI fatigue and cognitive impairment. Although the exact mechanism of action of modafinil is not fully understood, animal studies suggest that its promotion of wakefulness may be attributable to activation of hypocretin (orexin) neurons in the lateral hypothalamus (198), indirect, dose-dependent reduction GABA release in the cerebral cortex, medial preoptic area, and posterior hypothalamus (199, 200), and dose-dependent increases in glutamate release in the ventrolateral and the ventromedial thalamus (201). Some combination of these mechanisms in humans may increase arousal via activation of neurons of the arousal system, either directly via glutamatergic thalamic activation, indirectly via reduction of GABA function, or through the secondary effects of lateral hyopothalamic projections to regions involved in control of arousal and sleep-wake cycle (tubero-mammilary nucleus and the locus coeruleus) (202).

Studies of the effect of modafinil on fatigue and excessive sleepiness in patients with multiple sclerosis (203, 204) and Parkinson's disease (205) suggest that the beneficial effects of this agent are not exclusive to narcolepsy. Elovic (2000) (206) has suggested that modafinil may be of similar benefit in patients with TBI. Teitelman (2001) (207) described his use of modafinil among 10 outpatients with nonpenetrating traumatic brain injury and functionally significant excessive daytime sleepiness and in two patients with somnolence due to sedating psychiatric medications. The patients included in his report were between the ages of 42 to 72 years, all were outpatients, and were treated in an open-label fashion.

Doses of modafinil ranged between 100 mg to 400 mg daily. Nine patients reported marked improvements in excessive daytime sleepiness and three reported moderate improvements. Some of these patients reported subjective improvements in attention as other cognitive functions. Although this medication was generally well tolerated, Teitelman (2001) (207) observed treatment intolerance due to increased "emotional instability" in two women with brain injury complicated by multiple other medical conditions who were receiving multiple additional medications.

At the time of this writing there are no published formal clinical trials with which to evaluate the effectiveness or tolerability of modafinil for post-traumatic hypoarousal, hypersomnolence, fatigue, or other cognitive impairments. We have used this agent in the acute inpatient rehabilitation setting in persons with moderate-to-severe TBI in the lower Rancho Los Amigos stages (III-IV) for the treatment of hypoarousal or excessive daytime sleepiness with some success and without serious adverse effects; however, anecdotal reports such as this must be regarded with caution pending further study of this agent for this purpose.

If used in this population, modafinil should be started at 100 mg QAM, and can be increased to up to 400 mg/day administered in either a single daily dose or two divided doses (i.e., 200 mg in the morning, and 200 mg in the early afternoon). Higher doses (up to 600 mg daily) are sometimes used, but there is no evidence in any patient population that such doses offer benefit beyond that achieved with 400 mg daily.

Other Stimulant-like Medications

In general, prescription of tricyclic antidepressants should be avoided where possible among persons with significant posttraumatic cognitive impairments. The significant anticholinergic and antihistaminergic effects of these agents would be expected to further impair cognition in this population; such adverse effects of tricyclic antidepressants have been reported among persons with TBI and other neurologically-impaired populations (208, 209). Protriptyline, a secondary amine tricyclic agent, may be an exception in this regard. This agent has been suggested to have sufficient stimulant properties to permit its use for anergia and diminished motivation in TBI patients (210). However, this agent does not appear to confer any benefit on cognition beyond that afforded by improved arousal and motivation alone. Protriptyline should be considered as a treatment for posttraumatic hypoarousal, anergia, and apathy only when other standard psychostimulants have not proven effective or have produced intolerable side effects. Similarly, Reinhard and colleagues (1996) (211) administered amitriptyline (1 patient) and desipramine (2 patients) and found improvement in arousal and initiation after TBI. They hypothesized that the cognitive-enhancing effects of these agents resulted from the pro-noradrenergic effects of these agents. Again, these agents may be of some benefit on posttraumatic impairments in arousal but are probably best regarded as treatments of last resort when other stimulants have proven ineffective or intolerable. The side effects and drug-drug interactions of these agents are discussed in more detail in Chapter 52 (Pharmacotherapy of Neuropsychiatric Disturbances).

Showalter and Kimmel (2000) (212) report better-than-expected improvements in level of arousal in 9 of 13 severe (Rancho Los Amigos Scale I-III) TBI patients taking lamotrigine during the post-acute recovery period (up to 10 months). They suggested that this agent may permit more rapid emergence from deeper stages of diminished arousal (i.e., coma) following TBI than might occur spontaneously. Pachet et al. (2003) (213) also report improvements in cognition and other neurobehavioral functions (as assessed by the Functional Independence Measure) in a single case study of this agent in a 40 year-old man with severe TBI treated with lamotrigine for approximately four months in the late (1–1.5 years) period following his injury. The mechanism by which lamotrigine confers such benefits is unclear. Showalter and Kimmel (2000) (212) suggest that lamotrigine's ability to block of sodium channels and inhibit glutamate release may either prevent excitotoxic injury and/or facilitate recovery from injury. Additional studies are needed to ascertain the validity of this suggestion.

Cholinesterase Inhibitors

As described earlier in this chapter, posttraumatic cognitive impairments may, at least in part, result from chronic deficiencies of cerebral cholinergic function (7, 214). The common clinical observation of the susceptibility of TBI patients to exacerbation of cognitive impairments during treatment with anticholinergic medications, as well as animal studies echoing this observation (155, 159, 215), suggests that TBI results in reduced reserves of cerebral acetylcholine. As such, augmentation of cholinergic function may be an effective strategy by which to improve posttraumatic cognitive impairments.

Administration of the acetylcholine precursors, lecithin and choline, do not appear to reliably increase cerebral cholinergic function or confer cognitive benefits among persons with other neurological illnesses in which cholinergic deficits figure prominently (e.g., Alzheimer's disease) (216). Additionally, centrally-selective nicotinic or muscarinic receptor agonists are not presently available for use in this context.

At present, the principal pharmacologic means by which central cholinergic function may be augmented is cholinesterase inhibitors, of which there are several available for use in humans. These include physostigmine,

tacrine, donepezil, rivastigmine, and galantamine. Although these agents differ in their central (i.e., cerebral) selectivity and additional mechanisms of action – for example, prominent butyrylcholinestase inhibition by rivastigmine (217), and allosteric nicotinic modulation by galantamine and physostigmine (218) – all of these agents principally exert their clinical benefits via inhibition of synaptic acetylcholinesterase. This enzyme is the predominant synaptically-active cholinesterase, and is the principal mechanism by which acetylcholine is metabolized in cerebral synapses. Inhibition of synaptic acetylcholinesterase increases the availability of acetylcholine to both pre- and post-synaptic nicotinic and muscarinic receptors, and may thereby improve cholinergically-dependent cognitive functions such as arousal, attention, memory, language, and executive function.

Although there is considerable interest in the possible use of the cholinesterase inhibitors for the treatment of posttraumatic cognitive impairments, at the time of this writing there is published data for only physostigmine and donepezil. It is possible that the secondary mechanisms of action of both rivastigmine and galantamine may confer either greater or additional benefits on cognitive and neurobehavioral function among persons with TBI; however, reports describing both their effects and tolerability are needed before offering any formal recommendations regarding their use in this population.

Physostigmine

Physostigmine inhibits acetylcholinesterase both centrally and peripherally. Although it exerts its principal effects through inhibition of synaptic acetylcholinesterase, it also appears to allosterically modulate nicotinic receptors in a fashion similar to galantamine (218). Several reports describe cognitive improvements following administration of physostigmine, both in the acute (219) and post-acute (220, 221) injury period. Levin et al. (1986) (222) performed a double-blind, placebo-controlled study of combined oral physostigmine and lecithin in 16 patients with cognitive impairment following moderate to severe TBI. Sustained attention on the continuous performance test was more efficient under physostigmine than placebo, and lecithin did not appear to increase this effect. Cardenas et al. (1994) (223), in a double-blind, placebo-controlled, crossover design study of physostigmine, placebo, and scopolamine (a muscarinic receptor antagonist) in 36 males with memory impairment of at least 3 months duration following TBI, demonstrated improved memory scores on the long-term storage component of the Selective Reminding Test in 44% of subjects during treatment with oral physostigmine but not placebo or scopolamine.

Physostigmine is available in oral and intravenous preparations. Its absorption after oral administration is unpredictable, and its duration of action ranges from

30 minutes to 5 hours. Consequently, its use entails frequent dosing. Although physostigmine may be of benefit to cognitively impaired TBI survivors, both its lack of central selectivity and frequent administration produce systemic toxicity that limits its acceptability as a treatment for posttraumatic cognitive impairments (224). Given the availability of newer and generally better-tolerated cholinesterase inhibitors, we do not recommend routine use of physostigmine among persons with TBI. However, the benefits afforded by this agent do support the suggestion that cholinesterase inhibition may improve posttraumatic cognitive impairments in some patients, and may be used to support the use of the newer cholinesterase inhibitors in this population.

Donepezil

Donepezil is a cholinesterase inhibitor that exhibits relative central selectivity. Although it modestly inhibits butyrylcholinesterase (225), its predominant mechanism of action is believed to be inhibition of synaptic acetylcholinesterase (226). Taverni et al. (1998) (227) describe improvements in refractory memory impairments on the Rivermead Behavioral Memory Test and Ross Immediate Processing Assessment in the late (>3 years) post-injury period in two patients with severe TBI. These benefits were apparent after approximately three weeks of treatment with donepezil 5 mg per day. In a similarly small case series, Masanic et al. (2001) (228) treated four patients with persistent posttraumatic cognitive and neurobehavioral impairments with donepezil 5 mg per day for eight weeks followed by treatment with donepezil 10 mg per day for an additional four weeks. Patients were assessed pre- and post-treatment using the Rey Auditory Verbal Learning Test (RAVLT) and the Complex Figure Test (CFT). Items from the Rivermead Behavioral Learning Test (RBMT) and a test of semantic fluency were also administered. The Neuropsychiatric Inventory (NPI) was used to assess other neurobehavioral changes during treatment, and overall function was assessed using a clinician-based rating scale and the Functional Independence Measure (FIM). The authors reported modest but significant improvements in learning and short- and long-term recall on the RAVLT and more substantial improvements in short- and long-term recall on the CFT. Trends toward improvements were observed on the RBMT and the NPI. Given the small sample sizes, remoteness of injury, and the relatively severe injuries of the subjects in both studies, the observation of improvement in is encouraging of the possible benefits of donepezil for the treatment of posttraumatic memory impairments. However, the small sample sizes and uncontrolled nature of both studies limits the validity and generalizability of these treatment effects.

Kaye et al. (2003) (229) performed an 8-week open-label study of 10 persons with remote (1–5 years,

mean = 1.2 years) TBI in an outpatient setting using a forced titration protocol (5 mg per day for 4 weeks followed by 10 mg per day for 4 weeks). Subjects ranged in age from 26–60 years (mean age = 41 years), and included six with mild, one with moderate, and 3 with severe TBI. All subjects underwent pre- and post-treatment neuropsychiatric evaluations, including assessment of cognition using the Global Memory Scale (GMS) of the Memory Assessment Scale and two-independent clinician ratings of overall improvement using the Clinical Global Improvement scale (CGI). Eight subjects completed the study; one subject was dropped from the study due to treatment noncompliance, and one subject discontinued treatment due to intolerable gastrointestinal side effects. Among those completing the study, CGI ratings improved, although not necessarily as a function of improvements in memory. In fact, the authors observed no improvement on the GMS. Instead, the authors report that CGI improvements instead appeared to reflect the subject reports of improvements in "focus, attention, and clarity of thought." They note that several subjects reported being better able "to keep multiple ideas in mind simultaneously," and that subjects' family members frequently described "improved socialization." The authors note the limitations of the cognitive assessment used as a primary outcome measure in this study, and suggest that other measures better suited to assess cognitive flexibility, nonverbal abstract reasoning, learning from mistakes, and incidental visual memory might be more appropriate outcome measures in subsequent studies of this kind. They acknowledge that controlling for other variables such as age, severity of injury, time since injury, and baseline cognitive function, as well as the use of placebo control, is necessary to more rigorously assess the benefits of donepezil in the treatment of posttraumatic cognitive impairments. In spite of these limitations, they conclude their report by noting that seven of the eight subjects completing the study elected to continue treatment with donepezil given the subjective improvements they experienced during its use in this study. The eighth subject also reported such benefits, but elected not to continue treatment due to the development of treatment-emergent nausea.

Morey et al. (2003) (230) studied the effectiveness of donepezil for the treatment of chronic memory impairments in a group of seven patients with TBI. Subjects were on average 33 months post-injury (range = 20–65 months) and mean age was 31 years (range = 19–51). All subjects were without other medical, psychiatric, or physical problems that might interfere with ability to participate in neuropsychological assessment, and none were taking medications with anticholinergic properties. Measures of cognitive function included the Brief Visual Memory Test – Revised, Hopkins Verbal Learning Test, Digit Span and Letter-Number Sequence subtests of the Weschler Adult Intelligence Scale – Revised, Controlled Oral Word

Association Test, and the Memory Functioning Questionnaire, all of which were administered pre- and post-treatment during the two treatment phases of the study. These phases included donepezil 5 mg daily one month followed by donepezil 10 mg daily for an additional five months; following a six-week washout period, patients were treated for an additional six months with donepezil 5 mg daily. Treatment-emergent side effects (lethargy and somnolence) were observed in two subjects, prompting their discontinuation from the study. It is not clear in this report whether the final subject group in who cognitive testing was performed included seven or five subjects. Regardless, there were very few other complaints of side effects at either dose of donepezil. Improvements in immediate and delayed memory as assessed by the Brief Visual Memory Test – Revised were reported as a function of treatment with donepezil 10 mg per day but not 5 mg per day. No other significant effects on cognition were observed during treatment with this agent at either dose. Although this report suggests the possibility of benefit on visual memory during treatment with donepezil at 10 mg per day, lack of subject characterization data (i.e., severity of injury, presence of focal contusions vs. diffuse injury) and small sample size limit the generalizability of both positive and negative findings of this study.

Whelan et al. (2000) (231) performed an open-label study of donepezil in 53 outpatients and subsequent cognitive impairment who were receiving treatment for neuropsychiatric problems following TBI. All patients were assessed pre- and post-treatment using a clinician-based rating scale. Twenty-two of these patients were also assessed pre- and post-treatment using the Wechsler Adult Intelligence Scale-Revised (WAIS-R) and the Hooper Visual Organization Test. All of the patients were treated adjunctively with donepezil 5–10 mg daily for an average of 12 months. The authors reported improvements in full-scale IQ in the subset of patients in who cognitive assessments were performed, and improvements in clinician-based ratings in the sample as a whole. Although these improvements occurred well after the period during which spontaneous recovery and "practice effects" might offer better explanations for them, details regarding injury severity, specific neuropsychiatric comorbidities, other concurrent treatments, and changes in those treatments during the period of study are not fully described in that report, making interpretation of the reported findings challenging. Additionally, the cognitive assessment measures used are unusual in treatment studies of this kind. It is possible that modest improvements across the range of cognitive functions assessed by the WAIS-R contributed to the observed improvements while improvements in subscale scores were insufficient to rise to statistically significant levels. Alternatively, the sample size may have been inadequate to provide the statistical power needed to demonstrate a significant effect of

donepezil on the WAIS-R subscales. Given these considerations, this study is probably best interpreted as offering only a suggestion of a possible benefit of donepezil as an adjunctive treatment for persistent cognitive impairments among persons with other chronic neuropsychiatric disturbances following TBI.

More recently, Zhang et al. (2004) (232) reported findings from a 24-week, randomized, placebo-controlled, double-blind crossover trial of donepezil 10 mg daily in 18 subjects with TBI seen in two University-based hospitals. Patients were enrolled on the basis of a documented history of TBI (regardless of severity) 2–24 (4.6 ± .7) months prior to the study. Approximately two-thirds of the patients were male, ranged in age from 19–49 years, and had 10–17 years of education. Mean GCS scores at 24–48 hours post-injury were approximately 9 ± 1. All subjects demonstrated persistent attention as measured by the Paced Auditory Serial Addition Test (PASAT) and/or short-term memory impairment as measured by the Auditory Immediate Index (AII) or Visual Immediate Index (VII) of the Weschler Memory Scale-III. Subjects were excluded if they had cardiac arrhythmias on electrocardiogram (regardless of etiology), a history of cardiac contusion, uncontrolled posttraumatic seizures, uncorrected electrolyte imbalance, endocrine dysregulation, infection, or gastrointestinal bleeding. Subjects with severe cognitive and behavioral disturbances (i.e., Rancho Los Amigos functioning at level V or below), other neurologic or psychiatric problems (e.g., stroke, epilepsy, major depression, or neurodegenerative disorders), taking other psychotropic medications (e.g., antidepressants, anticonvulsants, antipsychotics, psychostimulants), or communication impairments (aphasia, dysarthria) that would interfere with neuropsychologic testing were excluded. Glasgow Outcome Scale scores were 4 or 5, and Rancho Los Amigos scores ranged from 7 to 8. In other words, the majority of subjects were functioned at an independent or a modified independent level but required some guidance and supervision from family members for daily activities.

Subjects were randomly assigned to two study groups consisting of 10 subjects each. The first group received donepezil 5 mg daily for two weeks followed by donepezil 10 mg daily for an additional 8 weeks; after a 4 week washout period, patients received placebo for 10 weeks. The second group received these preparations in the opposite order. Subjects were assessed using the PASAT, AII, and VII at baseline, and again at treatment weeks 10 and 24. Both study groups demonstrated significantly improved performance on these measures at treatment week 10 compared with baseline, and both groups demonstrated improvements at treatment week 10 compared to placebo week 10. The group treated with donepezil prior to placebo also demonstrated cognitive improvements at the end of the placebo phase when compared to baseline, suggesting a possible carry-over effect of donepezil on cognitive performance in this study population.

Although this is the most carefully performed study of donepezil for attention and memory impairments following TBI to-date, it suffers from several limitations. First, subjects were studied during the period in which spontaneous recovery may occur; while the placebo-controlled crossover design of the study offers some control over this confound, it cannot be entirely discounted as a contributor to the improvements observed in these subjects. Second, subjects with either mild injuries or more severe cognitive impairments were excluded from the study, limiting the generalizability of the study findings. Similarly, patients with common medical and neuropsychiatric comorbidities were excluded, as were patients taking other neuroactive medications prescribed commonly in this population. Both of these exclusions also limit the generalizability of the study findings. Nonetheless, this study offers reasonably strong evidence that donepezil improves attention and memory impairments in the post-acute injury period.

Cholinesterase Inhibitors in Clinical Practice

Collectively, these studies suggest that cholinesterase inhibitors may be of benefit for the treatment of posttraumatic cognitive impairments, and particularly posttraumatic attention and memory impairments. However, findings from the limited number of published studies are mixed with respect to the beneficial effects of these agents in this population. Given the ubiquitous role of acetylcholine in cognition and behavior, the cholinesterase inhibitors might be expected to improve a variety of cognitive impairments (e.g., hypoarousal, inattention, memory impairment, aphasia, executive dysfunction) and other neurobehavioral disturbances (e.g., apathy) in which cholinergic dysfunction is implicated.

The extent to which this type of treatment will be useful in an individual patient most likely depends on the extent to which cholinergic dysfunction in that patient contributes to his or her cognitive and behavioral impairments. Not all persons with TBI demonstrate postmortem (16, 162, 163) or *in vivo* electrophysiologic (24) evidence of posttraumatic cholinergic dysfunction. Consequently, it is unlikely that augmentation of cerebral cholinergic function will benefit all persons with posttraumatic cognitive impairments. However, findings from the published studies of cholinesterase inhibitor therapy among persons with TBI suggest that at least a portion of this population will benefit from such treatments. Multicenter, double-blind, placebo-controlled trials are needed to define both the types of benefits afforded by such treatments and the clinical profile of TBI patients most likely to experience such benefits.

For the present, cholinesterase inhibitors are among the pharmacotherapuetic options available to clinicians treating persons with posttraumatic cognitive impairments. Among these, donepezil is prescribed most commonly, although rivastigmine and galantamine are also sometimes used. When donepezil is prescribed, treatment begins with 5 mg daily. The relatively long half-life of donepezil makes it suitable for once-daily dosing (226). It is not clear whether increases to donepezil 10 mg daily affords additional benefits over 5 mg daily. When higher-dose donepezil is used, titration is generally undertaken at intervals of 2–4 weeks. Slower dose titration may limit the development of treatment-emergent side effects (usually gastrointestinal). Rivastigmine and galantamine have shorter half-lives, and require twice daily dosing. Rivastigmine is generally started at 1.5 mg BID and increased in 1.5 mg BID increments every four weeks until maximal benefits are attained or treatment intolerance develops. Galantamine is generally started at 4 mg BID and increased in 4 mg BID increments until maximal benefits are attained or treatment intolerance develops.

Although all of these agents may produce side effects such as headache, nausea, diarrhea, vomiting, fatigue, insomnia, muscle cramping, pain, and abnormal dreams, these side effects are generally related to overly rapid dose-escalation. Even in this context, such such effects are usually transient. When intolerable side effects develop and/or persist during treatment with any of these agents, dose reduction is prudent. Such reductions may reduce adverse effects and permit patients to continue treatment. Use of these agents should be avoided in women who are pregnant or who are breast feeding their children. Cardiac conduction abnormalities (first-degree A-V block) and symptomatic bradycardia are relative contradindications to the use of these medications. Concurrent administration of agents that inhibit hepatic metabolism via CYP450, 3A4, and 2D6 enzymatic pathways (e.g., ketoconazole and quinidine) may increase blood levels of donepezil. Inducers of hepatic metabolism (phenobarbital, phenytoin, carbamazepine, dexamethasone, rifampin) may decrease donepezil blood levels. To-date, there are no reports suggesting that the use of these agents in persons with traumatic brain injury is associated with a change (positive or negative) in seizure frequency.

CDP-Choline

Cytidine 5'-diphosphocholine (CDP-choline or citicoline) is an essential intermediate in the biosynthetic pathway of phospholipids incorporated into cell membranes. Orally ingested CDP-choline is metabolized into its two principal components, cytidine and choline. CDP-choline appears to activate the biosynthesis of structural phospholipids in neuronal membranes, increase cerebral metabolism, and enhance activity of dopamine, norepinephrine, and acetylcholine (157, 233). In light of these properties, CDP-choline might be expected to improve posttraumatic cognitive impairments.

Calatayud et al. (1991) (234) performed a single-blind randomized study of 216 patients with severe or moderate TBI during the acute post-injury period. They observed improvements in motor, cognitive, and psychiatric function during treatment with CDP-choline, and use of this agent was associated with decreased length of stay in the hospital. Levin (1991) (235) performed a double blind placebo-controlled study of 14 patients to evaluate the efficacy of CDP-choline for treating post-concussional symptoms in the first month after mild to moderate TBI. Oral CDP-choline (1 g daily) and placebo control groups were matched for age, education and severity of initial injury (as assessed by impairment of consciousness). CDP-choline reduced the severity of post-concussional symptoms and improved recognition memory for designs. Other aspects of neuropsychological performance were not significantly influenced by this treatment.

CDP-choline is available in the United States only as an over-the-counter nutritional supplement, and is most commonly formulated in 250 mg capsules. The content and purity of CDP-choline formulations may vary considerably, both within and between manufacturers. Patients electing to undertake treatment with CDP-choline should be cautioned about these problems and monitored carefully for both beneficial and adverse reactions during its use. A metanalysis of studies using CDP-choline in elderly patients suggests that its use is associated with fewer adverse effects than placebo (236), and there are no reports of serious adverse events related to treatment with this agent among persons with TBI. At present, the limited scope of the relevant literature and the lack of rigorous FDA scrutiny of the safety, tolerability, and efficacy of this agent preclude recommending routine use of CDP-choline in this population. However, for patients unwilling or unable to take other prescribed medications, CDP-choline may be a "nutritional supplement" that some patients may find acceptable and of modest benefit.

SUMMARY

Pharmacotherapy is one of several potentially useful strategies for the treatment of posttraumatic cognitive impairments. Prior to initiating any such treatment, following the basic principles of pharmacotherapy is imperative. Other neuropsychiatric conditions and other ongoing treatments should be evaluated in order to determine whether such may be contributing to an individual's apparent cognitive problems. The use of agents that are known to interfere with cognition in this population, including typical antipsychotics, anticonvulsants, and benzodiazepines, should be discontinued where possible.

If treatment with such medications is needed, those least likely to impair cognition should be used whenever possible. When pharmacotherapy of posttraumatic cognitive impairments is considered, the period over which an empiric trial of such medications will be undertaken should be defined prior to starting treatment. Specific target symptoms should be defined, and assessment of cognition using standardized bedside or formal neuropsychological measures before and during treatment should be performed. When treatment is initiated, using a start-low, go-slow approach that includes careful monitoring of adverse and drug-drug effects is recommended.

Our present understanding of the neurochemistry of cognition and the neurochemical consequences of TBI suggest that catecholaminergic and cholinergic function are likely to be the most useful neurochemical targets for pharmacologic intervention among persons with typical posttraumatic cognitive impairments such as hypoarousal, inattention, slowed processing speed, memory impairments, language disturbances, and executive dysfunction. It is possible that as more effective and tolerable NMDA receptor antagonists are developed, glutamatergic dysfunction in the acute, post-acute, and late post-injury periods may become a reasonable target for pharmacologic intervention as well.

Although there is less evidence of persistent catecholaminergic deficits among persons with TBI as a group, interindividual differences in the integrity of cerebral catacholaminergic systems post-injury and/or the metabolism of catecholamine neurotransmitters may offer some explanation for the apparent cognitive benefits afforded by catecholaminergically-active agents in this population. Although there is better evidence for persistent cerebral cholinergic dysfunction in association with cognitive impairments following TBI, the number of studies investigating cholinergic augmentation strategies and the strength of the evidence they provide are at present limited. Consequently, only preliminary treatment recommendations regarding the use of medications that increase cerebral cholinergic function can be offered.

In general, patients whose most troubling cognitive impairments include arousal, impaired speed of processing, and inattention may benefit from treatment with a psychostimulant such as methylphenidate. These agents may also improve posttraumatic language, praxis, and executive function impairments, and most of these agents appear to modestly improve some neurobehavioral functions such as apathy, agitation, and perseveration. The present evidence suggests that methylphenidate should be regarded as first-line therapy when an agent from this medication class is used. If methylphenidate proves ineffective or produces intolerable side effects, dextroamphetamine, amantadine, or bromocriptine may be useful alternative stimulant medications. In cases where none of these are effective, clinicians might consider use of modafanil, carbidopa/L-dopa, or other non-standard agents with stimulating properties such as protryptline or lamotrigine.

Use of psychostimulants in the acute rehabilitation setting may facilitate engagement in rehabilitation therapies, and it is possible that such treatment may hasten the recovery process (functionally, if not also neurobiologically). If used during the post-acute injury period (during which spontaneous recovery may occur), periodically decreasing the dose of these agents after maximal cognitive benefit has been achieved is recommended in order to determine if continued prescription of a psychostimulant is still necessary. When used in the late post-injury period, common clinical experience suggests that these medications maintain their effectiveness over the long-term and that abuse of and/or dependence on these agents is rare.

Among patients whose principal posttraumatic cognitive impairment is in the domain of memory (encoding, retrieval, or both), cholinesterase inhibitors may be of some benefit. Cholinergic augmentation would be predicted to have additional benefits on posttraumatic impairments in arousal, attention, language, executive function, and frontally-mediated behaviors, but the evidence in support of this prediction is at present preliminary. Among the cholinesterase inhibitors, donepezil is used most commonly and is for the present the agent with the most published evidence with which to support and guide its use. When patients respond to treatment with this agent, these benefits appear to be sustained during continued treatment over relatively long periods of time (i.e., months to years). It is not clear whether the other commonly used cholinesterase inhibitors (i.e., rivastigmine, galantamine) afford similar benefits, but there are theoretical reasons to expect comparable effects during treatment with these agents. Although the majority of reports describing the use of cholinesterase inhibitors in this population focus on the treatment of persons in the late post-injury period, these agents may be of use in the acute rehabilitation setting as well (237). If used during the period in which spontaneous recovery is likely to occur, periodic dose reduction and/or discontinuation of these agents is prudent in order to determine whether their use is still needed. In our experience, cognitive impairments that emerge following such dose reductions and/or medication discontinuations remain responsive to treatment once it is reinstituted.

In the absence of cost-effective and widely available *in vivo* markers of neurotransmitter function with which to guide the selection of a class of medication, pharmacologic treatment of posttraumatic cognitive impairments in an individual patient remains a matter of clinical judgment and empiric trial. Some patients respond robustly to catecholaminergic agents, others to cholinesterase inhibitors, some require treatment with some combination of these agents, and others respond poorly to all presently available medications. Additional studies are needed to clarify which agents are most effective for which types of posttraumatic cognitive impairments and better methods are needed to facilitate the identification of patients most likely to respond to such pharmacotherapies.

References

1. Waxweiler RJ, Thurman D, Sniezek J, Sosin D, O'Neil J. Monitoring the impact of traumatic brain injury: a review and update. *J Neurotrauma* 1995;12:509–516.
2. Kraus JF, Sorenson SB. Epidemiology. In Silver JM, Yudofsky SC, Hales RE (eds). *Neuropsychiatry of Traumatic Brain Injury.* Washington DC: American Psychiatric Press, Inc. 1994, pp. 3–41.
3. O'Shanick GJ, O'Shanick AM. Personality and Intellectual Changes. In Silver JM, Yudofsky SC, Hales RE (eds). *Neuropsychiatry of Traumatic Brain Injury.* Washington DC: American Psychiatric Press, Inc. 1994, pp. 163–188.
4. Lovell MR, Franzen MD. Neuropsychological Assessment. In Silver JM, Yudofsky SC, Hales RE (eds). *Neuropsychiatry of Traumatic Brain Injury.* Washington DC: American Psychiatric Press, Inc. 1994, pp. 133–160.
5. Fife D. Head injury with and without hospital admission: comparison of incidence and short–term disability. *Am J Public Health* 1987;77:810–812.
6. Spikman JM, Deelman BG, Van Zomeren AH. Executive functioning, attention and frontal lesions in patients with chronic CHI. *J Clin Exp Neuropsychol* 2000;22:325–338.
7. Arciniegas D, Adler L, Topkoff J, Cawthra E, Filley CM, Reite M. Attention and memory dysfunction after traumatic brain injury: cholinergic mechanisms, sensory gating, and a hypothesis for further investigation. *Brain Inj* 1999;13:1–13.
8. Novack TA, Dillon MC, Jackson WT. Neurochemical mechanisms in brain injury and treatment: a review. *J Clin Exp Neuropsychol* 1996;18:685–706.
9. Mesulam M-M. Attentional Networks, Confusional States, and Neglect Syndromes. In Mesulam M-M (ed). *Principles of Behavioral and Cognitive Neurology, 2nd ed.* Philadelphia: F.A. Davis 2000, pp. 174–256.
10. Mesulam M-M. Behavioral Neuroanatomy: Large-Scale Networks, Association Cortex, Frontal Syndromes, the Limbic System, and Hemispheric Specialization. In Mesulam M-M (ed.). *Principles of Behavioral and Cognitive Neurology, 2nd ed.* Philadelphia: F.A. Davis 2000, pp. 1–120.
11. Parizel PM, Makkat S, Jorens PG, Ozsarlak O, Cras P, Van Goethem JW, van den Hauwe L, Verlooy J, De Schepper AM. Brainstem hemorrhage in descending transtentorial herniation (Duret hemorrhage). *Intensive Care Med* 2002;28(1):85–88.
12. Jennett B, Adams JH, Murray LS, Graham DI. Neuropathology in vegetative and severely disabled patients after head injury. *Neurology* 2001;56(4):486–490.
13. Firsching R, Woischneck D, Klein S, Ludwig K, Dohring W.Brain stem lesions after head injury. *Neurol Res* 2002;24(2):145–146.
14. Polo MD, Newton P, Rogers D, Escera C, Butler S. ERPs and behavioural indices of long-term preattentive and attentive deficits after closed head injury. *Neuropsychologia* 2002;40(13):2350–2359.
15. McAllister TW. Neuropsychiatric sequelae of head injuries. *Psychiatr Clin North Am* 2002;15(2):395–413.
16. Murdoch I, Nicoll JA, Graham DI, Dewar D. Nucleus basalis of Meynert pathology in the human brain after fatal head injury. *J Neurotrauma* 2002;19(2):279–284.
17. Donnemiller E, Brenneis C, Wissel J, Schlerfler C, Poewe W, Riccabona G, Wenning GK. Impaired dopaminergic neurotransmission in patients with traumatic brain injury: a SPECT study using 123I-beta-CIT and 123I-IBZM. *Eur J Nuc Med* 2000;27:1410–1414.
18. Tang YP, Noda Y, Nabeshima T. Involvement of activation of dopaminergic neuronal system in learning and memory deficits

associated with experimental mild traumatic brain injury. *Euro J Neurosci* 1997;9:1720–1727.

19. Obrenovitch TP, Urenjak J. Is high extracellular glutamate the key to excitotoxicity in traumatic brain injury? *J Neurotrauma* 1997; 14(10):677–698.

20. Eghwrudjakpor PO, Miyake H, Kurisaka M, Mori K. Central nervous system bioaminergic responses to mechanical trauma. An experimental study. *Surg Neurol* 1991;35:273–279.

21. Pappius HM. Involvement of indoleamines in functional disturbances after brain injury. *Progress in Neuro-Psychopharmacology & Biological Psychiatry* 1989;13(3-4):353–361.

22. Hamill RW, Woolf PD, McDonald JV, Lee LA, Kelly M. Catecholamines predict outcome in traumatic brain injury. *Ann Neurol* 1987;21:438–443.

23. Woolf PD, Hamill RW, Lee LA, Cox C, McDonald JV. The predictive value of catecholamines in assessing outcome in traumatic brain injury. *J Neurosurg* 1987;66:875–882.

24. Arciniegas DB. The cholinergic hypothesis of cognitive impairment caused by traumatic brain injury. *Curr Psychiatry Rep* 2003; 5(5):391–399.

25. Arciniegas D, Olincy A, Topkoff J, McRae K, Filley CM, Reite M, Alder LE. Impaired auditory gating and P50 nonsuppression following traumatic brain injury. *J Neuropsych Clin Neurosci* 2000;12:77–85.

26. Arciniegas DB, Topkoff J, Rojas DC, Sheeder J, Teale P, Young D, Sandberg E, Reite ML, Adler LE. Reduced hippocampal volume in association with P50 nonsuppression following traumatic brain injury. *J Neuropsych Clin Neurosci* 2001;13:213–221.

27. LaBar KS, Gitelman DR, Parrish TB, Mesulam M. Neuroanatomic overlap of working memory and spatial attention networks: a functional MRI comparison within subjects. *Neuroimage* 1999; 10(6):695–704.

28. Booth JR, Burman DD, Meyer JR, Lei Z, Trommer BL, Davenport ND, Li W, Parrish TB, Gitelman DR, Mesulam MM. Neural development of selective attention and response inhibition. *Neuroimage* 2003;20(2):737–751.

29. Filley CM. The neuroanatomy of attention. *Semin Speech Lang* 2002;23(2):89–98.

30. Daffner KR, Mesulam MM, Holcomb PJ, Calvo V, Acar D, Chabrerie A, Kikinis R, Jolesz FA, Rentz DM, Scinto LF. Disruption of attention to novel events after frontal lobe injury in humans. *J Neurol Neurosurg Psychiatry* 2000;68(1):18–24.

31. Morecraft RJ, Geula C, Mesulam MM. Architecture of connectivity within a cingulo-fronto-parietal neurocognitive network for directed attention. *Arch Neurol* 1993;50(3):279–284.

32. Olincy A, Ross RG, Harris JG, Young DA, McAndrews MA, Cawthra E, McRae KA, Sullivan B, Adler LE, Freedman R. The P50 auditory event-evoked potential in adult attention-deficit disorder: comparison with schizophrenia. *Biol Psychiatry* 2000; 47(11):969–77.

33. Mapstone M, Weintraub S, Nowinski C, Kaptanoglu G, Gitelman DR, Mesulam MM. Cerebral hemispheric specialization for spatial attention: spatial distribution of search-related eye fixations in the absence of neglect. *Neuropsychologia* 2003;41(10): 1396–1409.

34. Gitelman DR, Nobre AC, Parrish TB, LaBar KS, Kim YH, Meyer JR, Mesulam M. A large-scale distributed network for covert spatial attention: further anatomical delineation based on stringent behavioural and cognitive controls. *Brain* 1999;122 (Pt 6): 1093–1106.

35. Konrad K, Gauggel S, Schurek J. Catecholamine functioning in children with traumatic brain injuries and children with attention-deficit/hyperactivity disorder. *Brain Res Cogn Brain Res* 2003; 16(3):425–433.

36. Grujic Z, Mapstone M, Gitelman DR, Johnson N, Weintraub S, Hays A, Kwasnica C, Harvey R, Mesulam MM. Dopamine agonists reorient visual exploration away from the neglected hemispace. *Neurology* 1998;51(5):1395–1398.

37. Manns JR, Squire LR. Perceptual learning, awareness, and the hippocampus. *Hippocampus* 2001;11(6):776–782.

38. Markowitsch HJ. Memory and Amnesia: In Mesulam M-M (ed.). *Principles of Behavioral and Cognitive Neurology, 2nd ed.* Philadelphia: F.A. Davis 2000, pp. 257–293.

39. Gabrieli JD. Cognitive neuroscience of human memory. *Annu Rev Psychol* 1998;49:87–115.

40. Wittenberg GM, Sullivan MR, Tsien JZ. Synaptic reentry reinforcement based network model for long-term memory consolidation. *Hippocampus* 2002;12(5):637–647.

41. Eichenbaum H. The hippocampus and declarative memory: cognitive mechanisms and neural codes. *Behav Brain Res* 2001; 127(1-2):199–207.

42. Redell JB, Moore AN, Dash PK. Expression of the prodynorphin gene after experimental brain injury and its role in behavioral dysfunction. *Exp Biol Med (Maywood)* 2003;228(3):261–269.

43. Albensi BC, Janigro D. Traumatic brain injury and its effects on synaptic plasticity. *Brain Inj* 2003;17(8):653–663.

44. Albensi BC. Models of brain injury and alterations in synaptic plasticity. *J Neurosci Res* 2001;65(4):279–283.

45. Phillips LL, Lyeth BG, Hamm RJ, Reeves TM, Povlishock JT. Glutamate antagonism during secondary deafferentation enhances cognition and axo-dendritic integrity after traumatic brain injury. *Hippocampus* 1998;8(4):390–401.

46. Bazan NG, Rodriguez de Turco EB, Allan G. Mediators of injury in neurotrauma: intracellular signal transduction and gene expression. *J Neurotrauma* 1995;12(5):791–814.

47. Dixon CE, Kochanek PM, Yan HQ, Schiding JK, Griffith RG, Baum E, Marion DW, DeKosky ST. One-year study of spatial memory performance, brain morphology, and cholinergic markers after moderate controlled cortical impact in rats. *J Neurotrauma* 1999;16(2):109–122.

48. Ciallella JR, Yan HQ, Ma X, Wolfson BM, Marion DW, DeKosky ST, Dixon CE. Chronic effects of traumatic brain injury on hippocampal vesicular acetylcholine transporter and M2 muscarinic receptor protein in rats. *Exp Neurol* 1998;152(1):11–19.

49. Gorman LK, Fu K, Hovda DA, Murray M, Traystman RJ. Effects of traumatic brain injury on the cholinergic system in the rat. *J Neurotrauma* 1996;13(8):457–463.

50. Hasselmo ME, Wyble BP, Wallenstein GV. Encoding and retrieval of episodic memories: role of cholinergic and GABAergic modulation in the hippocampus. *Hippocampus* 1996;6(6):693–708.

51. Barros DM, Izquierdo LA, Medina JH, Izquierdo I. Pharmacological findings contribute to the understanding of the main physiological mechanisms of memory retrieval. *Curr Drug Target CNS Neurol Disord* 2003;2(2):81–94.

52. Hasselmo ME, Wyble BP. Free recall and recognition in a network model of the hippocampus: simulating effects of scopolamine on human memory function. *Behav Brain Res* 1997;89(1-2):1–34.

53. Ogasawara T, Itoh Y, Tamura M, Ukai Y, Yoshikuni Y, Kimura K. NS-3, a TRH-analog, reverses memory disruption by stimulating cholinergic and noradrenergic systems. *Pharmacol Biochem Behav* 1996;53(2):391–399.

54. Murai S, Saito H, Masuda Y, Odashima J, Itoh T. AF64A disrupts retrieval processes in long-term memory of mice. *Neuroreport* 1995;6(2):349–352.

55. Ward H, Shum D, Wallace G, Boon J. Pediatric traumatic brain injury and procedural memory. *J Clin Exp Neuropsychol* 2002;24(4):458–470.

56. Nadeau SE. A paradigm shift in neurorehabilitation. *Lancet Neurol* 2002;1(2):126–130.

57. Rammsayer TH, Rodewald S, Groh D. Dopamine-antagonistic, anticholinergic, and GABAergic effects on declarative and procedural memory functions. *Brain Res Cogn Brain Res* 2000;9(1):61–71.

58. Damasio R, Damasio H. Aphasia and the Neural Basis of Language. In Mesulam M-M (ed.). *Principles of Behavioral and Cognitive Neurology, 2nd ed.* Philadelphia: F.A. Davis 2000, pp. 294–315.

59. Jurado MA, Mataro M, Verger K, Bartumeus F, Junque C. Phonemic and semantic fluencies in traumatic brain injury patients with focal frontal lesions. *Brain Inj* 2000;14(9):789–795.

60. Ferstl EC, Guthke T, von Cramon DY. Change of perspective in discourse comprehension: encoding and retrieval processes after brain injury. *Brain Lang* 1999;70(3):385–420.

61. Gil M, Cohen M, Korn C, Groswasser Z. Vocational outcome of aphasic patients following severe traumatic brain injury. *Brain Inj* 1996;10(1):39–45.

examined in one randomized, double-blind, placebo-controlled trial Zhang studied twenty patients with TBI who were randomized from two postacute rehabilitation clinics; 18 completed the trial. During the donepezil phase, the drug was administered at 5 mg/day for the first two weeks and 10 mg/day for the remaining eight weeks of the trial. Group analysis showed significant benefits of donepezil on neuropsychological functioning (52). Benefits of donepezil were sustained after the washout period. An early case series found that this medication did help in self-reported improvement of memory in two persons with acute TBI, yet this series was problematic in its design and control (48). An open label trial of 10 subjects with TBI treated with donezepil, patients noted a clinical global improvement (46). These agents have not yet been shown to assist in emergence from posttraumatic amnesia.

Dopamine Pathways

The dopamine neurons are generally located in the midbrain the periventricular areas of lateral ventricles including the very well known substantia nigra pathways. The most important dopaminergic pathways are the nigtostriatal, tuberoinfundibular, mesolimbic and mesocortical pathways (53, 54). Dopamine receptors exist as families of receptors with their designation in part being determined by their ability to activate adenyl cyclase (D1, D2, D3, D4, D5) see figure 54-3 (54). The D1 and D5 family of receptors activate adenyl cyclase while the D2, 3 and 4 family of receptors inhibit adenyl cyclase. These receptors all employ G proteins to inhibit or active processes (54). Dopamine is associated with motor movement and probably arousal. The pathways project to the hypothalamus and are associated with autonomic functions and hormonal levels.

In acute injury, a vast excitotoxic cascade occurs. It has been well established the increases in dopamine are correlated with increased cell death in the regions where dopamine acts as a neurotransmitter (55). Furthermore medications that block dopamine release or receptors have been implicated in slowing neuronal recovery (36, 56–58), these agents may affect hormonal levels through their affects on the hippocampal releasing hormones, and cause dysautonomia. Deficits associated with decreased

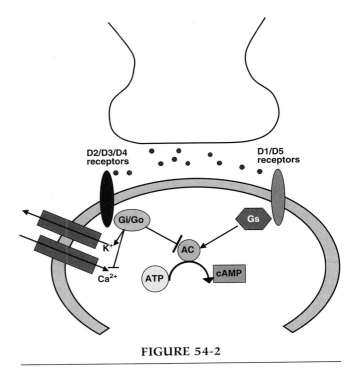

FIGURE 54-2

Dopamine receptor

dopamine such as movement disorders, and neuroleptic malignant syndrome is associated with blockade of the dopamine pathways as well (36).

Recovery

Patients who have had profound disruption of the dopamine pathways as noted in DAI and anoxic injury may forever be very susceptible to the side effects of medications that block the D1-D5 pathways (35, 36). For this reason these medications need to be judiciously utilized with preference to medications that block as few of these pathways as possible. For this reason medications that block the dopamine pathways are generally restricted in the early recovery stages of TBI due to their potential clinical effect.

Controversy

Typical antipsychotics and atypical antipsychotics carry varying degrees of dopamine blockade. Typical antipsychotics exist along a spectrum carrying various degrees of dopamine blockade (mostly D2) and anticholinergic activity (59). Atypical antipsychotics have activity not only via dopamine blockade but also on the serotonin system (59).

Typical antipsychotics have been used for the immediate control of aggression or agitation in TBI (60). These agents have the potential concern of lowered seizure threshold and clouded sensorium. As with other patient groups, neuroleptic malignant syndrome has been reported

TABLE 54-3 *Dopamine*		
RECEPTOR	**G-PROTEIN**	**EFFECTOR MECHANISM**
D1, D5	Gs	↑adenylyl cyclase; ↑cAMP
D2, D3, D4	Gi, Go	↓adenylyl cyclase; ↓cAMP; Ca2+/K+ channels

with the administration of typical and atypical antipsychotic agents. Presenting symptoms can include fever, leukocytosis, and muscle stiffness; this entity carries a potential mortality of 10% (61). The source of these adverse events appears to be the typical antipsychotic medications particular affinity for the D2 dopamine receptor. Atypical antipsychotic agents have less D2 activity and more 5HT2a activating thus theoretically reducing some of the undesirable effects and adrenergic blockade (59). Recently clinical concerns with cardiac dysfunction have been raised in the dementia population with the use of atypical and typical antipsychotic agents (62).

While numerous studies have been done in animal models there is a lack of clarity in optimal timing and in human data. Animal models of recovery after TBI consistently demonstrate a negative impact of dopamine blockers on recovery in the postacute period (57, 63). Yet not all animal models are clear on this issue. In an animal study evaluating the effects of antipsychotics on cognitive function after TBI, haloperidol was demonstrated to be harmful while olanzapine was not (64). Recent work has demonstrated a negative impact of chronic risperidone use (65). Perhaps these differences are explained by the relatively strong D2 receptor activity of risperidone (65).

While most rehabilitation clinicians treating those with TBI would attempt to avoid dopamine blockade the actual human evidence for this is rather weak. Rao et al studied the impact of haloperidol in a rehabilitation setting and noted no change in outcome but a longer length of posttraumatic amnesia in the haloperidol group (66). Maryinak et al demonstrated the successful use of the older antipsychotic methotrimeprazine in persons with TBI admitted to a rehabilitation unit (67). These authors noted that while those treated with the antipsychotic had a longer length of posttraumatic amnesia is likely reflected a greater injury severity (67). Other authors have noted that weaning antipsychotics in the chronic setting results in improved neuropsychological test scores (68). Of interest however is a recent study suggesting a benefit to the use of haloperidol in the ICU setting. Milbrandt and colleagues examined a total of 989 persons with ICU stays and mechanical ventilation of greater than 48 hours (69). Haloperidol use was associated with lower hospital mortality. While this retrospective study has limitations, this data appeared to remain consistent for those with trauma and neurological dysfunction. The authors postulated that at least acutely haloperidol inhibits the secretion of proinflammatory cytokines.

Medications that may increase dopamine have been postulated to enhance recovery from TBI (70, 71). The most studied of these medications is amantadine, which also may have effects on various neuronal growth factors. Other medications such as bromocriptine that demonstrate specific D1-D2 receptor pathway activity have also been useful (71).

The disruption of the dopaminergic pathways has also been implicated in the development of psychiatric disorders following TBI (35, 36). Delusions, hallucinations, and various behavioral dyscontrol syndromes have been implicated with TBI.

The role of dopamine enhancing medications in the potential recovery of persons with TBI remains an issue of great interest. These agents have been employed for aphasia, hemineglect, arousal, agitation and dysautonomic syndromes. Dixon and Klein have demonstrated the role of amantadine in the treatment of a laboratory model of chronic TBI (72). Bromocriptine has also been shown to improve lipid peroxidation after TBI (73). Other agents such as selegline have shown promise in the laboratory (74). Clearly, clinical trials are lacking and little level I evidence exists to guide clinicians in the use of these medications. Potential side effects of these medications include: dyskinesia, hypotension, lowered seizure threshold, hallucinations and behavioral dysfunction.

While many clinicians use neurostimulant medications for the treatment of hypoarousal in persons with TBI, unfortunately the literature to support their use is sparse (40). Amantadine has both pre and post dopaminergic activity as well as functioning as a NMDA antagonist (71). In a case report by Zafonte and colleagues, a male patient in a minimally conscious state regained full consciousness when placed on the dopaminergic agent amantadine but subsequently experienced a significant decline when the medication was withdrawn (76). A double blind placebo cross over study by Meyhthaler and colleagues, showed significant improvements in DRS scores and FIM-cognitive scores in groups taking amantadine were found, regardless of when it was started (71). Additionally, amantadine has shown promising results when given in the acute phase of TBI. Saniova et al. found decreased mortality rates and improved GCS scores in a small group of persons admitted to an ICU after severe TBI who were given a three-day course of amantadine (77). This agent is presently under evaluation in a multicenter trial to evaluate its impact on arousal. McDowell tested a group of 24 subjects with TBI using a double blind, placebo-controlled crossover trial (78). Bromocriptine was found to improve performance on some tasks served by prefrontal function, but not others. Dobkin had previously shown improvement in antegrade amnesia in a women with TBI (79). Substantial work still remains to identify the specific syndromes and characteristics of persons who respond to these medications.

Serotonergic Pathways

The serotonin pathways are found predominantly in the midbrain and brain stem but are distributed diffusely throughout the CNS. They have profound projections throughout the brain including to the frontal lobes and the hippocampus (80, 81). It has been theorized that these pathways are most disrupted by DAI. Serotonin (5-hydroxytryptamine or 5-HT) is likely the most phylogenetically ancient of currently known neurotransmitter molecules. Serotonergic neuronal cell bodies are organized in two distinct groups (81); caudal (in the medulla oblongata and the caudal half of the pons) and rostral (in the midbrain and rostral pons) (81). The rostral 5-HT neuron axons ascend toward the forebrain, while those from the caudal group descend to brainstem structures and the spinal cord. Numerous serotonin receptor types have been identified (82, 83) (Figure 54-4). The current classification system takes into account drug related properties, as well as information about amino acid sequencing of the receptor. It is the receptor interaction with the G protein that permits the particular receptor to modulate the activity of different effector systems such as ion channels, substances like adenyl cyclase. The 5HT1 family and 5HT2 family represent the major classes of serotonin receptors this family also includes the 5HT4, 5HT6 and 5HT7 all of whom are G protein dependent (83, 84). The 5HT3 receptor system is a gated ion channel dependent system and represents a separate functional family of receptors. These receptor differences create opportunity and hazards in drug development and clinical utility.

These widely distributed serotonergic pathways are involved in diverse cognitive functions. Data suggest that serotonergic neurotransmission plays a major role in stabilizing and modulating brain function (84, 85). The rostral part of the serotonergic raphe system consists of the caudal linear nucleus (in the midbrain), the dorsal raphe nucleus (extending from the caudal midbrain to rostral pontine levels), and the median raphe nucleus (superior central raphe nucleus found in the rostral pons) (80, 81). In the caudal division there are descending serotonergic neuronal projections found in the raphe magnus nucleus, raphe pallidus nucleus, and raphe obscurens nucleus. In addition there are serotonergic neuronal cell bodies present in the medullary reticular formation (involved in alertness and wakefulness) and other non-raphe regions such as the hippocampus (involved in memory functions) and the substantia nigra (involved with motor control) (80, 81) (see table 54-4).

Acute Injury

Very little work has been performed on the affects of acute serotonin disruption following TBI. However, increasing the levels in the first week following injury is hypothesized to have the same affect of causing increased neuronal cell death as with other excitatory neurotransmitters.

Unfortunately, projections of the serotonin system, including to the forebrain, limbic areas, and hippocampus,

TABLE 54-4
Serotonin

RECEPTOR	G-PROTEIN	EFFECTOR MECHANISM
5-HT1A,1B, 1D, 1E, 1F	Gi, Go	↓adenylyl cyclase; ↓cAMP; ↓Ca2+ influx/↑K+ efflux
5-HT2A, 2B, 2C	Gq, G1	↑PLC, ↑ phosphinositide hydrolysis; ↑IP3; ↑[Ca2+]i
5-HT3	NA	Ligand-gated ion channel; Na+/Ca2+ influx; K+ efflux
5-HT4, 6, 7	Gs	↑adenylyl cyclase; ↑cAMP
5-HT5	Unknown	Poorly Characterized

are prime sites of direct or secondary injury resulting from TBI. There is ample evidence that TBI impacts levels of serotonin in the central nervous system (CNS), but whether there is an elevation or depletion of serotonin is a matter of some debate. Several studies have documented elevations of serotonin in the CNS during the hours immediately after CNS injury, possibly extending for several days (85–88). Markianos, et al. found a significant negative correlation between CNS level of serotonin and the Glasgow Coma Scale score obtained at the time of assay, as well as an association of high serotonin levels with subsequent death (89). Under these conditions, serotonin has been suspected of worsening edema and contributing to vascular spasm (85–88). On the other hand, there are also studies that indicate diminished CNS serotonin levels within the first 24 hours after TBI (88–91), even in cases of mild injury (92). The decrease in serotonin level has been documented up to 60 days following TBI (60), suggesting a chronic down-regulation of the serotonergic system. In addition, there is evidence that serotonin may assist in controlling edema and serotonin receptor agonists may diminish the excitotoxic effects of glutamate release, or secondary inflammatory factors after neurotrauma (93, 94). Disruption of normal serotonin functioning has been documented on a chronic basis after even milder injury, based on a diminished prolactin response to buspirone, which activates serotonin receptors under normal conditions and results in prolactin release (90). Animal models also suggest that neuronal synthesis of serotonin may be inhibited even though extracellular levels of the substance may be high (95).

Recovery

Damaged serotonergic neurons can survive an injury and in time re-enervate target regions, reestablishing synaptic and neurotransmitter function and restoring behavior (1, 95–97). Mature adult neural circuitry can be remodeled and affected by the use of neurotrophic or neurotoxic factors (96). Serotonin facilitation may be involved in controlled neurogenesis. Pharmacological manipulation of neurotransmitter levels, including serotonin, may aid in the repair and reestablishment of useful neural pathways. Serotonin also plays a key role in sleep initiation.

Controversy

Animal data has suggested that 5HT agonist medications may be both helpful and harmful. Repinotan hydrochloride (repinotan) is a highly potent and selective 5-HT(1A) full receptor agonist. This agent has shown rapid uptake and a broad spectrum of neuroprotection in stroke and TBI (97). Kline has reported that 5-HT1A-receptor agonist 8-hydroxy-2-(di-n-propylamino)tetralin (8-OH-DPAT) attenuated traumatic brain injury (TBI)-induced cognitive deficits and histopathology(96). However Wilson studied the selective serotonin 5HT1a receptor agent fluoxetine that in a chronic administration did not impact motor or cognitive recovery (98). Boyeson 's team observed that high does of the phyenylpiperazine agents trazodone induced deficits in an animal model of TBI (99, 100).

Thus, there may be a period of time when introduction of serotonin agonist agents might be beneficial to recovery of the normal serotonin response. Selective serotonin reuptake inhibitors are among the most utilized medication s in North America. These agents have been employed to enhance arousal, improve behavior, and treat depression and emotional liability. An initial phase I study (101) examining the potential beneficial impact of serotonin agonists on recovery after TBI indicated that sertraline was safe, although the study may have been limited by a small subject pool and a short duration of treatment with an SSRI (2 weeks).

It has been theorized that disruption of these pathways is one of the causes of increased depression following TBI (102, 103). A single blind placebo run in trial by Fann et al demonstrated the potential utility of the SSRI Zoloft in the treatment of depression following mild TBI. These pathways have also been implicated in the development of the emotional liability and emotional incontinence noted to follow TBI (102). The use of SSRI antidepressants has become common during the rehabilitation phase following brain injury due to either stroke or TBI. In two studies, antidepressants were shown to aid in the management of behavioral disturbance. Kant and colleagues gave sertraline for eight weeks to 13 patients with TBI, resulting in decreased outbursts and irritability yet this study failed to clarify this issue (104). Bupropion was reported to improve psychomotor agitation and participation in therapies in a 20-year-old woman with TBI who had failed treatment with several other medications (105).

Trazodone, a triazolopyridine antidepressant, is a selective 5-HT reuptake inhibitor and 5-HT2 receptor antagonist and has been frequently used for its sedating effects. Used as an antidepressant, doses of up to 500mg/d are commonly required, however, at lower doses its sedative properties likely result from its antagonistic effect of the 5-HT2 receptors (106, 107). The effects of trazodone on sleep have been shown to occur after the first dose (107, 108). It has been found to closely mimic the natural sleep cycle by increasing the amount of total sleep, increasing the percentage of deep sleep (stages 3 and 4) and decreasing the number of intermittent awakenings (106, 108–114). Trazodone in one dose of 50 to 100 mg nightly to patients showed improvements in early sleep wakening, lack of sound sleep, and difficulty in initiating sleep at two weeks and six weeks with significant increases in total sleep time (111).

Mirtazapine is an alpha2-adrenoceptor antagonist as well as an indirect 5-HT agonist, increasing both synaptic norepinephrine and serotonin. Mirtazapine has been found to improve sleep continuity and increase latency to REM sleep, which may in part be due to its antihistamine properties (115). Yet concern exists regarding rapid weight gain have been noted. Further studies evaluating the role of mirtazapine in sleep disorders in the TBI population are warranted in order to evaluate potential cognitive sequelae.

These studies need to be expanded upon and several are underway at the current time. Whether increases in serotonin will improve the functional status following TBI, beyond that associated with affective disorders is not well understood. Just as important is a clearer understanding of the risks of these agents and their effectiveness in this population.

Norepinephrine Pathways

The excitatory norepinephrine pathways are widely distributed in the brain. However, they are most predominant in the neocortex. From a small cluster of neurons in the locus coeruleus axons are projected to vast areas diffusely throughout the central nervous system including the spinal cord, cerebellum, thalamus and cerebral cortex (116). These pathways have profound effects on behavior, affect, motor function and attention to name just a few of the wide effects of NE. As an example of the critical interactions between neurotransmitters a reduction of NE in the frontal cortex has been associated with attention deficits related to new learning (117). Hence, memory deficits may be related to reduced attention without deficits in the acetycholine pathways.

TABEL 54-5
Norepinephrine

RECEPTOR	G-PROTEIN	EFFECTOR MECHANISM
α1A, α1B, α1D	Gq	↑PLC, ↑ phosphinositide hydrolysis; ↑IP3; ↑[Ca2+]i
α2A, α2B, α2C	Gi, Go	↓adenylyl cyclase; ↓cAMP; ↓Ca2+ influx/ ↑K+ efflux
β1, β2, β3	Gs	↑adenylyl cyclase; ↑cAMP

Acute Injury

Increases of NE are discouraged in the first minutes, hours and days following TBI as the increase alone has been linked to increased neuronal cell death (118, 119). These increases play into the secondary injury cascade and appear to exacerbate other pathways. Indeed, blockade of some NE adrenergic pathways has been hypothesized to be useful in the first few days after injury (120–122).

Recovery

Long term reductions have been associated with an acquired attention deficit syndrome in TBI. This chronic decrement in response has been demonstrated in animal models (123, 124). Consequently, there has been research on the use of agents to increase NE in the weeks following TBI (125, 126).

Controversy

D-amphetamine enhances NE release and has been demonstrated to show benefits in dorsal frontal injury. Kline has demonstrated that chronic methylphenidate treatment enhances water maze performance in animal models of TBI (124).

The most commonly utilized medication is methylphenidate (125–127). Methylphenidate is believed to impact its action at least in part by activity at the dopamine transporter (DAT)(128). One group of investigators has conducted two randomized, double blind, placebo-controlled trials using crossover designs to evaluate the effects of methylphenidate on various aspects of attention after TBI (125). Methylphenidate's potential utility was demonstrated in a study of 34 adults with TBI and persistent deficits in attention (125). Significant benefits of methylphenidate were seen on speed of information processing, but not on divided attention, sustained attention or susceptibility to distraction. This well-designed study suggests the potential beneficial effects of methylphenidate on specific aspects of attention after TBI. While it's

role in arousing patients is not clear methylphenidate does appear to improve attention and processing speed. In a study of ICU persons with TBI, early use of methylphenidate was associated with reductions in ICU and hospital length of stay by 23% in severely TBI patients (128). Although concerns in using early methylphendiate therapy exist such as: increasing the excitability cascade and the proper timing of such therapies. Medications indicated for attention deficit, both on label and off label, have been frequently utilized in TBI patients to improve attention and processing speed in those patients with documented deficits. Since attention is related to so many neurocognitive function, there is a significant need to perform further research in this area. Further evaluation of the population specific benefits is also needed.

GABA Pathways

γ-Aminobutyric acid (GABA) is among the most prevalent neurotransmitter in the CNS. It invariably acts as an inhibitory pathway on excitatory neurotransmitters such as acetylcholine, dopamine, glutamate and norepinephrine. GABA pathways are distributed throughout the brain (116, 129).

GABA receptors have been classified into subtypes A, B and more recently C. The GABA–A receptor is the best understood and has three distinct subunits (116, 129, 130). GABA has been implicated in the inhibition of dopamine, norepinephrine, and cholinergic pathways in the brain. It also modulates the excitotoxicity of Glutamate (116). More recently, GABA has been implicated in the release of serotonin (131). As such GABA is the most widespread neurotransmitter and is invariably inhibitory (116).

Acute Injury

Because of GABA's effects via the G1 protein at Glutamate activated channels it has been considered to be a potentially neuroprotective agent in the first minutes, hours and days following TBI (116). Unfortunately, GABA is completely hydrophilic and does not cross membranes. This leads us to consider medications that indirectly increase its release.

TABLE 54-6
γ-Aminobutyric acid (GABA)

RECEPTOR	G-PROTEIN	EFFECTOR MECHANISM
GABA_A GABAc	NA	Cl- channel
GABA_B	Gi, Go	↓adenylyl cyclase; ↓cAMP; ↓Ca2+ influx/↑K+ efflux

One potential mechanism linked to the neuroprotective effects acute ETOH exposure following CNS injury is the blocking effects at Glutamate activated NMDA channels (132). However, chronic use of ETOH may actually down regulate the receptors thereby reducing the brain's ability to self protect itself from excitatory neurotransmitters (133–137).

Recovery

Use of GABA agonists has been implicated to reduce the rate of recovery following brain injury (138). This includes medications such as benzodiazepines and baclofen (139). The benzodiazepines are termed sedative hypnotics, they make you forget and/or they put you to sleep (138, 139). Both conditions are not conducive to recovery. It is felt that the first six months after injury from TBI are most critical to recovery. This means that these medications, often utilized for seizure prophylaxis, spasticity management and behavioral control should be restricted as much as possible.

Controversy

Bennzodiazepines, antiepileptic medications (AED's) and antipspasticity agents act via GABA yet their longterm impact of these agents is not well understood (138). Benzodiazepines are the oldest family of medications used for spasticity. Diazepam, the most commonly used agent, acts near the GABA$_A$ receptor to hyperpolarlize the cellular membrane, and thus increases presynaptic inhibition (140, 141). Work on the use of diazepam in spinal cord injury, cerebral palsy and multiple sclerosis demonstrated its efficacy in the treatment of spasticity over placebo (142–143). Diazepam has not shown functional improvement. Diazepam's major limitation is in its rather significant side effect profile is sedation it has limited tolerance of diazepam and thus limit its use in the TBI population (138, 140). Baclofen is active at the GABA b receptor both pre and postsynaptically. It has been employed for the treatment of spasticity in persons with SCI, cerebral palsy, multiple sclerosis, stroke and brain injury (138). Enteral baclofen therapy may be warranted for those with severe spasticity of cerebral origin who cannot tolerate dantrolene sodium and face the risk of severe contracture or loss of range of motion (140).

Baclofen has been noted to produce sedation, especially among those with cerebral disorders. Concerns with the use of this medication include: asthenia, depression, hallucinations, nausea, dizziness and paresthesias. Attention and memory induced deficits have been raised in animal models and observed with humans. GABA facilitory agents may impair recovery (145). Memory dysfunction has been associated with baclofen therapy in both animals and humans (145, 146). Additional concerns with baclofen include lowered seizure threshold, and withdrawal syndrome (146). Rapid withdrawal from baclofen therapy should be avoided and can induce seizures, altered mental status, hallucinations, hyperthermia and rigidity (138). Therefore concerns are raised regarding potential negative impact on neurorecovery. One implication of this concept is the long-term use of AED's, particularly those that may function via GABA, are discouraged in the long-term prophylaxis of seizures following TBI. There is considerable evidence they may impede recovery. Finally, inhibiting the effects of excitatory neurotransmitters such as glutamate via GABA invariably affects our ability to learn and adapt. Glutamate is necessary for neuroplasticity and learning and blockade invariably has the potential to reduce the rate and end-point of recovery. The timing of dosing of GABA agonists (early may be better than late) and amount of blockade by the various drugs may be critical.

CONCLUSION

While this is a brief discussion regarding some of the principles of neuropharmacology following TBI, there is much more to follow in the later chapters of the book. The primary purpose of this chapter is to give one a general outline of some of the major neurotransmitter systems that may affect the outcome from TBI. What has not been explored are therapeutic thresholds and toxicity levels for medications.

More research needs to be performed on the use of medications that modulate transmitter systems and the pharmacogenetics involved in treating such persons. When utilizing medications, thought should be given to their profound effects, often beyond the intended results. Randomized placebo controlled trials are needed to further define the potential benefits and risks of such therapy. In addition, a broad understanding of the "window of opportunity" for such medications is needed. As one reads further chapters in the textbook consider the untoward side effects presented as well as the beneficial uses of medications that may affect the CNS.

References

1. Meythaler JM, Peduzzi J, Eleftheriou E, Novack T. Current Concepts: Diffuse Axonal Injury – Associated Traumatic Brain Injury. *Arch Phys Med Rehabil* 2001;82:1461–71.
2. Graham DI. Neurpathology of head injury. In, *Neurotrauma*, Narayan RK, Wilburger JE, Povlishock JT. McGraw-Hill, New York, 1996, pp. 43–59.
3. Nelson JS, Parisi JE, and Schochet SS. *Principles and Practice of Neuropathology*. Mosby, St Louis, 1993.
4. Denny-Brown D, Russell WR. Experimental cerebral concussion. *Brain* 1941;64:93–164.
5. Frankowski RF, Annegers JF, Whitman S. The descriptive epidemiology of head trauma in the United States. In: Becker DP, Povlishock JT, EDS. Central nervous system research status report. Bethesda, MD: *NINCDS*, 1985:33–43.

6. Carus, J., Epidemiology of Head Injury In Head Injury, 3rd edition, Williams & Wilkins, 1993.

7. Horn J, Sherer M. Rehabilitation of traumatic brain injury. In Physical Medicine and Rehabilitation: The Complete Approach. Grabois M, Hart KA, Lehmkuhl LD, eds. Blackwell Science, Malden, Mass. 2000, pp.1281–1299.

8. Guerrero J, Thurman DJ, Sniezek JE. Emergency department visits association with traumatic brain injury: United States, 1995–1996. Brain Injury, 2000;14(2):181–6.

9. Thurman DJ, Guerrero J. Trends in hospitalization associated with traumatic brain injury. JAMA, 1999;282(10):954–7.

10. Unpublished data from Multiple Cause of Death Public Use Data from the National Center for Health Statistics, 1996. http://www.cdc.gov/ncipc/dacrrdp/tbi.htm Methods are described in Sosin DM, Sniezek JE, Waxweiler RJ. Trends in death associated with traumatic brain injury, 1979–1992. JAMA 1995; 273(22):1778–1780.

11. Analysis by the CDC National Center for Injury Prevention and Control, using data obtained from state health departments in Alaska, Arizona, California (reporting Sacramento County only), Colorado, Louisiana, Maryland, Missouri, New York, Oklahoma, Rhode Island, South Carolina, and Utah. Methods are described in:
a. *Centers for Disease Control and Prevention. Traumatic Brain Injury — Colorado, Missouri, Oklahoma, and Utah, 1990–1993. MMWR 1997;46(1):8–11.
b. *Thurman DJ, Sniezek JE, Johnson D, Greenspan A, Smith SM. Guidelines for Surveillance of Central Nervous System Injury. Atlanta: Centers for Disease Control and Prevention, 1995.

12. Thurman DJ, Alverson CA, Dunn KA, Guerrero J, Sniezek JE. Traumatic brain injury in the United States: a public health perspective. J Head Trauma Rehab, 1999;14(6):602–15.

13. Sandel ME, Finch M. The case for comprehensive residency training in traumatic brain injury: A commentary. Am J Phys Med Rehabil 1993;72:325–326.

14. Maxwell, WL, Povlishock, JT and Graham, DL. A mechanistic analysis of nondisruptive axonal injury: a review. J. Neurotrauma 1997;14:419–440.

15. Povlishock JT. Pathobiology of traumatically induced axonal injury in animals and man. Ann Emerg Med 1993;22:980-986.

16. Juurlink BH and Paterson PG. Review of oxidative stress in brain and spinal cord injury: Suggestions for pharmacological and nutritional management strategies. J Spinal Cord Med 1999;21:309–34.

17. Radi R, Rodriguez M, Castro L, Telleri R. Inhibition of mitochondrial electron transport by peroxynitrite. Arch Biochem Biophys 1994;24:369–80.

18. Young WY. Death by Calcium: A way of life. In, Neurotrauma, Narayan RK, Wilburger JE, Povlishock JT. McGraw-Hill, New York, 1996, pp. 1421–31.

19. Pike BR, Zhao X, Newcomb JK, Glenn CC, Anderson DK, Hayes RL. Stretch injury causes calpain and caspase-3 activation and necrotic and apoptotic cell death in septo-hippocampal cell cultures. J Neurotrauma 2000;17:283–98.

20. Brain Injury special Interest Group (AAPM&R-BI-SIG): Yablon SA, Meythaler JM, Englander J. A practice parameter recommendation of the American Academy of Physical Medicine and Rehabilitation. Antiepileptic drug (AED) prophylaxis of posttraumatic seizures (PTS). Approved by the Board of the American Academy of Physical Medicine and Rehabilitation. Arch Phys Med Rehabil 1998;79:594–7.

21. Bullock MR; Lyeth BG; Muizelaar JP. Current status of neuroprotection trials for traumatic brain injury: lessons from animal models and clinical studies. Neurosurgery 1999 Aug;45(2):207–17.

22. The Brain Trauma Foundation. The American Association of Neurological surgeons. The Joint Section on Neurotrauma and Critical care. Role of antiseizure prophylaxis following head injury. J Neurotrauma 2000;17:549–53.

23. Narayan, RK, Michel ME, Ansell B, Baethman A, Biegon A, Bracken MB, et al. Clinical trails in head injury. J Neurotrauma 2002;19:503–57.

24. Maxwell, WL, Povlishock, JT , Graham, DL. A mechanistic analysis of nondisruptive axonal injury: a review. J. Neurotrauma 1997;14:419–440.

25. Povlishock JT, Christman CW. The pathobiology of traumatically induced axonal injury in humans and animals: A review of current thoughts. In Traumatic Brain Injury: Bioscience and Mechanics. Bandak FA, Eppinger RH, Ommaya AK. Mary Ann Liebert, Inc. Larchmont, New York. 1996; pp. 51–60.

26. Bazan NG, Deturco EB, Allan G. Mediators of injury in neurotrauma: Intracellular signal transduction and gene expression. J Neurotrauma 1995;12:791–814.

27. Bates EJ. Eicosanoids, fatty acids and neutrophils: Their relevance to the pathophysiology of disease. Prostagland Leukotr Ess Fatty Acids 1955:53:75–86.

28. Henderson WR Jr. The role of leukotrienes in inflammation. Ann Int Med 1994;121:684–97.

29. Fern R, Ransom BR, and Waxman SG. Voltage-gated calcium channels in CNS white matter: role in anoxic injury. J Neurophys 1995, 74:369–377.

30. Saido TC, Sorimachi H, Suzuki K. Calpain: New perspectives in molecular diversity and physiological-pathological involvement. FASEB J 1994;8:814–22.

31. Campfl A, Posmanur RM, Zhao X, Schmutzhard E, Clifton GL, Hayes RL. Mechanisms of calpain proteolysis following traumatic brain injury: Implications for pathology and therapy: Review and update. J Neurotrauma 1997;14:121–34.

32. Ratan RR, Murphy TH, Baraban JM. Macromolecular synthesis inhibitors prevent oxidative stress-induced apoptosis in embryonic cortical neurons by shunting cysteine from protein synthesis to glutathione. J Neurosci 1994;14:4385–53.

33. Schallert T, Fleming SM, Woodlee MT. Should the injured and intact hemispheres be treated differently during the early phases of physical restorative therapy in experimental stroke or Parkinsonism? Harvey RL, Guest Editor. Motor Recovery After Stroke. W.B. Saunders, N Am Clinics of Phys Med Rehabil. 2003;14(S1) pp. S27–46.

34. Missal C, Nash SR, Robinson SW, Jaber M, Caron MG. Dopamine receptors: From structure to function. Physiol Rev 1998;78: 189–225.

35. Jaber M, Robinson SW, Missale C, Caron MG. Dopamine receptors and brain function. Neuropharmacol 1996;35:1503–19.

36. Wilkinson W, Meythaler JM, Guin-Renfroe S. Neuroleptic malignant syndrome induced by haloperidol following traumatic brain injury. Brain Injury 1999;13:1025–1031.

37. Shkryl VM, Nikolaenko LM, Kostyuk PG, Lukyanetz EA. High-threshold calcium channel activity in rat hippocampal neurons during hypoxia. Brain Res 1999;833:319–28.

38. Okuda T, Haga T. High affinity choline transporter. Neurochemical Res 2003;28:483–8.

39. Clader J, Wang Y. Muscarinic receptor agonists and antagonists in the treatment of Alzheimer's disease. Curr Pharm Des 2005;11:3353–61.

40. Gordon W, Zafonte R, Ciccerone K, Lombard L. TBI: State of the Science American Journal of Physical Medicine and Rehabilitation (in press).

41. Narajan, RK, Michel ME, and The Clinical Trials in Head Injury Study Group. Clinical Trials in Head Injury. J Neurotrauma 2002;19:503–57.

42. Solowij N, Stephens RS, Roffman RA,Babor T, Kadden R, Miller M, et al. Cognitive functioning of long-term heavy cannabis users seeking treatment. J Am Med Assoc 2002;287:1123–31.

43. Perry EK, Kilford L, Lees AJ, Burn DJ, Perry RH. Increased Alzheimer pathology in Parkinson's disease related to antimuscarinic drugs. Ann Neurol 2003;54:235–8.

44. Levy AI. Chronically mad as a hatter: Anticholinergic's and Alzheimer's disease Pathology. Annal Neurol 2003;54:144–6.

45. Morey CE, Cilo M, Berry J, Cusick C. The effect of Aricept in persons with persistent memory disorder following traumatic brain injury: a pilot study. Brain Injury 2003 Sep;17(9):809–15.

46. Kaye NS, Townsend JB 3rd, Ivins R. An open-label trial of donepezil (aricept) in the treatment of persons with mild traumatic brain injury. J Neuropsychiatry Clin Neurosci. 2003;15:383–4.

47. Blount PJ, Nguyen CD, McDeavitt JT. Clinical use of cholinomimetic agents: a review. J Head Trauma Rehabil 2002;17(4): 314–21.

48. Masanic CA, Bayley MT, VanReekum R, Simard M. Open-label study of donepezil in traumatic brain injury. Arch Phys Med Rehabil 2001;82(7):896–901.

49. Dempsey,RJ Raghavendra Rao VL. Cytidinediphosphocholine treatment to decrease traumatic brain injury induced hippocampal neuronal death, cortical contusion volume, and neurological dysfunction in rats. *J Neurosurg* Apr 2003;98(4):867–73.

50. Leon-Carrion J, Dominguez-Roldan JM, Murillo-Cabezas F, del Rosario Dominquez-Morales M, Munoz-Sanchez MA. The role of citicholine in neuropsychological training after traumatic brain injury. *NeuroRehabilitation* 2000;14(1):33–40.

51. Taverni JP, Seliger G, Lichtman SW. Donepezil mediated memory improvement in traumatic brain injury during post acute rehabilitation *Brain Inj* 1998;12(1):77–80.

52. Zhang L, Plotkin RC, Wang G, Sandel ME, Lee S. Cholinergic augmentation with donepezil enhances recovery in short-term memory and sustained attention after traumatic brain injury. *Arch Phys Med Rehabil* 2004;85(7):1050–55.

53. Smythies J. Section II. The dopamine system. *Int Rev Neurobiol* 2005;64:123–72.

54. Bonci A, Hopf F. The dopamine D2 receptor: new surprises from an old friend. *Neuron* 2005;47:335–8.

55. Willis C, Lybrand S, Bellamy N. Excitatory amino acid inhibitors for traumatic brain injury. *Cochrane Database Syst Rev* 2004;(1):CD003986.

56. Cardenas DD, McLean A. Psychopharmacologic management of traumatic brain injury. *Physical Med Rehabil Clinics N Am* 1992; 3:273-290.

57. Feeny DM, Gonzalez A, Law WA. Amphetamine, haloperidol and experience interact to affect rate of recovery after motor cortex surgery. *Science* 1982;217:855-857.

58. Vasconcellos J. Clinical evaluation of trifluoperazine in maximum-security brain-damaged patients with an organic brain disorder. *JAMA* 1978;240:380-382.

59. Elovic E, Lansang R, Li Y, Ricker J. The use of atypical antipsychotics in traumatic brain injury. *J Head Trauma Rehabil* 2003;18:177–95.

60. Fugate L, Spacek L , Kresty L, Levy C, Johnson J, Mysiw W. Measurement and treatment of agitation following traumatic brain injury:II. A survey of the Brain Injury Special Interest Group of the American Academy of Physical Medicine and Rehabilitation. *Arch Phys Med Rehabil* 1997;78;924–8.

61. Lombard L, Zafonte R. Agitation after traumatic brain injury: considerations and treatment options. *Am J Phys Med Rehabil* 2005;84;797–812.

62. Bullock, R. Treatment of behavioral and psychiatric symptoms in dementia: implications of recent safety warnings. *Curr Med Res Opin* Jan 2005;21(1):1–10.

63. Goldstein LB. Pharmacologic modulation of recovery after stroke: Clinical data. *J Neuro Rehab* 1991;5:129-140 .

64. Wilson M, Gibson C, Hamm R Haloperidol , but not olanzapine, impairs cognitive performance after traumatic brain injury in rats. *Am J Phys Med Rehabil* 2003;82;871–9.

65. Zafonte R, Dixon CE, Kline A . Chronic risperidone treatment after experimental traumatic brain injury negatively impacts functional outcome. *Arch Phys Med Rehabil* 2005;86:page e9.

66. Rao N, Jellienk H, Woolston D Agitation in closed head injury: haloperidol effect on rehabilitation outcome. *Arch Phys Med Rehabil* 1985;66;30–4.

67. Maryniak O, Manchanda R, Velani A. Methotrimeprazine in the treatment of agitation in acquired brain injury patients. *Brain Inj.* Feb 2001;15(2):167–174.

68. Stanislav SW, Childs A. Evaluating the usage of droperidol in acutely agitated persons with brain injury. *Brain Inj.* 2000;14(3):261–5.

69. Milbrandt E, Kersten A, Kong L, Weissfeld L, Clermont G, Fink M, Angus D. Haloperidol use is associated with lower hospital mortality in mechanically ventilated patients. *Crit Care Med* 2005;33;226–9.

70. Toide K. Effects of amantadine on dopaminergic neurons in discrete regions of the rat brain. *Pharm Res* 1990;7:670-67.

71. Meythaler JM, Brunner RC, Johnson A, Davis L, Novack T. Amantadine to Improve Neurorecovery in Traumatic Brain Injury associated Diffuse Axonal Injury: A pilot double-blind randomized trial. *J Head Trauma Rehabil* 2002;17:300–13.

72. Dixon CE, Kraus MF, Kline AE, Ma X, Yan HQ, Griffith RG, Wolfson BM, Marion DW. Amanatadine improves water maze

73. Kline AE, Massucci JL, Ma X, Zafonte RD, Dixon CE. Bromocriptine reduces lipid peroxidation and enahances spatial learning and hippocampal neuron survival in a rodent model of focal brain trauma. *J Neurotrauma* Dec 2004;21(12):1712–22.

74. Zhu J, Hamm RJ, Reeves TM, Povlishock JT, Phillips LL. Postinjury administration of L-deprenyl improves cognitive function and enhances neuroplasticity after traumatic brain injury. *Exp Neurol* 2000;200;166(1):136–52.

75. Whitaker-Azmitia PM. *The Neuropharmacology of serotonin. Current Concepts.* Upjohn Company, Kalamazoo, Michigan. 1992.

76. Zafonte RD, Watanabe T, Mann NR. Amantadine: a potential treatment for the minimally conscious state. *Brain Inj.* Jul 1998;12(7):617–21.

77. Snaiova B, Drobny M, Kneslova L, Minarik M. The outcome of patients with sever head injuries treated with amantadine sulphate. *J Neural Transm* Apr 2004;111(4):511–4.

78. McDowell S, Whyte J, D'Esposito M. Differential effect of a dopaminergic agonist of prefrontal function in traumatic brain injury patients. *Brain* Jun 1998;121(Pt 6):1155–64.

79. Dobkin BH, Hanlon R. Dopamine agonist treatment of antegrade amnesia from a mediobasal forebrain injury. *Ann Neurol* March 1993;33(3):313–6.

80. Azmitia EC. The serotonin-producing neurons of the midbrain median and dorsal raphe nuclei. In: Iverson I, Iverson S. Snyder S, Eds. *Handbook of Pharmacology.* New York, NY: Plenum Press; 1978;9:233–314.

81. Jacobs BL, Fornal CA, Wilkinson LO. Neurophysiological and neurochemical studies of brain serotonergic neurons in behaving animals. [Review] [30 refs]. *Annals of the New York Academy of Sciences* 1990;600:260–268.

82. Nayak AK, Mohanty S, Singh RK, Chansouria JP. Plasma biogenic amines in head injury. *Journal of the Neurological Sciences* 1980;47(2):211–219.

83. Salzman SK, Hirofuji E, Llados-Eckman C, MacEwen GD, Beckman AL. Monoaminergic responses to spinal trauma. Participation of serotonin in posttraumatic progression of neural damage. *Journal of Neurosurgery* 1987;66(3):431–439.

84. Sharma HS, Dey PK, Olsson Y. Brain edema blood brain barrier permeability and cerebral blood flow changes following intracarotid infusion of serotonin: Modification with cyproheptadine and indomethacin. In: Krieglstein J, editor. *Pharmacology of Cerebral Ischemia.* Boca Raton, FL: CRC Press, 1989:317–323.

85. Wester P, Bergstrom U, Eriksson A, Gezelius C, Hardy J, Winblad B. Ventricular cerebrospinal fluid monoamine transmitter and metabolite concentrations reflect human brain neurochemistry in autopsy cases. *Journal of Neurochemistry* 1990;54(4): 1148–1156.

86. van Woerkom T, Minderhoud J. Pharmacologic Interventions. In: Sandel M, Ellis D, editors. *Physical Medicine and Rehabilitation State of the Art Reviews.* Philadelphia: Hanley & Belfus, Inc, 1990:447–464.

87. Karakucuk EIPHPAOS. Endogenous neruopeptides in patients with acute traumatic head injury II: changes in the levels of cerebrospinal fluid substance P, serotonin and lipid peroxidations products in patients with head trauma. *Neuropeptides* 31[3], 259–62. 1997.

88. Pellegrino TC, Bayer BM. Role of central 5-HT (2) receptors in fluoxetine-induced decreases in T-lymphocyte activity. *Brain Behav Immun* 2002;16:87–103.

89. Markianos M, Seretis A, Kotsou S, Baltas I, Sacharogiannis H. CSF neurotransmitter metabolites and short-term outcome of patients in coma after head injury. *Acta Neurologica Scandinavica* 1992;86(2):190–193.

90. Mobayed M, Dinan TG. Buspirone/prolactin response in post head injury depression. *Journal of Affective Disorders* 1990;19(4): 237–241.

91. Singh S, Singh PM, Prasad GC, Udupa KN. Response and action of 5-hydroxytryptamine in experimental head injury. *Indian Journal of Experimental Biology* 1986;24(8):505–507.

92. Saran AS. Depression after minor closed head injury: role of dexamethasone suppression test and antidepressants. *Journal of Clinical Psychiatry* 1985;46(8):335–338.

93. Zauner A, Bullock R. The role of excitatory amino acids in severe brain trauma: Opportunities for therapy: A Review. In *Traumatic Brain Injury: Bioscience and Mechanics*. Bandak FA, Eppinger RH, Ommaya AK. Mary Ann Liebert, Inc. Larchmont, New York. 1996; pp. 97–104.

94. Whitaker-Azmitia PM, Shemer AV, Caruso J, Molino L, Azmitia EC. Role of high affinity serotonin receptors in neuronal growth. *Annals of the New York Academy of Sciences* 1990;600:315–330.

95. Fuller R, Wong D. Serotonin reuptake inhibitors without affinity for neuronal receptors. *Biochemistry and Pharmacology* 1987;7:14–20.

96. Kline AE, Yu J, Massucci JL, Zafonte RD, Dixon CE. Protective effects of the 5-HT1A receptor agonist 8-hydroxy-2-(di-n-propylamino)tetralin against traumatic brain injury-induced cognitive deficits and neuropathology in adult male rats. *Neurosci Lett* Nov 29 2002;333(3):179–82.

97. Mauler F, Horvath E. Neuroprotective efficacy of repinotan HCI, a 5–1A receptor agonist, in animal models of stroke and traumatic brain injury. *J Cereb Blood Flow Metab* Apr 2005;25(4):451–9.

98. Wilson M, Hamm R. Effects of fluoxetine on the 5HT1a receptor and recovery of cognitive function after TBI in rats. *Am J Phys Med Rehabil* 2002;81;364–72.

99. Boyeson MG, Harmon RL, Jones JL. Comparative effects of fluoxetine, amitriptyline and serotonin on functional motor recovery after sensorimotor cortex injury. *Am J Phys Med Rehabili* Apr 1994;73(2):76–83.

100. Boyeson MG, Harmon RL. Effects of trazodone and desipramine on motor recovery in brain-injured rats. *Am J Phys Med Rehabil* Oct 1993;72(5):286–93.

101. Meythaler JM, Depalma L, Devivo MJ, Guin-Renfroe S, Novack TA. Sertraline to improve arousal and alertness in severe traumatic brain injury secondary to motor vehicle crashes. *Brain Injury* 2001;15(4):321–331.

102. Fann J, Uomoto J, Katon W. Sertraline in the treatment of major depression following traumatic brain injury. *J Neuropsych Clin Neurosci* 2000;12;226–232.

103. Fann J, Uomoto J, Katon W. Cognitive improvement with treatment of depression following mild TBI. *Pscyhosomatics* 2001;42:48–54.

104. Kant R, Smith Seemiller L, Zeiler D. Treatment of aggression and irritability after head injury. *Brain Inj* Aug 1998;12(8):661–66.

105. Teng CJ, Bhalerao S, Lee Z, et al. The use of bupropion in the treatment of restlessness after a traumatic brain injury. *Brain Inj* 2001;15(5):463–7.

106. Haffmans, P.M. and M.S. Vos, The effects of trazodone on sleep disturbances induced by brofaromine. *Eur Psychiatry*, 1999. 14(3): pp. 167–71.

107. Bear MF, Connors BW, Paradiso. Neurotransmitter systems. *Neuroscience Exploring the Brain 2nd Ed*. Lippincott Williams and Wilkins, Philadelphia, PA. 2001.

108. Maj, J., W. Palider, and Rawlow, Trazodone, a central serotonin antagonist and agonist. *J Neural Transm*, 1979. 44(3): pp. 237–88.

109. Kaynak, H., et al., *The effects of trazodone on sleep in patients treated with stimulant antidepressants*. Sleep Med, 2004. 5(1): pp. 15–20.

110. Karli D, Burke D, Kim H, et al. Effects of dopaminergic combination therapy for frontal lobe dysfunction in traumatic brain injury rehabilitation. *Brain Injury* 1999;13:63–8.

111. Mashiko, H., et al., Effect of trazodone in a single dose before bedtime for sleep disorders accompanied by a depressive state: dose-finding study with no concomitant use of hypnotic agent. Psychiatry *Clin Neurosci*, 1999. 53(2): pp. 193–4.

112. Ware, J.C. and J.T. Pittard, Increased deep sleep after trazodone use: a double-blind placebo-controlled study in healthy young adults. *J Clin Psychiatry*, 1990. 51 Suppl: pp. 18–22.

113. Scharf, M.B. and B.A. Sachais, Sleep laboratory evaluation of the effects and efficacy of trazodone in depressed insomniac patients. *J Clin Psychiatry*, 1990. 51 Suppl: pp. 13–7.

114. Mouret, J., et al., Effects of trazodone on the sleep of depressed subjects—a polygraphic study. *Psychopharmacology (Berl)*, 1988. 95 Suppl: pp. S37–43.

115. Haddjeri, N., P. Blier, and C. de Montigny, Noradrenergic modulation of central serotonergic neurotransmission: acute and long-term actions of mirtazapine. *Int Clin Psychopharmacol*, 1995. 10 Suppl 4: pp. 11–7.

116. Bear MF, Connors BW, Paradiso. Neurotransmitter systems. *Neuroscience Exploring the Brain 2nd Ed*. Lippincott Williams and Wilkins, Philadelphia, PA 2001.

117. Karli D, Burke D, Kim H, et al. Effects of dopaminergic combination therapy for frontal lobe dysfunction in traumatic brain injury rehabilitation. *Brain Injury* 1999;13:63–8.

118. Zauner A, Bullock R. The role of excitatory amino acids in severe brain trauma: Opportunities for therapy: A Review. In *Traumatic Brain Injury: Bioscience and Mechanics*. Bandak FA, Eppinger RH, Ommaya AK. Mary Ann Liebert, Inc. Larchmont, New York. 1996; pp. 97–104.

119. Hamill RW, Woolf PD, McDaonald JV, Lee LA, Kelly M. Catecholamines predict outcome in traumatic brain injury. *Ann Neurol* 1987;21:438–443.

120. Nayak AK, Mohanty S, Singh RK, Chansouria JP. Plasma biogenic amines in head injury. *Journal of the Neurological Sciences* 1980;47(2):211–219.

121. Wester P, Bergstrom U, Eriksson A, Gezelius C, Hardy J, Winblad B. Ventricular cerebrospinal fluid monoamine transmitter and metabolite concentrations reflect human brain neurochemistry in autopsy cases. *Journal of Neurochemistry* 1990;54(4): 1148–1156.

122. Karakucuk EIPHPAOS. Endogenous neruopeptides in patients with acute traumatic head injury II: changes in the levels of cerebrospinal fluid substance P, serotonin and lipid peroxidations products in patients with head trauma. *Neuropeptides* 31[3], 259–263. 1997.

123. van Woerkom T, Minderhoud J. Pharmacologic Interventions. In: Sandel M, Ellis D, editors. *Physical Medicine and Rehabilitation State of the Art Reviews*. Philadelphia: Hanley & Belfus, Inc, 1990:447–464.

124. Kline AE, Yan HQ, Bao J, Marion DW, Dixon CE. Chronic methylphenidate treatment enhances water maze performance following traumatic brain injury in rats. *Neurosci Lett* Feb 25 2000;280(3):163.

125. Whyte J, Hart T, Schuster K, Fleming M, Polansky M, Coslett HB. Effects of methylphenidate on attentional function after traumatic brain injury. *Am J Phys Med Rehabil* 1997;76:440–50.

126. Evans RW, Gaultieri CT, Patterson D. Treatment of chronic closed head injury with psychostimulant drugs: A controlled case study and an appropriate evaluation procedure. *J Nerv Ment Disease* 1987;175:106–110.

127. Kaelin D, Whyte J, Sandel M. Methylphenidate effect on attention deficit in the acutely brain injured adult study. *Arch Phys Med Rehabil*. 1996;77:6–9.

128. Wagner AK, Chen, X, Kline AE, Li Y, Zafonte RD, Dixon CE. Gender and environmental enrichment impact dopamine transporter expression after experimental traumatic brain injury. *Exp Neurol* Oct 2005;195(2):475–83.

129. Moein H, Khalili HA, Keramatian K. Effect of methylphenidate on ICU and hospital length stay in patients with sever and moderate traumatic brain injury. *Clin Neurol Neurosurg* Oct 11 205.

130. Francisco GE, Kothari, S, Huls C. GABA agonists and Gabapentin for spastic hypertonia. Meythaler JM, Guest Editor. Spastic Hypertonia. W.B. Saunders, *N Am Clinics of Phys Med Rehabil*. 2001;12(Issue 4) pp. 875–88.

131. Meythaler JM, Roper JF, Davis L, Brunner RC. Cyproheptadine in intrathecal baclofen withdrawal: A case series. *Arch Phys Med Rehabil* 2003;84:638–42.

132. Kelly DF, Kozlowski DA, Haddad E, Echiverri A, Hovda DA, Lee SM. Ethanol reduces metabolic uncoupling following experimental head injury. *J Neurotrauma*. 2000;17:261–72.

133. Corrigan JD, Substance abuse as a medicating factor in outcome from traumatic brain injury. *Arch Phys Med Rehabil* 1995;76:302–9.

134. Jurkovich GJ, Rivara FP, Gurney JG, Fligner C, Ries R, Mueller BA, Copass M. The effect of acute alcohol intoxication and

chronic alcohol abuse on outcome from trauma. *J Am Med Assoc* 1993;270:51–56.

135. Zink BJ, Feustel PJ. Effects of ethanol on respiratory function in traumatic brain injury. *J Neurosurg* 1995;82:822–28.

136. Yamakami I, Vink R, Faden AI, Gennarelli TA, Lenkinski R, McIntosh TK. Effects of acute ethanol intoxication on experimental brain injru in the rat: neurobehavioral and phosphorus-31 nuclear magnetic resonance spectroscopy studies. *J Neurosurg* 1995;82:813–21.

137. Bombardier CH, Thurber CA. Blood alcohol level and early cognitive status after traumatic brain injury. *Brain Injury* 1998;12:725–34.

138. Zafonte R, Lombard L, Elovic E . Antispasticity medications ; uses and limitations of enteral therapy. *Am J Phys Med Rehabil* 2004;83;S50–8.

139. Meythaler JM. Use of intrathecally delivered medications for spasticity and dystonia in acquired brain injury. Yaksh, editor. *Spinal Drug Delivery*. Elsevier, New York. 1999, pp. 513–554.

140. Zafonte R, Elovic E, Lombard L. Acute management of post TBI spasticity. *J Head Trauma Rehabil* 2004;18:403–7.

141. Kelley AE, Andrzejewski ME, Baldwin AE, Hernandez PJ, Pratt WE. Glutamate-mediated plasticity in corticostriatal networks. *Annal New York Acad Sci* 2003;1003:159–68.

142. Naftchi NE, Schlosser W, Horst WD. Correlation of changes in the GABA-ergic system with the development of spasticity in paraplegic cats. *Adv Exp Med Biol.* 1979;123:431–450.

143. Wilson LA, McKechnie AA. Oral diazepam in the treatment of spasticity in paraplegia a double-blind trial and subsequent impressions. *Scott Med J.* Feb 1966;11(2):46–51.

144. Meythaler, J. M., W. Clayton, Orally delivered baclofen to control spastic hypertonia in acquired brain injury. *J Head Trauma Rehabil* 2004 19(2):101–4.

145. Terrence C, Fromm G, Roussan M. Baclofen its effect on seizure frequency. *Arch Neurol* 1983;40;28–9.

146. Sandyknb R, Gillman M. Baclofen induced memory impairment *Clin Neuropaharm* 1885;8;294–9.

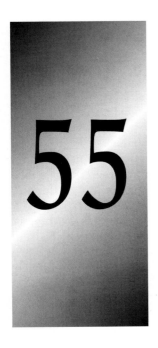

55 Nutraceuticals

Jeffrey S. Hecht

In surveys of various patient populations, it has been found that nutritional supplements not prescribed by (or known to) the attending physician are being used (1). Increasingly, physicians are being urged to ask about use of these non-traditional medications and become aware of the common and uncommon interactions with prescribed drugs. A huge and growing business exists for those purveyors of "health foods" and "health supplements"—with large sections of traditional pharmacies carrying them. The German government has long established a bureau to assure standard doses of these supplements, but the US has no such regulation at the present. However, in recent years the federal government, through the National Institute of Health, has established the National Center for Complementary and Alternative Medicine (NCCAM). The NCCAM has sponsored trials with nutritional supplements for dementia, but so far not in the area of traumatic brain injury.

The growing interest in nutritional supplements has lead to a growth of research in this area (2), a 1997 survey estimated that 12.1 percent of adults in the United States had used an herbal medicine in the previous 12 months (as compared with 2.5 percent in 1990), resulting in out-of-pocket payments of $5.1 billion, but little is specifically in the area of traumatic brain injury. Yet, some of the studies are relevant to problems experienced by the brain injured. These include the psychostimulants gingko and ephedra,

and the antidepressant St John's Wort (1, 3). One literature survey of particular value is that by Fugh-Berman and Cott in Psychosomatic Medicine (4).

NUTRITIONAL SUPPLEMENTS USED TO IMPROVE COGNITION

Choline Choline is an important component of the neurotransmitter acetylcholine. There is evidence that high doses of choline may improve memory in adults. (Doses up to 2500 mg po bid are used.) Choline is one of the B complex vitamins, and occurs in foods such as eggs, meat, fish, nuts, legumes, and soy.

Phosphatidylcholine Phosphatidylcholine is the most active ingredient found in soy lecithin. Every cell membrane in the body requires phosphatidylcholine (PC). Nerve and brain cells in particular need large quantities of PC for repair and maintenance. PC also aids in the metabolism of fats, regulates blood cholesterol, and is a component of myelin. PC is a major source of the neurotransmitter acetylcholine. Most of the choline normally present in our diet is in the form of lecithin where it occurs in seed oils and in unrefined foods containing oil.

Supplemental PC increases the amount of acetylcholine available for memory and thought processes. Increasing acetylcholine levels has been shown to improve performance by humans in a variety of intelligence and memory tests. Acetylcholine also is extremely important in maintaining brain cell structure.

CDP-Choline, Citidine, Citicoline, cytidine-5-diphosphate-choline, tidinediphosphocholine, Somazina, cytidine 5'-diphosphate choline

A medication that has been studied over 25 years with demonstrated efficacy in a variety of conditions including traumatic brain injury (TBI) is CDP-Choline. The drug is made of cytidine and choline moieties connected by a pyrophosphate bridge. Cytidine is incorporated into nucleic acids while choline ultimately "is in part converted into betaine, which in turn acts as methyl donor to homocysteine, yielding [14C]methionine, subsequently incorporated into proteins" (5).

Studies in animal models first suggested possible benefit of this drug. One study suggested inhibition of phospholipid breakdown by inhibition of an enzyme that is released following brain injury—phospholipase A2 (6).

Another study noted the strong polar nature of this drug, which prevents it from effectively crossing the blood-brain barrier (BBB). They studied a way to better cross the BBB by trapping citicoline in liposomes with the goal of improving its therapeutic effectiveness. The real therapeutic effectiveness of these citicoline liposome formulations was evaluated by biological assay with levels compared to the survival rate of ischemic reperfused male Wistar rats. Conjugated diene levels in the rat brains were measured, since this is an index of lipid peroxidation in rat cerebral cortex during post-ischemic reperfusion. The best mixture produced a reduction in diene levels of 60% and an increase in rat survival rate of about 24% and compared to the free drug (7). Other studies indicated that CDP-choline decreases edema formation and blood-brain barrier disruption following traumatic brain injury (TBI). One study of controlled cortical impact (CCI)-induced TBI in adult Wistar rats involved administration of the drug immediately post injury and once 6 hours post injury. The animals were sacrificed and the number of hippocampal neurons counted on the seventh post injury day. Treatment with CDP-choline significantly prevented TBI-induced neuronal loss in the hippocampus, decreased cortical contusion volume, and improved neurological recovery (8).

In another study, the authors examined the effect of CDP-Choline on brain edema and breakdown of the blood-brain barrier after TBI. Like the prior study, TBI was created using a CCI device. Half of the Sprague-Dawley rats received intraperitoneal injections of CDP-Choline twice following TBI. No significant benefit was noted at a low dose, but the higher doses (100 and 400 mg/kg) significantly decreased brain edema and BBB breakdown. Neuroprotective effects were demonstrated in the hippocampus as well as the directly injured cortex (9).

A Turkish study demonstrated significant neuroprotective effect of the drug and mortality reduction in rats following experimental cerebral ischemia (10).

A study from the department of neurosurgery at the University of Pittsburgh explored the role of CDP-choline in attenuating deficits in posttraumatic motor and spatial memory performance caused by direct trauma using a CCI model. They also explored whether CDP-choline increases acetylcholine (ACh) release in the dorsal hippocampus and neocortex.

The drug was first administered one day post injury and continued for 18 days. In the behavioral study, traumatic brain injury (TBI) was produced by lateral controlled cortical impact (2-mm deformation/6 m/sec) and administered CDP-choline (100 mg/kg) or saline daily for 18 days beginning 1-day post injury. Between 14–18 days post injury, CDP-choline-treated rats had significantly less cognitive (Morris water maze performance) deficits that injured saline-treated rats. CDP-choline treatment also attenuated the TBI-induced increased sensitivity to the memory-disrupting effects of scopolamine, a muscarinic antagonist. Microdialysis studies demonstrated a significant increase in extracellular levels of ACh in the dorsal hippocampus and neocortex in normal, awake, freely moving rats. The authors opined that this provides additional evidence that spatial memory performance deficits are, at least partially, associated with deficits in central cholinergic neurotransmission and that treatments that enhance ACh release in the chronic phase after TBI may attenuate cholinergic-dependent neurobehavioral deficits (11).

Clinical use of CDP-Choline in neurosurgery was first reported in the Japanese literature (12). Ogashiwa's article first reported both on the whole-body distribution of the drug in Wistar rats. It then went on to describe administration of CDP-choline to seven patients by intrathecal route to bypass the BBB. His second study reported benefit from 39 infusions given to 15 patients (13). Use of the drug in 60 cases of severe head injuries (wide-spread cerebral contusions and/or severe concussion) was reported by Cohadon and others in the French literature. They postulated that a shortening of the comatose period and an acceleration of neurological deficits recovery noted in the treated group was due to reduction of cerebral edema (14).

The authors of a Spanish single blind randomized study of 216 patients with moderate or severe brain injury study found "a trend towards a greater improvement in motor, cognitive and psychic alterations in the patients treated with CDP-choline, as well as a shortening of the stay in the hospital ward in the patients receiving this drug that initially presented with severe head injuries" (15).

By 2001, use of CDP-choline had apparently become part of standard neuro traumatology practice in Japan (16). The authors observed, "There appear to be two obvious differences in selection of pharmacological therapies among neurosurgeons in Japan and those in other countries; neurosurgeons in Japan prefer glycerol to mannitol for osmotic control of intracranial pressure, and barbiturate to morphine as sedatives. Two drugs are currently available in Japan for promoting the recovery from disturbance of consciousness after head trauma: cytidine diphosphate choline (CDP)-choline (Nicholin, Takeda Chemical Industries, Ltd., Osaka) and protirelin tartrate (Hirtonin; thyrotropin-releasing hormone (TRH) analogue, Takeda). Another TRH analogue, NS-3 (montirelin hydrate), is currently submitted to the Ministry of Health and Welfare for approval.

CDP-Choline has been the subject of double-blind placebo-controlled trials in humans in Japan with another type of brain insult—ischemic stroke—where it was found to be efficacious. Significant improvements in level of consciousness (Tazaki) and hemiplegia (Hazama) were noted in the studies (17, 18). In Spain, it has been reported to be effective in clinical trials of patients with Parkinson's Disease (19, 20) and Alzheimer's disease (21) CDP-Choline has been used late after brain injury as well as in the early stages. Harvey Levin, at the University of Texas in Galveston, reported it to be effective in a double-blind placebo-controlled trial of 14 patients with mild to moderate closed head injury who had postconcussional symptoms persisting for one month (22). Leon-Carrion and others, in Spain, reported that CDP-Choline improved cerebral blood flow of seven patients (by reversing brain injury-induced hypoperfusion) in the inferior left temporobasal region. Additionally, they noted an improved response to neuropsychological rehabilitation—specifically observing that the domains of "memory, learning processes and verbal fluency . . . improved significantly after treatment" (23). One case report suggesting positive effects on recovery was particularly interesting as it is autobiographical (24).

A review of the use of CDP-choline as well as other cholinomimetic agents is helpful. Their primary observation is that "preliminary data in traumatic brain injury suggest acetylcholine esterase inhibitors may play a significant role in the treatment of this patient population as well." (25)

Most published studies in animals(26, 27) and humans (28, 29) indicate that CDP-choline is safe. No side effects were observed in the studies on rats and dogs. One of the human tolerance studies of 2817 patients with neurological diseases on the medication for therapeutic reasons observed side effects in 5.01% of the patients: "the most frequently seen were digestive troubles, observed in 3.6% of the cases". The mean dose in that study was 6 ml/day. The other study of 12 adult healthy volunteers noted, "transient headaches were the only untoward events recorded", but the frequency was 33% in the "low dose" (600 mg/day) group and 42% in the "high dose" (1000 mg/day) group.

Gingko biloba. Gingko has been used to improve memory and attention. Gingko biloba extract is the most commonly prescribed plant remedy in the world. For thousands of years, Gingko has been part of the armamentarium of traditional Chinese herbal medicine. In Indian Aryeuvedic medicine, it is part of the elixir called Soma.

Modern studies have also demonstrated the effectiveness of this medication. A randomized, double-blind, placebo-controlled trial of 309 patients with Alzheimer's or multiinfarct dementia concluded that Gingko was beneficial in the treatment of dementia (30). The authors concluded that Gingko biloba "was safe and appears capable of stabilizing and, in a substantial number of cases, improving the cognitive performance and the social functioning of demented patients for six months to one year." Benefits were equivalent to Tacrine or Aricept—medications commonly prescribed to slow the progression of dementia. LeBars et al. found Gingko biloba extract effective, but with a side effect profile equivalent to placebo. This well-designed multicenter study showed significantly less decline in cognitive function among patients with dementia receiving gingko. They found the dose of 240 mg/day more effective than 120mg (31). They noted, "in contrast to narrow memory tests, broad cognitive assessments were more likely to detect the treatment effect." Beaubrun and Gray reviewed 40 controlled trials of gingko extracts in the treatment of dementia and found that 39 of 40 studies demonstrated clinically significant improvement in memory loss, concentration, fatigue, anxiety, and depressed mood (32). Wong and others found good evidence for the efficacy of gingko in the treatment of memory impairment caused by dementia (33). Other studies have also demonstrated significant benefit (34–36).

Side effects of gingko biloba are minimal. In a German post-marketing surveillance study of 10,815 patients treated with LI 1370 (another brand of standardized gingko), only 183 reported side effects. These side effects included nausea, headache, stomach problems, diarrhea, allergy, anxiety or restlessness, sleep disturbances, and in rare cases, serious bleeding problems. There have been five reports of bleeding associated with gingko treatment. These include two subdural hematomas, one with a documented increase in bleeding time, one intracerebral hemorrhage, and one subarachnoid hemorrhage. In most cases, patients were receiving concurrent anticoagulant drugs. Gingko reduces platelet aggregation by inhibiting platelet activation factor. Concurrent use of anticoagulants and gingko extracts should probably be avoided. It should also be avoided in patients with clotting problems. One case study reported ventricular arrhythmias with Gingko (37).

Cochrane reviews conclude there is "promising evidence of improvement in cognition and function associated with Gingko", but recommends larger controlled trials (38). Two randomized, placebo controlled and double blind trials of gingko biloba have been sponsored by the National Center for Complementary and Alternative Medicine (NCCAM). The Gingko Biloba Prevention Trial in Older Individuals was a stage III trial set up to determine the effect of 240mg/day Gingko biloba in decreasing the incidence of dementia and specifically Alzheimer's disease (AD), slowing cognitive decline and functional disability, reducing incidence of cardiovascular disease, and decreasing total mortality over five years. All subjects were 75 or older and without serious comorbidities. The study is now closed.

The other study, Preventing Cognitive Decline with Alternative Therapies, focuses on the oldest old who are at a particularly high risk for developing mild cognitive impairment (MCI), a precursor to dementia. The effect of standardized gingko biloba extract (GBE) on preventing or delaying cognitive decline in people age 85 years or older is studied over 42 months. Not yet closed, they plan to enroll 200 elderly cognitively healthy subjects and follow them for detection of conversion to MCI. The study hopes to definitively examine whether GBE has a disease modifying effect on the brain—distinct from a symptomatic effect. The magnitude of biological effect of the treatments will also be assessed with volumetric quantitative MRI, a complementary means of confirming whether there is a brain modifying effect (measured as a decrease in brain volume loss with treatment). Peripheral markers of oxidation status will measure possible anti-oxidant effects of GBE. The Principal Investigator is Dr. Jeffrey Kaye at the Oregon Health Sciences University in Portland.

Pyritinol Pyritinol is used by some to enhance neuronal metabolic function. The pyritinol molecule is structurally similar to vitamin B_6, but functions in the brain in a different way. The dose of pyritinol used in most of the human clinical studies is one 200-mg capsule taken three times a day.

Fischoff, et al. reported on a 12-week, double-blind clinical trial that was performed to investigate the benefit of pyritinol in the treatment of several forms of senile dementia (39). A total of 156 patients were allocated to either of two groups: the "senile dementia of the Alzheimer's type" group, or the "multi-infarct dementia (stroke)" group. The investigators noted, "The therapeutic efficacy of pyritinol was clearly demonstrated by confirmatory analysis as the drug was statistically significantly superior to placebo in all three target variables (of cognitive function). The EEG mapping demonstrated significant differences between placebo and pyritinol . . . it can be accepted that the therapeutic effect of pyritinol is superior to placebo in patients with mild to moderate dementia of both degenerative (Alzheimer's) and vascular (stroke) etiology."

A double-blind, placebo-controlled trial was carried out on 40 patients suffering from moderately advanced dementia. The patients were allocated randomly either pyritinol (800 mg daily) or identical placebo for three months. Assessments using a modified Crichton Geriatric Behavioral Rating Scale were made pre-treatment and monthly up to three months, and then at follow-up at six months. Patients on pyritinol showed significantly higher levels of improvement than did those on placebo. Laboratory tests conducted throughout remained within normal limits for both groups (40).

Another study, reported 26 patients with Alzheimer's disease who were randomly assigned in a double-blind trial of pyritinol versus placebo. The patients had a mild to moderate degree of dementia. The results of the study showed that "pyritinol was associated with a significant improvement in cognitive performance. Regional cerebral blood-flow data showed that treatment with pyritinol normalized the pattern of blood flow increase during activation and improved the score on the test used for activation (41). In the German journal Pharmacopsychiatry, the effects of pyritinol were investigated in a placebo-controlled, randomized, double-blind study in geriatric patients suffering from cerebral functional disorders, with a moderate to severe degree of chronic brain syndrome. In a previous study, a rise in the vigilance (wakefulness, alertness) level was demonstrated in patients undergoing pyritinol treatment. Data from 107 patients were included in the statistical analysis, 54 on pyritinol and 53 on placebo. No notable adverse drug reactions were observed. They noted "Statistically significant results were found in favor of pyritinol, compared with placebo, in both the level of clinical symptomatology and the performance level. Particularly impressive was the superiority of pyritinol in the factor 'social behavior'"(42).

One of the few studies that specifically used nutritional supplements in the brain-injured was carried out in the late 1970s by Kitamura in Tokyo. Two hundred and seventy patients suffering from the sequelae of different forms of brain injury were treated orally with pyritinol, 200 mg three times a day, for a period of six weeks. Compared with placebo therapy, pyritinol produced statistically significant improvements in the clinical and psycho neurological manifestations. It was concluded that pyritinol is a drug of therapeutic benefit in the treatment of the sequelae of cerebral trauma (43).

Piracetam (also nootropil) and Levirpiracetam (the S-enantomer) Piracetam has been the subject of multiple animal and human studies. It has been described as a "nootropic" drug due to it putative neuroprotective effects in rat models of brain injury. It has been reported as helpful in cognitive enhancement (44). It has been described as the "number one worldwide cognitive enhancer" on one web site that served to facilitate its procurement (the site has now been closed by federal agents.) A nonblinded polish study was reported in 1998 where the drug was administered IV or orally to patients with acute brain injury (45). Their conclusion that "the use of piracetam is recommended" is not supported by the study. Ricci reported on its use in acute ischemic stroke and found no demonstration of effectiveness, but a trend of increased mortality in the treatment group (46). Oosterveld reported on benefit in vestibular disorders following brain injury (47). Kessler and others reported in Stroke in 2000 that piracetam facilitates rehabilitation of post stroke aphasic patients (48). Yet, Greener and others, reporting in their Cochrane database review of use of piracetam for aphasia, found a trend toward increased mortality in the treatment group of Kessler's Study (49). Gualtieri and others questioned study design as the reason for some studies failing to demonstrate effectiveness of piracetam (50). Piracetam is available through foreign pharmacies and/or state side compounding pharmacies.

Acetyl-L-Carnitine and Vinpocetine Some nutrients with intriguing findings in human studies and possible value in humans, (44) but which need further study include vinpocetine (51, 52, 53, 54) and acetyl-L-carnitine.

Vinpocetine, Cavinton, vinpocetine-ethyl-apovincaminate, 14-ethoxycarbonyl-(3alpha,16alpha-ethyl)-14, 15-eburnamine, Apovincaminic acid

Another biological product with a variety of reputed CNS effects is vinpocetine. Originally synthesized in the late 1960s from an extract of the leaf of the lesser periwinkle plant (Vinca minor), vinpocetine was first commercially available in 1978. Marketed as Cavinton by the company Gedeon Richter Ltd in Budapest, the drug has been used widely in Eastern Europe. In fact, most of the literature is in Russian and other Slavic languages.

Vinpocetine is reported to have diverse effects. A Hungarian study noted:

> Early experiments with vinpocetine indicated five main pharmacological and biochemical actions: (1) selective enhancement of the brain circulation and oxygen utilization without significant alteration in parameters of systemic circulation, (2) increased tolerance of the brain toward hypoxia and ischemia, (3) anticonvulsant activity, (4) inhibitory effect on phosphodiesterase (PDE) enzyme and (5) improvement of rheological properties of the blood and inhibition of aggregation of thrombocytes. Later studies in various laboratories confirmed the above effects and clearly demonstrated that vinpocetine offers significant and direct neuroprotection both under in vitro and in vivo conditions (55).

Regarding mechanism, Nicholson summarizes a review of the literature with reference to vinpocetine that

"This compound attenuates cognitive deficits, reduces ischaemia-induced hippocampal cell loss and increases cerebral blood flow and glucose utilisation. These effects may be induced by modulation of cyclic nucleotide levels and adenosine re-uptake inhibition"(Nicholson, CD)(56).

Research published by the manufacturer reported that "vinpocetine is a potent inhibitor of the voltage-dependent Na(+) channels and a selective inhibitor of the Ca(2+)/caldmoduline-dependent phosphodiesterase 1." Their posititron emission tomography (PET) scan studies in monkeys and healthy humans using intravenously administered [11C]-labeled vinpocetine showed "the distribution pattern of vinpocetine in the brain was heterogeneous, with the highest uptake in the thalamus, basal ganglia and visual cortex."(57)

Is there a neuroprotective effect? A British study in normal subjects demonstrated a protective effect against memory impairments caused by exposure to benzodiazepines (58). A study of brain preservation in a rat model of ischemia showing a 42% reduction of infarct volume (59). The drug was even used in 162 victims of the accident at the Chernobyl Atomic Electric Power Station diagnosed with "dyscirculatory encephalopathy" (60). Hadjiev argues it is protective against cerebrovascular insufficiency in humans (61).

Does the drug really work in demented humans? A 2003 review article in Nutrition concluded that it is effective (62). A review of nontraditional medicines by Kidd observed that vinpocetine "is an excellent vasodilator and cerebral metabolic enhancer with proven benefits for vascular-based cognitive dysfunction."(63) One double-blind placebo controlled trial of the drug over nine months in 84 patients diagnosed with vascular dementia demonstrated the treatment group performed consistently "better in all evaluations of the effectiveness of treatment including measurements on the Clinical Global Impression (CGI) scale, the Sandoz Clinical Assessment-Geriatric (SCAG) scale, and the Mini-Mental Status Questionnaire (MMSQ)"(64). Yet, a yearlong Veterans Administration (VA) study of Alzheimer's patients found no benefit of vinpocetine at a variety of dosages (65).

A Cochrane database review in 2003 found three trials with a total of 583 people with degenerative or vascular dementia treated with vinpocetine (30–60 mg/day) or placebo (66). The number of patients treated for 6 months or more was small and only one study extended treatment to one year. They noted, "the evidence for beneficial effect of vinpocetine on patients with dementia is inconclusive and does not support clinical use." The conclusion was the same in a 2000 Cochrane review of its use in acute stroke (65).

The literature supporting the use of vinpocetine in traumatic brain injury (TBI) is even more sparse. One Russian study primarily reporting that diabetics do worse than others following TBI observed "inclusion of vasoactive agents Cavinton and Complamin into the scheme of complex therapy accelerates regression of the neurological symptomatology" (68). In an experimental study involving animals, Romodanov found that these vasoactive agents" promote regression of the changed cerebral blood flow" following TBI.

In summary, vinpocetine is of equivocal benefit, but there is little evidence of toxicity. Due to research suggesting effectiveness in some groups, further double-blind placebo-controlled studies of its use in specific patient populations is warranted.

DMAE (dimethylamino ethanol), Pantothenic acid, Lucidril, and Citicoline

Other nutrients are recommended on web sites with little evidence on effectiveness in humans. Based on animal studies (mostly Russian and Japanese from over twenty years ago), these include DMAE (dimethylamino ethanol), pantothenic acid, lucidril, and citicoline.

FOR BEHAVIORAL DISTURBANCES

Kava (Piper methysticum) Kava is widely used in Polynesia and Micronesia as a tranquilizing ceremonial beverage. Kava is one of the few herbs for which active constituents are well delineated. Some are centrally acting skeletal muscle relaxants and anticonvulsants. Their effects seem to be due to inhibition of sodium and calcium channels as well as effects on glutamate systems. Some are potent inhibitors of norepinephrine uptake (4).

A psychoactive member of the pepper family, kava is used to relieve anxiety and insomnia in Europe and the United States. It is formally approved in Germany for anxiety, tension, and agitation. In a randomized, double-blind, placebo-controlled trial, 58 patients with "anxiety and neurotic disorders" were randomly assigned to receive 70 mg of kava lactones or placebo three times daily for 4 weeks. Compared with the placebo group, the kava group demonstrated a significant reduction in anxiety (assessed by HAM-A) by the end of the first week; differences between the two groups increased during the course of the study. Side effects were minimal (69).

In a randomized, double-blind, placebo-controlled multicenter study, 101 outpatients with anxiety disorders (agoraphobia, specific phobia, generalized anxiety disorder, or adjustment disorder with anxiety) were treated with a kava extract for 24 weeks. Results showed significant reductions in HAM-A scores in the kava group beginning in the eighth week and increasing throughout the trial. Improvements were also seen in secondary outcome variables, which included Hamilton subscale scores for somatic and psychic anxiety, the Clinical Global Impression scale,

Self-Report Symptom Inventory, and the Adjective Mood scale (70). Side effects were greater in the placebo group than the kava group. Treatment with kava did not lead to tolerance. Several other controlled double-blind trials on kava extracts or the isolated compound DL-kawain have been published in the German literature (4).

Kava is reported to have potential adverse effects and interactions. Therapeutic doses may result in mild gastrointestinal complaints or allergic skin reactions (incidence, 1.5%) (4). Chronic use of kava up to 100 times the therapeutic dose results in an ichthyosiform eruption known as kava dermopathy, which is often accompanied by eye irritation. Abstaining from kava results in complete resolution of symptoms. Kava may potentiate the sedative affect of anesthetics (72).

Picamilon Picamilon is a vitamin-like compound consisting of a niacin analogue (n-nicotinyl) uniquely bonded to GABA (gamma aminobutyric acid). When niacin is bound to GABA, it readily penetrates the blood-brain barrier and enhances cerebral and peripheral circulation. Picamilon has reportedly been studied and used in Russia or its "tranquilizing influence on negative emotions". The effects of picamilon have been characterized as "a tranquilizing effect, without a sedative component but with elements of stimulant action." Doses are reported as 20–50 mg bid or tid. Picamilon has been reported to decrease cerebral blood-vessel tone and "increases intracranial circulation rate". Picamilon reportedly reduces anxiety and hyperesthesia (whereby normal touch creates pain) without sedative effects, and yet improved sleep. Studies in English are few.

Ginseng (Panax ginseng and others) Ginseng is a popular "tonic" herb that some take regularly for a "cumulative strengthening effect". There are several varieties of ginseng commonly used in herbal medicine: *P. ginseng*, grown in northeastern China and Korea; *P. quinquefolius*, grown in the United States and Canada; and *P. notoginseng*, grown in southwest China. Ginseng reportedly has many interesting effects, but its place in the treatment of psychiatric conditions or improving quality of life has not been demonstrated in clinical trials.

An 8-week, placebo-controlled study of a commercial ginseng among 60 patients admitted to the geriatric unit of a hospital found no differences between the treatment and control groups in length of stay, activities of daily living, cognitive function, or somatic symptoms (73, 80). Yet, a double-blind study of a multivitamin complex supplemented with ginseng vs. a multivitamin complex without ginseng in 625 patients complaining of stress or fatigue found significant improvement in the quality of life index at 4 months in those receiving ginseng (74). Hypoglycemia as well as bleeding complications have been reported with ginseng (72, 75).

Passionflower (Passiflora incarnata) Passionflower is used as a mild sedative. No clinical trials of its use as a single agent have been conducted. The German Commission E recommends 4 to 8 g of dried herb per day for "nervous unrest."

Passionflower contains flavonoids: a flavonoid derived from *Passiflora coerulea*, is a partial agonist of benzodiazepine receptors and has anxiolytic activity in mice without inducing sedation or muscle relaxation and could account for the activity of the plant (4).

In a double-blind trial in 182 patients with adjustment disorder with anxious mood, patients received a preparation containing six extracts (*Passiflora, Crataegus, Ballota, Valeriana, Cola,* and *Paullinia*) or placebo. HAM-A scores were improved in patients who took the herbal mixture compared with those who received a placebo (76).

Valerian (Valeriana officinalis) Valerian is a botanical medicine used for its mild sedative and tranquilizing properties. Valerian is an odoriferous plant that is a popular sleep remedy. In one study enrolling 166 subjects with various sleep difficulties, two different formulations of valerian were compared to placebo. Each person received three of each capsule, which were taken in random order on nonconsecutive nights. Only 128 patients completed the study, but only one patient withdrew because of side effects. Both valerian preparations improved sleep quality and reduced sleep latency scores. Night awakenings and dream recall were not affected by valerian, nor did valerian cause any somnolence the next morning (77). Beaubrun, in a review of the herbal medication literature, noted that: "Valerian has been shown to decrease sleep latency and nocturnal awakenings and improve subjective sleep quality, but placebo effects were marked in some studies, and in some cases the beneficial effects were not seen until two to four weeks of therapy" (Beaubrun G)(78).

Another study found efficacy of both valerian and melatonin (79). Dosing recommendations vary, but the German Commission E recommends 2 to 3 g of the dried root one or more times a day for "restlessness and nervous disturbance of sleep" (80).

A valerian withdrawal syndrome has been described. Garges reported a withdrawal reaction of delirium, and high output cardiac failure in a 58-year-old man hospitalized for congestive heart failure who received general anesthesia. After extubation, the patient developed sinus tachycardia, high output cardiac failure, oliguria, tremor, and signs of delirium. It was later discovered the patient had been taking valerian up to 2 g five times per day for years. A benzodiazepine was helpful in resolving many of his symptoms (81). Also, Valerian may potentiate the sedative effects of anesthetics (72).

Another problem with valerian is its unpleasant odor—one foul enough to be used as the aversive stimulus in a study of brain activation (71). This interferes with patient tolerance as well as the ability to do double-blinded trials.

Folic Acid, Vitamin B_{12}, S-adenosylmethionine (SAM or SAMe) and Mood Folic acid deficiency is one of the most common nutritional deficiencies in the world and has often been associated with neuropsychiatric disorders (82). Deficiencies of vitamin B_{12} and folate both cause similar neurological and psychiatric disturbances, including depression, dementia, and psychosis. Folate deficiency appears most tightly connected with depressive disorders, and cobalamin deficiency with psychosis (83). Contrary to intuition, vitamin deficiencies appear to occur infrequently with eating disorders. Hutto notes: "Clinicians should remain vigilant to the possibility of deficiencies of folate and cobalamin in diverse psychiatric populations" (Hutto)(83).

Normal hematological indices do not rule out B_{12} and folate deficiencies. This deficiency may be an overlooked and understudied risk factor for depression. Godfrey in London found that 41 (33%) of 123 patients with acute psychiatric disorders (DSM III diagnosis of major depression or schizophrenia) had borderline or definite folate deficiency (red-cell folate below 200 micrograms/l). These patients took part in a double-blind, placebo-controlled trial of methyl folate, 15 mg daily, for 6 months in addition to standard psychotropic treatment. Among both depressed and schizophrenic patients methyl folate significantly improved clinical and social recovery. The differences in outcome scores between methyl folate and placebo groups became greater with time. The authors wrote: "these findings add to the evidence implicating disturbances of methylation in the nervous system in the biology of some forms of mental illness" (Godfrey)(84).

Several studies have found that up to 35% of depressed patients are folate deficient (84). In elderly patients, the incidence of deficiency may even be higher.

Fava and others examined the relationships between levels of folate, vitamin B_{12}, and homocysteine and response to fluoxetine (20 mg/d for 8 weeks) treatment as measured by the 17-item HAM-D in 213 outpatients with major depressive disorder. Subjects with low folate levels were more likely to have melancholic depression and were significantly less likely to respond to fluoxetine (85).

Folate and vitamin B_{12} are required for the methylation of homocysteine to methionine and for the synthesis of S-adenosylmethionine. S-adenosylmethionine is involved in numerous methylation reactions involving proteins, phospholipids, DNA, and neurotransmitter metabolism. S-adenosylmethionine (SAM) has antidepressant properties. The commonest neuropsychiatric complication of severe folate deficiency is depression (86). Methylation in the nervous system may underlie the expression of mood and related processes and may be implicated in some affective disorders. Folate deficiency may specifically affect central monoamine metabolism and aggravate depressive disorders. The folate derivative necessary for the synthesis of serotonin and dopamine, tetrahydrobiopterin, has also been reported to have antidepressant activity (87). Folic acid may be helpful in bipolar disorders.

In a double-blind comparing a daily supplement of 200 mcg folic acid placebo in a group of 75 patients on lithium therapy, folate was shown to enhance the efficacy of lithium. During the trial the patients with the highest plasma folate concentrations showed a significant reduction in their affective morbidity. Patients who had their plasma folate increased to 13 µg/ml or above had a 40% reduction in their affective morbidity. The authors suggested that a daily supplement of 300–400 micrograms folic acid would be useful in long-term lithium prophylaxis (88).

Also called SAMe, S-adenosylmethionine is a methyl donor closely linked with folate and vitamin B_{12} (cyanocobalamin) metabolism. SAMe is required in numerous transmethylation reactions involving nucleic acids, proteins, phospholipids, monoamines, and other neurotransmitters. Bottiglieri at Baylor in Dallas wrote that deficiencies of either folate or B_{12} have been found to reduce the synthesis of SAMe (and thus its levels) in the central nervous system. They noted: "SAMe has antidepressant properties, and preliminary studies indicate that it may improve cognitive function in patients with dementia. Treatment with methyl donors (betaine, methionine and SAMe) is associated with re myelination in patients with inborn errors of folate and C-1 (one-carbon) metabolism"(Bottiglieri)(89).

Some feel this is relevant to brain injury rehabilitation. The administration of SAMe has antidepressant properties (91, 92). However, there are potential side effects of folic acid and same supplementation. In a randomized, double-blind, placebo-controlled trial of 15 inpatients with major depression, oral SAMe induced mania in one patient with no prior history of mania (90). In another study of SAM-treated patients with depression, 89% of bipolar patients switched from depression into an elevated mood state (hypomania, mania and euphoria) and the rest did not respond. Just over half of the endogenous unipolar patients improved and five did not (92). Anecdotally, methionine supplementation has been reported to aggravate schizophrenia. SAMe has been reported to cause mild and transient insomnia, nervousness, and lack of appetite, constipation, headaches, heart palpitations, nausea, dry mouth, sweating, and dizziness (93).

Folate has been reported to reduce the effectiveness of several anticonvulsants, potentially leading to seizures (94).

Tryptophan and 5-HTP   The amino acid, tryptophan, is a precursor of serotonin and has been used increase brain levels of serotonin. Tryptophan depletion can increase depressive symptoms in patients with major depression and seasonal affective disorder. Studies have shown tryptophan supplementation has positive effects in some depressed patients—particularly those with a relative tryptophan depletion (95). In most cases, tryptophan by itself may be insufficient to boost serotonin levels (96) Thus, SSRI antidepressants are much more efficacious overall. On the other hand, using tryptophan to supplement standard antidepressants has been more successful. Walinder found that 24 depressed patients started on clomipramine improved more rapidly in the symptoms of depressed mood, suicidal intent, depressive thought content, and anxiety with tryptophan supplementation (97). 5-HTP is an intermediate metabolite of the amino acid L-tryptophan in the serotonin pathway. Like tryptophan, 5-HTP is used for depression—in efforts to achieve a higher level in the CNS (98). Tryptophan is converted into 5-HTP by the enzyme tryptophan hydroxylase. This is the rate-limiting step in serotonin synthesis. 5-HTP is commercially produced by extraction from the seeds of an African plant, *Griffonia simplicifolia*—an extract available in the United States. However, there are significant concerns with tryptophan and 5-HTP supplementation. The severe complication of eosinophilic myositis (EMS) has occurred with contaminated tryptophan. It causes muscle pain and weakness (99). While contaminated L-tryptophan has been definitively associated with EMS, 5-HTP has been linked with several unusual cases of EMS-like symptoms. One study suggested that contamination may be difficult to avoid with L-tryptophan and 5-HTP preparations.

AGGRESSION AND DEPRESSION

Omega-3 Fatty Acids   Neuronal membranes contain high concentrations of the essential fatty acids arachidonic acid and DHA, which are crucial components of the phospholipid bilayer (each comprises approximately 25% of the phospholipid content.

It has been suggested that depletion of omega-3 polyunsaturated fatty acids, particularly DHA, impairs membrane function and may be of etiological importance in depression, aggression, schizophrenia, and other mental and neurological disorders. Hibbeln writes: "we propose that excessive phospholipase-A2 (PLA2) activity disrupts membrane fluidity, composition, and therefore, the activity, of membrane-dependent proteins. Similar disruptions in these proteins are documented in depressed patients and can be accounted for by excessive PLA2 activity"(Hibbeln)(100, 101).

The number of authors supporting this premise is limited. Yet, lipids and the membranes they inhabit may be very important. There are reports that rapid lowering of blood lipids by hydroxymethylglutaryl coenzyme A reductase inhibitors is associated with a large number of psychiatric disorders. In a national Norwegian database, 15% of psychiatric drug reactions were attributed to statins (102). Reactions included aggression, nervousness, depression, anxiety, and sleeping disorders. Cholesterol-lowering therapies and low cholesterol levels have been thought to increase the risk of suicide—possibly by lowering serotonin turnover. Therefore, some recommend omega-3 fatty acid supplementation as possibly helpful in brain disorders.

St John's Wort (Hypericum) St John's Wort (SJW), also called Hypericum, is one of the most widely-used supplements. In 1998, Wong reported that there was good evidence for the efficacy of St John's wort for the treatment of depression(33) There is data to suggest that St John's wort is more effective than placebo in the treatment of mild to moderate depression. The absolute increased response rate with the use of St John's wort ranged from 23% to 55% higher than with placebo, but ranged from 6% to 18% lower compared with tricyclic antidepressants (103). In 2000, Beaubrun and Gray reported on their review of herbal medicines for psychiatric disorders. They found nine controlled and standardized trials of St. John's wort. Of these, five showed the herb's superiority to placebo, and four found no differences in effectiveness when compared with antidepressant drugs (78). One author reported extensively on its neuropharmacology (3, 104).

Combination therapy may be helpful in combined anxiety and depression. Muller's open labeled study with SJW and valerian concluded that symptoms associated with anxiety that severely afflict patients can be clearly improved more quickly with a combination therapy of St John's wort extract and valerian extract than with St John's wort monotherapy (105). The combination therapy was well tolerated, no significant side-effects occurred. St. John's Wort is metabolized by the P450 system and thus has been reported to interact with several medications.

NUTRITIONAL SUPPLEMENTS FOR THE TREATMENT OF HEADACHE

Melatonin has been recommended for cluster headaches. In a double-blind, placebo-controlled clinical study of 20 patients, melatonin was reported to effectively reduce cluster headache in 50% of treated patients. In the paper's discussion, melatonin's biological functions are reviewed in relation to the putative mechanisms that cause cluster headache (106). In a more recent review of cluster headaches, Dodrick reported that melatonin may be a useful adjunctive therapy (112).

Petadolex, Petaxites hybridus, Butterbur root (a naturopathic agent)

Another agent used for headache is Petadolex (Petasites hybridus, an extract of Butterbur root). Petasites hybridus (PH) is much more commonly referenced for respiratory problems such as asthma than for headache (107). It is also used to reduce gastrointestinal and urogenital tract spasms. Reportedly, it active components are the petasines which inhibit the synthesis of leukotrienes (anti-inflammatory) and decrease the intracellular concentration of calcium (spasmolytic).

Still controversial, it has been recommended for migraine prophylaxis, but only one blinded study could be identified. A German group reported twice on the same randomized, group-parallel, placebo-controlled, double-blind clinical study of 60 patients. A "special CO_2 extract from the rhizome of Petasites hybridus" was administered at a dose of 50 mg b.i.d. for 12 weeks. Although no significant decrement in intensity and duration was observed, a significant 60% reduction in the frequency of migraine attacks was seen. No adverse events were reported (108, 109). Another unaffiliated group reanalyzed the data from that study (110). They looked at the data differently, but still noted a significant reduction in attack frequency—from 3.4 at baseline to 1.8 after three months. They concluded, "This small trial indicates that butterbur may be effective in the prophylaxis of migraine."

A German-language review article observed that toxicity is reportedly infrequent since the development of "extraction with supercritical CO_2 . . . (which reduced) the concentrations of the potentially hepatotoxic and carcinogenic pyrrolizidine alkaloids (to) below the detection limits"(111). Four cases of reversible cholestatic hepatitis have been associated with long-term administration of butterbur. Further side effects involve the gastrointestinal tract and are usually mild.

Other relatively unsupported recommendations for headache include green tea (which contains caffeine)(113) megadose vitamins C, (114, 115) and vitamin E, (116) lipoic acid, and Coenzyme Q at 150 mg/day (117). Gingko biloba has been anecdotally reported to be helpful for those patients suffering from migraine headaches. Another study found it helpful in preventing headache symptoms of acute mountain sickness (118). Oral magnesium is a complementary therapy for headache (119) that has documented efficacy in migraine prophylaxis for children (9mg/kg/day) (120). Recent studies using functional MRI suggest a drop in magnesium concentration may play a role in severe types of headaches (121, 122). In a Brooklyn, NY study, six of nine children with non-traumatic headaches had a deficiency in serium ionized magnesium, (123) but total magnesium levels were normal. The National Institute of Neurological Disorders and Stroke (NINDS) is sponsoring a phase III study of magnesium sulfate given within eight hours of a moderate or severe traumatic brain injury to look at the effect on survival, seizures, and outcome. http://www.edc.gsph.pitt.edu/neurotrauma/) .

NUTRITIONAL SUPPLEMENTS FOR VESTIBULAR DYSFUNCTION

Gingko biloba In an open label study of vertigo, gingko biloba given over three months improved symptoms of dizziness and also, on neuro-otologic testing, improved several parameter. Improvements were noted in saccadic velocities and smooth pursuit gain, nystagmus, vestibulo-ocular reflex and the visuovestibular –ocular reflex (124).

Pyritinol A reference in the French journal Ouest Med (29/1 1976), reports that pyritinol was tested on sixty patients who suffered from vertigo. They report "a cure rate of 83%, accompanied by an improvement in the patients' mental and social state. The drug was tolerated well by patients of all ages." The dose was 200 mg three times a day (125).

Piracetam A 1999 literature review of piracetam recommended doses of 2.4–4.8 gm daily for vertigo of central origin such as after brain injury (47).

Coenzyme Q10 (ubiquinone) Much of the extent of neurological impairment following brain injury depends upon secondary brain damage, with delayed neuronal death. Some stroke research suggests that secondary brain damage follows from secondary mitochondrial (and bioenergetic) failure after blood flow resumes.

Recent evidence points to programmed cell death as a major factor in delayed neuronal death. While this programmed cellular suicide normally disposes of aged cells, stroke may trigger it prematurely. Mitochondrial injury following ischemia leads to calcium overload, excitotoxicity, oxidative stress, and opening of the mitochondrial mega channels.

Medications that support normal cellular energy production and antioxidant defense could protect against this excitotoxic damage and subsequent programmed cell death. Some studies suggest CoQ10 may provide this protective effect (126–129).

Creatine Of all the nutritional supplements currently available, creatine appears to be the most effective for maintaining the ability of mitochondria to produce high-energy compounds such as adenosine triphosphate (ATP) and thus reduce "oxidative stress."

When ATP loses a phosphate molecule and becomes ADP, it must be converted back to ATP to once again be able to release energy. Creatine is stored in the human body as creatine phosphate (CP). Then ATP is depleted, it can be "recharged" by CP. CP donates a phosphate molecule to ADP allowing it to form a high-energy bond and reform ATP. An increased pool of CP means faster recharging of ATP, which means more work can be performed.

Creatine may protect the brain from neurotoxic agents, certain forms of injury and other insults. Neurons exposed to either glutamate, beta-amyloid (both highly toxic to neurons) are involved, (130) N-methyl-D-aspartate (NMDA) and malonate(131) (Another study found that feeding rats creatine helped protect them against tetrahydropyridine (MPTP), which produces parkinsonism in animals through impaired energy production (132). Another study found creatine protected neurons form ischemic damage (133).

NEUROPROTECTIVE ROLE OF CURCUMIN FROM CURCUMA LONGA ON ETHANOL-INDUCED BRAIN DAMAGE

Curcumin A widely used spice and coloring agent in food, curcumin has been shown to possess potent antioxidant, antitumor promoting and anti-inflammatory properties in vitro and in vivo. Curcumin is a small-molecular-weight compound that is isolated from the commonly used spice turmeric. In an animal study, curcumin was screened for neuroprotective activity using ethanol as a model of brain injury. Oral administration of curcumin to rats caused a significant reversal in lipid peroxidation of brain lipids and produced enhancement of glutathione, an antioxidant (134).

VITAMIN SUPPLEMENTATION TO FACILITATE NEUROLOGICAL RECOVERY

Vitamin (MVI) supplementation is controversial. Certainly the minimum daily requirement of MVI is needed for normal enzyme function. Earlier in this paper, effects of folic acid and vitamin B_{12} deficiencies and supplementation were discussed. However, some physicians feel that megavitamin supplementation of water-soluble vitamins is a waste – producing "only an expensive urine". Yet, the true need may vary between individuals and in disease states. High doses of Vitamin B6 (50–200 mg) are commonly used in carpal tunnel syndrome. By analogy, some physicians feel it is helpful in other types of nerve injury. Yet, in the example of Vitamin B_6, megadose (2000 mg+) can itself be neurotoxic (135).

Suggested supplements from physicians who prescribe for neural recovery following brain injury include vitamin B_1 (100 mg), vitamin B_6 (100 mg), vitamin B_{12} (1 mg), folic acid (1 mg) and vitamin C (500 mg). Also recommendations for myelin repair are octacosanol (2000–400 mg/day) with zinc, vitamin C and B_6. (Internet communication from

William Walsh, PhD re: study at Schwab Rehab Hospital—reportedly facilitating recovery after plateau in severe brain injury).

NUTRITIONAL SUPPLEMENT TO RETARD MUSCLE ATROPHY

In the setting of hypoglycemia, glutamine is the primary gluconeogenic amino acid. Aggressive glutamine supplementation is recommended to help maintain muscle mass for those critically ill or immobilized with severe brain injury.

However, extra caution is recommended in diabetics due to abnormal glutamine metabolism. Adding taurine may be beneficial.

WEB SITES OF INTEREST

Several studies looking at internet web sites for information about a variety of topics have determined that most offer limited and biased information of poor quality with most claiming to prevent, diagnose, treat, or cure specific diseases despite federal regulations prohibiting statements of this type (136, 137). Nevertheless, some sites have been determined to be particularly helpful in the investigation of dietary supplements. In a study conducted by the College of Pharmacy at the University of Michigan, the best electronic databases for providing information on herbal and dietary supplements were felt to be "Micro Medex" and the "Natural Medicine Comprehensive Database" (138). The best internet site was determined to be "The Natural Pharmacist". Another fine site is a review article on natural medications in Psychosomatic Medicine: http://www.psychosomaticmedicine.org/cgi/content/full/61/5/712

The interest in and use of nutritional supplements by the public has grown faster than the definitive medical knowledge of these drugs. Yet there is fairly extensive bench and some clinical research for many of them. Few studies have been done using these medications in patients with traumatic or anoxic brain injury. Yet much of what is known may be relevant to these populations. Desperate patients and families will look to their physicians for direction on optimal treatment. Greater physician knowledge of the benefits and results of the nutritional supplements will lead to better care.

References

1. Bennett J., Brown C. M., Use of herbal remedies by patients in a health maintenance organization. *J Am Pharm Assoc* (Wash) May–Jun, 2000;40(3):353–8.
2. De Smet P., Herbal remedies. *NEJM* 2002;347:246–250.
3. Bennett D. A Jr., Phun L., Polk J. F., Voglino S. A., Zlotnik V., Raffa R. B. *Neuropharmacology of St. John's Wort.* Ann Pharmacother. Nov, 1998 ;32(11):1201–8.
4. Fugh-Berman A., Cott J. M.. Dietary Supplements and Natural Products as Psychotherapeutic Agents. *Psychosomatic Medicine* (1999)61:712–728.
5. Galletti P., De Rosa M., Cotticelli M. G., Morana A., Vaccaro R., Zappia V. Biochemical rationale for the use of CDP choline in traumatic brain injury: pharmacokinetics of the orally administered drug. *J Neurol Sci.* Jul, 1991;103(Suppl):S19–25.
6. Arrigoni E., Averet N., Cohadon F. Effects of CDP-choline on phospholipase A2 and cholinephosphotransferase activities following a cryogenic brain injury in the rabbit. *Biochem Pharmacol.* Nov 1, 1987;36(21):3697–700.
7. Fresta M., Puglisi G., Di Giacomo C., Russo A. Liposomes as invivo carriers for citicoline: effects on rat cerebral post-ischaemic reperfusion. *J Pharm Pharmacol.* Dec, 1994;46(12):974–81.
8. Dempsey R. J., Raghavendra Rao V. L. Cytidinediphosphocholine treatment to decrease traumatic brain injury-induced hippocampal neuronal death, cortical contusion volume, and neurological dysfunction in rats. *J Neurosurg.* Apr, 2003;98(4):867–73.
9. Baskaya M. K., Dogan A., Rao A. M., Dempsey R. J. Neuroprotective effects of citicoline on brain edema and blood-brain barrier breakdown after traumatic brain injury. *J Neurosurg.* Mar, 2000;92(3):448–52.
10. Alkan T., Kahveci N., Goren B., et al. Ischemic brain injury caused by interrupted versus uninterrupted occlusion in hypotensive rats with subarachnoid hemorrhage: neuroprotective effects of citicoline. *Arch Physiol Biochem.* Apr, 2001;109(2):161–7.
11. Dixon C. E., Ma X., Marion D. W. Effects of CDP-choline treatment on neurobehavioral deficits after TBI and on hippocampal and neocortical acetylcholine release. *J Neurotrauma.* Mar, 1997;14(3):161–9.
12. Ogashiwa M., Takeuchi K., Hara M., Tanaka Y., et al. Studies on the intrathecal pharmacotherapy. Part I: CDP-choline. *Int J Clin Pharmacol Biopharm.* Oct, 1975;12(3):327–35.
13. Ogashiwa M., Takeuchi K. Intrathecal pharmacotherapy in coma. *Acta Neurochir* (Wien). 1976;34(1–4):37–44.
14. Cohadon F., Richer E., Poletto B. A precursor of phospholipids in the treatment of severe traumatic comas. *Neurochirurgie.* 1982;28(4):287–90.
15. Calatayud Maldonado V., Calatayud Perez J. B., Aso Escario J. Effects of CDP-choline on the recovery of patients with head injury. *J Neurol Sci.* Jul, 1991;103(Suppl):S15–8.
16. Maejima S., Katayama Y. Neurosurgical trauma in Japan. *World J Surg.* 2001 Sep;25(9):1205–9.
17. Tazaki Y., Sakai F., Otomo E., et al. Treatment of acute cerebral infarction with a choline precursor in a multicenter double-blind placebo-controlled study. *Stroke.* Feb, 1988;19(2):211–6.
18. Hazama T., Hasegawa T., Ueda S., Sakuma A. Evaluation of the effect of CDP-choline on poststroke hemiplegia employing a double-blind controlled trial. Assessed by a new rating scale for recovery in hemiplegia. *Int J Neurosci.* 1980;11(3):211–25.
19. Cubells J. M., Hernando C. Clinical trial on the use of cytidine diphosphate choline in Parkinson's disease. *Clin Ther.* 1988;10(6):664–71.
20. Marti Masso J. F., Urtasun M. Citicoline in the treatment of Parkinson's disease. *Clin Ther.* Mar–Apr, 1991;13(2):239–42.
21. Cacabelos R., Caamano J., Gomez M. J., et al. Therapeutic effects of CDP-choline in Alzheimer's disease. Cognition, brain mapping, cerebrovascular hemodynamics, and immune factors. *Ann N Y Acad Sci.* Jan 17, 1996;777:399–403.
22. Levin H. S. Treatment of postconcussional symptoms with CDP-choline. *J Neurol Sci.* Jul, 1991;103 Suppl:S39–42.
23. Leon-Carrion J., Dominguez-Roldan J. M., Murillo-Cabezas F., et al. The role of citicoline in neuropsychological training after traumatic brain injury. *NeuroRehabilitation.* 2000;14(1):33–40.
24. Spiers P. A., Hochanadel G. Citicoline for traumatic brain injury: report of two cases, including my own. *J Int Neuropsychol Soc.* Mar, 1999;5(3):260–4.
25. Blount P. J., Nguyen C. D., McDeavitt J. T. Clinical use of cholinomimetic agents: a review. *J Head Trauma Rehabil.* Aug, 2002;17(4):314–21.

26. Romero A., Grau T., Sacristan A., et al. Study of subacute toxicity of CDP-choline after 30 days of oral administration to rats. *Arzneimittelforschung.* 1983;33(7A):1035–8.

27. Romero A., Grau T., Sacristan A., et al. CDP-choline: 6-month study on toxicity in dogs. *Arzneimittelforschung.* 1983;33(7A):1038–42.

28. Lozano Fernandez R. Efficacy and safety of oral CDP-choline. Drug surveillance study in 2817 cases. *Arzneimittelforschung.* 1983;33(7A):1073–80.

29. Dinsdale J. R., Griffiths G. K., Castello J., et al. CDP-choline: repeated oral dose tolerance studies in adult healthy volunteers. *Arzneimittelforschung.* 1983;33(7A):1061–5.

30. Le Bars P. L., Katz M. M., Berman N., et al. A placebo-controlled, double-blind, randomized trial of an extract of *Gingko biloba* for dementia. *JAMA.* 1997;278:1327–32.

31. Le Bars P. L., Kastelan J. Efficacy and safety of a Gingko biloba extract. *Public Health Nutr.* Dec, 2000;3(4A):495–9.

32. Beaubrun G., Gray G. E. A review of herbal medicines for psychiatric disorders. *Psychiatr Serv.* Sep, 2000;51(9):1130–4.

33. Wong A. H., Smith M, Boon HS. Herbal remedies in psychiatric practice. *Arch Gen Psychiatry.* Nov, 1998;55(11):1033–44.

34. Kanowski S., Herrmann W. M., Stephan K., et al. Proof of efficacy of the Gingko biloba special extract EGb 761 in outpatients suffering from mild to moderate primary degenerative dementia of the Alzheimer type or multi-infarct dementia. *Pharmacopsychiatry.* 1996;29:47–56.

35. Hofferberth B. The efficacy of Egb 761 in patients with senile dementia of the Alzheimer type: a double-blind, placebo-controlled study on different levels of investigation. *Hum Psychopharmacol.* 1994;9;215–22.

36. Rai G. S., Shovlin C., Wesnes K. A. A double-blind, placebo-controlled study of Gingko biloba extract ('Tanakan') in elderly outpatients with mild to moderate memory impairment. *Curr Med Res Opin.* 1991;12;350–5.

37. Cianfrocca. Gingko biloba-induced frequent ventricular arrhythmia. *Ital Heart J.* Nov, 2002;3(11):689–91.

38. Birks J., Grumley E. V., Van Dongen M. Gingko biloba for cognitive impairment and dementia. *Cochrane Database Syst Rev.* 2002; (4):CD003120.

39. Fischoff P. K., Saleta B., Ruther E., et al. Therapeutic Efficacy of Pyritinol in Patients With Senile Dementia of the Alzhiemer Type (SDAT) and Multi-Infart Denentin (MID). *Neuro psychobiology.* 1992;26;65–70.

40. Cooper A. J., Magnus R. V. A Placebo-Controlled Study of Pyritinol ('Encephabol') in *Dementia Pharmatherapeutica.* 1980;2;317–22.

41. Knezevic S., Mubrin Z., Risberg J., et al. Pyritinal Treatment of SDAT Patients: Evaluation by psychiatric and neurological examination, psychometric testing, and rCBf measurements. *Int Clin Psycopharma Col*;1989;25–38.

42. Hermann, W. M., Kern U., Rohmel J. On the Effects of Pyritinol on Functional Deficits in Patients with Organic Mental Disorders. *Pharmacopsychiatry.* 1986;19:378–85.

43. Kitamura K.

44. *J Int Med Res.* 1981;9(3) (England) 1981; (3):215–221.

45. McDaniel M. A., Maier S. F., Einstein G. O. "Brain-specific" nutrients: a memory cure? *Nutrition.* 2003 Nov;19(11–12):957–75.

46. Goscinski I., Sliwonik S. Sondej T. Kwiatokowski S., Moskala M., et al. Piracetam in severe cranio-cerebral injuries. *Neurol Neurochir Pol.* Sep–Oct, 1998;32(5):1189–97. Polish.

47. Ricci S., Celani M. G., Cantisani A. T., et al. Piracetam for acute ischemic stroke. *Cochrane Database Syst Rev.* 2002;(4):CD000419. Review.

48. Oosterveld W. J. The effectiveness of piracetam in vertigo. *Pharmacopsychiatry.* Mar, 1999;32 Suppl 1:54–60. Review.

49. Kessler J. Thiel A., Karbe H., Heiss W. D. Piracetam improves activated blood flow and facilitates rehabilitation of poststroke aphasic patients. *Stroke.* Sep, 2000;31(9):2112–6.

50. Greener J., Enderby P., Whurr R. Pharmacological treatment for aphasia following stroke. *Cochrane Database Syst Rev.* 2001;(4):CD000424. Review.

51. Gualtieri F., Manetti D., Romanelli M. N., et al. Design and study of piracetam-like nootropics, controversial members of the problematic class of cognition-enhancing drugs. *Curr Pharm Des.* 2002;8(2):125–38. Review.

52. Szatmari S. Z., Whitehouse P. J. Vinpocetine for cognitive impairment and dementia. *Cochrane Database Syst Rev.* 2003;(1):CD003119.

53. Kidd P. M. A review of nutrients and botanicals in the integrative management of cognitive dysfunction. *Altern Med Rev.* Jun, 1999;4(3):144–61.

54. Sharman E. H., Vaziri N. D., Ni Z., et al. Reversal of biochemical and behavioral parameters of brain aging by melatonin and acetyl L-carnitine. *Brain Res.* Dec 13, 2002;957(2):223–30.

55. Kiss B., Karpati E. [Mechanism of action of vinpocetine] *Acta Pharm Hung.* Sep,1996;66(5):213–24.

56. Nicholson C. D. Pharmacology of nootropics and metabolically active compounds in relation to their use in dementia. *Psychopharmacology* (Berl). 1990;101(2):147–59.

57. Vas A., Gulyas B., Szabo Z., et al. Clinical and non-clinical investigations using positron emission tomography, near infrared spectroscopy and transcranial Doppler methods on the neuroprotective drug vinpocetine: a summary of evidences. *J Neurol Sci.* Nov 15, 2002;203–204:259–62.

58. Bhatti J. Z., Hindmarch I. Vinpocetine effects on cognitive impairments produced by flunitrazepam. *Int Clin Psychopharmacol.* Oct, 1987;2(4):325–31.

59. Dezsi L., Kis-Varga I., Nagy J., et al.Neuroprotective effects of vinpocetine in vivo and in vitro. Apovincamic acid derivatives as potential therapeutic tools in ischemic stroke *Acta Pharm Hung.* 2002;72(2):84–91.

60. Zozulia I. S., Iurchenko A. V. The adaptive potentials of those who worked in the cleanup of the aftermath of the accident at the Chernobyl Atomic Electric Power Station under the influence of different treatment methods. *Lik Sprava.* Apr–Jun, 2000;(3–4):18–21.

61. Hadjiev D. Asymptomatic ischemic cerebrovascular disorders and neuroprotection with vinpocetine. *Ideggyogy Sz.* May 20, 2003;56(5–6):166–72.

62. McDaniel M. A., Maier S. F., Einstein G. O. "Brain-specific" nutrients: a memory cure? *Nutrition.* Nov-Dec, 2003;19(11–12):957–75.

63. Kidd P. M. A review of nutrients and botanicals in the integrative management of cognitive dysfunction. *Altern Med Rev.* Jun, 1999;4(3):144–61.

64. Balestreri R., Fontana L., Astengo F. A double-blind placebo controlled evaluation of the safety and efficacy of vinpocetine in the treatment of patients with chronic vascular senile cerebral dysfunction. *J Am Geriatr Soc.* May, 1987;35(5):425–30.

65. Thal L. J., Salmon D. P., Lasker B., et al. The safety and lack of efficacy of vinpocetine in Alzheimer's disease. *J Am Geriatr Soc.* Jun, 1989;37(6):515–20.

66. Szatmari S. Z., Whitehouse P. J. Vinpocetine for cognitive impairment and dementia. *Cochrane Database Syst Rev.* 2003;(1):CD003119.

67. Bereczki D., Fekete I. Vinpocetine for acute ischaemic stroke. *Cochrane Database Syst Rev.* 2000;(2):CD000480.

68. Romodanov A. P., Potapov A. I., Dmitriev I. A. The characteristics of the clinical course of closed craniocerebral trauma in diabetics Zh Vopr Neirokhir Im N N Burdenko. Jul–Aug, 1991; (4):11–3.

69. Lehmann E., Kinzler E., Friedemann J. Efficacy of a special kava extract (Piper methysticum) in patients with states of anxiety, tension, and excitedness of nonmental origin—a double-blind placebo-controlled study of four weeks treatment. *Phytomedicine.* 1996;2;113–9.

70. Volz H. P., Kieser M. Kava-kava extract WS 1490 versus placebo in anxiety disorders—a randomized placebo-controlled 25-week outpatient trial. *Pharmacopsychiatry.* 1997;30;1–5.

71. Kline J. P., Blackhart G. C., Woodward K. M., et al.. Anterior electroencephalographic asymmetry changes in elderly women in response to a pleasant and an unpleasant odor. *Bio Psychol.* Apr, 2000;52(3):241–50.

72. Ang-Lee M. K., Moss J., Yuan C. S. Herbal Medicine and Perioperative Care. *JAMA.* 2001;286;208–16.

73. Thommessen B., Laake K. No identifiable effect of ginseng (Geri complex) as an adjuvant in the treatment of geriatric patients. *Aging Clin Exp Res.* 1996;8;417–20.

74. Marasco C., Ruiz V., Villagomez S., et al. Double-blind study of a multivitamin complex supplemented with ginseng extract. Drugs Exp Clin Res 1996;22;323–9.

75. Evans V. Herbs and the brain: friend or foe? The effects of gingko and garlic on warfarin use. *J Neurosci Nurs.* Aug, 2000;32:229–32.

76. Bourin M., Bougerol T., Guitton B., et al. A Combination of Plant Extracts in the Treatment of Outpatients with Adjustment Disorder with Anxious Mood; Controlled Study Versus Placebo. *Fundam Clin Pharmacol.* 1997;11;127–132.

77. Leathwood P. D., Chauffard F., Herck E., et al. Aqueous extract of valerian root improves sleep quality in man. *Pharmacol Biochem Behav.* 1982;17;65–71.

78. Beaubrun G., Gray G. E. A review of herbal medicines for psychiatric disorders. *Psychiatr Serv.* Sep, 2000;51(9):1130–4.

79. Wagner J., Wagner M. L., Hening W. A. Beyond benzodiazepines: alternative pharmacologic agents for the treatment of insomnia. *Ann Pharmacother.* 1998;32;680–91.

80. Blumenthal M. *The complete German Commission E monographs: therapeutic guide to herbal medicines.* Austin, TX: American Botanical Council; 1998.

81. Garges H. P., Varia I. Doraiswamy P. M. Cardiac complications and delirium associated with valerian root withdrawal. *JAMA.* 1998;280;1566–7.

82. Bottiglieri T. Folate, vitamin B_{12}, and neuropsychiatric disorders. *Nutr Rev* .1996;54;382–90.

83. Hutto B. R. Folate and cobalamin in psychiatric illness. *Compr Psychiatry.*1997;38;305–14.

84. Godfrey P. S., Toone B. K., Carney M. W., et al. Enhancement of recovery from psychiatric illness by methylfolate. *Lancet* .1990;336;392–5.

85. Fava M., Borus J. S., Alpert J. E., Nierenberg A. A., Rosenbaum J. F., Bottiglieri T. Folate, vitamin B_{12}, and homocysteine in major depressive disorder. *Am J Psychiatry.* 1997;154;426–8.

86. Reynolds E. H., Carney M. W., Toone B. K. Methylation and mood. *Lancet.* 1984;2;196–8.

87. Curtius H. C., Niederwieser A., Levine R. A., et al. Successful treatment of depression with tetrahydrobiopterin. *Lancet.* 1983;1;657–8.

88. Coppen A., Chaudhry S., Swade C. Folic acid enhances lithium prophylaxis. *J Affect Disord.*1986;10;9–13.

89. Bottiglieri T., Hyland K., Reynolds E. H. The clinical potential of ademetionine (*S*-adenosylmethionine) in neurological disorders. *Drugs.* 1994;48;137–52.

90. Kagan B. L., Sultzer D. L., Rosenlicht N., et al. Oral *S*-adenosylmethionine in depression: a randomized, double-blind, placebo-controlled trial. *Am J Psychiatry.* 1990;147;591–5.

91. Bressa G. M. *S*-Adenosyl-L-methionine (SAMe) as antidepressant: meta-analysis of clinical studies. *Acta Neurol Scand Suppl.* 1994;154;7–14.

92. Carney M. W., Chary T. K., Bottiglieri T., et al. The switch mechanism and the bipolar/unipolar dichotomy. *Br J Psychiatry.* 1989;154;48–51.

93. Fava M., Giannelli A., Rapisarda V., et al. Rapidity of onset of the antidepressant effect of parenteral *S*-adenosyl-L-methionine. *Psychiatry Res.* 1995;56;295–7.

94. Reynolds E. H. Mental effects of anticonvulsants and folic acid metabolism. *Brain.* 1968;91;197–214.

95. Moller S. E., Kirk L., Honore P. Relationship between plasma ratio of tryptophan to competing amino acids and the response to L-tryptophan treatment in endogenously depressed patients. *J Affect Disord* .1980;2;47–59.

96. van Praag H. M. Management of depression with serotonin precursors. *Biol Psychiatry.* 1981;16;291–310.

97. Walinder J., Skott A., Carlsson A., et al. Potentiation of the antidepressant action of clomipramine by tryptophan. *Arch Gen Psychiatry.* 1976;33;1384–9.

98. Byerley W. F., Judd L. L., Reimherr F. W., et al. 5-Hydroxytryptophan: a review of its antidepressant efficacy and adverse effects. *J Clin Psychopharmacol* .1987;7;127–37.

99. Hertzman P. A., Blevins W. L., Mayer J., Greenfield B., et al. Association of the eosinophilia-myalgia syndrome with the ingestion of tryptophan. *N Engl J Med.* 1990;322;869–73.

100. Hibbeln J. R., Palmer J. W., Davis J. M. Are disturbances in lipid-protein interactions by phospholipase-A2 a predisposing factor in affective illness? *Biol Psychiatry.* 1989;25;945–61.

101. Hibbeln J. R., Umhau J. C., George D. T., Salem N Jr. Do plasma polyunsaturates predict hostility and depression? *World Rev Nutr Diet.* 1997;82;175–86.

102. Buajordet I., Madsen S., Olsen H. Statins—the pattern of adverse effects with emphasis on mental reactions: data from a national and an international database. *Tidsskr Nor Laegeforen.* 1997;117;3210–3.

103. Gaster B., Holroyd J. St John's wort for depression: a systematic review. *Arch Intern Med.* Jan 24, 2000;160(2):152–6.

104. Butterwreck V. Mechanism of action of St. John's wort on depression: what is known. *CNS Drugs* 2003;17;539–562.

105. Muller D., Pfeil T., von den Driesch V. Treating depression comorbid with anxiety—results of an open, practice-oriented study with St John's wort WS 5572 and valerian extract in high doses. *Phytomedicine.* 2003;10 Suppl 4:25–30.

106. Leone M., D'Amico D., Moschianof, et al. Melatonin verses placebo in the prophyexis of cluster headache: a double-blind pilot study with parallel groups. *Cephalgia* 1996;16:494–496.

107. Danesch U. C. Petasites hybridus (Butterbur root) extract in the treatment of asthma – an open trial. *Altern Med Rev.* 2004 Mar;9(1):54–62.

108. Grossman W., Schmidramsl H. An extract of Petasites hybridus is effective in the prophylaxis of migraine. *Altern Med Rev.* 2001 Jun;6(3):303–10.

109. Grossmann M., Schmidramsl H. An extract of Petasites hybridus is effective in the prophylaxis of migraine. *Int J Clin Pharmacol Ther.* 2000 Sep;38(9):430–5.

110. Diener H. C., Rahlfs V. W., Danesch U. The first placebo-controlled trial of a special butterbur root extract for the prevention of migraine: reanalysis of efficacy criteria. *Eur Neurol.* 2004;51(2):89–97. .

111. Kalin P. The common butterbur (Petasites hybridus)—portrait of a medicinal herb. *Forsch Komplementarmed Klass Naturheilkd.* 2003 Apr;10 Suppl 1:41–4.

112. Dodick D. W., Capobianco D. J. Treatment and management of cluster headache. *Curr Pain Headache Rep.* 2001;5:83–91.

113. Ferra L., Montesano D., Senatove A. The distribution of minerals and flavonoids in the tea plant (cornellia sinenosis) *Farmaeco.* 2001;56;397–401.

114. Gaby A. R. Intravenous nutrient therapy: the "Myers' cocktail. *Altern Med Rev.* 2002, 7:389–403.

115. Bali L., Callaway E. Vitamin C and *Migraine*: A case report *N Engl J Med.* 1978;299:364.

116. Cox N. H., Vitamin E for dasone-individual headache. *Br J Dermatol.* 2002;146:174.

117. Rozen Td, Oshinsky M. L., Gebeline C. A., et al. Open label trial of coenzyme Q10 as a migraine preventative. *Cephalgia.* 2002; 22:137–141.

118. Gertsch J. H., Seto T. B., Mor J., et al. Gingko biloba for the prevention of severe acute mountain sickness (AMS) starting one day before rapid ascent. *High Alt Med Biol.* 2002;3:29–37.

119. Mauskop A. Alternative Therapies in Headache. Is there a role? *Med Clin North Am.* 2001;85–1007–84.

120. Wang F., Van Den Eeden S. K., Ackersen L. M., et al. Oral Magnesium Oxide Prophylaxis of Frequent Migrainous Headache in Children: A Randomized, Double-Blind, Placebo-Controlled Trial. *Headache.* 2003;43:601–610.

121. Tepper S. J., Rapoport A., Shftell F. The Pathophysiology of Migraine. *Neurology.* 2001;7:279–86.

122. Boska M. D., Welch K. M., Barker P. B., et al. Contrast in Cortical Magnesium, Phospholipid and Energy Metabolism between migraine syndromes. *Neurology.* 2002;58:1227–33.

123. Marcus J. C., Altura B. T., Altura B. M. Serum Ionized Magnesium in Post-traumatic Headaches. *J Pediatr.* 2001;139;459–62.

124. Cesarani A., Meloni F., Alpini D., et al. Gingko biloba (EGb761) in the treatment of equilibrium disorders. *Adv Ther.* 1998;15:291–304.

125. Pyritinol Hydrochloride for The Treatment of Vertigo. *Ouest Med.* France, 1976, 29/1 (43–46).

126. Ebadi M , Govitrapong P., Sharma S., et al. Ubiquinone (coenzyme q10) and mitochondria in oxidative stress of Parkinson's disease. *Biol Signals Recept*. May–Aug, 2001;10(3–4):224–53.

127. Favit A , Nicoletti F., Scapagnini U., et al. Ubiquinone protects cultured neurons against spontaneous and excitotoxin-induced degeneration. 1992. *J Cereb Blood Flow Metab*. 12;638–645.

128. Grieb P., Ryba M. S., Sawicki J., et al. Oral coenzyme Q10 administration prevents the development of ischemic brain lesions in a rabbit model of symptomatic vasospasm. *Acta Neuropathol* (Berl). Oct, 1997;94:363–368.

129. Matthews R. T., Yang L., Browne S., Baik M., et al. Coenzyme Q10 administration increases brain mitochondrial concentrations and exerts neuroprotective effects. 1998. *Proc Natl Acad Sci USA*. Jul 21, 1998;95(15):8892–8897.

130. Brewer G. J., Walliman T. W. Protective effect of energy precursor creatine against toxicity of glutamate and beta-amyloid in rat hippocampal neurons. *J Neurochem* 200;74:1968–78.

131. Malcon C., Kaddurah-Daoyk R., Beal M. F. Neuroprotective effects of creatine against NMDA and malonate toxicity. *Brain Res*. 2000;860;195–8.

132. Matthew R. T., et al. Creatine and cylcocreatine attenuate MPTP neurotoxicity. *Exp Neurol*. 1999;157:142–9.

133. Balestrino M., et al. Role of creatinine and phosphocreatine in neuronal protection from anoxic and ischemic damage. *Amino Acids Abstract*. 2002;23(1–3):221–229.

134. Phytother Res Nov, 1999;13(7):571–4.

135. Schaumburg H., Kaplan J., Windebark A., Vick n, Rasmus S., et al. Sensory neuropathy from pyridoxine abuse. A new megavitamin syndrome. *N Engl J Med* 1983;309:445–8.

136. Bulter L., Foster N. E. Back Pain Online: a cross-sectional survey on the quality of web-based information on low back pain. *Spine*. 2003;28;395–401.

137. Morris C. A., Avorn J. Internet Marketing of Herbal Products. *JAMA*. 2003;290;1519–20.

138. Sweet B. V., Gay W. E., Leady M. A., Stumpf J. L. Usefulness of Herbal and Dietary Supplement References. *Ann Pharmacother*. 2003;37;494–9.

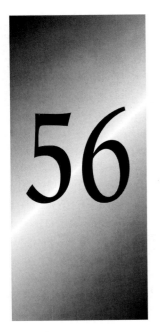

56 Traditional Chinese Medicine Theory in the Mechanism and Treatment of TBI

Gary G. Wang

INTRODUCTION

The theory of traditional Chinese medicine (TCM) is completely different from that of western medicine. The formation and development of TCM theory was greatly influenced by ancient Chinese philosophy. It is necessary to explain some basic TCM theories that developed over the past 3000 years before going into its specific applications in traumatic brain injury (TBI) management.

The theories of "*Yin-Yang*" and "The Five Elements" were two approaches to the study of nature in ancient China. Every object or phenomenon in the universe was thought to consist of two opposite yet interdependent parts known as *yin* and *yang*. The theory of the five elements on the other hand, held that wood, fire, earth, metal, and water constituted the physical world. Like *yin-yang*, the five elements were interdependent and inter-resistant. Both theories described the world in a state of constant change between balance and imbalance. Ancient Chinese physicians believed in the integration of the natural world with the bodies of human beings. Diseases were believed to be caused by imbalance among *yin-yang* and the five elements.

As with natural phenomena, ancient Chinese physicians classified human organs and emotions as belonging to one of the five elements. The laws pertaining to the inter-promoting, interacting, over-acting and counter-acting of the five elements were used to interpret the relationship between the physiology and pathology of the human body. "*Zang-fu*" refers to the gross anatomical entities of the internal organs. However, its meaning is different from that of modern anatomy. The term *zang-fu* is a generalization of the physiological functions of the human body. The heart, liver, spleen, lung, kidney and pericardium are known as the six *zang* organs. They are related to *yin*. Their main physiological functions are to manufacture and store essential substances including vital essence, *qi* (vital energy, pronounced "Chee"), blood, and body fluid. The small intestine, gall bladder, stomach, large intestine, urinary bladder, and *Sanjiao* are known collectively as the six fu organs. They are related to *yang*. *Sanjiao* is the name of a function without body shape structure. The main functions of fu organs are to receive and digest food, absorb nutrients, and transmit and excrete wastes.

The brain and uterus are two extraordinary fu organs. They are closely related to the other regular organs. According to TCM theory, the essence of the kidney produces the marrow that forms the brain as "a sea of marrow." The brain performs thinking and memorization functions. The heart is the main organ that dominates the mental activity of the brain. The heart, protected by pericardium, governs mental activities and generally handles the physiological function of the brain as it "houses the mind." Meanwhile the liver is also related to mental activities by regulating the unrestraint and patency of vital functions. The lung and spleen interfere with mental activity indirectly. The lung promotes the diffusion of *qi*, blood and body fluid into every portion of the body. The spleen supplies nourishment essential to heart and lung, keeps the blood circulating inside the vessels. Dysfunction of *zang* and *fu* will prevent the proper functioning of the brain. Conversely, disorders of the brain will also interfere with the function of *zang* and *fu*.

The channel doctrine is also essential for TCM theory. Meridian channels and the collaterals (Jing and Luo) are the pathways of *qi*, blood and fluid circulation. Meridian channels are the main routes while collaterals are the branches of the channels that connect internal organs as well as limbs to make the whole body into an entity. Each meridian channel comes from different *zang* or *fu* organs and distributes in the trunk and limbs. Channels and *zang fu* viscera are shown on the superficial human body at specific acupuncture points. Through these points, *qi* may be infused into the channels to promote balance in the body. The points are also the places where disease evils can easily pass through. This explains why acupuncture points are always selected as therapeutic locations. Acupuncture is a TCM therapy method to remove obstructions in the meridian channels and to regulate blood and *qi* by stimulating the points with needles. According to the philosophy of TCM, medications and treatment procedures facilitate the rebalance of the human body by altering its constituents.

Ancient Chinese physicians recognized and classified medications (most of these herbs) mainly by observing the effects of their clinical application. By performing numerous experiments, each medical herb was classified to either *yin* or *yang* and was characterized as belonging to one of the five elements with the ability to target different organs. The characteristics and functions of Chinese herbs were described in the book *Compendium of Materia Medica*, which was written by Li Shi-Zhen (1518–1593 A.D.). The process of prescribing the appropriate herbal prescription is a systematic technique developed over thousands of years starting with the analysis of clinical information collected from the patient by observation, auscultation, interrogation, and palpation of the pulse. A TCM physician will diagnose the location and nature of the major unbalanced elements and then prescribe an appropriate formula (combination) of herbs. There are several medical herbs in each formula and each of them may have a different function. Certain combinations of herbs work efficiently to target certain disease conditions and fulfill pharmacology functions. The effect of each formula has been documented through clinical verification and may be adjusted accordingly. A special name is given to each established formula. Thousands of

years of successful clinical treatment applications have produced many herb formulas that are still in use today.

Following, is an introduction to the classification of brain injury and TCM disease elements by organ system which includes prescription formulas available in China as pills widely used in the management of disorders related to TBI. The precise makeup of these prescriptions is too vast to include here, but can be researched using the name. Acupuncture management for traumatic brain injury will also be briefly discussed.

Acute Severe TBI: Consciousness and *Qi* Disturbance

TCM physicians differentiate and classify TBI patients into different syndromes according to their clinical symptoms. TCM physicians believe that traumatic injury will rupture the integrity of the natural protection system, permitting the invasion of evil factors, leaking essential *qi*, blood and fluids and inducing blood extravasation. All of these will directly disturb normal *qi* and blood circulation and induce pain. The brain is considered the cleanest organ. It is polluted by trauma, which facilitates the invasion of external pathogenic factors. After severe head trauma, evil factors will attack *zang-fu* organs, blocking the *qi* aperture of the heart and hurting the *qi* that acts as the primary motive force for life activities. TCM physicians usually differentiate and classify acute severe TBI patients into two syndrome-specific groups according to the patient's clinical symptoms, named *qibi* (blockage of *qi*) and *qituo* (exhaustion of *qi*). Because such cases are critical, the modern TCM physicians will usually suggest combined management with modern western medical methods.

Blockage of Qi *Qibi* symptoms include unresponsiveness, severe confusion, agitation, delirium, restlessness, flushed face, twitching, and tachypnea. A yellowish sticky film coats the tongue. The pulse is rapid and deep. The focus of treatment of *qibi* is to remove the pathogenic factors blocking the aperture of the heart. Some patients may have fever, flushed faces and be agitated. TCM believes that fever is caused by hot evil *qi* that blocks the function of the brain. An-Gong-Niu-Huang-Wan (安宫牛黄丸), Zi-Xiu-Dan (紫雪丹), and Zi-Bao-Dan (至宝丹) are the medications usually applied. These medications are also used for coma or severe agitation due to other etiologies such as stroke, high fever, meningitis, or encephalitis. An-Gong-Niu-Huang-Wan, is the pill most commonly prescribed. Its extracts for intravenous injection, named Xing-Nao-Jing (醒脑静), are available in China. Several preliminary controlled studies have shown the effectiveness of the intravenous application of Xing-Nao-Jing to treat the comatose state (1–3). As like other TCM medications, the chemical contents of An-Gong-Niu-Huang-Wan are

TABLE 56-1
TMC Diagnosis and Treatment of Acute Severe TBI

DIAGNOSIS	MANIFESTATION	TMC TREATMENT
Blockage of Qi	unresponsiveness, severe confusion, agitation, delirium, restlessness, flushed face, fever, yellowish tongue with sticky coat, rapid and deep pulse	*Decoction* An-Gong-Niu-Huang-Wan Zi-Xiu-Dan Zi-Bao-Dan *Acupuncture methods* Stimulating the points of the GV Channel on head combined with points on limbs, slightly bleeding the points on terminal digits.
Exhaustion of Qi	deep coma, loss of jaw control, lost bladder control, heavy perspiration, cooling distal limbs, whitish coat of tongue, weak pulse	*Decoction* Shen-Fu-Tang adding San-Qi *Acupuncture methods* Applying moxibustion and/or retaining needles to points of the Ren Channel adding stimulating at CV4, CV6, CV8.

complicated. The exact mechanisms of their effects on acute brain injury are not clear from Western biomedical views. However, recent scientific studies have provided some clues. For example, Niu-Huang (Bos Calculus), one of the major contents of An-Gong-Niu-Huang-Wan is bovine gallstone, a mixture of bilirubin metabolites and endogenous bile acids. After traumatic brain injury and stroke, massive bleeding could produce significant iron-mediated oxidative stress, programmed cell death (apoptosis), and neurodegeneration. Bilirubin metabolites were found to be potent endogenous antioxidants with neuroprotective effects (4–6). One of the major endogenous bile acids, tauroursodeoxycholic acid, was found to have the ability to modulate cell death by interrupting classic pathways of apoptosis and has wide-ranging neuroprotective effects after brain injury (7). However, because the formulation contains small amounts of arsine and mercury, the authors do not recommend the prolonged use of An-Gong-Niu-Huang-Wan.

The acupuncture methods for treating the syndrome of *qi* blockage promote resuscitation by stimulating the points of the Governor Vessel Meridian (GVChannel). Renzhong (GV 26) and Baihui (GV 20) are the two points most often selected. Usually, Yongquan (KI 1) is the point added to "conduct the evil factors down." The points at the distal fingers including Shaoshang (LU 11), Shaochong (HT 9), Shaoze (SI 1), Zhongchong (PC 9), Shangyang (LI 1), Guanchong (TE 1) are often selected for slight bleeding. In addition, Taichong (LR 3), Fenglong (ST 40), Laogong(PC 8) are sometimes stimulated.

Exhaustion of Qi Qituo by severe traumatic brain injury is a very serious and critical condition. The major

symptoms include deep coma with unresponsiveness, loss of jaw control with spontaneous mouth opening, heavy perspiration, lost of bladder control, and distal limb cooling. The tongue coat becomes whitish. The pulse is weak. Management of *qituo* is aimed at consolidating vital energy. TMC physicians prepare a formula by combining Shen-Fu-Tang (参附汤, a decoction of Ginseng and prepared Aconite) with powder of San-Qi (Radix Notoginseng). Acupuncture is also applied frequently for exhaustion of Qi to recapture *yang* and avert the collapsing status. Applying moxibustion to points of the Ren Channel is the traditional way. Guanyuan (CV 4), Qihai (CV6) and Shenjue (CV8) are the points for emergency measures to restore vital function. Continuous indirect moxibustion with salt and/or retaining needles for 30 minutes at these points is the traditional method.

Subacute TBI management with TCM

In TCM, diagnosis and treatment is based on clinical symptoms. Different diseases with similar clinical pictures usually are treated in similar ways. Meanwhile, the same disease with different clinical symptoms may be treated in different ways. Because of the clinical similarity, the management of TBI is quite similar to the treatment of stroke. After the crisis acute stage, in cases of prolonged comatose status, An-Gong-Niu-Huang-Wan and Su-He-Xiang-Wan (苏合香丸, Storax Pill) are often used for resuscitation. Acupuncture methods for coma cases are similar to that for *qi* blockage and additional appropriate points are added according to clinical symptoms present. TCM physicians will apply acupuncture by combining the local and distal points according to the courses of the

TABLE 56-2
TCM Management of Neural Deficits after Severe TBI

SYMPTOMS	DECOCTION	ACUPUNCTURE
Prolonged comatose status	An-Gong-Niu-Huang-Wan Su-He-Xiang-Wan	Similar to *qi* blockage
Aphasia	Ren-Shen-Zai-Zao-Wan	GV15, CV 23, HT 5
Paresis	Huo-Luo-Dan	GV 20, GV16, BL 7 and the points of *yang* Channels of the affected side. *upper limb paralysis* LI 15, LI 11, LI 10, TE 5, LI 4 *lower limb paralysis* GB 30, GB 34, ST 36, ST 41, BL 60 *facial paralysis* CV 17, ST 4, ST 6, GB 14, LI 4, SI 18, ST 7

channels. For example, because the Large Intestine Channel and Stomach Channel traverse the cheek, Jiache (ST 6), Xiaguan (ST 7) and Hegu (LI 4) are the points to be stimulated for those coma patients with clenched jaw. According to TCM theory, functionally the tongue is related to the heart. Aphasia is a symptom of heart function disorder. Ren-Shen-Zai-Zao-Wan (人参再造丸, Ginseng Restorative Bolus) is the often used to benefit heart *qi*, blood circulation, and promote recovery of aphasia. Yamen (GV15) and Lianquan (CV 23) are local and adjacent points of the tongue. Tongli (HT 5) is the Luo (connecting) point of the Heart Channel. These points are often selected to relieve stiffness of the tongue and treat aphasia and dysarthria. A small control study on TBI aphasia patients showed the functional recovery of the acupuncture treatment group was much better than that of the control group (8).

TCM believes that paresis is a mobility function deficit due to obstruction of *qi* and blood circulation in Channels. Huo-Luo-Dan (活络丹) is one of the popular TCM pills used in hemiplegia cases to remove obstruction and readjust *qi* and blood circulation. Acupuncture is widely used in China to promote the recovery of hemiplegia. The *Yang* Channels of the affected side are the main points to puncture. Points of the healthy side may be added also. Usually, TCM practitioners puncture the healthy side first and then the affected side. Moxibustion may be applied as a supplement. Baihau (GV 20), Fengfu (GV16), and Tongtian (BL 7) are commonly used for all paralysis cases. Jianyu (LI 15) Quchi (LI 11), Shousanli(LI 10), Waiguan (TE 5), and Hegu (LI 4) are usually selected for upper extremity affected cases. Huantiao (GB 30), Yanglingquan (GB 34), Zusanli (ST 36), Jiexi (ST 41), and Kunlun (BL 60) are used for lower limb paresis. Yifeng (CV 17), Dicang (ST 4), Jiache (ST 6), Yangbai (GB 14),

Hegu (LI 4), Quanliao (SI 18), and Xiaguan, (ST 7) are usually added for cases of facial paralysis.

Prescription of traditional Chinese medications is usually made according to a TCM diagnosis based on clinical symptoms. Following are the TCM diagnostic syndromes, most often seen in the subacute TBI cases. The prescriptions will be briefly introduced accordingly.

Stasis of Blood   Stasis of blood is one of the key etiologies in the TCM brain injury model. TCM theory dictates that the heart houses the mind. Traumatic brain injury may disturb the blood and *qi* circulation and interfere with heart function. Injury may directly induce the stasis of blood. The invasion of external pathogenic factors due to trauma may also interfere with blood circulation and induce stasis. Stasis of blood will interfere with *qi* movement. Pain usually comes from insufficiency or blockage of local *qi* circulation. As "the heart houses the mind", blood stasis results in a decreased level of consciousness. Consequently, these cases usually have headache and cognitive deficiency. Many TBI cases with symptoms of migraine-like headache are due to blood stasis. Usually, the patient complains of persistent pricking or stabbing headache in a fixed location. A purple tongue or purple spots on the tongue may be seen. The pulse is stringy and hesitant. Promoting blood flow to remove blood stasis is the focus of treatment. Xue-Fu-Zhu-Yu Tang (血府逐瘀汤) and Shu-Jing-Huo-Xie Tang (疏经活血汤) are among the most widely prescribed TCM formulas for those cases of blood stasis with headache and/or other neuralgia. Recent research has confirmed the beneficial effects of these groups of Chinese medicines on neural regeneration. It was reported that after the extracts of Shu-Jing-Huo-Xie Tang were added in a culture medium of neural cells, the neurite outgrowth induced by nerve growth factor (NGF) increased approximately 30-fold compared to NGF alone (9). Ci-Wu-Jia (Radix Acanthopanacis Sceticosi) is one of the herbs prescribed for this type of patient either individually or combined with other TCM medications. Animal studies have demonstrated the strong anti-inflammatory and antinociceptive activities of Acanthopanax Radix extract (10) and its effects as an agent in the prevention of multiple organ dysfunction (11). Acanthopanax Radix is also known to have healing and protective effects on stress-induced disturbances of mental status. Animal studies have suggested that Acanthopanax Radix may act by regulating noradrenaline (NA) and dopamine (DA) levels in specific brain regions related to the stress response (12).

Deficiency of Qi and Stagnancy of Blood   According to TCM theory, the brain is an organ belonging to *yin* and collecting clean *qi* of *yang*. The function of the brain depends on momentum of *yang-qi*. Some subacute TBI patients show weakness of *qi* as their major clinical phenomena. Deficiency of *qi* can induce stagnancy of blood. Fatigue and headache are the major complaints. The patients look tired with low voices. They have a dull headache, aggravated by fatigue, accompanied by lassitude, lack of strength, anorexia, palpitations, shortness of breath, and sometimes aversion to cold with cool limbs. The tongue shows a thin white coat. The pulses are "thready" and weak. Most TBI cases with hypopituitarism would be classified in this syndrome group. Promoting blood circulation by invigorating *qi* is the method of treatment. Bu-Yang-Huan-Wu-Tang (补阳还五湯), Yi-Qi-Hua-Yu-Tang (益气还五湯) and Taohong Siwu Tang (桃红四物汤, Decoction of Four Ingredients with Peach Seed and Safflower) are among the classic decoctions prescribed to TBI patients for promoting blood circulation by invigorating *qi*. A large-scale clinical case report on the management of subacute or chronic subdural hemorrhage patients with Yi-Qi-Hua-Yu-Tang showed significant therapeutic effects (13). It was reported that Bu-Yang-Huan-Wu showed beneficial effects on disturbance of the hypothalamus-pituitary-thyroid axis after brain ischemic injury (14). Animal studies found that Bu-Yang-Huan-Wu may protect brain neurons from apoptosis after cerebral ischemia. The mechanism may be related to its effects on the improvement of cerebral energy metabolism, regulation of nitric oxide synthesis and antagonism of toxic excitatory amino acids (15). The Taohong Siwu Decoction is effective in hydroxyl radical scavenging and is effective in inhibiting lipid peroxidation (16).

Astragalus root, Chinese angelica root, Ligusticum chuanxiong rhizome, and safflower are the common ingredients among these decoctions. Astragalus, Chinese Angelica, and Ligusticum Chuanxiong have demonstrated a wide range of immunopotentiating and immunomodulating effects (17–19). Angelica Sinensis, Ligusticum Chuanxong, and safflower have also showed anti-inflammatory and antioxidizing effects. They could improve brain microcirculation through inhibiting thrombus formation and platelet aggregation as well as blood viscosity active components (20–22). Laboratory studies have also suggested that chaunxiong and safflower have brain neuroprotective effects (23–25).

Kidney Insufficiency   Insufficiency of the kidney is a contributing factor in some of the post brain injury syndrome cases, especially among the geriatric population. Kidney insufficient patients usually complain of a constant dull headache, with a feeling of emptiness often worsening with exercise. Common accompanying symptoms include lassitude, debility, aching, weakness of the lower back and legs, forgetfulness, decreased intelligence and impotence. The patient often has a reddened tongue with little or no film. The pulses are deep, thready, and weak. There are two kinds of kidney insufficiency, *yin* and *yang*. Cases of the kidney *yin* insufficiency are usually accompanied by dizziness, tinnitus, dry mouth, flushed cheeks, and a hot sensation in the palms and soles. Liu-Wei-Di-Huang-Wan (六味地黄丸, Six Flavor Tea, Rehmannia Pill, LWDH) and Jin-Gui-Shen-Qi-Wan (金匮肾气丸) are the TCM decoctions given most widely. Insufficiency of the kidney-*yang*, is usually accompanied by aversion to cold, cold limbs, nocturia, and pale complexion. The tongue is pale and corpulent with a thick whitish coating. In these cases the TCM physician will usually prescribe kidney *yang* reinforcing medications such as You-Gui-Wan (右归丸) and Shen-Qi-Wan (肾气丸). The contents of LWDH are the main components for the formulas of all the kidney insufficiency prescriptions. LWDH has been widely studied. Recent animal studies have shown that LWDH possesses anti-amnesia effects and memory enhancing properties (26). It was suggested that LWDH corrects the abnormal expressions of hippocampal genes in dementia animals (27). Traditionally, kidney tonic Chinese medications containing LWDH are used widely for general health condition improvement. Those medications are able to enhance non-specific immunology activities (28). LWDH is able to improve immune function by regulating the ratio of T and B cells and control over-expression of cytokine genes from activated mononuclear cells (29–32). In addition, the compounds in LWDH may also protect tissues and organs from cytotoxic attack by noxious reagents (33–34). Dihuang (Radix Rehmanniae), one of the major ingredients of the kidney tonic formulas is also reported to have effects on intelligence enhancement (35).

Liver Dysfunction   The liver dominates unrestrained *qi* and maintains the patency of *qi* flow. Acute or subacute brain injury may alter liver function by changing the balance of liver-*yang* and of endogenous wind in the liver. Exuberance of liver-*yang* results in a headache characterized by cramping pain in the temple and vertex and is

TABLE 56-3
Subacute TBI TMC Differential Diagnosis and Decoctions Used Often

Diagnosis	Manifestations		Decoction
Stasis of blood	migraine-like headache and cognitive deficiency, purple or purple spots on the tongue, stringy and hesitant pulse		Xue-Fu-Zhu-Yu Tang Shu-Jing-Huo-Xie Tang
Deficiency of qi and stagnancy of blood	fatigue, dull headache, low voices, lassitude, anorexia, palpitations, shortness of breath, aversion to cold, cool limbs, thin whitish coated tongue, thready weak pulse		Bu-Yang-Huan-Wu-Tang Yi-Qi-Hua-Yu-Tang Taohong Siwu Tang
Kidney Insufficiency	constant dull headache with a feeling of emptiness, lassitude, debility, aching and weakness of the lower back and legs, forgetfulness, decreased intelligence	*kidney yin insufficiency* dizziness, tinnitus, dry mouth, flushed cheeks, and a hot sensation in the palms and soles, reddened tongue with little or no coat, deep and weak pulse	Liu-Wei-Di-Huang-Wan Jin-Gui-Shen-Qi-Wan
		kidney-yang insufficiency aversion to cold, cold limbs, listlessness, impotence, nocturia, pale complexion, spontaneous perspiration, pale and corpulent tongue with thick whitish coat, weak pulse	You-Gui-Wan Shen-Qi-Wan
Liver Dysfunction	cramping headache in temple and vertex aggravated by anger. faintness, giddiness, insomnia, bitterness in mouth, decreased self-control, irritability, restlessness, insomnia, tremors, twisting of the body, and localized or generalized convulsions, thin yellow coated tongue, a stringy rapid pulse		Tianma Gouteng Yin

aggravated by anger. The headache is often accompanied by faintness, giddiness, dizziness, insomnia, and bitterness in the mouth. Alterations of endogenous wind in the liver cause disturbances of emotions and body movements. Wind is always moving and changing reflecting the patient's symptoms of decreased self-control, irritability, restlessness, and insomnia. The patient may have abnormal body movements such as tremors, twisting of the body, and localized or generalized convulsions. Patients have a thin yellow tongue coating and a stringy rapid pulse. TMC management is oriented at subduing the exuberant *yang* of the liver in turn calming the internal wind. Tianma Gouteng Yin (天麻钩藤, Decoction of Gastrodia and Uncaria) is the formula most commonly prescribed for these patients. Tianma (Gastrodia elata Bl.) and Gouteng (Uncaria rhynchophylla Jack) are traditional Chinese herbs that are used to treat convulsive disorders such as epilepsy. Synergistic anticonvulsive effects were observed in animal studies (36). Gastrodia is widely used by TCM physicians to manage headache, dizziness, vertigo, dementia, and convulsions (37). Pharmacological studies have shown that the anticonvulsive properties and brain neuronal protective effects of the constituents of Gastrodia are related to their free radical scavenging activities and modulator effects on neurotransmission

(36, 38–41). The cognitive beneficial effects of Castrodia and its ability to improve learning and memory have been confirmed by animal studies (42–44). Interestingly, animal studies have also shown that motion sickness can be treated with Gastrodia (45).

Chronic Post-TBI Syndrome:

Patients suffering from brain concussion, brain contusion, and traumatic intracranial hemorrhage may have residual symptoms of post brain injury syndrome such as headache and dizziness. TCM physicians divide cases of post brain injury syndrome into several types according to the accompanying symptoms. The treatment methods may be the same for different diseases that share similar clinical pictures.

Qi, blood and body fluids are fundamental substances in the human body. They sustain normal vital activities. Their existence and function are generally manifest in the functional activities of various tissues and organs. Blood and *qi* are closely related. The formation and circulation of blood depends upon *qi*, while the formation and distribution of *qi* is intimately absorbed in blood. TCM physicians believe, as a result of endogenous injury, the chronic post brain injury syndrome is due to the unbalance of *qi*, blood, and body fluid. Trauma and prolonged morbid status would excessively consume *qi*, blood, and fluid essence and induce *qi* deficiency. Patients with *qi* deficiency will complain of a dull headache, which is aggravated by fatigue, accompanied by lassitude, lack of strength, anorexia, palpitations, and shortness of breath. A thin white tongue coating and thready weak pulse is usually found. Buzhong Yiqi Wan (补中益气丸) is the formula of choice to replenish *qi*. Post-brain injury patients with general blood deficiency usually have headache, dizziness, palpitations, insomnia, dreamful sleep, blurred vision, numbness of the limbs, pale tongue, and "thready" pulse. Siwu Tang (四物汤, Decoction of Four Ingredients) is the basic formula used to nourish the blood. Siwu Tang plus Flos Chrysanthemi (chrysanthemum flower) and Fructus Viticis (chastetree fruit) is a treatment for blood deficiency patients with headache as their major complaint. Those patients with symptoms of both *qi* and blood deficiency receive Renshen Yangyin Wan (人参养阴丸, Geinseng Nutrition Pill) and Shiquan Dabu Wan (十全大补丸, Bolus of Ten Powerful Tonics). Excessively consuming essence fluid of the kidney will induce kidney *yin* deficiency. For those post brain injury cases with *yin* deficient phenomena as described previously, Qi Ju Dihuang Wan (杞菊地黄丸, LWDH with Wolfberry and Chrysanthemum) is often prescribed.

Some cases with poor general health may also show symptoms similar to liver *yang* disturbance. Liver *yang* hyperactivity may be secondary to a relative *yin* deficiency. Nourishing *yin* and calming down *yang* is the strategy for treatment with Liu-Wei-Di-Huang-Wan and Zhengan Xifeng Wan (镇肝熄风丸). TCM physicians believe the liver aids the spleen and stomach in digestion and absorption. Trauma may disturb liver *qi* leading to digestive disorders manifested as nausea, anorexia, abdominal distention, acid regurgitation, loose stool, etc. Female patients may have irregular menstruation. For cases accompanied by liver-*yang* hyperactive symptoms described previously, Longdan Xiegan Wan (龙胆泻肝丸) is administered. Post-TBI patients with deficiency of the liver–*qi*, usually have a coexisting deficiency of blood in the liver. This manifests as pallor of the face and lips, lassitude, tinnitus, deafness, and liability to panic. Dan Zhi Xiaoyao Wan (丹栀消遥丸) is a medication often given (Table 56-4).

The acupuncture management strategies of post-TBI syndromes are also formulated according to clinical complaints and symptoms. Among the various post-TBI clinical symptoms, headache is one of the most common complaints. We hereby discuss headache as an example to introduce the basic acupuncture treatment methods of post-TBI symptoms. TMC theory relates that the head is the place where all the *yang* channels of the upper and

---

TABLE 56-4
Chronic Post-TBI Syndrome TCM Differentiation and Treatment

TYPES	MANIFESTATION	DECOCTION SUGGESTED
Qi deficiency	dull headache, aggravated by fatigue; lassitude, anorexia, palpitations, shortness of breath, thin white coated tongue, thready and weak pulse	Buzhong Yiqi Wan
Blood deficiency	headache, dizziness, palpitations, insomnia, dreamful sleep, blurred vision, numbness of the limbs, pale tongue, thready pulse	Siwu Tang
Both *qi* and blood deficiency	as above combined	Renshen Yangyin Wan Shiquan Dabu Wan
Kidney *yin* deficiency	lumbago, lassitude, dizziness, tinnitus, nocturnal emission, premature ejaculation, dry mouth, sore throat, flushed cheeks, hot sensation in palm and sole, reddened tongue with little or no coating, thread and rapid pulse	Qi Ju Dihuang Wan
Liver *yang* hyperactivity	cramping headache over temple and vertex, intermittent dizziness, giddiness, restessness, irritalbility, insominia, bitter taste, taut pulse	Liu-Wei-Di-Huang-Wan and Zhengan Xifeng Wan
Disturb liver *qi*	nausea, anorexia, abdominal distention, acid regurgitation, loose stool, irregular menstruation	Longdan Xiegan Wan
Deficiency of the liver–*qi*,	pallor of the face and lips, lassitude, tinnitus, deafness, liability to panic	Dan Zhi Xiaoyao Wan

TABLE 56-5
Acupuncture Point Selection for Chronic Post-TBI Headache

Region of Headache	Channel of Distal Point Selected	Prescription Example
Occipital	Urinary Bladder Channel of Foot – Taiyang	GB 20, BL 10, BL 60
Forehead and supraorbital	Stomach Channel of foot-Yangming.	ST 8, GV 24.5, LI 4, ST 44
Temporal	Gall bladder Channel of foot-Shaoyang.	GB 8, TE 5, GB 41
Parietal	Liver Channel of foot-Yueyin.	CV 20, SI 3, BL 67, LR 3

lower limbs meet. Attacks by trauma and other endogenous or exogenous factors may cause derangement of *qi* and blood in the head and retardation of circulation of *qi* in the channels that traverse the head. In such cases, headaches occur. Usually, the headache is differentiated according to its locality and its supplying channels (Table 56-5). The selection of acupuncture points is based on the combination of local points around the symptomatic area and distal points according to the channels affected. Pain at the occipital region and nape of the neck is believed to be Urinary Bladder Channel of Foot –Taiyang related. Fengchi (GB 20) and Tianzhu (BL 10) are the local points punctured. Kunlun (BL 60) is one of the distal points selected often. Pain at the forehead and supraorbital region is related to the Stomach Channel of foot-Yangming. Puncturing the local points of Touwei (ST 8) and Yintang (GV 24.5) combined with distal points Hegu (LI 4), Neiting (ST 44) is one of the popular methods. Headaches at the temporal region bilaterally or only one side are related to the Gall bladder Channel of foot-Shaoyang. Shauigu (GB 8), Waiguan (TE 5), and Zulinqi (GB 41) are the points to be punctured. Parietal region headache is related to the Liver Channel of foot-Yueyin. The points often selected include Baihui (CV 20), Houxi (SI 3), Zhiyin (BL 67), and Taichong (LR 3). For those with exuberance of liver-*yang*, add Xingjian. (LR 2) and Yanglingquan (GB 34). In cases of deficiency of *qi* and blood Qihai (CV 6) and Zusanli (ST 36) would be punctured also.

Post TBI cases are differentiated to Shi (solid) and Xu (insufficiency) types. Cases with symptoms of stasis of blood and exuberance of liver-*yang* belong to Shi types, while those with symptoms of insufficiency of *qi*, blood and kidney are grouped as Xu types. The acupuncture points are selected accordingly. For example, Laogong, (PC 8) and Yongquan (KI 1) are the points to be stimulated for Shi cases with syncope and dizziness. However, combining puncture and moxibustion at Baihui (GV 20),

Qihai (CV 6), and Zusanli (ST 36) is the treatment for those Xu cases with similar symptoms.

More and more evidence supports that acupuncture is able to stimulate the central nervous system to release chemicals, which influence the body's self-regulating systems and promote natural healing abilities. Most acupuncture points are located in the trunk and limbs. However, the points over the head play an important place in traditional TBI management with acupuncture. Scalp acupuncture is a newly developed promising method to treat severe TBI and its related symptoms (46–48). Future research may be aimed at scalp acupuncture and its effects on the release of neurotransmitters and neurohormones.

Discussion

Unlike the development of Western medicine, which is mainly based on the progress of biomedical sciences, the development of Traditional Chinese Medicine is based on the experience of numerous clinical applications of natural products and acupuncture. TCM has been used for at least 3,000 years and has accumulated rich clinical application experience. The chemical ingredients of natural products are complicated. The chemical contents of a TCM formula, made up of a combination of natural medicines, are even more complicated. Pharmacological research is needed to bring TCM from an experiential and historical level to current biopharmaceutical standards level. This is not to say that the chemical elements of TCM formulas should be extracted and purified into a single compound for administration in isolation.

Although there are increasing numbers of patients and physicians in western countries accepting TCM as an alternative form of medical treatment, there have been no large-scale, well-controlled studies done evaluating TCM management of TBI. Some "natural" ingredients may be harmful to humans. The issues of toxicity may be even more relevant following TBI when blood brain barrier permeability may be adversely impacted. Considering the complex contents of TCM medicines, it is certainly possible that some of them may interfere with the effects of prescribed pharmaceutical drugs. Most of the TCM medications mentioned in this chapter are available in the West as "natural food products". The authors recommend that patients who wish to use TCM medications for TBI related problems consult their physicians, and if such treatment is pursued, patients should ideally be under the guidance of TCM trained practitioners.

Acupuncture seems to have no obvious side effects; however, there are no large-scale controlled studies done yet on acupuncture management of TBI related problems. Clearly, this is an area of research that can meld TCM with Western medicine in an attempt to best optimize patient outcome following TBI.

How ultimately TCM will be integrated into the rehabilitative management of persons with traumatic brain injury is yet to be seen. Practitioners should remain open to treatment strategies such as TCM that potentially assist their patients' recovery and/or function and commensurately advocate for these areas of intervention to be more critically assessed through high quality controlled research studies.

ACKNOWLEDGEMENTS

We would like to thank Qu Yun, O.M.D. at Department of Rehabilitation Medicine, School of Medicine, Sichuan University in China for his help, suggestions and comments.

References

1. Hang Jie. Management of intracranial bleeding comatose patients with Xing-Nao-Jing intravenous injection, 25 cases clinical controlled study. *J Jiang-Xi-Zhong-Yi-Yao*. 2001, Dec. 32(6), 11.

2. Zhang Dongmei, Jin Beizi, Xiao Dexin. Clinical observation on diabetic comatose management with Xing-Nao-Jing injection. *J Zhong-Guo-Zhong-Yi-Ji-Zheng*, 2001, Oct. 10(5), 277.

3. Wu Yuebing, Qiu Jiansi. Case controlled study of management of 60 acute virus encephalitis patients with Xing-Nao-Jing injection. *J Zhong-Guo-Zhong-Xi-Yi Emergent Medicine*. 2000, Sept. 7(5), 272–74.

4. Dore S. Goto S. Sampei K. Blackshaw S. Hester LD. Ingi T. Sawa A. Traystman RJ. Koehler RC. Snyder SH. Heme oxygenase-2 acts to prevent neuronal death in brain cultures and following transient cerebral ischemia. *Neuroscience*. 2000;99(4):587–92.

5. Dore S. Snyder SH. Neuroprotective action of bilirubin against oxidative stress in primary hippocampal cultures. *Annals of the New York Academy of Sciences*. 1999;890:167–72.

6. Van Bergen P. Rauhala P. Spooner CM. Chiueh CC. Hemoglobin and iron-evoked oxidative stress in the brain:protection by bile pigments, manganese and S-nitrosoglutathione. *Free Radical Research*. 1999 Dec. 31(6):631–40.

7. Rodrigues CM. Sola S. Nan Z. Castro RE. Ribeiro PS. Low WC. Steer CJ. Tauroursodeoxycholic acid reduces apoptosis and protects against neurological injury after acute hemorrhagic stroke in rats. *Proceedings of the National Academy of Sciences of the United States of America*. 2003 May 13, 100(10):6087–92.

8. Liang Wei, Clinical study on acupuncture management of traumatic brain injury with aphasia, 24 case control study report. *Journal of New Chinese Medicine/Xin ZhongYi*, 2000;52(12) 42.

9. Kano Y. Takaguchi S. Nohno T. Hiragami F. Kawamura K. Iwama MK. Miyamoto K. Takehara M. Chinese medicine induces neurite outgrowth in PC12 mutant cells incapable of differentiation. *American Journal of Chinese Medicine*. 2002;30(2–3):287–95.

10. Jung HJ. Park HJ. Kim RG. Shin KM. Ha J. Choi JW. Kim HJ. Lee YS. Lee KT. In vivo anti-inflammatory and antinociceptive effects of liriodendrin isolated from the stem bark of Acanthopanax senticosus. *Planta Medica*. 2003 Jul. 69(7):610–6.

11. Yokozawa T. Rhyu DY. Chen CP. Protective effects of Acanthopanax Radix extract against endotoxemia induced by lipopolysaccharide. *Phytotherapy Research*. 2003 Apr. 17(4):353–7.

12. Fujikawa T. Soya H. Hibasami H. Kawashima H. Takeda H. Nishibe S. Nakashima K. Effect of Acanthopanax senticosus Harms on biogenic monoamine levels in the rat brain. *Phytotherapy Research*. 2002 Aug. 16(5):474–8.

13. Shi Ji, zhao Guangfu, Xie kejun:Study on management of subdual hemorrhage patients with Yi-qi-hua-yu. *Research Report of Nanjing University of Traditional Chinese Medicine*, 1986.

14. Huang Ting et al. Clinical studies on Bu-Yang-Huan-Wu Decoction on the Changes in hypothalamus-pituitary-thyroid axis in patients of cerebral infarction. *Zhejiang J Integrated Traditional Chinese and Western Medicine*. 2000;10(5) 213.

15. Liu Zhilong et al. Effect of Buyang Huanwu Decoction on neural cell apoptosis after cerebral ischemia in gerbils and tis mechanism. *J Guangzhou University of Traditional Chinese Medicine*. 2000;17(4):703.

16. Jin J. Inhibitory effect of taohong siwu decoction on collagen crosslinking, hyaluronic acid cleavaging and lipid peroxidation. *China J Chinese Materia Medica*. 1994 Nov. 19(11):680–3.

17. Sinclair S. Chinese herbs:a clinical review of Astragalus, Ligusticum, and Schizandrae. *Alternative Medicine Review*. 1998 Oct. 3(5):338–44.

18. Peng Z. Zhang Z. Xu Y. Effect of Angelica sinensis injection on CD11c and CD14 expression in alveolar macrophage membrane of chronic bronchitis patients. *Chinese J Integrated Traditional & Western Medicine*. 1999 May. 19(5):282–5.

19. Jin R. Zhang X. Chen C. Sun Z. Shen Y. Liu D. Hu Z. Studies on pharmacological junctions of hairy root of Astragalus membranaceus. *China J Chinese Materia Medica*. 1999 Oct. 24(10):619–21.

20. Li M. Handa S. Ikeda Y. Goto S. Specific inhibiting characteristics of tetramethylpyrazine, one of the active ingredients of the Chinese herbal medicine 'Chuanxiong,' on platelet thrombus formation under high shear rates. *Thrombosis Research*. 2001 Oct 1. 104(1):15–28.

21. Chen KJ. Chen K. Ischemic stroke treated with Ligusticum chuanxiong. *Chinese Medical Journal*. 1992 Oct.105(10):870–3.

22. Kuang PG. Zhou XF. Zhang FY. Lang SY. Yang ZL. Cerebral infarction improved by safflower treatment. *American J Chinese Medicine*. 1983;11(1–4):62–8.

23. Kanehira T. Takekoshi S. Nagata H. Osamura RY. Homma T. Kinobeon A as a potent tyrosinase inhibitor from cell culture of safflower:in vitro comparisons of kinobeon A with other putative inhibitors. *Planta Medica*. 2003;69(5):457–9.

24. Shih YH. Wu SL. Chiou WF. Ku HH. Ko TL. Fu YS. Protective effects of tetramethylpyrazine on kainate-induced excitotoxicity in hippocampal culture. *Neuroreport*. 2002 Mar 25. 13(4):515–9.

25. Romano C. Price M. Bai HY. Olney JW. Neuroprotectants in Honghua:glucose attenuates retinal ischemic damage. *Investigative Ophthalmology & Visual Science*. 1993 Jan. 34(1):72–80.

26. Hsieh MT. Cheng SJ. Lin LW. Wang WH. Wu CR. The ameliorating effects of acute and chronic administration of LiuWei Dihuang Wang on learning performance in rodents. *Biological & Pharmaceutical Bulletin*. 2003;26(2):156–61.

27. Wei XL. Studies on learning and memory function-related genes in the hippocampus and the relationship between the cognitive enhancing effect of liuwei dihuang decoction (LW) and gene expression. *Sheng Li Ko Hsueh Chin Chan (Progress in Physiological Sciences)*. 2000 Jul;31(3):227–30.

28. Liu XY. Ang NQ. Effect of Liu Wei Di Huang or Jin Gui Shen Qi Decoction as on adjuvant treatment in small cell lung cancer. *Chinese J Modern Developments in Traditional Medicine*. 1990 Dec; 10(12):720–2.

29. Nie W. Zhang Y. Ru X. Guiding-evaluation of immunomodulating activity of the Liuwei Dihuang Decoction during the stepwise fractionation. *Chinese J Integrated Traditional & Western Medicine*. 1998 May;18(5):287–9.

30. Yang S. Zhang YX. Lu XD. Study on immunomodulating mechanism of the active fraction of liuwei dihuang decoction. *Chinese J Integrated Traditional & Western Medicine* 2001 Feb. 21(2): 119–22.

31. Fang J. Zhang YX. Ru XB. Wei XL. Effect of liuwei dihuang decoction, on the cytokine expression in splenocytes in AA rats. *China J Chinese Materia Medica*. 2001 Feb;26(2):128–31.

32. Shen JJ. Lin CJ. Huang JL. Hsieh KH. Kuo ML. The effect of liuwei-di-huang wan on cytokine gene expression from human peripheral blood lymphocytes. *American J Chinese Medicine*. 2003;31(2):247–57.

33. Kim JS. Na CS. Pak SC. Kim YG. Effects of yukmi, an herbal formula, on the liver of senescence accelerated mice (SAM) exposed to oxidative stress. *American J Chinese Medicine*. 2000;28(3–4): 343–50.

34. Lee SC. Tsai CC. Chen JC. Lin JG. Lin CC. Hu ML. Lu S. Effects of "Chinese yam" on hepato-nephrotoxicity of acetaminophen in rats. *Acta Pharmacologica Sinica*. 2002 Jun. 23(6):503–8.

35. Cui Y. Yan ZH. Hou SL. Chang ZF. Intelligence enhancement of radix Rehmanniae praeparata and some comments on its research. *China J Chinese Materia Medica.* 2002 Jun. 27(6):404–6.

36. Hsieh CL. Tang NY. Chiang SY. Hsieh CT. Lin JG. Anticonvulsive and free radical scavenging actions of two herbs, Uncaria rhynchophylla (MIQ) Jack and Gastrodia elata Bl., in kainic acid-treated rats. *Life Sciences.* 1999;65(20):2071–82.

37. Huang ZL. Recent developments in pharmacological study and clinical application of Gastrodia elata in China. *Chinese J Modern Developments in Traditional Medicine.* 1985 Apr. 5(4):251–4.

38. Ha JH. Shin SM. Lee SK. Kim JS. Shin US. Huh K. Kim JA. Yong CS. Lee NJ. Lee DU. In vitro effects of hydroxybenzaldehydes from Gastrodia elata and their analogues on GABAergic neurotransmission, and a structure-activity correlation. *Planta Medica.* 2001 Dec. 67(9):877–80.

39. Kim HJ. Moon KD. Oh SY. Kim SP. Lee SR. Ether fraction of methanol extracts of Gastrodia elata, a traditional medicinal herb, protects against kainic acid-induced neuronal damage in the mouse hippocampus. *Neuroscience Letters.* 2001 Nov. 314(1–2): 65–8.

40. Hsieh CL. Chang CH. Chiang SY. Li TC. Tang NY. Pon CZ. Hsieh CT. Lin JG. Anticonvulsive and free radical scavenging activities of vanillyl alcohol in ferric chloride-induced epileptic seizures in Sprague-Dawley rats. *Life Sciences.* 2000;67(10):1185–95.

41. Hsieh CL. Chiang SY. Cheng KS. Lin YH. Tang NY. Lee CJ. Pon CZ. Hsieh CT. Anticonvulsive and free radical scavenging activities of Gastrodia elata Bl. in kainic acid-treated rats. *American Journal of Chinese Medicine.* 2001;29(2):331–41.

42. Hsieh MT. Wu CR. Chen CF. Gastrodin and p-hydroxybenzyl alcohol facilitate memory consolidation and retrieval, but not acquisition, on the passive avoidance task in rats. *J Ethnopharmacology.* 1997 Mar. 56(1):45–54.

43. Hsieh MT. Peng WH. Wu CR. Wang WH. The ameliorating effects of the cognitive-enhancing Chinese herbs on scopolamine-induced amnesia in rats. *Phytotherapy Research.* 2000 Aug; 14(5): 375–7.

44. Wu CR. Hsieh MT. Huang SC. Peng WH. Chang YS. Chen CF. Effects of Gastrodia elata and its active constituents on scopolamine-induced amnesia in rats. *Planta Medica.* 1996 Aug. 62(4):317–21.

45. Wang SP. Liu XM. Shang WF. Song J. Yu SR. Sun SM. Effect of Gastrodia on rotation induced motion sickness in mice. *Hangtian Yixue Yu Yixue Gongcheng/Space Medicine & Medical Engineering.* 1999 Oct. 12(5):342–5.

46. Tang W. Clinical observation on scalp acupuncture treatment in 50 cases of headache. *Chinese Medicine.* 2002;22(3):190–2.

47. Nakazawa H. Averil A. Scalp acupuncture. *Physical Medicine & Rehabilitation Clinics of North America.* 1999;10(3):555–62.

48. Li J. Xiao J. Clinical study on effect of scalp-acupuncture in treating acute cerebral hemorrhage. *Chinese Journal of Integrated Traditional & Western Medicine.* 1999;19(4):203–5.

*F*urther *R*eading

Tieh-Tao Teng (ed.). *Practical Diagnosis in Traditional Chinese Medicine.* Edinburgh: Churchill Livingstone 1999.

Cheng Xinnong (ed.). Chines Acupuncture and Moxibustion (Revised Edition). Chicago: Foreign Language Press 2002.

Deadman P, Al-Khafaji M, Baker K. A manual of acupuncture. Ann Arbor, MI: Cushing Malloy; 1998.

Zhu Mingqing. Zhu's Scalp Acupuncture. Hong Kong: Eight Dragons Publishing. 1992.

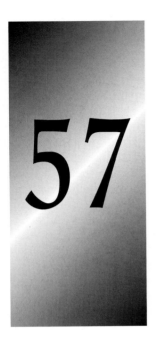

57 Complementary and Alternative Medicine

Jacinta McElligott, Alan M. Davis,
Jeffrey S. Hecht, Sunil Kothari,
John A. Muenz, Jr., Gary G. Wang

In the mid-1800's, medical and health care in the United States included a rich mixture of many different health care practices and philosophies from various cultures around the world. The introduction of the research control trial (RCT) and development of the scientific methodology and rigor which allowed for the proof of the efficiency of an intervention resulted in an explosion of effective medical treatments in the latter part of the nineteenth century. This successful biomedical approach continues to dominate the practice of medicine in western societies today. Traditional practices, although based on thousands of years of human experience, are now considered "complementary" or "alternative" therapies. Despite the predominance of the modern biomedical approach to medical practices the use of complementary and alternative medical practitioners in the United States and other Western societies continues to grow. Patients with brain injury may be particularly likely to seek treatment through CAM practitioners especially when there is a lack of effective treatment for many chronic impairments and symptoms associated with brain injury. The development of the research infrastructure, including centers of study and evidence-based scientific exploration has resulted in a growing body of literature related to the practices of CAM.

The purpose of this chapter is to explore the evolution of the modern biomedical approach to medicine from traditional to the scientific. We discuss the application and implications of the growing consumer use of CAM as it pertains to our current medical and rehabilitation management of patients with brain injury. We contend that CAM interventions can be most appropriately and successfully integrated into rehabilitation management of brain injury with the development of the scientific evidence to support such practices. We also discuss CAM interventions which may be of special interest to patients with brain injury along with the availability and accessible research literature relative to the integration of CAM into evidence-based practice.

Complementary and alternative therapy (CAM) is defined as the use and practice of therapies or diagnostic techniques that are not part of the current Western health care system. It was not until the latter part of the nineteenth century that the scientific research and rigor which forms the foundation of the modern biomedical approach to medical practice was introduced. With the success and preferential development and emphasis on the biomedical approach, traditional practices, often based on thousands of years of human experience may have been inadvertently left behind. Consider for example Ayurveda, practiced throughout the Indian subcontinent for more than 7000 years. Ayurveda promotes (1) an integrated approach to the prevention and treatment of disease with a healthy lifestyle of diet, herbs, exercise and yoga. Another of Asia's contributions to alternative medicine is Bencao Gangmu which was published during the Ming dynasty in China (1552–1558) (1). This text, by Li Shi-Zhen, lists 1,892 medical substances and contains more than 1,000 illustrations and 10,000 detailed descriptions. Chinese knowledge of botanic medicine dates back to 3,000 years B.C. with the discovery of Ma Huang, used as a stimulant and for respiratory afflictions. The active ingredient in Ma Huang was subsequently identified as ephedrine (1).

The modern biomedical approach to medical practice is based on an understanding of the pathophysiology of disease and scientific proof of the efficacy of an intervention. Some believe that this approach to medicine was established in the 2nd century AD by Galen, a Greek physician (1). Galen published a guide to the evaluation and treatment of patients which focused on anatomical knowledge and the use of visual and physical objectivity (1). In the 1800's, scholars in China also sought to move away from speculation and root their studies in "hard facts" (2) by practicing "Kaozhang" translated "practicing evidential research."

A landmark in the evolution of evidential research was the development of the randomized controlled trial. When James Lind (1716–1794) (3) was appointed as a ship's surgeon in Britain, scurvy was a crippling and prevalent disease among sailors. In his meticulous observations Lind included a simple account of what may have been the first prospective randomized controlled trial (RCT) ever undertaken in humans. With their full cooperation, Lind randomized sailors afflicted with scurvy into separate groups, each group receiving a different mode of treatment thought efficacious at that time. The results of the experiment were simply stated, "of the two men who had received 2 oranges and 1 lemon daily, one was fit for duty at the end of 6 days and one recovered to the point of attending the rest of the sick patients in the other groups". With this one concise clinical experiment Lind established the clear superiority of citrus fruits above all other supposed antiscorbotic remedies. Lind's work ultimately led to a government ordinance requiring the provision of citrus fruits to all sailors which in turn led to virtual eradication of this disease. Subsequently the continued systematic development of the scientific rigor which was so successful in proving the efficacy of interventions resulted in an explosion of effective preventative, diagnostic and therapeutic interventions. In medical education a report by Abraham Flexner early in the 20th century ultimately led to the disproportionate funding and development of medical schools which trained their students in the biomedical approach.

Despite the success and preferential development of the biomedical approach, patients in the United States and other Western societies are seeking treatment from traditional and alternative medical practitioners in growing numbers. Eisenberg et al. (4) performed a survey which documented the expanding use of CAM interventions by American Families. This survey identified an increase in the use of CAM from 33.8% of families in 1990 to 42.1% in 1997 (4). Extrapolating from the survey results the author's suggested a 47.3% increase in visits to alternative medicine practitioners, 427 million in 1990 to 629 million visits in 1997. Visits to alternative practitioners exceeded total visits to all U.S. primary care physicians with estimated expenditures for alternative medicine services in at $21.2 billion. CAM therapies were sought both for the maintenance of health and the prevention and treatment of illness. For conditions most pertinent to brain injury CAM interventions were sought for headache, neck problems, insomnia, depression and anxiety. An estimated 15 million adults in 1997 took prescription medications concurrently with herbal remedies and high dose megavitamins and less than 40% of patients disclosed this to their physicians (4).

Physicians attitude towards CAM was evaluated in a survey in 1997 by Sikand et al. (5). This survey was mailed to the fellows of the Michigan Chapter of the American Academy of Pediatrics (5). The majority of pediatricians responding believed a small percentage of their patients were seeking alternatives to conventional medicine. In addition, half of the physicians responding would consider referring patients for CAM, and most were interested in continuing medical education on CAM (5). In 1999 Spencer et al. reported that 63 US medical schools were offering courses and electives in CAM(6) however CAM therapies remained largely outside of most conventional medical school curriculums. The increasing use of CAM led to an awareness of the need for further research into CAM and may have prompted Congress to establish the Office of Alternative Medicine (OAM) at the National Institute of Health (6). Funds were appropriated to establish 11 centers of study and with the development of these centers the literature devoted to CAM has expanded and the number of research CAM databases has grown (6). Subsequently the World Health Organization designated the OAM as a collaborating center for traditional medicine (6).

There are inherent differences in the biomedical and CAM approach to medical practice. CAM interventions are often based on a philosophy and a holistic approach and often rely on verbal reports to evaluate effectiveness. Recognizing these fundamental differences Katz et al. (7) proposed a method of evidence mapping to evaluate the strength of the evidence in CAM. Evidence mapping systematically organizes the evidence available pertaining to a broad topic such as CAM. The breadth, depth, methodology and overall quality of pertinent evidence are characterized. Evidence mapping seeks to be broadly inclusive, performs abstractions and detailed assessments including systematic reviews and meta-analysis. The study objectives included, mapping the evidence underlying

CAM, identifying high priority areas of deficient evidence and conducting pilot studies in the areas where evidence is sparse. With this method of evidence mapping Katz et al. identified over 4,000 papers distributed to over 207 priority health care areas. Of conditions most pertinent to BI Katz et al. identified 7 RCT's relating to the use of CAM interventions in headache and 15 for the use of CAM in neck pain. Depression was considered one of the top 25 priority health care areas and 11 RCT were devoted to the study of relaxation and depression. There were a total of 112 studies in the use of vitamins and depression of which 41 were RCT. Fatigue was also included in the top 25 priority health care areas and 2 RCT were identified in the use of herbs for fatigue.

In a method similar to evidence mapping, consensus conferences draw from a broad body of experts to evaluate the evidence of therapeutic interventions, for example the NIH and the OAM sponsored a consensus conference evaluating the quality of research assessing the efficacy of acupuncture, unfortunately this conference concluded that generally the quality of the evidence was low with few well-designed studies assessing efficacy of acupuncture (8).

The development of research centers and internet access to electronic research databases set the stage for Gordan Guyatt at McMaster University in Canada to propose a paradigm shift in health care called evidence based medicine (EBM) (9). EBM is defined as the integration of best research evidence with clinical expertise and patient values. The agency for health care policy research (AHCPR) has sponsored several programs closely identified with evidence-based medicine in the United States (10). The Medical Treatment Effectiveness Program funds research on the efficacy, cost effectiveness, and appropriateness of clinical interventions. The AHPCR supports 12 Evidence Based Practice Centers, which include a mixture of academic centers and private organizations with national and international reputations for their work on systematic reviews, meta-analyses, and technology assessments. Several centers are devoted to complementary and alternative medicine including the following: Center for Alternative Medicine Research in Asthma and Immunology at the University of California at Davis: Center for Addiction and Alternative Medicine Research at the University of Minnesota: Complementary and Alternative medicine program in aging at Stanford University (10).

The Cochrane collaboration uses an evidence based approach including a registry of randomized control trials and systematic reviews. Systematic reviews critically appraise the qualitative aspects of the research literature and the strength of the evidence to support a particular intervention. Within the Cochrane database there is a complementary therapy research section. The Database of Abstracts of Reviews of Effectiveness (DARE) (11) published, in 2003, a systematic review of randomized control trials of complementary/alternative therapies in the treatment of tension-type and cervicogenic headache. Two reviewers used an 18-item quality protocol for adult headache sufferers. The participants in most studies were patients with tension type headache. A minority of patients suffered from cervicogenic or post-traumatic headache. Of the studies, which received a high quality, 1 RCT on the use of homeotherapy in 98 patients found no difference in efficacy of the treatments provided. One Research controlled trial (RCT) including 57 subjects found that Tiger Balm and paracetamol produced significantly greater pain relief for one episode of headache.

EBM has now been incorporated throughout health care curriculums and for clinicians trained in the biomedical approach, evidence based medicine is the safest and most effective means of incorporating the research available in complementary and alternative medicine into conventional clinical practice. EBM stresses the need for the clinician to examine the available information, or lack of information, from clinical research and to critically analyze the literature and incorporate the results of such analysis into clinical practice including the use of CAM. The expansion in the availability of health sciences electronic databases and libraries has supported the access and availability of pertinent research on CAM in real time to clinicians. The OAM, the creation of specialized centers and databases of systematic reviews of best evidence allows clinicians rapid access to concise summaries and evaluations of the evidence to support the therapeutic and diagnostic practices of CAM. See (Table 57-1) for electronic databases which contain literature applicable to CAM.

In the following sections of this chapter we explore some of the CAM techniques in common use in the US from a historical and traditional perspective, as well as the available research evidence to support the CAM practice especially as applicable to patients with brain injury.

HOMEOPATHY AND NATUROPATHY

Homeopathy is a 200-year-old therapeutic system that uses small doses of various substances to stimulate self-regulating and self-healing processes (12). Of the nearly 2.5 million patients using CAM in the United States in 1997 approximately 3.4% of patients used homeopathy and 0.7 % used naturopathy (13). Homeopathy remains one of the most controversial CAM's. *Similia similibus curentur* or, treating "like with like" is the basis of homeopathy. Homeopathists believe that patients complaining of particular symptoms can be cured with substances that can produce the same symptoms in healthy individuals. In addition to matching the symptoms of the disease, a homeopathist will select remedies based on the constitutional factors of the individual patient such as the patients' psychological state, environmental reactions, and habitus. Of the large number

TABLE 57-1
Evidence Based Databases and CAM

- The Cochrane Library: http://www.cochrane.org/index0.htm
  - Cochrane Central Register of Controlled Trials:
  - Cochrane Database of Systematic Reviews:
  - The Database of Abstracts of Reviews of Effects (DARE)

  Published by Wiley InterScience with new and updated Cochrane Reviews every three months.
- ACP Journal Club *http://www.acpjc.org/.*
- InfoPOEMS/InfoRetriever (*http://www.infopoems.com/*)
- PubMed (*http://www.ncbi.nlm.nih.gov/entrez/query.fcg*i searchers can apply the limit "Complementary Medicine"**
- Bandolier *http://www.jr2.ox.ac.uk/bandolier/booth/booths/altmed.html* **
- MD Consult-First Consult (*http://www.mdconsult.com/offers/standard.html*).
- EMBASE (*http://www.embase.com/*).
  - Alt HealthWatch (via EBSCOhost). *http://www.epnet.com/academic/althw.asp* MANTIS (see *http://www.healthindex.com/MANTISDatabaseOverview.html*) Natural Standard (see *http://www.naturalstandard.com/*)

- The TRIP Database (see http://www.tripdatabase.com/)
- AMED – Allied and Complementary Medicine Database (produced by the Health Care Information Service of the British Library) *http://www.bl.uk/collections/health/amed.html#net*
- Herbal database *http://www.herbmed.org/*: an interactive, electronic herbal database – provides hyperlinked access to the scientific data underlying the use of herbs for health. Evidence-based information resource provided by the nonprofit Alternative Medicine Foundation, Inc.

** available without subscription.

of homeopathic medicines which have been described, approximately 200 are in regular use (14) and about 60% of plant origin. Animal products, minerals, chemical salts, and disease products also may be used. Homeopathists believe that remedies retain biological activity if they are serially diluted and agitated between each dilution. The dilution most frequently used is designated "6c", which is a 10^{-12} dilution of the original "mother tincture". It is likely that a 6c dilution will contain a few molecules of the initial substance. These dilutions are said to produce effects even when diluted beyond Avogadro's number in which no original molecules of the starting substance remain. Many scientists believe that homoeopathy violates natural laws and thus any effect must be a placebo effect (15). However, because of the high dilution, homeopathy appears to be very safe, which is an important motivating factor amongst its patients. The public's belief in the effectiveness of homoeopathy is widespread (16). In the United States, patients who seek homeopathic care are more affluent and younger (17). As with other diseases and syndromes, the effectiveness of homeopathy for brain injury (BI) is quite questionable and controversial. A small pilot research study suggested that homeopathy is efficacious for certain symptoms related to brain injury such as headache (18, 19). Actually, there is insufficient evidence to show that homoeopathy is clearly efficacious for any single clinical condition. Reviews on homeopathic clinical trials have found that the majority of available studies have reported some positive results but the evidence is not convincing (20, 21).

There is no concise history of naturopathic medicine since the development of naturopathy has been strongly influenced by various cultures and religions and is therefore not a single discipline. Naturopathy and conventional medicine hold certain principles in common. Both emphasize disease prevention, patient education, seeking and treating the causes of disease, and both employ the therapeutic potential of the doctor-patient relationship. The basic principle of naturopathy dictates that nature acts powerfully through healing mechanisms in the body and mind to maintain and restore health. Naturopaths work to restore and support these inherent healing systems using non-invasive treatments believed to be in harmony with natural processes such as lifestyle modifications, nutrition, dietetics, herbs, education, and hydrotherapy. In addition, naturopaths may elect to use a variety of healing modalities including acupuncture, botanicals, homeopathy, massage, oriental medicine, and minor surgery (22). In general, naturopaths function as primary care providers with emphasis on prevention, education, and health maintenance (23, 24). It is vital that naturopathy be incorporated into conventional medical practices where treatment which has been proven to be effective is available, for example if a BI patient develops progressive hydrocephalus, a neurosurgical procedure may be appropriate to prevent further neural damage and facilitate functional recovery. It would not be appropriate to over-emphasize natural healing and natural treatment modalities in such situations.

Most of the modalities applied by naturopathy are relatively safe, however, they are not without any risks (25, 26). Naturopathy recommends administering vitamins and herbal medicines widely, even though more clinical trials are necessary to obtain evidence supporting their efficacy. For example, vitamins A, C, and E are considered necessary for protecting tissue free radical damage and are commonly used by naturopaths, however, there is not enough scientific data supporting their necessity in addition to what is consumed in a normal diet (27). Only a small fraction of the thousands of medicinal plants used worldwide have been tested rigorously in randomized controlled trials (28). Several clinical trials have shown that some herbal or natural medicines may have efficacy in BI related symptoms, for instance, use of hypericum perforatum (St. John's wort) for depression and Ginkgo biloba for dementia is supported by a significant amount of evidence (29–31). Results of randomized controlled trials also support the use of kava for anxiety and valerian for insomnia (32, 33). Although evidence for the use of vitamins and amino acids as sole agents for BI related neuropsychological symptoms is not strong, there is intriguing preliminary evidence for the use of folate, tryptophan, and phenylalanine as adjuncts to enhance the effectiveness of conventional antidepressants. Another product S-denosylmethionine seems to have some anti-depressant effects, while omega-3 polyunsaturated fatty acids, particularly docosahexaenoic acid, may have mood-stabilizing effects (34). It is important to note that scientific evidence is still lacking to support that the natural methods serve any therapeutic purpose better than conventional management. The scientific evidence is also lacking regarding what kind of natural foods the body can use for "reconstruction". Rehabilitation physicians should ask their BI patients about the ënatural products' they take and discuss their use in a frank and nonjudgmental manner. The potential side effects and drug-drug interactions should also be considered when initiating naturopathy (35, 36). Patients who seek alternative medical management may do so because the available standard pharmacological treatments are not effective for their symptoms however the evidence on the effectiveness of homeopathy for post BI patient is scant. Some of the natural herbs may have effects to relieve some BI related symptoms; however, there is inadequate evidence to support the natural methods as serving the therapeutic purposes better than conventional. Natural herbs also have potential side effects and may induce drug-herb reactions. Rehabilitation physicians should maintain open communication with their patients to help them understand the potential, sometimes adverse drug -herb interactions and to ensure patients are informed of effective therapies for serious diseases when the evidence for effective conventional therapy exists.

AROMATHERAPY

Aromatherapy is the therapeutic use of aroma-producing oils (essential oils) extracted from organic materials (flowers, leaves, stalks, bark, rind or roots), and utilized as a form of relaxation therapy. The oils are mixed with another substance such as an alcohol, oil, or a lotion, and are then applied to the skin, sprayed in the air, or inhaled. The oils can also be poured into a soaking bath to derive the therapeutic effect. Originating in Europe in the early 1900's, the philosophy behind aroma therapy is that specific plant oils produce aromas and fragrances that stimulate or relax the body, by acting on certain areas within the brain. Fragrances stimulate nasal nerves which then send impulses to the areas of the brain controlling memory and emotion. The oils themselves are thought to interact with the body's own naturally occurring hormones and enzymes to cause changes within autonomically-mediated reflexes, including the blood pressure and pulse. Theory suggests a fragrance stimulates glands to produce analgesic substances, perhaps prostaglandin stimulating substances, effecting relaxation pain relief. Practitioners utilize essential oils to treat physical conditions including inflammation and infection. Aroma therapy is used to treat mental health conditions, including anxiety, depression, and insomnia. Individuals with asthma, respiratory allergies, chronic lung disease, or certain skin allergies should use care participating in aromatherapy. Aromatherapy should be avoided in children under the age of five as their immune systems are not yet competent.

RELAXATION THERAPIES

Meditation is a relaxation therapy where one's attention is directed toward altering one's own state of consciousness. Meditation is a complex mental process involving changes in cognition, sensory perception, affect, hormones, and autonomic activity (37). The health benefits of meditation have been recognized in eastern philosophies for thousands of years with meditation now widely practiced in the west. There are two meditation techniques most commonly used: concentrative and mindful. In concentrative meditation, one focuses on a single image, sound, mantra (words spoken or sung in a pattern), or one's own breathing. Mindful meditation does not focus on a single purpose; rather, one is aware of all thoughts, feelings, sounds or images that pass through one's mind. Meditation usually involves slow regular breathing and quiet sitting, usually for durations of fifteen to twenty minutes. Meditation is used to help treat a wide range of physical and mental problems, including addictive behaviors; immune system diseases; anxiety, stress, depression; high cholesterol and high blood pressure; and, pain. There are believed to be no negative side effects or medical complications of meditation when combined with conventional medical treatment. Meditation alone is not considered appropriate or safe for acute or life-threatening situations.

Transcendental meditation (TM) is unique and fundamentally different from any other type of meditation. It was founded by the Maharishi Mahesh Yogi in 1957. TM is reportedly a very simple technique to learn and is simple to practice. Over 5 million people around the world, almost 200,000 in the United Kingdom, have learned the technique since it was founded in 1957. People learn TM for many reasons, including reducing stress, improving health, and increasing personal effectiveness. The first scientific research on TM was published in 1970, and now there are hundreds of published studies documenting the benefits for mind-body relationships and the environment. TM is neither mind control nor mental discipline. It is not concentration, eastern philosophy, or a way of life, and it does not exert control over breathing or muscles. Hypnosis is a state of focused concentration during which time a person becomes less aware of their immediate surroundings. The use of hypnosis and hypnotherapy have been recognized by the American Medical Association as a valid medical treatment since 1958. Hypnotherapy has been used to treat many physical or psychological conditions, and can be led by a therapist, or it can be taught to individuals, for self-hypnosis. It is thought that during hypnosis, a trancelike state, individuals have a heightened ability to accept suggestions. By suggesting changes in an individual's actions or behavior, an improved physical or mental condition is created. The hypnotherapist's goal is not to control a person, or give the person answers, but rather to help the person solve his or her own problems. Hypnosis does not work for everyone, as a person must be willing to directly focus his or her attention and follow the suggestions of the therapist. Hypnosis is covered in greater detail in another section of this chapter; but it is mentioned here as it is considered a powerful relaxation and self-improvement therapy (38).

Guided Imagery is a relaxation technique where a series of thoughts or suggestions direct a person's imagination toward a relaxed and focused state. An instructor, in person or on recorded media, guides the individual through the process of imagery. Guided imagery is based on the concept that one's mind and body share a unique connection. Using the special senses, one's body seems to respond as though what one is imagining is, indeed, occurring. A relaxed state may be achieved when it is imagined, in full detail. This relaxed state can then aid learning, healing, and performing. Guided imagery can

have one feeling in control of o.ne's emotions and thought processes, which then improves one's attitudes, health, and well-being. Guided imagery is especially useful in promoting relaxation. This relaxed state can lower blood pressure; reduce other stress-related problems, and enables one to reach other goals. Guided imagery is helpful in preparing for athletic events and for performance enhancement, including learning, weight loss, smoking cessation, and pain management. Guided imagery is safe, with no known associated risks, and it can be performed in any circumstance where improved performance is desired.

Autogenic training is a relaxation technique that teaches your body to respond to your own verbal commands. Using certain commands, a practitioner of autogenic training is able to tell their own body to relax, thus controlling breathing, blood pressure, heart rate and temperature. Autogenic training consists of six standard exercises that enable the body to feel relaxed, heavy, and warm. Each exercise has the individual assuming a simple posture, concentrating without goal, and then using visual imagery and verbal cluing to promote relaxation of the body in a specific way. The ultimate goal of autogenic training is to allow the individual to achieve a deep relaxation and stress reduction. Autogenic training is an effective treatment for chronic stress, as well as for other mental and emotional health issues. The mechanism of action is not fully understood, but the effects on the body are measurable. Experts believe that autogenic training works similarly to hypnosis, or self-hypnosis, or biofeedback. Helpful, with problems like generalized anxiety, fatigue, and irritability, some use autogenic training to manage pain, reduce sleep disorders, or increase their resistance to stress. Autogenic training has shown effectiveness in addressing: hyperventilation, asthma, gastrointestinal disorders, cardiovascular irregularities, autonomic dysfunction, headaches, and endocrine disorders. Some individuals have noticed a sharp change in their blood pressure when practicing autogenic training exercises; therefore, it is recommended that individuals with hypotension or hypertension have their individual physician's approval prior to participating in autogenic training. Autogenic training is not recommended for children under the age of five or in individuals with severe mental or emotional disorders (39).

Humor therapy, occasionally known as therapeutic humor, is a relaxation method that uses the power of smiles and laughter to help heal. Therapeutic humor, or humor therapy, simply means finding ways to make others, or yourself, smile and laugh more often. Laughter appears to actually change the brain chemistry, demonstrated on P.E.T. scans, and it may also boost the immune system, as well. Humor allows people to feel in greater control of their situations, can provide special perspective on problems, can allow the release of fear and anger, and it can eliminate stress that can create harm. Commonly, humor is used in the treatment of long-term and chronic diseases, especially those worsened by stress. Humor therapy is valuable as well as a preventative measure aiding the care-partners of people with chronic illness or disease, including stroke, heart attack and brain injury, as they are at high risk of becoming ill themselves.

Music therapy is a relaxation therapy used to promote physical and emotional healing and wellness. Generally, a trained and certified music therapist is able to offer therapy in school, healthcare facility, hospice mental health facility, and private practice setting. Sessions of therapy can involve passive listening, active music making, or both. Research is currently revealing how music works therapeutically on both body and mind. The rhythm and tone of music can stimulate or sedate; has positive effects on heart rate, oxygen saturation, blood pressure, and cognitive ability; and is a healthy, non-verbal mode of self-expression. It is socially connective and expressive; and it enhances verbal expression, fluency, and communication with self and with other individuals. Music therapy calms the body and mind, and with its rhythm, order and function, it organizes the mind. Sometimes, music therapy, combined with movement therapy, such as dance, is utilized as a combined therapy. Long-term and medium term memories appear stimulated with music therapy and it has been shown that newborn premature infants, in intensive care units, are better able to tolerate painful procedures when exposed to music therapy. There are no known risks to music therapy and more information can be obtained by visiting the American Music Therapy Association website at *www.musictherapy.org* (40).

Biofeedback is a relaxation therapy where an individual, utilizing physical and mental exercises, consciously seeks to control a bodily function in a manner normally autonomically regulated. The bodily function (under control) is measured and displayed on monitors, concurrent with the treatment, demonstrating the individual's self-control. Once an individual achieves the desired functional change, monitors flash lights or sound audible signals. Biofeedback is of two types. One device uses electromyography (EMG) as the principal device for measuring relaxation; the other device uses peripheral limb temperature for feedback. Learning biofeedback routinely requires multiple instructor- led sessions to achieve competence. Beyond relaxation, electroencephlographic (EEG) biofeedback has become a widely used alternative treatment for a variety of neurologic and non-neurologic conditions.

ELECTROENCEPHLOGRAPHIC BIOFEEDBACK

EEG biofeedback (also known as neurofeedback or neurotherapy is a widely used alternative treatment for variety of neurologic and in-neurologic and non-neurologic conditions. Based on the same principles as conventional (somatic) biofeedback. EEG biofeedback teaches individuals to modify, through the use of computerized feedback, the electrical activity of their own brains (41). As in other biofeedback modalities, the goal is to make normally unconscious or involuntary bodily processes perceptible so that they can be manipulated consciously. In conventional biofeedback, targets include such somatic processes as muscle tension, heart rate, and skin temperature. In EEG biofeedback, on the other hand, the target processes are certain characteristics of the patient's own EEG, such as frequency, amplitude, or cerebral localization.

During a typical EEG biofeedback session, the patient's brainwaves are recorded through scalp electrodes placed according to the "10–20" system used in traditional EEG recordings. The raw signal is amplified, filtered, and analyzed by specialized software which determines by how much the patient's EEG pattern deviates from target values that are determined ahead of time by the treating clinician. This information, in simplified form, is then communicated to the patient ("feedback"). Usually, the patient is only informed as to whether or not they are reaching their targets. This feedback can be delivered by something as simple as a light or sound that turns on only when patients are in the target range. Newer systems are characterized by more sophisticated and engaging modes of delivering feedback. For instance, one system utilizes a "Pacman" style video game: the "Pacman" character only moves (and thus scores points) when the EEG pattern is in target range. The costs of an EEG biofeedback session can range from $50 to $150 per session and most practitioners recommend an average of 40 (range 20–60) sessions for TBI, resulting in a total average cost of approximately four thousand dollars for a full course of treatment.

There are few, if any, dangerous side effects reported, although practitioners express concern about the possibility of triggering a seizure in patients with a known seizure disorder (this despite the fact that EEG biofeedback is considered a treatment for epilepsy). In general, the reported side effects already assume that EEG biofeedback is efficacious. For instance, practitioners will report concerns about "overshooting" and agitating a person with reduced initiation. Or, conversely, causing someone who is restless and anxious to become too sedated. Obviously, whether or not these side effects actually occur depends on whether EEG biofeedback can actually modify neurological or psychological symptoms.

The proposed mechanism of action of EEG biofeedback rests on two assumptions. First, it is assumed that EEG patterns are correlated with neurological or psychological states. For instance, the EEG of someone with anxiety disorder is thought to differ in predictable ways from the EEG of someone with depression. There is a fair degree of empirical support for this claim (42–44). There is also evidence for the second assumption, namely that individuals can be trained to modify features of their own EEG (45). Thus, one proposed explanation of how EEG biofeedback works is that patients are learning to "normalize" abnormal EEG patterns and that, as these patterns are normalized, the patient's symptoms improve or even resolve completely. Despite the empirical support for the assumptions that underlie this explanation, there is only limited evidence for the efficacy of EEG biofeedback in ameliorating clinical symptoms.

The FDA does not regulate either EEG biofeedback as a treatment modality or the equipment used (except generically as general biofeedback equipment). In addition, there are no local or national standards regulating the training or qualifications of those who provide this treatment. There are two national competency certifications offered by the Biofeedback Certification Institute of America as well as the Neurotherapy and Biofeedback Certification Board; however, these are strictly voluntary. Although anyone can provide these treatments, most providers tend to be professionals licensed in the fields of psychology, medicine, counseling, etc. It is estimated that approximately 3000 clinicians are currently providing EEG biofeedback treatment in the U.S. (46).

In fact, EEG biofeedback has been used for approximately 30 years to treat a variety of psychological conditions (including attention deficit disorders, depression, substance abuse, etc.) (47–52). There is a professional society entirely devoted to EEG biofeedback (International Society for Neuronal Regulation, with approximately 400 members) as well as an EEG Biofeedback Section (with approximately 600 members) in the well established Association for Applied Psychophysiology and Biofeedback. There are textbooks (53, 54) and a professional journal (*Journal of Neurotherapy*) devoted to the field. In addition, there are a growing number of dissertations being written on the topic. Finally, EEG biofeedback has become increasingly visible amongst consumers with TBI and their families. Recently, the Brain Injury Association of America published an article that discussed the modality in their national magazine (55). In addition, the state of Texas passed a law in 2001 mandating that commercial insurers must cover EEG biofeedback services for individuals with TBI (56).

The earliest and strongest evidence for the efficacy of EEG biofeedback is in the treatment of epilepsy. The intuition behind this research was the recognition that epilepsy was, by definition, a condition characterized by disordered electrophysiology. The goal was to teach individuals to modify those aspects of their EEG that most strongly correlated with seizure risk. Since 1972, there have been over 20 articles in peer-reviewed journals reporting on the use of EEG biofeedback to reduce seizure frequency in epilepsy; these have been recently summarized (57). Several of these articles reported the results of trials (including blinded, placebo controlled trials). The results were almost uniformly positive and supported the efficacy of EEG biofeedback in reducing seizure frequency. Indeed, even a recent review article that was skeptical of EEG biofeedback acknowledged its potential role in epilepsy (58).

Unfortunately, as noted by the same reviewer, the evidence of efficacy in the treatment of other neurological or psychological conditions is much more limited. Much of it has been in the form of case reports and case series (59) which have been systematically reviewed in several recent articles (60–65). Recently, however, several trials evaluating the efficacy of EEG biofeedback for attention deficit disorder (66–69), learning disabilities (70, 71), anxiety disorders (72–74), substance abuse (75), and fibromyalgia (76) have been published and all of them supported the efficacy of EEG biofeedback. Unfortunately, these studies all had significant methodological weaknesses that limit the conclusions that can be drawn from them. These weaknesses include: high risk of Type I error due to multiple outcomes and multiple statistical comparisons, small sample sizes, lack of blinded assessments, and lack of adequate controls (including the lack of blinded control groups) (77, 78). Recognizing these methodological flaws the two primary organizations in the field recently assembled a task force on "Methodology and Empirically Supported Treatments" which discussed some of the methodological problems unique to the field of EEG biofeedback (in contrast, for instance, to pharmaceutical research). These authors published a set of standards (79). These recommendations have been echoed by others (80).

With regards to TBI, the published literature is even more sparse. Here, too, all of the published accounts reported positive results. However, the number of articles in the peer-reviewed literature is very small and consists primarily of case reports (81) and case series (82–85) although two prospective trials (86, 87) have recently been published. Moreover, the published reports have almost exclusively involved individuals with mild TBI (88). There have been no published reports on individuals with primarily moderate or severe TBI.

The best designed prospective trial in TBI (89) still shares many of the methodological weaknesses of the studies discussed earlier. In this NIH funded study, 12 subjects with chronic, symptomatic, predominantly mild TBI were randomized into either an active treatment group or a wait-list control group. The treatment consisted of 25 sessions of neurotherapy over 8 weeks. Outcome measures, comprised of symptom rating scales and neuropsychological tests, were administered at baseline, post-treatment, and at three-month follow-up. Once the initial active treatment group finished treatment, the wait-list control underwent the same treatment protocol. At the conclusion of the study, two different types of statistical analyses were performed.

First, the results for the two different groups (active vs control) were compared in a "between-groups" analysis. Subsequently, the results of all subjects were pooled and their pre- and post-treatment outcomes were compared in a "within-groups" analysis. The analyses revealed that subjects experienced improvement in a variety of different domains (8 out of 26 measures in the between-groups analysis and 18 out of 26 measures in the within-groups analysis). The authors concluded that "taken as a whole, the findings of this study are strong enough to identify Flexyx Neurotherapy System as a promising new treatment for TBI, which merits further evaluation" (89).

Despite the promising results, there are several limitations of this study. These include a very small sample size (n=12), heterogeneous sample composition (9 mild and 3 moderate TBI), no mention of issues of subject retention/drop out, lack of a placebo control group, unblinded outcome assessments, no correction for practice effects seen in the neuropsychological measures, and multiple outcomes/statistical testing. The authors of the study recognized many of these weaknesses and correctly point out that many of them are inherent in the exploratory nature of the study. However, they are all issues that any future study must address.

In summary, there is insufficient evidence currently to support the use of EEG biofeedback in the treatment of TBI. However, the evidence of efficacy in other conditions is promising and more studies are clearly warranted. In the meantime, clinicians may choose to discuss this option with their patients, especially when there seem to be no further conventional treatments for relevant applicable symptoms. The relatively low risk and costs associated with EEG biofeedback make EEG biofeedback one of the more attractive options in alternative medicine. However, the clinician should stress the lack of research evidence supporting its use in TBI.

ENERGY-BASED THERAPIES

Bi-Aura therapy is an energy-based therapy which works to seek out, and remove, energy blockages from within the body and from within the body's energy field (aura or bio-field). Eastern medicine has long recognized the known energy and energy flow from the body, also known as Ch'I, Qi, and Prana. Bi-Aura therapy is a therapy in which a practitioner mostly through non-touch Bi-Aura techniques removes imbalances in the body's energy field. These imbalances can occur from trauma, physical and emotional distress, and from physical illness. Bi-Aura therapy seeks to locate energy imbalances, address them, and allow the body to return to health. Bi-Aura therapy can also function to help balance the mental and emotional state of the individual by clearing these bio-field blockages and restoring health. Light therapy, known also as phototherapy, involves the exposure to bright, non-full spectrum light. White light is considered optimal over narrow band wavelengths or ultraviolet light, both of which have been demonstrated to be toxic to skin and internal organs. It is believed that light therapy has an anti-depressant affect, that it may help balance certain brain chemicals, and that it may help reset proper circadian rhythms within the brain. Light therapy of 2,500 to 10,000 lux is generally considered safe and is considered one of the first lines of therapy for seasonal affective depression (SAD), a transient affective disorder affecting many during the cold and shortened daylight periods found in more northern latitudes, in the winter. The side effects of light therapy include visual disturbances with eyestrain, headaches, or skin irritation being the most common (90–92).

Healing touch therapy is an energy-based therapeutic approach to healing. Healing touch influences the energy system that is life itself. By assessing and treating the energy system, the practitioner helps the patient to self heal. Healing touch begins with the thought that people are naturally healthy, and that physical and emotional stress disturbs the natural energy, thereby causing illness. The goal in Healing touch is to restore wholeness through harmony and balance, through the "centered heart". It is non-invasive and economical (93). Healing touch is not considered appropriate or safe for acute life-threatening situations.

Reflexology is a type of energy-based therapy that predates the discovery of the new world. Reflexology presumes that there are specific areas in the hands and the feet, reflex points, that correlate to analogous organ systems in the body. Manipulation of these reflex points is believed to promote mental and physical relaxation-relaxation that then promotes healing. Reflexology is used to treat one of nine principle systems, each representing a major organ system, thereby aligning the harmony of the body. The results of reflexology have reportedly been most impressive in treating musculoskeletal disorders. Reiki is an ancient healing method that uses a hands-on approach to manipulate energy flows throughout the body. Reiki means "universal life energy and practitioners believe that there is an energy force in and around one's body, flowing between the person performing Reiki and the receiver of the treatment. It is thought that Reiki releases your own energy flow and allows your body's own natural healing ability to work. It is completely non-invasive, and the Reiki practitioner will put his or her hands over the body of the recipient at one of the main energy centers, called chakras. Reiki is occasionally utilized to assist sufferers with chronic pain. Some health professionals believe it may be useful in helping to acutely reduce stress and anxiety, which in effect may help to facilitate the natural healing process.

Massage therapy has a long history with many different types developed over centuries. These vary from light touch to very deep massage. Some forms focus on specific points or body areas. The many types and sub-types are beyond the scope of this chapter. Like other consumers of massage therapy, individuals with brain injury seek relief of pain and musculoskeletal symptoms using massage. Massage therapy has been successfully used in a number of post traumatic pain syndromes as well as chronic pain syndromes for patients both with and without brain injury. Massage therapy forms part of most physical therapy interventions for myofascial pain syndrome in conjunction with trigger point injections and stretching (94). Gam et al. (1998) (95) studied the long term effectiveness of massage, exercise, and ultrasound treatments for myofascial pain syndrome using a randomized controlled trial of 67 individuals. They found that exercise and massage, but not ultrasound, resulted in a decreased pain measured by visual analog scale and improved trigger point index scores when followed up six months later. In a survey of individuals with neck or back pain 54% used a complementary health care provider compared to 37% using a conventional provider. Of the 14% choosing massage, 65% found it "very helpful" compared to 27% receiving conventional care (96) (Wolsko 2003). Massage therapy has been shown to be effective in 2 randomized clinical trials as a treatment for chronic low back pain (97). Hernandez-Reif et al. (2001) (98) compared the effectiveness of relaxation therapy to massage therapy in 24 adults with nociceptive back pain of at least 6 months duration or longer. Patients were randomized to either relaxation therapy or 30 minutes of massage twice weekly for 5 weeks. Those individuals receiving massage had less pain, better sleep and higher dopamine and serotonin levels. A meta-analysis of randomized or quasi-randomized research trials for individuals with chronic or sub acute low back pain suggests that massage may be effective for pain relief especially when exercise and education are also included in the treatment plan (99). Massage has been applied to temporomandibular joint dysfunction (TMD). In a survey of complementary and alternative therapy (CAM) use by individuals with TMD, CAM with massage was the most frequently used, the most satisfactory and the most helpful (100).

The literature specific to traumatic brain injury is less substantial. Post-traumatic headache has been shown to respond to cervical massage better than cold packs in one prospective clinically controlled study (101). A case report successfully used massage therapy for hypersexuality after traumatic brain injury (102). In other patient populations massage produces relaxation, decreases anxiety and decreases pain (103). Massage was rated highly in survey of spinal cord injury patients for pain control (104). One mechanism of action that could account for better pain control, decreased anxiety, and the induction of relaxation could be increased parasympathetic activity. Parasympathetic activity can be assessed by analysis of heart rate variability. The respiratory sinus arrhythmia (the mild acceleration and deceleration of heart rate associated with breathing) has a parasympathetic component that can be isolated through analysis of heart rate variability. In a randomized controlled trial evaluating the short term autonomic effects of massage to the back, neck and shoulders on 30 healthy individuals, (105) noted significantly decreased systolic blood pressure and increased parasympathetic activity. Other possible mechanisms producing these effects could be soft tissue mobilization with passive stretching, stimulation of circulation to remove accumulated metabolic products in chronically tense muscles, and the effect of touch itself. In summary, the general literature supports the use of massage to reduce pain and anxiety in patients with post-traumatic pain syndromes such as neck and back pain, temporomandibular dysfunction, and myofascial pain syndrome. There is a smaller quantity of literature supporting its usefulness in other neurologic conditions such as spinal cord injury and stroke. Massage also forms an adjunct to other therapeutic interventions provided by physical therapists, occupational therapists, massage therapists and non-conventional body workers. The literature specific to brain injury is sparse, but for musculoskeletal post traumatic pain syndromes may be generalized to brain injured individuals.

CRANIOSACRAL MANIPULATION

William Garner Sutherland, DO, devised craniosacral manipulation, also known as osteopathy in the cranial Field, starting in 1939. Craniosacral osteopathy is used by osteopathic physicians (DO), allopathic medical doctors (MD), and dentists who attend research conferences and clinical courses presented by the Sutherland Cranial Teaching Foundation and the Cranial Academy. An extensive research bibliography is available from the Cranial Academy (106). A derivation called CranioSacral Therapy has been developed by John Upledger, DO, for massage therapists and other allied professionals who train at the Upledger Institute. Most CST practitioners are exposed to only a simplified version of the method, and chiropractors practice another variation called SacroOccipital Therapy.

After observing a disarticulated skull, Sutherland noted that bone and suture relationships were "beveled like the gills of a fish, indicating respiration" (107). Because this inherent pulsatile movement begins with embryonic development, well before the neonate's first breath of air, he called this phenomenon the Primary Respiratory Mechanism (PRM). The PRM provides the midline organization of structural and functional development. This impulse can be traced from the embryonic plate to the notochord, continuing in the adult as the oscillations between the lamina terminalis in the skull and the phylum terminale at the base of the spinal cord. In the same way that one can take a pulse to assess heart rate and count breaths to determine respiratory rate, one can learn to palpate subtle motions of the skull that correlate clinically with central nervous system motility. Research has only recently corroborated the millimeter-scale movements of the cranial vault that Sutherland identified with his hands (108). Even a cadaver's cranial bones move when typical craniosacral pressure is applied (109). Normal physiologic movements of the cranial vault are described as cycles of flexion and extension, occurring approximately six to fourteen cycles per minute. Sutherland called this the Cranial Rhythmic Impulse (CRI). Restrictions and alternations of the CRI include patterns of torsion, strain, and compression involving the craniofacial bones, membranes, and fluids and extending to the sacrum and the rest of the body. Sutherland stated five principles:

- Inherent motility of the brain and spinal cord
- Rhythmic fluctuation of the cerebrospinal fluid
- Motion of dural membranes
- Articulatory mobility of the cranial bones
- Articulatory mobility of the sacrum between the pelvic ilia.

Practitioners palpate subtle movements of the cranial vault and other structures to assess the cranial rhythmic impulse and to prompt its balancing. From the standpoint of osteopathic philosophy, return of wholeness to the person is the ultimate goal of this therapy. The physiologic effects of this therapy have yet to be clearly elucidated in the medical literature.

Individuals using craniosacral therapy typically seek relief from pain and functional problems such as balance deficits. There is very limited medical literature on craniosacral therapy and only one study of craniosacral therapy for brain injury. Most of the studies look at inter-rater reliability and reproducibility as well as documenting an abnormal cranial rhythm (110). Greenman et al. (1995) studied the cranial rhythmic impulse in 55 patients with traumatic brain injury as part of their assessment and treatment within an outpatient rehabilitation program. The author notes that cranial osteopathy has been empirically shown to be effective in the treatment of patients with traumatic brain injury. The study documents the cranial impulse slower than average with typically encountered cranial strain patterns noted in 97% of the patients. Three of the patients (5%) seized during treatment. Other unlikely adverse reactions reported include mild headache, exacerbation of vertigo, and visceral symptoms. Due to this seizure risk and adverse reactions, consideration of the practitioner and setting where craniosacral manipulation is performed should include preparedness for these events. Both the positive outcomes and adverse side effects suggest that cranial osteopathy affects the autonomic nervous system. Patients who have participated in

this treatment commonly report profound relaxation suggesting a parasympathetic activation. This was evaluated by Robbins (1996) (111) in a randomized controlled study of 6 normal individuals. Each subject underwent four interventions. The active treatments were cranial osteopathy on the head and cranial osteopathy on the sacrum. The control treatments were no touch and light touch to a different area of the body. The order of treatment and controls was randomized and each subject underwent the whole protocol twice with washout periods between interventions. Cranial therapy at the head, as opposed to treatment at the sacrum, produced significantly higher parasympathetic activity than no touch or light touch. In conclusion, despite patient reports of osteopathic cranial therapy and its variations having effectiveness in post traumatic headache, anxiety, and balance deficits, the paucity and quality of research on craniosacral therapy as reviewed by (112) Green (1999) do not support its effectiveness.

SPIRITUAL HEALING

Many individuals respond to illness and impairment by turning to prayer and requests for spiritual healing. Rehabilitation by its very nature seeks to motivate the patient and family members to produce the best possible functional outcome. Traumatic brain injury often occurs at a young age leaving people and their social support network with many years of living within a void replacing their previously functional lives. Maintaining hope in spite of this challenges the best of people. Prayer has been a traditional means of keeping a positive, constructive outlook in the face of despair. Prayer has an extensive literature that was reviewed in Larry Dossey's book *Healing Words* (113). In this book the author demonstrates the positive effect of prayerful intention on health across a number of clinical conditions. He notes that prayer is both non-local and not bound by time. Effective prayer may cross great distances or incredible boundaries. The time of prayer may be unrelated to the time of its need by the individual receiving prayer.

Harold Koenig wrote about spirituality and religion as a practical part of patient care (114). In this excellent book he addresses issues that arise when considering discussing patients' spirituality including boundaries, means to begin the discussion, and possible outcomes based on a review of medical literature. Three simple questionnaires discussed and in use today are the FICA spiritual assessment tool (115), the HOPE questionnaire (116), and the ACP Spiritual History (117). These tools can be used as part of the psychosocial history during patient interviews. Collecting this information serves as a means to let the patient know that their beliefs are valued and may strengthen the therapeutic relationship between the clinician and the patient. If the patient desires, the information is used to refer the patient to the hospital chaplain, a pastoral counselor, a clergy, or another person within their spiritual or religious community. Patients use religion and beliefs to cope with illness. In a review of more than 1200 articles from the 20th century evaluating the association between religion and health, Harold Koenig found that the vast majority of them showed a positive association (118). Medical literature suggests that patients do want to discuss how their spirituality and beliefs play a role in the recovery from illness and relief from impairment (119).

The shaman or community medicine man probably represents the oldest spiritual healing tradition dating back to pre-historic times. Historically the shaman represents a cross-cultural approach to the diagnosis and treatment of illness. This has traditionally been a culturally bound practice. Western contemporary shamanic practitioners may practice without a culturally bound approach. From the practitioner's perspective, the patient with traumatic brain injury who reports an abrupt personality change, a sense of loss or void, and depression suggests a profoundly spiritual component of illness. The practitioner may suggest that the patient had partial soul loss. During the traumatic event, the part of the person's soul fled as a survival mechanism. This would be described as dissociation in psychological terms. Another complaint of depression, loss of personal drive, lack of interest in life, and overall misfortune may be the result of spiritual power loss. The practitioner would approach these spiritual illnesses by attempting to retrieve them and reinstating them to the patient. Individuals with BI who have attempted these spiritual healing approaches have reported return of previous personality, relief of depression, increased sense of life's worth and improved energy level. Herbert Benson (120) proposes that spiritual healing could be a magnification of the placebo effect whereby, because the individual thinks that something will work, it is effective. This may be an appropriate mechanism for those interventions when a person knows something was done to them or for them. It doesn't explain non-local anonymous healing through prayer. Specific spiritual healing techniques besides prayer have little or no voice in the medical literature at present. Spiritual healing addresses the transpersonal element of returning to wellness. Individuals with brain injury commonly express a void in their life. This profound disconnection with the world is addressed through spiritual healing by re-connection to a whole greater than themselves. This affects individuals on a level responding to the questions of what happened to me; why did this happen to me; and does my life have any meaning anymore? By supporting the patient's spiritual and religious beliefs the physician expresses caring and compassion for the patient. In doing so the physician strengthens their relationship to the patient, opens the door to more effectively motivate the patient and their support system, and allows for healing outside of the medical model.

ELECTRICAL AND MAGNETIC THERAPIES

The relevance of magnetism to health care is only recently being explored in a scientific manner as demonstrated by the expansion of magnetic resonance imaging technology over the last twenty years. The history of magnetic and electrical therapy dates back into early recorded medical history. Dr. Frank Krusen, in his classic Physical Medicine and Rehabilitation (121) notes the medical reference to electrical therapy dated to about 2000 years ago:

> Electrotherapy was inaugurated in the reign of the Roman Emperor, Tiberius (14 to 37 CE). Anthero, a freedman, during a walk at the seashore, stepped on a torpedo (an electrified fish) and was thus "freed of gout."

About 50 CE, the physician Scribonius Largus recommended repeated applications of the electric-ray fish for the treatment of headache and neuralgia. In 78 CE, Pedanius Dioscorides recommended shocks from the torpedo fish for intractable headache, a procedure echoed by Galen in 200 CE. Moving away from the fish itself, Aetius in 450 CE recommended that a patient with gout hold a magnet as a treatment. Paracelsus (before 1541 CE) observed that the magnet has "power over the matter of all diseases." It was William Gilbert however who became the father of magnetic therapy, Gilbert published "De Magnete" (Of the Magnet) in 1600 CE and was appointed "chief physician in personal attendance on Queen Elizabeth" the next year. Gilbert also coined the term "electric", derived from the Greek name for amber. Magnets have been used in shoes and wristbands purportedly to help pain. Electromagnetic fields are commonly used to facilitate bone healing in the setting of a non-union, particularly of the tibia or spine. There is also limited research behind advocating magnets for various other medical conditions including wound healing, pain in the limbs, and muscle recovery after exercise (122). Unfortunately numerous claims in the lay literature that magnetism promotes healing are not supported in the available scientific literature to date.

Transcranial magnetic stimulation (TMS) is a widely available, painless and safe technique with a good sensitivity for both corticospinal and corticobulbar tract abnormalities. Owing to the low sensitivity of clinical signs in assessing upper motor neuron (UMN) disorders, there is a need for investigative tools capable of detecting abnormal function of the pyramidal tract. In TMS, an electromagnetic coil is placed on the scalp, high intensity electrical current is rapidly turned on and off in the coil, through the discharge of capacitors, with the stimulation produced by this discharge of electromagnetic capacitors then causing either an increase or a decrease in the excitability of the affected brain structures. TMS may contribute to the diagnosis of motor neuron disorders by reflecting a UMN dysfunction that is not clinically detectable (123–128).

Electrical stimulation was and is still used on the brain by psychiatrists (Electroconvulsive Therapy, ECT) to treat intractable depression. It has been speculated that the pathophysiology of depression may include synaptic hypoactivity of the left prefrontal cortex (129). Recently, transcranial magnetic stimulation (TMS) has been used to treat depression. TMS has been shown to be effective in double-blind, placebo-controlled trial (130, 131) and it was as effective as ECT in another controlled trial (132).

In 2001, a meta-analysis was performed on 12 published and unpublished sham-controlled studies of left or right prefrontal cortical repetitive transcranial magnetic stimulation (rTMS) in the treatment of depression (133). The study compared the decrease in Hamilton Depression Rating Scale (HDRS) achieved with rTMS and sham stimulation. The authors reported that rTMS was statistically superior to sham stimulation in the treatment of depression, showing a moderate to large effect size. However, the clinical significance of these results was modest and the differences in response to rTMS across studies was not clearly explained (134). A study by Triggs and others at the Human Motor Physiology Laboratory of the University of Florida Health Science Center at Gainesville looked for possible cognitive side effects associated with left prefrontal magnetic stimulation. They measured the effects of left prefrontal rapid TMS on mood, cognition, and motor evoked potential threshold in 10 patients with medication-resistant major depression. In a 2-week open trial of left prefrontal rapid TMS off antidepressant medications, scores on the Hamilton Rating Scale for Depression and the Beck Depression Inventory decreased by 41% and 40%, respectively. After resuming pre-TMS antidepressant medication, improvement in mood was still significant at 1 and 3 months later. In their study, TMS had no adverse effects on neuropsychological performance. Interestingly, TMS treatments were associated with significant decreases in motor evoked potential threshold in the 9 of 10 patients who remained off psychotropic medications during the 2-week treatment period (135).

In addition to its reported effect on mood, TMS has been studied in various types of motor pathology. From Italy, Cantello reported a use of TMS in movement disorders. Diseases for which TMS has been studied include Parkinson's disease, corticobasal degeneration, multiple system atrophy, progressive supranuclear palsy, essential tremor, dystonia, Huntington's chorea, myoclonus, the ataxias, Tourette's syndrome, restless legs syndrome, Wilson's disease, Rett syndrome, and stiff-person (stiff man) syndrome (136). In a controlled study from Spain, Gironell reported that TMS over the cerebellum is helpful in the treatment of essential tremor (137). From his Neuro Communication Research laboratory in Danbury, Connecticut, Sandyk has used TMS extensively in Parkinson's disease (138). Various aspects of Parkinson's disease were studied with TMS in a series of experiments conducted by Sandyk. All of Sandyk's studies were reported in the journal he established, the International Journal of Neuroscience. Sandyk reported improvements with weak electromagnetic fields using TMS in PD patients with speech impairments (139–144). Some would argue that his studies are quite controversial because of their publication in non-refereed journals, the weakness of the employed magnetic fields (in picotesla), generalization from case studies of just one subject or a limited number of subjects, and the lack of any attempt at blinding the patient and observer.

Heldmann reported in 2000 that repetitive Peripheral Magnetic Stimulation (RPMS) is useful in the treatment of sensory/right parietal lobe deficits by helping to overcome tactile extinction (145). Reporting from the Technical University of Munich, Germany, they studied 14 patients with lesions in the right-hemisphere and tactile extinction. Patients were randomly allocated to an experimental or a control group. The experimental group received one single RPMS treatment of the left forearm as well as a condition of attentional cueing known to improve visual extinction. The control group, with comparable tactile extinction scores, neither received RPMS nor verbal cueing. In the experimental group RPMS led to a significant reduction of left-sided extinctions in the recognition of different tactual surfaces, but had no effect on ipsilateral errors. They felt that these results showed that sensory inflow is an important modulatory factor in tactile extinction. Moser and others at the University of Iowa found improvements in cognition—reporting that rTMS improved executive functioning (146). In their study, the cognitive effects of active and sham repetitive transcranial magnetic stimulation (rTMS) were examined in 19 middle-aged and elderly patients with refractory depression. Patients received either active (n = 9) or sham (n = 10) rTMS targeted at the anterior portion of the left middle frontal gyrus. Patients in the active rTMS group improved significantly on a test of cognitive flexibility and conceptual tracking (Trail Making Test-B). Roth et al. studied rTMS on knowledge acquisition in 20 normal subjects and found no significant difference in a group of normal subjects treated with 25 minutes of high-frequency left dorsolateral prefrontal rTMS compared to a sham untreated group for any memory acquisition. In the area of motor functioning, Fraser et al. at the University Department of Gastroenterology in Salford, United Kingdom, reported that TMS can improve motor recovery following brain injury and speculated that the mechanism is improved plasticity of the motor cortex (147). They studied a group of acutely dysphagic stroke patients. TMS was used with varying patterns of input. They found that a specific pattern of magnetic stimulation induced the strongest cortical activation (and thus enhanced brain excitability) as measured by functional Magnetic Resonance Imaging (fMRI). This pattern was 5 Hz at 75% of the maximal tolerated intensity for 10 minutes. When this specific pattern of frequency, intensity, and duration of the magnetic stimulus was applied, a greater improvement in swallowing function was seen. This enhanced corticobulbar excitability was increased mainly in the undamaged hemisphere and correlated with recovery.

Others have likewise speculated upon and studied the mechanism of TMS. Conforto reported that TMS speeds central motor conduction time (148). As noted above, one study found that TMS treatments were associated with significant decreases in motor evoked potential threshold (149). Fraser and others wrote that TMS enhances plasticity of the motor cortex (150).

From the Max Planck Institute of Psychiatry in Munich, Keck and others reported that rTMS increases the release of dopamine in the mesolimbic and mesostriatal systems. These authors speculated that this increase in dopaminergic neurotransmission may contribute to the beneficial effects of rTMS in the treatment of affective disorders and Parkinson's disease. From the Montreal Neurological Institute at McGill University, Strafella and others reported that rTMS of the dorsolateral prefrontal cortex, but not the left occipital cortex, in healthy human subjects induces dopamine release in the ipsilateral caudate nucleus (151). They used [(11)C]raclopride and positron emission tomography to measure changes in extracellular dopamine concentration in vivo after repetitive transcranial magnetic stimulation (rTMS). In this study, there were no dopaminergic changes in the putamen, nucleus accumbens, or right caudate.

There is great controversy over the necessary intensity of the magnetic field for clinical effects to be seen. Sandyk uses electromagnetic fields that are so weak that some have questioned their efficacy. For cognitive deficits, he described using two successive transcranial applications, each of 20 minutes duration, with AC pulsed electromagnetic fields of 7.5 *pico*Tesla flux density and frequencies of 5Hz and 7Hz respectively (152). For perceptual deficits, he describes using "AC pulsed electromagnetic fields (EMFs) in the picotesla flux density applied transcranially" (153, 154). For word-fluency deficits, he describes five patients in which he used "electromagnetic fields (EMF) of extremely low intensity (in the picotesla range) and frequency (5–8Hz)" (155). Also using a relatively weak magnetic field, Baker-Price and others studied four subjects with a history of persistent or frequently intermittent

refractory depression following a closed head injury. They applied a "weak" field that was actually 100 times the strength of that used by Sandyk: 10^{-6} vs 10^{-8} to the head of each (156). A one microTesla complex, burst-firing magnetic field was applied to the temporoparietal regions of the head for five 30-minute sessions over five weeks. Their results showed that significant improvement of Beck depression scores, while other emotional and physical parameters did not change. They note that their results "support converging theoretical and empirical evidence that very weak, applied complex magnetic fields whose wave structure and pulse patterns are congruent with groups of neurons within specific regions of brain volume can improve neurocognitive function in human beings." (157) On the other hand, most authors recommend magnetic fields of higher intensity. In most cases, the magnetic field is quite powerful and is in the range of 1–2 Teslas or 10,000 to 20,000 Gauss. This was originally used for brain mapping to test the domains of brain function in the range of 2–3 cycles per second (Hz). More recent machines have used increased frequencies at ranges up to 50 Hz (158). Fraser's study improving dysphagia used 75% maximal tolerated intensity at 5 Hz for 10 min (159).

Since the general technology for magnetic stimulation may not be patented, several companies exist that fabricate the devices. Each has their own patents on their particular coils. Two of the largest include; *Neuronetics. magstim.com, www.neuronetics.com, www.magtim.com* Richards and others noted "there are EM effects on biology that are potentially both harmful and beneficial."(160) Certainly this is true, yet there have been few reported complications with TMS. A literature review revealed one study which reported one case of a "pseudoabsence seizure"(161). As mentioned above, one study specifically looking for complications found TMS had no adverse effects on neuropsychological performance (162). Regarding strength of the electromagnetic field, the FDA had ruled that a limit of 80% of the level, which would cause neuron depolarization, was the maximum levels considered safe for application. It has been suggested that the frequency and variation of the field is more important than its strength. This is an issue that needs to be addressed with further research.

TMS is a new frontier in brain injury and the efficacy remains controversial even in psychiatry (163) and Parkinson's disease—where it has most frequently been studied. Yet reports of its possible effectiveness with low morbidity are encouraging. Patients with brain injury certainly have many of the problems for which TMS has been purported to work: depression, movement disorders, tremor, and parietal lobe syndrome. Nevertheless the high power magnets are expensive and the procedure is a not yet a covered Medicare service, also the technology is not yet widely available. It remains to be seen whether what appears to be promising technology will be proven to be useful in brain injury.

Functional electrical stimulation (FES), sometimes referred to as functional neuromuscular stimulation (FNS) or neuromuscular stimulation (NMS), has both therapeutic and functional purposes, but excludes use in sensory systems. FES is used to stimulate nerves which innervate specific muscle groups to produce an effect similar to muscles in voluntary exercise. The clinical applications of FES in rehabilitation include muscle strengthening, improved range of motion, facilitation and re-education of voluntary motor function in orthotic training, and, inhibition of spasticity. It is believed that there are no absolute contraindications for FES though relative contraindications include individuals with cardiac arrhythmias, pregnancy, wounds that are healing (as stimulating muscle directly under healing tissues may be contraindicated), electrode sensitivity, or congestive heart failure. Occasionally these devices are implanted in the body to provide long-lasting effects, usually with electrodes at, or near, the spinal cord itself. FES is known to benefit paralysis of spasticity (UMN disorders) and is known to improve de-conditioned cardiovascular patients, and can function to facilitate improved limb movement. Neurogenic bowel and bladder have been shown to benefit from FES, as has sexual dysfunction, resulting from spinal cord injury, stroke, MS or closed head injury.

Transcutaneous electrical nerve stimulation (TENS) is a therapy that utilizes electrical current, usually direct current, delivered through electrodes which have been placed on the skin. . TENS is used for pain relief, electrical stimulation of the nerves has been shown to encourage the body to produce endorphins, which function to block the perception of pain, both centrally and peripherally. TENS is performed with a battery powered device, attached to two or four electrodes by small gauge insulated wires, that then conduct the electrical current from the TENS unit to the area of pain. The placement is frequently in a rectangle, surrounding the painful area and the current generated by the device creates a circuit of electrical impulses that, travel along the nerve fibers, reducing pain. The machine can be set for various wavelengths, and frequencies. The individual's physical therapist or physician usually determines the settings. Used most often to treat muscle, joint and bone problems occurring with neuromuscular or musculoskeletal problems, TENS is often utilized for acute or chronic pain including low back pain, neck pain, tendonitis, or bursitis. Though considered generally safe, the machine could cause harm if misused, so TENS use is currently restricted to application only after physician prescription.

Cranial electrical stimulation (CES) is an experimental and an investigational therapy used for the treatment of neuropsychological disorders. CES uses microcurrent, pulsed high frequency carrier waves (15,000 Hz) in a modulating action at low current levels to re-establish optimal neurotransmitter levels and functioning within the injured brain. The foundation of CES therapy is conversion of amino acids to neurotransmitters, improving the quality of neurotransmission (164). Its particular mode of functioning is as a corrective measure for brain dysrhythmia. After placement of electrode clips on each earlobe, the microcurrent pulses are thought to reach the brain via a perineuronal or vascular pathway, coursing via the auditory meatus to the thalamus, the primary center of activity. This cell membrane interaction occurs in a manner which then produces modifications in information transduction (physical energy conversion into nervous signal energy), as is associated with classical second messenger pathways, calcium channels and cyclic AMP (cAMP). Depression and anxiety have been shown to improve with CES use, as have hypertension and headaches. CES works in potentiating the effects of centrally-mediated analgesic drugs like fentanyl, morphine, and dextromoramide, thus aiding in chronic and cancer pain therapy. Neuroepileptic medication use in individuals with BI is decreased with CES therapies and the effects of general brain dysfunction and mood change subsequent to closed head injury appear responsive to CES (165). CES treatments are applied in the early hours, after awakening from sleep, avoiding use within three hours of scheduled sleep, to avoid a stimulative effect. Generally, CES is well tolerated, with no negative effects or major contraindications found for the use of CES, either in the US or in Europe. Rare paradoxical events occur, such as hyperexcitement, though this is unusual.

Electro-crystal therapy is a form of electrical therapy which involves the pulsing of electrical signals, through mineral crystals, in order to greatly amplify the crystals' inherent power. Crystal therapy works with the energy of specific crystals to clear blockages, both in the physical and auric bodies. This therapy uses resonance (one vibrating substance affecting the vibration in another vibrating substance) to re-establish balance in the ill or injured body, thus allowing the body the optimum opportunity of self-healing. Reportedly, after a crystal therapy session by a qualified crystal therapist, a great sense of relaxation and well-being is produced. A session alleviates tension and stress, bringing relief on the mental, emotional and physical plane. A tube of special crystals is placed over the area to be treated; then, the healing qualities of the specific crystals are magnified thousands of times by electrical signals passing through them. Electro-crystal therapy is believed to be beneficial in the treatment of stress and anxiety, headaches, musculoskeletal pain, spine pain, and chronic fatigue syndrome. There are no reported contraindications for the use of electro-crystal therapy and no reported adverse side effects are known.

Electro-homeopathy works according to the belief that there are two vital fluids present in the human body, the lymph system and the blood system. Practitioners believe that any blockages in either of those two systems causes disease and illness. It is believed then that electro-homeopathic medicines can regulate this lymph and blood problem, thereby assisting healing.

ALTERNATIVE MOVEMENT THERAPIES

The Alexander technique and Feldenkrais method are two popular contemporary alternative movement therapies used by individuals with BI. Both techniques are active treatment programs usually learned from a certified practitioner and performed by the patient. Both focus on awareness of movement and the person's inner emotional state associated with it. Frederic Matthias Alexander was a 19th century actor who lost his voice and developed his technique in response to observing how his uncoordinated movements and posture led to his voice loss. Alexander therapy consists of evaluating how common functional activities such as sitting, standing, and walking have muscular tension associated with them and then learning how to avoid triggering the muscular tension with the old pattern of movement. Attention initially focuses the individual's inner sense of movement and then progresses to shifting that sense to discover the release of tension with awareness of proper posture. By inhibiting those postural elements leading to tension the participant is able to recover greater fluidity of movement. No references were identified in a review of the medical literature specific to the application of Alexander technique to brain injury survivors. A randomized controlled clinical trial compared the Alexander technique, massage and no intervention on disability, depression, and attitude toward self, for patients with Parkinson's disease (166). The study showed statistically significant improvement in all three categories only in those patients treated with the Alexander technique.

Moshe Feldenkrais, a physicist, initially developed the Feldenkrais method based on his personal experience with severe knee injury. The therapy has evolved to a series of mat exercises and some touch-guided movement that together raise the awareness of the patient to their own movement patterns. Unlike traditional physical therapy techniques that desire a specific movement pattern as the outcome and train the patient toward the desired pattern, Feldenkrais's method seeks to support change through the deepest inner sense of the client's actual movement. A review of the medical literature did not provide any references specific to the application of the Feldenkrais method to brain injury survivors. The Feldenkrais method was compared to sham intervention for patients with multiple sclerosis using a crossover study design (167). Hand dexterity, anxiety, depression, self-efficacy, multiple sclerosis symptoms, performance, and perceived stress were measured. The Feldenkrais method significantly decreased perceived stress and anxiety, but did not improve self reported function or dexterity. Both the Alexander technique and the Feldenkrais method use awareness based learning rather than repetitive physical exercise. They seek to produce more fluid movement and more choices in movement with greater conscious awareness of the potential outcomes for chosen movement patterns. Traumatic brain injury patients using these therapies report a greater sense of comfort during activity, more solidity in their standing and walking, and fewer complaints related to their neurologic compromise such as vestibular hyper-reactivity and paresis. Based on the types of interventions and exercises applied, the mechanism could be postulated to result from greater body awareness of posture and movement. Through this awareness the individual may inhibit muscular tension, poor posture, and gait disturbances. A review of the medical literature provides no documented effectiveness in brain injury, but a limited literature shows some success in application to other neurologic conditions

HYPERBARIC OXYGEN THERAPY

Hyperbaric oxygen therapy (HBOT) is an established medical therapy for certain conditions and is increasingly being advocated for the treatment of neurological disorders such as cerebral palsy, multiple sclerosis, stroke, and traumatic brain injury (168). HBOT delivers 100% oxygen under pressure, which increases the amount of oxygen dissolved in the blood, thereby increasing the oxygen delivered to the body's tissues. HBOT may also enhance the formation of new blood vessels, decrease inflammation, and increase the volume of blood flow (168, 169).

Treatment sessions occur inside a sealed, pressurized space known as a hyperbaric chamber. The oxygen is delivered either by mask or directly into the chamber. The pressures used are expressed in units of atmospheric pressure and commonly range from 1.5 to 3 atmospheres. The sessions, often referred to as "dives", usually last from 30 to 90 minutes. Many practitioners recommend an average of 100 sessions (range 80–150) for the treatment of chronic, severe BI (168). Because the cost ranges from approximately $200- $400 a session, the total estimated cost of a full course of treatment is approximately twenty five thousand dollars. This amount is never covered by Medicare and rarely by commercial insurance. More the treatment of TBI is not recognized as an conceptual indication for HBOT.

Adverse events can be significant and are related to either the increased pressure or the high concentration of oxygen and include the possibility of seizures, pulmonary injury, and otic trauma. The incidence of seizures is thought to be about 1–2% in the non-neurological population and is related to the duration of treatment as well as the pressures utilized (170). Pulmonary injury includes aspiration, infiltrates, or direct barotrauma and has a reported incidence of 10% to 30 % (170) Otic complications such as pain or rupture of the tympanic membrane have an incidence of 5% to 10% (170) but may be prevented by temporary myringotomies. Additionally there is concern that a prolonged course of HBOT may result in subtle, long-term neurological deficits, although this has not been established (170).

Although the FDA regulates the hyperbaric chambers themselves as medical devices, there are no mandated national or local standards for the staffing or training of personnel. Even less regulation governs free-standing facilities because they are not covered under the regulations for hospitals. These issues are partially being addressed by a recent program of voluntary accreditation administered through the Undersea and Hyperbaric Medical Society. Treatment with HBOT requires a prescription from a physician. However, prescribing HBOT for the treatment of BI would be considered an "off-label" use, since BI, stroke, multiple sclerosis, and cerebral palsy are not FDA approved indications for HBOT. In fact, there are only thirteen FDA approved indications for HBOT among them carbon monoxide poisoning, air embolism, selected wounds, and decompression sickness.

Although many of these conditions are seen treated as HBOT for over 50 years, the use of HBOT has recently become even more common. There are over 500 HBOT centers currently operating in the United States. In addition, there is a major professional organization devoted to HBOT is the Undersea and Hyperbaric Medicine Society, which also publishes "Undersea and Hyperbaric Medicine". This organization, founded in 1967, now has over 2500 members. Board certification is offered by passing a subspecialty examination offered by the American Board of Preventive Medicine. Finally, there are two main textbooks in the field (168, 169). However, these organizations and publications focus almost exclusively on the accepted indications for HBOT and infrequently address the use of HBOT in the treatment of neurological conditions such as brain injury (BI).

The evidence for the efficacy of HBOT in the treatment of TBI, strokes, and cerebral palsy was extensively reviewed recently by the Agency for Healthcare Research and Quality (AHRQ) (170). The most authors of this report also published a separate review specifically addressing the evidence in TBI (171). The conclusions of these reviews were endorsed by the Undersea and Hyperbaric Medicine Society which also conducted their own review of the role of HBOT in the treatment of multiple sclerosis (172). In addition, a review of HBOT as a treatment for BI and stroke was also separately completed by an agency of the government of British Columbia (180). Finally, the Cochrane Database of Systematic Reviews

recently published their own reviews of the HBOT in TBI (174). All together, these reviews evaluated over one hundred papers that met their inclusion criteria.

In general, all of these reviews found that there was little evidence for the efficacy of HBOT for the conditions reviewed. In addition to TBI, the AHRQ report reviewed the role of HBOT in both stroke and cerebral palsy. For both these conditions, there were observational and uncontrolled studies that reported a significant benefit from HBOT. However, there were very few controlled trials (four in stroke and one in cerebral palsy) and none of them were rated better than "fair" by the AHRQ (on a scale of poor, fair, and good). Moreover, none of these trials demonstrated any benefit of HBOT treatment. Despite this, given the methodological limitations of the trials, the report concluded only that there was currently insufficient evidence of efficacy in these conditions (as opposed to evidence of lack of efficacy). The report by the agency of the provincial government of British Columbia reached a similar conclusion. The situation in multiple sclerosis is different to the extent that there have been many more controlled trials in this population (ten) and, with one exception, none demonstrated a benefit for HBOT treatment. Given the weight of the evidence, the review by the Undersea and Hyperbaric Society concluded that HBOT did not appear to be an effective treatment for multiple sclerosis (although they acknowledged that there may be subsets of patients who might benefit, especially with longer treatment periods).

In TBI, there has been only one controlled study in the past twenty five years (175). This trial was in the acute care setting and involved 168 severely brain injured patients randomized to receive either HBOT or standard treatment. The treatments, begun within 24 hours of injury, were 60 minutes in length and at 1.5 atmospheres. They were administered every 8 hours for two weeks or until the patient was either brain dead or could follow simple commands. On average, patients received 21 treatments. After one year, patients who received HBOT treatment had an almost 50% reduction in mortality (17% vs 31%). However, the proportion of those who were dead or severely disabled was unchanged (approximately 50% in each group). Thus, although mortality decreased, the rate of a favorable outcome was unchanged. This study was rated as "fair" by the AHRQ. The only other controlled trial, also in the acute care setting (176) was conducted in 1976. Unlike the later study, it did not find any statistically significant difference between the HBOT and control groups (although there was a trend towards better outcomes in the treatment group). This study was also rated as "fair" by the AHRQ task force. Unfortunately, it is difficult to apply the findings because the study was conducted when the care for TBI was substantially different than it is now.

There were also two uncontrolled acute care trials that reported on clinical endpoints (177, 178). Both reported benefits to HBOT treatment; however, both had serious methodological flaws and were rated as "poor" quality by the task force. The remainder of the studies in acute TBI was all observational studies or case reports. Although promising, most of these studies used intermediate endpoints such as cerebral blood flow, cerebral metabolism, CSF biochemistry, and intracranial pressure (179–184) thereby limiting their clinical applicability.

In chronic TBI, there have been no HBOT trials in the past twenty years. In fact, there are only three case reports and two case series (excluding abstracts or conference proceedings) (185–189). One case series reported a benefit for HBOT but reported only on intermediate outcomes (e.g. measures of cerebral metabolism) (185). The other case series found in evidence of clinical benefit in chronic TBI (186). Of the case reports, one reported a benefit to HBOT treatment but involved a patient only 6 weeks post-injury, thus making it difficult to separate out the effects of natural recovery (187). Another case report involved a patient approximately six months after BI and reported a benefit to HBOT treatment. However, the patient was also receiving rehabilitative intervention, thus making it difficult to separate the contributions of HBOT treatment from that of rehabilitation and natural recovery (188). Finally, one case report noted no benefit of HBOT treatment, but the focus was only on measures of gait and postural stability (189).

The previously published reviews (170–171) agree that there is insufficient evidence to recommend the use of HBOT for the treatment of BI. The Undersea and Hyperbaric Medical Society released a position paper on the use of HBOT for chronic brain injury, traumatic and non-traumatic. This paper concluded that "the weight of the currently available scientific literature is not felt to support an endorsement of HBOT for chronic brain injury" (172). Likewise, the evidence based review by the government of British Columbia also concluded that "the scientific literature as reviewed up until August 2001 does not support the use of hyperbaric oxygen in the treatment of head injury or stroke" (173) . This is in accord with the findings of the AHRQ. In the summary, there is little evidence currently to support the use of HBOT as a treatment for chronic BI, the evidence of benefit in acure BI in more formicity but too there clinical evidence. This situation marked accordingly patients about the use of HBOT more difficult. Indeed, BI clinicians may be facing a difficult dilemma as consumer demand for HBOT increases in the BI community. This increase in demand may be fueled by several different trends including the general population's interest in alternative treatments, the continued lack of many effective treatments for chronic BI, and the aggressive marketing by many HBOT facilities. The fact that most families will have to pay for the treatments themselves (due to lack of coverage of HBOT for BI) further underscores the importance of advising patients and families appropriately. Recently,

guidelines have been developed to help clinicians better address the ethical dilemmas this situation raises (190). In addition to supporting the evidence-based guidelines reviewed here, the authors also emphasize the importance of continued research to establish definitively the role of HBOT in the treatment of BI. Until definitive research is conducted, the authors recommend a full discussion with patients and families regarding the current lack of evidence of benefit as well as the risks involved, including the substantial financial commitment involved.

The use of CAM techniques to treat common associated sequelae of brain injury remains controversial. There is a lack of evidence to date supporting the safety and effectiveness of many CAM interventions. Nevertheless we may anticipate that brain injury survivors and their families will continue to seek CAM interventions to treat the multitude of symptomatic sequelae of brain injury, particularly where conventional medical practices may fail to provide effective relief. While the majority of CAM interventions are relatively safe the risk associated with and potential adverse effects of drug interactions and certain CAM interventions such as HBOT and some electrical therapies can be significant. With the expanding research focus on CAM interventions we anticipate further elucidation of the benefits and risks of CAM interventions and the incorporation of evidence- based CAM into conventional medical practices. It is important for physicians to recognize that their patients may pursue CAM interventions and that knowledge of the potential benefits and risk is essential in order to provide patients with the information they need for effective and safe use of CAM practices within Western health care systems.

*R*eferences

1. Spencer John W, Jacobs Joseph J. *Complementary/Alternative Medicine: An Evidence-Based Approach*. St. Louis. Mosby 1999.
2. Spence, Jonathan D. *Conquest and Consolidation: The Search from Modern China*, 1st edition. WW Norton & Co. 1990.
3. Lind J, *A Treatise on the Scurvy*. London 1772. Editorial comment and handbook.
4. Eisenberg, D M, Davis RB, Ettner SL, Appel S, Wilkey S, Von Rompay, Kessler RC. Trends in alternative medicine use in the United States, 1990–1997: results of a follow-up national survey. *JAMA* 1998;280(18):1569–1575.
5. Sikand A, Laken M. Pediatricians experience with and attitudes toward complementary/alternative medicine. *Arch Pediatr Adolesc Med* 1998;152:1059–1064.
6. Spencer John W, Jacobs Joseph J. *Complementary/Alternative Medicine: An Evidence-Based Approach*. St. Louis. Mosby 1999.
7. Katz D I, Williams A, Girard C, Goodman J, Comerford B, Behrman A, Bracken M B. The evidence base for complementary and alternative medicine: method of evidence mapping with application to CAM. *Alternative Therapies*. July/Aug 2003;9:4.
8. Spencer John W, Jacobs Joseph J. *Complementary/Alternative Medicine: An Evidence-Based Approach*. St. Louis. Mosby 1999.
9. Guyatt G. Evidence-based medicine working group. a new approach to teaching the practice of medicine. *JAMA* 1992; 268:2420–5.
10. Spencer John W, Jacobs Joseph J. *Complementary/Alternative Medicine: An eEvidence-Based Approach*. St. Louis. Mosby 1999.

11. *Database of Abstracts of Reviews of Effectiveness.* University of York. 2003. Volume (1). Ernst E, Rand J I, Barnes J, Stevinson C. Adverse effects profile of herbal antidepressant St. John's Wort (Hypericum perforatum L.) *Eur J Clin Pharmacol* 1998;54:589–594.

12. Brazier NC. Levine MA. Drug-herb interaction among commonly used conventional medicines: a compendium for health care professionals. *American Journal of Therapeutics.* 2003;10(3): 163–9.

13. Boon H. Stewart M. Kenard MA. Guimond J. Visiting family physicians and naturopathic practitioners. Comparing patient-practitioner interactions. *Canadian Family Physician.* 2003;49: 1481–7.

14. Chapman EH. Weintraub RJ. Milburn MA. Pirozzi TO. Woo E. Homeopathic treatment of mild traumatic brain injury: A randomized, double-blind, pacebo-controlled clinical trail. *Journal of Head Trauma Rehabilitation.* 1999;14(6):521–42

15. Cohen MH, Eisenberg DM. Potential physician malpractice liability associated with complementary and integrative medical therapies. *Ann Intern Med* 2002;136:596–603.

16. Dantas F. Rampes H. Do homeopathic medicines provoke adverse effects? A systematic review. *Homoeopathic Journal.* 2000;89 Suppl 1:S35–8.

17. D'Huyvetter K. Cohrssen A. Homeopathy. Primary Care; *Clinics in Office Practice.* 2002;29(2):407–18.

18. Eisenberg DM, Davis RB, Ettner SL, Appel S, Wilkey S, van Rompay M, Kessler RC. Trends in alternative medicine use in the United States, 1990–1997: results of a follow-up national survey. *JAMA* 1998;280:1569–75.

19. Eisenberg DM, Davis RB, Ettner SL, Appel S, Wilkey S, van Rompay M, Kessler RC. Trends in alternative medicine use in the United States, 1990–1997: results of a follow-up national survey. *JAMA* 1998;280:1569–75.

20. Linde, K, Clausius, N, Ramirez, G, Melchart, D, Eitel, F, Hedges, LV, & Jonas, WB: Are the clinical effects of homeopathy all placebo effects? A meta-analysis of randomized, placebo controlled trials. *Lancet* 1997;350:83443.

21. Linde K. Hondras M. Vickers A. ter Riet G. Melchart D. Systematic reviews of complementary therapies - an annotated bibliography. Part 3: homeopathy. *BMC Alternative Medicine.* 2001;1(1):4.

22. Smith MJ. Logan AC. Naturopathy. *Medical Clinics of North America.* 2002 ; 86(1):173–84.

23. Smith MJ. Logan AC. Naturopathy. *Medical Clinics of North America.* 2002 ; 86(1):173–84.

24. Eisenberg DM, Davis RB, Ettner SL, Appel S, Wilkey S, van Rompay M, Kessler RC. Trends in alternative medicine use in the United States, 1990–1997: results of a follow-up national survey. *JAMA* 1998;280:1569–75.

25. Eliopoulos C. Using complementary and alternative therapies wisely. *Geriatric Nursing.* 1999;20(3):139–42.

26. Cohen MH, Eisenberg DM. Potential physician malpractice liability associated with complementary and integrative medical therapies. *Ann Intern Med* 2002;136:596–603.

27. Meyers DG. Maloley PA. Weeks D. Safety of antioxidant vitamins. *Archives of Internal Medicine.* 1996;156(9):925–35.

28. Goldman P. Herbal medicines today and the roots of modern pharmacology. *Annals of Internal Medicine.* 2001;135(8 Pt 1):594–600.

29. Gupta RK. Moller HJ. St. John's Wort. An option for the primary care treatment of depressive patients?. *European Archives of Psychiatry & Clinical Neuroscience.* 2003;253(3):140–8.

30. Fugh-Berman A. Cott JM. Dietary supplements and natural products as psychotherapeutic agents. *Psychosomatic Medicine.* 1999;61(5):712–28.

31. Le Bars PL, Katz MM, Berman N, Itil TM, Freedman AM, Schatzberg AF. A placebo-controlled, double-blind, randomized trial of an extract of Ginkgo biloba for dementia. *JAMA* 1997; 278:1327–32.

32. Lehmann E, Kinzler E, Friedemann J. Efficacy of a special kava extract (Piper methysticum) in patients with states of anxiety, tension, and excitedness of nonmental origin—a double-blind placebo-controlled study of four weeks treatment. *Phytomedicine* 1996;2:113–9.

33. Volz HP, Kieser M. Kava-kava extract WS 1490 versus placebo in anxiety disorders—a randomized placebo-controlled 25-week outpatient trial. *Pharmacopsychiatry* 1997;30:1–5.

34. Fugh-Berman A. Cott JM. Dietary supplements and natural products as psychotherapeutic agents. *Psychosomatic Medicine.* 1999; 61(5):712–28.

35. Miller LG. Herbal medicinals: selected clinical considerations focusing on known or potential drug-herb interactions. *Archives of Internal Medicine.* 1998;158(20):2200–11.

36. Brazier NC. Levine MA. Drug-herb interaction among commonly used conventional medicines: a compendium for health care professionals. *American Journal of Therapeutics.* 2003;10(3):163–9.

37. Newberg AB, Iversen J, The neural basis of the complex mental task of meditation: neural transmitter and neurochemical considerations. *Med Hypotheses* 2003; August; 61 (2):282–91.

38. Vickers A, Zollman C. ABC of complementary medicine: Hypnosis and relaxation therapies. *BMJ,* 319:1346–1349.

39. Davis M, et al. *The Relaxation and Stress Reduction Workbook,* 5th ed., Oakland, CA: New Harbinger, 2000.

40. Larkin M. Music tunes up memory in dementia patients. *Lancet,* 2001;357:47.

41. Evans, J et al. *Quantitative EEG and Neurofeedback* 1999 San Diego: Academic Press.

42. Hughes, J et al. Conventional and quantitative electroencephalography in psychiatry. *Journal of Neuropsychiatry and Clinical Neuroscience* 1999;11(2):190–208.

43. Thornton K. Electrophysiology of the reasons the brain damaged subject can't recall what they hear. *Archives of Clinical Neuropsychology* 2002;17:1–17.

44. Thornton K. The electrophysiological effects of a brain injury on auditory memory functioning: the QEEG correlates of impaired memory. *Archives of Clinical Neuropsychology* 2003; 18:363–78.

45. Evans, J et al. *Quantitative EEG and Neurofeedback* 1999 San Diego: Academic Press.

46. Othmer, Sigfried Personal e-mail communication 2/10/03.

47. Duff J. The usefulness of QEEG and neurotherapy in the assessment and treatment of post-concussion syndrome. *Clinical EEG & Neuroscience* 2004;35(4):198–209.

48. Thatcher, R. EEG operant conditioning (biofeedback) and traumatic brain injury. *Clinical Electroencephalography* 2000;31(1): 38–44.

49. Rosenfeld, J. An EEG biofeedback protocol for affective disorders. *Clinical Electroencephalography* 2000;31(1):7–12.

50. Moore, N. A review of EEG biofeedback treatment of anxiety disorders. *Clinical Electroencephalography* 2000;31(1):1–6.

51. Trudeau, D. The treatment of addictive disorders by brain wave biofeedback: a review and suggestions for future research. *Clinical Electroencephalography* 2000;31(1):13–22.

52. Nash, J. Treatment of attention deficit hyperactivity disorder with neurotherapy. *Clinical Electroencephalography* 2000;31(1): 30–37.

53. Evans, J et al. *Quantitative EEG and Neurofeedback* 1999 San Diego: Academic Press.

54. Thompson, M et al. *The Neurofeedback Book* 2003 AAPB.

55. Thatcher, R. QEEG and traumatic brain injury: present and future. *Brain Injury Source* 1999;3(4):28–32.

56. Texas Department of Insurance Code: Subchapter W, §§21.3101– 21.3105.

57. Sterman, M. Basic concepts and clinical findings in the treatment of seizure disorders with EEG operant conditioning. *Clinical Electroencephalography* 2000;31(1):45–55.

58. Lohr, J et al. Neurotherapy does not qualify as an empirically supported behavioral treatment for psychological disorders. *Behavior Therapist* 2001;24(5):97–104.

59. "Comprehensive Neurofeedback Bibliography" at www.isnr.org.

60. Duff, J. The usefulness of QEEG and neurotherapy in the assessment and treatment of post-concussion syndrome. *Clinical EEG & Neuroscience* 2004;35(4):198–209.

61. Thatcher, R. EEG operant conditioning (biofeedback) and traumatic brain injury. *Clinical Electroencephalography* 2000;31(1): 38–44.

62. Rosenfeld, J. An EEG biofeedback protocol for affective disorders. *Clinical Electroencephalography* 2000;31(1):7–12.

63. Moore, N. A review of EEG biofeedback treatment of anxiety disorders. *Clinical Electroencephalography* 2000;31(1):1–6.

64. Trudeau, D. The treatment of addictive disorders by brain wave biofeedback: a review and suggestions for future research. *Clinical Electroencephalography* 2000;31(1):13–22.

65. Nash, J. Treatment of attention deficit hyperactivity disorder with neurotherapy. *Clinical Electroencephalography* 2000;31(1):30–37.

66. Monastra, V. et al. The effects of stimulant therapy, EEG biofeedback, and parenting style on the primary symptoms of attention deficit/hyperactivity disorder. *Applied Psychophysiology & Biofeedback* 2002;27(4):231–249.

67. Fuch, T. et al. Neurofeedback treatment for attention deficit/hyperactivity disorder in children: a comparison with methylphenidate. *Applied Psychophysiology & Biofeedback* 2003;28(1):1–12.

68. Rossiter, T. et al. A comparison of EEG biofeedback and psychostimulants in treating attention deficit/hyperactivity disorder. *Journal of Neurotherapy* 1995;1(1):48–59.

69. Linden, M. et al. A controlled study of the effects of EEG biofeedback on cognition and behavior of children with attention deficit disorder and learning disabilities. *Biofeedback and Self Regulation* 1996;21:31–49.

70. Linden, M. et al. A controlled study of the effects of EEG biofeedback on cognition and behavior of children with attention deficit disorder and learning disabilities. *Biofeedback and Self Regulation* 1996;21:31–49.

71. Fernandez, T. EEG and behavioral changes following neurofeedback treatment in learning disabled children. *Clinical Electroencephalography* 2003;34(3):145–150.

72. Peniston, E. et al. Alpha-theta brainwave neuro-feedback therapy with vietnam veterans with combat-related post-traumatic stress disorder. *Medical Psychotherapy* 1991;4:47–60.

73. Rice, K. et al. Biofeedback treatments of generalized anxiety disorder: preliminary results. *Biofeedback and Self-Regulation* 1993;18:93–105.

74. Vanathy, S. et al. The efficacy of alpha and theta neurofeedback training in the treatment of generalized anxiety disorder. *Indian Journal of Clinical Psychology* 1998;25:136–143.

75. Peniston, E. et al. Alcoholic personality and alpha-theta brainwave training. *Medical Psychotherapy*,3:37–55.

76. Mueller HH, Donaldson S, Nelson D et al. Treatment of fibromyalgia incorporating EEG-driven stimulation: a clinical outcomes study. *Journal of Clinical Psychology* 2001; 57(7):93–952.

77. Lohr, J. et al. Neurotherapy does not qualify as an empirically supported behavioral treatment for psychological disorders. *Behavior Therapist* 2001;24(5):97–104.

78. Kline, J. et al. A cacophony in the brainwaves: a critical appraisal of neurotherapy for attention-deficit disorders. *The Scientific Review of Mental Health Practice* 2002;1(1):44–54.

79. LaVaque, T. et al. Task force report on methodology and empirically supported treatments. *Applied Psychophysiology and Biofeedback* 2002;27(4):271–281.

80. Nelson, L. Neurotherapy and the challenge of empirical support: a call for a neurotherapy practice research network. *Journal of Neurotherapy* 2003;7(2):53–67.

81. Byers, A. Neurofeedback therapy for a mild head injury. *Journal of Neurotherapy* 1995;22–37.

82. Bounias, M. et al. EEG-neurobiofeedback treatment of patients with brain injury: Part 1: typological classification of clinical syndromes. *Journal of Neurotherapy* 2001;5(4):23–44.

83. Thornton, K. The improvement/rehabilitation of auditory memory functioning with EEG biofeedback. *NeuroRehabilitation* 2002;17:69–80.

84. Thornton, K. Improvement/rehabilitation of memory functioning with neurotherapy/QEEG biofeedback *Journal of Head Trauma Rehabilitation* 2000;15(6):1285–1296.

85. Walker JE, Norman CA, Weber RK. Impact of QEEG guided coherence training for patients with a mild closed head injury. *Journal of Neurotherapy* 6(2):31–43 2002.

86. Keller, I. Neurofeedback therapy of attention deficits in patients with traumatic brain injury. *Journal of Neurotherapy* 2001;5: 19–32 .

87. Schoenberger, N. et al. Flexyx neurotherapy system in the treatment of traumatic brain injury: an initial evaluation. *Journal of Head Trauma Rehabilitation* 2001;16(3):260–274.

88. Duff, J. The usefulness of QEEG and neurotherapy in the assessment and treatment of post-concussion syndrome. *Clinical EEG & Neuroscience* 2004;35(4):198–209.

89. Schoenberger, N. et al. Flexyx neurotherapy system in the treatment of traumatic brain injury: an initial evaluation. *Journal of Head Trauma Rehabilitation* 2001;16(3):260–274.

90. Lam RW, Levitt AJ. Canadian consensus guidelines for the treatment of seasonal affective disorder: A summary of the report of the Canadian consensus Group on SAD. *Canadian Journal of Diagnosis*. Vancouver, BC 2000.

91. Lewy AJ, et al. Morning versus evening light treatment of patients with winter depression. *Archives of General Psychiatry*, 1998; 55(10):890–896.

92. Terman M. et al. A controlled trial of timed bright light and negative air ionization for treatment of winter depression. *Archives of General Psychiatry*, 1998;55(10):875–882.

93. Astin JA, et al. The efficacy of "distant healing": A systematic review of randomized trials. *Annals of Internal Medicine* 2000;132:903–910.

94. Rubin D. Myofascial trigger point syndromes: an approach to management. *Arch Phys Med Rehabil* 1981 Mar; 62(3):107–10.

95. Gam AN, Warming S, Larsen LH, Jensen B, Hoydalsmo O, Allon I, Andersen B, Gotzsche NE, Petersen M, Mathiesen B. Treatment of myofascial trigger-points with ultrasound combined with massage and exercise—a randomised controlled trial. *Pain*. 1998 Jul;77(1):73–9.

96. Wolsko PM, Eisenberg DM, Davis RB, Kessler R, Phillips RS. Patterns and perceptions of care for treatment of back and neck pain: results of a national survey. *Spine*. 2003 Feb 1;28(3):292–7; discussion 298.

97. Cherkin D, Eisenberg D, Sherman KJ et al. Randomized trial comparing traditional Chinese medical acupuncture, therapeutic massage, and self care education for chronic with low back pain. *Arch Intern Med* 161:1081; 2001.

98. Hernandez-Reif M, Field T, Krasnegor J, Theakston H. Lower back pain is reduced and range of motion increased after massage therapy. *Int J Neurosci* 2001;106(3–4):131–45.

99. Furlan AD, Brosseau L, Imamura M, Irvin E. Massage for low-back pain: a systematic review within the framework of the Cochrane Collaboration Back Review Group. *Spine*. 2002 Sep 1; 27(17):1896–910.

100. DeBar LL, Vuckovic N, Schneider J, Ritenbaugh C. Use of complementary and alternative medicine for temporomandibular disorders. *J Orofac Pain*. 2003 Summer;17(3):224–36.

101. Jensen OK, Nielsen FF, Vosmar L. An open study comparing manual therapy with the use of cold packs in the treatment of post-traumatic headache. *Cephalalgia*. 1990 Oct;10(5):241–50.

102. Zencius A, Wesolowski MD, Burke WH, Hough S. Managing hypersexual disorders in brain-injured clients. *Brain Inj* 1990 Apr-Jun;4(2):175–81.

103. Ferrell T, Glick O. The use of therapeutic massage as a nursing intervention to modify anxiety and the perception of cancer pain. *Cancer Nurs* 1993;16:93.

104. Nayak S, The use of complementary and alternative therapies for chronic pain following spinal cord injury: a pilot survey. *J Spinal Cord Med* 2001;24(1):54.

105. Delaney JP, Leong KS, Watkins A, Brodie D. The short-term effects of myofascial trigger point massage therapy on cardiac autonomic tone in healthy subjects. *J Adv Nurs* 2002 Feb;37(4):364–71.

106. King HH, Jr., et al. A bibliography of research related to osteopathy in the cranial field June 1, 1999; version 1. *Cranial Academy Publications*, 1999.

107. Sutherland WG. *The Cranial Bowl*, Freeman Press, 1939.

108. Grietz, D., et al. Pulsatile brain movements and associated hydrodynamics studied by magnetic resonance phase imaging: the Monro-Kellie doctrine revisited. *Radiology*. 1992;34:370–380.

109. Kostopoulos DC, Keramidas G. Changes in elongation of falx cerebri during craniosacral therapy techniques applied on the skull of an embalmed cadaver. *Cranio*. 1992 Jan;10(1):9–12.

110. Greenman PE, McPartland JM. Cranial findings and iatrogenesis from craniosacral manipulation in patients with traumatic brain syndrome. *J Am Osteopath Assoc* 1995 Mar;95(3): 182–8; 191–2.

111. Robbins H. Evaluating the short-term effect of cranial osteopathy on spectral analysis of heart rate variability (unpublished data). Department of Physical Medicine and Rehabilitation. UMDNJ New Jersey Medical School (Newark). Medical Rehabilitation Fellowship 1996.

112. Green C, Martin CW, Bassett K, Kazanjian A. A systematic review of craniosacral therapy: biological plausibility, assessment reliability and clinical effectiveness. *Complement Ther Med* 1999 Dec;7(4):201–7.

113. Dossey, L. *Healing Words: The Power of Prayer and the Practice of Medicine* HarperSanFrancisco, 1993.

114. Koenig, HG. *Spirituality in Patient Care: Why, How, When and What.* Templeton Foundation Press Philadelphia 2002.

115. Puchalski CM, Romer AL. Taking a spiritual history allows clinicians to understand patients more fully. *J Palliative Medicine,* 2000;3:129–137.

116. Anandarajah G, Hight E. Spirituality and medical practice: using the HOPE questions as a practical tool for spiritual assessment. *American Family Physician,* 2001;63 (1): 82–88.

117. Lo B, Quill T, Tulsky J. Discussing palliative care with patients. *Annals Int Med,* 1999;130, 744–749.

118. Koenig HG, McCullough ME, Larson DB. *Handbook of Religion and Health.* New York: Oxford University Press 2001.

119. Ehman JW, Ott BB, Short TH, Ciampa RC, Hansen-Flaschen J. Do patients want physicians to inquire about their spiritual or religious beliefs if they become gravely ill? *Arch Intern Med* 1999; 159:1803–1806.

120. Benson H, Stark M. *Timeless Healing: The Power and Biology of Belief.* New York: Simon and Schuster 1996.

121. Krusen FH. *Physical Medicine: The Employment of Physical Agents for Diagnosis and Therapy.* Philadelphia: W B Saunders 1941.

122. Steizinger, C., Yerys, S., Scowcroft, N., Wygand, J., Otto, R. M. (1999). The effects of repeated magnet treatment on prolonged recovery from exercise induced delayed onset muscle soreness. *Medicine and Science in Sports and Exercise* 1999; 31(5), S208.

123. Sandyk R. Reversal of visuospatial deficit on the Clock Drawing Test in Parkinson's disease by treatment with weak electromagnetic fields. *Int J Neurosci* 1995; Jun;82(3–4): 255–68.

124. Sandyk R. Weak electromagnetic fields reverse visuospatial hemiinattention in Parkinson's disease. *Int J Neurosci* 1995 Mar; 81(1–2):67–82), and cognitive impairments.

125. Sandyk R. Reversal of cognitive impairment in an elderly Parkinsonian patient by transcranial application of picotesla electromagnetic fields. *Int J Neurosci* 1997 Sep;91(1–2):57–68.

126. Sandyk R. Improvement in short-term visual memory by weak electromagnetic fields in Parkinson's disease. *Int J Neurosci* 1994; Jul;77(1–2):23–46.

127. Heldmann B, Kerkhoff G, Struppler A, Havel P, Jahn T. Repetitive peripheral magnetic stimulation alleviates tactile extinction. *Neuroreport* 2000 Sep 28;1(14):3193–8.

128. Moser DJ, Jorge RE, Manes F, Paradiso S, Benjamin ML, Robinson RG. Improved executive functioning following repetitive transcranial magnetic stimulation. *Neurology* 2002 Apr 23; 58(8):1288–90.

129. Triggs WJ, McCoy KJ, Greer R, Rossi F, Bowers D, Kortenkamp S, Nadeau SE, Heilman KM, Goodman WK. Effects of left frontal transcranial magnetic stimulation on depressed mood, cognition, and corticomotor threshold. *Biol Psychiatry* 1999 Jun 1;45 (11):1440–6.

130. Klein E, Kreinin I, Chistyakov A, Koren D, Mecz L, Marmur S, Ben-Shachar D, Feinsod M. Therapeutic efficacy of right prefrontal slow repetitive transcranial magnetic stimulation in major depression: a double-blind controlled study. *Arch Gen Psychiatry* 1999 Apr;56 (4):315–20

131. George MS, Nahas Z, Molloy M, Speer AM, Oliver NC, Li XB, Arana GW, Risch SC, Ballenger JC. A controlled trial of daily left prefrontal cortex TMS for treating depression. *Biol Psychiatry* 2000 Nov 15:48 (10):962–70.

132. Dannon PN, Dolberg OT, Schrieber S, Grunhaus L. Three and six month outcome following courses of either ECT or rTMS in a population of severely depressed individuals—preliminary report. (*Biol Psychiatry* 2002 Nov 15;48(10):962–70.

133. Holtzheimer PE 3rd, Russo J, Avery DH. A meta-analysis of repetitive transcranial magnetic stimulation in the treatment of depression. *Pyschopharmacol Bull* 2001 Autumn;35(4):149–69.

134. Holtzheimer PE 3rd, Russo J, Avery DH. A meta-analysis of repetitive transcranial magnetic stimulation in the treatment of depression. *Pyschopharmacol Bull* 2001 Autumn;35(4):149–69.

135. Triggs WJ, McCoy KJ, Greer R, Rossi F, Bowers D, Kortenkamp S, Nadeau SE, Heilman KM, Goodman WK. Effects of left frontal transcranial magnetic stimulation on depressed mood, cognition, and corticomotor threshold. *Biol Psychiatry* 1999 Jun 1;45 (11):1440–6.

136. Cantello R. Applications of transcranial magnetic stimulation in movement disorders. *J Clin Neurophysiol* 2002; Aug; 19(4):272–93.

137. Gironell A, Kulisevsky J, Lorenzo J, Barbanoj M, Pascual-Sedano B, Otermin P. Transcranial magnetic stimulation of the cerebellum in essential tremor: a controlled study. *Arch Neurol* 2002; Mar;59(3):413–7.

138. Sandyk R. Reversal of body image disorder (macrosomatognosia) in Parkinson's disease by treatment with AC pulsed electromagnetic fields. *Int J Neurosci* 1998 Feb;93(1–2):43–54.

139. Sandyk R. Reversal of body image disorder (macrosomatognosia) in Parkinson's disease by treatment with AC pulsed electromagnetic fields. *Int J Neurosci* 1998 Feb;93(1–2):43–54.

140. Sandyk R. Improvement in word-fluency performance in Parkinson's disease by administration of electromagnetic fields. *Int J Neurosci* 1994 Jul;77(1–2):23–46) perceptual deficits.

141. Sandyk R. Reversal of visuospatial deficit on the Clock Drawing Testin Parkinson's disease by treatment with weak electromagnetic fields. *Int J Neurosci* 1995 Jun;82(3–4):255–68.

142. Sandyk R. Weak electromagnetic fields reverse visuospatial hemiinattention in Parkinson's disease. *Int J Neurosci* 1995 Mar; 81(1–2):67–82), and cognitive impairments.

143. Sandyk R. Reversal of cognitive impairment in an elderly parkinsonian patient by transcranial application of picotesla electromagnetic fields. *Int J Neurosci* 1997 Sep;91(1–2):57–68.

144. Sandyk R. Improvement in short-term visual memory by weak electromagnetic fields in Parkinson's disease. *Int J Neurosci* 1994; Jul;77(1–2):23–46.

145. Heldmann B, Kerkhoff G, Struppler A, Havel P, Jahn T. Repetitive peripheral magnetic stimulation alleviates tactile extinction. *Neuroreport* 2000 Sep 28;1(14):3193–8.

146. Moser DJ, Jorge RE, Manes F, Paradiso S, Benjamin ML, Robinson RG. Improved executive functioning following repetitive transcranial magnetic stimulation. *Neurology* 2002 Apr 23; 58(8):1288–90.

147. Fraser C, Power M, Hamdy S, Rothwell J, Hobday D, Hollander I, Tyrell P, Hobson A, Williams S, Thompson D. Driving plasticity in human adult motor cortex is associated with improved motor function after brain injury. *Neuron* 2002 May 30;34(5): 831–40.

148. Conforto AB, Marie SK, Cohen LG, Scaff M. Transcranial magnetic stimulation. *Arq Neuropsiquiatr.* 2003 Mar;61(1):146–52. *Epub* 2003; Apr 16.

149. Triggs WJ, McCoy KJ, Greer R, Rossi F, Bowers D, Kortenkamp S, Nadeau SE, Heilman KM, Goodman WK. Effects of left frontal transcranial magnetic stimulation on depressed mood, cognition, and corticomotor threshold. *Biol Psychiatry* 1999 Jun 1;45(11): 1440–6.

149. Fraser C, Power M, Hamdy S, Rothwell J, Hobday D, Hollander I, Tyrell P, Hobson A, Williams S, Thompson D. Driving plasticity in human adult motor cortex is associated with improved motor function after brain injury. *Neuron* 2002 May 30;34(5): 831–40.

150. Strafella AP, Paus T, Barrett J, Dagher A. Repetitive transcranial magnetic stimulation of the human prefrontal cortex induces dopamine release in the caudate nucleus. *J Neurosci* 2001 Aug 1; 21(15):RC157.

151. Sandyk R. Reversal of cognitive impairment in an elderly parkinsonian patient by transcranial application of picotesla electromagnetic fields. *Int J Neurosci* 1997 Sep;91(1–2):57–68.

152. Sandyk R. Reversal of body image disorder (macrosomatognosia) in Parkinson's disease by treatment with AC pulsed electromagnetic fields. *Int J Neurosci* 1998 Feb;93(1–2):43–54.

153. Sandyk R. Weak electromagnetic fields reverse visuospatial hemi-inattention in Parkinson's disease. *Int J Neurosci* 1995 Mar; 81(1–2):67–82), and cognitive impairments.

154. Sandyk R. Improvement in word-fluency performance in Parkinson's disease by administration of electromagnetic fields. *Int J Neurosci* 1994 Jul;77(1–2):23–46) perceptual deficits.

155. Baker-Price LA, Persinger MA. Weak, but complex pulsed magnetic fields may reduce depression following traumatic brain injury. *Percept Mot Skills* 1996 Oct;83(2):491–8.

156. Baker-Price LA, Persinger MA. Weak, but complex pulsed magnetic fields may reduce depression following traumatic brain injury. *Percept Mot Skills* 1996 Oct;83(2):491–8.

157. George MS, Wassermann EM, Williams WA, Steppel J, Pascual-Leone A, Basser P, Hallett M, Post RM. Changes in mood and hormone levels after rapid-rate transcranial magnetic stimulation (rTMS) of the prefrontal cortex. *J Neuropsychiatry Clin Neurosci* 1996 Spring 8(2):172–80.

158. Ferrell T, Glick O. The use of therapeutic massage as a nursing intervention to modify anxiety and the perception of cancer pain. *Cancer Nurs* 1993 16:93.

159. Richards TL, Lappin MS, Lawrie FW, Stegbauer KC. Bioelectromagnetic applications for multiple sclerosis. *Phys Med Rehabil Clin N Am* 1998; Aug 9(3)659–674.

161. Conca A, Konig P, Hausmann A. Transcranial magnetic stimulation induces 'psuedoabsence seizure'. *Acta Psychiatr Scand.* 2000 Mar;101 (3):246–8.

162. Triggs WJ, McCoy KJ, Greer R, Rossi F, Bowers D, Kortenkamp S, Nadeau SE, Heilman KM, Goodman WK. Effects of left frontal transcranial magnetic stimulation on depressed mood, cognition, and corticomotor threshold. *Biol Psychiatry* 1999 Jun 1;45(11): 1440–6.

163. George MS. Transcranial magnetic stimulation: applications in neuropsychiatry. *Arch Gen Psychiatry* 1999 Apr;56(4):300–11.

164. Keck ME, Welt T, Muller MB, Erhardt A, Ohl F, Toschi N, Holsboer F, Sillaber I. Repetitive transcranial magnetic stimulation increases the release of dopamine in the mesolimbic and mesostriatal system. *Neuropharmacology* 2002 Jul;43(1):101–9.

165. Strafella AP, Paus T, Barrett J, Dagher A. Repetitive transcranial magnetic stimulation of the human prefrontal cortex induces dopamine release in the caudate nucleus. *J Neurosci* 2001; Aug 1;21(15):RC157.

166. Stallibrass C, Sissons P, Chalmers C. Randomized controlled trial of the Alexander technique for idiopathic Parkinson's disease. *Clin Rehabil* 2002 Nov;16(7):695–708.

167. Greenman PE, McPartland JM. Cranial findings and iatrogenesis from craniosacral manipulation in patients with traumatic brain syndrome. *J Am Osteopath Assoc* 1995 Mar; 95(3): 182–8;191–2.

168. Jain KK (ed). *Textbook of Hyperbaric Medicine 3rd Ed* Kirkland, WA: Hogrete & Huber 1999.

169. Kindwall EP (ed). *Hyperbaric Medicine Practice 2nd Ed* Flagstaff, Az: Best Publishing 1999.

170. Agency for Healthcare Research and Quality *Hyperbaric Oxygen Therapy for Brain Injury, Cerebral Palsy, and Stroke* Rockville, MD: AHRQ Publications 2003.

171. McDonagh M, Helfland M, et al. Hyperbaric oxygen therapy for traumatic brain injury: A systematic review of the evidence, *Arch Phys Med & Rehab* 2004; 85(7): 1199–1204.

172. Undersea & Hyperbaric Society *Position Paper: The Treatment of Multiple Sclerosis with Hyperbaric Oxygen Therapy* www.uhms.org 2004.

173. The Alternative Therapy Evaluation Committee for the Insurance Corporation of British Columbia. A Review of the Scientific Evidence on the Treatment of Traumatic Brain Injuries and Strokes with Hyperbaric Oxygen. *Brain Injury* 2003;17(3): 225–236.

174. Rockswold GL, Ford SE, Anderson DC et al. *Hyperbaric Oxygen Therapy for the Adjunctive Treatment of Traumatic Brain Injury.* Cochrane Database of Systematic Reviews 2004;4: CD004C09.

175. Rockswold GL, Ford SE, Anderson DC et al. *Hyperbaric Oxygen Therapy for the Adjunctive Treatment of Traumatic Brain Injury.* Cochrane Database of Systematic Reviews 2004;4: CD004C09. Results of a Prospective Randomized Trial for Treatment of Severely Brain-Injured Patients with Hyperbaric Oxygen. *J. Neurosurg* 1992;76: 929–934.

176. Artru F, Chacornac R. Hyperbaric oxygenation for severe head injuries. *Eur. Neurol* 1976;14:310–318.

177. Ren H, Wang W, Zhaoming GE et al. Clinical, brain electric earth may, endothelin and transcranial ultrasonic doppler findings after hyperbaric oxygen treatment for severe brain injury. *Chinese Medical Journal* 2001;114(4):387–390.

178. Mogami H, Hayakawa T, Kanai N et al. Clinical application of hyperbaric oxygenation in the treatment of acute cerebral damage. *J. Neurosurg* 1969;31:636–643.

179. Rockswold SB, Rockswold GL, Vargo JM et al. Effects of hyperbaric oxygenation therapy on cerebral metabolism and intracranial pressure in severely brain injured patients. *J. Neurosurg* 2001;94:403–411.

180. Brown JA, Preul MC, Taha A. Hyperbaric oxygen in the treatment of elevated intracranial pressure after head injury. *Pediatric Neurosci* 1988;14:286–290.

181. Sukoff MH, Ragatz RE. Hyperbaric oxygenation for the treatment of acute cerebral edema. *Neurosurgery* 1982;10(1):29–38.

182. Artru F, Philippon B, Gau F et al. Cerebral blood flow, cerebral metabolism and cerebralspinal fluid biochemistry in brain-injured patients after exposure to hyperbaric oxygen. *Eur. Neurol* 1976;14:351–364.

183. Holbach KH, Schroder FK, Koster S. Alternations of cerebral metabolism in cases with acute brain injury during spontaneous respiration of air, oxygen, and hyperbaric oxygen. *European Neurology* 1972;8(1):158–160.

184. Hayakawa T, Kanai N, Kuroda R. Response of CSF pressure to hyperbaric oxygenation. *J Neurol Neurosurg Psychiatry* 1971; 34(5):580–586.

185. Golden ZL, Neubauer R, Golden CJ et al. Improvement in cerebral metabolism in chronic brain injury after hyperbaric oxygen therapy. *Intern. J. Neuroscience* 2002;112:119–131.

186. Barrett K, Masel B, Patterson J. Regional CBF in chronic stable TBI treated with hyperbaric oxygen. *Undersea & Hyperbaric Medicine* 2004;31(4):395–406.

187. Eltorai I, Montroy R. Hyperbaric oxygen therapy leading to recovery of a 6-week comatose patient afflicted by anoxic encephalopathy and posttraumatic edema. *Journal of Hyperbaric Medicine* 1991;6(3):189–197.

188. Neubauer RA, Gottlieb SF, Pevsner H. Hyperbaric oxygen for treatment of closed head injury. *Southern Medical Journal* 1994;87(9):933–936.

189. Wolley SM, Lawrence JA, Hornyak J. The effect of hyperbaric oxygen treatment on postural stability and gait of A brain injured patient. *Pediatric Rehabilitation* 1999;3(3):81–90.

190. Chan EC, Brody B. Ethical dilemmas in hyperbaric medicine. *Undersea and Hyperbaric Medicine* 2001;28(3):123–130.

XIV

PSYCHOSOCIAL AND VOCATIONAL ISSUES

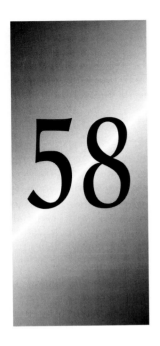

58 Community Re-entry Issues and Long-Term Care

Sally Kneipp
Allen Rubin

THE NEED FOR COMMUNITY RE-ENTRY SERVICES AND LONG-TERM CARE

A little more than two decades ago, following the creation of the National Head Injury Foundation in Framingham, Massachusetts (now the Brain Injury Association of America), post-acute services for persons with traumatic brain injury (TBI) began to develop, slowly at first and then at an increasingly rapid rate. Family members of individuals with traumatic brain injury and interested professionals first met informally, and later through formal associations, to identify the needs and potential service delivery systems for persons in the post-acute phases of recovery, including those with long-term needs. As more individuals with traumatic brain injury were discharged to community settings, efforts were made to design programs that would meet their short- and long-term needs. The diverse post-acute needs of persons with traumatic brain injury and the differing abilities of families to provide the support needed by individuals with traumatic brain injury over the long-term, resulted in a burgeoning of post-acute programs.

The Commission on Accreditation of Rehabilitation Facilities (CARF) established standards for brain injury programs, with growing recognition of the post-acute service delivery options in community settings. Managed care initiatives by insurance companies resulted in significant reductions in the length of stay in hospitals and facilities, resulting in much earlier discharges to post-acute programs (or to no additional treatment). Additionally, the 1979 Report of the United States General Accounting Office had emphasized the need for a redistribution in state and federal funds for persons with disabilities in institutionally-based programs (particularly, nursing homes) to services at home and in the community. In 1981, Medicaid Waiver Programs were initiated to reduce the cost of nursing home care and to foster more community-based services. By 1997, more than 500,000 persons with disabilities were reported to be receiving services through state Medicaid Waiver Programs. Twelve separate waiver programs had been established for persons with traumatic brain injury, and those states were serving 3,000 people in that category. Cusick, Gerhart, Mellick, et al. (1) reported that, among the Medicaid Waiver Programs, the expenditures were the smallest for the traumatic brain injury diagnostic group overall, but the amount spent on services per participant was greatest for that group because of the long-term sequelae of traumatic brain injury and the individuals' complex needs.

Venzie, Felicetti, and Cerra-Tyl (2) emphasized that, although legislative initiatives and managed care directives have been responsible in large part for the trend to more community-based programs, there has also been growing awareness of the clinical advantages of providing treatment in real-world settings. They discussed challenges inherent in, and recommendations for, the establishment of community integrative brain injury programs.

Post-acute programs whose purpose was to facilitate the individual's return to the community were variously referred to as community-based, community re-entry, community integration, community reintegration, community integrative, and community-integrated programs. For example, in the CARF medical rehabilitation standards (3), there are several accreditation categories that may address community re-entry issues and long-term care, the focus of this chapter. They include the brain injury outpatient rehabilitation programs, brain injury home- and community-based programs, brain injury residential rehabilitation programs, brain injury long-term residential services, and brain injury vocational services. There are many providers who have not sought CARF accreditation but have well-established programs to address community re-entry and long-term needs. (Most of the administrators of those programs have stated that, while they acknowledge the importance and value of accreditation, their budgets are inadequate to cover the direct and indirect costs associated with the accreditation process.)

The differences in terminology used to describe these programs has led to some confusion about their scope and purpose, particularly on the part of individuals seeking services, family members investigating services, and payers who are exploring options for cost-effective services. Given the extensive treatment and care provided to persons with traumatic brain injury by emergency medical personnel, and multidisciplinary professionals in a variety of acute care, acute and other post-acute rehabilitation settings, many third-party payers have asked why such a broad spectrum of post-acute programs is necessary at the point of community re-entry if earlier treatment was effective, and why such services are necessary for such long periods of time (frequently, for many years or lifelong). *Enabling America: Assessing the Role of Rehabilitation Science and Engineering*, the 1997 report of the Institute of Medicine established by the United States Congress to evaluate existing rehabilitation models (4), pertains to all disabilities and is not intended to be specific to traumatic brain injury. Nonetheless, the conclusions and recommendations of the report have particular relevance to persons with traumatic brain injury at the point of community re-entry and address the need for services at this point.

The 1997 Institute of Medicine report refers to the disability model proposed by Saad Nagi in the 1950s and refined in the 1991 Institute of Medicine report, *Disability in America*. Dr. Nagi's conceptualization of the disabling process included four components: pathology, impairment, functional limitation, and disability. Further refinement of this model appeared in the 1997 Institute of Medicine report. This differentiated model of pathology, impairment, functional limitation, and disability was revised to illustrate how biological, environmental (physical and social), and lifestyle/behavioral factors are involved in reversing the disabling process (i.e., rehabilitation, or the enabling process). The modified Institute of Medicine model presented the possibility of "no disabling condition," even in the presence of pathology, impairment, and functional limitation. The point made was that disability is not inherent in the individual; it can only be understood in relation to the interaction between an individual and his/her environment. It is precisely the challenge of achieving meaningful interaction with the environment that results in the need of individuals with traumatic brain injury for treatment to address community re-entry issues and long-term needs.

This point was underscored in 1998, when the National Institutes of Health (NIH) convened a consensus development conference on rehabilitation of persons with traumatic brain injury. The conference was followed by a press release and then a *NIH Consensus Statement* (5). As stated, the objective of the *NIH Consensus Statement* was to provide information on the findings of the conference to the biomedical research and clinical practice communities including, but not limited to, physicians representing many medical specialties, and psychologists. The Introduction of the *NIH Consensus Statement* emphasized that the greatest negative consequences following a traumatic brain injury are related to the individual's post-injury cognitive abilities and behavioral and emotional issues (rather than their physical impairments), since they compromise interpersonal relationships and impede participation in major life activities such as school and work.

Treatments mentioned for the cognitive, behavioral and emotional sequelae included cognitive rehabilitation therapy, assistive technology, psychotherapy, psychopharmacologic management, and manipulation of the environment to provide an optimal context for recovery and/or rehabilitation to occur. It was pointed out that treatments are provided in a wide range of settings, from rehabilitation hospitals to the home or community at large.

The significance of the consensus conference was that the conclusions were inclusive of the input of persons with traumatic brain injury, their family members, and nonmedical specialists in addition to medical specialists. The statement reflected the opinions of many persons associated with post-acute programs who had come to appreciate the importance, for positive outcomes to occur, of including many sources of input into the rehabilitation process. Some of the conclusions of the consensus conference relevant to this chapter were that:

1. the consequences of traumatic brain injury can be lifelong, even in cases of mild traumatic brain injury;
2. individually-tailored rehabilitation services should be modified to assure relevance as one's needs change over time;

3. extended care and rehabilitation for persons with traumatic brain injury should include community-based nonmedical services;

4. supportive services (e.g., respite care, counseling and in-home assistance) should be available to family members and significant others of individuals with traumatic brain injury;

5. modification of the individual's home, school, and work environments may be necessary to allow for increased participation in daily living;

6. the input of persons with traumatic brain injury, their family members, and significant others should be regarded as essential to the development and implementation of the rehabilitation program for each individual; and

7. consideration should be given to the timing of specific interventions, since the probability of a beneficial effect may be greater at some points in the rehabilitation process than at others. Moreover, recent investigation of the effects of aging following traumatic brain injury suggests the need for a service delivery system and specific treatments that can be provided when new clinical issues arise or become more pronounced as people age.

Program Design and Treatment Models

While some post-acute programs continue to base their treatment on a multidisciplinary model, treatment based on an interdisciplinary model has been the norm over the past decade, with a growing number of post-acute programs designing treatment using a transdisciplinary approach. From a conceptual standpoint, treatment using an interdiscplinary or transdisciplinary model is particularly relevant and appropriate at the point of community re-entry, and long-term, since the most pressing need at this time is for the individual to be able to integrate the knowledge and skills acquired or re-acquired during earlier phases of his/her rehabilitation. Additionally, treatment must be designed with relevance to the unique characteristics of the environment in which the individual will live and function. Depending on the intermittent or chronic needs of the individual, treatment may be provided by a team of rehabilitation practitioners or by a single-service provider. The individualized nature of rehabilitation treatment is more evident at the community re-entry stage of the rehabilitation process than at any other time. The value of a holistic treatment approach in maximizing potential outcomes has also been recognized.

Malec and Basford (6) summarized the state of the art in post-acute brain injury rehabilitation programs in the mid-1990s. While acknowledging limitations of the study from a research design standpoint, the authors provided a categorization of types of post-acute programs and presented a model of brain injury rehabilitation. This model, identified as an algorithm of level of rehabilitation care after traumatic brain injury, also appeared in a subsequent publication in 2003 (7). However, of concern is the component in the model designated "No services, or community-based services only." Particularly in the past decade, there has been growing awareness of the effectiveness of community-based services offered in the home and community (of the individual with traumatic brain injury), that are goal-oriented and ecologically valid treatment options. They are on a par with the other categories of the model (i.e., outpatient community re-entry, comprehensive/holistic day treatment, residential community reintegration and neurobehavioral) and should be clearly distinguished from "no services."

In describing the contributions of postacute neurorehabilitation to a national information system, Evans (8) explained that postacute providers frequently regarded the environment of the individual with TBI (i.e., the individual's home and where he/she spends time, such as in school, at the workplace, in the community at large) to be an extension of the treatment setting. Understanding the characteristics and dynamics of the individual's "world" was considered to be essential to the development of treatment approaches of optimal value. In these naturalistic settings, the concept of the treatment team was enlarged to include persons such as the individual's family members, teachers, employer, neighbors, etc. A shared information system is advocated as a means of facilitating the delivery of beneficial services and cost-effective outcomes.

In their article on the development of systems of care for persons with TBI over the past 20 years, Cope, Mayer and Cervelli (9) point out that the conceptualization of a comprehensive system of care now includes therapy and supported living in one's natural environment, perhaps throughout the individual's life. They identify cognitive and behavioral impairments as the focus of comprehensive therapy at this stage and acknowledge the benefits of treatment protocols delivered in the home and community of the individual with TBI to develop his or her ability to carry out activities of daily living and increase social opportunities. They recognize the use of a person-centered context to assist individuals to attain their life goals, and the value of community-based interventions such as "clubhouses" and peer support in improving long-term outcomes. They also recognize the role of psychopharmacologic and neuropharmacologic interventions.

Community re-entry and long-term needs must be addressed if an individual with traumatic brain injury is to achieve a satisfactory quality of life through purposeful, productive activity. Berube (10) explained that The Brain Injury Act, as amended in 2000, mandates exploration of interventions that will facilitate school and work re-entry and reintegration in the community. However, the process of meeting these needs is complicated by the extremely heterogeneous nature of traumatic brain injury, the prominent role of cognitive and psychosocial deficits in eventual rehabilitation outcome, and the fact that a traumatic brain injury in any family member will impact on the family system and others who relate to that individual to any degree.

When determining the optimal treatment program to address the community re-entry and/or long-term needs of an individual following TBI, the most fundamental question is whether a residential or non-residential brain injury program is indicated. In making this decision, an analysis of the individual's home environment and family system must be made, to assure the likelihood that the environment will be able to reinforce the goals of the therapy program and that the level of any supervision needed will be sufficient to assure the individual's safety. Within the scope of residential programs, a wide range of options is available to address the individual's short- and long-term needs. The spectrum of options may range from intense, highly-structured clinical protocols with 1:1 staff/client ratios for individuals with significant behavioral problems to comprehensive transitional living programs to prepare individuals for independent living, or supported living programs offering considerable flexibility, much less structure and only periodic check-ins by staff. Persons with brain injury who also have pre- or post-injury histories of alcohol or drug abuse may require residential treatment in a program designed specially to address those needs, with services provided by staff with particular expertise in substance abuse. Within the comprehensive program, there is typically flexibility to move the individual from one clinical program to the other, as may be needed. Although the services may be designed along a continuum, from the most intensive to least intensive therapeutic support, the reality is that rehabilitation following brain injury is not always linear and various treatment protocols may need to be tried.

Non-residential programs at the community re-entry or long-term stage may also offer an array of options (from comprehensive day programs offering such services as occupational therapy, physical therapy, speech therapy, psychotherapy, cognitive rehabilitation therapy, vocational services, recreational therapy, etc.) to very individualized, goal-directed programs carried out in the individual's milieu (i.e., home and community). These therapy programs have a rehabilitation focus and are different in purpose from home health programs, although home health services may also be indicated for some individuals due to needs for physical assistance with self-care and activities of daily living and/or the need for supervision due to cognitive-communication, behavioral and/or emotional issues.

Because of the highly heterogenous nature of traumatic brain injury, there must be an array of treatment options available to address community re-entry and

long-term needs. The state-federal vocational rehabilitation program, operated in accordance with a state plan, is a frequent resource for persons wishing to return to work. [*Note*: Employability and placeability are major concerns of persons with traumatic brain injury and their families; for more information on vocational issues, please refer to Chapter 61 in this book.] Incentives in relation to employment are available to persons receiving Social Security Disability Insurance (SSDI) and Supplemental Security Income (SSI) because of a disability or blindness. According to a home page of the Social Security Administration (SSA), *The Work Site* (11), the Ticket to Work and Work Incentives Improvement Act of 1999 led to the awarding of 119 cooperative agreements to community organizations to establish Benefits Planning, Assistance, and Outreach (BPAO) projects. The goal is to assist persons receiving SSDI or SSI to make informed decisions about working. Social Security Online also makes available, through its electronic booklet, "The Ticket to Work and Self-Sufficiency Program," answers to questions asked frequently by participants in this new SSA program (12).

The Brain Injury Association of America (BIAA) and its state affiliates offer an extensive array of services to persons with brain injuries, their family members, professionals and the community at large. Of particular value have been the support groups (normally held once a month at various locations), family support services and mentoring projects, and the *National Directory of Brain Injury Rehabilitation Services* (13).

Efficacy of Community-Based Programs

While the growth of community-based programs has been substantial, demonstrating the efficacy of such programs has been exceedingly difficult. Minnes, Carlson, McColls, et al. (14) acknowledged that community integration is an often-used outcome measure in rehabilitation research and underscored that is understandable since the aim of rehabilitation is to remove barriers to individuals' participation in daily living. They studied the relationship between community integration and salient variables that included impairment, activity, participation, quality of life, paid support and informal support. Their findings revealed the complexity of community integration and the difficulty of measuring it. They emphasized the importance of clearly defining community integration in research projects and recommended the use of subjective as well as objective measures. They also discussed the methodological difficulty of using questionnaires with research participants who have cognitive impairments and recommended that survey items be read aloud to the participants and that, with permission, collateral informants (e.g., family members) be present to increase the probability of accurate responses.

Goranson, Graves, Allison, and La Freniere (15) emphasized that the demand for accountability by payers is resulting in closer examination of the cost-effectiveness of traumatic brain injury programs offering cognitive rehabilitation therapy. They point out that functional outcomes and life satisfaction should be improved as a result of therapy to improve cognitive abilities and coping skills, but that it is difficult to establish the efficacy of such programs because of problems developing a suitable research methodology, the non-comparability of the outcome measures (given the heterogeneity of the population and the individualized treatment plans), and lack of a multidimensional analysis.

Dawson, Levine, Schwartz, and Stuss (16) acknowledged the extreme variance in outcomes and emphasized the importance of predicting real-world outcomes when establishing clinical goals. They advocated for more specific predictors of recovery (such as attention and memory and other salient variables such as coping style) rather than injury severity, and the need to find out if better long-term outcomes would be achieved by addressing process-specific variables (e.g., pre-injury personality characteristics) during the acute phase.

The difficulty conducting research with experimental or even quasi-experimental research designs during the community re-entry phase of rehabilitation has led to a limited amount of data demonstrating the efficacy of community re-entry programs. As a result, some third-party payers have denied funding for needed services on the basis that there is insufficient empirical evidence of the cost-effectiveness of the treatment. This is particularly true in relation to cognitive rehabilitation therapy, which has been a standard component of most brain injury rehabilitation programs, including community re-entry programs, for over two decades. In denying funding for cognitive rehabilitation therapy, some payers have described it as "investigative," "experimental" or "educational," failing to realize that addressing neurocognitive deficits is crucial to maximizing functional recovery following brain injury.

Treatment in Real-life Contexts

Cicerone, Dahlberg, Kalmar, et al. (17) pointed out that, even following moderate or good recovery neurologically, one's quality of life following traumatic brain injury may be severely compromised because of persistent cognitive deficits and maladaptive behavior. The real-life context for any given individual following traumatic brain injury must be taken into account in order to achieve a satisfactory interface between the individual and his/her environment. Cicerone and Tupper (18) emphasized that the goal of rehabilitation after brain injury must be improvement in the ability to function in real life (not just in a therapy setting) and requires learning new ways to perform daily activities in a variety of contexts. However, the individual's

cognitive deficits may impede the ability to benefit from traditional therapies, function successfully in daily living, and learn new ways to accomplish everyday tasks. There is a need for innovative therapeutic approaches in post-acute brain injury rehabilitation and for assurance that the approaches have true relevance to the individuals' lives, particularly at the point of community re-entry.

Gordon and Hibbard (19) concluded that evaluation studies and anecdotes confirm the benefits of cognitive rehabilitation and cognitive remediation if individualized to meet the specific needs of the individual and delivered systematically and creatively in an appropriate context. They emphasized that the treatment can be demanding for the individuals and team members, and that the intensity and duration can be significant, but that it is evident that the treatment helps individuals to adapt to challenges of daily living after a traumatic brain injury.

Funding for Community Re-entry Services

Funding for community re-entry services and long-term care comes from a variety of sources, which are frequently blended. Because the majority of traumatic brain injuries occur in motor vehicle accidents, the personal injury protection (PIP) portion of auto insurance policies is a major source of funding in many, if not most, states. Workers' compensation insurance is another large source of funding, following work-related accidents (e.g., falls). Funding for some community re-entry services is available through private long-term disability plans and some health insurance carriers, but not all. Examples of other typical sources of funding include money set aside in structured settlements for rehabilitation purposes, private pay, programs operated with state and federal funding (e.g., the Division of Developmental Disabilities, Medicaid Waiver Programs, other waiver programs, crime victims' boards, vocational rehabilitation agencies, recently-established traumatic brain injury funds), and voluntary agencies (brain injury associations).

Many insurance companies employ or contract with case managers (usually rehabilitation nurses) whose responsibility it is to assist the claims personnel in making decisions about the suitability of services recommended for the individual and the reasonableness of the costs for the services. They serve as external case managers to the programs offering the services; the programs may also employ internal case managers to assist program personnel in determining what services the individual will receive and assuring the availability of funding for reimbursement of costs for services rendered.

PREVALENT COMMUNITY RE-ENTRY ISSUES

Among the many community re-entry issues for individuals following traumatic brain injury, family adjustment, social isolation, limited community mobility, and barriers to employment are paramount. (Please see Chapter 61 for a discussion of vocational issues.) Even given the impetus of legislative initiatives such as the 1990 Americans with Disabilities Act, intended to facilitate the inclusion of persons with disabilities in society, the reality is that many individuals with traumatic brain injury remain homebound a large majority of the time, cared for by family members and significant others who are experiencing caregiver burden.

Family Adjustment

The normal developmental stages and transitions in family life are disrupted following the brain injury of any member of a family. Significant changes in the usual roles and functions occur, and are often permanent. If not addressed adequately, these issues (discussed by Sander in Chapter 60 of this book) result in a diminished quality of life for all persons involved. As stated in the *NIH Consensus Statement* (20), there are serious social consequences following traumatic brain injury at any level of severity. There are risks of prolonged unemployment, financial hardship, divorce, criminal activity, substance abuse, and suicide. In addition to the strain on families, the resources of social service agencies and legal systems are strained. The negative effects of the traumatic brain injury may become more evident, and more severe, following the individual's unsuccessful attempts to resume his/her usual roles and responsibilities. Psychosocial issues become evident in family members and significant others as well as the individual with the brain injury; family dynamics are frequently unsatisfactory and family functioning deteriorates. In some situations, particularly if not addressed, these problems worsen over time.

Results of a survey conducted by staff of a community re-entry program, and presented at a national brain injury symposium, supported the assertion of Williams and Kay (21) that, even at the point of community re-entry, after considerable treatment has been provided, family members are usually not prepared to cope with the persistent cognitive, psychosocial, and/or emotional problems of their family member with traumatic brain injury. Rider-Williams and Trout (22) identified the following characteristics of the individual's traumatic brain injury to be the greatest challenges for family members: problems remembering; social isolation; problems planning and organizing; poor judgment; mood swings; difficulty paying attention and concentrating; poor problem-solving; fatigue; problems with balance and coordination; poor decision-making; not being able to walk like before; and impulsivity. Rider-Williams and Trout concluded that much needs to be done to help individuals with TBI and their family members cope with the numerous long-term challenges of TBI. They emphasized that, given managed

care initiatives and the decreased inpatient stays in rehabilitation hospitals and facilities, there is insufficient time for hospital personnel to provide as much patient/family education as was typically provided in the past, prior to discharge. Moreover, even when patient and family education was available, family members and significant others may not have been able to process the information yet. Treatment providers must be sensitive to family members' needs for timely information throughout the rehabilitation process.

Laroi (23) discussed the value of family therapy sessions even after active rehabilitation treatment, to help the family be aware of, and seek attention for, any negative changes in the family system. Family therapy in the home was recommended as a way to facilitate timely changes following disruptions in the family system. Strongly advised were selection of a family therapist with expertise in brain injury rehabilitation and close collaboration between the family therapist and the professionals providing the individual's brain injury rehabilitation therapy.

Kosciulek and Pichette (24) conducted a survey of primary caregivers of individuals with TBI in an attempt to isolate factors that enhance care. They found that supportive friends; a positive family outlook; availability of family support; and family unity, loyalty, and cooperation were variables that had a positive correlation with care. The unavailability of respite services, an absence of vocational rehabilitation services, limited assistance for meeting day-to-day needs, inappropriate living situations, and emotional and behavioral problems in the injured family member were identified as variables impacting negatively on care. Kosciulek and Pichette concluded that family members of persons who have sustained a TBI require an array of support services if they are to provide a high quality of care over an extended period. They also suggested that family satisfaction may improve quality of life and contribute to positive rehabilitation outcomes.

Godfrey, Harnett, Knight, et al. (25) examined the impact on caregivers when personality changes in the individual with TBI are due to problems with emotional control or problems with motivation, and contribute to caregivers' distress, burden and depression. The Head Injury Behaviour Scale was found to have good internal consistency and reliability and to be a reliable and valid measure of caregiver distress.

Ponsford, Olver, Ponsford, and Nelms (26) also discussed the emotional burden of caregiving, the effect on family adjustment, and the need to develop models of long-term support that will help reduce caregiver burden on family members and relatives. To learn what will be most effective, they recommended studies of the attributes, values and coping styles of families who adjust well following the traumatic brain injury of a family member.

Social Isolation

Following a traumatic brain injury, many persons experience profound social isolation that severely compromises their quality of life. Burleigh, Farber and Gillard (27) pointed out that individuals with a TBI may have difficulty fulfilling or resuming an accepted social role, or simply may not be able to do so because of psychosocial deficits and/or emotional issues. They emphasized that rehabilitation treatment for these individuals should include the skills needed to develop and maintain interpersonal relationships, since otherwise they may become socially isolated and experience a low quality of life. They also pointed out that dissatisfaction with life could lead to psychological problems in addition to already-existing post-injury problems.

The goal of social integration should be part of the individual's treatment plan at the point of community reentry. A study by Brown, Gordon and Spielman (28), undertaken by a Research and Training Center on Community Integration of Individuals with Traumatic Brain Injury, focused on social and recreational activities of persons with traumatic brain injury (TBI) that required individuals leave their homes to engage in the activity and that addressed their social goals. Sample results of the study, based on self-report during interviews, revealed that the TBI sample (N = 279) was significantly less active than the no disability (ND) group (N = 244) on the composite measure of social-recreational activity and on each of the five indicators of social-recreational activity. The authors point out, however, that substantial within-group variance suggests the need to examine more closely what constitutes disadvantage in social participation. The authors also suggest that depression and fatigue, which frequently account for reduced social participation, should be addressed and that involvement in educational or work activity (either paid or volunteer) will provide additional opportunities for persons with traumatic brain injury to participate in social and recreational activities.

Limited Community Mobility

Following a traumatic brain injury, access to the community may be limited dramatically. Sequelae of traumatic brain injury may compromise the individual's ability to get around safely in the community by driving a motor vehicle, riding a bicycle, using public transportation (i.e., bus, train, taxi cabs or trolley), using specialized transportation (e.g., paratransit services), or simply walking. Physical or sensory impairments restricting community mobility may include gait and motor incoordination, balance problems, visual deficits, audiovestibular dysfunction, communication deficits, bladder and bowel dysfunction and conditions such as post-traumatic epilepsy. Cognitive deficits impeding community mobility may include such problems as distractibility; limited attention and concentration spans; poor memory; inadequate planning, organizing, decision-making and problem-solving skills; limited safety awareness and judgment; poor topographical orientation; impaired time awareness; and slow processing of information. Behavioral deficits such as apathy or lack of ability to initiate purposeful behavior, or behavioral excesses such as impulsivity or disinhibition, may also compromise one's community mobility. Limited stamina and endurance, and fatigue, are also moderating variables in one's ability to access the community.

Driving after Traumatic Brain Injury The sequelae of traumatic brain injury often make driving after a brain injury an unattainable, although highly desired, personal goal. The inability to drive a motor vehicle is a particularly distressing circumstance for late adolescents and young adults who comprise the greatest percentage of individuals with traumatic brain injury and who are frequently at important points in their career development. It is easy for anyone who drives to appreciate how an inability to drive can alter the ability to perform usual life roles. The inability to drive contributes to the major post-injury challenges of returning to work or school, resuming family roles, and reducing social isolation. The inability to drive can lead to lowered self-confidence and self-esteem and negative self-image, as it limits one's ability to function independently and access one's community. In rural areas, one's inability to drive is particularly problematic, since it usually results in a significant decrease in community involvement and/or significant demands on caregivers who must provide necessary transportation. Nonetheless, caregivers, as well as involved medical and non-medical professionals, must guard against making recommendations for driving based on sympathy for individuals whose attainment of personal goals is unquestionably complicated by the inability to drive. Decisions about one's driving privileges must take into account the public's right to a reasonable standard of safety. The public interest is protected, as well as the individual's, when there is a means for the individual to demonstrate the capacity to drive safely. Galski, et al. (29) summarize

> What is known about the residual effects of brain injury on driving has been derived from studies attempting to show the ways and extent to which specific deficits relate to driving performance. A basic but ever-growing compendium of deficits has been compiled, including, but not limited to, *sensory deficiencies*, such as defects in visual and auditory acuity, glare and contrast sensitivity, and motion perception; *motoric difficulties*, such as loss of or reduction in strength, coordination, and reaction speed; *cognitive impairments*, such as poor visual scanning of traffic and environment, difficulties in spatial perception and

orientation, slowness in information processing, and loss of attentional abilities; and *personality or behavior disturbances*, such as accident-proneness, anxiety, or confusion in the face of complex driving situations or problems (p. 896).

Executive functions (discussed by Cicerone in Chapter 41, and Eslinger in Chapters 42 of this book) are especially salient variables in driving. Self-awareness is crucial to one's ability to predict whether he or she will be able to drive safely. In studying the predictors of outcome after traumatic brain injury, Coleman, Rapport, Ergh, et al. (30) found that the significant other or caregiver is more likely than the individual with traumatic brain injury to determine whether and how much driving will be done post-injury. They concluded that family education provided in a rehabilitation setting could facilitate family members' and significant others' understanding of the abilities needed to drive safely; because driving is such a common activity, the complex cognitive demands may not be recognized. Of value would be helping them to make observations of the individual's behavior and its implication for driving. For example, family members and significant others who report that the individual is having post-injury problems with frustration, anger or impulsivity, could be helped to anticipate the potential risks of driving if exhibiting those behaviors. While it is expected that the implications of those behavioral excesses for driving would be easily understood (particularly with attention in the media to "road rage"), other behaviors, such as lack of initiation, mental inflexibility, and perseveration may need much more explanation.

In many states, physicians are regarded as possessing the knowledge to make reasonable decisions and implement statutory restrictions regarding an individual's fitness to operate a motor vehicle post-injury, whether compromised by recurrent seizures, physical impairment or only by cognitive impairment. State licensing statutes and regulations regarding driving after cerebral injuries vary, but typically require demonstration of adequate visual acuity, perceptual ability as required to respond in a timely manner to traffic control devices, knowledge of traffic laws, and skills to operate a motor vehicle. Krauss, et al. (31) provides two useful tables—one summarizing the state regulations regarding driving and epilepsy (see Table 58-1) and the other summarizing driving regulations in states with flexible driving restrictions (see Table 58-2). Physicians are strongly recommended to be aware of the regulations which apply in their region, and to discuss thoroughly the matter of driving with their patients and guardians. Some physicians may not possess the knowledge of driving capabilities per se or the ability to test driving competency in a real-life situation, and may be prone to inaccuracy when extrapolating from an office examination to a real-time driving experience. In such cases, the individual should be referred to a qualified driving evaluator with particular expertise in the assessment of driving capabilities following traumatic brain injury.

Such driving evaluations, consisting of driving simulations and then on-the-road ("behind-the-wheel") driving observation by a therapist or trainer sensitive to the issues of cerebral impairment, may be available through rehabilitation facilities. Following the driving evaluation, the physician analyzes recommendations in relation to his/her own medical knowledge of the individual, and thereby renders an opinion about fitness to drive.

Although requiring that a driver demonstrate adequate knowledge of pertinent laws and regulations, the standards of the state motor vehicle department may be relatively minimal in relation to physical abilities. For example, it may be minimally adequate to have visual acuity of 20/40, even if extemporaneous binocular or depth visual processing is impaired. It is likely that a state driving examiner will not anticipate the difficulties an individual with a brain injury may have in making rapid decisions, filtering complex simultaneous stimuli, or adapting in unpredictable situations. The physician, on the other hand, because of the understanding of brain function under the circumstances of challenge and duress, may need to take a more critical view of driving safety than does the state. The physician should be aware of possible adverse affects which treatment may have on driving, such as sedating side effects of medications, and make patients aware of these effects as potential restrictions to driving.

While physicians have a responsibility to protect third parties from potential harm, in some states issues of privacy and confidentiality may arise if the physician notifies legal authorities without the consent of the individual. Drazkowski (32) points out that the requirement to notify authorities may discourage patients from disclosing to their physicians the frequency and intensity of their seizures, and that could lead to inadequate medical care. Nonetheless, a physician's obligation to report patients who are engaging in illegal activity or pose the risk of danger or harm to the public at large takes precedence over issues of confidentiality.

With respect to seizures, Drazkowski recommends strongly that the physician take into account how antiepileptic drugs [AED] might affect driving capacity, the risk of AED non-compliance or discontinuation, initial reporting requirements at the time of diagnosis, and the need for adequate medical information to be provided subsequently to regulatory agencies, if called upon.

Although developed with specific reference to another medical condition with motoric, perceptual, cognitive, and executive function impairment (namely, Huntington's disease), the driving assessment developed by Rubin (33) may be useful to a physician (or other professionals) in arriving at an opinion of one's ability to

TABLE 58-1
*Driving and Epilepsy: Regulations and Practices of US States**

STATE	LEGAL SEIZURE-FREE RESTRICTION (MO)	RARE EXCEPTIONS TO SEIZURE-FREE INTERVAL BASED ON MITIGATING FACTORS†	REQUIRED MVA MEDICAL REVIEW, TYPE OR INTERVAL‡	MANDATORY PHYSICIAN REPORTING	MVA LICENSE APPEAL	PHYSICIAN LIABLE FOR DRIVING RECOMMENDATIONS§
Alabama	6	No	Annually for 5 y from last seizure	No	Yes	No
Alaska	6	No	Individual	No	Yes	Yes
Arizona	3	Nocturnal, auras, AED revision	Individual	No	Yes	No
Arkansas	12	No	Individual	No	Yes	Yes
California	3, 6, or 12//	Nocturnal, breakthrough, AED revision	Individual	Yes	Yes	Yes
Colorado	//	No	Individual	No	Yes	No
Connecticut	3//	No	Individual	No	Yes	Yes
District of Columbia	12	Nocturnal, AED revision, and solitary seizure	1 y (until seizure free for 5 y)	No	Yes	Yes
Delaware	//	No	Individual	Yes	Yes	No
Florida	24//	Nocturnal (must supply EEG)	Individual	No	Yes	No
Georgia	12	First seizure, nocturnal	Individual	No	Yes	No
Hawaii	//	No	Individual	No	Yes	Yes
Idaho	//	MD recommendation	1 y (or semiannually)	No	Yes	No
Illinois	//	No	Individual	No	Yes	No
Indiana	//	No	Individual	No	Yes	Yes
Iowa	6	Nocturnal	6 mo, then at every renewal	No	Yes	No
Kansas	6	Nocturnal, solitary seizure	1 y (until seizure free for 3 y)	No	Yes	No
Kentucky	3	No	1 y	No	Yes	No
Louisiana	6	AED revision	Individual	No	No	No
Maine	3//	Seizure 'breakthrough'	Individual	No	Yes	No
Maryland	3	AED revision	Individual	No	Yes	No
Massachusetts	6//	MAB recommendation	Individual	No	Yes	Yes
Michigan	6	AED revision	Individual	No	Yes	Yes
Minnesota	6	Acute illness, AED revision, first seizure	Every 6 mo (until seizure free for 1 y)	No	Yes	No
Mississippi	12	No	Individual	No	No	No
Missouri	6	MD recommendation	Individual	No	No	No
Montana	//	No	No (MVA may require)	No	Yes	No
Nebraska	3	No	No	No	Yes	Yes

(continued)

TABLE 58-1 (*continued*)

STATE	LEGAL SEIZURE-FREE RESTRICTION (MO)	RARE EXCEPTIONS TO SEIZURE-FREE INTERVAL BASED ON MITIGATING FACTORS†	REQUIRED MVA MEDICAL REVIEW, TYPE OR INTERVAL‡	MANDATORY PHYSICIAN REPORTING	MVA LICENSE APPEAL	PHYSICIAN LIABLE FOR DRIVING RECOMMENDATIONS§
Nevada	3	MD recommendation	1 y (for 3 y)	Yes	Yes	Yes
New Hampshire	12//	MD recommendation	No	No	Yes	Yes
New Jersey	12	Neurologic MAB recommendation	Every 6 mo for 2 y	Yes	Yes	Yes
New Mexico	12//	Nocturnal	Individual	No	Yes	No
New York	12//	AED revision, MD recommendation	Individual	No	Yes	No
North Carolina	6-12//	Nocturnal, auras, AED revision	1 y	No	Yes	No
North Dakota	6//	No	1 y (at least 3 y)	No	Yes	No
Ohio	//	No	6 and 12 mo, then annually	No	Yes	No
Oklahoma	12	Nocturnal	MVA determines	No	Yes	No
Oregon	6//	Nocturnal, auras, AED revision, acute illness	Individual	Yes	Yes	Yes
Pennsylvania	6	Nocturnal, auras, AED revision, acute illness	Individual	Yes	Yes	No
Rhode Island	//	MAB recommendation	Yes	No	Yes	No
South Carolina	6	No	6 mo, then 3 y annually	No	Yes	No
South Dakota	12//	No	Every 6 mo (until seizure free)	No	Yes	Yes
Tennessee	6	No	At discretion of MAB	No	Yes	Yes
Texas	6	AED revision	1 y	No	Yes	No
Utah	3//	Yes	6 mo (until seizure free for 1 y)	No	Yes	No
Vermont	//	No	Individual	Yes	Yes	Yes
Virginia	6	Nocturnal, auras, AED revision, acute illness	Individual	No	Yes	No
Washington	6	MD recommendation	Individual	No	Yes	Yes
West Virginia	12	Nocturnal, auras, AED revision, acute illness	Individual	No	Yes	No
Wisconsin	3	No	6 mo for 2 y	No	Yes	No
Wyoming	3	Nocturnal	1 y	No	Yes	Yes

*AED = antiepileptic drug; MAB = medical advisory board; MD = medical doctor; MVA = motor vehicle agency. Reprinted with permission from Krauss GL, Ampaw L, Krumholz A (28).

†Mitigating factors considered in permitting some patients to drive despite less than minimum seizure-free period: auras, nocturnal seizures only, seizure breakthrough during physician-directed AED change, solitary or first seizure, MD or MAB recommendation.

‡Individual = MVA medical review conducted on a case-by-case basis.

§No = physician legally immune or indemnified; Yes = physician possibly liable for driving recommendation.

//Seizure-free restriction frequently adjusted by MVA MAB and treating physicians (Table 58-2).

TABLE 58-2

Summary of Driving Regulations in States with Flexible Driving Restrictions for Patients with Epilepsy*

STATE	FLEXIBLE DRIVING RESTRICTIONS
California	6 mo seizure free; 3 mo if seizure occurs during physician-directed AED reduction or if previously seizure free 6 mo; 12 mo if repetitive seizure (several in 1–2 mo) after 6-12 mo seizure free
Colorado	Treating physician determines; 2-y restriction if not under physicianís care
Connecticut	Minimum 3 mo seizure free; MAB and treating physician determine; 6 mo without recommendation
Delaware	Treating physician determines; must have been under physicianís care for 3 mo
Florida	MAB usually shortens seizure-free period from 24 mo to 6 mo if under adequate medical treatment
Hawaii	MAB determines; usually 6 mo seizure free; treating physician indicates stable prognosis
Idaho	Treating physician recommends
Illinois	MAB determines; treating physician certifies patient is safe to drive; usually require 6 mo seizure free
Indiana	Treating physician determines; 12 mo seizure-free restriction without physician recommendation
Maine	Functional ability profile: driving generally permitted if >3 mo seizure free or 2 yr seizure free and off AED >3 mo
Massachusetts	6 mo seizure free; MAB may reduce interval if recommended by treating physician; MAB may increase seizure-free restriction
Montana	Treating physician recommends; must attest condition stable and would not interfere with safe driving
New Hampshire	12 mo seizure free; MVA frequently shortens interval on recommendation of treating physician
New Mexico	12 mo seizure free; MVA frequently shortens to 6 mo
New York	12 mo seizure free; MVA frequently shortens to 6 mo based on recommendation of treating physician
North Carolina	6-12 mo seizure free; determined by medical advisor
North Dakota	6 mo seizure free; temporary license for commuting to work or school frequently authorized by MAB if >3 mo seizure free with recommendation from treating physician
Ohio	Treating physician recommends
Oregon	6 mo seizure free usual; shorter intervals considered on recommendation of treating physician
Rhode Island	MAB determines
South Dakota	12 mo seizure free; MAB may give temporary license earlier with 6-mo reviews if physician verifies patientís statement that seizures are under control
Utah	Functional profile and treating physician recommendation (commonly 3 mo seizure free); may recommend limited driving (<40 mph, local roads, daytime only)
Vermont	MAB determines; usually 6 mo seizure free

*AED = antiepileptic drug; MAB = medical advisory board; MVA = motor vehicle agency. Reprinted with permission from Krauss GL, Ampaw L, Krumholz A (28).

drive safely and in communicating his/her opinion to the individual with brain injury, family members and/or significant other. A tabular presentation (see Table 58-3) may increase the likelihood that the basis for the physician's opinion is understood. In this assessment, the less obvious impairments which fall into the categories of efficiency and accuracy of information acquisition and processing, multi-tasking, problem-solving ability, response to simultaneous stimuli and a rapidly changing environment, as well as judgment, self-awareness, impulse control, and emotional status, are taken into account. Each observed quality is rated "normal," "sub-normal" (an abnormality is detected, but is considered acceptable for driving), or "impaired" (representing potential interference with safe driving). The logic of this assessment is that it allows for the recognition of some impairments for which compensatory actions may be possible, while an abundance of "sub-normal" findings, or a single "impaired" finding, would indicate that the physician should intercede to guard against the individual driving unless/until these component abilities recover adequately.

Schultheis, Hillary and Chute (34) compared the Neurocognitive Driving Test (NDT), a computer-based driving assessment tool, with a comprehensive hospital-based driver's evaluation of individuals with acquired brain injury (ABI). Participants included 15 adults with ABI and 15 matched healthy control (HC) participants. A significant relationship was found between the NDT and the comprehensive driving evaluation, and confirmed the value of the NDT in discriminating between the individuals who passed the comprehensive, hospital-based driving evaluation and those who failed. Additional research was recommended with larger sample sizes as was the inclusion of neuropsychological measures and

TABLE 58-3
Clinical Driving Assessment

Name _____ Date _____

Physician Evaluating: _____

❑ Normal   (no abnormality detected)
❑ Sub-normal   (an abnormality is detected, but considered acceptable for driving)
❑ Impaired   (feature is present and represents a potential interference with safe driving)

Alertness and attention:

Level of alertness	❑ Normal	❑ Sub-normal	❑ Impaired
Sustained attention, vigilance	❑ Normal	❑ Sub-normal	❑ Impaired

Primary sensation:

Visual acuity ∃ 20/40, reading	❑ Normal	❑ Sub-normal	❑ Impaired
Hearing	❑ Normal	❑ Sub-normal	❑ Impaired

Acquisition of visual information:

Functional visual field	❑ Normal	❑ Sub-normal	❑ Impaired
Eye movement	❑ Normal	❑ Sub-normal	❑ Impaired
Obligatory head use in gaze	❑ Normal	❑ Sub-normal	❑ Impaired

Processing of visual information:

Information processing ability	❑ Normal	❑ Sub-normal	❑ Impaired
Visual-spatial functioning	❑ Normal	❑ Sub-normal	❑ Impaired

Motor activation:

Foot strength	❑ Normal	❑ Sub-normal	❑ Impaired
Praxis	❑ Normal	❑ Sub-normal	❑ Impaired
Spasticity	❑ Normal	❑ Sub-normal	❑ Impaired
Coordination	❑ Normal	❑ Sub-normal	❑ Impaired
Intrusive involuntary movements of UE/LE	❑ Normal	❑ Sub-normal	❑ Impaired
Ability to perform several motor functions at once	❑ Normal	❑ Sub-normal	❑ Impaired
Other pertinent features of neurologic exam (specify)	❑ Normal	❑ Sub-normal	❑ Impaired

Motor response:

Response latency. Speed of reaction	❑ Normal	❑ Sub-normal	❑ Impaired
Problem-solving ability	❑ Normal	❑ Sub-normal	❑ Impaired
Response to simultaneous stimuli/changing environment	❑ Normal	❑ Sub-normal	❑ Impaired

Executive functions:

Judgment	❑ Normal	❑ Sub-normal	❑ Impaired
Ability to predict/anticipate	❑ Normal	❑ Sub-normal	❑ Impaired
Pertinent features on neuropsychological test (specify)	❑ Normal	❑ Sub-normal	❑ Impaired

Emotional status:

Impulse control	❑ Normal	❑ Sub-normal	❑ Impaired
Degree of risk-taking	❑ Normal	❑ Sub-normal	❑ Impaired
Suicidal depression or nihilism	❑ Normal	❑ Sub-normal	❑ Impaired
Other pertinent features on psychiatric exam (specify)	❑ Normal	❑ Sub-normal	❑ Impaired

Ability to compensate for an identified difficulty   (clarify)
Reliability in following a medical regimen   (comment)
Functional assessment: ADL   (attach)

TABLE 58-3 (*continued*)

Overall Assessment and Disposition:
(1) No clinical impediment to driving is suspected.
(2) Early or minor/acceptable difficulties are recognized. Reevaluate in six months. Patient able to compensate, adjust driving circumstances, or exercise adequate judgment to provide safety.
(3) Safe driving capacity is not definite. Patient instructed to obtain special assessment, and instructed not to drive until that assessment is obtained. If patient cannot or does not comply, see (4).
(4) Patient's driving constitutes a danger to public safety. Reporting may be obligatory in some states.

medical information in order to understand better the individual's cognitive impairments and the implications for driving performance.

Pietrapiana, Tamietto, Torrini et al. (35) described a study of 66 persons in Italy with severe traumatic brain injury, to explore the possibility of predicting post-injury fitness to drive. Predictor variables consisted of 16 measures representing demo/biographic, medicofunctional, neuropsychological and psychosocial domains. Driving outcomes were driving status (i.e., whether they returned to driving), driving safety (based on post-injury accidents) and driving violations. The findings were that the 50% resumed driving; the main difference was the shorter duration of coma in those individuals than the non-drivers. The variables that offered the best prediction of driving safety were the years post-injury, the number of pre-injury car accidents and driving violations, a pre-TBI risky-personality index, and pre-TBI risky-driving-style index. In combination, these four variables predicted 72.5% of the variance. The authors suggested that reports of pre-TBI histories be obtained from close relatives and/or significant others in making predictions about fitness to drive safely post-injury.

Although one's fitness to drive may be clearly evident in some cases, and the decision regarding driving is straightforward, in other cases one's fitness to drive may be marginal. In those cases, driver's training by an instructor with expertise in traumatic brain injury should be considered. The number of sessions would be determined based on the presenting issues, but should be provided at different times of the day and for sufficient lengths of time to be able to assess the possible effects of common sequelae such as fatigue and reduced physical and cognitive endurance on one's capacity to drive safely. Driver's training may also be recommended even in situations where the driver's evaluation clearly confirms one's capacity to drive, as a way for the individual, who may not have driven in quite some time post-injury, to have beneficial support and feedback while gradually returning to driving.

The Use of Public Transportation or Paratransit Services
While many persons would assume that public transportation or specialized transportation (i.e., paratransit services) offer persons with traumatic brain injuries a means to access the community, that is often not the reality. Physical, cognitive-communication, psychosocial and/or behavioral sequelae present enormous obstacles to the use of these systems. In rural areas, bus service may not be available or the nearest bus stop may be far enough away that non-drivers usually must walk to the bus stop. Persons with mobility impairments may be unable to walk that distance. In heavily trafficked areas, the individual may not be able to cross the street quickly enough to assure his or her safety. For individuals with cognitive impairments, inadequate time awareness and attentional deficits can lead to missing the bus, and poor problem-solving may result in impulsive behavior that puts the individual at risk.

Specialized transportation services are also often too complex for persons with traumatic brain injuries to utilize without assistance. Issues arise even when applying for such services since lack of awareness of one's disabilities may lead to inadequate information on application forms for eligibility, resulting in a decision that someone with no apparent mobility impairment does not require the services even when a significant cognitive impairment precludes his/her use of standard public transportation. If the individual *is* declared eligible for specialized services, cognitive-communication problems can undermine attempts to plan and schedule the trips. In particular, difficulty is encountered when transportation is not available at the time it is requested and the individual must consider, quickly, an alternative schedule. Moreover, when being picked up or dropped off by the transportation service, a 15-minute "window" is usual. Persons with attention deficits may become distracted and fail to be ready when the transporter does arrive. Many systems only allow this to happen twice before canceling one's eligibility for services. Trying to rectify some of these problems, the individual may attempt to contact the transportation service and encounter an automated telephone system with a menu of options that is too complicated for him or her to use successfully.

Cognitive rehabilitation therapy (offered by community re-entry programs) is strongly recommended to address these potential difficulties and should be individually tailored to enable the individual to handle the cognitive demands of the transportation systems he or she will actually use. While cognitive rehabilitation can be aimed at remediating functions (e.g., improving attentional abilities as required to signal a bus to stop), the focus is typically on ways to compensate for lost or reduced abilities. For example, compensatory strategies may include the development of structured forms and a telephone script to use when calling to schedule a trip, visual cues or electronic devices (e.g., a watch alarm or timer) to remind the individual to prepare to leave the house at a specified time in order to reach the bus stop on time, role-playing of appropriate verbal exchanges with the bus driver and other passengers, etc. Accompanying the individual on bus rides initially should be part of the therapy process, followed by shadowing, and then independent trips with strategies for problem-solving situations if necessary. Sufficient repetition and rehearsal is essential to mastery of the skills required for use of public transportation.

THE ROLE OF THE PHYSICIAN IN COMMUNITY RE-ENTRY AND LONG-TERM CARE

With respect to community re-entry programs and long-term care, the role of the physician can be discussed in relation to the responsibilities of medical management/medical consultation, and other professional activities, including education and training, research, and expert testimony. Discussion of these roles and responsibilities, in broad terms, follow.

Medical Management/Medical Consultation

Given the diversity in community integration programs, which may be residential or non-residential and based on multidisciplinary, interdisciplinary or transdisciplinary treatment models, the role of the physician will be dictated in large part by the specific focus of the program. Many community re-entry programs employ a medical director, on a full-time or part-time basis, whose responsibilities to the program include, in addition to patient care, functions such as strategic planning, program development, and program evaluation. In recent years, largely because of reductions in reimbursement and recognition of the growing extension of services into the community, many community re-entry programs have chosen to have physicians as consultants to these programs rather than employees. In either case, with respect to patient care, patients in some programs will have been discharged by their physician at an acute rehabilitation hospital (most often a physiatrist, neurologist or neuropsychiatrist) to follow-up by their primary care or family physician. In other

cases, the hospital-based physician may continue to follow the patient post-discharge, for an indefinite period of time. Moreover, physicians in private practice may interface informally with community re-entry providers, providing medical management/consultation on an as-needed basis. The physician serves as a guiding resource to the program or to other providers (medical and non-medical) to define and solve problems of patients or clients (the term preferred in many community re-entry programs) as they arise, with special emphasis on the problems which arise as a direct result of the brain dysfunction and the problems of secondary disruptions that result.

Zasler (36) emphasized that directing a brain injury rehabilitation program requires a shift from the traditional medical model with a disease orientation, to a holistic treatment approach with a functional orientation. In particular, he pointed out that the physician must understand how an individual's functional capabilities can be compromised by neurological and/or musculoskeletal impairments, and what may cause functional decline at various points post-injury. The physician must also recognize when other medical and/or psychological issues and non-injury factors are not directly related to the traumatic brain injury but may compound the disability resulting from TBI and impede the brain injury rehabilitation process.

Physicians with expertise in brain injury rehabilitation also perform a vital role in relation to the individual's return to work following traumatic brain injury. The individual's physician may be asked to provide an opinion of the suitability of a particular job for an individual and to delineate any work restrictions and reasonable accommodations. The need for work restrictions and/or accommodations may be related to physical or cognitive impairments. In some federal agencies, such as the United States Department of Labor's Office of Workers' Compensation Programs (OWCP), a physician's review of the potential job is a mandated part of the reemployment process. Physicians may also be hired by OWCP to evaluate workers' compensation claimants and provide a second opinion or independent medical examination (IME).

Zasler (37) discussed the neurologic sequelae that frequently impede one's ability to return to work, which may include post-traumatic epilepsy, post-traumatic hydrocephalus, olfactory dysfunction, visual deficits, audiovestibular dysfunction, oropharyngeal dysfunction, communication deficits, bladder and/or bowel dysfunction, visuoperceptual deficits, neuropsychological issues, sexuality issues, neurophysical deficits, and orthopedic issues. There is clearly a role for the physician to help agency personnel, employers, vocational rehabilitation personnel, and case managers, as well as the individual with TBI and his or her family members and significant others, to understand the vocational implications of traumatic brain injury sequelae.

Breed, Flanagan and Watson (38) studied 258 individuals with traumatic brain injury and 65 individuals without any disability, to compare the frequency with which they reported health problems and to explore the effects of age and traumatic brain injury on one's perception of his/her health. They pointed out that the limited amount of information on long-term health problems following traumatic brain injury is surprising, given the "central regulatory role" of the brain in physiologic functioning. The results of the study revealed that the individuals with traumatic brain injury reported more endocrine, genitourinary and neurologic problems, and had more complaints of joint pain and sleep disorders. The differences were statistically significant.

With respect to medical management and/or medical consultation, it is important to recognize that community re-entry models of rehabilitation draw primarily upon origins within a variety of pragmatic rehabilitation-related disciplines (e.g., neuropsychology, psychology, occupational therapy, speech pathology) rather than on medical management based on pathophysiology, diagnosis, and prognosis. As in the case of individuals with developmental disabilities, the role of the physician evolved historically through a secondary and consultative role that was problem-oriented and typically specific to the subspeciality area of concern (for example, orthopedic interventions, epilepsy or hydrocephalus management, interventions for depression and psychosis, plastic surgery, visual and auditory/vestibular dysfunctions). Those needs were addressed *ad seriatum* in the consultants' offices without integration to the rehabilitation program as a whole. Moreover, cognitive rehabilitation programs in the United States, developed initially with a focus on traumatic brain injury, have more recently included persons with non-traumatic cerebral injuries: anoxia-hypoxia, encephalitis, stroke and aneurysmal subarachnoid hemorrhage, and survivors of brain tumor resection. The design of intervention by most of the rehabilitative team draws on the clinical features which these disorders have in common rather than drawing on their pathophysiological differences. At times the physician must introduce knowledge and direction leading to program design recognizing differences between types of brain injury.

An integrated approach to residential and outpatient care requires the physician to broaden the scope of practice, and requires an evolution in treatment paradigm within residential and long-term rehabilitation programs. In presenting a neurological model of rehabilitation, Mills and Alexander (39) and Mills, Cassidy, and Katz (40) have outlined the necessary components to achieve suitably informed integration of treatment within an interdisciplinary program that encompasses neuroscience and neuromedical diagnosis and intervention. Diagnosis in rehabilitation ideally addresses the mechanisms and pathophysiology of impairment, and does not merely describe states or lists of functional impairments and disability. From a knowledge of pathophysiology, placed in the framework of neurological syndromes, predictions of improvement and outcome can be derived. That is, the physician is likely to bring to the treatment planning a critique which takes into account a more extensive knowledge of correlation between differentiated types of brain injury and consequent alterations of behavior. Moreover, the physician may articulate the rationale for a revision in expectations of recovery to higher or lower goal set-points, or a longer or shorter duration of treatment, to the treatment team who may define treatment needs in terms of observed functional deficits alone. The physician makes a pivotal contribution in defining the appropriate point of transition to long-term supervised situations for some, and in defining the need for redoubled rehabilitation-oriented efforts in others.

To some degree, all members of the rehabilitative team must be cognizant of premorbid personality and the premorbid endowment of abilities and limitations in defining an individual context for treatment planning. To this context is added behavioral analysis (which takes into account the environmental and interactive aspects of action) and symptom analysis (which generates hypotheses of involuntary and/or intentional generators of specific actions, expressions, or perceptions). The attribution of the meaning of both seemingly normal and seemingly disordered behaviors is drawn from these contexts, and placed in social, psychological, and biological frames of reference. In analyzing a given problematic behavior, understanding predisposing and precipitating factors, and the patient's manifest adaptive capacity, will be essential. The capacity of the individual with traumatic brain injury to adapt to his/her circumstances may reflect such factors as misperception, memory impairment, mental inflexibility, impulsivity, or hyper-reactivity. The physician or other professional who imports knowledge of mechanisms operant within specific neurological impairments will add an additional vital component. For example, a mechanistic view isolates perceptual errors, attribution errors, disconnection errors, overgeneralization errors, encoding vs. decoding errors in memory, and affect regulation vs. disinhibition errors. When grounded in a knowledge of the potentially reversible and potentially irreversible aspects of the brain injury, the rehabilitation strategy is transformed and redirected optimally. The presumed "natural history" of the disorder is then opened to interventions targeted to critical components.

In the modern era, the physician brings to the treatment team a perspective based on knowledge and practice of emerging neurochemistry, neurophysiology, functional neuroimaging, and cognitive neuroscience. These areas represented by the physician include psychopharmacology, cognitive-enhancing treatment, neuro-protective treatments, techniques of physiologic neurorehabilitation, and biomechanical interface. In addition, there are rapidly developing areas of study in neuroplasticity, intracerebral transplantation and regeneration, and hormonal and neurochemical aspects of brain injury and recovery. Many of these issues have been introduced in other chapters of this book.

In the phases of community re-entry, the opportunity arises for the physician to address components of the disordered behavior with a rapidly expanding repertoire of agents. Focusing on the neuropsychiatric and neurobehavioral domains in particular, the components which may yield to pharmacological intervention include inattention, states of hyper- or hypoarousal, depression, mood cycling or lability, aggression, obsessiveness and rigid inflexibility, sleep cycle disturbances and daytime somnolence and/or fatiguability, anxiety states (including posttraumatic stress disorder), pseudobulbar incontinence of emotional expression, hypersexuality or sexual dysfunction, psychosis (delusions, hallucinations), states of apathy, abulia, or failure of motivation and initiative. This is not an exhaustive list. At the same time, it is often the better strategy to integrate such interventions with non-pharmacological modalities, such as psychological support, cognitive rehabilitation therapy, structuring of routines, and education.

At present, many of the newer or experimental modalities of intervention are currently confined to the specialized outpatient clinics at university settings or research institutes, but it will be appropriate for the physician consulting in the community re-entry setting, in particular, to import these new modalities of treatment into the care of the individuals who are far into their post-acute recovery. In the future, rehabilitation may also include implantation of augmenting systems, for example, sensory devices for augmenting hearing and vision. At the present time, the physician is the representative of medical vigilance for such late complications as hydrocephalus, shunt failures, seizures, infections, endocrine disorders, and spasticity, as well as vigilance for adverse complications attributable to medications (SIADH, thrombocytopenia, extrapydramidal movement disorders, psychotoxic adverse side effects, and sedation being particularly common examples). In the population of individuals with traumatic brain injury, drug and alcohol abuse may be demographically over-represented. Accordingly, the physician's vigilance must extend to concerns over hepatitis, drug induced vasculitis, HIV infection, syphilis, tuberculosis, and vigilance for ongoing drug and alcohol abuse, including agents which may advance the degree of brain injury during the period of rehabilitation (toluene inhalation, and "recreational" psychostimulant abuse, for example).

In addition, non-traumatic factors such as late post radiation vasculopathy (in brain tumor survivors) and anoxic encephalopathy may also be present, the latter adding to impairments in movement (cerebellum and basal ganglia), perception (visual cortex), and memory (hippocampus), in addition to the above. (Discussion of the diagnosis and management of late complications of traumatic brain injury is found in chapter XX of this book, by Long.) The cumulative effects of neurologic aging, and the superimposed impairment of acquired brain neurodegenerative diseases in elderly persons, will also occur in those injured by trauma, and will require a refreshing of medical differential diagnosis when a progressive worsening of the pattern of impairments is detected. By far, the most prevalent late complications are those which fall into the neurobehavioral and neuropsychiatric domain, which are closely linked with the nature of the individual's emotional and neurocognitive deficits.

Structures of the brain which are known to be disproportionately vulnerable in brain trauma include the frontal and temporal lobes, but also the amygdala, hippocampus and basal ganglia. Late neuropsychiatric complications are at least equally prevalent though less well localized, and include depression, psychosis, a spectrum of disinhibited and unrealistic behaviors, and a persisting failure of insight, self-observation, or initiative. These represent disruption of the interface between the individual with brain injury and the environment which, at times by analogy or by comparison to recognized neurological and psychiatric syndromes, benefits from a medical understanding or intervention. The involvement of neurology, neuropsychology, and psychiatry in the understanding of the behavioral consequences which are intrinsic to these lesions, while built on a long history of the clinical pathological correlation of discrete lesions, has enjoyed an ascendence only in the last few decades, coincident with the emergence of the bridging subspecialties of behavioral neurology and neuropsychiatry.

Psychiatry, while historically not as often relying on clinical-pathological correlation, has allusion to a nosology of discrete syndromes which serve as reference points for intervention. The knowledge of the constellations of impairments which follow typically from traumatic brain injury should be known to any physician involved in the care of these individuals, including the broad range of other specialists and primary physicians.

Determining the Need for and Choice of Community-Based Treatment

After being discharged from the acute and subacute phases of rehabilitation, the status of treatment goals will determine the setting in which further recovery optimally will take place. Outpatient treatment and direct community re-entry will be possible if the individual with TBI has sufficient self-awareness of the need for it, and if outpatient resources are available to address persisting cognitive, behavioral, emotional, vocational, and physical needs. If self-awareness is sufficiently impaired to result in unsafe or disruptive behavior, the consideration for residential community treatment will be stronger.

Circumstances which may prompt a referral to a residential or nonresidential community re-entry program for persons with brain injuries include, but are not limited to, the following:

1) When community re-entry programs can provide essential, ecologically-valid observations and treatment that cannot be provided otherwise. Treatment rendered in a clinic, facility or office setting may not yield a clear picture of the sources of failure to function adequately. The importance of gaining a better understanding of the individual's needs is underscored when the individual is caught in a cascade or vicious cycle of repeated failures to function adequately and requires external reinforcement of adaptive and compensatory strategies, and/or continual feedback.

2) When intervention is required because of failed executive functioning. This circumstance may become apparent in relation to individuals who attempt living on their own following traumatic brain injury but who are unable to resume functioning at, or close to, their pre-injury level. Common problems for those individuals include inability to follow a prescribed medication regimen, to manage family, financial or personal responsibilities, or to maintain an environment conducive to satisfactory functioning. Crises of disorganization can result, exemplified by hoarding of possessions or accumulation of items/objects, leading to overwhelming clutter and chaos.

3) When the individual is unable to establish functional routines as needed to accomplish activities of daily living. Sequelae of traumatic brain injury may include memory problems, inadequate planning and organizing, difficulty making decisions and impaired ability to initiate purposeful activity, contributing to the inability to carry out daily routines. Other variables compromising one's ability to establish and maintain a productive daily activity pattern include apathy syndrome, severe obsessive disorder (whose rituals or unresolvable obsessions create "paralysis" of activity), depression, and anxiety. There may be repeated failures to resume work, school or social/leisure activity.

4) When outpatient programs are not available (for reasons of lack of funding, distance, or other reasons) or are not intensive enough to meet the individual's needs. This circumstance may be particularly problematic if the individual's family is unable to provide adequate support for, or reinforcement of, treatment interventions and when inadequate daily structure leads to maladaptive behavior.

5) When continued supervision is necessary. Once individuals are discharged home, other family members often anticipate they will be able to resume their usual roles (e.g., return to work) and do not fully appreciate the need for supervision that may be required by the individual with traumatic brain injury. Potential problems when adequate supervision is not provided include the use of alcohol or drugs, frontal syndrome with impulsivity and poor judgment, aggressive or disinhibited behavior, and frontal syndromes with anosognosia. Of paramount importance is the safety and well-being of the individual with traumatic brain injury and his/her family members. For example, memory problems may result in the individual forgetting to turn off the stove or oven, increasing the risk of fire. Fatigue is also common following traumatic brain injury and may result in the individual falling asleep while smoking. These possible scenarios underscore the need for supervision.

When the rehabilitative phase of post-TBI care yields to chronic maintenance or "custodial care," the physician's role remains vital. A number of factors, both physiological and psychological, may intrude and erode further the individual's quality of life and access to optimal level of functioning. It is also true that chronicity does not preclude the possibility of treatment targets that, when addressed, may improve function in the client who is many years beyond the scope of brain tissue recovery.

Other Physician Roles in Community Re-entry

Education and Training In patient care settings, education and training by the physician (often in collaboration with other professionals) may be directed to family or caretaking staff, to the programmatic design staff and/or to the patient himself or herself. When providing education to the individual with traumatic brain injury, the physician will attempt to help the individual understand the commonalities that persist despite cultural differences and, at the same time, represent the essential voice of culture in steering the rebuilding of self. The physician can be called on to recognize, or ideally to teach others to recognize, physiological disorders which mimic psychological disturbances. For example, a disorder of initiation, motivation, or "apathy" may arise from brain injury and may mimic amotivational or apathetic mood states. Dysfunction of cortical-subcortical circuits are particularly implicated in such amotivational states, including the medial prefrontal area, anterior cingulum, nucleus accumbens, ventral palladium or medial dorsal thalamus. It is essential that the treatment providers understand the difference, in order to select and render appropriate treatment methods. To assure optimal management of the patient, the treatment team must understand the pathophysiology of symptoms and signs of a given neurological disorder, and the natural history of both the disease and the impairments. When directing the treatment, the physician must assure that the team members understand the patient's impairment(s), diagnosis and prognosis, and how to implement the interdisciplinary treatment.

Mills and Alexander (41) identified four essential educational components for every team member: 1) the neurological diseases they will treat; 2) goal-setting and plan development for patients with complicated cognitive problems; 3) appreciation of the treatment outside his/her own specialty; and 4) development and use of cost-effective, affordable approaches to assessment and treatment.

Continuing education and training of other physicians and nonmedical personnel will also help to increase understanding of the needs of persons with traumatic brain injury. Conferences sponsored by professional associations are a frequent venue for such offerings. Because of the multidisciplinary nature of the field of rehabilitation, the American Congress of Rehabilitation Medicine (www.acrm.org) and the American Society for Neurorehabilitation (www.asnr.com) are particularly relevant.

Research   The National Institute on Disability and Rehabilitation Research (NIDRR), United States Department of Education, has been funding projects in the area of community integration through TBI Model System grants and Rehabilitation Research and Training Centers, which should provide valuable information to enhance understanding of the benefits of such programs, and opportunities for physicians to pursue research interests.

Expert Testimony   The physician may be called upon for a variety of official tasks. He or she will be called upon to mediate in medicolegal issues (e.g., designation of payee for entitlements, statements of capacity/competence, assessment for guardianship proceedings, driving licensure, designation of impairment for professional work, or letters of medical necessity) and may also provide expert testimony in personal injury cases. See Chapter 62 by Cantor on medicolegal aspects of traumatic brain injury and Chapter 63 by Ameis et al. on ethical issues in clinicolegal practice.

Manifestations of frontal dysfunction, which pervasively undermine normal adaptations to social environments, are difficult to represent to the legal system (42, 43). The physician may be called upon to justify continued compensation under auto insurance policies (e.g., personal injury protection [PIP] or workers' compensation policies). In the current era, the precertification of treatments may require the physician to act as advocate, at times in opposition to third party payers who would profit by nihilism.

Conclusion

There has been rapid growth in community re-entry services and long-term care for individuals with traumatic brain injury, spawned by greater understanding of their needs at this point in the rehabilitation process and augmented by legislative and managed care initiatives resulting in shorter hospital stays and earlier return to the community. While the methodological problems inherent in conducting empirical studies at this point, with such a highly heterogeneous population and extensive array of services, have resulted in limited scientific evidence of the efficacy of these programs and services, their value to the individual and his/her family cannot be questioned. Findings of studies that have been conducted and anecdotal reports support the value of these services in improving the functional outcomes and enhancing the quality of life for individuals with traumatic brain injury.

Services and supports at this point in the rehabilitation process are typically provided by nonmedical as well as medical personnel. There continues to be a vital role for the physician in relation to medical management and consultation as well as in relation to education, training and research.

It is through the familiarity with neurobehavioral constellations (which can be interpreted to the injured individual himself or herself and to the involved family) that the physician's involvement may impact uniquely upon rebuilding of personhood and the integrity of self, a goal of intervention distinct from, but no less valuable than, the more narrow focus of remission of medical problems. The concept of self has a grounding presence in the neurorehabilitation of those in whom the cerebral substrate of self has been undermined. Kircher (44) conceptualized the self as the sense of being a whole person constant over time but different from others, and the center of all our experience. A challenge, both cognitive and emotional, is frequently placed before the individual with brain injury to synthesize and evolve a novel posture from which to carry his or her transformed life forward. At times this new synthesis must encounter or master social developmental issues which may have, or may not have, been mastered prior to trauma, and frequently this new synthesis involves great losses or compromises of deeply set life goals and premorbid self-definitions. The brain's impairments may interfere with the adaptation, reframing, or flexibility, which would be required to escape a negative self-definition of incompetence, disappointment, or abandoned aspiration in an individual whose mental repertoire and capacity is forever altered. The physician may offer the important contribution to that individual of informed wisdom, both hopeful and realistic, about the brain's potential, and offer a continuing and long-term commitment to the individual's progress, even as that person shifts from setting to setting, and from one challenge to the next.

Note

National Directory of Brain Injury Rehabilitation Services 2005 Edition, Brain Injury Association of America, Inc., McLean, VA, 2005. This directory is published annually and includes listings of types of brain injury programs and service specialties, state and national resources, and information about military/veterans services through the Defense and Veterans Head Injury Program. Also included are explanations of common abbreviations in the field of brain injury rehabilitation as well as the Rancho Los Amigos Levels of Cognitive Functioning Scale and the Glasgow Coma Scale (GCS). In the 2005 edition, Appendix A consists of a guide to selecting and monitoring brain injury rehabilitation services, and Appendix B contains a glossary and definitions of commonly used terms. The directory can be purchased by calling the Brain Injury Association of American at 1-800-444-6443 or accessing the association's website (www.biausa.org).

References

1. Cusick CP, Gerhart KA, Mellick D, Breese P, Towle V, Whiteneck GC. Evaluation of the home and community-based services brain injury Medicaid Waiver Programme in Colorado. *Brain Injury* 2003;17(11):931–945.
2. Venzie DR, Felicetti T, Cerra-Tyl D. Planning considerations for community integrative brain injury programs. *J Head Trauma Rehabil* 1996;11(6):51–64.
3. Commission on Accreditation of Rehabilitation Facilities,*Medical Rehabilitation Standards Manual*,Tucson, AZ,2005.
4. Brandt EN, Pope AM (eds.). *Enabling America: Assessing the Role of Rehabilitation Science and Engineering*. Washington, DC: National Academy Press,1997.
5. *NIH Consensus Statement* (Volume 16, Number 1, October 26 to 28, 1998).
6. Malec JF, Basford JS. Postacute brain injury rehabilitation. *Arch Phys Med Rehabil* 1996;77:198–207.
7. Dobkin BH. *The Clinical Science of Neurologic Rehabilitation*. Oxford University Press, 2003;497–546.
8. Evans RW. Postacute Neurorehabilitation: Roles and responsibilities within a national information system. *Arch Phys. Med Rehabil* 1997;78(8, Suppl 4):S17-S25.
9. Cope DN, Mayer NH, Cervelli L. Development of systems of care for persons with traumatic brain injury. *J Head Trauma Rehabil* 2005;20(2):128–142.
10. Berube J. The Traumatic Brain Injury Act Amendments of 2000. *J Head Trauma Rehabil*. 2003;16(2):210–213.
11. Social Security Online, *The Work Site*, www.ssa.gov/work.
12. Social Security Online, *Electronic Booklets: The Ticket to Work and Self-Sufficiency Program*, www.ssa.gov/pubs.
13. *National Directory of Brain Injury Rehabilitation Services 2005 Edition*. Brain Injury Association of America, McLean, VA,2005.
14. Minnes P, Carlson P, McColls MA, Nolte MG, Johnston J, Buell K. Community integration: A useful construct, but what does it really mean? *Brain Injury* 2003;17(2):149–159.
15. Goranson TE, Graves RE, Allison D, La Freniere R. Community integration following multidisciplinary rehabilitation for traumatic brain injury. *Brain Injury* 2003;17(9):759–774.
16. Dawson DD, Levine B, Schwartz ML, Stuss DT. Acute predictors of real-world outcomes following traumatic brain injury: A prospective study. *Brain Injury* 2004;18(3):221–238.
17. Cicerone KD, Dahlberg C, Kalmar K,et al. Evidence-based cognitive rehabilitation: Recommendations for clinical practice. *Arch Phys Med Rehab* 2000;81:1596–1615.
18. Cicerone KD, Tupper DE. Neuropsychological rehabilitation: Treatment of errors in everyday functioning. In: Tupper ED, Cicerone KD (eds.). *The Neuropsychology of Everyday Life: Issues in Development and Rehabilitation*. Boston: Kluwer Academic Publishers, 1991.
19. Gordon WA, Hibbard MR. Cognitive Rehabilitation. In: Silver JM, McAllister TW, Yudofsky SC (eds.). *Textbook of Traumatic Brain Injury*. Washington, DC, American Psychiatric Publishing, 2005, 655–660.
20. *NIH Consensus Statement* (Volume 16,Number 1,October 26 to 28, 1998).
21. Williams JM, Kay T. *Head Injury: A Family Matter*. Baltimore, MD: Paul H. Brookes, 1991.
22. Rider-Williams B, Trout E. *Family Members' Adjustment to Traumatic Brain Injury Upon Community Re-entry*. Presentation at the Sixteenth Annual National Symposium sponsored by the Brain Injury Association, Inc., November 2,1997.
23. Laroi F. The family systems approach to treating families of persons with brain injury: A potential collaboration between family therapist and brain injury professional. *Brain Injury* 2003;17(2): 175–187.
24. Kosciulek JF, Pichette EF. Adaptation concerns of families of people with head injuries. *J Appl Rehabil Coun* 1996;27:8–13.
25. Godfrey HPD, Harnett MA, Knight RG,et al. Assessing distress in caregivers of people with a traumatic brain injury (TBI);a psychometric study of the Head Injury Behaviour Scale. *Brain Injury* 2003;17(5):427–435.
26. Ponsford J, Olver J, Ponsford M, Nelms R. Long-term adjustment of families following traumatic brain injury where comprehensive rehabilitation has been provided. *Brain Injury* 2003;17(6):453–468.
27. Burleigh SA, Farber RS, Gillard M. Community integration and life satisfaction after traumatic brain injury. Long-term findings. *Am J Occup Ther* 1998;52:45–52.
28. Brown M, Gordon WA, Spielman L. Participation in social and recreational activity in the community by individuals with traumatic brain injury. *Rehabilitation Psychology* 2003;48(4): 266–274.
29. Galski T, Ehle HT, McDonald MA, Mackevich J. Evaluating fitness to drive after cerebral injury: basic issues and recommendations for medical and legal communities. *J Head Trauma Rehabil* 2000;15(3):895–908.
30. Coleman RD, Rapport LJ, Ergh TC, Hanks RA, Ricker JH, Millis SR. Predictors of driving outcome after traumatic brain injury. *Arch Phys Med Rehabil* 2002;83:1415–1422.
31. Krauss GL, Ampaw L, Krumholz A. Individual state driving restrictions for people with epilepsy in the U.S. *Neurology*. 2001; 57:1780–1785.
32. Drazkowski JF. Symposium on seizures: Management of the social consequences of seizures. *Mayo Clin Proc*. 2003;78:641–649.
33. Rubin AJ. *Evaluating Driving Capacity in Huntington's Disease*. In McCormack MK, Rubin AJ, Lawler K, Grossman R, Schwartz RR, Dempsey KL. *Huntington's Disease: A Manual*. From the Samuel L. Baily Huntington's Disease Family Service Center of the University of Medicine and Dentistry of New Jersey School of Osteopathic Medicine and Robert Wood Johnson Medical School, Camden and New Brunswick, NJ and Cooper Hospital University Medical Center, Camden, NJ.
34. Schulteis MT, Hillary F, Chute DL. The Neurocognitive Driving Test: Applying Technology to the Assessment of Driving Ability Following Brain Injury. *Rehabilitation Psychology* 2003;48(4): 275–280.
35. Pietrapiana P, Tamietto M, Torrini G, Mezzanato T, Rago R, Perino C. Role of premorbid factors in predicting safe return to driving after severe TBI. *Brain Injury* 2005;19(3):197–211.
36. Zasler ND. Physiatric Assessment in Traumatic Brain Injury. In: Rosenthal M, Griffith ER, Kreutzer JS, Pentland B (eds.). *Rehabilitation of the Adult and Child with Traumatic Brain Injury* (Third Edition). Philadelphia: F.A. Davis, 1999;117–130.
37. Zasler ND. The Role of the Physiatrist. In: Wehman P, Kreutzer JS (eds.). *Vocational Rehabilitation: For Persons with Traumatic Brain Injury*. Rockville, MD: Aspen Publishers, 1990;71–87.
38. Breed ST, Flanagan SR, Watson KR. The relationship between age and the self-report of health symptoms in persons with traumatic brain injury. *Arch Phys Med Rehabil* 2004;85(Suppl 2):S61-S67.
39. Mills VM, Alexander MP. Cognitive rehabilitation: leadership and management of the clinical programme. In Stuss DT, Winocur G, Robertson IH (eds.). *Cognitive Neurorehabilitation*, Cambridge University Press,1999.
40. Mills VM, Cassidy JW, Katz DI. *Neurologic Rehabilitation: A Guide to Diagnosis, Prognosis, and Treatment Planning*,Blackwell Science,1997.
41. Mills VM, Alexander MP. Cognitive rehabilitation: leadership and management of the clinical programme. In Stuss DT, Winocur G,

Robertson IH (eds.). *Cognitive Neurorehabilitation.* Cambridge University Press, 1999.

42. Silver JM, McAllister TW. Forensic issues in the neuropsychiatric evaluation of the patient with mild traumatic brain injury. *J Neuropsychiatry Clin Neurosci* 1997;9(1):102–113.

43. Fogel BS. The significance of frontal system disorders for medical practice and health policy. *J. Neuropscyhiatry Clin Neurosci* 1994;6(4):343–347.

44. Kircher T, David A. *The Self in Neuropsychiatry and Psychiatry,* Cambridge University Press, 2003.

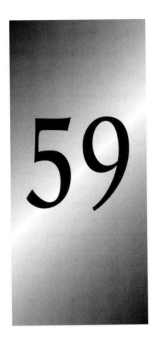

59 The Treatment of Substance Abuse in Persons with TBI

John D. Corrigan

THE TREATMENT OF ALCOHOL AND OTHER DRUG ABUSE IN PERSONS WITH TBI

Clinicians working with people who have incurred a traumatic brain injury (TBI) cannot avoid the issue of alcohol and other drug use. Whether consumption of these substances contributed to the cause of injury, or their use after injury places the individual at risk for medical complications, alcohol and other drug use must be addressed with adolescents and adults in order to preserve the benefits of rehabilitation. In addition to medical complications, substance abuse also limits outcomes by undermining environmental supports such as familial care or access to services. Indeed, alcohol and other drugs may be so detrimental to recovery of function and lifestyle and, in aggregate, to the case that can be made for the benefit to society of rehabilitation services, that it would be short-sighted not to do all we can to minimize their negative effects.

This chapter provides a review of current research on TBI and the use of alcohol and other drugs. There is far greater information describing this problem and its scope than there is research on treatment approaches to ameliorate use-related disorders. Studies of the risks of substance abuse after TBI are discussed, including who is at risk. A review of interventions and treatment approaches that have specifically addressed substance use following TBI precedes explication of a theoretical

model for the development of interventions to treat substance use disorders following TBI. Use of this model is intended to better focus both research and program development.

WHAT ARE THE RISKS OF SUBSTANCE USE AFTER TBI?

Persons with TBI and substance abuse problems are less likely to be working (1–3), have lower subjective well-being (4, 5), increased likelihood of suicide (6) and are at greater risk for seizure (7). There is also evidence from studies of incarcerated populations that the increased risk for aggressive behavior after TBI is further exacerbated by substance abuse. In addition to these psychosocial consequences, several studies have found an additive effect of negative consequences for both brain structure and function (8, 9).

Psychosocial Consequences

Numerous studies have observed that substance use problems preceding injury are often a significant predictor of post-injury unemployment. MacMillan , Hart, Martelli and Zasler (3) studied 45 adults two years after moderate or severe TBI. They hypothesized that severity of premorbid psychiatric and substance use disorders, as well as less social support following injury, would be associated with poorer post-injury employment, independent living and neurobehavioral symptom manifestation. They found that both pre-injury psychiatric and substance abuse histories predicted a lower likelihood of employment and that pre-injury substance abuse also was associated with less independence in living situation. Sherer, Bergloff, High, and Nick (2) studied 76 persons with moderate or severe TBI who received services through a specialized day treatment program. Employment status three months following discharge from this program was assessed, on average, two years post-injury. Predictors of employment status included severity of injury, premorbid education, pre-injury substance abuse, and need for physical, cognitive and behavioral supervision at discharge from acute rehabilitation. Multiple logistic regressions revealed that only level of pre-injury substance use was predictive of later productivity. Subjects with no history of pre-injury substance abuse were more than eight times as likely to be employed at follow-up.

Bogner and colleagues (4) investigated the relative contribution of substance abuse and violent injury etiology in a sample of 351 consecutive admissions for acute brain injury rehabilitation. At one year following injury prior history of substance use disorder was a significant predictor of post-injury employment, as were age, pre-injury employment and cognitive function at rehabilitation discharge. Despite the consistent finding that pre-injury substance abuse is associated with post-injury unemployment, the relationship with post-injury use may be more complex. Sander, Kreutzer and Fernandez (10) found that employed persons who had incurred moderate or severe TBI and were on the average 16 months post-injury reported consuming greater amounts of alcohol than similar subjects who were unemployed. This finding may be consistent with clinical observations that return to work can be a trigger for substance use because of having financial resources to purchase alcohol or other drugs, as well as increased stressors arising from the work environment.

Corrigan and colleagues (5) reported that a prior history of substance use disorder was highly associated with life satisfaction both one and two years after injury. At year one, prior substance abuse was the strongest independent predictor of life satisfaction and continued to be a significant predictor two years after injury, even after the effects of depressed mood, social integration and employment had been accounted for. Bogner and colleagues (4) considered whether life satisfaction was more affected by substance abuse history or violent injury etiology. As with employment, they found substance abuse history was the more important predictor, along with pre-injury employment and motor function at discharge.

In the general population there is a well documented relationship between depression and substance abuse (11),

and given the high rate of depression following TBI, the co-occurrence of depression and substance abuse would be expected in this population as well. Indeed, there has been some indication of an independent relationship between substance abuse and the likelihood of suicide following TBI. Teasdale and Engberg (6) examined suicide after TBI using the Danish population register for hospital admissions between 1979 and 1993. Standardized mortality ratios stratified by sex and age indicated the incidence of suicide relative to the general population was increased by 2.7 for concussions, 3.0 for cranial fractures and 4.1 for intracranial hemorrhage. When substance use diagnosis x TBI diagnosis was examined, standardized mortality ratios increased significantly. Silver, Kramer, Greenwald and Weissman (11) reported the relative risks of psychiatric problems for a randomly selected subgroup of the New Haven portion of the NIMH Epidemiologic Catchment Area study. TBI alone significantly increased the risk of suicide by an odds ratio of 5.7. After controlling for alcohol abuse and dependence, the likelihood of suicide attempt declined 4.5, suggesting that alcohol use accounted for approximately 20% of the risk of suicide after TBI.

Verma, Policherla and Buber (7) looked at the relationship between chronic abusers' withdrawal from alcohol and the occurrence of a seizure episode. They separated a sample of 54 adult male alcoholics who had experienced seizures into three groups—those for whom there was always a clear relationship between withdrawal and the seizure episode (the last drink occurring between 6 and 96 hours prior to seizure), those for whom some but not all seizure episodes were associated with withdrawal, and a third group in which none of the seizure episodes were associated with withdrawal. They found that a history of severe TBI preceding the onset of seizure disorder was present for none of those patients in the first group, approximately 40% of those in the second group, and more than 75% of those in the third. They concluded the lack of a constant relationship between alcohol withdrawal and seizure precipitation for the second and third groups appears to be a result of the higher incidence of prior TBI in those subjects, and that this relationship may account for the previously observed heterogeneity in the relationship between alcohol withdrawal and seizure episodes.

Finally, regarding substance abuse and poorer outcomes following TBI, there is mounting evidence of associations with aggression and criminal activity (12). Increased aggression following TBI has been reported in multiple studies (13–15). Persons with TBI are more likely to be involved with the criminal justice system (12, 16), and there is evidence of a high prevalence among prisoners. A sample of 1,000 consecutively admitted offenders to the Illinois state prison system found 25% had incurred at least one TBI (17). Of those reporting

60 A Cognitive-Behavioral Intervention for Family Members of Persons with TBI

Angelle M. Sander

The current Zeitgeist in the field of rehabilitation emphasizes the role of the environment in the ability of persons with impairments to participate fully in all societal roles and to integrate into their communities (1–4). The environmental context can foster the full integration of persons into the community or can provide barriers.

With the increasing emphasis on the importance of the environment, the role of the family in fostering the community integration of persons with TBI has gained more recognition. As the most basic unit of society, the individual's family has the potential to aid or impede recovery from TBI. Persons with TBI are frequently dependent upon family members in a variety of areas, including transportation, finances, leisure, and emotional support (5). A healthy family environment is likely to contribute to better adjustment for the person with injury. Unfortunately, there is ample evidence that TBI results in substantial emotional distress for family members. Family members who are distressed are less likely to be able to provide the support that persons with TBI need as they transition from the rehabilitation setting into the community. In spite of the evidence for family distress after injury, there has been relatively little focus on family intervention as part of the rehabilitation process. With the decreasing length of rehabilitation stays, the focus is often on training family members to care for the most immediate needs of the person with injury. There is minimal time to prepare family members for long-term cognitive and behavioral changes in the person with injury. There is even less time available to address the emotional needs of family members and to assist them in coping with the impact of injury on their life and relationships.

The purpose of the current chapter is to provide a framework for intervening with family members to assist them in managing injury-related stress and in helping the person with injury to compensate for difficulties in a way that will maximize participation. The chapter will begin with a brief review of the research on the impact of TBI on family members. A framework for conceptualizing the factors that contribute to family members' distress after injury will then be introduced. This framework will be used as a basis for proposing components of a family intervention program. Next, a theory-driven and comprehensive intervention program for family members will be introduced. The chapter will close with recommendations for future directions in conducting interventions with family members. The information in this chapter will be applicable to family members of persons with moderate to severe injury. There has been minimal research on the impact of mild TBI on the family.

WHAT IS THE IMPACT OF TBI ON THE FAMILY?

The research conducted over the past 30 years has been unequivocal in showing the emotional impact of TBI on family members (6–9). Family members report clinically significant amounts of depression and/or anxiety at the period between 3 months and 1 year post-injury (10–14). They also report significant levels of stress or "perceived burden" related to symptoms in the person with injury (13–17). While most persons with TBI show some improvement in symptoms over time, the research has shown that family distress actually persists and in certain cases increases over time. Substantial emotional distress has been noted in family members as long as 5 and 7 years after injury (12, 16–18). The persistence of distress is likely related to the type of symptoms that tend to endure in the person with injury. While substantial improvements are usually noted in physical, cognitive, and emotional symptoms over the first year after injury, some type of impairment often remains (19). The most enduring symptoms tend to be changes in emotions, social interaction, and higher level cognitive skills (e.g., organization, self-monitoring) (19). Changes in emotional functioning and social interaction skills have been shown to contribute most to family members' distress (20–23). Evidence of family members' emotional distress is manifested in the fact that they seek services for mental health problems more frequently after injury and they make greater use of alcohol and other drugs (24). There is evidence that a large proportion of family members have backgrounds that could predispose them toward having adjustment difficulties following injury. These backgrounds include pre-existing emotional difficulties and unhealthy family interactions (25).

Family members' emotional distress may be partially related to other types of changes that they experience after injury. Relationships among family members often change in a negative way after injury (12, 26, 27). The person with injury is often unable to resume the roles formerly held within the family. Some of the roles vacated by the person with injury may be action roles, such as earning money or performing chores, and others may be emotional, such as being the person who people turn to in times of trouble. The roles that the person with injury can no longer fill are usually taken over by another family member. The result is often that certain family members are attempting to fill too many roles, resulting in role strain. Role strain can have a negative impact on physical and mental health. Another type of change in relationships resulting from TBI is decreased communication among family members (12) Due to the increased time demands related to caring for the person with injury and taking over unfulfilled roles, there is typically less time for quality family interaction. Impaired communication,

particularly with regard to social skills and pragmatics, is common in persons with TBI and may impact the ability of family members to interact with one another. In certain cases, the person with TBI may have difficulty controlling verbally and/or physically aggressive behaviors, affecting the quality of family relationships.

Injury-related stress and changes in the person with injury may have a negative impact upon sharing of warmth and affection among family members (12) Especially for marital partners, injury often results in decreased intimacy and satisfaction with the relationship (26–28). Decreased intimacy can result from a combination of cognitive and behavioral changes in the person with injury, the emotional reaction of spouses or intimate partners to the injury, and environmental stressors, such as decreased finances and decreased time to devote to relationships. Spouses have reported that serving in the caregiving role for a person with TBI places them in a parent-like relationship that is incompatible with their role as an intimate partner (29). Partners often find changes in the person with TBI, such as dependent behaviors and disnhibited sexual comments, unattractive (30). Intimacy is further decreased by the fact that 1/3 to 1/2 of persons with TBI experience some form of sexual disturbance, including decreased drive and/or arousal, impaired physiological response, and decreased ability to achieve orgasm (31–34).

Another type of difficulty that family members often face after TBI is social isolation (6, 35) Immediately following the injury, family members typically experience an increase in social support. Friends, neighbors, church associates, and extended family typically rally during a catastrophic event such as a life-threatening injury. This immediate increase in support often wanes with time. Recovery from TBI is a long process, and for some persons, impairments endure for a lifetime. Sustaining social support for this length of time is rare for most family members. As time goes on, persons who initially provided support often visit and call less frequently. This decline in social support over time is a phenomenon that is typical following most catastrophic events. However, it may be compounded in the case of TBI due to emotional and behavioral deficits in the person with injury. Changes in social interaction skills are difficult for persons unfamiliar with the effects of TBI to understand. People who could provide support for family members may feel awkward interacting with the person who is injured, and may react by avoiding interactions with them and their family. In other cases, family members of persons with injury may withdraw from others because they are embarrassed by the social behaviors of the person with injury (6). In either case, the result is usually that the person with injury, as well as their family members, become isolated. This isolation usually occurs at longer post-injury intervals, when rehabilitation and other medical services have ended, further increasing isolation.

WHAT PREDICTS FAMILY MEMBERS' RESPONSE TO TBI?

Understanding what enables some family members to adjust relatively well to injury-related changes while others deteriorate physically or mentally is an important first step toward developing appropriate interventions. One possibility is that the family members of persons with more severe injuries and greater impairments will experience greater distress. However, this hypothesis has been only partially supported. While injury severity has been shown to be related to caregivers' distress at 3 to 6 months post-injury, little relationship has been found at longer follow-up periods (10, 11, 15, 21–23, 36). Regarding impairments in the person with injury, changes in emotional functioning and social interaction changes have been found to be related to caregivers' distress (14, 18, 20–23, 37). The relationship between caregivers' distress and cognitive deficits in the person with injury has generally been moderate (15, 22, 23). Physical impairments in the person with injury have not been found to contribute much to caregivers' distress (15, 22, 23).

There is some evidence that spouses of persons with TBI experience greater stress than do parents (22, 23). There are a couple of possible reasons for this. First, parents who care for adult children with TBI are returning to a caregiver role that is familiar to them. While they may not have been in that role with their child for many years, the familiarity of the role may reduce stress somewhat. In contrast, a husband or wife caring for an injured spouse is forced into a role that is likely unfamiliar and uncomfortable. Many family members describe the behavior of the person with injury as being more child-like. It is possible that parents may have an easier time accepting childlike behavior in their adult child than will a spouse. A second possible reason for decreased stress in parents relative to spouses may be that many parents will have a spouse or partner to assist them in the caregiving role. In contrast, a husband or wife caring for an injured spouse does not have the instrumental or emotional support of a partner. In addition, their relationship may have changed in a way that has them grieving for the loss of a significant partnership. It is important to realize that the research has not been conclusive in showing that parents experience less stress than spouses (10, 11, 21, 38). Many parents caring for an injured adult child may experience substantial stress on having their child return to a dependent role at a time in life when they were looking forward to retiring and relaxing. The switch in role may also lead to the emergence of dependence and autonomy struggles that had been earlier resolved during the child's transition to adulthood. Reemergence of these struggles can be very stressful for all involved.

There has also been some evidence that male family members experience greater stress in the caregiver role compared to females (39, 40). This finding may be partly due to the fact that the caregiving role may be more familiar for many females. Males may also be overwhelmed by the variety of roles they have to assume if their wife is injured. In many households, the wife typically bears the primary responsibility for childcare, household chores, and planning social activities. When the wife is injured, her husband is faced with taking over these roles, as well as maintaining employment. For many men, this results in substantial role strain. Finally, males may be less likely to seek emotional support or to share their emotions with others, making it more difficult for them to cope with stress.

The research to date has shown that injury-related characteristics and demographics only partially explain family members' response to TBI. Professionals who work with families after TBI realize that individual characteristics unique to different family members impact the way that they cope with the injury and related changes. Characteristics unique to individuals, such as coping style, cognitive appraisals of the caregiving situation, and social support can impact their response to stressful situations (41, 42). Coping skills, cognitive appraisals, and social support serve as a buffer between stressful events and family members' physical and mental health. This model has recently been adapted for caregivers of persons with TBI (40, 43). Due to its applicability to designing family interventions, the model and supporting evidence for caregivers of persons with TBI will be discussed in detail below.

A GUIDING MODEL FOR UNDERSTANDING FAMILY RESPONSE TO TBI

The model below has been adapted from previous research on stress and coping theory in individuals and in families (41, 42).

The model proposes that the relationship between the injury and family members' response, as operationalized by their physical and mental health, is not a direct one. Response to the injury is mediated by family members' coping styles, their perception or appraisal of the caregiving role, and the social support they have available. The model explains why 2 different family members who are caring for persons of similar injury severity with similar types of impairments can have different responses. Each individual is unique with regard to coping skills, the way they view events, and their social networks.

In the past 5 years, several studies have investigated the relationship of various components of this model to caregiver distress. Several studies have found that the coping style of caregivers is related to their distress (37, 40, 44, 45) Specifically, the use of strategies such as escape-avoidance (e.g., wishing that the problem would go away) and accepting responsibility or blaming oneself is related to higher levels of emotional distress in caregivers (46). Use of spiritual support, use of social support, and reframing of negative thoughts have been found to be associated with less stress and burden (45). The amount of social support that caregivers have available has also been shown to be related to distress (44, 47). However, one study indicated that it is caregivers' satisfaction with social support rather than the actual amount of support that predicts distress (40). The contribution of cognitive appraisals to caregiver distress has not received as much attention as the other components of the model. Struchen and colleagues (48) adapted a measure of caregiver appraisal, The Caregiver Appraisal Scale (49), that had been developed for use with caregivers of persons with dementia. They showed that the scale had validity for use with caregivers of persons with TBI and that negative appraisals were related to greater emotional distress. The subjective burden measure used by Brooks, McKinlay, and colleagues (15–17) can be conceptualized as an appraisal of the impact of injury, since it requires caregivers to rate the overall stress resulting from the injury. Sander and colleagues (40) found that scores on the subjective burden scale were significantly related to symptoms of emotional distress on a psychiatric inventory. They also provided evidence for the utility of the model shown in Figure 60-1. Level of impairment in the person with injury (stressful event), coping strategies, subjective burden, and social support accounted for more than half of the variance in emotional distress.

Implications of Research for Family Interventions

The research to date has shown that impairments in the person with injury contribute to family members' distress, and that impairments in emotional functioning and social behavior are most stressful for family members. However, family members' distress is also determined by characteristics unique to family members, including the coping strategies they use, how they perceive the injury and its consequences, and the social support they have and make use of. This information has implications regarding areas to target for intervention. Interventions may also be guided by the research on family needs conducted by Kreutzer and colleagues at the Medical College of Virginia. In a series of studies using their Family Needs Questionnaire, they documented that the needs rated as most important by family members were the needs to receive medical information (50, 51). Family members reported that they wished to receive information on the physical, cognitive, and emotional/behavioral changes in the person with injury. They also reported that they wished to have information presented in a clear and honest

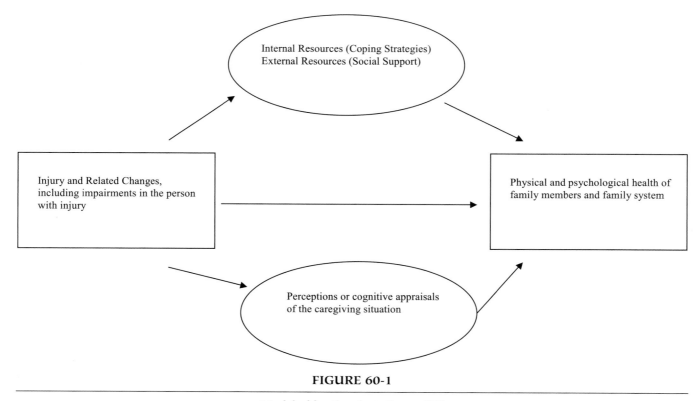

FIGURE 60-1

Model of family adaptation to TBI

manner. As part of these studies, family members were also asked to rate the extent to which various needs had been met. Family members routinely reported the majority of needs for medical information as being met. In contrast, they reported needs for emotional support and instrumental support (e.g., help with practical things like housekeeping) as primarily unmet. These needs were reported as unmet by most family members at long-term periods ranging up to 2 years post-injury (52). Unmet needs have been shown to be related to burden/stress for both African American and White caregiver of persons with TBI (53).

With funding from the National Institute on Disability and Rehabilitation Research, investigators at Baylor College of Medicine and The Institute for Rehabilitation and Research (TIRR) have developed an intervention for family members of persons with TBI. Guided by the research, they have proposed several crucial components of a family intervention program. The components are shown in Table 60-1.

The components shown in Table 60-1 address all of the areas that have emerged as important based on existing research, including provision of information, a focus on strengthening family relationships, improving coping skills, building support networks, and changing cognitive appraisals. These are all components that are proposed as important contributors to caregiver health, as shown in Figure 60-1. The interventions that have typically been offered in the acute and post-acute rehabilitation settings are usually focused on one only or two of these components. For example, education regarding the injury and its consequences, and how to manage cognitive and behavioral problems are a typical focus of many programs. Family members are usually referred to support groups in an attempt to meet their emotional needs. There is generally a lack of use of theory and research to guide interventions, with the result that there is not an integrated

program of intervention for family members that addresses all of the areas shown in Figure 60-1 to be important for family members' adjustment.

At Baylor College of Medicine and TIRR, investigators have developed an intervention program for family members that addresses each of the components shown in Table 60-1. An educational manual has been developed that provides information in all of these areas (54). The intervention has been carried out as a group treatment and as an individual treatment. The remainder of this chapter will be devoted to detailing this treatment and discussing caveats encountered when implementing the interventions.

A Cognitive-Behavioral Intervention for Family Members

As mentioned above, the treatment has been conducted in both group and individual settings. The research regarding the use of the treatment in individual settings is still ongoing. It is believed that the group approach to family intervention will be the most convenient and economical in acute and post-acute rehabilitation settings. For this reason, the discussion below will describe implementation of the intervention in the group setting.

The group intervention takes place across 6 sessions, occurring weekly for 2 hours each. The intervention is a combination of psychoeducational and cognitive-behavioral treatment approaches. The group is led by a Master's level therapist, such as a Licensed Social Worker or a Licensed Professional Counselor. Each session combines didactic training with group therapy. Thus, participants benefit from the instruction of a professional experienced in TBI, but also benefit from sharing their experiences with other family members and forming a social network that can endure beyond the group. The contents of each group session are described below.

Session 1 (Introduction)   Session 1 begins with a general introduction to the group. The therapist explains that the group is being conducted because TBI affects the entire family. Emphasis is placed on normalizing family members' experiences. The therapist commends family members for their efforts to cope with the injury, and provides examples from clinical experience and from the literature regarding difficulties that other family members have faced. Emphasis is placed on the importance of family members attending to their own needs in order to be able to provide adequate care for the person with injury. The importance of emphasizing this point derives from the findings of Kreutzer and colleagues that family members typically place more importance on information regarding the person with injury and less importance on their own emotional needs. Family members often feel selfish if they focus on their own needs when their loved one with

---

TABLE 60-1
Components of a Family Intervention Program

- General education regarding TBI and its consequences
- Direct training in management of physical, cognitive, and emotional/social impairments
- Discussion of changes in family relationships and strategies to improve communication and positive interactions within the family
- Training in stress management techniques for family members
  - Education regarding negative impact of stress
  - Teaching of a relaxation technique
  - Training in effective problem-solving
  - Training in positive reframing of negative thoughts
- Education regarding local and national community resources, including support groups

injury requires attention. Family members may feel less guilty about attending to their own needs if they are convinced that doing so will also have a positive impact on the person with injury. Following the general introduction by the therapist, each participant introduces him or herself and tells their story regarding the injury and the events that have led them to the group. The sharing of these stories is an important part of the group experience that allows participants to form a bond that will enable them to be comfortable sharing information in future sessions. Following the sharing of stories, the therapist presents a metaphor that will be used throughout the remainder of the sessions. The metaphor is borrowed from Marilyn Colter Maxwell's book *Missing Pieces: A Coping Guide for the Families of Head Injury Victims* (55). Ms. Maxwell is the wife of a man with a brain injury, and she stated that "Living with head injury is like trying to work a jigsaw puzzle without all the pieces." Group participants are asked if they have felt this way at any time since the injury, and they are asked to share their experiences. The therapist makes notes regarding experiences of individual family members that can be used to personalize concepts taught during later sessions. The first session ends with an overview of the next 5 sessions. All participants are provided an educational manual to take home.

Session 2 (General Education and Management of Specific Problems)   The second session contains the largest didactic portion of the intervention. The session begins with education regarding different types of TBI (closed versus penetrating) and the mechanisms of injury in each. The metaphor of jello floating in a container is used to illustrate what happens to the brain during injury. A neuroanatomically correct model of the brain is used to demonstrate the most common points of injury (frontal and temporal) and to describe coup-contrecoup lesions and the impact of diffuse axonal injury. Family members responded well to this portion of the intervention. For most participants, this was the first time the injury had been explained in such detail. Following the discussion of the cerebral changes resulting from injury, the therapist describes the most common changes occurring in the physical, cognitive, and emotional areas. Emphasis is placed on the fact that all human brains share many similarities, but each also has unique differences. Thus, participants are made aware that their family members' difficulties may share much in common with those of others, but may also be unique. The therapist discusses the typical pattern of improvement after TBI. Participants are told that the most rapid improvements occur within the first 6 months, with slower improvements occurring between 6 months and 1 year. They are informed that spontaneous improvement typically peaks between 1 and 2 years. However, they are provided with hope that daily functioning and quality of life can improve beyond 2 years

based on the implementation of compensatory strategies and environmental modifications to increase support. This is used as a segue to begin discussing strategies for specific problems in the person with injury. Participants are asked to complete a checklist of neurobehavioral symptoms observed in the person with injury. A checklist was developed as part of the educational manual, but any of the existing neurobehavioral inventories may be used. Once family members have completed the checklist, they are asked to pick 2 problems that result in the most stress for them and their families. The second half of the session is devoted to teaching family members specific strategies to assist the person with injury to compensate for deficits. The educational manual that was provided to family members during the first session contains strategies for all typical problems, so participants have access to help for difficulties that are not discussed during the session.

The strategies taught by the therapist are tailored to be specific to the needs of the participants and their particular family situation. For example, one of the problems that was particularly stressful for the wife of man with TBI was that her husband could not remember what to make for dinner. Her husband had been in charge of cooking dinner prior to injury, and apparently the family had very particular tastes with regard to meal plans. They were partial to certain combinations of food. For example, pork chops were always accompanied by applesauce, corn, and rice. Following the injury, this man no longer had accurate recall of the menu combinations, which was upsetting to his wife and daughter. Since flexibility in the meal plan was not an option that they would consider, the therapist suggested posting a weekly menu containing all the meal plans in the kitchen. The husband and wife wrote the menu together, and he successfully used it to independently prepare meals without having to call and interrupt his wife at work. Rather than attempting to change the dynamics of family interactions with regard to flexibility, which would require a family systems approach and more intensive therapy, the therapist was able to train this man's wife to compensate for the problem in a way that was satisfying to all involved.

The intervention has also shown success in teaching simple behavior management strategies to family members in the group setting. For example, the mother of a 20 year-old man with TBI experienced stress due to her son's perseveration on asking for money. He received a $50 allowance once per week, but would repeatedly ask for money in between allotments. He would phone his mother often while she was at work, and would begin asking for money as soon as she got home. The mother was exasperated by this behavior, but felt helpless to change it. The therapist presented a simple behavior management plan to her. The first time that her son asked for money after his allowance was given, he would be reminded that he was given money on Friday and would not be receiving more until the following Friday. He would be informed that the next time he asked for money, $5 would be deducted from the following week's allowance. Five dollars would subsequently be deducted each time he requested money. The therapist cautioned the mother that this behavior could result in an increase in requests at first, but encouraged her to remain firm in carrying out the plan. This young man stopped requesting extra money within one week, resulting in less stress on his mother and an improvement in their interactions.

The two examples discussed in the paragraphs above are typical of the types of difficulties reported as stressful by family members. While neither of these examples represented life-threatening changes, they resulted in significant daily hassles and stress for the family members. When family members experience a catastrophic event such as TBI, their resources to cope with daily hassles is restricted. Helping them to gain a sense of control by attacking small problems can instill feelings of self-efficacy that can allow them to tackle larger problems. Within the confines of a group therapy situation, it is important for therapists to acknowledge their limits. It will be difficult to change family dynamics or solve large problems. Therapists should be aware of when to refer group participants for individual or family therapy. For example, attempting to alter severely aggressive behavior in the person with injury via group therapy with family members would not be recommended. Altering this behavior would require the therapist to have a detailed understanding of the environmental antecedents of the behavior and contingencies supporting the behavior. The time required to change this behavior is greater than that which could be given during the group session. The danger of escalating aggressiveness during the initial stages of a behavior management plan is an issue that should be closely monitored and is beyond the scope of the group setting. On the other hand, the group setting has been effective for teaching simple behavior management to reduce mild to moderate cussing behavior.

Therapists should always caution family members that each strategy does not work for everyone. Successfully implementing a strategy often requires practice and persistence, and initial failures are common. Family members are encouraged to phone the therapist between sessions to discuss difficulties implementing strategies in the home. The first minutes of the remaining 4 group sessions are devoted to discussion of participants' experiences implementing the strategies. This allows other group members to benefit from hearing the experiences of others and the therapist's suggestions for remediating difficulties. Other family members in the group often offer their own suggestions for strategies that may work. Participants are encouraged to abandon strategies that do not seem to work after repeated attempts. They are referred to their educational manual for other strategies to try.

Session 3 (Relationships)   The goal of this session is not to alter family dynamics or to impact the overall family system. Individual family therapy sessions would be required to accomplish that goal. Rather, the goals of the session are to help family members accept that changes in relationships are a natural occurrence after TBI, to help them become aware of changes in their own family and process their feelings regarding these changes, and to help them develop ways to improve communication within their families and increase the quality of time spent together. The session begins with the therapist discussing some changes that family members have typically noted after TBI, including changes in roles, decreased communication. and less quality time together as a family. The therapist begins discussing common role changes within the family, including action roles (e.g., breadwinner, cooking, financial management) and emotional roles (e.g., the "rock" whom everyone turns to in times of trouble; the "clown" that makes everyone laugh in hard times). The therapist discusses the likelihood of role strain after injury and the negative impact that this can have on physical and mental health. Family members are encouraged to complete a chart stating the roles of different family members before and after injury. They are invited to share their stories about role changes in their families. The therapist assists them in finding ways that roles can be renegotiated to reduce strain on family members. Following the discussion of role changes, the therapist initiates discussion of changes in communication and positive interactions within the family. Changes in communication and interactions are explained as resulting from a combination of changes in roles and schedules, as well as the overwhelming nature of the injury and the prominence it has gained in dictating daily life. Participants are encouraged to share their stories regarding changes in communication and interaction within their families. The therapist assists them in developing ways to improve communication and time spent together. For example, family members are encouraged to spend some time together viewing old photos and reminiscing about happier times. Such activities reinforce their unity and emphasize the positive aspects of their relationships.

The topic of sexuality is addressed in an educational way within this session. The therapist mentions that many persons with TBI experience a disturbance in sexuality and explains some of the most common forms of sexual dysfunction. The therapist also explains how the self-esteem of persons with injury can be affected, and how this can impact their sexuality. Finally, the therapist normalizes the feeling that some partners may feel less attracted to a person with TBI.

The session on relationships is the least structured of all the sessions. Therapists should be sensitive to the level at which various participants have processed changes within their family relationships. Participants should not be pushed to acknowledge changes that they are not ready to process. Some family members may be using denial as a way to cope with negative relationship changes. Therapists should not attempt to break through this denial within the group setting. Sexuality is often a difficult subject for family members to discuss. Therapists should provide an atmosphere open to discussion of these topics by family members who are ready, but should not push them to disclose personal information. The goal is to normalize relationship changes within the context of TBI and to set the stage for later change if family members feel the need. The therapist emphasizes the positive impact of family therapy, including sexual therapy, for some families, and informs participants that they can request a referral at any time.

Session 4 (Stress Management I: Education, Relaxation, and Coping)

The goals of this session are to educate family members in the negative impact of stress on the mind and body, to train them to use a simple breathing exercise to relax, and to teach them to identify their coping strategies and evaluate their effectiveness. The therapist begins with a visualization exercise. Participants are asked to close their eyes and imagine themselves walking through a forest on a beautiful spring day. Various sensory aspects of the scene are described, and participants are encouraged to imagine themselves feeling completely relaxed. They are then instructed to visualize a snake, coiled and hissing, on the path in front of them. The therapist then leads them through a discussion of the physical changes they notice in their bodies (e.g., sweating, rapid heartbeat, rapid shallow breathing). This segues into a discussion of the adrenaline response and the negative impact of stress on the mind and body. Participants complete a stress symptom checklist to help them become aware of signs that can warn them of stress. Each participant shares their pattern of stress symptoms with the group.

The therapist then introduces a simple breathing exercise. This exercise was adapted from the workbook *Managing Stress Before It Manages You*, by Caudill (56). The exercise involves participants lying down on mats or sitting in a position that is comfortable for them. They are instructed to close their eyes and imagine a balloon in their abdomen. They are told to breathe in deeply and slowly and to imagine the balloon filling with air. They are then told to exhale slowly and fully, imagining the air seeping out of the balloon. The therapist encourages them to imagine the stress leaving their bodies like the air leaving the balloon. Participants complete a visual analogue scale to rate the amount of stress they are experiencing immediately prior to and immediately following the breathing exercise. They are encouraged to practice the exercise at least twice per day for the next week and to

rate their stress before and after each practice. In order to increase the possibility of them practicing the techniques, the therapist asks them to schedule specific times of day to perform relaxation exercises. The therapist emphasizes that learning to relax takes practice and encourages them not to give up if it doesn't seem to be working right away. They are also informed that not every relaxation exercise will work for everyone. They are referred to their educational manuals for other relaxation exercises that may work for them. The manual includes details about how to carry out progressive relaxation and visual imagery exercises. The breathing exercise was chosen over these others for implementation in the group because it is simple, brief, and can be used easily by family members in a variety of settings, even outside of the home.

The second half of session 4 focuses on the development of effective coping strategies. The therapist begins by pointing out that family members are all coping the best way that they know how. However, TBI is different from anything that they have experienced before, and not all of the coping strategies that they've used in other situations may work well in their new situation. The therapist presents several coping strategies that other family members have reported as helpful, as determined by Willer and colleagues (57). These strategies include taking time out for yourself, maintaining a sense of humor, being more assertive, trying to see things more realistically, being careful not to blame everything on the injury, and renegotiating roles and responsibilities. Group members are asked to discuss whether they've found any of these strategies to be helpful in coping with the results of TBI and are encouraged to provide additional strategies that they have found beneficial. The therapist next emphasizes the importance of evaluating coping strategies to make sure they are helpful. Participants are provided with a chart to use when evaluating coping strategies. The chart is shown in Appendix A. The goal of evaluation is for family members to learn to question whether the things they do to cope are leading to the results they desire. They are encouraged to think of alternative coping strategies for those that do not lead to the desired result. The therapist encourages family members to use the chart to evaluate strategies that they use to cope with stressful situations over the next week.

Session 5 (Stress Management II: Problem-Solving and Overcoming Negative Thinking)

The goals of session 5 are to train family members in a systematic approach to solving problems and to teach them to reframe negative thoughts into more positive, self-empowering thinking. The session begins with the therapist defining a problem as anything that requires a solution or decision. Thus, problems can be very small (e.g., deciding what to have

TABLE 60-2
Steps Toward Effective Problem-Solving

Identify the problem
Brainstorm solutions
Evaluate the alternatives
Choose a solution
Try the solution out
If the 1st solution doesn't work, try another one and repeat the evaluation procedure

for dinner) or very large (e.g., deciding which bill to pay when you only have the money to pay one). The therapist emphasizes that the injury has likely resulted in family members having to make so many decisions that they become overwhelmed. The therapist explains that when people feel overwhelmed, even making small decisions can become difficult. Participants are informed that the purpose of learning a systematic way to approach and solve problems is to help narrow down alternatives so that decision-making is easier. They are encouraged that effectively solving problems will lead to reduced stress and an increased confidence in their ability to solve larger problems. The therapist then introduces the problem-solving steps shown in Table 60-2.

When identifying the problem, participants are taught to break complex problems down into smaller steps in order to make it more manageable and to increase the probability of success. They are encouraged to choose the easiest problem first in order to build confidence for more difficult problems. Participants are taught to brainstorm all possible solutions to the problem, even ones that may appear unrealistic at first glance. They are then taught to generate pros and cons for each possible solution, and choose the solution that should lead to the best outcome. The therapist explains that the best solution is not always the one with the highest number of pros and the lowest number of cons. Some pros or cons carry more relative weight than others. When a solution does not seem to work, participants are encouraged to attempt to determine why. At times, this will lead to a new problem that requires a solution. At other time, it will lead to abandonment of the solution and the trying out of new solutions. The therapist emphasizes persistence in repeating the problem-solving steps until a satisfactory solution is achieved. A particular problem that was raised by a group participant during a previous session is then used by the therapist to illustrate working through the problem-solving steps. Family members are encouraged to practice the steps on a real-life problem during the following week.

The second half of session 5 focuses on training in overcoming negative thoughts. The session begins with a simple exercise aimed at helping group members become aware of the impact that thoughts can have on feelings and behaviors. The exercise follows:

> *Your friend says to you, "I found a great new hairstylist and I'll give you the number." How would you feel if you thought that your friend was implying that your hair is looking terrible, and you need some help? [Have them discuss how they would feel and how they might act toward the friend.] Now think about how you would feel if you thought that your friend was really excited about finding a great hairstylist and simply wanted to share it with people she cares about. [Have them discuss how they would feel and how they might act toward the friend.] In this situation, you would feel and act differently depending on the way you thought about what was being said.*

The therapist next explains the ABC model of the relationship between thoughts, feelings, and actions (58). The model specifies that an event or situation (A) does not directly impact feelings and actions (C). The event results in certain thoughts (B) that in turn impact feelings and actions. The therapist emphasizes that while family members may not be able to change the injury or its consequences, they do have power to change the way that they think about things. Participants are provided with a handout containing "The Ten Forms of Twisted Thinking", from David Burns' *Feeling Good Handbook*. (59) This handout describes common forms of irrational thinking that are considered counter-productive to combating stress. For example, overgeneralization is an irrational thought that occurs when someone views a single bad event as indicative of all past and future events. An example is thinking, "My husband's disability claim was denied the first time we tried. I guess we'll never be able to get any financial help." Group members are provided a chart with which to evaluate their thoughts in different situations. The chart is shown in Appendix B, along with an example. Family members are taught to reframe negative thoughts into positive thoughts that instill hope and self-confidence. As shown in Appendix B, the positive alternative thought for denial of the disability claim would be that many people are denied the first time and that better documentation of deficits may result in approval of the claim. Family members are encouraged to use the chart to evaluate their thoughts in different stressful situations over the next week. During the session, the therapist helps group members to identify one negative thought that they have often and to develop a positive alternative thought. They are provided with index cards, with the phrase "DON'T THINK _____; THINK _____." For example, a card may read "DON'T think we'll never get financial help; THINK we will gather more information in support of our claim and try again." These cards can be placed on their refrigerator, on their desk at work, or anywhere else they find convenient. The card will serve as a reminder to them to replace negative thoughts with positive ones.

Session 6 (Accessing Local and National Resources and Wrap-Up) The last session begins with the therapist reviewing the most common local and national resources family members can turn to for help. The therapist next reviews the highlights of the 6-week group in order to reinforce the material learned. Group members are encouraged to discuss their thoughts about the group, including which parts they found to be beneficial and what they were sorry to not see included. Participants are referred to local support groups in order to continue social support. Family members have also benefited from encouragement to become involved in state Brain Injury Associations and/or in local advocacy groups. The final session is also used to complete satisfaction surveys and any evaluative measures. Areas typically assessed include emotional distress, caregiver appraisals, coping skills, and social support before and after completion of the group.

Initial Experiences with the Group Intervention

As part of a NIDRR-funded project, the group intervention was piloted at 3 centers: The Institute for Rehabilitation and Research (TIRR) in Houston, Methodist Rehabilitation Center in Jackson, Mississippi, and The Mayo Clinic in Rochester, Minnesota. The groups were conducted with family members of persons who had sustained TBI 1 to 2 years prior. In all cases, the persons with injury had received comprehensive inpatient rehabilitation at the participating center. However, family members and the person with injury were not receiving any rehabilitative services at the time of their participation in the group. Two separate groups were conducted in Mississippi and Minnesota, and one was conducted in Houston. There were 3 to 4 participants in each of the groups. All group participants reported satisfaction with the contents of the group. In all cases, they reported that they learned information in the group that they had not heard previously regarding the injury and its consequences. While all family members had been participants in the inpatient rehabilitation process, they had obviously either not been exposed to this detailed information or had not been ready to process it at the time they had heard it. Some specific comments made by group members on the satisfaction survey were that they had learned not to feel guilty about wanting to take time for themselves and that they had learned that the behavior of the person with injury was due directly to brain injury and not to purposeful behavior. Family members also verbalized satisfaction with the social networking afforded by group participation. Some family members exchanged contact information in order to keep in touch after the group disbanded. At one center, one of the groups made plans to continue meeting after the therapist-led group was completed. While the intervention has shown success in small pilot groups, its effectiveness should be tested in clinical trials. Plans are currently underway to conduct this research.

Future Directions for Interventions with Family Members

Home-Based Therapies One of the reasons that the treatment groups described above were so small was that it was difficult to find a common time that was convenient for several family members to meet. The daily lives of families are particularly hectic in the months following TBI. Persons with injury and their family members often have difficulty attending facility-based treatments, even when they report on needs surveys that they desire services. This may be especially true for persons from low educational and/or socioeconomic backgrounds. Persons from these backgrounds often have difficulty obtaining transportation to appointments. In addition, they may feel less comfortable in a research facility or rehabilitation facility. On surveys conducted at TIRR, persons have often reported that they feel more comfortable receiving treatments in their own home or communities. Conducting treatments in the settings where people carry out their daily activities has been proposed as an important alternative to facility-based treatments (60). Conducting family interventions in the home has several advantages. First, it is convenient and economical for most family members. Second, it allows therapists to observe families and the person with injury within the home environment, where they can view problems as they occur. This allows therapists to suggest compensatory strategies that are truly tailored to the environment in which activities will be carried out. Third, facility-based interventions often result in uncertain generalizability to the home and community. Conducting therapy in the home has the potential to improve generalizability. Finally, intervening in the home environment often improves the rapport between the therapist and client. Trust and acceptance are more likely when the client sees the therapist as willing to enter their world and attempt to understand them in their own environment. A study is currently being conducted at TIRR to evaluate a family intervention conducted in the home setting. The family members are from primarily low education and low socioeconomic backgrounds. The rate of therapy completion using home-based treatments has been superior to that obtained when conducting facility-based treatments. Therapy members have generally welcomed research staff into their homes and the information gained through observation in the home setting has been invaluable. Given these advantages, it is recommended that family intervention be conducted in the home setting when possible.

Culturally Sensitive Interventions TBI is not a disorder that occurs equally among persons of different backgrounds. TBI is disproportionately represented among minorities and among persons of low socioeconomic status (SES) (61, 62). In spite of this, most persons from minority and low SES backgrounds do not have access to rehabilitation services. Family members in these groups are left to care for persons with injury at an early stage in the recovery process, with minimal training or assistance. Targeting interventions at this population of family members is very important. However, conducting therapy with these family members is often a challenge. They typically read below the 7th grade level, which renders many existing educational materials unhelpful. They often have difficulty relating to the language used by most therapists. For example, they may have difficulty describing their "feelings" about events and may focus more on concrete changes. They also may have difficulty trusting medical professionals due to previous difficulties and disappointments.

Family members from different racial/ethnic groups may hold beliefs that put them at odds with the practices of rehabilitation professionals. For example, many Hispanic persons place primary importance on physiological recovery and do not have a conceptual framework with which to discuss cognitive and emotional issues (63). Professionals should take extra time when providing education to these family members and should avoid using psychological terms. Hispanic persons also tend to subjugate their individual needs to the needs of the family (63). This belief may make it difficult for family members to express negative emotions regarding the injury and any negative feelings they may have toward the person with injury. Normalization of negative emotions will be especially important for these families. Another commonly held belief among Hispanic persons is that external agents (e.g., God) have a greater role in determining their future than they themselves do (63). This belief may result in difficulty understanding the importance of making changes in the environment of the person with injury and developing compensatory strategies. Consulting with experts in the areas of cultural sensitivity will be important for establishing rapport with these groups and for developing interventions that can serve the needs of these populations.

It is also possible that persons from different backgrounds have different priorities in terms of family needs. For example, many minority family members have extended family and support networks, which may result in less distress compared to Caucasian family members. Future development of family interventions that are tailored to the needs of diverse groups of people would be beneficial. Educational materials should be written at a 7th grade level or below. The use of the World-Wide web to disseminate materials to family members is likely to result in a cultural gap in access to information. In a recent survey conducted within the Houston Harris County Hospital District, family members from a low education and low socioeconomic background expressed a preference for receiving videotaped compared to written educational materials. Translation of materials into languages other than English is crucial for equal access. Finally, extensive outreach will be important in reaching persons from low education and/or low SES backgrounds. Family members in these groups often do not seek help within medical facilities, and they often fall between the cracks of traditional rehabilitation services. Reaching these family members will require actively reaching out within community settings, such as health care clinics and churches.

Timing of Interventions The group treatments conducted at TIRR have included family members of persons who sustained their injuries one to two years ago. Studies currently underway are investigating home-based interventions with family members at approximately 6 months post-injury. Conducting interventions beyond the acute period is important based on the research showing that family members' distress often increases with increasing time post-injury. This is thought to occur because during the initial 6 months after TBI, rapid improvements are usually noted. During this time, family members often hold out hope that things will return to normal. It is only when spontaneous recovery starts to peak and change becomes slower that family members begin to realize there may be permanent change. Unfortunately, this is also the time that rehabilitation services have usually been terminated and family members are caring for the person with injury on their own. Family members typically have many unanswered questions at this point. Providing education during the acute phases of recovery may not always prepare family members for long-term changes. Over the years, it has been noted that family members typically do not recall information that was provided to them early after injury. They tend to only process information that is applicable to the situation at the time. Furthermore, the shock and grief experienced by family members early in the recovery process may be an obstacle to learning information. Future interventions should be tailored to the phase of recovery that family members are experiencing. Recent studies have indicated that needs for information and involvement with care are predominant during the acute phases of recovery (64). Once persons are discharged and are living in the community, family members report needs for service delivery, advocacy/ empowerment issues, and social support (65). The research supports that family members need intervention at all time points after injury, including in the long-term. Development of outreach services will be crucial for meeting these needs.

APPENDIX A

Evaluating Coping Strategies

SITUATION	WHAT I DID TO COPE	WHAT HAPPENED	POSITIVE OR NEGATIVE?	OTHER STRATEGIES THAT MAY HAVE WORKED
We needed to see the Doctor because my family member ran out of medications, but there was a 2 month wait list.	Yelled at the receptionist and told her that was a ridiculous amount of time to wait.	Appointment time was not changed. My family member still didn't have his medicine.	Negative	
	Did nothing- just waited until the appointment.	Appointment time was not changed. My family member still didn't have his medicine.	Negative	
	Explained that he's out of medications and asked if he could get a temporary refill until the appointment.	Appointment was scheduled. Medication was refilled.	Positive	

APPENDIX B

Evaluation of Negative Thoughts

UPSETTING OR STRESSFUL SITUATION	NEGATIVE THOUGHTS	WHY THIS ISN'T REALISTIC	POSITIVE, REALISTIC THOUGHT
Example: Your family member's application for Disability benefits was denied.	"We will never be able to get any financial help." "They should have approved our application the first time." "No one cares about us."	One instance doesn't tell you how things will be in the future. People are just following the rules and may not understand the details of your situation. This situation has nothing to do with people's feelings for you or your family member.	Lots of people are denied the first time. We will try again and explain our situation in more detail. If we don't get approved, we will look for other sources of assistance.

References

1. Pope AM, Tarlov AR (eds.). *Disability in America: Toward a national agenda for prevention.* Washington, D.C.: National Academy Press 1991.
2. Brandt EN, Pope AM (eds.). *Enabling America: Assessing the role of rehabilitation science and engineering.* Washington, D.C.: National Academy Press 1997.
3. Geneva, World Health Organization. ICIDH-2: *International Classification of Functioning and Disability.* Beta-2 draft, Short Version. 1999.
4. U.S. Department of Education, Office of Special Education and Rehabilitation Services, National Institute on Disability and Rehabilitation Research. *Long-range plan 1999–2003.* Washington, D.C., 2000.
5. Jacobs HE. The Los Angeles Head Injury Survey: Procedures and initial findings. *Archives of Physical Medicine and Rehabilitation.* 1988;69:425–431.
6. Lezak M Living with the characterologically altered brain injured patient. *Journal of Clinical Psychiatry* 1978;39:592–598.
7. Lezak MD Brain damage is a family affair. *Journal of Clinical & Experimental Neuropsychology* 1988;10:111–123.
8. Florian V, Katz SLV. Impact of brain damamge on family dynamics and functioning: A review. *Brain Injury* 1989;3:219–233.
9. Brooks D. The head-injured family. *Journal of Clinical and Experimental Neuropsychology.* 1991;13:155–188.
10. Livingston MG, Brooks DN, Bond MR. Three months after severe head injury: Psychiatric and social impact on relatives. *Journal of Neurology, Neurosurgery, & Psychiatry* 1985:48: 870–875.
11. Livingston MG, Brooks DN, Bond MR. Patient outcome in the year following severe head injury and relatives' psychiatric and social functioning. *Journal of Neurology, Neurosurgery, & Psychiatry* 1985;48:876–881.
12. Kreutzer JS, Gervasio AH, Camplair PS. Primary caregivers' psychological status and family functioning after traumatic brain injury. *Brain Injury.* 1994;8:197–210.

13. Marsh NV, Kersel DA, Havill JH, Sleigh JW. Caregiver burden at 6 months following severe traumatic brain injury. *Brain Injury* 1998;12:225–238.

14. Marsh NV, Kersel DA, Havill JH, Sleigh JW. Caregiver burden 1 year following severe traumatic brain injury. *Brain Injury* 1998; 12:1045–1059.

15. McKinlay WW, Brooks DN, Bond MR. The short term outcome of severe blunt head injury as reported by the relatives of the injured person. *Journal of Neurology, Neurosurgery, & Psychiatry* 1981;44:527–533.

16. Brooks N, Campsie L, Symington C, Beattie A, McKinlay W. The five year outcome severe blunt head injury: A relative's view. *Journal of Neurology, Neurosurgery and Psychiatry*. 1986;49:764–770.

17. Brooks N, Campsie L, Symington C, Beattie A, McKinlay W. The effects of severe head injury on patient and relatives within seven years of injury. *Journal of Head Trauma Rehabilitation*. 1987; 2:1–13.

18. Ponsford J, Olver JP, Ponsford M, Nelms R. Long-term adjustment of families following traumatic brain injury where comprehensive rehabilitation has been provided. *Brain Injury* 2003; 453–468.

19. Levin H, Benton A, Grossman RG. *Neurobehavioral consequences of Closed Head Injury.* Nw York: Oxford University Press 1982.

20. Brooks DN, McKinlay. Personality and behavioral change after severe head injury – a relative's view. *Journal of Neurology, Neurosurgery, & Psychiatry* 1983;46:336–344.

21. Gillen R, Tennen H, Affleck G, Steinpreis R. Distress, Depressive Symptoms, and Depressive Disorder among Caregivers of Patients with Brain Injury. *Journal of Head Trauma Rehabilitation* 1998;13(3):31–43.

22. Kreutzer JS, Gervasio A, Camplair P. Patient correlates of caregiver distress and family functioning after traumatic brain injury. *Brain Injury* 1994;8:211–230.

23. Allen K, Linn RT, Gutierrez H, Willer BS. Family burden following traumatic brain injury. *Rehabilitation Psychology*. 1994; 39:29–48.

24. Hall KM, Karzmark P, Stevens M, Englander J, O'Hare P, Wright J. Family stressors in traumatic brain injury: A two-year follow-up. *Archives of Physical Medicine and Rehabilitation*. 1994;75: 876–884.

25. Sander AM, Sherer M, Malec JF, High WM Jr, Thompson RN, Moessner AN, Josey J. Preinjury emotional and family functioning in caregivers of persons with TBI. *Archives of Physical Medicine and Rehabilitation* 2003;84:197–2003.

26. Peters LC, Stambrook M, Moore AD. Psychosocial sequelae of closed head injury: Effects on the marital relationship. *Brain Injury* 1990;4:39–47.

27. Wood RL, Yurdakul LK. Changes in relationship status following traumatic brain injury. *Brain Injury* 1997;11:491–501.

28. Gosling J, Oddy M. Rearranged marriages: Marital relationships after head injury. *Brain Injury* 1999;13:785–796.

29. Chwalsiz K. The perceived stress model of caregiving burden: Evidence from spouses of persons with brain injuries. *Rehabilitation Psychology* 1996;41:91–114.

30. Gervasio AH, Griffith ER. Sexuality and sexual dysfunction. In: Rosenthal M, Griffith ER, Kreutzer JS, Pentland B (eds.). *Rehabilitation of the Adult and Child With Traumatic Brain Injury (3rd edition)*. Philadelphia: F.A. Davis Company 1999:479–502.

31. Sandel ME, Williams KS, Dellapietra L, Derogatis LR. Sexual functioning following traumatic brain injury. *Brain Injury* 1996; 10:719–728.

32. Kreutzer JS, Zasler ND. Psychosexual consequences of traumatic brain injury: Methodology and preliminary findings. *Brain Injury* 1989;3:177–186.

33. Kreuter M, Dahllof AG, Gudjonsson G, Sullivan M, Siosteen A. Sexual adjustment and its predictors after traumatic brain injury. *Brain Injury* 1998;12:349–368.

34. Ponsford J. Sexual changes associated with traumatic brain injury. *Neuropsychological Rehabilitation* 2003;13:275–289.

35. Thomsen IV Late outcome of very severe blunt head trauma: A 10–15 year second follow-up. *Journal of Neurology, Neurosurgery & Psychiatry* 1984;47:260–268.

36. Machamer J, Temkin N, & Dikmen S. Significant other burden and factors related to it in traumatic brain injury. *Journal of Clinical and Experimental Neuropsychology* 2002;4:420–433.

37. Knight RG, Devereuax R, Godfrey HPD. Caring for a family member with a traumatic brain injury. *Brain Injury* 1998;12: 467–481.

38. Oddy M, Humphrey M, Uttley D. Stresses upon the relatives of head-injured patients. *British Journal of Psychiatry* 1978;133: 507–513.

39. Gervasio AH, Kreutzer JS. Kinship and Family Members' Psychological Distress after Traumatic Brain Injury: A Large Sample Study. *Journal of Head Trauma Rehabilitation* 1997;12(3): 14–26.

40. Sander AM, High W, Hannay HJ, Sherer M. Predictors of psychological health in caregivers of patients with closed head injury. *Brain Injury* 1997;11(4):235–249.

41. McCubbin HI, Patterson JM. The family stress process: The double ABCX model of family adjustment and adaptation. In McCubbin HI, Sussman M, Patterson JM (Eds), *Social Stress and the Family: Advances and Developments in Family Stress Theory and Research*. 1983; New York: Haworth: pp. 7–37.

42. Lazarus R, Folkman S. *Stress, appraisal, and coping*. New York: Springer 1984.

43. Chwalisz K. Perceived stress and caregiver burden after brain injury. *Rehabilitation Psychology* 1992;37:189–203.

44. Douglas JM, Spellacy FJ. Indicators of long-term family functioning following severe traumatic brain injury in adults. *Brain Injury* 1996;10:819–839.

45. Minnes P, Graffi S, Nolte ML, Carlson P, Harrick L. Coping and stress in Canadian family caregivers of persons with traumatic brain injuries. *Brain Injury* 2000;14:737–748.

46. Sander AM. *Family needs, coping and psychological health following traumatic brain injury*. Unpublished manuscript.

47. Ergh TC, Rapport LJ, Coleman RD, Hanks RA. Predictors of caregiver and family functioning following traumatic brain injury: Social support moderates caregiver distress. *Journal of Head Trauma Rehabilitation* 2002;17:155–174.

48. Struchen MA, Atchison T, Roebuck T, Caroselli J,Sander AM. A multidomensional measure of caregiving appraisal: Validation of the Caregiver Appraisal Scale in Traumatic Brain Injury. *Journal of Head Trauma Rehabilitation* 2002;17:132–154.

49. Lawton MP, Kleban MH, Moss M, Rovine M, Glicksman A. Measuring caregiver appraisal. *Journal of Gerontology* 1989;44: 61–71.

50. Kreutzer JS, Serio CD,Bergquist S. Family needs after brain injury: A quantitative analysis. *Journal of Head Trauma Rehabilitation* 1994;9:104–115.

51. Serio CD, Kreutzer JS,Gervasio AH. Predicting family needs after brain injury: Implications for intervention. *Journal of Head Trauma Rehabilitation* 1995;10:32–45.

52. Witol AD, Sander AM,Kreutzer J. A longitudinal analysis of family needs following traumatic brain injury. *NeuroRehabilitation* 1996;7:175–187.

53. Nabors N, Seacat J, Rosenthal M. Predictors of caregiver burden following traumatic brain injury. *Brain Injury* 2002;16: 1039–1050.

54. Sander AM. *Picking up the pieces after TBI: A guide for family members*. Houston: Baylor College of Medicine, 2002.

55. Colter-Maxwell M. *Missing pieces: A coping guide for families of head injury victims*. Fort Collins, Colorado: MCM Books.

56. Caudill MA. *Managing pain before it manages you*. New York: Guilford Press 1995.

57. Willer BS, Allen KM, Liss M, Zicht MS. Problems and coping strategies of individuals with traumatic brain injury and their spouses. *Archives of Physical Medicine and Rehabilitation* 1991; 72:460–464.

58. Ellis A. *Reason and emotion in psychotherapy*. New York: Lyle Stuart 1962.

59. Burns DD. *The Feeling Good Handbook*. New York: Penguin Group 1989.

60. Frieden L. The John Stanley Coulter Memorial Lecture: Listening for footsteps. *Archives of Physical Medicine & Rehabilitation* 2002;83:150153.

61. Jager TE, Weiss HB, Coben JH, Pepe PE. Traumatic brain injuries evaluated in the U.S. emergency departments, 1992–1994. *Academy of Emergency Medicine* 2002;7:134–140.

62. Kraus JF, Fife D, Ramstein K, Conroy C, Cox P. The relationship of family income to the incidence, external causes, and outcomes of serious brain injury, San Diego County, California. *American Journal of Public Health* 1986;76:1345–1347.

63. Ponton MO, Monguio I. Rehabilitation of brain injury among Hispanic patients. In: Ponton MO, Leon-Carrion J (eds).

Neuropsychology and the Hispanic Patient. New Jersey: Lawrence Erlbaum Associates, Publishers 2001:307–319.

64. Bond AE, Draeger CRL, Mandleco B, Donnelly M. Needs of family members of patients with severe traumatic brain injury: Implications for evidence-based practice. *Critical Care Nurse* 2003; 23:63–72.

65. Leith KH, Phillips L, Sample PL. Exploring the needs and experiences of persons with TBI and their families: The South Carolina experience. *Brain Injury* 2004;18:1191–1208.

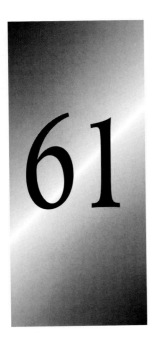

61 Return to Work Following TBI

Michael West
Pam Targett
Satoko Yasuda
Paul Wehman

INTRODUCTION

Vocational rehabilitation efforts in traumatic brain injury (TBI) have paralleled the increasing survival rate for those experiencing severe injury. Clearly, there have been more expanded efforts at ways of assessing and intervening vocational outcomes of persons with traumatic brain injury in the United States and worldwide. Work is increasingly viewed not only as an extremely worthwhile outcome economically, but therapeutically as an excellent means of enhancing cognitive and physical rehabilitation (1).

The natural course of work return as established by Dikmen et al. (2) suggests that 38 percent of adults with a severe injury, 66 percent of those with a moderate injury, and at least 80 percent of those with a mild TBI return to work within two years of injury. This particular study involved 366 consecutive admissions to a level 1 trauma center who considered their primary role activity to be working. Job retention, however, was not taken into consideration. Vocational rehabilitation intervention may or may not have occurred for this sample.

From the perspective of vocational rehabilitation research and demonstration projects with definite vocational intervention, most of these efforts are focused on adults experiencing a severe injury—Glasgow Coma Scale (GCS) score ≤ 8, post-traumatic amnesia >7 days, or duration of coma >24 hr. A summary of these studies suggests work access in the range of 50–80 percent, with

retention dropping into a range of 50–65 percent of those placed (3) with a second placement considered "almost normative." Wehman et al. (4) have suggested the use of a standard "monthly employment ratio" (percentage of months in which an individual worked half-time or more divided by months available for work) as a more standard manner of assessing employment success across projects. The reasons for variance in work return across studies, however, is a function of a range of study differences (e.g., lack of clear severity indicators, varying neuropsychological baseline measures, variance in time to rehabilitation and follow-up points, variance in defining outcome variables, etc.) (4).

There have been a wide and varied range of brain injury vocational rehabilitation research and demonstration efforts. Under private sector managed care, companies such as New Medico, Sunrise-Mediplex, Learning Centers, and others were unable (due to funding limitations) to sustain post-acute rehabilitation programs. As a result, a number of professionals who were focusing their energies in the TBI vocational rehabilitation field were forced to find other work endeavors. The Affirmative Industries (leased employee) work transition model, as described by Fraser et al. (5) at a Wisconsin New Medico program, was a benchmark program allowing *diverse, paid work evaluative experiences* for program participants in a residential program. This comprehensive program has not yet been replicated.

As has been noted, most of the existing vocational rehabilitation research has been focused on the moderate to severe injury cases. This is chiefly because most of the individuals involved in post-acute rehabilitation efforts, to include neuropsychologists and other rehabilitation staff, indicate that more than 80 percent of individuals with a mild traumatic brain injury or post-concussive syndrome concerns respond well to rehabilitation and have their issues resolved within a year of onset (6) or don't really need rehabilitation. Much of the concern here can really be the need for diagnostic specificity in mild TBI or post-concussive syndrome cases (e.g., a specific memory deficit, headaches, post-traumatic stress disorder concerns, etc.) and tailored intervention. In general, individuals with mild TBI are not referred to intensive vocational programs or relevant programs are simply not available.

In this chapter we will focus not only on specific return to work issues, but also those critical related factors such as health insurance, benefits planning, community supports, and career counseling in terms of work supports but community issues which affect employment. We begin with a review of the return to work (RTW) literature, with emphasis on those who experience more significant TBI.

Review of TBI Return to Work Literature

Traumatic brain injury can result in variety cognitive deficits, impaired psychosocial functioning, and physical or sensory functioning (7). As a result, individuals with TBI often experience difficulty becoming competitively employed post-injury and maintaining employment for extended periods of time (8–12). Young male adults have the highest risk in sustaining TBI (13), and because the survival rates after injury have dramatically increased due to medical advancements, they are anticipated to have long life expectancies and it becomes imperative that they become employed after recovery. However, high post-injury unemployment rates are continuously being reported. Post-injury employment rates range from 10 percent to 70 percent depending on the study, while pre-injury employment rates range from 61 percent to 75 percent (14–17). It is suggested that this variance in post-injury employment rates is mainly caused by various measures used for injury severity, method of return-to-work process, inconsistency among employment status, and absence of long-term follow-up (3, 14).

Numerous studies have been conducted in an attempt to determine variables that influence individuals returning to work after sustaining TBI. The relationship between injury severity and regaining employment has been examined extensively, but the findings vary depending on the measure used (17). The relationship between returning to work and duration of posttraumatic amnesia

has not been identified (18, 19). Those who returned to work were likely to have shorter duration of coma and were in inpatient rehabilitation for a shorter period (2, 19), Those who returned to work obtained better scores on standardized instruments at admission such as Glasgow Coma Scale (20).

Age at injury was a significant predictor of returning to work for individuals over age 60 (21). Age between 40 and above at the time of injury negatively affected returning to work (2, 17–19, 22–24). The age of individuals returning to work or to school was younger than those who did not (16, 19).

Marital status has been found to have significant relationship with returning to work (16). Individuals classified as married had a lower rate of returning to work compared to those classified as single. There is contradictory evidence regarding gender. While Ip et al. (16) reported no significant difference between gender and returning to work, McMordie et al. (17) reported that females are more likely to regain employment than males, possibly due to females sustaining less severe injury than males.

Educational level and occupation pre-injury has also been examined. Low education level negatively influenced returning to work (16, 18). Persons whose previous employment was either semi- or unskilled manual jobs were reported to have less success in regaining employment (25) and individuals who worked in structural occupations such as building and trades were more likely to return to their former occupation compared to those who were professional, managerial, clerical, or service workers (15). This contradicts studies that indicate greater likelihood of individuals with more education and technical skills having success in returning to work (26). Among those who regain work after TBI, more individuals start a new job rather than going back to their previous one. However, those who were hired by their previous employer remained successfully employed and had higher hourly wages than those who were employed by a new employer post-injury (27).

The effect of race on regaining work after TBI has only recently begun to be examined and the results are contradictory. For example, Greenspan et al. (28) reported that race appeared to be related to failure to regain employment one year post-injury, whereas O'Connell (29) found race to be not significant. Rosenthal et al. (30) examined whether minority status affected short-term and one year functional outcomes and community integration for TBI patients. Regaining employment after TBI was found to have a significant relationship with both pre- and post-injury employment status. This may be due to the relatively low percentage of pre-injury employment rate among minority subjects, if the assumption is made that pre-injury employment provides the skills and attitudes that are needed in post-injury employment (31) and may also be caused by differences in access to health care (32). Wright (33) summarizes that minorities with disabilities are less likely than whites to receive rehabilitative services, do not receive the same quality or quantity of services, and have poorer outcomes after rehabilitation.

A low level of social support is reported to have negative influence on returning to work (25, 34). Individuals with TBI receive a considerable amount of support while they are in post-acute care facility and also during return-to-work process from vocational rehabilitation personnel. However, after they are discharged and begin the return-to-work process, many require non-professional support, such as from families and community. This becomes an issue for persons sustaining TBI because many individuals with TBI are at a risk of becoming socially isolated (35).

Cognitive issues such as new learning and memory, impaired self-awareness, pre-existing and post-injury dysfunctional behaviors to impede return to work (4). However, not all impairments were identified as being barriers for persons with TBI to return to work or in maintaining employment. They became barriers if they affect achievement of their vocational goal and job maintenance for that particular individual (36). These included cognitive issues followed by emotional functioning, physical impairments such as hemi paresis, stamina or motor deficits, and characteristic and behavioral propensities that existed pre-injury.

Having a significant physical disability (37), psychosocial impairment (38), and cognitive impairment (39), history of alcohol abuse (16, 40) have been associated with impeding returning to work. Acquired deficits in the areas of social behavior, cognitive functioning and personality, all of which can result from TBI, also becomes barriers for persons with TBI to become successfully employed (14, 38). Cognitive deficits and personality change may have greater impact than physical impairment (18, 22, 41).

A combination of variables has been reported to increase the predictability of persons with TBI returning to work. These include: level of education, productivity status pre-injury, and overall functioning at discharge from acute rehabilitation (42); occupational category pre-injury (43); age, GCS score, and Disability Rating Scale score at rehabilitation admission (23); number of neuropsychological impairments (44); post-traumatic epilepsy, paralysis, visual field loss, verbal memory loss, psychological problems, and violent behavior (45).

Much of the prior research has focused on the symptoms and conditions of the individuals that influence retuning to work. It is becoming more imperative to examine retuning to work after TBI as an interaction between the needs and motivations of the individuals with TBI and the supports available within vocational, social and economic environments (46–48). Factors that lead to successful employment include socially inclusive work environments and availability of health insurance (48), level of social interaction on the job and return to jobs with greater decision-making latitude (47), and environmental modifications and focusing on vocational strengths of the individual (46).

Challenges in RTW

The preceding literature review indicates that investigators have typically focused on characteristics of individuals with TBI and the problems they exhibit, with a limited number of studies of the effects of workplace environment (e.g., Refs 47 and 48). However, it is important to realize that there are other influences on RTW that are often underestimated. Foremost among these is likely to be financial disincentives to RTW, such as when the individual is either pursuing or receiving public benefits such as Social Security disability benefits or other financial settlement. It is very likely that these individuals will be reluctant to pursue employment because they may believe that working negatively affect the financial well being of themselves and their families. This perception may seem contradictory and illogical, so some explanation is in order.

The Social Security Administration (SSA) administers disability benefits under two programs: the Disability Insurance (DI) program and the Supplemental Security Income (SSI) program. These two programs were designed to provide "safety net" levels of income and health care to individuals who are not capable of self-support due to disability. Unfortunately, SSI and DI are frequently cited as causes of high unemployment and underemployment of persons with significant disabilities. For example, Bowe (49) writes that these two programs are "dependence-oriented." To be eligible, individuals who seek benefits must prove themselves to be incapable of engaging in Substantial Gainful Activity (SGA), currently determined by earnings of over $800 per month. Fear of losing benefits, particularly medical coverage under Medicaid (typically tied to eligibility for SSI) or Medicare (tied to DI), persuades most beneficiaries to limit their earnings well below SGA or, more commonly, not enter the labor force at all. Further in this chapter, we will describe some of the ways in which SSA has attempted to counteract work disincentives and encourage their beneficiaries to attempt RTW. Understanding and accessing those work incentives is essential for convincing disability beneficiaries with TBI that attempting to return to work will not cause financial harm to themselves or their families.

In addition, a challenge that is common to many individuals across the range of disabilities is obtaining reliable and affordable transportation to and from work. This may be due to physical problems (i.e., vision, movement, etc.) that may preclude driving, lack of public transportation or paratransit services, or economic limitations that come with long-term unemployment and high medical costs. Accommodations or alternative work arrangements, such as allowing the individual to telework from home, might be used to mitigate this barrier.

THE CHANGING LANDSCAPE OF DISABILITY POLICY IN THE UNITED STATES

RTW services are delivered within a "landscape" of disability policy that defines such factors as eligibility criteria, types of services available, funding priorities and restrictions, mandates on providers and employers, and the rights and responsibilities of the recipient of services. Goodall and Ghiloni (50) present a thorough description of recent disability legislation in the United States that impact RTW for individuals with TBI, and brief summaries are provided in Table 61-1. We would like to focus on the most recent piece of legislation, the Ticket to Work and Work Incentives Improvement Act of 1999 because of the impact on Social Security Disability beneficiaries.

It is difficult to assess the participation in SSA disability programs by individuals with TBI because until recently SSA did not include TBI as a distinct impairment. SSA added TBI to its Listing of Impairments in August of 2000, and provided guidelines for disability assessment (51). The Listing of Impairments is used by SSA to determine if an individual's impairments are severe enough to prevent gainful activity. Because of this change, in the future it will be easier to estimate the numbers of individuals with TBI who receive SSA disability payments, engage in work activity while in disability status, and use Social Security's work incentives. Within our own RTW program, nearly 100 percent of supported employment participants enter the program as SSI or DI recipients. It would be a logical assumption the participation of individuals with TBI in SSI or DI is high as well, and particularly for those who have the desire and motivation to return to work.

Hennessey (52) undertook an examination of the factors that influence successful attempts to sustain work effort by 1,003 SSA Disability beneficiaries. The following factors were found by Hennessey to be most significantly related to RTW:

- The individual had a financial need to work (81.8 percent of successful RTWs);
- The individual wanted to work (55.2 percent); and
- The individual's health improved such that they could work (35.9 percent).

Other factors that were statistically significant included (a) knowledge of all the work incentives that were available to the beneficiary, (b) availability of job placement assistance, (c) flexible work scheduling as an accommodation, and (d) return to the same job and/or employer as before disability.

TABLE 61-1
Recent Disability-Related Legislation in the Individuals with TBI

NAME	YEAR	MAJOR PROVISIONS
Rehabilitation Act Amendments	1986	Added supported employment as a service option for individuals with the most severe disabilities who require ongoing employment support.
Individuals with Disabilities Education Act (IDEA) Amendments	1990	Adds TBI as a specific educational disability; mandated school-transitional services for students beginning age 16.
Americans with Disabilities Act (ADA)	1990	Title I prohibits discrimination against individuals with disabilities in hiring, termination, promotion; also mandates reasonable accommodations for otherwise qualified individuals with disabilities.
Workforce Investment Act	1998	Designed to consolidate, coordinate, and improve employment, training, literacy, and vocational rehabilitation programs in the United States; funds One-Stop Career Centers for local service coordination.
Ticket to Work and Work Incentives Improvement Act	1999	Created the Ticket to Work program for SSA Disability beneficiaries; created national networks of authorized employment service providers and benefits advisement centers; strengthened several work incentives for beneficiaries.

Although this study is certainly not conclusive, it provides insight into the practicalities of RTW for SSI and DI beneficiaries. First, successful RTW is dependent on motivation to work, through intrinsic desire to be productive, financial demands, or both. Knowledge of work incentives under SSA programs can help beneficiaries overcome their initial fears about returning to the workforce and the risk of failure. Returning to a comfortable, supportive and accommodating work situation is also critical.

Work Incentives

To remedy the concerns on the part of beneficiaries regarding employment and loss of benefit, Congress has enacted a number of work incentives for SSI and DI recipients (53, 54). Some of the more commonly used incentives are described in Table 61-2.

Increasing frustration with poor RTW within the SSI and DI programs led Congress to pass the Ticket to Work and Work Incentives Improvement Act of 1999 (TWWIIA, PL 106–170). This section will describe the enhanced Federal and State benefits programs and work incentives that either are or will soon be available to individuals with TBI and other significant disabilities receiving SSI or DI.

Benefits Planning and Assistance TWWIIA establishes a community-based benefits planning and assistance program designed to provide accurate information on work incentives to SSA beneficiaries. SSA has funded entities across the nation to provide benefits planning and assistance, and conduct ongoing outreach efforts to inform beneficiaries of available work incentives. That program, the Benefits Planning, Assistance, and Outreach Program (BPAO), will increase opportunities for beneficiaries to receive information and services needed to become employed and perhaps attain self-sufficiency. Additional information about the BPAO program, including lists of BPAO projects by state, can be found at The Work Site along with information regarding all work incentives (www.ssa.gov/work/).

Ticket to Work and Self-Sufficiency The Ticket to Work and Self-Sufficiency Program is a voluntary program that is designed to allow SSI and DI recipients the opportunity to direct their own employment services and choose the services and providers they feel they need to initiate or

TABLE 61-2
Most Commonly Used SSA Work Incentives

WORK INCENTIVE	AVAILABLE TO	DESCRIPTION
1619[a] and [b] Impairment	SSI recipients	These two options allow SSI/Medicaid recipients to retain either a cash benefit ([a]) or Medicaid coverage ([b]) for a period of time after achieving SGA.
Related Work Expenses (IRWE)	SSI and DI recipients	Certain expenses required for employment can be excluded from an SSI or DI beneficiary's earned income in determining monthly countable income. SSA must approve the work expenses.
Trial Work Period (TWP)	DI recipients	DI beneficiaries are given the opportunity to test ability to work without jeopardizing benefits. The TWP continues until a beneficiary accumulates nine months of work (not necessarily continuous work) in a rolling 60-month period.
Plan for Achieving Self-Support (PASS)	SSI recipients	Allows recipients to set aside income and/or resources to be used to achieve specific work goals. For example, money could be set aside for education, vocational training, transportation, or starting a business. The PASS must be approved by SSA.
Extended Period of Eligibility	DI recipients	Allows recipients to retain DI and Medicare eligibility while working.
Continued Payment Under a Vocational Rehabilitation Program	SSI and DI recipients	Allows for continuation of benefits while the recipient is engaged in Vocational Rehabilitation services.

return to work. SSI and DI recipients use a "ticket" or voucher to purchase needed services within an employment network, or EN. An EN can be a single provider agency, a one-stop delivery system, a group of providers that combines resources into a single delivery system, or even employers. If the individual enters and maintains employment above SGA, the EN will receive payment through one of two plans: (i) a fixed percentage of SSI or DI savings, or (ii) at achieved employment milestones.

Each EN in the ticket program serves a designated area and develops individualized work plans with beneficiaries from their service area who seek employment. A work plan will include statements of (i) the beneficiary's vocational goal; (ii) services and supports necessary to reach the goal; (iii) terms and conditions related to the provision of supports and services; (iv) rights and remedies available to the beneficiary; and (v) the beneficiary's right to modify the plan. Additional information about the ticket program is available at www.yourtickettowork.com.

Medicaid Buy-In   The Medicaid Buy-In provisions of TWWIIA address probably the most severe disincentive to employment of SSI or DI beneficiaries, the loss of health care coverage. Many, if not most individuals with significant disabilities will not enter the workforce in full-time positions with medical benefits, and therefore face the loss of health care when their earnings reach SGA. The Medicaid Buy-In component of TWWIIA will allow working individuals with disabilities (not just those receiving Social Security disability benefits) to purchase Medicaid services, just as if they were purchasing health care coverage through an employer-sponsored program.

A state can initiate a Medicaid Buy-In program through a relatively quick and simple amendment to its State plan that redefines eligible populations. This can be done through one or more of the following ways, such as raising income limits for eligible participants, disregarding g earned or unearned income of the beneficiary or his/her spouse, or exempting certain assets (such as work-related assets).

In addition to the Medicaid Buy-In, TWWIIA allows working DI recipients to extend premium-free Medicare Part A (hospitalization) coverage for an additional 4Ω years beyond current limits, to a potential duration of 8Ω years, under certain conditions. Because each state defines eligibility and limitations for the Buy-In, the state Medicaid agency or local BPAO would be the best source to receive information about the options available.

Other TWWIIA Incentives   TWWIIA contained two other major provisions that alleviate disincentives to work. Many beneficiaries are reluctant to attempt RTW out of fear that they would be unable to regain benefits should their physical or mental condition worsen and they would be unable to continue working. TWWIIA allows an individual to receive immediate reinstatement of benefits that were terminated due to earnings. To be eligible for reinstatement, an individual must request reinstatement within 60 months of termination of benefits.

Another major disincentive was the potential impact of work on a Continuing Disability Review (CDR). CDRs are periodic reviews to determine if an individual's medical condition has improved sufficient to terminate disability benefits. Any earnings reported to SSA might "trigger" a CDR before the individual is working at a self-sufficient level. TWWIIA addresses this concern by, first, disallowing CDRs for any beneficiary who is using a ticket, and second, disallowing CDRs triggered by work activity. CDRs that are regularly scheduled are allowed.

CAREER DEVELOPMENT OF PERSONS WITH TBI

Career development theories have evolved during the last ten years and the pressure to address the needs of racial and ethical minorities is making those more and more useful to people with disabilities. However, despite this fact, applicability of career development theories for people with disabilities remains a concern. Empirical research on the impact of disability on careers is at a relatively early stage. According to Szymanski et al. (55), outcome on career development for persons with disabilities has been strikingly similar to the study outcomes on racial and ethnic minority groups. Research has revealed that people with disabilities are underrepresented in the labor market and that certain contextual factors like education are related to employment. Outcomes have not indicated what mechanisms are involved in the career development of people with disabilities.

Szymanski et al. (55) also report, that there are some methodological problems inherent in studying the career development of people with disabilities. Various studies, and in particular those related to career indecision, have been plagued by poor design, conceptual ambiguities, methodological weakness, and low statistical power. Thus, it is not surprising that the data have resulted in conflicting findings. Even in light of these discouraging findings, career development theories can provide a conceptual framework that can be useful when providing career counseling to persons with disabilities. The key is to adjust the approach to the individual circumstances at hand (6).

Future research on career development for people with disabilities presents some interesting challenges. On the one hand, it is important to study this population due to their limited access to employment opportunities. On the other hand, it is important to recognize that there are inherent flaws in studying this or any population in isolation or in simple comparison with another group (33).

To better understand the career development of people with disabilities in a broader context future research should include people with disabilities and those from racial and ethnic minority groups in larger scale research. Qualitative research should also be considered to improve our knowledge of the complex interaction between disability and career development.

Career Interest Assessments

Career assessment interventions are important tools that allow people with or without disabilities to take control of their career planning. The 1992 Amendments to the Rehabilitation Act emphasize consumer involvement in the rehabilitation process, including vocational assessment; self-rating instruments and interviews appear to provide the individual with the disability with more involvement over the assessment process. In this section we will review several types of interventions that were selected by the authors due to their availability and applicability for people with Traumatic Brain Injury (TBI).

Many career assessment tools are available on the Internet. One of the most popular career interest inventories is the Self Directed Search designed by John Holland. There are three versions one for adults, one for college students, and one for secondary school students and adults with limited reading skills. It is based on Holland's theory that there are six basic personality types: Creative, Realistic, Investigative, Artistic, Social, and Enterprising. The theory assumes that there are six corresponding work environments, and that individuals will find "person-environment fit" in work environments that most closely match their personality (56).

The Strong Interest Inventory may also be useful in assessing career interests of individuals from middle school through adulthood. The instrument reports a score for the six areas of interest described by John Holland, as well as 23 basic interest scales and 207 occupational scales. Myers-Brigges provides information on personality type, and will give added perspective to self-exploration exercises. Both the Strong Interest Inventory and the Myers-Briggs are online at Career By Design at www.careers-by-design.com/.

The ability to reason is not a single process, but an extremely complex network of related processes. After a TBI, even simple tasks like completing an interest inventory, can require a great deal of thought. The inability to reason, make sound judgments and initiate, and plan or organize, may become virtually impossible, and this can affect a person's ability to independently perform career exploration activities. In such an instance a vocational specialist can provide the necessary support to enable the person to complete this type of activity.

Another popular career counseling strategy involves using computer assisted systems. These systems are able to handle vast quantities of information and assist with integration of information (78). Many computer assisted career guidance (CACG) systems are available: CHOICES, SIGI Plus, and DISCOVER to name a few (57). These interventions provide individuals with current, accurate, locally relevant occupational, and educational information.

Discover is a computer program that assists people with self-assessment and provides information related to making career decisions. SIGI Plus is similar, however it does not provide information on postsecondary education. Choices should be used under the guidance of a vocational counselor. It helps the jobseeker learn more about abilities and interests and how they may relate to different careers.

Some persons with TBI may be able to use these tools with out assistance, while others may need help with reading, writing and interpreting the results. In addition, to learning more about vocational interests and aptitudes the opportunity to work through a career search exercise with a person with a TBI can also provide valuable information about current physical, cognitive, and social skills.

A number of career planning books are available to assist persons with identifying their skills and abilities. For example, Melanie Witt's book *Job Strategies for People with Disabilities* (58) contains a wide range of self-assessment tools to help a person define their career direction. Another career planning book, *Coming Alive from Nine to Five* by Betty Michelozzi provides a number of self-assessment exercises that may be useful to person seeking a first job or switching career tracks. Again, some job seekers with TBI may require assistance with completing the assessments, as well as interpreting the results and translating this data into useful career search information.

Experiential Assessment

Work experience and similar interventions like volunteering or job shadowing may be useful for some people with TBI. If an individual has very limited experiences from which to make an informed career decisions, a work experience may help the person choose a career direction (55). Volunteering in various work settings may give some individuals with TBI ideas on abilities, preferences, and support needs. Job shadowing, can also serve this purpose. This strategy typically involves observing or "shadowing" a person who is performing a job. Some persons with TBI will need assistance with setting up and participating in either type of activity. A vocational rehabilitation specialist can assist an individual with contacting employers and making the necessary arrangements. Then while the activity is taking place, the vocational rehabilitation specialist can accompany the person to the jobsite and make notes on the person's likes and dislikes for certain types of jobs and work settings. This type of information can be very valuable in the future when the person is actively trying to determine an initial direction for the job search or making decisions about whether or not to accept a job offer. Please note that neither of these activities should be viewed as a prerequisite to going to work, instead both are time-limited career exploration activities.

Home Visits

Whenever a vocational rehabilitation specialist is involved with assisting a person with a TBI with locating work, a home visit can provide important vocational assessment and career search information. During the home visit the individual with the TBI is asked to share details on current abilities, work interests, and values. The person is also observed performing various tasks in their home environment, which demonstrates current physical, cognitive, and social skills. In addition, casual conversations about activities of daily living, tasks completed around the house, and leisure pursuits can also lead to some ideas on vocational abilities and interests (59).

Career Information Interviews

This approach provides a valuable means for learning more about an occupation or industry. It involves setting up an appointment with someone in a particular field and interviewing the person to learn more about a specific occupation or industry. Some people with TBI may need assistance with setting up and conducting the interview. In this instance, a vocational specialist assists the person with determining the businesses to contact, making contacts, coordinating the interview, formulating questions to ask, and actually conducting the interview. The person with a TBI is encouraged to participate in each activity as much as possible. The vocational specialist should assist as needed and if present at the interview should take notes, as well as make observations of the individual's abilities. This type of exploratory interview offers the job-seeker information on minimal qualifications, education or training needed, for certain types of work. Information on how a particular career choice might impact future earnings and quality of life can also be gleaned from an informational interview (59).

VOCATIONAL ASSESSMENT

Functional Assessment

As mentioned earlier, through the years, traditional evaluation practices that use aptitude batteries, work samples, and behavioral inventories have dominated vocational evaluations for persons with severe disabilities. However, problems related to reliability and validity has demanded

that the process of assessment be conceptualized once more, so persons with disabilities are not being considered "too disabled" and unable to work. The traditional evaluation process is a linear process that identifies interests, abilities, and aptitudes at one point in time and assumes that this will not change overtime. Then these outcomes are used to predict subsequent learning, performance and success at work. Simply said, they focus on what someone cannot do rather than tuning in to the power of workplace accommodations and on the job supports.

Since many persons with severe disabilities like TBI enter the vocational assessment or evaluation process with limited marketable skills, they are likely to be excluded from work. Instead, they may be told that they need a longer recovery period prior to seeking work, or that they are not likely to ever work again and should be resigned to staying at home and collecting government benefits. In the worse case scenario, they are advised to enter programs to "get ready" to work, offered pre-employment training for menial jobs, sent off to day activity centers, or to work in an enclave. An enclave involves having a small group of people with disabilities working together in a community-based job, while under the constant supervision of a vocational rehabilitation specialist. For example, a group of five people may work as a team to clean a department store.

Traditional vocational evaluations occur in artificial and simulated environments, which are not reliable or valid indicators of what someone can do in the real world. There are a number of limitations in traditional approaches to vocational evaluation for persons with significant disabilities. The authors strongly believe that the most fair and reliable way to assess a person's abilities is within the context of real work environments. And furthermore they believe that the focus of a vocational assessment should be on interests, abilities, supports available, and supports needed to succeed at work.

Consumer-Focused Alternatives to Traditional Vocational Assessment

An approach to career planning that is gaining more and more popularity, particularly in the medical community, are customized functional vocational assessments in real work environments (60). A functional vocational assessment provides a specific appraisal focusing on the needs, skills, and interest of the person within the context of future work environments.

This practical approach can provide valuable career development information to individuals with disabilities and particularly those with the most significant disabilities. All too often persons with severe disabilities are considered either too disabled to work or not ready for employment. This approach focuses on current strengths and abilities and the types of supports that will enable a person to succeed in the workplace. Since the assessment is customized, the design depends upon the person's previous work history and any current employment options. If the individual was working at the time of injury the assessment may be geared toward examining one of the following options: Return to Pre-injury Employer (includes self employment) performing pre-injury job (with or without accommodation), or return to Pre-injury Employer with reassignment to a different position (with or without accommodation). If the person does not have the option to return to the pre-injury employer, but desires information on whether or not he or she can use a specific skill set in the workplace, a Residual Skills Assessment may be warranted. If the person has limited or no work history or has been absent from the workplace for an extended period of time then a Career Exploration Assessment may be conducted. No matter which approach is used it is important that the evaluator is knowledgeable of any work medical work restrictions in advance to planning the assessment approach. A brief description of each approach will follow.

Accommodation and Support Needs

People with traumatic brain injury who are returning to work may need to perform their job in a different way or require modified workstations, compensatory strategies, or other accommodations or supports (61). In this approach a vocational rehabilitation specialist works closely with both the employer and employee to assess the person's vocational abilities by taking data on some specific vocational skill and if warranted recommend support strategies.

Once the person receives a release to return to work, the vocational rehabilitation specialist (with the employer's permission) accompanies the employee with TBI back to work and makes observations on the person's ability to perform the essential job functions. This criterion-referenced assessment measures the individuals' ability to do a specified task by collecting data on the steps of that task. Depending upon the nature and complexity of the job, other job-site personnel may need to be involved in planning and implementing the assessment. If difficulties arise, the specialist makes recommendations on ways to remove barriers and enhance independent performance.

For example, the returning employee and/or employer may need assistance with identifying and implementing accommodations like compensatory memory strategies. The return-to-work assessment is not used to determine whether or not someone can return to work but instead can provide ideas on types of possible accommodations and supports needed to enhance a successful return to work.

Residual Skills Assessment

While some individuals may have work to which they can return to, others may not, but may have a keen interest in pursuing an employment opportunity that requires the use of his/her specialized skills, training, or educational background. In order to make an informed decision about whether or not to return to this type of occupation, the individual may need information on his or her current skills, abilities, and possible accommodations. A customized vocational assessment specifically designed to explore current level of functioning in a previous line of work and support needs may prove useful, and instill the confidence the person needs to return to this type of work. Sometimes the assessment may also relate to using one's educational background in the workplace and might help someone determine whether or not to pursue a career in a specific field.

Depending on the nature and complexity of the occupation in question, a consultant who is actively engaged in such work may be needed to assist with designing and implementing the assessment. The consultant should be someone who could be considered an "expert" in the field or area that is under exploration. The vocational specialist usually takes responsibility for locating and securing the consultants' service, coordinating the effort, assisting with the assessment design and tools, and writing a report. The specialist may also actively participate in the assessment process by making observations and collecting data on the individual's abilities and support needs.

JOB SEARCH AND EMPLOYER NEGOTIATION STRATEGIES

Career development and planning are necessary first steps toward going to work and once a vocational direction has been established the job search should begin. As the search unfolds, the direction should be modified based on any new information that surfaces during this process. This section will review some of the issues that impact the job search and suggest strategies that may be useful when assisting persons with TBI with going to work.

Disability Issues

According to a recent Louis Harris and Associates (77) national survey of people with disabilities, more than 71 percent of working age adults with disabilities are unemployed, despite the fact that two-thirds of these individuals want to work. Moreover, in 1992, an extensive national longitudinal study of students with disabilities who had exited schools found that the employment rates of individuals with disabilities lagged significantly behind those of their peers without disabilities (62). Other studies confirm a continuing troublesome trend toward high rates of unemployment or underemployment for former recipients of special education services (63, 64).

These results suggest that the issue has never been whether or not persons with disabilities want to work, but instead has been on what is inhibiting their participation in the workforce. Several interrelated issues have made securing work a significant issue for persons with TBI. These include misperceptions and prejudice by employers, the general complexity involved in conducting a job search, and effectively representing one's abilities and support needs to an employer either during an interview or once hired.

Despite protections under the ADA, many people with disabilities remain unemployed. The law protects only qualified applicants or employees with disabilities. Some persons with significant disability may have a difficult time qualifying for an existing position or competing with all who apply for a given work opportunity. If an applicant or employee does not disclose that he or she has a disability he or she is not covered under the ADA. But at the same time, revealing this information may lead to being screened out of a job.

To avoid this conflict, it often pays to explore the "hidden job market". This requires learning about job opportunities before anyone else knows about them; these are the positions that are not being advertised. The best ways to tap into the hidden job market area by networking with personal contacts and contacting employers directly.

Individuals with TBI may have very limited personal networks due to social isolation (35). And in the instance where a personal network exists the individual may not be able to independently use his or her network to locate job opportunities. Memory problems can also make it difficult to manage the job search. For example, the person may not follow up for lead in a timely manner or may miss appointments with employers. Transportation can also be a problem. Some individuals may have difficulty getting to and from places of businesses without some assistance. Also, due to the myriad of cognitive problems that may result from a TBI some individuals may experience great difficulties with exploring occupations as well as conducting pre employment activities like completing employment applications, interviewing for a job, completing pre employment testing, and advocating for necessary on the job supports or accommodations.

It typically is the responsibility of the job applicant to best present his or her abilities to employers, and some people with TBI may have a difficult time doing so. Some individuals will not be able to explain to employers how their particular skills and abilities match the qualifications for the job. If the person is in need of an accommodation, he or she may experience difficulties explaining to the employer what is needed to allow him or her to succeed. Some persons with TBI may need to convince an employer to redesign task, location, or restructure a job that was originally designed with individuals without disabilities in mind. This may present difficulties for the applicant with a TBI if he or she has a myriad of cognitive difficulties and is unsure of what he or she may need to succeed on the job. If the job seeker is unclear on how his or her abilities can best match an employer's needs, it is unlikely that a job offer will surface.

Sometimes, employers may not see a "new or different" way to get a task done or may see the request for change as bothersome. Instead the company representative may simply choose to hire someone else who does not require any accommodation. On the other hand, many employers may be willing to hire individuals with TBI, but may need support to determine how best to make reasonable accommodation. Vocational rehabilitation specialists can be a valuable resource for employers in this area.

Vocational rehabilitation usually offers a range of job search and placement services, from the least to most intrusive approach. The approach selected generally depends upon the individual's abilities and support needs. We will review a couple of these approaches and then focus in on what the author's view as the most favorable strategy for assisting persons with severe TBI with gaining employment; a customized and tailored approach to this process.

Minimal Intervention

The first approach generally involves a minimum amount of intervention from a vocational rehabilitation specialist. For example, the jobseeker may simply need information on the labor market, insights concerning their interviewing skills, or leads on employment opportunities. Or perhaps the person simply needs information on adaptive aids or effective compensatory strategies. These individuals often know what they want, but need specific information to put their plan in to action. They may have pervious work history and have a good work ethic. These individuals are usually able to read, write, and can follow through on complex directives without assistance. They take the information given to them, generalize it, and apply it to their lives. There need for vocational assistance is often minimal. Unfortunately, vocational rehabilitation professionals, who are unfamiliar with TBI may feel that a person with an injury is much more capable than he or she truly is and may only offer minimal job search and placement assistance. Afterwards, in instances where the person does not follow through on specific directives this may be perceived, by the vocational rehabilitation provider, as a lack of motivation to work on the part of the individual with TBI and in some instances may lead to termination of services.

Education and Preparation Approach

The second vocational placement approach is for those individuals who appear to need some type of intervention, but not an extensive intervention. Usually, these individuals do not assimilate information quickly, and require assistance with carrying out a job search, but once employed may need no or limited assistance on the job. Often times, these individuals participate in classes designed to get ready or prepared for conducting either an independent job search or a job search with some limited assistance from a job placement specialist. This approach is usually not very effective for persons with significant TBI since most of the training takes place in a classroom type setting. Usually classes are conducted to teach job seeking and maintenance skills. For instance students learn about various occupations and how to analyze themselves and the job market to choose an appropriate career path, or receive information on how to complete employment applications or learn how to interview for a job.

Sometimes, particularly for persons with severe TBI, an inordinate amount of time is expended trying to get the person ready to conduct a job search, when in reality it is highly unlikely that the learning that takes place in the classroom will ever generalize into the real world. Instead, the authors feel that time could be better expended by providing individualized job placement assistance that is tailored to each job seekers specific needs and abilities.

Customized Approach

This approach can be helpful to anyone with a disability, but is particularly useful for people with more severe disabilities like TBI. Using this strategy the type and intensity of services and supports are adapted to each individual's needs and under some circumstances involve extensive intervention. Generally, individuals with significant cognitive impairments need more assistance with obtaining employment than those who have moderate physical or sensory disabilities. These individuals tend to learn best in the milieu where they will be expected to perform instead of learning away from that environment. Generally, they need one to one assistance with identifying their vocational strengths, support needs, and conducting a job search. Once employed, they may need assistance on the job. One vocational service option that offers individualized and intensive support services for both gaining and maintaining employment is Supported Employment. This approach encourages full inclusion of the person with the disability in his or her job search and offers reality-based activities. A person does not have to get ready to work instead a vocational support person sometimes called a job coach provides assistance with helping the person identify his or her abilities and support needs, contact employers to discuss hiring needs, and offers on the job assistance and long term follow along. This service option will be discussed in more detail in the next section.

WORKPLACE SUPPORTS

No two individuals with TBI are alike, nor are their abilities or disabilities similar. Add in the different types of occupations and the huge variances within work environments and you have a totally unique situation on hand. Therefore, individuals with TBI who are attempting to return to work will need supports that are customized to meet their individual needs at a specific workplace. The type, level, and intensity of support will vary depending on the person's abilities and the particular circumstances on hand. Some individuals with TBI may simply need information and guidance on how to conduct a job search or ways to compensate for memory deficits on the job, while others particularly those with severe disabilities will need more intensive intervention and one to one assistance. Furthermore, the type, level and intensity of support someone will need, does not remain static, but changes over time. For example, after learning how to do a job task, the individual may need additional instruction when new duties are introduced. Individuals with TBI, may benefit from a combination of workplace supports. Some examples follow. For example, someone who has a job to return to will not need assistance with locating a new occupation, however once back to work he or she may need assistance with learning how to get organized and manage their workload.

Accommodations

Some people with TBI will benefit from accessible building, particularly if the person has difficulty walking or uses a wheelchair for mobility. For example, a wheelchair lift was installed outside of the entrance of an inaccessible older historical building that allowed the employee who uses a wheelchair access. Those who have changes in vision post injury may also benefit from access supports. For example, raised letter directional signs may be posted in a building to help an employee identify restrooms or elevator controls.

A modified work schedule that allows an employee to get to work on time may also be necessary. For example, a person may be allowed to work 10 a.m. to 6 p.m. rather than 9 a.m. to 5 p.m. due to limitations on the availability of transportation to and from work. In other instances a person may need part-time work due to changes in one's stamina level or an increase in fatigue. Other people with TBI may be able to work full-time, but may need to have an opportunity to take additional scheduled breaks throughout the workday.

Job restructuring is another important accommodation. This involves having a non- essential (not major) work function or a marginal duty is removed from an employee's job description or a difficult task that the employee cannot do is exchanged for one that can be done. For example, a general worker at a retail store is not able to climb ladders to change the light bulbs. Management agrees to allow another employee to do this and in exchange the worker is responsible for checking the parking lot and returning customer carts to the building.

Sometimes, particularly if the person has a physical disability or slowed movements post injury it will be useful to purchase assistive equipment or devices to improve their ability to get the job done. More often existing items in the workplace may be modified or added on to accommodate the person. Assistive technology ranges from high tech to no tech, costly to no cost. Fortunately most auxiliary aids are not expensive.

For some individuals a change in where their work is performed may be helpful. This may simply involve allowing the employee to move to a different workstation or in some instances and if applicable allow telecommuting or working from home.

Some individuals with TBI may need support services. Examples of support services may include assisting the person with carrying out activities of daily living like eating or going to the restrooms, having a "buddy" assigned to alert the worker to an emergency situation, or helping the individual take notes during an employee training, or staff meeting.

Perhaps one of the most useful accommodations for workers with a TBI are internal or external compensatory strategies. Internal strategies require the use of a mental support system and do not rely on external devices. Examples include, making associations or drawing on analogies to remember how to do a task or using word mnemonics to remember a specific sequence. External strategies involve the use of objects like checklists or flow-charts to remember a sequence of steps to follow to complete a work activity. These strategies can serve multiple purposes. They not only promote learning, but can also serve as a reminder of what needs to be done and helps keep the worker organized, so the job can be completed in a proper and timely manner.

It is important to remember that all workplace supports and adaptive solutions that are used to compensate for functional limitations are highly individualized. In addition, the solution to the presenting problem will be highly dependent upon the user's willingness to use a strategy, as well as, the type of job tasks involved, the work environment, and the employers' consent to allow the use of the accommodation. Although, these examples were presented in isolation it is often the unique interplay and right combination of supports that will lead to success at work.

Table 61-3 below provides some examples of the types of workplace strategies used by employees with TBI, who used a Supported Employment approach to assist them with going to work post injury.

Sometimes there are existing cues in the workplace that the new employee can learn to attend to that will promote successful job performance. Consider the following examples, a landscaper who is required to mow the lawn in a large office complex, is given a diagram on a daily basis that illustrates what areas are to be cut that day. A patient transporter works in a hospital that has different colored signage that helps him find his way to the correct destination. A medical supply order puller receives a printout indicating where in the warehouse the items needed are located.

In other instances the necessary support will be simple ergonomic modifications to the workstation or a change in the way the work is performed. This might include adapting the layout of a workstation so that the task can be better sequenced, raising a worktable to accommodate a wheelchair or customized seat, or using jigs or adaptations to mitigate the employees limitations in vision, dexterity, judgment, etc.

Job Coaching

Most individuals with severe traumatic brain injury will need assistance with locating work, as well as assistance learning how to perform the job. One approach that has successfully been used to assist people with TBI with going to work is supported employment (4, 41). Using this approach a vocational rehabilitation specialist known as an "employment specialist" or "job coach" provides one to one individualized assistance to assist a person with a severe disability with finding a job, and once employed provides or facilitates the supports needed to help the person succeed at work. The type, level, and intensity of support varies depending upon the newly hired employee's abilities, the job, the work environment, existing supports in the workplace. Table 61-4 provides a brief overview of the role of the employment specialist, the person with a TBI, and other return to work process team members.

The level of involvement of the rehabilitation team will vary depending upon the time post injury and who is currently following the individual when he or she goes to work. The authors advocate for return to work as soon as possible. If a person has a job to return to it is important that some member of the team or family member act as a liaison with the employer to keep them abreast of the individual's progress in rehabilitation. In some instances the person may not be able to return to the same job, but there may be some other type of work within the organization. Some people maybe able to begin to return to work while involved in day rehabilitation on a part-time

TABLE 61-3
Examples of Workplace Supports

Position Title	Job-Related Functional Limitation	Presenting Issue	Workplace Support
Receptionist at small business	No use of arms or hands, unable to walk	Taking messages on the telephone	Tape records voice messages then uses voice activated software to type messages
Garment bagger at dry cleaners	Unsteady gait, loss of balance while walking or standing; becomes tired easily	Pulling bags over cleaned garments from a standing position; maintaining stamina	Fabricated metal stand to maintain balance while standing; has flip down seat to rest on when tired
Inventory clerk/order puller for retail store	Becomes frustrated when interrupted and yells at others	Appears angry when new coworkers ask for instructions on how to do the job	Created oversized document to refer new employee's questions
File clerk at insurance company	Becomes defensive or denies having any difficulty when given personal feedback	Appears angry when given constructive feedback on job performance	Uses self monitoring tool and discuss ways to improve performance
Cashier for fast food company	Socializing with strangers in an appropriate manner	Asked customers for their telephone numbers	Posted reminder "Don't creep me out" with picture of unhappy looking female on the phone
Activities assistant at nursing home	Remembering sequence of things to be done throughout the day to complete normal routine	Could not remember what order to complete various job duties	Organized master schedule of various duties to complete on certain days and a list of things to do once duties are done
Plant installer at green house/plant retail store	Remembering how to complete a certain task	Could not remember how to clean and care for various types of plants	Created manual with instructions and cross referenced by plant typical and phylum name
Houseman at hotel	Remembering what to do outside of normal routine	Could not remember what tasks to do outside of normal work routine	Manager on duty writes daily list of things to do in order of occurrence

basis. Some people will not have a job to return to or were unemployed at the time of injury. These individuals will need to seek new employment.

Again the composition of the team will vary depending upon a number of factors. For instance, if the person is involved in or has recently completed out patient rehabilitation the team is likely to be made up of the individual with a TBI, a physiatrist, an occupational therapist, a physical therapist, a neuropsychologist, a social worker, the parents or significant others, a state vocational rehabilitation counselor and if supported employment is being used, an employment specialist or job coach.

Over the years business have become more confident in their ability to manage a diverse workforce and more cognizant of the abilities of workers with disabilities. Also, with the passage of the ADA, larger companies are more open to making reasonable accommodations in the workplace. Thus, individuals who lack access to Supported Employment may still be able to achieve success at work, by simply working with the pre-injury employer or by seeking out flexible and accommodating employers.

INTERNATIONAL PERSPECTIVES

This chapter has focused largely on RTW programs, supports, and legislation within the United States. However, many of the European and other developed countries have well-established neurotrauma and neurosurgical management for traumatic brain injury (e.g. Refs. 65–69). These countries have comprehensive rehabilitation programs in place, with the emphasis on comprehensive interdisciplinary rehabilitation program that includes therapy to overcome the disability which are caused by physical,

TABLE 61-4

Overview of Supported Employment Services and Roles of Interdisciplinary Team Members

EMPLOYMENT SPECIALIST	INDIVIDUAL WITH TBI	OTHER TEAM MEMBER ROLES
Supported Employment Activity: Getting to know one another and establishing a direction for the job search		
• Conducts functional community based activities to get to know the jobseeker and observe current skills, abilities and potential support needs; • Interviews those who know the person best to determine the above; • Identifies jobseekers personal support network; • Discusses impact of earnings on benefits; • Discusses disclosure issues; • Provides feedback to others (i.e. family, team and funding source	• Becomes familiar with service option; • Gets to know the job coach; • Participates in activities to learn more about self and job market; • Expresses needs and wants related to employment; • Decide who will disclose disability to potential employers.	• Makes referral and introductions to SE; • Advocates for SE services with funding source if needed; • Shares information, current records, and insight on a person's abilities and support needs; • If returning to pre-injury job, is liaison between employer and SE provider; • Provides insight on family dynamics; • Develops questions for neuropsy evaluation and or assessment.
Supported Employment Activity: Conducting the job search, applying for jobs and interviewing		
• Locates work opportunities by tapping in to the hidden or unadvertised job market; • Meets with employers to describe SE services and job seeker's desires and abilities; • Analyzes workplace and job to determine pros and cons that may impact success at work and long term job retention; • Discusses above with job seeker; • Practices interviewing skills; • Arranges interviews; • Helps negotiate accommodations; • Provides feedback to others (i.e. family, team and funding source)	• Uses personal network and other resources to identify businesses to contact; • Decides whether or not to learn more about a work opportunity; • Completes applications for employment; • Attends job interviews; • Decides whether or not to accept job offer.	• Shares ideas on employers to contact; • Provides ideas on types of tasks or jobs that may maximize use of personal strengths; • Reviews job descriptions and • provide release for work if needed; • Makes suggestions on types of accommodations or strategies that mayprove useful;
Supported Employment Activity: Providing ongoing long-term job retention services.		
• Stays in touch with employer and employee to assist with any additional training needs or help resolve difficulties in the workplace; • Collects data on performance levels; • Provides additional services as indicated	• Asks for assistance if needed; • Expresses job satisfaction; • Helps problem solve.	• Helps problem solve.
Supported Employment Activity: Providing or facilitating off the job support case management services.		
• Assists with problem solving issues outside of work that if left unaddressed could adversely effect work; • Makes referrals to other resources	• Identifying problems outside of work that are effecting performance; • Helps problem solve	• Provides resources; • Makes referrals to other resources

communicative, cognitive, and behavioral impairments, providing assistance in community integration in terms of living situation, productivity, and social and recreational activities, and providing psychosocial support for patient and family members (e.g., Refs. 8, 23, 70, 71).

The importance of RTW after injury is being recognized, and these rehabilitation programs also offer similar types of vocational assistance, such as work trials, training at workshops, or work training organized on the open job market. However, some programs limit the provision of vocational rehabilitation to those who are eligible in terms of capabilities. For example, Rehab UK assesses the abilities and potential of the applicants before accepting them into the program, offering vocational rehabilitation opportunities only to those who have good cognitive skills (72).

In the developing countries, challenges that individuals with TBI are faced with are further magnified due to either short supply or unavailability of rehabilitation professionals, in addition to lack of service centers to cater for their requirements (73–75).

IMPROVING FUTURE OUTCOME THROUGH A TEAM APPROACH

Traumatic brain injury (TBI) results in disability that requires comprehensive and often lengthy rehabilitation efforts. It is expensive from the standpoint of rehabilitation costs, lost earnings, and therefore, loss to the gross national product, but moreover, costly due to human suffering. Although healthcare and vocational rehabilitation professionals are continually challenged in their efforts to return individuals with TBI to work, the likelihood of successful vocational rehabilitation for persons with traumatic brain injury can be enhanced by utilizing a team approach (76). Key members of the return to work team include the person with TBI; significant others; the employer; neuropsychologist; occupational, speech, and physical therapists; social worker; and vocational rehabilitation counselor or specialist often under the leadership and direction of a physiatrist. Through interdisciplinary collaboration, the team can communicate frequently and set mutual treatment goals for recovery.

The task before the team is to maximize the potential of the individual with brain injury to return to as high a level of pre-injury productivity as can be achieved. Further efforts related to return to work might focus upon establishing new and different life goals and activities. The overall goal of rehabilitation, therefore, involves an enormous effort on the part of both the survivor and rehabilitation team.

While there is no typical length of TBI rehabilitation, there is often a long and arduous process of treatment and therapies that assist the person with returning to pre-injury

lifestyles, including work. Much depends on the severity level of the TBI, the nature and extent of problems, availability of social support networks, accessible and available appropriate rehabilitation, and the circumstances surrounding re-employment and the current labor market. Fewer individuals return to work at the same level, for the same pay, and at the same number of hours per week as before the injury. Some return to a similar job at a full-to part-time level, with a reduced rate of pay, others do not pursue competitive employment. Psychosocial outcomes encompass a similar range, from those being able to resume a familiar social and family life to those who become divorced, separated, or experience shrinking social networks and eventual isolation.

In the best-case scenario, a psychiatrist will be integrally involved in and oversee the team efforts to assist the person with the returning to work. And once employed, the physiatrist and other team members continue to assist with either an advisory role or on an as needed basis.

As mentioned earlier, a neuropsychological evaluation is often used to assist in planning for employment or re-employment. A sound evaluation can provide valuable data to use when determining occupations or work settings that may be more suitable for the person with TBI to consider. The results of a good evaluation can help the person with TBI and team determine the best fit between cognitive assets and deficits, behavioral functioning, interpersonal propensities, overlearned skills or old learning ability, with specific job tasks and work environment for the person with TBI. The results can generate probability statements about the type of job, sort of tasks that may be most appropriate, as well as the types of environmental factors, and supports that may promote the person's success at work.

However, the relationship between neuropsychological test scores and the demands of daily life can be weak. These is why the evaluation should include more than just testing, but also involve gathering other relevant historical, medical, psychosocial, and vocational information from the person, significant other, and team members.

The return to work team can make suggestions on what specific information needs to be obtained from the neuropsychological evaluation and provide other relevant information. For example, inquiring about the personal assets can often be more helpful than dwelling on what the person is unable to do, particularly when planning for a return to work. Also, whenever deficits are mentioned, asking what areas are amenable to remediation and to what extent training or supports can contribute to change is critical. For example, the neuropsychologist may be able to state functions that are expected to improve due to spontaneous recovery or can be assisted by compensatory strategies or other means like job restructuring or environmental modifications.

The use of simple assistive technology is often pivotal to a successful return to work. Technology can help eliminate difficulties in physically accomplishing work activities or improve cognitive functions, like the ability to attend, organize, sequence, and evaluate the result of work activities. Often the process and effort involved in identifying an appropriate intervention can be more involved and costly than the intervention itself. Thus, consultation with experienced team members is very important, as it can not only expedite this, but enhance probability of success.

Using assistive technology at work may be the first time the person is offered assistance that does not appear to be typically clinical. Such interventions are often very empowering and can contribute significantly to the person's ability to be productive at work, as well as more effective in other activities of daily living.

A TBI interferes with a person's identity and social roles. The results of the injury and particularly the inability to work often disrupt a person's sense of purpose, productivity, and self-worth. Therefore, counseling may prove beneficial and help a person with reestablishing a satisfactory level of self-sufficiency. Also, after returning to work, the individual may experience depression or increased frustration at not being able to do things as easy as pre-injury levels. Furthermore, not being accepted by peers or rejection from coworkers can lead to problems. In some instances counseling may be warranted, in others medication may be helpful. The psychiatrist can recommend interventions to assist here. As illustrated, the role of the team, under the direction of a physiatrist, cannot be over emphasized (76). Unfortunately, however, in some instances, a physiatrist may not be accessible. In such an instance a competent general medical practitioner, who is willing to consult with a physiatrist, can lead the team.

Note: Preparation of this chapter was supported in part by Cooperative Agreement No. H133B9800036 from the National Institute on Disability and Rehabilitation Research (NIDRR), U.S. Department of Education. This support does not constitute official endorsement of the information or views presented here.

References

1. Wehman, P., West, M., Johnson, A., Cifu, D. Vocational rehabilitation for individuals with traumatic brain injury. In M. Rosenthal, E.R. Griffith, J.S. Kreutzer, B. Pentland (Eds.), *Rehabilitation of the Adult and Child with Traumatic Brain Injury*, third edition (pp. 326–341). Philadelphia: F.A. Davis, 1999.
2. Dikmen, S. S., Temkin, N. R., Machamer, J. E., et al. Employment following traumatic head injuries. *Arch Neurol* 1994;51,177–186.
3. Fraser, R. T., Wehman, P. Traumatic brain injury rehabilitation: Issues in vocational outcome. *Neuro Rehabil* 1995;5:39–48.
4. Wehman, P. H., West, M, D., Kregel, J., et al. Return to work for persons with severe traumatic brain injury: A data-based approach to program development. *J Head Trauma Rehabil* 1995;10(1): 27–39.
5. Fraser, R.T., Wehman, P., McMahon, B.T. *Traumatic Brain Injury Vocational Rehabilitation: Job Placement Models*. Monograph #4, TBI Series. Delray Beach, FL: St. Lucie Press, 1992.
6. Harrington, D. E., Malec, J., Cicerone, K., Katz, H. T. Current perceptions of rehabilitation professionals towards mild traumatic brain injury. *Arch Phys Med Rehabil* 1993;74:579–586.
7. Horn, I. J., Sherer, M. Rehabilitation of traumatic brain injury. In M. Grabois, S. J. Garrison, K. A. Hart, L. D. Lehmkuhl (Eds.), *Physical Medicine and Rehabilitation: The Complete Approach* (pp. 1281–1304). Cambridge, MA: Blackwell Science, 1999.
8. Asikainen, L., Kaste, M., Sarna, S. Predicting late outcome for patients with traumatic brain injury referred to a rehabilitation programme: A study of 508 Finnish patients 5 years or more after injury *Brain Inj* 1998;12(2):95–107.
9. Curl, R. M., Fraser, R. T., Cook, R. G., Clemmons, D. Traumatic brain injury vocational rehabilitation: Preliminary findings for the coworkers as trainer project. *J Head Trauma Rehabil* 1996;11(1): 75–85.
10. Keyser-Marcus, L., Bricout, J., Wehman, P., et al. Acute predictors of return to employment after traumatic brain injury: A longitudinal follow-up. *Arch Phys Med Rehabil* 2002;83:635–641.
11. Kreutzer, J., Morto, M. V. Traumatic brain injury: Supported employment and compensatory strategies for enhancing vocational outcomes. In P. Wehman, S. Moon (Eds), *Vocational Rehabilitation and Supported Employment* (pp. 291–311). Baltimore: PH Brookes, 1988.
12. McMordie, W. R., Barker, S. L. The financial trauma of head injury. *Brain Inj* 1988;2:357–364.
13. Abrams, D., Barker, L. T., Haffey, W., et al. The economics of return to work for survivors of traumatic brain injury: Vocational services are worth the investment. *J Head Trauma Rehabil* 1993;8:59–76.
14. Ben-Yishay, Y., Silver, S. M., Piasetsky, E., et al. Relationship between employability and vocational outcome after intensive holistic cognitive rehabilitation. *J Head Trauma Rehabil* 1987; 2(1):35–48.
15. Fraser, R. T., Dikmen, S., McLean, A., et al. Employability of head injury survivors: First year post-injury. *Rehabil Counsel Bull* 1988;31:276–284.
16. Ip, R. Y., Dornan, J., Schentag, C. Traumatic brain injury: Factor predicting return to work or school. *Brain Inj* 1995;9:517–532.
17. McMordie, W. R., Barker, S. L., Paolo, T. M. Return to work after head injury. *Brain Inj* 1990;4:57–69.
18. Brooks, N., McKinlay, W., Symington, C., Beattie, A., Campsie, L. Return to work within the first seven years of severe head injury *Brain Inj* 1993;1:5–19.
19. Rao, N., Rosenthal, M., Cronin-Stubbs, D., et al. Return to work after rehabilitation following traumatic brain injury. *Brain Inj* 1990;4:49–56.
20. Cifu, D. X., Keyser-Marcus, L., Lopez, E., et al. Acute predictors of successful return to work 1 year after traumatic brain injury: A multicenter analysis. *Arch Phys Med Rehabil* 1997;78:125–131.
21. Crepeau, F., Scherzer, P. Predictors and indicators of work status after traumatic brain injury: A meta-analysis. *Neuropsychol Rehabil* 1993;3,5–35.
22. Humphrey, M., Oddy, M. Return to work after head injury: A review of post-war studies. *Brain Inj* 1980;12:107–114.
23. Ponsford, J. L., Oliver, J. H., Curran, C., et al. Prediction of employment status 2 years after traumatic brain injury. *Brain Inj* 1995;9:11–20.
24. Sander, A., Kreutzer, J., Rosenthal, M., et al. A multicenter longitudinal investigation of return to work and community integration following traumatic brain injury. *J Head Trauma Rehabil* 1996;11(5):70–84.
25. Mackenzie, E., Shapiro, S., Smith, R., Siegel, J., Moody, M., Pitt, A. Factors influencing return to work following hospitalization for traumatic injury. *Amer Journal Pub Health* 1987;77:329–334.
26. Vogenthaler, D. R., Smith, K. R., Goldfader, P. Head injury a multivariate study: Predicting long-term productivity and independent living outcome. *Brain Inj* 1989;3:369–385.
27. Fabiano, R. J., Crewe, N., Goran, D. A. Differences between elapsed time to employment and employer selection in vocational outcome following severe traumatic brain injury. *J App Rehabil Counsel* 1995;26(4):17–20.
28. Greenspan, A. I., Wrigley, J. M., Kresnow, M., et al. Factors influencing failure to return to work due to traumatic brain injury. *Brain Inj* 1996;10(3):207–218.

29. O'Connel, M. J. Prediction of return to work following traumatic brain injury: Intellectual, memory, and demographic variables. *Rehabil Psychol* 2000;45(2):212–217.

30. Rosenthal, M., Dijkers, M., Harrison-Felix, C., et al. Impact of minority status on functional outcome and community integration following traumatic brain injury. *J Head Trauma Rehabil* 1996;11(5):40–57.

31. Skord, K. G., Miranti, S. V. Towards a more integrated approach to job placement and retention for persons with traumatic brain injury and premorbid disadvantages. *Brain Inj* 1994;8:383–392.

32. Lillie-Blanton, M., Alfaro-Correa, A. *In the Nation's Interest: Equality in Access to Health Care: Project on the Health Care Needs of Hispanics and African Americans*. Summary report from the Joint Center for Political and Economic Studies. Washington, DC: Joint Center for Political and Economic Studies, 1995.

33. Wright, T. J. Enhancing the professional preparation of rehabilitation counselors for improved services to ethnic minorities with disabilities. *J Appl Rehabil Counsel* 1988;19(4):4–9.

34. Oddy, M., Coughlan, T., Tyerman, A., et al. Social adjustment after closed head injury: A further follow-up seven years later. *J Neurol Neurosurg Psych* 1985;48:564–568.

35. Morton, M. V., Wehman, P. Psychosocial and emotional sequelae of individuals with traumatic brain injury: A literature review and recommendations. *Brain Inj* 1995;9(1):81–92.

36. Fraser, R., Baarlag-Benson, R. Crossdisciplinary collaboration in the removal of work barriers after traumatic brain injury. *Top Language Disorders* 1994;15:55–67.

37. McKinlay, W., Brooks, D., Bond, M. Post-concussional symptoms, financial compensation and outcome of severe blunt head injury. *J Neurol Neurosurg Psych* 1983;46:1084–1091.

38. Thompsen, I. V. Late outcome of very severe blunt head trauma. A 10–15 year second follow-up. *J Neurol Neuropsychol Psych* 1984;47:260–268.

39. Martin-Tamer, P. Differential vocational outcome following traumatic head injury. *Dissertation Abstract International* 1988;49:5,508B.

40. Sherer, M., Bergloff, P., High, W., et al. Contribution of functional ratings to prediction of long-term employment outcome after traumatic brain injury. *Brain Inj* 1999;13(1):973–981.

41. Wehman, P. H., Kregel, J., Kreutzer, J. S., et al. Return to work for persons following severe traumatic brain injury: Supported employment outcome after five years. *Amer J Phys Med Rehabil* 1993;76(6):355–363.

42. Gollaher, K., High, W., Shere, M., et al. Prediction of employment outcome one to three years following traumatic brain injury. *Brain Inj* 1998;12(4):255–263.

43. Orr, M. R., Walker, W. C., Marwitz, J. H., Kreutzer, J. Occupational categories and return to work after traumatic brain injury. *Arch Phys Med Rehabil* 2003;84(9):E:5.

44. Godfrey, H., Bisharo, S., Partridge, F., et al. Neuropsychological impairment and return to work following severe closed head injury: Implementations for clinical management. *NZ Med J* 1993;106:310–393.

45. Schwab, K., Grafman, J., Salazar, A., et al. Residual impairments and work status 15 years after penetrating head injury: Report from the Vietnam head injury study. *Neurology*, 1993;43:96–103.

46. Kowalske, K., Plenger, P. M., Lusby, B., et al. Vocational reentry following TBI: An enablement model. *J Head Trauma Rehabil* 2000;15:989–999.

47. Ruffolo, C. F., Friedland, J. F., Dawson, D. R., et al. Mild traumatic brain injury from motor vehicle accidents: Factors associated with return to work. *Arch Phys Med Rehabil* 1999;80:392–398.

48. West, M. Aspects of the workplace and return to work for persons with brain injuries in supported employment. *Brain Inj* 1995;9:301–313.

49. Bowe, F. G. Statistics, politics, and employment of people with disabilities. *J Disability Policy Studies* 1993;4:83–91.

50. Goodall, P., Ghiloni, C. T. The changing face of publicly funded employment services. *J Head Trauma Rehabil* 2001;16(1):94–106.

51. Federal Register. *Revised Medical Criteria for Evaluating Mental Disorders and Traumatic Brain Injury: Final Rules* 2000, August 21;65(162):50745.

52. Hennessey, J. C. Factors affecting the work efforts of disabled-worker beneficiaries. *Soc Sec Bull* 1997;60(3):3–20.

53. Social Security Administration. *2003 Red Book*. Baltimore, 2003.

54. Social Security Administration. *SSI Recipients Who Work*. Baltimore, March 2000.

55. Szymanski, E. M., Turner, K. D., Hershenson, D. Career development of people with disabilities: Theoretical perspectives. In F. R. Rusch, L. DeStefano, J. Chadsey-Rusch, et al. (Eds), *Transition from School to Adult Life: Models, Linkages, and Policy* (pp. 391–406). Sycamore, IL: Sycamore.

56. Holland, J. *The Self-Directed Search*. San Antonio, TX: Psychological Corporation, 1994.

57. Taylor, K. M. Advances in career-planning systems. In W. B. Walsh, S. H. Osipow (Eds.), *Career Decision Making* (pp. 137–211). Hillsdale, NJ: Erlbaum, 1988.

58. Witt, Melanie Astaire. *Job Strategies for People with Disabilities*. Princeton, N. J.: Peterson's Guides, 1992.

59. Targett, P. S., Witting, K. M. Functional vocational assessment. In P. Wehman, P. S. Targett, *Vocational Curriculum for Individuals with Special Needs* (pp. 25–61), Austin, TX: Pro-Ed, 1999.

60. Targett, P. S., Ferguson, S. S., McLaughlin, J. Consumer involvement in vocational evaluation. In P. Wehman, J. Kregel (Eds), *More Than a Job: Securing Satisfying Careers for People with Disabilities* (pp. 95–117). Baltimore: Paul H. Brookes, 1998.

61. Targett, P., Wehman, P., Petersen, R., & Gorton, S. Enhancing work outcomes for three persons with traumatic brain injury. *Int J Rehabil Res* 1995;21:41–50.

62. Wagner, M., D'Amico, R., Marder, C., Newman, L., Blackorby, J. *What Happens Next? Trends in Post-School Outcomes of Youth with Disabilities*. Menlo Park, CA: SRI International, 1992.

63. Colley, D. A., Jamison, D. Post-school results for youth with disabilities: Key indicators and policy implications. *Career Development for Exceptional Individuals* 1998;21:145–160.

64. Rogan, P. *Review and Analysis of Post-School Follow-Up Results: 1996–1997 Indiana Post-School Follow-Up Study*. Indianapolis: Indiana Department of Education, Division of Special Education, 1997.

65. Atkinson, L., Merry, G. Advances in neurotrauma in Australia 1970–2000. *World J Surg* 2001;25:1224–1229.

66. Firsching, R., Woischneck, D. Present status of neurosurgical trauma in Germany. *World J Surg* 2001;25:1221–1223.

67. Kay, A., Teasdale, G. Head injury in the United Kingdom. *World J Surg* 2001;25:1210–1220.

68. Kelly, D., Becker, D. Advances in management of neurosurgical trauma: USA and Canada. *World J Surg* 2001;25:1179–1185.

69. Maejima, S., Katayama, Y. Neurosurgical trauma in Japan. *World J Surg* 2001;25:1205–1209.

70. Queen Elizabeth's Foundation Brain Injury Centre. 2003. Available on-line: *http://www.qefd.org/braininjury/vocationalrehabprog.htm*

71. Schmidt, S., Oort-Marburger, D., Meijman, T. Employment after rehabilitation for musculoskeletal impairments: The impact of vocational rehabilitation and working on a trial basis. *Arch Phys Med Rehabil* 1995;76:950–954.

72. Rehab UK. 2003. Available on-line: *http://www.rehabuk.org*

73. Gururaj, G. Need and scope of rehabilitation services for traumatic brain injury survivors. *ActionAid Disability News* 1998;9:27–31.

74. Gururaj, G. Epidemiology of traumatic brain injuries: Indian scenario. *Neurol Res* 2002;24(1):24–28.

75. Raja, I., Vohra, A., Ahmed, M. Neurotrauma in Pakistan. *World J Surg* 2001;25:1230–1237.

76. Zasler, N. D. The role of medical rehabilitation in vocational reentry. *J Head Trauma Res* 1997;12(5):42–56.

77. Louis Harris and Associates. *The ICD Survey III: Employing Disabled Americans*. Washington, DC: National Organization on Disability, 1998.

78. Sampson, J. P., Jr. Computer applications and issues in using tests in counseling. In C. E. Watkins, Jr., V. L. Campbell (Eds.), *Testing in Counseling Practice* (pp. 475–480). Hillsdale, NJ: Erlbaum, 1990.

XV

MEDICOLEGAL AND ETHICAL ISSUES

62 Medicolegal Aspects of TBI

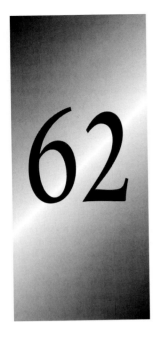

Irvin V. Cantor

INTRODUCTION

According to the Brain Injury Association, each year at least 1.5 million Americans sustain a traumatic brain injury ("TBI"). TBI has been called "the silent epidemic" of our society. Associated with this epidemic is a myriad of legal issues specific to persons who have sustained TBI's and their families. Since it would be far too ambitious a task to analyze all of these legal issues in the space available, this chapter is intended as a basic outline and discussion of some of the pertinent medicolegal aspects of TBI.

SPECTRUM OF MEDICOLEGAL ISSUES OF TBI

There exits a vast array of traumatic brain injuries in our society. The contexts in which TBI's may arise are many, including motor vehicle collisions, recreational accidents, watercraft accidents, workplace accidents, defective products, and medical malpractice. The injury to the brain may be mild, moderate or severe. The mechanism of injury to the brain may involve blunt trauma, acceleration—deceleration of the head, or a metabolic process which may result in hypoxic or ischemic insult to the brain. TBI's may cause physical, cognitive and emotional dysfunction. Unlike most other injuries to the human body, an injury to the brain may not be noticeable to others. All of these factors result in an enormous spectrum of medicolegal issues.

The issues discussed in this chapter are intended to reflect a basic and broad discussion of the medical legal aspects of TBI:

1. Finding the Right Attorney
2. Competency and Capacity Issues
3. Right To Die and Do Not Resuscitate Laws
4. Anatomy of a Worker's Compensation TBI Case
5. Anatomy of a Personal Injury TBI Case
6. Anatomy of a Medical Malpractice ABI Case
7. Independent Medical Examinations
8. Expert Witness Testimony in a TBI Case
9. Lay Witness Testimony in a TBI Case
10. Demonstrative Evidence in a TBI Case
11. Protection and Preservation of the TBI Client's Recovery After Settlement, Verdict, or Award

There are several books which have been written on the subject of the legal aspects of TBI, which provide a detailed discussion of many of the issues addressed in this chapter (1–4).

FINDING THE RIGHT ATTORNEY

Traumatic brain injury litigation is one of the most complex areas of trial law. It requires a working knowledge of the anatomy and function of the human brain combined with an understanding of how best to present evidence to prove or disprove the mechanism, nature and extent of the TBI. In recent years, there has evolved the field of neuro-law, comprised of trial lawyers who have training and experience in traumatic brain injury litigation. It is usually advisable for someone seeking legal help for a TBI to seek out an attorney who has knowledge and experience in handling such cases.

The context of the TBI is a key element in finding the right attorney. The four primary areas of law involving TBI litigation are: (1) Personal injury, where the injury was caused by a motor vehicle or other type of accident; (2) Worker's Compensation, where the injury occurred in a workplace accident; (3) Medical Malpractice, where the injury was due to the negligence of a hospital, physician, or other healthcare provider; and (4) Products Liability, where the injury was due to the use of a defective product. Generally speaking, trial attorneys specialize in one or more of these areas of law. However, just because an attorney regularly handles TBI cases stemming from motor vehicle collisions, for example, does not mean he or she has any experience with worker's compensation or medical malpractice cases. It is almost always advisable for the person seeking legal help to choose an attorney who specializes in the particular area of law in which his or her case arises.

The best way to locate the right attorney is often to seek referrals from healthcare professionals who regularly are involved in TBI litigation or others who are knowledgeable of those attorneys in the community who regularly handle TBI cases. The Brain Injury Association of America (5), the statewide brain injury associations and the local brain injury associations, are also excellent referral sources. The Brain Injury Association of America publishes a book, *National Directory of Brain Injury Rehabilitation Services*, which lists attorneys who regularly handle TBI cases in each state in the United States (6). Likewise, the American Trial Lawyers Association (ATLA) (7) and the statewide and local trial lawyers associations often will provide names of attorneys who regularly handle TBI cases. Martindale-Hubble, a national legal directory which lists attorneys in every locality in the United States, includes information about the attorney and his or her areas of practice, including TBI litigation and neurolaw (8).

Most importantly, the person seeking legal help for his or her TBI case must feel comfortable and confident with the attorney chosen. TBI litigation is often a long, tedious and uncomfortable process, in which a strong relationship between the client and the attorney is invaluable.

COMPETENCE AND CAPACITY ISSUES

Issues involving competency and capacity often arise following traumatic brain injuries. Cognitive dysfunction caused by injuries to the brain may range from mild problems with attention, concentration or memory, at one extreme, to being in a comatose or vegetative condition, in the other extreme. Consequently, it is important to determine the ability of the person who has sustained a TBI to understand and comprehend the consequences of his or her actions.

"Competency" generally refers to someone's ability to perform an act or understand the consequences of an act. "Capacity" is generally a legal term, describing one's adjudicated ability to perform an act or form an intent regarding an act. The adjudication of incompetency by a court determines one's capacity. This adjudication is issue specific, limited to only those acts or actions which the person is unable to do or comprehend. For example, one may be adjudicated incapacitated to handle his or her own financial affairs, but fully capable of making his or her own decisions about medical care. The law is designed to protect incompetent individuals. Minors under the age of 18 are generally deemed incompetent. Adults are presumed to be competent. In the author's home state of Virginia, Virginia Code Section 37.1–134.6 defines "Incapacitated Person" as:

> . . . an adult who has been found by a court to be incapable of receiving and evaluating information effectively or responding to people, events, or environments to such an extent that the individual lacks the capacity to: (i) meet the essential requirements for his health, care, safety or therapeutic needs without the assistance or protection of a guardian or (ii) manage the property or financial affairs or provide for his or her support or for the support of his legal dependents without the assistance or protection of a conservator. A finding that the individual displays poor judgment, alone, shall not be considered sufficient evidence that the individual is an incapacitated person within the meaning of this definition. A finding that the person is incapacitated shall be construed as a finding that the person is "mentally incompetent . . . [for the acts and actions listed in the court's order].

Health care providers often treat TBI patients who are obviously incompetent, but have not yet been adjudicated incapacitated. In these situations, the patient's next of kin are typically vested with the statutory authority to make health care decisions for the patient. This surrogate decision-making by family members is usually the determinative factor when it comes to decisions involving do not resuscitate orders or terminating life support efforts.

Attorneys who are requested to represent the interests of the TBI patient must be sure the patient is competent to manage his or her affairs. If not, the attorney must quickly take steps to have the patient adjudicated incapacitated and have a legal fiduciary appointed. Only the duly appointed fiduciary has the authority to actually engage the attorney to represent the incapacitated person. Additionally, since the fiduciary may serve as the patient's surrogate for medical decisions, the attorney should advise the patient's family of the applicable right to die and related medical decision—making statutes.

One commonly overlooked area of TBI litigation is the competency of the TBI litigant to manage any funds recovered as a result of the litigation. It is not uncommon for the TBI litigant to be fully competent to hire counsel, initiate a lawsuit, and make his or her own medical decisions, yet be incompetent to manage his or her financial affairs. In such situations, the attorney must be careful to have a court order the proper disposition of the funds. Typically, this will result in the court having the funds placed in trust for the TBI litigant.

RIGHT TO DIE AND DO NOT RESUSCITATE LAWS

When someone suffers a catastrophic brain injury, there are tremendous consequences not only to the patient, but also to the family, the healthcare providers, and many others who have a connection to the patient. Hopelessness, futility, and despair are common emotions felt by these persons. In this framework, ethical and moral dilemmas abound.

There is a wide disparity of recovery after severe brain injury, ranging from the person who substantially regains his or her pre-morbid level of functioning to the person who has remained in a vegetative state for a prolonged time. Moreover, predicting outcome after traumatic brain injury can be difficult. Consequently, extreme caution should be employed by those who consider the quality of the patient's life and issues involving the patient's right to die.

One's quality of life is a personal and subjective determination. Obviously, the patient's awareness of his or her environment is a key factor in this determination. In patients in permanent vegetative state, questions arise on both personal and societal levels. Should the patient be kept alive by artificial means or be allowed to die? Does it make sense to continue to provide the enormous costs necessary to keep the patient alive or should our limited societal resources be used for others who have a better medical and functional prognosis? Such questions have also come up in legal challenges involving patients in a minimally conscious state, where there is clearly more ethical debate in the medical community at large regarding issues of medical futility. Non-vegetative patients who demonstrate low level neurobehavioral response, such as those in a minimally conscious state ("MCS"), by definition, have some level of awareness. Such severe disability may seem like a poor quality of life to one person, but quite acceptable to another person given the potential of

death. Consequently, decisions to allow MCS patients to die are extremely emotional, controversial decisions to make.

One significant area of debate in vegetative state cases is whether or not a patient should be made a "DNR" (do not resuscitate), and if so, when. There actually exists a continuum of medical orders which will and/or could result in death to the patient in VS: (1) do not resuscitate orders ("DNR"); (2) withholding medical treatment such as antibiotics or surgery; (3) removal of a feeding tube; (4) removal from a respirator; and (5) withholding or withdrawing other life sustaining care, noting that withdrawing care reaches a greater level of potential moral and ethical compromise than withholding care. The decision to take such actions, first and foremost, belongs to the patient, and if the patient is incapable of making an informed decision, or had no advance directive, then to his surrogate, usually his family. Most states have laws regarding one's right to die based upon the person's living will or advance directive, such that any decision to withhold or withdraw medical treatment is based upon the patient's previously expressed preferences. Most states further provide that the attending physician may withhold or withdraw medical treatment upon compliance with the applicable state law and the proper authorization of the patient's surrogate. In the author's home state of Virginia, Va. Code Section 54.1–2986 enumerates an order of priority of persons who may be such surrogate, beginning with the patient's guardian or committee and then to the patient's next of kin. The Virginia statute dictates that where the patient has not previously expressed a preference regarding withholding or withdrawing medical treatment, the surrogate "shall (i) prior to giving consent, make a good faith effort to ascertain the risks and benefits of and alternatives to the treatment and the religious beliefs and basic values of the patient receiving treatment. . . and (ii) base his decision on the patient's religious beliefs and basic values and any preferences previously expressed by the patient regarding such treatment to the extent they are known, and if unknown or unclear, on the patient's best interests." Va. Code Section 54.1–2986(A). Virginia Code Section 54.1–2987.1, Virginia's Durable Do Not Resuscitate Order statute, provides, among other things, that a physician may issue a durable do not resuscitate order "for his patient with whom he has a bona fide physician/patient relationship as defined in the guidelines of the Board of Medicine, and only with the consent of the patient or, if the patient is a minor or is otherwise incapable of making an informed decision regarding consent for such an order, upon the request of and with the consent of the person authorized to consent on the patient's behalf".

In *Cruzan v. Director, Missouri Department of Health.* 497 U.S. 261, 110 S. Ct. 2841 (1990), the U.S. Supreme Court stated that a person has a constitutionally protected right to refuse lifesaving medical care, including hydration and nutrition. With regard to an incompetent person, such as Nancy Cruzan who was presumptively in a vegetative state (although experts on the two sides debated this), the State of Missouri had a statutory scheme which allowed a surrogate to elect to withdraw hydration and nutrition and thus cause death upon clear and convincing proof that such withdrawal was what the incompetent desired. The Supreme Court upheld the statute as constitutional in a case where the surrogates, Nancy Cruzan's parents, requested withdrawal of hydration and nutrition, but failed to meet the clear and convincing standard embodied in the Missouri statute. In a dissenting opinion, Justice Brennan argued that the incompetent should not have such "improperly biased procedural obstacles" preventing her from dying with dignity. *Id* at 302. He pointed out that "Missouri is virtually the only state to have fashioned a rule that lessens the likelihood of accurate determinations" because of its heightened evidentiary standard. *Id* at 326.

Virginia, like most other states, has a statute which does not contain a heightened evidentiary standard such as Missouri's statute, which was the subject of *Cruzan*. Rather, Virginia's statute simply provides the surrogate shall "make a good faith effort" in analyzing the factors enumerated in the statute. Va. Code Section 54.1–2986(A). The statute further provides that anyone may petition the court to enjoin the withdrawal of medical care "upon finding by a preponderance of the evidence that the action is not lawfully authorized by this article or by other state or federal law." Va. Code Section 54.1–2986(E).

In two 1997 cases, *Washington v. Glucksberg*, 521 U.S. 702, 117 S. Ct. 2258 and *Vacco v. Quill*, 521 U.S. 793, 117 S. Ct. 2293, the U.S. Supreme Court held that state statutes banning assisted suicide are constitutional. In both cases, Chief Justice Rehnquist, citing *Cruzan*, *supra*, emphasized that there was a "distinction between letting a patient die and making that patient die." *Washington*, *supra*, at 715; *Vacco*, *supra*, at 802–803.

Although a constitutionally protected framework exists in most states for the patient's family to elect to withdraw medical care of the incompetent patient, it is still extremely difficult for the family to make such an election. The family members often cannot emotionally accept the futility of the situation even if they intellectually understand it. This may be true even where the family has been previously told by the patient that he or she would want to be allowed to die if in a vegetative condition. The conflict experienced by the family may be immense. There may be disagreement among family members regarding termination of treatment. Many states, such as Virginia, set forth a priority of persons, based upon kinship, who have the authority to make the decision. Nonetheless, as a practical matter, even if the ultimate decision maker wants to terminate treatment,

he or she will often defer to those other family members who do not want to terminate treatment. In one highly publicized case in Virginia, *Gilmore v. Finn*, 259 Va. 448, 527 S.E. 2nd 426 (2000), the Governor of Virginia, James Gilmore, actually filed a petition to enjoin the withdrawal of hydration and nutrition to a patient in a vegetative condition where there was disagreement between the patient's wife and guardian and the patient's parents and sibling regarding whether or not the patient should be allowed to die. Ultimately, the court held that while the Governor had the right to intervene in the case in order to seek an "authoritative construction" of Virginia's right to die statute, the patient's wife and guardian indeed had the authority to direct her husband's physicians to withdraw hydration and nutrition for him since she was the first person in priority as enumerated in Virginia Code Section 54.1–2986. *Id*. at 455, 458.

Perhaps the most highly publicized case has been the Terri Schiavo case. As in *Finn*, there was a controversy between the spouse of a vegetative patient who wanted his wife to die and the parents who did not. Ms. Schiavo collapsed in her home in 1990, suffering from heart failure causing a severe anoxic brain injury, which left Ms. Schiavo in a vegetative state. Ms. Schiavo remained in a vegetative state for 15 years. During this time period, the parties litigated the case in the state and federal court system. After Ms. Schiavo's husband prevailed in the Florida courts, the Florida legislature actually passed legislation, authorizing the Governor to issue a one-time stay of withdrawals of life sustaining measures where the patient did not have a written advance directive and a family member had challenged such withdrawal. Immediately after the legislation was enacted, Governor Jeb Bush issued a stay against the withdrawal of nutrition and hydration for Ms. Sciavo. In September, 2004, the Florida Supreme Court ruled that this legislation was unconstitutional. After this ruling, Ms. Schiavo's parents pursued every available judicial and legislative avenue to avoid having Ms. Schiavo's feeding tube removed. In March, 2005, the U.S. Congress passed a law, signed by President Bush, to allow Ms. Schiavo's parents to seek redress in the federal courts to prevent removal of Ms. Schiavo's feeding tube. Subsequent thereto, the parents filed a petition in federal court to enjoin the removal of the feeding tube, which was denied in the U.S. District Court for the Middle District of Florida, the 11th Circuit Court of Appeals, and the U.S. Supreme Court. With no other forums left to seek an injunction of removal of the feeding tube, Ms. Schiavo's tube was removed, and she died on March 31, 2005. The controversy surrounding the case was covered extensively by the media worldwide. As a result of the Terri Schiavo case, the debate regarding a person's right to die has intensified to a level never previously seen. Only time will tell if the debate results in revisions of the states' right to die laws.

In the context of the dilemmas which arise in such cases, the clinician should be honest and direct in conveying diagnostic and prognostic information to the family. If the physician is not comfortable providing such information, then an adequately qualified professional should be consulted. Likewise, the trial attorney, too, should be forthright in his discussions with the family about the legal directives which are in place. At the same time, both the clinician and trial attorney must be sensitive to the family's emotional needs and dynamics. For a discussion of the medical and ethical issues facing a clinician in severe traumatic brain injury cases, see "Medicolegal Aspects of Severe Traumatic Brain Injury", co-authored by Dr. Nathan Zasler and Irvin V. Cantor (10).

ANATOMY OF A WORKER'S COMPENSATION TBI CASE

Worker's compensation is a statutorily created program which exists in each state to compensate workers who get injured in the workplace. Unlike the general tort system, where liability is generally determined by fault, worker's compensation is not a fault-based program, but rather compensates the injured worker so long as the injury arose out of the job while the worker was in the scope of his employment. If an injury is deemed compensable, then the worker is usually entitled to indemnity benefits for his lost wages and medical benefits for any medical expenses incurred as a result of the injury.

Many TBI's arise as a result of workplace accidents. Most of the worker's compensation litigation involving TBI's deals with either: (1) causation, whether or not the injury to the brain was caused by the workplace accident, or (2) the extent of damages, what sequelae are attributable to the TBI. Some states provide for lifetime benefits for workers who suffer TBI's. The central issue in lifetime benefit litigation is whether or not the worker is permanently unable to work as a result of the TBI. For example, Virginia Code Section 65.2–503(C)(3) provides for lifetime awards "when there is injury to the brain which is so severe as to render the employee permanently unemployable in gainful employment."

The worker's compensation case is generally initiated by the filing of a claim by the employee or employer. If the case is not contested, then generally the employer's worker's compensation carrier will voluntarily provide benefits to the worker. In most states, the worker's compensation carrier has the right to designate the treating physician for the injured worker. If the case is contested, then generally the claimant and the employer will be represented by counsel, who will litigate the case in the worker's compensation system.

The worker's compensation system is typically administered outside of the state's general court system, usually by a Worker's Compensation Commission. Worker's compensation cases are generally heard by an administrative judge or deputy commissioner, and not by juries. Pre-trial discovery is typically allowed in worker's compensation cases, including subpoenas of documents, interrogatories, and depositions. Attendance at the hearing of the case may be compelled by subpoena. Most states provide that the expert witness fees for the professionals who testify in worker's compensation cases must be approved by the Worker's Compensation Commission.

The percentage of TBI worker's compensation cases that are contested is much higher than other types of injuries. This is due primarily to the fact that disagreements between the parties in TBI cases often arise over causation, extent of damages, and whether or not the claimant is permanently unemployable. Consequently, TBI healthcare providers often are called to testify in worker's compensation cases. It is usually a wise idea for the healthcare provider who is asked to testify in a worker's compensation case to clarify at the outset with the attorney requesting his or her testimony what the rules are regarding the format of the testimony and the payment of the fees for testifying.

ANATOMY OF A PERSONAL INJURY TBI CASE

TBI's resulting from motor vehicle collisions, recreational accidents, use of defective products, trips and falls at dangerous premises, and many other sources are the subject of personal injury cases. These cases are litigated in the traditional court system and usually by a jury.

TBI personal injury cases are becoming increasingly prevalent as society and the legal community is being made more aware of the silent epidemic of traumatic brain injuries. The vast majority of TBI litigation in the United States involves mild TBI's. The most contested issues in TBI personal injury cases are the same as in worker's compensation cases, namely causation and extent of damages.

The TBI personal injury case is initiated by the plaintiff filing a lawsuit, usually called a Complaint. The defendant responds to the lawsuit, usually with an Answer. The parties then engage in pre-trial discovery of the lawsuit. Discovery typically consists of interrogatories between the parties, subpoenaed documents from the parties and others, including the treating healthcare providers of the plaintiff, depositions of the parties and others, including the treating healthcare providers of the plaintiff, and independent medical examinations of the plaintiff by healthcare providers selected by the defendant or the court. Discovery is usually a lengthy process, often taking many months and sometimes years.

Discovery in TBI cases is usually more extensive than in other types of injury cases. The defense often wants to know everything it can about the plaintiff's pre-morbid condition, in order to determine if the plaintiff's problems can be attributed to conditions or events that existed before the incident in question. Additionally, it is not at all uncommon for the defense to request multiple independent medical examinations of the plaintiff, including examinations by a physician and neuropsychologist.

After discovery is completed, the case is scheduled for trial. Trial of a personal injury case typically consists of the following segments: (1) voir dire, where the prospective jurors are questioned by the court and counsel; (2) selection of the jury by counsel; (3) opening statements by counsel; (4) presentation of the plaintiff's case, the plaintiff proceeding first since the plaintiff has the burden of proof; (5) presentation of the defendant's case; (6) presentation of rebuttal evidence by the plaintiff regarding new matters raised by the defendant's case; (7) instructions of the jury by the court; (8) closing argument by counsel; and (9) deliberation by the jury. Trial of a TBI case usually takes longer than trials of other types of injury cases. This is due, in large part, to the fact that the court and the jury must be educated about traumatic brain injury, often resulting in counsel spending more time in talking to the jury, calling more lay and expert witnesses to the stand, and presenting more demonstrative evidence.

ANATOMY OF A MEDICAL MALPRACTICE ABI CASE

Medical malpractice cases involve claims of negligence in providing medical care, brought by a patient or patient's representative against a health care provider. Most states have statutes which define "health care provider" and set forth procedures for bringing and litigating medical negligence claims. Like personal injury cases, medical malpractice cases are generally litigated in the traditional court system and usually decided by a jury.

The plaintiff must prove three basic elements to prevail in a medical malpractice case: (1) the health care provider deviated from the standard of care in his medical treatment; (2) the deviation of the standard of care caused the injury suffered by the plaintiff; and (3) the plaintiff suffered damages as a result of the injury caused by the deviation of the standard of care. Standard of care is generally "that degree of skill and diligence practiced by a reasonably prudent practitioner in the field of practice or specialty" of the defendant. (Va. Code Section 8.01–580.20, which definition is typical of most state statutes in the United States.) In order to prove a breach of the standard of care, it is almost always necessary for the plaintiff to present one or more expert witnesses to testify at trial that the defendant's actions constituted such a breach. It is also usually necessary for the plaintiff to present one or more expert witnesses to testify on the subject of causation and damages. As a practical matter: (1) it is often quite difficult for plaintiffs to locate good, qualified expert witnesses to give the testimony required to prevail and (2) physicians, nurses, and other health care providers are often well liked and respected in their community and by the juries in their community. Consequently, over 70% of all medical malpractice cases taken to trial in the U.S. result in defense verdicts.

Many states have statutes which provide for certain screening procedures and caps on damages applicable only to medical malpractice cases. Among these statutes are: (1) requirements that a plaintiff have a qualified expert witness provide an opinion that the medical care provided deviated from the standard of care as a condition precedent to filing a lawsuit; (2) requirements that the case be reviewed by a medical malpractice review panel before the case can proceed to trial; (3) requirements that certain allegations of medical negligence (such as birth related injury claims) be brought as administrative proceedings outside of the traditional tort system; and (4) caps on damages, wherein the plaintiff may not recover more than a certain maximum recovery, determined legislatively.

Brain injuries are the subject of many medical malpractice cases. Birth injury cases resulting in either anoxic/hypoxic/ischemic or structural injury to the brain are probably the most prevalent type of acquired brain injury ("ABI") medical malpractice case. Cases involving hypoxic-isclemic brain injuries ("HIBI") caused by alleged negligence in surgery, anesthesia, or other circumstances of intubation or extubation are perhaps the second most prevalent type of ABI medical malpractice case. Other types of ABI medical malpractice cases brought with some frequency include allegations of negligent surgery resulting in structural injury to the brain and failure to diagnose malignant brain tumors and meningeomas.

As a general rule, medical malpractice cases involve a much higher percentage of severe brain injuries than personal injury cases. This is due primarily to the fact that so many of these cases involve anoxic, hypoxic or ischemic injuries resulting in profound sequelae for the patient.

The discovery and trial of a medical malpractice case are generally the same as that for personal injury cases, as set forth in the previous section. ABI medical malpractice trials are usually quite complicated for the jury, for not only does the jury need to understand the medical procedures in question, but also the mechanism of the brain injury. The voir dire questioning of jurors in ABI medical malpractice cases often takes a longer period of time than in other types of negligence cases. There are usually more expert witnesses called to trial in ABI medical malpractice cases than in other types of cases. Also, counsel in ABI medical malpractice cases frequently use demonstrative illustrations, models, and charts to aid the jury on understanding the issues in the case.

INDEPENDENT MEDICAL EXAMINATIONS

The rules of civil procedure in federal court and in almost all state courts provide that a party in a lawsuit involving the physical or mental condition of a person may request an examination of the person by a physician or health care provider of the party's choosing. Federal Rules of Civil Procedure, Rule 35 (11), which serves as the model for many states' procedures, provides as follows:

(a) Order For Examination

When the mental or physical condition (including the blood group) of a party or of a person in the custody or under the legal control of a party, is in controversy, the court in which the action is pending may order the party to submit to a physical or mental examination by a suitably licensed or certified examiner or to produce for examination the person in the party's custody or legal control. The order may be made only on motion for good cause shown and upon notice to the person to be examined and to all parties and shall specify the time, place, manner, conditions, and scope of the examination and the person or persons by whom it is to be made.

(b) Report of Examiner

If requested by the party against whom an order is made under Rule 35(a) or the person examined, the party causing the examination to be made shall deliver to the requesting party a copy of the detailed written report of the examiner setting out the examiner's findings, including results of all tests made, diagnoses and conclusions, together with like reports of all earlier examinations of the same condition. . . .

These examinations are commonly referred to as "independent medical examinations" ("IME's"). The physician or other health care provider who performs such an examination does not have a traditional physician-patient relationship with the examinee. On the contrary, the examiner's role is to serve as an independent resource to provide an unbiased forensic opinion regarding the mental or physical condition of the examinee. The AMA ethics guidelines (12) define the IME physician—patient relationship as follows:

. . . .IME's are responsible for administering an objective medical evaluation but not for monitoring patients' health over time, treating patients, or fulfilling many other duties traditionally held by physicians. Consequently, a limited patient—physician relationship should be considered to exist. IME's still are expected to evaluate objectively patients' health or disability, maintain confidentiality, and disclose potential or perceived conflicts of interest. In addition, upon discovering important health information or abnormalities during the course of the examination, IME's are expected to inform the patient about the condition, ensure that they understand fully the diagnosis, and suggest that they seek care from a qualified physician.

Ideally, even though the examiner is chosen and paid by the party requesting the examination, he or she should resist the temptation to try to please the party who engaged his or her services. The written report prepared by the examiner should be thorough and complete, listing all of the written materials reviewed by the examiner, the results of all of the examinations and/or testing conducted by the examiner, the opinions of the examiner, and the basis for each such opinion.

IME examiners should realize that once they undertake an IME, they will in all likelihood have to give a deposition, usually requested by the examinee's attorney, and if the case does not settle, testify at trial. Sometimes in lieu of testifying at trial, the deposition of the IME examiner, usually taken by audio-visual means, may be used. The deposition which is used as evidence at trial is often referred to as a "de bene esse" deposition. If there is a reason the IME examiner is unable or unwilling to attend trial, he or she should make that known at the outset to the attorney requesting the IME.

In TBI cases especially involving mild TBI's, there is often disagreement between the parties about: (1) whether or not the plaintiff suffered a TBI; (2) the extent of the TBI and the true sequelae resulting from it; and (3) the cause of the deficits and problems suffered by the plaintiff. Consequently, IME's are routinely requested in mild TBI cases. In fact, it is not at all uncommon for the defense in TBI cases to request multiple IME's, including an examination by a physician specializing in neurorehabilitation and a full battery of testing by a neuropsychologist.

A frequently litigated issue in mild TBI cases is what role does the plaintiff's pre-morbid history play versus the traumatic event, such as a motor vehicle collision, as a causative factor in the plaintiff's post-accident functioning. When faced with this issue, the IME examiner should request and review all available pre-morbid records of the plaintiff, including medical, educational and vocational records, and be sure to list in the IME report all of the documents so reviewed. It is wise for the IME examiner to pay close attention to documents dealing with the level of functioning of the plaintiff to determine if there is a discernible difference between the pre-morbid and post-accident performance. In the event the IME examiner is of the opinion that the deficits suffered by the plaintiff are multifactorial in nature, then he or she should set out in detail in the IME report each of those factors and how they have impacted the plaintiff.

In TBI cases there seems to be an unusually high number of experts who are overly dependent financially on medico-legal cases in their practice. These "professional" expert witnesses sometimes derive a very large percentage of their income from certain attorneys or sides in the litigation who hire them. Unfortunately, there are some experts who routinely find in favor of the party that hires them. It is strongly recommended that those experts who make themselves available for IME's do not compromise their impartiality and objectivity. For a discussion regarding the ethical considerations in IME's following TBI, there are several in-depth articles, co-written by Nathan Zasler, M.D. and Michael Martelli, Ph.D. (13–16).

EXPERT WITNESS TESTIMONY IN A TBI CASE

As a general rule, only expert witnesses, qualified as such by the court, are permitted to give opinion testimony at trial. Rule 702, Federal Rules of Evidence (17), upon which many state statutes are based, reads as follows:

> *Rule 702. Testimony by Experts*
> If scientific, technical, or other specialized knowledge will assist the trier of fact to understand the evidence or to determine a fact in issue, a witness qualified as an expert by knowledge, skill, experience, training, or education may testify thereto in the form of an opinion or otherwise, if (1) the testimony is based upon sufficient facts or data, (2) the testimony is the product of reliable principles and methods, and (3) the witness has applied the principles and methods reliably to the facts of the case.

It is not necessary that a person be a practitioner of a science or technical profession in order to qualify as an expert. Rather, the person must have sufficient expertise in his or her field that the expert's opinion will be of benefit to the trier of fact. The court has discretion to qualify the person as an expert in a particular field so long as the person is shown to possess sufficient expertise in the professional field.

An expert's opinion testimony must be based upon reliable facts and assumptions. Testimony which is speculative, based upon faulty assumptions, or is otherwise determined to be "junk science" is inadmissible. In *Daubert v. Merrell Dow Pharmaceuticals, Inc.*, 509 U.S. 579 (1993), the Supreme Court of the United States, applying Rule 702 of the Federal Rules of Evidence, set forth the following factors for the trial judge, as the "gatekeeper" for the admissibility of such evidence, to determine if the expert's testimony possessed requisite scientific validity:

1. The theories and techniques employed by the scientific expert have been tested;
2. The theories and techniques have been subjected to peer review and publication;
3. The techniques employed by the expert have a known error rate;
4. The techniques employed by the expert are subject to standards governing their application; and
5. The theories and techniques employed by the expert enjoy widespread acceptance.

Using this test, the Supreme Court remanded a birth injury case back to the trial court so that the trial judge could decide if the proferred expert testimony, regarding whether or not the mother's prenatal ingestion of the drug, Bendectin, was shown to cause birth defects, was admissible. Prior to the five-prong test of *Daubert*, the rule was that expert opinion based upon a scientific technique was inadmissible unless the technique is generally accepted as reliable in the relevant scientific community. *Frye v. United States*, 54 App. DC 46, 293F. 1013 (1923). Since 1993, the *Daubert* test has been used by a multitude of trial judges to determine the admissibility of scientific expert testimony. This litigation has resulted in a complicated, often contradictory set of results. A useful website dedicated to the rule espoused in *Daubert* and links to post-*Daubert* cases, articles, tactics and other materials regarding determination of the scientific validity of expert testimony is "Daubert On The Web", www.daubertontheweb.com (18).

TBI cases, perhaps more than any other type of injury case, typically involve multiple expert witnesses. This is due primarily to the fact that the court and the jury are generally unfamiliar with brain anatomy and function. A sampling of expert witnesses often involved in TBI cases includes neurologists, neurosurgeons, physiatrists, neuropsychiatrists, neuropsychologists, neuroradiologists, nuclear medicine specialists, speech language therapists, physical therapists, occupational therapists, vocational specialists, life care planners, accident reconstructionists, forensic engineers, and economists.

TBI physicians, as a general rule, have little trouble qualifying as expert witnesses and giving opinion testimony at trial. For example, since it is well established in the medical literature that complete loss of consciousness is not a prerequisite for a diagnosis of TBI, opinion testimony from a TBI physician to that effect is uniformly permitted. However, when the physician bases his or her opinions on assumptions that are controversial and speculative, then such specific opinions may not be allowed. One area of much litigation is the reliance by the physician on abnormal functional imaging studies of the brain to diagnose TBI, discussed in more detail herein on pages 30–31.

Non-physician experts in TBI cases are much more likely to have their testimony excluded as unreliable. Some of the experts in TBI cases whose opinions have been disallowed include accident reconstructionists, who try to determine the speed of crash vehicles by crush analysis, and forensic engineers, who try to determine the amount of force exerted on an occupant of a vehicle in a collision. In most states, neuropsychologists are permitted to give their opinion as to whether or not a person suffered a TBI. However, a recent Virginia case, *John v. Im*, 263 Va. 315, 559 S.E. 2d 694 (2002), held that since the neuropsychologist was not a medical doctor, he was "not qualified to state an expert medical opinion" regarding the cause of the patient's brain injury.

Expert witnesses generally bill hourly for the time they spend on medico-legal matters. The party who has hired the expert generally pays the expert's fees. The opposing party is required to pay the expert for the fees incurred in responding to pre-trial discovery, whether by deposition or interrogatories. Rule 35(b) (4)(c)(i), Federal Rules of Procedure, states that:

> (i) the court shall require that the party seeking discovery pay the expert a reasonable fee for time spent in responding to discovery. . . .

A "reasonable fee" generally includes the customary hourly fee the expert charges for medico-legal work. It is strongly suggested that the expert keep detailed, accurate records of his or her time in a case. This is especially true in TBI cases where the expert may have voluminous records to review and longer than usual depositions to give.

Some practical tips for expert witnesses are:

1. Always maintain your impartiality and objectivity.
2. At the outset of a case, clearly communicate with the attorney who has engaged your services about the scope of your role, your availability for litigation, and the financial terms of your engagement.
3. Carefully and thoroughly record your examination results, observations, or other notes in a legible, preferably typewritten, manner.
4. Review all pertinent records and data.
5. Accurately keep and record the time you spend on the case.
6. Always remain courteous and professional with all litigants and their attorneys.
7. Thoroughly review all relevant records and data prior to any deposition or trial.
8. Understand the disparate roles of the participants: your role as the expert is to provide objective scientific or technical opinions, whereas the role of the attorneys and the litigants is to win.

LAY WITNESS TESTIMONY IN A TBI CASE

While much time and attention is given to the testimony of expert witnesses in TBI litigation, the most important evidence usually is the testimony of the plaintiff and those persons who best know the plaintiff. Invariably, if you ask trial attorneys who regularly handle TBI cases what is the most critical element in a TBI case, they will tell you it is the quality of the plaintiff and his or her lay witnesses. The reason for this seems obvious: the jury, whose job it is to decide if, and how, the plaintiff is affected by the TBI, is most influenced by: (1) how the plaintiff presents at trial

and (2) what those who best know the plaintiff say about how the plaintiff has been affected by the TBI.

Despite this seemingly obvious focus, health care providers and attorneys often fail to consider the reports of those closest to the person who sustained a TBI. This emphasis on opinions by experts, to the exclusion of reports by lay witnesses, not only fails to provide a comprehensive view of the case, but typically results in an unsatisfactory outcome at trial.

Individuals who sustain TBI's usually do not have good insight about their deficits. This phenomenon is probably due to the nature of the injury, itself, (e.g. frontal lobe dysfunction) or to the fact that the patient is in denial over his or her condition or to a combination of these factors. The most accurate description of the TBI patient typically comes from a spouse, a sibling, a child, a best friend or someone else who best knows the patient.

In diagnosing a TBI and the resulting deficits suffered by the patient, the physician, neuropsychologist, or other health care provider should make an effort to learn the reports of family, friends, co-workers, and others close to the patient about the ways the TBI has affected the patient. It is helpful if the health care provider talks to those who know and regularly interact with the patient. It is also wise for the health care provider to obtain school records, job evaluation reports, or other documents which memorialize the observations of others about the TBI patient. Without consideration of the reports and observations by others of the TBI patient, it is very difficult for the health care providers to accurately determine the pre-morbid and post-traumatic conditions of the patient. Moreover, if the health care provider has not considered the reports of lay witnesses prior to reaching his or her opinions, then the health care provider will be quite vulnerable to attack in cross-examination at deposition or trial.

The trial attorney should make sure to discover and develop lay witness testimony about the TBI patient. Without such testimony, the jury will be left with many unanswered questions and will not be motivated to render a verdict in favor of the party who disregarded such testimony.

Sometimes the inquiry regarding lay witness observations of the TBI patient will result in the discovery that the patient had complained of similar deficits many times before the traumatic event. Other times, the inquiry will result in the discovery that the patient's life has been completely altered as a result of the TBI. In all cases, proper analysis of the TBI case can only be achieved if due consideration is given to the reports by those who best know the TBI patient-plaintiff.

DEMONSTRATIVE EVIDENCE IN A TBI CASE

Individuals who suffer TBI's frequently appear perfectly fine. They often do not have any disfigurement, no scars, no limp, and no visible sign of impairment. It is no wonder TBI victims are referred to as "the walking wounded." Consequently, in the trial of TBI cases, there is much use of visual aids to assist the jury to understand the TBI and its sequelae. This type of evidence is commonly referred to as "demonstrative evidence" because it is used to demonstrate and clarify testimony. There is perhaps no other type of injury case which necessitates the use of demonstrative evidence more than the trial of a TBI.

Since the TBI was caused by a traumatic event, evidence to explain how the forces of the accident were exerted on the plaintiff's head and brain are often used. In motor vehicle collisions, photographs of the vehicle are almost always introduced into evidence. Such photographs may include not only the body damage to the vehicles, but also a bent steering wheel, a broken headrest or seat, or a shattered windshield. In many cases, photographs of the interior and exterior of a windshield, which has a spider web pattern as a result of contact with the plaintiff's head, are introduced into evidence.

A simple but powerful way to demonstrate an acceleration/deceleration injury to the brain is for the physician to use a model of the skull and brain in his or her testimony. While using the model, the physician can explain that the skull is a rigid structure, but the brain has the consistency of jelled gelatin, and that rapid changes in direction of movement of the skull and brain can cause stretching and shearing of tissue and fibers to the brain. There are some interesting short animated films available to depict this process. Two such films are: (1) "Closed Head Injury", produced by Technical Medical Animation Corporation, Denver, Colorado (19) and (2) "Understanding Mild Traumatic Brain Injury", produced by Body Mind Publications, Olympia, Washington (20). Another excellent source for video animations of types of TBI, brain functioning and mechanics of TBI is the Traumatic Brain Injury Resources Guide website, www.neuroskills.com (21).

Structural imaging tests of the brain, x-rays, CT Scans, and MRI's, are routinely used in TBI trials, especially where the plaintiff has suffered a skull fracture, an intracranial or extracranial bleed, or other discernible brain lesion. Sometimes it is helpful to construct 3-D models from the CT and MRI computer tapes since these 3-D models can show shape, form and color for the jury.

Functional imaging studies, testing brain activity, are also used quite often in TBI cases. This is due in large part to the fact that structural imaging studies of persons sustaining mild TBI's generally are negative. The most often used studies are PET Scans (Positron Emission Tomography), SPECT Scans (Single Photon Emission Computerized Tomography), EEG (Electroencephalography) and QEEG studies (Quantitative Electroencephalography).

Abnormalities in brain function are not diagnostic of brain injury in and of themselves. Many clinical conditions can produce abnormalities on PET and SPECT. Consequently, caution must be exercised when using abnormal functional imaging studies in TBI litigation. The use of such tests at trial depends upon several factors: (1) the type of equipment used in the test procedures; (2) the credentials, expertise and experience of the technician conducting the test procedures; (3) the credentials, expertise and experience of the clinician interpreting the test results; and (4) the manner in which the test results are used in the clinician's analysis. The admissibility of functional imaging tests of the brain have been the subject of much litigation throughout the country, where the focus of the courts has been on whether or not the test results are "reliable scientific evidence". The overwhelming majority of these cases hold that the results of functional imaging tests are admissible at trial for a qualified expert to use as a factor (as opposed to "the sole factor") in arriving at his or her opinion about the TBI. Consequently, when an expert intends to use a functional imaging test in his or her testimony, it is strongly recommended that the expert make it clear that the results of the functional imaging test are being used as a confirmatory factor in his or her opinion about the TBI and the resulting brain function. When a PET or SPECT Scan is used at trial, as with CT's and MRI's, it is often helpful to have 3-D models made from the computer tape of the PET or SPECT.

Most TBI trials include testimony from neuropsychologists who have performed neuropsychological evaluations of the plaintiff. Often the plaintiff has undergone multiple neuropsychological evaluations prior to trial. Many times these serial evaluations will result in clear patterns of test performance. When a clear pattern is demonstrated, sometimes graphs and charts depicting test performance are used to help the jury understand the person's deficits or lack thereof. Such visual aides of neuropsychological test results should be used only when such results are significant, correlate with the clinical examinations of the person, and are otherwise not subject to attack on cross-examination.

There are a myriad of other types of demonstrative evidence commonly used in TBI cases. Some of these are: (1) illustrations of the brain and its network of neurons; (2) "day in the life" videos of the plaintiff, depicting some of the problems the plaintiff experiences on a daily basis; (3) surveillance videos, surreptitiously taken by the defense, to show the plaintiff actually engages in activities inconsistent with his or her claimed deficits; and (4) blow-ups of academic records and job evaluations.

A knowledge of the use of demonstrative evidence in TBI cases is helpful for the clinician or expert witness involved in a TBI case to interact with counsel or the injured plaintiff.

PROTECTION AND PRESERVATION OF THE TBI CLIENT'S RECOVERY AFTER SETTLEMENT, VERDICT OR AWARD

The TBI case is not over just because the plaintiff has achieved a settlement or verdict. Rather, attention must be given to how the monetary proceeds achieved in litigation should be received and structured. Failure to properly structure these funds is a trap for the unwary and may result in the loss of benefits otherwise available to the injured person.

Individuals who sustain a TBI are often eligible for Social Security, Medicare, and Medicaid benefits. Social Security and Medicare benefits are generally available to the person (or his relative) who has made the requisite payments of FICA taxes to the federal government. These benefits provide monthly income and medical coverage. If the person does not qualify for Medicare, he or she still may be eligible for Supplemental Security Income (SSI) and Medicaid benefits. SSI provides monthly income benefits and Medicaid provides medical benefits. SSI and Medicaid are "needs based" programs, insofar as the individual must meet an asset-based test in order to qualify. In addition to monthly income and medical benefits, SSI and Medicaid recipients are also eligible for long-term care and various rehabilitation programs. For the TBI victim facing substantial long-term care expenses, SSI and Medicaid benefits are a vital resource.

The creation of a properly drafted trust to hold the funds recovered by the plaintiff in a TBI case can serve to protect the plaintiff's eligibility for needs based programs. Assets held in these trusts, often referred to as "Special Needs Trusts" or "Settlement Trusts", are not considered available to the beneficiary because title to the assets does not vest in the beneficiary until and unless the trust is terminated. The beneficiary of such a trust, having retained his or her eligibility for needs based benefits, continues to receive SSI and Medicaid benefits, and uses the funds held in trust to pay for needs not covered by SSI and Medicaid, hence the name "Special Needs Trust."

Special Needs/Settlement Trusts not only preserve the beneficiary's eligibility for needs based benefits, but typically also provide for professional investment management of the trust funds, a function many TBI victims are unable to properly perform. The trust must be created by a court. The court's jurisdiction is based upon the incapacity of the beneficiary to reasonably understand and/or manage the proper disbursement of the TBI case proceeds.

The constantly evolving laws regarding trusts and federal and state benefits are quite complex. Consequently, it is generally wise for a competent trust attorney to draft the Special Needs/Settlement Trust. A complete understanding and working knowledge of these laws is usually not within the province of the plaintiff's trial attorney.

The proper use of a Special Needs/Settlement Trust can maximize the funds and benefits available to the TBI victim. This can often result in a dramatic enhancement of the life of the person who has sustained a TBI.

CONCLUSION

The epidemic of TBI in our society has spawned an ever-increasing myriad of legal issues. These issues are vast and complex. Hopefully, this chapter has shed some light on some of the pertinent medico-legal aspects of TBI.

References

1. Roberts, A.C., M.D. (ed.), *Head Trauma Cases: Law and Medicine*, 2nd Edition, Wiley Law Publications, New York, N.Y., 1991.
2. Roberts, A.C., M.D. (ed.), *Litigating Head Trauma Cases*, Wiley Law Publications, New York, N.Y., 1994.
3. Simkins, Charles N. (ed.), *Analysis, Understanding and Presentation of Cases Involving Traumatic Brain Injury*, National Head Injury Foundation, Washington, D.C., 1994.
4. Taylor, J.S. (ed.), *Neurolaw: Brain and Spinal Cord Injuries*, West Publishing, Eagan, Minnesota, 1997.
5. *Brain Injury Association of America* (BIA), 8201 Greensboro Drive, Suite 611, McLean, VA 22102, 800-444-6443, www.biausa.org.
6. Brain Injury Association of America, *National Directory of Brain Injury Rehabilitation Services*, 2003-2004 Edition.
7. *American Trial Lawyers Association* (ATLA), 1050 31st Street, N.W., Washington, D.C., 20007, 800-424-2725, www.atla.org.
8. *Martindale-Hubble Legal Directory*, 121 Chanlon Road, New Providence, N.J. 07974 (U.S. residents), 800-526-4902 (U.S. residents); Holden House, 57 Rathbone Place, London W1 T 1JU (Outside U.S.), +44 20 7868 4885 (Outside U.S.), www.martindale.com.
9. "Terri Schindler-Schiavo Foundation", 4615 Gulf Boulevard, #104, St. Petersburg Beach, Florida 33706, www.terrisfight.org.
10. "Medicolegal Aspects of Severe Traumatic Brain Injury", Nathan D. Zasler, M.D. and Irvin V. Cantor, *The Journal of the Virginia Trial Lawyers Association*, Winter, 2004.
11. *Federal Rules of Civil Procedure*—may be accessed on the web by going to Legal Information Institute, www.law.cornell.edu/rules/frcp.
12. "Patient -Physician Relationship in the context of work related and Independent Medical Examinations", *American Medical Association, Reports of the Council on Ethical and Judicial Affairs*, 1998.
13. Martelli, Bush and Zasler, "Identifying, Avoiding and Addressing Ethical Misconduct In Neuropsychological Medicolegal Practice", *International Journal of Forensic Psychology*, 2003.
14. Martelli, Zasler and Johnson-Greene, "Promoting Ethical and Objective Practice in the Medicolegal Arena of Disability Evaluation", *Physical Medicine and Rehabilitation Clinics of North America*, Volume 12, No. 3, 2001.
15. Martelli, Zasler and Grayson, "Ethics and Medicolegal Evaluation of Impairment After Brain Injury", *Attorney's Guide To Ethics In Forensic Science and Medicine*, Schiffman, M. (ed.), Springfield, Illinois, 2000.
16. Martelli, Zasler and Grayson, "Ethical Consideration In Impairment and Disability Evaluations Following Injury", *Guide To Functional Capacity Evaluation with Impairment Rating Applications*, May and Martelli (eds.), NADEP Publications, Richmond, Virginia, 1999.
17. *Federal Rules of Evidence*—may be accessed on the web by going to Legal Information Institute, www. law.cornell.edu/rules/fre.
18. "Daubert On The Web", www.daubertontheweb.com, is a website dedicated to the rule espoused in *Daubert v. Merrell Dow Pharmaceuticals, Inc.*, 509 US 579 (1993), and links to cases, articles, tactics and other material regarding determination of the scientific validity of expert testimony.

19. *"Closed Head Injury"*, Technical Medical Animation Corporation (TMAC), 3100 Umatilla Street, Denver, Colorado 80211, 800-618-2740.

20. *"Understanding Mild Traumatic Brain Injury"*, Body Mind Publications, 7631 Forest Park Drive, N.W., Olympia, Washington 98502, 800-295-3346.

21. *Traumatic Brain Injury Resources Guide*, www.neuroskills.com, offers a website where you can click on "Multi-Media Center" and purchase digital animations of types of TBI, brain functioning, and mechanics of TBI or download video snippets of such videos.

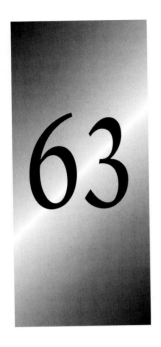

63 Ethical Issues in Clinicolegal Practice

Arthur Ameis
Nathan D. Zasler
Michael F. Martelli
Shane S. Bush

INTRODUCTION

The general requirement for ensuring ethical conduct in any form of clinicolegal evaluation is rendered even more imperative when confronted by the complex, often subtle range of effects and severities of impairments of the traumatized brain. The clinicolegal evaluator must be especially cognizant of rules and guidelines for assigning causation for singular etiologies, or relative attribution for multifactorial circumstances; of the pathomechanics of various traumatic scenarios; of the differential diagnosis of psychological versus neurological disorders; and of the interplay of emotional states and needs with psychological functions and cognition.

Pronouncements on the severity or even existence of any impairment must be rigorously supported by objective evidence and strictly limited to reasonable inference.

If *'the past is often prologue'* then it becomes critically important to establish an accurate, complete prior history of all injuries or illnesses capable of affecting the brain. It is equally critical to clarify all potentially relevant comorbidities, especially social/situational distress, sleep deficit, pain, OTC and prescription medication 'side'effects, and surreptitious substance use/abuse.

The evaluator must be fully aware of active controversies concerning the therapeutic efficacy of various interventions, for both minor and severe brain injury: while long, expensive programs of care can lead in some cases to profound improvements in insight, impairment control and quality of life, in other cases the result may be financially profligate, devoid of discernible benefit, or even tainted by serious iatrogenic harm.

Setting the bar high, creating specific, rigorous criteria for ethical and competent evaluation and testimony, with suitable tests and benchmarks, appears to be the trend in the courts (1), wherein clinicolegal expertise is most needed. It behooves each clinician to know where the risks lie, and to avoid falling into practice patterns of substandard work, or permitting exposure to real or even apparent ethical misconduct. A key risk area concerns lack of familiarity with relevant, and especially with recent important developments including: court rulings; new diagnostic procedures and measures of functional capacity; improved validity and reliability data for currently used clinical tests and outcome measures; and changes in relevant ethics codes (e.g. the 1999 AMA Ethics Guidelines on Physician/Patient Relationships in the Context of Independent Medical Evaluation, and the 2003 NAN position paper on independent and court-order forensic neuropsychological examinations (2–4).

Similarly, it is appropriate to expect health care professionals to take a proactive role in individual professional as well as general quality assurance. When lack of competence, apparent or actual ethical misconduct is observed in one's colleagues, the evaluator is obligated to take appropriate steps to defend the consumers of our services and thereby safeguard the public's trust in the healing professions in general and in independent expert evaluation in particular.

Ongoing education is required at all levels, from student to practitioner to academic, on the application of ethical principles to clinicolegal practice, in order to create and sustain ethical professional behavior in ourselves and in our colleagues; and as a legacy for the generation of evaluators who will surely follow us.

SPECIAL ETHICAL CHALLENGES OF THE ADVERSARIAL ENVIRONMENT

The Practice Paradigm Shift

The adversarial clinicolegal environment contrasts sharply with that in which health caregivers train and work. Within the health care environment the emphasis is on selfless aspects of professionalism including personal sacrifice, devotion to duty and to public health; with the primacy of the fiduciary 'duty of care' reflected in patient advocacy. These principles shape the attitude of each healthcare professional when assessing and treating in his/her clinical practice.

However, the clinicolegal environment is typically dominated by adversarial polarization. The person, already having (inadvertently) assumed a *sick role* by being rendered a *patient* through loss of health secondary to injury or illness, acquires (by having taken legal action) some of the typical characteristics of certain sociolegalistic identities or roles: with labels such as *Client, Litigant, Victim, Claimant, Disabled Person* and/or *Evaluee*.

Advocacy, by parties supporting or opposing the litigation, tends to be a common basis of request for services, including professional evaluation, caregiving reports, and court testimony. Infrequently, the request may be 'neutral', an invitation for a substantive review expressly for the objective education of the triers of fact. Thus, for many clinicians, upon accepting a request for expert examination of a litigant, the transition from the classroom or treatment clinic to the evaluation setting or courtroom will require a substantial and abrupt perceptual paradigm shift from fiduciary duty to forensic functions; and a corresponding, often ill-informed struggle with novel, sometimes subtle ethical, moral, and legal issues.

As with any anticipated paradigm shift, preventative measures are preferable to remedial actions. Effective professional education can create a heightened appreciation of and corresponding sensitivity to the pitfalls that may be created when conflicting interests encroach upon the clinician who is suddenly challenged to apply general guidelines of routine practice ethics in unfamiliar clinicolegal circumstances.

Unfortunately, many, if not most, clinicians who evaluate and/or treat persons with traumatic brain injury,

as well as those serving on panels that establish policy involving training and certification of professional competency, would acknowledge having had insufficient education/training in the prevalence and nature of special ethic challenges and ethical guidelines specific to the clinicolegal setting.

Prevalence of Ethical Challenges

The results of a 1992 survey of the membership of the American Psychological Association (APA) regarding ethical concerns in clinical psychology (5) are generally applicable to all evaluating clinicians. Critical incidents were separated into 23 categories of ethical dilemmas. Issues involving forensic psychology ranked fifth, due to concerns about the presentation of false testimony, the attorney's role in eliciting desirable (but possibly false) testimony, the rendering of conclusions that are not grounded in objective data or scientific principles, and the potential for unintentional harm that could result from reporting inaccurate data.

Specifically pertinent to TBI casework is a survey of the membership of the National Academy of Neuropsychology (NAN) which revealed that the majority of the respondents were concerned about examiner competence (64%), inappropriate use of tests (61%), and conflict between the law and ethics (55%) (6).

Adapting General Biomedical Ethics to TBI Casework

Building upon the universal commitment of the clinician to his/her patient, four core bioethical Principles have been described: *Autonomy, Non-Maleficence, Beneficence,* and *Justice* (7).

Autonomy refers to self-determination; that is, the ability to make healthcare-related decisions independently.

Non-Maleficence is closely related to the Oath of Hippocrates, loosely translated from Greek into Latin as: *primum non nocere* (First, Do No Harm!).

The concept of *Beneficence* is more proactive, requiring that there is a promotion of that which is in the best interest of the patient.

In healthcare, the concept of *Justice* typically concerns the equitable distribution of the burdens and benefits of care.

Common to these four Principles is the expectation of a fundamental obligation to respect the patient at all times. Certainly, the fundamental obligation of respect applies equally to when the interaction is solely one of evaluator-examinee, with no clinician-patient relationship. Clinicians are expected to provide equal measures of respect to a person, whether seen in the context of patient or that of evaluee, including courtesy, dignity and fairness; and spending adequate time during the assessment process.

While the concepts of non-maleficence, beneficence and justice remain closely tied to the universal commitment of respect for the person, there is a need for adaptation to the special circumstances of the medico-legal context, in which the person's goals are those of a litigant, potentially unrelated to his/her concurrent goals as a patient. Although an examiner must recognize and respect the responsibility to bring no direct harm to the examinee during the examination, certain forms of examinations may need to be provocative in order to evoke and test symptoms and signs, including pain, or emotional distress. Thus, the psychiatric interview or neuropsychological testing may result in temporary frustration from challenging cognitive tasks, or in changes in mood due to emotionally sensitive query.

Moreover, although potentially true (tangentially) of the treating clinician examination, findings from a clinicolegal evaluation may have the potential of significantly and directly impacting upon the examinee's diagnostic label, future financial status, treatment or vocational options, environmental modifications, and/or even level of credibility. The successful reconciliation of these three Principles to the clinicolegal environment rests with the appreciation that the duty is owed – as it is with the judiciary – equally impartially to all litigating parties. It is the evaluator's task to conduct the evaluation in a fair manner and to present the results objectively, fully and dispassionately. The court or other party requesting the examination will then have the responsibility to see that the outcome is just. Outcome must never be a factor in the presentation of findings, conclusions or opinions by a clinicolegal evaluator.

An examinee who is denied services or monies based in full or in part on the results of an independent examination may believe that he/she was not treated justly and that the examination did indeed cause harm. However, the evaluator who has treated that individual respectfully and with dignity and has facilitated a meaningful interview, (including listening carefully and reasonably patiently to the examinee's expressed concerns), and then spent sufficient time in examination and in report preparation, will be less likely to be perceived as unfair or acting with maleficence.

With independent examinations, the principle of beneficence does not apply directly to the examinee. The examiner's role is an impartial one, favouring neither the examinee nor the opposing party. Unlike caregiving situations, promotion of the examinee's well-being is not a primary goal. Instead, the examiner's evaluation is conducted to inform the referring party and by extension is for the benefit of the trier of fact or other decision-making body to whom the parties turn for dispute resolution. The examinee, like the other parties to a clinico-legal dispute, may benefit in whole or in part, or may not benefit at all, from the results of the evaluation and any decisions based upon the results. The examiner has no responsibility to the examinee, and to his/her needs or wishes, beyond courtesy, expertise, thoroughness and objectivity, and must take no interest in the process or outcome, of settlement negotiations or judicial determinations.

As a corollary, the ethical examiner must not be drawn into making partial decisions on the basis of 'universal' axioms such as: *benefit of the doubt always goes to the patient*. That axiom certainly belongs within 'when in doubt' decision algorithms relating to patient safety, such as the management of acute chest pain complaints. It does not necessarily apply equally to circumstances where parties have opposing interests in causation or settlements, and have a right to expect an evaluator to function without any decision bias. An inherent, consistent preference for one position or party, no matter how beneficent in intent, not only projects the appearance of bias but may in fact cross the ethical boundary of neutrality, as well as, reduce the utility of the evaluator's conclusions.

There is another aspect to beneficence, related to the clinician's universal societal-legal obligations, from which there is no exemption created within a clinicolegal context. A physician who discovers a clinical condition that could be harmful to the individual or to others has a direct obligation to report that condition to the appropriate body: in the case of unsafe driving (in some jurisdictions), to a driver's licensing authority (e.g. impaired vision / cognition, or seizures); in the case of child neglect/abuse to a children's aide agency. Typically, where mandatory reporting exists, special protocols are created by the authority / agency to safeguard anonymity, in addition to legislation to protect the reporting clinician from lawsuit. Typically the attending clinician or clinicolegal evaluator has no concurrent obligation to the evaluee, to disclose the fact of reporting.

AVOIDING ETHICAL MISCONDUCT

Proactivity

Clinicians, whether they are placed in or place themselves in clinicolegal situations, must make themselves aware of potential ethical pitfalls and must actively take steps to avoid them. Passive reliance on a sincere belief, that by performing competent work one is *a priori* assured of being perceived as 'ethical', is not sufficient protection in the face of the complex and wide range of potential ethical dilemmas, and will not necessarily safeguard against a perception of boundary-crossing leading to an accusation of ethical misconduct. The clinician must instead be assertive in seeking out knowledge, skills, and feedback related to ethical practice; constantly vigilant for evolving dilemmas; and briskly proactive in avoiding or remediating same.

Developing and Maintaining Reliable Expert Qualifications

It is axiomatic that one's qualifications and expertise must be consistent with or exceed currently accepted professional guidelines. Clinicians should strive to maintain high standards of competence in their work, including recognition of and deference to the boundaries of their competencies and the limitations of their expertise, and to provide only those services and use only those techniques for which they are qualified by education, training, or experience.

While variability in education, training, and experience remain, the achievement of eligibility for Board certification (e.g. diplomate or fellowship status) is an accepted basic standard for clinical specialist expertise. This standard is superceded only by acquisition of formal Board specialty or subspecialty certification, which is conferred only through successful completion of a rigorous examination process.

In general, the attainment of Board specialty or subspecialty certification provides the clearest single universal evidence of competence in the relevant area of specialty. Given that Board eligibility is a widely recognized basic standard for expert witness qualifications, it is recommended that clinicians not opting for Board certification should have their credentials independently evaluated by appropriate bodies to verify meeting Board eligibility threshold requirements.

Many organizations offer 'Board certification'. The criteria for attainment of these "Board certifications" vary from merely paying a fee, through varying levels of training, practical experience, written and oral examination. Prior to expending time, effort and funds towards such certification, it is important for the clinician to carefully investigate the organization as well as it's certification's inclusionary and exclusionary criteria, including both the stringency of the eligibility requirements and the thoroughness and applicability of the examination processes. Affiliation with an organization which offers certification examination to virtually any applicant, notwithstanding possession of a suitable professional background, or whose certification examination has a 100% pass rate, offers no real validation to one's knowledgable peers or to a critical court system.

It can be recommended that clinicians involved with clinicolegal evaluation of persons with complex conditions such as TBI: (a) seek rigorous peer review to ensure competence in the general area of assessment, as well as, any special areas of interest, and obtain supervision and documentation that any identified deficiencies have been remediated, (b) obtain Board certification as the most rigorous mechanism of peer review, and (c) exercise care to practice only within the boundaries of competence, and seek consultation from other experts when appropriate.

Continuing education is critical for maintaining expertise. Given the rapidly evolving field of TBI and of brain function research in general, clinicians must maintain a reasonable level of awareness of current general scientific theory and applied practice knowledge. This should include awareness of general trends in the relevant literature, the state of current knowledge, and the significant limitations in said knowledge. Documented, regular attendance at specialty-focused professional conferences and seminars formally signals a significant investment in furthering one's knowledge.

Additional professional activities may demonstrate expertise in specific areas of knowledge or skill. Publications, lectures or seminars given, academic appointments, and administrative positions may all reflect high levels of expertise. However, as with board certification, the manner in which these credentials are obtained can vary considerably. Publications in peer-reviewed media with stringent acceptance criteria represent the highest standard of publication.

Professionals making presentations at national or international conferences are often regarded as accepted authorities in their field, as inferred from the fact of invitation from highly credentialed and merit-discriminating peer conference organizers, particularly those who have a broad spectrum of choice of experts. Faculty or administrative appointments should be evaluated on the manner in which they are earned and the degree of selectivity of the process.

Neutrality and Sphere of Expertise

The American Medical Association's (AMA) Council on Ethical and Judicial Affairs publishes a Code of Medical Ethics (8). The AMA Ethics Code is fairly general; however, it does state that medical experts should "have recent and substantive experience in the area in which they testify and should limit testimony to their sphere of medical expertise." The code further stipulates that the "medical witness must not become an advocate or partisan in the legal proceeding." It further suggests that the medical witness inform attorneys of "all favorable and unfavorable information developed by the physician's evaluation of the case." The latter is of course a universal criterion. Failure to make full disclosure has the appearance of deliberate selectivity, from which flows the inevitable inference of an unbalanced, partial evaluation.

The lay-person is at a significant disadvantage with respect to appreciating the subtleties of the various subspecialty scopes of practice, and the significance of 'positive' (what was found that should not be there) and 'negative' (what should have been there and was not found) findings. Thus, in the assessment of apparent hysterical blindness after a head injury, appreciation of the distinction between the abilities of a general ophthalmologist and a neuro-ophthalmologist, or between a general psychiatrist and a neuro-psychiatrist, may be critical to appreciating the relative value of various 'expert' findings of normality or abnormality. Moreover, a notation that a patient with TBI could not read a sample text is of little value in the absence of clarification of the potential modifying conditions such as prior literacy; or the confirmation that the eyes did not suffer from corneal opacity or medication-induced loss of acuity, uncorrected/poorly corrected vision or poor fitting contact lenses or retinopathies; or that there were no cranial nerve palsies creating diplopia, etc.

Material Contribution to Case Resolution

The American Academy of Physical Medicine and Rehabilitation (9) published a 'white paper' with recommendations for expert witness testimony. This document indicates that the expert witness should serve to educate the court as a whole, rather than representing one side or the other, notwithstanding that the expert may have been retained by one party. The document suggests that the ultimate test for accuracy and impartiality is a willingness to prepare reports or offer testimony that could be presented without alteration for use by either the plaintiff or the defendant. As a corollary, judges have remarked that the ability to accurately discern the identity of the requesting party, merely from reading reports or reviewing transcripts of testimony, potentially signals a lack of genuine neutrality on the part of the evaluator. Three additional recommendations are emphasized: (a) the physician should identify opinions which are personal and not necessarily held by other physicians, (b) a distinction should be made between medical malpractice and medical maloccurrence when analyzing case evidence, and (c) there should be a willingness to submit transcripts of depositions and/or courtroom testimony for peer review.

The American Academy of Neurology and the American Board of Medical Specialties have presented the following guidelines for the physician expert witness: (a) the physician expert witness should be fully trained in a specialty or a diplomate of a specialty board recognized by the American Board of Medical Specialties, and qualified by experience or demonstrated competence in the subject of the case; the specialty of the physician should be appropriate to the subject matter in the case, and (b) the physician expert witness should be familiar with the clinical practice of the specialty for the subject matter of the case at the time of the occurrence, and should be actively involved in the clinical practice of the specialty for the subject matter of the case for three of the previous five years at the time of the testimony. Similar guidelines have also been published by the American Academy of Psychiatry and the Law (10).

Avoidance of Relational Conflict Issues

The ethical guidelines governing the relationship between an examiner and an evaluee are special adaptations of universal clinical practice 'caregiver' guidelines in which the primary concern is for the safety and welfare of the patient. The caregiver role is 'active', involving a 'fiduciary' 'duty of care' with a predominant focus on *individual outcome*.

In clinical practice, given the perceived power differential between doctor and patient, entering into any personal, scientific, financial, or other relationships with a caregiver has the potential of being exploitative to the patient. Clinical training emphasizes the need for avoidance of excessively intimate personal relationships with a current patient (and sometimes even a former patient).

Building on the Hippocratic Oath, the AMA explicitly expresses the concerns of the profession towards any blurring of the boundaries between the personal and professional relationships of the physician, where boundary violations "may exploit the vulnerability of the patient" or "may obscure the physician's objective judgment concerning the patient's health care". The AMA formalizes its proscription against exploitation of any former patient by declaring any post-caregiving relationship unethical: "if the physician uses or exploits trust, knowledge, emotions or influence derived from the previous professional relationship" and: "At a minimum, a physician's ethical duties include terminating the physician-patient relationship before initiating a dating, romantic or sexual relationship".

In direct contrast, the role of the clinicolegal evaluator is 'passive' in relationship to the evaluee and his/her family. The evaluator neither seeks nor accepts any duty of care, and must also firmly and unambiguously discourage any expectation of care. The value of clinicolegal work lies not only in the examiner's clinical expertise, but equally in impartiality and objectivity, and the extent to which critical powers are applied to case evidence and scientific knowledge – making a material contribution to case resolution.

The guidelines for clinicolegal practice should be adhered to as rigorously as those applicable to the most worrisome of clinical practice circumstances. To ensure that neither real nor apparent conflict of interest enters into the clinico-legal evaluation, an examiner must decline any evaluation involving an evaluee with whom the examiner has, or has had, a personal, social or therapeutic relationship. The examiner should also decline any evaluation involving an evaluee who has a personal relationship with any member of the examiner's immediate family. In essence, safeguarding the perception of neutrality requires that an examiner decline any evaluation circumstance in which he/she can not be entirely free of pressure in regard to presenting candid, complete opinions on issues such as causation, entitlement to benefits, disability, or prognosis; or circumstances in which an observer could develop a reasonable concern.

Clearly, for the clinicolegal examiner, ethical guidelines for encounters and relationships are simple and unequivocal. Aside from the provision of urgent therapeutic services, there must be absolutely no advice or caregiving during the encounter, and no contact or relationship of any kind in the future with an evaluee or his/her immediate family, until at least the formal conclusion of all clinicolegal proceedings. Clearly, violation of such boundaries carries considerable risk of appearance, if not actual, conflicts of interest. Otherwise, the evaluator could be placed in a position of considerable power and potential exploitation; ironically, the reverse could also be true since the evaluee or family member might attain a position of considerable influence over the evaluator.

This raises the question of associated or prior relationships. Concerning the former, it is readily evident that the evaluator should avoid any case in which subtle influence might be exerted on him/her, such as when the evaluee or immediate family is somehow connected through employment, friendship, social or professional group, acquaintance or family relationships. For example, given the likelihood of social encounters it might be prudent to avoid evaluating the parent of a child who is in the same school class as one's own child.

For the purposes of clinicolegal evaluation, any pre-existing relationship that was more than a casual acquaintanceship creates the potential for real or apparent conflict of interest (11). As a general rule therefore, any relationship that may be seen by others, as well as by the parties involved, as having the potential to bias the opinion of the examiner should eliminate that professional from consideration as an examiner (12). However, exceptions may be required, particularly when no other expert in a particular field is readily available and where entitlement to benefit issues requires urgent evaluation. Prioritizing provision of a needed service may outweigh many potential objections. When any such exception is required, the nature of any pre-existing relationship and its potential ramifications on the results of the clinico-legal examination must be disclosed to all parties prior to conducting the examination and should be clearly documented in the subsequent written clinico-legal report. In addition, all safeguards that will be employed to ensure objectivity should be described. As a final corollary, should circumstances change outside of the control of the examiner, as might happen during the course of a clinicolegal case that lasts many years, such that the examiner no longer feels that neutrality and freedom from influence exists, the examiner should notify all parties and offer to withdraw from the case.

Professional Role Distinctions

The ethical codes discussed to this point emphasize proscription of creation of dual relationships in which the examiner had/has both a professional and a nonprofessional relationship with an evaluee. Avoiding conflicts between differing professional roles is of equal importance given the potential for undermining the professional's objectivity and credibility, negatively affecting the parties served.

Equally applicable to physicians and other professionals, Blau (13, 14), identified three different and conflicting professional roles for professionals working in clinicolegal settings: Treating Doctor, Expert Witness, and Trial Consultant.

The *Treating Doctor* is in an active role, with a duty of care. The clinician tends to seek or accept an empathic bond with the patient, and is expected to advocate for the patient in ways intended to improve mental or physical health, or facilitate stable, supportive circumstances. When offering testimony, the Treating Doctor is a special type of fact witness, relying on expertise in helping the triers of fact while describing the symptoms and signs, the investigations done, the treatments provided, and the course and impact of the condition. As a fact witness, the Treating Doctor's reports and testimony must be anchored in his/her findings, diagnoses and treatment records. However, the Treating Doctor is also capable of service as an expert resource to the court, subject to qualifications being reviewed and a determination made as to the limits of testimony for each individual professional. Unlike the lay person, who as a fact witness cannot offer expert opinion but rather can only describe what was personally seen or heard, clinical professionals may be permitted to offer the court more general information about differential diagnosis, natural history of diseases, investigations, treatment paradigms, and prognosis, drawing on professional training and experience. It is of course understood by all parties that any such testimony may be potentially influenced by the underlying treating relationship, but it is expected that when so requested, the clinician will strive to assist the court with full disclosure and cooperation, careful consideration of responses, and avoidance of argumentativeness or disproportionate, impassioned advocacy. The triers of fact will later assign appropriate weight to the testimony. It is never appropriate for a Treating Doctor to enter into contractual arrangements for fee-for-service evaluations of a current or former patient on any basis other than that of the physician-patient relationship.

The *Expert Witness*, having no prior direct knowledge of the examinee, is obligated to obtain special and often exceptionally complete information in order to render an expert opinion. In order to facilitate objectivity, no emotional or other bond can exist with the examinee. All clinical evidence must be evenhandedly reviewed with an approach founded in critical appraisal. It is appropriate to approach the case from a perspective of reasonable skepticism, testing all evidence for reliability and applicability.

The *Trial Consultant* is retained to assist with the critical scrutiny of expert opinions. Given the realities of the adversarial process, the trial consultant may be expected to identify experts on the opposing side who are potentially susceptible to impeachment and to then lay the groundwork for that effort. Clearly, an objective and dispassionate status towards the evaluee, and towards all other professionals involved in the case, is essential to trial consultancy, in order to offer sound, unemotional advice to retaining counsel.

A further role existing in some circumstances is that of *Case Reviewer*, retained to review the case evidence without direct assessment (evidentiary review), and/or to critically evaluate the assessing evaluators and treating clinicians (peer review). Not all clinicians are comfortable with performing an evidentiary review solely confined to documentation, and leading to expert opinions about a claimant that one has not interviewed and examined. The peer review involves at least the potential of having to state findings critical of one's colleagues' knowledge, clinical acumen, ethics or practices. The Case Reviewer must always declare at the outset of the report precisely what information (such as specific documentation) was relied upon, and that the opportunity for a direct evaluation was not provided. It is appropriate to state whether a direct evaluation might alter the opinion being presented. It is necessary to state whether the documentation was found to be clear and complete, and to indicate the limits of scope and certainty of the opinions that could be derived. For example, a Reviewer might be asked to determine the total percent Impairment of the Whole Person by applying documented clinical findings to the AMA Guides to the Evaluation of Permanent Impairment (15). While the Reviewer is able to offer expert analysis of the proper Chapters, Tables and Figures and Combined Values, the opinion remains entirely dependent on other clinicians' work for the comprehensiveness of the list of diagnoses and impairments and the reliability of the clinical findings. Oftentimes, in the context of a review, incomplete records are provided to the clinician – yet opinions are requested based on the information available. It can be argued that any ethical clinician should never provide opinions without first requesting an opportunity to review all relevant materials. Lastly, given that there is, by definition, no opportunity availed to the clinician to directly examine the injured party in the context of a review, clinicians must be careful, on ethical clinicolegal grounds, regarding opining as to specific impairment and disability related issues.

In general these four roles are separate and distinct and represent differing interests and obligations. Failure to clarify the limits of one's role for both oneself and the other parties involved may lead to inappropriate mixing of roles, with a resultant loss of objectivity and professional accuracy. Notwithstanding which role the clinician is asked to assume, any fixed-outcome oriented solicitation should be promptly and firmly responded to in unequivocal terms, with clear instruction to the requesting party concerning the ethical limits which govern the professional's participation. Similarly, the professional should decline any request in which remuneration is made contingent on 'satisfactory' outcome (as defined by an interested party) or in which the final fee paid may differ according to settlement terms.

For the Treating Doctor, role conflicts may be further avoided by providing the patient's treatment record instead of a report or testimony (16).

Any role conflicts that do nevertheless arise should be acknowledged in reports and in testimony.

Immunity of Clinicolegal Work and Expert Testimony

Illustrative of the special role of the Expert Witness is an Ontario court ruling which arose from a class action law suit for damages by several plaintiffs against two clinicians whose clinicolegal evaluations were in compliance with dispute resolution requirements of Ontario's no-fault auto insurance legislation. In dismissing the lawsuit the judge reviewed prior court decisions on point and concluded that the *only* relationship between the plaintiffs and their evaluators involved the assessment of and report on each of the plaintiffs by one or both of the defendants. The legislated dispute resolution process required the defendants to intervene as evaluators, which they did. The ruling set out that clinicolegal evaluators cannot be sued for carrying out their statutory duty because they owe no duty of care to the plaintiffs. They cannot be sued for malpractice because their contact with the plaintiffs was not sufficient to create a medical duty of care to the plaintiffs. They cannot be sued for breach of fiduciary duty because the assessment relationship lacks the element of expectation that the assessor will act in the interests of the plaintiff and so does not give rise to a fiduciary duty in favor of the plaintiffs, and such a duty would be inconsistent with their neutral position. Lastly, they cannot be sued for what they say in their reports because such reports are absolutely protected by witness immunity.

We would note, however, that not all judicial systems act as logically as the Ontario Courts, and one of the authors (Zasler) has personal knowledge of several claims that have come out of clinicolegal expert testimony involvement where experts were sued for, among other things, claims of slander consequential to claiming that someone was symptom magnifying or malingering. Another author (Ameis) has had personal experience with cases in which regulatory bodies have held formal reviews of clinicians in response to complainants objecting to medicolegal reports containing similarly 'provocative' terms. Clinicians should not assume, therefore, that they are totally immune for their actions in the capacity as an expert witness.

There are ways to protect oneself from the effects of such claims, such as by carrying additional insurance (most malpractice policies do not cover clinicolegal work).

Medical Boards and professional peers may also take various actions against unethical clinicolegal conduct when observed with fellow professionals although all too often such conduct is left to fester and propagate as professionals would rather "not get involved" due to potential personal and political ramifications.

ETHICAL CLINICAL OFFICE PRACTICES

Use of Objectively Validated Assessment/Reporting

Professionals demonstrate nonmaleficence and beneficence and promote justice in clinico-legal settings by conducting unbiased examinations and testifying honestly. Sweet and Moulthrop (17) have offered relevant and pointed self-examination questions that should be utilized when conducting assessments in adversarial contexts. These contain questions for procedural conduct, including, for example, favorability of findings to referral source, comparison of current findings with base-rates, and presence of emotions and actions suggesting advocacy. They also contain questions for written reports which include whether a panel of peers / experts would agree with findings and conclusions; whether contradictory facts and evidence were included or excluded; and whether exaggerated or dramatic descriptors were employed. Thus, the merits of a report might be determined in part by whether opinions flow logically from findings or seem to be pre-formed, whether equivocal test results (i.e., from high false-positive radiological, laboratory or neuropsychological tests) are appropriately employed to inform or merely selectively chosen, overweighted and exploited to persuade; and whether terminology was dispassionate, measured and proportionate; or emotionally charged and inflammatory.

Lees-Haley (18) has suggested that, in addition to self-examination, examiners should develop and employ externally validated safeguards to increase the probability of objectivity. Until such safeguards are developed, proposed guidelines (14, 19–22) offer good starting points for attempting to maintain examiner objectivity.

Avoidance of Outcome Dependency

When the definition of success of two groups of professionals differs dramatically, their ability to work together on a project will be very limited. Hence when plaintiff lawyers define success as the development of a case capable of attracting a large settlement, no matter how modest the TBI impairment sequelae and how high functioning the claimant, then the report of the clinician who defines success solely by expertise, objectivity, and candor, will not be well received.

Attorneys must answer to their clients, who require them to be advocates and to maximize the benefits at outcome: it is natural that such attorneys will seek out experts whose viewpoints are more likely to be strongly supportive of their clients' cases, irrespective of case merits. Therefore, unless the referral is by mutual consent of the parties, or arises from the court itself, or unless the identity of the referral source is masked, the examiner must deal with the reality of being cognizant of the referral and payment source, and associated potential disincentives to full candor.

Unfavorable examination findings may trigger an undesirable set of consequences such as the attorney's inability or refusal to pay for services provided if the case is 'lost', or loss of further referrals by that attorney and perhaps his/her colleagues, with consequent decreased clinico-legal income. Given the restrictions in reimbursement in other areas of healthcare, there are considerable pressures and reinforcements that serve as disincentives to producing 'unfavorable' findings. Consequently, subtle processes, such as suggesting limited reliability/credibility to contradictory information sources and making selective interpretations in unclear situations, would seem especially vulnerable to influence. Subtle- to not-so-subtle influences involving the preference/need of the referring attorney may also predispose examiners to unidirectionally interpreting all findings or to advancing unusually firm or unequivocal views. Such influences represent threats to objective, ethical practice and to professional credibility.

Many jurisdictions have made, or at least contemplated, practical attempts to neutralize the potential for influence related to outcome. In 1996 the Provincial legislature of Ontario created a system of Designated Assessment Centres (DACs). An impartial governmental team would randomly assign a case to Center, where expert evaluators were expected to make benefit determinations while adhering to standards of neutrality, transparency, cost-efficiency and timeliness. Competence and cost were monitored, and Center administrators were held accountable for quality assurance, always subject to loss of designation. Within this system, evaluator selection was independent of either party; fees were predetermined and payment was assured. Evaluators were highly insulated from outcome, by virtue of a random referral process in which determinations had no influence on future referrals, payment arrangements or income. The primary determinants of case load related to delisting from DAC rosters for persistent failure to maintain expertise, timeliness or neutrality. Unfortunately, the DAC system fell victim to political 'reforms' and was eliminated in March 2006 in favor of an Insurer Examination system.

Neutrality and Selectivity in Office Practices

Avoiding the *appearance* of lack or loss of Neutrality is often as important as the actual state of neutrality. Both perception and existence of neutrality require active as well as passive measures, more easily achieved in group practices than for the individual practitioner. A balanced and fair, written referral policy is a reliable passive approach. The appearance of neutrality of a clinician is reinforced by the appreciation that the clinician is prepared to evenhandedly accept suitable cases from plaintiff and defense.

High selectivity in case acceptance can indicate the clinician's commitment to working strictly within scope of practice, and general or special expertise. However, it can also work against positive perception. Thus, a consistent policy of accepting only severe TBI cases, evenhandedly from plaintiff and defence, signals a neutral interest in a specific condition suitably challenging to the clinician's expertise, while by contrast an indiscriminate policy of accepting 'all comers', including cases of dubious brain trauma or impairment, or worse, a selective policy of taking primarily dubious claimant cases, may signal a pattern of self-marketing, as an advocate and "case builder".

Clearly, perceived neutrality is enhanced by the degree of perceived distance between the referring party and the clinician. Thus, selectivity within a group practice may be particularly significant. While the group may have an open policy on acceptance of referrals, there may be an internal agreement (1) to randomly assign cases, or (2) to 'stream' on the basis of individual member expertise and experience. Additionally clinical examiner groups may have their staff mask all information about the referral source, substituting a briefing paper, which sets out the goals of the evaluation without specifying whether the referral is for plaintiff or defense sides.

In some cases, in order to resolve clinical ambiguities, establish the current scientific understanding, or otherwise clarify issues before trial, the presiding judge may select an examiner and order an expert examination, or may order the parties to jointly select a mutually agreeable examiner. Either approach may significantly advance the process of settlement through neutralization of the expert referral process.

Attorneys who recognize the potential that their act of referral may itself 'taint' the expert should carefully craft the referral request in neutral terms to identify the issues that remain in dispute, and fairly set out the difficulties existing between the parties owing to their understandings and positions, requesting diagnostic or management opinion or clarification of existing opinion so as to best inform the parties and the triers of fact.

Unfortunately, a clinician's commitment to neutrality may be compromised by a selection process which is intended to 'take advantage' of clinical proclivities; the clinician then becoming the unwitting tool of advocacy. Attorneys are often well versed on which clinicians consistently favor a certain scientific theory or a particular threshold, or test finding. Thus, in order to garner support for a weak case, an attorney may refer to a clinician known to uncritically accept all complaints and claims as entirely reliable. Similarly, in order to attack a strong case, an attorney may refer to a clinician who is an unremitting skeptic of all subjective matters and prefers to rely solely on the results of MRI and objective clinical findings.

Toward the goal of maintaining examiner objectivity, Brodsky (19) suggested that examiners calculate an *objectivity quotient* in order to quantify the degree to which the expert clinician's findings have been in agreement with, or different from, a referring attorney's position. The objectivity quotient is calculated by dividing the number of cases in which findings support the referring attorney's position by the total number of cases the clinician has been involved in as a consultant and/or expert. A cutoff score of 0.7 has been proposed for potential examiner bias.

Expert Witness: Trial Consultant Role Boundaries

Experts must be vigilant against the possibility that their assistance of the retaining party in the clinico-legal aspects of a case could extend into ethically questionable behavior. Expert Witnesses must not go beyond providing their own independent and objective opinion about the examinee. There should be no crossing of the line that separates disinterest in outcome from outcome promotion.

It is proper for the Trial Consultant to focus on outcome and to work towards optimization of outcome terms satisfactory to the referring party, but nevertheless based on the evidence and merits of a case. He/she is expected to assist with strategic or tactical "trial preparation" by participating in efforts to accumulate a complete case database, and to effectively cross-examine concerning the procedures, opinions or other testimony of clinician witnesses. However, partisan criticism against experts and advocacy for the adversarial attorney team in its battle to "win" through impeachment (e.g., by preparing deposition or trial questions or strategy or discussing stylistics or cases beyond the current one) strains ethical clinical boundaries. An ethical Trial Consultant assists with identification of the strengths and weaknesses of all opinions, and advises in balanced fashion on the current science.

It is ethically inappropriate for any professional to participate in preparation of *ad hominum* personal attacks, or in selective, misrepresentative citations of literature, or misuse of statistical analysis, with the ultimate intention of confusing or misinforming the triers of fact.

CONDUCTING THE CLINICO-LEGAL EXAMINATION

Establishing Ground Rules in Advance

Most commonly, referrals of a strictly clinico-legal nature come from attorneys, insurance companies, and other third party payors and are clearly intended for use in litigation. The clinician has a clear opportunity to decide on involvement. By contrast clinical referrals from physicians or other referral sources may start out as requests for consultation or for participation in caregiving, with the clinician's caregiver involvement making inevitable some linkage to any subsequent litigation process. Indeed, a 'Trojan horse' phenomenon is sometimes seen, in which the clinical referral for consultation is in fact instigated or influenced by a plaintiff lawyer, whose intent is either to later obtain a relatively inexpensive expert clinicolegal report, or ensure the clinician's involvement in an eventual trial, or at least ensure that no other party can obtain that clinician's services as Expert Witness in the case.

In a clinicolegal referral it is critically important to establish the basis of the referral and the parameters of anticipated or permissible interaction with the evaluee, since many patients confuse the roles and may resent or even actively complain to regulatory boards about perceived failure to give the advice or care expected. This is particularly important for the patient with impairments of cognition, where concrete thought or memory deficits reduce the ability to appreciate the distinction between caregiving and independent assessment.

Equally, prior to carrying out an independent evaluation, it is important to ensure that the referral source appreciates that no therapeutic relationship of advice or care will exist. The evaluator should not be expected to provide direct advice or care to the examinee at the time of the evaluation or at any time thereafter, and there is no ongoing relationship or obligation to the evaluee beyond normal ethical and professional behaviour. As a corollary, it is improper for an evaluator to offer direct advice following an IME, and instead this potentially disrupts existing therapeutic relationships and thus is an ethical violation.

In parallel, the source of funding for the referral must be carefully established. Seeking concurrent fees from both a clinicolegal referral source who requested an independent examination along with billing any other party such as a health care insurer, has been referred to as 'double billing' or 'double dipping', and is unethical.

Communicating Ground Rules to the Examinee

Examinees very often present for independent examinations with ambivalence, anxiety, or even distrust (19, 21–23). For the TBI patient, such psycho-emotional states may be superimposed on neurological impairments of cognition, emotion, or behavior; physical impairments; and/or financial, vocational and/or interpersonal difficulties that are the reasons for the examination. Apprehension may be due in part to inaccurate or incomplete information provided to them by their attorney, family members, treating health professionals, or others regarding the purpose and nature of the independent examination.

Not uncommonly, the referral by an insurance company for clinicolegal examination is interpreted by the evaluee as hostile in nature, implying or even seeming to overtly accuse the evaluee of unreliability or deception, or the attending clinicians of incompetence. For example, the lack of proper understanding of the nature of an independent clinicolegal evaluation accounts for the majority of all complaints to the College of Physicians and Surgeons of Ontario, with the most common complaint involving the perceived improper behaviour of the physician in either not offering or refusing to provide, on request, advice or prescription.

The examiner who provides accurate information about the purpose of the examination and the procedures to be employed at the outset of the evaluation will likely help to reduce the examinee's anxiety and distrust and to increase his or her cooperation. Recognizing the potential for anxiety that is inherent in such examinations and emphasizing the objective nature of the examination should serve to increase the examinee's comfort level and perception of fairness, while fostering reliable performance. Clearly, as Binder and Thompson (24) have noted, in the case of the neuropsychologist but with general application to all clinicians, one must attempt to minimize any potential discomfort associated with the examination.

The Canadian Society of Medical Evaluators has developed educational pamphlets specifically for dissemination by clinicians or insurers to evaluees. Separate pamphlets were prepared to meet the somewhat differing circumstances of physical medicine and psychiatric independent examinations. By anecdotal reports, its use by CSME members has been associated with a marked decrease in regulatory body complaints, and/or facilitation of complaint resolution.

Response Bias

Response bias is the deliberate or inadvertent presentation of oneself as more or less impaired than one actually is. Its presence must always be considered, assessed and commented upon as it might pertain to the clinician's findings, and in regard to the findings of other clinicians. This provides the report's readers with a reference point as to how fairly and competently this confounding element was assessed, what finding was made, and whether the implications were considered and applied to the balance of the report. It may serve to provide a basis of understanding for some differing clinical opinions.

Employing formal and informal means of assessing response bias, followed by formal, structured reporting of related findings is a critically important component of a comprehensive TBI evaluation. The official position paper of the National Academy of Neuropsychology on symptom validity testing now posits both that response bias assessment, and any specific symptom validity tests deemed necessary for evaluation of symptom validity, is medically necessary (NAN Position paper reference) National Academy of Neuropsychology Position Paper: Symptom validity assessment: Practice issues and medical necessity: Official Statement of the National Academy of Neuropsychology, Approved by the Board of Directors 2/28/05. www.nanonline.org/downloads/paio/Position/NANsvt.pdf. Retrieved 4/21/06 (25). However, the examiner should exercise caution in regard to going further, by inferring motivation - the intent and goal of the evaluee. The evaluator should instead discuss the differential diagnostic list of potential sources of the unreliability detected: including inadvertency, medication, pain, fatigue, personality or pathopsycho-emotional mechanisms. As a corollary of a careful assessment for response bias, the examiner will be in an enhanced position to consider the reliability and validity of the apparently abnormal findings of those clinicians who did not look for inconsistencies or otherwise allow for response bias. (See Chapter by Martelli, et al. in this text on response bias assessment, and National Academy of Neuropsychology Position Paper on symptom validity testing) National Academy of Neuropsychology Position Paper: Symptom validity assessment: Practice issues and medical necessity: Official Statement of the National Academy of Neuropsychology, Approved by the Board of Directors 2/28/05. www.nanonline.org/ downloads/paio/Position/NANsvt.pdf. Retrieved 4/21/06 (26).

As a further quality control measure, prior to examination the evaluee should be given an explanation of the anticipated examination process; as a component of this description, the examiner should emphasize the importance of displaying one's real capacities, including consistently putting forth one's best efforts throughout the examination. It should also be explained that the consistency and extent of the examinee's effort and degree of disclosure will be assessed and may impact on the examiner's rating of reliability.

It is ethically necessary to give the evaluee notice before the evaluation that response bias and reliability may be tested. It is not necessary or even advisable to disclose the nature of the testing, or that there may be use of informal, as well as, formal means. However, it is imperative that the evaluee also understand that pain, fatigue, confusion, memory lapses, or other neurological impairments will not be regarded solely as evidence of lack of cooperation or effort.

Perceived Control and Quality Assurance

It is important for the evaluee undergoing a clinicolegal examination to retain a sense of control over the proceedings, including to a reasonable extent the right to control its pace, and the right to ask why a particular question is being posed or test procedure performed. The evaluee has an absolute right to decline to proceed with a given question, exam procedure and/or the evaluation itself. Within reason, accommodations should be made for breaks to use the restroom, or to rest due to fatigue and/or the need to take medication. It is often instructive to encourage the evaluee to comment during and particularly towards the end of the evaluation if any element of questioning or testing was new, unfamiliar, or omitted. The examinee should be informed of the importance of reporting any sense of difficulty or distress to the examiner in 'real-time', not later.

It may also be necessary to notify the evaluee of "zero tolerance" rules regarding any inappropriate verbal or physical behavior, and of potential negative inferences from lack of cooperation, or from premature termination of the evaluation, without reasonable basis. The expert examiner must always allow for the possibility that in TBI evaluation, response bias, lack of consistent cooperation, or problematic verbal or physical behaviors may be the inadvertent and uncontrollable consequences of pain, fatigue, medication, seizure, or behavioral disinhibition.

Confidentiality Issues

The clinicolegal evaluation is one in which a limited duty of confidentiality is owed to the evaluee. The referring party is entitled to full disclosure of anything learned by the examiner at any time during the evaluation. The evaluee should be under no misapprehension that the evaluator can be held to instructions of 'strict confidence', including disclosures involving sexual orientation; sexual, physical or substance abuse history; STDs or abortion.

The absence of a therapeutic relationship does not prevent the examiner from communicating verbally or in writing with a treating clinician, regarding any concerns or suggestions, particularly emerging issues such as suicidal rumination or inappropriate regimen or dose of medication. A memo must be made of the date, name and content of any verbal communication. Written communication by mail, fax or email, must be retained with the file. The appropriate means of communication will depend upon the nature and priority of the circumstance; a note should not be entrusted to the evaluee if there is any doubt as to whether and when it will be delivered or concern over the evaluee reading the contents.

Informed Consent

Once the examinee understands the purpose of the examination, the process of the examination, rules of disclosure, expectations for cooperation and effort, evaluee rights, and the extent of feedback regarding the results of the examination, the examiner should invite questions and provide further clarification as needed. Only after these issues are seen to be clearly understood by the examinee should his or her informed consent to participate be sought. Consent forms are necessary to document the examiner's efforts to inform and the examinee's consequent understanding and agreement. In addition, consent forms can facilitate communication between examiner and examinee. A checklist can be incorporated into the consent form, allowing examinees to systematically consider, seek clarification if necessary, and then indicate their understanding of each major point by initialing each point on the list and/or signing the bottom of the form along with a witness.

Clearly, informed consent cannot be obtained and should not be sought directly from evaluees with marked cognitive or communication disorders or from minor children. In such situations, consent must be obtained from the individual's legal guardian. In some circumstances the evaluator should seek written proof of guardianship.

Third Party Observers—Direct and Indirect

The issue of allowing a person other than the examiner and examinee into the examination session is complicated. Without exception, the physician examiner should consider use of a staff person as chaperone, to assist and to attest that no inappropriate conversation or action took place. In many jurisdictions it is the right of the evaluee to designate another, suitable third party to be present for his/her comfort and/or as an observer, a witness to what transpires.

Where the evaluator retains a veto right, persuasive pro and con arguments can be considered: a 'pro' argument may exist when the claimant can be expected to be exceptionally apprehensive unless accompanied. In fact, the issue often benefits from avoiding the polarization of the "either/or" proposition, and instead clarification of who should be able to observe and in which settings and with what relative benefit to evaluator or evaluee. The evaluator should however bear in mind that, oftentimes, skilled third party witnesses such as nurses are specifically designated owing to their ability to testify as credible observers about what happened during the examination. Evaluators should always keep in mind that they almost always retain the option of declining the referral if any of the imposed conditions of evaluation appear unacceptable, including designation of a third party.

A claimant-designated third party is, ideally, a passive witness to the procedural events, with no role beyond reassurance of the claimant. No third party should ever be permitted to participate, advise or interfere unless invited to do so, and no third party disruption that compromises the quality of the evaluation should ever be tolerated.

Several authors have presented reasons why the presence of a third party may be contra-indicated during examinations in which standardized tests are used. These reasons include (a) compromise of test security and subsequent misuse of tests, (b) invalidation of results due to tests not having been standardized for third party presence,

and (c) invalidation of results due to social facilitation, (27–31). A policy statement from the American Academy of Clinical Neuropsychology made the distinction between involved observers and uninvolved observers (32). An involved third party observer is someone who has some investment in the outcome of the examination, whereas an uninvolved third party has no stake in the outcome, and instead is strictly a source of emotional support to the evaluee. In contrast, a NAN policy statement distinguished between settings, with third party observers being acceptable in clinical settings for training purposes but unacceptable in forensic settings (29). Issues of observer training, observer involvement, and examination context have all been considered relevant in the debate on the appropriateness of having a third person present during neuropsychological examinations.

The Canadian Society of Medical Evaluators (CSME) has developed guidelines for assisting in the determination of 'who and when' for the presence of a third-party, where there is a choice. The Society recommends that it's members maintain a written protocol, not only to assist them but also to demonstrate to others the rational basis and consistency of their decisions. Thus, one's protocol might set out that a chaperone will always be present; in addition, a first order family member is mandatory for examining any minor. The Society notes that a medical professional such as a nurse is preferable to a non-family lay third party, as an evaluee-designated observer, owing to insight into what constitutes acceptable questions and routine examination practices. Any third party must agree to be placed outside the visual field of the evaluee, to prevent any cueing or other interaction.

We would also note that there is both extensive experience and now some recent literature to support the position that despite best intentions and circumstances, examinee performance may be adversely affected by observers, even or especially when they are their own family, friend or case representative (e.g., case manager or lawyer). Negative consequences of third party observers become difficult if not impossible to factor out when considering apportionment of sub-optimal or otherwise misleading performance.

Videotaping and audiotaping are seemingly less intrusive means of monitoring the examination process. However, these methods of observation can also introduce atypical dynamics into the examination process (analogous to the abruptly altered behaviours evident in home movies or the 'frozen' look of one's colleagues, stuttering into a reporter's microphone. Evaluees may 'act out' for the future audience, or may withhold candor anticipating abreactions of family viewers. At particular disadvantage may be certain TBI evaluees, who are anxious about being perceived as abnormal, embarrassed by paretic facial appearance or speech impairments, or behaviourally disinhibited.

Examiners too may experience alteration of well-established, efficient and effective routines, due to inadvertent effects on body language, tonality, questioning style, or pace (unnaturally slow or hurried).

The setting too is usually not ideal, since the medical office is neither a recording studio nor a well-lit television studio complete with camera- and soundmen. People mumble, tummies rumble, clothes brush on microphones, clocks tick, computers hum, tapes run out and batteries fail. Voices may be non-uniformly distorted in tonality or nasality, or unnaturally amplified or suppressed, subtly influencing the viewer long accustomed to the quality of TV and movie. Voice activation, ambient noise suppression mechanisms, static, activity outside the microphone or camera range, or involving soft speech, shadows or reflections, may cause an audio or video to fail to clearly capture words or events that the examiner observed and found sufficiently relevant to make notes about. This may create a 'Hobson's choice' dilemma for the reviewer, compelled to assign relative weight to the electronic record and to the version of events noted and/or recollected by the examiner.

Preliminary studies suggest that formal testing results may be negatively affected by the presence of observers or recording devices, in a selective, non-uniform fashion. In one study, audio recording appeared to negatively affect verbal learning and recall but not motor performance (33). In another, video recording negatively affected immediate and delayed memory performance but not motor performance or recognition memory (34). Such studies indicate that both direct observation and indirect observation via recording devices may have a negative effect on psychological test results, posing a threat to the validity of tests developed without scrutiny for such variables, and placing in jeopardy the reliability of the test results and the relevance to the specific evaluee of subsequent interpretations of test results.

Selection of Assessment Procedures

It is routine for TBI assessment reports to be closely scrutinized by all parties, and actively critiqued, particularly by opposing counsel who may retain professionals for that specific and sole purpose. The examiner should be aware that every aspect, including the selection of questions and tests, the method of carrying out the tests, the findings, and their interpretation, will be subject to retrospective analysis and possibly to aggressive criticism. Clinicolegal examiners do not have the option of citing as excuses the practical exigencies of daily practice; examiners are expected to set aside as much time as necessary to carry out all relevant testing, to review all potentially significant documentation, to seek a complete data base and only then to comprehensively analyze data and formulate opinions without urgency. Nevertheless, even the most thorough and methodical approach is not safe from criticism.

Due to differences of opinion regarding optimal methods of investigation, no set of medical, psychological or neuropsychological test procedures is beyond the critic's reach. However, criticism is far less successfully applied to tests and assessment procedures that are standardized, have a strong research base for relevance, validity and reliability, are well accepted and commonly taught and used within the profession for the same general or specific purpose, and have a history of acceptance in the courts.

Testing must comply with accepted standards and protocols; to further ensure the perception of even-handedness the clinician may benefit from consistently applying the same test protocols to all patients seen with the same condition. (e.g., a medical evaluation of functional recovery, for all TBI claimants whose residual symptoms include excess daytime fatigue, might routinely include an Epworth Sleepiness Scale for severity quantification, and a differential diagnostic screening for comorbid but non-traumatic nocturnally disruptive conditions such as sleep apnea or benign prostatic hypertrophy).

It is appropriate to omit or take particular precautions with administering, considering and, reporting tests that have poor validity and reliability – which nevertheless remain in widespread usage. To a reasonable extent the clinician may need to explain why each such commonly used test was not employed, and what other tests was substituted and with what advantages.

Not uncommonly, rather than developing and defending their own protocols, examiners rely reflexively upon published authorities, without ensuring familiarization with both strengths and weaknesses. One widely used reference is the American Medical Association Guides to the Evaluation of Permanent Impairment (GEPI) (35), which throughout its' five editions to date (2001), has provided, in substantial detail, sets of standardized measurement procedures; describes means of determining the tolerances of intra-observer variability; and offers alternative methods to direct measurements – such as Diagnosis Related Estimates (DRE). Critics of the GEPI complain that the authors do not adequately acknowledge the limitations inherent in consensus-based guidelines, the dearth of strictly validated sets of test processes for impairment measurement in the various bodily Systems, lack of specific identification, correlation and weighting of impairments to various instrumental and personal activities of daily living (ADL), or the perpetuation of confusion regarding such terms as impairment and disability, among numerous other limitations.

The examiner should acknowledge limitations in current knowledge. Moreover, if, under special circumstances, experimental procedures or normative data not representative of the examinee's condition are used, test results must be interpreted cautiously, and clear documentation of these procedures and the rationale for their use and potential for erroneous labelling (e.g. selectivity and specificity) should be provided.

There is a danger in utilizing test procedures that are anecdotal in origin, such as those one might develop over the years within one's own practice, or might acquire from mentors and colleagues. Proving validity and reliability may require blind testing of substantial groups of subjects, with comparison of results and interpretation to tests of established reliability. Caution should be employed in the use of tests which may be well accepted in certain domains of impairment evaluation, but have no known reliability or usefulness in other domains. For example, JAMAR grip testing is routinely employed in functional capacity testing for chronic pain and orthopaedic impairment cases; consistent, full effort is required for the results to be valid for peak strength. Falsification is a serious concern. The Rapid Exchange Grip (REG) test (rapidly alternating right and left hand grips) has been found to be very difficult to falsify and REG results are considered relevant to the question of whether full effort was consistently exerted, and thus whether the measurements obtained on routine JAMAR grip testing were representative of peak strength. However, the typical test subject has no neurolegical impairment of coordination, pace, propioception, or motor tone. The validity and reliability, for applying the REG to TBI patients with hemiparesis, spasticity, or apraxia, remains insufficiently tested and thus unknown.

Delegation in Testing

Delegation of testing to one's subordinates is a source of potentially critical flaws. Delegation may be found in certain procedures such as electromyography, neuropsychology, or even interview taking, test administration and/or physical examinations. However, delegation of interpretation is never acceptable. Standardizing methods, order and choice of procedures, ensuring training and maintenance of competence, and minimizing or excluding subjective input are all elementary requirements of appropriate delegation.

It is self-evident that delegation of interviewing not only reduces the evaluator's total contact time with the evaluee but also reduces the dynamic interview element of following leads created by hesitation or special comment, facial expression, vagueness and/or ambiguity. On the other hand, the accusation that the interviewer rushed the interview or selected questions that precluded the evaluee from providing complete or balanced information is offset when an assessment is allotted a standard amount of time and pace, and a standardized, core set of questions and checklists is employed, an essential approach to TBI cases.

While it would seem that there is no 'right' answer applicable to all clinicians, or all circumstances, the general principles remain applicable: the evaluator is ultimately responsible for the comprehensiveness and validity of all data collection, and for its interpretation. When it can be shown that more direct evaluation or testing

time, with either a more standardized or a more dynamic, responsive approach, would have led to a better outcome then valid criticism can be applied; and the weight given to the examiner's opinion proportionately diminished.

TBI CLINICOLEGAL REPORTING

Critical Components

The report of any comprehensive independent examination should include the following: demographic details; referral source; party responsible for payment; basis of report (file review alone, claimant alone, family interview etc.); documents requested and reviewed; documents requested but not received; history of present illness; past medical history; family medical history; psychosocial history; educational history; vocational history, including military history if applicable; legal history, including both civil and criminal, as applicable; review of medical systems; comprehensive review of examination findings, including pertinent negative findings; validity of findings, including results of response validity assessments; diagnostic impressions; opinions regarding current and expected future status; maximum medical improvement (MMI) and prognostic opinions; causality and apportionment opinions; risk and restrictions as related to the injury or disease in question; recommendations for treatment or further diagnostic studies; degree of confidence in findings and conclusions; and relevant appendices, clauses and caveats. All opinions should be qualified by degree of certainty (e.g. likelihood with greater than 50% confidence is termed 'probable', while 50:50 or less is termed 'possible'; strong qualifiers of confidence in common clinical use include 'balance of probabilities' and 'reasonable medical certainty').

Review of Documentation

A critically important component of the report is the thoughtful review of specific findings and opinions from medical records. Although some readers with access to all medical records may find this integration of information to be repetitive, the independent examination report is sometimes the only place where a comprehensive integration of the totality of relevant information can be found. A review of background information and medical opinions serves to (a) demonstrate that the records were reviewed, (b) establish the temporal relationship of complaints to sthe reported injury, (c) facilitate an analysis of the symptom profile in relation to the type of injury being claimed, (d) evaluate the consistency of symptom reporting over time and across contexts, (e) evaluate indicators suggestive of recovery, if present, over time, and (f) provide clear delineation of the inferential reasoning process employed.

It is important to identify and discuss the potential relevance of any materials or other sources of information not available to the examiner for review. Not uncommonly in TBI case work, this may include prior records which might indicate fetal problems, birth trauma, childhood trauma or infection. School records of achievement and behaviour, as well as any learning deficit, and any intelligence, personality or aptitude testing, can all be of enormous value in appreciating acquired deficits.

There may be situations in which the examiner is not provided with all consultant, treatment or investigative records related to a case. Such restrictions limit the confidence that the examiner can place in his or her own findings. It is relevant to realize that the same shortcomings of database were likely in effect when other professionals reviewed the case, and the same reservations can be fairly applied to the balance of opinions already advanced by others and thus to be found in the file.

Materials not provided can be ranked as to potential importance to report completion. Thus, material may be deemed either Critically Required for a competent evaluation, or merely of Potential Value to clarification or confirmation of existing evidence.

Critically required documentation contains data expected to be of considerable importance, such that without access it would be impossible and improper for the ethical, expert examiner to offer informed, authoritative final conclusions. Thus, certain past medical records may contain information critical to establishing date of onset or other causation-related facts; disinterested clinical or other observer records may enhance one's understanding of the nature and sequence of an event, or provide independent sources of information about daily function, to supplement the narrative interview of the evaluee or family members. As a specific illustration, when a student suffers a TBI and claims subsequent impairment of academic abilities, corroboration or clarification may be critically influenced by a direct review of prior as well as subsequent academic records of attendance, behaviour and marks, essays and test answers.

Materials of potential value might include documents whose review would be prudent, to ensure thoroughness. For example, one or more 'silent periods' in which there are no entries in either prior or post-injury medical records provided, out of keeping with established care-seeking patterns and/or spanning long periods of time, might well be corroborative of claims of interim good health or stoic self-reliance; alternatively these chronological 'black holes' may reflect undisclosed health care in the same or another community, or even episodes of incarceration. Completion of the healthcare record may reveal unsuspected premorbid or comorbid social, familial, legal, vocational, financial, psychiatric or physical problems - including instances of prior traumatic, vascular, infectious or other brain injury.

It may also be prudent, and sometimes it is critically important, for examiners to request (where appropriate to scope of practice) raw data from certain testing procedures or hard copies of pertinent radiologic studies and to consider seeking opportunities for corroboratory interviews to round out information collection.

Regarding the overall analysis of assembled information, including examination findings already carried out and documented in prior records, it is reasonable for the examiner to comment on the appropriateness of diagnostic procedures and processes employed, and the consequent reliability and validity of the findings, including estimation of the degree to which the measures used were specific and sensitive to the condition being examined, and the degree of confidence that can be placed in the interpretations and opinions presented. Many examiners feel uncomfortable commenting on the methods and/or conclusions of their colleagues, especially in the absence of the raw data. However, balanced, expert, critical reviews are essential to promotion of thoroughness and objectivity and thus are essential to quality assurance in examinations in clinicolegal settings. Each step in the examination process should be open to critical evaluation in the context of the case and the research literature. The reviewer needs to establish that there has been appropriate choice and administration of tests, proper and balanced interpretation of all of the test data, appropriate data assembly, and sufficient and unbiased reporting of all data. However, in the absence of required raw data, informed critical review may not be possible and report completion may have to be suspended.

Completeness of Records and Disclosure of Findings

Clinicolegal examinations require complete documentation of all procedures conducted and results obtained. The examiner must create appropriate documentation in the expectation that one's records will be critically reviewed by independent professionals both within and outside of one's areas of professional specialty. In addition to formal reports, all information generated during an examination, including handwritten notes and test protocols, may be subject to review by others. Some practitioners advocate for inclusion of all handwritten notes as part of their final report, including copies of all testing results (sans any copyrighted materials). Notes must be legible and abbreviations universal or otherwise unequivocal in interpretation.

Drafts and Final Reports

Ethical practice requires that examination findings be presented objectively, fully and carefully in a report, that no inaccurate documentation be generated, especially for information not obtained or findings not made, with no salient information excluded. Notably, distinct from internal drafts, some professionals will release preliminary reports prior to preparing a final report. Like most other areas of practice, the reasons for such procedures and the manner in which they are handled determine the degree to which these may potentially challenge ethical principles. Certainly, offering the referring party one or more drafts and soliciting 'feedback' will introduce potential for perception of, as well as actual, biasing of the final report.

Distinct from the above might be a circumstance in which a preliminary report is released to apprise the parties of the status of a continuing evaluation, including justification for requests for further visits, tests or documents. Similarly, a preliminary draft may be released to the referring party along with a specific request for confirmation that all issues of concern have been addressed fully and clearly. It follows that no material alteration in the findings or conclusions, reflecting the referring party's censorial or advocatorial preferences should appear in the subsequent final report.

A report may be released in stages, involving independent components. Any released report component should be considered final for its purpose. Thus, while pending neuropsychological testing or current school year marks prevents completion of a report on spectrum and severity of impairment from TBI, an initial report may be released in which the evaluator addresses questions of causation, mechanism, and diagnosis.

The temptation to request 'tweaking' (alteration to enhance value) of the final report can be irresistible to advocatorial referring/paying parties. Once a final report is issued, the examiner must carefully consider whether and how to respond to any subsequent requests for alterations by the referring party, the evaluee or others. The examiner should always insist on first receiving any such request in writing. Some requests for changes are fully justifiable, including typographical, chronological or factual errors. It is also appropriate to respond to requests for clarification or amplification or requests of similarly constructive nature, while avoiding altering or debating the findings or opinions. Common instances include requests for clarification of technical terms or reasoning for the court, or for the clinician's opinion to be stated in accord with the formulaic language of legislation – as an example, it may be required that the report unequivocally establish whether impairments meet a verbal threshold such as 'substantial', 'permanent' or 'severe'; an opinion regarding a treatment may require specific reference to whether it is both 'necessary and reasonable'.

Options for rectification of factual errors include: 1) attaching an amended page to the report, 2) marking through the incorrect portion of the report by putting a single line through the incorrect material so that the original can still be read, and then writing (and initialling) the correction in the space above the line, or 3) producing a corrected version of the report and documenting the

rationale within a cover letter. All draft and amended versions of reports, (other than those which fall under solicitor-expert privilege such as notes and other work-products made solely for purposes of discussion with the referring party), should be maintained and produced upon request, as a proof of credibility. Self-tweaking an unsupported conclusion in advance of report release is not ethical; the examiner's report should closely correspond to his/her written records.

Use of Disclaimer Statements

It is recommended that examiners have a disclaimer at the beginning or end of their reports reiterating the basis of the report and the opinions, as related to his/her qualifications. It should be noted that all opinions were provided with the strength of "probability", (greater than 50%) unless otherwise indicated. It is also advisable that examiners include a statement noting that their conclusions are based, in part, on the assumption that the materials provided for review are complete and correct and that if any additional information becomes available at a later date, opinions may be subject to change. It will be relevant to state, in the case of a file review, whether the opportunity for direct clinical assessment was offered, and to what extent such an opportunity might have resulted in a different set of conclusions and recommendations. It is relevant to state the nature and source of the referral, and any special instructions. For example, the examiner may wish to clarify that referral originated with plaintiff's counsel, relating to an MVA claim of a certain date, and that the referral request included a specific request for, or direction to deal only with, the management and prognosis of post-TBI seizures.

It is relevant to declare the absence of any known conflict of interest, or to explain how any potential conflicts were identified and addressed. For example, where two physicians work in an assessment centre, and one has been a treating practitioner, the second – in the role of independent examiner – should state that the case was never discussed between them; that the provision of a second opinion is common in medical practice; and that the examiner felt no reservations about discussing in his/her report any area of disagreement over diagnosis involving his colleagues.

USE OF EXPERT WITNESSES

Expert Witness Fees

Examiners are typically entitled to be paid at higher rates for clinico-legal work than for routine clinical services, owing to factors such as (a) requirements for an expanded, and specialized scope of knowledge and assessment skills; (b) special stressors and exceptional rigor required in maintaining the standards and following guidelines associated with the litigation process; (c) the exceptional impact of such work on clinical responsibilites, including detraction from normal patient scheduling, and need for arranging clinical coverage, under circumstances of deadlines and unpredictable scheduling, etc.; (d) requirements for careful reading and note taking of substantial amounts of material; and (e) special precision in note taking and record keeping, report structure and preparation, proofing, correction, issuance, privacy issues, etc.

However, the creation of differential fee structures also creates a set of serious ethical issues. The primary concern, from the perspective of perception if not reality, is that differential fees introduce financial incentives, capable of exerting at least a subtle influence on the assessment process and formulation of opinions. The aforementioned must be counteracted by avoidance of any contingencies to the payment arrangement. Neither the size of the fee nor the timing and assurance of payment should ever be contingent upon the outcome of the case. The prospects of future referrals should not be contingent on favourability of opinion to the referring party. Such factors introduce bias, and such behavior is clearly proscribed in professional ethics codes.

Professional fees and terms should be agreed upon at the outset, involving mutual understanding of the feasibility and level of challenge of the type and scope of assessment contemplated. It is preferrable that there be clarification of whether the fee is fixed or can be adjusted by the evaluator according to actual time, effort, and complications encountered during the assessment. Clearly, the establishment of fixed fees carries a greater perception of disinterest in individual cases; however, in order to avoid a negative bias against the referral source it is important to ensure appropriate adjustments for unanticipated and specially onerous circumstances such as urgency, need to seek further documentation, special research, language barriers, multiple or last minute cancellations and rebookings, or the especially difficult to examine evaluee. A reasonable compromise may involve either a set of standard fees that factor in exigencies, or a set of fee ranges, with terms for payment that do not change for particular referring parties.

The ethical burden can be somewhat alleviated by consistently referring to or utilizing published fee schedules and application guidelines from professional organizations. Ultimately the ethical test will be one of justification: can the evaluator explain how a fee and terms were developed within the context of a specific case. Clear records for that case and for comparable cases must be kept and kept available. Ethical behaviour therefore includes both internal consistency within one's own practice, and general consistency to the practices of one's ethical colleagues. In the latter context, ethical standards for medical experts can be expressed in terms of "reasonableness" and "consistency" of fees (36). In this case,

"reasonableness" is defined as the degree of similarity to fees charged by other examiners in similar specialties and localities; "consistency" is defined as the degree to which fees are compatible with other medical procedures of similar demand provided by the practitioner or his peer group, as well as for similar time units.

Court-Selected and Court-Hired Experts

The use of court-nominated examiners is a potential solution to problems of partiality or advocacy. Recently, judges in Virginia have begun playing an increased role in the selection of experts for independent evaluations. Specifically, the presiding trier of fact may solicit a list or panel of experts from one or both counsel, from which the judge, or the judge in collaboration with opposing counsel, selects the professional to perform an independent evaluation. Although initially applied in situations where opposing counsel protested or attempted to block utilization of a particular expert, this practice seems to be expanding to other contexts.

Ideally, this approach to neutrality would find the trier of fact supervising or making the referral decisions, after a consensus process which ensures through careful selection that the experts will provide the court with objective, reliable, complete information. However, the experts must be commensurately remunerated for their consensually agreed upon capability, objectivity and ethics, and as a corollary their commitment to avoid the various degrees of "scientific perjury" which some other referral systems may encourage. Joint commitment to funding also ensures that payment is never contingent on outcome, and will not be subject to delay/discount/ bonus. There is the further attraction that the expert and the court are relieved of the time consuming and stressful process of impeaching experts by opposing counsel.

Admissibility of Expert Witness TBI Testimony

The type of testimony that is admissible in court depends on the type of professional role that the expert plays in a given case (e.g., treating doctor/fact witness or expert witness). The treating doctor is permitted to present information related to clinical assessment and treatment conducted based on medical judgment of necessity and reasonableness. In contrast, the expert witness (in federal court and those state courts which accept Daubert (1)) may now be held to the Daubert standard (1) that scientific testimony must be supported by valid scientific theory or techniques. Specifically, Daubert requires that the scientific strategy or procedure has been tested, published under peer review, and is well accepted in the scientific community. Because the skills that make a good expert witness are not always consistent with reliance on "good science", the Daubert ruling seems to offer attorneys and the court a useful strategy for evaluating the merit of expert testimony. Given the complexity of many diagnostic procedures, particularly in TBI, scrutiny of the scientific methodology on which diagnoses are based is warranted, indeed essential.

Monitoring Bias in Examiners and Examinees

In the context of personal injury examinations, clinical attribution bias refers to the consistent and predictable tendency to incorrectly attribute current symptoms to the injury or to the event in question. It typically results in a confounding of accurate diagnosis and appropriate treatment. Patients demonstrate inadvertent attribution bias when they incorrectly interpret periodic, common cognitive inefficiencies as being pathological, entirely attributable to a resolved Mild TBI. Ironically, attribution bias may interact with true neurogenic symptoms to increase impairment. Attribution bias can be influenced by others (e.g., family, attorneys or healthcare professionals) and, unfortunately, can also occur intentionally.

An examinee's presentation and approach to test taking exists on a continuum ranging from valid to response biased. Due to the financial incentive to misrepresent one's optimal performance during examinations in clinicolegal contexts, evaluation of the examinee's response validity is a necessary component of the examination. The examiner must ensure that assessments, recommendations, reports, and diagnostic or evaluative statements are substantiated by sufficient information and techniques. Formal assessment of response validity is essential in order to increase the likelihood that interpretation of test data will be based on reliable results of valid tests; that is, the results will reflect the examinee's true abilities and deficits.

Examiner misattribution bias represents a problematic source of error that can violate the core ethical principle of avoiding harm. Clinicians sensitized to the signs and symptoms of their particular specialty may misdiagnose or over-diagnose problems, with inadequate attention to competing explanations. For example, a Neurologist and a Psychiatrist, when confronted with a same symptom set, may be prone to speciality-specific diagnoses of, respectively, either brain injury or psychosocial distress (37). Inadequate rigor in developing appropriate diagnosis causes increased medical costs, inappropriate treatment, treatment failures and even chronic disability in the injured person. These errors can be prevented in TBI patients by comprehensive assessment that integrates data from observation, history, examination, radiological and neuropsychological testing and collateral sources, with a critical appraisal of base-rates of relevant symptoms (38–40) and careful differential diagnosis of all possible explanations for symptoms.

Chapman and Elstein (41) have discussed how biases can occur in the face of uncertainty in medical decision-making. Examiners can signal decision bias through any predictable tendencies: such as consistently discounting certain complaints as either not credible or unimportant; or to the contrary, consistently accepting all complaints uncritically, as self-validating (42). Compelling evidence of perceived expert witness bias is offered from a Federal Judiciary Committee sanctioned study, by Johnson, Krafka and Cecil (43), of active Federal judges and lead attorneys who presented the docket cases before them. For 1991 to 1998, the primary problem with expert testimony was experts who "abandon objectivity and become advocates for the side that hired them" (p. 5). Mean rating of partisan bias of experts on a 1–5 Likert rating scale was approximately 3.7. Clearly, there is a need for development, dissemination and universal acceptance of bias-avoidance guidelines, and of active promotion of objectivity and ethical conduct in clinico-legal contexts. However, when seious ethical violations are observed in colleagues, carefully deliberated action is indicated.

ADDRESSING ETHICAL VIOLATIONS

Consistent with previously mentioned survey results, it is not uncommon in clinicolegal practice to observe apparently unethical work by colleagues. In order to protect patients, referral sources, and payors, and to preserve the reputation of one's profession, it is necessary to actively but appropriately address potential ethical violations, when they are observed (44). Perhaps nothing so diminishes a profession's reputation as the disclosure that the 'community' has known and tolerated or even covered up a colleague's substance abuse, patient abuse, incompetence or unethical clinicolegal behaviour over an extended period of time.

Competency and objectivity may be the most frequently violated ethical standards. However, caution must be exercised in order to ensure that perceptions of incompetence or non-objectivity in a colleague are not overly reflective of professional or ideological differences. Certainly, there exist widespread differences of opinion in a number of areas of practice. Sensitivity to such differences is paramount.

However, the clinician who practices or makes judgments outside of even these diverse positions is at risk for justifiable implication of ethical misconduct if such practices or judgments cannot be defended through referral to published standards and guidelines, and recent research literature.

It is important to consider that consistent attribution bias may merely reflect a particular, sincere viewpoint rather than crass claim advocacy. In such instances, the identical attribution pattern can be expected no matter which side made the referral, or how sizable was the fee.

The authors acknowledge that the decision regarding whether or not to confront the poor judgment or apparent ethical misconduct of a colleague may be one of the more difficult professional decisions. That difficulty may be related to a number of factors, including uncertainty about the nature of the behavior and whether or not it occurred, as well as personal feelings toward the colleague, fear of retaliation, and uncertainty about how to address potential misconduct. However, the clinician must be candid with him/herself, as to whether such explanations and excuses are merely self-justifications for an attitude of complacency, or truly necessitate exemption from responsible actions.

Regulatory professional Boards and Colleges may bear some responsibility in this regard: by excess tolerance of either unethical behaviour or revealed instances of collegial complacency; or by lack of mechanisms for efficiently and confidentially receiving notifications of ethical violation concerns by professional colleagues and then promptly and professionally investigating them.

CONCLUSIONS

Given the potentially devastating impact on all facets of life, TBI represent an very important subset of overall clinicolegal casework. Sadly, as with clinicolegal casework in general, TBI casework offers considerable potential for apparent or real ethical misconduct. The potential for harm is commensurately increased with patient vulnerability, particularly true of the TBI patient.

The ability to identify, for oneself, any areas of particular risk is the essential first step in avoiding not only actual ethical misconduct, but also the appearance of same. For competent professionals, the *loss of objectivity* is the primary risk factor for ethically compromised behavior.

In addition to competency and objectivity, a *lack of awareness and familiarity*: with relevant recent legal cases e.g., Daubert vs. Merrell Dow (1), with new methods and procedures, and with changes in relevant ethics codes, place the examiner at an ethical disadvantage. Thus, ongoing education on the application of ethical principles to clinicolegal practice is required for ethical professional behavior.

In order to promote consistently high levels of competent and ethical clinico-legal practice, the legal system must continue to establish *contingencies* and to use reliable *indices*, in order to genuinely increase the likelihood of objective examinations and testimony.

Proactivity is the proper response, when ethical misconduct is observed in one's colleagues. Appropriate steps need to be taken to prevent the abuse of the consumers of clinico-legal services and to promote the public's perception of fairness and consequent trust in the clinicolegal process. Ultimately, this is also of great service to one's profession, to one's professional colleagues, and to the generation of clinicians who will follow, emulate and ultimately replace us.

References

1. Daubert v. Merrell Pharmaceuticals, 61 U.S.L. W 4805 (U.S. June 29, 1993).
2. American Medical Association Policy: *E-10.03 Patient-Physician Relationship in the Context of Work-Related and Independent Medical Examinations.* Adopted June 1999. American Medical Association Website (AMA Policy). June 16, 2004. *www.ama-assn.org.*
3. National Academy of Neuropsychology Position Paper: *Independent and Court Ordered Forensic Neuropsychological Examinations: Official Statement of the National Academy of Neuropsychology Approved by the Board of Directors 10/14/03. www.nanonline.org/paio/IME.shtm.* Retrieved 27/07/04.
4. National Academy of Neuropsychology Position Paper: Symptom validity assessment: Practice issues and medical necessity: Official Statement of the National Academy of Neuropsychology, Approved by the Board of Directors 2/28/05. www.nanonline.org/downloads/paio/Position/NANsvt.pdf. Retrieved 4/21/06.
5. Pope K.S., Vetter V.A., Ethical Dilemmas encountered by Members of the American Psychological Association: A National Survey. *American Psychologist* 1992;47(3):397–411.
6. Brittain J.L., Frances J.P., and Barth J.T. Ethical Issues and Dilemmas in Neuropsychological Practice Reported by ABCN Diplomates. *Advances in Medical Psychotherapy* 1995;8:1–22.
7. Beauchamp Tom L., James F. Childress. *Principles of Biomedical Ethics, 4th ed.* New York: Oxford University Press, 1994.
8. American Medical Association, Council on Ethical and Judicial Affairs. *Code of Medical Ethics: Current Opinions with Annotations.* 1996, Washington, D.C.
9. American Academy of Physical Medicine and Rehabilitation. *Expert Witness Testimony.* 1992: White Paper.
10. American Academy of Psychiatry and the Law. Ethical Guidelines for the Practice of Forensic Psychiatry. *American Academy of Psychiatry and the Law x–xiii:* Bloomfield CT: Author. 1989.
11. Greenberg S.A., and Shulman D.W., Irreconcilable Conflict Between Therapeutic and Forensic Roles. *Professional Psychology: Research and Practice* 1997;28(1):50–57.
12. Shulman D.W., Greenberg S.A., Heilbrun K., and Foote W.E. An Immodest Proposal: Should treating Mental Health Professionals Be Barred From Testifying About Their Patients? *Behavioural Sciences and the Law* 1998;16:509–523.
13. Blau, T. *The Psychologist as Expert Witness* New York: John Wiley & Sons, 1984.
14. Blau,T. The Psychologist as Expert Witness. *Workshop Presented at the National Academy of Neuropsychology Annual Meeting.* Reno Nevada: 1992.
15. American Medical Association. *American Medical Association Guides to the Evaluation of Permanent Impairment 4th ed.* Chicago: American Medical Association, 1993.
16. Strasburger H., Gutheil T.G. Brodsky B.A. On Wearing Two Hats: Role Conflict In Serving as Both Psychotherapist and Expert Witness. *American Journal of Psychiatry* 1997;154 (4):48–56.
17. Sweet J.J., Moulthrop M.A., Self-Examination Questions as a Means of Identifying Bias in Adversarial Assessments. *Journal of Forensic Neuropsychology* 1998;(1):73–88.
18. Lees-Haley P. Commentary on Sweet and Moulthrop's De-Biasing Procedures. *Journal of Forensic Neuropsychology* 1999;1(3):43–47.
19. Brodsky S.L. *Testifying in Court: Guidelines and Maxims for the Expert Witness* Washington, D.C.: American Psychological Association, 1991.
20. Martelli M.F., Zasler N.D., and Grayson, R. Ethical Considerations in Medicolegal Evaluation of Neurologic Injury and Impairment. *Neurorehabilitation: An Interdisciplinary Journal* 1999a; 13(1):45–66.
21. Weiner (ed.). R.B Martelli M.F., and Zasler N.D. Ethics and Objectivity in Medicolegal Contexts: Recommendations for

Experts. *Pain Management: A Practical Guide For Clinicians* Boca Ratan Florida: St. Lucie Press, 2001a.

22. Martelli M.F., Zasler N.D., and Johnson-Green D. Promoting Ethical and Objective Practice in the Medicolegal Arena of Disability Evaluation. *Disability Evaluation: Physical Medicine and Rehabilitation Clinics of North America* 2001b;12(3): 571–584.

23. May, R.V., Martelli M.F. (eds.). Martelli M.F., Zasler N.D., and Grayson R. Ethical Considerations in Impairment and Disability Evaluations Following Acquired Brain Injury. *Guide to Functional Capacity Evaluation With Impairment Rating Applications* Richmond: NADEP Publications, 1999(b).

24. Binder L.M., and Thompson L.L. The Ethics Code and Neuropsychological Assessment Practices. *Archives of Clinical Neuropsychology* 1995;10(1):27–46.

25. National Academy of Neuropsychology Position Paper: Symptom validity assessment: Practice issues and medical necessity: Official Statement of the National Academy of Neuropsychology, Approved by the Board of Directors 2/28/05. www.nanonline.org/downloads/paio/Position/NANsvt.pdf. Retrieved 4/21/06.

26. National Academy of Neuropsychology Position Paper: Symptom validity assessment: Practice issues and medical necessity: Official Statement of the National Academy of Neuropsychology, Approved by the Board of Directors 2/28/05. www.nanonline.org/downloads/paio/Position/NANsvt.pdf. Retrieved 4/21/06.

27. Binder J.T., Johnson-Greene D. Observer effects on Neuropsychological Performance: A Case Report. *The Clinical Neuropsychologist*, 1995;9:74–78.

28. McCaffrey R.J., Fisher J.M., Gold G.A. and Lynch J.K. The Presence of Third Parties During Neuropsychological Evaluations: Who is Evaluating Whom? *The Clinical Neuropsychologist* 1996; 10(40):435–449.

29. National Academy of Neuropsychology, Policy and Planning Committee. Presence of Third Party Observers During Neuropsychological Testing: Official Statement of the National Academy of Neuropsychology. *Archives of Clinical Neuropsychology* 2000a;15(5):379–380.

30. National Academy of Neuropsychology, Policy and Planning Committee. The Use of Neuropsychology Test Technicians in Clinical Practice: Official Statement of the National Academy of Neuropsychology. *Archives of Clinical Neuropsychology* 2000b;15(5): 381–382.

31. National Academy of Neuropsychology, Policy and Planning Committee. Test Security: Official Statement of the National Academy of Neuropsychology 2003. Retrieved 17/02/04 from http://nanonline.prg/paio/security_update.htm

32. Hamsher K., Baron I.S. and Lee G.P. *Third Party Observers: Policy Statement for The American Academy of Clinical Neuropsychology,* 1999.

33. Constantinou M. Ashendorf L., McCaffrey R.J. When the Third Party Observer of a Neuropsychological Evaluation is an Audio-Recorder. *Clin Neuropsycholog* 2002;16(3):407–12.

34. Constantinou M, McCaffrey R.J. The Effects of 3rd Party Observation: When the Observer is a Video *Camera.Archives of Clinical Neuropsychology* 2003:18(7):788–789.

35. *American Medical Association Guides to the Evaluation of Permanent Impairment 5th ed.*American Medical Association. Chicago, Illinois: 2001.

36. Shiffman M.A. Medical Expert Witness Fees and Court. *The Forensic Examiner* 1997;6(5–6):26.

37. May, R.V., Martelli, M.F. Richmond (Eds.) Martelli M.F., Zasler, N.D., Grayson R. Ethical Considerations in Impairment and Disability Evaluations Following Acquired Brain Injury. *Guide to Functional Capacity Evaluation With Impairment Rating Applications* NADEP Publications, 1999(b).

38. Sweet J.J. (ed.). Gouvier W.D. Base Rates and Clinical Decision Making in Neuropsychology *Forensic Neuropsychology: Fundamentals and Practice.* Lisse, NL: Swets & Zeitlinger Publishers, 1999.

39. Lees-Haley P., and Brown R. Neuropsychological Complaint Base Rates of 170 Personal Injury Claimants. *Archives of Clinical Neuropsychology* 1993;8:203–209.

40. Lees-Haley P., and Courtney J.C. Isn't Everything in Forensic Neuropsychology Controversial? *Neurorehabilitation* 2001;16(4): 267–274.

41. Chapman G.B., Sonnenberg F.A., and Frank A. (Eds.) Chapman G.B., and Elstein A.S. Cognitive Processes and Biases in Medical Decision Making. *Decision Making in Health Care: Theory, Psychology, and Applications. Cambridge Series on Judgment and Decision Making* New York, New York: Cambridge University Press, 2000:183–210.

42. McBeath J.G. Labelling of Post Concussion Patients as Malingering and Litigious: A Common Practice in Need of Criticism. *Headache* 2000;40:609–10.

43. Johnson M.T., Krafka C., and Cecil J.S. Expert Testimony in Federal Civil Trials: A Preliminary Analysis. *Federal Judicial Center* 2000.

44. Grote C.L., Lewin J.L., Gould J.W. and Van Gorp W.G. Responses to Perceived Unethical Practices in Clinical Neuropsychology: Ethical and Legal Considerations. *The Clinical Neuropsychologist* 2000;14(10):119–134.

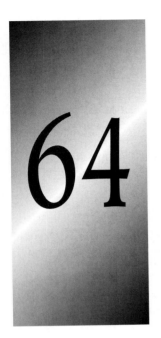

64

Assessment of Response Bias in Clinical and Forensic Evaluations of Impairment Following TBI

Michael F. Martelli
Keith Nicholson
Nathan D. Zasler
Mark C. Bender

INTRODUCTION

Evaluation of neurologic impairments and associated disability presents a significant diagnostic challenge. In cases of more catastrophic or functionally disabling injuries, the evaluations and opinions of different medical practitioners are often fairly consistent. In other cases, however, the evaluations and opinions of practitioners may vary widely.

Impairment and disability evaluation following neurologic injury typically involves such contexts as social security disability application, personal injury litigation, worker's compensation claims, disability insurance policy application, other health care insurance policy coverage, and determination of competence to handle finances or other important life functions (e.g., parenting) or decisions. Traditionally, these evaluations have fallen within the purview of the general fields of physical medicine and rehabilitation, neurology, neurosurgery, psychiatry, psychology and neuropsychology. More recently, and especially in cases of less catastrophic and more subtle cognitive impairment and disability, practitioners who specialize in brain injury evaluation and treatment are increasingly relied upon.

Impairment and disability evaluation may be one of the more misunderstood areas of work as it applies to assessment and treatment of persons with injury residua and/or functional limitations due to injury. The task of making determinations regarding impairment and disability in persons with neurologic impairment and injury is fraught with potential obstacles and confounding issues. This is due in part to the frequently subtle yet complex nature of the deficits involved, as well as the lack of formal, scientifically validated "rating systems" for many of the deficits associated with these disorders. There are multiple possible types of problems associated with brain or other neurologic injury and there are often a number of other associated problems such as chronic pain or psychoemotional problems. Disentangling the multiple contributors to cognitive dysfunction and to impairment and disability presents a diagnostic challenge and requires careful scrutiny (1).

IMPORTANCE OF RESPONSE BIAS IN BRAIN INJURY EXAMINATION

Persons with brain injury may present with some response bias to report or demonstrate impairment or related disability. Response bias, in this chapter, is defined as a class of behaviors that reflect less than fully truthful, accurate or valid symptom report and presentation. Importantly, response bias is a ubiquitous phenomenon affecting almost any domain of human self-report. Some forms of response bias may be associated with conscious manipulation or intent to deceive but many, or most, are not. However, in the context of impairment and disability evaluations, or insurance related evaluations, the importance of conscious or other bias becomes more acute (2–4).

Given the frequent incentives to distort performance during impairment and disability examinations, assessment of examinee motivation to provide full effort to do well during assessment becomes a necessary component of such evaluations. The importance of detecting response biases is critical with regard to providing accurate diagnosis. Accurate diagnosis is prerequisite to provision of appropriate and timely treatment, to obtaining optimal recovery, to prevention of iatrogenic impairment and disability reinforcement, and to appropriate legal compensation decisions. The impairment / disability context and other internal or environmental variables make ensuring accurate representation of a patient's functional status essential. In order to ensure accuracy, a number of factors must be considered including decisions regarding validity of observed impairment and disability, symptomatology displayed during the examination, sensitivity and specificity of assessment measures, and generalizability of test findings to functioning in everyday life.

Blau (5) has expounded on the importance of determining response biases and measuring true levels of impairment in medicolegal situations. Essentially, in this arena, an alleged victim of a wrongful act or omission attempts to establish (a) causality to demonstrate entitlement to compensation for damages, which is awarded based on (b) level of damages suffered. In cases of less obvious, clear cut and significant trauma with psychologic, neurologic or soft tissue damage, causality and level of current and future damages are more difficult to prove and expert evaluation and opinion is heavily relied upon for making legal determinations. In the parallel insurance situation, the insured attempts to access entitlements to health care treatment and disability benefits, and expert evaluation and opinion are relied upon for making policy determinations. In both cases, financial and other incentives clearly represent motivational factors that increase the likelihood of response bias in the form of exaggerated or feigned symptoms.

RESPONSE BIAS ASSESSMENT

Examinee Response Biases

Examinee response bias can take several forms. Bias ranges from symptoms that may be minimized to those that are exaggerated or feigned. Exaggeration or accentuation of symptoms is usually associated with other psychological factors such as catastrophizing and are less often associated with conscious deception for the purposes of obtaining financial or other compensation, i.e., feigning or malingering. Symptoms may be accurately or inaccurately attributed to different events. For instance, pre-existing symptoms may suddenly be attributed to an accident, or pre-existing problems previously not noticed can suddenly be given more prominence due to attention and anxiety. Similarly, an accident may cause an aging person to do a self-inventory of health that reveals age related symptoms that were previously minimized or ignored. As awareness of these symptoms or difficulties, many of which may well be "normal" or common in the general population, are temporally related to an accident or injury, they are frequently misattributed to such an event. In addition, social realities also exert influence over response to injury and symptoms. For example, the vastly different consequences for diagnoses of cancer versus mild traumatic brain injury (MTBI) or back injury produce differential reinforcement. The former is clearly undesirable, negative and highly stressful, while the latter can result in desirable consequences (e.g., monetary compensation, avoidance of stressful work demands).

Martelli, Zasler, Mancini and MacMillan (6) reviewed the literature and found several injury context variables associated with poorer post-injury adaptation and recovery and increased likelihood of response bias. These are listed in Table 64-1.

These variables represent vulnerability factors, which can reduce effective coping with post injury impairments and increase the likelihood of maladaptive coping and response bias. They are not mutually exclusive and, as with the variables presented below, more than one can contribute to symptom report and presentation.

Additional review of the literature (7–15), combined with clinical experience, indicate several other sources of poor post-injury adaptation and increased likelihood of significant response bias that may be encountered during examinations. These are included in Table 64-2.

A frequently overlooked form of bias is that which is iatrogenic to an increasingly restrictive insurance and adversarial medicolegal system. In an effort to elucidate expectancy influences and bias for persons who have sustained injuries, Martelli and colleagues (6, 36) conducted convenience attitudinal surveys of professionals who evaluate and treat injured workers, rehabilitation and worker's compensation (WC) case managers, and injured workers. They found an overall 25% estimate of exaggerating or malingering WC patients, with highest estimates from WC case managers (29%), suggesting a general skepticism and distrust faced by injured workers. Furthermore, the majority of professionals and case managers filling out the survey believed that they would personally be treated unfairly by the WC system if they were injured, suggesting an even stronger general skepticism and distrust of the extant systems that fund evaluation and treatment of injury and disability. Although these data are preliminary, the findings are characteristic of the levels of diffuse distrust often observed by the authors in impairment and disability evaluation situations across the United States and Canada. These findings highlight the

TABLE 64-1

Variables Associated with Poor Post-Injury Adaptation and Response Bias

• Anger, resentment, or perceived mistreatment	• Fear of losing disability status, benefits, and safety net
• Fear of failure or rejection (e.g. damaged goods; fear of being fired after injury)	• Perceptions of high compensability for injury
• Loss of self-confidence and self-efficacy associated with residual impairments	• Pre-injury job (task, work environment) dissatisfaction
• External (health, pain) locus of control	• Collateral injuries (especially if "silent")
• Irrational fear of injury extension, re-injury, or pain	• Inadequate and inaccurate medical information
• Discrepancies between personality / coping style and injury consequences (e.g., highly physically active person with few intellectual resources who has a back injury)	• Misdiagnosis, late diagnosis, or delays in instituting treatment
• Insufficient residual coping resources and skills	
	• Insurance resistance to authorizing treatment or delays in paying bills
• Prolonged inactivity resulting in disuse atrophy	• Retention of an attorney
• Greater reinforcement for "illness" vs. "wellness" behavior	

importance of considering the motivational factors that operate on examinees that present for impairment and disability evaluations.

In an interesting conceptualization of a major type of response bias in chronically disabled workers, Matheson (7, 10–12) defined symptom magnification as a conscious or unconscious self destructive and socially reinforced pattern of behavior or symptom production intended to control life circumstances of the sufferer, but which impede health care efforts. He further defined three major subtypes. The Type I "refugee" displays illness behavior that provides escape or avoidance of life situations perceived as unsolvable. Somatization, conversion, psychogenic pain, and hypochondriacal disorders are conceptualized as extreme subcategories for this type. The Type II "game player" employs symptoms for positive gain. Although this type seems associated with malingering, Matheson argues that true malingering is a medicolegal concept, while the Type II symptom magnifier is a treatable self-destructive syndrome. The Type III "identified patient" is motivated by maintenance of the patient role as a means of life survival. Associated psychiatric diagnoses include factitious disorder.

Main and Spanswick (15) examined the response bias of simulated or exaggerated incapacity in persons claiming physical disability. They identified a list of features associated with and suggestive of simulated or exaggerated incapacity associated with chronic pain. These include: failure to comply with reasonable treatment; report of severe pain with no associated psychological effects; marked inconsistencies in effects of pain on general activities; poor work record; previous litigation. Features that they found to be not primarily suggestive of response bias included: mismatch between physical findings and reported symptoms; report of severe or

continuous pain; anger; poor response to treatment; behavioral signs / symptoms.

Attribution and Bias

Several sources of attribution bias which require assessment during evaluation of physical, sensory and neurocognitive impairments need to be considered.

Examinee attribution biases can confound accurate diagnosis. Examples include mistaking physical, cognitive, and motivation problems associated with depression and sleep disturbance for neurologic injury or sequelae. This can occur due to misattribution, over-attribution, retrospective attribution, illusory correlation, or to heightened awareness due to vigilance biases. Importantly, the previously mentioned conditions (e.g., depression, sleep disturbance) are reversible and may have been present prior to the injury without producing significant limitations. Furthermore, the emotional states or fatigue may be interacting with actual physical injury symptoms to increase impairment.

Examiner misattribution can similarly occur. Only methodical neurologic, psychologic and other assessment can differentiate sequelae secondary to brain injury from factors with overlapping presentations such as cranial/cranial adnexal and cervical trauma impairments, chronic pain, motivational factors and/or other psychological sequelae or other non-neurologic factors. When "abnormal" neurocognitive findings and/or non-specific somatic complaints are obtained, tendencies toward "over-diagnosis" of neurologic disorders, such as MTBI, can only be avoided through careful differential diagnosis. Brain injury specialists sensitized to neurologic symptoms have

---

TABLE 64-2

Additional Variables Associated with Poor Post Injury Adaptation and/or Response Bias

---

Cultural Differences. For example, different cultures mix emotional and physical pain and symptoms at a conceptual and phenomenological level in different ways. Also, some cultures see failure to impose severe penalty / extract significant compensation for harm as a sign of weakness and disgrace in God's eyes.

Conditioned Avoidance Pain Related Disability (CAPRD). CAPRD represents phobic reactions associated with fear of pain wherein behavior, either gross motor activity (kinesiophobia) or cognitive exertion (cogniphobia), is avoided due to fear of exacerbation of pain. Such behavioral reactions are typically beyond or minimally within the realm of conscious awareness and control.

Desperation Induced Malingering/ Symptom Exaggeration. Individuals that are particularly prone to these types of response bias may include the following: insecure immigrant workers, immigrants who attempt cultural assimilation but feel resentful that they were not rewarded, aging workers, tired workers, workers insecure about work changes, workers fearing their own limited or declining abilities, persons whose premorbid coping was tenuous and who feel too overwhelmed and unable to cope with an additional stress, those with real or imagined abuse from others, such as employers, family, etc., immigrants who feel rejected by the culture and feel entitled, immigrants who feel disillusioned because the new land was not everything they had hoped (i.e., those who believe this to be a viable solution to a desperate situation). A second group of patients represented by this category are those making desperate pleas for help and those who, upon confronting tests that seem different and maybe easier than the real life situations where they have problems, reduce effort to highlight their problems. Again, in some individuals such responses may not be within conscious awareness or control but, in others, there may be more explicit and conscious attempts at deception.

Sociopathic, Manipulative and Opportunistic personality traits. These personality traits can be found in all groups, but may be associated with a greater incidence of conscious dissimulation.

Passive Aggressive, Impatient, or Rebellious personality traits. Such individuals tend to resent others for not listening to them and believing them. They tend to resent imposed evaluations or doctor's visits, especially ones that examine psychological function or motivation. They may play games with doctors by withholding or undermining procedures or treatments, and may alter performance on tests that seem non-challenging or do not appear face valid.

Factitious and Somatoform Disorders. Individuals with factitious disorder and somatoform disorders (i.e., conversion disorders including non-epileptic seizures [pseudo-seizures], somatoform pain disorder, somatization disorder, and undifferentiated somatoform disorder) may present symptoms that represent a combination of several items in this table or other factors.

Psychological Decompensation. These individuals usually display conspicuous psychological distress and pathology that differentiates them from others.

Skepticism. Many individuals are very skeptical of doctors, examinations and examination procedures, and may be poorly motivated to comply with the conditions required for valid assessment.

Diagnosis Threat. This refers to the effect of negative expectations on cognitive test performance. Suhr and Gustad (13, 14) demonstrated that subjects with a history of mild head injury performed significantly worse on general intellectual and memory measures, and rated themselves as putting forth less effortful performance, when attention was called to their head injury ("diagnosis threat"). This effect may play an important role in many situations where response bias and poor adaptation are noted.

Iatrogenic bias. A frequently overlooked form of bias is that which is iatrogenic to the nature of the insurance and adversarial legal system. Preliminary attitudinal data gathered from injured workers and the individuals who treat and case manage them (6, 36) indicates a strong and prevalent skepticism and distrust faced by injured persons in the extant insurance systems. This real or perceived mistrust reflects fear and expected unfair treatment from doctor's and insurance companies that can result in a deliberate and reactive magnification of symptoms. Persons most vulnerable to this type of bias may be persons or groups with tendencies toward suspiciousness, including immigrants, outcasts, outsiders, and those who feel chronically underprivileged, "slighted" or "short-changed". As indicate above, the increased attention called to head injuries can undoubtedly produce a "diagnosis threat" effect.

---

been observed by the authors to often misdiagnose chronic pain sequelae as post-concussive symptoms, which may result in an escalation of medical costs, prolongation of inappropriate treatment, and eventual treatment failure which may contribute to a sense of helplessness and chronic disability in the injured person. Conversely, similar observations have been made for psychiatrists and psychologists prone to infer psychiatric or psychological etiologies for all pathology, including brain injury or actual physical injury (1, 6, 16).

Response Bias Assessment

Formal response bias assessment procedures, which may be lacking or only haphazardly attended to in clinical examinations, must be employed in order to increase the probability that clinical examination findings are accurate and valid reflections of impairment. Response bias exists on a continuum that extends through denial and unawareness of impairments, symptom minimization, no bias to symptom magnification and malingering. While many examinees approach testing in a forthright and adequately motivated manner, it is necessary to examine the potential for response bias with each patient.

Anosognosia or unawareness of one's deficits is a neurologic phenomenon owing to dysfunction of brain operations subserving awareness (6, 16). This condition is usually more pronounced early after injury, is typically associated with more significant neurologic insults, and can lead to chronic under appreciation of deficits.

Symptom minimization, in contrast, may be a consciously or unconsciously motivated phenomenon. It is usually motivated by either a desire to engage in activities that might otherwise be restricted or to maintain a positive view of oneself and ones life (e.g., persons high in trait "social desirability"). *Denial* is a psychological defense employed unconsciously to protect one from facing painful realizations about losses that may be overwhelming and threaten the integrity of the self. Failure to detect such biases can result in failure to identify important impairments and an overestimation of abilities that could potentially endanger the welfare of the examinee.

Symptom magnification, in contrast, refers to accentuation or exaggeration of impairment. This can occur in relation to multiple factors, can represent an attempt to inflate financial compensation, and can serve a wide range of psychological needs. Some examples include efforts to legitimize latent dependency needs; resolve pre-existing life conflicts; retaliate against employer or spouse or other; reduce anxiety; fulfill self-denigrating or self-abasement personality patterns; exert a "plea for help"; or solicit acknowledgment of perceived difficulties. Symptom exaggeration can also occur in patients with pre-morbid histories of psychiatric and psychoemotional problems who "latch on" to a specific diagnosis which not only becomes responsible for all life problems, but also promotes passivity, helplessness, and an external locus of control. When patients are assessed for claims of major disability following uncomplicated mild and often even more significant brain injury, non-neurologic contributors should be closely scrutinized. Depression, post traumatic stress disorder and other anxiety conditions or other psychiatric syndromes or psychological processes such as catastrophizing can produce symptoms that are mistaken for neurologic impairment.

Misdiagnosis of these conditions serves to promulgate misperceptions and amplify functional disability and health care costs.

Malingering is deliberate symptom production for purposes of secondary gain, especially financial compensation. Malingering in the examination setting will often be associated with unexpectedly poor performance (6). Measures of response bias should always be administered regardless of the context of the evaluation. However, this should be considered imperative in cases of medicolegal presentation or suspicion of any incentive to make less than fully effortful or accurate presentation.

Importantly, the identification of unambiguous cases of malingering is difficult. Whereas the most convincing evidence of certain or definite malingering is a confession or admission, this seldom occurs and may not be truthful. A secondary form of evidence, also unreliable, is when the person or examinee is detected, via surveillance, performing an act that they reported that they could not do. Many persons will sometimes report being unable to do certain things which may represent a response bias to report problems, negative self-evaluations or poor self-judgment A third form of evidence comes from corroboratory report, i.e., third party contradiction of what the examinee claims. There are also various problems associated with this evidence as is true of many situations when there is a discrepancy between what one party and another reports. Finally, a variety of instruments and examination procedures are available as indicators of response bias. Any of several measures designed to assess atypical, worse than chance performance, or non-organic responses can be employed to assess response bias in cognitive, motor, sensory or physical performances or self report. However, again, most of these measures also require careful clinical interpretation as there may be a number of possible alternative explanations for performance. *Importantly, the presence of response bias, although required, is not sufficient evidence of malingering as this is a probabilistic evaluation predicated on converging evidence from a thorough analysis and integration of history, contextual information, behavioral observation, interview data, examination and test data, collaborative data, and personality and emotional status data. It requires thoughtful analysis of all data (e.g., consideration of both secondary gain and secondary losses), as well as competent differential diagnosis to consider alternative explanations (16). It also* requires cautious and critical consideration of the probability of malingering vis-à-vis the limitations of the assessment and response bias measures and the potential consequences of incorrect impressions. *Measures of response bias provide valuable information for estimating the degree to which a person was presenting accurately, exerting full effort and the degree to which test results are reliable and valid and reflect actual abilities. They do not provide reliable evidence of malingering.*

Evaluating clinicians should be familiar with psychological syndromes that may present as organic disorders, including factitious disorder and somatoform disorders (e.g., conversion disorders including non-epileptic seizures [pseudo-seizures], somatoform pain disorder, somatization disorder, and undifferentiated somatoform disorder), which may be important in the differential diagnosis of malingering. Of course, the presence of a psychological syndrome and/or response bias does not necessarily exclude the diagnosis of an actual neurological syndrome or malingering. This certainly complicates the process of disentangling multiple clinical entities that sometimes co-exist. Unfortunately, the art and science of methodical differential diagnosis is too often under-appreciated in the evaluation process (1).

Examination Strategies

Physicians should be familiar with examination strategies designed to evaluate non-organic musculoskeletal and neurologic disorders, including the use of specialized bedside examination techniques for physical and cognitive dissimulation. Examples include such strategies as Hoover's test for evaluation of malingered lower extremity weakness, sideways/backwards walking for assessment of feigned gait disturbance, and a positive Stenger's test on audiologic assessment for non-organic hearing loss. Other tests that might be of value in the context of response bias detection on the physical examination include: Mankopf's maneuver, strength reflex test, arm and/or wrist drop test, hip adductor test, axial loading test, Gordon-Welberry toe test, Bowlus and Currier test, Burns bench test, Magnuson's test, and others (1, 17).

Examination findings that suggest a possible non-neurological basis for the observed impairments include patchy sensory loss, pain in an improbable nondermatomal distribution (such as a midline sensory demarcation), non-pronator drift, and/or astasia-abasia (18). Motor and other impairment inconsistencies that fluctuate or disappear under hypnosis, drug assisted interviews, or "presumed" non-observation may also suggest some psychophysiological or functional substrate and cast doubt on a hard-wired or intractable organic deficit. Importantly, some non-organic or non-neurologic signs such as hemisensory loss may be in response to central psychophysiological factors associated with actual changes in brain function (19). Both feigned and conversional hemiparesis are typically more common on the left side (18–20), perhaps due to the fact that most persons are right hand dominant. Consistency regarding laterality of symptoms, particularly with neurologic impairment and/or referred pain, should be evaluated.

When of central (versus peripheral) origin, pain complaints should be assessed, in part, by concurrently assessing temperature perception, given that the same neural pathways mediate these sensations. When temperature sensation is preserved in the presence of a loss of pain sensation, after either brain or spinal cord injury, the deficit is not likely to reflect direct CNS impairment (the loss should occur contralateral to and below the level of the lesion). This point also reinforces the need to understand the neuropathology/pathology of the lesion based on imaging studies and to appreciate the implications that these findings have for anticipated clinical exam findings. Alleged pain imperception can be evaluated, as can nearly any reported neurological impairment for that matter, with appropriately designed forced choice testing (21). Additionally, examiners should realize that alleged pain imperception or loss of sensation is difficult to fake upon repeated bilateral stimulation. This is due to the fact that examinees that exaggerate rely on subjective strategies rather than truly responding to the strength of the stimuli. Therefore, assessments with such techniques as Von Frey hairs could be utilized in the aforementioned scenario to provide further objective evidence of the validity of reported symptoms.

Defining pain and its possible deception is extremely challenging. The standard accepted definition of pain describes it as a physiologic and psychologic response to noxious stimuli, the latter being defined as a stimulus that may or does produce tissue damage (22). One must, however, differentiate between psychic and physical pain, or pain and suffering, in the context of performing an Independent Medical Evaluation (IME). These may be inextricably intertwined with each other as well as with affective conditions such as depression and anxiety. Examiners must understand that multiple variables may impact on pain reporting and behavior and be totally valid yet potentially appear invalid. For example, arousal, stress, tension and anger all may exacerbate subjective reporting of pain and pain behavior, as may depression, through psychophysiological effects. Psychoemotional and psychosocial concomitants of chronic pain must be appreciated, including loss of self-esteem, lowered frustration tolerance, depression, sexual dysfunction, including decreased libido, anger, and guilt.

A very recently disproved screening procedure frequently used by physical therapists, physicians, and chiropractors for estimating when psychological factors are significantly influencing pain related responses is the assessment for Waddell's Non Organic signs (23, 24). These signs include: Overreaction (guarding/limping, bracing, rubbing affected area, grimacing, sighing); Tenderness (widespread sensitivity to light touch of superficial tissue); Axial Loading (light pressure to skull of standing patient should not significantly increase low back symptoms); Rotation (back pain reported when shoulders and pelvis are passively rotated in the same plane); Straight Leg

Raising (marked difference between leg raising in the supine and seated position); Motor and Sensory (giving way or cog wheeling to motor testing or regional sensory loss in a stocking or non dermatomal distribution, when peripheral nerve dysfunction has been ruled out). Additional non-organic signs that have been considered have included: lower extremity give-away, no pain-free spells in the past year, intolerance of treatments, and emergency admissions to hospital with back trouble (15, 20, 23).

Initially thought to indicate degree of non-organic or psychological contribution to pain experience, the Waddell signs were never intended to exclude physical components as a cause of low back pain, or imply that psychological factors were a cause versus result of pain. More recent evidence indicates that the Waddell signs are not valid measures of non-organicity. In a structured, evidence based review of all available evidence, Fishbain (24) concludes that Waddell signs are neither correlated with psychological distress or secondary gain and do not discriminate organic from nonorganic problems. In fact, they may represent an organic phenomenon and are associated with greater pain levels and poorer treatment outcomes.

This finding has significant implications. By demonstrating the invalidity of one of the most heavily relied upon methods for making inferences and medical diagnostic conclusions about nonorganicity, it calls into question the general diagnostic validity of many physical and medical evaluations. Moreover, it almost certainly limits the utility of all commonly used psychological measures that were developed to predict medical diagnoses that relied on these invalid measures.

With regard to assessment of psychological and neuropsychological impairments and chronic pain, response bias represents an especially important threat to validity. As these assessments usually begin with an interview about self-reported symptoms and subsequently rely heavily on standardized measures of performance on well-normed tests, the validity of the results requires the veracity, cooperation, and motivation of the patient. Recent evidence, however, suggests that some patients seen for presumptive brain injury-related impairments over-report pre-injury functional status (25). This may be especially true with post-concussive deficits since these symptoms appear with similar frequency in the general population (26). In addition, the demonstrated ability of neuropsychologists to accurately detect malingering in test protocols has been less than impressive (e.g., 27). Finally, the common practice of utilizing technicians to administer tests, as previously noted, has been called into question for reasons that include adequacy to detect and manage response bias issues (28). Nonetheless, various instruments, techniques and strategies are available which have demonstrated at least some utility in detecting response bias, as a means of increasing confidence in the validity of assessment findings.

In Table 64-3, what have often been considered as hallmarks signs of response bias are presented (29). The signs can be applied to most aspects of a medical examination. However, as noted, caveats exist for most.

Notably, in the evaluation of response bias, as in evaluation of all aspects of pre- and post-injury status, the following investigative tools may be used in conjunction with client interviews and testing: 1) school records; 2) medical records; 3) driver records; 4) military records 5) criminal records; 6) employment records; 7) evaluations from other psychologists; 8) interviews with family members, friends, teachers and employers, etc.; and 9) all materials available to the attorney through formal discovery or otherwise.

These guidelines and strategies are presented as important possible indicators for interpreting patient examination data. Integration of contextual information, history, behavioral observation, interview data, collaborative data, and personality data, with measures of effort and neuropsychological test data provides the best information for estimating the degree to which a person was exerting full effort and the degree to which test results are reliable and valid and reflect actual abilities.

The recent increase in attention to response bias assessment and malingering may reflect a pendulum like overcompensation to earlier times when such issues were not properly appreciated and when excessive compensation packages or awards may have been made due to an assessment of disability that did not take into account response bias. In the current and increasingly restrictive healthcare environment, where services and benefits are more critically evaluated, and where legal and decision making policies favor either-or and black or white conceptualizations, there are tendencies to consider response bias as dichotomous and to consider response bias and malingering as synonymous. In fact, response bias measures are often erroneously referred to in many publications as "malingering measures". This undoubtedly contributes to what the authors note as too frequently haphazard and overzealous application of poorly validated detection procedures, failure to critically and objectively evaluate both the weaknesses, as well as strengths, of these procedures, and tendencies to overinterpret or overgeneralize them.

Again, it is especially important to realize that response bias and malingering are not synonymous. For example, Moore and Donders (30) showed that psychiatric history and financial compensation seeking were associated with a similar increase in likelihood of invalid responding on cognitive symptom validity and neuropsychological measures. Grillo, Brown, Hilsabeck, Price and Lees-Haley (31), using several indicators of response bias that included the Fake Bad Scale (FBS), offered evidence that characterologic / personality

TABLE 64-3
Response Bias: Typical Hallmark Signs

I. Inconsistencies Within and Between:
1. Reported Symptoms
2. Examination / Test Performance
3. Clinical Presentation
4. Known Diagnostic Patterns
5. Observed Behavior (in another setting)
6. Reported Symptoms & Exam / Test Performance
7. Measures of Similar Abilities (inter-test scatter)
8. Similar Tasks or Items Within the Same Exam or Test (intra test scatter) - especially when difficult tasks are performed more easily than easy ones
9. Different Testing Sessions

Caveat: The potential contributions of significant psychiatric, attentional, comprehension, or other problems that often involve inconsistent presentations should be considered in evaluating inconsistency.

II. Overly Impaired Performance (vs. expected)
1. Very Poor Performance on Easy Tasks Presented as Difficult
2. Failing Tasks That All But those with Severe Impairment Perform Easily
3. Poorer Performance than Normative Data For Similar Injury/Illness.
4. Below Chance Level Performance

Caveat: Unusually poor level of performance may be due to actual interference effects associated with various psychologic, sleep or other disturbances; statistically significant levels of below chance performance may be expected in 1/20 cases with the usual significance levels.

III. Lack of Specific Diagnostic Signs of Impairment
Caveat: Many disorders do not have unambiguous diagnostic signs.

IV. Specific Signs of Response Bias on Psychological or Neuropsychological Tests
1. MMPI-2 Scales: F, F-K, L, VRIN, TRIN, Fb
2. MMPI-2 "Fake Bad Scale" (FBS) (103)
3. Malingering Detection Tests
4. Actuarial formulas for clinical neuropsychological tests (e.g., WCST, CVLT)

Caveat: Many of these signs are not unambiguous or have not been thoroughly validated.

V. Interview Evidence
1. Atypical temporal relationship of symptoms to injury
2. Psychological symptoms, or symptoms which are improbable, absurd, overly specific or of unusual frequency or severity (e.g., triple vision)
3. Disparate examinee history or complaints across interviews or examiners
4. Disparate corroboratory interview data versus examinee report

Caveat: Other explanations are possible for disparate or atypical interview data.

VI. Physical Exam Findings
1. Non-organic sensory findings
2. Non-organic motor findings
3. Pseudoneurologic findings in the absence of anticipated associated pathologic findings
4. Inconsistent exam findings
5. Failure on physical exam procedures designed to specifically assess malingering

Caveat: As indicated above, non-organic sensory findings may have a psychophsyiological basis as may psychogenic movement disorders or other pseudoneurologic presentations.

disorder factors, rather than "malingering" contributes to exaggerated results in a forensic setting. Ample other evidence indicates that psychiatric or functional disorders can produce response bias or actual performance deficits related to poor adaptation and maladaptive coping versus malingering (e.g., 32–35). There is also evidence that negative expectancy (e.g., "diagnosis threat"), independent of impairment, can reduce cognitive performance (13, 14).

Based on a critical evaluation of the current state of the art, it appears necessary to caution that malingering: 1) should not be considered dichotomous, as *either / or* (i.e., present or not present, black or white); 2) should not be considered something that clinicians can reliably or validly assess or diagnose with a high degree of probability, even when serious efforts are made; and 3) should not be considered a discrete entity assessed by often used response bias measures. Further, it should not be assumed that response bias measures have a high degree of reliability and validity in predicting valid examination performance on other measures or functional ability in other settings, or that patients take the examination process as seriously as examiners do.

A summary of some of the major limitations and problems with current response bias procedures include (8, 9, 19, 36–40):

- Psychometric research Inadequacies (i.e., basic test construction issues such as reliability and validity; sensitivity and specificity).
- Limited generalizability of analogue research (e.g., unknown differences between simulated and real malingerers).
- Variable Group Membership (wide variability in samples for both simulators and symptom disorder groups).
- Differential Vulnerability to Response Bias (some tests are more obvious or subtle, sensitive or specific).
- Questionable Generalizability of Findings (e.g., from analogue simulation studies to real life situations, from one response bias measure to another, to other tests, to actual symptoms, or across time).
- Absence of Mutual Exclusivity (poor effort can occur in presence of real disorders).
- "Law of the Instrument" bias wherein "malingering" becomes what "malingering" tests measure. Specifically, the definitions of "effort", and validation studies to examine the construct, are often lacking. Further "effort" cannot be assumed uniform for individuals, individuals within diagnostic groups or for nonlitigating and litigating situations.
- Questionable Specificity: The effects of fatigue, pain, disinterest, non-attended (e.g., computer) administration, mixing cognitive tests and SVT's in a battery with unknown validity, and other factors on response bias tests, are not understood and have not been addressed.
- Frequently High Misclassification (i.e., false positive or false negative) rates, especially in the very few studies that examined ecological or real world validity (38, 39).
- Incautious use of most current SVT Indexes with regard to diagnosis and decision making may violate APA ethics and "APA Standards for Educational and Psychological Tests", given the aforementioned psychometric limitations.

These limitations emphasize: 1) caution with regard to over-interpretation of response bias procedures; and 2) the importance of employing multiple data sources and making thoughtful inferences only after integration of thorough historical information, interview, assessment, behavioral observations, collaborative interview and data sources, and so on.

In order to caution against simplistic and dichotomous conceptualizations with regard to diagnosis, the following table is presented. Notably, Table 64-4 represents just 64 of the possibilities with regard to injury-related presentations. The represented possibilities range from (a) persons with real, uncomplicated disorders with impairments on exam and in functional status and without exaggeration on either (but possible minimization or denial) to (b) persons with complicated, misattributed or non existent disorders with only exaggerated or feigned impairments on exam and/or in functional status. In an ongoing review of medicolegal report findings that will be submitted for future publication, the authors have examined the frequency of possible diagnostic conclusions in reports from cases in which they have been involved. Findings have consistently indicated that a preponderance of conclusions reflect only a few of these possibilities and reach mostly black or white diagnostic inferences regarding presence or absence of neurologic dysfunction and malingering.

A cautious approach is indicated with regard to estimating the probabilities regarding presence or absence of physical impairment and response bias. For instance, if a person has both actual symptoms and is exaggerating difficulty, inferences must be generated not only about the degree of deliberateness and the degree of physical impairment, but also the degree of awareness of

TABLE 64-4
Diagnostic Possibilities in Brain Injury Assessment

Brain Injury Impairment	Residual Functional Impairments	Residual Impairments on Examination
1. Yes	1. Yes & Exaggerated	1. Yes & Not Exaggerated
2. Mixed	2. Yes & Not Exaggerated	2. Yes & Exaggerated
3. Indeterminate	3. No & Exaggerated	3. No & Exaggerated
4. No	4. No & Not Exaggerated	4. No & Not Exaggerated

exaggeration on the part of the subject. Has the person adopted a sick role and talked themselves into believing they cannot perform certain tasks and lack certain abilities (e.g., somatoform disorder), with conscious withholding of effort due to intention of demonstrating what they believe to be true disabilities? Or, are they less conscious and aware, as in a conversion disorder? Or are they completely aware, but coping in a way that may be adaptive? An example of the latter is the case of an aging worker with a chronic history of back failures who has low self-esteem and a poor relationship with his or her employer. This employee may have a belief that another back injury is inevitable and will be cumulatively painful and disabling, will require uncomfortable interactions with others, may result in being fired despite conviction that the company did not make obvious safety precautions to prevent their injury, and that no other job options are realistic.

Table 64-5 presents a summary of major response bias detection strategies and techniques that may indicate that the validity of medical examination and psychological test data should be carefully considered. This table was prepared on the basis of a comprehensive review of existing literature (see 6–15, 17–21, 23–150). Multiple sources were used for most of the indicators. Special attention was given to reviews of specific empirical indicators such as those offered by Nies and Sweet (41) and Trueblood and Schmidt (57), which served as a model for this effort. Notably, this table illustrates the utility of a constellation or profiling approach to response bias detection. This multiaxial conceptual model is presented as a methodological approach for constructing a profile of motivation and response bias, which incorporates a wide array of findings from common instruments and procedures during evaluation. Empirical support exists indicating that each of these indicators has at least some utility in detecting sub-optimal effort or other response bias (e.g., 41, 45, 46).

Importantly, review of original test manuals and studies should be conducted before employing any of these instruments. Also, as noted previously, numerous pitfalls and limitations of each of these procedures, both conceptual and methodological, exist. However, some increasing evidence exists for improved discrimination and increased reliability when multiple measures are employed (54). The proposed conceptual approach is one in which multiple factors are integrated as an optimal method for estimating the degree of effort and the degree to which examination findings are reliable and valid. This conceptual model and procedure (MAP) for estimating motivation economically incorporates currently available instruments and methods and the available published research for direct and indirect measurement of effort and response bias. For review of these instruments and methods, the reader is referred to several good reviews

in textbooks of neuropsychology or the many previous reports and reviews of this literature (e.g., 9, 41, 45, 46, 54, 56, 104, 141, 148, 149).

Most major objective personality measures and many neuropsychological measures have scales or indices that can be calculated, (e.g., Memory Assessment Scales (60) and the Rey Complex Figure Test and Recognition Trial (61)) that provide data on the performance of simulators. The advantages inherent in such procedures include: reduced need for administering and charging for very long tests designed solely for detection of potential motivation problems (especially if negative), and for which numerous generalization difficulties exit; limiting the amount of available time for administering other relevant measures and conducting more comprehensive interview (examinee, collaborative others); potential enhancement of face validity of measures to examinees.

The techniques or strategies suggested in Table 64-5 should not be utilized singly or simple mindedly. They are not intended to support a simple dualistic model that equates response bias or other phenomena (e.g. actual interference effects associated with pain, psychoemotional distress, etc) to malingering and then considers examinee responses as either accurate or malingered. Evidence of response bias on any one test does not necessarily imply absence of impairment or in real world abilities. It cannot be concluded that failure on specific indicators represents inadequate performance or response bias. Rather, the strategies are offered with the following suggestions.

1. Examination responses can be influenced by multiple factors that affect the reliability and validity of examination presentations and performances (e.g., deliberate and nondeliberate effort, psychiatric disorders).
2. The degree to which presentations and performances displayed on examination accurately reflect genuine functional abilities exists on a continuum (versus a dichotomy) and can be estimated by the extent to which indicators of response bias are present.
3. Because the interpretation of findings and diagnostic impressions are dependent upon the reliability and validity of examination results, the reliability and validity of interpretations and impressions is reduced to the extend that indicators of response bias are present.

It should again be emphasized that "failure" on one measure of response bias does not mean that the entire set of complaints is biased or invalid. Ethical guidelines caution against overzealous interpretation of limited test data and, in this regard, with erroneously considering response bias and malingering as synonymous or dichotomous, or neglecting how psychiatric or other factors affect response bias measures. At present, the authors are

TABLE 64-5

Motivation Assessment Profile—Brain Injury Evaluations (MAP–BI)

Performance Patterns on Existing Neuropsychological Tests

Full Scale IQ	
Low (vs. expected, estimated, etc.)	Age Scale Score < 5
Digit Span (Floor Effect)	Non-improvement with "chunking"
Digit Span: Testing Limits with "Chunking"	"Near-miss" (Ganser errors)
Arithmetic and Orientation scale Performance	Attention-Concentration Index Score < General Memory
WMS-R Malingering Index: Attention/ Concentration	Index(AC-GMI)
Index versus Memory Index	Hard Items ≥ Easy Items
Paired Associate learning: Easy vs. Hard item Performance	GNDS Score < 44
General Neuropsych Deficit Scale (35)	>17 errors (Poor)
Speech Sounds Perception Test Performance	>8 errors (Poor)
Seashore Rhythm Test Performance	Unusually low w/o gross motor deficit
Finger Tapping Test	Errors bilaterally vs. laterally
Tactual Stimulation Performance	>5
Finger Tip Number Writing – Errors	>3
Finger Agnosia – Errors	Unusually low w/o gross motor deficit
Grip Strength	Rare or "spike three" errors; Or > 1 Error on Trials I or II
Category Test Performance	Discrepant # Perseverative vs. # Category Errors
Wisconsin Card Sorting Test Errors	< 6
Recognition memory (RAVLT)	< 13
Recognition memory (CVLT)	Abnormal patterns
List Learning Serial Order Effects	Score < 38 (RMW), < 26 (RMF)
Warrington Recognition Memory Test (RMT)	Atypical Recognition Errors (≥2); Recognition
Rey Complex Figure Recognition Trial	Failure Errors
	Poor or unusual performance
Word Stem Priming Task Performance	

Instruments to Specifically Evaluate Level of Cognitive Effort/Response Bias

Symptom Validity Testing (SVT)	sig *< 50% chance level responding
Hiscock Forced Choice Procedure (HFCP)	sig < 50% chance level responding, <66 correct
Victoria Symptom Validity Test (VSVT)	sig < 50% chance level responding, <16 on easy and/or
	hard items
Portland Digit Recognition Test (PDRT)	sig < 50%, chance responding
21-Item Test	<5 on free recall, <3 on free recall, <13 on recognition,
	<9 on recognition
Test of Memory Malingering (TOMM)	<45 trial 2 or recognition
Forced Choice test of Nonverbal Ability (61)	sig < 50% chance level responding
Dot Counting Test (DCT)	Correct/incorrect responses
Computer Assessment of Response Bias (CARB),	< 89% raises suspicion
Word Memory Test (WMT) IR, DR, Consistency	<89% raises suspicion
Autobiographical Interview (36)	>3 errors
Memorization of 16 Items Test (MSIT)	>8 Omissions, >6 Omissions, <6 Total Correct
Rey Word Recognition List (WRL)	<6 correct, <5 (total correct minus false positives)
Rey Memory for 15 Items Test (MFIT)	<3 complete sets, <9 items (38))
Word Completion Memory Test (WCMT)	R < 9 or Inclusion <15

*sig = statistically significantly

Personality Instruments with Built-in Detection Designs

Personality Assessment Inventory (PAI) (104)
- Inconsistency (INC), Infrequency (INF), Positive Impression Management (PIM), and Negative Impression Management (NIM) scales.
- 8 score patterns thought to comprise a "Malingering Index".
- >2 patterns malingering suspected
- >4 patterns likely malingering

TABLE 64-5 (*continued*)

Minnesota Multiphasic Personality Inventory (MMPI-2)

- Validity indices (L, F, Fb, Fp, Ds, K, VRIN, TRIN, F-K) (44, 103, 105)
- The Fake Bad Scale (105)

Rogers (37) – cutoff scores:
Liberal:
  1. *F-Scale raw score > 23*
  2. *F-Scale T-Score > 81*
  3. *F-K Index > 10*
  4. *Obvious – subtle score > 83*
  5. *Conservative:*
  6. *F-scale raw > 30*

F-K index > 25

Qualitative Variables in Assessing Response Bias

Time /Response Latency Comparisons Across Similar Tasks
Inconsistencies across tasks
Performance on Easy Tasks Presented as Hard
Remote Memory Report

Personal Information
Comparison Between Test Performance & Behavioral Observations
Inconsistencies in History and/or Complaints, Performance
Comparisons for Inconsistencies Within Testing Session (Quantitative & Qualitative):

Comparisons Across Testing Sessions (Qualitative, Quantitative)
Symptom Self Report: Complaints

Low scores or unusual errors
Difficulties, especially if < recent memory, or severely impaired in absence of gross amnesia
Very poor personal information in absence of gross amnesia
Discrepancies

Inconsistencies across time, interviewer, etc.
A. Within Tasks (e.g., Easy vs. Hard Items)
B. Between Tasks (e.g., Easy vs. Hard)
C. Across Repetitions of same/parallel tasks (R/O fatigue)
D. Across similar tasks under different motivational sets
Poorer/inconsistent performance on re-testing

High frequency of complaints; patient complaints > significant others'

Main & Spanswick Indicators (15)

- Failure to comply with reasonable treatment
- Report of severe pain with no associated psychological effects
- Marked inconsistencies in effects of pain on general activities
- Poor work record and history of persistent awards
- Previous litigation

Symptom Self Report: Early vs. Late Symptom Complaint
Early Symptoms reported late

Neuromedical Indicators

Hoover's test	Test for feigned lower extremity weakness associated with normal crossed hip extensor response
Astasia abasia	"Drunken type" non-organic gait with near-falls but no actual falls to ground
Non-organic sensory impairments	Patchy sensory loss, midline sensory loss, large scotoma in visual field, tunnel vision (Note: usually not, but sometimes, organic)
Non-neurologic upper extremity drift	Long tract involvement results in pronator type drift. Proximal shoulder girdle weakness and malingering typically present with non-pronator drift.
Stenger's Test	Test for malingered hearing loss during audiologic evaluation.
Gait discrepancies when observed versus not observed	If organic should be consistent regardless of whether observed or not.
Gait discrepancies relative to direction of requested ambulation	Gait should present with same impairments in all directions. Malingerers do not as a rule practice a feigned gait in all directions.
Forearm pronation, hand clasping and forearm supination test for digit/finger sensory loss	Malingered finger sensory loss is difficult to maintain in this perceptually confusing, intertwined hand/finger position

TABLE 64-5 (continued)

Pain versus temperature discrepancies	Due to the fact that both sensory modalities run in the spinothalamic tract, they should be found to be commensurately impaired contralateral to the side of the CNS lesion.
Lack of atrophy in a chronically paretic/paralytic limb	Lack of atrophy in a paralyzed/paretic limb suggests the limb is being used or is getting regular electrical stimulation to maintain mass.
Impairment diminishes under influence of sodium amytal, hypnosis or lack of observation	All these observations are most consistent with non-organic presentations including consideration of malingering or conversion disorder.
Incongruence between neuroanatomical imaging and neurologic examination	Lack of any static imaging findings on brain CT or MRI in the presence of a dense motor or sensory deficit suggests non-organicity.
Arm drop test	An aware patient malingering profound alteration in consciousness or significant arm paresis will not let their own hand, when held over their head, drop onto their face.
Presence of ipsilateral findings when implied neuroanatomy would dictate contralateral findings	An examinee claiming severe right brain damage who claims right eye blindness and right-sided weakness and sensory loss.
Tell me "when I'm not touching" responses	An examinee with claimed sensory loss who endorses that he does not feel you touch him when you ask him to tell you "if you do not feel this".
Lack of shoe wear in presence of gait disturbance	An examinee with claimed longer term gait deviation due to orthopedic or neurologic causes should demonstrate commensurate wear on shoes (if worn with any frequency)
Calluses on hands in "totally disabled" examinee	An examinee who is unable to work should not present with signs of ongoing evidence of physical labor
Assistive device "wear and tear" signs	In any examinee using assistive devices for any period of time e.g. cane, crutches, there should be commensurate wear on the device consistent with their claimed impairment and disability.
Mankopf's maneuver	Increase in heart rate commensurate with nociceptive stimulation during exam (there is some controversy on whether this always occurs).
Lack of atrophy in a limb that is claimed to be significantly impaired	If side to side measurements and/or inspection do not bear out atrophy consider other causes aside from one being claimed.
Sudden motor give-away or ratchitiness on manual strength testing	Considered to normally be a sign of incomplete effort or symptom exaggeration.
Weakness on manual muscle testing without commensurate asymmetry of DTRs or muscle bulk.	Suggests simulated muscle weakness if longstanding.
Toe test for simulated low back pain	Flexion of hip and knee with movement only of toes should not produce an increase in low back pain.
Magnuson's test	Have examinee point to area several times over period of examination; inconsistencies suggest increased potential for non-organicity.
Delayed response sign	Pain reaction temporally delayed relative to application of perceived nociceptive stimulus.
Wrist drop test	In an examinee with claimed wrist extensor loss, have them pronate forearm, extend elbow and flex shoulder . . . if on making a fist in this position they also extend wrist then non-organicity should be suspected.
Object drop test	Examinee claims inability to bend down yet does so to pick up a light object "inadvertently" dropped by examiner
Hip adductor test	Test for claimed paralysis of lower extremity, similar to Hoover's test yet looks for crossed adductor response
Disparity between tested range of motion and observed range of motion of any joint	When ROM under testing is significantly disparate (e.g. less) from observed, spontaneous ROM suspect functional contributors
Straight leg raise (SLR) disparities dependent on examinee positioning	Differences in SLR between sitting, standing and/or bending may suggest a functional overlay to low back complaints
Grip strength testing via Dynamometer • 3 Repitions • 5 Positions	• Three repetitions at any given setting should not vary more than 20% and/or • Bell shaped curve should be generated if all 5 positions are tested.

	TABLE 64-5 (*continued*)
Sensory "flip" test	Sensory findings should be the same if testing upper extremity in supination or pronation or lower extremity in internal versus external rotation. Differences may suggest a functional overlay.
Pinch test for low back pain	Pinching the lumbar fat pad should not reproduce pain due to axial structure involvement; if test is positive suspect a functional overlay.

Important Considerations
Caveats:
1. *The potential contributions of significant psychiatric, attentional, comprehension, or other disorders that often involve inconsistent presentations should be considered in evaluating inconsistency.*
2. *Unusually poor level of performance may be due to actual interference effects associated with various psychologic, sleep or other disturbances, especially heightened anxiety or fear of pain.*
3. *Many disorders do not have unambiguous diagnostic signs*
4. *Many of these indicators are not unambiguous and have not been thoroughly validated.*
5. *Non-organic sensory findings may have a psychophsyiological basis as may psychogenic movement disorders or other pseudoneurologic presentations.*
6. *Other explanations are possible for disparate or atypical interview data.*

preparing a paper that documents a group of severe TBI clinical subjects who are not in litigation or receiving compensation where large numbers "fail" response bias measures (i.e., score below recommended cut offs) despite very strong external reinforcement for performing well. In addition, several other researchers have submitted or are preparing papers that demonstrate similar results and/or document a proportion of subjects who fail response bias tests but perform adequately on neuropsychological measures.

A practical approach to considering the numerous indicators of response discussed in this chapter is presented in the flow chart in Figure 64-1. This flowchart is intended to facilitate the integration of these measures in deriving meaningful inferences regarding the presence and extent of response bias. This in turn serves the ultimate purpose of estimating the effect of response biases on performance and impairments noted on self report and examination.

Practitioners should recognize that a great disparity exists between the adversarial legal process where attorneys are advocates for their clients and the IME setting where the doctor must be dispassionate and objective. The danger of attorney "coaching" based on utilization of this material cannot be underestimated. This, of course, would then represent a form of "stealth" threat to the validity of examination data. This threat, or expected consequence of collision between the disparate legal and scientific ethics, has been documented in a publication noting a case of attorney client coaching (146). However, compared to simpler models where only a couple of isolated response bias measures are used, it seems more unlikely that the multiple measures employed in the MAP approach could be understood and manipulated.

Finally, enhancing response bias detection as a means of optimizing interpretability of examination results, critical as it is, should not be considered the final step. Decreasing the potential for response bias is a more efficacious and economic approach to enhancing utility of assessment. The following recommendations for enhancing motivation, assessing response bias, and increasing efficiency, utility and ecological validity of examination procedures are offered.

RECENT DEVELOPMENTS

Recent efforts to identify response bias and malingering have been problematic. Malingering, or the act of willful, deliberate, and fraudulent feigning, or gross exaggeration, is only one variant of response bias, and an extreme one. The presence of response bias is much more easily documented than malingering. However, the two are often confounded and used synonymously in professional neuropsychological publications and practice, where response bias measures are frequently referred to, explicitly or implicitly, as "malingering tests". Inferences about malingering, especially in a restrictive health care environment with strong gate keeping pressures, are inherently challenging. In the absence of dependent measures or clinical methods with demonstrated validity for assessment of malingering, inferences about malingering using current measures and procedures necessarily produce fallible judgments with unknown false positive rates.

Two of the major obstacles to developing highly reliability and valid measures of malingering are: the absence of an accepted gold standard, which accounts for the absence of any blinded studies comparing malingerers

Flowchart for Reponse Bias Assessment

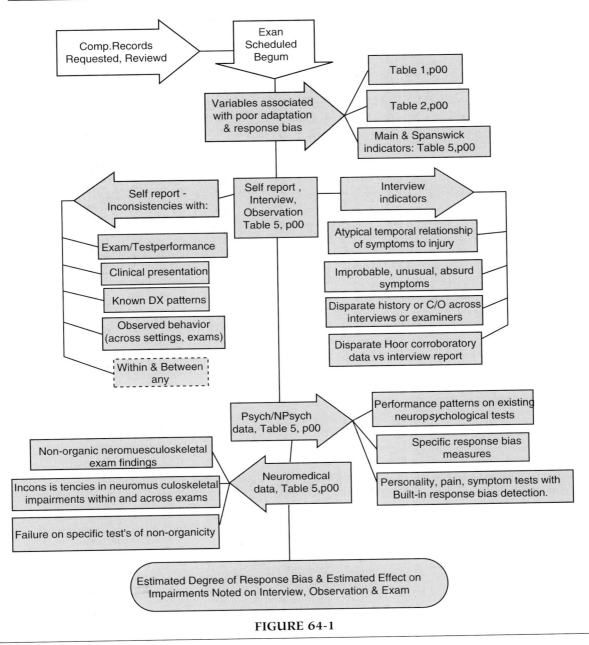

FIGURE 64-1

Flow chart for response bias assessment

and non malingerers; 2) nearly exclusive reliance on simulation studies (i.e., non-injured persons instructed to feign deficits) for establishing reliability and validity (129). In one of the only large group studies that examined the validity of symptom validity instruments for identifying cognitive malingering, the results suggested high false positive rates (38). A research design which attempts to circumvent obstacles relating to simulation studies and absence of a valid gold standard criterion for malingering is one that attempts to employ known

groups. That is, this design examines criterion groups of patients and purported or assumed malingerers and systematically analyzes differences between the groups. This approach may benefit from recent proposals for specifying criteria for malingering (129).

Drawing on previous research, Slick, Sherman and Iverson (151) have proposed diagnostic criteria for malingered neurocognitive dysfunction (MND), defined as volitional exaggeration or fabrication of cognitive dysfunction for the purpose of secondary environmental gain (e.g., compensation or avoidance). The Slick et al. criteria allow for estimations of three probabilities of MND, including:

- Definite MND: presence of (1) substantial external incentive, (2) definite negative response bias on neuropsychological testing, and (3) definite negative response bias is not fully accounted for by psychiatric, neurological or developmental factors.
- Probable MND: presence of: (1) substantial external incentive; 2) evidence from neuropsychological testing, excluding definite negative response bias, and one or more types of evidence from self-report, and (3) information or data utilized for criterion #2 are not fully accounted for by psychiatric, neurological or developmental factors.
- Possible MND: presence of (1) substantial external incentive; 2) evidence from self-report; 3) information or data utilized for criterion #2 are not fully accountable by psychiatric, neurological, or developmental factors.

Slick et al. (151) urge that inferences regarding malingering be preceded by thorough consideration of differential diagnostic considerations of other types of response bias and psychological, neurologic and developmental contributors, and adoption of a "reasonable doubt" strategy that considers the limitations of assessment methodology, and the cost of false positive errors.

The Slick et al. Proposed Diagnostic criteria for malingering are helpful in delineating the need for multiple indicators for poor effort, and consideration of other, non-SVT factors to be considered in reaching a somewhat less dichotomous diagnosis of definite, probable or possible malingered neurocognitive deficit. However, they nonetheless still suffer from a somewhat limited consideration of factors that can contribute to poor symptom validity test scores, as well as all of the previously noted limitations of available symptom validity measures. Regarding the latter, Ranks (152) recently examined a series of individual cases using detailed analysis of symptom validity measures with the best currently available research support. His presentations, which are being prepared in a manuscript, demonstrate the problems of symptom validity assessment in individual cases using instruments that appear much stronger when examining data from group studies. In findings from a recent investigation by Loring, Lee and Meador (153), the Victoria Symptom Validity Test (VSVT) was found to identify cases of incomplete effort in patients being evaluated for strictly clinical purposes in which no external incentive to perform poorly has been identified. It was also noted that the older patients appeared to be at increased risk for suboptimal performance. Gorissen, Sanz and Schmand (154) investigated schizophrenia patients and

reported that suboptimal performances on symptom validity tests reflected core components of that psychopathology. This suggests that effort is a component of many neurologic disorders and false positives can be expected on tests of effort and motivation, especially in the case of executive impairments.

Evidence from these and other studies (e.g., 152–154) indicate that true base rates for effort test scores (for which there may be a wide range of possible base rates for an individual) have not been established, and that at least some norms from samples that have been offered are unlikely to be representative. Hence, statements from test authors that anyone who is not severely demented can pass such tests appear overly exuberant or misleadingly presumptuous. The search for simple solutions has a long and illustrious history in psychology and medicine where initially positive signs or tests are widely and prematurely and incautiously adopted. Examples such as using the MMPI "conversion V" (58) or the Waddell nonorganic physical signs (23) to purportedly discriminate organic from nonorganic physical etiologies, represent just two examples. In both cases, the professions have shown slow and recalcitrant willingness to abandon these false safety blankets after proving to be invalid indicators. This has been despite the immense potential for negative consequences, and in seeming disregard for core bioethical principles that dictate nonmaleficence (i.e., "First do no harm").

Sreenivasan, Kirkish and Garrick (155) have recently offered an interesting practical model for the assessment of amplified neuropsychological and psychiatric deficits in civil litigants in cases of MTBI. They proposed a more comprehensive and detailed checklist intended to assist with differentiating between subtle brain dysfunction, symptom amplification, psychological causes for the presence of cognitive and other deficits, or frank malingering. The checklist included examination and rating of patterns for greater consistency with either genuine injury or symptom exaggeration in the following areas:

I. Neuropsychological testing issues, including: (a) base rates for brain injury, (b) testing consistency with severity of injury and (c) findings on motivational tests:
II. Congruence of testing data and observed behavior during testing (within and between) with: (a) CNS process; (b) across serial testing; (c) with medical reports; and (d) with occupational and/or or school functioning;
III. Congruence of symptoms or signs with clinical data, including consistency of symptoms/signs with clinical interview (within and between) with: (a) clinical course; (b) past records; (c) physical exam; (d) objective laboratory and test findings; (e) collateral or surveillance data; (f) medication response for natural

history of CNS disease; (g) social, occupational, and/or school functioning;

IV. Nonclinical factors, including: whether there is: (a) decline in income/business versus pre-injury; (b) pending pre-injury lawsuits; (c) pre-injury work related burn out, job actions, co-worker conflicts and skills problems (d) compensation less than pre-injury income; (e) repeated evaluations with same tests; (f) evaluation context impacting presentation; (g) reasonableness of expectations for recovery;

In addition, it allows for evaluation of the presence or absence of:

V. Psychiatric and other conditions that may contribute to amplified or atypical symptoms, including: (a) depression/anxiety; (b) personality disorder; (c) conversion/somatization; (d) substance abuse; (e) cumulative concussion; (f) impact of chronic pain; (g) impact of medications; (h) impact of medical comorbidities

VI. Miscellaneous history, including: (a) prior history of litigation; (b) prior history of lying, malingering; (c) prior criminal activity; (d) prior job track record; (e) prior responses to injury

This model appears to warrant closer consideration, especially with regard to its attention to differential diagnosis and specification of the alternative contributors to failure on symptom validity measures. Future efforts to identify factors predictive of response bias and symptom invalidity should also pay more attention to not only indicators suggesting response bias, but also ones that are inconsistent with response bias and secondary gain, including secondary losses.

Recommendations for Enhancing Validity in Impairment and Disability Assessment Findings

1. Establish rapport and a basic working relationship with patients and examinees. Even in cases of independent evaluations where the referral source and expectation is adversarial, valid data collection requires a collaborative effort. The possibility of dissimulation might be reduced given better rapport (9, 130, 131), understanding of reported symptoms or complaints and communication of that understanding, as well as explanation, feedback and clarification given any suggestion of uncertain motivation. Spend time with patients and try to get to know them as individual persons. We cannot assume that everyone takes our exams and procedures seriously, is as honest or effortful as we would like, or that we will not have to work at getting them interested or invested in doing their best.

2. Ensure that emotional variables affecting motivation are adequately assessed during an interview that is conducted prior to the exam. Specifically, assess the impact of anger or blame and feelings of resentment or victimization (130, 131), as well as the other variables shown in the literature to be associated with poor recovery and adaptation to impairment (6). Assess pain, fatigue or other factors that may actually interfere with optimal performance. Always assess interest/disinterest in the testing process and any obstacles or impediments to optimal effort and performance. Prepare patients / examinees before beginning testing. Employ understanding, as well as education to help prepare persons to perform to the best of their ability.

3. Make efforts to maximize validity of exam procedures. Where possible, utilize instruments with built-in symptom validity measures. Where possible, utilize comparisons with published patterns and indices indicating sub-optimal test performance for available tests for which there are data for symptom validity indicators (e.g., hand dynamometer; finger tapping; the Wechsler Memory Scale–Revised General Memory vs. Attention/ Concentration index). For example, in addition to comparison of three repeated trials at the same position and comparison of assessment at all five positions, repeat testing with the hand dynamometer allows analysis of consistency of performance patterns across time. Further, measurement of completion time for similar tasks also allows analysis of consistency. Additionally, validity indicators should be developed for existing assessment procedures and symptom validity measures should be built in to newly developed cognitive assessment tests and procedures. Finally, most measures of symptom validity have limitations and caution is advised. Efforts should be made to avoid making strong inferences from instruments for which there are not available data regarding sensitivity and specificity in clinical samples. Instruments with disputed or disproved validity (e.g., Waddell signs) should not be employed or given credibility.

4. Employ shorter symptom validity tests in order to minimize possibility of negative reactions owing to the nature of protracted participation in easy, boring, or atypical tasks. Where possible, employ procedures that both appear more credible and are not well-known. Vary measures and procedures that are employed in order to prevent discrimination of ability measures from symptom validity measures. Publicization of these tests has led to increased recognition by attorneys, clients, support groups, internet groups, and so on. Finally, do not freely share information about symptom validity measures to non-medical professionals. Other professionals adhere to a completely different set of professional

ethics and recent law publications indicate a practice of preparing clients for testing by counseling them with this information (125, 146).

5. Validity of examinations will likely be enhanced when conducted by clinicians who treat persons with brain injury, which also helps to assure more adequate clinical skills for detecting and modifying sub-optimal performance, as well as collection of internalized tracking data to allow validation of previous inferences across time. More experienced brain injury clinicians are more capable of: a) integrating history, interview, corroboratory interview / reports, collateral data, test findings, and personality and emotional status data with more sophisticated clinical observations during examination; (b) adapting more creative modifications of exam procedures and instructions given suspicion of low motivation, to increase motivation and optimize effort; (c) benefiting from the probability that examinees will be more forthcoming and more trusting of an experienced 'doctor'.

6. Remain aware that, in science and medicine, situations are rarely either-or, clear-cut, or one-dimensional. Avoid simplistic conceptual models that are compatible with dichotomous approaches to assessing effort and response bias. Such approaches usually rely on a couple of measures with cut off scores. Cut off scores, by their nature, always entail judgment (150), inherently result in misclassification and impose an artificial dichotomy on essentially continuous variables. "True" cut off scores do not exist. Employ sophisticated, continuous conceptualizations of effort and response bias by using multiple independent measures of estimated effort. Employ a model that conceptualizes motivation and effort as continuous variables that can vary across exam procedures, settings, and occasions. Performance data provides the best information for estimating the degree of effort exerted, and the degree to which test results are reliable and valid.

7. Utilize and devise models that measure the degree of apparent motivation and effort, using multiple data sources, and estimate confidence levels of inferences, given consideration of the multiple factors that contribute to exam findings. Employ similarly sophisticated models for assessing persistent impairments, adaptation to impairments, and disability. Probability statements based on multiple measures are the most appropriate. Integration of contextual information, history, behavioral observations, interview and collaborative data, personality and coping data with multiple measures of effort or performance and current tests exam and qualitative data provides the best information for estimating the degree of effort exerted, and the degree to which test results are reliable and valid.

CONCLUSION

Evaluation of impairments following brain injury presents a significant challenge with numerous potential obstacles and confounding issues. In addition to frequently subtle but complex deficits, the lack of validated "rating systems" for many residual impairments, and the multiple contributors to impairment and disability, persons with brain injury may present with some bias to report or demonstrate impairment or related disability. Given frequent incentives to distort symptoms during examinations, assessment of examinee motivation is necessary to providing accurate diagnosis. This is prerequisite to provision of appropriate and timely treatment, promotion of optimal recovery, prevention of iatrogenic impairment and disability reinforcement, and appropriate legal compensation and treatment access decision making. In the current chapter, the importance of response bias was reviewed. Response bias assessment procedures relevant to brain injury assessment and treatment were considered and elucidated and appropriate cautions were indicated. Finally, recommendations for enhancing validity in impairment and disability evaluations were offered.

References

1. Zasler ND, Martelli MF. Assessing Mild Traumatic Brain Injury. *AMA Guides Newsletter* 1998; November / December, 1–5.
2. Rohling ML, Binder LM. Money matters: A meta-analytic review of the association between financial compensation and the experience and treatment of chronic pain. *Health Psychol* 1995; 14:537–547.
3. Youngjohn JR, Burrows L, Erdal K. Brain damage or compensation neurosis? The controversial post-concussion syndrome. *Clin Neuropsychol* 1995;2:112–123.
4. Binder LM, Rohling ML. Money matters: a meta-analytic review of the effects of financial incentives on recovery after closed-head injury. *Am J Psychiatry* 1996;153:7–10.
5. Blau T. *The Psychologist as Expert Witness* New York: John Wiley & Sons, 1984.
6. Martelli MF, Zasler ND, Mancini A, MacMillan PJ. Psychological assessment and applications in impairment and disability evaluations. In: May RV, Martelli MF (eds.). *Guide to Functional Capacity Evaluation with Impairment Rating Applications*, Richmond: VA: NADEP Publications, 1999:3–84.
7. Matheson L. Symptom magnification syndrome: A modern tragedy and its treatment – Part one: Description and definition. *Industrial Rehabilitation Quarterly* 1990;3:1–23.
8. Hayes JS. Hilsabeck RC, Gouvier WD. Malingering Traumatic Brain Injury: Current Issues and Caveats in Assessment and Classification. In Varney R, Roberts RJ (eds.). *The Evaluation and Treatment of Mild Traumatic Brain Injury* Mahwah, NJ: Lawrence Ehrlbaum and Associates, 1999;240–290.
9. Martelli MF, Zasler ND, Nicholson, K, Pickett TC, May VR. Assessing the veracity of pain complaints and associated disability. In Weiner RB (ed.). *Pain Management: A Practical Guide for Clinicians* 6th edition Boca Raton: FL: St. Lucie Press, 2001; 789–805.
10. Matheson L. Symptom magnification syndrome. In: Isernhagen S (ed.). *Work Injury* Rockville: MD: Aspen Publishers, 1988; 48–91.
11. Matheson L. Symptom magnification syndrome: A modern tragedy and it's treatment – Part two: Techniques of identification. *Ind Rehabil Q* 1991;4;1:1–17.

12. Matheson L. Symptom magnification syndrome: A modern tragedy and it's treatment - Part three: Techniques of treatment. *Ind Rehabil Q* 1991;4:2:1–24.

13. Suhr JA, Gunstad J. Further exploration of the effect of "diagnosis threat" on cognitive performance in individuals with mild head injury. *Journal of the International neuropsychological Society*, 2005;11:1, 23–29.

14. Suhr JA, Gunstad J. "Diagnosis Threat": the effect of negative expectations on cognitive performance in head injury. Journal of Clinical and Experimental *Neuropsychology*, 2002;24:4, 448–57.

15. Main CJ, Spanswick CC. Functional overlay and illness behaviour in chronic pain: distress or malingering? Conceptual difficulties in medico-legal assessment of personal injury claims. *J Psychosom Res* 1995;39:737–754.

16. Martelli MF, Bush, SS, Zasler ND. Identifying and avoiding ethical misconduct in medicolegal contexts. *International Journal of Forensic Psychology* 2003;1(1): 26–44. http://ijfp.psych.uow.au/ IJFPArticlesIssue1/Martelli.pdf

17. Babitsky S, Brigham CR, Mangraviti JJ. *symptom magnification, deception and malingering: iidentification through distraction and other tests and techniques* VHS video. Falmouth: MA: SEAK, Inc., 2000.

18. Kaufman DM. *Clinical Neurology for Psychiatrists* Philadelphia, PA: W.B. Saunders, 1995.

19. Mailis A, Papagapiou M, Umana M, Cohodarevic T, Nowak J, Nicholson K. Unexplainable nondermatomal somatosensory deficits in patients with chronic nonmalignant pain in the context of litigation/compensation: a role for involvement of central factors? *Journal of Rheumatology* 2001;28:1385–93.

20. Hall HV, Pritchard DA. *Detecting Malingering and Deception: Forensic Distortion Analysis* Delray Beach: FL: St. Lucie Press, 1996.

21. Ruchinskas R, Maitin I. The detection of exaggerated sensory symptoms. In Zasler ND, Martelli, MF, eds. *Physical Medicine and Rehabilitation: State of the Art Reviews Functional Disorders*. Philadelphia: Hanley and Belfus, 2002:113–118.

22. Nicholson K, Martelli MF, Zasler ND. Myths and misconceptions about chronic pain: The problem of mind body dualism. In Weiner RB (ed.). *Pain Management: A Practical Guide for Clinicians* 6th edition Boca Raton: FL: St. Lucie Press, 2001:465–474.

23. Waddell G, Main CJ, Morris EW, Paola MD, Gray IC. Chronic low back pain, psychologic distesss, and illness behavior, *Spine* 1984;9:209–213.

24. Fishbain DA, Cole B, Cutler RB, Lewis J, Rosomoff HL, Rosomoff RS. A structured evidence-based review on the meaning of nonorganic physical signs: Waddell signs. *Pain Med.* 2003 Jun;4(2): 141–81.

25. Lees-Haley PR, Williams CW, Zasler ND, Margulies S, English LT, Steven KB. Response bias in plaintiff's histories. *Brain Inj* 1997;11:791–799

26. Lees-Haley, P, Brown RS. Neuropsychological complaint base rates of 170 personal injury claimants. *Arch Clin Neuropsychol* 1993;8:203–210.

27. Loring DW. Psychometric Detection of Malingering. Paper presented at the Annual Meeting of the *American Academy of Neurology*, Seattle: WA, 1995.

28. Cummings JL., et al., Report of the Therapeutics and Technology Assessment Subcommittee of the American Academy of Neurology: Assessment: Neuropsychological testing of adults, *Neurology* 1996;47:592–599.

29. Rogers R. ed. *Clinical assessment of malingering and deception*. New York, NY: Guilford Press, 1988.

30. BA Moore, J Donders. Predictors of invalid neuropsychological test performance after traumatic brain injury. *Brain Injury*, 2004; 18:975- 984

31. Grillo J, Brown RS, Hilsabeck R, Price JR, Lees-Haley PR. Raising doubts about claims of malingering: implications of relationships between MCMI-II and MMPI-2 performances. *Journal of Clinical Psychology*, 1994;50:651–655.

32. Heilbronner RL, Martelli MF, Nicholson K, Zasler ND. Masquerades of Brain Injury. Part IV: Functional Disorders. *The Journal of Controversial Medical Claims*, 2002;9(3):1–7.

33. MacMillan PJ, Martelli MF, Hart RP, Zasler, N.D. Pre-injury status and Adaptation Following Traumatic Brain Injury. *Brain Injury*, 2002;16(1):41–49.

34. Martelli MF, Zasler ND, MacMillan P. Mediating the relationship between injury, impairment and disability: A vulnerability, stress & coping model of adaptation following–brain injury. NeuroRehabilitation: *An interdisciplinary journal*, 1998;11(1): 51–66.

35. Binder LM, Campbell KA. Medically unexplained symptoms and neuropsychological assessment. *J Clin Exp Neuropsychol*, 2004;26:369–92.

36. Martelli MF, Zasler ND, Nicholson K, Hart RP, Heilbronner RL. Masquerades of Brain Injury. Part III: Critical Examination of Symptom Validity Testing and Diagnostic Realities in Assessment, *J Controversial Med Claims* 2002;9:19–21.

37. Reynolds CR, ed. Detection of malingering during head iniury litigation. NY: Oxford University Press, 1998.

38. Vanderploeg RD, Curtiss G. Malingering Assessment: Evaluation of Validity of Performance. *NeuroRehabilitation: Interdisciplinary J* 2001;4:245–251.

39. Senior G, Douglas L. Misconceptions and misuse of the MMPI-2 in assessing personal injury claimants. *NeuroRehabilitation: Interdisciplinary J* 2001;4:203–214.

40. Williams AD. Psychometric concerns in neuropsychological testing. *NeuroRehabilitation: Interdisciplinary J* 2001;4:221–224.

41. Nies K, Sweet J. Neuropsychological assessment and malingering: A critical review of past and present strategies. *Arch Clin Neuropsychol* 1994;9:501–552.

42. Simmonds MJ. Kumar S, Lechelt E. Psychosocial factors in disabling low back pain: Causes or consequences? *Disabil Rehabil* 1998;18:161–168.

43. Martelli MF, Zasler ND. Assessment of motivation and response bias following aquired brain injury (ABI). *J Legal Nurse Consult* 2002;13:7–14.

44. Bernard LC, McGrath MJ, Houston. Discriminating between simulated malingering and closed head injury on the Wechsler Memory Scale Revised. *Arch Clin Neuropsychol* 1993;8:539–551.

45. Trueblood W. Qualitative and Quantitative characteristics of malingered and other invalid WAIS-R and clinical memory data. *J Clin Exp Neuropsychol* 1994;16:597–607.

46. Vickery CD, Berry DTR, Inman TH, Harris MJ, Orey SA. Detection of inadequate effort on neuropsychological testing: A meta-analytic review of selected procedures. *Archives of Clinical Neuropsychology* 2001;16:45–73.

47. Strauss E, Spellacy F, Hunter M, Berry T. Assessing believable deficits on measures of attention and information processing capacity. *Arch Clin Neuropsychol* 1994;9:483–490.

48. Martens M, Donders J, Millis SR. Evaluation of invalid response sets after traumatic head injury. *Journal of Forensic Neuropsychology*, 2001;2:1–18.

49. Mittenberg W, Theroux-Fichera S, Zielinski RE, Heilbronner RL. Identification of malingered head injury on the Wechsler Adult Intelligence Scale – Revised. *Prof Psychol* 1995;26:491–498.

50. Mittenberg W, Arzin R, Millsaps C, Heilbronner R. Identification of malingered head injury on the Wechsler Memory Scale. *Psychol Assess* 1993;5:34–40.

51. Rogers R. ed. Clinical assessment of malingering and deception, 2nd ed New York, NY: Guilford Press, 1997.

52. Reitan RM, Wolfson D. Influence of age and education on neuropsychological test results. *Clin Neuropsychol* 1995;9:151–158.

53. Millis SR, Putnam SH, Adams KM, Ricker JH. The California verbal learning test in the detection of incomplete effort in neuropsychological evaluation. *Psychol Assess* 1995;7:463–471.

54. Nelson NW, Boone K, Dueck A, Wagener L, Lu P, Grills C. Relationships between eight measures of suspect effort. *Clinical Neuropsychologist* 2003, 17(2): 263–72.

55. Wiggins EC, Brandt J. The detection of simulated amnesia. *Law Hum Behav* 1988;12:57–78.

56. Lezak M. *Neuropsychological assessment* 3rd ed NewYork, NY: Oxford University Press, 1996.

57. Trueblood W, Schmidt M. Malingering and other validity considerations in the neuropsychological evaluation of mild head injury. *J Clin Exp Neuropsychol* 1993;15:578–590.

58. Martelli MF, Zasler, ND. Survey of indicators suggestive on non-organic presentations and somatic, psychologic, and cognitive response biases. In Zasler ND, Martelli, MF, eds. *Physical Medicine and Rehabilitation: State of the Art Reviews Functional Disorders*. Philadelphia: Hanley and Belfus, 2002:169–173.

59. Goebel RA. Detection of faking on the Halstead-Reitan neuropsychological test battery. *J Clin Psychol* 1983;39: 731–742.

60. Williams JM. *The Memory Assessment Scales* Odessa, FL: Psychological Assessment Resources, 1992.

61. Meyers JE, Meyers KR. *Rey Complex Figure and Recognition Trial* Odessa: FL: Psychological Assessment Resources, 1995.

62. Beetar JT, Williams JM. Malingering response styles on the Memory Assessment Scales and symptom validity tests. *Arch Clin Neuropsychol* 1995;10:57–65.

63. Allen LM, Cox DR. *Computerized Assessment of Response Bias: Revised edition* Durham, NC: CogniSyst, Inc., 1995.

64. Benton A, Spreen O. Visual memory test: The simulation of mental incompetence, *Archives of General Psychiatry* 1961;4:79–83.

65. Bernard LC. Prospects for faking believable memory deficits on neuropsychological tests and the use of incentives in simulation research. *J Clin Exp Neuropsychol* 1990;12:715–728.

66. Bernard LC. The detection of faked deficits on the Rey auditory verbal learning test: the effects of serial position. *Arch Clin Neuropsychol* 1991;6:81–88.

67. Bernard LC, Houston W, Natoli L. Malingering on neuropsychological memory tests: Potential objective indicators. *J Clin Psychol* 1993;49:45–53.

68. Delis D. *The California Verbal Learning Test* San Antonio, TX: The Psychological Corporation, 1987.

69. Arnett PA, Hammeke TA, Schwartz, L. Quantitative and qualitative performance on Rey's 15-Item Test in neurological patients and dissimulators. *Clin Neuropsychol* 1995;9:17–22.

70. Green P, Allen L, Astner K. *The Word Memory Test: A manual for the oral and computerized forms* Durham, NC: CogniSyst, Inc., 1996.

71. Green P, Gervais R, Astner K, Kiss I, Allen L. *CARB malingering test results in 210 accident/ compensation cases with and without head injury*. Paper presented at the annual meeting of the National Academy of Neuropsychology, Phoenix: Az, 1993.

72. Green P, Iverson G, Allen L. Detecting malingering in head injury litigation with the Word Memory Test. *Brain Inj* 1999;13: 813–819.

73. Guilmette TJ, Hart KJ, Giuliano AJ. Malingering detection: The use of a forced-choice method in identifying organic versus simulated memory impairment. *Clin Neuropsychol* 1993;7:59–69.

74. Iverson GL. Qualitative aspects of malingered memory deficits. *Brain Inj* 1995;9:35–40.

75. Iverson GL, Franzen MD, The Recognition Memory Test, Digit Span, and Knox Cube Test as markers of malingered memory impairment. *Assessment* 1994;1:323–34.

76. Iverson GL, Franzen MD, McCracken LM. Evaluation of an objective assessment technique for the detection of malingered memory deficits. *LawHum Behav* 1991;15:667–676.

77. Iverson GL, Franzen MD, McCracken LM. Application of a forced-choice memory procedure designed to detect experimental malingering. *Arch Clin Neuropsychol* 1994;9:437–450.

78. Iverson GL, Slick DJ, Franzen MD. Evaluation of a WMS-R malingering index n a non-litigating clinical sample. Paper presented at the annual meeting of the National Academy of Neuropsychology, New Orleans: LA, 1996.

79. Frederick RI, Foster HG. Multiple measures of malingering on a forced-choice test of cognitive ability. *Psychol Assess* 1991;3: 596–602.

80. Bigler ED. Neuropsychology and malingering: Comment on Faust, Hart, and Guilmette (1988). *J Consult Clin Psychol* 1990;58: 244–247.

81. Binder LM, Pankratz L. Neuropsychological evidence of a factitious memory complaint. *J Clin Exp Neuropsychol* 1987;9: 167–171.

82. Binder LM, Willis SC. Assessment of motivation after a financially compensable minor head trauma. *Psychol Assess* 1991;3: 175–181.

83. Binder LM. Forced-choice testing provides evidence of malingering. *Arch Phys Med Rehab* 1992;73:377–80 .

84. Binder LM. Assessment of malingering after mild head trauma with the Portland Digit Recognition Test (published erratum appears in J Clin Exp Neuropsychol, Nov, 15(6), 852). *J Clin Exp Neuropsychol* 1993;15:170–182.

85. Cercy SP, Schretlen DJ, Brandt J. Simulated amnesia and the pseudo-memory phenomena. In: Rogers R (ed.). *Clinical assessment of malingering and deception* 2nd ed. NewYork, NY: Guilford Press, 1997:108–129.

86. Brandt J, Rubinsky E, Lassen G. Uncovering malingered amnesia. *Ann N Y Acad Sci* 1985;44:502–503.

87. Cliffe MJ. Symptom-validity testing of feigned sensory or memory deficits: a further elaboration for subjects who understand the rationale. *B J Clin Psychol* 1992;31:207–209.

88. Dalby JT. Detecting faking in the pretrial psychological assessment. *Am J Forensic Psychol* 1988;6:49–55.

89. Daniel AE, Resnick PJ. Mutism, malingering, and competency to stand trial. *Bull Am Acad Psychiatry Law* 1987;15:301–308.

90. Dush DM, Simons LE, Platt M, Nation PC, Ayres SY. Psychological profiles distinguishing litigating and nonlitigating pain patients: subtle, and not so subtle. *J Pers Assess* 1994;62:299–313

91. Ensalada LH. Illness Behavior. *The AMA Guides Newsletter* May/June. 1998:4–6.

92. Faust D. The detection of deception. (Review). *Neurol Clin* 1995;13:255–265.

93. Faust D, Guilmette T J. To say it's not so doesn't prove that it isn't: research on the detection of malingering. Reply to Bigler, *J Consult Clin Psychol* 1990;58:248–250.

94. Cullum C, Heaton, R, Grant, I. Psychogenic factors influencing neuropsychological performance: Somatoform disorders, factitious disorders and malingering. In: Doerr HO, Carlin AS (eds.). *Forensic neuropsychology* New York, NY: Guilford Press, 1991.

95. Braverman M. Post-injury malingering is seldom a calculated ploy. *Occup Health Saf* 1978;47:36–40.

96. Franzen MD, Iverson GL, McCracken, LM. The detection of malingering in neuropsychological assessment. *Neuropsychol Rev* 1990;1:247–279.

97. Frederick RI, Sarfaty SD, Johnston JD, Powel J. Validation of a detector of response bias on a forced-choice test of nonverbal ability. *Neuropsychology* 1994;8:118–125.

98. Gilbertson AD, Torem M, Cohen R, Newman I. Susceptibility of common self-report measures of dissociation to malingering. *Dissociation: Progress in the Dissociative Disorders* 1992; 5:216–220.

99. Greiffenstein MF, Baker WJ, Gola T. Validation of malingered amnesia measures with a large clinical sample. *Psychol Assess* 1994;6:218–224.

100. Heaton RK, Smith HH, Lehman RA, Vogt AT. Prospects for faking believable deficits on neuropsychological testing. *J Consult Clin Psychol* 1978;46:892–900.

101. Hiscock M, Hiscock C. Redefining the forced choice method for the detection of malingering. *J Clin Exp Neuropsychol* 1989;11: 967–974.

102. Hiscock CK, Branham JD, Hiscock M. Detection of feigned cognitive impairment: The two-alternative forced-choice method compared with selected conventional tests. *J Psychopathol Behav Assess* 1994;16:95–110.

103. Rose, FE, Hall S, Szalda P, Allen D. Portland Digit Recognition Test - computerized: Measuring response latency improves the detection of malingering. *Clin Neuropsychol* 1995;9:124–134.

104. Sweet, JJ. Malingering: Differential Diagnosis. In Sweet, JJ ed, *Forensic Neuropsychology: Fundamentals and Practice*. Lisse: Swets & Zeitlinger, 1999:255–285.

105. Slick D, Hopp G, Strauss E, Hunter M, Pinch D. Detecting dissimulation: profiles of simulated malingerers, traumatic brain-injury patients, and normal controls on a revised version of Hiscock and Hiscock's Forced-Choice Memory Test. *J Clin Exp Neuropsychol* 1994;16:472–481.

106. Meyers J, Volbrecht M. Detection of Malingerers using the Rey Complex Figure and Recognition Trial. *App Neuropsychol* 1999; 6:201–207.

107. Meyers J, Galinsky A, Volbrecht M. Malingering and Mild Brain Injury: How Low is too Low. *App Neuropsychol* 1999;6: 208–216.

108. Larrabee GJ. On modifying recognition memory tests for detection of malingering. *Neuropsychology* 1992;6:23–27.

109. Lee GP, Loring DW, Martin RC. Rey's 15-item visual memory test for the detection of malingering: Normative observations on patients with neurological disorders. *Psychol Assess* 1992; 4:43–46.

110. Sbordone RJ, Seyranian GD, Ruff RM. The use of significant others to enhance the detection of malingerers from traumatically brain injured patients. *Arch Clin Neuropsychol* 2000; 15:465–477.

111. Schacter DL. On the relation between genuine and simulated amnesia. *Behav Sci Law* 1086;4:47–64.

112. Horton KD, Smith SA, Barghout NK, Connolly DA. The use of indirect memory tests to assess malingered amnesia: a study of metamemory. *J Exp Psychol Gen* 1992;121:326–351.

113. Iverson G, Green P, Gervais R. Using the Word Memory Test to detect biased responding in head injury litigation. *J Cogn Rehabil* March/April. 1999;2–6.

114. Rogers R. Development of a new classificatory model of malingering. *Bull Am Acad Psychiatry Law* 1990;18:323–333.

115. Jacobsen RR. The Post-Concussional Syndrome: Physiogenesis, psychogenesis and malingering. An integrative model. *J Psychosom Res* 1995;39:675–693.

116. Lees-Haley P, Brown RS. Biases in perception and reporting of following a perceived toxic exposure. *Percept Mot Skills* 1992;75:533–544.

117. Pankratz L, Fausti SA, Peed S. A forced-choice technique to evaluate deafness in the hysterical or malingering patient. *J Consult Clin Psychology* 1975;43:421–422.

118. Pankrantz L. Symptom validity testing and symptom retraining: procedures for the assessment and treatment of functional sensory deficits. *J Consult Clin Psychol* 1979;47:409–410.

119. Lees-Haley P, Brown RS. Neuropsychological complaint base rates of 170 personal injury claimants. *Arch Clin Neuropsychol* 1993;8:203–210.

120. Lees-Haley, PR, Brown RS. Biases in perception and reporting following a perceived toxic exposure. *Percept Mot Skills* 1992; 75:531–544.

121. Berry DT, Baer RA, Harris MJ. Detection of malingering on the MMPI: A meta-analysis. *Clin Psychol Rev* 1991;11:585–591.

122. Morey LC. *Interpretive Guide to the Personality Assessment Inventory (PAI)* Odessa, FL: Psychological Assessment Resources, 1996.

123. Gough HG. Some common misperceptions about neuroticism. *J Consult Psychol* 1954;18:287–292.

124. Lees-Haley. PR, English LT, Glenn WJ. A fake bad scale on the MMPI-2 for personal injury claimants. *Psychol Rep* 1991;68: 203–210.

125. Lees-Haley P. Attorneys influence expert evidence in forensic psychological and neuropsychological cases. *Assessment* 1997;4: 321–324.

126. Hart RP Martelli MF, Zasler ND. Chronic pain and neuropsychological functioning. *Neuropsychol Rev* 2000;10: 131–149.

127. Lees-Haley PR, Iverson GL, Lange RT, Fox DD, Allen LM. Malingering in forensic neuropsychology: *Daubert* and the MMPI-2. *Journal of Forensic Neuropsychology*, 2002, 3, 167–203.

128. Brady JP, Lind DL. Experimental analysis of hysteria. *Arch Gen Psychiatry* 1961;4:331–339.

129. Larrabee GJ. Assessment of Malingering. In GJ Larrabee, ed, *Forensic Neuropsychology:A Scientific Approach*. New York: Oxford University Press, 2005.

130. Martelli MF, Bush S, Zasler ND. Assessment of response bias impairment and disability evaluations following brain injury. In J Leon and G Zitnay, eds, *Practices in Brain Injury*. Philadelphia: Hanley and Belfus, in press.

131. Martelli MF, Zasler ND, Grayson R. Ethics and medicolegal evaluation of impairment after brain injury. In Schiffman M, ed, *Attorney's Guide to Ethics in Forensic Science and Medicine*. Springfield, Ilinois: Charles C. Thomas, 2000.

132. May RV. Symptom Magnification Syndrome. In: May RV, Martelli MF, eds, *Guide to Functional Capacity Evaluation with Impairment Rating Applications*. Richmond, VA: NADEP Publications, 1998:2:1–22.

133. Millis S. Recognition Memory Test in the detection of malingered and exaggerated memory deficits. *Clin Neuropsychol* 1992;6: 406–414.

134. Millis SR. Assessment of motivation and memory with the Recognition Memory Test after financially compensable mild head injury. *J Clin Psychol* 1994;50:601–605.

135. Millis SR, Kler S. Limitations of the Rey Fifteen-Item Test in the detection of malingering. *Clin Neuropsychol* 1995;9:241–244.

136. Martelli MF, Zasler ND, Hart, Nicholson K, Hart RP, Heilbronner RL. Masquerades of Brain Injury. Part II: Response bias assessment in Medicolegal Examinees and Examiners. *J Controversial Med Claims* 2001;8(3):13–23.

137. Palmer BW, Boone KB, Allman L, Castro DB. Co-occurrence of brain lesions and cognitive deficit exaggeration. *Clin Neuropsychol* 1995;9:68–73.

138. Ross SR, Millis SR, Krukowski RA, Putnam SH, Adams, KM. Detecting probable malingering on the MMPI-2: An examination of the Fake-Bad Scale in mild head injury. *Journal of Clinical and Experimental Neuropsychology* 2002;26:115–121

139. Resnick, PJ. Malingering of Posttraumatic Disorders. In R. Rogers, ed., *Clinical assessment of malingering and deception*. New York: Guilford Press, 1997:130–152.

140. Armstrong, JG, High, JR. Guidelines for Differentiating Malingering from PTSD. NC-PTSD Clinical Quarterly Volume 8 (3) Summer 1999, 46–48.

141. Bender SD, Rogers R. Detection of neurocognitive feigning: development of a multi-strategy assessment. *Arch Clin Neuropsychol.* 2004;9(1):49–60.

142. Teichner G, Wagner MT. The Test of Memory Malingering (TOMM): normative data from cognitively intact, cognitively impaired, and elderly patients with dementia. *Arch Clin Neuropsychology.* 2004 Apr;19(3):455–64.

143. Larrabee GJ. Detection of malingering using atypical performance patterns on standard neuropsychological tests. *Clin Neuropsychololgy,* 2003;17(3):410–25.

144. Rogers R, Harrell EH, Liff CD. Feigning neuropsychological impairment: A critical review of methodological and clinical considerations. *Clin Psychol Rev* 1993;13:255–274.

145. Wedding D, Faust D. Clinical judgement and decision-making in neuropsychology. *Arch Clin Neuropsychology* 1998;233–265.

146. Youngjohn JR. Confirmed attorney coaching prior to neuropsychological evaluation. *Assessment* 1995;2:279–283.

147. Rutherford, WH. Postconcussion Symptoms: relationship to acute neurological indices, individual differences, and circumstances of injury. In: Levin HS, Eisenberg HM, Benton AL, eds. *Mild Head Injury* New York, NY: Oxford University Press, 1989:229–244.

148. Hom J, Denney RL, eds. Detection of response bias in forensic neuropsychology: Part I. *Journal of Forensic Neuropsychology*, 2002, 2:1–166.

149. Hom J, Denney RL, eds. Detection of response bias in forensic neuropsychology: Part II. *Journal of Forensic Neuropsychology*, 2002, 3:167–314.

150. Dwyer CA. Cut Scores & Testing: Statistics, Judgment, Truth, and Error. *Psychol Assess* 1996;8:360–362.

151. Slick DJ, Sherman EMS, Iverson GL: Diagnostic criteria for malingered neurocognitive dysfunction: Proposed standards for clinical practice and research. *The Clinical Neuropsychologist* 1999;13:545–561.

152. Ranks D: The Problem of analyzing symptom invalidity. *Presentation to the Reitan Society*, June, 2005

153. Loring DW, Lee GP, Meador, KJ: Victoria Symptom Validity Test Performance in Non-Litigating Epilepsy Surgery Candidates. *Journal of Clinical and Experimental Neuropsychology* 2005; 27:610–617.

154. Gorissen M, Sanz JC, Schmand B: Effort and cognition in schizophrenia patients. *Schizophrenia Research* 2005;78:199–208.

155. Sreenivasan S, Eth S, Kirkish P, Garrick T: A practical method for the evaluation of symptom exaggeration in minor head trauma among civil litigants. *J Am Acad Psychiatry Law* 2003;31(2):220–31.

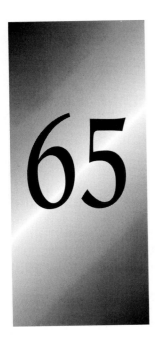

65 Decision-Making Capacity After TBI: Clinical Assessment and Ethical Implications

Sunil Kothari
Kristi Kirschner

he ability to assess decision-making capacity is one of the "core competencies" of brain injury rehabilitation. Questions about the presence or absence of this capacity lie at the root of many of our recurring clinical and ethical dilemmas. The extent to which a patient can make health care decisions, decide to live without supervision, participate in research, enter into contracts or even engage in sexual activity depends on the nature and extent of their decisional capacity. Unfortunately, many brain injury clinicians feel uncomfortable and ill-prepared to evaluate these abilities. The situation is compounded by the fact that the standard bioethical model of decision-making capacity has limitations when applied to brain injury.

The result is that, "quite frequently", inadequate attention is paid to assessing decision-making capacity or obtaining legitimate consent in brain injury rehabilitation (1). Even when attempts are made to assess decision-making capacity, there are significant discrepancies between the assessments made by rehabilitation clinicians and those performed by trained experts (2). These difficulties may partly account for the findings of a congressional investigation that brain injury rehabilitation centers often infringed on patients' autonomy (3). Rehabilitation clinicians do recognize their shortcomings in this area and have ranked as amongst their highest priorities further

education on decision-making capacity as well as the patient's role in decision making (4).

The objective of this chapter is to enable brain injury clinicians to assess the decision-making capacity of their patients as well as to understand the ethical implications of their findings. Although patients face many types of decisions after a brain injury, we will focus on the capacity to make health care decisions. It is in this realm that questions about decision-making capacity first arise after a brain injury. Moreover, we believe that the model for assessing the capacity to make health care decisions is, with some modification, directly transferable to other contexts (such as deciding to live without supervision, engaging in sexual activity, or entering into contractual relationships).

The chapter is arranged in sections as follows:

- Foundations: balancing autonomy and beneficence
- Decision-making capacity: key principles
- The standard model of assessing decision-making capacity
- Clinical application of the standard model
- The role of neuropsychological testing
- Limitations of the standard model in brain injury
- Choosing an alternate decision maker
- Beyond consent: assent and dissent
- Surrogate decision-making: the special case of withdrawal of care

FOUNDATIONS: BALANCING AUTONOMY WITH BENEFICENCE

Although our society has long protected the right of individuals to make and act on their own decisions, Anglo-American medicine had been slow to honor this right or even the principle of autonomy underlying it (5). Now, however, autonomy is the foundational value in both bioethics and health care law. The practical consequence of our commitment to this ideal is that patients, and not family members or health care professionals, have the right to make the final decisions regarding their care.

The value of respecting a patient's autonomy is based partly on the presumption that the patient is in the best position to judge what is in her best interest. However, respecting a patient's wishes has value even when she chooses a course of action detrimental to her own welfare. That is, even if a person's choice is not in her best interest, the legal and ethical consensus is that her free exercise of will is more important than preventing any harm that may result to her from the choice made. Of course, the possibility that *others* may be harmed might justify overriding a patient's choice.

If autonomy is so valuable, why shouldn't we honor the choices of all our patients, including those with brain injuries? The answer has to do with the concept of competence. For a patient's choice to be counted as autonomous, and thereby respected, it must be the product of an adequate capacity to reason and choose. But it is precisely this capacity that can be impaired in people with brain injuries. Therefore, the determination as to whether or a not a person's choice is to be honored depends crucially on whether the person is competent to make that decision.

When a person is found to be competent, then the value of autonomy outweighs all other considerations. That is, it is only under extraordinary circumstances that we can override a patient's choice, no matter how much we believe it might harm them. On the other hand, if a person lacks decision-making capacity, then the value of beneficence, which represents a commitment to protecting and even enhancing a person's welfare, is paramount. Although we may still choose to honor the patient's wishes for other reasons, we can now offer a justification (the patient's welfare) for overriding their choices.

Thus, the concern with assessing decision-making capacity is motivated both by a concern with autonomy *and* a concern with beneficence. If a person is competent, we want to make sure that we do not infringe on their ethical and legal right to control their own life. On the other hand, if a person is incompetent, we are obligated to recognize this so that we can prevent or mitigate any harm that may come to them as a result of their choices. This is why it is so important that our assessment of a patient's decision-making capacity be accurate.

DECISION-MAKING CAPACITY: KEY PRINCIPLES

Whenever a medical decision is to be made, the first step is to determine if the patient has the capacity to make that decision. (Figure 65-1) If so, the patient's wishes must ultimately be honored. If not, an alternate decision maker must be found. Most of this chapter focuses on how to assess whether a patient has decision-making capacity. Near the end however, we will discuss how to identify the appropriate decision maker when a patient is found to lack decision-making capacity.

The model of decision-making capacity that we present represents by far the most widely accepted account, both in bioethics and in the law (6). It should be noted, however, that there is some disagreement about the details of the model, even in the law, where different judicial opinions have occasionally relied on different theories of competence (7). In the text, we have indicated when there are alternatives to the views we present. We start by outlining some general principles which will frame the rest of our discussion. (Figure 65-2) First, it should be noted that, strictly speaking, "competency" is a *legal* category. This means that only a court can find someone incompetent in a particular area. The terms, "decision-making capacity" or "decisional capacity" are used to refer to the *same* set of abilities, as assessed clinically. Therefore, as clinicians, we assess the decision making capacities of our patients, not their competence. Although the legal system does rely heavily on assessments provided by clinicians, the ultimate determination is a judicial one. However, this does not mean that clinicians must rely on the courts every time there is a question about a person's capacity to make decisions; this would overwhelm the legal system. In the vast majority of cases, these assessments can and should be made by clinicians.

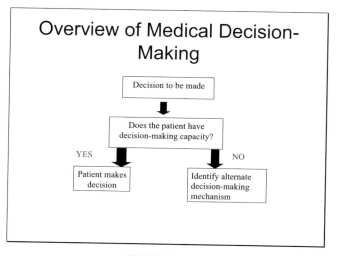

FIGURE 65-1

Overview of medical decision-making

1. Competency is a *legal* category; decision-making capacity is its clinical correlate.
2. Decision making is a *process*. Assess *how* the decision is made, *not what* is decided.
3. Evaluation should involve *direct observation* of a person's decision making abilities. Avoid inferring from the diagnosis or specific cognitive deficits.
4. Decision-making capacity is *domain specific*. One can be incompetent in some areas (e.g. financial management) but not others (e.g. medical decision making).
5. The decision making abilities required will *vary* with the demands of the situation. Consider how the patient's abilities match up with the demands of the particular decision to be made.
6. The more significant the consequences of a decision, the greater the evidence of competency required ("sliding scale" model).

FIGURE 65-2

Fundamental principles of competency

Later in the chapter, we will discuss when recourse to the courts might be necessary. For now, the key point is that competence and incompetence are *legal* terms and are most appropriately used to describe judicial determinations. However, because it is common in everyday clinical situations to use the terms "competence" and "decision-making capacity" interchangeably, we will occasionally do the same. Readers should be aware of the distinction, however.

Another key principle is that the focus of an assessment should be on the process by which a decision is made rather than the decision itself. If the process by which a decision is made is sound, then the decision is considered valid, regardless of the clinician's opinion of its merit. Theoretically, the emphasis on the decision making process might lead to a situation in which a particular patient is determined to lack decision-making capacity even while another patient, making the same decision under identical circumstances, is considered competent. This would happen when the process by which one of the patients reached her decision was impaired, while the other's was satisfactory. Further detail on how to assess the decision making process in actual clinical situations will be provided in the next section.

The importance of evaluating the actual decision making process also means that one cannot infer the presence of decision-making capacity from a patient's diagnosis or cognitive deficits. Clearly not everyone with a brain injury or impaired memory lacks decision-making capacity. For this reason, we need to assess patients individually, in the context of the particular decision being made. Ideally, we should observe them as they engage in the process of making the decision that is at issue. This

way we can directly assess their ability to understand, appreciate, and reason with the relevant information (components of decisional capacity that we elaborate on below).

In addition, an assessment of decision-making capacity is distinct from an evaluation of cognitive capacities such as memory, attention, cognitive flexibility, etc. Although these processes affect or even underlie decision-making capacity, deficits in these areas do not automatically preclude the presence of decision-making capacity. Therefore, their evaluation should never supplant (although it can supplement) the direct observation of a person's decision making abilities. This issue will be discussed further in the section on the role of neuropsychological testing.

Decision-making capacity is rarely an all-or-nothing phenomenon; a person may lack the capacity to make certain decisions but not others. In other words, decision-making capacity is domain specific. This is also true of legal determinations of competency. For instance, someone may be found to be incompetent to manage her financial affairs but competent to make medical decisions. In the same way, a clinician may decide that a patient has the capacity to make decisions regarding her place of residence but not about whether to undergo a medical procedure.

Moreover, even *within* a domain, the decision-making capacity required will vary with the particular decision being made. This is because different decisions make different cognitive demands on the patient. Even with regard to medical decision making, patients may be able to make some decisions but not others. For instance, someone may be able to make a simple decision where the risks are low and the benefits high (for instance, to undergo surgery for acute appendicitis) but be unable to make a more complicated decision involving intermediate risks and different categories of outcomes (for instance, trading off a low risk of death for a moderate improvement in functional status). Thus, all assessments of decision-making capacity must be done in the context of the specific decision being made. This principle is well summarized by Grisso and Appelbaum, when they write that ". . . competence is not simply dependent on a person's abilities, but on the *match or mismatch between the patient's abilities and the decision-making demands of the situation that the patient faces.*" (From Ref. 6, p. 23)

Another corollary of the context dependence of assessing decision-making capacity is that the potential consequences of a decision should affect how thoroughly we investigate a patient's abilities. This is known as the "sliding scale" model of assessment. The idea is this: the more significant the consequences of a particular decision, the more evidence we should require that a person has decisional capacity. For example, we would require stronger evidence that a patient has decision-making capacity when she chooses to forgo life sustaining treatment than when she refuses an antacid to treat gastric reflux. The greater the risk to the patient, the more we need to be certain that the decision represents an autonomous choice.

THE STANDARD MODEL OF ASSESSING DECISION-MAKING CAPACITY

We have stressed the importance, in assessing decision-making capacity, of contextual features such as the nature, demands, and consequences of the decision being made. We now turn to the specific abilities that constitute decisional capacity. (Figure 65-3) Although the terminology used to describe these skills varies, there is agreement in the bioethical and legal literature about the nature of the abilities themselves. In what follows, we adopt the terminology used by Grisso and Appelbaum (6).

The first and most basic ability required is the ability to *express a choice*. A person who is not able to express (either verbally or behaviorally) a preference lacks decision-making capacity. This would certainly be the case early after a brain injury, before a patient has recovered consciousness. Even after patients have regained the ability to express preferences, however, it is important to recognize that the ability to express a choice is by itself insufficient to establish decision-making capacity. Patients must also possess the other abilities discussed below. The importance of expressing a choice lies in its absence, signaling unequivocal lack of the capacity to make decisions.

A second ability required in order to make decisions is the ability to *understand* relevant information. In the context of medical decision making, this information would include the nature and rationale of the treatment and its risks and benefits as well alternatives to the proposed treatment (as well as their risks and benefits). (Figure 65-4) Of course, this assumes that the clinician herself know what the risks and benefits are; there is considerable

evidence that rehabilitation clinicians have difficulty in estimating patients' risks for activities such as walking, living alone, etc (8).

Of course, simply understanding the information is not enough; one must acknowledge that it is relevant to one's situation. We refer specifically to an *appreciation* of one's condition, with a special emphasis on how the intervention(s) being proposed applies to one's own circumstances. This ability is often impaired in people with brain injuries and manifests itself as decreased insight into any deficits that are present. As a result, a patient may evince complete understanding of the information outlined in Figure 65-4 and yet be unable to relate it meaningfully to her own situation.

In addition to understanding and appreciating the relevant information, patients must also be able to *reason* appropriately. The information must be processed by the patient in a logical and coherent manner. For one, a patient needs to relate the various possible outcomes to their own values. For example, is the value the patient places on physical independence reflected in their thinking and the choices they make? Patients also need to able to imagine what the consequences of the various options would be. Ideally, patients would be able to go beyond simply verbalizing consequences to being able to describe the potential effects on their life (for instance, to appreciate the impact on their life of possible impotence after prostate surgery). These are just some of the factors that we all consider in making these sorts of decisions.

CLINICAL APPLICATION OF THE STANDARD MODEL

How does one assess whether or not a person has the required abilities to choose, understand, appreciate and reason? While the evaluation of some of these abilities seems fairly straightforward (e.g. is a person capable of expressing a preference?), the assessment of others seems to be more complicated (e.g. how to assess reasoning ability?). In what follows, we offer suggestions on how clinicians can evaluate a patient's decisional capacity. Our

---

1. The ability to *express a choice*
2. The ability to *understand* information relevant to treatment decision making
3. The ability to *appreciate* the significance of that information for one's own situation, especially concerning one's illness and the probable consequences of one's treatment options
4. The ability to *reason* with relevant information so as to engage in a logical process of weighing treatment options.

Adapted from *Assessing Competence to Consent to Treatment* by Grisso and Applebaum, 1998, Oxford University Press

FIGURE 65-3

Components of decision-making capacity

- Nature and rationale of treatment
- Risks and benefits of treatment (including their likelihood)
- Risks and benefits of the alternatives (including no treatment)

Adapted from *Assessing Competence to Consent to Treatment* by Grisso and Applebaum, 1998, Oxford University Press

FIGURE 65-4

Relevant information that patients must understand

focus throughout is on a "bedside" evaluation which can be performed without the aid of more formal tools. However, we should note that such tools are now being developed, including one developed by Grisso and Appelbaum (6). In addition, we address the role of neuropsychological testing in the next section.

As we mentioned earlier, one of the key principles of assessing decisional capacity is that we operationalize our assessment. This means that we should evaluate the abilities described above when a patient is actively involved in the process of making a decision. During this process, we can engage the patient through a series of questions. (Figure 65-5) The point is that we are not inferring the patient's capacities from either their diagnosis or cognitive deficits (e.g. impaired memory); we are directly examining the abilities in question.

The questions outlined in Figure 65-5 for assessing appreciation, understanding, and expressing a choice are self explanatory. As we mentioned above, assessing the component of reasoning is the least straightforward. The strategy here is to ask the person to "think out loud". That is, one asks them to retrace for the examiner the process by which they reached their decision. The examiner observes for a logical and coherent thought process. Of special interest are issues such as: how does the person understand and weigh risks (including their likelihood), is the person making a choice consistent with the values that they profess, is the person able to imagine the consequences of the various options, etc.

ABILITY TO EXPRESS A CHOICE
  "Please tell me what your decision is."

ABILITY TO UNDERSTAND THE RELEVANT INFORMATION
  "Can you tell me, in your own words, what you know about:
  • Your condition.
  • The treatment recommended
  • The risks and benefits of this treatment
  • The risks and benefits of other options (including no treatment at all)."

ABILITY TO APPRECIATE ONE'S OWN SITUATION
  "Can you tell me what you believe is wrong with you?"
  "Do you believe that you need some sort of treatment?"

ABILITY TO REASON WITH THE RELEVANT INFORMATION
  "Tell me how you reached your decision"
  "What factors did you consider?"

Adapted from *Assessing Competence to Consent to Treatment* by Grisso and Appelbaum, 1998, Oxford University Press

FIGURE 65-5

Questions to ask in assessing decision-making abilities

The assessment of a patient's decision-making capacity is not limited to an evaluation of their abilities to understand, appreciate, and reason. As discussed previously, the context in which these capacities are exercised is crucial. In particular, one needs to understand the specific decisional task the patient is confronting. This is because different tasks make different demands on understanding and reasoning. We should adjust the degree of understanding and reasoning we expect based on the inherent nature and complexity of the decision. For example, certain treatments in acute care medicine may result in a somewhat higher risk of death initially but a better functional outcome for survivors. These outcomes and the resulting necessity to balance values such as death and functional status make greater demands on understanding and reasoning abilities than, for instance, deciding to undergo a minimally risky treatment that should lead to a cure.

In addition to taking into account the complexity of the decision to be made, one should also keep in mind the possible consequences of the decision. This is because, the more significant the consequences, the more evidence of decision-making capacity we should require. For instance, if a patient refuses a low risk, potentially life saving intervention, we would require that they more thoroughly demonstrate evidence of their decision-making capacity than if they refused a high risk intervention with little chance of success. We should adjust the questions that we ask and the answers we deem acceptable based on the likely impact on the patient's welfare.

Although we have stressed the indispensable role of direct observation of a person's decision making abilities, there is a role for supplementary information. Specifically, in addition to the assessment outlined in Figure 65-5, one should also solicit information from third parties including caregivers and family members. As a result of the time that they spend with the patient, they often have a richer knowledge of the patient's decision making abilities than can be gathered from the clinician's formal assessment. For instance, their observations of how the patient reasons through other decisions or situations will have some bearing on how they deliberate in the present situation. More importantly, there are factors that may be relevant to decision-making capacity that may only be gleaned from direct observation of behavior in other realms.

For instance, as we will discuss below, it is entirely possible that a person could satisfactorily answer the questions asked in a formal assessment, and yet not behave in a way consistent with their answers. This "verbal-behavioral dissociation" is often seen in people with brain injuries but, by its very nature, can easily be missed in the verbally and cognitively biased assessment that we have outlined. Supplementary information in the form of observations by family members and other third parties is crucial in these cases. Of course, one must always keep in mind the possibility of conflicts of interest between family members and the patient that might affect the information provided.

Finally, a few logistical points should be made about the assessment. First, because cognitive capacities can fluctuate after brain injury, multiple evaluations are often necessary to ensure that a person's best performance is observed. Performing such serial assessments also allows one to establish the consistency of a patient's choices over time. The absence of such consistency (for instance, when a patient changes her decision from day to day) raises serious questions about a patient's decision-making abilities. Moreover, one must also be mindful of any potentially reversible factors that might influence a person's ability to make decisions. Examples would include medication effects and the impact of fatigue. As much as possible, one should attempt to minimize the effects of such factors in the interests of maximizing a patient's performance.

It is also important to ensure that the optimal mode of communication has been established. Communication impairments are ubiquitous in brain injury, ranging from specifically linguistic problems (i.e. aphasias) to higher order impairments (e.g. pragmatic deficits). As a result, it is crucial that adequate communication exists such that there is little doubt that information is being appropriately conveyed to and from the patient. Also, adequate time needs to be spent with the patient to ensure that all the relevant information is provided and that all questions are addressed. Any ancillary means to enhance the disclosure of information should be utilized (e.g. written explanations, visual aids, augmentative communication, etc.).

THE ROLE OF NEUROPSYCHOLOGICAL TESTING

Neuropsychological testing often plays a significant role in the evaluation of decision-making capacity. We believe, however, that its proper function can be misunderstood. In particular, we are concerned that testing can become a substitute for the direct clinical assessment of decisional capacity, resulting in less accurate and potentially inappropriate conclusions. Neuropsychological testing should play a *supplementary* role in the assessment of decisional capacity; the determination of intact or impaired decision-making capacity should rarely be based solely on the results of such an evaluation. We want to stress that our concerns are limited to *formal testing* only and not assessments performed by neuropsychologists. In fact, by virtue of their training and skills, neuropsychologists are ideally suited to perform the clinical assessment described earlier in the chapter.

It is easy to see why the formal assessment of cognitive deficits is thought to be central to the evaluation of decisional capacity. After all, impairments in decision-making

capacity are a direct result of the neuropsychological sequelae of brain injury. The cognitive, affective, and behavioral domains affected by brain injury form the substrate of most of our everyday tasks, including our ability to make decisions. Since discrete cognitive capacities such as attention, memory, language, etc. underlie the ability to make decisions, it seems only natural that these be formally assessed whenever decisional capacity is in question. However, the desire to base conclusions regarding decision-making capacity purely on formal testing is based on a misunderstanding of the nature of decision making abilities and the ways in which they are affected by cognitive deficits.

Although impairments in decision-making capacity are a *consequence* of neuropsychological deficits (whether cognitive, affective, or volitional), they are not identical with them. The ability to make decisions is best understood by analogy to other abilities in rehabilitation medicine, such as walking. In the case of walking, the inability to walk is the consequence of a complex interaction between various physical deficits (e.g., weakness in different muscle groups, spasticity, deconditioning, residual abilities in other parts of the body, presence of neglect, etc.) as well as the context in which one walks (e.g., level surfaces, carpet, incline, etc.). Although one could theoretically devise a model that incorporates all of these variables to predict whether a particular patient will walk, it is far easier to perform a direct assessment by standing them up and attempting to walk with them. Moreover, given the complexity of walking and its dependence on context, no model will ever be as accurate as direct assessment.

Similarly, the ability to make decisions is the consequence of a complex interaction between various mental capacities (memory, abstract reasoning, attention, etc.) and the context of the decision to be made (whom to vote for, whether to undergo surgery, to engage in sexual activity, etc.). Once again, given the number of variables involved and the complexity of their potential interaction, it would be far easier to directly assess decision-making capacity (as outlined earlier) than attempt to infer its presence or absence from what are, at best, surrogate markers. In addition, the importance of taking the context into account can not be over-emphasized: a particular cognitive deficit might impair the capacity to make one decision but not another.

Because decision-making capacity is not identical with the capacities that underlie it, there is no clear way to determine what pattern of test findings preclude adequate decision making. Even with isolated deficits, there is rarely a one to one correspondence between a deficit and the ability to make a particular decision, much less the ability to make all decisions. For instance, while it is clear that impaired attention can affect most of the components of decisional capacity mentioned above (for instance, understanding or reasoning), it is not clear, except in cases of extreme impairment, what degree of attentional deficit precludes adequate decision making. We have to return to the direct assessment outlined above (Fig. 65-5) in order to confirm that a patient's inattention is significantly affecting their ability to process information.

The problem is compounded by the fact that, as mentioned above, decision making tasks of differing complexity require different levels of understanding or reasoning abilities. Therefore, a person with impaired attention may have the capacity to make a simple decision but not a more complex one. Once again, we would have to assess the person's abilities directly. Finally, because one can compensate for attentional deficits to a certain extent, the same degree of attentional impairment may result in a patient having decision-making capacity at some times and not others (depending on whether the information is presented in a quiet, distraction-free environment, repeated several times, etc.). There are cases described of patients believed to lack decision-making capacity solely because they had certain deficits on testing (e.g. aphasia), who were found, on a more direct assessment, to actually have decisional capacity (especially when compensatory strategies were employed) (9).

The inability to "read off" a person's decision making status from their cognitive impairments is the primary obstacle to relying *exclusively* on neuropsychological testing; however, there are other limitations as well. It is difficult to test certain capacities that have a direct bearing on decision-making capacity. The best known of these are the so called frontal lobe capacities such as cognitive flexibility, the ability to plan, the ability to consider hypothetical situations, etc. Frontal lobe function can only be incompletely tested at the present time and patients can do well on formal testing even though they have frontal lobe dysfunction directly affecting their decisional capacity (10, 11). This is not as much of an issue when one is directly assessing decision-making capacity because one is directly observing the effects of possible frontal lobe deficits on the patient's reasoning. That is, one can directly observe the patient's ability to consider consequences, recognize and weigh alternatives, assess the ability of a particular decision to realize their goals, etc., all in the context of the decision in question. Once again, direct assessment will usually be superior to a formal assessment of certain neuropsychological domains.

Indeed, we believe that the actual determination of a person's decision-making capacity can often be made independently of a formal neuropsychological evaluation. This is because, as we have outlined above, the components of decision-making capacity (evincing a choice, understanding, appreciation, and reasoning) can be *directly* assessed (Fig. 65-5), without having to evaluate the cognitive capacities that underlie these abilities. While it is true that cognitive functions such as attention or memory form the basis of decision-making capacity, it is *not*

necessary to know how and to what extent they are affected in order to determine whether or not a patient has adequate decision making abilities for a particular situation. Since we are primarily concerned with the *effects* of cognitive deficits on decision-making capacity, we would be better off assessing the decision making abilities directly, rather than inferring them from neuropsychological test results.

In fact, studies that have investigated the correlation between neuropsychological test results and decision-making capacity acknowledge that the clinical assessment of decision-making capacity is the "gold standard" (11, 12). The aim of these studies was to determine whether testing by itself could match the accuracy of direct clinical assessments. Not surprisingly, while neuropsychological test results were correlated with the presence or absence of decision-making capacity, testing by itself was never as accurate as direct clinical assessment (13–16).

Despite its limitations, formal testing does have an important role to play. There are at least two purposes it can serve. First, the presence of deficits on testing can alert us to the possibility that a patient's decision-making capacity may be impaired. For instance, the identification of a short-term memory problem, while not enough to determine that a person lacks decision-making capacity, can prompt a direct assessment to make that determination.

More importantly, neuropsychological testing allows us to determine *why* a person's decision-making capacity may be impaired. The "direct" assessment that we outlined earlier simply allows us to determine whether or not a person has decisional capacity adequate to the task at hand. It rarely allows an identification of the cognitive impairments that underlie a particular patient's difficulties. For example, a person's inability to understand the information provided by a clinician may be caused by inattention or a language deficit. While knowing the cause does not alter the determination that the person lacks decision-making capacity, it does allow the clinician to target interventions to either correct the underlying deficit (e.g. discontinuing a sedating medication) or compensate for it (e.g. provide verbal explanations for someone with alexia).

LIMITATIONS OF THE PROPOSED MODEL IN BRAIN INJURY

If forced to choose one method of evaluation, the direct assessment of decisional capacity is superior to neuropsychological testing. However, the two approaches complement each other and are best used together. Unfortunately, even this combination is sometimes not enough, especially in the case of brain injury. This is primarily because both direct assessment as well as neuropsychological testing have a strong cognitive bias. That is, they are heavily weighted towards evaluating the cognitive aspects of decision making while virtually ignoring the affective, volitional, and behavioral domains which are often impaired in people with brain injuries. As is well known, cognitive abilities can often dissociate from these other domains. As a result, someone whose cognitive functions are preserved may be thought to have adequate decision-making capacity when, in reality, deficits in emotion, volition, or behavior may be impairing their ability to make decisions.

The most obvious example is the person who is unable to conform their behavior to their professed beliefs and desires. There are many people with brain injuries who are able to reply appropriately to questions about how they would act in particular situations but are unable to do so when they are actually confronted with them (17). Unfortunately, an assessment that limits itself to purely verbal or written responses (such as in a clinical interview or formal testing) will not be able to identify these problems precisely because they arise only when the patient is performing an action. For instance, in assessing whether someone has the capacity to decide to live on their own, one would ask how the patient would respond to different scenarios (for instance, smelling a gas leak). Even if the patient responded appropriately, one can not automatically assume they will act in the way they described. This might be because they have difficulty with impulse control which circumvents their ability to act in ways they might have intended. Or, the patient may have an amotivational syndrome that affects their ability to act on any of their beliefs or desires. These examples underscore the point made earlier about the importance of supplementing interview-based data with behavioral information obtained both through one's own observations as well as those of others.

Despite its significance in many contexts, the dissociation between cognition and behavior is not quite as relevant for decisions regarding health care. This is because for these decisions the patient rarely has to act; rather, they are passive recipients of others' actions (as in undergoing surgery). Since there is rarely behavior on the patient's part following a health care decision, a cognitively oriented evaluation should be adequate. For those decisions that do have a prominent behavioral component (such as the decision to engage in sexual activity), such an evaluation would have to be supplemented by knowledge of a patients' behavior.

Information about verbal-behavioral dissociations is often relatively easy to collect. Unfortunately, there are other non-cognitive impairments that may be more difficult to detect, thus increasing the chances that someone might be thought to have decisional capacity when, in fact, they don't. The most common of these impairments involve disorders of affect such as moderate to severe depression. Although it is known that depression can

directly affect cognition (for instance, information processing efficiency, short term memory, etc.)(6), these effects should be detectable by a direct assessment such as the one outlined in this chapter (at least in so far as these deficits compromise decision making ability for the decision at hand).

However, disorders of affect can compromise decision making in more subtle, but still significant ways (7). For instance, depression can alter how one values certain outcomes. Consider a severely depressed patient who is faced with a potentially life saving intervention with relatively low risk and minimal discomfort. The patient may have full understanding of the intervention, an appreciation of her medical situation, and adequate reasoning or information processing skills. She may still choose to refuse the intervention because she no longer wishes to live and sees her condition as offering an opportunity to die (18, 19). According to our original model, one would consider this patient to have intact decision-making capacity because she has the requisite cognitive capacities that are the focus of the evaluation. What is impaired is her ability to *value* appropriately; her depression causes her to favor outcomes that she would not have favored prior to the onset of her mood disorder.

The impact of emotions on decision making extends beyond the classical disorders of affect, however. Brain injury can affect emotions in other ways, most notably in the form of the hypoemotionality that can be seen after ventromedial frontal lobe injury (20). According to Damasio, certain frontal lobe injuries can result in an impairment in ". . . assigning different values to different options,. . . [thereby making one's] decision-making landscape hopelessly flat." (from 20, p. 57) He elaborates: ". . . the process of emotion and feeling are indispensable for rationality. At their best, feelings point us in the proper direction, take us to the appropriate place in a decision-making space, where we may put the instruments of logic to good use." (from 20, p.58) In the case of depression, patients still have the capacity to value; however, their valuations are inappropriate and different from what they would have been in the past. In the case of hypoemotionality, however, the capacity to value *any* outcome is impaired, thereby compromising decisional capacity in the way outlined by Damasio.

Impairments of hypo-emotionality are often difficult to identify on standard neuropsychological assessments. Indeed, one patient that Damasio discusses did well on all neuropsychological tests, even those specific for frontal lobe dysfunction. Yet, this patient had profound deficits in making decisions in "real life" situations, attributed to his affective impairments (20). For similar reasons, the assessment of decision-making capacity that we have presented, focused as it is on cognitive skills such as understanding and reasoning, may also fail to identify these sorts of impairments.

Decision making not only involves the ability to value outcomes appropriately but also the ability to respond appropriately to risks. This goes beyond simply understanding the quantitative aspects of risk, which can be impaired in depression (21). It also involves the appropriate emotional reaction to risk (such as being averse to risk unless the potential benefits outweigh the risks involved). Unfortunately, brain injury can also distort risk taking behavior, potentially changing the decisions patients might otherwise have made. For instance, depression after a brain injury can cause people to become more risk averse (22). This might prevent a depressed patient from choosing a moderately risky but highly beneficial medical intervention which they might normally have chosen before they became depressed. Yet, the patient's ability to express a choice, understand, appreciate, and reason would be found to be intact, leading one to conclude that the patient's decision-making capacity was not compromised. Other disorders of affect may cause similar distortions of our perception and response to risks. For instance, anxiety may also cause a state of risk aversion while mania or hypomania can cause one to be risk seeking. Regardless of whether one becomes more or less risk averse, these classical disorders of emotion can affect decision making in a way that would be difficult to detect by either direct assessment or formal testing.

In cases of hypoemotionality, there is evidence that individuals may lose the ability to feel *any* emotional response to the presence of risk. For instance, studies have shown that many patients with frontal lobe injuries do not manifest the normal activation of the sympathetic nervous system when confronted by risk (20, 23). These patients subsequently demonstrated increased risk taking behavior (23). The implications for decision making are clear. In the case of behaviors, not having the appropriate emotional response in the presence of risk will probably lead to increased risk taking with implications for a person's capacity to decide to, for instance, engage in sexual activity. Even for decisions that don't necessarily lead to overt actions on the part of the patient (such as medical decision making), the lack of the affective component of risk perception may lead patients to decide on risky interventions that they might otherwise have avoided. Once again, purely cognitive evaluations such as direct clinical assessments or formal testing will be unable to detect the influence of this type of affective impairment on decision making.

These evaluations will also fail to identify other impairments in decision making that can occur after frontal lobe injury. For instance, there is evidence that patients with ventromedial injuries discount the future excessively and, as a consequence, distort their decision-making by placing undue weight on short term gains or losses at the expense of future gains or losses (23). In the context of medical decision making, this might lead to a patient deciding against an intervention that might have some temporary discomfort early on but significant benefits in the long-term. Or the reverse might happen: the patient may choose an intervention that provides some short-term gains but may actually be deleterious in the future. It would be difficult to identify this sort of impairment through direct clinical assessment or testing. One would have to rely on behavioral evidence based on one's own observations or reports from others. Unfortunately, this evidence is often not available in the first few months after brain injury since patients have not yet been in contexts where they have had to make many of their own decisions. This type of temporal "myopia" can also affect behavior such that patients might choose short–term pleasure (e.g. not using contraception) over long-term risks (e.g. an unwanted pregnancy).

Finally, there is evidence that frontal lobe injury can result in a lack of sensitivity to behavioral reinforcers (24). This might lead someone to repeat poor decisions because the aversive consequences of that decision are limited in their ability to change the patient's behavior. This sort of deficit is more relevant to decisions involving actions (such as those involving sexual activity) than those that involve health care decisions. When assessing for the presence of this type of deficit, one can often rely on evidence of past behaviors.

In summary, there are a variety of affective or behavioral impairments that can directly affect decision making and yet not be detected by either direct assessment of decisional capacity or formal testing: lack of sensitivity to behavioral reinforcers, temporal myopia and changes in valuation and risk perception (whether caused by classical disorders of affect or hypoemotionality). Of these, only those deficits related to classical disorders of affect (such as depression, anxiety, and mania) are readily accessible to routine clinical examination (whether in the form of interview or formal questionnaires). One should supplement all evaluations of decision making with these assessments to probe for the presence of any significant affective symptomology. If present, more time will need to be spent determining the effects of these affective symptoms on valuation and risk perception. Unfortunately, it is more difficult to assess for the effects of hypoemotionality on valuation and risk perception, the presence of temporal myopia, or the lack of responsiveness to behavioral reinforcers. At the present time, other than finding clues from knowledge of past behaviors and the clinical interview, there is little guidance available on how to directly assess for these deficits.

Even after taking into account volitional, affective, and behavioral issues, there is another situation encountered after brain injury that challenges our traditional methods of assessing decision making. This situation arises when a moderate or severe brain injury seems to cause a fundamental change in the patient's identity.

Family members often comment on these types of changes by statements such as "She's a different person", "He's not the man I married", or "I'm living with a stranger". This phenomenon has significant implications for the status of the decisions made by someone with a brain injury.

For instance, consider someone who seems to have full decision-making capacity as outlined above (i.e. no significant deficits in understanding, appreciation, reasoning, or expressing their choices) *and* no significant affective, volitional, or behavioral deficits. However, they now make decisions that they clearly would not have made prior to their injury. For example, what they value and consider important may have changed so that they now spend their money on activities that they would not have before their injury. These sorts of changes are undoubtedly part of the phenomenon that the family describes when they note that the patient is "a different person". Moreover, families often see the patient's new choices as *prima facie* evidence that the patient has lost decision-making capacity.

In these situations, the clinician is faced with a difficult situation: someone whose decision-making capacity appears to be intact but who is now choosing courses of action that she may not have chosen prior to the injury. Should the person's decisions be honored? This is a controversial question which has been most extensively discussed in the context of dementia (25, 26). In someone with a brain injury, our belief is that, as long as the person currently has intact decision-making capacity, their decisions should always be honored. The patient who is being treated is the patient as they are *now*. We feel that it would be unfair to the patient as they are now to sacrifice their autonomy and interests for the sake of their former self.

Finally, although not unique to people with brain injuries, it is important to be aware of any psychodynamic issues that might be affecting a patient's decision making. We have been struck by how often a person's decision is determined not by the information at hand (e.g. the risks and benefits of the treatment and its alternatives, etc.) but rather by underlying psychological factors that may or may not be apparent to the patient. Unless explicitly addressed, the examiner will almost always miss the presence and significance of these factors. Yet, these psychological issues often represent the "missing piece of the puzzle" that makes sense of what might appear to be a perplexing decision. This is particularly true when there appears to be a "gap" between the patient's apparently intact cognitive capacities and the seemingly "irrational" choice they make.

For instance, a young adult may refuse a relatively innocuous medication simply because her family also wants her to take it and she is trying to establish independence from them. Her decision is determined by the conflict with her family and *not* by the indications and effects of the medication itself. However, the patient may articulate her refusal in terms of her fear of the side effects. Even when reassured about the side effects, she might still maintain her refusal, suggesting to the family and clinician that her decision-making capacity might be impaired. Or, a patient may be very anxious about her symptoms and demand that "everything be done" to evaluate the cause, despite reassurance by the clinician of the benign nature of her condition. Further exploration might reveal that the patient had a family member who became very ill or died after developing similar symptoms.

In both cases, a direct assessment of decisional capacity may fail to reveal any significant deficits. Rather than simply acquiesce, however, clinicians should spend time exploring psychodynamic issues when faced with these dissociations between intact decision-making capacity and seemingly irrational decisions. Recognition of these psychological factors provides an opportunity to address what is really motivating the decision and, hopefully, result in a situation where patients base their decision solely on information that is directly relevant to the treatment.

WHEN SOMEONE LACKS DECISION-MAKING CAPACITY: CHOOSING AN ALTERNATE DECISION-MAKER

When it is determined that a patient lacks decision-making capacity for a particular decision, we must rely on alternate methods of making that decision. (Figure 65-1) Most states specify an order which must be followed in identifying another mechanism of decision making. (Figure 65-6) Assuming that the patient does not currently have a guardian, it is important to establish whether or not the patient has retained the capacity to execute a durable power of attorney for health care (DPAHC, which may go by different names in other states). As discussed in further detail below, such a document allows patients to designate another person to make health care decisions for them. Although it might seem odd that a patient who is considered incapacitated from making medical decisions might still retain the capacity to appoint

- Current guardian
- Establish if patient has the capacity to execute a DPAHC
- Advance directive
- Surrogate decision maker (designated by state statute)
- Appoint guardian

FIGURE 65-6

Example of alternate healthcare decision-making (Texas) listed in order of priority

a surrogate decision maker, this is clearly in line with the emphasis placed earlier on the context specific nature of decision-making capacity.

What is required to execute a DPAHC is that a patient must *appreciate* why they need someone to make decisions for them, *understand* the nature, benefits, and risks of a DPAHC, its alternatives, and of the person they might designate, and *reason* with this information in a logical and coherent manner. There are patients who either understand or accept that they are unable to make medical decisions and who have strong feelings about who they want to be making decisions in their stead. As long as these patients understand the nature and implications of a DPAHC and alternatives and have logical and appropriate reasons for preferring a particular person, they should be allowed to designate a surrogate decision maker by executing a DPAHC. In fact, in our experience, courts have favored this approach since it represents the "least restrictive" limitation of a patient's autonomy.

If a patient does not currently have the capacity to execute a DPAHC, one should ascertain whether they had executed one prior to their injury. This would represent one type of an advance directive, known as a proxy directive. The other type of advance directive is known as a decision directive (6, 26). In contrast to the proxy directive, a decision directive does not identify a surrogate decision maker. Rather, it specifies what decisions a patient would want made under particular circumstances. For instance, a person may specify in advance that they do not want to be placed on a ventilator if terminally ill. Thus, a decision directive attempts to anticipate possible scenarios and outlines patients' wishes should they be unable to express them. The familiar "living will" is one example of a decision directive.

Although very useful in some situations, decision directives have limited applicability in the context of brain injury. The primary reason for this is that very few people have executed advance directives of this sort, especially in the age groups often affected. Even when they exist, decision directives rarely address the situations most often encountered in the rehabilitation setting; rather, they almost always focus on terminal illness. It is true that some states recognize decision directives that apply in cases of permanent unconsciousness or severe disability; however, even these will only apply to a subset of the patients encountered in most rehabilitation settings (26).

More useful in brain injury rehabilitation are proxy directives. Rather than attempt to anticipate the myriad decisions that need to be made, these types of advance directives allow a person to designate a proxy to serve as the decision-maker. As discussed earlier, the Durable Power of Attorney for Health Care (DPAHC) is the legally recognized method for designating a health care proxy. The advantage of such a proxy directive is that it allows the designated decision-maker to make all healthcare decisions that the patient could have made, unless limited by the patient in the directive. Unfortunately, as with decision directives, proxy advance directives are rarely available in the context of brain injury rehabilitation.

The decision-maker designated by a proxy directive is one example of a surrogate decision-maker. A surrogate decision-maker is one who is morally and/or legally empowered to speak on behalf of another person. In the case of a proxy directive, the surrogate's authority derives from the fact that the patient explicitly designated them as the proxy. However, there are other methods of choosing a surrogate decision-maker, should the patient not have specified someone in advance. These include a person recognized through state surrogate statutes or a court appointed guardian.

The vast majority of patients do not have either a guardian or an advance directive. To address this situation, many states have adopted statutes that specify, in order of priority, who should serve as the surrogate decision-maker for an incapacitated patient. While the order may vary slightly depending on the individual state statute, the hierarchy usually formalizes the conventionally recognized "next of kin" as the decision-maker. For example, a spouse would precede the adult child, who would precede the parent, who would precede siblings, etc. If no family exists, then even a close friend or clergyman may be recognized as the surrogate decision-maker in some states.

Being familiar with the statute in one's state is critical. Many surrogate statutes have restrictions on the circumstances under which they are applicable as well as on the types of decisions that surrogates are allowed to make (particularly regarding withholding or withdrawing life-sustaining treatments). In addition, most statutes require a court hearing if another family member challenges the decisions of the surrogate decision-maker recognized by the statute.

If there is no state surrogate statute, most jurisdictions require the appointment of a guardian. A guardian may also be required in states with statutes when the legally recognized decision-maker is being challenged by other family members. Another case in which appeal to the courts may be required is if no one knows the patient or agrees to serve as a surrogate. Other situations that usually require a guardian are the need to make any non-medical decisions (for instance, about financial matters) or when it is obvious that the duration of the patient's incapacity will be prolonged. Deciding whether to petition for guardianship after a brain injury can be difficult and complex; the reader is referred to several useful reviews of the subject (27, 28).

To summarize, once it is determined that a person lacks decisional capacity, the first step is to identify a surrogate decision-maker. (Fig. 65-1) If the patient lacks the capacity to designate their own surrogate by executing a DPAHC, one should ascertain whether or not an advance directive exists. If one doesn't (or if it is inapplicable), then the person identified by the relevant state statute is recognized as the decision-maker. If there is no surrogate statute (or if other family members disagree with the decision-maker recognized by a statute), then a guardian will need to be appointed. A guardian will also need to be appointed for all non-healthcare related decisions, since both advance directives as well as state surrogate statutes almost always apply only to healthcare decision-making.

While identifying a surrogate decision-maker is a necessary first step, the clinician also has an ongoing responsibility to ensure that the decisions made by the surrogate are appropriate. This means, first, that the clinician recognizes the limits to the types of decisions the surrogate can make (as specified in the laws of their jurisdiction). In addition, however, the clinician should also focus on the actual decisions made in order to ensure their appropriateness. In other words, the fact that the surrogate is legally empowered to make decisions on behalf of the patient does *not* mean that the surrogate is free to make any decision at all. There are ethical and legal guidelines that constrain the choices that a surrogate can make, and the clinician should be aware of whether these are being followed.

In general, there are two different principles that should guide the decisions made by a surrogate. These are known as the "substituted judgment" standard and the "best interests" standard. In exercising substituted judgment, surrogates are asked to make a decision as they think the patient would have made it. They are asked to put aside their own thoughts and feelings and choose as they believe the patient would have chosen based on their presumed knowledge of the patient's values, beliefs, desires, etc. Although a widely accepted standard, there are certain difficulties encountered in exercising substituted judgment.

First, there is a growing body of evidence documenting the difficulty that surrogates have in accurately predicting patients' wishes in particular situations (29–35). Even when the surrogates felt confident that they knew what their family members would want, these studies revealed a poor correlation between the surrogate's decisions and the patient's actual preferences. Although disturbing, these findings do not necessarily undermine the substituted judgment standard itself.

They do highlight, however, another important issue: what is the evidence for a patient's prior wishes? For instance, was the substituted judgment based on explicit and repeated statements by the patient or a single casual remark? Or does the substituted judgment simply represent an inference based on the patient's past behaviors or presumed values? In general, the most reliable evidence of a patient's wishes are prior statements by

the patient that are explicit and well considered. These statements are especially valid if it is known that the patient had direct or indirect knowledge of the condition in question (through the care of a family member, for instance). In addition, because evidence shows that preferences change over time, more recent statements are especially likely to be representative (36). For all these reasons, it becomes important to ask a surrogate how they came to their decision regarding what the patient would have wanted.

Even when one is confident about the patient's *previous* wishes, however, another, more fundamental problem may arise. Specifically, a person may change their mind after a brain injury. For instance, impairments that may have seemed intolerable to them prior to their injury may now come to be accepted (26). This shift may simply represent the fact that we did not really know what living with certain conditions was like. We all find it difficult, beforehand, to accurately imagine a condition significantly different from our own. In particular, there is a large body of evidence that documents how the able-bodied, including clinicians, significantly underestimate the quality of life possible after a disability, (26, 37–40) even when they live with someone with a severe disability (41).

Another reason that a person's preferences may seem to change after a brain injury is that their fundamental values, beliefs, and desires might, in fact, have been altered by the injury. This change in identity that some patients undergo was discussed earlier. In this context, it raises a fundamental issue: is it even appropriate to appeal to past wishes in making decisions for patients? We alluded to the controversy that surrounds this issue previously; the reader is again referred to several detailed examinations of this issue (25, 26, 34, 35).

Given some of the difficulties in exercising substituted judgment, another criterion is often utilized in evaluating a surrogate's decisions: the "best interest" standard. According to this standard, the criterion for making decisions is to do what is in the best interest of the patient. The primary role for the best interest standard is when the patient's previous wishes are not known. This is often the case in brain injury rehabilitation because few people anticipate having a brain injury, much less discuss with family members in advance what they would want done. In these cases, the decision that is made should be the one that is in the best interests of the patient, regardless of how the surrogate may actually feel about a particular decision.

Although intuitively appealing, the best interest standard faces its own set of difficulties. Specifically, what a person's best interests are and what would advance those interests is often a source of disagreement. One potential danger is that a family member, while well intentioned, may unconsciously project her own beliefs or values into the situation. This can be especially problematic when seen in the light of the difficulty, discussed above, that we all have in imagining unfamiliar situations. In particular, the tendency of the able-bodied to underestimate the quality of life of the disabled can significantly distort the decisions of surrogates.

Another issue is the proper role of the family or caregivers' interests in decision-making. The rationale for both the substituted judgment and best interest standards is that they place the *patient's* interests first. Certainly, clinicians should be sensitive to any evidence that the family is making decisions based primarily on potential gain to themselves (e.g. financially). Yet, because the family or caregivers are greatly affected by the consequences of any decision made, it seems unreasonable to expect that their interests should have no role in decision-making.

As in many other difficult cases, the exact role that the families' interests play will vary from case to case and, even then, may be a source of reasonable and legitimate disagreement (34, 35). For instance, the placement of a patient in a nursing facility solely so that the family can have use of the patient's home is clearly wrong. On the other hand, it seems understandable when the same decision is made because the family member is a single, working parent unable to provide 24 hour care. It is important to acknowledge that these issues are not merely personal but also ones that have public policy and social implications. The lack of readily available social support systems, financial remuneration for caregivers, and viable community-based living alternatives for persons with brain injuries adds layers of complexity to any surrogate decision-making process.

In conclusion, after identifying the appropriate surrogate decision-maker, the clinician still has an ongoing responsibility to evaluate the decisions made to ensure that they represent what the patient herself would have wanted or, at least, are in the patient's best interests. If the clinician feels that the decisions made by a surrogate are not appropriate, every effort should be made to address and resolve this issue in discussions with the surrogate and other involved parties. Ethics committee consultations and/or consultation with legal counsel may also be needed to mediate conflicts and ensure adequate protection for vulnerable patients. If an ethics committee mechanism is used, it is desirable to ensure that persons who are knowledgeable about life with brain injury be included in the process. If these measures don't resolve the concerns, then appeal to the legal system may be necessary.

BEYOND CONSENT: ASSENT AND DISSENT IN BRAIN INJURY REHABILITATION

While accurate, the process depicted in Figure 65-1 omits a crucial moral dimension of our approach to patients whose decision-making capacity is at question: the content and quality of the conversations and interactions that precede the final decision. This is especially clear if we approach the process from the point of view of patients who decline or "dissent" from our recommendations. While it is true that we must ultimately honor the wishes of those patients who possess decision-making capacity, we are also morally obliged to engage them in conversation intended to understand their perspective and persuade them to re-consider their choice. Likewise, for patients who lack decisional capacity, it is still morally important that we attempt to secure their agreement or "assent" to the decisions that are made. In both cases, our commitment to our patients' welfare obliges us to make a significant effort, short of manipulation or coercion, to persuade them of the treatment plan. Although consent is the central concept in approaching decision-making capacity after brain injury, clinicians also need to be aware of the moral significance of assent and dissent (42).

By "assent", we refer to securing the agreement of a patient who does not have the decisional capacity to provide full informed consent. The concept of assent was first developed in the field of pediatrics, where it was recognized that children, although unable to give full consent, should still play some role in the decision making that surrounds their care. In fact, it has been urged that clinicians always attempt to secure the assent of children for treatment decisions, even though the parents have both the ethical and legal authority to make the actual decisions (43).

We believe that the concept of assent is also relevant to brain injury rehabilitation and that we should always make an attempt to secure the assent of decisionally incapacitated patients. This reflects a basic respect for and acknowledgement of the patient, despite the impairments in their decision-making. At a more practical level, a patient's assent is likely to increase patient compliance, especially with those treatments that require their active participation. Of course, there are situations in which assent is not relevant, such as in the minimally conscious patient. And there will be situations in which, in spite of the best efforts of the treatment team, patients may still refuse to give their assent to the treatment plan.

In these situations, it is generally acceptable to proceed with treatment, at least in the inpatient setting, especially if not proceeding leads to significant harm to the patient. Clearly, this only applies to those decisions where the patient is a passive recipient of treatment (for instance, receiving medications). If the treatment involves the active participation of the patient (such as engaging in physical therapy), forcing treatment is usually impossible and often morally repugnant. Addressing these issues in the outpatient setting is more complex and other legal considerations might apply (for instance, by virtue of the fact that the patient is no longer in a health care facility) and legal consultation may need to be obtained.

SURROGATE DECISION-MAKING: THE SPECIAL CASE OF WITHDRAWAL OR WITHHOLDING LIFE-SUSTAINING TREATMENT FOR PERSONS WITH BRAIN INJURY

Surrogate decision making in the context of withdrawal of care raises issues that are not found for other health care decisions. Prior to the 1970's, disputes regarding the use of life-sustaining technologies were rare; indeed, in many cases these technologies were non-existent. With the growth and increased availability of technologies such as ventilators and gastrostomy tubes, questions about how and when to apply these technologies became commonplace (and, in fact, account for the impetus behind the growth in bioethics as a discipline). Patients with brain injuries were often front and center in such discussions. No case probably symbolizes the beginning of this era more than that of Karen Ann Quinlan.

Philosophers, theologians, ethicists, and health care professionals have disagreed over the years about whether there is a moral difference between withholding life-sustaining treatment (i.e. not initiating the life saving treatment) and withdrawing life-sustaining treatment, or taking away the treatment that is believed to be sustaining life (44). In general, there has been more recent consensus in the United States that they are morally equivalent acts (45, 46). In fact some would argue that to withhold the initiation of life-sustaining treatment because of a fear that a withdrawal decision may arise is dangerous, unwise, and not in the best interest of the patient. Sometimes (and brain injury is often one of these cases) only through the initiation of life-sustaining treatment can better prognostic information be clarified thus allowing a more considered decision about the on-going role of life-sustaining treatment if needed.

In the next section, we will briefly review some of the salient and often very public legal cases regarding persons with brain injuries in which questions of withdrawal of life-sustaining treatment arose. These cases have been chosen as we believe they help to illustrate some of the common law guidelines, cultural mores, and evolving moral discussions in this always complex, and often contentious, area of decision-making.

Karen Ann Quinlan

In 1975, Karen Ann Quinlan, at the age of 21, sustained cardiac arrest and anoxic brain injury, resulting in permanent vegetative state (PVS). (We will use this phraseology to delineate a condition in which the patient lacks awareness of their environment and recovery is highly unlikely). In 1976, her father sought legal guardianship with specific authority to direct the withdrawal of her mechanical ventilation (47). The Supreme Court of

New Jersey granted him guardianship as requested and indicated that he could exercise on her behalf her right to privacy (i.e., to be free of unwanted medical treatment). In essence, if Mr. Quinlan and her family believed that Ms. Quinlan would not want to have her life supported by a ventilator, they could choose to have the ventilator withdrawn. The Court further stated that this decision was clearly based upon her *poor medical prognosis*—i.e. her state of PVS, believing that the "overwhelming majority of [society] would, we think, in similar circumstances, exercise such a choice in the same way for themselves or for those closest to them."(47)

Nancy Beth Cruzan

In 1983, Nancy Beth Cruzan was in a motor vehicle crash. She was also judged to be in a permanent vegetative state, and was fed via a gastrostomy tube. In 1986, her parents, acting as her guardians, initiated proceedings "to terminate her artificial nutrition and hydration." Their request was based upon her poor medical prognosis for improvement as well as statements that she had made to a friend that "if sick or injured she would not wish to continue her life unless she could live at least halfway normally." In essence, this case weighed 2 aspects of the due process clause of the 14th amendment to the Constitution: States are prohibited from "depriving any person of life, liberty, or property without due process of law."(48) In other words, the first aspect was her *liberty right* to be free of unwanted medical treatment and the second was her *right to life*. The argument of the appellants (Nancy Cruzan's parents) was rejected by the Supreme Court of Missouri as not meeting the State's standard of "clear and convincing evidence"[1] of the incompetent person's wishes.

This case was reviewed by the U.S. Supreme Court in 1990 (49). The U.S. Supreme Court upheld a state's right to decide the standard of proof required before life-sustaining treatment can be withdrawn (most though not all have chosen the clear and convincing standard of proof). The Court also specifically commented on the role of surrogate decision-makers in the process, noting the difficulty that surrogates might have in executing decisions:

> Close family members may have a strong feeling—a feeling not at all ignoble or unworthy, but not entirely disinterested, either—that they do not wish to witness the continuation of the life of a loved one which they regard as hopeless, meaningless, and even degrading. But

---

[1] Clear and convincing standard of proof has been defined as "proof sufficient to persuade the trier of fact that the patient held a firm and settled commitment to the termination of life supports under the circumstances like those presented" *In re Westchester County Medical Center on behalf of O'Connor*, 72 N.Y. 2d 517, 531, N.E. 2d 606, 613 (1988).

there is no automatic assurance that the view of close family members will necessarily be the same as the patient's would have been had she been confronted with the prospect of her situation while competent. Furthermore, "the State may also properly decline to make judgments about the "quality" of a particular individual's life and simply assert an unqualified interest in the preservation of human life to be weighed against the constitutionally protected interests of the individual" (49).

Michael Martin

In 1987, Michael Martin sustained a head injury, leaving him with extensive cognitive and physical impairments. (50) He had a colostomy and a gastrostomy for nutrition and hydration. He was unable to take food orally. Mr. Martin lived in a nursing home, and communicated with head nods and gestures. In 1992, while being treated for a bowel obstruction, Mary Martin, his wife and guardian, contacted the hospital's bioethics committee to determine whether Mr. Martin's nutrition and hydration could be withdrawn. Based upon prior conversations, Mr. Martin was reported to say to his wife that he would rather die than be dependent on people or machines. In casual conversations on 2 occasions with co-workers he said he would not want to live if he were in a "vegetative state." The hospital ethic's committee issued a statement that withdrawal of treatment was both medically and ethically appropriate, but that it must be authorized by the court before the hospital would assist in withdrawal of treatment.

In contrast to Karen Ann Quinlan and Nancy Beth Cruzan, Michael Martin was *not* in a permanent vegetative state. Though he could understand short, simple questions, the medical experts all agreed that he lacked decisional capacity. Furthermore, Mr. Martin's sister contested Mary Martin's request and asked that she be removed as his guardian and conservator. Though Mary Martin was upheld as the guardian and conservator, the Michigan Supreme Court reversed the Court of Appeals decision in favor of withdrawal of medical treatment, concluding that there was not clear and convincing evidence that withdrawal of food and fluid is what Mr. Martin would want in his *current* condition: "To end the life a patient who still derives meaning and enjoyment from life or to condemn persons to lives from which they cry out for release is nothing short of barbaric. If we are to err, however, we must err in preserving life." (from 50 at 401–2).

Michael Martin's case is particularly interesting because he was neither terminally ill nor in a permanent vegetative state, which have been referred to as "condition-based thresholds" that some argue must be present before a non-treatment decision can be made. Though he had made some compelling statements about not wanting to live on machines or if in a vegetative state, he seemed content and did not indicate after his brain injury a desire to die. The Michigan Supreme Court ruled that to be clear and convincing, the statements previously made needed to be a "serious, well thought out, consistent decision to refuse treatment under these exact circumstances, or circumstances highly similar to the current" (50).

Robert Wendland

Robert Wendland, like Michael Martin had an extensive brain injury (in 1993 from a drunk driving accident) but was clearly not in a vegetative state. He was conscious but unable to talk. He was fed and given water through a gastrostomy tube and needed assistance with his activities of daily living. He lived in a nursing home in California. In 1995 his wife and conservator, Rose Wendland, petitioned the court for permission to withdraw his nutrition and hydration based upon statements that Mr. Wendland had made while competent that led her to believe he would not want to be sustained in his current state.

Like the prior cases, there was no written advance directive. The request was challenged by Mr. Wendland's mother and sister who brought suit to remove Rose Wendland as his conservator (51). Two critical issues emerged in this case: the threshold issue (and notably, for the first time, the language of "minimally conscious state" was being applied in court to describe the neurological state of the patient), and 2. the clear and convincing evidence standard was again challenged. Mr. Wendland died before the case could be decided by the California Supreme Court, but given the importance of the case they chose to issue a ruling clarifying and confirming that a "clear and convincing" evidence standard was necessary.

The case sparked a great deal of interest and a large number of amicus curiae briefs on both sides. Substantial support in favor of allowing Rose Wendland to withdraw Mr. Wendland's nutrition and hydration and thus lower the standard of evidence from clear and convincing to a preponderance of the evidence included the California Medical Association, the American Civil Liberties Union, and 41 bioethicists (52). Those opposed included a number of disability activists organizations including Not Dead Yet, ADAPT, the ARC, Brain Injury Association, Inc., the Disability Rights Center, The National Council on Independent Living, and the National Spinal Injury Association.[2]

---

[2] Not Dead Yet is a national grassroots organization of people with disabilities formed in 1996 to advocate against legalization of physician assisted suicide and euthanasia. ADAPT is composed of people with disabilities whose purpose is to advocate for the civil rights of people with disabilities to live in their homes and communities. The ARC is devoted to the welfare of persons with mental retardation and their families, and was instrumental in framing the ADA. The Disability Rights Center was established in 1978 to enable people with disabilities to live in society and secure their human and civil rights. The National Council on Independent Living is the oldest cross-disability grass roots organization run by and for people with disabilities.

Terri Schiavo

In 1990, at the age of 26, Terri Schiavo sustained a cardiac arrest resulting in anoxic brain injury. In May of 1998, Michael Schiavo, Terri's husband and guardian, filed a petition in Florida to remove her gastrostomy tube. In support of the petition, Ms. Schiavo's husband presented testimony about statements Ms. Schiavo made before her arrest that he believed indicated she would not want to live in her current state (like the other cases reviewed, she did not have a written advance directive). Ms. Schiavo's parents, the Schindlers, who opposed the petition, objected to this testimony and also sought to have Mr. Schiavo removed as her guardian. In contrast to Nancy Beth Cruzan, Ms. Schiavo's neurological diagnosis of permanent vegetative state has been the subject of dispute, with medical experts on both sides disagreeing about her diagnosis and prognosis for improvement with further rehabilitation efforts (53). Specifically, the court placed the burden on the Schindlers to "establish that new treatment offers sufficient promise of increased cognitive function in Mrs. Schiavo's cerebral cortex—significantly improving the quality of Mrs. Schiavo's life—so that she herself would elect to undergo this treatment and would reverse the prior decision to withdraw life-prolonging procedures." The Second District Court of Appeals of Florida determined that there was not sufficient evidence presented to question her diagnosis of vegetative state or her poor prognosis for improvement (54). The appellate court also addressed the issue of family involvement in such decisions:

> But in the end, this case is not about the aspirations that loving parents have for their children. It is about Teresa Schiavo's right to make her own decision, independent of her parents and independent of her husband. In circumstances such as these, when families cannot agree, the law has opened the doors of the circuit courts to permit trial judges to serve as surrogates or proxies to make decisions about life-prolonging procedures. It is the trial judge's duty not to make the decision that the judge would make for himself or herself or for a loved one. Instead, the trial judge must make a decision that the clear and convincing evidence show the ward would have made for herself (54).

After multiple appeals, legislative maneuvering, and much public dissension, Ms. Schiavo's nutrition and hydration was withdrawn and she died 13 days later on March 31, 2005 in a Florida hospice.

SUMMARY

There are no simple guidelines for decision-making regarding the withdrawal and/or withholding of life sustaining treatment for persons with brain injury. The only case of the five presented above that was reviewed by the U.S. Supreme Court, and thus has clear federal jurisdiction, is that of Nancy Beth Cruzan. The other cases were tried in the various states of New Jersey, Michigan, California and Florida, and are thus subject to the laws of each state. As each State is likely to have specific laws governing such decisions, it is imperative to be well-versed in state law and to consider consultation with legal counsel and ethics committees in the decision-making process. Many people will also find guidance from spiritual advisers or religious leaders to be very helpful and these resources should always be offered. Nonetheless, there are some generalizations and guidelines that we feel might be helpful in negotiating this difficult terrain:

1. It is important to know whether the person with a brain injury ever executed an advance directive. Are there written statements regarding the person's wishes for care and medical treatment? Did the person stipulate who they trusted to make decisions on his/her behalf if incompetent? Such directives have great moral and legal authority in this country, and in most instances are considered sufficient to satisfy evidence of "clear and convincing evidence" of a person's wishes. That is not to say, though, that an advance directive should be considered absolute and binding (26, 55). Specifically, while competency is required to make an advance directive, it is not necessarily a requirement for negating one. Thus, if a person with brain injury is able to reliably indicate that they no longer wish for their advance directive to be followed, then (in general) it should not be followed. (There are rare exceptions. For example, the Declaration for Mental Health Treatment in Illinois allows a person to sign an advance directive indicating they wish treatment including hospitalization, medication, electroconvulsive therapy, etc. if they have a mental condition requiring such treatment in the future, *even if they would refuse it at the time*) (56).

2. One of the critical questions in considering the withdrawal of life sustaining treatments involving persons with brain injury is: when is life with disability worse than death? These decisions inherently involve quality of life determinations by third parties, often invoking considerations of concepts of pain and suffering, the meaning of human life and personhood, concepts of "dignity," and economic considerations. While there is growing consensus among the legal, medical and bioethics communities that withdrawing life sustaining treatment is permissible when a person has permanent vegetative state in the US, there are still substantial minority voices that oppose this practice. There is also not a clear social consensus regarding whether withdrawal or withholding of treatment is

permissible in the absence of an advance directive when a person is not permanently unconscious; i.e., is minimally conscious or otherwise has severe brain injury.

3. It is imperative to establish a careful neurological diagnosis and provide the most accurate prognostic information possible. It is unlikely that a single, brief bedside neurological examination can establish with a high degree of certainty a diagnosis such as permanent vegetative state (PVS), and indeed, there is substantial evidence to show that an erroneous diagnosis of PVS is not an infrequent occurrence. (57, 58)

4. Given the complexities of brain injury, it is extremely important that health care providers with extensive experience with this condition (and in particular the rehabilitation phase) be involved in evaluating patients and providing information to families. For example, speech language therapists can help ferret out problems with communication that are due to sensory or motor impairments and not due to unconsciousness. Information about how people with brain injury (in general) adjust and experience their lives is also critical information, yet often missing from discussions of prognosis. While the experiences of a group cannot allow us to predict the experience of a single individual, it does provide a more complete, balanced and holistic view than a list of likely impairments.

5. Try to present information to families and surrogates in as balanced (i.e., neutral) a fashion as possible and avoid value-laden terminology. For example, the Glasgow Outcome Scale categories are highly value-laden, and thus potentially problematic. Only level five is considered a "good recovery," with moderate disability, severe disability, PVS, and death constituting the other four categories. These categories also are very broad and focus on the level of disability and not the level of handicap or life satisfaction, both of which are critically important to one's adjustment to brain injury (40).

6. Do not assume that all families feel equipped to provide care for their family member with a brain injury. In the U.S., it is not uncommon that families are expected to assume the responsibility for being caregivers—often at great personal expense, being asked to sacrifice jobs, other family responsibilities, and financial resources to meet the person's needs. It may be important to provide permission to the family member *not* to assume this role and to explore with families alternatives to support the person with brain injury in getting his/her needs met.

References

1. Fowles G.P., Fox B.A. Competency to Consent to Treatment and Informed Consent in Neurobehavioral Rehabilitation. *The Clinical Neuropsychologist* 1995;9(3):251–257.

2. Auerbach V.S., Banja J.D. Assessing Client Competence to Participate in Rehabilitation Decision Making. *Neurorehabilitation* 1996;6:123–132.

3. U.S. House of Representatives:Committee on Government Operations *Fraud And Abuse In The Head Injury Rehabilitation Industry* 1992.

4. Kirschner K, Stocking C et al. Ethical Issues Identified by Rehabilitation Clinicians. *Arch Phys Med Rehabil* 2001;82 (Suppl 2):S2-S8.

5. Jonsen A, Siegler M, Winslade W *Clinical Ethics 4th Ed.* New York:McGraw-Hill, 1998.

6. Grisso T, Appelbaum P.S. *Assessing Competence To Consent To Treatment: A Guide For Physicians And Other Health Professionals.* New York:Oxford University Press, 1998.

7. Gert B, Culver C.M., Clouser K.D. *Bioethics:A Return To Fundamentals.* New York: Oxford University Press, 1997.

8. Macciocchi S, Stringer A. Assessing Risk and Harm: The Convergence of Ethical and Empirical Considerations. *Arch Phys Med Rehabil* 2001;82 (Suppl 2):S15–S19.

9. Alexander M.P. Clinical Determination of Mental Competence: A Theory and a Retrospective Study. *Arch Neurol* 1988;45:23–26.

10. Lezak M *Neuropsychological Assessment.* New York:Oxford University Press, 2004.

11. Reid-Proctor G, Galin K et al. Evaluation of Legal Competency in Patients with Frontal Lobe Injury. *Brain Injury* 2001;15(5):377–386.

12. Rutman D, Silberfeld M. A Preliminary Report on the Discrepancy Between Clinical and Test Evaluations of Competence. *Canadian J of Psychiatry* 1992;37(9):634–639.

13. Holzer J.C., Gansler DA et al. Cognitive Functions in the Informed Consent Evaluation Process: A Pilot Study. *J Am Acad Psychiatry Law* 1997;25(4):531–540.

14. Bassett S. Attention:Neuropsychological Predictor of Competency in Alzheimer's Disease. *Psychiatry Neurol* 1999;12:200–205.

15. Marson D, Harrell L. "Executive Dysfunction and Loss of Capacity to Consent to Medical Treatment in Patients With Alzheimer's Disease". Seminars in Clin Neuropsych 1999;4(1):41–49.

16. Marson D.C., Chatterjee A, et al. Toward a Neurologic Model of Competency: Cognitive Predictors Of Capacity to Consent in Alzheimer's Disease Using Three Different Legal Standards. *Neurology* 1996;46:666–672.

17. McCullough L.B., Molinari V et al. Implications of Impaired Executive Control Functions for Patient Autonomy and Surrogate Decision Making. *J Clinical Ethics* 2001;12(4):397–405.

18. Elliott C. Caring About Risks:Are Severely Depressed Patients Competent to Consent to Research?. *Arch Gen Psychiatry* 1997; 54:115–116.

19. Lee M.A., Ganzini L. Depression in the Elderly:Effect on Patient Attitudes Toward Life-Sustaining Therapy. *J Am Geriatr Soc* 1992;40:983–988.

20. Damasio A.R. *Descartes' Error:Emotion, Reason, And The Human Brain:* New York, Avon Books, 1994.

21. Bursztajn H.J., Harding HP et al. Beyond Cognition:The Role of Disordered Affective States in Impairing Competence to Consent to Treatment. *Bull Am Acad Psychiatry* Law 1991;19:383–388.

22. Yuen K, Lee T. Could Mood State Affect Risk-Taking Decisions? *J of Affective Disorders* 2003;75:11–18.

23. Bechara A, Tranel D et al. Characterization of the Decision-Making Deficit of Patients with Ventromedial Prefrontal Cortex Lesions. *Brain* 2000;123:2189–2202.

24. Schlund MW, Pace GM et al. Relations Between Decision-Making Deficits and Discriminating Contingencies Following Brain Injury. *Brain Injury* 2001;15:1061–1071.

25. Dworkin R. *Life's Dominion* New York:Vintage Books, 1994.

26. Stein J. The Ethics of Advance Directives:A Rehabilitation Perspective. *Am J Phys Med Rehabil* 2003;82(2):1–14.

27. Anderson T.P., Fearey M.S.Legal Guardianship in Traumatic Brain Injury Rehabilitation:Ethical Implications. *J Head Trauma Rehabil* 1989;4(1):57–64.

28. Wolf L.R., Colenda C.C. The Role of Guardianship in the Care and Management of Patients Following Head Trauma. *Psychiatric Medicine* 1989;7(1):51–57.

29. Emanuel E.J., Emanuel L.L. Proxy Decision Making for Incompetent Patients: An Ethical and Empirical Analysis. *JAMA* 1992; 267:2067–2071.

30. Seckler A.B., Meier D.B., et al. Substituted Judgment:How Accurate Are Proxy Predictions? *Ann Intern Med* 1991;115: 92–98.

31. Hare J, Pratt C et al. Agreement Between Patients and Their Self-Selected Surrogates on Difficult Medical Decisions. *Arch Int Med* 1992;152:1049–1054.

32. Zwiebel NR, Cassel CK. Treatment Choices at the End of Life: A Comparisons of Decisions by Older Patients and Their Physician-Selected Proxies. *Gerontologist* 1989;29:615–621.

33. Terry P.B., Vettese M et al. End-of-Life Decision Making: When Patients and Surrogates Disagree. *J Clin Ethics* 1999;10: 286–293.

34. Nelson J, Frader J. Brain Trauma and Surrogate Decision Making: Dogmas, Challenges, and Response. *J Clin Ethics* 2004;15(4): 264–276.

35. Gill C. Depolarizing and Complicating the Ethics of Treatment Decision Making in Brain Injury: A Disability Rights Response to Nelson and Frader. *J Clin Ethics* 2004;15(4):277–288.

36. Emanuel L.L., Emanuel E.J., et al. Advance Directives: Stability of Patients' Treatment Choices. *Arch Intern Med* 1994;154: 209–217.

37. Gerhart K.A., Koziol-McLain J, et al. Quality of Life Following Spinal Cord Injury:Knowledge and Attitudes of Emergency Care Providers. *Ann Emer Med* 1994;23(4):807–812.

38. Bach J.R., Tilton M.C. Life Satisfaction and Well-Being Measures in Ventilator Assisted Individuals with Traumatic Tetraplegia. *Arch Phys Med Rehabil* 1994;75:626–632.

39. Kothari S. Clinical Misjudgments of Quality of Life after Disability. *J Clin Ethics* 2004;15(4):300–307.

40. Kothari S, Sander AM, Contant C et al. The Relation Between Level of Disability and Satisfaction with Life in Individuals with Traumatic Brain Injury. *Arch Phys Med Rehabil* 2001;82(10): 1490

41. Gething L. Perceptions of Disability of Persons with Cerebral Palsy, Their Close Relatives and Able Bodied Persons. *Soc Sci Med* 1985;20:561–565.

42. Kothari S, Kirschner K. Beyond Consent:Assent and Empowerment in Brain Injury rehabilitation. *J Head Trauma Rehabil* 2003;18(4):379–382.

43. American Academy of Pediatrics. Informed Consent, Parental Permission, and Assent in Pediatric Practice. *Pediatrics* 1995;95(2): 314–317.

44. Sulmasy D.P., Sugarman J. Are Withholding and withdrawing therapy always morally equivalent? *J Med Ethics* 1994;20: 218–222.

45. American Medical Association Council on Ethical and Judicial Affairs. *Code of Medical Ethics,* 2002–3 Edition.

46. Beauchamp T.L., Childress J.F. *Principles Of Biomedical Ethics, 4th Ed.* New York:Oxford University Press, 1994.

47. *In Re Quinlan,* Supreme Court of New Jersey. 70 N.J. 10, 355 A2d 647 (decided March 31, 1976).

48. U.S. Constitution, Amendment XIV

49. *Cruzan v. Director,* Department of Health, 58 U.S. L.W. 4916 (6/26/90).

50. *In re Michael Martin* (Nos. 99699, 99700) Supreme Court of Michigan, August 22, 1995.

51. *Conservatorship of Wendland* 26 Cal 4th 519, 2001.

52. Conservatorship of Wendland, Supreme Court of California, S087265.

53. *Schindler v. Schiavo,* 780 So. 2d 176 (Fla. 2d DCA 2001), 792 So. 2d.551 (Fla. 2d DCA 2001), 800 So. 2d 640 (Fla. 2d DCA 2001).

54. *In re:guardianship of Theresa Marie Schiavo,* Case No. 2D02–5394; filed June 6, 2003.

55. Kirschner KL. When written advance directives are not enough. *Clinics in Geriatric Medicine* 2005;21:193–209.

56. IL Declaration for Mental Health Treatment

57. Andrews K, Murphy L, et al. Misdiagnosis of the vegetative state:retrospective study in a rehabilitation unit. Br Med J. 1996;313(7048):13–16.

58. Childs NL, Mercer WN, et al. Accuracy of diagnosis of persistent vegetative state. Neurology 1993;43(8):1465–1467.

Life Care Planning After TBI: Clinical and Forensic Issues

Roger O. Weed
Debra E. Berens

INTRODUCTION

This chapter presents an overview of the tenets, methodologies, topics, and issues to be considered when evaluating the future medical, or life care, needs of the patient with acquired brain injury (ABI). Commonly known as a life care plan, the plan can be relatively short, with very little "medical" needs, or very complex and detailed, with multiple medical and rehabilitation needs outlined. For example, a patient may or may not have experienced a loss of consciousness, yet still exhibit clinical signs and symptoms suggesting long-term follow-up that affect vocational and social functioning but require little or no physician or medical needs (1,2). Although information relating to a wide range of brain injury conditions is included in this chapter, most details will be geared toward the patient who has multiple future care needs that justify an assessment for life care plan development.

A generally accepted and working definition for life care plan is:

> A *life care plan* is a dynamic document based upon published standards of practice, comprehensive assessment, data analysis and research, which provides an organized concise plan for current and future needs with associated costs, for individuals who have experienced catastrophic injury or have chronic health care needs.

Source: Combined definition of the University of Florida and Intelicus annual life care planning conference and the American Academy of Nurse Life Care Planners (now known as the International Academy of Life Care Planners) presented at the Forensic Section meeting, National Association of Rehabilitation Professionals in the Private Sector (NARPPS) annual conference, Colorado Springs, CO, and agreed upon April 3, 1998 (3).

As a "dynamic document," medication changes and other updates can be expected over time. As will be seen below, however, life care plans, when completed according to established procedures, are a reliable document.

HISTORY

Life care planning first appeared in the legal publication, *Damages in Tort Action* (4), which established the guidelines for determining damages in civil litigation cases. By 1985, the life care plan was introduced to the health care industry in *A Guide to Rehabilitation* (5). One of the first rehabilitation professional training programs was organized by Dr. Paul Deutsch and offered on September 16–17, 1986, in Hilton Head, SC, where more than 100 rehabilitation professionals from throughout the United States, including one of this chapter's authors, assembled to begin the process of setting standards for development of life care plans.

In the fall of 1992, five rehabilitation professionals—Richard Bonfiglio, MD; Paul Deutsch, Ph.D.; Julie Kitchen, CDMS; Susan Riddick, RN; and Roger Weed, Ph.D.—met to discuss issues associated with the life care planning industry. Concerned that fragmentation and poor standardization would result in an overall decline of the industry, the group developed a concentrated training program representing the various aspects of life care planning (3).

After designing the program, a management company (Rehabilitation Training Institute) was contracted to set up training programs throughout the United States. Before the announcements were fully distributed, the first of the organized tracks was filled. It appeared obvious that there was a number of rehabilitation professionals interested in pursuing advanced education related to life care planning, and several participants requested official recognition for their educational efforts. Dr. Horace Sawyer of the University of Florida agreed to pursue an official certificate of completion through the University of Florida's Continuing Education Department. As a result, a private/public partnership between the Rehabilitation Training Institute and the University of Florida was formed and named Intelicus. The five founders donated the program content to Intelicus. Some even continue today as faculty, although they no longer have control over program content or management. Over the years, these courses have been adjusted to focus on the roles and responsibilities that more specifically identify with life care planners based on research and participant comments. Most recently, the Intelicus life care planning training program was purchased by MediPro Seminars, LLC, to continue to offer life care planning advanced training, as well as the annual international life care planning conference. (See www.mediproseminars.com.)

Although the certificate from the University of Florida added value to obtaining education specific to this specialty practice, it did not provide the assurance of ethical practice or the professional identity desired by people who had invested thousands of dollars and many hours of their time in the training process. Ultimately, the Commission on Disability Examiner Certification (now known as the Commission on Health Care Certification, or CHCC) based in Midlothian, Virginia, and directed by V. Robert May, Rh.D., assumed the responsibility in leading the way to certification. Because of his efforts, the first national certification in life care planning (i.e., Certified Life Care Planner) was offered in 1996. Currently, several organizations have approval of the certification Board to provide training leading to certification and/or continuing education training for certification maintenance. Also, in the 1990s, the International Academy of Life Care Planners was formed (previously known as the American Academy of Nurse Life Care Planners), and in 2002, the *Journal of Life Care Planning* and the Foundation for Life Care Planning Research were launched. Life Care Planning Summits also have been held bi-annually since 2000 to discuss and reach consensus on many topics of importance to ethical life care planning practice.

Over the years, life care plans have been expanding into a variety of fields including but not limited to managed care, workers' compensation, civil litigation, mediation, reserve setting for insurance companies, estate trust fund planning, gerontology care, and federal vaccine injury fund cases, all of which include individuals with brain injury in the patient population (6–11).

The range of future care needs can differ significantly depending on a mild, moderate, or severe brain injury. Individuals with mild brain injury, for instance, may not require a comprehensive life care plan and may be less likely to need all of the care commonly considered for a life care plan. Nevertheless, there may be value in utilizing the standardized approach in these cases to assure a comprehensive evaluation is done. For details with regard to definitions and functional deficits for individuals with mild acquired brain injury, the reader is referred to Goldberg's chapter on Post-Concussive Disorders found elsewhere in this book.

Patients with mild or moderate brain injury can have few, if any, physical problems. Therefore, the physician or medical team may not be an integral part of the future care planning. Instead, the case manager, neuropsychologist, vocational expert and, perhaps, the family or other support system, will be the most relevant participants in the life care planning process. However, it is not uncommon for an individual with mild to moderate head injury to also have musculoskeletal problems including fractures, facial damage (which may or may not be repairable), seizures, and other physiological deficits (12). On the other hand, patients with more severe brain injury often have multiple and obvious physical impairments as well as more severe cognitive deficits and require multiple physicians, life-long medical care, and multiple supply, medication and equipment needs. Obviously, an effective life care plan will include items for all treatable deficits that are related to or a result of the ABI.

In order to assure that the rehabilitation consultant addresses all appropriate issues for earning capacity analysis, it is helpful to utilize a standard methodology such as RAPEL (2, 3, 8, 9, 13). RAPEL is a mnemonic to help ensure the relevant "damages" of a case are evaluated. Adapted for pediatric cases, PEEDS-RAPEL© expands the RAPEL method and analyzes relevant data specific to the child with a disability, i.e., P (parental/family occupations), E (educational attainment), E (evaluation results), D (developmental stage), and S (synthesis). For further discussion on PEEDS-RAPEL© for pediatric case evaluation, the reader is referred to Neulicht & Berens (14).

Although all sections of RAPEL will be discussed in this chapter, only one part, the Rehabilitation plan, is directly related to the life care plan.

RAPEL APPROACH

When developing a reasonable opinion for forensic cases, it is expected that the rehabilitation consultant follow a standardized assessment approach to provide the appropriate information for the patient, patient's family, attorney, and economist. Certain specific requirements are necessary in order to satisfy all of these issue and although methods for determining the cost for future care as well as vocational and hedonic damages have been published

(6, 15, 16), it appeared that a comprehensive "common sense" approach encompassing both needs was lacking. The RAPEL method, representing five primary issues relating to future care needs and earnings capacity analysis (see Table 66-1), was designed to address rehabilitation needs and provide a "road map" of care, as well as generate a "bottom line" figure based on future care needs and earnings capacity analysis for persons with a catastrophic injury, including ABI.

The first of the RAPEL topics is as follows:

R = Rehabilitation Plan. The patient's vocational and functional limitations, strengths, emotional functioning, and cognitive capabilities are assessed utilizing information gathered from treating professionals or other experts listed in this chapter. This may include additional future testing, counseling, training fees, rehabilitation technology, job analysis, job coaching, placement, and

---

TABLE 66-1

The RAPEL Method: A Common Sense Approach To Future Care and Earnings Capacity Analysis

Rehabilitation plan	Determine the rehabilitation plan based on the patient's vocational and functional limitations, vocational strengths, emotional functioning, and cognitive capabilities. This may include testing, counseling, training fees, rehab technology, job analysis, job coaching, placement, and other needs for increasing employment potential. Also consider reasonable accommodation. A life care plan is appropriate for catastrophic injuries.
Access to the labor market	Determine the patient's access to the labor market. Methods include skilltrait (www.skilltrait.com) or various other computer programs, transferability of skills (or worker trait) analysis, disability statistics, and experience. This may also represent the patient's loss of choice and is particularly relevant if earnings potential is based on very few positions.
Placeability	This represents the likelihood that the patient could be successfully placed in a job. This is where the "rubber meets the road". Consider the employment statistics for people with disabilities, employment data for the specific medical condition (if available), economic situation of the community (may include a labor market survey), availability (not just existence) of jobs in chosen occupations. Note that the patient's attitude, personality, and other factors will influence the ultimate outcome.
Earnings capacity	Based on the above, what is the pre-incident capacity to earn compared to the post-incident capacity to earn. Methods include analysis of the specific job titles or class of jobs that a person could have engaged in pre- vs. post-incident, the ability to be educated (sometimes useful for people with acquired brain injury), family history for pediatric injuries, and computer analysis based on the individual's worker traits. Special consideration applies to children, women with limited or no work history, people who choose to work below their capacity (e.g., highly educated who are farmers), and military trained.
Labor force participation	This represents the patient's work life expectancy. Determine the amount of time that is lost, if any, from the labor force as a result of the disability. Issues include longer time to find employment, part-time vs. full-time employment, medical treatment or follow up, earlier retirement, etc. Display data using specific dates or percentages. For example, an average of four hours a day may represent a 50% loss.

Reprinted with permission from Ref. 17.

other needs for improving the patient's potential for employment. Future medical care is also addressed here and typically is displayed in a life care plan for individuals with a catastrophic injury.

One commonly observed problem for forensic cases is the lack of specific data to conscientiously determine a complete lifetime cost. Many professionals who write reports expect that a re-evaluation will take place in one to two years, at which time additional recommendations will be made. However, in personal injury litigation, it is important to determine, as much as possible at the time of plan development, all of the issues that are expected to be addressed throughout the patient's lifetime. Generally, it is recommended that the rehabilitation consultant meet or communicate with the patient's treatment team (if able) or other appropriate experts associated with the case to discuss the case in detail, rather than rely upon written reports or other records. Extensive rehabilitation plans may best be addressed through a detailed assessment of lifetime needs; i.e., the life care plan. The life care plan is a published format designed to outline appropriate future care details (3, 4, 6, 9, 10).

ELEMENTS OF THE LIFE CARE PLAN

First, it is important to understand that a variety of formats have been developed to display patient needs. In the original texts and books, the topics listed below were suggested and are still used today. The important aspect is to assure that all topics below are considered, as appropriate, in effective life care planning.

1. *Projected Evaluations.* Intended to describe non-physician evaluations that will occur on a periodic basis. These may include evaluations in physical therapy, speech therapy, recreational therapy, occupational therapy, music therapy, dietary assessment, audiology, vision screening, swallow studies, and others. The information displays specific recommendations, frequency over lifetime, and expected costs.

2. *Projected Therapeutic Modalities.* After projected evaluations have been completed, recommendations for ongoing treatment will be offered. With patients who have a catastrophic brain injury, it is common to include physical therapy, speech therapy, occupational therapy, family education, counseling, etc. This page identifies which non-physician treatment is recommended, over a specific period of time, at what frequency, and what cost.

3. *Diagnostic Testing/Educational Assessment.* Generally speaking, people with a catastrophic brain injury will undergo a variety of diagnostic testing, including neuropsychological, psychological, vocational evaluation, and, in the case of children, psycho-educational testing. Often evaluations will occur at specific points in a patient's life which would be identified by listing the years at which the evaluation would take place. For example, a child might be tested psychologically at ages that coincide with certain developmental stages or specific educational milestones. Such milestones may be the beginning of school, onset of puberty, beginning of high school, and entering employment or transitioning to adulthood. Consideration also should be given to additional evaluations that may be indicated as the patient ages, such as between age 50–60.

4. *Wheelchair Needs.* This page includes the type and configuration of wheelchairs the patient requires. For example, people who are tetraplegic often require a power wheelchair that reclines or tilts in space. The individual accesses and controls the wheelchair in a variety of ways, including joystick, sip and puff, head tilting, voice control, and others. The specifications will allow the life care planner to research costs from a variety of vendors (18). Some patients with hemiparesis may prefer a scooter for mobility assistance and some with less severe brain injuries may be ambulatory for short distances but need a light-weight manual wheelchair for longer distances.

5. *Wheelchair Accessories and Maintenance.* Each wheelchair requires certain accessories such as cushions for skin care, lap tables, carry bags, and other potential custom features. In addition, the wheelchair, depending on amount of use, requires maintenance. Maintenance can be very expensive for power wheelchairs, like the iBOT™, or inexpensive for wheelchairs which are used only for back-up purposes and are lightly used.

6. *Aids for Independent Function.* Many individuals with a brain injury have restricted ability to use their bodies and can make use of certain items for independence. A common example is the environmental control unit (ECU) or system that allows the patient to turn lights on and off, open and close doors, start and stop computers, turn on/off televisions, radios, fans, etc. Some less expensive adaptive aides may include reachers which will allow an individual to grasp items on a shelf or on the floor without having to stand up or bend over.

7. *Orthotics and Prosthetics.* With regard to significant brain injury, many patients will require braces or ankle/foot orthosis (AFO) to help with contractures, decrease spasticity, etc. Sometimes these braces, when custom designed, are costly and, over an individual's lifetime, can add up to a significant amount of money. Prosthetics generally are needed for individuals with one or more amputations. Prostheses

also require accessories (e.g., socks, liners, cosmetic covers, etc.) and will need replacement and ongoing maintenance over the patient's lifetime. The cost for all of these items, as well as applicable maintenance and replacement schedules, will be included on this page.

8. *Home Furnishing and Accessories.* Often a patient living at home will have need for a specialty bed and skin care mattress or powered lift and recline, portable ramps for accessibility, patient lift systems, etc. This section will require a specific inventory of the patient's needs at home or in their place of residence.

9. *Drug and Supply Needs.* This page includes prescription and non-prescription medication and supplies as related to or a result of the brain injury. As an example, a patient who is in a persistent vegetative state will likely need catheters or adult diapers, skin care products, and medications for various injury related problems or complications.

10. *Home Care/Facility Care.* Philosophically, it is more desirable to have a patient live in the least restrictive setting possible. This alternative also is a way to reduce complications from diseases from other patients that are common in a facility setting, as well as to improve the emotional status of the patient. However, this may not be the most cost effective alternative nor, in some cases, the most medically appropriate. Facility care, generally, is not as responsive to an individual as a custom-designed home care program; however, some individuals have no capability of living at home, or their needs exceed those which are available in a home environment. In this situation, facilities for individuals with serious behavioral disorder or those in persistent vegetative state as a result of acquired brain injury may be the most appropriate. There also may be need for specialty programs such as yearly summer camps, especially for children and adolescents. The level of in-home care also should be identified. For example, some individuals need only occasional home care or a time specific amount each day (i.e., 4 hours per day) while other patients need 24-hour, high-tech, nursing care.

11. *Future Medical Care: Routine.* Probably the most common routine medical care for individuals with acquired brain injury is provided by a physiatrist. The frequency of visits will depend on the medications, complications and severity of the injury. A person on antiseizure medication may be seen several times per year to evaluate the blood level and efficacy of the drug. Routine medical care also may include annual evaluations by the various specialty(ies) that may be appropriate for the severity of the brain injury. For instance, in dual diagnosis cases where the individual has both a brain injury

and a spinal cord injury, the patient may need a routine annual evaluation by physiatry, urology, dermatology, orthopedics, neurology, and others, as well as X-rays and lab work or diagnostic tests (e.g., urodynamics). This page summarizes those needs.

12. *Transportation.* Transportation needs vary substantially from patient to patient. Some individuals need little or no modification to their vehicles and may only require mileage reimbursement for injury-related appointments. Others may have a need for adding hand controls to their present vehicle. Yet other individuals may need a custom-designed van with lift and wheelchair tie-downs and rely on a driver for all driving activities or be able to drive with highly sophisticated technology such as the Digi Drive system (19).

13. *Health and Strength Maintenance.* This page, titled Recreation and Leisure Time Activities in the original literature, is designed to identify specialty recreation needs, adaptive games, and devices that will allow patients to be as active as possible and engage in health improving therapeutic action. Activity is very important to the physical and emotional well-being of a patient and such activities are often adjunctive to, and less expensive than, hiring a physical or occupational therapist. Specialty sports-related wheelchairs (such as basketball, tennis, and other custom-designed chairs) should not go on this page, but instead should be placed on the Wheelchair page. For more information on Health and Strength Maintenance, see *Support for Recreation and Leisure Time Activities in Life Care Plans* (20).

14. *Architectural Renovations.* If the patient is to be cared for at home, significant and comprehensive architectural renovations often will be required depending on the extent of the injury and the patient's functional limitations. For example, a patient who uses a wheelchair for mobility will need ramps (preferably at two entries into the home), hallways may need to be widened, the kitchen may require modification, fire or smoke detection will be needed, specialized floor coverings may be installed, bathrooms may be enlarged, equipment and attendant rooms may be added, and an emergency exit out of or near the bedroom may be added. Hablutzel and McMahon (21) published architectural renovation standards based on the Americans with Disability Act for those who wish to read more about this area.

15. *Potential Complications.* Costs of Potential Complications are not included in the total cost of the life care plan, presumably because effective life care planning will reduce potential complications as it provides the structure for quality care. On the other hand, it is important for people to understand what common

complications are involved with a particular disability (i.e., acquired brain injury). In the case of people with significant ABI, they are at higher risk to reinjure themselves due to poor balance or judgment and lack of safety awareness. Also, individuals with severe brain injury or who are in a persistent vegetative state often have skin breakdown, cardiovascular difficulty, pulmonary diseases, etc. Individuals on long-term Dilantin anti-seizure medication often have gum disease or other dental problems. Poor psychological adjustment to the person's disability often is the direct result of poor environment, poor care, or inability to engage in meaningful activities (22).

16. *Future Medical Care/Surgical Intervention or Aggressive Treatment.* In some situations the patient will have known needs for aggressive care. Commonly known problems for people with a brain injury include plastic surgery, dental restoration, time-limited rehabilitation programs, and short-term inpatient brain injury "tune-ups" (episodic one to four week rehabilitation programs). To be placed on this page, it is expected that these services are more probable than not to occur and occasional or time-limited treatment.

17. *Orthopedic Equipment Needs.* Some patients will need specific orthopedic equipment, such as body support equipment, walkers, or standing table. This is frequently termed "durable medical equipment."

18. *Vocational/Educational Plan.* This page was not included in the original life care planning literature and was later added to specifically address future vocational and educational or training needs. The professional involved in developing the life care plan may not be responsible for addressing this portion of the patient's future care if he/she is not qualified to assess these issues. Additionally, other qualified professionals may choose to complete a narrative report and a specific rehabilitation plan that focuses on vocational issues in a separate document. It is the authors' opinion that this page should be included in the life care plan in the same way that allied health recommendations are included, since overlap or "falling between the cracks" can otherwise result. This page obviously should include recommendations for vocationally-related items such as job coaching, supported employment, vocational counseling, tuition/fees, books and supplies for training programs, rehabilitation technology, and/or specialized educational programs, as well as the cost of each item.

The Life Care Planning Team

In many ways, developing a comprehensive life care plan is much like completing a puzzle and making sure all the pieces fit together to complete the picture (11). The following individuals and professionals commonly have a role to play in the life care planning process and may or may not be involved in any given case. (Note: in forensic cases when developing a defense plan, the treating team, patient and others may not be available to the life care planner.)

- **Patient** (i.e., the person with the disability). Assuming that the patient is accessible (i.e., legally permitted) and capable of appropriate interaction, interview and listen to him or her. Legally permitted in this context refers to the potential that defense experts in some states do not always have the "right" to interview patients and, therefore, do not have access to meet or talk with them. In cases where the patient is interviewed, it is the authors' experience that during the interview, patients often will demonstrate deficits or discuss their problems in reasonable detail. For cases where an interview does not occur, one possible alternative is to have the attorney ask standard interview questions via deposition. A videotaped "Day in the Life" of the patient also is helpful to review. An important point to make is that defense "consultants" are not disclosed and, therefore, will not interview patients.
It is also recommended that the patient interview take place in the person's residence (home or facility). In the authors' opinion, patients are less inconvenienced and more comfortable in their normal setting. Secondly, for patients with numerous supplies, medications and equipment requirements, this procedure maximizes the potential for a comprehensive assessment of needs, including a review of potential architectural needs.
- **Family members/caregivers.** Similar to the patient interview, life care planners commonly interview and listen to the family (if legally permitted) involved in the patient's care. It is not uncommon for patients with a brain injury to be unable to describe in adequate detail the difficulties that they experience, and the family can help to "paint the picture." In addition, family support often is very important to ultimate outcome.
- **Medical evaluation.** Medical evaluation(s) with appropriate medical specialists should include an assessment of the patient's functional limitations, expected future medical treatment including referral to other specialties, a review of medications, supplies, and/or durable medical equipment, as well as related topics (see Table 66-2 for suggested questions).
- **Physiatrist.** Many patients with mild to moderate brain injury will have few, if any, long term *medical* needs. However, for major injuries, a physiatrist who specializes in long term brain injury rehabilitation can be designated the team leader for many of the

---

TABLE 66-2

Example Questions for Physicians: Life Care Plan Only

---

1. Future Care (Distinguish what is reasonable and appropriate vs. medically necessary vs. desirable.)
   - How long will the patient need follow-up?
   - When will the patient reach maximum medical improvement?
   - How long and how often will treatment be needed? (Include frequency and duration, e.g., every six months for 2 years then once per year thereafter, etc.)
   - What treatment is expected? (Follow-up visits, routine evaluations, etc.)
   - How much will each visit cost?
   - Are X-rays or lab work needed? If so, how often and how much will each cost?
   - Do you anticipate any further surgeries or aggressive medical treatment; e.g., several years from now due to complications? If so, what, when, and how much will each cost?

2. Possible Complications
   What complications are possible/expected? (Traumatic arthritis, contractures, adverse reactions to medications, seizures, spasticity, earlier onset of aging-related dementia, maladaptive behaviors, additional injury due to reduced physical skills or poor judgement, etc.)

3. Recommended Medical Follow-up By Other Specialties
   - Orthopedist?
   - Neurology?
   - Physiatrist?
   - Cosmetic Surgeon?
   - Dermatology?
   - Psychology/Neuropsychology?
   - Occupational Therapist, Physical Therapist, Speech Therapy, Dietary, Recreation Therapy?
   - Other?
   If you recommend any of the above, do you have an opinion regarding what treatment will be needed, how often it will be needed, and expected costs?

Partially adapted and reprinted with permission from Ref. 17.

---

specialties listed below, and a team may be assembled which includes physicians who address specific areas, such as plastic surgery, pulmonology, orthopedics, etc. As cited in Weed (3), in general, the physiatrist will be the best physician to establish a medical foundation for a life care plan (23, 24). As noted by Zasler (24), "All too often physicians may not be fully versed in life care planning. It is therefore critical that life care planners communicate in an appropriate and timely manner to assure that their role in a particular case is understood" (p. 57). One way to assure that future care information is properly solicited is to utilize the example questions checklist in this chapter. For physicians, if recommending a life care plan for a patient, or if meeting with an already assigned life care planner for one of his/her patients, it is recommended that the person conducting the life care planning assessment be asked if he/she is board certified as a life care planner (specifically if they are a CLCP). The goal of this questioning is to increase the likelihood that the life care plan is developed according to existing standards.

- **Neuropsychologist.** The neuropsychologist can play an invaluable role in evaluating the long-term effects of the brain injury on the patient's ability to

function (25). It is within the role of the life care planner to refer a patient for a neuropsychological evaluation in cases where there is documented or suspected brain injury/impairment (26). A specialized list of questions to help the life care planner prepare a life care plan, including address future vocational/educational issues, has been developed to assure that the appropriate questions are asked during the evaluation (see Table 66-3). Asking the right questions is important because many neuropsychological evaluations do not seem to be geared toward identifying long-term future care needs or rehabilitation strategies to maximize the patient's ability to function in society or participate in gainful work.

- **Occupational therapist.** The occupational therapist may be an appropriate referral for an assessment for seating and positioning, adaptive aids, safety in the residence, and other vocationally-related issues (27). For some patients, activities of daily living training, including household safety, would be included.

- **Speech and language pathologist** (may also be called Communication Disorders Specialist). The qualified speech and language pathologist is instrumental in assessing augmentative communications for patients with more severe communications disorder, as well

---

TABLE 66-3
Neuropsychologist Questions
(with credit to Robert Fraser, Ph.D.)

In addition to the standard evaluation report, add the following as appropriate.
1. Please describe, in lay terms, the damage to the brain.
2. Please describe the effects of the accident on the patient's ability to function.
3. Please provide an opinion to the following topics:
    a. Intelligence level? (include pre- vs. post-incident if able)
    b. Personality style with regard to the workplace and home?
    c. Stamina level?
    d. Functional limitations and assets?
    e. Ability for education/training?
    f. Vocational implications - style of learning?
    g. Level of insight into present functioning?
    h. Ability to compensate for deficits?
    i. Ability to initiate action?
    j. Memory impairments (short-term, long-term, auditory, visual, etc.)?
    k. Ability to identify and correct errors?
    l. Recommendations for compensation strategies?
    m. Need for companion or attendant care?
4. What is the proposed treatment plan?
    a. Counseling? (individual and family)
    b. Cognitive therapy?
    c. Re-evaluations?
    d. Referral to others? (e.g., physicians)
    e. Other?
5. How much and how long? (Include the cost per session or hour and re-evaluations.)

Reprinted with permission from Ref. 17.

---

as assessing receptive/expressive speech and language abilities, and identifying cognitive remediation professionals (28).

- **Physical therapist.** A physical therapist is often the most appropriate referral to determine the patient's true physical capabilities by compiling a functional capacity assessment that is more detailed than most physicians can report (29). For example, Ergos™ equipment has become quite sophisticated, as has Lido™, Cybex™, and other equipment designed to identify the individual's physical and functional capabilities.

- **Educational consultant.** For the school-aged patient, an educational consultant can be very important to maximize the patient's educational potential. Under the federal Individuals with Disabilities Education Act (IDEA), the public school system is responsible for providing specialized services to eligible school-age children with disabilities through age 21, if appropriate. Additionally, each state offers early intervention programs for children from birth to age 3. However, many of these school-aged children are poorly served for a variety of reasons. One may be that the child has not been adequately assessed in order to identify deficits that would meet the criteria for specialized education. Another is that the child may meet the eligibility requirements but the school's funding is inadequate and the school fails to provide appropriate support. Another potential for dispute may be the school's contention that therapy is required for "medical" purposes rather than "educational" and the school, therefore, will not provide the services. Educational consultants who are familiar with the rules often can negotiate the appropriate education protocol which would then be included in the life care plan.

- **Vocational evaluator** (if there is work potential). A vocational evaluator can establish standardized protocols for assessing the patient's vocational capabilities, including aptitudes, interests, temperaments, and other related information (25). For the patient with a brain injury, a "real work" situational assessment or on-the-job evaluation may be more appropriate than formal timed or time-limited testing. The evaluator should have at least a Master's degree and experience working with individuals with a brain injury. A Certified Vocational Evaluator (CVE) is the recommended specialty for this assessment.

- **Rehabilitation counselor.** A rehabilitation counselor with a Master's degree or higher from an accredited rehabilitation counselor training program should be involved to assist in arranging for a job analysis, labor market surveys, vocational guidance and counseling, selective job placement, and/or supported employment, and is often the true coordinator of services (25, 30). Indeed, for purposes of this chapter, the rehabilitation consultant for the patient with a mild to moderate brain injury is likely the prime candidate to take the information generated by the specialties listed above and develop it into a rehabilitation plan and earnings capacity analysis. A Certified Rehabilitation Counselor (CRC) is recommended, although a CVE (see above) may also have the expertise to provide this service.

- **Economist.** In most situations, the life care planner or expert witness, in forensic cases, will work with an economist. The economist will rely upon the base costs in the life care plan to project the cost of care throughout the patient's life expectancy (16). This specialized industry is sophisticated and complex. The rehabilitation professional who does not have an education in economic forecasting is sometimes requested to project life care plan costs in personal injury litigation cases, and it is the authors' opinion that this is a dangerous practice in most instances. It is important to know, for example, what the different rates of inflation are for medical and non-medical care, as well as discounts to present value methodologies. In most cases, the economist will be necessary as they are well-versed and educated in inflation rules and investment strategies. On the other hand, there are a few states that endorse the "Alaska Rule" which assumes that inflation and reasonable investment rates are essentially equal and "wash out" each other such that an economist may not be needed in those cases. In summary, it is strongly recommended that the life care planner defer to an economist or other trained and qualified professional for the ultimate cost of the life care plan, unless he or she has specific training in this specialized area.

As a general rule, in order for an economist to project the cost of care, certain details must be included. In the authors' experience, many health care providers offer opinions that a patient will require follow-up services for "a long time;" however, it is not possible to identify specific costs for patient needs when the time frame is not quantified. In order to obtain a "bottom line" cost for the care plan, the professional must obtain the following information:

a. expected type and amount of treatment (frequency)
b. date to start treatment
c. date to stop treatment
d. base cost of treatment (in today's dollars)

See Table 66-4 for an example entry that contains the minimum required data to calculate future costs.

TABLE 66-4
Example Minimum Information Needed for Economist to Project Costs

Psychological Evaluation 6/2005 at a cost of $600.

Expect counseling to start 7/2005, one time per week, one hour session each for 26 weeks at a cost of $100 per hour.

Expect group counseling one time per week for 2 years, beginning 1/2006 at a cost of $40 per session.

Expect medical follow-up four times per year by psychiatrist at a cost of $150 for the initial visit, then $75 each visit until 1/2007.

Medication prescribed is Prozac, one 20 mg. per day, from 7/2005-1/2007, at a cost of $53.86 for 30 pills.

Occasionally, identifying the frequency and duration of activities can be very complex. Pediatric brain injury cases often will include needs for periodic speech, occupational, and physical therapy which may begin and end at specific developmental periods in the child's life (27-29). Although these therapies may be provided through the school system while the child is in school, private or medically based therapies often are indicated to address the child's needs outside the education setting for the following reasons: (1) to augment school-based services, (2) to address the child's needs at home and in the community, (3) to prevent or reduce medical complications, and 4) to provide continuation of therapies throughout the summer to assure maintenance and carry over of skills into the next developmental stage. By knowing what services are provided by the school system, the life care planner can better determine what additional services the child needs outside the school environment to achieve short and long-term goals (31). For instance, occupational therapy may be needed for activities of daily living for a six-year-old child and then be discontinued throughout school years until the child is ready to enter the work world at which time an occupational therapist may rejoin the treatment team in order to furnish assistive devices for work-related activity. A challenge for life care planning is that sometimes treatment team professionals fail to consider the life-time needs of a patient, since they are most often involved in care lasting only one to two years.

To continue with an explanation of the RAPEL method previously described:

A = Access to Labor Market. In many cases involving individuals with ABI, the patient may very well be able to return to a job that is custom-designed around his/her disability or with an employer who is interested in hiring an employee with mild to moderate cognitive deficits. However, the patient may not have access to the same number or level of vocational choices as he or she did prior to the injury. In essence, it may be that the patient would appear to have no particular loss of earnings capacity, but at the same time be at high risk for losing a job and then having a significant problem locating alternate suitable employment. Access to labor market can be determined through the services of a qualified rehabilitation consultant and is beyond the scope of this chapter.

P = Placeability. Placeability represents the likelihood that the patient will be successfully placed in a job with or without rehabilitation or rehabilitation consultant assistance. One may need to conduct a labor market survey, job analysis, or, in pediatric cases, rely upon statistical data to opine about ultimate placeability as an adult. In some situations, the economic condition of the community also may be a factor. It is important that the rehabilitation consultant recognize that the patient's personality, cognitive limitations, and other factors certainly influence the ultimate outcome. For adults, the rehabilitation consultant generally should include an opinion about jobs that are available (actual openings) in addition to jobs that exist but are not currently available to the patient.

E = Earnings Capacity. Based on the rehabilitation or life care plan, access to the labor market, and placeability factors, the patient may or may not be employable in the labor market. If employment is likely, an estimate of the earnings potential is included as a mitigating factor in determining damages. In addition, identifying the pre-incident earnings capacity is a necessary element of determining what is included in the life care plan since jurisdiction "rules" will determine certain needs. For example, if the life care plan is being prepared for a patient related to a vaccine injury fund case, then general living costs (housing, food, transportation, etc.) will be part of the plan, whereas these costs generally are not included in personal injury cases.

L = Labor Force Participation. This category represents an opinion about the patient's expected work life expectancy or amount of time expected to be in the work force. Usually an individual who has a reduced life expectancy also will be expected to have a reduced work life expectancy. At the other end of the spectrum, the patient's participation in the labor force may be unchanged after the brain injury. Or, an individual may have the capacity to work six hours per day rather than eight hours per day, which represents a 25% loss of normal work life expectancy. Other patients may require a longer period of time to find a job or have longer time off between jobs as a result of the ABI and this could have an impact on their worklife expectancy. Further, some patients, pre-injury, may have demonstrated consistent extra income by working overtime hours or at a second job and this situation should be considered in the analysis as well.

In summary, the RAPEL method identifies the minimum data needed for determining damages in personal injury litigation and provides the data needed for economists to arrive at a bottom line figure.

GENERAL LIFE CARE PLANNING PROCEDURES

As a first step, the life care planner must request and receive all medical records and consultations (9, 18, 32, 33). If the individual is involved in litigation, depositions of health care professionals often are available and useful to review as related to damages and/or future care needs. If information is unclear, confirmation of diagnosis is essential. As previously noted, if the patient resides at home, it is recommended that the interview take place in the residence rather than in an office or other location so that a complete inspection of the individual's needs can be done. It is unlikely that the patient and/or family member(s) will remember all of the drugs and supplies, and an on-site inventory is the most effective way to determine the patient's current needs. In addition to an inventory of medications, supplies, and equipment during the initial interview, information is obtained with respect to the patient's pre-incident medical and social history, family history, current physical and emotional status (including limitations), medical treatment, socioeconomic status, employment history, and long-term plans. A thorough assessment usually requires several hours to complete.

Subsequent to the review of medical records and patient/family interview, the life care planner begins the process of identifying long-term care issues and options, including considerations for aging (32). If the care planner is retained by the plaintiff, the treatment team is usually consulted and is encouraged to take an active role in development of the life care plan. In fact, if the life care planner has access to relevant treatment members and fails to communicate with them, a serious breach of professional responsibility is likely. However, it is recognized that there are cases where it is not permissible to contact treatment team members. (For additional information on this topic see 34). The life care planner acts to coordinate and communicate information to and from all members of the treatment team, patient and family. Generally, the life care planner will be the author of the document, although many people, including the patient, provide opinions and recommendations. The life care plan will identify the source of each recommendation(s), frequency, and treatment areas consistent with appropriate and reasonable care. The life care planner needs to have enough knowledge about the disability to participate in the planning process by knowing which questions to ask, who to invite to participate, how to fill in gaps of information, and when participants' contributions are unreasonable (either excessive or deficient).

Similarly, the clinician on whom the life care planner relies needs to be competent and confident in their opinions with regard to future needs as the reliability and validity of the life care plan rests on the foundation of each individual entry. The physician or health care provider must know the patient's particular situation and the literature with regard to probable needs. For example, does a person with a brain injury really need EEGs every year to life and is there reasonable support or foundation for the recommendation? Obviously, there is a shared responsibility between the health care clinician and life care planner and the life care planner must be acutely familiar with the patient and his/her disability to know if the clinician is offering recommendations that are reasonable and resemble an accepted standard of care. For example, one of the authors met with the treating physician for a patient with tetraplegia. After a few recommendations were elicited, it was obvious the doctor was not well-versed about the long-term implications of spinal cord injury as related to future care needs. It was eventually revealed that the physician had treated only one tetraplegic patient in his career, and he happily supported the author's recommendation to refer the patient to a specialty spinal center to obtain the required information. In addition, it is the physician's or health care professional's responsibility to make sure the life care planner is qualified with which to collaborate on development of the life care plan. One way for the clinician to be sure of the life care planner's qualifications is to ask if the life care planner has completed specific training and/or achieved certification in this specialty profession (i.e., Certified Life Care Planner/CLCP).

Once an initial life care plan is developed based on adequate foundation for the entries, investigation into resources, cost research, and availability of services begins. The process of identifying resources can be a long and arduous task, involving research and personal contact with community and national resources, catalogs, and Internet databases. Upon a complete and thorough investigation, the life care plan is usually presented and reviewed by the patient/family (if clinically appropriate) and perhaps the treatment team. The plan can provide the patient, family, and treatment providers the opportunity to coordinate and execute effective care options with a clear understanding of the financial resources necessary for providing the service(s). Caveat: In the event the author of the life care plan has solicited and received written recommendations from the medical/therapeutic providers, or a consultation has been properly documented in the file, it may not be necessary to specifically send the life care plan back to the provider(s) for review. However, it is the authors' experience that having the physician or physicians who participated in development of the plan to review and sign off or endorse the medically-based recommendations as being a reasonable plan of care can be helpful and important for case documentation.

CLINICAL AND FORENSIC ISSUES

1. The rehabilitation expert is expected to provide an opinion in personal injury cases about what is "more probable than not" within rehabilitation certainty, as represented by the standards of the profession (7, 9, 35, 36). If a patient *might* need additional plastic surgery, then this does not represent what is more probable than not and cost for such items should not be included in the plan totals. It should not make a difference as to whether the expert is retained by the plaintiff or the defense since qualified professionals should arrive at similar conclusions if the data is appropriately analyzed (37). However, there may be occasions where there are philosophical differences or, perhaps, an attorney has provided information that is biased, and it is within the rehabilitation consultant's ethics to attempt, to the best of his or her ability, to fairly and objectively develop a plan which would accurately represent the patient's needs in order to help *resolve* litigation.

2. Replacement schedules for equipment can be dependent on a variety of conditions[38]. When possible, the source which supplied the product (assuming the patient already has it) should be contacted to obtain an opinion based on the individual patient. Contact with manufacturers also may be an acceptable source, although in the authors' experience, replacement schedules as promoted by the manufacturer may be less often than what it is in practical terms. Factors to consider include age, activity level, anticipated amount of use, patient's weight, and quality of product. For example, a younger individual who requires the use of a wheelchair may be very active, participate in wheelchair sports, live in a rural area that is "hard" on wheelchairs, etc., and each of these factors must be considered. Another example may be that of a patient who is 70 years of age, very sedentary, and never leaves the residential facility where he/she lives. Replacement schedules based on the above examples obviously differ for the reasons stated. An overview of basic guidelines to consider when determining replacement schedules can be reviewed in Amsterdam's chapter (38).

3. Items included in the life care plan should represent what is considered reasonable quality of care and presumes fewer complications than would otherwise be expected. The life care plan should identify potential complications based on research, patient's

history of complications, records reviewed, or expert opinion. For example, as discussed earlier in this chapter, people with ABI commonly have a higher risk of re-injury due to poor judgment and/or physical skills, among other factors. However, unless one can identify the nature of the re-injury, severity, frequency or duration, or the likelihood that re-injury has a better than 50% probability of occurrence, costs should not be included in the plan totals.

4. The life care plan generally should not include needs that are not directly related to the patient's disability. (Note: There are occasions where this rule does not apply, such as family trusts and vaccine injury fund cases). For example, a person with pre-existing diabetes would not have the cost of medication, glucose monitor, or physician visits related to diabetes included in the plan. Assuming that damages related to earnings capacity is a part of the case, costs associated with normal living expenses also would be excluded. For example, the cost of an individual's vehicle would be deducted from the cost of a handicapped van so that the plan would only include those costs associated with the need to modify the van as a result of the injury. The additional costs associated with van maintenance (only for those parts that have been modified, i.e., wheelchair lift, hand controls or other driving modifications, swivel seats, etc.), mileage to injury-related medical/therapy appointments, and increased insurance as a result of insuring a more costly, modified van would be included. Routine maintenance, fuel, etc. would not be included in the plan as the patient would have been expected to incur those costs associated with owning a regular vehicle had the injury not occurred (although an allowance for increased mileage may be added as appropriate). Similarly, the cost of home modifications as a result of the injury are reasonable to include in the plan, but the entire cost of a house is not (again, for the reason that the patient would have been expected to live somewhere had the injury not occurred). In the event the existing home is not modifiable, the value of the existing home, or the average value of a comparable home in the local community should be deducted from the value of purchasing or building an accessible home. Another example is that individuals who reside in a facility usually receive food and housing as part of the per diem cost. If a part of the patient's damages includes earning capacity, then the economist should be instructed to deduct the average yearly cost of food and housing that the patient would have expected to incur even without the injury. For patients who receive nutrition via enteral feeding, the average yearly cost of regular food should be deducted from the cost of their liquid nutrition. However, the life care planner must be cognizant of the nature of the case which may dictate what is properly included and accepted in the life care plan. As noted previously, special rules apply to litigation cases such as federal vaccine injury fund, Federal Employees Liability Act (FELA), or one of many other jurisdictions that may have special requirements.

5. For a child with a brain injury who attends public school, an individually designed educational program that includes occupational therapy, physical therapy, speech/language therapy, vision therapy, special education, and/or other resource services is available through the school at no additional cost to the family. Typically no cost for these school-based services should be included in the life care plan. However, what is defined as "educationally related" vs. "medically related" can form the basis for conflict and may determine what or whether the child receives school-based services. As suggested previously in this chapter, it may be wise to include the services of an educational consultant or expert in the life care plan to help negotiate the best school-based program. In some rare situations, a private specialty school may clinically be the best option for the patient, in which event the costs for the private specialty school will be included in the life care plan.

6. Personal injury cases in some states have collateral source rules which mean that certain patient needs, if covered by another entity, should not be a part of the life care plan. Although the life care planner must take this issue into account, the retaining attorney would know when this rule applies and should inform the expert.

7. The method for obtaining recommendations from treating professionals or other experts can take many forms. For life care planners who are retained by the plaintiff, direct contact with the treatment team is recommended. An in-person meeting with the physiatrist, for example, can assure that the life care planner has the full attention of the physician. Phone contact may also be a reasonable option, especially where distance and/or scheduling issues dictate alternate means of communication other than face-to-face. It is recommended that the life care planner take notes during such communications, then send the written notes back to the physician so that he/she can review, sign and return them to the life care planner for documentation, along with any corrections or refinements that are indicated. Another method is to send the entire life care plan to the physician(s) for review, endorsement, and signature. A third approach is to submit a letter with specific questions on which the physician can handwrite recommendations or can dictate responses typed on the doctor's letterhead. The important

factor is that written documentation verifies the medical foundation for life care plan entries.

8. For patients who require attendant care, the life care planner is expected to research agency costs (typically minimum of three sources). Some experts assert that privately hired attendants are less expensive. However, the life care planner needs to be certain that the family infrastructure for private hiring is in place. Second, the costs associated with private hire are not as low as it may seem on the surface. Costs for advertising, interviewing, hiring, bonding, background checks, training costs, back-up provision, insurance, payroll expenses, taxes, etc. are in addition to the hourly rate paid to the private caregiver (see Kitchen & Brown, 39, for additional details).

9. The concept of "medically necessary" is one which the physician and allied health professionals are familiar. In the authors' experience, a common tenet in personal injury cases is that the injured party has a "right" to be made whole (reasonably). So, what may be "medically necessary" in Medicare may not meet the same threshold in personal injury litigation. The reader should discuss this issue with the referral source to refine the definition and be sure all necessary items are included in the plan.

10. *Qualified* life care planners are trained to conduct their assessments in the same manner (i.e., following the same methodology and procedures) regardless of who pays the bill. One test is to inquire about the percentage of plaintiff vs. defense cases on which the professional has worked. Some life care planners are noted for providing close to 100% defense work, while others are close to 100% plaintiff work. One can easily assume there is a reason. It is recognized that there is no "law" that requires life care planners to be licensed or certified (unlike physicians) and that there are some who are considered very good but who also are not certified. However, it is the authors' opinion that certification in life care planning at least assures that the planner has knowledge about standards and procedures. As with most certifications, no competence can be assured, but minimum knowledge has been demonstrated in the testing process. Incidentally, unlike most rehabilitation related certifications, there was no "grandfathering" in the CLCP certification so all individuals who sit for the exam from the first administration in 1996 forward, has had to achieve a passing score on the test to become certified.

11. Life expectancy can be a significant factor for life care planning and controversy exists over who is qualified to render a life expectancy opinion. It is clear that a life care plan is designed to provide the needs for the patient's life expectancy; however, for some children who are severely or significantly impaired, they will not live to be an adult. In these and other cases of individuals with a reduced life expectancy, the age of life expectancy becomes a critical point in assessing a patient's future. Typically, the life care planner will rely on a physician or medical expert to render the life expectancy opinion (23, 40, 41) and the life care plan needs will be adjusted accordingly. However, there are life expectancy experts who are not physicians or medical specialists who have been involved in research and have successfully been qualified in court to opine about how long a person will live (42-45). Obviously, this topic can be a battleground in forensic cases since each year that a person lives costs more. In some cases, an expert for the plaintiff may claim that a child would live to age 60 and the defense expert may opine to age 20, resulting in millions of dollars in differences. Also, in a few jurisdictions, a normal life expectancy table may be specifically required. The theory is that the defendant who is responsible for an injury that shortens one's life should not receive "credit" for the reduction and would therefore be required to pay for damages to a normal life expectancy.

12. The Health Insurance Portability and Accountability Act of 1996 (HIPAA) will have an effect on how health care providers, life care planners, insurance companies, law firms, etc. interact with regard to medical information pertaining to an individual with a disability. The authors are beginning to see some of its effects in their own practices and some challenges that are being created as a result. Although details are beyond the scope of this chapter, many life care planners will need to sign business associate agreements with law firms and/or insurance companies and additional safeguards for "protected health information" will be required. Some life care planners have reported more difficulty interfacing with physicians and medical providers to access their patient's medical information and research their health care needs even with a properly signed and executed information release form. As a recent example, one of the authors researched a patient's medication costs to include in the life care plan and, as part of routine practice, asked the patient's pharmacist for a printout of the medications and supplies. Rather than complying as had been done numerous times in the past, the pharmacist informed the life care planner that the request and information release form signed by the patient had to be sent to an outside "HIPAA compliance vendor" for review and authorization before the pharmacy would release the information. Implications of this are that the new procedure could potentially add weeks onto the research portion of the plan and

would delay obtaining the patient's actual medication history. In other instances, pharmacies have required that the patient/family personally pick up the medication history rather than send it directly to the life care planner.

BASIC ETHICAL ISSUES

The efficacy and value of the life care plan is dependent in large part on the ethics of the person developing the plan[46, 47, 48]. Several common issues arise in this domain which deserve brief mention (Weed & Berens, 49, reprinted here with permission).

Professional Preparation

The qualifications of professional rehabilitation practitioners depend on experience and academic preparation. It is imperative that one's credentials be represented accurately, and that current licensure and/or credentialing be maintained. Life care planning practitioners are held to the ethical standards of their professional discipline(s). Therefore, the life care planner should belong to a relevant organization that has ethics and/or should be certified as a life care planner (see the International Academy of Life Care Planners at www.IALCP.com and the Commission on Health Care Certification at www.CHCC1.com).

Who Is the Patient? (A.K.A. Client)

Common within the field of rehabilitation service delivery and for purposes of this chapter, the patient is the person with a disability. The life care planner is expected to provide objective, independent opinions, limited to his or her field of expertise, and demonstrate no conflict of interest. It is important that their contract for services clarifies the responsibilities and duties of the life care planner. Ultimately, the goal is to develop a document that provides for the needs of the patient over his/her lifetime in a manner that preserves quality of life, reduces potential complications, and also provides quality, appropriate, efficient and cost-effective services.

Informed Consent

In most cases, patient consent is required for the review of confidential medical records, for patient interviews, and communication with providers of goods and services. The patient or their legal representative must understand and consent to these services. He or she is free to withdraw consent from any or all portions of services at any time. In some cases, the life care planner may act as a consultant to an insurance company or attorney, in which case, different rules may apply since direct contact may

be limited or non-existent. The life care planner must know which rules apply in the cases on which they provide services.

Confidentiality

Protection of patient confidentiality must be maintained at all times, within legal and ethical parameters. Case managers and life care planners may release records of their work with proper authorization from the patient or his/her legal representative. Written summaries and recommendations should be addressed to the referral source who can then be responsible for distribution of copies to insurers, the patient, and service providers. Special care should be taken with the use of computerized files, electronic mail, and facsimile transmission of information in order to protect confidentiality.

Written Reports

In personal injury litigation, it is not uncommon for the life care planner to decline to provide written opinions, probably at the request of the attorney who retained their services. Obviously, written reports represent the most common way of expressing opinions and making recommendations in all rehabilitation industries. Failure to do so in litigation related cases is inviting criticism of the life care planning process as a whole. It is the authors' opinion that the life care planner have some form of written documentation in their file.

Use Existing Standards

Again, in personal injury litigation, certain trends are developing with regard to how life care plans are compiled. In the past, some rehabilitation consultants have chosen to use their own "private logic" when outlining future care needs. Under the Daubert[50] ruling (1993), it is important for the expert to develop opinions subject to published and peer reviewed methods, procedures and standards. One publication that focuses exclusively on this topic is the *Journal of Life Care Planning*, 2002, 1(1) (available through Elliott & Fitzpatrick, www.elliottfitzpatrick.com). Another resource for consensus on life care planning issues is the 2000 Life Care Planning Summit Proceedings[51].

CONCLUSIONS

In general, determining lifetime future care needs for a patient with ABI can be a challenge. Oftentimes, deficits are subtle and require significant expertise to identify not only what the deficits are but strategies to assist the patient with becoming as functional and independent as possible over his/her lifetime. These cases can require a remarkable amount of information gathering, records review, and diligent coordination among rehabilitation professionals as well as research of necessary items and services. If the evaluation is thorough, a life care plan with a reasonable estimate of financial damages can be attained and will assist in resolving the case so the patient can "get on with his or her life" (i.e., have the services in the life care plan implemented).

References

1. Deutsch, P. & Fralish, K. *Innovations in Head Injury*. New York, NY: Matthew Bender, 1989.
2. Weed, R. Life care planning and earnings capacity analysis for brain injured patients involved in personal injury litigation utilizing the RAPEL method. *Journal of NeuroRehabilitation*, 1996a; 7(2):119–135.
3. Weed. R (Ed.) *Life Care Planning and Case Management Handbook*, 2nd ed. Boca Raton, FL: St. Lucie/CRC Press, LLC, 2004.
4. Deutsch, P. & Raffa, J. *Damages in Tort Action*, Vol. 8 and 9. New York, NY: Matthew Bender, 1981.
5. Deutsch, P. & Sawyer, H. *A Guide to Rehabilitation*. New York, NY: Matthew Bender, 1985.
6. Deutsch, P. & Sawyer, H. *A Guide to Rehabilitation*. White Plains, NY: Ahab Press, 1994, 2003.
7. Weed, R. Life care plans as a managed care tool. *Medical Interface*, 1995c; 8(2):111–118.
8. Weed, R. Life care planning: An overview. *Directions in Rehabilitation*, (1998b); 9(11):135–147.
9. Weed, R. & Field, T. *The Rehabilitation Consultant's Handbook*, 3rd ed. Athens, GA: E&F Vocational Services, 2001.
10. Weed, R. & Riddick, S. Life care plans as a case management tool. *The Individual Case Manager Journal*, 1992; 3(1):26–35.
11. Riddick, S. & Weed, R. The life care planning process for managing catastrophically impaired patients. In S. Bancett & D. Flarey (Eds.), *Case Studies in Nursing Case Management*, 61–91. Gaithersburg, MD: Aspen, 1996.
12. Ripley, D. & Weed, R. Life care planning for acquired brain injury. In R. Weed (Ed.) *Life Care Planning and Case Management Handbook*. Boca Raton, FL: CRC Press, LLC, 2004.
13. Weed, R. Forensic rehabilitation. In A. E. Dell Orto & R. P. Marinelle (Eds.). *Encyclopedia of Disability and Rehabilitation*, 326–330. New York, NY: Macmillan, 1995a.
14. Neulicht, A. T. & Berens, D. E. PEEDS-RAPEL©: A case conceptualization model for evaluating pediatric cases. *Journal of Life Care Planning*, 2005, 4(1):27–36.
15. Brookshire, M. & Smith, S. *Economic/Hedonic Damages: The Practice Book for Plaintiff and Defense Attorneys*. Cincinnati, OH: Anderson Publishing Co., 1990.
16. Dillman, E. *Economic Damages and Discounting Methods*. Athens, GA: Elliott & Fitzpatrick, 1989.
17. Weed, R. & Field, T. *The Rehabilitation Consultant's Handbook*. 2nd ed. Athens, GA: E&F Vocational Services, 1994.
18. Weed, R. Life care plan development. *Topics in Spinal Cord Injury*, 2002a; 7(4):5–20.
19. Weed, R. O. & Englehart, L. R. Factors affecting the cost of vehicle modifications: Some considerations for life care planners. *Journal of Life Care Planning*, 2005, 4(2):115–126.
20. Weed, R. Support for recreation and leisure activities in life care plans. *The Rehab Consultant*, 1991; 3(1):1–3.
21. Hablutzel H. & McMahon, B. *The Americans with Disabilities Act: Access and Accommodations*, 129–138. Orlando, FL: P. M. Deutsch Press, 1992.
22. Blackwell, T., Sluis-Powers, A. & Weed, R. *Life Care Planning for the Brain Injured* (Foreword by James S. Brady). Athens, GA: E & F Vocational Services, 1994.
23. Bonfiglio, R. The role of the physiatrist in life care planning. In R. Weed (Ed) *Life Care Planning and Case Management Handbook*. Boca Raton, FL: CRC Press, LLC, 2004.
24. Zasler, N. A physiatric perspective on life care planning. *Journal of Private Sector Rehabilitation*, 1994; 9(2 & 3):57–61.
25. Berens, D. & Weed, R. The role of the vocational counselor in life care planning. In R. Weed (Ed.). *Life Care Planning and Case Management Handbook*. Boca Raton, FL: CRC Press, LLC, 2004.
26. Evans, R. The role of the neuropsychologist in life care planning. In R. Weed (Ed.). *Life Care Planning and Case Management Handbook*. Boca Raton, FL: CRC Press, LLC, 2004.
27. McCaigue, I. The role of the occupational therapist in life care planning. In R. Weed (Ed.). *Life Care Planning and Case Management Handbook*. Boca Raton, FL: CRC Press, LLC, 2004.
28. Higdon, C. The role of the speech language pathologist in life care planning. In R. Weed (Ed.). *Life Care Planning and Case Management Handbook*. Boca Raton, FL: CRC Press, LLC, 2004.
29. Peddle, A. The role of the physical therapist in life care planning. In R. Weed (Ed.). *Life Care Planning and Case Management Handbook*. Boca Raton, FL: CRC Press, LLC, 2004.
30. Blackwell, T., Conrad, D. & Weed, R. *Job Analysis and the ADA: A Step-by-Step Guide*. Athens, GA: E & F Vocational Services, 1992.
31. Neulicht, A.T. & Berens, D.E. (2004). The role of the vocational counselor in life care planning. In S. Riddick-Grisham (Ed), *Pediatric Life Care Planning and Case Management*. Boca Raton, FL: CRC Press, LLC, 2004.
32. Weed, R. Future care planning for persons with acquired brain injury (feature article). *re-Learning* [Newsletter by Learning Services, Inc.], 1996b; 3(4):5–6.
33. Weed, R. Aging with a brain injury: The effects on life care plans and vocational opinions. *The Rehabilitation Professional*, 1998a; 6(5):30–34.
34. Weed, R. The life care planner: Secretary, know-it-all, or general contractor? One person's perspective. *Journal of Life Care Planning*, 2002b; 1(2):173–177.
35. Weed, R. The role of the rehabilitation expert. In PESI, *Georgia proof of personal injury damages*. Eau Claire, WI: Professional Educational Systems, 1990a.
36. Weed, R. Presenting the rehabilitation consultant at trial. *Trial Diplomacy Journal*, 1990b; 13(4):212–226.
37. Sutton, A., Deutsch, P., Weed, R., & Berens, D. Reliability of life care plans: A comparison of original and updated plans. *Journal of Life Care Planning*, 2002, 1(3):187–194.
38. Amsterdam, P. Medical equipment choices and the role of the rehab equipment specialist in life care planning. In R. Weed (Ed), *Life care planning and case management handbook*. Boca Raton, FL: CRC Press, LLC, 2004.
39. Kitchen, J. & Brown, E. Life care planning resources. In R. Weed (Ed), *Life care planning and case management handbook*. Boca Raton, FL: CRC Press, LLC, 2004.
40. Weed, R. & Berens, D. Ethics in life care planning. In R. Weed (Ed.). *Life Care Planning and Case Management Handbook*. Boca Raton, FL: CRC Press, LLC, 2004.
41. Winkler, T. & Weed, R. Life care planning for the spinal cord injured. In R. Weed (Ed.). *Life Care Planning and Case Management Handbook*. Boca Raton, FL: CRC Press, LLC, 2004.
42. Strauss, D.J., DeVivo, M.J. & Shavelle, R.M. Long-term mortality risk after spinal cord injury. *Journal of Insurance Medicine*, 2000, 32:11–16.
43. Shavelle, R. & Strauss, D. Comparative mortality of adults with traumatic brain injury in California, 1988–97. *Journal of Insurance Medicine*, 2000, 32:163–166.
44. Strauss, D., Ashwal, S., Day, S. & Shavelle, R. Life expectancy of children in vegetative and minimally conscious states. *Pediatric Neurology*, 2000, 23:312–319.
45. Shavelle, R., Strauss, D., Whyte, J., Day, S. & Yu, Y. Long-term causes of death after traumatic brain injury. *American Journal of Physical Medicine & Rehabilitation*, 2001, 80:510–516.
46. Weed, R. Ethics in rehabilitation opinions and testimony. *Rehabilitation Counseling Bulletin*, 2000; 43(4):215–218, 245.
47. Weed, R. Objectivity in life care planning. *Inside Life Care Planning*, 1995b; 1(1):1–5.
48. Weed, R., Berens, D. & Pataky, S. Malpractice and ethics issues in private sector rehabilitation practice: An update for the 21st century. *RehabPro*, 2003; 11(1):47–54.

49. Weed, R. & Berens, D. Ethics in life care planning. In P. Deutsch (Ed.). *The Expert's Role as an Educator Continues: Meeting the Demands Under Daubert*, 59–67. White Plains, NY: Ahab Press, 2003.
50. *Daubert v. Merrell Dow*, (1993), 125 L Ed 2d 469.
51. Weed, R. & Berens, D. (Eds.). *Life Care Planning Summit 2000 Proceedings*. Sponsored by Intelicus, International Academy of Life Care Planners, International Association of Rehabilitation Professionals, and the Commission on Disability Examiner Certification, April 12, 2000, Dallas, TX. Monograph printed by Elliott & Fitzpatrick, Inc., Athens, GA, 2000.

CASE STUDY*

Rehabilitation Plan and Vocational Worksheet Using Rapel Method and Approved by Physiatrist and Others Involved in Client's Treatment

Re:	Losta Newron
Address:	XXXX, Chicago, IL
Date of Report	5/6/03
Date of Birth:	4/11/99
Date of Injury:	11/11/01

Description of Injury

Apparently, the patient was pulling on a chain when the counter to which the chain was attached fell on her. The mother states the counter weighed between 200-300 pounds and required two men to pull it off. Reportedly, the patient was unconscious and had blood coming from her ears, mouth and nose. She was diagnosed with severe closed head injury with multiple skull fractures and facial lacerations. She had a very good recovery based on the initial extent of injuries. However, several life long sequelae were expected and are outlined in the life care plan below.

Rehabilitation Plan (see Life Care Plan)

Potential Complications

Potential complications include, but are not limited to:

1. Seizure disorder.
2. Risk of re-injury due to reduced judgment, intelligence, physical skills, and visual perception.

Anticipated Length of Rehabilitation Program: Through childhood and potentially lifetime.

RECOMMENDATION	DATES	FREQUENCY	EXPECTED COST
Comprehensive neuropsychological evaluation	2004 (age 5) through 2017	Once in 2004, then yearly through 2010 (age 11), 2013, 2017 (age 18)	$600 (2004) then $1,000 each
Psychological a. Individual or couples therapy for parents	2003–2005	Expect once per week for 6–8 mos.	$90–110 per hour
b. Family and individual client counseling	Begin 2005	Once per week for one year, twice per week from age 12 to14, twice per week from age 16 to 18, once per week from age 18 to 21	$90–110 per hour
Physiatric evaluation	2003–2017	Yearly	$75–100 each
Occupational therapy	To 2004 (age 5)	Once or twice per week	$100 each visit
Physical therapy evaluation	Est. September 2003	Once only (also see comprehensive eval.)	$100
Neurological evaluation	2003–2010	Yearly	$80 each (does not include EEG or CT scans or other diagnostic studies, if needed)
Ophthalmologic evaluation for strabismus related to ABI	June 2003 to life expectancy	Yearly	$35–55 each (does not include dilation or corrective lenses, if necessary)
Speech/language evaluation	2003 and 2004 at age 5 (included in comprehensive evaluation)	Once in 2003, 2004	$100 (2003) 2004 cost included in comp. eval.

*For purposes of this chapter, the below case study is in an abbreviated form.

RECOMMENDATION	DATES	FREQUENCY	EXPECTED COST
Comprehensive team evaluation (include medical, P.T., O.T., speech/language, etc.)	2004 (age 5)	Once only	$1,800
Special education Option 1: Private school for children with disabilities. Also consider summer education or camp.	2003–2017	36 weeks per year (40 weeks per year if summer school)	$10,000 per school year (recommended for maximum outcome)
			4 weeks @ $350–$1,000 per week (summer)
Option 2: Public school system covered by the Individuals with Disabilities Education Act (IDEA). Include 13 years of learning disability consulting, 3 days per week for school year and summer school.			$0 for public school.
			$40/hour learning disability consulting 36 weeks per year regular school or 40 weeks per year with summer school
Neurobehavior development consultant	2003–2017	3 contacts with school and patient per year to enhance educational achievement	Expect 2 hr per occasion at $100/hr (total 6 hr per year)
Health and strength maintenance (including pool therapy, walking, and recreational activities to encourage motor coordination, perceptual training and strengthening)	2003 through entrance into school, 2004 (age 5)		No additional expected cost.
Driving evaluation	2014 (age 15)	1 X only	$400
Vocational a. Pre-vocational evaluation	2015 (age 16)	Once only	$600
b. Vocational evaluation	2017 (age 18)	Once only	$600
c. Vocational counseling, guidance, placement assistance, and follow-up. (Note: Costs for job coaching and supported employment, which may be appropriate, are not included.)	2016–2019	150 hours over three years	$65/hour
d. Post-high school education or vocational-technical training			Unknown

Note: This plan does not include costs associated with the patient's case management services nor her reduced ability to work outside of the home.

3. More significant psychological reaction to injury than expected.
4. Poorer educational/vocational achievement than expected.
5. Medical treatment and follow-up which is more extensive than expected.

Access To The Labor Market

Vocational Considerations

The limitations listed below are consistent with the U. S. Department of Labor definitions:

Physical Demands

Jobs which require significant amounts of functioning in following categories:

Standing   Balancing
Reaching upward   Stooping
Crouching   Fingering
Sitting   Visual perception
Eye/hand/foot coordination
Operating controls with right hand/arm or right foot/leg

Cognitive

Significant visual-spatial perception disturbance
Problems with attention, concentration, memory
Reduced frustration tolerance
Difficulties following through on tasks
Slowed thought process
Trouble following directions
Distractibility
Reduced intelligence
Reduced ability to be educated/trained (According to the neuropsychologist's report, auditory learning is recommended)

Emotional

No current significant emotional difficulties noted. Expect moderate emotional difficulties upon entrance into formal education program (2004, age 5) and various developmental periods to adulthood.

Conclusion

The patient has experienced a mild to moderate impact on the range of job alternatives available to her and has reduced ability to be educated or trained. Her loss of access to the *competitive* labor market is expected to be in excess of 98%.

Placeability

The patient has experienced an impact on her ability to be placed in a job as a result of the ABI. Cognitive retraining and special educational services will be needed. Additionally, vocational guidance/career counseling, job skills training, and selective placement is expected to decrease the impact of the injury on the patient's ability to be placed in the *competitive* labor market. Job placement will depend to a large extent on the success of the patient's rehabilitation program and her ability to complete a minimum of a high school education. Employment, if likely, should maximize the patient's strength in auditory skills.

Earnings Capacity

Pre-Incident	A review of the patient's family history suggests the capacity for college education or master's level education. Earnings potential to be determined by economist.
Post-Incident	High school or its equivalent and possibly technical school training. Earnings potential to be determined by economist.

Diminution of earnings capacity: To be computed by an economist.

Labor Force Participation (Work Life Expectancy)

Although clearly not employable in the manner as before the accident, the patient will have no reduction in labor force participation assuming no complications and excellent rehabilitation/education program. Expect entry into labor force at age 20 (2019).

Index

Brain Injury
Medicine

*Principles
and Practice*